Place-of-Service Codes for Professional Claims

Listed below are place-of-service codes and descriptions. These codes should be used on professional claims to specify the entity where service(s) were rendered. Check with individual payers (eg, Medicare, Medicaid, other private insurance) for reimbursement policies regarding these codes. If you would like to comment on a code(s) or description(s), please send your request to posinfo@cms.hhs.gov.

Place of Service Code(s)	Place of Service Name	Place of Service Description
01	Pharmacy	A facility or location where drugs and other medically related items and services are sold, dispensed, or otherwise provided directly to patients. (Effective 10/1/03)
02	Telehealth	The location where health services and health related services are provided or received, through a telecommunication system. (Effective 1/1/17)
03	School	A facility whose primary purpose is education.
04	Homeless Shelter	A facility or location whose primary purpose is to provide temporary housing to homeless individuals (eg, emergency shelters, individual or family shelters).
05	Indian Health Service Free-Standing Facility	A facility or location, owned and operated by the Indian Health Service, which provides diagnostic, therapeutic (surgical and non-surgical), and rehabilitation services to American Indians and Alaska Natives who do not require hospitalization.
06	Indian Health Service Provider-Based Facility	A facility or location, owned and operated by the Indian Health Service, which provides diagnostic, therapeutic (surgical and non-surgical), and rehabilitation services rendered by, or under the supervision of, physicians to American Indians and Alaska Natives admitted as inpatients or outpatients.
07	Tribal 638 Free-Standing Facility	A facility or location owned and operated by a federally recognized American Indian or Alaska Native tribe or tribal organization under a 638 agreement, which provides diagnostic, therapeutic (surgical and non-surgical), and rehabilitation services to tribal members who do not require hospitalization.
08	Tribal 638 Provider-Based Facility	A facility or location owned and operated by a federally recognized American Indian or Alaska Native tribe or tribal organization under a 638 agreement, which provides diagnostic, therapeutic (surgical and non-surgical), and rehabilitation services to tribal members admitted as inpatients or outpatients.
09	Prison/Correctional Facility	A prison, jail, reformatory, work farm, detention center, or any other similar facility maintained by either Federal, State, or local authorities for the purpose of confinement or rehabilitation of adult or juvenile criminal offenders. (Effective 7/1/06)
10	Unassigned	N/A
11	Office	Location, other than a hospital, skilled nursing facility (SNF), military treatment facility, community health center, State or local public health clinic, or intermediate care facility (ICF), where the health professional routinely provides health examinations, diagnosis, and treatment of illness or injury on an ambulatory basis.
12	Home	Location, other than a hospital or other facility, where the patient receives care in a private residence.
13	Assisted Living Facility	Congregate residential facility with self-contained living units providing assessment of each resident's needs and on-site support 24 hours a day, 7 days a week, with the capacity to deliver or arrange for services including some health care and other services. (Effective 10/1/03)
14	Group Home	A residence, with shared living areas, where clients receive supervision and other services such as social and/or behavioral services, custodial service, and minimal services (eg, medication administration). (Effective 10/1/03)
15	Mobile Unit	A facility/unit that moves from place-to-place equipped to provide preventive, screening, diagnostic, and/or treatment services.
16	Temporary Lodging	A short term accommodation such as a hotel, camp ground, hostel, cruise ship or resort where the patient receives care, and which is not identified by any other POS code. (Effective 1/1/08)
17	Walk-in Retail Health Clinic	A walk-in health clinic, other than an office, urgent care facility, pharmacy, or independent clinic, and not described by any other Place of Service code, that is located within a retail operation and provides, on an ambulatory basis, preventive and primary care services. (Effective 5/1/10)
18	Place of Employment—Worksite	A location, not described by any other POS code, owned or operated by a public or private entity where the patient is employed, and where a health professional provides on-going or episodic occupational medical, therapeutic or rehabilitative services to the individual. (This code is available for use effective January 1, 2013 but no later than May 1, 2013.)
19	Off Campus—Outpatient Hospital	A portion of an off-campus hospital provider based department which provides diagnostic, therapeutic (both surgical and nonsurgical), and rehabilitation services to sick or injured persons who do not require hospitalization or institutionalization. (Effective January 1, 2016)
20	Urgent Care Facility	Location, distinct from a hospital emergency room, an office, or a clinic, whose purpose is to diagnose and treat illness or injury for unscheduled, ambulatory patients seeking immediate medical attention. (Effective 1/1/03)
21	Inpatient Hospital	A facility, other than psychiatric, which primarily provides diagnostic, therapeutic (both surgical and non-surgical), and rehabilitation services by, or under, the supervision of physicians to patients admitted for a variety of medical conditions.
22	On Campus—Outpatient Hospital	A portion of a hospital's main campus which provides diagnostic, therapeutic (both surgical and non-surgical), and rehabilitation services to sick or injured persons who do not require hospitalization or institutionalization. (Description change effective January 1, 2016)
23	Emergency Room—Hospital	A portion of a hospital where emergency diagnosis and treatment of illness or injury is provided.
24	Ambulatory Surgical Center	A free-standing facility, other than a physician's office, where surgical and diagnostic services are provided on an ambulatory basis.
25	Birthing Center	A facility, other than a hospital's maternity facilities or a physician's office, which provides a setting for labor, delivery, and immediate postpartum care as well as immediate care of newborn infants.
26	Military Treatment Facility	A medical facility operated by one or more of the Uniformed Services. Military Treatment Facility (MTF) also refers to certain former U.S. Public Health Service (USPHS) facilities now designated as Uniformed Service Treatment Facilities (USTF).
27-30	Unassigned	N/A

31	Skilled Nursing Facility	A facility which primarily provides inpatient skilled nursing care and related services to patients who require medical, nursing, or rehabilitative services but does not provide the level of care or treatment available in a hospital.
32	Nursing Facility	A facility which primarily provides to residents skilled nursing care and related services for the rehabilitation of injured, disabled, or sick persons, or, on a regular basis, health-related care services above the level of custodial care to other than individuals with intellectual disabilities.
33	Custodial Care Facility	A facility that provides room, board, and other personal assistance services, generally on a long-term basis, and which does not include a medical component.
34	Hospice	A facility, other than a patient's home, in which palliative and supportive care for terminally ill patients and their families are provided.
35-40	Unassigned	N/A
41	Ambulance—Land	A land vehicle specifically designed, equipped and staffed for lifesaving and transporting the sick or injured.
42	Ambulance—Air or Water	An air or water vehicle specifically designed, equipped, and staffed for lifesaving and transporting the sick or injured.
43-48	Unassigned	N/A
49	Independent Clinic	A location, not part of a hospital and not described by any other Place of Service code, that is organized and operated to provide preventive, diagnostic, therapeutic, rehabilitative, or palliative services to outpatients only. (Effective 10/1/03)
50	Federally Qualified Health Center	A facility located in a medically underserved area that provides Medicare beneficiaries preventive primary medical care under the general direction of a physician.
51	Inpatient Psychiatric Facility	A facility that provides inpatient psychiatric services for the diagnosis and treatment of mental illness on a 24-hour basis, by or under the supervision of a physician.
52	Psychiatric Facility—Partial Hospitalization	A facility for the diagnosis and treatment of mental illness that provides a planned therapeutic program for patients who do not require full time hospitalization, but who need broader programs than are possible from outpatient visits to a hospital-based or hospital-affiliated facility.
53	Community Mental Health Center	A facility that provides the following services: outpatient services, including specialized outpatient services for children, the elderly, individuals who are chronically ill, and residents of the CMHC's mental health services area who have been discharged from inpatient treatment at a mental health facility; 24 hour a day emergency care services; day treatment, other partial hospitalization services, or psychosocial rehabilitation services; screening for patients being considered for admission to State mental health facilities to determine the appropriateness of such admission; and consultation and education services.
54	Intermediate Care Facility/Individuals with Intellectual Disabilities	A facility which primarily provides health-related care and services above the level of custodial care to individuals with intellectual disabilities but does not provide the level of care or treatment available in a hospital or SNF.
55	Residential Substance Abuse Treatment Facility	A facility which provides treatment for substance (alcohol and drug) abuse to live-in residents who do not require acute medical care. Services include individual and group therapy and counseling, family counseling, laboratory tests, drugs and supplies, psychological testing, and room and board.
56	Psychiatric Residential Treatment Center	A facility or distinct part of a facility for psychiatric care which provides a total 24-hour therapeutically planned and professionally staffed group living and learning environment.
57	Non-residential Substance Abuse Treatment Facility	A location which provides treatment for substance (alcohol and drug) abuse on an ambulatory basis. Services include individual and group therapy and counseling, family counseling, laboratory tests, drugs and supplies, and psychological testing. (Effective 10/1/03)
58-59	Unassigned	N/A
60	Mass Immunization Center	A location where providers administer pneumococcal pneumonia and influenza virus vaccinations and submit these services as electronic media claims, paper claims, or using the roster billing method. This generally takes place in a mass immunization setting, such as, a public health center, pharmacy, or mall but may include a physician office setting.
61	Comprehensive Inpatient Rehabilitation Facility	A facility that provides comprehensive rehabilitation services under the supervision of a physician to inpatients with physical disabilities. Services include physical therapy, occupational therapy, speech pathology, social or psychological services, and orthotics and prosthetics services.
62	Comprehensive Outpatient Rehabilitation Facility	A facility that provides comprehensive rehabilitation services under the supervision of a physician to outpatients with physical disabilities. Services include physical therapy, occupational therapy, and speech pathology services.
63-64	Unassigned	N/A
65	End-Stage Renal Disease Treatment Facility	A facility other than a hospital, which provides dialysis treatment, maintenance, and/or training to patients or caregivers on an ambulatory or home-care basis.
66-70	Unassigned	N/A
71	Public Health Clinic	A facility maintained by either State or local health departments that provides ambulatory primary medical care under the general direction of a physician.
72	Rural Health Clinic	A certified facility which is located in a rural medically underserved area that provides ambulatory primary medical care under the general direction of a physician.
73-80	Unassigned	N/A
81	Independent Laboratory	A laboratory certified to perform diagnostic and/or clinical tests independent of an institution or a physician's office.
82-98	Unassigned	N/A
99	Other Place of Service	Other place of service not identified above.

current procedural terminology

cpt® 2019

Professional Edition

AMA
AMERICAN MEDICAL ASSOCIATION

*Member of the CPT Executive Committee
†New Panel Member

Executive Vice President, Chief Executive Officer: James L. Madara, MD
Chief Operating Officer: Bernard L. Hengesbaugh
Senior Vice President, Health Solutions: Laurie A.S. McGraw
Vice President, Coding and Reimbursement Policy and Strategy: Jay Ahlman
Director, CPT Coding and Regulatory Services: Marie Mindeman
Manager, CPT Editorial Panel Processes: Desiree Rozell
Manager, CPT Content Management and Development: Karen E. O'Hara
Vice President, Operations: Denise C. Foy
Manager, Book and Product Development and Production: Nancy Baker
Senior Developmental Editor: Lisa Chin-Johnson
Production Specialist: Mary Ann Albanese
Vice President, Sales: Lori Prestesater
Director, Channel Sales: Erin Kalitowski
Executive, Key Account Manager: Mark Daniels
Vice President, Marketing and Strategic Initiatives: Dave Sosnow
Product Manager, Print and Digital Products: Carol Brockman
Marketing Manager: Vanessa Prieto

Printed in the United States of America. 18 19 20 / BD-RD / 9 8 7 6 5 4 3 2 1

Professional ISBN: 978-1-62202-752-1
ISSN: 0276-8283

1st Edition printed 1966
2nd Edition printed 1970
3rd Edition printed 1973
4th Edition printed 1977
Revised: 1978, 1979, 1980, 1981, 1982, 1984, 1985, 1986, 1987, 1988, 1989, 1990, 1991, 1992, 1993, 1994, 1995, 1996, 1997, 1998, 1999, 2000, 2001, 2002, 2003, 2004, 2005, 2006, 2007, 2008, 2009, 2010, 2011, 2012, 2013, 2014, 2015, 2016, 2017, 2018

To purchase additional CPT products, contact the American Medical Association Customer Service at 800 621-8335 or AMA|Store at **amastore.com**.
Refer to product number EP054119.

To request a license for distribution of products containing or reprinting CPT codes and/or guidelines, please see our website at www.ama-assn.org/go/cpt, or contact the American Medical Association CPT/DBP Intellectual Property Services, 330 North Wabash Avenue, Suite 39300, Chicago, IL 60611, 312 464-5022.

AC36:EP054119:9/18

About CPT

Current Procedural Terminology (CPT®), Fourth Edition, is a listing of descriptive terms and identifying codes for reporting medical services and procedures performed by physicians and other qualified health care professionals. The purpose of the terminology is to provide a uniform language that will accurately describe medical, surgical, and diagnostic services, and will thereby provide an effective means for reliable nationwide communication among physicians and other qualified health care professionals, patients, and third parties. *CPT 2019* is the most recent revision of a work that first appeared in 1966.

CPT descriptive terms and identifying codes currently serve a wide variety of important functions in the field of medical nomenclature. The CPT code set is useful for administrative management purposes such as claims processing and for the development of guidelines for medical care review. The uniform language is also applicable to medical education and outcomes, health services, and quality research by providing a useful basis for local, regional, and national utilization comparisons. The CPT code set is the most widely accepted nomenclature for the reporting of physician and other qualified health care professional procedures and services under government and private health insurance programs. In 2000, the CPT code set was designated by the Department of Health and Human Services as the national coding standard for physician and other health care professional services and procedures under the Health Insurance Portability and Accountability Act (HIPAA). This means that for all financial and administrative health care transactions sent electronically, the CPT code set will need to be used.

The changes that appear in this revision have been prepared by the CPT Editorial Panel with the assistance of physicians and representatives of other health care professions representing all specialties of medicine, and with important contributions from many third-party payers and governmental agencies.

The American Medical Association trusts that this revision will continue the usefulness of its predecessors in identifying, describing, and coding medical, surgical, and diagnostic services.

Maintenance and Authorship of the CPT Code Set

The CPT Editorial Panel (Panel) is tasked with ensuring that CPT codes remain up to date and reflect the latest medical care provided to patients. In order to do this, the Panel maintains an open process and convenes meetings at a minimum three times per year.

The Panel wishes to sincerely thank the many national medical specialty societies, health insurance organizations and agencies, and individual physicians and other health professionals who have made contributions. In particular the Panel acknowledges the efforts of the following Panel Organizational and Coding Liaison Participants:

Claudia Bonnell, *Blue Cross and Blue Shield Association*

Sue Bowman, RHIA, *American Health Information Management Association*

Raemarie Jiminez, CPC, *American Academy of Professional Coders*

Nelly Leon-Chisen, *American Hospital Association*

Also key to authorship of the code set and resulting *CPT Professional Edition* codebook is AMA CPT staff. This experienced team prepares agenda materials for each panel meeting, facilitates the application process, compiles and reviews advisor comments, reconciles differences in opinions, and ultimately compiles all resulting information into a codebook filled with informative guidelines, practical tips, and procedural illustrations.

AMA CPT Staff

Jay T. Ahlman
Thilani Attale, MS
Jennifer Bell, BS, RHIT, CPC, CPMA, CPC-I, CEMC
Andrei Besleaga, BS, RHIT
Judy Connelly
Caitlin Dale
Martha Espronceda
Desiree D. Evans, BS
DeHandro Hayden, BS
Zach Hochstetler, MPP, MBA, CPC
Janette Meggs, RHIA
Marie L. Mindeman, BA, RHIT
Karen E. O'Hara, BS, CCS-P
Michael Pellegrino
Gary Pilacinski, ACHE, LSSMBB
Desiree Rozell, MPA
Nancy Spector, BSN, MSC
Lianne Stancik, BA, RHIT
Keisha A. Sutton, MHA, CPC
Ada Walker, CCA
Arletrice Watkins, MHA, RHIA
Rejina L. Young

AMA CPT Advisory Committee

American Academy of Child & Adolescent Psychiatry
Benjamin N. Shain, MD, PhD
Jason V. Chang, MD

American Academy of Dermatology
Alexander Miller, MD
Ann F. Haas, MD

American Academy of Disability Evaluating Physicians
Douglas W. Martin, MD, FAADEP, FACOEM
James B. Talmage, MD

American Academy of Family Physicians
Bradley P. Fox, MD, FAAFP
Samuel L. Church, MD, MPH, CPC, CRC, FAAFP

American Academy of Neurology
Bruce H. Cohen, MD, FAAN
Neil A. Busis, MD

American Academy of Ophthalmology
Michael X. Repka, MD, MBA
John M. Haley, MD

American Academy of Orthopaedic Surgeons
Frank R. Voss, MD
Louis S. Stryker, MD

American Academy of Otolaryngic Allergy
Paul T. Fass, MD, FACS

American Academy of Otolaryngology Head and Neck Surgery
Lawrence M. Simon, MD, FAAP

American Academy of Pain Medicine
Eduardo M. Fraifeld, MD
Gregory R. Polston, MD‡

American Academy of Pediatrics
Joel F. Bradley, Jr, MD, FAAP
David M. Kanter, MD, MBA, CPC, FAAP

American Academy of Physical Medicine and Rehabilitation
Annie D. Purcell, DO
Scott I. Horn, DO

American Association for Clinical Chemistry
William A. Clark, PhD, MBA

American Association for Thoracic Surgery
Kirk R. Kanter, MD
Richard K. Freeman, II, MD

American Association of Clinical Endocrinologists
Eric A. Orzeck, MD, FACP, FACE
William C. Biggs, MD, FACE, ECNU

American Association of Neurological Surgeons
Joseph S. Cheng, MD, MS, FACS, FAANS
Jeffrey W. Cozzens, MD, FACS

American Association of Neuromuscular and Electrodiagnostic Medicine
John C. Kincaid, MD
Earl J. Craig, MD

American Clinical Neurophysiology Society
Marc R. Nuwer, MD, PhD, FAAN, FACP
Susan T. Herman, MD

American College of Allergy, Asthma and Immunology
James L. Sublett, MD‡
Gary N. Gross, MD

American College of Cardiology
Randall C. Thompson, MD
Anthony A. Hilliard, MD, FACC

American College of Chest Physicians
Steve G. Peters, MD
Michael E. Nelson, MD, FCCP

American College of Emergency Physicians
Jacob Mark J. Meredith, III, MD, MMM, FACEP
Michael J. Lemanski, MD, FACEP, FAAFP

American College of Gastroenterology
Christopher Y. Kim, MD, MBA, FACG, FASGE, AGAF, FACP
Daniel C. DeMarco, MD, FACP

American College of Medical Genetics and Genomics
David B. Flannery, MD

American College of Medical Quality
Joel Grossman, MD

American College of Mohs Surgery
David B. Pharis, MD, PC

American College of Nuclear Medicine
Scott C. Bartley, MD
Gary L. Dillehay, MD, FACNP, FACR

American College of Occupational and Environmental Medicine
Lee S. Glass, MD, JD

American College of Phlebology
Bruce R. Hoyle, MD
Thomas F. Wright, MD, FACP

American College of Physicians
Jeannine Z. Engel, MD, FACP
Tiffany R. Groover, MD, MPH

American College of Preventive Medicine
Brian J. Miller, MD, MBA, MPH

American College of Radiation Oncology
Shelia Rege, MD, FACRO
Andy W. Su, MD

American College of Radiology
Mark D. Alson, MD, FACR, RCC‡
Timothy A. Crummy, MD, RCC

American College of Rheumatology
Timothy J. Laing, MD
Joseph E. Huffstutter, MD‡

American College of Surgeons
Samuel D. Smith, MD
Megan E. McNally, MD, FACS

American Congress of Obstetricians and Gynecologists
Judith K. Volkar, MD, MBA
Mark R. Hoffman, MD

American Dental Association
Joshua E. Everts, DDS, MD
Adam S. Pitts, DDS, MD

American Gastroenterological Association
Braden Kuo, MD‡

‡New Advisors

American Geriatrics Society
Robert A. Zorowitz, MD, MBA, FACP, AGSF, CMD

American Institute of Ultrasound in Medicine
James M. Shwayder, MD, JD

American Medical Directors Association
Michelle F. Bellantoni, MD, CMD

American Orthopaedic Association
Blair C. Filler, MD

American Orthopaedic Foot and Ankle Society
John A. DiPreta, MD
Aaron J. Guyer, MD

American Osteopathic Association
James M. Bailey, DO, PhD

American Psychiatric Association
Jeremy S. Musher, MD, DFAPA
Gregory G. Harris, MD, MPH

American Roentgen Ray Society
Dana H. Smetherman, MD, MPH, FACR
Eric M. Rubin, MD‡

American Society for Aesthetic Plastic Surgery, Inc.
Paul R. Weiss, MD

American Society for Clinical Pathology
Lee H. Hilborne, MD, MPH, FASCP

American Society for Dermatologic Surgery
Murad Alam, MD, MBA
Jeremy S. Bordeaux, MD, MPH

American Society for Gastrointestinal Endoscopy
Glenn D. Littenberg, MD, MACP
Daniel C. DeMarco, MD, FACP‡

American Society for Metabolic and Bariatric Surgery
Matthew L. Brengman, MD

American Society for Radiation Oncology
William F. Hartsell, MD
Corbin R. Johnson, MD

American Society for Reproductive Medicine
Beth W. Rackow, MD, FACOG

American Society for Surgery of the Hand
Steven H. Goldberg, MD, FAAOS‡
Daniel J. Nagle, MD

American Society of Addiction Medicine
Stuart Gitlow, MD, MPH, MBA
Joel V. Brill, MD, FACP, AGAF‡

American Society of Anesthesiologists
Peter A. Goldzweig, DO
Padma Gulur, MD

American Society of Breast Surgeons
Richard E. Fine, MD, FACS
Eric R. Whitacre, MD, FACS

American Society of Cataract and Refractive Surgery
Parag D. Parekh, MD, MPA‡

American Society of Clinical Oncology
Christian A. Thomas, MD
Joseph J. Merchant, MD‡

American Society of Colon and Rectal Surgeons
William J. Harb, MD, FACS
Stephen M. Sentovich, MD, MBA, FACS, FASCRS

American Society of Cytopathology
Carol A. Filomena, MD

American Society of Dermatopathology
Jonathan S. Ralston, MD
Aleodor A. Andrea, MD, MBA

American Society of Echocardiography
Michael L. Main, MD

American Society of General Surgeons
George K. Gillian, MD, FACS
Christopher C. Smith, MD

American Society of Hematology
Samuel M. Silver, MD, PhD, MACP, FAHA, FASCO‡

American Society of Interventional Pain Physicians
Vikram B. Patel, MD, DABA
Sachin Jha, MD, MS

American Society of Neuroradiology
Raymond K. Tu, MD, FACR

American Society of Ophthalmic Plastic and Reconstructive Surgery
L. Neal Freeman, MD, MBA, CCS-P, FACS

American Society of Plastic Surgeons
Deborah S. Bash, MD
Daniel T. Ness, MD

American Society of Retina Specialists
Ankoor R. Shah, MD

American Thoracic Society
Stephen P. Hoffmann, MD
Michael E. Nelson, MD, FCCP

American Urological Association
Ronald P. Kaufman, Jr, MD, FACS
Jonathan R. Rubenstein, MD‡

Association of University Radiologists
Robert K. Zeman, MD, FACR
Richard Duszak, Jr., MD, FACR

College of American Pathologists
Ronald W. McLawhon, MD, PhD

Congress of Neurological Surgeons
Henry H. Woo, MD, FACS, FAANS

Heart Rhythm Society
JoEllyn C. Moore, MD, FACC
Steven C. Hao, MD, FACC, FHRS‡

Infectious Disease Society of America
Steven K. Schmitt, MD

International Society for the Advancement of Spine Surgery
James J. Yue, MD
Morgan L. Lorio, MD, FACS

National Association of Medical Examiners
John S. Denton, MD

North American Spine Society
William Mitchell, MD
David R. O'Brien, Jr, MD

Radiological Society of North America
Timothy A. Crummy, MD
Eric M. Rubin, MD

Renal Physicians Association
Chester A. Amedia, Jr, MD, FACP
Timothy A. Pflederer, MD

Society for Cardiovascular Angiography and Interventions
Arthur C. Lee, MD, FSCAI
Sergio Bartakian, MD, FSCAI‡

Society for Investigative Dermatology
Stephen P. Stone, MD

Society for Vascular Surgery
Sean P. Roddy, MD, FACS
Robert J. Feezor, MD, FACS

Society of American Gastrointestinal Endoscopic Surgeons
John S. Roth, MD, FACS
Kevin E. Wasco, MD, FACS

Society of Critical Care Medicine
George A. Sample, MD, FCCP

Society of Interventional Radiology
Timothy L. Swan, MD
Clifford M. Hawkins, MD

Society of Nuclear Medicine and Molecular Imaging
Gary L. Dillehay, MD, FACNP, FACR

Society of Thoracic Surgeons
Francis C. Nichols, III, MD
Jeffrey P. Jacobs, MD, FACS, FACC, FCCP

The Endocrine Society
Carol H. Wysham, MD

The Spinal Intervention Society
Scott I. Horn, DO
Luis A. Guerrero, MD

The Triological Society
Richard W. Waguespack, MD, FACS

United States and Canadian Academy of Pathology
Michael O. Idowu, MD, MPH
David S. Wilkinson, MD, PhD

AMA Health Care Professionals Advisory Committee (HCPAC)

Kenneth P. Brin, MD, PhD, MACC*, Co-Chair
AMA CPT Editorial Panel
Leslie F. Davidson, PhD, OTR/L, FAOTA, Co-Chair
AMA CPT Editorial Panel

Academy of Nutrition and Dietetics
Keith-Thomas Ayoob, EdD, RN, FADA, CSP
Jessie M. Pavlianc, MS, RD, CSR, LD

American Academy of Audiology
Brad A. Stach, PhD
Annette A. Burton, AuD

American Academy of Physician Assistants
Patrick J. Cafferty, MPAS, PA-C

American Association of Naturopathic Physicians
Eva Miller, ND
Amy E. Hobson, ND

American Association for Respiratory Care
Susan Rinaldo-Gallo, MEd, RRT, FAARC, CTTS

American Chiropractic Association
Leo Bronston, DC, MAppSc

American Massage Therapy Association
Nancy M. Porambo, BA, MS, LMT, NCTMB
Clark E. Simpson, MBA, Med, ATC‡

American Nurses Association
Jamesetta A. Newland, PhD, RN, FNP-BC, FAANP, DPNAP
Jill Olmstead, MSN, NP-C, ANP-BC, FAANP‡

American Occupational Therapy Association
Mary Jo McGuire, MS, OTR/L, FAOTA
Jeremy R. Furniss, OTD/OTR/L, BCG, CDP

American Optometric Association
Rebecca H. Wartman, OD
Harvey B. Richman, OD, FAAO

American Physical Therapy Association
Kathleen M. Picard, PT

American Podiatric Medical Association
Ira H. Kraus, DPM
Phillip E. Ward, DPM

American Psychological Association
Neil H. Pliskin, PhD, ABPP-CN
Randy E. Phelps, PhD

American Speech-Language-Hearing Association
Stuart G. Trembath, MA, CCC-A

National Athletic Trainers' Association
Karen D. Fennell, MS, ATC
Joseph J. Greene, MS, ATC‡

National Association of Social Workers
Mirean F. Coleman, LICSW
Doris F. Tomer, LCSW, BCD

National Society of Genetic Counselors
Karen E. Lewis, MS, MM, CGC

Pharmacy Health Information Technology Collaborative
Daniel E. Buffington, PharmD, MBA
Brian J. Isetts, PhD, BCPS, FAPhA

*Member of the CPT Executive Committee
‡New Advisors

Contents

About CPT v
Maintenance and Authorship of the CPT Code Set v
AMA CPT Staff v

Introduction xii
Section Numbers and Their Sequences xii
Instructions for Use of the CPT Codebook xii
Format of the Terminology xiii
Requests to Update the CPT Nomenclature xiii
Application Submission Requirements xiii
General Criteria for Category I, II, and III Codes . . . xiii
Category-Specific Requirements xiv
Guidelines xiv
Add-on Codes xv
Modifiers xv
Place of Service and Facility Reporting xv
Unlisted Procedure or Service xv
Results, Testing, Interpretation, and Report xvi
Special Report xvi
Time xvi
Code Symbols xvi
Alphabetical Reference Index xvi
CPT 2019 in Electronic Formats xvii
References to AMA Resources xvii

Illustrated Anatomical and Procedural Review xviii
Prefixes, Suffixes, and Roots xviii
Numbers xviii
Surgical Procedures xviii
Conditions xviii
Directions and Positions xix
Additional References xix
Medical Dictionaries xix
Anatomy References xix
Lists of Illustrations xix
Anatomical Illustrations xix
Procedural Illustrations xx
Evaluation and Management Tables xxiii

Evaluation and Management (E/M) Services Guidelines 4
Classification of Evaluation and Management (E/M) Services 4
Definitions of Commonly Used Terms 4
Unlisted Service 8
Special Report 8
Clinical Examples 8
Instructions for Selecting a Level of E/M Service 9

Evaluation and Management 11
Office or Other Outpatient Services 11
Hospital Observation Services 13
Hospital Inpatient Services 15
Consultations 19
Emergency Department Services 22
Critical Care Services 23
Nursing Facility Services 25
Domiciliary, Rest Home (eg, Boarding Home), or Custodial Care Services 28
Domiciliary, Rest Home (eg, Assisted Living Facility), or Home Care Plan Oversight Services 30
Home Services 30
Prolonged Services 32
Case Management Services 35
Care Plan Oversight Services 36
Preventive Medicine Services 37
Non-Face-to-Face Services 39
Special Evaluation and Management Services 42
Newborn Care Services 43
Delivery/Birthing Room Attendance and Resuscitation Services 43
Inpatient Neonatal Intensive Care Services and Pediatric and Neonatal Critical Care Services 44
Cognitive Assessment and Care Plan Services 48
Care Management Services 49
Psychiatric Collaborative Care Management Services . . . 52
Transitional Care Management Services 54
Advance Care Planning 55
General Behavioral Health Integration Care Management 56
Other Evaluation and Management Services 56

Anesthesia Guidelines 60
Time Reporting 60
Anesthesia Services 60
Supplied Materials 60
Separate or Multiple Procedures 60
►Unlisted Service or Procedure◄ 60
Special Report 61
Anesthesia Modifiers 61
Qualifying Circumstances 61

Anesthesia 62
Head 62
Neck 62
Thorax (Chest Wall and Shoulder Girdle) 63
Intrathoracic 63
Spine and Spinal Cord 63
Upper Abdomen 64

►◄ = Contains new or revised text

Lower Abdomen ... 64
Perineum ... 65
Pelvis (Except Hip) ... 65
Upper Leg (Except Knee) ... 66
Knee and Popliteal Area ... 66
Lower Leg (Below Knee, Includes Ankle and Foot) ... 66
Shoulder and Axilla ... 67
Upper Arm and Elbow ... 67
Forearm, Wrist, and Hand ... 67
Radiological Procedures ... 68
Burn Excisions or Debridement ... 68
Obstetric ... 68
Other Procedures ... 69

Surgery Guidelines ... 72
Services ... 72
CPT Surgical Package Definition ... 72
Follow-Up Care for Diagnostic Procedures ... 72
Follow-Up Care for Therapeutic Surgical Procedures ... 72
Supplied Materials ... 72
Reporting More Than One Procedure/Service ... 72
Separate Procedure ... 72
Unlisted Service or Procedure ... 73
Special Report ... 74
Imaging Guidance ... 74
Surgical Destruction ... 74

Surgery ... 77
General ... 77
Integumentary System ... 78
Musculoskeletal System ... 116
Respiratory System ... 187
Cardiovascular System ... 214
Hemic and Lymphatic Systems ... 290
Mediastinum and Diaphragm ... 295
Digestive System ... 300
Urinary System ... 357
Male Genital System ... 381
Reproductive System Procedures ... 387
Intersex Surgery ... 387
Female Genital System ... 391
Maternity Care and Delivery ... 401
Endocrine System ... 404
Nervous System ... 412
Eye and Ocular Adnexa ... 447
Auditory System ... 464
Operating Microscope ... 468

Radiology Guidelines (Including Nuclear Medicine and Diagnostic Ultrasound) ... 472
Subject Listings ... 472
Separate Procedures ... 472
Unlisted Service or Procedure ... 472
Special Report ... 473
►Supervision and Interpretation, Imaging Guidance◄ ... 473
Administration of Contrast Material(s) ... 473
Written Report(s) ... 473

Radiology ... 474
Diagnostic Radiology (Diagnostic Imaging) ... 474
Diagnostic Ultrasound ... 493
Radiologic Guidance ... 499
Breast, Mammography ... 500
Bone/Joint Studies ... 502
Radiation Oncology ... 502
Nuclear Medicine ... 510

Pathology and Laboratory Guidelines ... 536
Services in Pathology and Laboratory ... 536
Separate or Multiple Procedures ... 536
Unlisted Service or Procedure ... 536
Special Report ... 536

Pathology and Laboratory ... 537
Organ or Disease-Oriented Panels ... 537
Drug Assay ... 539
Therapeutic Drug Assays ... 546
Evocative/Suppression Testing ... 548
Consultations (Clinical Pathology) ... 550
Urinalysis ... 550
Molecular Pathology ... 551
Genomic Sequencing Procedures and Other Molecular Multianalyte Assays ... 578
Multianalyte Assays with Algorithmic Analyses ... 581
Chemistry ... 583
Hematology and Coagulation ... 594
Immunology ... 597
Transfusion Medicine ... 603
Microbiology ... 604
Anatomic Pathology ... 612
Cytopathology ... 612
Cytogenetic Studies ... 614
Surgical Pathology ... 615
In Vivo (eg, Transcutaneous) Laboratory Procedures ... 620
Other Procedures ... 621
Reproductive Medicine Procedures ... 621
Proprietary Laboratory Analyses ... 623

Medicine Guidelines ... 631
Add-on Codes ... 631
Separate Procedures ... 631
Unlisted Service or Procedure ... 631

Special Report 632
Imaging Guidance....632
Supplied Materials....632

Medicine 633
Immune Globulins, Serum or Recombinant Products....633
Immunization Administration for Vaccines/Toxoids 633
Vaccines, Toxoids....634
Psychiatry 639
Biofeedback 643
Dialysis....643
Gastroenterology 646
Ophthalmology....648
Special Otorhinolaryngologic Services....653
Cardiovascular 657
Noninvasive Vascular Diagnostic Studies 686
Pulmonary....689
Allergy and Clinical Immunology 692
Endocrinology....695
Neurology and Neuromuscular Procedures 695
Medical Genetics and Genetic Counseling Services....709
►Adaptive Behavior Services◄ 709
Central Nervous System Assessments/Tests (eg, Neuro-Cognitive, Mental Status, Speech Testing) 712
Health and Behavior Assessment/Intervention....716
Hydration, Therapeutic, Prophylactic, Diagnostic Injections and Infusions, and Chemotherapy and Other Highly Complex Drug or Highly Complex Biologic Agent Administration....717
Photodynamic Therapy....722
Special Dermatological Procedures....723
Physical Medicine and Rehabilitation 724
Medical Nutrition Therapy....731
Acupuncture....731
Osteopathic Manipulative Treatment 732
Chiropractic Manipulative Treatment 732
Education and Training for Patient Self-Management 733
Non-Face-to-Face Nonphysician Services 734
Special Services, Procedures and Reports....734
Qualifying Circumstances for Anesthesia 736
Moderate (Conscious) Sedation....736
Other Services and Procedures 738
Home Health Procedures/Services 739
Medication Therapy Management Services 740

Category II Codes....743
Modifiers 744
Composite Codes 744
Patient Management 745
Patient History 746
Physical Examination 749
Diagnostic/Screening Processes or Results 750
Therapeutic, Preventive, or Other Interventions 756
Follow-up or Other Outcomes 761
Patient Safety....762
Structural Measures....762
Nonmeasure Code Listing 762

Category III Codes 764

Appendix A—Modifiers....791

Appendix B—Summary of Additions, Deletions, and Revisions 798

Appendix C—Clinical Examples 805
Office or Other Outpatient Service....805
Hospital Inpatient Services 815
Subsequent Hospital Care 818
Consultations 821
Emergency Department Services....827
Critical Care Services....828
Prolonged Services....828
Care Plan Oversight Services....829
Prolonged Clinical Staff Services with Physician or Other Qualified Health Care Professional Supervision 829
Inpatient Neonatal Intensive Care Service and Pediatric and Neonatal Critical Care Services 829

Appendix D—Summary of CPT Add-on Codes....830

Appendix E—Summary of CPT Codes Exempt from Modifier 51....831

Appendix F—Summary of CPT Codes Exempt from Modifier 63....832

Appendix G—Summary of CPT Codes That Include Moderate (Conscious) Sedation 833

Appendix H—Alphabetical Clinical Topics Listing (AKA – Alphabetical Listing)....833

Appendix I—Genetic Testing Code Modifiers....833

Appendix J—Electrodiagnostic Medicine Listing of Sensory, Motor, and Mixed Nerves 834

Appendix K—Product Pending FDA Approval....837

Appendix L—Vascular Families....838

Appendix M—Renumbered CPT Codes–Citations Crosswalk 848

Appendix N—Summary of Resequenced CPT Codes....854

Appendix O—Multianalyte Assays with Algorithmic Analyses 858

Appendix P—CPT Codes That May Be Used For Synchronous Telemedicine Services....869

Index....871

► ◄ = Contains new or revised text

Introduction

Current Procedural Terminology (CPT®), Fourth Edition, is a set of codes, descriptions, and guidelines intended to describe procedures and services performed by physicians and other health care professionals, or entities. Each procedure or service is identified with a five-digit code. The use of CPT codes simplifies the reporting of procedures and services. In the CPT code set, the term "procedure" is used to describe services, including diagnostic tests.

Inclusion of a descriptor and its associated five-digit code number in the CPT Category I code set is based on whether the procedure or service is consistent with contemporary medical practice and is performed by many practitioners in clinical practice in multiple locations. Inclusion in the CPT code set of a procedure or service, or proprietary name, does not represent endorsement by the American Medical Association (AMA) of any particular diagnostic or therapeutic procedure or service or proprietary test or manufacturer. Inclusion or exclusion of a procedure or service, or proprietary name, does not imply any health insurance coverage or reimbursement policy.

The CPT code set is published annually in late summer or early fall as both electronic data files and books. The release of CPT data files on the Internet typically precedes the book by several weeks. In any case, January 1, is the effective date for use of the updated CPT code set. The interval between the release of the update and the effective date is considered an implementation period and is intended to allow physicians and other providers, payers, and vendors to incorporate CPT changes into their systems. Changes to the CPT code set are meant to be applied prospectively from the effective date. The exceptions to this schedule of release and effective dates are CPT Category III codes, vaccine product codes, and CPT Category II codes. CPT Category III codes and vaccine product codes are released twice a year on January 1 or July 1, with effective dates six months after release depending on specific payer implementation period and coverage policy. CPT Category II codes are released three times a year with an effective date of three months after release.

The main body of the Category I section is listed in six sections. Each section is divided into subsections with anatomic, procedural, condition, or descriptor subheadings. The procedures and services with their identifying codes are presented in numeric order with one exception—the entire **Evaluation and Management** section (99201-99499) appears at the beginning of the listed procedures. These items are used by most physicians in reporting a significant portion of their services.

Section Numbers and Their Sequences

Evaluation and Management 99201-99499

Anesthesiology 00100-01999, 99100-99140

Surgery 10021-69990

Radiology (Including Nuclear Medicine and Diagnostic Ultrasound) 70010-79999

Pathology and Laboratory 80047-89398, 0001U-0061U

Medicine (except Anesthesiology) 90281-99199, 99500-99607

The first and last code numbers and the subsection name of the items appear at the top margin of most pages (eg, "10140-11006 Surgery/Integumentary System"). The continuous pagination of the CPT codebook is found on the lower margin of each page along with explanation of any code symbols that are found on that page.

Instructions for Use of the CPT Codebook

Select the name of the procedure or service that accurately identifies the service performed. Do not select a CPT code that merely approximates the service provided. If no such specific code exists, then report the service using the appropriate unlisted procedure or service code. In surgery, it may be an operation; in medicine, a diagnostic or therapeutic procedure; in radiology, a radiograph. Other additional procedures performed or pertinent special services are also listed. When necessary, any modifying or extenuating circumstances are added. Any service or procedure should be adequately documented in the medical record.

It is equally important to recognize that as techniques in medicine and surgery have evolved, new types of services, including minimally invasive surgery, as well as endovascular, percutaneous, and endoscopic interventions have challenged the traditional distinction of Surgery vs Medicine. Thus, the listing of a service or procedure in a specific section of this book should not be interpreted as strictly classifying the service or procedure as "surgery" or "not surgery" for insurance or other purposes. The placement of a given service in a specific section of the book may reflect historical or other considerations (eg, placement of the percutaneous peripheral vascular endovascular interventions in the Surgery/Cardiovascular System section, while the percutaneous coronary interventions appear in the Medicine/Cardiovascular section).

When advanced practice nurses and physician assistants are working with physicians, they are considered as working in the exact same specialty and exact same subspecialties as the physician. A "physician or other qualified health care professional" is an individual who is qualified by education, training, licensure/regulation (when applicable), and facility privileging (when applicable) who performs a professional service within his/her scope of practice and independently reports that professional service. These professionals are distinct from "clinical staff." A clinical staff member is a person who works under the supervision of a physician or other qualified health care professional and who is allowed by law, regulation, and facility policy to perform or assist in the performance of a specified professional service, but who does not individually report that professional service. Other policies may also affect who may report specific services.

Throughout the CPT code set the use of terms such as "physician," "qualified health care professional," or "individual" is not intended to indicate that other entities may not report the service. In selected instances, specific instructions may define a service as limited to professionals or limited to other entities (eg, hospital or home health agency).

Instructions, typically included as parenthetical notes with selected codes, indicate that a code should not be reported with another code or codes. These instructions are intended to prevent errors of significant probability and are not all inclusive. For example, the code with such instructions may be a component of another code and therefore it would be incorrect to report both codes even when the component service is performed. These instructions are not intended as a listing of all possible code combinations that should not be reported, nor do they indicate all possible code combinations that are appropriately reported. When reporting codes for services provided, it is important to assure the accuracy and quality of coding through verification of the intent of the code by use of the related guidelines, parenthetical instructions, and coding resources, including *CPT Assistant* and other publications resulting from collaborative efforts of the American Medical Association with the medical specialty societies (ie, *Clinical Examples in Radiology*).

Format of the Terminology

The CPT code set has been developed as stand-alone descriptions of medical procedures. However, some of the procedures in the CPT codebook are not printed in their entirety but refer back to a common portion of the procedure listed in a preceding entry. This is evident when an entry is followed by one or more indentations. This is done in an effort to conserve space.

Example

25100 Arthrotomy, wrist joint; with biopsy

25105 with synovectomy

Note that the common part of code 25100 (the part before the semicolon) should also be considered part of code 25105. Therefore, the full procedure represented by code 25105 should read:

25105 Arthrotomy, wrist joint; with synovectomy

Requests to Update the CPT Nomenclature

The effectiveness of the CPT nomenclature depends on constant updating to reflect changes in medical practice. This can only be accomplished through the interest and timely suggestions of practicing physicians and other qualified health care professionals, specialty/professional societies, state medical associations, organizations, agencies, individual users of the CPT code set, and other stakeholders. Accordingly, the AMA welcomes correspondence, inquiries, and suggestions concerning CPT coding and nomenclature for old and new procedures and services, as well as any matters relating to the CPT code set.

For information on submission of an application to add, delete, or revise codes contained in the CPT code set, please see www.ama-assn.org/go/cpt-processfaq or contact:

CPT Editorial Research & Development
American Medical Association
330 North Wabash Avenue
Suite 39300
Chicago IL 60611-5885

Code change applications are available at the AMA's CPT website at www.ama-assn.org/go/cpt-application.

All proposed changes to the CPT code set will be considered by the CPT Editorial Panel, in consultation with medical specialty societies as represented by the CPT Advisory Committee, other health care professional societies as represented by the Health Care Professionals Advisory Committee (HCPAC), and other interested parties.

Application Submission Requirements

All complete CPT code change applications are reviewed and evaluated by the CPT staff, the CPT/HCPAC Advisory Committee, and the CPT Editorial Panel. Strict conformance with the following is required for review of a code change application:

- Submission of a complete application, including all necessary supporting documents;
- Adherence to all posted deadlines;
- Cooperation with requests from the CPT staff and/or Editorial Panel members for clarification and information; ***and***
- Compliance with CPT Lobbying Policy.

General Criteria for Category I, II, and III Codes

All Category I, II, and III code change applications must satisfy each of the following criteria:

- The proposed descriptor is unique, well-defined, and describes a procedure or service that is clearly identified and distinguished from existing procedures and services already in the CPT code set;
- The descriptor structure, guidelines, and instructions are consistent with the current CPT Editorial Panel standards for maintenance of the code set;
- The proposed descriptor for the procedure or service is neither a fragmentation of an existing procedure or service nor currently reportable as a complete service by one or more existing codes (with the exclusion of unlisted codes). However, procedures and services frequently performed together may require new or revised codes;
- The structure and content of the proposed code descriptor accurately reflects the procedure or service as typically performed. If always or frequently performed with one or more other procedures or services, the descriptor structure and content will reflect the typical combination or complete procedure or service;
- The descriptor for the procedure or service is not proposed as a means to report extraordinary circumstances related to the performance of a procedure or service already described in the CPT code set; ***and***

- The procedure or service satisfies the category-specific criteria set forth below.

Category-Specific Requirements

Category I Criteria

A proposal for a new or revised Category I code must satisfy all of the following criteria:

- All devices and drugs necessary for performance of the procedure or service have received FDA clearance or approval when such is required for performance of the procedure or service;
- The procedure or service is performed by many physicians or other qualified health care professionals across the United States;
- The procedure or service is performed with frequency consistent with the intended clinical use (ie, a service for a common condition should have high volume, whereas a service commonly performed for a rare condition may have low volume);
- The procedure or service is consistent with current medical practice; and
- The clinical efficacy of the procedure or service is documented in literature that meets the requirements set forth in the CPT code change application.

Category II Criteria

The following criteria are used by the CPT/HCPAC and the CPT Editorial Panel for evaluating Category II code applications:

- Measurements that were developed and tested by a national organization;
- Evidence-based measurements with established ties to health outcomes;
- Measurements that address clinical conditions of high prevalence, high risk, or high cost; and
- Well-established measurements that are currently being used by large segments of the health care industry across the country.

In addition, all of the following are required:

- Definition or purpose of the measure is consistent with its intended use (quality improvement and accountability, or solely quality improvement)
- Aspect of care measured is substantially influenced by the physician (or other qualified health care professional or entity for which the code may be relevant)
- Reduces data collection burden on physicians (or other qualified health care professionals or entities)
- Significant
  - o Affects a large segment of health care community
  - o Tied to health outcomes
  - o Addresses clinical conditions of high prevalence, high costs, high risks
- Evidence-based
  - o Agreed upon
  - o Definable
  - o Measurable
- Risk-adjustment specifications and instructions for all outcome measures submitted or compelling evidence as to why risk adjustment is not relevant
- Sufficiently detailed to make it useful for multiple purposes
- Facilitates reporting of performance measure(s)
- Inclusion of select patient history, testing (eg, glycohemoglobin), other process measures, cognitive or procedure services within CPT, or physiologic measures (eg, blood pressure) to support performance measurements
- Performance measure–development process that includes
  - o Nationally recognized expert panel
  - o Multidisciplinary
  - o Vetting process

Category III Criteria

The following **criteria** are used by the CPT/HCPAC Advisory Committee and the CPT Editorial Panel for evaluating Category III code **applications**:

- The procedure or service is currently or recently performed in humans; ***and***

At least one of the following additional criteria has been met:

- The application is supported by at least one CPT or HCPAC advisor representing practitioners who would use this procedure or service; ***or***
- The actual or potential clinical efficacy of the specific procedure or service is supported by peer reviewed literature, which is available in English for examination by the CPT Editorial Panel; ***or***
- There is (a) at least one Institutional Review Board–approved protocol of a study of the procedure or service being performed; (b) a description of a current and ongoing United States trial outlining the efficacy of the procedure or service; or (c) other evidence of evolving clinical utilization.

Guidelines

Specific guidelines are presented at the beginning of each of the sections. These guidelines define items that are necessary to appropriately interpret and report the procedures and services contained in that section. For example, in the **Medicine** section, specific instructions are provided for handling unlisted services or procedures, special reports, and supplies and materials provided. Guidelines also provide explanations regarding terms that apply only to a particular section. For instance, **Radiology Guidelines** provide a definition of the unique term, "radiological supervision and interpretation." While in **Anesthesia**, a discussion of reporting time is included.

A written report (eg, handwritten or electronic) signed by the interpreting individual should be considered an integral part of a radiologic procedure or interpretation. Please see the guidelines regarding Imaging Guidance in each individual section.

Add-on Codes

Some of the listed procedures are commonly carried out in addition to the primary procedure performed. These additional or supplemental procedures are designated as add-on codes with the ✚ symbol and they are listed in **Appendix D** of the CPT codebook. Add-on codes in CPT 2019 can be readily identified by specific descriptor nomenclature that includes phrases such as "each additional" or "(List separately in addition to primary procedure)."

The add-on code concept in CPT 2019 applies only to add-on procedures or services performed by the same physician. Add-on codes describe additional intra-service work associated with the primary procedure, eg, additional digit(s), lesion(s), neurorrhaphy(s), vertebral segment(s), tendon(s), joint(s).

Add-on codes are always performed in addition to the primary service or procedure and must never be reported as a stand-alone code. All add-on codes in the CPT code set are exempt from the multiple procedure concept (see the modifier 51 definition in **Appendix A**).

Modifiers

A modifier provides the means to report or indicate that a service or procedure that has been performed has been altered by some specific circumstance but not changed in its definition or code. Modifiers also enable health care professionals to effectively respond to payment policy requirements established by other entities. The judicious application of modifiers obviates the necessity for separate procedure listings that may describe the modifying circumstance. Modifiers may be used to indicate to the recipient of a report that:

- A service or procedure had both a professional and technical component.
- A service or procedure was performed by more than one physician or other health care professional and/or in more than one location.
- A service or procedure was increased or reduced.
- Only part of a service was performed.
- An adjunctive service was performed.
- A bilateral procedure was performed.
- A service or procedure was provided more than once.
- Unusual events occurred.

Example

A physician providing diagnostic or therapeutic radiology services, ultrasound, or nuclear medicine services in a hospital would add modifier 26 to report the professional component.

73090 with modifier 26 = Professional component only for an X ray of the forearm

Example

Two surgeons may be required to manage a specific surgical problem. When two surgeons work together as primary surgeons performing distinct part(s) of a procedure, each surgeon should report his/her distinct operative work by adding modifier 62 to the procedure code and any associated code(s) for that procedure as long as both surgeons continue to work together as primary surgeons. Each surgeon should report the co-surgery once using the same procedure code. Modifier 62 would be applicable. For instance, a neurological surgeon and an otolaryngologist are working as co-surgeons in performing transphenoidal excision of a pituitary neoplasm.

The first surgeon would report:

61548 62 = Hypophysectomy or excision of pituitary tumor, transnasal or transseptal approach, nonstereotactic + two surgeons modifier

and the second surgeon would report:

61548 62 = Hypophysectomy or excision of pituitary tumor, transnasal or transseptal approach, nonstereotactic + two surgeons modifier

If additional procedure(s) (including add-on procedure[s]) are performed during the same surgical session, separate code(s) may also be reported with modifier 62 added. It should be noted that if a co-surgeon acts as an assistant in the performance of additional procedure(s) during the same surgical session, those services may be reported using separate procedure code(s) with modifier 80 or modifier 82 added, as appropriate. A complete listing of modifiers is found in **Appendix A**.

Place of Service and Facility Reporting

Some codes have specified places of service (eg, evaluation and management codes are specific to a setting). Other services and procedures may have instructions specific to the place of service (eg, therapeutic, prophylactic, and diagnostic injections and infusions). The CPT code set is designated for reporting physician and other qualified health care professional services. It is also the designated code set for reporting services provided by organizations or facilities (eg, hospitals) in specific circumstances. Throughout the CPT code set, the use of terms such as "physician," "qualified health care professional," or "individual" is not intended to indicate that other entities may not report the service. In selected instances, specific instructions may define a service as limited to professionals or limited to other entities (eg, hospital or home health agency). The CPT code set uses the term "facility" to describe such providers and the term "nonfacility" to describe services settings or circumstances in which no facility reporting may occur. Services provided in the home by an agency are facility services. Services provided in the home by a physician or other qualified health care professional who is not a representative of the agency are nonfacility services.

Unlisted Procedure or Service

It is recognized that there may be services or procedures performed by physicians or other qualified health care professionals that are not found in the CPT code set. Therefore, a number of specific code numbers have been designated for reporting unlisted procedures. When an unlisted procedure number is used, the service or procedure should be described (see specific section guidelines). Each of these unlisted procedural code numbers (with the appropriate accompanying topical entry) relates to a specific section of the book and is presented in the guidelines of that section.

In some cases alternative coding and procedural nomenclature as contained in other code sets may allow appropriate reporting of a more specific code. CPT references to use an unlisted procedure code do not preclude the reporting of an appropriate code that may be found in other code sets.

Results, Testing, Interpretation, and Report

Results are the technical component of a service. Testing leads to results; results lead to interpretation. Reports are the work product of the interpretation of test results. Certain procedures or services described in CPT involve a technical component (eg, tests), which produces "results" (eg, data, images, slides). For clinical use, some of these results require interpretation. Some CPT descriptors specifically require interpretation and reporting in order to report that code.

Special Report

A service that is rarely provided, unusual, variable, or new may require a special report. Pertinent information should include an adequate definition or description of the nature, extent, and need for the procedure and the time, effort, and equipment necessary to provide the service.

Time

The CPT code set contains many codes with a time basis for code selection. The following standards shall apply to time measurement, unless there are code or code-range–specific instructions in guidelines, parenthetical instructions, or code descriptors to the contrary. Time is the face-to-face time with the patient. Phrases such as "interpretation and report" in the code descriptor are not intended to indicate in all cases that report writing is part of the reported time. A unit of time is attained when the mid-point is passed. For example, an hour is attained when 31 minutes have elapsed (more than midway between zero and sixty minutes). A second hour is attained when a total of 91 minutes have elapsed. When codes are ranked in sequential typical times and the actual time is between two typical times, the code with the typical time closest to the actual time is used. See also the **Evaluation and Management (E/M) Services Guidelines**. When another service is performed concurrently with a time-based service, the time associated with the concurrent service should not be included in the time used for reporting the time-based service. Some services measured in units other than days extend across calendar dates. When this occurs a continuous service does not reset and create a first hour. However, any disruption in the service does create a new initial service. For example, if intravenous hydration (96360, 96361) is given from 11 PM to 2 AM, 96360 would be reported once and 96361 twice. For facility reporting on a single date of service or for continuous services that last beyond midnight (ie, over a range of dates), report the total units of time provided continuously.

Code Symbols

A summary listing of additions, deletions, and revisions applicable to the CPT codebook is found in **Appendix B**. New procedure numbers added to the CPT codebook are identified throughout the text with the ● symbol placed before the code number. In instances where a code revision has resulted in a substantially altered procedure descriptor, the ▲ symbol is placed before the code number. The ▶ ◀ symbols are used to indicate new and revised text other than the procedure descriptors. These symbols indicate CPT Editorial Panel actions. The AMA reserves the right to correct typographical errors and make stylistic improvements.

CPT add-on codes are annotated by the ✚ symbol and are listed in **Appendix D**. The symbol ⊘ is used to identify codes that are exempt from the use of modifier 51 but have not been designated as CPT add-on procedures or services. A list of codes exempt from modifier 51 usage is included in **Appendix E**. The ⚡ symbol is used to identify codes for vaccines that are pending FDA approval (see **Appendix K**). The # symbol is used to identify codes that are listed out of numerical sequence (see **Appendix N**). The ★ symbol is used to identify codes that may be used to report telemedicine services when appended by modifier 95 (see **Appendix P**).

Resequenced codes that are not placed numerically are identified with the # symbol, and a reference placed numerically (ie, Code is out of numerical sequence. See…) as a navigational alert to direct the user to the location of the out-of-sequence code (see **Appendix N**). Resequencing is utilized to allow placement of related concepts in appropriate locations within the families of codes regardless of the availability of numbers for sequential numerical placement.

▶Duplicate proprietary laboratory analyses (PLA) tests are annotated by the ⋈ symbol. PLA codes describe proprietary clinical laboratory analyses and can be either provided by a single ("sole-source") laboratory or licensed or marketed to multiple providing laboratories (eg, cleared or approved by the Food and Drug Administration [FDA]). All codes that are included in the PLA section are also included in Appendix O, with the procedure's proprietary name. In some instances, the descriptor language of PLA codes may be identical and the code may only be differentiated by the listed proprietary name in Appendix O. When more than one PLA test has an identical descriptor, the codes will be denoted by the symbol ⋈.◀

Alphabetical Reference Index

This codebook features an expanded alphabetical index that includes listings by procedure and anatomic site. Procedures and services commonly known by their eponyms or other designations are also included.

CPT 2019 in Electronic Formats

CPT 2019 procedure codes and descriptions are available as downloadable data files. The CPT data files are available in ASCII and EBCDIC formats and provide a convenient way to import the 2019 CPT codes and descriptions into existing documentation or into any billing and claims reporting software that accepts a text (.TXT) file format. The data files contain the complete official AMA CPT guidelines, descriptor package, and new descriptors for consumers and clinicians.

The *CPT Professional* codebook is also available as an e-book. For more information about CPT electronic formats, call 800 621-8335 or visit **amastore.com**.

References to AMA Resources

The symbols ➔ ➔ and ➔ appear after many codes throughout this codebook, which indicate that the AMA has published reference material regarding that particular code.

The symbol ➔ refers to the *CPT Changes: An Insider's View*, an annual book with all of the coding changes for the current year, the ➔ refers to the *CPT Assistant* monthly newsletter. The symbol ➔ refers to the quarterly newsletter *Clinical Examples in Radiology*.

Example

36598 Contrast injection(s) for radiologic evaluation of existing central venous access device, including fluoroscopy, image documentation and report

➔ *CPT Changes: An Insider's View* 2006

➔ *Clinical Examples in Radiology* Winter 2006:15

In this example, the blue reference symbol indicates that in the 2006 edition of *CPT Changes: An Insider's View* information is available that may assist in understanding the application of the code. The red reference symbol indicates that the 2006 Winter issue of *Clinical Examples in Radiology* (page 15) should be consulted.

CPT Assistant and *Clinical Examples in Radiology* are available online. Benefits exclusive to the online versions include:

- Monthly (*CPT Assistant*) and quarterly (*Clinical Examples in Radiology*) updates! The home screen notifies you when a new issue is available and you can review the latest issue in its entirety.
- Unlimited access to every archived issue and article dating back to when the newsletters first published.
- A historical CPT code list that references when a code was added, deleted, and/or revised since 1990.
- Simple search capabilities, including intuitive menus and a cumulative index of article titles.
- Anatomical illustrations, charts, and graphs for quick reference.
- A full archive of *CPT Assistant* articles (1990-2018) is also available in the *CPT Professional Print and Digital* app bundle (see the following information about the *CPT QuickRef* app).

The *CPT QuickRef* app is available for iOS (Apple) and Android devices (smart phones and tablets). The *QuickRef* app contains important coding and billing tools, including:

- The entire CPT 2019 code set (full codes, descriptions, icons, illustrations, and parenthetical notes), plus the entire 2018 code set to facilitate the year-end code set transition.
- Facility and non-facility RVUs and Global Days.
- Medicare Physician Fee Schedule calculator that can be set to a specific geographic region (GPCI)
- E/M Code Selection Wizard with the option to apply CPT, CMS '95, or CMS '97 guidelines.
- *CPT Assistant* Archive: all content and every issue of *CPT Assistant* from 1990 through 2017, linked to the pertinent CPT codes and available for browsing.
- Official AMA CPT coding guidelines linked to each CPT code.
- Up to 4,200 clinical examples/vignettes.
- More than 200 AMA-created colorized procedural and anatomical illustrations
- Modifiers
- Keyword and code number search
- Favorites capability, to store most-frequently used codes or modifiers for easy access.

For more information, call 800 621-8335.

Illustrated Anatomical and Procedural Review

It is essential that coders have a thorough understanding of medical terminology and anatomy to code accurately. The following section reviewing the basics of vocabulary and anatomy can be used as a quick reference to help you with your coding. It is not intended as a replacement for up-to-date medical dictionaries and anatomy texts, which are essential tools for accurate coding.

Prefixes, Suffixes, and Roots

Although medical terminology may seem complex, many medical terms can be broken into component parts, which makes them easier to understand. Many of these terms are derived from Latin or Greek words, but some include the names of physicians.

Prefixes are word parts that appear at the beginning of a word and modify its meaning; suffixes are found at the end of words. By learning what various prefixes and suffixes mean, it is possible to decipher the meaning of a word quickly. The following lists are a quick reference for some common prefixes and suffixes.

Numbers

Prefix	Meaning	Example
mono-, uni-	one	monocyte, unilateral
bi-	two	bilateral
tri-	three	triad
quadr-	four	quadriplegia
hex-, sex-	six	hexose
diplo-	double	diplopia

Surgical Procedures

Suffix	Meaning	Example
-centesis	puncture a cavity to remove fluid	amniocentesis
-ectomy	surgical removal (excision)	appendectomy
-ostomy	a new permanent opening	colostomy
-otomy	cutting into (incision)	tracheotomy
-orrhaphy	surgical repair/suture	herniorrhaphy
-opexy	surgical fixation	nephropexy
-oplasty	surgical repair	rhinoplasty
-otripsy	crushing, destroying	lithotripsy

Conditions

Prefix	Meaning	Example
ambi-	both	ambidextrous
aniso-	unequal	anisocoria
dys-	bad, painful, difficult	dysphoria
eu-	good, normal	euthanasia
hetero-	different	heterogeneous
homo-	same	homogeneous
hyper-	excessive, above	hypergastric
hypo-	deficient, below	hypogastric
iso-	equal, same	isotonic
mal-	bad, poor	malaise
megalo-	large	megalocardia

Suffix	Meaning	Example
-algia	pain	neuralgia
-asthenia	weakness	myasthenia
-emia	blood	anemia
-iasis	condition of	amebiasis
-itis	inflammation	appendicitis
-lysis	destruction, break down	hemolysis
-lytic	destroy, break down	hemolytic
-oid	like	lipoid
-oma	tumor	carcinoma
-opathy	disease of	arthropathy
-orrhagia	hemorrhage	menorrhagia
-orrhea	flow or discharge	amenorrhea
-osis	abnormal condition of	tuberculosis
-paresis	weakness	hemiparesis
-plasia	growth	hyperplasia
-plegia	paralysis	paraplegia
-pnea	breathing	apnea

Directions and Positions

Prefix	Meaning	Example
ab-	away from	abduction
ad-	toward	adduction
ecto, exo-	outside	ectopic, exocrine
endo-	within	endoscope
epi-	upon	epigastric
infra-	below, under	infrastructure
ipsi-	same	ipsilateral
meso-	middle	mesopexy
meta-	after, beyond, transformation	metastasis
peri-	surrounding	pericardium
retro-	behind, back	retroversion
trans-	across, through	transvaginal

Word	Meaning
anterior or ventral	at or near the front surface of the body
posterior or dorsal	at or near the back surface of the body
superior	above
inferior	below
lateral	side
distal	farthest from center
proximal	nearest to center
medial	middle
supine	face up or palm up
prone	face down or palm down
sagittal	vertical body plane, divides the body into equal right and left sides
transverse	horizontal body plane, divides the body into top and bottom sections
coronal	vertical body plane, divides the body into front and back sections

Additional References

For best coding results, you will need to use other reference materials in addition to your CPT® coding books. These references include medical dictionaries and anatomy books.

Medical Dictionaries

Dorland's Illustrated Medical Dictionary, 32nd ed.
Philadelphia, PA: Elsevier; 2011.

Stedman's CPT® Dictionary, 2nd ed.
Chicago, IL: American Medical Association; 2009.
OP:300609

Stedman's Medical Dictionary. 28th ed.
Philadelphia, PA: Lippencott; 2005.

Anatomy References

Bernard, SP. *Netter's Atlas of Human Anatomy for CPT® Surgery.*
Chicago, IL: American Medical Association; 2015.
OP495015

Kirschner, CG. *Netter's Atlas of Human Anatomy for CPT® Coding*, 2nd ed.
Chicago, IL: American Medical Association; 2009.
OP490609

Netter, FH. *Atlas of Human Anatomy*, 6th ed.
Philadelphia, PA; Elsevier; 2014.
OP936714

Lists of Illustrations

To further aid coders in properly assigning CPT codes, the codebook contains a number of anatomical and procedural illustrations.

Anatomical Illustrations

Thirty-one anatomical illustrations are located on the following pages:

Page	Illustration Title
xxii	Body Planes—3/4 View
xxii	Body Aspects—Side View
xxii	Body Planes—Front View
75	Structure of Skin
109	Skeletal System
110	Skull—Front and Lateral Views
110	Thoracic Vertebra—Superior View
110	Lumbar Vertebra—Superior View
110	Lumbar Vertebrae—Lateral View
112	Bones, Muscles, and Tendons of Hand
113	Bones and Muscles of Foot
114	Muscular System—Front
115	Muscular System—Back
185	Paranasal Sinuses
186	Respiratory System
207	Aortic Anatomy
208	Cardiac Anatomy, Heart Blood Flow
210	Circulatory System, Arteries
211	Circulatory System, Veins
212	Brachial Artery
213	Lymphatic System
298	Digestive System
356	Urinary System
380	Male Genital System
389	Female Genital System
410	Nervous System
411	Brain Anatomy
411	Sagittal Section of Brain and Brain Stem
446	Eye Anatomy
463	Ear Anatomy
473	Endocrine System
706	Cranial Nerves

Procedural Illustrations

Procedural illustrations are placed throughout the codebook and are associated with the following specific CPT codes.

CPT Code(s)	Illustration Title
11005	Debridement of Abdominal Wall
11200, 11201	Removal of Skin Tags
11423, 11600, 11606, 11642	Measuring and Coding the Removal of a Lesion
11719-11765	Lateral Nail View
11719-11765	Dorsal Nail View
14000-14061	Adjacent Tissue Repairs
15730	Midface Flap Surgery
15731	Axial Pattern Forehead Flap
16000-16030	Lund-Browder Diagram and Classification Method Table for Burn Estimations
17004	Destruction, Benign or Premalignant Lesions
20552, 20553	Trigger Point Injection
20610	Arthrocentesis, Aspiration, or Injection of Major Joint or Bursa
20664	Halo Application for Thin Skull Osteology
20690	Uniplane External Fixation System
20692	Multiplane External Fixation System
21196	Reconstruction of Mandibular Rami
22510	Percutaneous Vertebroplasty
22548	Arthrodesis (Anterior Transoral Technique)
22554	Anterior Approach for Cervical Fusion
22558	Anterior Approach for Lumbar Fusion (Anterior Retroperitoneal Exposure)
22840	Non-Segmental Spinal Instrumentation
22842-22844	Segmental Spinal Instrumentation
22853, 22854, 22859	Spinal Prosthetic Devices
27125	Partial Hip Replacement With or Without Bipolar Prosthesis
27130	Total Hip Replacement
27235	Percutaneous Treatment of Femoral Fracture
27236	Open Treatment of Femoral Fracture
27405, 27427	Posterolateral Corner of the Knee
28289	Hallux Rigidus Correction
28291	Hallux Rigidus Correction with Implant
28292	Hallux Valgus Correction
28292	Hallux Valgus Correction with Proximal Phalanx Base Resection
28295	Hallux Valgus Correction with Proximal First Metatarsal Osteotomy
28296	Hallux Valgus Correction with Distal First Metatarsal Osteotomy
28297	Hallux Valgus Correction with Metatarsal-Medial Cuneiform Joint Arthrodesis
28298	Hallux Valgus Correction with Proximal Phalanx Osteotomy
28299	Hallux Valgus Correction with Double Osteotomy
29824	Arthroscopy, Shoulder, Distal Claviculectomy (Mumford Procedure)

CPT Code(s)	Illustration Title
29866-29887	Arthroscopy of the Knee
29894-29899	Arthroscopy of the Ankle
30465	Surgical Repair of Vestibular Stenosis
31070	Sinusotomy, Frontal
31231-31294	Sinus Endoscopy
31622-31661	Bronchoscopy
32554, 32555	Thoracentesis
32601-32665	Thoracoscopy
32674	Mediastinal Lymph Nodes: Station Number and Descriptions
32994	Cryoablation Therapy of Pulmonary Tumors
33210	Temporary Pacemaker
33212, 33214	A. Implanted Pacemaker—Single Chamber
33212, 33214	B. Implanted Pacemaker—Two Chambers
33224-33226	Biventricular Pacing
33510-33516	A. Coronary Artery Bypass—Venous Grafting Only—Single Graft
33510-33516	B. Coronary Artery Bypass—Venous Grafting Only—Three Coronary Grafts
33517-33530	Coronary Artery Bypass—Combined Arterial-Venous Grafting
33517-33530	Coronary Artery Bypass—Sequential Combined Arterial-Venous Grafting
33621	Initial Hybrid Palliation
33622	Hybrid Reconstruction
33820	Patent Ductus Arteriosus
33864	Aortic Root Remodeling: Coronary Arteries Reimplanted
33927-33929	Total Heart Implantation Device
33979	Insertion of Implantable Single Ventricle Assist Device
34705, 34706, 34709, 34710, 34711	Endovascular Repair
35371-35372	Thromboendarterectomy
35571	Bypass Graft, Vein
35600	Harvest of Upper Extremity Artery
36002	Injection Procedure (eg, Thrombin) for Percutaneous Treatment of Extremity Pseudoaneurysm
36222-36228	Angiography, Carotid Artery
36555-36556	Insertion of Non-Tunneled Centrally Inserted Central Venous Catheter
36557-36558	Insertion of Tunneled Central Venous Catheter
36570, 36571, 36576, 36578	Implantable Venous Access Port
36572	Peripherally Inserted Central Catheter
36821	Arteriovenous Anastomosis, Direct
36825-36830	Arteriovenous Fistula
37191	Vena Cava Filter
37220, 37222	Transluminal Ballon Angioplasty
37220-37235	Iliac and Lower Extremity Arterial Anatomy Territory
37246	Transluminal Balloon Angioplasty
37700	Ligation and Division of Long Saphenous Vein
38230	Bone Marrow Harvesting for Transplantation

CPT Code(s)	Illustration Title
38746	Mediastinal Lymph Nodes: Station Number and Descriptions
43235	Esophagogastroduodenoscopy
43260	Endoscopic Retrograde Cholangiopancreatography (ERCP)
43280	Laparoscopic Fundoplasty
43284	Laparoscopic Esophageal Sphincter Augmentation
43327, 43328	Nissen Fundoplasty
43753	Gastric Intubation
43846	Gastric Bypass for Morbid Obesity
44127	Enterectomy, Resection for Congenital Atresia
44140	Colectomy, Partial
44160	Colectomy With Removal of Terminal Ileum and Ileocolostomy
45171-45172	Rectal Tumor Excision
45378	Colonoscopy
45385, 45388	Colonoscopy With Lesion Ablation or Removal
46020	Placement of Seton
46250-46262	Hemorrhoidectomy of Internal Prolapsed Hemorrhoid Columns
47533, 47534, 47538, 47539, 47540	Percutaneous Biliary Stent(s) and Drain Placement
47562	Laparoscopic Cholecystectomy
49320	Laparoscopy
50020	Drainage of Renal Abscess
50060-50075	Nephrolithotomy With Calculus Removal
50432	Introduction of Catheter Into Renal Pelvis
50545	Laparoscopic Radical Nephrectomy
50546	Laparoscopic Nephrectomy
50590	Lithotripsy
50605	Indwelling Ureteral Stent
50820	Ureteroileal Conduit
50947	Laparoscopic Ureteroneocystostomy
51798	Measurement of Postvoiding
51990	Laparoscopic Sling Suspension Urinary Incontinence
52005	Cystourethroscopy With Ureteral Catheterization
52601	Transurethral Resection of Prostate, Complete
52648	Contact Laser Vaporization of Prostate
53855	Temporary Prostatic Urethral Stent Insertion
54692	Laparoscopic Orchiopexy
57106	Vaginectomy, Partial Removal of Vaginal Wall
57111	Vaginectomy, Complete Removal of Vaginal Wall (Radical Vaginectomy)
57426	Laparoscopic Revision of Prosthetic Vaginal Graft
58563	Hysteroscopy
59001	Amniocentesis, Therapeutic Amniotic Fluid Reduction
59150	Laparoscopic Treatment of Ectopic Pregnancy
59400-59410	Vaginal Delivery
59510-59515	Cesarean Delivery
60220	Thyroid Lobectomy
60512	Posterior View of the Pharynx

CPT Code(s)	Illustration Title
60650	Laparoscopic Adrenalectomy
61700	Intracranial Aneurysm, Intracranial Approach
61867-61868, 61885	Placement of Cranial Neurostimulator
62223	Cerebrospinal Fluid (CSF) Shunt (Ventricular Peritoneal)
62362	Intrathecal or Epidural Drug Infusion Pump Implantation
63005	Lumbar Laminectomy
63650	Percutaneous Implantation of Neurostimulator Electrodes
63655	Placement of Neurostimulator Electrodes Through Laminectomy
64568-64570	Implantation Neurostimulator Electrodes, Cranial Nerve (Vagus Nerve Stimulation)
64581	Incisional Implantation of Sacral Nerve Neurostimulator
64642	Chemodenervation of Extremity
65450	Cryotherapy of Lesion on Cornea
67027	Intravitreal Drug Delivery System
67107	Repair of Retinal Detachment
67311-67346	Extraocular Muscles of Right Eye
67311-67312	Strabismus Surgery—Horizontal Muscles
67314-67316	Strabismus Surgery—Vertical Muscles
67320	Transposition Procedure
67335	Strabismus Surgery—Adjustable Sutures
67820-67825	Trichiasis
68761	Closure of Lacrimal Punctum by Plug
68816	Probing of Nasolacrimal Duct
69433-69436	Tympanostomy
69635-69646	Tympanoplasty
69930	Cochlear Device Implantation
69990	Operating Microscope
72275	Epidurography
75600-75630	Aortography
75820-75822	Venography
77067	Screening Mammography
91034	Esophageal Acid Reflux Test
92225, 92226	Extended Ophthalmoscopy
92235	Fluorescein Angiography
92601-92604	A View of the Outer Cochlear Implant
92978	Intravascular Ultrasound (Coronary Vessel or Graft)
93312-93318	Transesophageal Echocardiography (TEE)
93451	Right Heart Catheterization
93452	Left Heart Catherization
93454	Coronary Angiography Without Concomitant Left Heart Catheterization
93571	Intravascular Distal Blood Flow Velocity
95951	Electroencephalographic (EEG) Monitoring and Video Recording
97810-97811	Acupuncture, Needle

Figure 1A

Body Planes — 3/4 View

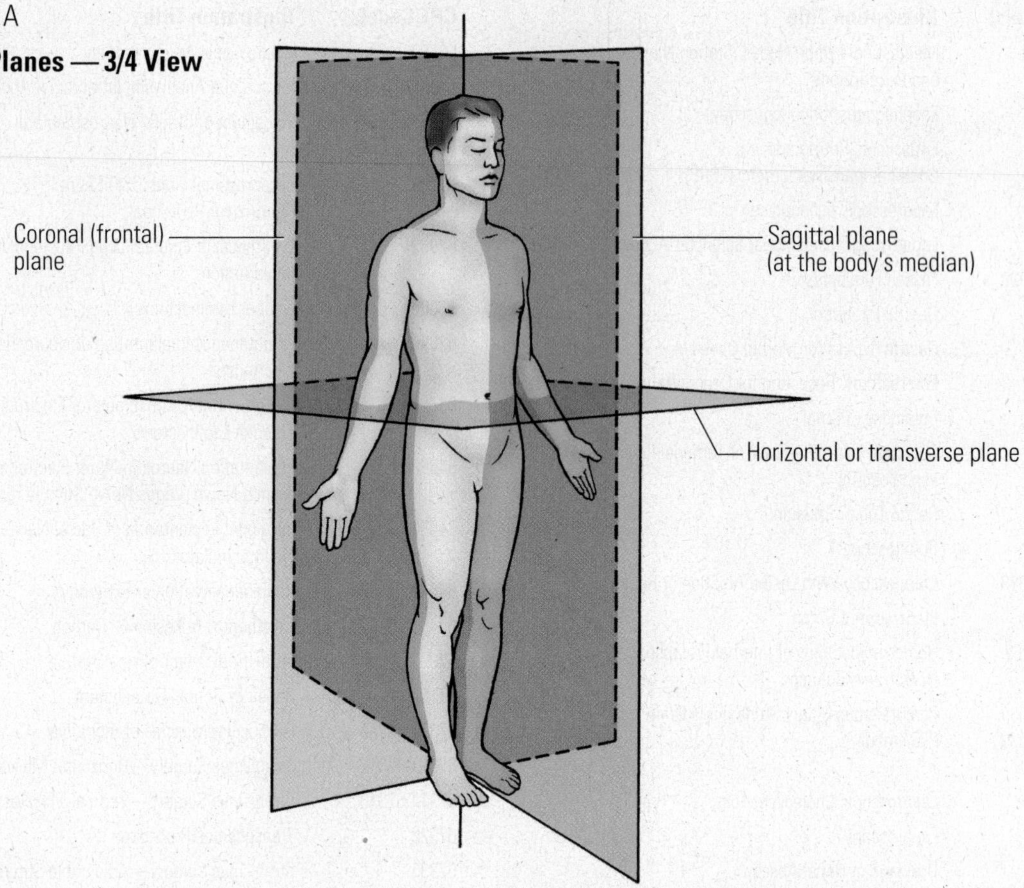

Figure 1B

Body Aspects — Side View

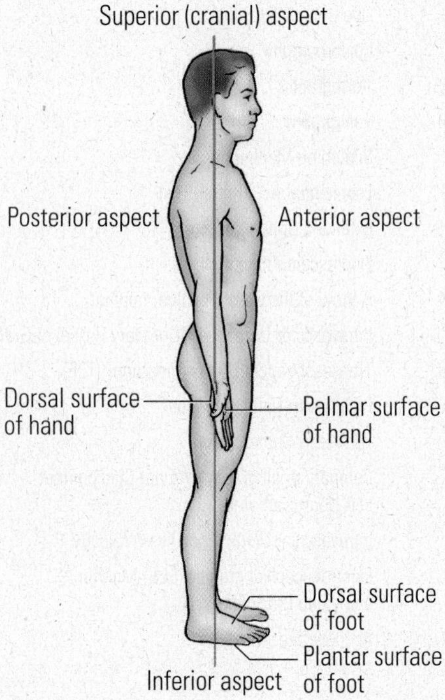

Figure 1C

Body Planes — Front View

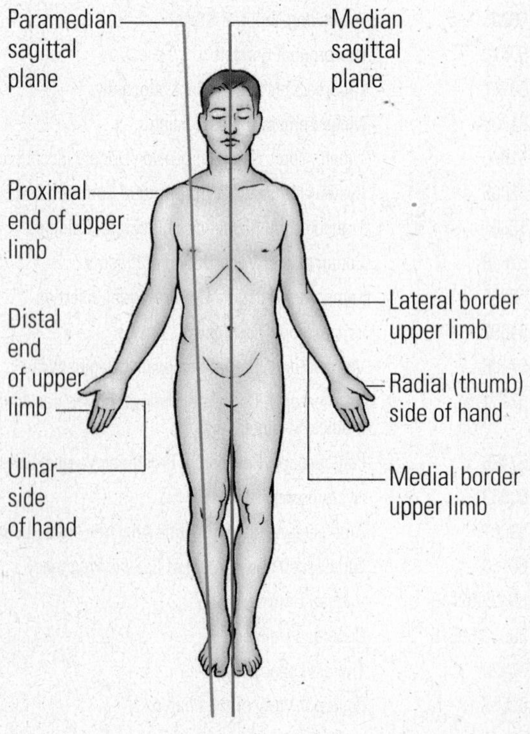

Evaluation and Management Tables

Office or Other Outpatient Services

Patient: New					
Required Components: 3/3					
Code	**99201**	**99202**	**99203**	**99204**	**99205**
REQUIRED KEY COMPONENTS					
History and Examination (#1 and #2)					
Problem-Focused	X				
Expanded Problem-Focused		X			
Detailed			X		
Comprehensive				X	X
Medical Decision Making (Complexity) (#3)					
Straightforward	X	X			
Low			X		
Moderate				X	
High					X
CONTRIBUTORY FACTORS					
Presenting Problem (Severity) (#1)					
Self-limited or Minor	X				
Low to Moderate		X			
Moderate			X		
Moderate to High				X	X
Counseling (#2) See E/M Guidelines					
Coordination of Care (#3) See E/M Guidelines					
Typical Face-to-Face Time (#4)					
Minutes	10	20	30	45	60

Initial Observation Care

Patient: New or Established			
Required Components: 3/3			
Code	**99218**	**99219**	**99220**
REQUIRED KEY COMPONENTS			
History and Examination (#1 and #2)			
Detailed or Comprehensive	X		
Comprehensive		X	X
Medical Decision Making (Complexity) (#3)			
Straightforward or Low	X		
Moderate		X	
High			X
CONTRIBUTORY FACTORS			
Presenting Problem (Severity) (#1)			
Low	X		
Moderate		X	
High			X
Counseling (#2) See E/M Guidelines			
Coordination of Care (#3) See E/M Guidelines			
Bedside/Unit/Floor Time (#4)			
Minutes	30	50	70

Subsequent Observation Care

Patient: New or Established			
Required Components: 2/3			
Code	**99224**	**99225**	**99226**
REQUIRED KEY COMPONENTS			
Interval History and Examination (#1 and #2)			
Problem-Focused	X		
Expanded Problem-Focused		X	
Detailed			X
Medical Decision Making (Complexity) (#3)			
Straightforward or Low	X		
Moderate		X	
High			X
CONTRIBUTORY FACTORS			
Presenting Problem (Severity) (#1)			
Stable/Recovering/ Improving	X		
Inadequate Response to Therapy/ Minor Complication Development		X	
Unstable/Significant Complication/ Significant New Problem			X
Counseling (#2) See E/M Guidelines			
Coordination of Care (#3) See E/M Guidelines			
Bedside/Unit/Floor Time (#4)			
Minutes	15	25	35

Office or Other Outpatient Services

Patient: Established					
Required Components: 2/3					
Code	**99211**	**99212**	**99213**	**99214**	**99215**
REQUIRED KEY COMPONENTS					
History and Examination (#1 and #2)					
Problem-Focused	N/A	X			
Expanded Problem-Focused			X		
Detailed				X	
Comprehensive					X
Medical Decision Making (Complexity) (#3)					
Straightforward	N/A	X			
Low			X		
Moderate				X	
High					X
CONTRIBUTORY FACTORS					
Presenting Problem (Severity) (#1)					
Minimal	X				
Self-Limited or Minor		X			
Low to Moderate			X		
Moderate to High				X	X
Counseling (#2) See E/M Guidelines					
Coordination of Care (#3) See E/M Guidelines					
Typical Face-to-Face Time (#4)					
Minutes	5	10	15	25	40

Initial Hospital Care

Patient: New or Established			
Required Components: 3/3			
Code	**99221**	**99222**	**99223**
REQUIRED KEY COMPONENTS			
History and Examination (#1 and #2)			
Detailed or Comprehensive	X		
Comprehensive		X	X
Medical Decision Making (Complexity) (#3)			
Straightforward or Low	X		
Moderate		X	
High			X
CONTRIBUTORY FACTORS			
Presenting Problem (Severity) (#1)			
Low	X		
Moderate		X	
High			X
Counseling (#2) See E/M Guidelines			
Coordination of Care (#3) See E/M Guidelines			
Bedside/Unit/Floor Time (#4)			
Minutes	30	50	70

Subsequent Hospital Care

Patient: New or Established			
Required Components: 2/3			
Code	**99231**	**99232**	**99233**
REQUIRED KEY COMPONENTS			
Interval History and Examination (#1 and #2)			
Problem-Focused	X		
Expanded Problem-Focused		X	
Detailed			X
Medical Decision Making (Complexity) (#3)			
Straightforward or Low	X		
Moderate		X	
High			X
CONTRIBUTORY FACTORS			
Presenting Problem (Severity) (#1)			
Stable/Recovering/Improving	X		
Responding Inadequately/ Minor Complication		X	
Unstable/Significant Complication/ New Problem			X
Counseling (#2) See E/M Guidelines			
Coordination of Care (#3) See E/M Guidelines			
Bedside/Unit/Floor Time (#4)			
Minutes	15	25	35

Office or Other Outpatient Consultations

Patient: New or Established

Required Components: 3/3

Code	99241	99242	99243	99244	99245
REQUIRED KEY COMPONENTS					
History and Examination (#1 and #2)					
Problem-Focused	X				
Expanded Problem-Focused		X			
Detailed			X		
Comprehensive				X	X
Medical Decision Making (Complexity) (#3)					
Straightforward	X	X			
Low			X		
Moderate				X	
High					X
CONTRIBUTORY FACTORS					
Presenting Problem (Severity) (#1)					
Self-limited or Minor	X				
Low		X			
Moderate			X		
Moderate to High				X	X
Counseling (#2) See E/M Guidelines					
Coordination of Care (#3) See E/M Guidelines					
Typical Face-to-Face Time (#4)					
Minutes	15	30	40	60	80

Inpatient Consultations

Patient: New or Established

Required Components: 3/3

Code	99251	99252	99253	99254	99255
REQUIRED KEY COMPONENTS					
History and Examination (#1 and #2)					
Problem-Focused	X				
Expanded Problem-Focused		X			
Detailed			X		
Comprehensive				X	X
Medical Decision Making (Complexity) (#3)					
Straightforward	X	X			
Low			X		
Moderate				X	
High					X
CONTRIBUTORY FACTORS					
Presenting Problem (Severity) (#1)					
Self-limited or Minor	X				
Low		X			
Moderate			X		
Moderate to High				X	X
Counseling (#2) See E/M Guidelines					
Coordination of Care (#3) See E/M Guidelines					
Bedside/Unit/Floor Time (#4)					
Minutes	20	40	55	80	110

Subsequent Nursing Facility Care

Patient: New or Established

Required Components: 2/3

Code	99307	99308	99309	99310
REQUIRED KEY COMPONENTS				
History and Examination (#1 and #2)				
Problem-Focused	X			
Expanded Problem-Focused		X		
Detailed			X	
Comprehensive				X
Medical Decision Making (Complexity) (#3)				
Straightforward	X			
Low		X		
Moderate			X	
High				X
CONTRIBUTORY FACTORS				
Presenting Problem (Severity) (#1)				
Stable/Recovering/Improving	X			
Responding Inadequately to Therapy/Minor Complication		X		
Significant Complication/ Significant New Problem			X	
Unstable/Significant New Problem Requiring Immediate Physician Attention				X
Counseling and Coordination of Care (#2 and #3) Counseling and/or coordination of care with other physicians, other qualified health care professionals, or agencies are provided consistent with the nature of the problem(s) and the patient's and/or family's needs.				
Bedside/Unit/Floor Time (#4)				
Minutes	10	15	25	35

Observation or Inpatient Care Services (Including Admission and Discharge Services)

Patient: New or Established

Required Components: 3/3

Code	99234	99235	99236
REQUIRED KEY COMPONENTS			
History and Examination (#1 and #2)			
Detailed or Comprehensive	X		
Comprehensive		X	X
Medical Decision Making (Complexity) (#3)			
Straightforward or Low	X		
Moderate		X	
High			X
CONTRIBUTORY FACTORS			
Presenting Problem (Severity) (#1)			
Low	X		
Moderate		X	
High			X
Counseling (#2) See E/M Guidelines			
Coordination of Care (#3) See E/M Guidelines			
Bedside/Unit/Floor Time (#4)			
Minutes	40	50	55

Initial Nursing Facility Care

Patient: New or Established

Required Components: 3/3

Code	99304	99305	99306
REQUIRED KEY COMPONENTS			
History and Examination (#1 and #2)			
Detailed or Comprehensive	X		
Comprehensive		X	X
Medical Decision Making (Complexity) (#3)			
Straightforward or Low	X		
Moderate		X	
High			X
CONTRIBUTORY FACTORS			
Presenting Problem (Severity) (#1)			
Low	X		
Moderate		X	
High			X
Counseling and Coordination of Care (#2 and #3) Counseling and/or coordination of care with other physicians, other qualified health care professionals, or agencies are provided consistent with the nature of the problem(s) and the patient's and/or family's needs.			
Bedside/Unit/Floor Time (#4)			
Minutes	25	35	45

Emergency Department Services

Patient: New or Established

Required Components: 3/3

Code	99281	99282	99283	99284	99285
REQUIRED KEY COMPONENTS					
History and Examination (#1 and #2)					
Problem-Focused	X				
Expanded Problem-Focused		X	X		
Detailed				X	
Comprehensive					X
Medical Decision Making (Complexity) (#3)					
Straightforward	X				
Low		X			
Moderate			X	X	
High					X
CONTRIBUTORY FACTORS					
Presenting Problem (Severity) (#1)					
Self-limited or Minor	X				
Low to Moderate		X			
Moderate			X		
High				X	
High Severity/ Immediate Significant Threat to Life or Physiological Function					X
Counseling and Coordination of Care (#2 and #3) Counseling and/or coordination of care with other physicians, other qualified health care professionals, or agencies are provided consistent with the nature of the problem(s) and the patient's and/or family's needs.					
Typical Time (#4)					
N/A					

Domiciliary, Rest Home (eg, Boarding Home), or Custodial Care Services

Patient: New
Required Components: 3/3

Code	99324	99325	99326	99327	99328
REQUIRED KEY COMPONENTS					
History and Examination (#1 and #2)					
Problem-Focused	X				
Expanded Problem-Focused		X			
Detailed			X		
Comprehensive				X	X
Medical Decision Making (Complexity) (#3)					
Straightforward	X				
Low		X			
Moderate			X	X	
High					X
CONTRIBUTORY FACTORS					
Presenting Problem (Severity) (#1)					
Low	X				
Moderate		X			
Moderate to High			X		
High				X	
Unstable/Significant New Problem Requiring Immediate Physician Attention					X
Counseling (#2) See E/M Guidelines					
Coordination of Care (#3) See E/M Guidelines					
Typical Time (#4)					
Minutes	20	30	45	60	75

Domiciliary, Rest Home (eg, Boarding Home), or Custodial Care Services

Patient: Established
Required Components: 2/3

Code	99334	99335	99336	99337
REQUIRED KEY COMPONENTS				
History and Examination (#1 and #2)				
Problem-Focused	X			
Expanded Problem-Focused		X		
Detailed			X	
Comprehensive				X
Medical Decision Making (Complexity) (#3)				
Straightforward	X			
Low		X		
Moderate			X	
Moderate to High				X
CONTRIBUTORY FACTORS				
Presenting Problem (Severity) (#1)				
Self-limited or Minor	X			
Low to Moderate		X		
Moderate to High			X	
Moderate to High/Unstable/ Significant New Problem				X
Counseling (#2) See E/M Guidelines				
Coordination of Care (#3) See E/M Guidelines				
Typical Time (#4)				
Minutes	15	25	40	60

Neonatal and Pediatric Critical/Intensive Care

Initial Inpatient Neonatal and Pediatric Critical Care

Code	99468	99471	99475	99291–99292
Age	28 days or less	29 days to 24 mos	2–5 yrs	6 yrs +

Subsequent Inpatient Neonatal and Pediatric Critical Care

Code	99469	99472	99476	99291–99292
Age	28 days or less	29 days to 24 mos	2–5 yrs	6 yrs +

Initial Neonatal Intensive Care

Code	99477
Age	28 days of age or younger
Presenting Problem	Requires intensive observation, frequent interventions/other intensive care services

Continuing Neonatal and Infant Inpatient Low Birth-Weight Intensive Care

Code	99478	99479	99480	99231–99233
Weight	1500 gms or less	1500–2500 gms	2501–5000 gms	+5000 gms
Presenting Problem	Recovering			

Home Services

Patient: New
Required Components: 3/3

Code	99341	99342	99343	99344	99345
REQUIRED KEY COMPONENTS					
History and Examination (#1 and #2)					
Problem-Focused	X				
Expanded Problem-Focused		X			
Detailed			X		
Comprehensive				X	X
Medical Decision Making (Complexity) (#3)					
Straightforward	X				
Low		X			
Moderate			X	X	
High					X
CONTRIBUTORY FACTORS					
Presenting Problem (Severity) (#1)					
Low	X				
Moderate		X			
Moderate to High			X		
High				X	
Unstable/Significant New Problem					X
Counseling (#2) See E/M Guidelines					
Coordination of Care (#3) See E/M Guidelines					
Typical Face-to-Face Time (#4)					
Minutes	20	30	45	60	75

Home Services

Patient: Established
Required Components: 2/3

Code	99347	99348	99349	99350
REQUIRED KEY COMPONENTS				
History and Examination (#1 and #2)				
Problem-Focused	X			
Expanded Problem-Focused		X		
Detailed			X	
Comprehensive				X
Medical Decision Making (Complexity) (#3)				
Straightforward	X			
Low		X		
Moderate			X	
Moderate to High				X
CONTRIBUTORY FACTORS				
Presenting Problem (Severity) (#1)				
Self-limited or Minor	X			
Low to Moderate		X		
Moderate to High			X	
Moderate to High/Unstable/ Significant New Problem				X
Counseling (#2) See E/M Guidelines				
Coordination of Care (#3) See E/M Guidelines				
Typical Time (#4)				
Minutes	15	25	40	60

Critical Care Time Reporting

Total Duration of Critical Care	CPT Codes
Less than 30 minutes	Appropriate E/M codes
30–74 minutes (1/2 hour–1 hour 14 minutes)	99291 X 1
75–104 minutes (1 hour 15 minutes–1 hour 44 minutes)	99291 X 1 and 99292 X 1
105–134 minutes (1 hour 45 minutes–2 hours 14 minutes)	99291 X 1 and 99292 X 2
135–164 minutes (2 hours 15 minutes–2 hours 44 minutes)	99291 X 1 and 99292 X 3
165–194 minutes (2 hours 45 minutes–3 hours 14 minutes)	99291 X 1 and 99292 X 4
195 minutes or more (3 hours 15 minutes or more)	99291 and 99292 as appropriate

Evaluation and Management (E/M) Services Guidelines

The following is a listing of headings and subheadings that appear within the Evaluation and Management section of the CPT codebook. The subheadings or subsections denoted with asterisks (*) below have special instructions unique to that subsection. Where these are indicated, special notes or guidelines will be presented preceding those procedural terminology listings, referring to that subsection specifically.

Classification of Evaluation and Management (E/M) Services* 4

Definitions of Commonly Used Terms* 4

New and Established Patient* 4

Chief Complaint* 5

Concurrent Care and Transfer of Care* 5

Counseling* 6

Family History* 6

History of Present Illness* 6

Levels of E/M Services* 6

Nature of Presenting Problem* 7

Past History* 7

Social History* 7

System Review (Review of Systems)* 7

Time* 7

Unlisted Service* 8

Special Report* 8

Clinical Examples* 8

Instructions for Selecting a Level of E/M Service* 9

Review the Reporting Instructions for the Selected Category or Subcategory* 9

Review the Level of E/M Service Descriptors and Examples in the Selected Category or Subcategory* 9

Determine the Extent of History Obtained* 9

Determine the Extent of Examination Performed* 9

Determine the Complexity of Medical Decision Making* 10

Select the Appropriate Level of E/M Services Based on the Following* 10

Evaluation and Management

Office or Other Outpatient Services* (99201-99215) 11

New Patient (99201-99205) 11

Established Patient (99211-99215) 12

Hospital Observation Services* (99217-99220, 99224-99226) 13

Observation Care Discharge Services* (99217) 14

Initial Observation Care (99218-99220) 14

  New or Established Patient* (99218-99220) 14

Subsequent Observation Care* (99224-99226) 15

Hospital Inpatient Services* (99221-99223, 99231-99239) 15

Initial Hospital Care (99221-99223) 16

  New or Established Patient* (99221-99223) 16

Subsequent Hospital Care* (99231-99233) 17
Observation or Inpatient Care Services (Including Admission and Discharge Services)* (99234-99236) 18
Hospital Discharge Services* (99238-99239) 18

Consultations* (99241-99255) 19
Office or Other Outpatient Consultations (99241-99245) 19
New or Established Patient* (99241-99245) 19
Inpatient Consultations (99251-99255) 21
New or Established Patient* (99251-99255) 21

Emergency Department Services (99281-99288) 22
New or Established Patient* (99281-99285) 22
Other Emergency Services* (99288) 23

Critical Care Services* (99291-99292) 23

Nursing Facility Services* (99304-99318) 25
Initial Nursing Facility Care (99304-99306) 26
New or Established Patient* (99304-99306) 26
Subsequent Nursing Facility Care* (99307-99310) 27
Nursing Facility Discharge Services* (99315-99316) 27
Other Nursing Facility Services (99318) 28

Domiciliary, Rest Home (eg, Boarding Home), or Custodial Care Services* (99324-99337) 28
New Patient (99324-99328) 28
Established Patient (99334-99337) 29

Domiciliary, Rest Home (eg, Assisted Living Facility), or Home Care Plan Oversight Services (99339-99340) 30

Home Services* (99341-99350) 30
New Patient (99341-99345) 30
Established Patient (99347-99350) 31

Prolonged Services (99354-99360, 99415, 99416) 32
Prolonged Service With Direct Patient Contact* (99354-99357) 32
Prolonged Service Without Direct Patient Contact* (99358-99359) 33
Prolonged Clinical Staff Services With Physician or Other Qualified Health Care Professional Supervision* (99415, 99416) 34
Standby Services* (99360) 34

Case Management Services* (99366-99368) 35
Anticoagulant Management 35
Medical Team Conferences* (99366-99368) 35
Medical Team Conference, Direct (Face-to-Face) Contact With Patient and/or Family (99366) 35
Medical Team Conference, Without Direct (Face-to-Face) Contact With Patient and/or Family (99367-99368) 36

Care Plan Oversight Services* (99374-99380) 36

Preventive Medicine Services* (99381-99429) 37
New Patient (99381-99387) 37
Established Patient (99391-99397) 38

Counseling Risk Factor Reduction and Behavior Change Intervention (99401-99429)........38
New or Established Patient* (99401-99416)........38
Preventive Medicine, Individual Counseling (99401-99404)........38
Behavior Change Interventions, Individual (99406-99409)........39
Preventive Medicine, Group Counseling (99411, 99412)........39
Other Preventive Medicine Services (99429)........39
Non-Face-to-Face Services (99441-99457)........39
Telephone Services* (99441-99443)........39
On-Line Medical Evaluation* (99444)........40
►Interprofessional Telephone/Internet/Electronic Health Record Consultations*◄ (99446-99449, 99451, 99452)........40
►Digitally Stored Data Services/Remote Physiologic Monitoring*◄ (99453, 99454, 99091)........41
►Remote Physiologic Monitoring Treatment Management Services*◄ (99457)........42
Special Evaluation and Management Services* (99450-99456)........42
Basic Life and/or Disability Evaluation Services (99450)........42
Work Related or Medical Disability Evaluation Services (99455-99456)........43
Newborn Care Services* (99460-99463)........43
Delivery/Birthing Room Attendance and Resuscitation Services (99464-99465)........43
Inpatient Neonatal Intensive Care Services and Pediatric and Neonatal Critical Care Services (99466-99486)........44
Pediatric Critical Care Patient Transport* (99466, 99467, 99485, 99486)........44
Inpatient Neonatal and Pediatric Critical Care* (99468-99476)........45
Initial and Continuing Intensive Care Services* (99477-99480)........47
Cognitive Assessment and Care Plan Services* (99483)........48
Care Management Services* (99487, 99489, 99490-99491)........49
Chronic Care Management Services* (99490-99491)........50
Complex Chronic Care Management Services* (99487, 99489)........51
Psychiatric Collaborative Care Management Services* (99492-99494)........52
Transitional Care Management Services* (99495-99496)........54
Advance Care Planning* (99497-99498)........55
General Behavioral Health Integration Care Management* (99484)........56
Other Evaluation and Management Services (99499)........56

Evaluation and Management (E/M) Services Guidelines

In addition to the information presented in the Introduction, several other items unique to this section are defined or identified here.

Classification of Evaluation and Management (E/M) Services

The E/M section is divided into broad categories such as office visits, hospital visits, and consultations. Most of the categories are further divided into two or more subcategories of E/M services. For example, there are two subcategories of office visits (new patient and established patient) and there are two subcategories of hospital visits (initial and subsequent). The subcategories of E/M services are further classified into levels of E/M services that are identified by specific codes. This classification is important because the nature of work varies by type of service, place of service, and the patient's status.

The basic format of the levels of E/M services is the same for most categories. First, a unique code number is listed. Second, the place and/or type of service is specified, eg, office consultation. Third, the content of the service is defined, eg, comprehensive history and comprehensive examination. (See "Levels of E/M Services," page 6, for details on the content of E/M services.) Fourth, the nature of the presenting problem(s) usually associated with a given level is described. Fifth, the time typically required to provide the service is specified. (A detailed discussion of time is provided on page 7.)

Definitions of Commonly Used Terms

Certain key words and phrases are used throughout the E/M section. The following definitions are intended to reduce the potential for differing interpretations and to increase the consistency of reporting by physicians in differing specialties. E/M services may also be reported by other qualified health care professionals who are authorized to perform such services within the scope of their practice.

New and Established Patient

Solely for the purposes of distinguishing between new and established patients, **professional services** are those face-to-face services rendered by physicians and other qualified health care professionals who may report evaluation and management services reported by a specific CPT code(s). A new patient is one who has not received any professional services from the physician/qualified health care professional or another physician/qualified health care professional of the **exact** same specialty **and subspecialty** who belongs to the same group practice, within the past three years.

An established patient is one who has received professional services from the physician/qualified health care professional or another physician/qualified health care professional of the **exact** same specialty **and subspecialty** who belongs to the same group practice, within the past three years. See Decision Tree.

In the instance where a physician/qualified health care professional is on call for or covering for another physician/qualified health care professional, the patient's encounter will be classified as it would have been by the physician/qualified health care professional who is not available. When advanced practice nurses and physician assistants are working with physicians they are considered as working in the exact same specialty and exact same subspecialties as the physician.

No distinction is made between new and established patients in the emergency department. E/M services in the emergency department category may be reported for any new or established patient who presents for treatment in the emergency department.

The Decision Tree on page 5 is provided to aid in determining whether to report the E/M service provided as a new or an established patient encounter.

Coding Tip

Instructions for Use of the CPT Codebook

When advanced practice nurses and physician assistants are working with physicians they are considered as working in the exact same specialty and exact same subspecialties as the physician. A "physician or other qualified health care professional" is an individual who is qualified by education, training, licensure/regulation (when applicable), and facility privileging (when applicable) who performs a professional service within his or her scope of practice and independently reports that professional services. These professionals are distinct from "clinical staff." A clinical staff member is a person who works under the supervision of a physician or other qualified health care professional, and who is allowed by law, regulation and facility policy to perform or assist in the performance of a specific professional service, but does not individually report that professional service. Other policies may also affect who may report specific services.

CPT Coding Guidelines, Introduction, Instructions for Use of the CPT Codebook

Chief Complaint

A chief complaint is a concise statement describing the symptom, problem, condition, diagnosis, or other factor that is the reason for the encounter, usually stated in the patient's words.

Concurrent Care and Transfer of Care

Concurrent care is the provision of similar services (eg, hospital visits) to the same patient by more than one physician or other qualified health care professional on the same day. When concurrent care is provided, no special reporting is required. Transfer of care is the process whereby a physician or other qualified health care professional who is providing management for some or all of a patient's problems relinquishes this responsibility to another physician or other qualified health care professional who explicitly agrees to accept this responsibility and who, from the initial encounter, is not providing consultative services. The physician or other qualified health care professional transferring care is then no longer providing care for these problems though he or she may continue providing care for other conditions when appropriate. Consultation codes should not be reported by the physician or other qualified health care professional who has agreed to accept transfer of care before an initial evaluation but are appropriate to report if the decision to accept transfer of care cannot be made until after the initial consultation evaluation, regardless of site of service.

Decision Tree for New vs Established Patients

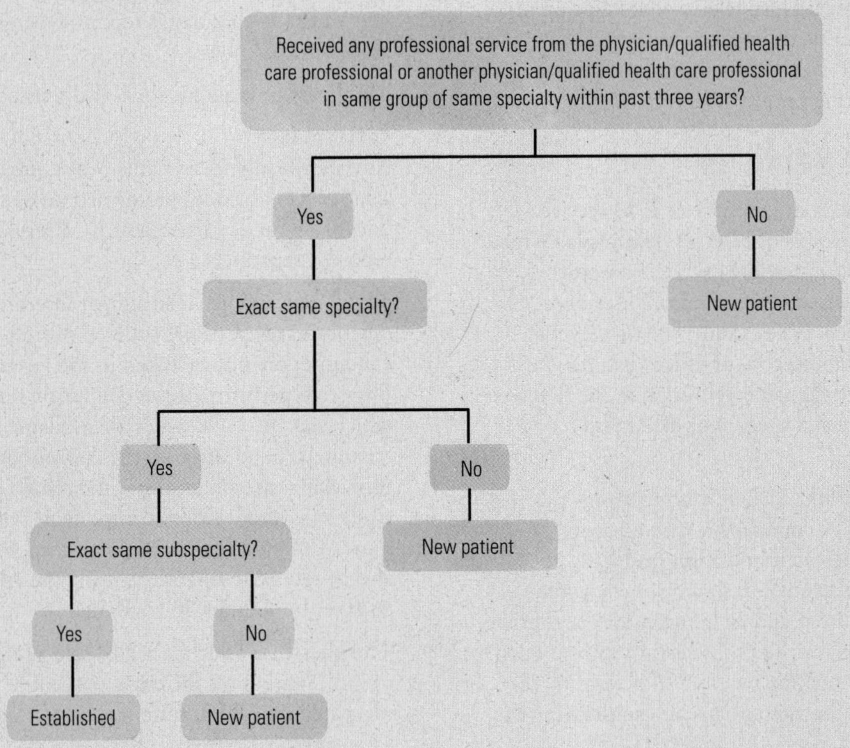

Counseling

Counseling is a discussion with a patient and/or family concerning one or more of the following areas:

- Diagnostic results, impressions, and/or recommended diagnostic studies
- Prognosis
- Risks and benefits of management (treatment) options
- Instructions for management (treatment) and/or follow-up
- Importance of compliance with chosen management (treatment) options
- Risk factor reduction
- Patient and family education

(For psychotherapy, see 90832-90834, 90836-90840)

Family History

A review of medical events in the patient's family that includes significant information about:

- The health status or cause of death of parents, siblings, and children
- Specific diseases related to problems identified in the Chief Complaint or History of the Present Illness, and/or System Review
- Diseases of family members that may be hereditary or place the patient at risk

History of Present Illness

A chronological description of the development of the patient's present illness from the first sign and/or symptom to the present. This includes a description of location, quality, severity, timing, context, modifying factors, and associated signs and symptoms significantly related to the presenting problem(s).

Levels of E/M Services

Within each category or subcategory of E/M service, there are three to five levels of E/M services available for reporting purposes. Levels of E/M services are **not** interchangeable among the different categories or subcategories of service. For example, the first level of E/M services in the subcategory of office visit, new patient, does not have the same definition as the first level of E/M services in the subcategory of office visit, established patient.

The levels of E/M services include examinations, evaluations, treatments, conferences with or concerning patients, preventive pediatric and adult health supervision, and similar medical services, such as the determination of the need and/or location for appropriate care. Medical screening includes the history, examination, and medical decision making required to determine the need and/or location for appropriate care and treatment of the patient (eg, office and other outpatient setting, emergency department, nursing facility). The levels of E/M services encompass the wide variations in skill, effort, time, responsibility, and medical knowledge required for the prevention or diagnosis and treatment of illness or injury and the promotion of optimal health. Each level of E/M services may be used by all physicians or other qualified health care professionals.

The descriptors for the levels of E/M services recognize seven components, six of which are used in defining the levels of E/M services. These components are:

- History
- Examination
- Medical decision making
- Counseling
- Coordination of care
- Nature of presenting problem
- Time

The first three of these components (history, examination, and medical decision making) are considered the **key** components in selecting a level of E/M services. (See "Determine the Extent of History Obtained," page 9.)

The next three components (counseling, coordination of care, and the nature of the presenting problem) are considered **contributory** factors in the majority of encounters. Although the first two of these contributory factors are important E/M services, it is not required that these services be provided at every patient encounter.

Coordination of care with other physicians, other health care professionals, or agencies without a patient encounter on that day is reported using the case management codes.

The final component, time, is discussed in detail on page 7.

Any specifically identifiable procedure (ie, identified with a specific CPT code) performed on or subsequent to the date of initial or subsequent E/M services should be reported separately.

The actual performance and/or interpretation of diagnostic tests/studies ordered during a patient encounter are not included in the levels of E/M services. Physician performance of diagnostic tests/studies for which specific CPT codes are available may be reported separately, in addition to the appropriate E/M code. The physician's interpretation of the results of diagnostic tests/studies (ie, professional component) with preparation of a separate distinctly identifiable signed written report may also be reported separately, using the appropriate CPT code with modifier 26 appended.

The physician or other health care professional may need to indicate that on the day a procedure or service identified by a CPT code was performed, the patient's condition required a significant separately identifiable E/M service above and beyond other services provided or beyond the usual preservice and postservice care associated with the procedure that was performed. The E/M service may be caused or prompted by the symptoms or condition for which the procedure and/or service was provided. This circumstance may be reported by adding modifier 25 to the appropriate level of E/M service. As such, different diagnoses are not required for reporting of the procedure and the E/M services on the same date.

Nature of Presenting Problem

A presenting problem is a disease, condition, illness, injury, symptom, sign, finding, complaint, or other reason for encounter, with or without a diagnosis being established at the time of the encounter. The E/M codes recognize five types of presenting problems that are defined as follows:

Minimal: A problem that may not require the presence of the physician or other qualified health care professional, but service is provided under the physician's or other qualified health care professional's supervision.

Self-limited or minor: A problem that runs a definite and prescribed course, is transient in nature, and is not likely to permanently alter health status OR has a good prognosis with management/compliance.

Low severity: A problem where the risk of morbidity without treatment is low; there is little to no risk of mortality without treatment; full recovery without functional impairment is expected.

Moderate severity: A problem where the risk of morbidity without treatment is moderate; there is moderate risk of mortality without treatment; uncertain prognosis OR increased probability of prolonged functional impairment.

High severity: A problem where the risk of morbidity without treatment is high to extreme; there is a moderate to high risk of mortality without treatment OR high probability of severe, prolonged functional impairment.

Past History

A review of the patient's past experiences with illnesses, injuries, and treatments that includes significant information about:

- Prior major illnesses and injuries
- Prior operations
- Prior hospitalizations
- Current medications
- Allergies (eg, drug, food)
- Age appropriate immunization status
- Age appropriate feeding/dietary status

Social History

An age appropriate review of past and current activities that includes significant information about:

- Marital status and/or living arrangements
- Current employment
- Occupational history
- Military history
- Use of drugs, alcohol, and tobacco
- Level of education
- Sexual history
- Other relevant social factors

System Review (Review of Systems)

An inventory of body systems obtained through a series of questions seeking to identify signs and/or symptoms that the patient may be experiencing or has experienced. For the purposes of the CPT codebook the following elements of a system review have been identified:

- Constitutional symptoms (fever, weight loss, etc)
- Eyes
- Ears, nose, mouth, throat
- Cardiovascular
- Respiratory
- Gastrointestinal
- Genitourinary
- Musculoskeletal
- Integumentary (skin and/or breast)
- Neurological
- Psychiatric
- Endocrine
- Hematologic/lymphatic
- Allergic/immunologic

The review of systems helps define the problem, clarify the differential diagnosis, identify needed testing, or serves as baseline data on other systems that might be affected by any possible management options.

Time

The inclusion of time in the definitions of levels of E/M services has been implicit in prior editions of the CPT codebook. The inclusion of time as an explicit factor beginning in *CPT 1992* is done to assist in selecting the most appropriate level of E/M services. It should be recognized that the specific times expressed in the visit code descriptors are averages and, therefore, represent a range of times that may be higher or lower depending on actual clinical circumstances.

Time is **not** a descriptive component for the emergency department levels of E/M services because emergency department services are typically provided on a variable intensity basis, often involving multiple encounters with several patients over an extended period of time. Therefore, it is often difficult to provide accurate estimates of the time spent face-to-face with the patient.

Studies to establish levels of E/M services employed surveys of practicing physicians to obtain data on the amount of time and work associated with typical E/M services. Since "work" is not easily quantifiable, the codes must rely on other objective, verifiable measures that correlate with physicians' estimates of their "work." It has been demonstrated that estimations of **intraservice** time (as explained on the next page), both within and across specialties, is a variable that is predictive of the "work" of E/M services. This same research has shown there is a strong relationship between intraservice time and total time for E/M services. Intraservice time, rather than total time, was chosen for inclusion with the codes because of its relative ease of measurement and because of its direct correlation with measurements of the total amount of time and work associated with typical E/M services.

Intraservice times are defined as **face-to-face** time for office and other outpatient visits and as **unit/floor** time for hospital and other inpatient visits. This distinction is necessary because most of the work of typical office visits takes place during the face-to-face time with the patient, while most of the work of typical hospital visits takes place during the time spent on the patient's floor or unit. When prolonged time occurs in either the office or the inpatient areas, the appropriate add-on code should be reported.

Face-to-face time (office and other outpatient visits and office consultations): For coding purposes, face-to-face time for these services is defined as only that time spent face-to-face with the patient and/or family. This includes the time spent performing such tasks as obtaining a history, examination, and counseling the patient.

Time is also spent doing work before or after the face-to-face time with the patient, performing such tasks as reviewing records and tests, arranging for further services, and communicating further with other professionals and the patient through written reports and telephone contact.

This **non-face-to-face** time for office services—also called pre- and postencounter time—is not included in the time component described in the E/M codes. However, the pre- and post-non-face-to-face work associated with an encounter was included in calculating the total work of typical services in physician surveys.

Thus, the face-to-face time associated with the services described by any E/M code is a valid proxy for the total work done before, during, and after the visit.

Unit/floor time (hospital observation services, inpatient hospital care, initial inpatient hospital consultations, nursing facility): For reporting purposes, intraservice time for these services is defined as unit/floor time, which includes the time present on the patient's hospital unit and at the bedside rendering services for that patient. This includes the time to establish and/or review the patient's chart, examine the patient, write notes, and communicate with other professionals and the patient's family.

In the hospital, pre- and post-time includes time spent off the patient's floor performing such tasks as reviewing pathology and radiology findings in another part of the hospital.

This pre- and postvisit time is not included in the time component described in these codes. However, the pre- and postwork performed during the time spent off the floor or unit was included in calculating the total work of typical services in physician surveys.

Thus, the unit/floor time associated with the services described by any code is a valid proxy for the total work done before, during, and after the visit.

Unlisted Service

An E/M service may be provided that is not listed in this section of the CPT codebook. When reporting such a service, the appropriate unlisted code may be used to indicate the service, identifying it by "Special Report," as discussed in the following paragraph. The "Unlisted Services" and accompanying codes for the E/M section are as follows:

99429 **Unlisted preventive** medicine service

99499 **Unlisted evaluation and management** service

Special Report

An unlisted service or one that is unusual, variable, or new may require a special report demonstrating the medical appropriateness of the service. Pertinent information should include an adequate definition or description of the nature, extent, and need for the procedure and the time, effort, and equipment necessary to provide the service. Additional items that may be included are complexity of symptoms, final diagnosis, pertinent physical findings, diagnostic and therapeutic procedures, concurrent problems, and follow-up care.

Clinical Examples

Clinical examples of the codes for E/M services are provided to assist in understanding the meaning of the descriptors and selecting the correct code. The clinical examples are listed in Appendix C. Each example was developed by the specialties shown.

The same problem, when seen by different specialties, may involve different amounts of work. Therefore, the appropriate level of encounter should be reported using the descriptors rather than the examples.

Instructions for Selecting a Level of E/M Service

Review the Reporting Instructions for the Selected Category or Subcategory

Most of the categories and many of the subcategories of service have special guidelines or instructions unique to that category or subcategory. Where these are indicated, eg, "Inpatient Hospital Care," special instructions will be presented preceding the levels of E/M services.

Review the Level of E/M Service Descriptors and Examples in the Selected Category or Subcategory

The descriptors for the levels of E/M services recognize seven components, six of which are used in defining the levels of E/M services. These components are:

- History
- Examination
- Medical decision making
- Counseling
- Coordination of care
- Nature of presenting problem
- Time

The first three of these components (ie, history, examination, and medical decision making) should be considered the **key** components in selecting the level of E/M services. An exception to this rule is in the case of visits that consist predominantly of counseling or coordination of care (see numbered paragraph 3, page 10).

The nature of the presenting problem and time are provided in some levels to assist the physician in determining the appropriate level of E/M service.

Determine the Extent of History Obtained

The extent of the history is dependent upon clinical judgment and on the nature of the presenting problem(s). The levels of E/M services recognize four types of history that are defined as follows:

Problem focused: Chief complaint; brief history of present illness or problem.

Expanded problem focused: Chief complaint; brief history of present illness; problem pertinent system review.

Detailed: Chief complaint; extended history of present illness; problem pertinent system review extended to include a review of a limited number of additional systems; **pertinent** past, family, and/or social history **directly related to the patient's problems.**

Comprehensive: Chief complaint; extended history of present illness; review of systems that is directly related to the problem(s) identified in the history of the present illness plus a review of all additional body systems; **complete** past, family, and social history.

The comprehensive history obtained as part of the preventive medicine E/M service is not problem-oriented and does not involve a chief complaint or present illness. It does, however, include a comprehensive system review and comprehensive or interval past, family, and social history as well as a comprehensive assessment/history of pertinent risk factors.

Determine the Extent of Examination Performed

The extent of the examination performed is dependent on clinical judgment and on the nature of the presenting problem(s). The levels of E/M services recognize four types of examination that are defined as follows:

Problem focused: A limited examination of the affected body area or organ system.

Expanded problem focused: A limited examination of the affected body area or organ system and other symptomatic or related organ system(s).

Detailed: An extended examination of the affected body area(s) and other symptomatic or related organ system(s).

Comprehensive: A general multisystem examination or a complete examination of a single organ system. **Note:** The comprehensive examination performed as part of the preventive medicine E/M service is multisystem, but its extent is based on age and risk factors identified.

For the purposes of these CPT definitions, the following body areas are recognized:

- Head, including the face
- Neck
- Chest, including breasts and axilla
- Abdomen
- Genitalia, groin, buttocks
- Back
- Each extremity

For the purposes of these CPT definitions, the following organ systems are recognized:

- Eyes
- Ears, nose, mouth, and throat
- Cardiovascular
- Respiratory
- Gastrointestinal
- Genitourinary
- Musculoskeletal
- Skin
- Neurologic
- Psychiatric
- Hematologic/lymphatic/immunologic

Determine the Complexity of Medical Decision Making

Medical decision making refers to the complexity of establishing a diagnosis and/or selecting a management option as measured by:

- The number of possible diagnoses and/or the number of management options that must be considered
- The amount and/or complexity of medical records, diagnostic tests, and/or other information that must be obtained, reviewed, and analyzed
- The risk of significant complications, morbidity, and/or mortality, as well as comorbidities, associated with the patient's presenting problem(s), the diagnostic procedure(s), and/or the possible management options

Four types of medical decision making are recognized: straightforward, low complexity, moderate complexity, and high complexity. To qualify for a given type of decision making, two of the three elements in Table 1 must be met or exceeded.

Comorbidities/underlying diseases, in and of themselves, are not considered in selecting a level of E/M services *unless* their presence significantly increases the complexity of the medical decision making.

Select the Appropriate Level of E/M Services Based on the Following

1. For the following categories/subcategories, **all of the key components,** ie, history, examination, and medical decision making, must meet or exceed the stated requirements to qualify for a particular level of E/M service: office, new patient; hospital observation services; initial hospital care; office consultations; initial inpatient consultations; emergency department services; initial nursing facility care; domiciliary care, new patient; and home, new patient.
2. For the following categories/subcategories, **two of the three key components** (ie, history, examination, and medical decision making) must meet or exceed the stated requirements to qualify for a particular level of E/M services: office, established patient; subsequent hospital care; subsequent nursing facility care; domiciliary care, established patient; and home, established patient.
3. When counseling and/or coordination of care dominates (more than 50%) the encounter with the patient and/or family (face-to-face time in the office or other outpatient setting or floor/unit time in the hospital or nursing facility), then **time** shall be considered the key or controlling factor to qualify for a particular level of E/M services. This includes time spent with parties who have assumed responsibility for the care of the patient or decision making whether or not they are family members (eg, foster parents, person acting in loco parentis, legal guardian). The extent of counseling and/or coordination of care must be documented in the medical record.

Table 1
Complexity of Medical Decision Making

Number of Diagnoses or Management Options	Amount and/or Complexity of Data to be Reviewed	Risk of Complications and/or Morbidity or Mortality	Type of Decision Making
minimal	minimal or none	minimal	**straightforward**
limited	limited	low	**low complexity**
multiple	moderate	moderate	**moderate complexity**
extensive	extensive	high	**high complexity**

Evaluation and Management

Office or Other Outpatient Services

The following codes are used to report evaluation and management services provided in the office or in an outpatient or other ambulatory facility. A patient is considered an outpatient until inpatient admission to a health care facility occurs.

To report services provided to a patient who is admitted to a hospital or nursing facility in the course of an encounter in the office or other ambulatory facility, see the notes for initial hospital inpatient care (page 16) or initial nursing facility care (page 26).

For services provided in the emergency department, see 99281-99285.

For observation care, see 99217-99226.

For observation or inpatient care services (including admission and discharge services), see 99234-99236.

Coding Tip

Determination of Patient Status as New or Established Patient

Solely for the purposes of distinguishing between new and established patients, **professional services** are those face-to-face services rendered by physicians and other qualified health care professionals who may report evaluation and management services reported by a specific CPT code(s). A new patient is one who has not received any professional services from the physician/qualified health care professional or another physician/qualified health care professional of the **exact** same specialty and subspecialty who belongs to the same group practice, within the past three years.

An established patient is one who has received professional services from the physician/qualified health care professional or another physician/qualified health care professional of the exact same specialty and subspecialty who belongs to the same group practice, within the past three years.

In the instance where a physician/qualified health care professional is on call for or covering for another physician/qualified health care professional, the patient's encounter will be classified as it would have been by the physician/qualified health care professional who is not available. When advanced practice nurses and physician assistants are working with physicians they are considered as working in the **exact** same specialty and exact same **subspecialties** as the physician.

CPT Coding Guidelines, Evaluation and Management, Definitions of Commonly Used Terms, New and Established Patient

New Patient

★ 99201 **Office or other outpatient visit** for the evaluation and management of a new patient, which requires these 3 key components:

- **A problem focused history;**
- **A problem focused examination;**
- **Straightforward medical decision making.**

Counseling and/or coordination of care with other physicians, other qualified health care professionals, or agencies are provided consistent with the nature of the problem(s) and the patient's and/or family's needs.

Usually, the presenting problem(s) are self limited or minor. Typically, 10 minutes are spent face-to-face with the patient and/or family.

➲ *CPT Changes: An Insider's View* 2011, 2013, 2017

➲ *CPT Assistant* Winter 91:11, Spring 92:13, 24, Summer 92:1, 24, Spring 93:34, Summer 93:2, Fall 93:9, Spring 95:1, Summer 95:4, Fall 95:9, Jul 98:9, Sep 98:5, Jun 99:8, Feb 00:3, 9, 11, Aug 01:2, Oct 04:11, Mar 05:11, Apr 05:1, May 05:1, Jun 05:11, Dec 05:10, Feb 06:14, May 06:1, Jun 06:1, Aug 06:12, Oct 06:15, Apr 07:11, Sep 07:1, Nov 08:10, Mar 09:3, Aug 09:5, Dec 09:9, Jul 10:10, Jan 11:3, Jan 12:5, Mar 12:4, 8, Apr 12:10, Jan 13:9, Jun 13:3, Aug 13:13, 14, Aug 14:3, Oct 14:3, Nov 14:14, Jan 15:12, Mar 16:11, Sep 16:6, Apr 18:10

➲ *Clinical Examples in Radiology* Winter 12:9

★ 99202 **Office or other outpatient visit** for the evaluation and management of a new patient, which requires these 3 key components:

- **An expanded problem focused history;**
- **An expanded problem focused examination;**
- **Straightforward medical decision making.**

Counseling and/or coordination of care with other physicians, other qualified health care professionals, or agencies are provided consistent with the nature of the problem(s) and the patient's and/or family's needs.

Usually, the presenting problem(s) are of low to moderate severity. Typically, 20 minutes are spent face-to-face with the patient and/or family.

➲ *CPT Changes: An Insider's View* 2013, 2017

➲ *CPT Assistant* Winter 91:11, Spring 92:13, 24, Summer 92:1, 24, Spring 93:34, Summer 93:2, Fall 93:9, Spring 95:1, Summer 95:4, Fall 95:9, Jul 98:9, Sep 98:5, Feb 00:11, Aug 01:2, Apr 02:14, Oct 04:10, Apr 05:1, 3, Jun 05:11, Dec 05:10, May 06:1, Jun 06:1, Oct 06:15, Apr 07:11, Sep 07:1, Mar 09:3, Aug 09:5, Dec 09:9, Jan 11:3, Mar 12:4, 8, Jan 13:9, Jun 13:3, Aug 13:13, 14, Jan 15:12, Mar 16:11, Sep 16:6, Apr 18:10

➲ *Clinical Examples in Radiology* Winter 12:9

★ **99203** **Office or other outpatient visit** for the evaluation and management of a new patient, which requires these 3 key components:

- **A detailed history;**
- **A detailed examination;**
- **Medical decision making of low complexity.**

Counseling and/or coordination of care with other physicians, other qualified health care professionals, or agencies are provided consistent with the nature of the problem(s) and the patient's and/or family's needs.

Usually, the presenting problem(s) are of moderate severity. Typically, 30 minutes are spent face-to-face with the patient and/or family.

➲ *CPT Changes: An Insider's View* 2013, 2017

➲ *CPT Assistant* Winter 91:11, Spring 92:14, 24, Summer 92:1, 24, Spring 93:34, Summer 93:2, Fall 93:9, Spring 95:1, Summer 95:4, Fall 95:9, Jul 98:9, Sep 98:5, Feb 00:11, Aug 01:2, Apr 02:14, Oct 04:10, Feb 05:9, Apr 05:1, 3, Jun 05:11, Dec 05:10, May 06:1, Jun 06:1, Oct 06:15, Apr 07:11, Sep 07:1, Mar 09:3, Aug 09:5, Dec 09:9, Jan 11:3, Mar 12:4, 8, Jan 13:9, Jun 13:3, Aug 13:13, 14, Jan 15:12, Mar 16:11, Sep 16:6, Apr 18:10

➲ *Clinical Examples in Radiology* Winter 12:9

★ **99204** **Office or other outpatient visit** for the evaluation and management of a new patient, which requires these 3 key components:

- **A comprehensive history;**
- **A comprehensive examination;**
- **Medical decision making of moderate complexity.**

Counseling and/or coordination of care with other physicians, other qualified health care professionals, or agencies are provided consistent with the nature of the problem(s) and the patient's and/or family's needs.

Usually, the presenting problem(s) are of moderate to high severity. Typically, 45 minutes are spent face-to-face with the patient and/or family.

➲ *CPT Changes: An Insider's View* 2013, 2017

➲ *CPT Assistant* Winter 91:11, Spring 92:14, 24, Summer 92:1, 24, Spring 93:34, Summer 93:2, Fall 93:9, Spring 95:1, Summer 95:4, Fall 95:9, Jul 98:9, Sep 98:5, Feb 00:11, Aug 01:2, Apr 02:14, May 02:1, Oct 04:10, Apr 05:1, 3, Jun 05:11, Dec 05:10, May 06:1, Jun 06:1, Oct 06:15, Apr 07:11, Sep 07:1, Mar 09:3, Aug 09:5, Dec 09:9, Jan 11:3, Mar 12:4, 8, Jan 13:9, Jun 13:3, Aug 13:13, 14, Jan 15:12, Mar 16:11, Sep 16:6, Apr 18:10

➲ *Clinical Examples in Radiology* Winter 12:9

★ **99205** **Office or other outpatient visit** for the evaluation and management of a new patient, which requires these 3 key components:

- **A comprehensive history;**
- **A comprehensive examination;**
- **Medical decision making of high complexity.**

Counseling and/or coordination of care with other physicians, other qualified health care professionals, or agencies are provided consistent with the nature of the problem(s) and the patient's and/or family's needs.

Usually, the presenting problem(s) are of moderate to high severity. Typically, 60 minutes are spent face-to-face with the patient and/or family.

➲ *CPT Changes: An Insider's View* 2013, 2017

➲ *CPT Assistant* Winter 91:11, Spring 92:14, 24, Summer 92:1, 24, Spring 93:34, Summer 93:2, Fall 93:9, Spring 95:1, Summer 95:4, Fall 95:9, Jul 98:9, Sep 98:5, Feb 00:11, Aug 01:2, Apr 02:2, May 02:1, Oct 04:10, Apr 05:1, 3, Jun 05:11, Dec 05:10, May 06:1, Jun 06:1, Oct 06:15, Apr 07:11, Sep 07:1, Mar 09:3, Aug 09:5, Dec 09:9, Jul 10:4, Jan 11:3, Jan 12:3, Mar 12:4, 8, Jan 13:9, Jun 13:3, Aug 13:13, 14, Jan 15:12, Mar 16:11, Sep 16:6, Apr 18:10

➲ *Clinical Examples in Radiology* Winter 12:9

Established Patient

99211 **Office or other outpatient visit** for the evaluation and management of an established patient, that may not require the presence of a physician or other qualified health care professional. Usually, the presenting problem(s) are minimal. Typically, 5 minutes are spent performing or supervising these services.

➲ *CPT Changes: An Insider's View* 2013

➲ *CPT Assistant* Winter 91:11, Spring 92:14, 24, Summer 92:1, 24, Spring 93:34, Summer 93:2, Fall 93:9, Spring 95:1, Summer 95:4, Fall 95:9, Oct 96:10, Feb 97:9, May 97:4, Jul 98:9, Sep 98:5, Oct 99:9, Feb 00:11, Aug 01:2, Jan 02:2, Oct 04:10, Feb 05:15, Mar 05:11, Apr 05:1, 3, May 05:1, Jun 05:11, Nov 05:1, Dec 05:10, Feb 06:14, May 06:1, Jun 06:1, Jul 06:19, Oct 06:15, Nov 06:21, Apr 07:11, Jul 07:1, Sep 07:1, Dec 07:9, Mar 08:3, Aug 08:13, Mar 09:3, Aug 09:5, Apr 10:10, Jan 11:3, Jan 12:3, Mar 12:4, 8, Apr 12:10, Jan 13:9, Mar 13:13, Jun 13:3, Aug 13:13, 14, Nov 13:3, Mar 14:14, Jan 15:12, Mar 16:11, Sep 16:6, Mar 17:10, Apr 18:10

★ **99212** **Office or other outpatient visit** for the evaluation and management of an established patient, which requires at least 2 of these 3 key components:

- **A problem focused history;**
- **A problem focused examination;**
- **Straightforward medical decision making.**

Counseling and/or coordination of care with other physicians, other qualified health care professionals, or agencies are provided consistent with the nature of the problem(s) and the patient's and/or family's needs.

Usually, the presenting problem(s) are self limited or minor. Typically, 10 minutes are spent face-to-face with the patient and/or family.

➲ *CPT Changes: An Insider's View* 2013, 2017

➲ *CPT Assistant* Winter 91:11, Spring 92:14, 24, Summer 92:1, 24, Spring 93:34, Summer 93:2, Fall 93:9, Spring 95:1, Summer 95:4, Fall 95:9, Jul 98:9, Sep 98:5, Feb 00:11, Jun 00:11, Aug 01:2, Jan 02:2, May 02:3, Apr 04:14, Oct 04:10, Apr 05:1, 3, Jun 05:11, Dec 05:10, May 06:1, Jun 06:1, 11, Sep 06:8, Oct 06:15, Apr 07:11, Jul 07:1, Sep 07:1, Mar 08:3, Mar 09:3, Aug 09:5, Feb 10:13, Jul 10:4, Sep 10:4, Jan 11:3, Jun 11:3, Mar 12:4, 8, Apr 12:17, Jan 13:9, Mar 13:13, Jun 13:3, Aug 13:13, 14, Feb 14:11, Jan 15:12, Mar 16:11, Sep 16:6, Dec 16:12, Oct 17:6, Apr 18:10

★ **99213** **Office or other outpatient visit** for the evaluation and management of an established patient, which requires at least 2 of these 3 key components:

- **An expanded problem focused history;**
- **An expanded problem focused examination;**
- **Medical decision making of low complexity.**

Counseling and coordination of care with other physicians, other qualified health care professionals, or agencies are provided consistent with the nature of the problem(s) and the patient's and/or family's needs.

Usually, the presenting problem(s) are of low to moderate severity. Typically, 15 minutes are spent face-to-face with the patient and/or family.

➲ *CPT Changes: An Insider's View* 2013, 2017

➲ *CPT Assistant* Winter 91:11, Spring 92:14, 24, Summer 92:1, 24, Spring 93:34, Summer 93:2, Fall 93:9, Spring 95:1, Summer 95:4, Fall 95:9, Jan 97:10, Jul 98:9, Sep 98:5, Aug 01:2, May 02:3, Oct 03:5, Apr 04:14, Oct 04:10, Mar 05:11, Apr 05:1, 3, Jun 05:11, Dec 05:10, May 06:1, Jun 06:1, 11, Sep 06:8, Oct 06:15, Apr 07:11, Jul 07:1, Sep 07:1, Mar 08:3, Mar 09:3, Aug 09:5, Sep 10:4, Jan 11:3, Jun 11:3, Mar 12:4, 8, Jan 13:9, Mar 13:13, Jun 13:3, Aug 13:13, 14, Jan 15:12, Mar 16:11, Sep 16:6, Apr 18:10

★ **99214** **Office or other outpatient visit** for the evaluation and management of an established patient, which requires at least 2 of these 3 key components:

- **A detailed history;**
- **A detailed examination;**
- **Medical decision making of moderate complexity.**

Counseling and/or coordination of care with other physicians, other qualified health care professionals, or agencies are provided consistent with the nature of the problem(s) and the patient's and/or family's needs.

Usually, the presenting problem(s) are of moderate to high severity. Typically, 25 minutes are spent face-to-face with the patient and/or family.

➲ *CPT Changes: An Insider's View* 2013, 2017

➲ *CPT Assistant* Winter 91:11, Spring 92:15, 24, Summer 92:1, 24, Spring 93:34, Summer 93:2, Fall 93:9, Spring 95:1, Summer 95:4, Fall 95:9, May 97:4, Jul 98:9, Sep 98:5, Aug 01:2, Jan 02:2, May 02:1-2, Oct 03:5, Apr 04:14, Oct 04:10, Apr 05:1, 3, Jun 05:11, Dec 05:10, May 06:1, Jun 06:1, 11, Sep 06:8, Oct 06:15, Apr 07:11, Jul 07:1, Sep 07:1, Mar 08:3, Mar 09:3, Aug 09:5, Sep 10:4, Jan 11:3, Jun 11:3, Mar 12:4, 8, Jan 13:9, Mar 13:13, Jun 13:3, Aug 13:13, 14, Jan 15:12, Oct 15:3, Mar 16:11, Sep 16:6, Apr 18:10

★ **99215** **Office or other outpatient visit** for the evaluation and management of an established patient, which requires at least 2 of these 3 key components:

- **A comprehensive history;**
- **A comprehensive examination;**
- **Medical decision making of high complexity.**

Counseling and/or coordination of care with other physicians, other qualified health care professionals, or agencies are provided consistent with the nature of the problem(s) and the patient's and/or family's needs.

Usually, the presenting problem(s) are of moderate to high severity. Typically, 40 minutes are spent face-to-face with the patient and/or family.

➲ *CPT Changes: An Insider's View* 2013, 2017

➲ *CPT Assistant* Winter 91:11, Spring 92:15, 24, Summer 92:1, 24, Spring 93:34, Summer 93:2, Fall 93:9, Spring 95:1, Summer 95:4, Fall 95:9, Jan 97:10, Jul 98:9, Sep 98:5, Aug 01:2, Jan 02:2, May 02:1, 3, Apr 04:14, Oct 04:10, Mar 05:11, Apr 05:1, 3, Jun 05:11, Dec 05:10, May 06:1, Jun 06:1, 11, Sep 06:8, Oct 06:15, Apr 07:11, Jul 07:1, Sep 07:1, Mar 08:3, Mar 09:3, Aug 09:5, Jul 10:4, Sep 10:4, Jan 11:3, Jun 11:3, Jan 12:3, Mar 12:4, 8, Apr 12:10, Jan 13:9, Mar 13:13, Jun 13:3, Aug 13:13, 14, Nov 13:3, Aug 14:3, Oct 14:3, Nov 14:14, Jan 15:12, Mar 16:11, Sep 16:6, Apr 18:10

Hospital Observation Services

The following codes are used to report evaluation and management services provided to patients designated/admitted as "observation status" in a hospital. It is not necessary that the patient be located in an observation area designated by the hospital.

If such an area does exist in a hospital (as a separate unit in the hospital, in the emergency department, etc.), these codes are to be utilized if the patient is placed in such an area.

For definitions of key components and commonly used terms, please see **Evaluation and Management Services Guidelines.**

Coding Tip

The Significance of Time as a Factor in Selection of an Evaluation and Management Code

The inclusion of time as an explicit factor beginning in CPT 1992 is done to assist in selecting the most appropriate level of E/M services. It should be recognized that the specific times expressed in the visit code descriptors are averages and, therefore, represent a range of times that may be higher or lower depending on actual clinical circumstances.

Intraservice times are defined as **face-to-face** time for office and other outpatient visits and as **unit/floor** time for hospital and other inpatient visits. This distinction is necessary because most of the work of typical office visits takes place during the face-to-face time with the patient, while most of the work of typical hospital visits takes place during the time spent on the patient's floor or unit.

Unit/floor time (hospital observation services, inpatient hospital care, initial inpatient hospital consultations, nursing facility):

For reporting purposes, intraservice time for these services is defined as unit/floor time, which includes the time present on the patient's hospital unit and at the bedside rendering services for that patient. This includes the time to establish and/or review the patient's chart, examine the patient, write notes, and communicate with other professionals and the patient's family.

In the hospital, pre- and post-time includes time spent off the patient's floor performing such tasks as reviewing pathology and radiology findings in another part of the hospital.

This pre- and postvisit time is not included in the time component described in these codes. However, the pre- and post-work performed during the time spent off the floor or unit was included in calculating the total work of typical services in physician surveys.

Thus, the unit/floor time associated with the services described by any code is a valid proxy for the total work done before, during, and after the visit.

CPT Coding Guidelines, Evaluation and Management, Definitions of Commonly Used Terms, Time

Observation Care Discharge Services

Observation care discharge of a patient from "observation status" includes final examination of the patient, discussion of the hospital stay, instructions for continuing care, and preparation of discharge records. For observation or inpatient hospital care including the admission and discharge of the patient on the same date, see codes 99234-99236 as appropriate.

99217 **Observation care discharge** day management (This code is to be utilized to report all services provided to a patient on discharge from outpatient hospital "observation status" if the discharge is on other than the initial date of "observation status." To report services to a patient designated as "observation status" or "inpatient status" and discharged on the same date, use the codes for Observation or Inpatient Care Services [including Admission and Discharge Services, 99234-99236 as appropriate.])

CPT Changes: An Insider's View 2013, 2018

CPT Assistant Nov 97:2, Mar 98:1, May 98:3, Sep 98:5, Sep 00:3, May 05:1, Nov 05:10, Sep 06:8, Dec 06:14, Sep 10:4, Jun 11:3, Jul 12:10, 11, 14, Jan 13:9, Jun 13:3, Nov 14:14

Initial Observation Care

New or Established Patient

The following codes are used to report the encounter(s) by the supervising physician or other qualified health care professional with the patient when designated as outpatient hospital "observation status." This refers to the initiation of observation status, supervision of the care plan for observation and performance of periodic reassessments. For observation encounters by other physicians, see office or other outpatient consultation codes (99241-99245) or subsequent observation care codes (99224-99226) as appropriate.

To report services provided to a patient who is admitted to the hospital after receiving hospital observation care services on the same date, see the notes for initial hospital inpatient care (page 15). For observation care services on other than the initial or discharge date, see subsequent observation services codes (99224-99226). For a patient admitted to the hospital on a date subsequent to the date of observation status, the hospital admission would be reported with the appropriate initial hospital care code (99221-99223). For a patient admitted and discharged from observation or inpatient status on the same date, the services should be reported with codes 99234-99236 as appropriate. Do not report observation discharge (99217) in conjunction with a hospital admission (99221-99223).

When "observation status" is initiated in the course of an encounter in another site of service (eg, hospital emergency department, office, nursing facility) all evaluation and management services provided by the supervising physician or other qualified health care professional in conjunction with initiating "observation status" are considered part of the initial observation care when performed on the same date. The observation care level of service reported by the supervising physician or other qualified health care professional should include the services related to initiating "observation status" provided in the other sites of service as well as in the observation setting.

Evaluation and management services including new or established patient office or other outpatient services (99201-99215), emergency department services (99281-99285), nursing facility services (99304-99318), domiciliary, rest home, or custodial care services (99324-99337), home services (99341-99350), and preventive medicine services (99381-99429) on the same date related to the admission to "observation status" should not be reported separately.

These codes may not be utilized for post-operative recovery if the procedure is considered part of the surgical "package." These codes apply to all evaluation and management services that are provided on the same date of initiating "observation status."

99218 **Initial observation care,** per day, for the evaluation and management of a patient which requires these 3 key components:

- **A detailed or comprehensive history;**
- **A detailed or comprehensive examination; and**
- **Medical decision making that is straightforward or of low complexity.**

Counseling and/or coordination of care with other physicians, other qualified health care professionals, or agencies are provided consistent with the nature of the problem(s) and the patient's and/or family's needs.

Usually, the problem(s) requiring admission to outpatient hospital "observation status" are of low severity. Typically, 30 minutes are spent at the bedside and on the patient's hospital floor or unit.

CPT Changes: An Insider's View 2012, 2013, 2018

CPT Assistant Spring 93:34, Fall 95:9, Nov 97:2, Mar 98:1, Sep 98:5, Sep 00:3, Jan 03:10, Aug 04:11, May 05:1, Nov 05:10, Sep 06:8, Dec 06:14, Sep 10:4, Oct 10:6, Jun 11:3, Jul 12:11, 14, Jan 13:9, Jun 13:3, Aug 13:13, Mar 15:3, Jul 15:3

99219 **Initial observation care,** per day, for the evaluation and management of a patient, which requires these 3 key components:

- **A comprehensive history;**
- **A comprehensive examination; and**
- **Medical decision making of moderate complexity.**

Counseling and/or coordination of care with other physicians, other qualified health care professionals, or agencies are provided consistent with the nature of the problem(s) and the patient's and/or family's needs.

Usually, the problem(s) requiring admission to outpatient hospital "observation status" are of moderate severity. Typically, 50 minutes are spent at the bedside and on the patient's hospital floor or unit.

➲ *CPT Changes: An Insider's View* 2012, 2013, 2018

➲ *CPT Assistant* Spring 93:34, Fall 95:16, Nov 97:2, Mar 98:1, Sep 98:5, Sep 00:3, Jan 03:10, Aug 04:11, Nov 05:10, Sep 06:8, Dec 06:14, Sep 10:4, Oct 10:6, Jun 11:3, Jul 12:11, 14, Jan 13:9, Jun 13:3, Aug 13:13

99220 **Initial observation care,** per day, for the evaluation and management of a patient, which requires these 3 key components:

- **A comprehensive history;**
- **A comprehensive examination; and**
- **Medical decision making of high complexity.**

Counseling and/or coordination of care with other physicians, other qualified health care professionals, or agencies are provided consistent with the nature of the problem(s) and the patient's and/or family's needs.

Usually, the problem(s) requiring admission to outpatient hospital "observation status" are of high severity. Typically, 70 minutes are spent at the bedside and on the patient's hospital floor or unit.

➲ *CPT Changes: An Insider's View* 2012, 2013, 2018

➲ *CPT Assistant* Spring 93:34, Fall 95:16, Nov 97:2, Mar 98:1, Sep 98:5, Sep 00:3, Jan 03:10, Aug 04:11, Nov 05:10, Sep 06:8, Dec 06:14, Sep 10:4, Oct 10:6, Jun 11:3, Jul 12:11, Jan 13:9, Jun 13:3, Aug 13:13, Nov 14:14

Subsequent Observation Care

All levels of subsequent observation care include reviewing the medical record and reviewing the results of diagnostic studies and changes in the patient's status (ie, changes in history, physical condition, and response to management) since the last assessment.

 # 99224 **Subsequent observation care,** per day, for the evaluation and management of a patient, which requires at least 2 of these 3 key components:

- **Problem focused interval history;**
- **Problem focused examination;**
- **Medical decision making that is straightforward or of low complexity.**

Counseling and/or coordination of care with other physicians, other qualified health care professionals, or agencies are provided consistent with the nature of the problem(s) and the patient's and/or family's needs.

Usually, the patient is stable, recovering, or improving. Typically, 15 minutes are spent at the bedside and on the patient's hospital floor or unit.

➲ *CPT Changes: An Insider's View* 2011, 2013

➲ *CPT Assistant* Jun 11:3, Aug 11:11, Jul 12:10, 11, Jun 13:3, Aug 13:13, Nov 14:14

 # 99225 **Subsequent observation care,** per day, for the evaluation and management of a patient, which requires at least 2 of these 3 key components:

- **An expanded problem focused interval history;**
- **An expanded problem focused examination;**
- **Medical decision making of moderate complexity.**

Counseling and/or coordination of care with other physicians, other qualified health care professionals, or agencies are provided consistent with the nature of the problem(s) and the patient's and/or family's needs.

Usually, the patient is responding inadequately to therapy or has developed a minor complication. Typically, 25 minutes are spent at the bedside and on the patient's hospital floor or unit.

➲ *CPT Changes: An Insider's View* 2011, 2013

➲ *CPT Assistant* Jun 11:3, Aug 11:11, Jul 12:10, 11, Jan 13:9, Jun 13:3, Aug 13:13

 # 99226 **Subsequent observation care,** per day, for the evaluation and management of a patient, which requires at least 2 of these 3 key components:

- **A detailed interval history;**
- **A detailed examination;**
- **Medical decision making of high complexity.**

Counseling and/or coordination of care with other physicians, other qualified health care professionals, or agencies are provided consistent with the nature of the problem(s) and the patient's and/or family's needs.

Usually, the patient is unstable or has developed a significant complication or a significant new problem. Typically, 35 minutes are spent at the bedside and on the patient's hospital floor or unit.

➲ *CPT Changes: An Insider's View* 2011, 2013

➲ *CPT Assistant* Jun 11:3, Aug 11:11, Jul 12:10, 11, Jan 13:9, Jun 13:3, Aug 13:13, Nov 14:14

Hospital Inpatient Services

The following codes are used to report evaluation and management services provided to hospital inpatients. Hospital inpatient services include those services provided to patients in a "partial hospital" setting. These codes are to be used to report these partial hospitalization services. See also psychiatry notes in the full text of the CPT code set.

For definitions of key components and commonly used terms, please see **Evaluation and Management Services Guidelines.** For Hospital Observation Services, see 99218-99220, 99224-99226. For a patient admitted and discharged from observation or inpatient status on the same date, the services should be reported with codes 99234-99236 as appropriate.

Coding Tip

The Significance of Time as a Factor in Selection of an Evaluation and Management Code

The inclusion of time as an explicit factor beginning in CPT 1992 is done to assist in selecting the most appropriate level of E/M services. It should be recognized that the specific times expressed in the visit code descriptors are averages and, therefore, represent a range of times that may be higher or lower depending on actual clinical circumstances.

Intraservice times are defined as **face-to-face** time for office and other outpatient visits and as **unit/floor** time for hospital and other inpatient visits. This distinction is necessary because most of the work of typical office visits takes place during the face-to-face time with the patient, while most of the work of typical hospital visits takes place during the time spent on the patient's floor or unit.

Unit/floor time (hospital observation services, inpatient hospital care, initial inpatient hospital consultations, nursing facility):

For reporting purposes, intraservice time for these services is defined as unit/floor time, which includes the time present on the patient's hospital unit and at the bedside rendering services for that patient. This includes the time to establish and/or review the patient's chart, examine the patient, write notes, and communicate with other professionals and the patient's family.

In the hospital, pre- and post-time includes time spent off the patient's floor performing such tasks as reviewing pathology and radiology findings in another part of the hospital.

This pre- and postvisit time is not included in the time component described in these codes. However, the pre- and post-work performed during the time spent off the floor or unit was included in calculating the total work of typical services in physician surveys.

Thus, the unit/floor time associated with the services described by any code is a valid proxy for the total work done before, during, and after the visit.

CPT Coding Guidelines, Evaluation and Management, Definitions of Commonly Used Terms, Time

Initial Hospital Care

New or Established Patient

The following codes are used to report the first hospital inpatient encounter with the patient by the admitting physician.

For initial inpatient encounters by physicians other than the admitting physician, see initial inpatient consultation codes (99251-99255) or subsequent hospital care codes (99231-99233) as appropriate.

For admission services for the neonate (28 days of age or younger) requiring intensive observation, frequent interventions, and other intensive care services, see 99477.

When the patient is admitted to the hospital as an inpatient in the course of an encounter in another site of service (eg, hospital emergency department, observation status in a hospital, office, nursing facility) all evaluation and management services provided by that physician in conjunction with that admission are considered part of the initial hospital care when performed on the same date as the admission. The inpatient care level of service reported by the admitting physician should include the services related to the admission he/she provided in the other sites of service as well as in the inpatient setting.

Evaluation and management services including new or established patient office or other outpatient services (99201-99215), emergency department services (99281-99285), nursing facility services (99304-99318), domiciliary, rest home, or custodial care services (99324-99337), home services (99341-99350), and preventive medicine services (99381-99397) on the same date related to the admission to "observation status" should **not** be reported separately. For a patient admitted and discharged from observation or inpatient status on the same date, the services should be reported with codes 99234-99236 as appropriate.

99221 **Initial hospital care,** per day, for the evaluation and management of a patient, which requires these 3 key components:

- **A detailed or comprehensive history;**
- **A detailed or comprehensive examination; and**
- **Medical decision making that is straightforward or of low complexity.**

Counseling and/or coordination of care with other physicians, other qualified health care professionals, or agencies are provided consistent with the nature of the problem(s) and the patient's and/or family's needs.

Usually, the problem(s) requiring admission are of low severity. Typically, 30 minutes are spent at the bedside and on the patient's hospital floor or unit.

➔ *CPT Changes: An Insider's View* 2013

➔ *CPT Assistant* Winter 91:11, Spring 92:14, 24, Summer 92:10, 24, Fall 92:1, Spring 93:34, Spring 95:1, Fall 95:9, Jul 96:11, Sep 96:10, Nov 97:2, Mar 98:1, Sep 98:5, Jan 02:2-3, Apr 03:26, Apr 04:14, Aug 04:11, May 05:1, Sep 06:8, Jul 07:12, Jul 12:12, Jan 13:9, Jun 13:3, Aug 13:13, Feb 14:11, May 14:4, Nov 14:14, Dec 15:16, Mar 16:11

99222 **Initial hospital care,** per day, for the evaluation and management of a patient, which requires these 3 key components:

- **A comprehensive history;**
- **A comprehensive examination; and**
- **Medical decision making of moderate complexity.**

Counseling and/or coordination of care with other physicians, other qualified health care professionals, or agencies are provided consistent with the nature of the problem(s) and the patient's and/or family's needs.

Usually, the problem(s) requiring admission are of moderate severity. Typically, 50 minutes are spent at the bedside and on the patient's hospital floor or unit.

➔ *CPT Changes: An Insider's View* 2013

➔ *CPT Assistant* Winter 91:11, Spring 92:14, 24, Summer 92:10, 24, Fall 92:1, Spring 93:34, Spring 95:1, Fall 95:9, Jul 96:11, Sep 96:10, Nov 97:2, Mar 98:1, Sep 98:5, Jan 02:2-3, Apr 03:26, Apr 04:14, Aug 04:11, Sep 06:8, Jul 07:12, Jul 12:12, Jan 13:9, Jun 13:3, Aug 13:13, Mar 15:3, Dec 15:16, Mar 16:11

99223 **Initial hospital care,** per day, for the evaluation and management of a patient, which requires these 3 key components:

- **A comprehensive history;**
- **A comprehensive examination; and**
- **Medical decision making of high complexity.**

Counseling and/or coordination of care with other physicians, other qualified health care professionals, or agencies are provided consistent with the nature of the problem(s) and the patient's and/or family's needs.

Usually, the problem(s) requiring admission are of high severity. Typically, 70 minutes are spent at the bedside and on the patient's hospital floor or unit.

➔ *CPT Changes: An Insider's View* 2013

➔ *CPT Assistant* Winter 91:11, Spring 92:14, 24, Summer 92:10, 24, Fall 92:1, Spring 93:34, Spring 95:1, Fall 95:9, Jul 96:11, Sep 96:10, Nov 97:2, Mar 98:1, Sep 98:5, Jan 02:2-3, Apr 03:26, Apr 04:14, Aug 04:11, Sep 06:8, Jul 07:12, Jul 12:12, Jan 13:9, Jun 13:3, Aug 13:13, May 14:4, Nov 14:14, Dec 15:16, Mar 16:11

99224 Code is out of numerical sequence. See 99219-99222

99225 Code is out of numerical sequence. See 99219-99222

99226 Code is out of numerical sequence. See 99219-99222

Subsequent Hospital Care

All levels of subsequent hospital care include reviewing the medical record and reviewing the results of diagnostic studies and changes in the patient's status (ie, changes in history, physical condition and response to management) since the last assessment.

★ **99231** **Subsequent hospital care,** per day, for the evaluation and management of a patient, which requires at least 2 of these 3 key components:

- **A problem focused interval history;**
- **A problem focused examination;**
- **Medical decision making that is straightforward or of low complexity.**

Counseling and/or coordination of care with other physicians, other qualified health care professionals, or agencies are provided consistent with the nature of the problem(s) and the patient's and/or family's needs.

Usually, the patient is stable, recovering or improving. Typically, 15 minutes are spent at the bedside and on the patient's hospital floor or unit.

➔ *CPT Changes: An Insider's View* 2013, 2017

➔ *CPT Assistant* Winter 91:11, Spring 92:14, 24, Summer 92:10, 24, Fall 92:1, Spring 93:34, Spring 95:1, Fall 95:16, Nov 97:2, Sep 98:5, Jan 99:10, Nov 99:5, Aug 01:2, Jan 02:2-3, Apr 04:14, Aug 04:11, Mar 05:11, May 05:1, May 06:1, 16, Jul 06:4, Mar 07:9, Jul 07:1, Mar 09:3, Dec 09:9, Jun 11:3, Jul 12:12, Jan 13:9, Jun 13:3, Aug 13:14, Sep 13:18, May 14:4, Nov 14:14

★ **99232** **Subsequent hospital care,** per day, for the evaluation and management of a patient, which requires at least 2 of these 3 key components:

- **An expanded problem focused interval history;**
- **An expanded problem focused examination;**
- **Medical decision making of moderate complexity.**

Counseling and/or coordination of care with other physicians, other qualified health care professionals, or agencies are provided consistent with the nature of the problem(s) and the patient's and/or family's needs.

Usually, the patient is responding inadequately to therapy or has developed a minor complication. Typically, 25 minutes are spent at the bedside and on the patient's hospital floor or unit.

➔ *CPT Changes: An Insider's View* 2013, 2017

➔ *CPT Assistant* Winter 91:11, Spring 92:14, 24, Summer 92:10, 24, Fall 92:1, Spring 93:34, Spring 95:1, Fall 95:16, Nov 97:2, Sep 98:5, Jan 99:10, Nov 99:5, Jan 00:11, Aug 01:2, Apr 04:14, Aug 04:11, May 06:1, 16, Jul 06:4, Mar 07:9, Jul 07:1, Mar 09:3, Dec 09:9, Jun 11:3, Jul 12:12, Jan 13:9, Jun 13:3, Aug 13:14, Oct 16:8

★ **99233** **Subsequent hospital care,** per day, for the evaluation and management of a patient, which requires at least 2 of these 3 key components:

- **A detailed interval history;**
- **A detailed examination;**
- **Medical decision making of high complexity.**

Counseling and/or coordination of care with other physicians, other qualified health care professionals, or agencies are provided consistent with the nature of the problem(s) and the patient's and/or family's needs.

Usually, the patient is unstable or has developed a significant complication or a significant new problem. Typically, 35 minutes are spent at the bedside and on the patient's hospital floor or unit.

CPT Changes: An Insider's View 2013, 2017

CPT Assistant Winter 91:11, Spring 92:14, 24, Summer 92:10, 24, Fall 92:1, Spring 93:34, Spring 95:1, Fall 95:16, Nov 97:2, Sep 98:5, Jan 99:10, Nov 99:5, Aug 01:2, Apr 04:14, Aug 04:11, May 06:1, 16, Jul 06:4, Mar 07:9, Jul 07:1, Mar 09:3, Dec 09:9, Jun 11:3, Jul 12:12, Jan 13:9, Jun 13:3, Aug 13:13, 14, May 14:4, Nov 14:14, Oct 16:8

Observation or Inpatient Care Services (Including Admission and Discharge Services)

The following codes are used to report observation or inpatient hospital care services provided to patients admitted and discharged on the same date of service. When a patient is admitted to the hospital from observation status on the same date, only the initial hospital care code should be reported. The initial hospital care code reported by the admitting physician or other qualified health care professional should include the services related to the observation status services he/she provided on the same date of inpatient admission.

When "observation status" is initiated in the course of an encounter in another site of service (eg, hospital emergency department, office, nursing facility) all evaluation and management services provided by the supervising physician or other qualified health care professional in conjunction with initiating "observation status" are considered part of the initial observation care when performed on the same date. The observation care level of service should include the services related to initiating "observation status" provided in the other sites of service as well as in the observation setting when provided by the same individual.

For patients admitted to observation or inpatient care and discharged on a different date, see codes 99217, 99218-99220, 99224-99226, or 99221-99223, 99238 and 99239.

99234 **Observation or inpatient hospital care,** for the evaluation and management of a patient including admission and discharge on the same date, which requires these 3 key components:

- **A detailed or comprehensive history;**
- **A detailed or comprehensive examination; and**
- **Medical decision making that is straightforward or of low complexity.**

Counseling and/or coordination of care with other physicians, other qualified health care professionals, or agencies are provided consistent with the nature of the problem(s) and the patient's and/or family's needs.

Usually the presenting problem(s) requiring admission are of low severity. Typically, 40 minutes are spent at the bedside and on the patient's hospital floor or unit.

CPT Changes: An Insider's View 2013

CPT Assistant Nov 97:2, Mar 98:2, May 98:1, Sep 98:5, Jan 00:11, Sep 00:3, Jan 02:2, Jun 02:10, Jan 03:10, May 05:1, Nov 05:10, Sep 06:8, Dec 06:14, Sep 10:4, Jun 11:3, Jul 12:14, Jun 13:3, Apr 18:10

99235 **Observation or inpatient hospital care,** for the evaluation and management of a patient including admission and discharge on the same date, which requires these 3 key components:

- **A comprehensive history;**
- **A comprehensive examination; and**
- **Medical decision making of moderate complexity.**

Counseling and/or coordination of care with other physicians, other qualified health care professionals, or agencies are provided consistent with the nature of the problem(s) and the patient's and/or family's needs.

Usually the presenting problem(s) requiring admission are of moderate severity. Typically, 50 minutes are spent at the bedside and on the patient's hospital floor or unit.

CPT Changes: An Insider's View 2013

CPT Assistant Nov 97:2, Mar 98:2, May 98:1, Sep 98:5, Jan 00:11, Sep 00:3, Jan 02:2, Jun 02:10, Jan 03:10, Nov 05:10, Sep 06:8, Dec 06:14, Sep 10:4, Jun 11:3, Jul 12:14, Jun 13:3, Apr 18:10

99236 **Observation or inpatient hospital care,** for the evaluation and management of a patient including admission and discharge on the same date, which requires these 3 key components:

- **A comprehensive history;**
- **A comprehensive examination; and**
- **Medical decision making of high complexity.**

Counseling and/or coordination of care with other physicians, other qualified health care professionals, or agencies are provided consistent with the nature of the problem(s) and the patient's and/or family's needs.

Usually the presenting problem(s) requiring admission are of high severity. Typically, 55 minutes are spent at the bedside and on the patient's hospital floor or unit.

CPT Changes: An Insider's View 2013

CPT Assistant Nov 97:2, Mar 98:2, May 98:1, Sep 98:5, Jan 00:11, Sep 00:3, Jan 02:2, Jun 02:10, Jan 03:10, Nov 05:10, Sep 06:8, Dec 06:14, Sep 10:4, Jun 11:3, Jul 12:14, Jun 13:3, Apr 18:10

Hospital Discharge Services

The hospital discharge day management codes are to be used to report the total duration of time spent by a physician for final hospital discharge of a patient. The codes include, as appropriate, final examination of the patient, discussion of the hospital stay, even if the time spent by the physician on that date is not continuous, instructions for continuing care to all relevant caregivers, and preparation of discharge records, prescriptions and referral forms. For a patient admitted and discharged from observation or inpatient status on the same date, the services should be reported with codes 99234-99236 as appropriate.

99238 **Hospital discharge day management;** 30 minutes or less

CPT Assistant Fall 92:1, Spring 93:4, Nov 97:4, Mar 98:3, 11, May 98:2, Jan 99:10, Jan 02:2, Aug 04:11, May 05:1, Sep 06:8, Nov 09:10, Dec 09:9, Jul 11:16, Jul 12:10, 12, Jun 13:3, Aug 13:13

99239 more than 30 minutes

CPT Assistant Nov 97:4, Mar 98:3, 11, May 98:2, Jan 99:10, Jan 02:2, Aug 04:11, Sep 06:8, Nov 09:10, Dec 09:9, Jul 11:16, Jul 12:12, Jun 13:3, Aug 13:13

(These codes are to be utilized to report all services provided to a patient on the date of discharge, if other than the initial date of inpatient status. To report services to a patient who is admitted as an inpatient and discharged on the same date, see codes 99234-99236 for observation or inpatient hospital care including the admission and discharge of the patient on the same date. To report concurrent care services provided by an individual other than the physician or qualified health care professional performing the discharge day management service, use subsequent hospital care codes [99231-99233] on the day of discharge.)

(For Observation Care Discharge, use 99217)

(For observation or inpatient hospital care including the admission and discharge of the patient on the same date, see 99234-99236)

(For Nursing Facility Care Discharge, see 99315, 99316)

(For discharge services provided to newborns admitted and discharged on the same date, use 99463)

Consultations

A consultation is a type of evaluation and management service provided at the request of another physician or appropriate source to either recommend care for a specific condition or problem or to determine whether to accept responsibility for ongoing management of the patient's entire care or for the care of a specific condition or problem.

A physician consultant may initiate diagnostic and/or therapeutic services at the same or subsequent visit.

A "consultation" initiated by a patient and/or family, and not requested by a physician or other appropriate source (eg, physician assistant, nurse practitioner, doctor of chiropractic, physical therapist, occupational therapist, speech-language pathologist, psychologist, social worker, lawyer, or insurance company), is not reported using the consultation codes but may be reported using the office visit, home service, or domiciliary/rest home care codes as appropriate.

The written or verbal request for consult may be made by a physician or other appropriate source and documented in the patient's medical record by either the consulting or requesting physician or appropriate source. The consultant's opinion and any services that were ordered or performed must also be documented in the patient's medical record and communicated by written report to the requesting physician or other appropriate source.

If a consultation is mandated (eg, by a third-party payer) modifier 32 should also be reported.

Any specifically identifiable procedure (ie, identified with a specific CPT code) performed on or subsequent to the date of the initial consultation should be reported separately.

If subsequent to the completion of a consultation the consultant assumes responsibility for management of a portion or all of the patient's condition(s), the appropriate **Evaluation and Management** services code for the site of service should be reported. In the hospital or nursing facility setting, the consultant should use the appropriate inpatient consultation code for the initial encounter and then subsequent hospital or nursing facility care codes. In the office setting, the consultant should use the appropriate office or other outpatient consultation codes and then the established patient office or other outpatient services codes.

To report services provided to a patient who is admitted to a hospital or nursing facility in the course of an encounter in the office or other ambulatory facility, see the notes for Initial Hospital Inpatient Care (page 16) or Initial Nursing Facility Care (page 26).

For definitions of key components and commonly used terms, please see **Evaluation and Management Services Guidelines.**

Office or Other Outpatient Consultations

New or Established Patient

The following codes are used to report consultations provided in the office or in an outpatient or other ambulatory facility, including hospital observation services, home services, domiciliary, rest home, or emergency department (see the preceding consultation definition above). Follow-up visits in the consultant's office or other outpatient facility that are initiated by the consultant or patient are reported using the appropriate codes for established patients, office visits (99211-99215), domiciliary, rest home (99334-99337), or home (99347-99350). If an additional request for an opinion or advice regarding the same or a new problem is received from another physician or other appropriate source and documented in the medical record, the office consultation codes may be used again. Services that constitute transfer of care (ie, are provided for the management of the patient's entire care or for the care of a specific condition or problem) are reported with the appropriate new or established patient codes for office or other outpatient visits, domiciliary, rest home services, or home services.

Coding Tip

Definition of Transfer of Care

Transfer of care is the process whereby a physician or other qualified health care professional who is providing management for some or all of a patient's problems relinquishes this responsibility to another physician or other qualified health care professional who explicitly agrees to accept this responsibility and who, from the initial encounter, is not providing consultative services. The physician or other qualified health care professional transferring care is then no longer providing care for these problems though he or she may continue providing care for other conditions when appropriate. Consultation codes should not be reported by the physician or other qualified health care professional who has agreed to accept transfer of care before an initial evaluation but are appropriate to report if the decision to accept transfer of care cannot be made until after the initial consultation evaluation, regardless of site of service.

CPT Coding Guidelines, Evaluation and Management, Definitions of Commonly Used Terms, Concurrent Care and Transfer of Care

★ **99241** **Office consultation** for a new or established patient, which requires these 3 key components:

- **A problem focused history;**
- **A problem focused examination; and**
- **Straightforward medical decision making.**

Counseling and/or coordination of care with other physicians, other qualified health care professionals, or agencies are provided consistent with the nature of the problem(s) and the patient's and/or family's needs.

Usually, the presenting problem(s) are self limited or minor. Typically, 15 minutes are spent face-to-face with the patient and/or family.

➲ *CPT Changes: An Insider's View* 2013, 2017

➲ *CPT Assistant* Winter 91:11, Spring 92:4, 23-24, Summer 92:12, Spring 93:4, Spring 95:1, Oct 97:1, Sep 98:5, Jun 99:10, Apr 00:10, Aug 01:3, Jan 02:2, Jul 02:2, Sep 02:11, May 05:1, Dec 05:10, Jan 06:46, May 06:1, 16, Jun 06:1, Sep 06:8, Jan 07:28, Apr 07:11, Jul 07:1, May 08:13, Nov 08:10, Aug 09:9, Jan 10:3, Jul 10:4, Jun 11:3, Apr 12:10, Jan 13:9, Jun 13:3, Aug 14:3, Sep 14:13, Nov 14:14, Jan 15:12, Dec 15:18, Sep 16:6, Apr 18:10

➲ *Clinical Examples in Radiology* Summer 09:3

★ **99242** **Office consultation** for a new or established patient, which requires these 3 key components:

- **An expanded problem focused history;**
- **An expanded problem focused examination; and**
- **Straightforward medical decision making.**

Counseling and/or coordination of care with other physicians, other qualified health care professionals, or agencies are provided consistent with the nature of the problem(s) and the patient's and/or family's needs.

Usually, the presenting problem(s) are of low severity. Typically, 30 minutes are spent face-to-face with the patient and/or family.

➲ *CPT Changes: An Insider's View* 2000, 2013, 2017

➲ *CPT Assistant* Winter 91:11, Spring 92:4, 23-24, Summer 92:12, Spring 93:2, 34, Spring 95:1, Oct 97:1, Sep 98:5, Aug 01:3, Jan 02:2, Jul 02:2, Sep 02:11, Dec 05:10, May 06:1, 16, Jun 06:1, Sep 06:8, Apr 07:11, Jul 07:1, Jan 10:3, Jun 11:3, Jan 13:9, Jun 13:3, Sep 14:13, Jan 15:12, Sep 16:6, Apr 18:10

➲ *Clinical Examples in Radiology* Summer 09:3

★ **99243** **Office consultation** for a new or established patient, which requires these 3 key components:

- **A detailed history;**
- **A detailed examination; and**
- **Medical decision making of low complexity.**

Counseling and/or coordination of care with other physicians, other qualified health care professionals, or agencies are provided consistent with the nature of the problem(s) and the patient's and/or family's needs.

Usually, the presenting problem(s) are of moderate severity. Typically, 40 minutes are spent face-to-face with the patient and/or family.

➲ *CPT Changes: An Insider's View* 2013, 2017

➲ *CPT Assistant* Winter 91:11, Spring 92:4, 23-24, Summer 92:12, Spring 93:2, 34, Spring 95:1, Oct 97:1, Sep 98:5, Aug 01:3, Jan 02:2, Jul 02:2, Sep 02:11, Oct 03:5, Dec 05:10, May 06:1, 16, Jun 06:1, Sep 06:8, Apr 07:11, Jul 07:1, Jan 10:3, Jun 11:3, Jan 13:9, Jun 13:3, Sep 14:13, Jan 15:12, Sep 16:6, Apr 18:10

➲ *Clinical Examples in Radiology* Summer 09:3

★ **99244** **Office consultation** for a new or established patient, which requires these 3 key components:

- **A comprehensive history;**
- **A comprehensive examination; and**
- **Medical decision making of moderate complexity.**

Counseling and/or coordination of care with other physicians, other qualified health care professionals, or agencies are provided consistent with the nature of the problem(s) and the patient's and/or family's needs.

Usually, the presenting problem(s) are of moderate to high severity. Typically, 60 minutes are spent face-to-face with the patient and/or family.

➲ *CPT Changes: An Insider's View* 2013, 2017

➲ *CPT Assistant* Winter 91:11, Spring 92:3, 23-24, Summer 92:12, Spring 93:2, 34, Spring 95:1, Oct 97:1, Sep 98:5, Aug 01:3, Jan 02:2, Jul 02:2, Sep 02:11, Oct 03:5, Dec 05:10, May 06:1, 16, Jun 06:1, Sep 06:8, Apr 07:11, Jul 07:1, Jan 10:3, Jun 11:3, Jan 13:9, Jun 13:3, Aug 13:12, Sep 14:13, Jan 15:12, Sep 16:6, Apr 18:10

➲ *Clinical Examples in Radiology* Summer 09:2, 3

★ **99245** **Office consultation** for a new or established patient, which requires these 3 key components:

- **A comprehensive history;**
- **A comprehensive examination; and**
- **Medical decision making of high complexity.**

Counseling and/or coordination of care with other physicians, other qualified health care professionals, or agencies are provided consistent with the nature of the problem(s) and the patient's and/or family's needs.

Usually, the presenting problem(s) are of moderate to high severity. Typically, 80 minutes are spent face-to-face with the patient and/or family.

➲ *CPT Changes: An Insider's View* 2013, 2017

➲ *CPT Assistant* Winter 91:11, Spring 92:4, 23-24, Summer 92:12, Spring 93:2, 34, Spring 95:1, Oct 97:1, Sep 98:5, Aug 01:2, Jan 02:2, Jul 02:2, Sep 02:11, Dec 05:10, May 06:1, 16, Jun 06:1, Sep 06:8, Apr 07:11, Jul 07:1, Jan 10:3, Jul 10:4, Jun 11:3, Apr 12:10, Jan 13:9, Jun 13:3, Aug 14:3, Sep 14:13, Jan 15:12, Sep 16:6, Apr 18:10

➲ *Clinical Examples in Radiology* Summer 09:3

Inpatient Consultations

New or Established Patient

The following codes are used to report physician or other qualified health care professional consultations provided to hospital inpatients, residents of nursing facilities, or patients in a partial hospital setting. Only one consultation should be reported by a consultant per admission. Subsequent services during the same admission are reported using subsequent hospital care codes (99231-99233) or subsequent nursing facility care codes (99307-99310), including services to complete the initial consultation, monitor progress, revise recommendations, or address a new problem. Use subsequent hospital care codes (99231-99233) or subsequent nursing facility care codes (99307-99310) to report transfer of care services (see page 5, Concurrent Care and Transfer of Care definitions).

When an inpatient consultation is performed on a date that a patient is admitted to a hospital or nursing facility, all evaluation and management services provided by the consultant related to the admission are reported with the inpatient consultation service code (99251-99255). If a patient is admitted after an outpatient consultation (office, emergency department, etc), and the patient is not seen on the unit on the date of admission, only report the outpatient consultation code (99241-99245). If the patient is seen by the consultant on the unit on the date of admission, report all evaluation and management services provided by the consultant related to the admission with either the inpatient consultation code (99251-99255) or with the initial inpatient admission service code (99221-99223). Do not report both an outpatient consultation (99241-99245) and inpatient consultation (99251-99255) for services related to the same inpatient stay. When transfer of care services are provided on a date subsequent to the outpatient consultation, use the subsequent hospital care codes (99231-99233) or subsequent nursing facility care codes (99307-99310).

★ 99251 **Inpatient consultation** for a new or established patient, which requires these 3 key components:

- **A problem focused history;**
- **A problem focused examination; and**
- **Straightforward medical decision making.**

Counseling and/or coordination of care with other physicians, other qualified health care professionals, or agencies are provided consistent with the nature of the problem(s) and the patient's and/or family's needs.

Usually, the presenting problem(s) are self limited or minor. Typically, 20 minutes are spent at the bedside and on the patient's hospital floor or unit.

➲ *CPT Changes: An Insider's View* 2007, 2013, 2017

➲ *CPT Assistant* Winter 91:11, Spring 92:16, 23-24, Summer 92:12, Spring 93:34, Spring 95:1, Oct 97:1, Sep 98:5, Aug 01:3, Sep 02:11, May 05:1, May 06:1, 16, Jun 06:1, Jul 06:19, Jul 07:1, Jan 10:3, Jan 13:9, Jun 13:3

➲ *Clinical Examples in Radiology* Summer 09:3

★ 99252 **Inpatient consultation** for a new or established patient, which requires these 3 key components:

- **An expanded problem focused history;**
- **An expanded problem focused examination; and**
- **Straightforward medical decision making.**

Counseling and/or coordination of care with other physicians, other qualified health care professionals, or agencies are provided consistent with the nature of the problem(s) and the patient's and/or family's needs.

Usually, the presenting problem(s) are of low severity. Typically, 40 minutes are spent at the bedside and on the patient's hospital floor or unit.

➲ *CPT Changes: An Insider's View* 2007, 2013, 2017

➲ *CPT Assistant* Winter 91:11, Spring 92:16, 23-24, Summer 92:12, Summer 93:34, Spring 95:1, Oct 97:1, Sep 98:5, Aug 01:4, Sep 02:11, May 06:1, 16, Jun 06:1, Jul 06:19, Jul 07:1, Jan 10:3, Jan 13:9, Jun 13:3

➲ *Clinical Examples in Radiology* Summer 09:3

★ 99253 **Inpatient consultation** for a new or established patient, which requires these 3 key components:

- **A detailed history;**
- **A detailed examination; and**
- **Medical decision making of low complexity.**

Counseling and/or coordination of care with other physicians, other qualified health care professionals, or agencies are provided consistent with the nature of the problem(s) and the patient's and/or family's needs.

Usually, the presenting problem(s) are of moderate severity. Typically, 55 minutes are spent at the bedside and on the patient's hospital floor or unit.

➲ *CPT Changes: An Insider's View* 2007, 2013, 2017

➲ *CPT Assistant* Winter 91:11, Spring 92:16, 23-24, Summer 92:12, Summer 93:34, Spring 95:1, Oct 97:1, Sep 98:5, Aug 01:4, Sep 02:11, May 06:1, 16, Jun 06:1, Jul 06:19, Jul 07:1, Jan 10:3, Jan 13:9, Jun 13:3

➲ *Clinical Examples in Radiology* Summer 09:3

★ **99254** **Inpatient consultation** for a new or established patient, which requires these 3 key components:

- **A comprehensive history;**
- **A comprehensive examination; and**
- **Medical decision making of moderate complexity.**

Counseling and/or coordination of care with other physicians, other qualified health care professionals, or agencies are provided consistent with the nature of the problem(s) and the patient's and/or family's needs.

Usually, the presenting problem(s) are of moderate to high severity. Typically, 80 minutes are spent at the bedside and on the patient's hospital floor or unit.

➲ *CPT Changes: An Insider's View* 2007, 2013, 2017

➲ *CPT Assistant* Winter 91:11, Spring 92:16, 23-24, Summer 92:12, Summer 93:34, Spring 95:1, Oct 97:1, Sep 98:5, Aug 01:4, Sep 02:11, May 06:1, 16, Jun 06:1, Jul 06:19, Jul 07:1, Jan 10:3, Jan 13:9, Jun 13:3

➲ *Clinical Examples in Radiology* Summer 09:3

★ **99255** **Inpatient consultation** for a new or established patient, which requires these 3 key components:

- **A comprehensive history;**
- **A comprehensive examination; and**
- **Medical decision making of high complexity.**

Counseling and/or coordination of care with other physicians, other qualified health care professionals, or agencies are provided consistent with the nature of the problem(s) and the patient's and/or family's needs.

Usually, the presenting problem(s) are of moderate to high severity. Typically, 110 minutes are spent at the bedside and on the patient's hospital floor or unit.

➲ *CPT Changes: An Insider's View* 2007, 2013, 2017

➲ *CPT Assistant* Winter 91:11, Spring 92:16, 23-24, Summer 92:12, Summer 93:34, Spring 95:1, Oct 97:1, Sep 98:5, Aug 01:4, Sep 02:11, May 06:1, 16, Jun 06:1, Jul 06:19, Jul 07:1, Jan 10:3, Jan 13:9, Jun 13:3, Nov 14:14

➲ *Clinical Examples in Radiology* Summer 09:3

Emergency Department Services

New or Established Patient

The following codes are used to report evaluation and management services provided in the emergency department. No distinction is made between new and established patients in the emergency department.

An emergency department is defined as an organized hospital-based facility for the provision of unscheduled episodic services to patients who present for immediate medical attention. The facility must be available 24 hours a day.

For critical care services provided in the emergency department, see Critical Care notes and 99291, 99292.

For evaluation and management services provided to a patient in an observation area of a hospital, see 99217-99220.

For observation or inpatient care services (including admission and discharge services), see 99234-99236.

Coding Tip

Time as a Factor in the Emergency Department Setting

Time is **not** a descriptive component for the emergency department levels of E/M services because emergency department services are typically provided on a variable intensity basis, often involving multiple encounters with several patients over an extended period of time. Therefore, it is often difficult for physicians to provide accurate estimates of the time spent face-to-face with the patient.

CPT Coding Guidelines, Evaluation and Management, Definitions of Commonly Used Terms, Time

99281 **Emergency department visit** for the evaluation and management of a patient, which requires these 3 key components:

- **A problem focused history;**
- **A problem focused examination; and**
- **Straightforward medical decision making.**

Counseling and/or coordination of care with other physicians, other qualified health care professionals, or agencies are provided consistent with the nature of the problem(s) and the patient's and/or family's needs.

Usually, the presenting problem(s) are self limited or minor.

➲ *CPT Changes: An Insider's View* 2013

➲ *CPT Assistant* Winter 91:11, Spring 92:24, Summer 92:18, Spring 93:34, Spring 95:1, Feb 96:3, Sep 98:5, Jan 00:11, Feb 00:11, Sep 00:3, Apr 02:14, Jul 02:2, Nov 05:10, Feb 06:14, Dec 06:14, Dec 07:13, Jan 13:9, Jun 13:3, Nov 14:14, Jan 15:12

99282 **Emergency department visit** for the evaluation and management of a patient, which requires these 3 key components:

- **An expanded problem focused history;**
- **An expanded problem focused examination; and**
- **Medical decision making of low complexity.**

Counseling and/or coordination of care with other physicians, other qualified health care professionals, or agencies are provided consistent with the nature of the problem(s) and the patient's and/or family's needs.

Usually, the presenting problem(s) are of low to moderate severity.

➲ *CPT Changes: An Insider's View* 2013

➲ *CPT Assistant* Winter 91:11, Spring 92:24, Summer 92:18, Spring 93:34, Spring 95:1, Summer 95:1, Feb 96:3, Sep 98:5, Jan 00:11, Feb 00:11, Sep 00:3, Apr 02:14, Jul 02:2, Nov 05:10, Feb 06:14, Dec 06:14, Dec 07:13, Jan 13:9, Jun 13:3, Jan 15:12

99283 **Emergency department visit** for the evaluation and management of a patient, which requires these 3 key components:

- **An expanded problem focused history;**
- **An expanded problem focused examination; and**
- **Medical decision making of moderate complexity.**

Counseling and/or coordination of care with other physicians, other qualified health care professionals, or agencies are provided consistent with the nature of the problem(s) and the patient's and/or family's needs.

Usually, the presenting problem(s) are of moderate severity.

➲ *CPT Changes: An Insider's View* 2013

➲ *CPT Assistant* Winter 91:11, Spring 92:24, Summer 92:18, Spring 93:34, Spring 95:1, Summer 95:1, Feb 96:3, Sep 98:5, Jan 00:11, Feb 00:11, Sep 00:3, Apr 02:14, Jul 02:2, Nov 05:10, Feb 06:14, Dec 06:14, Dec 07:13, Jan 13:9, Jun 13:3, Jan 15:12

99284 **Emergency department visit** for the evaluation and management of a patient, which requires these 3 key components:

- **A detailed history;**
- **A detailed examination; and**
- **Medical decision making of moderate complexity.**

Counseling and/or coordination of care with other physicians, other qualified health care professionals, or agencies are provided consistent with the nature of the problem(s) and the patient's and/or family's needs.

Usually, the presenting problem(s) are of high severity, and require urgent evaluation by the physician, or other qualified health care professionals but do not pose an immediate significant threat to life or physiologic function.

➲ *CPT Changes: An Insider's View* 2013

➲ *CPT Assistant* Winter 91:11, Spring 92:24, Summer 92:18, Spring 93:34, Spring 95:1, Summer 95:1, Feb 96:3, Sep 98:5, Jan 00:11, Feb 00:11, Sep 00:3, Apr 02:14, Jul 02:2, Nov 05:10, Feb 06:14, Dec 06:14, Dec 07:13, Jan 13:9, Jun 13:3, Jan 15:12

99285 **Emergency department visit** for the evaluation and management of a patient, which requires these 3 key components within the constraints imposed by the urgency of the patient's clinical condition and/or mental status:

- **A comprehensive history;**
- **A comprehensive examination; and**
- **Medical decision making of high complexity.**

Counseling and/or coordination of care with other physicians, other qualified health care professionals, or agencies are provided consistent with the nature of the problem(s) and the patient's and/or family's needs.

Usually, the presenting problem(s) are of high severity and pose an immediate significant threat to life or physiologic function.

➲ *CPT Changes: An Insider's View* 2000, 2013

➲ *CPT Assistant* Winter 91:11, Spring 92:24, Summer 92:18, Spring 93:34, Spring 95:1, Summer 95:1, Feb 96:3, Aug 98:8, Sep 98:5, Nov 99:23, Jan 00:11, Feb 00:11, Sep 00:3, Apr 02:14, Jul 02:2, Sep 02:11, Mar 05:11, Nov 05:10, Feb 06:14, Dec 06:14, Dec 07:13, Jan 13:9, Jun 13:3, Nov 14:14, Jan 15:12

Coding Tip

Emergency Department Classification of New vs Established Patient

No distinction is made between new and established patients in the emergency department. E/M services in the emergency department category may be reported for any new or established patient who presents for treatment in the emergency department.

CPT Coding Guidelines, Evaluation and Management, Definitions of Commonly Used Terms, New and Established Patient

Other Emergency Services

In directed emergency care, advanced life support, the physician or other qualified health care professional is located in a hospital emergency or critical care department, and is in two-way voice communication with ambulance or rescue personnel outside the hospital. Direction of the performance of necessary medical procedures includes but is not limited to: telemetry of cardiac rhythm; cardiac and/or pulmonary resuscitation; endotracheal or esophageal obturator airway intubation; administration of intravenous fluids and/or administration of intramuscular, intratracheal or subcutaneous drugs; and/or electrical conversion of arrhythmia.

99288 **Physician or other qualified health care professional direction of** emergency medical systems (EMS) emergency care, advanced life support

➲ *CPT Changes: An Insider's View* 2013

➲ *CPT Assistant* Summer 92:18, May 05:1, Nov 07:5, May 13:6

Critical Care Services

Critical care is the direct delivery by a physician(s) or other qualified health care professional of medical care for a critically ill or critically injured patient. A critical illness or injury acutely impairs one or more vital organ systems such that there is a high probability of imminent or life threatening deterioration in the patient's condition. Critical care involves high complexity decision making to assess, manipulate, and support vital system function(s) to treat single or multiple vital organ system failure and/or to prevent further life threatening deterioration of the patient's condition. Examples of vital organ system failure include, but are not limited to: central nervous system failure, circulatory failure, shock, renal, hepatic, metabolic, and/or respiratory failure. Although critical care typically requires interpretation of multiple physiologic parameters and/or application of advanced technology(s), critical care may be provided in life threatening situations when these elements are not present. Critical care may be provided on multiple days, even if no changes are made in the treatment rendered to the patient, provided that the patient's condition continues to require the level of attention described above.

Providing medical care to a critically ill, injured, or post-operative patient qualifies as a critical care service only if both the illness or injury and the treatment being provided meet the above requirements. Critical care is usually, but not always, given in a critical care area, such as the coronary care unit, intensive care unit, pediatric intensive care unit, respiratory care unit, or the emergency care facility.

Inpatient critical care services provided to infants 29 days through 71 months of age are reported with pediatric critical care codes 99471-99476. The pediatric critical care codes are reported as long as the infant/young child qualifies for critical care services during the hospital stay through 71 months of age. Inpatient critical care services provided to neonates (28 days of age or younger) are reported with the neonatal critical care codes 99468 and 99469. The neonatal critical care codes are reported as long as the neonate qualifies for critical care services during the hospital stay through the 28th postnatal day. The reporting of the pediatric and neonatal critical care services is not based on time or the type of unit (eg, pediatric or neonatal critical care unit) and it is not dependent upon the type of physician or other qualified health care professional delivering the care. To report critical care services provided in the outpatient setting (eg, emergency department or office), for neonates and pediatric patients up through 71 months of age, see the critical care codes 99291, 99292. If the same individual provides critical care services for a neonatal or pediatric patient in both the outpatient and inpatient settings on the same day, report only the appropriate neonatal or pediatric critical care code 99468-99472 for all critical care services provided on that day. Also report 99291-99292 for neonatal or pediatric critical care services provided by the individual providing critical care at one facility but transferring the patient to another facility. Critical care services provided by a second individual of a different specialty not reporting a per day neonatal or pediatric critical care code can be reported with codes 99291, 99292. For additional instructions on reporting these services, see the Neonatal and Pediatric Critical Care section and codes 99468-99476.

Services for a patient who is not critically ill but happens to be in a critical care unit are reported using other appropriate E/M codes.

Critical care and other E/M services may be provided to the same patient on the same date by the same individual.

▶For reporting by professionals, the following services are included in critical care when performed during the critical period by the physician(s) providing critical care: the interpretation of cardiac output measurements (93561, 93562), chest X rays (71045, 71046), pulse oximetry (94760, 94761, 94762), blood gases, and collection and interpretation of physiologic data (eg, ECGs, blood pressures, hematologic data); gastric intubation (43752, 43753); temporary transcutaneous pacing (92953); ventilatory management (94002-94004, 94660, 94662); and vascular access procedures (36000, 36410, 36415, 36591, 36600). Any services performed that are not included in this listing should be reported separately. Facilities may report the above services separately.◀

Codes 99291, 99292 should be reported for the attendance during the transport of critically ill or critically injured patients older than 24 months of age to or from a facility or hospital. For transport services of critically ill or critically injured pediatric patients 24 months of age or younger, see 99466, 99467.

Codes 99291, 99292 are used to report the total duration of time spent in provision of critical care services to a critically ill or critically injured patient, even if the time spent providing care on that date is not continuous. For any given period of time spent providing critical care services, the individual must devote his or her full attention to the patient and, therefore, cannot provide services to any other patient during the same period of time.

Time spent with the individual patient should be recorded in the patient's record. The time that can be reported as critical care is the time spent engaged in work directly related to the individual patient's care whether that time was spent at the immediate bedside or elsewhere on the floor or unit. For example, time spent on the unit or at the nursing station on the floor reviewing test results or imaging studies, discussing the critically ill patient's care with other medical staff or documenting critical care services in the medical record would be reported as critical care, even though it does not occur at the bedside. Also, when the patient is unable or lacks capacity to participate in discussions, time spent on the floor or unit with family members or surrogate decision makers obtaining a medical history, reviewing the patient's condition or prognosis, or discussing treatment or limitation(s) of treatment may be reported as critical care, provided that the conversation bears directly on the management of the patient.

▶Time spent in activities that occur outside of the unit or off the floor (eg, telephone calls whether taken at home, in the office, or elsewhere in the hospital) may not be reported as critical care since the individual is not immediately available to the patient. Time spent in activities that do not directly contribute to the treatment of the patient may not be reported as critical care, even if they are performed in the critical care unit (eg, participation in administrative meetings or telephone calls to discuss other patients). Time spent performing separately reportable procedures or services should not be included in the time reported as critical care time.◄

Code 99291 is used to report the first 30-74 minutes of critical care on a given date. It should be used only once per date even if the time spent by the individual is not continuous on that date. Critical care of less than 30 minutes total duration on a given date should be reported with the appropriate E/M code.

Code 99292 is used to report additional block(s) of time, of up to 30 minutes each beyond the first 74 minutes. (See the following table.)

The following examples illustrate the correct reporting of critical care services:

Total Duration of Critical Care	Codes
less than 30 minutes	appropriate E/M codes
30-74 minutes (30 minutes - 1 hr. 14 min.)	99291 X 1
75-104 minutes (1 hr. 15 min. - 1 hr. 44 min.)	99291 X 1 AND 99292 X 1
105-134 minutes (1 hr. 45 min. - 2 hr. 14 min.)	99291 X 1 AND 99292 X 2
135-164 minutes (2 hr. 15 min. - 2 hr. 44 min.)	99291 X 1 AND 99292 X 3
165-194 minutes (2 hr. 45 min. - 3 hr. 14 min.)	99291 X 1 AND 99292 X 4
195 minutes or longer (3 hr. 15 min. - etc.)	99291 and 99292 as appropriate (see illustrated reporting examples above)

99291 **Critical care, evaluation and management** of the critically ill or critically injured patient; first 30-74 minutes

➲ *CPT Assistant* Summer 92:18, Summer 93:1, Summer 95:1, Jan 96:7, Apr 97:3, Dec 98:6, Nov 99:3, Apr 00:6, Sep 00:1, Dec 00:15, Jul 02:2, Feb 03:15, Oct 03:2, Aug 04:7, 10, Oct 04:14, May 05:1, Jul 05:15, Nov 05:10, Jul 06:4, Dec 06:13, Nov 07:5, Jan 09:5, Mar 09:3, Jul 09:10, Aug 11:10, Sep 11:3, Jul 12:13, Feb 13:17, May 13:6, May 14:4, Aug 14:5, Oct 14:14, Feb 15:10, May 16:3, Aug 16:9, Oct 16:8

+ 99292 each additional 30 minutes (List separately in addition to code for primary service)

➲ *CPT Assistant* Summer 92:18, Summer 93:1, Summer 95:1, Jan 96:7, Apr 97:3, Dec 98:6, Nov 99:3, Apr 00:6, Sep 00:1, Dec 00:15, Feb 03:15, Oct 03:2, Aug 04:10, Oct 04:14, Jul 05:15, Nov 05:10, Jul 06:4, Dec 06:13, Nov 07:5, Jan 09:5, Mar 09:3, Aug 11:10, Sep 11:3, Feb 13:17, May 13:6, May 14:4, Aug 14:5, Oct 14:14, Feb 15:10, May 16:3, Aug 16:9

(Use 99292 in conjunction with 99291)

Coding Tip

Services Included in Critical Care Services

For reporting by professionals, the following services are included in critical care when performed during the critical period by the physician(s) providing critical care: the interpretation of cardiac output measurements (93561, 93562), chest X rays (71045, 71046), pulse oximetry (94760, 94761, 94762), blood gases, and collection and interpretation of physiologic data (eg, ECGs, blood pressures, hematologic data); gastric intubation (43752, 43753); temporary transcutaneous pacing (92953); ventilatory management (94002-94004, 94660, 94662); and vascular access procedures (36000, 36410, 36415, 36591, 36600). Any services performed that are not listed above should be reported separately. Facilities may report the above services separately

CPT Coding Guideline, Critical Care

Nursing Facility Services

The following codes are used to report evaluation and management services to patients in nursing facilities (formerly called skilled nursing facilities [SNFs], intermediate care facilities [ICFs], or long-term care facilities [LTCFs]).

These codes should also be used to report evaluation and management services provided to a patient in a psychiatric residential treatment center (a facility or a distinct part of a facility for psychiatric care, which provides a 24-hour therapeutically planned and professionally staffed group living and learning environment). If procedures such as medical psychotherapy are provided in addition to evaluation and management services, these should be reported in addition to the evaluation and management services provided.

Nursing facilities that provide convalescent, rehabilitative, or long term care are required to conduct comprehensive, accurate, standardized, and reproducible assessments of each resident's functional capacity using a Resident Assessment Instrument (RAI). All RAIs include the Minimum Data Set (MDS), Resident Assessment Protocols (RAPs), and utilization guidelines. The MDS is the primary screening and assessment tool; the RAPs trigger the identification of potential problems and provide guidelines for follow-up assessments.

Physicians have a central role in assuring that all residents receive thorough assessments and that medical plans of care are instituted or revised to enhance or maintain the residents' physical and psychosocial functioning. This role includes providing input in the development of the MDS and a multi-disciplinary plan of care, as required by regulations pertaining to the care of nursing facility residents.

Two major subcategories of nursing facility services are recognized: Initial Nursing Facility Care and Subsequent Nursing Facility Care. Both subcategories apply to new or established patients.

For definitions of key components and commonly used terms, please see **Evaluation and Management Services Guidelines.**

(For care plan oversight services provided to nursing facility residents, see 99379-99380)

Initial Nursing Facility Care

New or Established Patient

When the patient is admitted to the nursing facility in the course of an encounter in another site of service (eg, hospital emergency department, office), all evaluation and management services provided by that physician in conjunction with that admission are considered part of the initial nursing facility care when performed on the same date as the admission or readmission. The nursing facility care level of service reported by the admitting physician should include the services related to the admission he/she provided in the other sites of service as well as in the nursing facility setting.

Hospital discharge or observation discharge services performed on the same date of nursing facility admission or readmission may be reported separately. For a patient discharged from inpatient status on the same date of nursing facility admission or readmission, the hospital discharge services should be reported with codes 99238, 99239 as appropriate. For a patient discharged from observation status on the same date of nursing facility admission or readmission, the observation care discharge services should be reported with code 99217. For a patient admitted and discharged from observation or inpatient status on the same date, see codes 99234-99236.

(For nursing facility care discharge, see 99315, 99316)

Coding Tip

The Significance of Time as a Factor in Selection of an Evaluation and Management Code

The inclusion of time as an explicit factor beginning in CPT 1992 is done to assist in selecting the most appropriate level of E/M services. It should be recognized that the specific times expressed in the visit code descriptors are averages and, therefore, represent a range of times that may be higher or lower depending on actual clinical circumstances.

Intraservice times are defined as **face-to-face** time for office and other outpatient visits and as **unit/floor** time for hospital and other inpatient visits. This distinction is necessary because most of the work of typical office visits takes place during the face-to-face time with the patient, while most of the work of typical hospital visits takes place during the time spent on the patient's floor or unit.

Unit/floor time (hospital observation services, inpatient hospital care, initial inpatient hospital consultations, nursing facility):

For reporting purposes, intraservice time for these services is defined as unit/floor time, which includes the time present on the patient's hospital unit and at the bedside rendering services for that patient. This includes the time to establish and/or review the patient's chart, examine the patient, write notes, and communicate with other professionals and the patient's family.

In the hospital, pre- and post-time includes time spent off the patient's floor performing such tasks as reviewing pathology and radiology findings in another part of the hospital.

This pre- and postvisit time is not included in the time component described in these codes. However, the pre- and post-work performed during the time spent off the floor or unit was included in calculating the total work of typical services in physician surveys.

Thus, the unit/floor time associated with the services described by any code is a valid proxy for the total work done before, during, and after the visit.

CPT Coding Guidelines, Evaluation and Management, Definitions of Commonly Used Terms, Time

99304 Initial nursing facility care, per day, for the evaluation and management of a patient, which requires these 3 key components:

- **A detailed or comprehensive history;**
- **A detailed or comprehensive examination; and**
- **Medical decision making that is straightforward or of low complexity.**

Counseling and/or coordination of care with other physicians, other qualified health care professionals, or agencies are provided consistent with the nature of the problem(s) and the patient's and/or family's needs.

Usually, the problem(s) requiring admission are of low severity. Typically, 25 minutes are spent at the bedside and on the patient's facility floor or unit.

➲ *CPT Changes: An Insider's View* 2006, 2008, 2010, 2013

➲ *CPT Assistant* Jul 10:4, Jan 11:3, Jun 11:3, Jan 12:3, Jul 12:12, Jan 13:9, Jun 13:3, Nov 14:14

99305 Initial nursing facility care, per day, for the evaluation and management of a patient, which requires these 3 key components:

- **A comprehensive history;**
- **A comprehensive examination; and**
- **Medical decision making of moderate complexity.**

Counseling and/or coordination of care with other physicians, other qualified health care professionals, or agencies are provided consistent with the nature of the problem(s) and the patient's and/or family's needs.

Usually, the problem(s) requiring admission are of moderate severity. Typically, 35 minutes are spent at the bedside and on the patient's facility floor or unit.

➲ *CPT Changes: An Insider's View* 2006, 2008, 2010, 2013

➲ *CPT Assistant* Jan 11:3, Jun 11:3, Jul 12:12, Jan 13:9, Jun 13:3

99306 Initial nursing facility care, per day, for the evaluation and management of a patient, which requires these 3 key components:

- **A comprehensive history;**
- **A comprehensive examination; and**
- **Medical decision making of high complexity.**

Counseling and/or coordination of care with other physicians, other qualified health care professionals, or agencies are provided consistent with the nature of the problem(s) and the patient's and/or family's needs.

Usually, the problem(s) requiring admission are of high severity. Typically, 45 minutes are spent at the bedside and on the patient's facility floor or unit.

➲ *CPT Changes: An Insider's View* 2006, 2008, 2010, 2013

➲ *CPT Assistant* Jan 11:3, Jun 11:3, Jan 12:3, Jul 12:12, Jan 13:9, Jun 13:3

Subsequent Nursing Facility Care

All levels of subsequent nursing facility care include reviewing the medical record and reviewing the results of diagnostic studies and changes in the patient's status (ie, changes in history, physical condition, and response to management) since the last assessment by the physician or other qualified health are professional.

★ **99307** Subsequent nursing facility care, per day, for the evaluation and management of a patient, which requires at least 2 of these 3 key components:

- **A problem focused interval history;**
- **A problem focused examination;**
- **Straightforward medical decision making.**

Counseling and/or coordination of care with other physicians, other qualified health care professionals, or agencies are provided consistent with the nature of the problem(s) and the patient's and/or family's needs.

Usually, the patient is stable, recovering, or improving. Typically, 10 minutes are spent at the bedside and on the patient's facility floor or unit.

➲ *CPT Changes: An Insider's View* 2006, 2008, 2010, 2013, 2017

➲ *CPT Assistant* May 06:1, 16, Jun 06:1, 19, Mar 07:9, Jul 07:1, Jul 09:3, 8, Jan 11:3, Jan 12:3, Jul 12:12, Jan 13:9, Jun 13:3

★ **99308** Subsequent nursing facility care, per day, for the evaluation and management of a patient, which requires at least 2 of these 3 key components:

- **An expanded problem focused interval history;**
- **An expanded problem focused examination;**
- **Medical decision making of low complexity.**

Counseling and/or coordination of care with other physicians, other qualified health care professionals, or agencies are provided consistent with the nature of the problem(s) and the patient's and/or family's needs.

Usually, the patient is responding inadequately to therapy or has developed a minor complication. Typically, 15 minutes are spent at the bedside and on the patient's facility floor or unit.

➲ *CPT Changes: An Insider's View* 2006, 2008, 2010, 2013, 2017

➲ *CPT Assistant* May 06:1, 16, Jun 06:1, 19, Mar 07:9, Jul 07:1, Jul 09:3, 8, Jan 11:3, Jul 12:12, Jan 13:9, Jun 13:3

★ **99309** Subsequent nursing facility care, per day, for the evaluation and management of a patient, which requires at least 2 of these 3 key components:

- **A detailed interval history;**
- **A detailed examination;**
- **Medical decision making of moderate complexity.**

Counseling and/or coordination of care with other physicians, other qualified health care professionals, or agencies are provided consistent with the nature of the problem(s) and the patient's and/or family's needs.

Usually, the patient has developed a significant complication or a significant new problem. Typically, 25 minutes are spent at the bedside and on the patient's facility floor or unit.

➲ *CPT Changes: An Insider's View* 2006, 2008, 2010, 2013, 2017

➲ *CPT Assistant* May 06:1, 16, Jun 06:1, 19, Mar 07:9, Jul 07:1, Jul 09:3, 8, Jan 11:3, Jul 12:12, Jan 13:9, Jun 13:3

★ **99310** Subsequent nursing facility care, per day, for the evaluation and management of a patient, which requires at least 2 of these 3 key components:

- **A comprehensive interval history;**
- **A comprehensive examination;**
- **Medical decision making of high complexity.**

Counseling and/or coordination of care with other physicians, other qualified health care professionals, or agencies are provided consistent with the nature of the problem(s) and the patient's and/or family's needs.

The patient may be unstable or may have developed a significant new problem requiring immediate physician attention. Typically, 35 minutes are spent at the bedside and on the patient's facility floor or unit.

➲ *CPT Changes: An Insider's View* 2006, 2008, 2010, 2013, 2017

➲ *CPT Assistant* May 06:1, 16, Jun 06:1, 19, Mar 07:9, Jul 07:1, Jul 09:3, 8, Jul 10:4, Jan 11:3, Jan 12:3, Jul 12:12, Jan 13:9, Jun 13:3

Nursing Facility Discharge Services

The nursing facility discharge day management codes are to be used to report the total duration of time spent by a physician or other qualified health care professional for the final nursing facility discharge of a patient. The codes include, as appropriate, final examination of the patient, discussion of the nursing facility stay, even if the time spent on that date is not continuous. Instructions are given for continuing care to all relevant caregivers, and preparation of discharge records, prescriptions and referral forms.

99315 Nursing facility discharge day management; 30 minutes or less

CPT Assistant Nov 97:5-6, Sep 98:5, May 02:19, Nov 02:11, May 05:1, Jul 09:3, Jan 11:3, Jan 12:3, Jul 12:12, Jan 13:9, Jun 13:3

99316 more than 30 minutes

CPT Assistant Nov 97:5-6, Sep 98:5, May 02:19, Nov 02:11, Jul 09:3, Jan 11:3, Jul 12:12, Jan 13:9, Jun 13:3

Other Nursing Facility Services

99318 Evaluation and management of a patient involving an annual nursing facility assessment, which requires these 3 key components:

- **A detailed interval history;**
- **A comprehensive examination; and**
- **Medical decision making that is of low to moderate complexity.**

Counseling and/or coordination of care with other physicians, other qualified health care professionals, or agencies are provided consistent with the nature of the problem(s) and the patient's and/or family's needs.

Usually, the patient is stable, recovering, or improving. Typically, 30 minutes are spent at the bedside and on the patient's facility floor or unit.

CPT Changes: An Insider's View 2006, 2008, 2010, 2013

CPT Assistant Jan 11:3, Jan 12:3, Jan 13:9, Jun 13:3, Nov 14:14

(Do not report 99318 on the same date of service as nursing facility services codes 99304-99316)

Domiciliary, Rest Home (eg, Boarding Home), or Custodial Care Services

The following codes are used to report evaluation and management services in a facility which provides room, board and other personal assistance services, generally on a long-term basis. These codes include evaluation and management services provided in an assisted living facility, group home, custodial care, and intermediate care facilities.

The facility's services do not include a medical component.

For definitions of key components and commonly used terms, please see **Evaluation and Management Services Guidelines.**

(For care plan oversight services provided to a patient in a domiciliary facility under the care of a home health agency, see 99374, 99375, and for hospice agency, see 99377, 99378. For care plan oversight provided to a patient under hospice or home health agency care, see 99339, 99340)

New Patient

99324 Domiciliary or rest home visit for the evaluation and management of a new patient, which requires these 3 key components:

- **A problem focused history;**
- **A problem focused examination; and**
- **Straightforward medical decision making.**

Counseling and/or coordination of care with other physicians, other qualified health care professionals, or agencies are provided consistent with the nature of the problem(s) and the patient's and/or family's needs.

Usually, the presenting problem(s) are of low severity. Typically, 20 minutes are spent with the patient and/or family or caregiver.

CPT Changes: An Insider's View 2006, 2013

CPT Assistant Jan 06:1, Jun 06:1, Jul 09:8, Aug 09:5, Jan 11:3, Jan 12:3, Apr 12:10, Jan 13:9, Jun 13:3, Oct 14:3, Nov 14:14

99325 Domiciliary or rest home visit for the evaluation and management of a new patient, which requires these 3 key components:

- **An expanded problem focused history;**
- **An expanded problem focused examination; and**
- **Medical decision making of low complexity.**

Counseling and/or coordination of care with other physicians, other qualified health care professionals, or agencies are provided consistent with the nature of the problem(s) and the patient's and/or family's needs.

Usually, the presenting problem(s) are of moderate severity. Typically, 30 minutes are spent with the patient and/or family or caregiver.

CPT Changes: An Insider's View 2006, 2013

CPT Assistant Jan 06:1, Jun 06:1, Jul 09:8, Aug 09:5, Jan 11:3, Jan 13:9, Jun 13:3

99326 Domiciliary or rest home visit for the evaluation and management of a new patient, which requires these 3 key components:

- **A detailed history;**
- **A detailed examination; and**
- **Medical decision making of moderate complexity.**

Counseling and/or coordination of care with other physicians, other qualified health care professionals, or agencies are provided consistent with the nature of the problem(s) and the patient's and/or family's needs.

Usually, the presenting problem(s) are of moderate to high severity. Typically, 45 minutes are spent with the patient and/or family or caregiver.

➔ *CPT Changes: An Insider's View* 2006, 2013

➔ *CPT Assistant* Jan 06:1, Jun 06:1, Jul 09:8, Aug 09:5, Jan 11:3, Jan 13:9, Jun 13:3

99327 Domiciliary or rest home visit for the evaluation and management of a new patient, which requires these 3 key components:

- **A comprehensive history;**
- **A comprehensive examination; and**
- **Medical decision making of moderate complexity.**

Counseling and/or coordination of care with other physicians, other qualified health care professionals, or agencies are provided consistent with the nature of the problem(s) and the patient's and/or family's needs.

Usually, the presenting problem(s) are of high severity. Typically, 60 minutes are spent with the patient and/or family or caregiver.

➔ *CPT Changes: An Insider's View* 2006, 2013

➔ *CPT Assistant* Jan 06:1, Jun 06:1, Jul 09:8, Aug 09:5, Jan 11:3, Jan 13:9, Jun 13:3

99328 Domiciliary or rest home visit for the evaluation and management of a new patient, which requires these 3 key components:

- **A comprehensive history;**
- **A comprehensive examination; and**
- **Medical decision making of high complexity.**

Counseling and/or coordination of care with other physicians, other qualified health care professionals, or agencies are provided consistent with the nature of the problem(s) and the patient's and/or family's needs.

Usually, the patient is unstable or has developed a significant new problem requiring immediate physician attention. Typically, 75 minutes are spent with the patient and/or family or caregiver.

➔ *CPT Changes: An Insider's View* 2006, 2013

➔ *CPT Assistant* Jan 06:1, Jun 06:1, Jul 09:8, Aug 09:5, Jan 11:3, Jan 12:3, Jan 13:9, Jun 13:3

Established Patient

99334 Domiciliary or rest home visit for the evaluation and management of an established patient, which requires at least 2 of these 3 key components:

- **A problem focused interval history;**
- **A problem focused examination;**
- **Straightforward medical decision making.**

Counseling and/or coordination of care with other physicians, other qualified health care professionals, or agencies are provided consistent with the nature of the problem(s) and the patient's and/or family's needs.

Usually, the presenting problem(s) are self-limited or minor. Typically, 15 minutes are spent with the patient and/or family or caregiver.

➔ *CPT Changes: An Insider's View* 2006, 2013

➔ *CPT Assistant* Jan 06:1, Jun 06:1, Jul 07:1, Jul 09:8, Aug 09:5, Jan 11:3, Jan 12:3, Jan 13:9, Jun 13:3, Nov 13:3

99335 Domiciliary or rest home visit for the evaluation and management of an established patient, which requires at least 2 of these 3 key components:

- **An expanded problem focused interval history;**
- **An expanded problem focused examination;**
- **Medical decision making of low complexity.**

Counseling and/or coordination of care with other physicians, other qualified health care professionals, or agencies are provided consistent with the nature of the problem(s) and the patient's and/or family's needs.

Usually, the presenting problem(s) are of low to moderate severity. Typically, 25 minutes are spent with the patient and/or family or caregiver.

➔ *CPT Changes: An Insider's View* 2006, 2013

➔ *CPT Assistant* Jan 06:1, Jun 06:1, Jul 07:1, Jul 09:8, Aug 09:5, Jan 11:3, Jan 13:9, Jun 13:3

99336 Domiciliary or rest home visit for the evaluation and management of an established patient, which requires at least 2 of these 3 key components:

- **A detailed interval history;**
- **A detailed examination;**
- **Medical decision making of moderate complexity.**

Counseling and/or coordination of care with other physicians, other qualified health care professionals, or agencies are provided consistent with the nature of the problem(s) and the patient's and/or family's needs.

Usually, the presenting problem(s) are of moderate to high severity. Typically, 40 minutes are spent with the patient and/or family or caregiver.

➔ *CPT Changes: An Insider's View* 2006, 2013

➔ *CPT Assistant* Jan 06:1, Jun 06:1, Jul 07:1, Jul 09:8, Aug 09:5, Jan 11:3, Jan 13:9, Jun 13:3

99337 Domiciliary or rest home visit for the evaluation and management of an established patient, which requires at least 2 of these 3 key components:

- **A comprehensive interval history;**
- **A comprehensive examination;**
- **Medical decision making of moderate to high complexity.**

Counseling and/or coordination of care with other physicians, other qualified health care professionals, or agencies are provided consistent with the nature of the problem(s) and the patient's and/or family's needs.

Usually, the presenting problem(s) are of moderate to high severity. The patient may be unstable or may have developed a significant new problem requiring immediate physician attention. Typically, 60 minutes are spent with the patient and/or family or caregiver.

➔ *CPT Changes: An Insider's View* 2006, 2013

➔ *CPT Assistant* Jan 06:1, Jun 06:1, Jul 07:1, Jul 09:8, Aug 09:5, Jan 11:3, Jan 12:3, Apr 12:10, Jan 13:9, Jun 13:3, Nov 13:3, Oct 14:3, Nov 14:14

Domiciliary, Rest Home (eg, Assisted Living Facility), or Home Care Plan Oversight Services

(For instructions on the use of 99339, 99340, see introductory notes for 99374-99380)

(For care plan oversight services for patients under the care of a home health agency, hospice, or nursing facility, see 99374-99380)

(Do not report 99339, 99340 for time reported with 98966-98969, 99441-99444)

99339 Individual physician supervision of a patient (patient not present) in home, domiciliary or rest home (eg, assisted living facility) requiring complex and multidisciplinary care modalities involving regular physician development and/or revision of care plans, review of subsequent reports of patient status, review of related laboratory and other studies, communication (including telephone calls) for purposes of assessment or care decisions with health care professional(s), family member(s), surrogate decision maker(s) (eg, legal guardian) and/or key caregiver(s) involved in patient's care, integration of new information into the medical treatment plan and/or adjustment of medical therapy, within a calendar month; 15-29 minutes

➲ *CPT Changes: An Insider's View* 2006

➲ *CPT Assistant* Jan 06:1, Dec 06:4, Mar 07:11, Sep 08:3, Jul 09:5, 10, Jan 12:3, Apr 13:3, Jun 13:3, Sep 13:15, Nov 13:3, Oct 14:3

99340 30 minutes or more

➲ *CPT Changes: An Insider's View* 2006

➲ *CPT Assistant* Jan 06:1, Dec 06:4, Mar 07:11, Sep 08:3, Jul 09:5, 10, Jan 12:3, Apr 13:3, Jun 13:3, Sep 13:15, Nov 13:3, Oct 14:3

(Do not report 99339, 99340 for patients under the care of a home health agency, enrolled in a hospice program, or for nursing facility residents)

(Do not report 99339, 99340 during the same month with 99487-99489)

(Do not report 99339, 99340 when performed during the service time of codes 99495 or 99496)

Home Services

►The following codes are used to report evaluation and management services provided in a home. Home may be defined as a private residence, temporary lodging, or short term accommodation (eg, hotel, campground, hostel, or cruise ship).◄

For definitions of key components and commonly used terms, please see **Evaluation and Management Services Guidelines.**

(For care plan oversight services provided to a patient in the home under the care of a home health agency, see 99374, 99375, and for hospice agency, see 99377, 99378. For care plan oversight provided to a patient under hospice or home health agency care, see 99339, 99340)

New Patient

99341 **Home visit** for the evaluation and management of a new patient, which requires these 3 key components:

- **A problem focused history;**
- **A problem focused examination; and**
- **Straightforward medical decision making.**

Counseling and/or coordination of care with other physicians, other qualified health care professionals, or agencies are provided consistent with the nature of the problem(s) and the patient's and/or family's needs.

Usually, the presenting problem(s) are of low severity. Typically, 20 minutes are spent face-to-face with the patient and/or family.

➲ *CPT Changes: An Insider's View* 2013

➲ *CPT Assistant* Winter 91:11, Spring 92:24, Summer 92:12, Spring 93:34, Spring 95:1, Jun 97:6, Nov 97:6-8, Oct 98:6, Oct 03:7, May 05:1, Jan 06:1, Jul 09:8, Aug 09:5, Jan 11:3, Jan 12:3, Apr 12:10, Jan 13:9, Jun 13:3, Oct 14:3, Nov 14:14

99342 **Home visit** for the evaluation and management of a new patient, which requires these 3 key components:

- **An expanded problem focused history;**
- **An expanded problem focused examination; and**
- **Medical decision making of low complexity.**

Counseling and/or coordination of care with other physicians, other qualified health care professionals, or agencies are provided consistent with the nature of the problem(s) and the patient's and/or family's needs.

Usually, the presenting problem(s) are of moderate severity. Typically, 30 minutes are spent face-to-face with the patient and/or family.

➲ *CPT Changes: An Insider's View* 2013

➲ *CPT Assistant* Winter 91:11, Spring 92:24, Summer 92:12, Spring 93:34, Spring 95:1, Jun 97:6, Nov 97:6-8, Oct 98:6, Jan 06:1, Jul 09:8, Aug 09:5, Jan 11:3, Jan 13:9, Jun 13:3

99343 **Home visit** for the evaluation and management of a new patient, which requires these 3 key components:

- **A detailed history;**
- **A detailed examination; and**
- **Medical decision making of moderate complexity.**

Counseling and/or coordination of care with other physicians, other qualified health care professionals, or agencies are provided consistent with the nature of the problem(s) and the patient's and/or family's needs.

Usually, the presenting problem(s) are of moderate to high severity. Typically, 45 minutes are spent face-to-face with the patient and/or family.

➔ *CPT Changes: An Insider's View* 2013

➔ *CPT Assistant* Winter 91:11, Spring 92:24, Summer 92:12, Spring 93:34, Spring 95:1, Jun 97:6, Nov 97:6-8, Oct 98:6, Jan 06:1, Jul 09:8, Aug 09:5, Jan 11:3, Jan 13:9, Jun 13:3

99344 **Home visit** for the evaluation and management of a new patient, which requires these 3 key components:

- **A comprehensive history;**
- **A comprehensive examination; and**
- **Medical decision making of moderate complexity.**

Counseling and/or coordination of care with other physicians, other qualified health care professionals, or agencies are provided consistent with the nature of the problem(s) and the patient's and/or family's needs.

Usually, the presenting problem(s) are of high severity. Typically, 60 minutes are spent face-to-face with the patient and/or family.

➔ *CPT Changes: An Insider's View* 2013

➔ *CPT Assistant* Nov 97:6-8, Oct 98:6, Jan 06:1, Jul 09:8, Aug 09:5, Jan 11:3, Jan 13:9, Jun 13:3

99345 **Home visit** for the evaluation and management of a new patient, which requires these 3 key components:

- **A comprehensive history;**
- **A comprehensive examination; and**
- **Medical decision making of high complexity.**

Counseling and/or coordination of care with other physicians, other qualified health care professionals, or agencies are provided consistent with the nature of the problem(s) and the patient's and/or family's needs.

Usually, the patient is unstable or has developed a significant new problem requiring immediate physician attention. Typically, 75 minutes are spent face-to-face with the patient and/or family.

➔ *CPT Changes: An Insider's View* 2013

➔ *CPT Assistant* Nov 97:6-8, Oct 98:6, Jan 06:1, Jul 09:8, Aug 09:5, Jan 11:3, Jan 12:3, Jan 13:9, Jun 13:3

Established Patient

99347 **Home visit** for the evaluation and management of an established patient, which requires at least 2 of these 3 key components:

- **A problem focused interval history;**
- **A problem focused examination;**
- **Straightforward medical decision making.**

Counseling and/or coordination of care with other physicians, other qualified health care professionals, or agencies are provided consistent with the nature of the problem(s) and the patient's and/or family's needs.

Usually, the presenting problem(s) are self limited or minor. Typically, 15 minutes are spent face-to-face with the patient and/or family.

➔ *CPT Changes: An Insider's View* 2013

➔ *CPT Assistant* Nov 97:6-8, Oct 98:6, May 05:1, Jan 06:1, Jul 07:1, Jul 09:8, Aug 09:5, Jan 11:3, Jan 12:3, Jan 13:9, Jun 13:3, Nov 13:3

99348 **Home visit** for the evaluation and management of an established patient, which requires at least 2 of these 3 key components:

- **An expanded problem focused interval history;**
- **An expanded problem focused examination;**
- **Medical decision making of low complexity.**

Counseling and/or coordination of care with other physicians, other qualified health care professionals, or agencies are provided consistent with the nature of the problem(s) and the patient's and/or family's needs.

Usually, the presenting problem(s) are of low to moderate severity. Typically, 25 minutes are spent face-to-face with the patient and/or family.

➔ *CPT Changes: An Insider's View* 2013

➔ *CPT Assistant* Nov 97:6-8, Oct 98:6, Jan 06:1, Jul 07:1, Jul 09:8, Aug 09:5, Jan 11:3, Jan 13:9, Jun 13:3

99349 **Home visit** for the evaluation and management of an established patient, which requires at least 2 of these 3 key components:

- **A detailed interval history;**
- **A detailed examination;**
- **Medical decision making of moderate complexity.**

Counseling and/or coordination of care with other physicians, other qualified health care professionals, or agencies are provided consistent with the nature of the problem(s) and the patient's and/or family's needs.

Usually, the presenting problem(s) are moderate to high severity. Typically, 40 minutes are spent face-to-face with the patient and/or family.

➔ *CPT Changes: An Insider's View* 2013

➔ *CPT Assistant* Nov 97:6-8, Oct 98:6, Jan 06:1, Jul 07:1, Jul 09:8, Aug 09:5, Jan 13:9, Jun 13:3

99350 **Home visit** for the evaluation and management of an established patient, which requires at least 2 of these 3 key components:

- **A comprehensive interval history;**
- **A comprehensive examination;**
- **Medical decision making of moderate to high complexity.**

Counseling and/or coordination of care with other physicians, other qualified health care professionals, or agencies are provided consistent with the nature of the problem(s) and the patient's and/or family's needs.

Usually, the presenting problem(s) are of moderate to high severity. The patient may be unstable or may have developed a significant new problem requiring immediate physician attention. Typically, 60 minutes are spent face-to-face with the patient and/or family.

➔ *CPT Changes: An Insider's View* 2013

➔ *CPT Assistant* Nov 97:6-8, Oct 98:6, Oct 03:7, Jan 06:1, Jul 07:1, Jul 09:8, Aug 09:5, Jan 12:3, Apr 12:10, Jan 13:9, Jun 13:3, Nov 13:3, Oct 14:3, Nov 14:14

Prolonged Services

Prolonged Service With Direct Patient Contact

Codes 99354-99357 are used when a physician or other qualified health care professional provides prolonged service(s) involving direct patient contact that is provided beyond the usual service in either the inpatient or outpatient setting. Direct patient contact is face-to-face and includes additional non-face-to-face services on the patient's floor or unit in the hospital or nursing facility during the same session. This service is reported in addition to the primary procedure (ie, the designated evaluation and management services at any level, code 90837, *Psychotherapy, 60 minutes with patient*, 90847, *Family psychotherapy [conjoint psychotherapy] [with patient present], 50 minutes*), and any other services provided at the same session. Appropriate codes should be selected for supplies provided or other procedures performed in the care of the patient during this period.

Codes 99354-99355 are used to report the total duration of face-to-face time spent by a physician or other qualified health care professional on a given date providing prolonged service in the office or other outpatient setting, even if the time spent by the physician or other qualified health care professional on that date is not continuous. Codes 99356-99357 are used to report the total duration of time spent by a physician or other qualified health care professional at the bedside and on the patient's floor or unit in the hospital or nursing facility on a given date providing prolonged service to a patient, even if the time spent by the physician or other qualified health care professional on that date is not continuous.

Time spent performing separately reported services other than the E/M or psychotherapy service is not counted toward the prolonged services time.

Code 99354 or 99356 is used to report the first hour of prolonged service on a given date, depending on the place of service.

Either code should be used only once per date, even if the time spent by the physician or other qualified health care professional is not continuous on that date. Prolonged service of less than 30 minutes total duration on a given date is not separately reported because the work involved is included in the total work of the evaluation and management or psychotherapy codes.

Code 99355 or 99357 is used to report each additional 30 minutes beyond the first hour, depending on the place of service. Either code may also be used to report the final 15-30 minutes of prolonged service on a given date. Prolonged service of less than 15 minutes beyond the first hour or less than 15 minutes beyond the final 30 minutes is not reported separately.

The use of the time based add-on codes requires that the primary evaluation and management service have a typical or specified time published in the CPT codebook.

For E/M services that require prolonged clinical staff time and may include face-to-face services by the physician or other qualified health care professional, use 99415, 99416. Do not report 99354, 99355 with 99415, 99416.

The following table illustrates the correct reporting of prolonged physician or other qualified health care professional service with direct patient contact in the office setting beyond the usual service time.

Total Duration of Prolonged Services	Code(s)
less than 30 minutes	Not reported separately
30-74 minutes (30 minutes - 1 hr. 14 min.)	99354 X 1
75-104 minutes (1 hr. 15 min. - 1 hr. 44 min.)	99354 X 1 AND 99355 X 1
105 or more (1 hr. 45 min. or more)	99354 X 1 AND 99355 X 2 or more for each additional 30 minutes.

Coding Tip

Reporting Service of Less than 30 Minutes

Prolonged service of less than 30 minutes total duration on a given date is not separately reported because the work involved is included in the total work of the evaluation and management codes.

CPT Coding Guidelines, Evaluation and Management, Prolonged Physician Service with Direct (Face-to-Face) Patient Contact

★+ 99354 Prolonged evaluation and management or psychotherapy service(s) (beyond the typical service time of the primary procedure) in the office or other outpatient setting requiring direct patient contact beyond the usual service; first hour (List separately in addition to code for office or other outpatient **Evaluation and Management** or psychotherapy service)

➔ *CPT Changes: An Insider's View* 2009, 2012, 2016, 2017

➔ *CPT Assistant* Spring 94:30, 32, May 97:3, Sep 98:5, Sep 00:2, Jul 01:2, May 05:1, Nov 05:10, Jun 08:12, Sep 08:3, Jul 09:8, Apr 12:10, Aug 12:3, 4, 5, May 13:12, Jun 13:3, Oct 13:11, Apr 14:6, Jun 14:14, Oct 15:3, 9

(Use 99354 in conjunction with 90837, 90847, 99201-99215, 99241-99245, 99324-99337, 99341-99350, 99483)

(Do not report 99354 in conjunction with 99415, 99416)

★+ 99355 each additional 30 minutes (List separately in addition to code for prolonged service)

➔ *CPT Changes: An Insider's View* 2009, 2012, 2016, 2017

➔ *CPT Assistant* Spring 94:30, 32, May 97:3, Sep 98:5, Sep 00:2, Jul 01:2, Nov 05:10, Jun 08:12, Sep 08:3, Jul 09:8, Apr 12:10, Aug 12:3, 4, 5, May 13:12, Jun 13:3, Oct 13:11, Apr 14:6, Jun 14:14, Oct 15:3, 9

(Use 99355 in conjunction with 99354)

(Do not report 99355 in conjunction with 99415, 99416)

+ 99356 Prolonged service in the inpatient or observation setting, requiring unit/floor time beyond the usual service; first hour (List separately in addition to code for inpatient **Evaluation and Management** service)

➔ *CPT Changes: An Insider's View* 2009, 2012

➔ *CPT Assistant* Spring 94:30, 32, Apr 97:3, May 97:3, Sep 98:5, Sep 00:2, Jul 01:2, Nov 05:10, Jun 08:12, Sep 08:3, Jul 09:8, Jun 11:3, Aug 11:11, Jul 12:11, Aug 12:3, 4, 5, May 13:12, Jun 13:3, Oct 13:11, Apr 14:6, Jun 14:14, Oct 15:3, 9

(Use 99356 in conjunction with 90837, 90847, 99218-99220, 99221-99223, 99224-99226, 99231-99233, 99234-99236, 99251-99255, 99304-99310)

+ 99357 each additional 30 minutes (List separately in addition to code for prolonged service)

➔ *CPT Changes: An Insider's View* 2009, 2012

➔ *CPT Assistant* Spring 94:34, Apr 97:3, May 97:3, Sep 98:5, Sep 00:2, Jul 01:2, Nov 05:10, Jun 08:12, Sep 08:3, Jul 09:8, Jun 11:3, Aug 11:11, Jul 12:11, Aug 12:3, 4, 5, May 13:12, Jun 13:3, Oct 13:11, Apr 14:6, Jun 14:14, Oct 15:3, 9

(Use 99357 in conjunction with 99356)

Prolonged Service Without Direct Patient Contact

Codes 99358 and 99359 are used when a prolonged service is provided that is neither face-to-face time in the office or outpatient setting, nor additional unit/floor time in the hospital or nursing facility setting during the same session of an evaluation and management service and is beyond the usual physician or other qualified health care professional service time.

This service is to be reported in relation to other physician or other qualified health care professional services, including evaluation and management services at any level. This prolonged service may be reported on a different date than the primary service to which it is related. For example, extensive record review may relate to a previous evaluation and management service performed earlier and commences upon receipt of past records. However, it must relate to a service or patient where (face-to-face) patient care has occurred or will occur and relate to ongoing patient management. A typical time for the primary service need not be established within the CPT code set.

Codes 99358 and 99359 are used to report the total duration of non-face-to-face time spent by a physician or other qualified health care professional on a given date providing prolonged service, even if the time spent by the physician or other qualified health care professional on that date is not continuous. Code 99358 is used to report the first hour of prolonged service on a given date regardless of the place of service. It should be used only once per date.

Prolonged service of less than 30 minutes total duration on a given date is not separately reported because the work involved is included in the total work of the evaluation and management or psychotherapy codes.

Code 99359 is used to report each additional 30 minutes beyond the first hour regardless of the place of service. It may also be used to report the final 15 to 30 minutes of prolonged service on a given date.

Prolonged service of less than 15 minutes beyond the first hour or less than 15 minutes beyond the final 30 minutes is not reported separately.

Do not report 99358, 99359 for time spent in care plan oversight services (99339, 99340, 99374-99380), home and outpatient INR monitoring (93792, 93793), medical team conferences (99366-99368), or on-line medical evaluations (99444).

99358 **Prolonged evaluation and management service** before and/or after direct patient care; first hour

➔ *CPT Changes: An Insider's View* 2010, 2012

➔ *CPT Assistant* Spring 94:34, Nov 98:3, Sep 00:3, Nov 05:10, Jun 08:12, Sep 08:3, Aug 12:3, 4, 5, Apr 13:3, Oct 13:11, Nov 13:3, Oct 14:3

+ 99359 each additional 30 minutes (List separately in addition to code for prolonged service)

➔ *CPT Changes: An Insider's View* 2010, 2012

➔ *CPT Assistant* Spring 94:34, Sep 00:3, Nov 05:10, Jun 08:12, Sep 08:3, Aug 12:3, 4, 5, Apr 13:3, Oct 13:11, Nov 13:3, Oct 14:3

(Use 99359 in conjunction with 99358)

►(Do not report 99358, 99359 during the same month with 99484, 99487-99489, 99490, 99491, 99492, 99493, 99494)◄

(Do not report 99358, 99359 when performed during the service time of codes 99495 or 99496)

Total Duration of Prolonged Services Without Direct Face-to-Face Contact	**Code(s)**
less than 30 minutes	Not reported separately
30-74 minutes (30 minutes - 1 hr. 14 min.)	99358 X 1
75-104 minutes (1 hr. 15 min. - 1 hr. 44 min.)	99358 X 1 AND 99359 X 1
105 or more (1 hr. 45 min. or more)	99358 X 1 AND 99359 X 2 or more for each additional 30 minutes.

Prolonged Clinical Staff Services With Physician or Other Qualified Health Care Professional Supervision

Codes 99415, 99416 are used when a prolonged evaluation and management (E/M) service is provided in the office or outpatient setting that involves prolonged clinical staff face-to-face time beyond the typical face-to-face time of the E/M service, as stated in the code description. The physician or qualified health care professional is present to provide direct supervision of the clinical staff. This service is reported in addition to the designated E/M services and any other services provided at the same session as E/M services.

Codes 99415, 99416 are used to report the total duration of face-to-face time spent by clinical staff on a given date providing prolonged service in the office or other outpatient setting, even if the time spent by the clinical staff on that date is not continuous. Time spent performing separately reported services other than the E/M service is not counted toward the prolonged services time.

Code 99415 is used to report the first hour of prolonged clinical staff service on a given date. Code 99415 should be used only once per date, even if the time spent by the clinical staff is not continuous on that date. Prolonged service of less than 45 minutes total duration on a given date is not separately reported because the clinical staff time involved is included in the E/M codes. The typical face-to-face time of the primary service is used in defining when prolonged services time begins. For example, prolonged clinical staff services for 99214 begin after 25 minutes, and 99415 is not reported until at least 70 minutes total face-to-face clinical staff time has been performed. When face-to-face time is noncontiguous, use only the face-to-face time provided to the patient by the clinical staff.

Code 99416 is used to report each additional 30 minutes of prolonged clinical staff service beyond the first hour. Code 99416 may also be used to report the final 15-30 minutes of prolonged service on a given date. Prolonged service of less than 15 minutes beyond the first hour or less than 15 minutes beyond the final 30 minutes is not reported separately.

Codes 99415, 99416 may be reported for no more than two simultaneous patients. The use of the time-based add-on codes requires that the primary E/M service has a typical or specified time published in the CPT code set.

For prolonged services by the physician or qualified health care professional, use 99354, 99355. Do not report 99415 or 99416 with 99354 or 99355.

Facilities may not report 99415, 99416.

#+ 99415 Prolonged clinical staff service (the service beyond the typical service time) during an evaluation and management service in the office or outpatient setting, direct patient contact with physician supervision; first hour (List separately in addition to code for outpatient **Evaluation and Management** service)

➲ *CPT Changes: An Insider's View* 2016

➲ *CPT Assistant* Oct 15:3, Feb 16:13

(Use 99415 in conjunction with 99201, 99202, 99203, 99204, 99205, 99211, 99212, 99213, 99214, 99215)

(Do not report 99415 in conjunction with 99354, 99355)

#+ 99416 each additional 30 minutes (List separately in addition to code for prolonged service)

➲ *CPT Changes: An Insider's View* 2016

➲ *CPT Assistant* Oct 15:3, Feb 16:13

(Use 99416 in conjunction with 99415)

(Do not report 99416 in conjunction with 99354, 99355)

The Total Duration of Prolonged Services Table illustrates the correct reporting of prolonged services provided by clinical staff with physician supervision in the office setting beyond the initial 45 minutes of clinical staff time:

Total Duration of Prolonged Services	Code(s)
less than 45 minutes	Not reported separately
45-74 minutes (45 minutes - 1 hr. 14 min.)	99415 X 1
75-104 minutes (1 hr. 15 min. - 1 hr. 44 min.)	99415 X 1 AND 99416 X 1
105 minutes or more (1 hr. 45 min. or more)	99415 X 1 AND 99416 X 2 or more for each additional 30 minutes.

Standby Services

Code 99360 is used to report physician or other qualified health care professional standby services that are requested by another individual and that involve prolonged attendance without direct (face-to-face) patient contact. Care or services may not be provided to other patients during this period. This code is not used to report time spent proctoring another individual. It is also not used if the period of standby ends with the performance of a procedure, subject to a surgical package by the individual who was on standby.

Code 99360 is used to report the total duration of time spent on a given date on standby. Standby service of less than 30 minutes total duration on a given date is not reported separately.

Second and subsequent periods of standby beyond the first 30 minutes may be reported only if a full 30 minutes of standby was provided for each unit of service reported.

99360 **Standby service,** requiring prolonged attendance, each 30 minutes (eg, operative standby, standby for frozen section, for cesarean/high risk delivery, for monitoring EEG)

➲ *CPT Changes: An Insider's View* 2013

➲ *CPT Assistant* Spring 94:32, Apr 97:10, Aug 97:18, Nov 97:8, Nov 99:5-6, Aug 00:3, Sep 00:3, May 05:1, Nov 05:10, Nov 06:23, Mar 08:14, Feb 11:3, May 13:8, Apr 14:5, 11

(For hospital mandated on call services, see 99026, 99027)

(99360 may be reported in addition to 99460, 99465 as appropriate)

(Do not report 99360 in conjunction with 99464)

Case Management Services

Case management is a process in which a physician or another qualified health care professional is responsible for direct care of a patient and, additionally, for coordinating, managing access to, initiating, and/or supervising other health care services needed by the patient.

Anticoagulant Management

(99363, 99364 have been deleted. To report, see 93792, 93793)

Medical Team Conferences

Medical team conferences include face-to-face participation by a minimum of three qualified health care professionals from different specialties or disciplines (each of whom provide direct care to the patient), with or without the presence of the patient, family member(s), community agencies, surrogate decision maker(s) (eg, legal guardian), and/or caregiver(s). The participants are actively involved in the development, revision, coordination, and implementation of health care services needed by the patient. Reporting participants shall have performed face-to-face evaluations or treatments of the patient, independent of any team conference, within the previous 60 days.

Physicians or other qualified health care professionals who may report evaluation and management services should report their time spent in a team conference with the patient and/or family present using evaluation and management (E/M) codes (and time as the key controlling factor for code selection when counseling and/or coordination of care dominates the service). These introductory guidelines do not apply to services reported using E/M codes (see E/M services guidelines). However, the individual must be directly involved with the patient, providing face-to-face services outside of the conference visit with other physicians, and qualified health care professionals, or agencies.

Reporting participants shall document their participation in the team conference as well as their contributed information and subsequent treatment recommendations.

No more than one individual from the same specialty may report 99366-99368 at the same encounter.

Individuals should not report 99366-99368 when their participation in the medical team conference is part of a facility or organizational service contractually provided by the organization or facility.

The team conference starts at the beginning of the review of an individual patient and ends at the conclusion of the review. Time related to record keeping and report generation is not reported. The reporting participant shall be present for all time reported. The time reported is not limited to the time that the participant is communicating to the other team members or patient and/or family. Time reported for medical team conferences may not be used in the determination of time for other services such as care plan oversight (99374-99380), home, domiciliary, or rest home care plan oversight (99339-99340), prolonged services (99354-99359), psychotherapy, or any E/M service. For team conferences where the patient is present for any part of the duration of the conference, nonphysician qualified health care professionals (eg, speech-language pathologists, physical therapists, occupational therapists, social workers, dietitians) report the team conference face-to-face code 99366.

Medical Team Conference, Direct (Face-to-Face) Contact With Patient and/or Family

99366 **Medical team conference** with interdisciplinary team of health care professionals, face-to-face with patient and/or family, 30 minutes or more, participation by nonphysician qualified health care professional

➲ *CPT Changes: An Insider's View* 2008

➲ *CPT Assistant* Apr 13:3, Jun 14:3, Oct 14:3

(Team conference services of less than 30 minutes duration are not reported separately)

(For team conference services by a physician with patient and/or family present, see Evaluation and Management services)

(Do not report 99366 during the same month with 99487-99489)

(Do not report 99366 when performed during the service time of codes 99495 or 99496)

Evaluation / Management 99201-99499

Medical Team Conference, Without Direct (Face-to-Face) Contact With Patient and/or Family

99367 **Medical team conference** with interdisciplinary team of health care professionals, patient and/or family not present, 30 minutes or more; participation by physician

➔ *CPT Changes: An Insider's View* 2008

➔ *CPT Assistant* Apr 13:3, Jun 14:3

99368 participation by nonphysician qualified health care professional

➔ *CPT Changes: An Insider's View* 2008

➔ *CPT Assistant* Apr 13:3, Jun 14:3, Oct 14:3

(Team conference services of less than 30 minutes duration are not reported separately)

(Do not report 99367, 99368 during the same month with 99487-99489)

(Do not report 99367, 99368 when performed during the service time of codes 99495 or 99496)

Care Plan Oversight Services

Care plan oversight services are reported separately from codes for office/outpatient, hospital, home, nursing facility or domiciliary, or non-face-to-face services. The complexity and approximate time of the care plan oversight services provided within a 30-day period determine code selection. Only one individual may report services for a given period of time, to reflect the sole or predominant supervisory role with a particular patient. These codes should not be reported for supervision of patients in nursing facilities or under the care of home health agencies unless they require recurrent supervision of therapy.

The work involved in providing very low intensity or infrequent supervision services is included in the pre- and post-encounter work for home, office/outpatient and nursing facility or domiciliary visit codes.

(For care plan oversight services of patients in the home, domiciliary, or rest home [eg, assisted living facility], see 99339, 99340, and for hospice agency, see 99377, 99378)

(Do not report 99374-99380 for time reported with 98966-98969, 99441-99444)

(Do not report 99374-99378 during the same month with 99487-99489)

(Do not report 99374-99380 when performed during the service time of codes 99495 or 99496)

99374 **Supervision** of a patient under care of home health agency (patient not present) in home, domiciliary or equivalent environment (eg, Alzheimer's facility) requiring complex and multidisciplinary care modalities involving regular development and/or revision of care plans by that individual, review of subsequent reports of patient status, review of related laboratory and other studies, communication (including telephone calls) for purposes of assessment or care decisions with health care professional(s), family member(s), surrogate decision maker(s) (eg, legal guardian) and/or key caregiver(s) involved in patient's care, integration of new information into the medical treatment plan and/or adjustment of medical therapy, within a calendar month; 15-29 minutes

➔ *CPT Changes: An Insider's View* 2002, 2013

➔ *CPT Assistant* Summer 94:9, Nov 97:8-9, May 05:1, Dec 06:4, Mar 07:11, Mar 08:6, Sep 08:3, Jul 09:5, 10, Apr 13:3, Jul 13:11, Sep 13:15, Nov 13:3, Feb 14:11, Oct 14:3

99375 30 minutes or more

➔ *CPT Changes: An Insider's View* 2013

➔ *CPT Assistant* Summer 94:9, Nov 97:8-9, Dec 06:4, Mar 07:11, Mar 08:6, Sep 08:3, Jul 09:5, 10, Apr 13:3, Jul 13:11, Sep 13:15

99377 **Supervision** of a hospice patient (patient not present) requiring complex and multidisciplinary care modalities involving regular development and/or revision of care plans by that individual, review of subsequent reports of patient status, review of related laboratory and other studies, communication (including telephone calls) for purposes of assessment or care decisions with health care professional(s), family member(s), surrogate decision maker(s) (eg, legal guardian) and/or key caregiver(s) involved in patient's care, integration of new information into the medical treatment plan and/or adjustment of medical therapy, within a calendar month; 15-29 minutes

➔ *CPT Changes: An Insider's View* 2001, 2002, 2013

➔ *CPT Assistant* Nov 97:8-9, Dec 06:4, Mar 07:11, Sep 08:3, Jul 09:5, 10, Apr 13:3, Jul 13:11, Sep 13:15

99378 30 minutes or more

➔ *CPT Changes: An Insider's View* 2013

➔ *CPT Assistant* Nov 97:8-9, Dec 06:4, Mar 07:11, Mar 08:6, Sep 08:3, Jul 09:5, 10, Apr 13:3, Jul 13:11, Sep 13:15

99379 **Supervision** of a nursing facility patient (patient not present) requiring complex and multidisciplinary care modalities involving regular development and/or revision of care plans by that individual, review of subsequent reports of patient status, review of related laboratory and other studies, communication (including telephone calls) for purposes of assessment or care decisions with health care professional(s), family member(s), surrogate decision maker(s) (eg, legal guardian) and/or key caregiver(s) involved in patient's care, integration of new information into the medical treatment plan and/or adjustment of medical therapy, within a calendar month; 15-29 minutes

➔ *CPT Changes: An Insider's View* 2002, 2013

➔ *CPT Assistant* Dec 06:4, Mar 08:6, Sep 08:3, Jul 09:5, Apr 13:3, Jul 13:11, Sep 13:15

99380 30 minutes or more

➔ *CPT Changes: An Insider's View* 2013

➔ *CPT Assistant* Nov 97:8-9, Dec 06:4, Mar 08:6, Sep 08:3, Jul 09:5, Apr 13:3, Jul 13:11, Sep 13:15, Nov 13:3, Oct 14:3

Preventive Medicine Services

The following codes are used to report the preventive medicine evaluation and management of infants, children, adolescents, and adults.

The extent and focus of the services will largely depend on the age of the patient.

If an abnormality is encountered or a preexisting problem is addressed in the process of performing this preventive medicine evaluation and management service, and if the problem or abnormality is significant enough to require additional work to perform the key components of a problem-oriented E/M service, then the appropriate Office/Outpatient code 99201-99215 should also be reported. Modifier 25 should be added to the Office/Outpatient code to indicate that a significant, separately identifiable evaluation and management service was provided on the same day as the preventive medicine service. The appropriate preventive medicine service is additionally reported.

An insignificant or trivial problem/abnormality that is encountered in the process of performing the preventive medicine evaluation and management service and which does not require additional work and the performance of the key components of a problem-oriented E/M service should not be reported.

The "comprehensive" nature of the Preventive Medicine Services codes 99381-99397 reflects an age and gender appropriate history/exam and is **not** synonymous with the "comprehensive" examination required in Evaluation and Management codes 99201-99350.

Codes 99381-99397 include counseling/anticipatory guidance/risk factor reduction interventions which are provided at the time of the initial or periodic comprehensive preventive medicine examination. (Refer to 99401, 99402, 99403, 99404, 99411, and 99412 for reporting those counseling/anticipatory guidance/risk factor reduction interventions that are provided at an encounter separate from the preventive medicine examination.)

(For behavior change intervention, see 99406, 99407, 99408, 99409)

Vaccine/toxoid products, immunization administrations, ancillary studies involving laboratory, radiology, other procedures, or screening tests (eg, vision, hearing, developmental) identified with a specific CPT code are reported separately. For immunization administration and vaccine risk/benefit counseling, see 90460, 90461, 90471-90474. For vaccine/toxoid products, see 90476-90749.

New Patient

99381 **Initial comprehensive preventive medicine** evaluation and management of an individual including an age and gender appropriate history, examination, counseling/anticipatory guidance/risk factor reduction interventions, and the ordering of laboratory/diagnostic procedures, new patient; infant (age younger than 1 year)

➔ *CPT Changes: An Insider's View* 2002, 2009

➔ *CPT Assistant* Winter 91:11, Spring 93:14, 34, Spring 95:1, Aug 97:1, Jul 98:9, Sep 98:5, Nov 98:3-4, May 02:1, May 05:1, Aug 05:15, Oct 06:15, Mar 09:3, Jul 09:7, Aug 09:5, Jan 13:9, Dec 14:18, Mar 16:7

99382 early childhood (age 1 through 4 years)

➔ *CPT Changes: An Insider's View* 2009

➔ *CPT Assistant* Winter 91:11, Spring 93:14, 34, Spring 95:1, Aug 97:1, Jul 98:9, Sep 98:5, Nov 98:3-4, May 02:1, Aug 05:15, Oct 06:15, Jul 09:5, Aug 09:5, Jan 13:9, Dec 14:18, Mar 16:7

99383 late childhood (age 5 through 11 years)

➔ *CPT Changes: An Insider's View* 2009

➔ *CPT Assistant* Winter 91:11, Spring 93:14, 34, Spring 95:1, Aug 97:1, Jul 98:9, Sep 98:5, Nov 98:3-4, May 02:1, Aug 05:15, Oct 06:15, Jul 09:7, Aug 09:5, Jan 13:9, Dec 14:18, Mar 16:7

99384 adolescent (age 12 through 17 years)

➔ *CPT Changes: An Insider's View* 2009

➔ *CPT Assistant* Winter 91:11, Spring 93:14, 34, Spring 95:1, Aug 97:1, Jul 98:9, Sep 98:5, Nov 98:3-4, May 02:1, Aug 05:15, Oct 06:15, Jul 09:7, Aug 09:5, Jan 13:9, Dec 14:18, Jan 15:12, Mar 16:7

99385 18-39 years

➔ *CPT Changes: An Insider's View* 2009

➔ *CPT Assistant* Winter 91:11, Spring 93:14, 34, Spring 95:1, Aug 97:7, Jul 98:9, Sep 98:5, Nov 98:3-4, May 02:1, Aug 05:15, Oct 06:15, Jul 09:5, Aug 09:5, Jan 13:9, Dec 14:18, Jan 15:12, Mar 16:7

99386 40-64 years

➔ *CPT Changes: An Insider's View* 2009

➔ *CPT Assistant* Winter 91:11, Spring 93:14, 34, Spring 95:1, Aug 97:1, Jul 98:9, Sep 98:5, Nov 98:3-4, May 02:1, Aug 05:15, Oct 06:15, Jul 09:7, Aug 09:5, Jan 13:9, Dec 14:18, Jan 15:12, Mar 16:7

99387 65 years and older

➔ *CPT Changes: An Insider's View* 2009

➔ *CPT Assistant* Winter 91:11, Spring 93:14, 34, Spring 95:1, Aug 97:1, Jul 98:9, Sep 98:5, Nov 98:3-4, May 02:1, Aug 05:15, Oct 06:15, Jul 09:7, Aug 09:5, Jan 13:9, Dec 14:18, Mar 16:7

Established Patient

99391 **Periodic comprehensive preventive medicine** reevaluation and management of an individual including an age and gender appropriate history, examination, counseling/anticipatory guidance/risk factor reduction interventions, and the ordering of laboratory/diagnostic procedures, established patient; infant (age younger than 1 year)

➔ *CPT Changes: An Insider's View* 2002, 2009

➔ *CPT Assistant* Winter 91:11, Spring 93:14, 34, Spring 95:1, Aug 97:1, Jul 98:9, Sep 98:5, Nov 98:3-4, May 02:1, May 05:1, Aug 05:15, Oct 06:15, Mar 09:3, Jul 09:7, Aug 09:5, Jan 13:9, Dec 14:18, Mar 16:7

99392 early childhood (age 1 through 4 years)

➔ *CPT Changes: An Insider's View* 2009

➔ *CPT Assistant* Winter 91:11, Spring 93:14, 34, Spring 95:1, Aug 97:1, Jul 98:9, Sep 98:5, Nov 98:3-4, May 02:1, Aug 05:15, Oct 06:15, Jul 09:7, Jan 13:9, Dec 14:18, Mar 16:7

99393 late childhood (age 5 through 11 years)

➔ *CPT Changes: An Insider's View* 2009

➔ *CPT Assistant* Winter 91:11, Spring 93:14, 34, Spring 95:1, Aug 97:1, Jul 98:9, Sep 98:5, Nov 98:3-4, May 02:1, Aug 05:15, Oct 06:15, Jul 09:7, Jan 13:9, Dec 14:18, Mar 16:7

99394 adolescent (age 12 through 17 years)

➔ *CPT Changes: An Insider's View* 2009

➔ *CPT Assistant* Winter 91:11, Spring 93:14, 34, Spring 95:1, Aug 97:1, Jul 98:9, Sep 98:5, Nov 98:3-4, May 02:1, Aug 05:15, Oct 06:15, Jul 09:7, Jan 13:9, Dec 14:18, Jan 15:12, Mar 16:7

99395 18-39 years

➔ *CPT Changes: An Insider's View* 2009

➔ *CPT Assistant* Winter 91:11, Spring 93:14, 34, Spring 95:1, Aug 97:1, Jul 98:9, Sep 98:5, Nov 98:3-4, May 02:1, Aug 05:15, Oct 06:15, Mar 08:3, Jul 09:7, Jan 13:9, Dec 14:18, Jan 15:12, Mar 16:7

99396 40-64 years

➔ *CPT Changes: An Insider's View* 2009

➔ *CPT Assistant* Winter 91:11, Spring 93:14, 34, Spring 95:1, Aug 97:1, Jul 98:9, Sep 98:5, Nov 98:3-4, May 02:1, Aug 05:15, Oct 06:15, Jul 09:7, Mar 12:4, Jan 13:9, Dec 14:18, Jan 15:12, Mar 16:7, Sep 17:11

99397 65 years and older

➔ *CPT Changes: An Insider's View* 2009

➔ *CPT Assistant* Winter 91:11, Spring 93:14, 34, Spring 95:1, Aug 97:1, Jul 98:9, Sep 98:5, Nov 98:3-4, May 02:1, Aug 05:15, Oct 06:15, Jul 09:7, Jan 13:9, Dec 14:18, Mar 16:7

Counseling Risk Factor Reduction and Behavior Change Intervention

New or Established Patient

These codes are used to report services provided face-to-face by a physician or other qualified health care professional for the purpose of promoting health and preventing illness or injury. They are distinct from evaluation and management (E/M) services that may be reported separately with modifier 25 when performed. Risk factor reduction services are used for persons without a specific illness for which the counseling might otherwise be used as part of treatment.

Preventive medicine counseling and risk factor reduction interventions will vary with age and should address such issues as family problems, diet and exercise, substance use, sexual practices, injury prevention, dental health, and diagnostic and laboratory test results available at the time of the encounter.

Behavior change interventions are for persons who have a behavior that is often considered an illness itself, such as tobacco use and addiction, substance abuse/misuse, or obesity. Behavior change services may be reported when performed as part of the treatment of condition(s) related to or potentially exacerbated by the behavior or when performed to change the harmful behavior that has not yet resulted in illness. Any E/M services reported on the same day must be distinct and reported with modifier 25, and time spent providing these services may not be used as a basis for the E/M code selection. Behavior change services involve specific validated interventions of assessing readiness for change and barriers to change, advising a change in behavior, assisting by providing specific suggested actions and motivational counseling, and arranging for services and follow-up.

For counseling groups of patients with symptoms or established illness, use 99078.

Health and Behavior Assessment/Intervention services (96150-96155) should not be reported on the same day as codes 99401-99412.

Preventive Medicine, Individual Counseling

99401 **Preventive medicine counseling** and/or risk factor reduction intervention(s) provided to an individual (separate procedure); approximately 15 minutes

➔ *CPT Assistant* Aug 97:1, Jan 98:12, May 05:1, Aug 07:9, Oct 10:3, Dec 10:3, Jan 13:9, Aug 14:5, Mar 16:7

99402 approximately 30 minutes

➔ *CPT Assistant* Aug 97:1, Jan 98:12, May 05:1, Oct 10:3, Dec 10:3, Jan 13:9, Mar 16:7

99403 approximately 45 minutes

➔ *CPT Assistant* Aug 97:1, Jan 98:12, May 05:1, Oct 10:3, Dec 10:3, Jan 13:9, Mar 16:7

99404 approximately 60 minutes

➔ *CPT Assistant* Aug 97:1, Jan 98:12, May 05:1, Oct 10:3, Dec 10:3, Jan 13:9, Aug 14:5, Mar 16:7

Behavior Change Interventions, Individual

★ **99406** Smoking and tobacco use cessation counseling visit; intermediate, greater than 3 minutes up to 10 minutes

➔ *CPT Changes: An Insider's View* 2008, 2017

➔ *CPT Assistant* Jan 08:1, Sep 09:11, Oct 10:3, Dec 10:3, Jan 13:9, Mar 16:7

★ **99407** intensive, greater than 10 minutes

➔ *CPT Changes: An Insider's View* 2008, 2017

➔ *CPT Assistant* Jan 08:1, Sep 09:11, Oct 10:3, Dec 10:3, Jan 13:9, Mar 16:7

(Do not report 99407 in conjunction with 99406)

★ **99408** Alcohol and/or substance (other than tobacco) abuse structured screening (eg, AUDIT, DAST), and brief intervention (SBI) services; 15 to 30 minutes

➔ *CPT Changes: An Insider's View* 2008, 2017

➔ *CPT Assistant* Oct 10:3, Dec 10:3, Jan 13:9, Mar 16:7, Nov 16:5

(Do not report services of less than 15 minutes with 99408)

★ **99409** greater than 30 minutes

➔ *CPT Changes: An Insider's View* 2008, 2017

➔ *CPT Assistant* Oct 10:3, Dec 10:3, Jan 13:9, Mar 16:7, Nov 16:5

(Do not report 99409 in conjunction with 99408)

(Do not report 99408, 99409 in conjunction with 96160, 96161)

(Use 99408, 99409 only for initial screening and brief intervention)

Preventive Medicine, Group Counseling

99411 **Preventive medicine counseling** and/or risk factor reduction intervention(s) provided to individuals in a group setting (separate procedure); approximately 30 minutes

➔ *CPT Assistant* Aug 97:1, Jan 98:12, Sep 98:5, May 05:1, Oct 10:3, Dec 10:3, Jan 13:9, Mar 16:7

99412 approximately 60 minutes

➔ *CPT Assistant* Aug 97:1, Jan 98:12, Sep 98:5, May 05:1, Aug 07:9, Oct 10:3, Dec 10:3, Jan 13:9, Mar 16:7

99415 Code is out of numerical sequence. See 99358-99366

99416 Code is out of numerical sequence. See 99358-99366

Other Preventive Medicine Services

(99420 has been deleted. To report, see 96160, 96161)

99429 **Unlisted preventive** medicine service

➔ *CPT Assistant* Sep 98:5, May 05:1, Oct 10:3, Dec 10:3, Jan 13:9, Mar 16:7

Non-Face-to-Face Services

Telephone Services

Telephone services are non-face-to-face evaluation and management (E/M) services provided to a patient using the telephone by a physician or other qualified health care professional, who may report evaluation and management services. These codes are used to report episodes of patient care initiated by an established patient or guardian of an established patient. If the telephone service ends with a decision to see the patient within 24 hours or next available urgent visit appointment, the code is not reported; rather the encounter is considered part of the preservice work of the subsequent E/M service, procedure, and visit. Likewise if the telephone call refers to an E/M service performed and reported by that individual within the previous seven days (either requested or unsolicited patient follow-up) or within the postoperative period of the previously completed procedure, then the service(s) are considered part of that previous E/M service or procedure. (Do not report 99441-99443 if 99441-99444 have been reported by the same provider in the previous seven days.)

(For telephone services provided by a qualified nonphysician who may not report evaluation and management services [eg, speech-language pathologists, physical therapists, occupational therapists, social workers, dietitians], see 98966-98968)

99441 Telephone evaluation and management service by a physician or other qualified health care professional who may report evaluation and management services provided to an established patient, parent, or guardian not originating from a related E/M service provided within the previous 7 days nor leading to an E/M service or procedure within the next 24 hours or soonest available appointment; 5-10 minutes of medical discussion

➔ *CPT Changes: An Insider's View* 2008, 2013

➔ *CPT Assistant* Mar 08:6, Apr 13:3, Oct 13:11, Nov 13:3, Oct 14:3, Mar 18:7

99442 11-20 minutes of medical discussion

➔ *CPT Changes: An Insider's View* 2008, 2013

➔ *CPT Assistant* Mar 08:6, Apr 13:3, Oct 13:11, Mar 18:7

99443 21-30 minutes of medical discussion

➔ *CPT Changes: An Insider's View* 2008, 2013

➔ *CPT Assistant* Mar 08:6, Apr 13:3, Oct 13:11, Nov 13:3, Oct 14:3, Mar 18:7

(Do not report 99441-99443 when using 99339-99340, 99374-99380 for the same call[s])

(Do not report 99441-99443 for home and outpatient INR monitoring when reporting 93792, 93793)

(Do not report 99441-99443 during the same month with 99487-99489)

(Do not report 99441-99443 when performed during the service time of codes 99495 or 99496)

On-Line Medical Evaluation

An on-line electronic medical evaluation is a non-face-to-face evaluation and management (E/M) service by a physician to a patient using Internet resources in response to a patient's on-line inquiry. Reportable services involve the physician's personal timely response to the patient's inquiry and must involve permanent storage (electronic or hard copy) of the encounter. This service is reported only once for the same episode of care during a seven-day period, although multiple physicians could report their exchange with the same patient. If the on-line medical evaluation refers to an E/M service previously performed and reported by the physician within the previous seven days (either physician requested or unsolicited patient follow-up) or within the postoperative period of the previously completed procedure, then the service(s) are considered covered by the previous E/M service or procedure. A reportable service encompasses the sum of communication (eg, related telephone calls, prescription provision, laboratory orders) pertaining to the on-line patient encounter.

(For an on-line medical evaluation provided by a qualified nonphysician health care professional, use 98969)

99444 Online evaluation and management service provided by a physician or other qualified health care professional who may report evaluation and management services provided to an established patient or guardian, not originating from a related E/M service provided within the previous 7 days, using the Internet or similar electronic communications network

➲ *CPT Changes: An Insider's View* 2008, 2013

➲ *CPT Assistant* Nov 12:13, Apr 13:3, Oct 13:11, Nov 13:3, Oct 14:3, Mar 18:7

(Do not report 99444 when using 99339, 99340, 99374-99380 for the same communication[s])

(Do not report 99444 for home and outpatient INR monitoring when reporting 93792, 93793)

(Do not report 99444 during the same month with 99487-99489)

(Do not report 99444 when performed during the service time of codes 99495 or 99496)

▸Interprofessional Telephone/Internet/Electronic Health Record Consultations◂

▸The consultant should use codes 99446, 99447, 99448, 99449, 99451 to report interprofessional telephone/Internet/electronic health record consultations. An interprofessional telephone/Internet/electronic health record consultation is an assessment and management service in which a patient's treating (eg, attending or primary) physician or other qualified health care professional requests the opinion and/or treatment advice of a physician with specific specialty expertise (the consultant) to assist the treating physician or other qualified health care professional in the diagnosis and/or management of the patient's problem without patient face-to-face contact with the consultant.

The patient for whom the interprofessional telephone/Internet/electronic health record consultation is requested may be either a new patient to the consultant or an established patient with a new problem or an exacerbation of an existing problem. However, the consultant should not have seen the patient in a face-to-face encounter within the last 14 days. When the telephone/Internet/electronic health record consultation leads to a transfer of care or other face-to-face service (eg, a surgery, a hospital visit, or a scheduled office evaluation of the patient) within the next 14 days or next available appointment date of the consultant, these codes are not reported.

Review of pertinent medical records, laboratory studies, imaging studies, medication profile, pathology specimens, etc is included in the telephone/Internet/electronic health record consultation service and should not be reported separately when reporting 99446, 99447, 99448, 99449, 99451. The majority of the service time reported (greater than 50%) must be devoted to the medical consultative verbal or Internet discussion. If greater than 50% of the time for the service is devoted to data review and/or analysis, 99446, 99447, 99448, 99449 should not be reported. However, the service time for 99451 is based on total review and interprofessional-communication time.

If more than one telephone/Internet/electronic health record contact(s) is required to complete the consultation request (eg, discussion of test results), the entirety of the service and the cumulative discussion and information review time should be reported with a single code. Codes 99446, 99447, 99448, 99449, 99451 should not be reported more than once within a seven-day interval.

The written or verbal request for telephone/Internet/electronic health record advice by the treating/requesting physician or other qualified health care professional should be documented in the patient's medical record, including the reason for the request. Codes 99446, 99447, 99448, 99449 conclude with a verbal opinion report and written report from the consultant to the treating/requesting physician or other qualified health care professional. Code 99451 concludes with only a written report.

Telephone/Internet/electronic health record consultations of less than five minutes should not be reported. Consultant communications with the patient and/or family may be reported using 98966, 98967, 98968, 98969, 99441, 99442, 99443, 99444, and the time related to these services is not used in reporting 99446, 99447, 99448, 99449. Do not report 99358, 99359 for any time within the service period, if reporting 99446, 99447, 99448, 99449, 99451.

When the sole purpose of the telephone/Internet/electronic health record communication is to arrange a transfer of care or other face-to-face service, these codes are not reported.

The treating/requesting physician or other qualified health care professional may report 99452 if spending 16-30 minutes in a service day preparing for the referral and/or communicating with the consultant. Do not report 99452 more than once in a 14-day period. The treating/requesting physician or other qualified health care professional may report the prolonged service codes 99354, 99355, 99356, 99357 for the time spent on the interprofessional telephone/Internet/electronic health record discussion with the consultant (eg, specialist) if the time **exceeds 30 minutes** beyond the typical time of the appropriate E/M service performed and the patient is present (on-site) and accessible to the treating/requesting physician or other qualified health care professional. If the interprofessional telephone/Internet/electronic health record assessment and management service occurs when the patient is not present and the time spent in a day **exceeds 30 minutes,** then the non-face-to-face prolonged service codes 99358, 99359 may be reported by the treating/requesting physician or other qualified health care professional.◀

(For telephone services provided by a physician to a patient, see 99441, 99442, 99443)

(For telephone services provided by a qualified health care professional to a patient, see 98966, 98967, 98968)

(For an on-line medical evaluation provided by a physician to a patient, use 99444)

(For an on-line assessment and management service provided by a qualified health care professional to a patient, use 98969)

▲ **99446** Interprofessional telephone/Internet/electronic health record assessment and management service provided by a consultative physician, including a verbal and written report to the patient's treating/requesting physician or other qualified health care professional; 5-10 minutes of medical consultative discussion and review

➲ *CPT Changes: An Insider's View* 2014, 2019

➲ *CPT Assistant* Jun 14:14

▲ **99447** 11-20 minutes of medical consultative discussion and review

➲ *CPT Changes: An Insider's View* 2014, 2019

➲ *CPT Assistant* Jun 14:14

▲ **99448** 21-30 minutes of medical consultative discussion and review

➲ *CPT Changes: An Insider's View* 2014, 2019

➲ *CPT Assistant* Jun 14:14

▲ **99449** 31 minutes or more of medical consultative discussion and review

➲ *CPT Changes: An Insider's View* 2014, 2019

➲ *CPT Assistant* Jun 14:14

#● **99451** Interprofessional telephone/Internet/electronic health record assessment and management service provided by a consultative physician, including a written report to the patient's treating/requesting physician or other qualified health care professional, 5 minutes or more of medical consultative time

➲ *CPT Changes: An Insider's View* 2019

#● **99452** Interprofessional telephone/Internet/electronic health record referral service(s) provided by a treating/requesting physician or other qualified health care professional, 30 minutes

➲ *CPT Changes: An Insider's View* 2019

▸Digitally Stored Data Services/ Remote Physiologic Monitoring◂

▶Codes 99453 and 99454 are used to report remote physiologic monitoring services (eg, weight, blood pressure, pulse oximetry) during a 30-day period. To report 99453, 99454, the device used must be a medical device as defined by the FDA, and the service must be ordered by a physician or other qualified health care professional. Code 99453 may be used to report the set-up and patient education on use of the device(s). Code 99454 may be used to report supply of the device for daily recording or programmed alert transmissions. Codes 99453, 99454 are not reported if monitoring is less than 16 days. Do not report 99453, 99454 when these services are included in other codes for the duration of time of the physiologic monitoring service (eg, 95250 for continuous glucose monitoring requires a minimum of 72 hours of monitoring).

Code 99091 should be reported no more than once in a 30-day period to include the physician or other qualified health care professional time involved with data accession, review and interpretation, modification of care plan as necessary (including communication to patient and/or caregiver), and associated documentation.

If the services described by 99091 are provided on the same day the patient presents for an Evaluation and Management (E/M) service, these services should be considered part of the E/M service and not reported separately.

Do not report 99091 in the same calendar month as care plan oversight services (99374, 99375, 99377, 99378, 99379, 99380), home, domiciliary, or rest home care plan oversight services (99339, 99340), and remote physiologic monitoring services (99457). Do not report 99091 if other more specific codes exist (eg, 93227, 93272 for cardiographic services; 95250 for continuous glucose monitoring). Do not report 99091 for transfer and interpretation of data from hospital or clinical laboratory computers.

Code 99453 is reported for each episode of care. For coding remote monitoring of physiologic parameters, an episode of care is defined as beginning when the remote monitoring physiologic service is initiated, and ends with attainment of targeted treatment goals.◄

#● **99453** Remote monitoring of physiologic parameter(s) (eg, weight, blood pressure, pulse oximetry, respiratory flow rate), initial; set-up and patient education on use of equipment

➔ *CPT Changes: An Insider's View* 2019

►(Do not report 99453 more than once per episode of care)◄

►(Do not report 99453 for monitoring of less than 16 days)◄

#● **99454** device(s) supply with daily recording(s) or programmed alert(s) transmission, each 30 days

➔ *CPT Changes: An Insider's View* 2019

►(For physiologic monitoring treatment management services, use 99457)◄

►(Do not report 99454 for monitoring of less than 16 days)◄

►(Do not report 99453, 99454 in conjunction with codes for more specific physiologic parameters [eg, 93296, 94760])◄

#▲ **99091** Collection and interpretation of physiologic data (eg, ECG, blood pressure, glucose monitoring) digitally stored and/or transmitted by the patient and/or caregiver to the physician or other qualified health care professional, qualified by education, training, licensure/regulation (when applicable) requiring a minimum of 30 minutes of time, each 30 days

➔ *CPT Changes: An Insider's View* 2002, 2013, 2019

➔ *CPT Assistant* May 02:19, Jun 03:10, Aug 06:6, Sep 06:15, Jan 07:30, Apr 09:7, Dec 09:6, Apr 13:3, Nov 13:3, Oct 14:3, Feb 18:7, Mar 18:5

►(Do not report 99091 in conjunction with 99457)◄

►(Do not report 99091 if it occurs within 30 days of 99339, 99340, 99374, 99375, 99377, 99378, 99379, 99380, 99457)◄

►Remote Physiologic Monitoring Treatment Management Services◄

►Remote physiologic monitoring treatment management services are provided when clinical staff/physician/other qualified health care professional use the results of remote physiological monitoring to manage a patient under a specific treatment plan. To report remote physiological monitoring, the device used must be a medical device as defined by the FDA, and the service must be ordered by a physician or other qualified health care professional. Use 99457 for time spent managing care when patients or the practice do not meet the requirements to report more specific services. Code 99457 may be reported during the same service period as chronic care management services (99487, 99489, 99490), transitional care management services (99495, 99496), and behavioral health integration services (99484, 99492, 99493, 99494). However, time spent performing these services should remain separate and no time should be counted toward the required time for both services in a single month. Code 99457 requires a live, interactive communication with the patient/caregiver and 20 minutes or more of clinical staff/physician/other qualified health care professional time in a calendar month. Report 99491 one time regardless of the number of physiologic monitoring modalities performed in a given calendar month.

Do not count any time on a day when the physician or other qualified health care professional reports an E/M service (office or other outpatient services 99201, 99202, 99203, 99204, 99205, 99211, 99212, 99213, 99214, 99215, domiciliary, rest home services 99324, 99325, 99326, 99327, 99328, 99334, 99335, 99336, 99337, home services 99341, 99342, 99343, 99344, 99345, 99347, 99348, 99349, 99350). Do not count any time related to other reported services (eg, 93290).◄

#● **99457** Remote physiologic monitoring treatment management services, 20 minutes or more of clinical staff/physician/other qualified health care professional time in a calendar month requiring interactive communication with the patient/caregiver during the month

➔ *CPT Changes: An Insider's View* 2019

►(Report 99457 once each 30 days, regardless of the number of parameters monitored)◄

►(Do not report 99457 in conjunction with 99091)◄

Special Evaluation and Management Services

The following codes are used to report evaluations performed to establish baseline information prior to life or disability insurance certificates being issued. This service is performed in the office or other setting, and applies to both new and established patients. When using these codes, no active management of the problem(s) is undertaken during the encounter.

If other evaluation and management services and/or procedures are performed on the same date, the appropriate E/M or procedure code(s) should be reported in addition to these codes.

Basic Life and/or Disability Evaluation Services

99450 **Basic life** and/or disability examination that includes:

- **Measurement of height, weight, and blood pressure;**
- **Completion of a medical history following a life insurance pro forma;**
- **Collection of blood sample and/or urinalysis complying with "chain of custody" protocols; and**

- **Completion of necessary documentation/ certificates.**

CPT Assistant Summer 95:14, Sep 98:5, May 05:1

99451 Code is out of numerical sequence. See 99448-99455

99452 Code is out of numerical sequence. See 99448-99455

99453 Code is out of numerical sequence. See 99448-99455

99454 Code is out of numerical sequence. See 99448-99455

Work Related or Medical Disability Evaluation Services

99455 **Work related** or medical disability examination by the treating physician that includes:

- **Completion of a medical history commensurate with the patient's condition;**
- **Performance of an examination commensurate with the patient's condition;**
- **Formulation of a diagnosis, assessment of capabilities and stability, and calculation of impairment;**
- **Development of future medical treatment plan; and**
- **Completion of necessary documentation/ certificates and report.**

CPT Assistant Summer 95:14, Sep 98:5, May 05:1, Aug 13:13

99456 **Work related** or medical disability examination by other than the treating physician that includes:

- **Completion of a medical history commensurate with the patient's condition;**
- **Performance of an examination commensurate with the patient's condition;**
- **Formulation of a diagnosis, assessment of capabilities and stability, and calculation of impairment;**
- **Development of future medical treatment plan; and**
- **Completion of necessary documentation/ certificates and report.**

CPT Assistant Summer 95:14, Sep 98:5, Aug 13:13

(Do not report 99455, 99456 in conjunction with 99080 for the completion of Workman's Compensation forms)

99457 Code is out of numerical sequence. See 99448-99455

Newborn Care Services

The following codes are used to report the services provided to newborns (birth through the first 28 days) in several different settings. Use of the normal newborn codes is limited to the initial care of the newborn in the first days after birth prior to home discharge.

Evaluation and Management (E/M) services for the newborn include maternal and/or fetal and newborn history, newborn physical examination(s), ordering of diagnostic tests and treatments, meetings with the family, and documentation in the medical record.

When delivery room attendance services (99464) or delivery room resuscitation services (99465) are required, report these in addition to normal newborn services Evaluation and Management codes.

For E/M services provided to newborns who are other than normal, see codes for hospital inpatient services (99221-99233) and neonatal intensive and critical care services (99466-99469, 99477-99480). When normal newborn services are provided by the same individual on the same date that the newborn later becomes ill and receives additional intensive or critical care services, report the appropriate E/M code with modifier 25 for these services in addition to the normal newborn code.

Procedures (eg, 54150, newborn circumcision) are not included with the normal newborn codes, and when performed, should be reported in addition to the newborn services.

When newborns are seen in follow-up after the date of discharge in the office or outpatient setting, see 99201-99215, 99381, 99391 as appropriate.

99460 Initial hospital or birthing center care, per day, for evaluation and management of normal newborn infant

CPT Changes: An Insider's View 2009

99461 Initial care, per day, for evaluation and management of normal newborn infant seen in other than hospital or birthing center

CPT Changes: An Insider's View 2009

99462 Subsequent hospital care, per day, for evaluation and management of normal newborn

CPT Changes: An Insider's View 2009

99463 Initial hospital or birthing center care, per day, for evaluation and management of normal newborn infant admitted and discharged on the same date

CPT Changes: An Insider's View 2009

(For newborn hospital discharge services provided on a date subsequent to the admission date, see 99238, 99239)

Delivery/Birthing Room Attendance and Resuscitation Services

99464 Attendance at delivery (when requested by the delivering physician or other qualified health care professional) and initial stabilization of newborn

CPT Changes: An Insider's View 2009, 2013

(99464 may be reported in conjunction with 99460, 99468, 99477)

(Do not report 99464 in conjunction with 99465)

99465 Delivery/birthing room resuscitation, provision of positive pressure ventilation and/or chest compressions in the presence of acute inadequate ventilation and/or cardiac output

➲ *CPT Changes: An Insider's View* 2009

(99465 may be reported in conjunction with 99460, 99468, 99477)

(Do not report 99465 in conjunction with 99464)

(Procedures that are performed as a necessary part of the resuscitation [eg, intubation, vascular lines] are reported separately in addition to 99465. In order to report these procedures, they must be performed as a necessary component of the resuscitation and not as a convenience before admission to the neonatal intensive care unit)

Inpatient Neonatal Intensive Care Services and Pediatric and Neonatal Critical Care Services

Pediatric Critical Care Patient Transport

Codes 99466, 99467 are used to report the physical attendance and direct face-to-face care by a physician during the interfacility transport of a critically ill or critically injured pediatric patient 24 months of age or younger. Codes 99485, 99486 are used to report the control physician's non-face-to-face supervision of interfacility transport of a critically ill or critically injured pediatric patient 24 months of age or younger. These codes are not reported together for the same patient by the same physician. For the purpose of reporting 99466 and 99467, face-to-face care begins when the physician assumes primary responsibility of the pediatric patient at the referring facility, and ends when the receiving facility accepts responsibility for the pediatric patient's care. Only the time the physician spends in direct face-to-face contact with the patient during the transport should be reported. Pediatric patient transport services involving less than 30 minutes of face-to-face physician care should not be reported using 99466, 99467. Procedure(s) or service(s) performed by other members of the transporting team may not be reported by the supervising physician.

Codes 99485, 99486 may be used to report control physician's non-face-to-face supervision of interfacility pediatric critical care transport, which includes all two-way communication between the control physician and the specialized transport team prior to transport, at the referring facility and during transport of the patient back to the receiving facility. The "control" physician is the physician directing transport services. These codes do not include pretransport communication between the control physician and the referring facility before or following patient transport. These codes may only be reported for patients 24 months of age or younger who are critically ill or critically injured. The control physician provides treatment advice to a specialized transport team who are present and delivering the hands-on patient care. The control physician does not report any services provided by the specialized transport team. The control physician's non-face-to-face time begins with the first contact by the control physician with the specialized transport team and ends when the patient's care is handed over to the receiving facility team. Refer to 99466 and 99467 for face-to-face transport care of the critically ill/injured patient. Time spent with the individual patient's transport team and reviewing data submissions should be recorded. Code 99485 is used to report the first 16-45 minutes of direction on a given date and should only be used once even if time spent by the physician is discontinuous. Do not report services of 15 minutes or less or any time when another physician is reporting 99466, 99467. Do not report 99485 or 99486 in conjunction with 99466, 99467 when performed by the same physician.

For the definition of the critically injured pediatric patient, see the **Neonatal and Pediatric Critical Care Services** section.

The non-face-to-face direction of emergency care to a patient's transporting staff by a physician located in a hospital or other facility by two-way communication is not considered direct face-to-face care and should not be reported with 99466, 99467. Physician-directed non-face-to-face emergency care through outside voice communication to transporting staff personnel is reported with 99288 or 99485, 99486 based upon the age and clinical condition of the patient.

Emergency department services (99281-99285), initial hospital care (99221-99223), critical care (99291, 99292), initial date neonatal intensive (99477) or critical care (99468) may only be reported after the patient has been admitted to the emergency department, the inpatient floor, or the critical care unit of the receiving facility. If inpatient critical care services are reported in the referring facility prior to transfer to the receiving hospital, use the critical care codes (99291, 99292).

►The following services are included when performed during the pediatric patient transport by the physician providing critical care and may not be reported separately: routine monitoring evaluations (eg, heart rate, respiratory rate, blood pressure, and pulse oximetry), the interpretation of cardiac output measurements (93562), chest X rays (71045, 71046), pulse oximetry (94760, 94761, 94762), blood gases and information data stored in computers (eg, ECGs, blood pressures, hematologic data), gastric intubation (43752, 43753), temporary transcutaneous pacing (92953), ventilatory management (94002, 94003, 94660, 94662), and vascular access procedures (36000, 36400, 36405, 36406, 36415,

36591, 36600). Any services performed which are not listed above should be reported separately.◀

Services provided by the specialized transport team during non-face-to-face transport supervision are not reported by the control physician.

Code 99466 is used to report the first 30 to 74 minutes of direct face-to-face time with the transport pediatric patient and should be reported only once on a given date. Code 99467 is used to report each additional 30 minutes provided on a given date. Face-to-face services of less than 30 minutes should not be reported with these codes.

Code 99485 is used to report the first 30 minutes of non-face-to-face supervision of an interfacility transport of a critically ill or critically injured pediatric patient and should be reported only once per date of service. Only the communication time spent by the supervising physician with the specialty transport team members during an interfacility transport should be reported. Code 99486 is used to report each additional 30 minutes beyond the initial 30 minutes. Non-face-to-face interfacility transport of 15 minutes or less is not reported.

(For total body and selective head cooling of neonates, use 99184)

99466 **Critical care** face-to-face services, during an interfacility transport of critically ill or critically injured pediatric patient, 24 months of age or younger; first 30-74 minutes of hands-on care during transport

➔ *CPT Changes: An Insider's View* 2009, 2013

➔ *CPT Assistant* Sep 11:3, May 13:6, May 14:4

+ 99467 each additional 30 minutes (List separately in addition to code for primary service)

➔ *CPT Changes: An Insider's View* 2009, 2013

➔ *CPT Assistant* Sep 11:3, May 13:6, May 14:4

(Use 99467 in conjunction with 99466)

(Critical care of less than 30 minutes total duration should be reported with the appropriate E/M code)

 # 99485 Supervision by a control physician of interfacility transport care of the critically ill or critically injured pediatric patient, 24 months of age or younger, includes two-way communication with transport team before transport, at the referring facility and during the transport, including data interpretation and report; first 30 minutes

➔ *CPT Changes: An Insider's View* 2013

➔ *CPT Assistant* May 13:6, May 14:4

#+ 99486 each additional 30 minutes (List separately in addition to code for primary procedure)

➔ *CPT Changes: An Insider's View* 2013

➔ *CPT Assistant* May 13:6, May 14:4

(Use 99486 in conjunction with 99485)

(For physician direction of emergency medical systems supervision for a pediatric patient older than 24 months of age, or at any age if not critically ill or injured, use 99288)

(Do not report 99485, 99486 with any other services reported by the control physician for the same period)

(Do not report 99485, 99486 in conjunction with 99466, 99467 when performed by the same physician)

Inpatient Neonatal and Pediatric Critical Care

The same definitions for critical care services apply for the adult, child, and neonate.

Codes 99468, 99469 may be used to report the services of directing the inpatient care of a critically ill neonate or infant 28 days of age or younger. They represent care starting with the date of admission (99468) for critical care services and all subsequent day(s) (99469) that the neonate remains in critical care. These codes may be reported only by a single individual and only once per calendar day, per patient. Initial inpatient neonatal critical care (99468) may only be reported once per hospital admission. If readmitted for neonatal critical care services during the same hospital stay, then report the subsequent inpatient neonatal critical care code (99469) for the first day of readmission to critical care, and 99469 for each day of critical care following readmission.

The initial inpatient neonatal critical care code (99468) can be used in addition to 99464 or 99465 as appropriate, when the physician or other qualified health care professional is present for the delivery (99464) or resuscitation (99465) is required. Other procedures performed as a necessary part of the resuscitation (eg, endotracheal intubation [31500]) may also be reported separately, when performed as part of the pre-admission delivery room care. In order to report these procedures separately, they must be performed as a necessary component of the resuscitation and not simply as a convenience before admission to the neonatal intensive care unit.

Codes 99471-99476 may be used to report the services of directing the inpatient care of a critically ill infant or young child from 29 days of postnatal age through 5 years of age. They represent care starting with the date of admission (99471, 99475) for pediatric critical care services and all subsequent day(s) (99472, 99476) that the infant or child remains in critical condition. These codes may only be reported by a single individual and only once per calendar day, per patient. Services for the critically ill or critically injured child 6 years of age or older would be reported with the time-based critical care codes (99291, 99292). Initial inpatient critical care (99471, 99475) may only be reported once per hospital admission. If readmitted to the pediatric critical care unit during the same hospital stay, then report the subsequent inpatient pediatric critical care code 99472 or 99476 for the first day of readmission to critical care and 99472 or 99476 for each day of critical care following readmission.

The pediatric and neonatal critical care codes include those procedures listed for the critical care codes (99291, 99292). In addition, the following procedures are also included (and are not separately reported by professionals, but may be reported by facilities) in the pediatric and neonatal critical care service codes (99468-99472, 99475, 99476) and the intensive care services codes (99477-99480).

Any services performed that are not included in these listings may be reported separately. For initiation of selective head or total body hypothermia in the critically ill neonate, report 99184. Facilities may report the included services separately.

Invasive or non-invasive electronic monitoring of vital signs

Vascular access procedures

- Peripheral vessel catheterization (36000)
- Other arterial catheters (36140, 36620)
- Umbilical venous catheters (36510)
- Central vessel catheterization (36555)
- Vascular access procedures (36400, 36405, 36406)
- Vascular punctures (36420, 36600)
- Umbilical arterial catheters (36660)

Airway and ventilation management

- Endotracheal intubation (31500)
- Ventilatory management (94002-94004)
- Bedside pulmonary function testing (94375)
- Surfactant administration (94610)
- Continuous positive airway pressure (CPAP) (94660)

Monitoring or interpretation of blood gases or oxygen saturation (94760-94762)

Car Seat Evaluation (94780-94781)

Transfusion of blood components (36430, 36440)

Oral or nasogastric tube placement (43752)

Suprapubic bladder aspiration (51100)

Bladder catheterization (51701, 51702)

Lumbar puncture (62270)

Any services performed which are not listed above may be reported separately.

When a neonate or infant is not critically ill but requires intensive observation, frequent interventions, and other intensive care services, the Continuing Intensive Care Services codes (99477-99480) should be used to report these services.

To report critical care services provided in the outpatient setting (eg, emergency department or office) for neonates and pediatric patients of any age, see the Critical Care codes 99291, 99292. If the same individual provides critical care services for a neonatal or pediatric patient less than 6 years of age in both the outpatient and inpatient settings on the same day, report only the appropriate Neonatal or Pediatric Critical Care codes 99468-99476 for all critical care services provided on that day. Critical care services provided by a second individual of a different specialty not reporting a per-day neonatal or pediatric critical care code can be reported with 99291, 99292.

When critical care services are provided to neonates or pediatric patients less than 6 years of age at two separate institutions by an individual from a different group on the same date of service, the individual from the referring institution should report their critical care services with the time-based critical care codes (99291, 99292) and the receiving institution should report the appropriate initial day of care code 99468, 99471, 99475 for the same date of service.

Critical care services to a pediatric patient 6 years of age or older are reported with the time based critical care codes 99291, 99292.

When the critically ill neonate or pediatric patient improves and is transferred to a lower level of care to another individual in another group within the same facility, the transferring individual does not report a per day critical care service. Subsequent hospital care (99231-99233) or time-based critical care services (99291-99292) is reported, as appropriate based upon the condition of the neonate or child. The receiving individual reports subsequent intensive care (99478-99480) or subsequent hospital care (99231-99233) services, as appropriate based upon the condition of the neonate or child.

When the neonate or infant becomes critically ill on a day when initial or subsequent intensive care services (99477-99480), hospital services (99221-99233), or normal newborn services (99460, 99461, 99462) have been performed by one individual and is transferred to a critical care level of care provided by a different individual in a different group, the transferring individual reports either the time-based critical care services performed (99291, 99292) for the time spent providing critical care to the patient, the intensive care service (99477-99480), hospital care services (99221-99233), or normal newborn service (99460, 99461, 99462) performed, but only one service. The receiving individual reports initial or subsequent inpatient neonatal or pediatric critical care (99468-99476), as appropriate based upon the patient's age and whether this is the first or subsequent admission to the critical care unit for the hospital stay.

When a newborn becomes critically ill on the same day they have already received normal newborn care (99460, 99461, 99462), and the same individual or group assumes critical care, report initial critical care service (99468) with modifier 25 in addition to the normal newborn code.

When a neonate, infant, or child requires initial critical care services on the same day the patient already has received hospital care or intensive care services by the same individual or group, only the initial critical care service code (99468, 99471, 99475) is reported.

Time-based critical care services (99291, 99292) are not reportable by the same individual or different individual of the same specialty and same group, when neonatal or pediatric critical care services (99468-99476) may be reported for the same patient on the same day. Time-based critical care services (99291, 99292) may be reported by an individual of a different specialty from either the same or different group on the same day that neonatal or pediatric critical care services are reported. Critical care interfacility transport face-to-face (99466, 99467) or supervisory (99485, 99486) services may be reported by the same or different individual of the same specialty and same group, when neonatal or pediatric critical care services (99468-99476) are reported for the same patient on the same day.

99468 **Initial inpatient neonatal critical care,** per day, for the evaluation and management of a critically ill neonate, 28 days of age or younger

➲ *CPT Changes: An Insider's View* 2009

➲ *CPT Assistant* Nov 11:5, May 14:4, Feb 15:10, Oct 15:8, May 16:3

99469 **Subsequent inpatient neonatal critical care,** per day, for the evaluation and management of a critically ill neonate, 28 days of age or younger

➲ *CPT Changes: An Insider's View* 2009

➲ *CPT Assistant* Nov 11:5, May 14:4, Feb 15:10, Oct 15:8, May 16:4

99471 **Initial inpatient pediatric critical care,** per day, for the evaluation and management of a critically ill infant or young child, 29 days through 24 months of age

➲ *CPT Changes: An Insider's View* 2009

➲ *CPT Assistant* Nov 11:5, Feb 15:10, May 16:3

99472 **Subsequent inpatient pediatric critical care,** per day, for the evaluation and management of a critically ill infant or young child, 29 days through 24 months of age

➲ *CPT Changes: An Insider's View* 2009

➲ *CPT Assistant* Nov 11:5, Feb 15:10, May 16:4

99475 **Initial inpatient pediatric critical care,** per day, for the evaluation and management of a critically ill infant or young child, 2 through 5 years of age

➲ *CPT Changes: An Insider's View* 2009

➲ *CPT Assistant* Feb 15:10, May 16:3

99476 **Subsequent inpatient pediatric critical care,** per day, for the evaluation and management of a critically ill infant or young child, 2 through 5 years of age

➲ *CPT Changes: An Insider's View* 2009

➲ *CPT Assistant* Feb 15:10, May 16:4

Initial and Continuing Intensive Care Services

Code 99477 represents the initial day of inpatient care for the child who is not critically ill but requires intensive observation, frequent interventions, and other intensive care services. Codes 99478-99480 are used to report the subsequent day services of directing the continuing intensive care of the low birth weight (LBW 1500-2500 grams) present body weight infant, very low birth weight (VLBW less than 1500 grams) present body weight infant, or normal (2501-5000 grams) present body weight newborn who does not meet the definition of critically ill but continues to require intensive observation, frequent interventions, and other intensive care services. These services are for infants and neonates who are not critically ill but continue to require intensive cardiac and respiratory monitoring, continuous and/or frequent vital sign monitoring, heat maintenance, enteral and/or parenteral nutritional adjustments, laboratory and oxygen monitoring, and constant observation by the health care team under direct supervision of the physician or other qualified health care professional. Codes 99477-99480 may be reported by a single individual and only once per day, per patient in a given facility. If readmitted to the intensive care unit during the same hospital stay, report 99478-99480 for the first day of intensive care and for each successive day that the child requires intensive care services.

These codes include the same procedures that are outlined in the **Neonatal and Pediatric Critical Care Services** section and these services should not be separately reported.

The initial day neonatal intensive care code (99477) can be used in addition to 99464 or 99465 as appropriate, when the physician or other qualified health care professional is present for the delivery (99464) or resuscitation (99465) is required. In this situation, report 99477 with modifier 25. Other procedures performed as a necessary part of the resuscitation (eg, endotracheal intubation [31500]) are also reported separately when performed as part of the pre-admission delivery room care. In order to report these procedures separately, they must be performed as a necessary component of the resuscitation and not simply as a convenience before admission to the neonatal intensive care unit.

The same procedures are included as bundled services with the neonatal intensive care codes as those listed for the neonatal (99468, 99469) and pediatric (99471-99476) critical care codes.

When the neonate or infant improves after the initial day and no longer requires intensive care services and is transferred to a lower level of care, the transferring individual does not report a per day intensive care service. Subsequent hospital care (99231-99233) or subsequent normal newborn care (99460, 99462) is reported as appropriate based upon the condition of the neonate or infant. If the transfer to a lower level of care occurs on the same day as initial intensive care services were provided by the transferring individual, 99477 may be reported.

When the neonate or infant is transferred after the initial day within the same facility to the care of another individual in a different group, both individuals report subsequent hospital care (99231-99233) services. The receiving individual reports subsequent hospital care (99231-99233) or subsequent normal newborn care (99462).

When the neonate or infant becomes critically ill on a day when initial or subsequent intensive care services (99477-99480) have been reported by one individual and is transferred to a critical care level of care provided by a different individual from a different group, the transferring individual reports either the time-based critical care services performed (99291, 99292) for the time spent providing critical care to the patient or the initial or subsequent intensive care (99477-99480) service, but not both. The receiving individual reports initial or subsequent inpatient neonatal or pediatric critical care (99468-99476) based upon the patient's age and whether this is the first or subsequent admission to critical care for the same hospital stay.

When the neonate or infant becomes critically ill on a day when initial or subsequent intensive care services (99477-99480) have been performed by the same individual or group, report only initial or subsequent inpatient neonatal or pediatric critical care (99468-99476) based upon the patient's age and whether this is the first or subsequent admission to critical care for the same hospital stay.

For the subsequent care of the sick neonate younger than 28 days of age but more than 5000 grams who does not require intensive or critical care services, use codes 99231-99233.

99477 **Initial hospital care,** per day, for the evaluation and management of the neonate, 28 days of age or younger, who requires intensive observation, frequent interventions, and other intensive care services

➲ *CPT Changes: An Insider's View* 2008

➲ *CPT Assistant* Jan 08:8, Jul 08:10, Mar 09:3, Nov 11:5, May 14:4

(For the initiation of inpatient care of the normal newborn, use 99460)

(For the initiation of care of the critically ill neonate, use 99468)

(For initiation of inpatient hospital care of the ill neonate not requiring intensive observation, frequent interventions, and other intensive care services, see 99221-99223)

99478 **Subsequent intensive care,** per day, for the evaluation and management of the recovering very low birth weight infant (present body weight less than 1500 grams)

➲ *CPT Changes: An Insider's View* 2009

99479 **Subsequent intensive care,** per day, for the evaluation and management of the recovering low birth weight infant (present body weight of 1500-2500 grams)

➲ *CPT Changes: An Insider's View* 2009

99480 **Subsequent intensive care,** per day, for the evaluation and management of the recovering infant (present body weight of 2501-5000 grams)

➲ *CPT Changes: An Insider's View* 2009

➲ *CPT Assistant* May 14:4, Jul 15:3

Cognitive Assessment and Care Plan Services

Cognitive assessment and care plan services are provided when a comprehensive evaluation of a new or existing patient, who exhibits signs and/or symptoms of cognitive impairment, is required to establish or confirm a diagnosis, etiology and severity for the condition. This service includes a thorough evaluation of medical and psychosocial factors, potentially contributing to increased morbidity. Do not report cognitive assessment and care plan services if any of the required elements are not performed or are deemed unnecessary for the patient's condition. For these services, see the appropriate evaluation and management code. A single physician or other qualified health care professional should not report 99483 more than once every 180 days.

Services for cognitive assessment and care plan include a cognition-relevant history, as well as an assessment of factors that could be contributing to cognitive impairment, including, but not limited to, psychoactive medication, chronic pain syndromes, infection, depression and other brain disease (eg, tumor, stroke, normal pressure hydrocephalus). Medical decision making includes current and likely progression of the disease, assessing the need for referral for rehabilitative, social, legal, financial, or community-based services, meal, transportation, and other personal assistance services.

99483 Assessment of and care planning for a patient with cognitive impairment, requiring an independent historian, in the office or other outpatient, home or domiciliary or rest home, with all of the following required elements:

- Cognition-focused evaluation including a pertinent history and examination;
- Medical decision making of moderate or high complexity;
- Functional assessment (eg, basic and instrumental activities of daily living), including decision-making capacity;
- Use of standardized instruments for staging of dementia (eg, functional assessment staging test [FAST], clinical dementia rating [CDR]);
- Medication reconciliation and review for high-risk medications;

- Evaluation for neuropsychiatric and behavioral symptoms, including depression, including use of standardized screening instrument(s);
- Evaluation of safety (eg, home), including motor vehicle operation;
- Identification of caregiver(s), caregiver knowledge, caregiver needs, social supports, and the willingness of caregiver to take on caregiving tasks;
- Development, updating or revision, or review of an Advance Care Plan;
- Creation of a written care plan, including initial plans to address any neuropsychiatric symptoms, neuro-cognitive symptoms, functional limitations, and referral to community resources as needed (eg, rehabilitation services, adult day programs, support groups) shared with the patient and/or caregiver with initial education and support.

Typically, 50 minutes are spent face-to-face with the patient and/or family or caregiver.

➲ *CPT Changes: An Insider's View* 2018

➲ *CPT Assistant* Apr 18:9

▶(Do not report 99483 in conjunction with E/M services [99201, 99202, 99203, 99204, 99205, 99211, 99212, 99213, 99214, 99215, 99241, 99242, 99243, 99244, 99245, 99324, 99325, 99326, 99327, 99328, 99334, 99335, 99336, 99337, 99341, 99342, 99343, 99344, 99345, 99347, 99348, 99349, 99350, 99366, 99367, 99368, 99497, 99498]; psychiatric diagnostic procedures [90785, 90791, 90792]; brief emotional/behavioral assessment [96127]; health risk assessment administration [96160, 96161]; medication therapy management services [99605, 99606, 99607])◀

99484 Code is out of numerical sequence. See 99497-99499

99485 Code is out of numerical sequence. See 99466-99469

99486 Code is out of numerical sequence. See 99466-99469

Care Management Services

▶Care management services are management and support services provided by clinical staff, under the direction of a physician or other qualified health care professional, or may be provided personally by a physician or other qualified health care professional to a patient residing at home or in a domiciliary, rest home, or assisted living facility. Services include establishing, implementing, revising, or monitoring the care plan, coordinating the care of other professionals and agencies, and educating the patient or caregiver about the patient's condition, care plan, and prognosis. The physician or other qualified health care professional provides or oversees the management and/or coordination of services, as needed, for all medical conditions, psychosocial needs, and activities of daily living.◀

A plan of care must be documented and shared with the patient and/or caregiver. A care plan is based on a physical, mental, cognitive, social, functional, and environmental assessment. It is a comprehensive plan of care for all health problems. It typically includes, but is not limited to, the following elements: problem list, expected outcome and prognosis, measurable treatment goals, symptom management, planned interventions, medication management, community/social services ordered, how the services of agencies and specialists unconnected to the practice will be directed/coordinated, identification of the individuals responsible for each intervention, requirements for periodic review, and, when applicable, revision of the care plan.

▶Codes 99487, 99489, 99490, 99491 are reported only once per calendar month and may only be reported by the single physician or other qualified health care professional who assumes the care management role with a particular patient for the calendar month.

For 99487, 99489, 99490 the face-to-face and non-face-to-face time spent by the clinical staff in communicating with the patient and/or family, caregivers, other professionals, and agencies; creating, revising, documenting, and implementing the care plan; or teaching self-management is used in determining the care management clinical staff time for the month. Only the time of the clinical staff of the reporting professional is counted. Only count the time of one clinical staff member when two or more clinical staff members are meeting about the patient. For 99491, only count the time personally spent by the physician or other qualified health care professional. Do not count any of the clinical staff time spent on the day of an initiating visit (the creation of the care plan, initial explanation to the patient and/or caregiver, and obtaining consent).

Care management activities performed by clinical staff, or personally by the physician or other qualified health care professional, typically include:◀

- communication and engagement with patient, family members, guardian or caretaker, surrogate decision makers, and/or other professionals regarding aspects of care;
- communication with home health agencies and other community services utilized by the patient;
- collection of health outcomes data and registry documentation;
- patient and/or family/caregiver education to support self-management, independent living, and activities of daily living;
- assessment and support for treatment regimen adherence and medication management;
- identification of available community and health resources;
- facilitating access to care and services needed by the patient and/or family;

- management of care transitions not reported as part of transitional care management (99495, 99496);
- ongoing review of patient status, including review of laboratory and other studies not reported as part of an E/M service, noted above;
- development, communication, and maintenance of a comprehensive care plan.

The care management office/practice must have the following capabilities:

- provide 24/7 access to physicians or other qualified health care professionals or clinical staff including providing patients/caregivers with a means to make contact with health care professionals in the practice to address urgent needs regardless of the time of day or day of week;
- provide continuity of care with a designated member of the care team with whom the patient is able to schedule successive routine appointments;
- provide timely access and management for follow-up after an emergency department visit or facility discharge;
- utilize an electronic health record system so that care providers have timely access to clinical information;
- use a standardized methodology to identify patients who require care management services;
- have an internal care management process/function whereby a patient identified as meeting the requirements for these services starts receiving them in a timely manner;
- use a form and format in the medical record that is standardized within the practice;
- be able to engage and educate patients and caregivers as well as coordinate care among all service professionals, as appropriate for each patient.

►E/M services may be reported separately by the same physician or other qualified health care professional during the same calendar month. A physician or other qualified health care professional who reports codes 99487, 99489, 99490, may not report care plan oversight services (99339, 99340, 99374-99380), prolonged services without direct patient contact (99358, 99359), home and outpatient INR monitoring (93792, 93793), medical team conferences (99366, 99367, 99368), education and training (98960, 98961, 98962, 99071, 99078), telephone services (99366, 99367, 99368, 99441, 99442, 99443), on-line medical evaluation (98969, 99444), preparation of special reports (99080), analysis of data (99091), transitional care management services (99495, 99496), medication therapy management services (99605, 99606, 99607) and, if performed, these services may not be reported separately during the month for which 99487, 99489, 99490 are reported. All other services may be reported. Do not report 99487, 99489, 99490, 99491 if reporting ESRD services (90951-90970) during the same month. If the care management services are performed within the postoperative period of a reported surgery, the same individual may not report 99487, 99489, 99490, 99491.

Care management may be reported in any calendar month during which the clinical staff time or physician or other qualified health care professional personal time requirements are met. If care management resumes after a discharge during a new month, start a new period or report transitional care management services (99495, 99496) as appropriate. If discharge occurs in the same month, continue the reporting period or report Transitional Care Management Services. Do not report 99487, 99489, 99490 for any post-discharge care management services for any days within 30 days of discharge, if reporting 99495, 99496.

When behavioral or psychiatric collaborative care management services are also provided, 99484, 99492, 99493, 99494 may be reported in addition.◄

Chronic Care Management Services

►Chronic care management services are provided when medical and/or psychosocial needs of the patient require establishing, implementing, revising, or monitoring the care plan. Patients who receive chronic care management services have two or more chronic continuous or episodic health conditions that are expected to last at least 12 months, or until the death of the patient, and that place the patient at significant risk of death, acute exacerbation/decompensation, or functional decline. Code 99490 is reported when, during the calendar month, at least 20 minutes of clinical staff time is spent in care management activities. Code 99491 is reported when 30 minutes of physician or other qualified health care professional personal time is spent in care management activities. Do not report 99490 in the same month as 99491.◄

 # 99490 Chronic care management services, at least 20 minutes of clinical staff time directed by a physician or other qualified health care professional, per calendar month, with the following required elements:

- multiple (two or more) chronic conditions expected to last at least 12 months, or until the death of the patient;
- chronic conditions place the patient at significant risk of death, acute exacerbation/decompensation, or functional decline;
- comprehensive care plan established, implemented, revised, or monitored.

➲ *CPT Changes: An Insider's View* 2015

➲ *CPT Assistant* Oct 14:3, Feb 15:3, Feb 18:7, Mar 18:5

(Chronic care management services of less than 20 minutes duration, in a calendar month, are not reported separately)

►(Do not report 99490 in the same calendar month as 99487, 99489, 99491)◄

#● 99491 Chronic care management services, provided personally by a physician or other qualified health care professional, at least 30 minutes of physician or other qualified health care professional time, per calendar month, with the following required elements:

- multiple (two or more) chronic conditions expected to last at least 12 months, or until the death of the patient;
- chronic conditions place the patient at significant risk of death, acute exacerbation/decompensation, or functional decline;
- comprehensive care plan established, implemented, revised, or monitored.

➲ *CPT Changes: An Insider's View* 2019

▶(Do not report 99491 in the same calendar month as 99487, 99489, 99490)◀

▶(Do not report 99491 in conjunction with 99339, 99340)◀

Complex Chronic Care Management Services

Complex chronic care management services are provided during a calendar month that includes criteria for chronic care management services as well as establishment or substantial revision of a comprehensive care plan; medical, functional, and/or psychosocial problems requiring medical decision making of moderate or high complexity; and clinical staff care management services for at least 60 minutes, under the direction of a physician or other qualified health care professional. Physicians or other qualified health care professionals may not report complex chronic care management services if the care plan is unchanged or requires minimal change (eg, only a medication is changed or an adjustment in a treatment modality is ordered). Medical decision making as defined in the Evaluation and Management (E/M) guidelines is determined by the problems addressed by the reporting individual during the month.

Patients who require complex chronic care management services may be identified by practice-specific or other published algorithms that recognize multiple illnesses, multiple medication use, inability to perform activities of daily living, requirement for a caregiver, and/or repeat admissions or emergency department visits. Typical adult patients who receive complex chronic care management services are treated with three or more prescription medications and may be receiving other types of therapeutic interventions (eg, physical therapy, occupational therapy). Typical pediatric patients receive three or more therapeutic interventions (eg, medications, nutritional support, respiratory therapy). All patients have two or more chronic continuous or episodic health conditions that are expected to last at least 12 months, or until the death of the patient, and that place the patient at significant risk of death, acute exacerbation/decompensation, or functional decline. Typical patients have complex diseases and morbidities and, as a result, demonstrate one or more of the following:

- need for the coordination of a number of specialties and services;
- inability to perform activities of daily living and/or cognitive impairment resulting in poor adherence to the treatment plan without substantial assistance from a caregiver;
- psychiatric and other medical comorbidities (eg, dementia and chronic obstructive pulmonary disease or substance abuse and diabetes) that complicate their care; and/or
- social support requirements or difficulty with access to care.

Total Duration of Staff Care Management Services	Complex Chronic Care Management
Less than 60 minutes	Not reported separately
60 to 89 minutes (1 hour - 1 hr. 29 min.)	99487 X 1
90 - 119 minutes (1 hr. 30 min. - 1 hr. 59 min.)	99487 X 1 and 99489 X 1
120 minutes or more (2 hours or more)	99487 X 1 and 99489 X 2 and 99489 for each additional 30 minutes

99487 Complex chronic care management services, with the following required elements:

- multiple (two or more) chronic conditions expected to last at least 12 months, or until the death of the patient,
- chronic conditions place the patient at significant risk of death, acute exacerbation/decompensation, or functional decline,
- establishment or substantial revision of a comprehensive care plan,
- moderate or high complexity medical decision making;
- 60 minutes of clinical staff time directed by a physician or other qualified health care professional, per calendar month.

➲ *CPT Changes: An Insider's View* 2013, 2015

➲ *CPT Assistant* Apr 13:3, Sep 13:15, Nov 13:3, Feb 14:3, Jun 14:3, 5, Oct 14:3, Apr 17:9, Feb 18:7, Mar 18:5

(Complex chronic care management services of less than 60 minutes duration, in a calendar month, are not reported separately)

+ 99489 each additional 30 minutes of clinical staff time directed by a physician or other qualified health care professional, per calendar month (List separately in addition to code for primary procedure)

➲ *CPT Changes: An Insider's View* 2013, 2015

➲ *CPT Assistant* Apr 13:3, Sep 13:15, Nov 13:3, Jun 14:5, Oct 14:3, Apr 17:9, Feb 18:7, Mar 18:5

(Report 99489 in conjunction with 99487)

(Do not report 99489 for care management services of less than 30 minutes additional to the first 60 minutes of complex chronic care management services during a calendar month)

►(Do not report 99487, 99489, 99490 during the same month with 90951-90970, 93792, 93793, 98960-98962, 98966-98969, 99071, 99078, 99080, 99091, 99339, 99340, 99358, 99359, 99366-99368, 99374-99380, 99441-99444, 99495, 99496, 99605-99607)◄

Coding Tip

If the physician personally performs the clinical staff activities, his or her time may be counted toward the required clinical staff time to meet the elements of the code.

99490 Code is out of numerical sequence. See 99480-99489

99491 Code is out of numerical sequence. See 99480-99489

Psychiatric Collaborative Care Management Services

►Psychiatric collaborative care services are provided under the direction of a treating physician or other qualified health care professional (see definitions below) during a calendar month. These services are reported by the treating physician or other qualified health care professional and include the services of the treating physician or other qualified health care professional, the behavioral health care manager (see definition below), and the psychiatric consultant (see definition below), who has contracted directly with the treating physician or other qualified health care professional, to provide consultation. Patients directed to the behavioral health care manager typically have behavioral health signs and/or symptoms or a newly diagnosed behavioral health condition, may need help in engaging in treatment, have not responded to standard care delivered in a nonpsychiatric setting, or require further assessment and engagement, prior to consideration of referral to a psychiatric care setting.

These services are provided when a patient requires a behavioral health care assessment; establishing, implementing, revising, or monitoring a care plan; and provision of brief interventions.

The following definitions apply to this section:◄

Definitions

Episode of care patients are treated for an episode of care, which is defined as beginning when the patient is directed by the treating physician or other qualified health care professional to the behavioral health care manager and ending with:

- the attainment of targeted treatment goals, which typically results in the discontinuation of care management services and continuation of usual follow-up with the treating physician or other qualified health care professional; or
- ►failure to attain targeted treatment goals culminating in referral to a psychiatric care provider for ongoing treatment of the behavioral health condition; or◄
- lack of continued engagement with no psychiatric collaborative care management services provided over a consecutive six month calendar period (break in episode).

A new episode of care starts after a break in episode of six calendar months or more.

Health care professionals refers to the treating physician or other qualified health care professional who directs the behavioral health care manager and continues to oversee the patient's care, including prescribing medications, providing treatments for medical conditions, and making referrals to specialty care when needed. Evaluation and management (E/M) and other services may be reported separately by the same physician or other qualified health care professional during the same calendar month.

Behavioral health care manager refers to clinical staff with a masters-/doctoral-level education or specialized training in behavioral health who provides care management services as well as an assessment of needs, including the administration of validated rating scales, the development of a care plan, provision of brief interventions, ongoing collaboration with the treating physician or other qualified health care professional, maintenance of a registry, all in consultation with a psychiatric consultant. Services are provided both face-to-face and non-face-to-face and psychiatric consultation is provided minimally on a weekly basis, typically non-face-to-face.

The behavioral health care manager providing other services in the same calendar month, such as psychiatric evaluation (90791, 90792), psychotherapy (90832, 90833, 90834, 90836, 90837, 90838), psychotherapy for crisis (90839, 90840), family psychotherapy (90846, 90847), multiple family group psychotherapy (90849), group psychotherapy (90853), smoking and tobacco use cessation counseling (99406, 99407), and alcohol and/or substance abuse structured screening and brief intervention services (99408, 99409), may report these services separately. Activities for services reported separately are not included in the time applied to 99492, 99493, 99494.

Psychiatric consultant refers to a medical professional, who is trained in psychiatry or behavioral health, and qualified to prescribe the full range of medications. The psychiatric consultant advises and makes recommendations, as needed, for psychiatric and other medical care, including psychiatric and other medical differential diagnosis, treatment strategies regarding appropriate therapies, medication management, medical management of complications associated with treatment

Type of Service	Total Duration of Collaborative Care Management Over Calendar Month	Code(s)
Initial - 70 minutes	Less than 36 minutes	Not reported separately
	36-85 minutes (36 minutes - 1 hr. 25 minutes)	99492 X 1
Initial plus each additional increment up to 30 minutes	86-115 minutes (1 hr. 26 minutes - 1 hr. 55 minutes)	99492 X 1 AND 99494 X 1
Subsequent - 60 minutes	Less than 31 minutes	Not reported separately
	31-75 minutes (31 minutes - 1 hr. 15 minutes)	99493 X 1
Subsequent plus each additional increment up to 30 minutes	76-105 minutes (1 hr. 16 minutes - 1 hr. 45 minutes)	99493 X 1 AND 99494 X 1

of psychiatric disorders, and referral for specialty services, which are typically communicated to the treating physician or other qualified health care professional through the behavioral health care manager. The psychiatric consultant typically does not see the patient or prescribe medications, except in rare circumstances.

The psychiatric consultant may provide services in the calendar month described by other codes, such as evaluation and management (E/M) services and psychiatric evaluation (90791, 90792). These services may be reported separately by the psychiatric consultant. Activities for services reported separately are not included in the services reported using 99492, 99493, 99494.

Do not report 99492 and 99493 in the same calendar month.

99492 **Initial psychiatric collaborative care management,** first 70 minutes in the first calendar month of behavioral health care manager activities, in consultation with a psychiatric consultant, and directed by the treating physician or other qualified health care professional, with the following required elements:

- outreach to and engagement in treatment of a patient directed by the treating physician or other qualified health care professional;
- initial assessment of the patient, including administration of validated rating scales, with the development of an individualized treatment plan;
- review by the psychiatric consultant with modifications of the plan if recommended;
- entering patient in a registry and tracking patient follow-up and progress using the registry, with appropriate documentation, and participation in weekly caseload consultation with the psychiatric consultant; and
- provision of brief interventions using evidence-based techniques such as behavioral activation, motivational interviewing, and other focused treatment strategies.

➲ *CPT Changes: An Insider's View* 2018
➲ *CPT Assistant* Nov 17:3, Feb 18:7, Mar 18:5

99493 **Subsequent psychiatric collaborative care management,** first 60 minutes in a subsequent month of behavioral health care manager activities, in consultation with a psychiatric consultant, and directed by the treating physician or other qualified health care professional, with the following required elements:

- tracking patient follow-up and progress using the registry, with appropriate documentation;
- participation in weekly caseload consultation with the psychiatric consultant;
- ongoing collaboration with and coordination of the patient's mental health care with the treating physician or other qualified health care professional and any other treating mental health providers;
- additional review of progress and recommendations for changes in treatment, as indicated, including medications, based on recommendations provided by the psychiatric consultant;
- provision of brief interventions using evidence-based techniques such as behavioral activation, motivational interviewing, and other focused treatment strategies;
- monitoring of patient outcomes using validated rating scales; and
- relapse prevention planning with patients as they achieve remission of symptoms and/or other treatment goals and are prepared for discharge from active treatment.

➲ *CPT Changes: An Insider's View* 2018
➲ *CPT Assistant* Nov 17:3, Feb 18:7, Mar 18:5

+ 99494 **Initial or subsequent psychiatric collaborative care management,** each additional 30 minutes in a calendar month of behavioral health care manager activities, in consultation with a psychiatric consultant, and directed by the treating physician or other qualified health care professional (List separately in addition to code for primary procedure)

➲ *CPT Changes: An Insider's View* 2018
➲ *CPT Assistant* Nov 17:3, Feb 18:7, Mar 18:5

(Use 99494 in conjunction with 99492, 99493)

Coding Tip

If the treating physician or other qualified health care professional personally performs behavioral health care manager activities and those activities are not used to meet criteria for a separately reported code, his or her time may be counted toward the required behavioral health care manager time to meet the elements of 99492, 99493, 99494.

Transitional Care Management Services

Codes 99495 and 99496 are used to report transitional care management services (TCM). These services are for a new or established patient whose medical and/or psychosocial problems require moderate or high complexity medical decision making during transitions in care from an inpatient hospital setting (including acute hospital, rehabilitation hospital, long-term acute care hospital), partial hospital, observation status in a hospital, or skilled nursing facility/nursing facility to the patient's community setting (home, domiciliary, rest home, or assisted living). TCM commences upon the date of discharge and continues for the next 29 days.

TCM is comprised of one face-to-face visit within the specified timeframes, in combination with non-face-to-face services that may be performed by the physician or other qualified health care professional and/or licensed clinical staff under his/her direction.

Non-face-to-face services provided by clinical staff, under the direction of the physician or other qualified health care professional, may include:

- communication (with patient, family members, guardian or caretaker, surrogate decision makers, and/or other professionals) regarding aspects of care,
- communication with home health agencies and other community services utilized by the patient,
- patient and/or family/caretaker education to support self-management, independent living, and activities of daily living,
- assessment and support for treatment regimen adherence and medication management,
- identification of available community and health resources,
- facilitating access to care and services needed by the patient and/or family

Non-face-to-face services provided by the physician or other qualified health care provider may include:

- obtaining and reviewing the discharge information (eg, discharge summary, as available, or continuity of care documents);
- reviewing need for or follow-up on pending diagnostic tests and treatments;
- interaction with other qualified health care professionals who will assume or reassume care of the patient's system-specific problems;
- education of patient, family, guardian, and/or caregiver;
- establishment or reestablishment of referrals and arranging for needed community resources;
- assistance in scheduling any required follow-up with community providers and services.

TCM requires a face-to-face visit, initial patient contact, and medication reconciliation within specified time frames. The first face-to-face visit is part of the TCM service and not reported separately. Additional E/M services provided on subsequent dates after the first face-to-face visit may be reported separately. TCM requires an interactive contact with the patient or caregiver, as appropriate, within two business days of discharge. The contact may be direct (face-to-face), telephonic, or by electronic means. Medication reconciliation and management must occur no later than the date of the face-to-face visit.

These services address any needed coordination of care performed by multiple disciplines and community service agencies. The reporting individual provides or oversees the management and/or coordination of services, as needed, for all medical conditions, psychosocial needs and activity of daily living support by providing first contact and continuous access.

Medical decision making and the date of the first face-to-face visit are used to select and report the appropriate TCM code. For 99496, the face-to-face visit must occur within 7 calendar days of the date discharge and medical decision making must be of high complexity. For 99495, the face-to-face visit must occur within 14 calendar days of the date of discharge and medical decision making must be of at least moderate complexity.

Type of Medical Decision Making	Face-to-Face Visit Within 7 Days	Face-to-Face Visit Within 8 to 14 Days
Moderate Complexity	99495	99495
High Complexity	99496	99495

Medical decision making is defined by the E/M Services Guidelines. The medical decision making over the service period reported is used to define the medical decision making of TCM. Documentation includes the timing of the initial post discharge communication with the patient or caregivers, date of the face-to-face visit, and the complexity of medical decision making.

Only one individual may report these services and only once per patient within 30 days of discharge. Another TCM may not be reported by the same individual or group for any subsequent discharge(s) within the 30 days. The same individual may report hospital or observation discharge services and TCM. However, the discharge service may not constitute the required face-to-face visit. The same individual should not report TCM services provided in the postoperative period of a service that the individual reported.

►A physician or other qualified health care professional who reports codes 99495, 99496 may not report care plan oversight services (99339, 99340, 99374-99380), prolonged services without direct patient contact (99358, 99359), home and outpatient INR monitoring (93792, 93793), medical team conferences (99366-99368), education and training (98960-98962, 99071, 99078), telephone services (98966-98968, 99441-99443), end stage renal disease services (90951-90970), online medical evaluation services (98969, 99444), preparation of special reports (99080), analysis of data (99091), complex chronic care coordination services (99487-99489), medication therapy management services (99605-99607), during the time period covered by the transitional care management services codes.◄

★ **99495** **Transitional Care Management Services** with the following required elements:

- Communication (direct contact, telephone, electronic) with the patient and/or caregiver within 2 business days of discharge
- Medical decision making of at least moderate complexity during the service period
- Face-to-face visit, within 14 calendar days of discharge

➔ *CPT Changes: An Insider's View* 2013, 2017

➔ *CPT Assistant* Apr 13:3, Jul 13:11, Aug 13:13, Sep 13:15, Nov 13:3, Dec 13:11, Mar 14:13, Oct 14:3, Feb 18:7, Mar 18:5

★ **99496** **Transitional Care Management Services** with the following required elements:

- Communication (direct contact, telephone, electronic) with the patient and/or caregiver within 2 business days of discharge
- Medical decision making of high complexity during the service period
- Face-to-face visit, within 7 calendar days of discharge

➔ *CPT Changes: An Insider's View* 2013, 2017

➔ *CPT Assistant* Apr 13:3, Jul 13:11, Aug 13:13, Sep 13:15, Nov 13:3, Mar 14:13, Oct 14:3, Feb 18:7, Mar 18:5

(Do not report 99495, 99496 in conjunction with 93792, 93793)

►(Do not report 90951-90970, 98960-98962, 98966-98969, 99071, 99078, 99080, 99091, 99339, 99340, 99358, 99359, 99366-99368, 99374-99380, 99441-99444, 99487-99489, 99605-99607, when performed during the service time of codes 99495 or 99496)◄

Coding Tip

If another individual provides TCM services within the postoperative period of a surgical package, modifier 54 is not required.

The required contact with the patient or caregiver, as appropriate, may be by the physician or qualified health care professional or clinical staff. Within two business days of discharge is Monday through Friday except holidays without respect to normal practice hours or date of notification of discharge. The contact must include capacity for prompt interactive communication addressing patient status and needs beyond scheduling follow-up care. If two or more separate attempts are made in a timely manner, but are unsuccessful and other transitional care management criteria are met, the service may be reported.

Advance Care Planning

Codes 99497, 99498 are used to report the face-to-face service between a physician or other qualified health care professional and a patient, family member, or surrogate in counseling and discussing advance directives, with or without completing relevant legal forms. An advance directive is a document appointing an agent and/or recording the wishes of a patient pertaining to his/her medical treatment at a future time should he/she lack decisional capacity at that time. Examples of written advance directives include, but are not limited to, Health Care Proxy, Durable Power of Attorney for Health Care, Living Will, and Medical Orders for Life-Sustaining Treatment (MOLST).

When using codes 99497, 99498, no active management of the problem(s) is undertaken during the time period reported.

Codes 99497, 99498 may be reported separately if these services are performed on the same day as another Evaluation and Management service (99201-99215, 99217, 99218, 99219, 99220, 99221, 99222, 99223, 99224, 99225, 99226, 99231, 99232, 99233, 99234, 99235, 99236, 99238, 99239, 99241, 99242, 99243, 99244, 99245, 99251, 99252, 99253, 99254, 99255, 99281, 99282, 99283, 99284, 99285, 99304, 99305, 99306, 99307, 99308, 99309, 99310, 99315, 99316, 99318, 99324, 99325, 99326, 99327, 99328, 99334, 99335, 99336, 99337, 99341, 99342, 99343, 99344, 99345, 99347, 99348, 99349, 99350, 99381-99397, 99495, 99496).

99497 Advance care planning including the explanation and discussion of advance directives such as standard forms (with completion of such forms, when performed), by the physician or other qualified health care professional; first 30 minutes, face-to-face with the patient, family member(s), and/or surrogate

➔ *CPT Changes: An Insider's View* 2015

➔ *CPT Assistant* Dec 14:11, Feb 16:7

+ 99498 each additional 30 minutes (List separately in addition to code for primary procedure)

➲ *CPT Changes: An Insider's View* 2015

➲ *CPT Assistant* Dec 14:11, Feb 16:7

(Use 99498 in conjunction with 99497)

(Do not report 99497 and 99498 on the same date of service as 99291, 99292, 99468, 99469, 99471, 99472, 99475, 99476, 99477, 99478, 99479, 99480, 99483)

General Behavioral Health Integration Care Management

General behavioral health integration care management services (99484) are reported by the supervising physician or other qualified health care professional. The services are performed by clinical staff for a patient with a behavioral health (including substance use) condition that requires care management services (face-to-face or non-face-to-face) of 20 or more minutes in a calendar month. A treatment plan as well as the specified elements of the service description is required. The assessment and treatment plan is not required to be comprehensive and the office/practice is not required to have all the functions of chronic care management (99487, 99489, 99490). Code 99484 may be used in any outpatient setting, as long as the reporting professional has an ongoing relationship with the patient and clinical staff and as long as the clinical staff is available for face-to-face services with the patient.

The reporting professional must be able to perform the evaluation and management (E/M) services of an initiating visit. General behavioral integration care management (99484) and chronic care management services may be reported by the same professional in the same month, as long as distinct care management services are performed. Behavioral health integration care management (99484) and psychiatric collaborative care management (99492, 99493, 99494) may not be reported by the same professional in the same month. Behavioral health care integration clinical staff are not required to have qualifications that would permit them to separately report services (eg, psychotherapy), but, if qualified and they perform such services, they may report such services separately, as long as the time of the service is not used in reporting 99484.

 # 99484 Care management services for behavioral health conditions, at least 20 minutes of clinical staff time, directed by a physician or other qualified health care professional, per calendar month, with the following required elements:

- initial assessment or follow-up monitoring, including the use of applicable validated rating scales;
- behavioral health care planning in relation to behavioral/psychiatric health problems, including revision for patients who are not progressing or whose status changes;
- facilitating and coordinating treatment such as psychotherapy, pharmacotherapy, counseling and/or psychiatric consultation; and
- continuity of care with a designated member of the care team.

➲ *CPT Changes: An Insider's View* 2018

➲ *CPT Assistant* Feb 18:7, Mar 18:5

(Do not report 99484 in conjunction with 99492, 99493, 99494 in the same calendar month)

(E/M services, including care management services [99487, 99489, 99490, 99495, 99496], and psychiatric services [90785-90899] may be reported separately by the same physician or other qualified health care professional on the same day or during the same calendar month, but activities used to meet criteria for another reported service do not count toward meeting criteria for 99484)

Coding Tips

If the treating physician or other qualified health care professional personally performs behavioral health care manager activities and those activities are not used to meet the criteria for a separately reported code, his or her time may be counted toward the required behavioral health care manager time to meet the elements of 99484, 99492, 99493, 99494.

Clinical staff time spent coordinating care with the emergency department may be reported using 99484, but time spent while the patient is inpatient or admitted to observation status may not be reported using 99484.

Other Evaluation and Management Services

99499 **Unlisted evaluation and management** service

➲ *CPT Assistant* Apr 96:11, Mar 05:11, May 05:1, Jan 06:46, Sep 06:8, Jan 07:30, May 11:7, Apr 12:10, Jul 12:10, 11, Nov 12:13, Oct 14:9

Notes

Notes

Anesthesia Guidelines

The following is a listing of headings and subheadings that appear within the Anesthesia section of the CPT codebook. The subheadings or subsections denoted with asterisks (*) below have special instructions unique to that subsection. Where these are indicated, special notes or guidelines will be presented preceding those procedural terminology listings, referring to that subsection specifically.

Time Reporting 60
Anesthesia Services 60
Supplied Materials 60
Separate or Multiple Procedures 60
▸Unlisted Service or Procedure◂ 60
Special Report 61
Anesthesia Modifiers 61
Physical Status Modifiers 61
Qualifying Circumstances 61

Anesthesia

Head (00100-00222) 62
Neck (00300-00352) 62
Thorax (Chest Wall and Shoulder Girdle) (00400-00474) 63
Intrathoracic (00500-00580) 63
Spine and Spinal Cord (00600-00670) 63
Upper Abdomen (00700-00797) 64
Lower Abdomen (00800-00882) 64
Perineum (00902-00952) 65
Pelvis (Except Hip) (01112-01173) 65
Upper Leg (Except Knee) (01200-01274) 66
Knee and Popliteal Area (01320-01444) 66
Lower Leg (Below Knee, Includes Ankle and Foot) (01462-01522) 66
Shoulder and Axilla* (01610-01680) 67
Upper Arm and Elbow (01710-01782) 67
Forearm, Wrist, and Hand (01810-01860) 67
Radiological Procedures (01916-01936) 68
Burn Excisions or Debridement (01951-01953) 68
Obstetric (01958-01969) 68
Other Procedures (01990-01999) 69

Anesthesia Guidelines

Services involving administration of anesthesia are reported by the use of the anesthesia five-digit procedure code (00100-01999) plus modifier codes (defined under "Anesthesia Modifiers" later in these Guidelines).

The reporting of anesthesia services is appropriate by or under the responsible supervision of a physician. These services may include but are not limited to general, regional, supplementation of local anesthesia, or other supportive services in order to afford the patient the anesthesia care deemed optimal by the anesthesiologist during any procedure. These services include the usual preoperative and postoperative visits, the anesthesia care during the procedure, the administration of fluids and/or blood and the usual monitoring services (eg, ECG, temperature, blood pressure, oximetry, capnography, and mass spectrometry). Unusual forms of monitoring (eg, intra-arterial, central venous, and Swan-Ganz) are not included.

Items used by all physicians in reporting their services are presented in the **Introduction.** Some of the commonalities are repeated in this section for the convenience of those physicians referring to this section on **Anesthesia.** Other definitions and items unique to anesthesia are also listed.

To report moderate (conscious) sedation provided by a physician also performing the service for which conscious sedation is being provided, see codes 99151, 99152, 99153. P. 736

When a second physician other than the health care professional performing the diagnostic or therapeutic services provides moderate (conscious) sedation in the facility setting (eg, hospital, outpatient hospital/ambulatory surgery center, skilled nursing facility), the second physician reports the associated moderate sedation procedure/service 99155, 99156, 99157; when these services are performed by the second physician in the nonfacility setting (eg, physician office, freestanding imaging center), codes 99155, 99156, 99157 would not be reported. Moderate sedation does not include minimal sedation (anxiolysis), deep sedation, or monitored anesthesia care (00100-01999).

To report regional or general anesthesia provided by a physician also performing the services for which the anesthesia is being provided, see modifier 47 in Appendix A.

Time Reporting

Time for anesthesia procedures may be reported as is customary in the local area. Anesthesia time begins when the anesthesiologist begins to prepare the patient for the induction of anesthesia in the operating room (or in an equivalent area) and ends when the anesthesiologist is no longer in personal attendance, that is, when the patient may be safely placed under postoperative supervision.

Anesthesia Services

Services rendered in the office, home, or hospital; consultation; and other medical services are listed in the **Evaluation and Management Services** section (99201-99499 series) on page 11. "Special Services and Reporting" (99000-99091 series) are listed in the **Medicine** section.

Supplied Materials

Supplies and materials provided (eg, sterile trays, drugs) over and above those usually included with the office visit or other services rendered may be listed separately. Drugs, tray supplies, and materials provided should be listed and identified with 99070 or the appropriate supply code.

Separate or Multiple Procedures

When multiple surgical procedures are performed during a single anesthetic administration, the anesthesia code representing the most complex procedure is reported. The time reported is the combined total for all procedures.

▸Unlisted Service or Procedure◂

▶A service or procedure may be provided that is not listed in this edition of the CPT codebook. When reporting such a service, the appropriate "Unlisted Procedure" code may be used to indicate the service, identifying it by "Special Report" as discussed in the section below. The "Unlisted Procedures" and accompanying code for **Anesthesia** is as follows:◀

01999 Unlisted anesthesia procedure(s)

Special Report

A service that is rarely provided, unusual, variable, or new may require a special report. Pertinent information should include an adequate definition or description of the nature, extent, and need for the procedure and the time, effort, and equipment necessary to provide the service.

Anesthesia Modifiers

All anesthesia services are reported by use of the anesthesia five-digit procedure code (00100-01999) plus the addition of a physical status modifier. The use of other optional modifiers may be appropriate.

Physical Status Modifiers

Physical Status modifiers are represented by the initial letter 'P' followed by a single digit from 1 to 6 as defined in the following list:

P1: A normal healthy patient

P2: A patient with mild systemic disease

P3: A patient with severe systemic disease

P4: A patient with severe systemic disease that is a constant threat to life

P5: A moribund patient who is not expected to survive without the operation

P6: A declared brain-dead patient whose organs are being removed for donor purposes

These six levels are consistent with the American Society of Anesthesiologists (ASA) ranking of patient physical status. Physical status is included in the CPT codebook to distinguish among various levels of complexity of the anesthesia service provided.

Example: 00100-P1

Qualifying Circumstances

More than one qualifying circumstance may be selected.

Many anesthesia services are provided under particularly difficult circumstances, depending on factors such as extraordinary condition of patient, notable operative conditions, and/or unusual risk factors. This section includes a list of important qualifying circumstances that significantly affect the character of the anesthesia service provided. These procedures would not be reported alone but would be reported as additional procedure numbers qualifying an anesthesia procedure or service.

+ 99100 Anesthesia for patient of extreme age, younger than 1 year and older than 70 (List separately in addition to code for primary anesthesia procedure)

(For procedure performed on infants younger than 1 year of age at time of surgery, see 00326, 00561, 00834, 00836)

+ 99116 Anesthesia complicated by utilization of total body hypothermia (List separately in addition to code for primary anesthesia procedure)

+ 99135 Anesthesia complicated by utilization of controlled hypotension (List separately in addition to code for primary anesthesia procedure)

+ 99140 Anesthesia complicated by emergency conditions (specify) (List separately in addition to code for primary anesthesia procedure)

(An emergency is defined as existing when delay in treatment of the patient would lead to a significant increase in the threat to life or body part)

Anesthesia

Head

00100 Anesthesia for procedures on salivary glands, including biopsy
➲ *CPT Assistant* Feb 97:4, Nov 99:6, Feb 06:9, Mar 06:15, Nov 07:8, Oct 11:3, Jul 12:13, Aug 14:6, Dec 17:8
➲ *Clinical Examples in Radiology* Summer 11:2, Spring 13:5, Summer 13:5, Winter 13:5, Spring 14:7, Winter 16:4

00102 Anesthesia for procedures involving plastic repair of cleft lip
➲ *CPT Changes: An Insider's View* 2000
➲ *CPT Assistant* Nov 99:6

00103 Anesthesia for reconstructive procedures of eyelid (eg, blepharoplasty, ptosis surgery)
➲ *CPT Changes: An Insider's View* 2000
➲ *CPT Assistant* Nov 99:6

00104 Anesthesia for electroconvulsive therapy

00120 Anesthesia for procedures on external, middle, and inner ear including biopsy; not otherwise specified

00124 otoscopy
➲ *CPT Assistant* Nov 99:7

00126 tympanotomy

00140 Anesthesia for procedures on eye; not otherwise specified

00142 lens surgery

00144 corneal transplant

00145 vitreoretinal surgery
➲ *CPT Changes: An Insider's View* 2001

00147 iridectomy

00148 ophthalmoscopy

00160 Anesthesia for procedures on nose and accessory sinuses; not otherwise specified

00162 radical surgery

00164 biopsy, soft tissue

00170 Anesthesia for intraoral procedures, including biopsy; not otherwise specified

00172 repair of cleft palate

00174 excision of retropharyngeal tumor

00176 radical surgery

00190 Anesthesia for procedures on facial bones or skull; not otherwise specified
➲ *CPT Changes: An Insider's View* 2001

00192 radical surgery (including prognathism)

00210 Anesthesia for intracranial procedures; not otherwise specified

00211 craniotomy or craniectomy for evacuation of hematoma
➲ *CPT Changes: An Insider's View* 2009

00212 subdural taps

00214 burr holes, including ventriculography
➲ *CPT Changes: An Insider's View* 2000
➲ *CPT Assistant* Nov 99:7

00215 cranioplasty or elevation of depressed skull fracture, extradural (simple or compound)
➲ *CPT Changes: An Insider's View* 2001

00216 vascular procedures

00218 procedures in sitting position

00220 cerebrospinal fluid shunting procedures

00222 electrocoagulation of intracranial nerve
➲ *CPT Assistant* Jul 12:13

Neck

00300 Anesthesia for all procedures on the integumentary system, muscles and nerves of head, neck, and posterior trunk, not otherwise specified
➲ *CPT Assistant* Nov 99:7, Mar 06:15, Oct 11:3, Jul 12:13

00320 Anesthesia for all procedures on esophagus, thyroid, larynx, trachea and lymphatic system of neck; not otherwise specified, age 1 year or older
➲ *CPT Changes: An Insider's View* 2003

00322 needle biopsy of thyroid

(For procedures on cervical spine and cord, see 00600, 00604, 00670)

00326 Anesthesia for all procedures on the larynx and trachea in children younger than 1 year of age
➲ *CPT Changes: An Insider's View* 2003
➲ *CPT Assistant* Dec 17:8

(Do not report 00326 in conjunction with 99100)

00350 Anesthesia for procedures on major vessels of neck; not otherwise specified

00352 simple ligation
➲ *CPT Assistant* Nov 07:8, Jul 12:13

(For arteriography, use 01916)

Thorax (Chest Wall and Shoulder Girdle)

00400 Anesthesia for procedures on the integumentary system on the extremities, anterior trunk and perineum; not otherwise specified
➔ *CPT Assistant* Mar 06:15, Nov 07:8, Oct 11:3, Jul 12:13

00402 reconstructive procedures on breast (eg, reduction or augmentation mammoplasty, muscle flaps)

00404 radical or modified radical procedures on breast

00406 radical or modified radical procedures on breast with internal mammary node dissection

00410 electrical conversion of arrhythmias

00450 Anesthesia for procedures on clavicle and scapula; not otherwise specified

00454 biopsy of clavicle

00470 Anesthesia for partial rib resection; not otherwise specified

00472 thoracoplasty (any type)

00474 radical procedures (eg, pectus excavatum)
➔ *CPT Assistant* Nov 07:8, Jul 12:13

Intrathoracic

00500 Anesthesia for all procedures on esophagus
➔ *CPT Assistant* Mar 06:15, Nov 07:8, Oct 11:3, Jul 12:13

00520 Anesthesia for closed chest procedures; (including bronchoscopy) not otherwise specified
➔ *CPT Changes: An Insider's View* 2000
➔ *CPT Assistant* Nov 99:7

00522 needle biopsy of pleura

00524 pneumocentesis

00528 mediastinoscopy and diagnostic thoracoscopy not utilizing 1 lung ventilation
➔ *CPT Changes: An Insider's View* 2000, 2003, 2004
➔ *CPT Assistant* Nov 99:7

(For tracheobronchial reconstruction, use 00539)

00529 mediastinoscopy and diagnostic thoracoscopy utilizing 1 lung ventilation
➔ *CPT Changes: An Insider's View* 2004
➔ *CPT Assistant* Jun 04:3

00530 Anesthesia for permanent transvenous pacemaker insertion
➔ *CPT Changes: An Insider's View* 2001

00532 Anesthesia for access to central venous circulation

00534 Anesthesia for transvenous insertion or replacement of pacing cardioverter-defibrillator
➔ *CPT Changes: An Insider's View* 2001

(For transthoracic approach, use 00560)

00537 Anesthesia for cardiac electrophysiologic procedures including radiofrequency ablation
➔ *CPT Changes: An Insider's View* 2001

00539 Anesthesia for tracheobronchial reconstruction
➔ *CPT Changes: An Insider's View* 2003

00540 Anesthesia for thoracotomy procedures involving lungs, pleura, diaphragm, and mediastinum (including surgical thoracoscopy); not otherwise specified

00541 utilizing 1 lung ventilation
➔ *CPT Changes: An Insider's View* 2003

(For thoracic spine and cord anesthesia procedures via an anterior transthoracic approach, see 00625-00626)

00542 decortication

00546 pulmonary resection with thoracoplasty

00548 intrathoracic procedures on the trachea and bronchi
➔ *CPT Assistant* Nov 97:10

00550 Anesthesia for sternal debridement
➔ *CPT Changes: An Insider's View* 2001

00560 Anesthesia for procedures on heart, pericardial sac, and great vessels of chest; without pump oxygenator
➔ *CPT Changes: An Insider's View* 2002

00561 with pump oxygenator, younger than 1 year of age
➔ *CPT Changes: An Insider's View* 2005
➔ *CPT Assistant* Dec 17:8

(Do not report 00561 in conjunction with 99100, 99116, and 99135)

00562 with pump oxygenator, age 1 year or older, for all noncoronary bypass procedures (eg, valve procedures) or for re-operation for coronary bypass more than 1 month after original operation
➔ *CPT Changes: An Insider's View* 2009

00563 with pump oxygenator with hypothermic circulatory arrest
➔ *CPT Changes: An Insider's View* 2001

00566 Anesthesia for direct coronary artery bypass grafting; without pump oxygenator
➔ *CPT Changes: An Insider's View* 2001, 2009

00567 with pump oxygenator
➔ *CPT Changes: An Insider's View* 2009

00580 Anesthesia for heart transplant or heart/lung transplant
➔ *CPT Assistant* Nov 07:8, Jul 12:13

Spine and Spinal Cord

00600 Anesthesia for procedures on cervical spine and cord; not otherwise specified
➔ *CPT Assistant* Mar 06:15, May 07:9, Nov 07:8, Oct 11:3, Jul 12:13

(For percutaneous image-guided spine and spinal cord anesthesia procedures, see 01935, 01936)

00604 procedures with patient in the sitting position
➔ *CPT Changes: An Insider's View* 2001

00620 Anesthesia for procedures on thoracic spine and cord, not otherwise specified
➔ *CPT Assistant* Mar 07:9

00625 Anesthesia for procedures on the thoracic spine and cord, via an anterior transthoracic approach; not utilizing 1 lung ventilation
➔ *CPT Changes: An Insider's View* 2007
➔ *CPT Assistant* Mar 07:9

00626 utilizing 1 lung ventilation
➔ *CPT Changes: An Insider's View* 2007
➔ *CPT Assistant* Mar 07:9

(For anesthesia for thoracotomy procedures other than spinal, see 00540-00541)

00630 Anesthesia for procedures in lumbar region; not otherwise specified

00632 lumbar sympathectomy

00635 diagnostic or therapeutic lumbar puncture
➔ *CPT Changes: An Insider's View* 2001

00640 Anesthesia for manipulation of the spine or for closed procedures on the cervical, thoracic or lumbar spine
➔ *CPT Changes: An Insider's View* 2003

00670 Anesthesia for extensive spine and spinal cord procedures (eg, spinal instrumentation or vascular procedures)
➔ *CPT Changes: An Insider's View* 2001
➔ *CPT Assistant* Nov 07:8, Jul 12:13

Upper Abdomen

00700 Anesthesia for procedures on upper anterior abdominal wall; not otherwise specified
➔ *CPT Assistant* Mar 06:15, Nov 07:8, Oct 11:3, Jul 12:13

00702 percutaneous liver biopsy

00730 Anesthesia for procedures on upper posterior abdominal wall

00731 Anesthesia for upper gastrointestinal endoscopic procedures, endoscope introduced proximal to duodenum; not otherwise specified
➔ *CPT Changes: An Insider's View* 2018
➔ *CPT Assistant* Dec 17:8

00732 endoscopic retrograde cholangiopancreatography (ERCP)
➔ *CPT Changes: An Insider's View* 2018
➔ *CPT Assistant* Dec 17:8

(For combined upper and lower gastrointestinal endoscopic procedures, use 00813)

(00740 has been deleted. To report, see 00731, 00732)

00750 Anesthesia for hernia repairs in upper abdomen; not otherwise specified

00752 lumbar and ventral (incisional) hernias and/or wound dehiscence

00754 omphalocele

00756 transabdominal repair of diaphragmatic hernia

00770 Anesthesia for all procedures on major abdominal blood vessels

00790 Anesthesia for intraperitoneal procedures in upper abdomen including laparoscopy; not otherwise specified

00792 partial hepatectomy or management of liver hemorrhage (excluding liver biopsy)
➔ *CPT Changes: An Insider's View* 2001

00794 pancreatectomy, partial or total (eg, Whipple procedure)

00796 liver transplant (recipient)

(For harvesting of liver, use 01990)

00797 gastric restrictive procedure for morbid obesity
➔ *CPT Changes: An Insider's View* 2002
➔ *CPT Assistant* Nov 07:8, Jul 12:13

Lower Abdomen

00800 Anesthesia for procedures on lower anterior abdominal wall; not otherwise specified
➔ *CPT Assistant* Mar 06:15, Nov 07:8, Oct 11:3, Jul 12:13

00802 panniculectomy

(00810 has been deleted. To report, see 00811, 00812, 00813)

00811 Anesthesia for lower intestinal endoscopic procedures, endoscope introduced distal to duodenum; not otherwise specified
➔ *CPT Changes: An Insider's View* 2018
➔ *CPT Assistant* Dec 17:8

00812 screening colonoscopy
➔ *CPT Changes: An Insider's View* 2018
➔ *CPT Assistant* Dec 17:8

(Report 00812 to describe anesthesia for any screening colonoscopy regardless of ultimate findings)

00813 Anesthesia for combined upper and lower gastrointestinal endoscopic procedures, endoscope introduced both proximal to and distal to the duodenum
➔ *CPT Changes: An Insider's View* 2018
➔ *CPT Assistant* Dec 17:8

00820 Anesthesia for procedures on lower posterior abdominal wall

00830 Anesthesia for hernia repairs in lower abdomen; not otherwise specified

00832 ventral and incisional hernias

(For hernia repairs in the infant 1 year of age or younger, see 00834, 00836)

00834 Anesthesia for hernia repairs in the lower abdomen not otherwise specified, younger than 1 year of age
➲ *CPT Changes: An Insider's View* 2003
➲ *CPT Assistant* Dec 17:8

(Do not report 00834 in conjunction with 99100)

00836 Anesthesia for hernia repairs in the lower abdomen not otherwise specified, infants younger than 37 weeks gestational age at birth and younger than 50 weeks gestational age at time of surgery
➲ *CPT Changes: An Insider's View* 2003
➲ *CPT Assistant* Dec 17:8

(Do not report 00836 in conjunction with 99100)

00840 Anesthesia for intraperitoneal procedures in lower abdomen including laparoscopy; not otherwise specified

00842 amniocentesis

00844 abdominoperineal resection

00846 radical hysterectomy

00848 pelvic exenteration

00851 tubal ligation/transection
➲ *CPT Changes: An Insider's View* 2002
➲ *CPT Assistant* Oct 14:14

00860 Anesthesia for extraperitoneal procedures in lower abdomen, including urinary tract; not otherwise specified

00862 renal procedures, including upper one-third of ureter, or donor nephrectomy

00864 total cystectomy

00865 radical prostatectomy (suprapubic, retropubic)

00866 adrenalectomy

00868 renal transplant (recipient)

(For donor nephrectomy, use 00862)

(For harvesting kidney from brain-dead patient, use 01990)

00870 cystolithotomy

00872 Anesthesia for lithotripsy, extracorporeal shock wave; with water bath

00873 without water bath

00880 Anesthesia for procedures on major lower abdominal vessels; not otherwise specified

00882 inferior vena cava ligation

Perineum

(For perineal procedures on integumentary system, muscles and nerves, see 00300, 00400)

00902 Anesthesia for; anorectal procedure
➲ *CPT Changes: An Insider's View* 2001
➲ *CPT Assistant* Mar 06:15, Oct 11:3, Jul 12:13

00904 radical perineal procedure

00906 vulvectomy

00908 perineal prostatectomy

00910 Anesthesia for transurethral procedures (including urethrocystoscopy); not otherwise specified

00912 transurethral resection of bladder tumor(s)

00914 transurethral resection of prostate

00916 post-transurethral resection bleeding

00918 with fragmentation, manipulation and/or removal of ureteral calculus
➲ *CPT Changes: An Insider's View* 2000
➲ *CPT Assistant* Nov 99:8, Apr 09:8

00920 Anesthesia for procedures on male genitalia (including open urethral procedures); not otherwise specified
➲ *CPT Changes: An Insider's View* 2001
➲ *CPT Assistant* Sep 12:16

00921 vasectomy, unilateral or bilateral
➲ *CPT Changes: An Insider's View* 2003

00922 seminal vesicles

00924 undescended testis, unilateral or bilateral

00926 radical orchiectomy, inguinal

00928 radical orchiectomy, abdominal

00930 orchiopexy, unilateral or bilateral

00932 complete amputation of penis

00934 radical amputation of penis with bilateral inguinal lymphadenectomy

00936 radical amputation of penis with bilateral inguinal and iliac lymphadenectomy

00938 insertion of penile prosthesis (perineal approach)

00940 Anesthesia for vaginal procedures (including biopsy of labia, vagina, cervix or endometrium); not otherwise specified

00942 colpotomy, vaginectomy, colporrhaphy, and open urethral procedures
➲ *CPT Changes: An Insider's View* 2001, 2002

00944 vaginal hysterectomy

00948 cervical cerclage

00950 culdoscopy

00952 hysteroscopy and/or hysterosalpingography
➲ *CPT Changes: An Insider's View* 2000
➲ *CPT Assistant* Nov 99:8, Jul 12:13

Pelvis (Except Hip)

01112 Anesthesia for bone marrow aspiration and/or biopsy, anterior or posterior iliac crest
➲ *CPT Changes: An Insider's View* 2001
➲ *CPT Assistant* Mar 06:15, Oct 11:3, Jul 12:13

01120 Anesthesia for procedures on bony pelvis

01130 Anesthesia for body cast application or revision

01140 Anesthesia for interpelviabdominal (hindquarter) amputation

01150 Anesthesia for radical procedures for tumor of pelvis, except hindquarter amputation

01160 Anesthesia for closed procedures involving symphysis pubis or sacroiliac joint

01170 Anesthesia for open procedures involving symphysis pubis or sacroiliac joint

01173 Anesthesia for open repair of fracture disruption of pelvis or column fracture involving acetabulum

➔ *CPT Changes: An Insider's View* 2004

➔ *CPT Assistant* Jun 04:3-4

(01180, 01190 have been deleted)

Upper Leg (Except Knee)

01200 Anesthesia for all closed procedures involving hip joint

➔ *CPT Assistant* Mar 06:15, Nov 07:8, Jul 12:13

01202 Anesthesia for arthroscopic procedures of hip joint

01210 Anesthesia for open procedures involving hip joint; not otherwise specified

01212 hip disarticulation

01214 total hip arthroplasty

➔ *CPT Changes: An Insider's View* 2001, 2002

01215 revision of total hip arthroplasty

➔ *CPT Changes: An Insider's View* 2001, 2002

01220 Anesthesia for all closed procedures involving upper two-thirds of femur

01230 Anesthesia for open procedures involving upper two-thirds of femur; not otherwise specified

01232 amputation

01234 radical resection

01250 Anesthesia for all procedures on nerves, muscles, tendons, fascia, and bursae of upper leg

01260 Anesthesia for all procedures involving veins of upper leg, including exploration

01270 Anesthesia for procedures involving arteries of upper leg, including bypass graft; not otherwise specified

01272 femoral artery ligation

01274 femoral artery embolectomy

➔ *CPT Assistant* Nov 07:8, Jul 12:13

Knee and Popliteal Area

01320 Anesthesia for all procedures on nerves, muscles, tendons, fascia, and bursae of knee and/or popliteal area

➔ *CPT Assistant* Mar 06:15, Nov 07:8, Oct 11:3, Jul 12:13

01340 Anesthesia for all closed procedures on lower one-third of femur

01360 Anesthesia for all open procedures on lower one-third of femur

01380 Anesthesia for all closed procedures on knee joint

01382 Anesthesia for diagnostic arthroscopic procedures of knee joint

➔ *CPT Changes: An Insider's View* 2003

01390 Anesthesia for all closed procedures on upper ends of tibia, fibula, and/or patella

01392 Anesthesia for all open procedures on upper ends of tibia, fibula, and/or patella

01400 Anesthesia for open or surgical arthroscopic procedures on knee joint; not otherwise specified

➔ *CPT Changes: An Insider's View* 2003

01402 total knee arthroplasty

➔ *CPT Changes: An Insider's View* 2002

01404 disarticulation at knee

01420 Anesthesia for all cast applications, removal, or repair involving knee joint

01430 Anesthesia for procedures on veins of knee and popliteal area; not otherwise specified

01432 arteriovenous fistula

01440 Anesthesia for procedures on arteries of knee and popliteal area; not otherwise specified

01442 popliteal thromboendarterectomy, with or without patch graft

01444 popliteal excision and graft or repair for occlusion or aneurysm

➔ *CPT Assistant* Nov 07:8, Jul 12:13

Lower Leg (Below Knee, Includes Ankle and Foot)

01462 Anesthesia for all closed procedures on lower leg, ankle, and foot

➔ *CPT Assistant* Mar 06:15, Nov 07:8, Oct 11:3, Jul 12:13

01464 Anesthesia for arthroscopic procedures of ankle and/or foot

➔ *CPT Changes: An Insider's View* 2003

01470 Anesthesia for procedures on nerves, muscles, tendons, and fascia of lower leg, ankle, and foot; not otherwise specified

01472 repair of ruptured Achilles tendon, with or without graft

01474 gastrocnemius recession (eg, Strayer procedure)

01480 Anesthesia for open procedures on bones of lower leg, ankle, and foot; not otherwise specified

01482 radical resection (including below knee amputation)
CPT Changes: An Insider's View 2001

01484 osteotomy or osteoplasty of tibia and/or fibula

01486 total ankle replacement

01490 Anesthesia for lower leg cast application, removal, or repair

01500 Anesthesia for procedures on arteries of lower leg, including bypass graft; not otherwise specified

01502 embolectomy, direct or with catheter

01520 Anesthesia for procedures on veins of lower leg; not otherwise specified

01522 venous thrombectomy, direct or with catheter
CPT Assistant Nov 07:8, Jul 12:13

Shoulder and Axilla

Includes humeral head and neck, sternoclavicular joint, acromioclavicular joint, and shoulder joint.

01610 Anesthesia for all procedures on nerves, muscles, tendons, fascia, and bursae of shoulder and axilla
CPT Assistant Mar 06:15, Nov 07:8, Oct 11:3, Jul 12:13

01620 Anesthesia for all closed procedures on humeral head and neck, sternoclavicular joint, acromioclavicular joint, and shoulder joint

01622 Anesthesia for diagnostic arthroscopic procedures of shoulder joint
CPT Changes: An Insider's View 2003

01630 Anesthesia for open or surgical arthroscopic procedures on humeral head and neck, sternoclavicular joint, acromioclavicular joint, and shoulder joint; not otherwise specified
CPT Changes: An Insider's View 2003

01634 shoulder disarticulation

01636 interthoracoscapular (forequarter) amputation

01638 total shoulder replacement

01650 Anesthesia for procedures on arteries of shoulder and axilla; not otherwise specified

01652 axillary-brachial aneurysm

01654 bypass graft

01656 axillary-femoral bypass graft

01670 Anesthesia for all procedures on veins of shoulder and axilla

01680 Anesthesia for shoulder cast application, removal or repair, not otherwise specified

(01682 has been deleted)

Upper Arm and Elbow

01710 Anesthesia for procedures on nerves, muscles, tendons, fascia, and bursae of upper arm and elbow; not otherwise specified
CPT Assistant Mar 06:15, Nov 07:8, Oct 11:3, Jul 12:13

01712 tenotomy, elbow to shoulder, open

01714 tenoplasty, elbow to shoulder

01716 tenodesis, rupture of long tendon of biceps

01730 Anesthesia for all closed procedures on humerus and elbow

01732 Anesthesia for diagnostic arthroscopic procedures of elbow joint
CPT Changes: An Insider's View 2003

01740 Anesthesia for open or surgical arthroscopic procedures of the elbow; not otherwise specified
CPT Changes: An Insider's View 2003

01742 osteotomy of humerus

01744 repair of nonunion or malunion of humerus

01756 radical procedures

01758 excision of cyst or tumor of humerus

01760 total elbow replacement

01770 Anesthesia for procedures on arteries of upper arm and elbow; not otherwise specified

01772 embolectomy

01780 Anesthesia for procedures on veins of upper arm and elbow; not otherwise specified

01782 phleborrhaphy
CPT Assistant Nov 07:8, Jul 12:13

Forearm, Wrist, and Hand

01810 Anesthesia for all procedures on nerves, muscles, tendons, fascia, and bursae of forearm, wrist, and hand
CPT Assistant Mar 06:15, Nov 07:8, Oct 11:3, Jul 12:13

01820 Anesthesia for all closed procedures on radius, ulna, wrist, or hand bones

01829 Anesthesia for diagnostic arthroscopic procedures on the wrist
CPT Changes: An Insider's View 2003

01830 Anesthesia for open or surgical arthroscopic/endoscopic procedures on distal radius, distal ulna, wrist, or hand joints; not otherwise specified
CPT Changes: An Insider's View 2003

01832 total wrist replacement

01840 Anesthesia for procedures on arteries of forearm, wrist, and hand; not otherwise specified

01842 embolectomy

01844 Anesthesia for vascular shunt, or shunt revision, any type (eg, dialysis)

01850 Anesthesia for procedures on veins of forearm, wrist, and hand; not otherwise specified

01852 phleborrhaphy

01860 Anesthesia for forearm, wrist, or hand cast application, removal, or repair
➲ *CPT Assistant* Nov 07:8, Jul 12:13

Radiological Procedures

01916 Anesthesia for diagnostic arteriography/venography
➲ *CPT Changes: An Insider's View* 2002
➲ *CPT Assistant* Nov 07:8, Oct 11:3, Jul 12:13

(Do not report 01916 in conjunction with therapeutic codes 01924-01926, 01930-01933)

01920 Anesthesia for cardiac catheterization including coronary angiography and ventriculography (not to include Swan-Ganz catheter)

01922 Anesthesia for non-invasive imaging or radiation therapy

01924 Anesthesia for therapeutic interventional radiological procedures involving the arterial system; not otherwise specified
➲ *CPT Changes: An Insider's View* 2002

01925 carotid or coronary
➲ *CPT Changes: An Insider's View* 2002

01926 intracranial, intracardiac, or aortic
➲ *CPT Changes: An Insider's View* 2002

01930 Anesthesia for therapeutic interventional radiological procedures involving the venous/lymphatic system (not to include access to the central circulation); not otherwise specified
➲ *CPT Changes: An Insider's View* 2002

01931 intrahepatic or portal circulation (eg, transvenous intrahepatic portosystemic shunt[s] [TIPS])
➲ *CPT Changes: An Insider's View* 2002, 2008
➲ *CPT Assistant* Apr 08:3

01932 intrathoracic or jugular
➲ *CPT Changes: An Insider's View* 2002

01933 intracranial
➲ *CPT Changes: An Insider's View* 2002

01935 Anesthesia for percutaneous image guided procedures on the spine and spinal cord; diagnostic
➲ *CPT Changes: An Insider's View* 2008
➲ *CPT Assistant* Apr 08:3

01936 therapeutic
➲ *CPT Changes: An Insider's View* 2008
➲ *CPT Assistant* Apr 08:3, Jul 12:13

Burn Excisions or Debridement

01951 Anesthesia for second- and third-degree burn excision or debridement with or without skin grafting, any site, for total body surface area (TBSA) treated during anesthesia and surgery; less than 4% total body surface area
➲ *CPT Changes: An Insider's View* 2001, 2002
➲ *CPT Assistant* Mar 06:15, Oct 11:3, Jul 12:13

01952 between 4% and 9% of total body surface area
➲ *CPT Changes: An Insider's View* 2001, 2002

+ 01953 each additional 9% total body surface area or part thereof (List separately in addition to code for primary procedure)
➲ *CPT Changes: An Insider's View* 2001
➲ *CPT Assistant* Jun 11:13, Jul 12:13

(Use 01953 in conjunction with 01952)

Obstetric

01958 Anesthesia for external cephalic version procedure
➲ *CPT Changes: An Insider's View* 2004
➲ *CPT Assistant* Jun 04:5-6, Oct 11:3, Jul 12:13

01960 Anesthesia for vaginal delivery only
➲ *CPT Changes: An Insider's View* 2002
➲ *CPT Assistant* Dec 01:3

01961 Anesthesia for cesarean delivery only
➲ *CPT Changes: An Insider's View* 2002, 2003

01962 Anesthesia for urgent hysterectomy following delivery
➲ *CPT Changes: An Insider's View* 2002, 2003

01963 Anesthesia for cesarean hysterectomy without any labor analgesia/anesthesia care
➲ *CPT Changes: An Insider's View* 2002, 2003

01965 Anesthesia for incomplete or missed abortion procedures
➲ *CPT Changes: An Insider's View* 2006

01966 Anesthesia for induced abortion procedures
➲ *CPT Changes: An Insider's View* 2006

01967 Neuraxial labor analgesia/anesthesia for planned vaginal delivery (this includes any repeat subarachnoid needle placement and drug injection and/or any necessary replacement of an epidural catheter during labor)
➲ *CPT Changes: An Insider's View* 2002
➲ *CPT Assistant* Dec 01:3, Oct 14:14

+ 01968 Anesthesia for cesarean delivery following neuraxial labor analgesia/anesthesia (List separately in addition to code for primary procedure performed)
➲ *CPT Changes: An Insider's View* 2002, 2003
➲ *CPT Assistant* Dec 01:3, Jun 11:13, Oct 14:14

(Use 01968 in conjunction with 01967)

+ 01969 Anesthesia for cesarean hysterectomy following neuraxial labor analgesia/anesthesia (List separately in addition to code for primary procedure performed)

➔ *CPT Changes: An Insider's View* 2002, 2003

➔ *CPT Assistant* Dec 01:3, Jun 11:13, Jul 12:13

(Use 01969 in conjunction with 01967)

Other Procedures

01990 Physiological support for harvesting of organ(s) from brain-dead patient

➔ *CPT Assistant* Mar 06:15, Nov 07:8, Oct 11:3, Jul 12:13

01991 Anesthesia for diagnostic or therapeutic nerve blocks and injections (when block or injection is performed by a different physician or other qualified health care professional); other than the prone position

➔ *CPT Changes: An Insider's View* 2003, 2013

01992 prone position

➔ *CPT Changes: An Insider's View* 2003, 2013

(Do not report 01991 or 01992 in conjunction with 99151, 99152, 99153, 99155, 99156, 99157)

(When regional intravenous administration of local anesthetic agent or other medication in the upper or lower extremity is used as the anesthetic for a surgical procedure, report the appropriate anesthesia code. To report a Bier block for pain management, use 64999)

(For intra-arterial or intravenous therapy for pain management, see 96373, 96374)

01996 Daily hospital management of epidural or subarachnoid continuous drug administration

➔ *CPT Changes: An Insider's View* 2003

➔ *CPT Assistant* Feb 97:5, Nov 97:10, May 99:6, Jul 12:5, Oct 12:14, May 15:10

(Report code 01996 for daily hospital management of continuous epidural or subarachnoid drug administration performed after insertion of an epidural or subarachnoid catheter)

01999 Unlisted anesthesia procedure(s)

➔ *CPT Assistant* Feb 97:4, Feb 06:9, Mar 06:15, Jan 07:30, Nov 07:8, Oct 11:3, Jul 12:13, Aug 14:6, 14, May 15:10, Dec 17:8

➔ *Clinical Examples in Radiology* Summer 11:2, Spring 13:5, Summer 13:5, Winter 13:5, Spring 14:7, Winter 16:4

Notes

Surgery Guidelines

Services 72
CPT Surgical Package Definition 72
Follow-Up Care for Diagnostic Procedures 72
Follow-Up Care for Therapeutic Surgical Procedures 72
Supplied Materials 72
Reporting More Than One Procedure/Service 72
Separate Procedure 72
Unlisted Service or Procedure 73
Special Report 74
Imaging Guidance 74
Surgical Destruction 74

Surgery Guidelines

Guidelines to direct general reporting of services are presented in the **Introduction.** Some of the commonalities are repeated here for the convenience of those referring to this section on **Surgery.** Other definitions and items unique to Surgery are also listed.

Services

Services rendered in the office, home, or hospital, consultations, and other medical services are listed in the **Evaluation and Management Services** section (99201-99499) beginning on page 11. "Special Services and Reports" (99000-99091) are listed in the **Medicine** section.

CPT Surgical Package Definition

By their very nature, the services to any patient are variable. The CPT codes that represent a readily identifiable surgical procedure thereby include, on a procedure-by-procedure basis, a variety of services. In defining the specific services "included" in a given CPT surgical code, the following services related to the surgery when furnished by the physician or other qualified health care professional who performs the surgery are included in addition to the operation per se:

- Evaluation and Management (E/M) service(s) subsequent to the decision for surgery on the day before and/or day of surgery (including history and physical)
- Local infiltration, metacarpal/metatarsal/digital block or topical anesthesia
- Immediate postoperative care, including dictating operative notes, talking with the family and other physicians or other qualified health care professionals
- Writing orders
- Evaluating the patient in the postanesthesia recovery area
- Typical postoperative follow-up care

Follow-Up Care for Diagnostic Procedures

Follow-up care for diagnostic procedures (eg, endoscopy, arthroscopy, injection procedures for radiography) includes only that care related to recovery from the diagnostic procedure itself. Care of the condition for which the diagnostic procedure was performed or of other concomitant conditions is not included and may be listed separately.

Follow-Up Care for Therapeutic Surgical Procedures

Follow-up care for therapeutic surgical procedures includes only that care which is usually a part of the surgical service. Complications, exacerbations, recurrence, or the presence of other diseases or injuries requiring additional services should be separately reported.

Supplied Materials

Supplies and materials (eg, sterile trays/drugs), over and above those usually included with the procedure(s) rendered are reported separately. List drugs, trays, supplies, and materials provided. Identify as 99070 or specific supply code.

Reporting More Than One Procedure/Service

When more than one procedure/service is performed on the same date, same session or during a post-operative period (subject to the "surgical package" concept), several CPT modifiers may apply (see Appendix A for definition).

Separate Procedure

Some of the procedures or services listed in the CPT codebook that are commonly carried out as an integral component of a total service or procedure have been identified by the inclusion of the term "separate procedure." The codes designated as "separate procedure" should not be reported in addition to the code for the total procedure or service of which it is considered an integral component.

However, when a procedure or service that is designated as a "separate procedure" is carried out independently or considered to be unrelated or distinct from other procedures/services provided at that time, it may be reported by itself, or in addition to other procedures/services by appending modifier 59 to the specific "separate procedure" code to indicate that the procedure is not considered to be a component of another procedure, but is a distinct, independent procedure. This may represent a different session, different procedure or surgery, different site or organ system, separate incision/excision, separate lesion, or separate injury (or area of injury in extensive injuries).

Unlisted Service or Procedure

A service or procedure may be provided that is not listed in this edition of the CPT codebook. When reporting such a service, the appropriate "Unlisted Procedure" code may be used to indicate the service, identifying it by "Special Report" as discussed in the section below. The "Unlisted Procedures" and accompanying codes for **Surgery** are as follows:

15999	Unlisted procedure, excision pressure ulcer
17999	Unlisted procedure, skin, mucous membrane and subcutaneous tissue
19499	Unlisted procedure, breast
20999	Unlisted procedure, musculoskeletal system, general
21089	Unlisted maxillofacial prosthetic procedure
21299	Unlisted craniofacial and maxillofacial procedure
21499	Unlisted musculoskeletal procedure, head
21899	Unlisted procedure, neck or thorax
22899	Unlisted procedure, spine
22999	Unlisted procedure, abdomen, musculoskeletal system
23929	Unlisted procedure, shoulder
24999	Unlisted procedure, humerus or elbow
25999	Unlisted procedure, forearm or wrist
26989	Unlisted procedure, hands or fingers
27299	Unlisted procedure, pelvis or hip joint
27599	Unlisted procedure, femur or knee
27899	Unlisted procedure, leg or ankle
28899	Unlisted procedure, foot or toes
29799	Unlisted procedure, casting or strapping
29999	Unlisted procedure, arthroscopy
30999	Unlisted procedure, nose
31299	Unlisted procedure, accessory sinuses
31599	Unlisted procedure, larynx
31899	Unlisted procedure, trachea, bronchi
32999	Unlisted procedure, lungs and pleura
33999	Unlisted procedure, cardiac surgery
36299	Unlisted procedure, vascular injection
37501	Unlisted vascular endoscopy procedure
37799	Unlisted procedure, vascular surgery
38129	Unlisted laparoscopy procedure, spleen
38589	Unlisted laparoscopy procedure, lymphatic system
38999	Unlisted procedure, hemic or lymphatic system
39499	Unlisted procedure, mediastinum
39599	Unlisted procedure, diaphragm
40799	Unlisted procedure, lips
40899	Unlisted procedure, vestibule of mouth
41599	Unlisted procedure, tongue, floor of mouth
41899	Unlisted procedure, dentoalveolar structures
42299	Unlisted procedure, palate, uvula
42699	Unlisted procedure, salivary glands or ducts
42999	Unlisted procedure, pharynx, adenoids, or tonsils
43289	Unlisted laparoscopy procedure, esophagus
43499	Unlisted procedure, esophagus
43659	Unlisted laparoscopy procedure, stomach
43999	Unlisted procedure, stomach
44238	Unlisted laparoscopy procedure, intestine (except rectum)
44799	Unlisted procedure, small intestine
44899	Unlisted procedure, Meckel's diverticulum and the mesentery
44979	Unlisted laparoscopy procedure, appendix
45399	Unlisted procedure, colon
45499	Unlisted laparoscopy procedure, rectum
45999	Unlisted procedure, rectum
46999	Unlisted procedure, anus
47379	Unlisted laparoscopic procedure, liver
47399	Unlisted procedure, liver
47579	Unlisted laparoscopy procedure, biliary tract
47999	Unlisted procedure, biliary tract
48999	Unlisted procedure, pancreas
49329	Unlisted laparoscopy procedure, abdomen, peritoneum and omentum
49659	Unlisted laparoscopy procedure, hernioplasty, herniorrhaphy, herniotomy
49999	Unlisted procedure, abdomen, peritoneum and omentum
50549	Unlisted laparoscopy procedure, renal
50949	Unlisted laparoscopy procedure, ureter
51999	Unlisted laparoscopy procedure, bladder
53899	Unlisted procedure, urinary system

54699	Unlisted laparoscopy procedure, testis
55559	Unlisted laparoscopy procedure, spermatic cord
55899	Unlisted procedure, male genital system
58578	Unlisted laparoscopy procedure, uterus
58579	Unlisted hysteroscopy procedure, uterus
58679	Unlisted laparoscopy procedure, oviduct, ovary
58999	Unlisted procedure, female genital system (nonobstetrical)
59897	Unlisted fetal invasive procedure, including ultrasound guidance, when performed
59898	Unlisted laparoscopy procedure, maternity care and delivery
59899	Unlisted procedure, maternity care and delivery
60659	Unlisted laparoscopy procedure, endocrine system
60699	Unlisted procedure, endocrine system
64999	Unlisted procedure, nervous system
66999	Unlisted procedure, anterior segment of eye
67299	Unlisted procedure, posterior segment
67399	Unlisted procedure, extraocular muscle
67599	Unlisted procedure, orbit
67999	Unlisted procedure, eyelids
68399	Unlisted procedure, conjunctiva
68899	Unlisted procedure, lacrimal system
69399	Unlisted procedure, external ear
69799	Unlisted procedure, middle ear
69949	Unlisted procedure, inner ear
69979	Unlisted procedure, temporal bone, middle fossa approach

Special Report

A service that is rarely provided, unusual, variable, or new may require a special report. Pertinent information should include an adequate definition or description of the nature, extent, and need for the procedure, and the time, effort, and equipment necessary to provide the service.

Imaging Guidance

▶When imaging guidance or imaging supervision and interpretation is included in a surgical procedure, guidelines for image documentation and report, included in the guidelines for Radiology (Including Nuclear Medicine and Diagnostic Ultrasound), will apply. Imaging guidance should not be reported for use of a nonimaging-guided tracking or localizing system (eg, radar signals, electromagnetic signals). Imaging guidance should only be reported when an imaging modality (eg, radiography, fluoroscopy, ultrasonography, magnetic resonance imaging, computed tomography, or nuclear medicine) is used and is appropriately documented.◀

Surgical Destruction

Surgical destruction is a part of a surgical procedure and different methods of destruction are not ordinarily listed separately unless the technique substantially alters the standard management of a problem or condition. Exceptions under special circumstances are provided for by separate code numbers.

Surgery

The following is a listing of headings and subheadings that appear within the Integumentary System section of the CPT codebook. The subheadings or subsections denoted with asterisks (*) below have special instructions unique to that subsection. Where these are indicated, special notes or guidelines will be presented preceding those procedural terminology listings, referring to that subsection specifically.

General (10004-10021) 77

►Fine Needle Aspiration (FNA) Biopsy*◄ (10004-10021) 77

Integumentary System (10030-19499) 78

Skin, Subcutaneous, and Accessory Structures (10030-11646) 78

- Introduction and Removal (10030-10036) 78
- Incision and Drainage (10040-10180) 78
- Debridement* (11000-11047) 79
- Paring or Cutting (11055-11057) 80
- Biopsy* (11102-11107) 80
- Removal of Skin Tags* (11200-11201) 82
- Shaving of Epidermal or Dermal Lesions* (11300-11313) 82
- Excision—Benign Lesions* (11400-11471) 83
- Excision—Malignant Lesions* (11600-11646) 85

Nails (11719-11765) 86

Pilonidal Cyst (11770-11772) 87

Introduction (11900-11983) 87

Structure of Skin

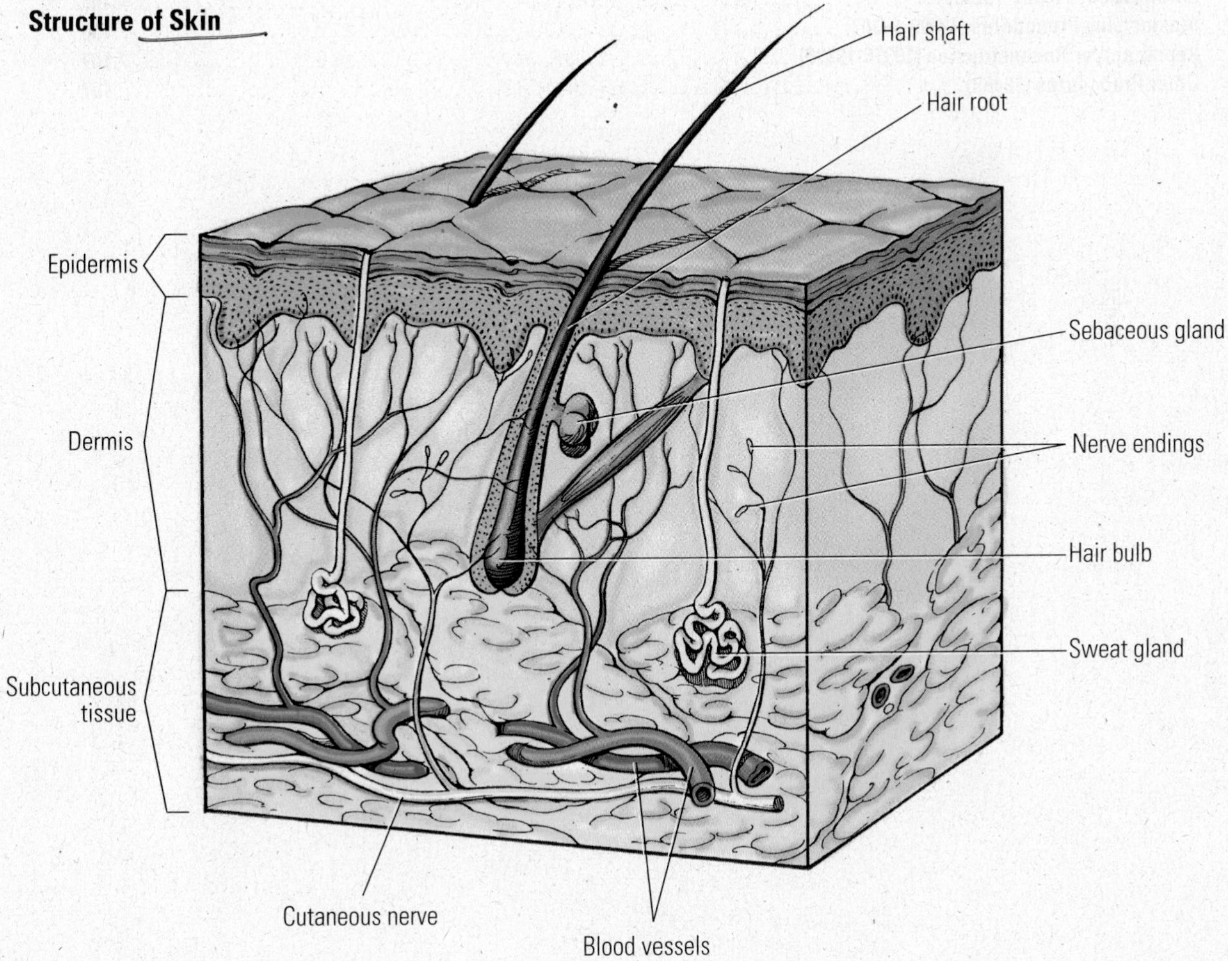

Repair (Closure)* (12001-16036) 88
- **Repair—Simple* (12001-12021)** 88
- **Repair—Intermediate* (12031-12057)** 89
- **Repair—Complex* (13100-13160)** 90
- **Adjacent Tissue Transfer or Rearrangement* (14000-14350)** 90
- **Skin Replacement Surgery* (15002-15278)** 91
  - **Definitions*** 92
  - **Surgical Preparation (15002-15278)** 93
    - *Autografts/Tissue Cultured Autograft (15040-15261)* *93*
    - *Skin Substitute Grafts* (15271-15278)* *95*
- **Flaps (Skin and/or Deep Tissues)* (15570-15738)** 95
- **Other Flaps and Grafts* (15740-15777)** 97
- **Other Procedures (15780-15879)** 97
- **Pressure Ulcers (Decubitus Ulcers) (15920-15999)** 98
- **Burns, Local Treatment* (16000-16036)** 99

Destruction* (17000-17999) 99
- **Destruction, Benign or Premalignant Lesions (17000-17250)** 101
- **Destruction, Malignant Lesions, Any Method (17260-17286)** 102
- **Mohs Micrographic Surgery* (17311-17315)** 102
- **Other Procedures (17340-17999)** 103

Breast (19000-19499) 103
- **Incision (19000-19030)** 103
- **Excision* (19081-19272)** 103
- **Introduction* (19281-19298)** 105
- **Mastectomy Procedures (19300-19307)** 106
- **Repair and/or Reconstruction (19316-19396)** 107
- **Other Procedures (19499)** 107

Surgery

General

▸Fine Needle Aspiration (FNA) Biopsy◂

▶A **fine needle aspiration** (FNA) biopsy is performed when material is aspirated with a fine needle and the cells are examined cytologically. A **core needle biopsy** is typically performed with a larger bore needle to obtain a core sample of tissue for histopathologic evaluation. FNA biopsy procedures are performed with or without imaging guidance. Imaging guidance codes (eg, 76942, 77002, 77012, 77021) may not be reported separately with 10004, 10005, 10006, 10007, 10008, 10009, 10010, 10011, 10012, 10021. Codes 10004, 10005, 10006, 10007, 10008, 10009, 10010, 10011, 10012, 10021 are reported once per lesion sampled in a single session. When more than one FNA biopsy is performed on separate lesions at the same session, same day, same imaging modality, use the appropriate imaging modality add-on code for the second and subsequent lesion(s). When more than one FNA biopsy is performed on separate lesions, same session, same day, using different imaging modalities, report the corresponding primary code with modifier 59 for each additional imaging modality and corresponding add-on codes for subsequent lesions sampled. This instruction applies regardless of whether the lesions are ipsilateral or contralateral to each other, and/or whether they are in the same or different organs/structures. When FNA biopsy and core needle biopsy both are performed on the same lesion, same session, same day using the same type of imaging guidance, do not separately report the imaging guidance for the core needle biopsy. When FNA biopsy is performed on one lesion and core needle biopsy is performed on a separate lesion, same session, same day using the same type of imaging guidance, both the core needle biopsy and the imaging guidance for the core needle biopsy may be reported separately with modifier 59. When FNA biopsy is performed on one lesion and core needle biopsy is performed on a separate lesion, same session, same day using different types of imaging guidance, both the core needle biopsy and the imaging guidance for the core needle biopsy may be reported with modifier 59.◂

10004 Code is out of numerical sequence. See 10021-10035

10005 Code is out of numerical sequence. See 10021-10035

10006 Code is out of numerical sequence. See 10021-10035

10007 Code is out of numerical sequence. See 10021-10035

10008 Code is out of numerical sequence. See 10021-10035

10009 Code is out of numerical sequence. See 10021-10035

10010 Code is out of numerical sequence. See 10021-10035

10011 Code is out of numerical sequence. See 10021-10035

10012 Code is out of numerical sequence. See 10021-10035

▲ **10021** Fine needle aspiration biopsy, without imaging guidance; first lesion

➔ *CPT Changes: An Insider's View* 2002, 2019

➔ *CPT Assistant* Aug 02:10, Mar 05:11

➔ *Clinical Examples in Radiology* Fall 08:4, Fall 10:3, 8, Spring 14:3, Winter 17:4

▶(10022 has been deleted. To report, see 10005, 10006, 10007, 10008, 10009, 10010, 10011, 10012)◀

#+● **10004** each additional lesion (List separately in addition to code for primary procedure)

➔ *CPT Changes: An Insider's View* 2019

▶(Use 10004 in conjunction with 10021)◀

▶(Do not report 10004, 10021 in conjunction with 10005, 10006, 10007, 10008, 10009, 10010, 10011, 10012 for the same lesion)◀

▶(For evaluation of fine needle aspirate, see 88172, 88173, 88177)◀

#● **10005** Fine needle aspiration biopsy, including ultrasound guidance; first lesion

➔ *CPT Changes: An Insider's View* 2019

#+● **10006** each additional lesion (List separately in addition to code for primary procedure)

➔ *CPT Changes: An Insider's View* 2019

▶(Use 10006 in conjunction with 10005)◀

▶(Do not report 10005, 10006 in conjunction with 76942)◀

▶(For evaluation of fine needle aspirate, see 88172, 88173, 88177)◀

#● **10007** Fine needle aspiration biopsy, including fluoroscopic guidance; first lesion

➔ *CPT Changes: An Insider's View* 2019

#+● **10008** each additional lesion (List separately in addition to code for primary procedure)

➔ *CPT Changes: An Insider's View* 2019

▶(Use 10008 in conjunction with 10007)◀

▶(Do not report 10007, 10008 in conjunction with 77002)◀

▶(For evaluation of fine needle aspirate, see 88172, 88173, 88177)◀

#● **10009** Fine needle aspiration biopsy, including CT guidance; first lesion

➔ *CPT Changes: An Insider's View* 2019

#+● **10010** each additional lesion (List separately in addition to code for primary procedure)

CPT Changes: An Insider's View 2019

►(Use 10010 in conjunction with 10009)◄

►(Do not report 10009, 10010 in conjunction with 77012)◄

►(For evaluation of fine needle aspirate, see 88172, 88173, 88177)◄

#● **10011** Fine needle aspiration biopsy, including MR guidance; first lesion

CPT Changes: An Insider's View 2019

#+● **10012** each additional lesion (List separately in addition to code for primary procedure)

CPT Changes: An Insider's View 2019

►(Use 10012 in conjunction with 10011)◄

►(Do not report 10011, 10012 in conjunction with 77021)◄

►(For evaluation of fine needle aspirate, see 88172, 88173, 88177)◄

(For percutaneous needle biopsy other than fine needle aspiration, see 19081-19086 for breast, 20206 for muscle, 32400 for pleura, 32405 for lung or mediastinum, 42400 for salivary gland, 47000 for liver, 48102 for pancreas, 49180 for abdominal or retroperitoneal mass, 50200 for kidney, 54500 for testis, 54800 for epididymis, 60100 for thyroid, 62267 for nucleus pulposus, intervertebral disc, or paravertebral tissue, 62269 for spinal cord)

►(For percutaneous image-guided fluid collection drainage by catheter of soft tissue [eg, extremity, abdominal wall, neck], use 10030)◄

Integumentary System

Skin, Subcutaneous, and Accessory Structures

Introduction and Removal

10030 Image-guided fluid collection drainage by catheter (eg, abscess, hematoma, seroma, lymphocele, cyst), soft tissue (eg, extremity, abdominal wall, neck), percutaneous

CPT Changes: An Insider's View 2014, 2017

CPT Assistant May 14:3, 9, Aug 17:9

Clinical Examples in Radiology Fall 13:6, Summer 14:9, Spring 15:8, Winter 16:10

(Report 10030 for each individual collection drained with a separate catheter)

(Do not report 10030 in conjunction with 75989, 76942, 77002, 77003, 77012, 77021)

(For image-guided fluid collection drainage, percutaneous or transvaginal/transrectal of visceral, peritoneal, or retroperitoneal collections, see 49405-49407)

Soft tissue-marker placement with imaging guidance is reported with 10035 and 10036. If a more specific site descriptor than soft tissue is applicable (eg, breast), use the site-specific codes for marker placement at that site. Report 10035 and 10036 only once per target, regardless of how many markers (eg, clips, wires, pellets, radioactive seeds) are used to mark that target.

10035 Placement of soft tissue localization device(s) (eg, clip, metallic pellet, wire/needle, radioactive seeds), percutaneous, including imaging guidance; first lesion

CPT Changes: An Insider's View 2016

CPT Assistant Jun 16:3

Clinical Examples in Radiology Winter 16:4

+ **10036** each additional lesion (List separately in addition to code for primary procedure)

CPT Changes: An Insider's View 2016

CPT Assistant Jun 16:3

Clinical Examples in Radiology Winter 16:5

(Use 10036 in conjunction with 10035)

(Do not report 10035, 10036 in conjunction with 76942, 77002, 77012, 77021)

(To report a second procedure on the same side or contralateral side, use 10036)

Incision and Drainage

(For excision, see 11400, et seq)

10040 Acne surgery (eg, marsupialization, opening or removal of multiple milia, comedones, cysts, pustules)

CPT Assistant Fall 92:10, Feb 08:8

10060 Incision and drainage of abscess (eg, carbuncle, suppurative hidradenitis, cutaneous or subcutaneous abscess, cyst, furuncle, or paronychia); simple or single

CPT Assistant Sep 12:10

10061 complicated or multiple

CPT Assistant Sep 12:10

10080 Incision and drainage of pilonidal cyst; simple

CPT Assistant Fall 92:13, Dec 06:15, May 07:5

10081 complicated

CPT Assistant Fall 92:13, Dec 06:15, May 07:5

(For excision of pilonidal cyst, see 11770-11772)

10120 Incision and removal of foreign body, subcutaneous tissues; simple

CPT Assistant Sep 12:10, Apr 13:10, Dec 13:16

10121 complicated

CPT Assistant Spring 91:7, Dec 06:15, Sep 12:10, Dec 13:16

(To report wound exploration due to penetrating trauma without laparotomy or thoracotomy, see 20100-20103, as appropriate)

(To report debridement associated with open fracture(s) and/or dislocation(s), use 11010-11012, as appropriate)

10140 Incision and drainage of hematoma, seroma or fluid collection
➲ *CPT Changes: An Insider's View* 2002
➲ *CPT Assistant* Nov 14:5

10160 Puncture aspiration of abscess, hematoma, bulla, or cyst
➲ *CPT Changes: An Insider's View* 2002
➲ *CPT Assistant* Aug 17:9
➲ *Clinical Examples in Radiology* Fall 09:8, Summer 14:9, Spring 15:8, Winter 16:10

(If imaging guidance is performed, see 76942, 77002, 77012, 77021)

10180 Incision and drainage, complex, postoperative wound infection
➲ *CPT Assistant* Nov 14:5

(For secondary closure of surgical wound, see 12020, 12021, 13160)

Debridement

Wound debridements (11042-11047) are reported by depth of tissue that is removed and by surface area of the wound. These services may be reported for injuries, infections, wounds and chronic ulcers. When performing debridement of a single wound, report depth using the deepest level of tissue removed. In multiple wounds, sum the surface area of those wounds that are at the same depth, but do not combine sums from different depths. For example: When bone is debrided from a 4 sq cm heel ulcer and from a 10 sq cm ischial ulcer, report the work with a single code, 11044. When subcutaneous tissue is debrided from a 16 sq cm dehisced abdominal wound and a 10 sq cm thigh wound, report the work with 11042 for the first 20 sq cm and 11045 for the second 6 sq cm. If all four wounds were debrided on the same day, use modifier 59 with either 11042, or 11044 as appropriate.

(For dermabrasions, see 15780-15783)

(For nail debridement, see 11720-11721)

(For burn(s), see 16000-16035)

(For pressure ulcers, see 15920-15999)

Coding Tip

Use of Depth and Surface Area For Reporting Debridement of Wounds

When performing debridement of a single wound, report depth using the deepest level of tissue removed. In multiple wounds, sum the surface area of those wounds that are at the same depth, but do not combine sums from different depths.

CPT Coding Guidelines, Debridement

11000 Debridement of extensive eczematous or infected skin; up to 10% of body surface
➲ *CPT Assistant* May 99:10, Oct 12:3, Feb 18:10

(For abdominal wall or genitalia debridement for necrotizing soft tissue infection, see 11004-11006)

+ 11001 each additional 10% of the body surface, or part thereof (List separately in addition to code for primary procedure)
➲ *CPT Changes: An Insider's View* 2009
➲ *CPT Assistant* May 99:10, Oct 12:3, Feb 18:10

(Use 11001 in conjunction with 11000)

11004 Debridement of skin, subcutaneous tissue, muscle and fascia for necrotizing soft tissue infection; external genitalia and perineum
➲ *CPT Changes: An Insider's View* 2005
➲ *CPT Assistant* Jan 12:6, Oct 12:3, Oct 13:15, Feb 18:10

11005 abdominal wall, with or without fascial closure
➲ *CPT Changes: An Insider's View* 2005
➲ *CPT Assistant* Jan 12:6, Oct 12:3, Oct 13:15, Feb 18:10

11006 external genitalia, perineum and abdominal wall, with or without fascial closure
➲ *CPT Changes: An Insider's View* 2005
➲ *CPT Assistant* Jan 12:6, Oct 12:3, Oct 13:15

(If orchiectomy is performed, use 54520)

(If testicular transplantation is performed, use 54680)

Debridement of Abdominal Wall
11005

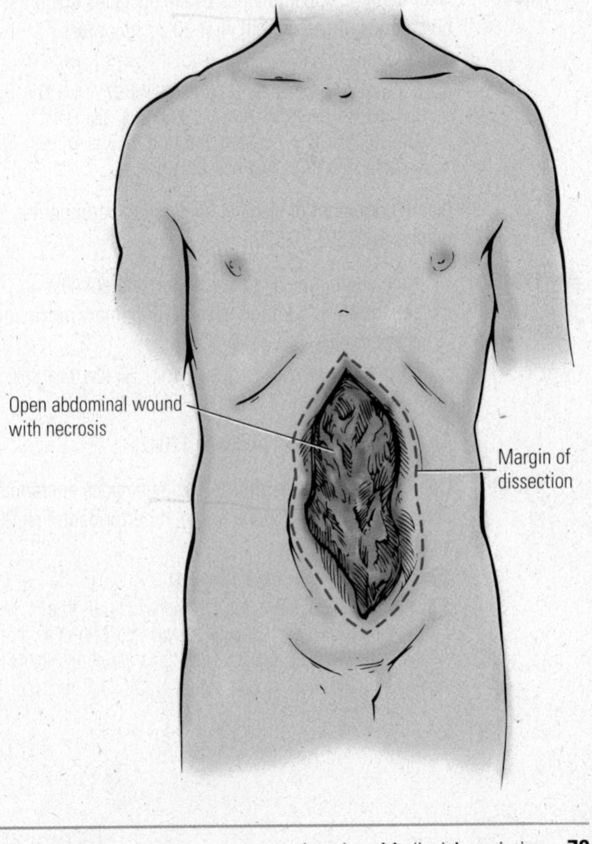

Integumentary 10021-19499

+ 11008 Removal of prosthetic material or mesh, abdominal wall for infection (eg, for chronic or recurrent mesh infection or necrotizing soft tissue infection) (List separately in addition to code for primary procedure)

➔ *CPT Changes: An Insider's View* 2005, 2008

➔ *CPT Assistant* Jan 12:6, Oct 12:3

(Use 11008 in conjunction with 10180, 11004-11006)

(Report skin grafts or flaps separately when performed for closure at the same session as 11004-11008)

(When insertion of mesh is used for closure, use 49568)

11010 Debridement including removal of foreign material at the site of an open fracture and/or an open dislocation (eg, excisional debridement); skin and subcutaneous tissues

➔ *CPT Changes: An Insider's View* 2011

➔ *CPT Assistant* Mar 97:2, Apr 97:10, Aug 97:6, Oct 03:10, May 11:3, Oct 12:13

11011 skin, subcutaneous tissue, muscle fascia, and muscle

➔ *CPT Changes: An Insider's View* 2011

➔ *CPT Assistant* Mar 97:2, Apr 97:10, Aug 97:6, May 11:3, Oct 12:13

11012 skin, subcutaneous tissue, muscle fascia, muscle, and bone

➔ *CPT Changes: An Insider's View* 2011

➔ *CPT Assistant* Mar 97:2, Apr 97:10, Aug 97:6, Oct 03:10, May 11:3, Oct 12:13

(For debridement of skin [ie, epidermis and/or dermis only], see 97597, 97598)

(For active wound care management, see 97597, 97598)

(For debridement of burn wounds, see 16020-16030)

11042 Debridement, subcutaneous tissue (includes epidermis and dermis, if performed); first 20 sq cm or less

➔ *CPT Changes: An Insider's View* 2011

➔ *CPT Assistant* Winter 92:10, May 96:6, Feb 97:7, Aug 97:6, Jun 05:1, 10, Oct 07:15, Nov 10:9, May 11:3, Sep 11:11, Jan 12:6, Mar 12:3, Oct 12:13, Feb 13:16, Sep 13:17, Oct 13:15, Nov 14:5, Feb 16:14, Aug 16:9, Oct 16:3

(For debridement of skin [ie, epidermis and/or dermis only], see 97597, 97598)

#+ 11045 each additional 20 sq cm, or part thereof (List separately in addition to code for primary procedure)

➔ *CPT Changes: An Insider's View* 2011

➔ *CPT Assistant* May 11:3, Sep 11:11, Jan 12:6, Mar 12:3, Oct 12:13, Nov 14:5, Aug 16:9, Oct 16:3

(Use 11045 in conjunction with 11042)

11043 Debridement, muscle and/or fascia (includes epidermis, dermis, and subcutaneous tissue, if performed); first 20 sq cm or less

➔ *CPT Changes: An Insider's View* 2011

➔ *CPT Assistant* May 96:6, Feb 97:7, Apr 97:11, Aug 97:6, Dec 99:10, Jun 05:1, 10, Oct 07:15, Nov 10:9, May 11:3, Sep 11:11, Jan 12:6, Mar 12:3, Oct 12:13, Feb 13:16, Nov 14:5, Aug 16:9, Oct 16:3

#+ 11046 each additional 20 sq cm, or part thereof (List separately in addition to code for primary procedure)

➔ *CPT Changes: An Insider's View* 2011

➔ *CPT Assistant* May 11:3, Sep 11:11, Jan 12:6, Mar 12:3, Oct 12:13, Feb 13:16, Nov 14:5, Aug 16:9, Oct 16:3

(Use 11046 in conjunction with 11043)

11044 Debridement, bone (includes epidermis, dermis, subcutaneous tissue, muscle and/or fascia, if performed); first 20 sq cm or less

➔ *CPT Changes: An Insider's View* 2011

➔ *CPT Assistant* Fall 93:21, Mar 96:10, May 96:6, Feb 97:7, Apr 97:11, Aug 97:6, Jun 05:1, 10, Oct 07:15, Nov 10:9, May 11:3, Sep 11:11, Jan 12:6, Mar 12:3, Oct 12:13, Feb 13:16, Nov 14:5, Aug 16:9, Oct 16:3

11045 Code is out of numerical sequence. See 11012-11047

11046 Code is out of numerical sequence. See 11012-11047

+ 11047 each additional 20 sq cm, or part thereof (List separately in addition to code for primary procedure)

➔ *CPT Changes: An Insider's View* 2011

➔ *CPT Assistant* May 11:3, Sep 11:11, Jan 12:6, Mar 12:3, Oct 12:13, Nov 14:5, Aug 16:9, Oct 16:3

(Do not report 11042-11047 in conjunction with 97597-97602 for the same wound)

(Use 11047 in conjunction with 11044)

Paring or Cutting

(To report destruction, see 17000-17004)

11055 Paring or cutting of benign hyperkeratotic lesion (eg, corn or callus); single lesion

➔ *CPT Assistant* Nov 97:11, Jan 99:11

11056 2 to 4 lesions

➔ *CPT Assistant* Nov 97:11, Jan 99:11, Sep 10:9

11057 more than 4 lesions

➔ *CPT Assistant* Nov 97:11, Jan 99:11, May 99:10

Biopsy

►The use of a biopsy procedure code (eg, 11102, 11103, 11104, 11105, 11106, 11107) indicates that the procedure to obtain tissue solely for diagnostic histopathologic examination was performed independently, or was unrelated or distinct from other procedures/services provided at that time. Biopsies performed on different lesions or different sites on the same date of service may be reported separately, as they are not considered components of other procedures.

During certain surgical procedures in the integumentary system, such as excision, destruction, or shave removals, the removed tissue is often submitted for pathologic examination. The obtaining of tissue for pathology during the course of these procedures is a routine component of such procedures. This obtaining of tissue is not considered a separate biopsy procedure and is not separately reported.

Partial-thickness biopsies are those that sample a portion of the thickness of skin or mucous membrane and do not penetrate below the dermis or lamina propria. Full-thickness biopsies penetrate into tissue deep to the dermis or lamina propria, into the subcutaneous or submucosal space.

Sampling of stratum corneum only, by any modality (eg, skin scraping, tape stripping) does not constitute a skin biopsy procedure and is not separately reportable.

An appropriate biopsy technique is selected based on optimal tissue-sampling considerations for the type of neoplastic, inflammatory, or other lesion requiring a tissue diagnosis. Biopsy of the skin is reported under three distinct techniques:

Tangential biopsy **(eg, shave, scoop, saucerize, curette)** is performed with a sharp blade, such as a flexible biopsy blade, obliquely oriented scalpel or curette to remove a sample of epidermal tissue with or without portions of underlying dermis. The intent of a tangential biopsy (11102, 11103) is to obtain a tissue sample from a lesion for the purpose of diagnostic pathologic examination. Biopsy of lesions by tangential technique (11102, 11103) is not considered an excision. Tangential biopsy technique may be represented by a superficial sample and does not involve the full thickness of the dermis, which could result in portions of the lesion remaining in the deeper layers of the dermis.

For therapeutic removal of epidermal or dermal lesion(s) using shave technique, see 11300-11313.

An indication for a shave removal (11300-11313) procedure may include a symptomatic lesion that rubs on waistband or bra, or any other reason why an elevated lesion is being completely removed with the shave technique, suggesting a therapeutic intent. It is the responsibility of the physician or qualified health care professional performing the procedure to clearly indicate the purpose of the procedure.

Punch biopsy requires a punch tool to remove a full-thickness cylindrical sample of skin. The intent of a punch biopsy (11104, 11105) is to obtain a cylindrical tissue sample of a cutaneous lesion for the purpose of diagnostic pathologic examination. Simple closure of the defect is included in the service. Manipulation of the biopsy defect to improve wound approximation is included in simple closure.

Incisional biopsy requires the use of a sharp blade (not a punch tool) to remove a full-thickness sample of tissue via a vertical incision or wedge, penetrating deep to the dermis, into the subcutaneous space. The intent of an incisional biopsy (11106, 11107) is to obtain a full-thickness tissue sample of a skin lesion for the purpose of diagnostic pathologic examination. This type of biopsy may sample subcutaneous fat, such as those performed for the evaluation of panniculitis. Although closure is usually performed on incisional biopsies, simple closure is not separately reported.

(For complete lesion excision with margins, see 11400-11646)

When multiple biopsy techniques are performed during the same encounter, only one primary lesion biopsy code (11102, 11104, 11106) is reported. Additional biopsy codes should be selected based on the following convention:

If multiple biopsies of the same type are performed, the primary code for that biopsy should be used along with the corresponding add-on code(s).

If an incisional biopsy is performed, report 11106 in combination with a tangential (11103), punch (11105), or incisional biopsy (11107) for the additional biopsy procedures.

If a punch biopsy is performed, report 11104 in combination with a tangential (11103), or punch (11105), for the additional biopsy procedures.

If multiple tangential biopsies are performed, report tangential biopsy (11102) in combination with 11103 for the additional tangential biopsy procedures.

When two or more biopsies of the same technique (ie, tangential, punch, or incisional) are performed on separate/additional lesions, use the appropriate add-on code (11103, 11105, 11107) to specify each additional biopsy. When two or three different biopsy techniques (ie, tangential, punch, or incisional) are performed to sample separate/additional lesions, select the appropriate biopsy code (11102, 11104, 11106) plus an additional add-on code (11103, 11105, 11107) for each additional biopsy performed.

The following table provides an illustration of the appropriate use of these codes for multiple biopsies:

Procedures Performed	CPT Code(s) Reported
2 tangential biopsies	11102 X 1, 11103 X 1
3 punch biopsies	11104 X 1, 11105 X 2
2 incisional biopsies	11106 X 1, 11107 X 1
1 incisional biopsy, 1 tangential biopsy and 1 punch biopsy	11106 X 1, 11103 X 1, 11105 X 1
1 punch biopsy and 2 tangential biopsies	11104 X 1, 11103 X 2◄

►(For biopsy of nail unit, use 11755)◄

►(For biopsy, intranasal, use 30100)◄

►(For biopsy of lip, use 40490)◄

►(For biopsy of vestibule of mouth, use 40808)◄

Integumentary 10021-19499

►(For biopsy of tongue, anterior two-thirds, use 41100)◄

►(For biopsy of floor of mouth, use 41108)◄

►(For biopsy of penis, use 54100)◄

►(For biopsy of vulva or perineum, see 56605, 56606)◄

►(For biopsy of eyelid skin including lid margin, use 67810)◄

►(For biopsy of conjunctiva, use 68100)◄

►(For biopsy of ear, use 69100)◄

►(11100 has been deleted. To report, see 11102, 11104, 11106)◄

►(11101 has been deleted. To report, see 11103, 11105, 11107)◄

● **11102** Tangential biopsy of skin (eg, shave, scoop, saucerize, curette); single lesion

CPT Changes: An Insider's View 2019

+● **11103** each separate/additional lesion (List separately in addition to code for primary procedure)

CPT Changes: An Insider's View 2019

►(Report 11103 in conjunction with 11102, 11104, 11106, when different biopsy techniques are performed to sample separate/additional lesions for each type of biopsy technique used)◄

● **11104** Punch biopsy of skin (including simple closure, when performed); single lesion

CPT Changes: An Insider's View 2019

+● **11105** each separate/additional lesion (List separately in addition to code for primary procedure)

CPT Changes: An Insider's View 2019

►(Report 11105 in conjunction with 11104, 11106, when different biopsy techniques are performed to sample separate/additional lesions for each type of biopsy technique used)◄

● **11106** Incisional biopsy of skin (eg, wedge) (including simple closure, when performed); single lesion

CPT Changes: An Insider's View 2019

+● **11107** each separate/additional lesion (List separately in addition to code for primary procedure)

CPT Changes: An Insider's View 2019

►(Report 11107 in conjunction with 11106)◄

Removal of Skin Tags

Removal by scissoring or any sharp method, ligature strangulation, electrosurgical destruction or combination of treatment modalities, including chemical destruction or electrocauterization of wound, with or without local anesthesia.

11200 Removal of skin tags, multiple fibrocutaneous tags, any area; up to and including 15 lesions

CPT Assistant Winter 90:3, Nov 97:11-12, Nov 02:11, Aug 09:7, Jun 11:13

Removal of Skin Tags
11200,11201

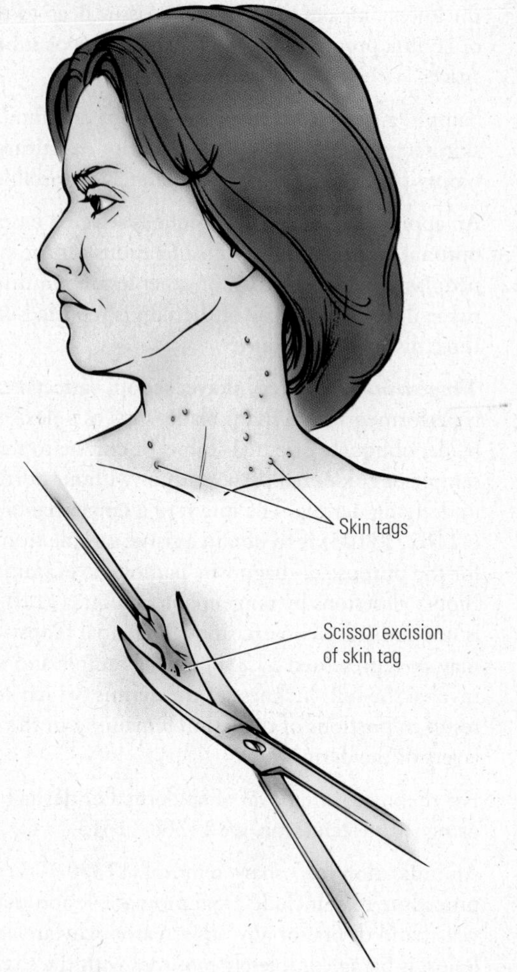

+ **11201** each additional 10 lesions, or part thereof (List separately in addition to code for primary procedure)

CPT Changes: An Insider's View 2009

CPT Assistant Winter 90:3, Nov 97:11-12, Nov 02:11, Jun 11:13

(Use 11201 in conjunction with 11200)

Shaving of Epidermal or Dermal Lesions

Shaving is the sharp removal by transverse incision or horizontal slicing to remove epidermal and dermal lesions without a full-thickness dermal excision. This includes local anesthesia, chemical or electrocauterization of the wound. The wound does not require suture closure.

11300 Shaving of epidermal or dermal lesion, single lesion, trunk, arms or legs; lesion diameter 0.5 cm or less

CPT Assistant Feb 00:11, Nov 02:11, Feb 08:1, Dec 17:14, Feb 18:10

11301 lesion diameter 0.6 to 1.0 cm

CPT Assistant Feb 00:11, Feb 08:1, Dec 17:14, Feb 18:10

11302 lesion diameter 1.1 to 2.0 cm

CPT Assistant Feb 00:11, Feb 08:1, Dec 17:14, Feb 18:10

11303 lesion diameter over 2.0 cm

CPT Assistant Feb 00:11, Feb 08:1, Dec 17:14, Feb 18:10

11305 Shaving of epidermal or dermal lesion, single lesion, scalp, neck, hands, feet, genitalia; lesion diameter 0.5 cm or less

CPT Assistant Feb 00:11, Feb 08:1, Dec 17:14, Feb 18:10

11306 lesion diameter 0.6 to 1.0 cm

CPT Assistant Feb 00:11, Feb 08:1, Dec 17:14, Feb 18:10

11307 lesion diameter 1.1 to 2.0 cm

CPT Assistant Feb 00:11, Feb 08:1, Dec 17:14, Feb 18:10

11308 lesion diameter over 2.0 cm

CPT Assistant Feb 00:11, Feb 08:1, Dec 17:14, Feb 18:10

11310 Shaving of epidermal or dermal lesion, single lesion, face, ears, eyelids, nose, lips, mucous membrane; lesion diameter 0.5 cm or less

CPT Assistant Feb 00:11, Feb 08:1, Feb 13:16, Mar 13:6, Dec 17:14, Feb 18:10

11311 lesion diameter 0.6 to 1.0 cm

CPT Assistant Feb 00:11, Feb 08:1, Feb 13:16, Mar 13:6, Feb 18:10

11312 lesion diameter 1.1 to 2.0 cm

CPT Assistant Feb 00:11, Feb 08:1, Feb 13:16, Mar 13:6, Feb 18:10

11313 lesion diameter over 2.0 cm

CPT Assistant Feb 00:11, Feb 08:1, Feb 13:16, Mar 13:6, Feb 18:10

Excision—Benign Lesions

Excision (including simple closure) of benign lesions of skin (eg, neoplasm, cicatricial, fibrous, inflammatory, congenital, cystic lesions), includes local anesthesia. See appropriate size and area below. For shave removal, see 11300 et seq, and for electrosurgical and other methods see 17000 et seq.

Excision is defined as full-thickness (through the dermis) removal of a lesion, including margins, and includes simple (non-layered) closure when performed. Report separately each benign lesion excised. Code selection is determined by measuring the greatest clinical diameter of the apparent lesion plus that margin required for complete excision (lesion diameter plus the most narrow margins required equals the excised diameter). The margins refer to the most narrow margin required to adequately excise the lesion, based on individual judgment. The measurement of lesion plus margin is made prior to excision. The excised diameter is the same whether the surgical defect is repaired in a linear fashion, or reconstructed (eg, with a skin graft).

The closure of defects created by incision, excision, or trauma may require intermediate or complex closure. Repair by intermediate or complex closure should be

Measuring and Coding the Removal of a Lesion

Measuring lesion removal.

A. Example: excision, malignant lesion of the back, 1.0 cm. Code 11606.

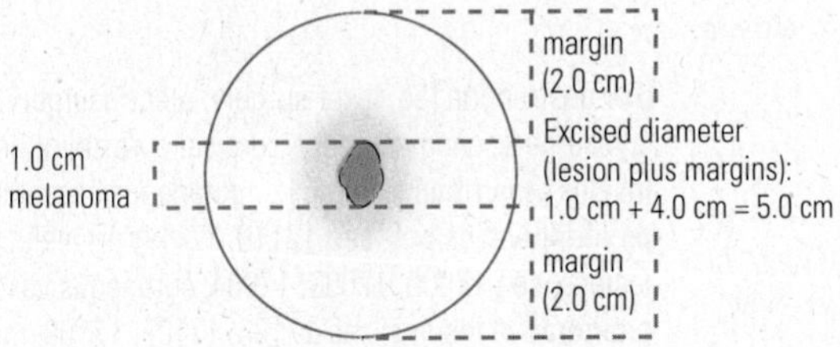

B. Example: Excision of benign lesion of the neck, 1.0 cm by 2.0 cm. Code 11423.

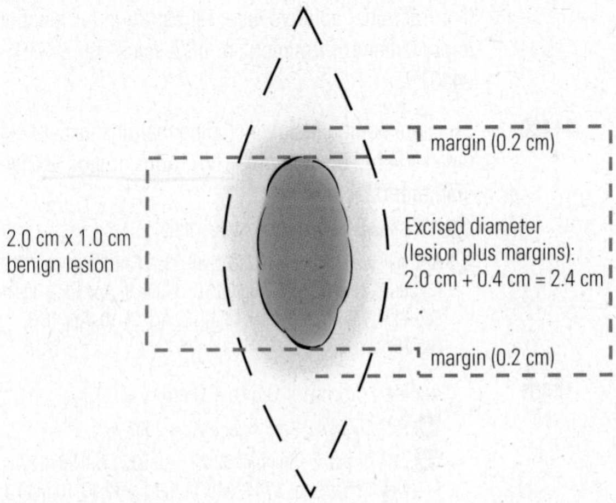

C. Example: Excision, malignant lesion of the nose, 0.9 cm. Code 11642.

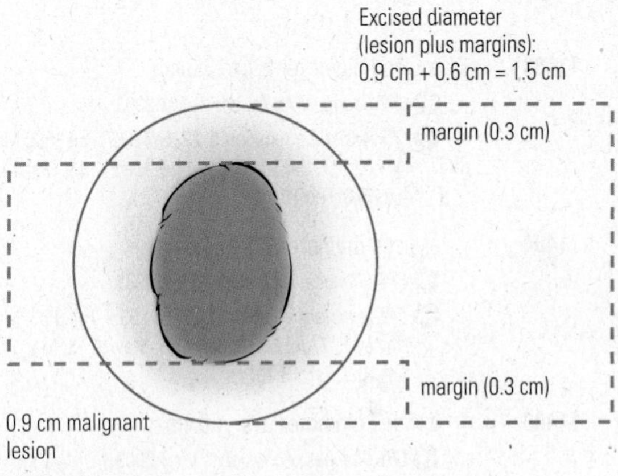

reported separately. For excision of benign lesions requiring more than simple closure, ie, requiring intermediate or complex closure, report 11400-11446 in addition to appropriate intermediate (12031-12057) or complex closure (13100-13153) codes. For reconstructive closure, see 15002-15261, 15570-15770. For excision performed in conjunction with adjacent tissue transfer, report only the adjacent tissue transfer code (14000-14302). Excision of lesion (11400-11446) is not separately reportable with adjacent tissue transfer. See page 88 for the definition of *intermediate* or *complex* closure.

(For destruction [eg, laser surgery, electrosurgery, cryosurgery, chemosurgery, surgical curette] of benign lesions other than skin tags or cutaneous vascular proliferative lesions, see 17110, 17111; premalignant lesions, see 17000, 17003, 17004; cutaneous vascular proliferative lesions, see 17106, 17107, 17108; malignant lesions, see 17260-17286)

(For excision of cicatricial lesion[s] [eg, full thickness excision, through the dermis], see 11400-11446)

(For incisional removal of burn scar, see 16035, 16036)

(For fractional ablative laser fenestration for functional improvement of traumatic or burn scars, see 0479T, 0480T)

11400 Excision, benign lesion including margins, except skin tag (unless listed elsewhere), trunk, arms or legs; excised diameter 0.5 cm or less

CPT Changes: An Insider's View 2003

CPT Assistant Summer 92:22, Fall 93:7, Fall 95:3, May 96:11, Aug 00:5, Nov 02:5, 7, Aug 06:10, Jul 08:5, Apr 10:3, Jul 10:10, Jan 11:9, May 12:13, Mar 14:4, 12, Apr 14:10, Apr 16:3, Feb 18:10

11401 excised diameter 0.6 to 1.0 cm

CPT Changes: An Insider's View 2003

CPT Assistant Summer 92:22, Fall 93:7, Fall 95:3, May 96:11, Nov 02:5, 7, Jul 10:10, Jan 11:9, May 12:13, Mar 14:4, 12, Apr 16:3, Feb 18:10

11402 excised diameter 1.1 to 2.0 cm

CPT Changes: An Insider's View 2003

CPT Assistant Summer 92:22, Fall 93:7, Fall 95:3, May 96:11, Nov 02:5, 7, Jul 10:10, Jan 11:9, May 12:13, Mar 14:4, 12, Apr 16:3, Feb 18:10

11403 excised diameter 2.1 to 3.0 cm

CPT Changes: An Insider's View 2003

CPT Assistant Summer 92:22, Fall 93:7, Fall 95:3, May 96:11, Nov 02:5, 7, Jul 10:10, Jan 11:9, May 12:13, Mar 14:4, 12, Apr 16:3, Feb 18:10

11404 excised diameter 3.1 to 4.0 cm

CPT Changes: An Insider's View 2003

CPT Assistant Summer 92:22, Fall 93:7, Fall 95:3, May 96:11, Nov 02:5, 7, Jul 10:10, Jan 11:9, May 12:13, Mar 14:4, 12, Apr 16:3, Feb 18:10

11406 excised diameter over 4.0 cm

CPT Changes: An Insider's View 2003

CPT Assistant Summer 92:22, Fall 93:7, Fall 95:3, May 96:11, Nov 02:5, 7, Jul 10:10, Jan 11:9, May 12:13, Mar 14:4, 12, Apr 14:10, Apr 16:3, Feb 18:10

(For unusual or complicated excision, add modifier 22)

11420 Excision, benign lesion including margins, except skin tag (unless listed elsewhere), scalp, neck, hands, feet, genitalia; excised diameter 0.5 cm or less

CPT Changes: An Insider's View 2003

CPT Assistant Summer 92:22, Fall 95:3, Jul 08:5, Jul 10:10, May 12:13, Jan 13:15, Mar 14:4, 12, Apr 16:3, Feb 18:10

11421 excised diameter 0.6 to 1.0 cm

CPT Changes: An Insider's View 2003

CPT Assistant Summer 92:22, Fall 95:3, May 96:11, Jul 10:10, May 12:13, Jan 13:15, Mar 14:4, 12, Apr 16:3, Feb 18:10

11422 excised diameter 1.1 to 2.0 cm

CPT Changes: An Insider's View 2003

CPT Assistant Summer 92:22, Fall 95:3, May 96:11, Aug 00:5, Jul 10:10, Mar 12:4, May 12:13, Jan 13:15, Mar 14:4, 12, Apr 16:3, Feb 18:10

11423 excised diameter 2.1 to 3.0 cm

CPT Changes: An Insider's View 2003

CPT Assistant Summer 92:22, Fall 95:3, May 96:11, Jul 10:10, May 12:13, Jan 13:15, Mar 14:4, 12, Apr 16:3, Feb 18:10

11424 excised diameter 3.1 to 4.0 cm

CPT Changes: An Insider's View 2003

CPT Assistant Summer 92:22, Fall 95:3, May 96:11, Jul 10:10, May 12:13, Jan 13:15, Mar 14:4, 12, Apr 16:3, Feb 18:10

11426 excised diameter over 4.0 cm

CPT Changes: An Insider's View 2003

CPT Assistant Summer 92:22, Fall 95:3, May 96:11, Jul 10:10, May 12:13, Jan 13:15, Mar 14:4, 12, Apr 16:3, Feb 18:10

(For unusual or complicated excision, add modifier 22)

11440 Excision, other benign lesion including margins, except skin tag (unless listed elsewhere), face, ears, eyelids, nose, lips, mucous membrane; excised diameter 0.5 cm or less

CPT Changes: An Insider's View 2003

CPT Assistant Summer 92:22, Fall 95:3, May 96:11, Jul 08:5, Jul 10:10, May 12:13, Mar 14:4, 12, Apr 16:3, Feb 18:10

11441 excised diameter 0.6 to 1.0 cm

CPT Changes: An Insider's View 2003

CPT Assistant Summer 92:22, Fall 95:3, May 96:11, Jul 10:10, May 12:13, Mar 14:4, 12, Apr 16:3, Feb 18:10

11442 excised diameter 1.1 to 2.0 cm

CPT Changes: An Insider's View 2003

CPT Assistant Summer 92:22, Fall 95:3, May 96:11, Aug 00:5, Jun 08:14, Jul 10:10, May 12:13, Mar 14:4, 12, Apr 16:3, Feb 18:10

11443 excised diameter 2.1 to 3.0 cm

CPT Changes: An Insider's View 2003

CPT Assistant Summer 92:22, Fall 95:3, May 96:11, Jul 10:10, May 12:13, Mar 14:4, 12, Apr 16:3, Feb 18:10

11444 excised diameter 3.1 to 4.0 cm

CPT Changes: An Insider's View 2003

CPT Assistant Summer 92:22, Fall 95:3, May 96:11, Jul 10:10, May 12:13, Mar 14:4, 12, Apr 16:3, Feb 18:10

11446 excised diameter over 4.0 cm

CPT Changes: An Insider's View 2003

CPT Assistant Summer 92:22, Fall 95:3, May 96:11, Aug 06:10, Jul 08:5, Apr 10:3, Jul 10:10, May 12:13, Mar 14:4, 12, Apr 16:3, Feb 18:10

(For unusual or complicated excision, add modifier 22)

(For eyelids involving more than skin, see also 67800 et seq)

11450 Excision of skin and subcutaneous tissue for hidradenitis, axillary; with simple or intermediate repair

CPT Assistant May 12:13, Aug 16:9, Feb 18:10

11451 with complex repair

CPT Assistant May 12:13, Aug 16:9, Feb 18:10

11462 Excision of skin and subcutaneous tissue for hidradenitis, inguinal; with simple or intermediate repair

CPT Assistant May 12:13, Aug 16:9, Feb 18:10

11463 with complex repair

CPT Assistant May 12:13, Aug 16:9, Feb 18:10

11470 Excision of skin and subcutaneous tissue for hidradenitis, perianal, perineal, or umbilical; with simple or intermediate repair

CPT Assistant May 12:13, Aug 16:9, Feb 18:10

11471 with complex repair

CPT Assistant May 12:13, Aug 16:9, Feb 18:10

(When skin graft or flap is used for closure, use appropriate procedure code in addition)

(For bilateral procedure, add modifier 50)

Excision—Malignant Lesions

Excision (including simple closure) of malignant lesions of skin (eg, basal cell carcinoma, squamous cell carcinoma, melanoma) includes local anesthesia. (See appropriate size and body area below.) For destruction of malignant lesions of skin, see destruction codes 17260-17286.

Excision is defined as full-thickness (through the dermis) removal of a lesion including margins, and includes simple (non-layered) closure when performed. Report separately each malignant lesion excised. Code selection is determined by measuring the greatest clinical diameter of the apparent lesion plus that margin required for complete excision (lesion diameter plus the most narrow margins required equals the excised diameter). The margins refer to the most narrow margin required to adequately excise the lesion, based on the physician's judgment. The measurement of lesion plus margin is made prior to excision. The excised diameter is the same whether the surgical defect is repaired in a linear fashion, or reconstructed (eg, with a skin graft).

The closure of defects created by incision, excision, or trauma may require intermediate or complex closure. Repair by intermediate or complex closure should be reported separately. For excision of malignant lesions requiring more than simple closure, ie, requiring intermediate or complex closure, report 11600-11646 in addition to appropriate intermediate (12031-12057) or complex closure (13100-13153) codes. For reconstructive closure, see 15002-15261, 15570-15770. For excision performed in conjunction with adjacent tissue transfer, report only the adjacent tissue transfer code (14000-14302). Excision of lesion (11600-11646) is not separately reportable with adjacent tissue transfer. See page 88 for the definition of *intermediate* or *complex* closure.

When frozen section pathology shows the margins of excision were not adequate, an additional excision may be necessary for complete tumor removal. Use only one code to report the additional excision and re-excision(s) based on the final widest excised diameter required for complete tumor removal at the same operative session. To report a re-excision procedure performed to widen margins at a subsequent operative session, see codes 11600-11646, as appropriate. Append modifier 58 if the re-excision procedure is performed during the postoperative period of the primary excision procedure.

11600 Excision, malignant lesion including margins, trunk, arms, or legs; excised diameter 0.5 cm or less

CPT Changes: An Insider's View 2003

CPT Assistant Fall 95:3, May 96:11, Nov 02:5, Oct 04:4, Feb 08:8, Feb 10:3, Apr 10:3, May 12:13, Jul 12:12, Mar 14:4, 12

Measuring and Coding the Removal of a Lesion

11600

Example: Excision, malignant lesion, 0.4 cm. Code 11600.

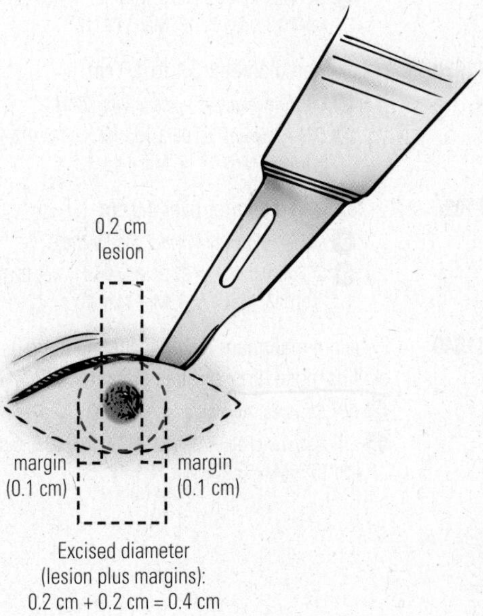

Integumentary 10021-19499

11601 excised diameter 0.6 to 1.0 cm
➔ *CPT Changes: An Insider's View* 2003
➔ *CPT Assistant* Fall 95:3, May 96:11, Nov 02:5, Feb 10:3, Mar 12:7, May 12:13, Jul 12:12, Mar 14:4, 12

11602 excised diameter 1.1 to 2.0 cm
➔ *CPT Changes: An Insider's View* 2003
➔ *CPT Assistant* Fall 95:3, May 96:11, Nov 02:5, Feb 08:8, Feb 10:3, Apr 10:3, Mar 12:4, May 12:13, Jul 12:12, Mar 14:4, 12

11603 excised diameter 2.1 to 3.0 cm
➔ *CPT Changes: An Insider's View* 2003
➔ *CPT Assistant* Fall 95:3, May 96:11, Nov 02:5, Feb 08:8, Feb 10:3, May 12:13, Jul 12:12, Mar 14:4, 12

11604 excised diameter 3.1 to 4.0 cm
➔ *CPT Changes: An Insider's View* 2003
➔ *CPT Assistant* Fall 95:3, May 96:11, Nov 02:5, Feb 08:8, Feb 10:3, May 12:13, Jul 12:12, Mar 14:4, 12

11606 excised diameter over 4.0 cm
➔ *CPT Changes: An Insider's View* 2003
➔ *CPT Assistant* Fall 91:6, Fall 95:3, May 96:11, Nov 02:5, Feb 08:8, Feb 10:3, May 12:13, Jul 12:12, Mar 14:4, 12

11620 Excision, malignant lesion including margins, scalp, neck, hands, feet, genitalia; excised diameter 0.5 cm or less
➔ *CPT Changes: An Insider's View* 2003
➔ *CPT Assistant* Fall 95:3, Nov 02:5, Oct 04:4, Feb 08:8, Feb 10:3, May 12:13, Jul 12:12, Mar 14:4, 12

11621 excised diameter 0.6 to 1.0 cm
➔ *CPT Changes: An Insider's View* 2003
➔ *CPT Assistant* Fall 95:3, May 96:11, Nov 02:5, Feb 08:8, Feb 10:3, May 12:13, Mar 14:4, 12

11622 excised diameter 1.1 to 2.0 cm
➔ *CPT Changes: An Insider's View* 2003
➔ *CPT Assistant* Fall 95:3, May 96:11, Nov 02:5, Feb 08:8, Feb 10:3, May 12:13, Mar 14:4, 12

11623 excised diameter 2.1 to 3.0 cm
➔ *CPT Changes: An Insider's View* 2003
➔ *CPT Assistant* Fall 95:3, May 96:11, Nov 02:5, Feb 08:8, Feb 10:3, May 12:13, Mar 14:4, 12

11624 excised diameter 3.1 to 4.0 cm
➔ *CPT Changes: An Insider's View* 2003
➔ *CPT Assistant* Fall 95:3, May 96:11, Nov 02:5, Feb 08:8, Feb 10:3, May 12:13, Mar 14:4, 12

11626 excised diameter over 4.0 cm
➔ *CPT Changes: An Insider's View* 2003
➔ *CPT Assistant* Fall 95:3, May 96:11, Nov 02:5, Feb 08:8, Feb 10:3, May 12:13, Mar 14:4, 12

11640 Excision, malignant lesion including margins, face, ears, eyelids, nose, lips; excised diameter 0.5 cm or less
➔ *CPT Changes: An Insider's View* 2003
➔ *CPT Assistant* Fall 95:3, May 96:11, Nov 02:5, Oct 04:4, Feb 08:8, Feb 10:3, May 12:13, Mar 14:4, 12

11641 excised diameter 0.6 to 1.0 cm
➔ *CPT Changes: An Insider's View* 2003
➔ *CPT Assistant* Fall 95:3, May 96:11, Feb 08:8, Feb 10:3, May 12:13, Mar 14:4, 12

11642 excised diameter 1.1 to 2.0 cm
➔ *CPT Changes: An Insider's View* 2003
➔ *CPT Assistant* Fall 95:3, May 96:11, Feb 08:8, Feb 10:3, May 12:13, Mar 14:4, 12

11643 excised diameter 2.1 to 3.0 cm
➔ *CPT Changes: An Insider's View* 2003
➔ *CPT Assistant* Fall 95:3, May 96:11, Feb 08:8, Feb 10:3, May 12:13, Mar 14:4, 12

11644 excised diameter 3.1 to 4.0 cm
➔ *CPT Changes: An Insider's View* 2003
➔ *CPT Assistant* Fall 95:3, May 96:11, Feb 08:8, Feb 10:3, May 12:13, Mar 14:4, 12

11646 excised diameter over 4.0 cm
➔ *CPT Changes: An Insider's View* 2003
➔ *CPT Assistant* Fall 95:3, May 96:11, Feb 08:8, Feb 10:3, Apr 10:3, May 12:13, Mar 14:4, 12

(For eyelids involving more than skin, see also 67800 et seq)

Nails

(For drainage of paronychia or onychia, see 10060, 10061)

11719 Trimming of nondystrophic nails, any number
➔ *CPT Assistant* Nov 97:12, Dec 02:4

11720 Debridement of nail(s) by any method(s); 1 to 5
➔ *CPT Assistant* Nov 96:3, Dec 02:4

11721 6 or more
➔ *CPT Assistant* Nov 96:3, Dec 02:4

11730 Avulsion of nail plate, partial or complete, simple; single
➔ *CPT Assistant* Mar 96:10, Dec 02:4, Dec 03:11

+ 11732 each additional nail plate (List separately in addition to code for primary procedure)
➔ *CPT Assistant* Dec 02:4

(Use 11732 in conjunction with 11730)

Lateral Nail View
11719-11765

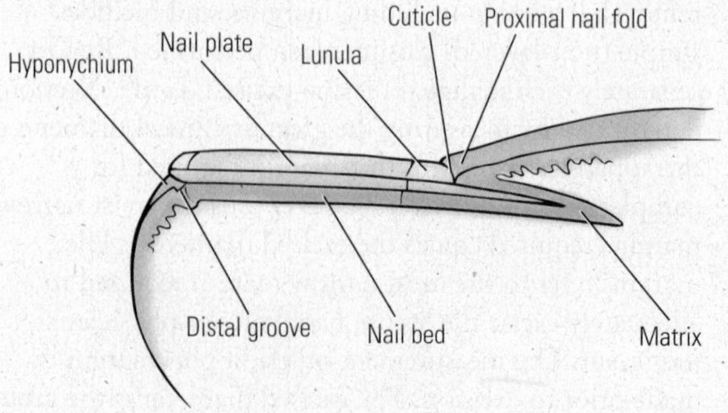

11740 Evacuation of subungual hematoma
➔ *CPT Assistant* Dec 02:4

11750 Excision of nail and nail matrix, partial or complete (eg, ingrown or deformed nail), for permanent removal
➔ *CPT Assistant* Dec 02:4

(11752 has been deleted. To report, see 26236, 28124, 28160)

(For pinch graft, use 15050)

11755 Biopsy of nail unit (eg, plate, bed, matrix, hyponychium, proximal and lateral nail folds) (separate procedure)
➔ *CPT Changes: An Insider's View* 2002
➔ *CPT Assistant* Mar 96:11, Dec 02:4, Oct 04:14

11760 Repair of nail bed
➔ *CPT Assistant* Dec 02:4

11762 Reconstruction of nail bed with graft
➔ *CPT Assistant* Dec 02:4

11765 Wedge excision of skin of nail fold (eg, for ingrown toenail)
➔ *CPT Assistant* Dec 02:4

Dorsal Nail View
11719-11765

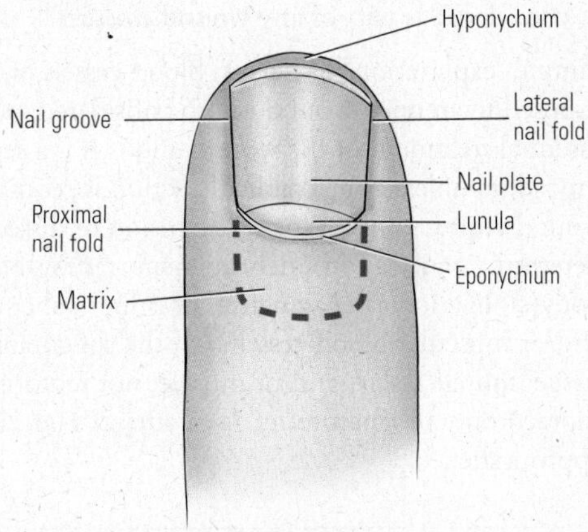

Pilonidal Cyst

11770 Excision of pilonidal cyst or sinus; simple

11771 extensive

11772 complicated
➔ *CPT Assistant* Sep 15:12

(For incision of pilonidal cyst, see 10080, 10081)

Introduction

11900 Injection, intralesional; up to and including 7 lesions
➔ *CPT Assistant* Sep 96:5, May 98:10, Nov 99:8, Feb 00:11, Sep 04:12, Nov 13:14

11901 more than 7 lesions
➔ *CPT Assistant* Sep 96:5, May 98:10, Nov 99:8, Feb 00:11, Sep 04:12

(11900, 11901 are not to be used for preoperative local anesthetic injection)

(For veins, see 36470, 36471)

(For intralesional chemotherapy administration, see 96405, 96406)

11920 Tattooing, intradermal introduction of insoluble opaque pigments to correct color defects of skin, including micropigmentation; 6.0 sq cm or less
➔ *CPT Assistant* Aug 16:9

11921 6.1 to 20.0 sq cm
➔ *CPT Assistant* Aug 16:9

+ 11922 each additional 20.0 sq cm, or part thereof (List separately in addition to code for primary procedure)
➔ *CPT Changes: An Insider's View* 2009

(Use 11922 in conjunction with 11921)

11950 Subcutaneous injection of filling material (eg, collagen); 1 cc or less
➔ *CPT Assistant* Jun 12:15

11951 1.1 to 5.0 cc
➔ *CPT Assistant* Jun 12:15

11952 5.1 to 10.0 cc
➔ *CPT Assistant* Jun 12:15

11954 over 10.0 cc
➔ *CPT Assistant* Jun 12:15

11960 Insertion of tissue expander(s) for other than breast, including subsequent expansion
➔ *CPT Assistant* Winter 91:2

(For breast reconstruction with tissue expander(s), use 19357)

11970 Replacement of tissue expander with permanent prosthesis
➔ *CPT Assistant* Aug 05:1, Jan 13:15

11971 Removal of tissue expander(s) without insertion of prosthesis
➔ *CPT Assistant* Jun 05:11

11976 Removal, implantable contraceptive capsules

11980 Subcutaneous hormone pellet implantation (implantation of estradiol and/or testosterone pellets beneath the skin)
➔ *CPT Changes: An Insider's View* 2000
➔ *CPT Assistant* Nov 99:8

11981 Insertion, non-biodegradable drug delivery implant
➔ *CPT Changes: An Insider's View* 2002
➔ *CPT Assistant* Apr 11:12

11982 Removal, non-biodegradable drug delivery implant
➔ *CPT Changes: An Insider's View* 2002

11983 Removal with reinsertion, non-biodegradable drug delivery implant
➔ *CPT Changes: An Insider's View* 2002

Integumentary 10021-19499

Repair (Closure)

Use the codes in this section to designate wound closure utilizing sutures, staples, or tissue adhesives (eg, 2-cyanoacrylate), either singly or in combination with each other, or in combination with adhesive strips. Wound closure utilizing adhesive strips as the sole repair material should be coded using the appropriate E/M code.

Definitions

The repair of wounds may be classified as Simple, Intermediate, or Complex.

Simple repair is used when the wound is superficial; eg, involving primarily epidermis or dermis, or subcutaneous tissues without significant involvement of deeper structures, and requires simple one layer closure. This includes local anesthesia and chemical or electrocauterization of wounds not closed.

Intermediate repair includes the repair of wounds that, in addition to the above, require layered closure of one or more of the deeper layers of subcutaneous tissue and superficial (non-muscle) fascia, in addition to the skin (epidermal and dermal) closure. Single-layer closure of heavily contaminated wounds that have required extensive cleaning or removal of particulate matter also constitutes intermediate repair.

Complex repair includes the repair of wounds requiring more than layered closure, viz., scar revision, debridement (eg, traumatic lacerations or avulsions), extensive undermining, stents or retention sutures. Necessary preparation includes creation of a limited defect for repairs or the debridement of complicated lacerations or avulsions. Complex repair does not include excision of benign (11400-11446) or malignant (11600-11646) lesions, excisional preparation of a wound bed (15002-15005) or debridement of an open fracture or open dislocation.

Instructions for listing services at time of wound repair:

1. The repaired wound(s) should be measured and recorded in centimeters, whether curved, angular, or stellate.
2. When multiple wounds are repaired, add together the lengths of those in the same classification (see above) and from all anatomic sites that are grouped together into the same code descriptor. For example, add together the lengths of intermediate repairs to the trunk and extremities. Do not add lengths of repairs from different groupings of anatomic sites (eg, face and extremities). Also, do not add together lengths of different classifications (eg, intermediate and complex repairs).

   When more than one classification of wounds is repaired, list the more complicated as the primary procedure and the less complicated as the secondary procedure, using modifier 59.
3. Decontamination and/or debridement: Debridement is considered a separate procedure only when gross contamination requires prolonged cleansing, when appreciable amounts of devitalized or contaminated tissue are removed, or when debridement is carried out separately without immediate primary closure.

   (For extensive debridement of soft tissue and/or bone, not associated with open fracture(s) and/or dislocation(s) resulting from penetrating and/or blunt trauma, see 11042-11047.)

   (For extensive debridement of subcutaneous tissue, muscle fascia, muscle, and/or bone associated with open fracture(s) and/or dislocation(s), see 11010-11012.)
4. Involvement of nerves, blood vessels and tendons: Report under appropriate system (Nervous, Cardiovascular, Musculoskeletal) for repair of these structures. The repair of these associated wounds is included in the primary procedure unless it qualifies as a complex repair, in which case modifier 59 applies.

   Simple ligation of vessels in an open wound is considered as part of any wound closure.

Simple "exploration" of nerves, blood vessels or tendons exposed in an open wound is also considered part of the essential treatment of the wound and is not a separate procedure unless appreciable dissection is required. If the wound requires enlargement, extension of dissection (to determine penetration), debridement, removal of foreign body(s), ligation or coagulation of minor subcutaneous and/or muscular blood vessel(s) of the subcutaneous tissue, muscle fascia, and/or muscle, not requiring thoracotomy or laparotomy, use codes 20100-20103, as appropriate.

Repair—Simple

Sum of lengths of repairs for each group of anatomic sites.

12001 Simple repair of superficial wounds of scalp, neck, axillae, external genitalia, trunk and/or extremities (including hands and feet); 2.5 cm or less

CPT Assistant Jun 96:7, Feb 98:11, Jan 00:11, Feb 00:10, Apr 00:8, Jul 00:10, Jan 02:10, Feb 07:10, Feb 08:8, Mar 12:5, Dec 17:15

12002 2.6 cm to 7.5 cm

CPT Assistant Feb 00:10, Jan 02:10, Feb 08:8, Oct 14:14

12004 7.6 cm to 12.5 cm

CPT Assistant Feb 00:10, Jan 02:10, Feb 08:8

12005 12.6 cm to 20.0 cm

CPT Assistant Feb 00:10, Jan 02:10, Feb 08:8

12006 20.1 cm to 30.0 cm
➲ *CPT Assistant* Feb 98:11, Feb 00:10, Jan 02:10, Feb 08:8

12007 over 30.0 cm
➲ *CPT Assistant* Feb 00:10, Jan 02:10, Feb 08:8

12011 Simple repair of superficial wounds of face, ears, eyelids, nose, lips and/or mucous membranes; 2.5 cm or less
➲ *CPT Assistant* Feb 00:10, May 00:8, Jan 02:10, Feb 08:8, May 14:5

12013 2.6 cm to 5.0 cm
➲ *CPT Assistant* Feb 00:10, Jan 02:10, Feb 08:8

12014 5.1 cm to 7.5 cm
➲ *CPT Assistant* Feb 00:10, Jan 02:10, Feb 08:8

12015 7.6 cm to 12.5 cm
➲ *CPT Assistant* Feb 00:10, Jan 02:10, Feb 08:8

12016 12.6 cm to 20.0 cm
➲ *CPT Assistant* Feb 00:10, Jan 02:10, Feb 08:8

12017 20.1 cm to 30.0 cm
➲ *CPT Assistant* Feb 00:10, Jan 02:10, Feb 08:8

12018 over 30.0 cm
➲ *CPT Assistant* Feb 00:10, Jan 02:10, Feb 07:10, Feb 08:8, May 14:5

12020 Treatment of superficial wound dehiscence; simple closure
➲ *CPT Assistant* Feb 00:10, Jan 02:10, Feb 08:8

12021 with packing
➲ *CPT Assistant* Feb 00:10, Jan 02:10, Feb 08:8

(For extensive or complicated secondary wound closure, use 13160)

Repair—Intermediate

Sum of lengths of repairs for each group of anatomic sites.

12031 Repair, intermediate, wounds of scalp, axillae, trunk and/or extremities (excluding hands and feet); 2.5 cm or less
➲ *CPT Changes: An Insider's View* 2009
➲ *CPT Assistant* Sep 97:11, Feb 00:10, Apr 00:8, Jan 02:10, Aug 06:1, Feb 07:10, Apr 10:3

12032 2.6 cm to 7.5 cm
➲ *CPT Changes: An Insider's View* 2009
➲ *CPT Assistant* May 96:6, Jun 96:8, Feb 00:10, Jan 02:10, Feb 07:10

12034 7.6 cm to 12.5 cm
➲ *CPT Changes: An Insider's View* 2009
➲ *CPT Assistant* Fall 91:6, Feb 00:10, Jan 02:10, Feb 07:10

12035 12.6 cm to 20.0 cm
➲ *CPT Changes: An Insider's View* 2009
➲ *CPT Assistant* Feb 00:10, Jan 02:10, Feb 07:10

12036 20.1 cm to 30.0 cm
➲ *CPT Changes: An Insider's View* 2009
➲ *CPT Assistant* Feb 00:10, Jan 02:10, Feb 07:10

12037 over 30.0 cm
➲ *CPT Changes: An Insider's View* 2009
➲ *CPT Assistant* Feb 00:10, Jan 02:10, Feb 07:10

12041 Repair, intermediate, wounds of neck, hands, feet and/or external genitalia; 2.5 cm or less
➲ *CPT Changes: An Insider's View* 2009
➲ *CPT Assistant* Sep 97:11, Feb 00:10, Apr 00:8, Jan 02:10, Feb 07:10, Jan 13:15

12042 2.6 cm to 7.5 cm
➲ *CPT Changes: An Insider's View* 2009
➲ *CPT Assistant* Feb 00:10, Apr 00:9, Jan 02:10, Feb 07:10, Jan 13:15

12044 7.6 cm to 12.5 cm
➲ *CPT Changes: An Insider's View* 2009
➲ *CPT Assistant* Feb 00:10, Jan 02:10, Feb 07:10, Jan 13:15

12045 12.6 cm to 20.0 cm
➲ *CPT Changes: An Insider's View* 2009
➲ *CPT Assistant* Feb 00:10, Jan 02:10, Feb 07:10, Jan 13:15

12046 20.1 cm to 30.0 cm
➲ *CPT Changes: An Insider's View* 2009
➲ *CPT Assistant* Feb 00:10, Jan 02:10, Feb 07:10, Jan 13:15

12047 over 30.0 cm
➲ *CPT Changes: An Insider's View* 2009
➲ *CPT Assistant* Feb 00:10, Jan 02:10, Feb 07:10, Jan 13:15

12051 Repair, intermediate, wounds of face, ears, eyelids, nose, lips and/or mucous membranes; 2.5 cm or less
➲ *CPT Changes: An Insider's View* 2009
➲ *CPT Assistant* Sep 97:11, Feb 00:10, Apr 00:8, Jan 02:10, Feb 07:10, May 14:5

12052 2.6 cm to 5.0 cm
➲ *CPT Changes: An Insider's View* 2009
➲ *CPT Assistant* Feb 00:10, Aug 00:9, Jan 02:10, Feb 07:10, Jul 08:5

12053 5.1 cm to 7.5 cm
➲ *CPT Changes: An Insider's View* 2009
➲ *CPT Assistant* Feb 00:10, Jan 02:10, Feb 07:10

12054 7.6 cm to 12.5 cm
➲ *CPT Changes: An Insider's View* 2009
➲ *CPT Assistant* Feb 00:10, Jan 02:10, Feb 07:10

12055 12.6 cm to 20.0 cm
➲ *CPT Changes: An Insider's View* 2009
➲ *CPT Assistant* Feb 00:10, Jan 02:10, Feb 07:10

12056 20.1 cm to 30.0 cm
➲ *CPT Changes: An Insider's View* 2009
➲ *CPT Assistant* Feb 00:10, Jan 02:10, Feb 07:10

12057 over 30.0 cm
➲ *CPT Changes: An Insider's View* 2009
➲ *CPT Assistant* Feb 00:10, Jan 02:10, Feb 07:10, Apr 10:3, May 14:5

Repair—Complex

Reconstructive procedures, complicated wound closure.

Sum of lengths of repairs for each group of anatomic sites.

(For full thickness repair of lip or eyelid, see respective anatomical subsections)

13100 Repair, complex, trunk; 1.1 cm to 2.5 cm

➲ *CPT Assistant* Sep 97:11, Dec 98:5, Nov 99:9-10, Feb 00:10, Apr 00:8, Feb 10:3, Apr 10:3, May 11:4, Jan 12:8, Dec 12:6, Apr 17:9

(For 1.0 cm or less, see simple or intermediate repairs)

13101 2.6 cm to 7.5 cm

➲ *CPT Assistant* Dec 98:5, Nov 99:9-10, Feb 00:10, Apr 00:9, Feb 10:3, May 11:4, Jan 12:8, Dec 12:6, Apr 17:9

+ 13102 each additional 5 cm or less (List separately in addition to code for primary procedure)

➲ *CPT Changes: An Insider's View* 2000

➲ *CPT Assistant* Nov 99:9-10, Feb 00:10, Apr 00:9, Feb 10:3, May 11:4, Jan 12:8, Dec 12:6, Apr 17:9

(Use 13102 in conjunction with 13101)

13120 Repair, complex, scalp, arms, and/or legs; 1.1 cm to 2.5 cm

➲ *CPT Assistant* Sep 97:11, Apr 99:11, Nov 99:9-10, Feb 00:10, Apr 00:8, Feb 10:3, May 11:4, Jan 12:8, Dec 12:6

(For 1.0 cm or less, see simple or intermediate repairs)

13121 2.6 cm to 7.5 cm

➲ *CPT Assistant* Dec 98:5, Nov 99:9-10, Feb 00:10, Feb 10:3, Apr 10:3, May 11:4, Jan 12:8, Dec 12:6

+ 13122 each additional 5 cm or less (List separately in addition to code for primary procedure)

➲ *CPT Changes: An Insider's View* 2000

➲ *CPT Assistant* Nov 99:10, Feb 10:3, May 11:4, Jan 12:8, Dec 12:6

(Use 13122 in conjunction with 13121)

13131 Repair, complex, forehead, cheeks, chin, mouth, neck, axillae, genitalia, hands and/or feet; 1.1 cm to 2.5 cm

➲ *CPT Assistant* Fall 93:7, Sep 97:11, Dec 98:5, Nov 99:10, Feb 00:10, Apr 00:8, Feb 10:3, May 11:4, Jan 12:8, Dec 12:6, Jan 13:15, Apr 17:9

(For 1.0 cm or less, see simple or intermediate repairs)

13132 2.6 cm to 7.5 cm

➲ *CPT Assistant* Fall 93:7, Dec 98:5, Nov 99:10, Dec 99:10, Feb 00:10, Apr 00:9, Aug 00:9, Feb 10:3, May 11:4, Jan 12:8, Dec 12:6, Jan 13:15, Oct 14:14, Apr 17:9

+ 13133 each additional 5 cm or less (List separately in addition to code for primary procedure)

➲ *CPT Changes: An Insider's View* 2000

➲ *CPT Assistant* Fall 93:7, Feb 00:10, Apr 00:9, Feb 10:3, May 11:4, Jan 12:8, Dec 12:6, Jan 13:15, Apr 17:9

(Use 13133 in conjunction with 13132)

(For 1.0 cm or less, see simple or intermediate repairs)

13151 Repair, complex, eyelids, nose, ears and/or lips; 1.1 cm to 2.5 cm

➲ *CPT Changes: An Insider's View* 2014

➲ *CPT Assistant* Dec 98:5, Nov 99:10, Feb 00:10, Feb 10:3, May 11:4, Jan 12:8, Dec 12:6, Mar 14:12, May 14:3, 5

13152 2.6 cm to 7.5 cm

➲ *CPT Changes: An Insider's View* 2014

➲ *CPT Assistant* Dec 98:5, Nov 99:10, Feb 00:10, Feb 10:3, May 11:4, Jan 12:8, Dec 12:6, May 14:3, Oct 14:14

+ 13153 each additional 5 cm or less (List separately in addition to code for primary procedure)

➲ *CPT Changes: An Insider's View* 2000, 2014

➲ *CPT Assistant* Nov 99:10, Feb 00:10, Feb 10:3, Apr 10:3, May 11:4, Jan 12:8, Dec 12:6, May 14:3, 5

(Use 13153 in conjunction with 13152)

13160 Secondary closure of surgical wound or dehiscence, extensive or complicated

➲ *CPT Assistant* Sep 97:11, Dec 98:5, Apr 00:8, May 11:4, Dec 12:6

(For packing or simple secondary wound closure, see 12020, 12021)

Adjacent Tissue Transfer or Rearrangement

For full thickness repair of lip or eyelid, see respective anatomical subsections.

Codes 14000-14302 are used for excision (including lesion) and/or repair by adjacent tissue transfer or rearrangement (eg, Z-plasty, W-plasty, V-Y plasty, rotation flap, random island flap, advancement flap). When applied in repairing lacerations, the procedures listed must be performed by the surgeon to accomplish the repair. They do not apply to direct closure or rearrangement of traumatic wounds incidentally resulting in these configurations. Undermining alone of adjacent tissues to achieve closure, without additional incisions, does not constitute adjacent tissue transfer, see complex repair codes 13100-13160. The excision of a benign lesion (11400-11446) or a malignant lesion (11600-11646) is not separately reportable with codes 14000-14302.

Skin graft necessary to close secondary defect is considered an additional procedure. For purposes of code selection, the term "defect" includes the primary and secondary defects. The primary defect resulting from the excision and the secondary defect resulting from flap design to perform the reconstruction are measured together to determine the code.

14000 Adjacent tissue transfer or rearrangement, trunk; defect 10 sq cm or less

➲ *CPT Assistant* Sep 96:11, Jul 99:3, Jul 00:10, Jan 06:47, Dec 06:15, Jul 08:5, Mar 10:4, Apr 10:3, Jan 12:8, May 12:13, Nov 12:13, Dec 12:6, Apr 14:10, Feb 15:10, Sep 15:12, Oct 17:9

14001 defect 10.1 sq cm to 30.0 sq cm

➔ *CPT Assistant* Aug 96:8, Jul 99:3, Jan 06:47, Dec 06:15, Jul 08:5, Mar 10:4, Jan 12:8, May 12:13, Nov 12:13, Dec 12:6, Apr 14:10, Feb 15:10, Oct 17:9

14020 Adjacent tissue transfer or rearrangement, scalp, arms and/or legs; defect 10 sq cm or less

➔ *CPT Assistant* Jul 99:3, Jan 06:47, Dec 06:15, Jul 08:5, Mar 10:4, Jan 12:8, May 12:13, Nov 12:13, Dec 12:6

14021 defect 10.1 sq cm to 30.0 sq cm

➔ *CPT Assistant* Jul 99:3, Jan 06:47, Dec 06:15, Jul 08:5, Mar 10:4, Jan 12:8, May 12:13, Nov 12:13, Dec 12:6

14040 Adjacent tissue transfer or rearrangement, forehead, cheeks, chin, mouth, neck, axillae, genitalia, hands and/or feet; defect 10 sq cm or less

➔ *CPT Assistant* Jul 99:3, Jul 00:10, Jan 06:47, Dec 06:15, Jul 08:5, Mar 10:4, Jan 12:8, May 12:13, Nov 12:13, Dec 12:6

14041 defect 10.1 sq cm to 30.0 sq cm

➔ *CPT Assistant* Jul 99:3, Jan 06:47, Dec 06:15, Jul 08:5, Mar 10:4, Jan 12:8, May 12:13, Nov 12:13, Dec 12:6

14060 Adjacent tissue transfer or rearrangement, eyelids, nose, ears and/or lips; defect 10 sq cm or less

➔ *CPT Assistant* Fall 93:7, Jul 99:3, Jan 06:47, Dec 06:15, Jul 08:5, Mar 10:4, Jan 12:8, May 12:13, Aug 12:13, Nov 12:13, Dec 12:6

14061 defect 10.1 sq cm to 30.0 sq cm

➔ *CPT Assistant* Jul 99:3, Jan 06:47, Dec 06:15, Jul 08:5, Mar 10:4, Jan 12:8, May 12:13, Nov 12:13, Dec 12:6

(For eyelid, full thickness, see 67961 et seq)

14301 Adjacent tissue transfer or rearrangement, any area; defect 30.1 sq cm to 60.0 sq cm

➔ *CPT Changes: An Insider's View* 2010

➔ *CPT Assistant* May 12:13, Nov 12:13, Dec 12:6, Apr 17:9

+ 14302 each additional 30.0 sq cm, or part thereof (List separately in addition to code for primary procedure)

➔ *CPT Changes: An Insider's View* 2010

➔ *CPT Assistant* May 12:13, Nov 12:13, Dec 12:6

(Use 14302 in conjunction with 14301)

14350 Filleted finger or toe flap, including preparation of recipient site

➔ *CPT Assistant* Jan 06:47, Jul 08:5, Mar 10:4, May 12:13, Dec 12:6

Skin Replacement Surgery

Skin replacement surgery consists of ***surgical preparation*** and topical placement of an ***autograft*** (including tissue cultured autograft) or ***skin substitute graft*** (ie, homograft, allograft, xenograft). The graft is anchored using the individual's choice of fixation. When services are performed in the office, routine dressing supplies are not reported separately.

The following definition should be applied to those codes that reference "100 sq cm or 1% of body area of infants and children" when determining the involvement of body

Adjacent Tissue Repairs

14000-14061

Repair of primary and secondary defects requires assignment of a code based upon the location and the approximate description (as demonstrated below) of the area required.

A. Advancement Flap

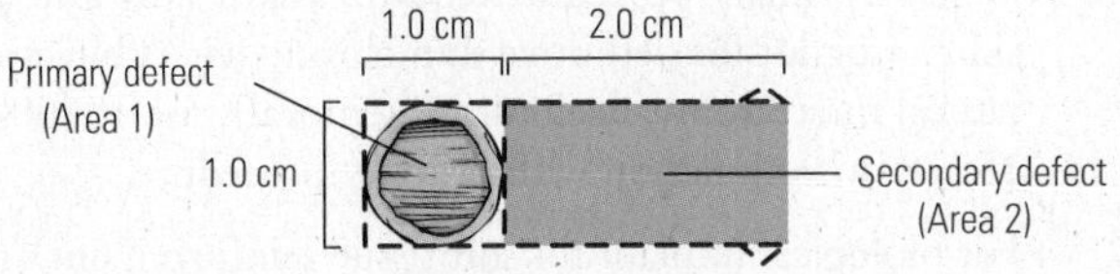

Area 1: 1.0 cm x 1.0 cm = 1.0 sq cm
Area 2: 1.0 cm x 2.0 cm = 2.0 sq cm
(Area 1) + (Area 2) = 1.0 sq cm + 2.0 sq cm = 3.0 sq cm

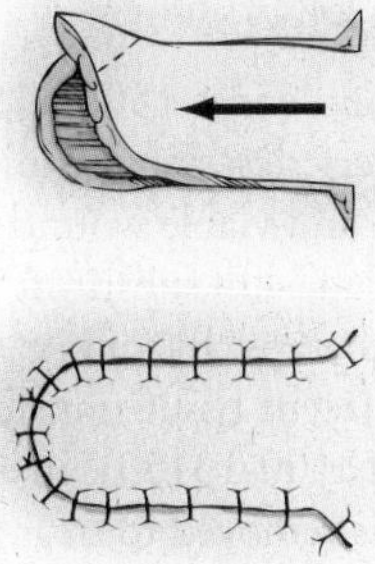

B. Rotation Flap

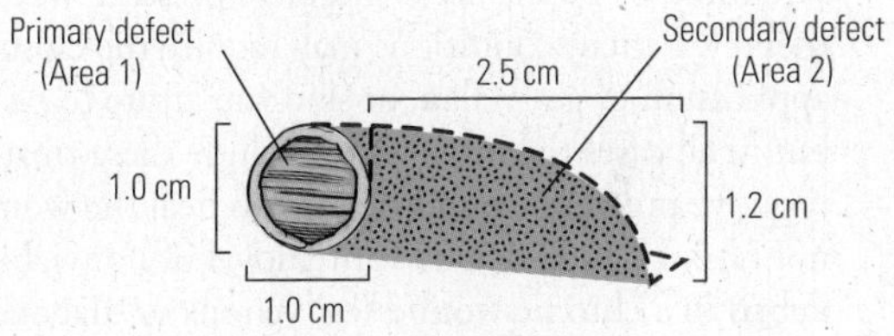

Area 1: 1.0 cm x 1.0 cm = 1.0 sq cm
Area 2: 2.5 cm x 1.2 cm = 3.0 sq cm
(Area 1) + (Area 2) = 1.0 sq cm + 3.0 sq cm = 4.0 sq cm

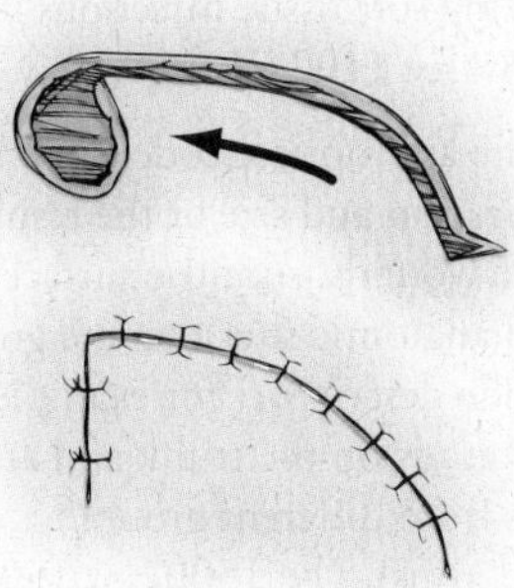

size: The measurement of 100 sq cm is applicable to adults and children 10 years of age and older; and percentages of body surface area apply to infants and children younger than 10 years of age. The measurements apply to the size of the recipient area.

Procedures involving wrist and/or ankle are reported with codes that include arm or leg in the descriptor.

When a primary procedure requires a skin substitute or skin autograft for definitive skin closure (eg, orbitectomy, radical mastectomy, deep tumor removal), use 15100-15278 in conjunction with primary procedure.

For biological implant for soft tissue reinforcement, use 15777 in conjunction with primary procedure.

The supply of skin substitute graft(s) should be reported separately in conjunction with 15271-15278.

Definitions

Surgical preparation codes 15002-15005 for skin replacement surgery describe the initial services related to preparing a clean and viable wound surface for placement of an autograft, flap, skin substitute graft or for negative pressure wound therapy. In some cases, closure may be possible using adjacent tissue transfer (14000-14061) or complex repair (13100-13153). In all cases, appreciable nonviable tissue is removed to treat a burn, traumatic wound or a necrotizing infection. The clean wound bed may also be created by incisional release of a scar contracture resulting in a surface defect from separation of tissues. The intent is to heal the wound by primary intention, or by the use of negative pressure wound therapy. Patient conditions may require the closure or application of graft, flap, or skin substitute to be delayed, but in all cases the intent is to include these treatments or negative pressure wound therapy to heal the wound. Do not report 15002-15005 for removal of nonviable tissue/debris in a chronic wound (eg, venous or diabetic) when the wound is left to heal by secondary intention. See active wound management codes (97597, 97598) and debridement codes (11042-11047) for this service. For necrotizing soft tissue infections in specific anatomic locations, see 11004-11008.

Select the appropriate code from 15002-15005 based upon location and size of the resultant defect. For multiple wounds, sum the surface area of all wounds from all anatomic sites that are grouped together into the same code descriptor. For example, sum the surface area of all wounds on the trunk and arms. Do not sum wounds from different groupings of anatomic sites (eg, face and arms). Use 15002 or 15004, as appropriate, for excisions and incisional releases resulting in wounds up to and including 100 sq cm of surface area. Use 15003 or 15005 for each additional 100 sq cm or part thereof. For example: Surgical preparation of a 20 sq cm wound on the right hand and a 15 sq cm wound on the left hand would be reported with a single code, 15004. Surgical preparation of a 75 sq cm wound on the right thigh and a 75 sq cm wound on the left thigh would be reported with 15002 for the first 100 sq cm and 15003 for the second 50 sq cm. If all four wounds required surgical preparation on the same day, use modifier 59 with 15002, and 15004.

Autografts/tissue cultured autografts include the harvest and/or application of an autologous skin graft. Repair of donor site requiring skin graft or local flaps is reported separately. Removal of current graft and/or simple cleansing of the wound is included, when performed. Do not report 97602. Debridement is considered a separate procedure only when gross contamination requires prolonged cleansing, when appreciable amounts of devitalized or contaminated tissue are removed, or when debridement is carried out separately without immediate primary closure.

Select the appropriate code from 15040-15261 based upon type of autograft and location and size of the defect. The measurements apply to the size of the recipient area. For multiple wounds, sum the surface area of all wounds from all anatomic sites that are grouped together into the same code descriptor. For example, sum the surface area of all wounds on the trunk and arms. Do not sum wounds from different groupings of anatomic sites (eg, face and arms).

►***Skin substitute grafts*** include non-autologous human skin (dermal or epidermal, cellular and acellular) grafts (eg, homograft, allograft), non-human skin substitute grafts (ie, xenograft), and biological products that form a sheet scaffolding for skin growth. These codes are not to be reported for application of non-graft wound dressings (eg, gel, powder, ointment, foam, liquid) or injected skin substitutes. Application of non-graft wound dressings is not separately reportable. Removal of current graft and/or simple cleansing of the wound is included, when performed. Do not report 97602. Debridement is considered a separate procedure only when gross contamination requires prolonged cleansing, when appreciable amounts of devitalized or contaminated tissue are removed, or when debridement is carried out separately without immediate primary closure.

Select the appropriate code from 15271-15278 based upon location and size of the defect. For multiple wounds, sum the surface area of all wounds from all anatomic sites that are grouped together into the same code descriptor. For example, sum the surface area of all wounds on the trunk and arms. Do not sum wounds from different groupings of anatomic sites (eg, face and arms). The supply of skin substitute graft(s) should be reported separately in conjunction with 15271, 15272, 15273, 15274, 15275, 15276, 15277, 15278. For biologic implant for soft tissue reinforcement, use 15777 in conjunction with code for primary procedure.◄

Surgical Preparation

15002 Surgical preparation or creation of recipient site by excision of open wounds, burn eschar, or scar (including subcutaneous tissues), or incisional release of scar contracture, trunk, arms, legs; first 100 sq cm or 1% of body area of infants and children

CPT Changes: An Insider's View 2007

CPT Assistant Jan 12:6, Oct 12:13, Dec 12:6, Feb 13:16, Mar 14:12, Oct 16:3

(For linear scar revision, see 13100-13153)

+ 15003 each additional 100 sq cm, or part thereof, or each additional 1% of body area of infants and children (List separately in addition to code for primary procedure)

CPT Changes: An Insider's View 2007, 2009

CPT Assistant Jan 12:6, Oct 12:13, Feb 13:16, Mar 14:12, Oct 16:3

(Use 15003 in conjunction with 15002)

15004 Surgical preparation or creation of recipient site by excision of open wounds, burn eschar, or scar (including subcutaneous tissues), or incisional release of scar contracture, face, scalp, eyelids, mouth, neck, ears, orbits, genitalia, hands, feet and/or multiple digits; first 100 sq cm or 1% of body area of infants and children

CPT Changes: An Insider's View 2007

CPT Assistant Jan 12:6, Oct 12:13, Feb 13:16, Mar 14:12, Oct 16:3

+ 15005 each additional 100 sq cm, or part thereof, or each additional 1% of body area of infants and children (List separately in addition to code for primary procedure)

CPT Changes: An Insider's View 2007, 2009

CPT Assistant Jan 12:6, Oct 12:13, Feb 13:16, Mar 14:12, Oct 16:3

(Use 15005 in conjunction with 15004)

Autografts/Tissue Cultured Autograft

15040 Harvest of skin for tissue cultured skin autograft, 100 sq cm or less

CPT Changes: An Insider's View 2006

CPT Assistant Aug 06:10, Oct 06:1, Feb 08:3, Apr 10:3, Jan 12:6

15050 Pinch graft, single or multiple, to cover small ulcer, tip of digit, or other minimal open area (except on face), up to defect size 2 cm diameter

CPT Assistant Apr 97:4, Sep 97:2, Nov 98:6, Jan 12:6, Jun 16:8

15100 Split-thickness autograft, trunk, arms, legs; first 100 sq cm or less, or 1% of body area of infants and children (except 15050)

CPT Changes: An Insider's View 2002, 2006

CPT Assistant Fall 93:7, Apr 97:4, Aug 97:6, Sep 97:3, Nov 98:6, Sep 02:3, Oct 06:1, Feb 08:3, Mar 11:9, Jan 12:6, Oct 12:3, Jun 16:8

+ 15101 each additional 100 sq cm, or each additional 1% of body area of infants and children, or part thereof (List separately in addition to code for primary procedure)

CPT Changes: An Insider's View 2002

CPT Assistant Apr 97:4, Nov 98:6, Sep 02:3, Feb 08:3, Mar 11:9, Jan 12:6, Oct 12:3, Jun 16:8

(Use 15101 in conjunction with 15100)

15110 Epidermal autograft, trunk, arms, legs; first 100 sq cm or less, or 1% of body area of infants and children

CPT Changes: An Insider's View 2006

CPT Assistant Feb 08:3, Mar 11:9, Jan 12:6, Oct 12:3

+ 15111 each additional 100 sq cm, or each additional 1% of body area of infants and children, or part thereof (List separately in addition to code for primary procedure)

CPT Changes: An Insider's View 2006

CPT Assistant Feb 08:3, Mar 11:9, Jan 12:6, Oct 12:3

(Use 15111 in conjunction with 15110)

15115 Epidermal autograft, face, scalp, eyelids, mouth, neck, ears, orbits, genitalia, hands, feet, and/or multiple digits; first 100 sq cm or less, or 1% of body area of infants and children

CPT Changes: An Insider's View 2006

CPT Assistant Feb 08:3, Mar 11:9, Jan 12:6, Oct 12:3

+ 15116 each additional 100 sq cm, or each additional 1% of body area of infants and children, or part thereof (List separately in addition to code for primary procedure)

CPT Changes: An Insider's View 2006

CPT Assistant Feb 08:3, Mar 11:9, Jan 12:6, Oct 12:3

(Use 15116 in conjunction with 15115)

15120 Split-thickness autograft, face, scalp, eyelids, mouth, neck, ears, orbits, genitalia, hands, feet, and/or multiple digits; first 100 sq cm or less, or 1% of body area of infants and children (except 15050)

CPT Changes: An Insider's View 2002, 2006

CPT Assistant Apr 97:4, Aug 97:6, Sep 97:3, Nov 98:6, Jan 99:4, Sep 02:3, Feb 08:3, Jul 08:5, Mar 11:9, Jan 12:6, Oct 12:3, Jun 16:8

+ 15121 each additional 100 sq cm, or each additional 1% of body area of infants and children, or part thereof (List separately in addition to code for primary procedure)

CPT Changes: An Insider's View 2002

CPT Assistant Apr 97:4, Aug 97:6, Sep 97:3, Nov 98:6, Jan 99:4, Sep 02:3, Feb 08:3, Mar 11:9, Jan 12:6, Oct 12:3, Jun 16:8

(Use 15121 in conjunction with 15120)

(For eyelids, see also 67961-67975)

15130 Dermal autograft, trunk, arms, legs; first 100 sq cm or less, or 1% of body area of infants and children

CPT Changes: An Insider's View 2006

CPT Assistant Feb 08:3, Mar 11:9, Jan 12:6, Oct 12:3

+ 15131 each additional 100 sq cm, or each additional 1% of body area of infants and children, or part thereof (List separately in addition to code for primary procedure)
CPT Changes: An Insider's View 2006
CPT Assistant Feb 08:3, Mar 11:9, Jan 12:6, Oct 12:3

(Use 15131 in conjunction with 15130)

15135 Dermal autograft, face, scalp, eyelids, mouth, neck, ears, orbits, genitalia, hands, feet, and/or multiple digits; first 100 sq cm or less, or 1% of body area of infants and children
CPT Changes: An Insider's View 2006
CPT Assistant Feb 08:3, Mar 11:9, Jan 12:6, Oct 12:3

+ 15136 each additional 100 sq cm, or each additional 1% of body area of infants and children, or part thereof (List separately in addition to code for primary procedure)
CPT Changes: An Insider's View 2006
CPT Assistant Mar 11:9, Jan 12:6, Oct 12:3

(Use 15136 in conjunction with 15135)

15150 Tissue cultured skin autograft, trunk, arms, legs; first 25 sq cm or less
CPT Changes: An Insider's View 2006, 2012
CPT Assistant Oct 06:1, Feb 08:3, Mar 11:9, Jan 12:6, Oct 12:3

+ 15151 additional 1 sq cm to 75 sq cm (List separately in addition to code for primary procedure)
CPT Changes: An Insider's View 2006, 2012
CPT Assistant Oct 06:1, Feb 08:3, Mar 11:9, Jan 12:6, Oct 12:3

(Do not report 15151 more than once per session)

(Use 15151 in conjunction with 15150)

+ 15152 each additional 100 sq cm, or each additional 1% of body area of infants and children, or part thereof (List separately in addition to code for primary procedure)
CPT Changes: An Insider's View 2006, 2012
CPT Assistant Oct 06:1, Feb 08:3, Mar 11:9, Jan 12:6, Oct 12:3

(Use 15152 in conjunction with 15151)

15155 Tissue cultured skin autograft, face, scalp, eyelids, mouth, neck, ears, orbits, genitalia, hands, feet, and/or multiple digits; first 25 sq cm or less
CPT Changes: An Insider's View 2006, 2012
CPT Assistant Oct 06:1, Feb 08:3, Mar 11:9, Jan 12:6, Oct 12:3

+ 15156 additional 1 sq cm to 75 sq cm (List separately in addition to code for primary procedure)
CPT Changes: An Insider's View 2006, 2012
CPT Assistant Oct 06:1, Feb 08:3, Mar 11:9, Jan 12:6, Oct 12:3

(Do not report 15156 more than once per session)

(Use 15156 in conjunction with 15155)

+ 15157 each additional 100 sq cm, or each additional 1% of body area of infants and children, or part thereof (List separately in addition to code for primary procedure)
CPT Changes: An Insider's View 2006, 2012
CPT Assistant Oct 06:1, Feb 08:3, Apr 10:3, Mar 11:9, Jan 12:6, Oct 12:3

(Use 15157 in conjunction with 15156)

15200 Full thickness graft, free, including direct closure of donor site, trunk; 20 sq cm or less
CPT Changes: An Insider's View 2002
CPT Assistant Aug 96:11, Aug 97:6, Sep 97:3, Feb 08:3, Mar 08:14, Jan 12:6, Oct 12:3, Jun 16:8

+ 15201 each additional 20 sq cm, or part thereof (List separately in addition to code for primary procedure)
CPT Changes: An Insider's View 2002, 2009
CPT Assistant Apr 97:4, Aug 97:6, Sep 97:3, Feb 08:3, Mar 08:14, Jan 12:6, Oct 12:3, Jun 16:8

(Use 15201 in conjunction with 15200)

15220 Full thickness graft, free, including direct closure of donor site, scalp, arms, and/or legs; 20 sq cm or less
CPT Changes: An Insider's View 2002
CPT Assistant Apr 97:4, Aug 97:6, Sep 97:3, Aug 98:9, Feb 08:3, Mar 08:14, Jan 12:6, Oct 12:3, Jun 16:8

+ 15221 each additional 20 sq cm, or part thereof (List separately in addition to code for primary procedure)
CPT Changes: An Insider's View 2002, 2009
CPT Assistant Apr 97:4, Aug 97:6, Sep 97:3, Aug 98:9, Feb 08:3, Mar 08:14, Jan 12:6, Oct 12:3, Jun 16:8

(Use 15221 in conjunction with 15220)

15240 Full thickness graft, free, including direct closure of donor site, forehead, cheeks, chin, mouth, neck, axillae, genitalia, hands, and/or feet; 20 sq cm or less
CPT Changes: An Insider's View 2002
CPT Assistant Apr 97:4, Aug 97:6, Sep 97:3, Nov 00:10, Feb 08:3, Mar 08:14, Jan 12:6, Oct 12:3, Jun 16:8

(For fingertip graft, use 15050)

(For repair of syndactyly, fingers, see 26560-26562)

+ 15241 each additional 20 sq cm, or part thereof (List separately in addition to code for primary procedure)
CPT Changes: An Insider's View 2002, 2009
CPT Assistant Apr 97:4, Aug 97:6, Sep 97:3, Feb 08:3, Mar 08:14, Jan 12:6, Oct 12:3, Jun 16:8

(Use 15241 in conjunction with 15240)

15260 Full thickness graft, free, including direct closure of donor site, nose, ears, eyelids, and/or lips; 20 sq cm or less
CPT Changes: An Insider's View 2002
CPT Assistant Fall 91:7, Fall 93:7, Apr 97:4, Aug 97:6, Sep 97:3, Jul 99:3, Feb 08:3, Mar 08:14, Jan 12:6, Oct 12:3, Jun 16:8

+ 15261 each additional 20 sq cm, or part thereof (List separately in addition to code for primary procedure)
CPT Changes: An Insider's View 2002, 2009
CPT Assistant Fall 91:7, Apr 97:4, Aug 97:6, Sep 97:3, Feb 08:3, Mar 08:14, Apr 10:3, Jan 12:6, Oct 12:3, Jun 16:8

(Use 15261 in conjunction with 15260)

(For eyelids, see also 67961-67975)

(Repair of donor site requiring skin graft or local flaps is considered a separate procedure)

Skin Substitute Grafts

The supply of skin substitute graft(s) should be reported separately in conjunction with 15271-15278. For biologic implant for soft tissue reinforcement, use 15777 in conjunction with code for primary procedure.

15271 Application of skin substitute graft to trunk, arms, legs, total wound surface area up to 100 sq cm; first 25 sq cm or less wound surface area
- *CPT Changes: An Insider's View* 2012
- *CPT Assistant* Jan 12:6, Oct 12:3, Jun 14:14, Oct 17:9

+ 15272 each additional 25 sq cm wound surface area, or part thereof (List separately in addition to code for primary procedure)
- *CPT Changes: An Insider's View* 2012
- *CPT Assistant* Jan 12:6, Oct 12:3, Oct 13:15, Jun 14:14

(Use 15272 in conjunction with 15271)

(For total wound surface area greater than or equal to 100 sq cm, see 15273, 15274)

(Do not report 15271, 15272 in conjunction with 15273, 15274)

15273 Application of skin substitute graft to trunk, arms, legs, total wound surface area greater than or equal to 100 sq cm; first 100 sq cm wound surface area, or 1% of body area of infants and children
- *CPT Changes: An Insider's View* 2012
- *CPT Assistant* Jan 12:6, Oct 12:3, Oct 13:15, Nov 13:14, Jun 14:14

+ 15274 each additional 100 sq cm wound surface area, or part thereof, or each additional 1% of body area of infants and children, or part thereof (List separately in addition to code for primary procedure)
- *CPT Changes: An Insider's View* 2012
- *CPT Assistant* Jan 12:6, Oct 12:3, Oct 13:15, Nov 13:14, Jun 14:14

(Use 15274 in conjunction with 15273)

(For total wound surface area up to 100 sq cm, see 15271, 15272)

15275 Application of skin substitute graft to face, scalp, eyelids, mouth, neck, ears, orbits, genitalia, hands, feet, and/or multiple digits, total wound surface area up to 100 sq cm; first 25 sq cm or less wound surface area
- *CPT Changes: An Insider's View* 2012
- *CPT Assistant* Jan 12:6, Oct 12:3, Oct 13:15, Jun 14:14

+ 15276 each additional 25 sq cm wound surface area, or part thereof (List separately in addition to code for primary procedure)
- *CPT Changes: An Insider's View* 2012
- *CPT Assistant* Jan 12:6, Oct 12:3, Oct 13:15, Jun 14:14

(Use 15276 in conjunction with 15275)

(For total wound surface area greater than or equal to 100 sq cm, see 15277, 15278)

(Do not report 15275, 15276 in conjunction with 15277, 15278)

15277 Application of skin substitute graft to face, scalp, eyelids, mouth, neck, ears, orbits, genitalia, hands, feet, and/or multiple digits, total wound surface area greater than or equal to 100 sq cm; first 100 sq cm wound surface area, or 1% of body area of infants and children
- *CPT Changes: An Insider's View* 2012
- *CPT Assistant* Jan 12:6, Oct 12:3, Oct 13:15, Nov 13:14, Jun 14:14

+ 15278 each additional 100 sq cm wound surface area, or part thereof, or each additional 1% of body area of infants and children, or part thereof (List separately in addition to code for primary procedure)
- *CPT Changes: An Insider's View* 2012
- *CPT Assistant* Jan 12:6, Oct 12:3, Oct 13:15, Nov 13:14, Jun 14:14

(Use 15278 in conjunction with 15277)

(For total wound surface area up to 100 sq cm, see 15275, 15276)

(Do not report 15271-15278 in conjunction with 97602)

Flaps (Skin and/or Deep Tissues)

The regions listed refer to the recipient area (not the donor site) when a flap is being attached in a transfer or to a final site.

The regions listed refer to a donor site when a tube is formed for later transfer or when a "delay" of flap occurs prior to the transfer. Codes 15733-15738 are described by donor site of the muscle, myocutaneous, or fasciocutaneous flap.

Codes 15570-15738 do not include extensive immobilization (eg, large plaster casts and other immobilizing devices are considered additional separate procedures).

A repair of a donor site requiring a skin graft or local flaps is considered an additional separate procedure.

(For microvascular flaps, see 15756-15758)

(For flaps without inclusion of a vascular pedicle, see 15570-15576)

(For adjacent tissue transfer flaps, see 14000-14302)

15570 Formation of direct or tubed pedicle, with or without transfer; trunk
- *CPT Assistant* Nov 02:7, Mar 10:4, Apr 10:3, Dec 12:6

15572 scalp, arms, or legs
- *CPT Assistant* Mar 10:4, Dec 12:6

15574 forehead, cheeks, chin, mouth, neck, axillae, genitalia, hands or feet
- *CPT Assistant* Mar 10:4, Dec 12:6

Integumentary 10021-19499

15576 eyelids, nose, ears, lips, or intraoral
➔ *CPT Assistant* Mar 10:4, Dec 12:6

15600 Delay of flap or sectioning of flap (division and inset); at trunk
➔ *CPT Assistant* Nov 99:10, Mar 10:4, Dec 12:6

15610 at scalp, arms, or legs
➔ *CPT Assistant* Mar 10:4, Dec 12:6

15620 at forehead, cheeks, chin, neck, axillae, genitalia, hands, or feet
➔ *CPT Assistant* Mar 10:4, Dec 12:6

15630 at eyelids, nose, ears, or lips
➔ *CPT Assistant* Mar 10:4, Dec 12:6

15650 Transfer, intermediate, of any pedicle flap (eg, abdomen to wrist, Walking tube), any location
➔ *CPT Assistant* Mar 10:4, Dec 12:6

(For eyelids, nose, ears, or lips, see also anatomical area)

(For revision, defatting or rearranging of transferred pedicle flap or skin graft, see 13100-14302)

15730 Midface flap (ie, zygomaticofacial flap) with preservation of vascular pedicle(s)
➔ *CPT Changes: An Insider's View* 2018
➔ *CPT Assistant* Nov 17:6, Apr 18:10

Midface Flap Surgery
15730

Midface muscles surrounding eye [skin and muscle flap procedures]

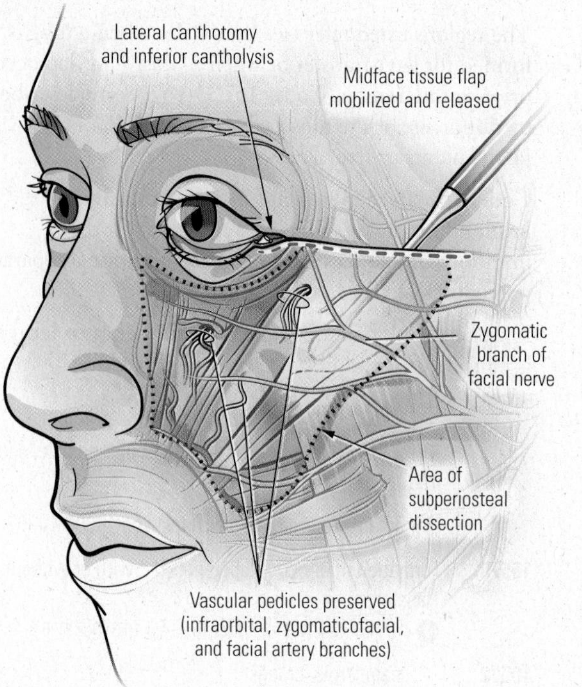

15731 Forehead flap with preservation of vascular pedicle (eg, axial pattern flap, paramedian forehead flap)
➔ *CPT Changes: An Insider's View* 2007
➔ *CPT Assistant* Dec 12:6, Nov 17:6

(For muscle, myocutaneous, or fasciocutaneous flap of the head or neck, use 15733)

(15732 has been deleted. To report myocutaneous or fasciocutaneous flap, use 15733)

Axial Pattern Forehead Flap
15731

Reconstruction of a nasal defect with a forehead flap based on the left supratrochlear vessels

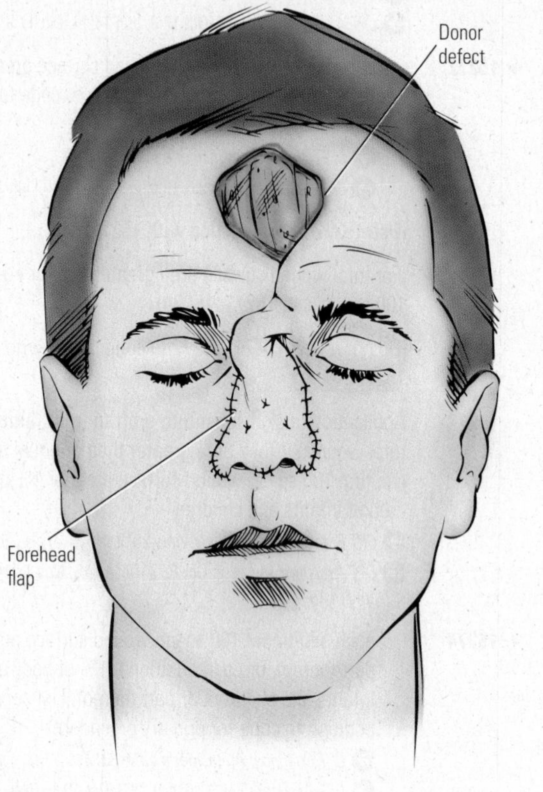

15733 Muscle, myocutaneous, or fasciocutaneous flap; head and neck with named vascular pedicle (ie, buccinators, genioglossus, temporalis, masseter, sternocleidomastoid, levator scapulae)
➔ *CPT Changes: An Insider's View* 2018
➔ *CPT Assistant* Nov 17:6, Apr 18:10

(For forehead flap with preservation of vascular pedicle, use 15731)

(For anterior pericranial flap on named vascular pedicle, for repair of extracranial defect, use 15731)

(For repair of head and neck defects using non-axial pattern advancement flaps [including lesion] and/or repair by adjacent tissue transfer or rearrangement [eg, Z-plasty, W-plasty, V-Y plasty, rotation flap, random island flap, advancement flap], see 14040, 14041, 14060, 14061, 14301, 14302)

15734 trunk
CPT Changes: An Insider's View 2018
CPT Assistant Dec 12:6, Oct 13:15, Apr 14:10, Nov 17:6

15736 upper extremity
CPT Changes: An Insider's View 2018
CPT Assistant Dec 12:6, Mar 13:13, Nov 17:6

15738 lower extremity
CPT Changes: An Insider's View 2018
CPT Assistant Sep 03:15, Apr 10:3, Dec 12:6, Nov 17:6

Other Flaps and Grafts

Code 15740 describes a cutaneous flap, transposed into a nearby but not immediately adjacent defect, with a pedicle that incorporates an anatomically named axial vessel into its design. The flap is typically transferred through a tunnel underneath the skin and sutured into its new position. The donor site is closed directly.

Neurovascular pedicle procedures are reported with 15750. This code includes not only skin but also a functional motor or sensory nerve(s). The flap serves to reinnervate a damaged portion of the body dependent on touch or movement (eg, thumb).

Repair of donor site requiring skin graft or local flaps should be reported as an additional procedure.

For random island flaps, V-Y subcutaneous flaps, advancement flaps, and other flaps from adjacent areas without clearly defined anatomically named axial vessels, see 14000-14302.

15740 Flap; island pedicle requiring identification and dissection of an anatomically named axial vessel
CPT Changes: An Insider's View 2013
CPT Assistant Mar 04:11, Sep 04:12, Oct 04:15, Apr 10:3, Dec 12:6, Dec 17:14

15750 neurovascular pedicle
CPT Assistant Dec 17:14

15756 Free muscle or myocutaneous flap with microvascular anastomosis
CPT Changes: An Insider's View 2003
CPT Assistant Apr 97:5, Nov 97:12, Nov 98:6

(Do not report code 69990 in addition to code 15756)

15757 Free skin flap with microvascular anastomosis
CPT Assistant Apr 97:5, Nov 98:6, Apr 16:8

(Do not report code 69990 in addition to code 15757)

15758 Free fascial flap with microvascular anastomosis
CPT Assistant Apr 97:5, Nov 98:6

(Do not report code 69990 in addition to code 15758)

15760 Graft; composite (eg, full thickness of external ear or nasal ala), including primary closure, donor area
CPT Assistant Sep 97:3

15770 derma-fat-fascia
CPT Assistant Sep 97:3, Apr 10:3

15775 Punch graft for hair transplant; 1 to 15 punch grafts
CPT Assistant Sep 97:3

15776 more than 15 punch grafts
CPT Assistant Sep 97:3

(For strip transplant, use 15220)

+ 15777 Implantation of biologic implant (eg, acellular dermal matrix) for soft tissue reinforcement (ie, breast, trunk) (List separately in addition to code for primary procedure)
CPT Changes: An Insider's View 2012, 2014
CPT Assistant Jan 12:10, Oct 13:15

(For implantation of biologic implants for soft tissue reinforcement in tissues other than breast and trunk, use 17999)

(For bilateral breast procedure, report 15777 with modifier 50)

(For implantation of mesh or other prosthesis for open incisional or ventral hernia repair, use 49568 in conjunction with 49560-49566)

(For insertion of mesh or other prosthesis for closure of a necrotizing soft tissue infection wound, use 49568 in conjunction with 11004-11006)

(For topical application of skin substitute graft to a wound surface, see 15271-15278)

(For repair of anorectal fistula with plug (eg, porcine small intestine submucosa [SIS]), use 46707)

(For insertion of mesh or other prosthesis for repair of pelvic floor defect, use 57267)

(For implantation of non-biologic or synthetic implant for fascial reinforcement of the abdominal wall, use 0437T)

(The supply of biologic implant should be reported separately in conjunction with 15777)

Other Procedures

15780 Dermabrasion; total face (eg, for acne scarring, fine wrinkling, rhytids, general keratosis)
CPT Assistant Apr 03:27

15781 segmental, face

15782 regional, other than face

15783 superficial, any site (eg, tattoo removal)
CPT Assistant Apr 03:27

15786 Abrasion; single lesion (eg, keratosis, scar)

+ 15787 each additional 4 lesions or less (List separately in addition to code for primary procedure)

(Use 15787 in conjunction with 15786)

Integumentary 10021-19499

15788 Chemical peel, facial; epidermal

15789 dermal

15792 Chemical peel, nonfacial; epidermal

15793 dermal

15819 Cervicoplasty

15820 Blepharoplasty, lower eyelid;
➔ *CPT Assistant* Feb 04:11, May 04:12, Feb 05:16

15821 with extensive herniated fat pad
➔ *CPT Assistant* Feb 04:11, May 04:12, Feb 05:16

15822 Blepharoplasty, upper eyelid;
➔ *CPT Assistant* Feb 04:11, May 04:12, Feb 05:16

15823 with excessive skin weighting down lid
➔ *CPT Assistant* Sep 00:7, Feb 04:11, May 04:12, Feb 05:16, Aug 11:8

(For bilateral blepharoplasty, add modifier 50)

15824 Rhytidectomy; forehead
➔ *CPT Assistant* Apr 17:9

(For repair of brow ptosis, use 67900)

15825 neck with platysmal tightening (platysmal flap, P-flap)
➔ *CPT Assistant* Apr 17:9

15826 glabellar frown lines

15828 cheek, chin, and neck

15829 superficial musculoaponeurotic system (SMAS) flap

(For bilateral rhytidectomy, add modifier 50)

15830 Excision, excessive skin and subcutaneous tissue (includes lipectomy); abdomen, infraumbilical panniculectomy
➔ *CPT Changes: An Insider's View* 2007

(Do not report 15830 in conjunction with 12031-12037, 13100-13102, 14000, 14001, 14302 for the same wound)

15832 thigh

15833 leg

15834 hip

15835 buttock

15836 arm

15837 forearm or hand

15838 submental fat pad

15839 other area

(For bilateral procedure, add modifier 50)

15840 Graft for facial nerve paralysis; free fascia graft (including obtaining fascia)

(For bilateral procedure, add modifier 50)

15841 free muscle graft (including obtaining graft)

15842 free muscle flap by microsurgical technique
➔ *CPT Changes: An Insider's View* 2001

(Do not report code 69990 in addition to code 15842)

15845 regional muscle transfer

(For intravenous fluorescein examination of blood flow in graft or flap, use 15860)

(For nerve transfers, decompression, or repair, see 64831-64876, 64905, 64907, 69720, 69725, 69740, 69745, 69955)

+ 15847 Excision, excessive skin and subcutaneous tissue (includes lipectomy), abdomen (eg, abdominoplasty) (includes umbilical transposition and fascial plication) (List separately in addition to code for primary procedure)
➔ *CPT Changes: An Insider's View* 2007

(Use 15847 in conjunction with 15830)

(For abdominal wall hernia repair, see 49491-49587)

(To report other abdominoplasty, use 17999)

15850 Removal of sutures under anesthesia (other than local), same surgeon
➔ *CPT Assistant* Spring 93:34, Nov 97:22

15851 Removal of sutures under anesthesia (other than local), other surgeon
➔ *CPT Assistant* Spring 93:34, Nov 97:22

15852 Dressing change (for other than burns) under anesthesia (other than local)

15860 Intravenous injection of agent (eg, fluorescein) to test vascular flow in flap or graft
➔ *CPT Changes: An Insider's View* 2002

15876 Suction assisted lipectomy; head and neck

15877 trunk
➔ *CPT Assistant* Oct 99:10, Feb 05:14

15878 upper extremity

15879 lower extremity

(Do not report 15876, 15877, 15878, 15879 in conjunction with 0489T, 0490T)

(For harvesting of adipose tissue for autologous adipose-derived regenerative cell therapy, see 0489T, 0490T)

Pressure Ulcers (Decubitus Ulcers)

15920 Excision, coccygeal pressure ulcer, with coccygectomy; with primary suture

15922 with flap closure

15931 Excision, sacral pressure ulcer, with primary suture;

15933 with ostectomy

15934 Excision, sacral pressure ulcer, with skin flap closure;

15935 with ostectomy

15936 Excision, sacral pressure ulcer, in preparation for muscle or myocutaneous flap or skin graft closure;
➔ *CPT Assistant* Nov 98:6-7

15937 with ostectomy

(For repair of defect using muscle or myocutaneous flap, use code(s) 15734 and/or 15738 in addition to 15936, 15937. For repair of defect using split skin graft, use codes 15100 and/or 15101 in addition to 15936, 15937)

15940 Excision, ischial pressure ulcer, with primary suture;

15941 with ostectomy (ischiectomy)

15944 Excision, ischial pressure ulcer, with skin flap closure;

15945 with ostectomy

15946 Excision, ischial pressure ulcer, with ostectomy, in preparation for muscle or myocutaneous flap or skin graft closure
➔ *CPT Assistant* Nov 98:6-7, Jun 02:10, Jan 03:23

(For repair of defect using muscle or myocutaneous flap, use code(s) 15734 and/or 15738 in addition to 15946. For repair of defect using split skin graft, use codes 15100 and/or 15101 in addition to 15946)

15950 Excision, trochanteric pressure ulcer, with primary suture;

15951 with ostectomy

15952 Excision, trochanteric pressure ulcer, with skin flap closure;

15953 with ostectomy

15956 Excision, trochanteric pressure ulcer, in preparation for muscle or myocutaneous flap or skin graft closure;
➔ *CPT Assistant* Nov 98:6-7

15958 with ostectomy
➔ *CPT Assistant* Nov 98:6-7

(For repair of defect using muscle or myocutaneous flap, use code(s) 15734 and/or 15738 in addition to 15956, 15958. For repair of defect using split skin graft, use codes 15100 and/or 15101 in addition to 15956, 15958)

15999 Unlisted procedure, excision pressure ulcer

(For free skin graft to close ulcer or donor site, see 15002 et seq)

Burns, Local Treatment

Procedures 16000-16036 refer to local treatment of burned surface only. Codes 16020-16030 include the application of materials (eg, dressings) not described in codes 15100-15278.

List percentage of body surface involved and depth of burn.

For necessary related medical services (eg, hospital visits, detention) in management of burned patients, see appropriate services in **Evaluation and Management** and **Medicine** sections.

For the application of skin grafts or skin substitutes, see codes 15100-15777.

(For fractional ablative laser fenestration for functional improvement of traumatic or burn scars, see 0479T, 0480T)

16000 Initial treatment, first degree burn, when no more than local treatment is required
➔ *CPT Assistant* Aug 97:6, Oct 12:3

16020 Dressings and/or debridement of partial-thickness burns, initial or subsequent; small (less than 5% total body surface area)
➔ *CPT Changes: An Insider's View* 2006
➔ *CPT Assistant* Aug 97:6, Oct 12:3

16025 medium (eg, whole face or whole extremity, or 5% to 10% total body surface area)
➔ *CPT Changes: An Insider's View* 2006
➔ *CPT Assistant* Aug 97:6, Jun 08:14, Oct 12:3

16030 large (eg, more than 1 extremity, or greater than 10% total body surface area)
➔ *CPT Changes: An Insider's View* 2006
➔ *CPT Assistant* Aug 97:6, Jun 08:14, Oct 12:3

16035 Escharotomy; initial incision
➔ *CPT Changes: An Insider's View* 2001
➔ *CPT Assistant* Aug 97:6, Oct 12:3

+ 16036 each additional incision (List separately in addition to code for primary procedure)
➔ *CPT Changes: An Insider's View* 2001
➔ *CPT Assistant* Oct 12:3

(Use 16036 in conjunction with 16035)

(For debridement, curettement of burn wound, see 16020-16030)

Destruction

Destruction means the ablation of benign, premalignant or malignant tissues by any method, with or without curettement, including local anesthesia, and not usually requiring closure.

Any method includes electrosurgery, cryosurgery, laser and chemical treatment. Lesions include condylomata, papillomata, molluscum contagiosum, herpetic lesions, warts (ie, common, plantar, flat), milia, or other benign, premalignant (eg, actinic keratoses), or malignant lesions.

(For destruction of lesion(s) in specific anatomic sites, see 40820, 46900-46917, 46924, 54050-54057, 54065, 56501, 56515, 57061, 57065, 67850, 68135)

(For laser treatment for inflammatory skin disease, see 96920-96922)

(For paring or cutting of benign hyperkeratotic lesions (eg, corns or calluses), see 11055-11057)

(For sharp removal or electrosurgical destruction of skin tags and fibrocutaneous tags, see 11200, 11201)

(For cryotherapy of acne, use 17340)

Lund-Browder Diagram and Classification Method Table for Burn Estimations

The Lund-Browder Classification Method is used for estimating the extent, depth, and percentage of burns, allowing for the varying proportion of body surface in persons of different ages.

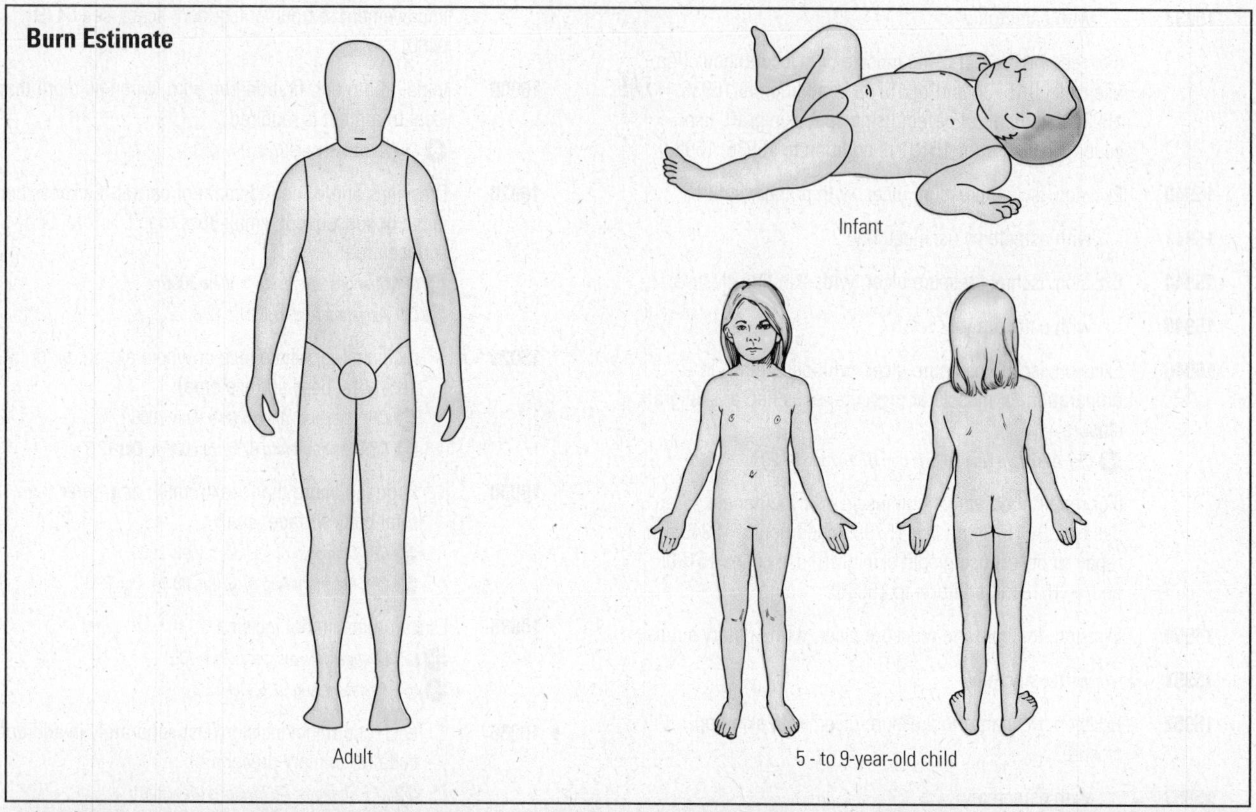

Area	Birth 1 year	1-4 years	5-9 years	10-14 years	15 years	Adult	2 degrees	3 degrees	Total	Donor areas
Head	19	17	13	11	9	7				
Neck	2	2	2	2	2	2				
Ant. trunk	13	13	13	13	13	13				
Post. trunk	13	13	13	13	13	13				
R. buttock	2 1/2	2 1/2	2 1/2	2 1/2	2 1/2	2 1/2				
L. buttock	2 1/2	2 1/2	2 1/2	2 1/2	2 1/2	2 1/2				
Genitalia	1	1	1	1	1	1				
R. U. arm	4	4	4	4	4	4				
L. U. arm	4	4	4	4	4	4				
R. L. arm	3	3	3	3	3	3				
L. L. arm	3	3	3	3	3	3				
R. hand	2 1/2	2 1/2	2 1/2	2 1/2	2 1/2	2 1/2				
L. hand	2 1/2	2 1/2	2 1/2	2 1/2	2 1/2	2 1/2				
R. thigh	5 1/2	6 1/2	8	8 1/2	9	9 1/2				
L. thigh	5 1/2	6 1/2	8	8 1/2	9	9 1/2				
R. leg	5	5	5 1/2	6	6 1/2	7				
L. leg	5	5	5 1/2	6	6 1/2	7				
R. foot	3 1/2	3 1/2	3 1/2	3 1/2	3 1/2	3 1/2				
L. foot	3 1/2	3 1/2	3 1/2	3 1/2	3 1/2	3 1/2				
Total										

(For initiation or follow-up care of topical chemotherapy (eg, 5-FU or similar agents), see appropriate office visits)

(For shaving of epidermal or dermal lesions, see 11300-11313)

(For excision of cicatricial lesion[s] [eg, full thickness excision, through the dermis], see 11400-11446)

(For incisional removal of burn scar, see 16035, 16036)

(For fractional ablative laser fenestration for functional improvement of traumatic or burn scars, see 0479T, 0480T)

Destruction, Benign or Premalignant Lesions

17000 Destruction (eg, laser surgery, electrosurgery, cryosurgery, chemosurgery, surgical curettement), premalignant lesions (eg, actinic keratoses); first lesion

➲ *CPT Changes: An Insider's View* 2002, 2007

➲ *CPT Assistant* Winter 90:3, Nov 97:12, Jun 99:10, May 06:19, Feb 07:10, Aug 09:7, Mar 10:10, Mar 12:7, May 12:13, Dec 17:14

+ 17003 second through 14 lesions, each (List separately in addition to code for first lesion)

➲ *CPT Assistant* Nov 97:12, Jun 99:10, May 06:19, Feb 07:10, Aug 09:7, Mar 10:10, Dec 17:14

(Use 17003 in conjunction with 17000)

(For destruction of common or plantar warts, see 17110, 17111)

⊘ 17004 Destruction (eg, laser surgery, electrosurgery, cryosurgery, chemosurgery, surgical curettement), premalignant lesions (eg, actinic keratoses), 15 or more lesions

➲ *CPT Changes: An Insider's View* 2002, 2007

➲ *CPT Assistant* Nov 97:12, Nov 98:7, Jun 99:10, Mar 03:21, Feb 07:10, Aug 09:7, Mar 10:10, Dec 17:14

(Do not report 17004 in conjunction with 17000-17003)

17106 Destruction of cutaneous vascular proliferative lesions (eg, laser technique); less than 10 sq cm

➲ *CPT Assistant* Winter 90:3, Apr 07:11, Jun 08:14, Aug 09:7, Dec 17:14

17107 10.0 to 50.0 sq cm

➲ *CPT Assistant* Winter 90:3, Apr 07:11, Jun 08:14, Aug 09:7, Dec 17:14

17108 over 50.0 sq cm

➲ *CPT Assistant* Winter 90:3, Apr 07:11, Jun 08:14, Aug 09:7, Dec 17:14

17110 Destruction (eg, laser surgery, electrosurgery, cryosurgery, chemosurgery, surgical curettement), of benign lesions other than skin tags or cutaneous vascular proliferative lesions; up to 14 lesions

➲ *CPT Changes: An Insider's View* 2002, 2007, 2008

➲ *CPT Assistant* Nov 97:13, Feb 07:10, Apr 07:11, Nov 08:10, Aug 09:7, Apr 16:3, Dec 17:14

Destruction, Benign or Premalignant Lesions
17004

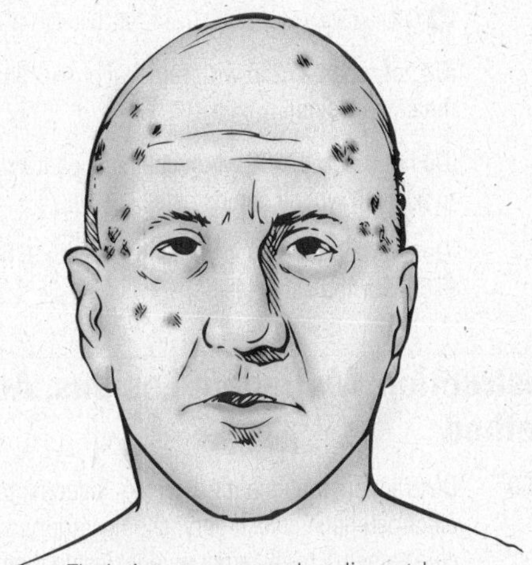

The lesions, seen as rough scaling patches scattered over the face, scalp, and ears, are destroyed by cryosurgery or other surgical means.

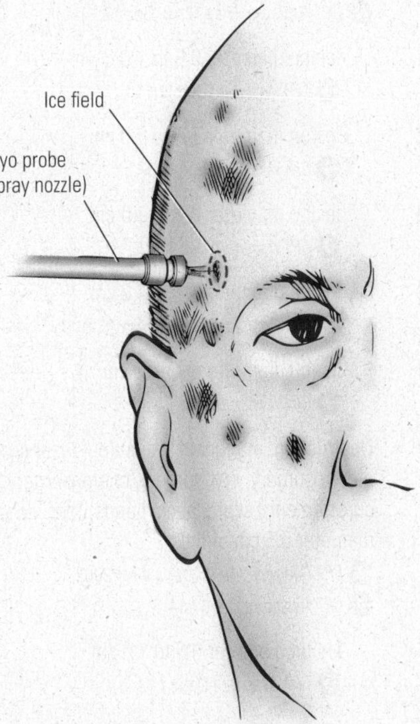

17111 15 or more lesions

➲ *CPT Assistant* Nov 97:13, Feb 07:10, Apr 07:11, Nov 08:10, Aug 09:7, Apr 16:3, Dec 17:14

(For destruction of extensive cutaneous neurofibroma over 50-100 lesions, see 0419T, 0420T)

17250 Chemical cauterization of granulation tissue (ie, proud flesh)
➲ *CPT Changes: An Insider's View* 2018
➲ *CPT Assistant* May 12:13, Dec 12:15, Dec 17:14

(Do not report 17250 with removal or excision codes for the same lesion)

(Do not report 17250 when chemical cauterization is used to achieve wound hemostasis)

(Do not report 17250 in conjunction with 97597, 97598, 97602 for the same lesion)

Destruction, Malignant Lesions, Any Method

17260 Destruction, malignant lesion (eg, laser surgery, electrosurgery, cryosurgery, chemosurgery, surgical curettement), trunk, arms or legs; lesion diameter 0.5 cm or less
➲ *CPT Changes: An Insider's View* 2002
➲ *CPT Assistant* May 12:13, Dec 17:14

17261 lesion diameter 0.6 to 1.0 cm
➲ *CPT Assistant* Dec 17:14

17262 lesion diameter 1.1 to 2.0 cm
➲ *CPT Assistant* Dec 17:14

17263 lesion diameter 2.1 to 3.0 cm
➲ *CPT Assistant* Dec 17:14

17264 lesion diameter 3.1 to 4.0 cm
➲ *CPT Assistant* Dec 17:14

17266 lesion diameter over 4.0 cm
➲ *CPT Assistant* Dec 17:14

17270 Destruction, malignant lesion (eg, laser surgery, electrosurgery, cryosurgery, chemosurgery, surgical curettement), scalp, neck, hands, feet, genitalia; lesion diameter 0.5 cm or less
➲ *CPT Changes: An Insider's View* 2002
➲ *CPT Assistant* Dec 17:14

17271 lesion diameter 0.6 to 1.0 cm
➲ *CPT Assistant* Dec 17:14

17272 lesion diameter 1.1 to 2.0 cm
➲ *CPT Assistant* Dec 17:14

17273 lesion diameter 2.1 to 3.0 cm
➲ *CPT Assistant* Dec 17:14

17274 lesion diameter 3.1 to 4.0 cm
➲ *CPT Assistant* Dec 17:14

17276 lesion diameter over 4.0 cm
➲ *CPT Assistant* Dec 17:14

17280 Destruction, malignant lesion (eg, laser surgery, electrosurgery, cryosurgery, chemosurgery, surgical curettement), face, ears, eyelids, nose, lips, mucous membrane; lesion diameter 0.5 cm or less
➲ *CPT Changes: An Insider's View* 2002
➲ *CPT Assistant* Dec 17:14

17281 lesion diameter 0.6 to 1.0 cm
➲ *CPT Assistant* Dec 17:14

17282 lesion diameter 1.1 to 2.0 cm
➲ *CPT Assistant* Dec 17:14

17283 lesion diameter 2.1 to 3.0 cm
➲ *CPT Assistant* Dec 17:14

17284 lesion diameter 3.1 to 4.0 cm
➲ *CPT Assistant* Dec 17:14

17286 lesion diameter over 4.0 cm
➲ *CPT Assistant* Dec 17:14

Mohs Micrographic Surgery

Mohs micrographic surgery is a technique for the removal of complex or ill-defined skin cancer with histologic examination of 100% of the surgical margins. It requires the integration of an individual functioning in two separate and distinct capacities: surgeon and pathologist. If either of these responsibilities is delegated to another physician or other qualified health care professional who reports the services separately, these codes should not be reported. The Mohs surgeon removes the tumor tissue and maps and divides the tumor specimen into pieces, and each piece is embedded into an individual tissue block for histopathologic examination. Thus a tissue block in Mohs surgery is defined as an individual tissue piece embedded in a mounting medium for sectioning.

►If repair is performed, use separate repair, flap, or graft codes. If a biopsy of a suspected skin cancer is performed on the same day as Mohs surgery because there was no prior pathology confirmation of a diagnosis, then report a diagnostic skin biopsy (11102, 11104, 11106) and frozen section pathology (88331) with modifier 59 to distinguish from the subsequent definitive surgical procedure of Mohs surgery.◄

(If additional special pathology procedures, stains or immunostains are required, see 88311-88314, 88342)

(Do not report 88314 in conjunction with 17311-17315 for routine frozen section stain (eg, hematoxylin and eosin, toluidine blue) performed during Mohs surgery. When a nonroutine histochemical stain on frozen tissue is utilized, report 88314 with modifier 59)

(Do not report 88302-88309 on the same specimen as part of the Mohs surgery)

17311 Mohs micrographic technique, including removal of all gross tumor, surgical excision of tissue specimens, mapping, color coding of specimens, microscopic examination of specimens by the surgeon, and histopathologic preparation including routine stain(s) (eg, hematoxylin and eosin, toluidine blue), head, neck, hands, feet, genitalia, or any location with surgery directly involving muscle, cartilage, bone, tendon, major nerves, or vessels; first stage, up to 5 tissue blocks
➲ *CPT Changes: An Insider's View* 2007
➲ *CPT Assistant* Feb 14:10, Oct 14:14

+ **17312** each additional stage after the first stage, up to 5 tissue blocks (List separately in addition to code for primary procedure)
➔ *CPT Changes: An Insider's View* 2007

(Use 17312 in conjunction with 17311)

17313 Mohs micrographic technique, including removal of all gross tumor, surgical excision of tissue specimens, mapping, color coding of specimens, microscopic examination of specimens by the surgeon, and histopathologic preparation including routine stain(s) (eg, hematoxylin and eosin, toluidine blue), of the trunk, arms, or legs; first stage, up to 5 tissue blocks
➔ *CPT Changes: An Insider's View* 2007

+ **17314** each additional stage after the first stage, up to 5 tissue blocks (List separately in addition to code for primary procedure)
➔ *CPT Changes: An Insider's View* 2007

(Use 17314 in conjunction with 17313)

+ **17315** Mohs micrographic technique, including removal of all gross tumor, surgical excision of tissue specimens, mapping, color coding of specimens, microscopic examination of specimens by the surgeon, and histopathologic preparation including routine stain(s) (eg, hematoxylin and eosin, toluidine blue), each additional block after the first 5 tissue blocks, any stage (List separately in addition to code for primary procedure)
➔ *CPT Changes: An Insider's View* 2007
➔ *CPT Assistant* May 12:13, Feb 14:10, Oct 14:14

(Use 17315 in conjunction with 17311-17314)

Other Procedures

17340 Cryotherapy (CO2 slush, liquid N2) for acne
➔ *CPT Assistant* May 12:13

17360 Chemical exfoliation for acne (eg, acne paste, acid)

17380 Electrolysis epilation, each 30 minutes

(For actinotherapy, use 96900)

17999 Unlisted procedure, skin, mucous membrane and subcutaneous tissue
➔ *CPT Assistant* Dec 98:9, May 99:11, Jun 05:11, Nov 08:10, Mar 11:9, May 12:13, Oct 13:15, May 16:13, Dec 17:13
➔ *Clinical Examples in Radiology* Winter 10:15

Breast

Incision

19000 Puncture aspiration of cyst of breast;
➔ *CPT Assistant* Fall 94:18, Apr 05:6, Nov 08:10, Dec 13:17

+ **19001** each additional cyst (List separately in addition to code for primary procedure)
➔ *CPT Assistant* Fall 94:18, Apr 05:6, Dec 13:17

(Use 19001 in conjunction with 19000)

(If imaging guidance is performed, see 76942, 77021)

19020 Mastotomy with exploration or drainage of abscess, deep
➔ *CPT Assistant* Apr 05:6, Dec 14:16

19030 Injection procedure only for mammary ductogram or galactogram
➔ *CPT Assistant* Jul 04:8, Apr 05:6

(For radiological supervision and interpretation, see 77053, 77054)

Excision

Excisional breast surgery includes certain biopsy procedures, the removal of cysts or other benign or malignant tumors or lesions, and the surgical treatment of breast and chest wall malignancies. Biopsy procedures may be percutaneous or open, and they involve the removal of differing amounts of tissue for diagnosis.

Breast biopsies, without image guidance are reported with 19100 and 19101. Image-guided breast biopsies, including the placement of localization devices when performed, are reported using codes 19081-19086. The image-guided placement of localization devices without image-guided biopsy are reported with 19281-19288. When more than one biopsy or localization device placement is performed using the same imaging modality, use an add-on code whether the additional service(s) is on the same or contra-lateral breast. If additional biopsies or localization device placements are performed using different imaging modalities, report another primary code for each additional biopsy or localization device placement performed using a different image guidance modality. When an open incisional biopsy is performed after image-guided placement of a localization device, 19101 is reported and the appropriate image-guided localization device placement code is reported. The open excision of breast lesions (eg, lesions of the breast ducts, cysts, benign or malignant tumors), without specific attention to adequate surgical margins, with or without the preoperative placement of radiological markers, is reported using codes 19110-19126. Partial mastectomy procedures (eg, lumpectomy, tylectomy, quadrantectomy, or segmentectomy) describe open excisions of breast tissue with specific attention to adequate surgical margins.

Partial mastectomy procedures are reported using codes 19301 or 19302 as appropriate. Documentation for partial mastectomy procedures includes attention to the removal of adequate surgical margins surrounding the breast mass or lesion. Intraoperative placement of clip(s) is not separately reported.

Total mastectomy procedures include simple mastectomy, complete mastectomy, subcutaneous mastectomy, modified radical mastectomy, radical mastectomy, and more extended procedures (eg, Urban type operation). Total mastectomy procedures are reported using codes 19303-19307 as appropriate. Intraoperative placement of clip(s) is not separately reported.

Excisions or resections of chest wall tumors including ribs, with or without reconstruction, with or without mediastinal lymphadenectomy, are reported using codes 19260, 19271, or 19272. Codes 19260-19272 are not restricted to breast tumors and are used to report resections of chest wall tumors originating from any chest wall component. (For excision of lung or pleura, see 32310 et seq.)

When more than one breast biopsy is performed using the same imaging modality, use an add-on code whether the additional service(s) is on the same or contra-lateral breast. If additional biopsies are performed using different imaging modalities, report another primary code for each additional modality.

To report bilateral image-guided breast biopsies, report 19081, 19083, or 19085 for the initial biopsy. The contra-lateral and each additional breast image guided biopsy are then reported with code 19082, 19084 or 19086.

(To report bilateral procedures for codes 19100-19120, report modifier 50 with the procedure code)

19081 Biopsy, breast, with placement of breast localization device(s) (eg, clip, metallic pellet), when performed, and imaging of the biopsy specimen, when performed, percutaneous; first lesion, including stereotactic guidance

- *CPT Changes: An Insider's View* 2014
- *CPT Assistant* May 14:3, Jun 14:14, Mar 15:5, May 15:8, Jun 16:3
- *Clinical Examples in Radiology* Spring 14:4, 10, Winter 17:5

+ 19082 each additional lesion, including stereotactic guidance (List separately in addition to code for primary procedure)

- *CPT Changes: An Insider's View* 2014
- *CPT Assistant* May 14:3, Jun 14:14, Mar 15:5, May 15:8, Jun 16:3
- *Clinical Examples in Radiology* Winter 17:5

(Use 19082 in conjunction with 19081)

19083 Biopsy, breast, with placement of breast localization device(s) (eg, clip, metallic pellet), when performed, and imaging of the biopsy specimen, when performed, percutaneous; first lesion, including ultrasound guidance

- *CPT Changes: An Insider's View* 2014
- *CPT Assistant* May 14:3, Jun 14:14, Mar 15:5, May 15:8, Jun 16:3
- *Clinical Examples in Radiology* Spring 14:2, 3, Winter 17:5, Spring 18:13

+ 19084 each additional lesion, including ultrasound guidance (List separately in addition to code for primary procedure)

- *CPT Changes: An Insider's View* 2014
- *CPT Assistant* May 14:3, Jun 14:14, Mar 15:5, May 15:8, Jun 16:3
- *Clinical Examples in Radiology* Spring 14:10, Winter 17:5

(Use 19084 in conjunction with 19083)

19085 Biopsy, breast, with placement of breast localization device(s) (eg, clip, metallic pellet), when performed, and imaging of the biopsy specimen, when performed, percutaneous; first lesion, including magnetic resonance guidance

- *CPT Changes: An Insider's View* 2014
- *CPT Assistant* May 14:3, Jun 14:14, Mar 15:5, May 15:8, Jun 16:3
- *Clinical Examples in Radiology* Winter 17:5

+ 19086 each additional lesion, including magnetic resonance guidance (List separately in addition to code for primary procedure)

- *CPT Changes: An Insider's View* 2014
- *CPT Assistant* May 14:3, Jun 14:14, Mar 15:5, May 15:8, Jun 16:3
- *Clinical Examples in Radiology* Spring 14:4, Winter 17:5

(Use 19086 in conjunction with 19085)

(Do not report 19081-19086 in conjunction with 19281-19288, 76098, 76942, 77002, 77021 for same lesion)

19100 Biopsy of breast; percutaneous, needle core, not using imaging guidance (separate procedure)

- *CPT Changes: An Insider's View* 2001
- *CPT Assistant* Spring 93:35, Fall 94:18, Apr 96:8, Mar 97:4, Nov 97:24, Nov 98:7, Jan 01:10, May 02:18, Apr 05:6, Dec 06:10, Nov 08:10, May 14:3
- *Clinical Examples in Radiology* Fall 10:3, Spring 14:10, Winter 17:5

►(For fine needle aspiration biopsy, see 10004, 10005, 10006, 10007, 10008, 10009, 10010, 10011, 10012, 10021)◄

19101 open, incisional

- *CPT Changes: An Insider's View* 2001
- *CPT Assistant* Spring 93:35, Fall 94:19, Nov 97:24, Jan 01:8, May 02:18, Apr 05:6, May 14:3
- *Clinical Examples in Radiology* Spring 14:10

(For placement of percutaneous localization clip with imaging guidance, see 19281-19288)

19105 Ablation, cryosurgical, of fibroadenoma, including ultrasound guidance, each fibroadenoma

- *CPT Changes: An Insider's View* 2007

(Do not report 19105 in conjunction with 76940, 76942)

(For adjacent lesions treated with 1 cryoprobe insertion, report once)

19110 Nipple exploration, with or without excision of a solitary lactiferous duct or a papilloma lactiferous duct

- *CPT Assistant* Apr 05:6

19112 Excision of lactiferous duct fistula

- *CPT Assistant* Apr 05:6

19120 Excision of cyst, fibroadenoma, or other benign or malignant tumor, aberrant breast tissue, duct lesion, nipple or areolar lesion (except 19300), open, male or female, 1 or more lesions

- *CPT Changes: An Insider's View* 2001, 2007
- *CPT Assistant* Feb 96:9, Nov 97:14, Jan 01:8, May 01:10, Apr 05:6, 13, Mar 14:13, Mar 15:5

19125 Excision of breast lesion identified by preoperative placement of radiological marker, open; single lesion
➔ *CPT Changes: An Insider's View* 2001
➔ *CPT Assistant* Fall 94:18, Mar 98:10, Jan 01:8, Apr 05:6, Mar 09:10, Mar 15:5

+ 19126 each additional lesion separately identified by a preoperative radiological marker (List separately in addition to code for primary procedure)
➔ *CPT Changes: An Insider's View* 2001
➔ *CPT Assistant* Fall 94:18, Mar 98:10, Jan 01:8, Apr 05:6

(Use 19126 in conjunction with 19125)

(Intraoperative placement of clip[s] is not separately reported)

19260 Excision of chest wall tumor including ribs
➔ *CPT Assistant* Apr 05:6, 7, Apr 10:3

19271 Excision of chest wall tumor involving ribs, with plastic reconstruction; without mediastinal lymphadenectomy
➔ *CPT Assistant* Apr 05:6, 7

19272 with mediastinal lymphadenectomy
➔ *CPT Assistant* Apr 05:6, 7

(Do not report 19260, 19271, 19272 in conjunction with 32100, 32503, 32504, 32551, 32554, 32555)

Introduction

Breast biopsies without image guidance are reported with 19100 and 19101. Image-guided breast biopsies, including the placement of localization devices when performed, are reported using 19081-19086. The image-guided placement of localization devices without image-guided biopsy are reported with 19281-19288. When more than one biopsy or localization device placement is performed using the same imaging modality, use an add-on code whether the additional service(s) is on the same or contra-lateral breast. If additional biopsies or localization device placements are performed using different imaging modalities, report another primary code for each additional biopsy or localization device placement performed using a different image guidance modality. When an open incisional biopsy is performed after image-guided placement of a localization device, 19101 is reported and the appropriate image-guided localization device placement code is reported.

When more than one breast localization device placement is performed using the same imaging modality, use an add-on code whether the additional service(s) is on the same or contra-lateral breast. If additional localization devices are placed using different imaging modalities, report another primary code for each additional modality. When an open incisional biopsy is performed after image-guided placement of a localization device, 19101 is reported and the appropriate image-guided localization device placement code is reported.

To report bilateral image-guided placement of localization devices report 19281, 19283, 19285, or 19287 for the initial lesion localized. The contra-lateral and each additional breast image-guided localization device placement is reported with code 19282, 19284, 19286 or 19288.

Code 19294 is used to report the preparation of the tumor cavity with placement of an intraoperative radiation therapy applicator concurrent with partial mastectomy (19301, 19302).

19281 Placement of breast localization device(s) (eg, clip, metallic pellet, wire/needle, radioactive seeds), percutaneous; first lesion, including mammographic guidance
➔ *CPT Changes: An Insider's View* 2014
➔ *CPT Assistant* May 14:3, Jun 14:14, May 15:8, Jun 16:3
➔ *Clinical Examples in Radiology* Spring 14:8, Spring 18:3

+ 19282 each additional lesion, including mammographic guidance (List separately in addition to code for primary procedure)
➔ *CPT Changes: An Insider's View* 2014
➔ *CPT Assistant* May 14:3, Jun 14:14, May 15:8, Jun 16:3
➔ *Clinical Examples in Radiology* Spring 18:3

(Use 19282 in conjunction with 19281)

19283 Placement of breast localization device(s) (eg, clip, metallic pellet, wire/needle, radioactive seeds), percutaneous; first lesion, including stereotactic guidance
➔ *CPT Changes: An Insider's View* 2014
➔ *CPT Assistant* May 14:3, May 15:8, May 16:13, Jun 16:3
➔ *Clinical Examples in Radiology* Spring 18:3

+ 19284 each additional lesion, including stereotactic guidance (List separately in addition to code for primary procedure)
➔ *CPT Changes: An Insider's View* 2014
➔ *CPT Assistant* May 14:3, May 15:8, May 16:13, Jun 16:3
➔ *Clinical Examples in Radiology* Spring 18:3

(Use 19284 in conjunction with 19283)

19285 Placement of breast localization device(s) (eg, clip, metallic pellet, wire/needle, radioactive seeds), percutaneous; first lesion, including ultrasound guidance
➔ *CPT Changes: An Insider's View* 2014
➔ *CPT Assistant* May 14:3, May 15:8, May 16:13, Jun 16:3
➔ *Clinical Examples in Radiology* Spring 18:3

+ 19286 each additional lesion, including ultrasound guidance (List separately in addition to code for primary procedure)
➔ *CPT Changes: An Insider's View* 2014
➔ *CPT Assistant* May 14:3, May 15:8, May 16:13, Jun 16:3
➔ *Clinical Examples in Radiology* Spring 18:3

(Use 19286 in conjunction with 19285)

19287 Placement of breast localization device(s) (eg clip, metallic pellet, wire/needle, radioactive seeds), percutaneous; first lesion, including magnetic resonance guidance

➔ *CPT Changes: An Insider's View* 2014

➔ *CPT Assistant* May 14:3, May 16:13, Jun 16:3

➔ *Clinical Examples in Radiology* Spring 18:3

+ 19288 each additional lesion, including magnetic resonance guidance (List separately in addition to code for primary procedure)

➔ *CPT Changes: An Insider's View* 2014

➔ *CPT Assistant* May 14:3, May 16:13, Jun 16:3

➔ *Clinical Examples in Radiology* Spring 14:8, Spring 18:3

(Use 19288 in conjunction with 19287)

(Do not report 19281-19288 in conjunction with 19081-19086, 76942, 77002, 77021 for same lesion)

(For surgical specimen radiography, use 76098)

(To report image-guided placement of breast localization devices during image-guided biopsy, see 19081-19086. To report image-guided placement of breast localization devices without image-guided biopsy, see 19281-19288)

+ 19294 Preparation of tumor cavity, with placement of a radiation therapy applicator for intraoperative radiation therapy (IORT) concurrent with partial mastectomy (List separately in addition to code for primary procedure)

➔ *CPT Changes: An Insider's View* 2018

(Use 19294 in conjunction with 19301, 19302)

19296 Placement of radiotherapy afterloading expandable catheter (single or multichannel) into the breast for interstitial radioelement application following partial mastectomy, includes imaging guidance; on date separate from partial mastectomy

➔ *CPT Changes: An Insider's View* 2005, 2009

➔ *CPT Assistant* Apr 05:6-8, Nov 05:15, Apr 09:3, Dec 09:9, Mar 10:10

+ 19297 concurrent with partial mastectomy (List separately in addition to code for primary procedure)

➔ *CPT Changes: An Insider's View* 2005, 2009

➔ *CPT Assistant* Apr 05:6-8, Nov 05:15, Apr 09:3, Mar 10:10

(Use 19297 in conjunction with 19301 or 19302)

19298 Placement of radiotherapy after loading brachytherapy catheters (multiple tube and button type) into the breast for interstitial radioelement application following (at the time of or subsequent to) partial mastectomy, includes imaging guidance

➔ *CPT Changes: An Insider's View* 2005, 2017

➔ *CPT Assistant* Apr 05:6-7, 9, 16, Nov 05:15, Apr 09:3, Mar 10:10

Mastectomy Procedures

19300 Mastectomy for gynecomastia

➔ *CPT Changes: An Insider's View* 2007

➔ *CPT Assistant* Feb 07:4, Mar 14:13

19301 Mastectomy, partial (eg, lumpectomy, tylectomy, quadrantectomy, segmentectomy);

➔ *CPT Changes: An Insider's View* 2007

➔ *CPT Assistant* Feb 07:4, Dec 07:8, Sep 08:5, Mar 10:10, Nov 13:14, Mar 15:5, Oct 17:9

19302 with axillary lymphadenectomy

➔ *CPT Changes: An Insider's View* 2007

➔ *CPT Assistant* Feb 07:4, Dec 07:8, Sep 08:5, Mar 10:10, Mar 15:5

(For placement of radiotherapy afterloading balloon/brachytherapy catheters, see 19296-19298)

(Intraoperative placement of clip[s] is not separately reported)

(For the preparation of tumor cavity with placement of an intraoperative radiation therapy applicator concurrent with partial mastectomy, use 19294)

19303 Mastectomy, simple, complete

➔ *CPT Changes: An Insider's View* 2007

➔ *CPT Assistant* Feb 07:4, Mar 15:5

(Intraoperative placement of clip[s] is not separately reported)

(For immediate or delayed insertion of implant, see 19340, 19342)

(For gynecomastia, use 19300)

19304 Mastectomy, subcutaneous

➔ *CPT Changes: An Insider's View* 2007

➔ *CPT Assistant* Feb 07:4, Dec 07:7, 8

(Intraoperative placement of clip[s] is not separately reported)

(For immediate or delayed insertion of implant, see 19340, 19342)

19305 Mastectomy, radical, including pectoral muscles, axillary lymph nodes

➔ *CPT Changes: An Insider's View* 2007

➔ *CPT Assistant* Feb 07:4, Sep 08:5

(Intraoperative placement of clip[s] is not separately reported)

(For immediate or delayed insertion of implant, see 19340, 19342)

19306 Mastectomy, radical, including pectoral muscles, axillary and internal mammary lymph nodes (Urban type operation)

➔ *CPT Changes: An Insider's View* 2007

➔ *CPT Assistant* Feb 07:4, Sep 08:5

(Intraoperative placement of clip[s] is not separately reported)

(For immediate or delayed insertion of implant, see 19340, 19342)

19307 Mastectomy, modified radical, including axillary lymph nodes, with or without pectoralis minor muscle, but excluding pectoralis major muscle

➲ *CPT Changes: An Insider's View* 2007

➲ *CPT Assistant* Feb 07:4, Sep 08:5, Mar 15:5

(Intraoperative placement of clip[s] is not separately reported)

(For immediate or delayed insertion of implant, see 19340, 19342)

Repair and/or Reconstruction

(To report bilateral procedure, report modifier 50 with the procedure code)

(For biologic implant for soft tissue reinforcement, use 15777 in conjunction with primary procedure)

19316 Mastopexy

➲ *CPT Assistant* Jan 03:7, Apr 05:6, Feb 12:11

19318 Reduction mammaplasty

➲ *CPT Assistant* Jan 03:7, Apr 05:6, Apr 14:10

19324 Mammaplasty, augmentation; without prosthetic implant

➲ *CPT Assistant* Apr 05:6

19325 with prosthetic implant

➲ *CPT Assistant* Apr 05:6

(For flap or graft, use also appropriate number)

19328 Removal of intact mammary implant

➲ *CPT Assistant* Apr 05:6

19330 Removal of mammary implant material

➲ *CPT Assistant* Nov 01:11, Apr 05:6

19340 Immediate insertion of breast prosthesis following mastopexy, mastectomy or in reconstruction

➲ *CPT Assistant* Aug 96:8, Apr 05:6, Aug 05:1, Mar 10:9, Dec 15:18

19342 Delayed insertion of breast prosthesis following mastopexy, mastectomy or in reconstruction

➲ *CPT Assistant* Aug 96:8, Apr 05:6, Aug 05:1, Jan 13:15, Nov 15:10

(For supply of implant, use 99070)

(For preparation of custom breast implant, use 19396)

19350 Nipple/areola reconstruction

➲ *CPT Assistant* Aug 96:11, Apr 05:6, Jan 13:15, Aug 16:9

19355 Correction of inverted nipples

➲ *CPT Assistant* Apr 05:6

19357 Breast reconstruction, immediate or delayed, with tissue expander, including subsequent expansion

➲ *CPT Assistant* Winter 91:2, Apr 05:6, Aug 05:1, Mar 10:9, Oct 13:15, Feb 15:10

19361 Breast reconstruction with latissimus dorsi flap, without prosthetic implant

➲ *CPT Changes: An Insider's View* 2007

➲ *CPT Assistant* Apr 05:6, Aug 05:1, Mar 10:9, Feb 15:10

(For insertion of prosthesis, use also 19340)

19364 Breast reconstruction with free flap

➲ *CPT Assistant* Aug 96:8, Nov 98:7, Apr 05:6, Aug 05:1, Jun 10:8, Dec 11:14, Jul 12:12, Mar 13:13, Apr 14:10, Feb 15:10

(Do not report code 69990 in addition to code 19364)

(19364 includes harvesting of the flap, microvascular transfer, closure of the donor site, and inset shaping the flap into a breast)

19366 Breast reconstruction with other technique

➲ *CPT Assistant* Aug 96:8, Nov 98:7, Apr 05:6, Dec 11:14, Apr 14:10, Feb 15:10

(For operating microscope, use 69990)

(For insertion of prosthesis, use also 19340 or 19342)

19367 Breast reconstruction with transverse rectus abdominis myocutaneous flap (TRAM), single pedicle, including closure of donor site;

➲ *CPT Assistant* Nov 98:7, Apr 05:6, Aug 05:1, Feb 15:10

19368 with microvascular anastomosis (supercharging)

➲ *CPT Assistant* Nov 98:7, Apr 05:6, Aug 05:1, Feb 15:10

(Do not report code 69990 in addition to code 19368)

19369 Breast reconstruction with transverse rectus abdominis myocutaneous flap (TRAM), double pedicle, including closure of donor site

➲ *CPT Assistant* Oct 00:3, Apr 05:6, Aug 05:1, Feb 15:10

19370 Open periprosthetic capsulotomy, breast

➲ *CPT Assistant* Aug 96:8, Apr 05:6, Dec 15:18

19371 Periprosthetic capsulectomy, breast

➲ *CPT Assistant* Aug 96:8, Nov 01:11, Apr 05:6, Jan 13:15

19380 Revision of reconstructed breast

➲ *CPT Assistant* Apr 05:6, Dec 15:18, Dec 17:13

19396 Preparation of moulage for custom breast implant

➲ *CPT Assistant* Jan 03:7, Apr 05:6

Other Procedures

19499 Unlisted procedure, breast

➲ *CPT Assistant* Apr 05:6, Dec 09:9, Nov 13:14, Dec 14:16, Dec 16:16

➲ *Clinical Examples in Radiology* Fall 08:4, Summer 09:15

Notes

Surgery

Musculoskeletal System* (20100-29999) ... **116**

The following is a listing of headings and subheadings that appear within the Musculoskeletal System section of the CPT codebook. The subheadings or subsections denoted with asterisks (*) below have special instructions unique to that subsection. Where these are indicated, special notes or guidelines will be presented preceding those procedural terminology listings, referring to that subsection specifically.

General (20100-20999) ... 117

Incision ... **117**

Wound Exploration—Trauma (eg, Penetrating Gunshot, Stab Wound)* (20100-20103) ... **117**

Excision (20150-20251) ... **117**

Introduction or Removal (20500-20697) ... **118**

Replantation (20802-20838) ... **121**

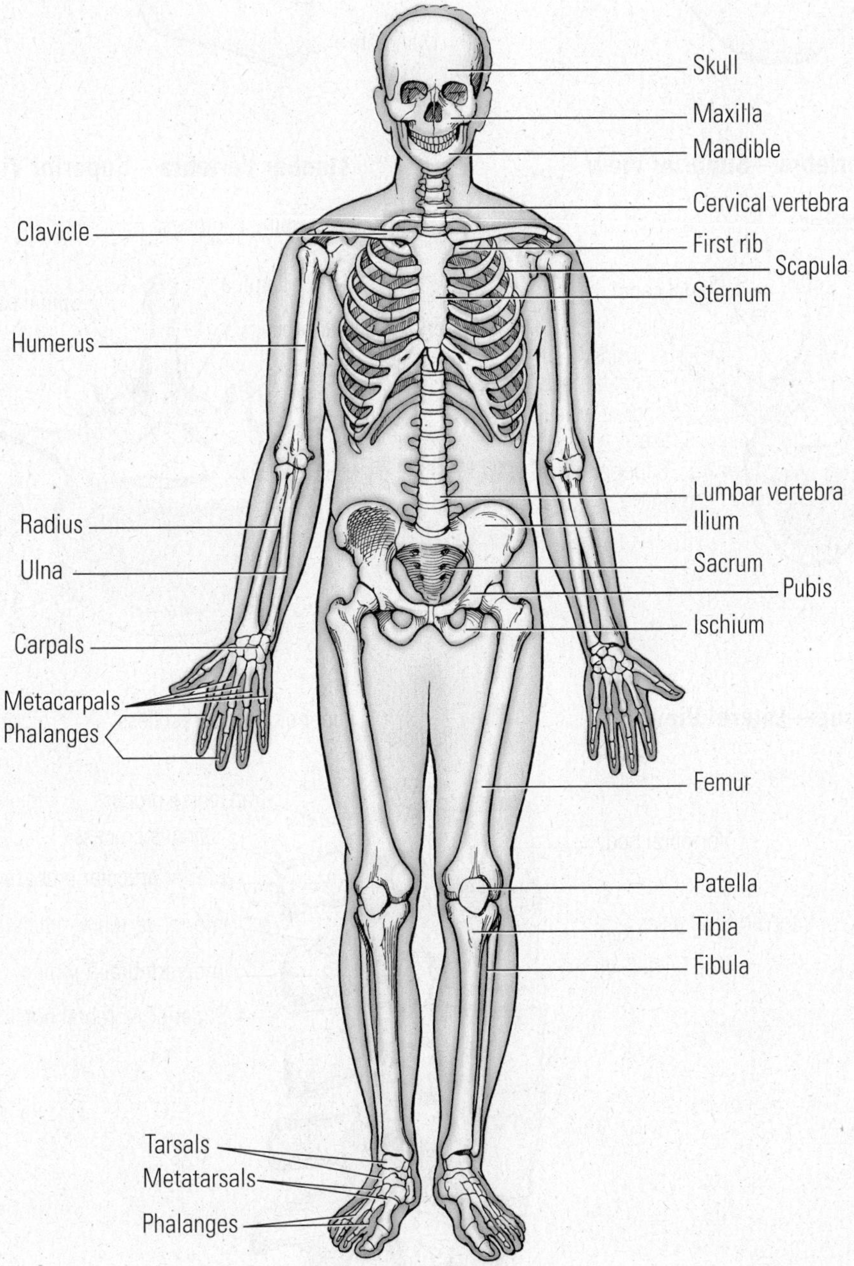

Skeletal System

Skull, Frontal View

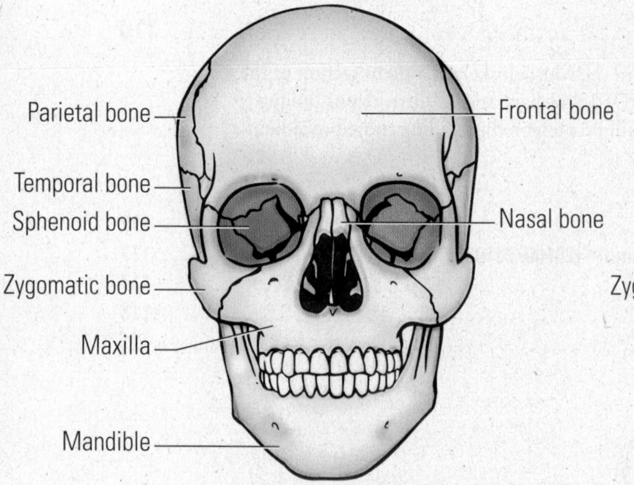

Skull, Lateral View

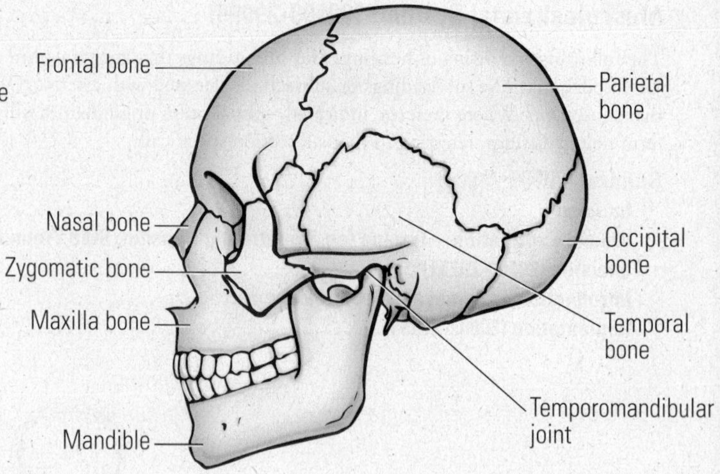

Thoracic Vertebra—Superior View

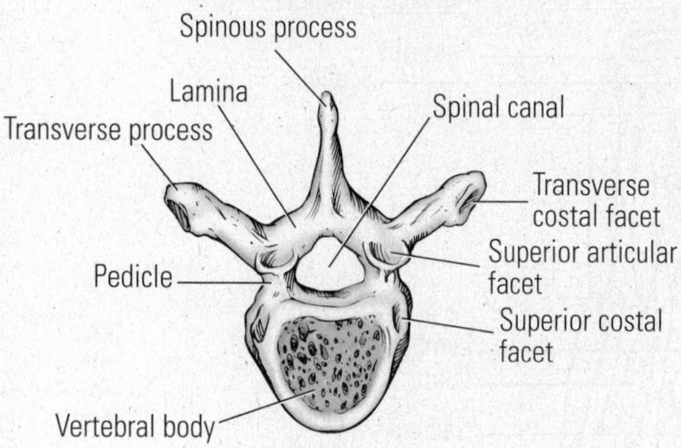

Lumbar Vertebra—Superior View

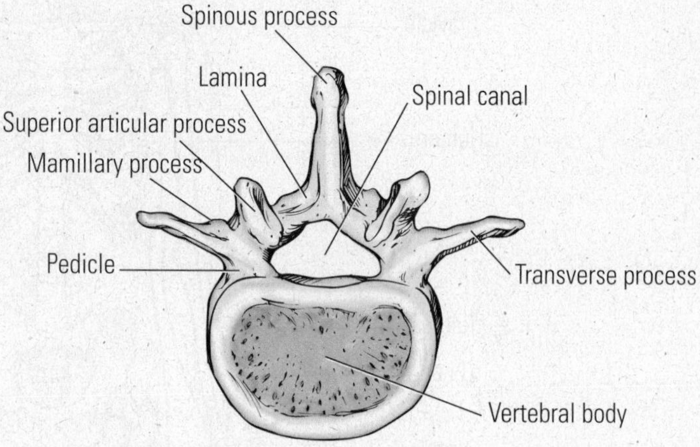

Lumbar Vertebrae—Lateral View

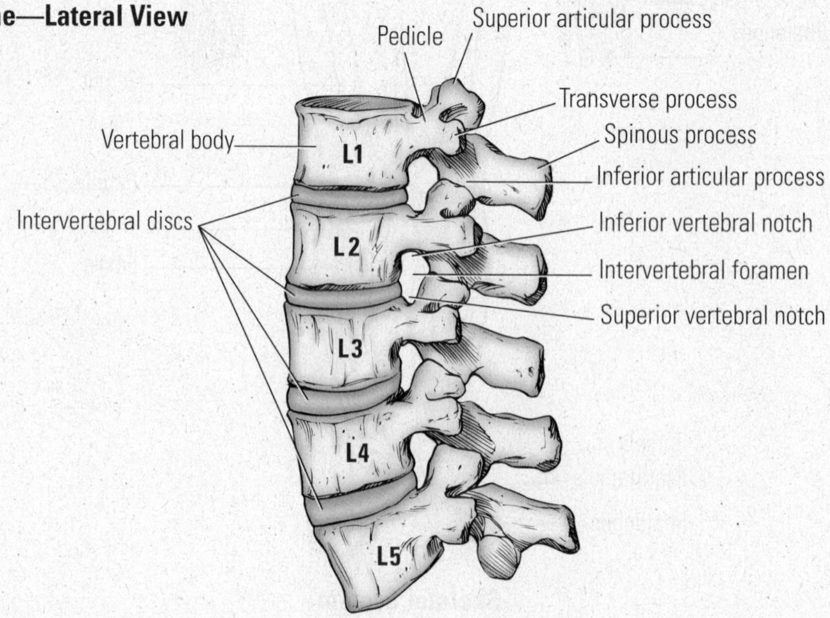

Grafts (or Implants)* (20900-20939) ... 122
Other Procedures (20950-20999) ... 123

Head* (21010-21499) ... 124
Incision (21010) ... 124
Excision (21011-21070) ... 124
Manipulation (21073) ... 125
Head Prosthesis* (21076-21089) ... 125
Other Procedures (21089) ... 125
Introduction or Removal (21100-21116) ... 125
Repair, Revision, and/or Reconstruction (21120-21296) ... 125
Other Procedures (21299) ... 127
Fracture and/or Dislocation (21310-21497) ... 127
Other Procedures (21499) ... 128

Neck (Soft Tissues) and Thorax (21501-21899) ... 128
Incision (21501-21510) ... 128
Excision (21550-21632) ... 129
Repair, Revision, and/or Reconstruction (21685-21750) ... 129
Fracture and/or Dislocation (21811-21825) ... 129
Other Procedures (21899) ... 130

Back and Flank (21920-21936) ... 130
Excision (21920-21936) ... 130

Spine (Vertebral Column)* (22010-22899) ... 130
Incision (22010-22015) ... 131
Excision* (22100-22116) ... 131
Osteotomy* (22206-22226) ... 131
Fracture and/or Dislocation* (22310-22328) ... 132
Manipulation (22505) ... 133
Percutaneous Vertebroplasty and Vertebral Augmentation* (22510-22515) ... 133
Percutaneous Augmentation and Annuloplasty (22526-22527) ... 134
Arthrodesis* (22532-22819) ... 134
Lateral Extracavitary Approach Technique (22532-22534) ... 134
Anterior or Anterolateral Approach Technique* (22548-22586) ... 134
Posterior, Posterolateral or Lateral Transverse Process Technique* (22590-22634) ... 136
Spine Deformity (eg, Scoliosis, Kyphosis)* (22800-22819) ... 137
Exploration* (22830) ... 137
Spinal Instrumentation* (22840-22870) ... 137
Other Procedures (22899) ... 141

Abdomen (22900-22999) ... 141
Excision (22900-22905) ... 141
Other Procedures (22999) ... 141

Shoulder* (23000-23929) ... 141
Incision (23000-23044) ... 141
Excision (23065-23220) ... 142
Introduction or Removal (23330-23350) ... 142
Repair, Revision, and/or Reconstruction (23395-23491) ... 143
Fracture and/or Dislocation (23500-23680) ... 144
Manipulation (23700) ... 144
Arthrodesis (23800-23802) ... 144
Amputation (23900-23921) ... 145
Other Procedures (23929) ... 145

Humerus (Upper Arm) and Elbow* (23930-24999) ... 145
Incision (23930-24006) ... 145
Excision (24065-24155) ... 145
Introduction or Removal (24160-24220) ... 146
Repair, Revision, and/or Reconstruction (24300-24498) ... 146
Fracture and/or Dislocation (24500-24685) ... 147
Arthrodesis (24800-24802) ... 148
Amputation (24900-24940) ... 148
Other Procedures (24999) ... 148

Forearm and Wrist* (25000-25999) 148
Incision (25000-25040) 148
Excision (25065-25240) 148
Introduction or Removal (25246-25259) 149
Repair, Revision, and/or Reconstruction (25260-25492) 149
Fracture and/or Dislocation (25500-25695) 151
Arthrodesis (25800-25830) 152
Amputation (25900-25931) 152
Other Procedures (25999) 152
Hand and Fingers (26010-26989) 152
Incision (26010-26080) 152
Excision (26100-26262) 152
Introduction or Removal (26320) 153
Repair, Revision, and/or Reconstruction (26340-26596) 153

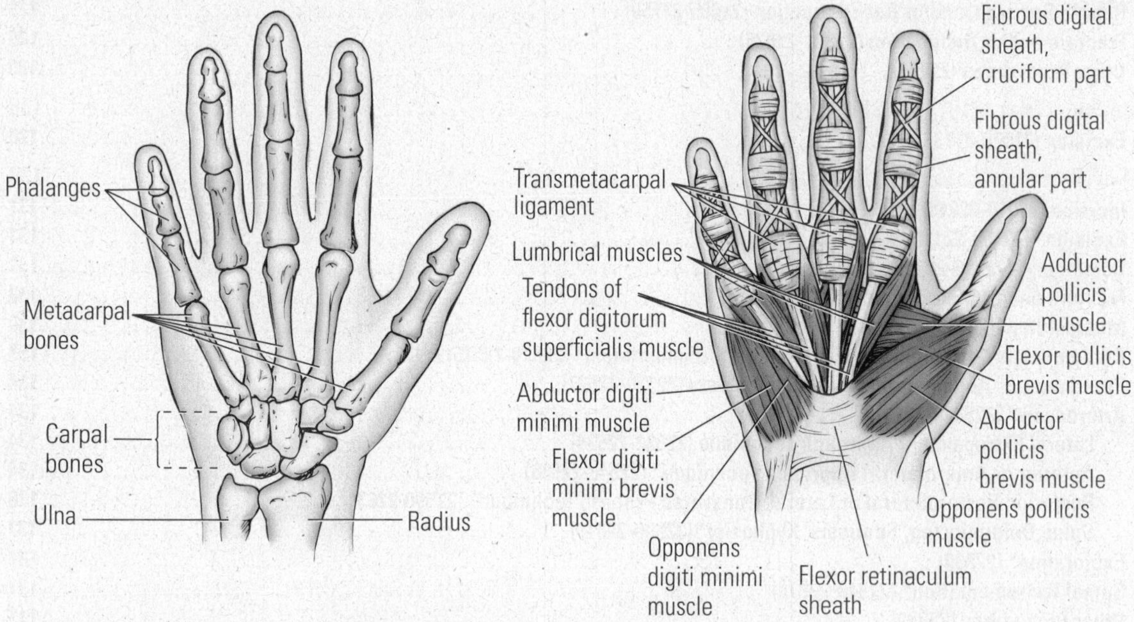

Bones, Muscles, and Tendons of Hand

Fracture and/or Dislocation (26600-26785) 156
Arthrodesis (26820-26863) 157
Amputation (26910-26952) 157
Other Procedures (26989) 157
Pelvis and Hip Joint* (26990-27299) 157
Incision (26990-27036) 157
Excision (27040-27080) 158
Introduction or Removal (27086-27096) 158
Repair, Revision, and/or Reconstruction (27097-27187) 159
Fracture and/or Dislocation (27197-27269) 160
Manipulation (27275) 162
Arthrodesis (27279-27286) 162
Amputation (27290-27295) 162
Other Procedures (27299) 162
Femur (Thigh Region) and Knee Joint* (27301-27599) 162
Incision (27301-27310) 162
Excision (27323-27365) 163
Introduction or Removal (27369-27372) 163
Repair, Revision, and/or Reconstruction (27380-27499) 164
Fracture and/or Dislocation (27500-27566) 166

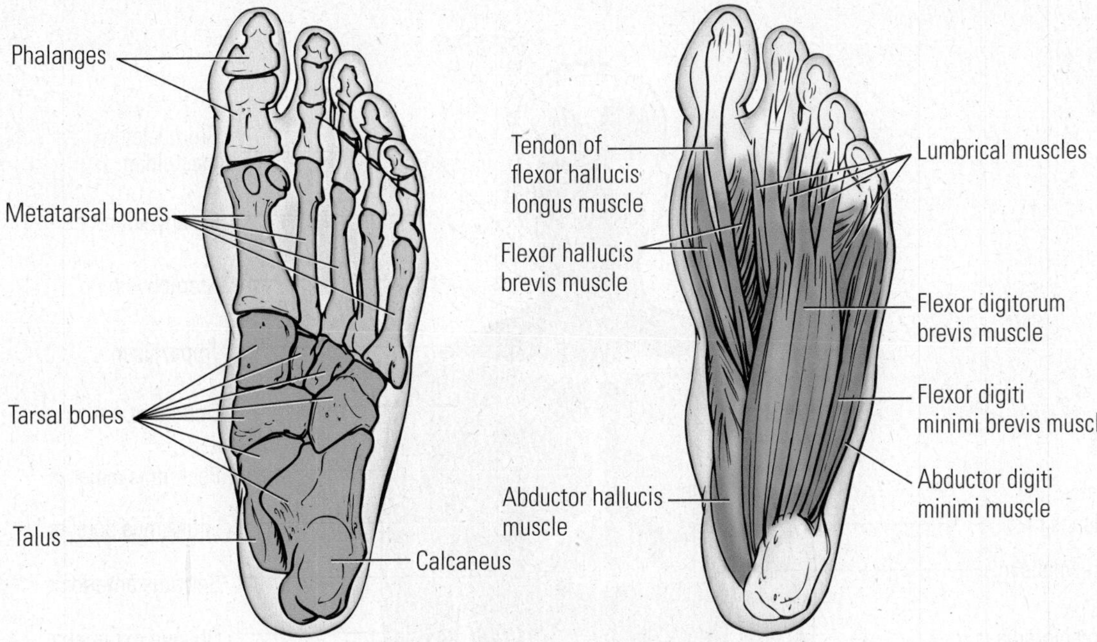

Bones and Muscles of Foot

Manipulation (27570) 167
Arthrodesis (27580) 167
Amputation (27590-27598) 167
Other Procedures (27599) 167

Leg (Tibia and Fibula) and Ankle Joint (27600-27899) 167
Incision (27600-27612) 167
Excision (27613-27647) 167
Introduction or Removal (27648) 168
Repair, Revision, and/or Reconstruction (27650-27745) 168
Fracture and/or Dislocation (27750-27848) 169
Manipulation (27860) 170
Arthrodesis (27870-27871) 170
Amputation (27880-27889) 170
Other Procedures (27892-27899) 170

Foot and Toes (28001-28899) 171
Incision (28001-28035) 171
Excision (28039-28175) 171
Introduction or Removal (28190-28193) 172
Repair, Revision, and/or Reconstruction (28200-28360) 172
Fracture and/or Dislocation (28400-28675) 176
Arthrodesis (28705-28760) 177
Amputation (28800-28825) 177
Other Procedures (28890-28899) 177

Application of Casts and Strapping* (29000-29799) 178
Body and Upper Extremity (29000-29280) 178
Casts (29000-29086) 178
Splints (29105-29131) 178
Strapping—Any Age (29200-29280) 178
Lower Extremity (29305-29584) 179
Casts (29305-29450) 179
Splints (29505-29515) 179
Strapping—Any Age (29520-29584) 179
Removal or Repair* (29700-29750) 179
Other Procedures (29799) 180

Endoscopy/Arthroscopy* (29800-29999) 180

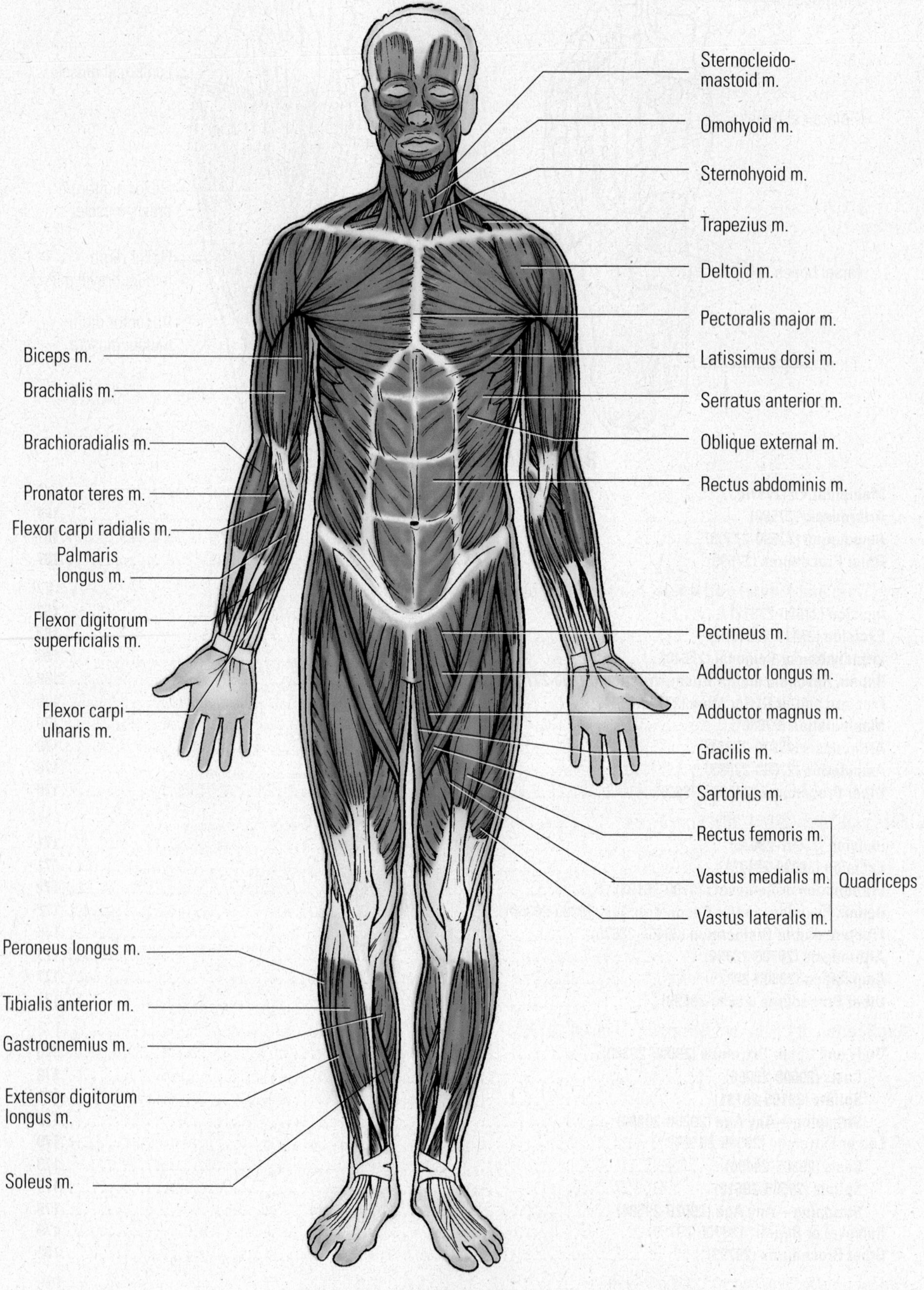

Muscular System, Front

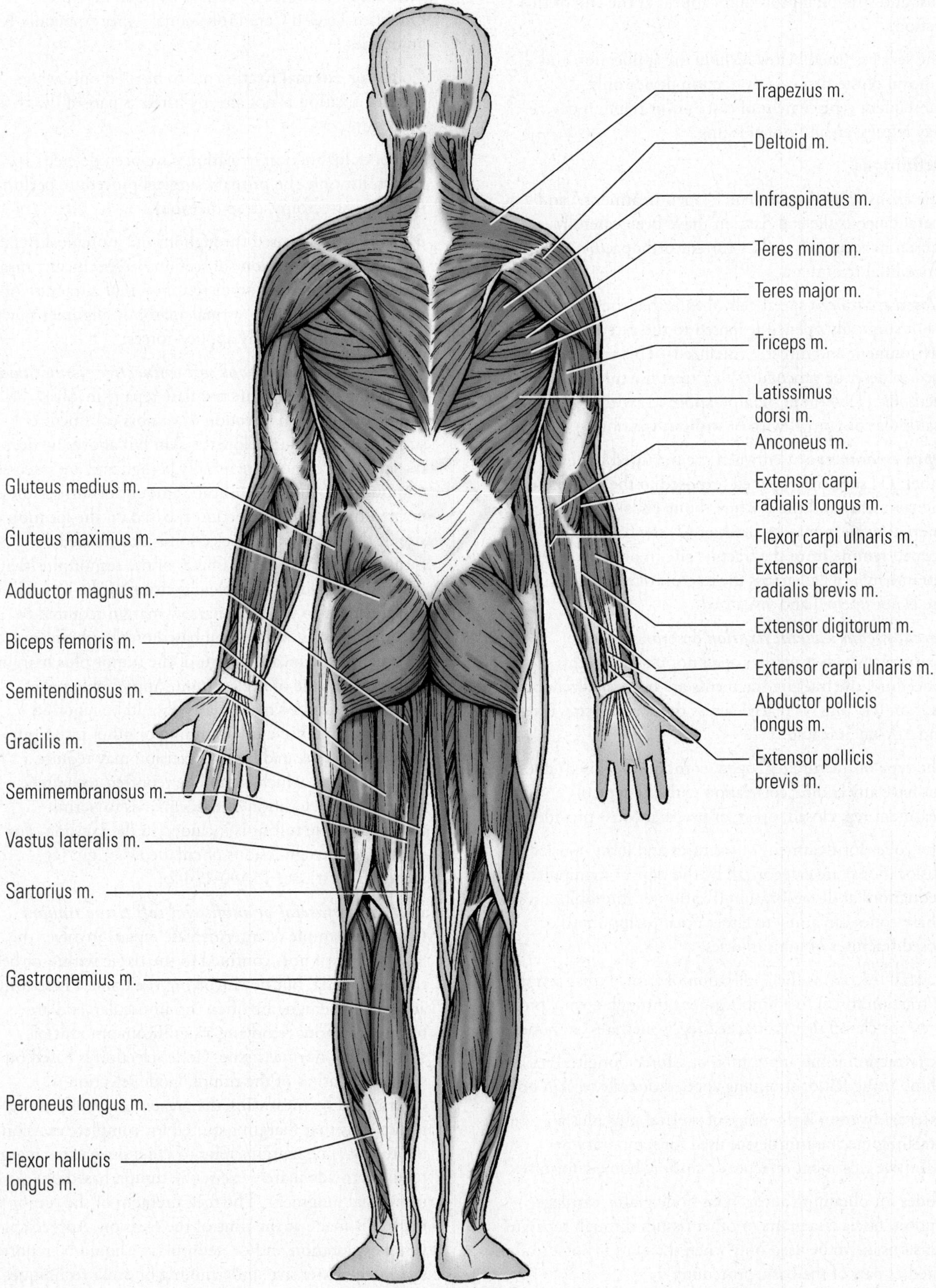

Muscular System, Back

Musculoskeletal System

Cast and strapping procedures appear at the end of this section.

The services listed below include the application and removal of the first cast or traction device only. Subsequent replacement of cast and/or traction device may require an additional listing.

Definitions

The terms "closed treatment," "open treatment," and "percutaneous skeletal fixation" have been carefully chosen to accurately reflect current orthopaedic procedural treatments.

Closed treatment specifically means that the fracture site is not surgically opened (exposed to the external environment and directly visualized). This terminology is used to describe procedures that treat fractures by three methods: (1) without manipulation; (2) with manipulation; or (3) with or without traction.

Open treatment is used when the fractured bone is either: (1) surgically opened (exposed to the external environment) and the fracture (bone ends) visualized and internal fixation may be used; or (2) the fractured bone is opened remote from the fracture site in order to insert an intramedullary nail across the fracture site (the fracture site is not opened and visualized).

Percutaneous skeletal fixation describes fracture treatment which is neither open nor closed. In this procedure, the fracture fragments are not visualized, but fixation (eg, pins) is placed across the fracture site, usually under X-ray imaging.

The type of fracture (eg, open, compound, closed) does not have any coding correlation with the type of treatment (eg, closed, open, or percutaneous) provided.

The codes for treatment of fractures and joint injuries (dislocations) are categorized by the type of manipulation (reduction) and stabilization (fixation or immobilization). These codes can apply to either open (compound) or closed fractures or joint injuries.

Skeletal traction is the application of a force (distracting or traction force) to a limb segment through a wire, pin, screw, or clamp that is attached (eg, penetrates) to bone.

Skin traction is the application of a force (longitudinal) to a limb using felt or strapping applied directly to skin only.

External fixation is the usage of skeletal pins plus an attaching mechanism/device used for temporary or definitive treatment of acute or chronic bony deformity.

Codes for obtaining autogenous bone grafts, cartilage, tendon, fascia lata grafts or other tissues through separate incisions are to be used only when the graft is not already listed as part of the basic procedure.

Re-reduction of a fracture and/or dislocation performed by the primary physician or other qualified health care professional may be identified by the addition of modifier 76 to the usual procedure number to indicate "Repeat Procedure or Service by Same Physician or Other Qualified Health Care Professional." (See Appendix A guidelines.)

Codes for external fixation are to be used only when external fixation is not already listed as part of the basic procedure.

All codes for suction irrigation have been deleted. To report, list only the primary surgical procedure performed (eg, sequestrectomy, deep incision).

Manipulation is used throughout the musculoskeletal fracture and dislocation subsections to specifically mean the attempted reduction or restoration of a fracture or joint dislocation to its normal anatomic alignment by the application of manually applied forces.

Excision of subcutaneous soft connective tissue tumors (including simple or intermediate repair) involves the simple or marginal resection of tumors confined to subcutaneous tissue below the skin but above the deep fascia. These tumors are usually benign and are resected without removing a significant amount of surrounding normal tissue. Code selection is based on the location and size of the tumor. Code selection is determined by measuring the greatest diameter of the tumor plus that margin required for complete excision of the tumor. The margins refer to the most narrow margin required to adequately excise the tumor, based on the physician's judgment. The measurement of the tumor plus margin is made at the time of the excision. Appreciable vessel exploration and/or neuroplasty should be reported separately. Extensive undermining or other techniques to close a defect created by skin excision may require a complex repair which should be reported separately. Dissection or elevation of tissue planes to permit resection of the tumor is included in the excision. For excision of benign lesions of cutaneous origin (eg, sebaceous cyst), see 11400-11446.

Excision of fascial or subfascial soft tissue tumors (including simple or intermediate repair) involves the resection of tumors confined to the tissue within or below the deep fascia, but not involving the bone. These tumors are usually benign, are often intramuscular, and are resected without removing a significant amount of surrounding normal tissue. Code selection is based on size and location of the tumor. Code selection is determined by measuring the greatest diameter of the tumor plus that margin required for complete excision of the tumor. The margins refer to the most narrow margin required to adequately excise the tumor, based on individual judgment. The measurement of the tumor plus margin is made at the time of the excision. Appreciable vessel exploration and/or neuroplasty should be reported separately. Extensive undermining or other techniques to close a defect created by skin excision may require a complex repair which should be reported separately.

Dissection or elevation of tissue planes to permit resection of the tumor is included in the excision.

Digital (ie, fingers and toes) subfascial tumors are defined as those tumors involving the tendons, tendon sheaths, or joints of the digit. Tumors which simply abut but do not breach the tendon, tendon sheath, or joint capsule are considered subcutaneous soft tissue tumors.

Radical resection of soft connective tissue tumors (including simple or intermediate repair) involves the resection of the tumor with wide margins of normal tissue. Appreciable vessel exploration and/or neuroplasty repair or reconstruction (eg, adjacent tissue transfer[s], flap[s]) should be reported separately. Extensive undermining or other techniques to close a defect created by skin excision may require a complex repair which should be reported separately. Dissection or elevation of tissue planes to permit resection of the tumor is included in the excision. Although these tumors may be confined to a specific layer (eg, subcutaneous, subfascial), radical resection may involve removal of tissue from one or more layers. Radical resection of soft tissue tumors is most commonly used for malignant connective tissue tumors or very aggressive benign connective tissue tumors. Code selection is based on size and location of the tumor. Code selection is determined by measuring the greatest diameter of the tumor plus that margin required for complete excision of the tumor. The margins refer to the most narrow margin required to adequately excise the tumor, based on individual judgment. The measurement of the tumor plus margin is made at the time of the excision. For radical resection of tumor(s) of cutaneous origin (eg, melanoma), see 11600-11646.

Radical resection of bone tumors (including simple or intermediate repair) involves the resection of the tumor with wide margins of normal tissue. Appreciable vessel exploration and/or neuroplasty and complex bone repair or reconstruction (eg, adjacent tissue transfer[s], flap[s]) should be reported separately. Extensive undermining or other techniques to close a defect created by skin excision may require a complex repair which should be reported separately. Dissection or elevation of tissue planes to permit resection of the tumor is included in the excision. It may require removal of the entire bone if tumor growth is extensive (eg, clavicle). Radical resection of bone tumors is usually performed for malignant tumors or very aggressive benign tumors. If surrounding soft tissue is removed during these procedures, the radical resection of soft tissue tumor codes should not be reported separately. Code selection is based solely on the location of the tumor, **not** on the size of the tumor or whether the tumor is benign or malignant, primary or metastatic.

General

Incision

►(20005 has been deleted)◄

►(For incision and drainage of subfascial soft tissue abscess, see appropriate incision and drainage for specific anatomic sites)◄

Wound Exploration—Trauma (eg, Penetrating Gunshot, Stab Wound)

20100-20103 relate to wound(s) resulting from penetrating trauma. These codes describe surgical exploration and enlargement of the wound, extension of dissection (to determine penetration), debridement, removal of foreign body(s), ligation or coagulation of minor subcutaneous and/or muscular blood vessel(s), of the subcutaneous tissue, muscle fascia, and/or muscle, not requiring thoracotomy or laparotomy. If a repair is done to major structure(s) or major blood vessel(s) requiring thoracotomy or laparotomy, then those specific code(s) would supersede the use of codes 20100-20103. To report simple, intermediate, or complex repair of wound(s) that do not require enlargement of the wound, extension of dissection, etc, as stated above, use specific Repair code(s) in the **Integumentary System** section.

20100 Exploration of penetrating wound (separate procedure); neck

➔ *CPT Assistant* Jun 96:7, Aug 96:10, Sep 06:13

20101 chest

➔ *CPT Assistant* Jun 96:7, Sep 06:13

20102 abdomen/flank/back

➔ *CPT Assistant* Jun 96:7, Sep 06:13

20103 extremity

➔ *CPT Assistant* Jun 96:7, Aug 96:10, Sep 06:13

Excision

20150 Excision of epiphyseal bar, with or without autogenous soft tissue graft obtained through same fascial incision

20200 Biopsy, muscle; superficial

20205 deep

20206 Biopsy, muscle, percutaneous needle

➔ *Clinical Examples in Radiology* Summer 08:5, Fall 10:7, Winter 17:5

(If imaging guidance is performed, see 76942, 77002, 77012, 77021)

►(For fine needle aspiration biopsy, see 10004, 10005, 10006, 10007, 10008, 10009, 10010, 10011, 10012, 10021)◄

(For evaluation of fine needle aspirate, see 88172-88173)

(For excision of muscle tumor, deep, see specific anatomic section)

20220 Biopsy, bone, trocar, or needle; superficial (eg, ilium, sternum, spinous process, ribs)
➔ *CPT Assistant* Winter 92:17, Jul 98:4
➔ *Clinical Examples in Radiology* Summer 08:5, Fall 10:7, Winter 17:5

20225 deep (eg, vertebral body, femur)
➔ *CPT Changes: An Insider's View* 2002
➔ *CPT Assistant* Winter 92:17, Jul 98:4, Jun 12:10, Jan 15:8
➔ *Clinical Examples in Radiology* Fall 10:8, Winter 17:5

(Do not report 20225 in conjunction with 22510, 22511, 22512, 22513, 22514, 22515, 0200T, 0201T, when performed at the same level)

(For bone marrow biopsy[ies] and/or aspiration[s], see 38220, 38221, 38222)

(For radiologic supervision and interpretation, see 77002, 77012, 77021)

20240 Biopsy, bone, open; superficial (eg, sternum, spinous process, rib, patella, olecranon process, calcaneus, tarsal, metatarsal, carpal, metacarpal, phalanx)
➔ *CPT Changes: An Insider's View* 2004, 2017
➔ *CPT Assistant* Winter 92:17, Jul 98:4, Aug 04:11, Aug 05:13

20245 deep (eg, humeral shaft, ischium, femoral shaft)
➔ *CPT Changes: An Insider's View* 2017
➔ *CPT Assistant* Winter 92:17, Jul 98:4

20250 Biopsy, vertebral body, open; thoracic
➔ *CPT Assistant* Winter 92:17, Jul 98:4

20251 lumbar or cervical
➔ *CPT Assistant* Winter 92:17, Jul 98:4

(For sequestrectomy, osteomyelitis or drainage of bone abscess, see anatomical area)

Introduction or Removal

(For injection procedure for arthrography, see anatomical area)

(For injection of autologous adipose-derived regenerative cells, see 0489T, 0490T)

20500 Injection of sinus tract; therapeutic (separate procedure)
➔ *Clinical Examples in Radiology* Summer 15:8

20501 diagnostic (sinogram)

(For radiological supervision and interpretation, use 76080)

(For contrast injection[s] and radiological assessment of gastrostomy, duodenostomy, jejunostomy, gastro-jejunostomy, or cecostomy [or other colonic] tube including fluoroscopic imaging guidance, use 49465)

20520 Removal of foreign body in muscle or tendon sheath; simple

20525 deep or complicated

20526 Injection, therapeutic (eg, local anesthetic, corticosteroid), carpal tunnel
➔ *CPT Changes: An Insider's View* 2002
➔ *CPT Assistant* Mar 02:7

20527 Injection, enzyme (eg, collagenase), palmar fascial cord (ie, Dupuytren's contracture)
➔ *CPT Changes: An Insider's View* 2012
➔ *CPT Assistant* Jul 12:8, 14

(For manipulation of palmar fascial cord (ie, Dupuytren's cord) post enzyme injection (eg, collagenase), use 26341)

20550 Injection(s); single tendon sheath, or ligament, aponeurosis (eg, plantar "fascia")
➔ *CPT Changes: An Insider's View* 2002, 2003, 2004
➔ *CPT Assistant* Jan 96:7, Jun 98:10, Mar 02:7, Aug 03:14, Sep 03:13, Dec 03:11, Jan 09:6, Jul 12:14, Oct 14:9
➔ *Clinical Examples in Radiology* Winter 10:14

(For injection of Morton's neuroma, see 64455, 64632)

20551 single tendon origin/insertion
➔ *CPT Changes: An Insider's View* 2002, 2004
➔ *CPT Assistant* Mar 02:7, Sep 03:13, Oct 14:9, Dec 17:16
➔ *Clinical Examples in Radiology* Fall 10:10, Winter 10:14

(Do not report 20550, 20551 in conjunction with 0232T, 0481T)

(For harvesting, preparation, and injection[s] of platelet-rich plasma, use 0232T)

20552 Injection(s); single or multiple trigger point(s), 1 or 2 muscle(s)
➔ *CPT Changes: An Insider's View* 2002, 2003, 2004
➔ *CPT Assistant* Mar 02:7, May 03:19, Sep 03:11, Feb 10:9, Feb 11:5, Jul 11:16, Apr 12:19, Oct 14:9, Jun 17:10, Dec 17:16
➔ *Clinical Examples in Radiology* Winter 10:14, Fall 11:10

20553 single or multiple trigger point(s), 3 or more muscles
➔ *CPT Changes: An Insider's View* 2002, 2003
➔ *CPT Assistant* Mar 02:7, May 03:19, Sep 03:11, Jun 08:8, Feb 10:9, Feb 11:5, Jul 11:16, Oct 14:9, Jun 17:10
➔ *Clinical Examples in Radiology* Winter 10:14

(If imaging guidance is performed, see 76942, 77002, 77021)

20555 Placement of needles or catheters into muscle and/or soft tissue for subsequent interstitial radioelement application (at the time of or subsequent to the procedure)
➔ *CPT Changes: An Insider's View* 2008
➔ *CPT Assistant* Feb 08:8

(For placement of devices into the breast for interstitial radioelement application, see 19296-19298)

(For placement of needles, catheters, or devices into muscle or soft tissue of the head and neck, for interstitial radioelement application, use 41019)

(For placement of needles or catheters for interstitial radioelement application into prostate, use 55875)

(For placement of needles or catheters into the pelvic organs or genitalia [except prostate] for interstitial radioelement application, use 55920)

(For interstitial radioelement application, see 77770, 77771, 77772, 77778)

(For imaging guidance, see 76942, 77002, 77012, 77021)

Trigger Point Injection
20552, 20553

Insertion of needle into muscle trigger point for injection of therapeutic agent

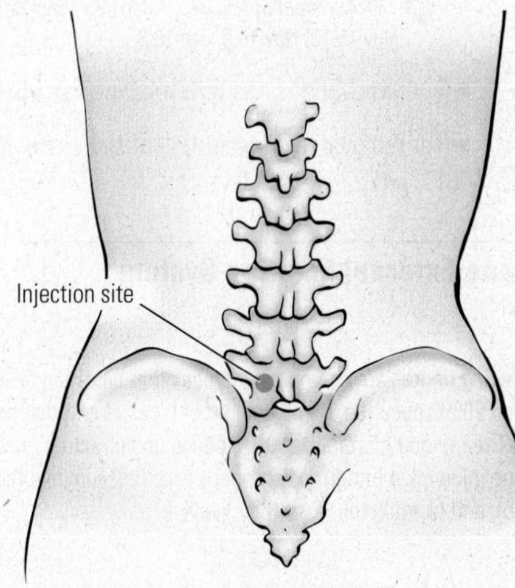

Cross section through the body wall at level of lumbar vertebra

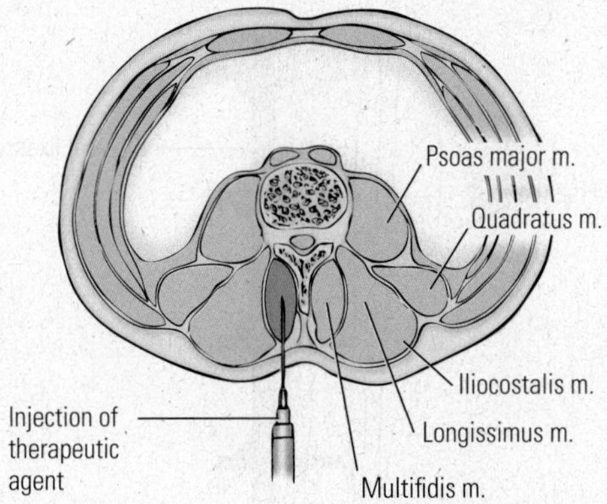

20600 Arthrocentesis, aspiration and/or injection, small joint or bursa (eg, fingers, toes); without ultrasound guidance
- *CPT Changes: An Insider's View* 2003, 2015
- *CPT Assistant* Dec 07:10, Feb 15:6, Nov 15:10, Aug 17:9
- *Clinical Examples in Radiology* Spring 15:6

20604 with ultrasound guidance, with permanent recording and reporting
- *CPT Changes: An Insider's View* 2015
- *CPT Assistant* Feb 15:6, Jul 15:10
- *Clinical Examples in Radiology* Spring 15:6

(Do not report 20600, 20604 in conjunction with 76942, 0489T, 0490T)

(If fluoroscopic, CT, or MRI guidance is performed, see 77002, 77012, 77021)

20605 Arthrocentesis, aspiration and/or injection, intermediate joint or bursa (eg, temporomandibular, acromioclavicular, wrist, elbow or ankle, olecranon bursa); without ultrasound guidance
- *CPT Changes: An Insider's View* 2003, 2015
- *CPT Assistant* Dec 07:10, Feb 15:6, Nov 15:10, Aug 17:9
- *Clinical Examples in Radiology* Spring 15:6

20606 with ultrasound guidance, with permanent recording and reporting
- *CPT Changes: An Insider's View* 2015
- *CPT Assistant* Feb 15:6, Jul 15:10
- *Clinical Examples in Radiology* Spring 15:6

(Do not report 20605, 20606 in conjunction with 76942)

(If fluoroscopic, CT, or MRI guidance is performed, see 77002, 77012, 77021)

20610 Arthrocentesis, aspiration and/or injection, major joint or bursa (eg, shoulder, hip, knee, subacromial bursa); without ultrasound guidance
- *CPT Changes: An Insider's View* 2015
- *CPT Assistant* Spring 92:8, Mar 01:10, Apr 04:15, Jul 06:1, Dec 07:10, Jul 08:9, Mar 12:6, Jun 12:14, Dec 14:18, Feb 15:6, Aug 15:6, Nov 15:10, Apr 17:10
- *Clinical Examples in Radiology* Spring 13:11, Spring 15:7

Arthrocentesis, Aspiration, or Injection of Major Joint or Bursa
20610

Insertion of needle into major joint or bursa for injection of therapeutic or diagnostic agent, aspiration, or arthrocentesis

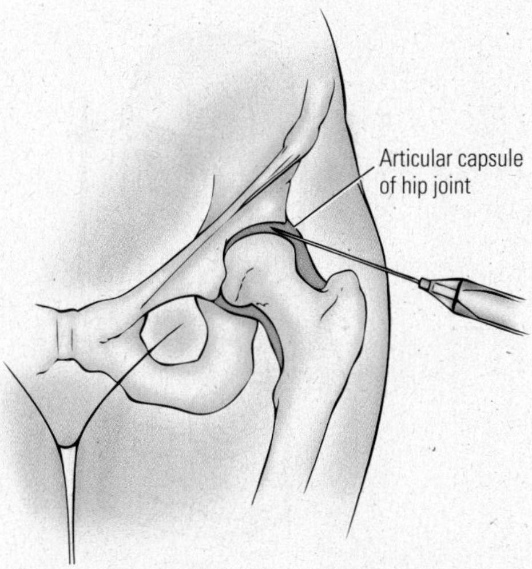

20611 with ultrasound guidance, with permanent recording and reporting
- *CPT Changes: An Insider's View* 2015
- *CPT Assistant* Feb 15:6, Jul 15:10, Aug 15:6, Nov 15:10
- *Clinical Examples in Radiology* Spring 15:7

►(Do not report 20610, 20611 in conjunction with 27369, 76942)◄

(If fluoroscopic, CT, or MRI guidance is performed, see 77002, 77012, 77021)

Musculoskeletal 20100-29999

20612 Aspiration and/or injection of ganglion cyst(s) any location

➔ *CPT Changes: An Insider's View* 2003

(To report multiple ganglion cyst aspirations/injections, use 20612 and append modifier 59)

20615 Aspiration and injection for treatment of bone cyst

20650 Insertion of wire or pin with application of skeletal traction, including removal (separate procedure)

20660 Application of cranial tongs, caliper, or stereotactic frame, including removal (separate procedure)

➔ *CPT Changes: An Insider's View* 2008

➔ *CPT Assistant* Jun 96:10, Nov 97:14, Jan 06:46, Dec 06:10, Feb 08:8, Jul 08:10, Nov 09:6, Apr 12:11, Aug 12:14

20661 Application of halo, including removal; cranial

➔ *CPT Assistant* Nov 97:14, Aug 12:14

20662 pelvic

20663 femoral

20664 Application of halo, including removal, cranial, 6 or more pins placed, for thin skull osteology (eg, pediatric patients, hydrocephalus, osteogenesis imperfecta)

➔ *CPT Changes: An Insider's View* 2011

➔ *CPT Assistant* Nov 97:14, Aug 12:5, Aug 13:12

Halo Application for Thin Skull Osteology
20664

A cranial halo is placed on the head of a child whose skull is unusually thin due to congenital or developmental problems.

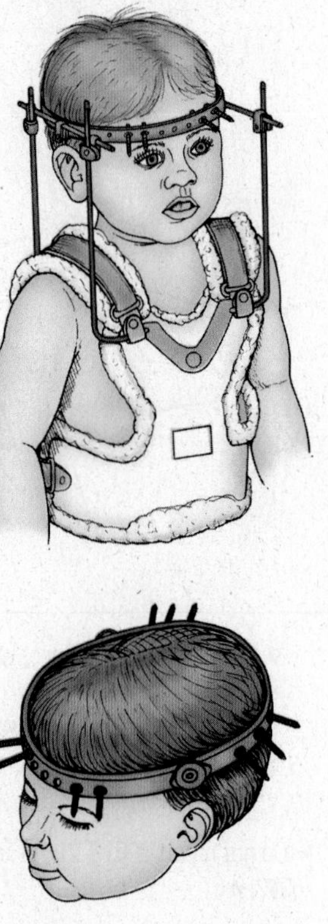

20665 Removal of tongs or halo applied by another individual

➔ *CPT Changes: An Insider's View* 2013

➔ *CPT Assistant* Apr 12:12

20670 Removal of implant; superficial (eg, buried wire, pin or rod) (separate procedure)

➔ *CPT Assistant* Dec 07:7, 8, Jun 09:7, Apr 12:17

20680 deep (eg, buried wire, pin, screw, metal band, nail, rod or plate)

➔ *CPT Assistant* Spring 92:11, Jun 09:7, Sep 12:16, Mar 14:4, Nov 15:10, Nov 16:9, Jan 18:3

►(For removal of sinus tarsi implant, use 0510T)◄

►(For removal and reinsertion of sinus tarsi implant, use 0511T)◄

Uniplane External Fixation System
20690

The following figures are examples of types of stabilization devices. Codes 20690 and 20692 describe the placement of types of external fixation devices. The method of stabilization depends upon fracture grade (degree of soft tissue injury/skin integrity disruption), type (eg, comminuted, spiral, impacted), and location (eg, extremity, pelvis).

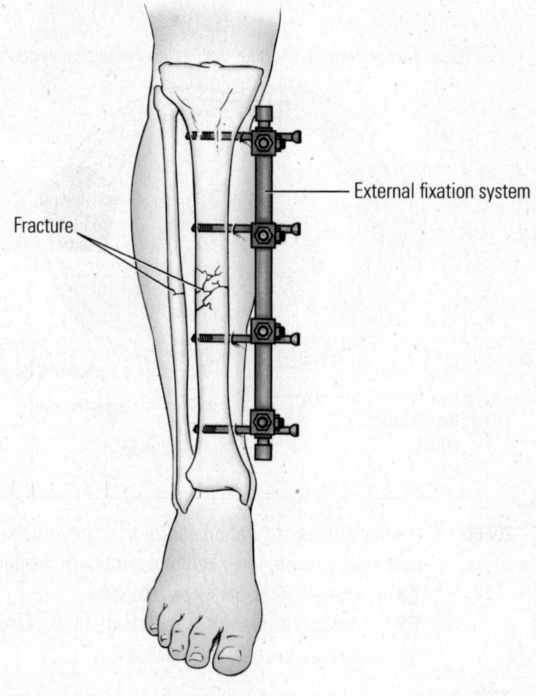

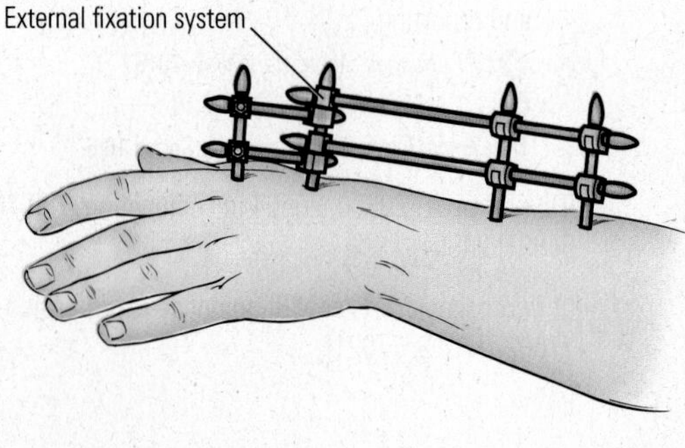

20690 Application of a uniplane (pins or wires in 1 plane), unilateral, external fixation system

➲ *CPT Changes: An Insider's View* 2008

➲ *CPT Assistant* Winter 90:4, Winter 92:11, Fall 93:21, Oct 99:5, Jan 04:27, Jun 05:12, Oct 07:7, Jan 08:4, Feb 08:9, Jun 09:7, Jan 18:3

20692 Application of a multiplane (pins or wires in more than 1 plane), unilateral, external fixation system (eg, Ilizarov, Monticelli type)

➲ *CPT Changes: An Insider's View* 2008

➲ *CPT Assistant* Winter 90:4, Fall 93:21, Oct 99:5, Jul 00:11, Feb 08:9, Jun 09:7, Jan 18:3

Multiplane External Fixation System
20692

The following figure is an example of a type of multiplane stabilization device. Codes 20690 and 20692 describe the placement of types of external fixation devices. The method of stabilization depends upon fracture grade (degree of soft tissue injury/skin integrity disruption), type (eg, comminuted, spiral, impacted), and location (eg, extremity, pelvis).

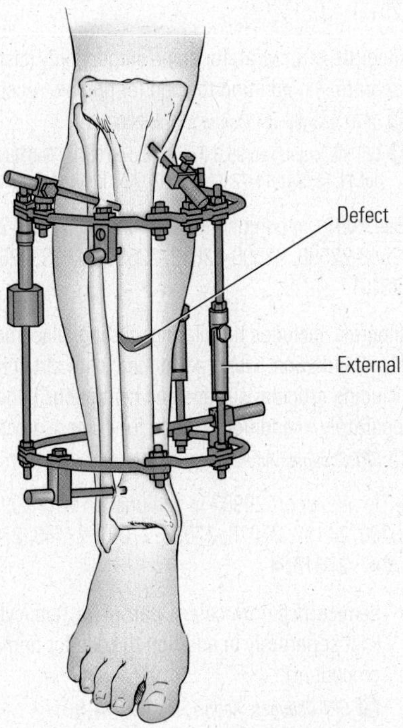

20693 Adjustment or revision of external fixation system requiring anesthesia (eg, new pin[s] or wire[s] and/or new ring[s] or bar[s])

➲ *CPT Assistant* Fall 93:21, Oct 99:5, Jul 00:11, Jun 09:7, Jan 18:3

20694 Removal, under anesthesia, of external fixation system

➲ *CPT Assistant* Winter 92:10, Fall 93:21, Oct 99:5, Jul 00:11, Jan 18:3

20696 Application of multiplane (pins or wires in more than 1 plane), unilateral, external fixation with stereotactic computer-assisted adjustment (eg, spatial frame), including imaging; initial and subsequent alignment(s), assessment(s), and computation(s) of adjustment schedule(s)

➲ *CPT Changes: An Insider's View* 2009

➲ *CPT Assistant* Jan 18:3

(Do not report 20696 in conjunction with 20692, 20697)

⊘ **20697** exchange (ie, removal and replacement) of strut, each

➲ *CPT Changes: An Insider's View* 2009

➲ *CPT Assistant* Jan 18:3

(Do not report 20697 in conjunction with 20692, 20696)

Replantation

20802 Replantation, arm (includes surgical neck of humerus through elbow joint), complete amputation

(To report replantation of incomplete arm amputation, see specific code[s] for repair of bone[s], ligament[s], tendon[s], nerve[s], or blood vessel[s] with modifier 52)

20805 Replantation, forearm (includes radius and ulna to radial carpal joint), complete amputation

(To report replantation of incomplete forearm amputation, see specific code[s] for repair of bone[s], ligament[s], tendon[s], nerve[s], or blood vessel[s] with modifier 52)

20808 Replantation, hand (includes hand through metacarpophalangeal joints), complete amputation

(To report replantation of incomplete hand amputation, see specific code[s] for repair of bone[s], ligament[s], tendon[s], nerve[s], or blood vessel[s] with modifier 52)

20816 Replantation, digit, excluding thumb (includes metacarpophalangeal joint to insertion of flexor sublimis tendon), complete amputation

➲ *CPT Assistant* Oct 96:11

(To report replantation of incomplete digit amputation, excluding thumb, see specific code[s] for repair of bone[s], ligament[s], tendon[s], nerve[s], or blood vessel[s] with modifier 52)

20822 Replantation, digit, excluding thumb (includes distal tip to sublimis tendon insertion), complete amputation

(To report replantation of incomplete digit amputation, excluding thumb, see specific code[s] for repair of bone[s], ligament[s], tendon[s], nerve[s], or blood vessel[s] with modifier 52)

20824 Replantation, thumb (includes carpometacarpal joint to MP joint), complete amputation

(To report replantation of incomplete thumb amputation, see specific code[s] for repair of bone[s], ligament[s], tendon[s], nerve[s], or blood vessel[s] with modifier 52)

20827 Replantation, thumb (includes distal tip to MP joint), complete amputation

(To report replantation of incomplete thumb amputation, see specific code[s] for repair of bone[s], ligament[s], tendon[s], nerve[s], or blood vessel[s] with modifier 52)

(To report replantation of complete leg amputation, see specific code[s] for repair of bone[s], ligament[s], tendon[s], nerve[s], or blood vessel[s] with modifier 52)

(To report replantation of incomplete leg amputation, see specific code[s] for repair of bone[s], ligament[s], tendon[s], nerve[s], or blood vessel[s] with modifier 52)

20838 Replantation, foot, complete amputation

(To report replantation of incomplete foot amputation, see specific code[s] for repair of bone[s], ligament[s], tendon[s], nerve[s], or blood vessel[s] with modifier 52)

Grafts (or Implants)

Codes for obtaining autogenous bone, cartilage, tendon, fascia lata grafts, bone marrow, or other tissues through separate skin/fascial incisions should be reported separately, unless the code descriptor references the harvesting of the graft or implant (eg, includes obtaining graft).

Do not append modifier 62 to bone graft codes 20900-20938.

(For spinal surgery bone graft[s] see codes 20930-20938)

20900 Bone graft, any donor area; minor or small (eg, dowel or button)
➲ *CPT Changes: An Insider's View* 2008
➲ *CPT Assistant* Dec 00:15, Jul 11:18

20902 major or large
➲ *CPT Changes: An Insider's View* 2008
➲ *CPT Assistant* Dec 00:15, Jul 11:18

20910 Cartilage graft; costochondral
➲ *CPT Changes: An Insider's View* 2008
➲ *CPT Assistant* Jan 13:15

20912 nasal septum
➲ *CPT Changes: An Insider's View* 2008

(For ear cartilage, use 21235)

20920 Fascia lata graft; by stripper
➲ *CPT Changes: An Insider's View* 2008
➲ *CPT Assistant* Aug 99:5, Jan 05:8

20922 by incision and area exposure, complex or sheet
➲ *CPT Changes: An Insider's View* 2008
➲ *CPT Assistant* Jan 05:8

20924 Tendon graft, from a distance (eg, palmaris, toe extensor, plantaris)
➲ *CPT Changes: An Insider's View* 2008

20926 Tissue grafts, other (eg, paratenon, fat, dermis)
➲ *CPT Changes: An Insider's View* 2008
➲ *CPT Assistant* Summer 91:12, Aug 99:5, Nov 99:10, May 06:16, Jun 12:15, Oct 16:11

(Do not report 20926 in conjunction with 0489T, 0490T)

(For harvesting of adipose tissue for autologous adipose-derived regenerative cell therapy, see 0489T, 0490T)

(For injection of autologous adipose-derived regenerative cells, see 0489T, 0490T)

(For harvesting, preparation, and injection[s] of platelet-rich plasma, use 0232T)

+ 20930 Allograft, morselized, or placement of osteopromotive material, for spine surgery only (List separately in addition to code for primary procedure)
➲ *CPT Changes: An Insider's View* 2008, 2011
➲ *CPT Assistant* Feb 96:6, Mar 96:4, Sep 97:8, Nov 99:10, Feb 02:6, Jan 04:27, Dec 07:1, Feb 08:8, Nov 10:8, Jul 11:18, Dec 11:15, Apr 12:14, Jun 12:11, Jul 13:3

(Use 20930 in conjunction with 22319, 22532, 22533, 22548-22558, 22590-22612, 22630, 22633, 22634, 22800-22812)

+ 20931 Allograft, structural, for spine surgery only (List separately in addition to code for primary procedure)
➲ *CPT Changes: An Insider's View* 2008, 2011
➲ *CPT Assistant* Feb 96:6, Feb 02:6, Feb 05:15, Feb 08:8, Nov 10:8, Jul 11:18, Sep 11:12, Dec 11:15, Apr 12:14, Jun 12:11, Jul 13:3

(Use 20931 in conjunction with 22319, 22532-22533, 22548-22558, 22590-22612, 22630, 22633, 22634, 22800-22812)

+● 20932 Allograft, includes templating, cutting, placement and internal fixation, when performed; osteoarticular, including articular surface and contiguous bone (List separately in addition to code for primary procedure)
➲ *CPT Changes: An Insider's View* 2019

►(Do not report 20932 in conjunction with 20933, 20934, 23200, 24152, 27078, 27090, 27091, 27448, 27646, 27647, 27648)◄

+● 20933 hemicortical intercalary, partial (ie, hemicylindrical) (List separately in addition to code for primary procedure)
➲ *CPT Changes: An Insider's View* 2019

►(Do not report 20933 in conjunction with 20932, 20934, 23200, 24152, 27078, 27090, 27091, 27448, 27646, 27647, 27648)◄

+● 20934 intercalary, complete (ie, cylindrical) (List separately in addition to code for primary procedure)
➲ *CPT Changes: An Insider's View* 2019

►(Do not report 20934 in conjunction with 20932, 20933, 20955, 20956, 20957, 20962, 23146, 23156, 23200, 24116, 24126, 24152, 25126, 25136, 27078, 27090, 27091, 27130, 27132, 27134, 27138, 27236, 27244, 27356, 27448, 27638, 27646, 27647, 27648, 28103, 28107)◄

►(Insertion of joint prosthesis may be separately reported)◄

►(Use 20932, 20933, 20934 in conjunction with 23210, 23220, 24150, 25170, 27075, 27076, 27077, 27365, 27645, 27704)◄

+ 20936 Autograft for spine surgery only (includes harvesting the graft); local (eg, ribs, spinous process, or laminar fragments) obtained from same incision (List separately in addition to code for primary procedure)
- *CPT Changes: An Insider's View* 2008
- *CPT Assistant* Feb 96:6, Sep 97:8, Feb 02:6, Feb 08:8, Dec 11:15, Apr 12:14, Jun 12:11, Jul 13:3

(Use 20936 in conjunction with 22319, 22532, 22533, 22548-22558, 22590-22612, 22630, 22633, 22634, 22800-22812)

+ 20937 morselized (through separate skin or fascial incision) (List separately in addition to code for primary procedure)
- *CPT Changes: An Insider's View* 2008
- *CPT Assistant* Feb 96:6, Sep 97:8, Dec 99:2, Feb 02:6, Feb 08:8, Dec 11:15, Apr 12:11, Jun 12:11, Jul 13:3

(Use 20937 in conjunction with 22319, 22532, 22533, 22548-22558, 22590-22612, 22630, 22633, 22634, 22800-22812)

+ 20938 structural, bicortical or tricortical (through separate skin or fascial incision) (List separately in addition to code for primary procedure)
- *CPT Changes: An Insider's View* 2008
- *CPT Assistant* Feb 96:6, Mar 96:5, Sep 97:8, Feb 02:6, Feb 08:8, Jul 11:18, Dec 11:15, Apr 12:12, May 12:11, Jun 12:11, Jul 13:3

(Use 20938 in conjunction with 22319, 22532, 22533, 22548-22558, 22590-22612, 22630, 22633, 22634, 22800-22812)

(For aspiration of bone marrow for bone grafting, spine surgery only, use 20939)

+ 20939 Bone marrow aspiration for bone grafting, spine surgery only, through separate skin or fascial incision (List separately in addition to code for primary procedure)
- *CPT Changes: An Insider's View* 2018
- *Clinical Examples in Radiology* Spring 18:6

(Use 20939 in conjunction with 22319, 22532, 22533, 22534, 22548, 22551, 22552, 22554, 22556, 22558, 22590, 22595, 22600, 22610, 22612, 22630, 22633, 22634, 22800, 22802, 22804, 22808, 22810, 22812)

(For bilateral procedure, use 20939 with modifier 50)

(For aspiration of bone marrow for the purpose of bone grafting, other than spine surgery and other therapeutic musculoskeletal applications, use 20999)

(For bone marrow aspiration[s] for platelet-rich stem cell injection, use 0232T)

(For diagnostic bone marrow aspiration[s], see 38220, 38222)

Other Procedures

20950 Monitoring of interstitial fluid pressure (includes insertion of device, eg, wick catheter technique, needle manometer technique) in detection of muscle compartment syndrome
- *CPT Assistant* Sep 07:10

20955 Bone graft with microvascular anastomosis; fibula
- *CPT Assistant* Apr 97:4

20956 iliac crest
- *CPT Assistant* Apr 97:4

20957 metatarsal
- *CPT Assistant* Apr 97:4

20962 other than fibula, iliac crest, or metatarsal
- *CPT Assistant* Apr 97:4

(Do not report code 69990 in addition to codes 20955-20962)

20969 Free osteocutaneous flap with microvascular anastomosis; other than iliac crest, metatarsal, or great toe
- *CPT Assistant* Apr 97:4

20970 iliac crest
- *CPT Assistant* Apr 97:4

20972 metatarsal
- *CPT Assistant* Apr 97:4

20973 great toe with web space
- *CPT Assistant* Apr 97:4

(Do not report code 69990 in addition to codes 20969-20973)

(For great toe, wrap-around procedure, use 26551)

⊘ 20974 Electrical stimulation to aid bone healing; noninvasive (nonoperative)
- *CPT Assistant* Sep 96:11, Nov 00:8

⊘ 20975 invasive (operative)
- *CPT Assistant* Nov 00:8

20979 Low intensity ultrasound stimulation to aid bone healing, noninvasive (nonoperative)
- *CPT Changes: An Insider's View* 2000
- *CPT Assistant* Nov 99:10, Nov 00:8

20982 Ablation therapy for reduction or eradication of 1 or more bone tumors (eg, metastasis) including adjacent soft tissue when involved by tumor extension, percutaneous, including imaging guidance when performed; radiofrequency
- *CPT Changes: An Insider's View* 2004, 2015, 2017
- *CPT Assistant* Jul 15:8, Sep 15:12
- *Clinical Examples in Radiology* Spring 15:3

20983 cryoablation
- *CPT Changes: An Insider's View* 2015, 2017
- *CPT Assistant* Jul 15:8
- *Clinical Examples in Radiology* Spring 15:2

Musculoskeletal 20100-29999

(Do not report 20982, 20983 in conjunction with 76940, 77002, 77013, 77022)

+ 20985 Computer-assisted surgical navigational procedure for musculoskeletal procedures, image-less (List separately in addition to code for primary procedure)
➲ *CPT Changes: An Insider's View* 2008, 2009
➲ *CPT Assistant* Jul 11:12

(Do not report 20985 in conjunction with 61781-61783)

(20986, 20987 have been deleted)

(For computer-assisted navigational procedures with image guidance based on pre-operative and intraoperatively obtained images, see 0054T, 0055T)

20999 Unlisted procedure, musculoskeletal system, general
➲ *CPT Assistant* Sep 03:13, Jul 15:8
➲ *Clinical Examples in Radiology* Spring 15:3

Head

Skull, facial bones, and temporomandibular joint.

Incision

►(For incision and drainage procedures, cutaneous/subcutaneous, see 10060, 10061)◄

(For removal of embedded foreign body from dentoalveolar structure, see 41805, 41806)

21010 Arthrotomy, temporomandibular joint

(To report bilateral procedure, report 21010 with modifier 50)

Excision

21011 Excision, tumor, soft tissue of face or scalp, subcutaneous; less than 2 cm
➲ *CPT Changes: An Insider's View* 2010
➲ *CPT Assistant* Feb 10:3, Apr 10:3

21012 2 cm or greater
➲ *CPT Changes: An Insider's View* 2010
➲ *CPT Assistant* Feb 10:3, Apr 10:3

(For excision of benign lesions of cutaneous origin [eg, sebaceous cyst], see 11420-11426)

21013 Excision, tumor, soft tissue of face and scalp, subfascial (eg, subgaleal, intramuscular); less than 2 cm
➲ *CPT Changes: An Insider's View* 2010
➲ *CPT Assistant* Feb 10:3, Apr 10:3

21014 2 cm or greater
➲ *CPT Changes: An Insider's View* 2010
➲ *CPT Assistant* Feb 10:3, Apr 10:3

21015 Radical resection of tumor (eg, sarcoma), soft tissue of face or scalp; less than 2 cm
➲ *CPT Changes: An Insider's View* 2010, 2014
➲ *CPT Assistant* Feb 10:3, Apr 10:3

(To report excision of skull tumor for osteomyelitis, use 61501)

21016 2 cm or greater
➲ *CPT Changes: An Insider's View* 2010, 2014
➲ *CPT Assistant* Feb 10:3, Apr 10:3

(For radical resection of tumor[s] of cutaneous origin [eg, melanoma], see 11620-11646)

21025 Excision of bone (eg, for osteomyelitis or bone abscess); mandible
➲ *CPT Assistant* Oct 11:10

21026 facial bone(s)

21029 Removal by contouring of benign tumor of facial bone (eg, fibrous dysplasia)

21030 Excision of benign tumor or cyst of maxilla or zygoma by enucleation and curettage
➲ *CPT Changes: An Insider's View* 2003
➲ *CPT Assistant* Nov 03:9

21031 Excision of torus mandibularis

21032 Excision of maxillary torus palatinus

21034 Excision of malignant tumor of maxilla or zygoma
➲ *CPT Changes: An Insider's View* 2003
➲ *CPT Assistant* Nov 03:9

21040 Excision of benign tumor or cyst of mandible, by enucleation and/or curettage
➲ *CPT Changes: An Insider's View* 2003
➲ *CPT Assistant* Nov 03:9

(For enucleation and/or curettage of benign cysts or tumors of mandible not requiring osteotomy, use 21040)

(For excision of benign tumor or cyst of mandible requiring osteotomy, see 21046-21047)

21044 Excision of malignant tumor of mandible;

21045 radical resection

(For bone graft, use 21215)

21046 Excision of benign tumor or cyst of mandible; requiring intra-oral osteotomy (eg, locally aggressive or destructive lesion[s])
➲ *CPT Changes: An Insider's View* 2003
➲ *CPT Assistant* Nov 03:9

21047 requiring extra-oral osteotomy and partial mandibulectomy (eg, locally aggressive or destructive lesion[s])
➲ *CPT Changes: An Insider's View* 2003
➲ *CPT Assistant* Nov 03:9

21048 Excision of benign tumor or cyst of maxilla; requiring intra-oral osteotomy (eg, locally aggressive or destructive lesion[s])
➲ *CPT Changes: An Insider's View* 2003
➲ *CPT Assistant* Nov 03:9

21049 requiring extra-oral osteotomy and partial maxillectomy (eg, locally aggressive or destructive lesion[s])
➲ *CPT Changes: An Insider's View* 2003
➲ *CPT Assistant* Nov 03:9

21050 Condylectomy, temporomandibular joint (separate procedure)

(For bilateral procedures, report 21050 with modifier 50)

21060 Meniscectomy, partial or complete, temporomandibular joint (separate procedure)

(For bilateral procedures, report 21060 with modifier 50)

21070 Coronoidectomy (separate procedure)

(For bilateral procedures, report 21070 with modifier 50)

Manipulation

21073 Manipulation of temporomandibular joint(s) (TMJ), therapeutic, requiring an anesthesia service (ie, general or monitored anesthesia care)
➲ *CPT Changes: An Insider's View* 2008
➲ *CPT Assistant* Feb 08:9, Jan 18:3

(For TMJ manipulation without an anesthesia service [ie, general or monitored anesthesia care], see 97140, 98925-98929, 98943)

(For closed treatment of temporomandibular dislocation, see 21480, 21485)

Head Prosthesis

Codes 21076-21089 describe professional services for the rehabilitation of patients with oral, facial, or other anatomical deficiencies by means of prostheses such as an artificial eye, ear, or nose or intraoral obturator to close a cleft. Codes 21076-21089 should only be used when the physician or other qualified health care professional actually designs and prepares the prosthesis (ie, not prepared by an outside laboratory).

(For application or removal of caliper or tongs, see 20660, 20665)

21076 Impression and custom preparation; surgical obturator prosthesis

21077 orbital prosthesis

21079 interim obturator prosthesis
➲ *CPT Assistant* Winter 90:5, Sep 06:13, Dec 06:10

21080 definitive obturator prosthesis
➲ *CPT Assistant* Winter 90:5, Sep 06:13, Dec 06:10

21081 mandibular resection prosthesis
➲ *CPT Assistant* Winter 90:5, Sep 06:13, Dec 06:10

21082 palatal augmentation prosthesis
➲ *CPT Assistant* Winter 90:5, Sep 06:13, Dec 06:10

21083 palatal lift prosthesis
➲ *CPT Assistant* Winter 90:5, Sep 06:13, Dec 06:10

21084 speech aid prosthesis
➲ *CPT Assistant* Winter 90:5, Sep 06:13, Dec 06:10

21085 oral surgical splint
➲ *CPT Assistant* Winter 90:5, Sep 06:13, Dec 06:10, Sep 17:14

21086 auricular prosthesis
➲ *CPT Assistant* Winter 90:5, Sep 06:13, Dec 06:10

21087 nasal prosthesis
➲ *CPT Assistant* Winter 90:5, Sep 06:13, Dec 06:10

21088 facial prosthesis
➲ *CPT Assistant* Winter 90:5, Sep 06:13, Dec 06:10

Other Procedures

21089 Unlisted maxillofacial prosthetic procedure
➲ *CPT Assistant* Winter 90:5, Sep 06:13, Dec 06:10

Introduction or Removal

21100 Application of halo type appliance for maxillofacial fixation, includes removal (separate procedure)

21110 Application of interdental fixation device for conditions other than fracture or dislocation, includes removal
➲ *CPT Assistant* Mar 97:10, Dec 13:16

(For removal of interdental fixation by another individual, see 20670-20680)

21116 Injection procedure for temporomandibular joint arthrography
➲ *CPT Assistant* Aug 15:6, May 16:13

(For radiological supervision and interpretation, use 70332. Do not report 77002 in conjunction with 70332)

Repair, Revision, and/or Reconstruction

(For cranioplasty, see 21179, 21180 and 62120, 62140-62147)

21120 Genioplasty; augmentation (autograft, allograft, prosthetic material)

21121 sliding osteotomy, single piece

21122 sliding osteotomies, 2 or more osteotomies (eg, wedge excision or bone wedge reversal for asymmetrical chin)

21123 sliding, augmentation with interpositional bone grafts (includes obtaining autografts)

21125 Augmentation, mandibular body or angle; prosthetic material

21127 with bone graft, onlay or interpositional (includes obtaining autograft)

21137 Reduction forehead; contouring only

21138 contouring and application of prosthetic material or bone graft (includes obtaining autograft)

21139 contouring and setback of anterior frontal sinus wall

21141 Reconstruction midface, LeFort I; single piece, segment movement in any direction (eg, for Long Face Syndrome), without bone graft

21142 2 pieces, segment movement in any direction, without bone graft

21143 3 or more pieces, segment movement in any direction, without bone graft

21145 single piece, segment movement in any direction, requiring bone grafts (includes obtaining autografts)

21146 2 pieces, segment movement in any direction, requiring bone grafts (includes obtaining autografts) (eg, ungrafted unilateral alveolar cleft)

21147 3 or more pieces, segment movement in any direction, requiring bone grafts (includes obtaining autografts) (eg, ungrafted bilateral alveolar cleft or multiple osteotomies)

21150 Reconstruction midface, LeFort II; anterior intrusion (eg, Treacher-Collins Syndrome)

21151 any direction, requiring bone grafts (includes obtaining autografts)

21154 Reconstruction midface, LeFort III (extracranial), any type, requiring bone grafts (includes obtaining autografts); without LeFort I

21155 with LeFort I

21159 Reconstruction midface, LeFort III (extra and intracranial) with forehead advancement (eg, mono bloc), requiring bone grafts (includes obtaining autografts); without LeFort I

21160 with LeFort I

21172 Reconstruction superior-lateral orbital rim and lower forehead, advancement or alteration, with or without grafts (includes obtaining autografts)

(For frontal or parietal craniotomy performed for craniosynostosis, use 61556)

21175 Reconstruction, bifrontal, superior-lateral orbital rims and lower forehead, advancement or alteration (eg, plagiocephaly, trigonocephaly, brachycephaly), with or without grafts (includes obtaining autografts)

(For bifrontal craniotomy performed for craniosynostosis, use 61557)

21179 Reconstruction, entire or majority of forehead and/or supraorbital rims; with grafts (allograft or prosthetic material)

21180 with autograft (includes obtaining grafts)

(For extensive craniectomy for multiple suture craniosynostosis, use only 61558 or 61559)

21181 Reconstruction by contouring of benign tumor of cranial bones (eg, fibrous dysplasia), extracranial

21182 Reconstruction of orbital walls, rims, forehead, nasoethmoid complex following intra- and extracranial excision of benign tumor of cranial bone (eg, fibrous dysplasia), with multiple autografts (includes obtaining grafts); total area of bone grafting less than 40 sq cm

21183 total area of bone grafting greater than 40 sq cm but less than 80 sq cm

➔ *CPT Changes: An Insider's View* 2002

21184 total area of bone grafting greater than 80 sq cm

➔ *CPT Changes: An Insider's View* 2002

(For excision of benign tumor of cranial bones, see 61563, 61564)

21188 Reconstruction midface, osteotomies (other than LeFort type) and bone grafts (includes obtaining autografts)

21193 Reconstruction of mandibular rami, horizontal, vertical, C, or L osteotomy; without bone graft

➔ *CPT Assistant* Apr 96:11

21194 with bone graft (includes obtaining graft)

➔ *CPT Assistant* Apr 96:11

21195 Reconstruction of mandibular rami and/or body, sagittal split; without internal rigid fixation

➔ *CPT Assistant* Apr 96:11

21196 with internal rigid fixation

➔ *CPT Assistant* Apr 96:11, Mar 97:11

Reconstruction of Mandibular Rami
21196

The mandibular ramus is reconstructed to lengthen, set back, or rotate the mandible.

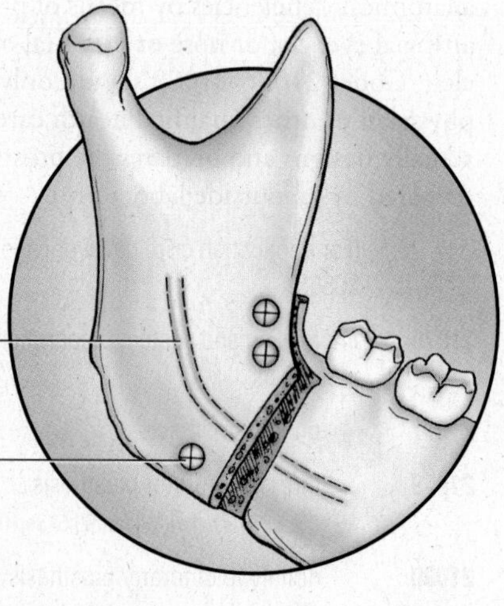

21198 Osteotomy, mandible, segmental;

➔ *CPT Changes: An Insider's View* 2001

➔ *CPT Assistant* Dec 13:16

21199 with genioglossus advancement

➔ *CPT Changes: An Insider's View* 2001

(To report total osteotomy of the maxilla, see 21141-21160)

21206 Osteotomy, maxilla, segmental (eg, Wassmund or Schuchard)

21208 Osteoplasty, facial bones; augmentation (autograft, allograft, or prosthetic implant)

21209 reduction

21210 Graft, bone; nasal, maxillary or malar areas (includes obtaining graft)

(For cleft palate repair, see 42200-42225)

21215 mandible (includes obtaining graft)

21230 Graft; rib cartilage, autogenous, to face, chin, nose or ear (includes obtaining graft)

21235 ear cartilage, autogenous, to nose or ear (includes obtaining graft)

(To report graft augmentation of facial bones, use 21208)

21240 Arthroplasty, temporomandibular joint, with or without autograft (includes obtaining graft)

21242 Arthroplasty, temporomandibular joint, with allograft

21243 Arthroplasty, temporomandibular joint, with prosthetic joint replacement

21244 Reconstruction of mandible, extraoral, with transosteal bone plate (eg, mandibular staple bone plate)

21245 Reconstruction of mandible or maxilla, subperiosteal implant; partial

21246 complete

21247 Reconstruction of mandibular condyle with bone and cartilage autografts (includes obtaining grafts) (eg, for hemifacial microsomia)

21248 Reconstruction of mandible or maxilla, endosteal implant (eg, blade, cylinder); partial

21249 complete

(To report midface reconstruction, see 21141-21160)

21255 Reconstruction of zygomatic arch and glenoid fossa with bone and cartilage (includes obtaining autografts)

21256 Reconstruction of orbit with osteotomies (extracranial) and with bone grafts (includes obtaining autografts) (eg, micro-ophthalmia)

21260 Periorbital osteotomies for orbital hypertelorism, with bone grafts; extracranial approach

21261 combined intra- and extracranial approach

21263 with forehead advancement

21267 Orbital repositioning, periorbital osteotomies, unilateral, with bone grafts; extracranial approach

21268 combined intra- and extracranial approach

21270 Malar augmentation, prosthetic material

(For malar augmentation with bone graft, use 21210)

21275 Secondary revision of orbitocraniofacial reconstruction

21280 Medial canthopexy (separate procedure)

(For medial canthoplasty, use 67950)

21282 Lateral canthopexy

21295 Reduction of masseter muscle and bone (eg, for treatment of benign masseteric hypertrophy); extraoral approach

21296 intraoral approach

Other Procedures

21299 Unlisted craniofacial and maxillofacial procedure

Fracture and/or Dislocation

(For operative repair of skull fracture, see 62000-62010)

(To report closed treatment of skull fracture, use the appropriate Evaluation and Management code)

21310 Closed treatment of nasal bone fracture without manipulation

➔ *CPT Assistant* Jan 18:3

21315 Closed treatment of nasal bone fracture; without stabilization

➔ *CPT Assistant* Jan 18:3

21320 with stabilization

21325 Open treatment of nasal fracture; uncomplicated

21330 complicated, with internal and/or external skeletal fixation

21335 with concomitant open treatment of fractured septum

21336 Open treatment of nasal septal fracture, with or without stabilization

21337 Closed treatment of nasal septal fracture, with or without stabilization

21338 Open treatment of nasoethmoid fracture; without external fixation

21339 with external fixation

21340 Percutaneous treatment of nasoethmoid complex fracture, with splint, wire or headcap fixation, including repair of canthal ligaments and/or the nasolacrimal apparatus

21343 Open treatment of depressed frontal sinus fracture

21344 Open treatment of complicated (eg, comminuted or involving posterior wall) frontal sinus fracture, via coronal or multiple approaches

21345 Closed treatment of nasomaxillary complex fracture (LeFort II type), with interdental wire fixation or fixation of denture or splint

21346 Open treatment of nasomaxillary complex fracture (LeFort II type); with wiring and/or local fixation

21347 requiring multiple open approaches

21348 with bone grafting (includes obtaining graft)

21355 Percutaneous treatment of fracture of malar area, including zygomatic arch and malar tripod, with manipulation

21356 Open treatment of depressed zygomatic arch fracture (eg, Gillies approach)

21360 Open treatment of depressed malar fracture, including zygomatic arch and malar tripod

21365 Open treatment of complicated (eg, comminuted or involving cranial nerve foramina) fracture(s) of malar area, including zygomatic arch and malar tripod; with internal fixation and multiple surgical approaches

21366 with bone grafting (includes obtaining graft)

21385 Open treatment of orbital floor blowout fracture; transantral approach (Caldwell-Luc type operation)

21386 periorbital approach

21387 combined approach

21390 periorbital approach, with alloplastic or other implant

21395 periorbital approach with bone graft (includes obtaining graft)

21400 Closed treatment of fracture of orbit, except blowout; without manipulation

21401 with manipulation

21406 Open treatment of fracture of orbit, except blowout; without implant

21407 with implant

21408 with bone grafting (includes obtaining graft)

21421 Closed treatment of palatal or maxillary fracture (LeFort I type), with interdental wire fixation or fixation of denture or splint

21422 Open treatment of palatal or maxillary fracture (LeFort I type);

21423 complicated (comminuted or involving cranial nerve foramina), multiple approaches

21431 Closed treatment of craniofacial separation (LeFort III type) using interdental wire fixation of denture or splint

21432 Open treatment of craniofacial separation (LeFort III type); with wiring and/or internal fixation

21433 complicated (eg, comminuted or involving cranial nerve foramina), multiple surgical approaches

21435 complicated, utilizing internal and/or external fixation techniques (eg, head cap, halo device, and/or intermaxillary fixation)

(For removal of internal or external fixation device, use 20670)

21436 complicated, multiple surgical approaches, internal fixation, with bone grafting (includes obtaining graft)

21440 Closed treatment of mandibular or maxillary alveolar ridge fracture (separate procedure)

21445 Open treatment of mandibular or maxillary alveolar ridge fracture (separate procedure)

21450 Closed treatment of mandibular fracture; without manipulation

21451 with manipulation

21452 Percutaneous treatment of mandibular fracture, with external fixation

21453 Closed treatment of mandibular fracture with interdental fixation

➲ *CPT Assistant* Dec 07:7, 8

21454 Open treatment of mandibular fracture with external fixation

21461 Open treatment of mandibular fracture; without interdental fixation

21462 with interdental fixation

21465 Open treatment of mandibular condylar fracture

21470 Open treatment of complicated mandibular fracture by multiple surgical approaches including internal fixation, interdental fixation, and/or wiring of dentures or splints

➲ *CPT Assistant* Nov 02:10

21480 Closed treatment of temporomandibular dislocation; initial or subsequent

21485 complicated (eg, recurrent requiring intermaxillary fixation or splinting), initial or subsequent

21490 Open treatment of temporomandibular dislocation

(For interdental wire fixation, use 21497)

(To report treatment of closed fracture of larynx, use the applicable Evaluation and Management codes)

21497 Interdental wiring, for condition other than fracture

➲ *CPT Assistant* Mar 97:10

Other Procedures

21499 Unlisted musculoskeletal procedure, head

(For unlisted craniofacial or maxillofacial procedure, use 21299)

Neck (Soft Tissues) and Thorax

(For cervical spine and back, see 21920 et seq)

(For injection of fracture site or trigger point, use 20550)

Incision

(For incision and drainage of abscess or hematoma, superficial, see 10060, 10140)

21501 Incision and drainage, deep abscess or hematoma, soft tissues of neck or thorax;

➲ *CPT Assistant* Dec 14:16

(For posterior spine subfascial incision and drainage, see 22010-22015)

21502 with partial rib ostectomy

21510 Incision, deep, with opening of bone cortex (eg, for osteomyelitis or bone abscess), thorax

Excision

(For bone biopsy, see 20220-20251)

21550 Biopsy, soft tissue of neck or thorax

(For needle biopsy of soft tissue, use 20206)

21552 Code is out of numerical sequence. See 21550-21558

21554 Code is out of numerical sequence. See 21550-21558

21555 Excision, tumor, soft tissue of neck or anterior thorax, subcutaneous; less than 3 cm
➔ *CPT Changes: An Insider's View* 2010
➔ *CPT Assistant* Oct 02:11

 # 21552 3 cm or greater
➔ *CPT Changes: An Insider's View* 2010

(For excision of benign lesions of cutaneous origin [eg, sebaceous cyst], see 11420-11426)

21556 Excision, tumor, soft tissue of neck or anterior thorax, subfascial (eg, intramuscular); less than 5 cm
➔ *CPT Changes: An Insider's View* 2010

 # 21554 5 cm or greater
➔ *CPT Changes: An Insider's View* 2010

21557 Radical resection of tumor (eg, sarcoma), soft tissue of neck or anterior thorax; less than 5 cm
➔ *CPT Changes: An Insider's View* 2010, 2014
➔ *CPT Assistant* Apr 10:11

21558 5 cm or greater
➔ *CPT Changes: An Insider's View* 2010, 2014

(For radical resection of tumor[s] of cutaneous origin [eg, melanoma], see 11600-11620)

21600 Excision of rib, partial
➔ *CPT Assistant* Jul 12:12, Mar 13:13

(For radical resection of chest wall and rib cage for tumor, use 19260)

(For radical debridement of chest wall and rib cage for injury, see 11044, 11047)

21610 Costotransversectomy (separate procedure)

21615 Excision first and/or cervical rib;
➔ *CPT Assistant* Mar 14:13

21616 with sympathectomy

21620 Ostectomy of sternum, partial

21627 Sternal debridement
➔ *CPT Assistant* May 11:3

(For debridement and closure, use 21750)

21630 Radical resection of sternum;

21632 with mediastinal lymphadenectomy

Repair, Revision, and/or Reconstruction

(For superficial wound, see **Integumentary System** section under Repair—Simple)

21685 Hyoid myotomy and suspension
➔ *CPT Changes: An Insider's View* 2004
➔ *CPT Assistant* Aug 04:11

21700 Division of scalenus anticus; without resection of cervical rib

21705 with resection of cervical rib
➔ *CPT Assistant* Mar 14:13

21720 Division of sternocleidomastoid for torticollis, open operation; without cast application

(For transection of spinal accessory and cervical nerves, see 63191, 64722)

21725 with cast application

21740 Reconstructive repair of pectus excavatum or carinatum; open
➔ *CPT Changes: An Insider's View* 2003

21742 minimally invasive approach (Nuss procedure), without thoracoscopy
➔ *CPT Changes: An Insider's View* 2003

21743 minimally invasive approach (Nuss procedure), with thoracoscopy
➔ *CPT Changes: An Insider's View* 2003

21750 Closure of median sternotomy separation with or without debridement (separate procedure)
➔ *CPT Changes: An Insider's View* 2002
➔ *CPT Assistant* May 11:3

Fracture and/or Dislocation

(To report closed treatment of an uncomplicated rib fracture, use the Evaluation and Management codes)

(21805 has been deleted)

21811 Open treatment of rib fracture(s) with internal fixation, includes thoracoscopic visualization when performed, unilateral; 1-3 ribs
➔ *CPT Changes: An Insider's View* 2015
➔ *CPT Assistant* Aug 15:3

(For bilateral procedure, report 21811 with modifier 50)

21812 4-6 ribs
➔ *CPT Changes: An Insider's View* 2015
➔ *CPT Assistant* Aug 15:3

(For bilateral procedure, report 21812 with modifier 50)

21813 7 or more ribs
➔ *CPT Changes: An Insider's View* 2015
➔ *CPT Assistant* Aug 15:3

Musculoskeletal 20100-29999

(For bilateral procedure, report 21813 with modifier 50)

21820 Closed treatment of sternum fracture

21825 Open treatment of sternum fracture with or without skeletal fixation

(For sternoclavicular dislocation, see 23520-23532)

Other Procedures

21899 Unlisted procedure, neck or thorax
➔ *CPT Assistant* Aug 15:3

Back and Flank

Excision

21920 Biopsy, soft tissue of back or flank; superficial

21925 deep

(For needle biopsy of soft tissue, use 20206)

21930 Excision, tumor, soft tissue of back or flank, subcutaneous; less than 3 cm
➔ *CPT Changes: An Insider's View* 2010

21931 3 cm or greater
➔ *CPT Changes: An Insider's View* 2010

(For excision of benign lesions of cutaneous origin [eg, sebaceous cyst], see 11400-11406)

21932 Excision, tumor, soft tissue of back or flank, subfascial (eg, intramuscular); less than 5 cm
➔ *CPT Changes: An Insider's View* 2010

21933 5 cm or greater
➔ *CPT Changes: An Insider's View* 2010

21935 Radical resection of tumor (eg, sarcoma), soft tissue of back or flank; less than 5 cm
➔ *CPT Changes: An Insider's View* 2010, 2014

21936 5 cm or greater
➔ *CPT Changes: An Insider's View* 2010, 2014

(For radical resection of tumor[s] of cutaneous origin [eg, melanoma], see 11600-11606)

Spine (Vertebral Column)

Cervical, thoracic, and lumbar spine.

Within the spine section, bone grafting procedures are reported separately and in addition to arthrodesis. For bone grafts in other Musculoskeletal sections, see specific code(s) descriptor(s) and/or accompanying guidelines.

To report bone grafts performed after arthrodesis, see 20930-20938. Do not append modifier 62 to bone graft codes 20900-20938.

Example:

Posterior arthrodesis of L5-S1 for degenerative disc disease utilizing morselized autogenous iliac bone graft harvested through a separate fascial incision.

Report as 22612 and 20937.

Within the spine section, instrumentation is reported separately and in addition to arthrodesis. To report instrumentation procedures performed with definitive vertebral procedure(s), see 22840-22855, 22859. Instrumentation procedure codes 22840-22848, 22853, 22854, 22859 are reported in addition to the definitive procedure(s). Modifier 62 may not be appended to the definitive or add-on spinal instrumentation procedure code(s) 22840-22848, 22850, 22852, 22853, 22854, 22859.

Example:

Posterior arthrodesis of L4-S1, utilizing morselized autogenous iliac bone graft harvested through separate fascial incision, and pedicle screw fixation.

Report as 22612, 22614, 22842, and 20937.

Vertebral procedures are sometimes followed by arthrodesis and in addition may include bone grafts and instrumentation.

When arthrodesis is performed in addition to another procedure, the arthrodesis should be reported in addition to the original procedure with modifier 51 (multiple procedures). Examples are after osteotomy, fracture care, vertebral corpectomy, and laminectomy. Bone grafts and instrumentation are never performed without arthrodesis.

Example:

Treatment of a burst fracture of L2 by corpectomy followed by arthrodesis of L1-L3, utilizing anterior instrumentation L1-L3 and structural allograft.

Report as 63090, 22558-51, 22585, 22845, and 20931.

When two surgeons work together as primary surgeons performing distinct part(s) of a single reportable procedure, each surgeon should report his/her distinct operative work by appending modifier 62 to the single definitive procedure code. If additional procedure(s) (including add-on procedure[s]) are performed during the same surgical session, separate code(s) may be reported by each co-surgeon, with modifier 62 appended (see Appendix A).

Example:

A 42-year-old male with a history of posttraumatic degenerative disc disease at L3-4 and L4-5 (internal disc disruption) underwent surgical repair. Surgeon A performed an anterior exposure of the spine with mobilization of the great vessels. Surgeon B performed anterior (minimal) discectomy and fusion at L3-4 and L4-5 using anterior interbody technique.

Report surgeon A: 22558 append modifier 62, 22585 append modifier 62

Report surgeon B: 22558 append modifier 62, 22585 append modifier 62, 20931

(Do not append modifier 62 to bone graft code 20931)

(For injection procedure for myelography, use 62284)

(For injection procedure for discography, see 62290, 62291)

(For injection procedure, chemonucleolysis, single or multiple levels, use 62292)

(For injection procedure for facet joints, see 64490-64495, 64633-64636)

(For needle or trocar biopsy, see 20220-20225)

Incision

22010 Incision and drainage, open, of deep abscess (subfascial), posterior spine; cervical, thoracic, or cervicothoracic
➔ *CPT Changes: An Insider's View* 2006

22015 lumbar, sacral, or lumbosacral
➔ *CPT Changes: An Insider's View* 2006

(Do not report 22015 in conjunction with 22010)

(Do not report 22015 in conjunction with instrumentation removal, 10180, 22850, 22852)

(For incision and drainage of abscess or hematoma, superficial, see 10060, 10140)

Excision

For the following codes, when two surgeons work together as primary surgeons performing distinct part(s) of partial vertebral body excision, each surgeon should report his/her distinct operative work by appending modifier 62 to the procedure code. In this situation, modifier 62 may be appended to the procedure code(s) 22100-22102, 22110-22114 and, as appropriate, to the associated additional vertebral segment add-on code(s) 22103, 22116 as long as both surgeons continue to work together as primary surgeons.

(For bone biopsy, see 20220-20251)

(To report soft tissue biopsy of back or flank, see 21920-21925)

(For needle biopsy of soft tissue, use 20206)

(To report excision of soft tissue tumor of back or flank, use 21930)

22100 Partial excision of posterior vertebral component (eg, spinous process, lamina or facet) for intrinsic bony lesion, single vertebral segment; cervical
➔ *CPT Assistant* Jul 13:3

22101 thoracic
➔ *CPT Assistant* Jul 13:3

22102 lumbar
➔ *CPT Assistant* Jul 13:3

(For insertion of posterior spinous process distraction devices, see 22867, 22868, 22869, 22870)

+ 22103 each additional segment (List separately in addition to code for primary procedure)
➔ *CPT Assistant* Feb 96:6

(Use 22103 in conjunction with 22100, 22101, 22102)

22110 Partial excision of vertebral body, for intrinsic bony lesion, without decompression of spinal cord or nerve root(s), single vertebral segment; cervical
➔ *CPT Assistant* Jul 13:3

22112 thoracic
➔ *CPT Assistant* Jul 13:3

22114 lumbar
➔ *CPT Assistant* Jul 13:3

+ 22116 each additional vertebral segment (List separately in addition to code for primary procedure)
➔ *CPT Assistant* Feb 96:6

(Use 22116 in conjunction with 22110, 22112, 22114)

(For complete or near complete resection of vertebral body, see vertebral corpectomy, 63081-63091)

(For spinal reconstruction with bone graft [autograft, allograft] and/or methylmethacrylate of cervical vertebral body, use 63081 and 22554 and 20931 or 20938)

(For spinal reconstruction with bone graft [autograft, allograft] and/or methylmethacrylate of thoracic vertebral body, use 63085 or 63087 and 22556 and 20931 or 20938)

(For spinal reconstruction with bone graft [autograft, allograft] and/or methylmethacrylate of lumbar vertebral body, use 63087 or 63090 and 22558 and 20931 or 20938)

(For spinal reconstruction following vertebral body resection, use 63082 or 63086 or 63088 or 63091, and 22585)

(For harvest of bone autograft for vertebral reconstruction, see 20931 or 20938)

(For cervical spinal reconstruction with prosthetic replacement of resected vertebral bodies, see codes 63081 and 22554 and 20931 or 20938 and 22853, 22854, 22859)

(For thoracic spinal reconstruction with prosthetic replacement of resected vertebral bodies, see codes 63085 or 63087 and 22556 and 20931 or 20938 and 22853, 22854, 22859)

(For lumbar spinal reconstruction with prosthetic replacement of resected vertebral bodies, see codes 63087 or 63090 and 22558 and 20931 or 20938 and 22853, 22854, 22859)

(For osteotomy of spine, see 22210-22226)

Osteotomy

To report arthrodesis, see codes 22590-22632. (Report in addition to code[s] for the definitive procedure with modifier 51.)

To report instrumentation procedures, see 22840-22855, 22859. (Report in addition to code[s] for the definitive procedure[s].) Do not append modifier 62 to spinal instrumentation codes 22840-22848, 22850, 22852, 22853, 22854, 22859.

To report bone graft procedures, see 20930-20938. (Report in addition to code[s] for the definitive procedure[s].) Do not append modifier 62 to bone graft codes 20900-20938.

For the following codes, when two surgeons work together as primary surgeons performing distinct part(s) of an anterior spine osteotomy, each surgeon should report his/her distinct operative work by appending modifier 62 to the procedure code. In this situation, modifier 62 may be appended to the procedure code(s) 22210-22214, 22220-22224 and, as appropriate, to associated additional segment add-on code(s) 22216, 22226 as long as both surgeons continue to work together as primary surgeons.

Spinal osteotomy procedures are reported when a portion(s) of the vertebral segment(s) is cut and removed in preparation for re-aligning the spine as part of a spinal deformity correction. For excision of an intrinsic lesion of the vertebra without deformity correction, see 22100-22116. For decompression of the spinal cord and/or nerve roots, see 63001-63308.

The three columns are defined as anterior (anterior two-thirds of the vertebral body), middle (posterior third of the vertebral body and the pedicle), and posterior (articular facets, lamina, and spinous process).

22206 Osteotomy of spine, posterior or posterolateral approach, 3 columns, 1 vertebral segment (eg, pedicle/vertebral body subtraction); thoracic
➲ *CPT Changes: An Insider's View* 2008
➲ *CPT Assistant* Feb 08:9, Jul 13:3

(Do not report 22206 in conjunction with 22207)

22207 lumbar
➲ *CPT Changes: An Insider's View* 2008
➲ *CPT Assistant* Feb 08:9, Jul 13:3

(Do not report 22207 in conjunction with 22206)

+ 22208 each additional vertebral segment (List separately in addition to code for primary procedure)
➲ *CPT Changes: An Insider's View* 2008
➲ *CPT Assistant* Feb 08:9

(Use 22208 in conjunction with 22206, 22207)

(Do not report 22206, 22207, 22208 in conjunction with 22210-22226, 22830, 63001-63048, 63055-63066, 63075-63091, 63101-63103, when performed at the same level)

22210 Osteotomy of spine, posterior or posterolateral approach, 1 vertebral segment; cervical
➲ *CPT Assistant* Jul 13:3

22212 thoracic
➲ *CPT Assistant* Dec 07:1, Jul 13:3

22214 lumbar
➲ *CPT Assistant* Dec 07:1, Jul 13:3, Dec 14:16

+ 22216 each additional vertebral segment (List separately in addition to primary procedure)
➲ *CPT Assistant* Dec 07:1

(Use 22216 in conjunction with 22210, 22212, 22214)

22220 Osteotomy of spine, including discectomy, anterior approach, single vertebral segment; cervical
➲ *CPT Assistant* Feb 02:4, Jul 13:3

22222 thoracic
➲ *CPT Assistant* Feb 02:4

22224 lumbar
➲ *CPT Assistant* Feb 02:4, Jul 13:3

+ 22226 each additional vertebral segment (List separately in addition to code for primary procedure)
➲ *CPT Assistant* Feb 96:6, Feb 02:4

(Use 22226 in conjunction with 22220, 22222, 22224)

(For vertebral corpectomy, see 63081-63091)

Fracture and/or Dislocation

To report arthrodesis, see codes 22590-22632. (Report in addition to code[s] for the definitive procedure with modifier 51.)

To report instrumentation procedures, see 22840-22855, 22859. (Report in addition to code[s] for the definitive procedure[s].) Do not append modifier 62 to spinal instrumentation codes 22840-22848, 22850, 22852, 22853, 22854, 22859.

To report bone graft procedures, see 20930-20938. (Report in addition to code[s] for the definitive procedure[s].) Do not append modifier 62 to bone graft codes 20900-20938.

For the following codes, when two surgeons work together as primary surgeons performing distinct part(s) of open fracture and/or dislocation procedure(s), each surgeon should report his/her distinct operative work by appending modifier 62 to the procedure code. In this situation, modifier 62 may be appended to the procedure code(s) 22318-22327 and, as appropriate, the associated additional fracture vertebrae or dislocated segment add-on code 22328 as long as both surgeons continue to work together as primary surgeons.

(22305 has been deleted. To report, see the appropriate evaluation and management codes)

22310 Closed treatment of vertebral body fracture(s), without manipulation, requiring and including casting or bracing
➲ *CPT Assistant* Jun 12:10, Jul 13:3, Jul 14:8

(Do not report 22310 in conjunction with 22510, 22511, 22512, 22513, 22514, 22515, when performed at the same level)

22315 Closed treatment of vertebral fracture(s) and/or dislocation(s) requiring casting or bracing, with and including casting and/or bracing by manipulation or traction
➔ *CPT Changes: An Insider's View* 2011
➔ *CPT Assistant* Apr 12:11, Jun 12:10, Jul 13:3

(Do not report 22315 in conjunction with 22510, 22511, 22512, 22513, 22514, 22515, when performed at the same level)

(For spinal subluxation, use 97140)

22318 Open treatment and/or reduction of odontoid fracture(s) and or dislocation(s) (including os odontoideum), anterior approach, including placement of internal fixation; without grafting
➔ *CPT Changes: An Insider's View* 2000
➔ *CPT Assistant* Nov 99:11, Apr 12:13, Jul 13:3

22319 with grafting
➔ *CPT Changes: An Insider's View* 2000
➔ *CPT Assistant* Nov 99:11, Apr 12:16, Jul 13:3

22325 Open treatment and/or reduction of vertebral fracture(s) and/or dislocation(s), posterior approach, 1 fractured vertebra or dislocated segment; lumbar
➔ *CPT Assistant* Sep 97:8, Jun 12:10, Jul 13:3, Aug 17:9

(Do not report 22325 in conjunction with 22511, 22512, 22514, 22515 when performed at the same level)

22326 cervical
➔ *CPT Assistant* Sep 97:8, Jul 13:3

(Do not report 22326 in conjunction with 22510, 22512, when performed at the same level)

22327 thoracic
➔ *CPT Assistant* Sep 97:8, Jun 12:10, Jul 13:3

(Do not report 22327 in conjunction with 22510, 22512, 22513, 22515 when performed at the same level)

+ 22328 each additional fractured vertebra or dislocated segment (List separately in addition to code for primary procedure)
➔ *CPT Assistant* Feb 96:6

(Use 22328 in conjunction with 22325-22327)

(For treatment of vertebral fracture by the anterior approach, see corpectomy 63081-63091, and appropriate arthrodesis, bone graft and instrument codes)

(For decompression of spine following fracture, see 63001-63091; for arthrodesis of spine following fracture, see 22548-22632)

Manipulation

(For spinal manipulation without anesthesia, use 97140)

22505 Manipulation of spine requiring anesthesia, any region
➔ *CPT Assistant* Mar 97:11, Jan 99:11

Percutaneous Vertebroplasty and Vertebral Augmentation

Codes 22510, 22511, 22512, 22513, 22514, 22515 describe procedures for percutaneous vertebral augmentation that include vertebroplasty of the cervical, thoracic, lumbar, and sacral spine and vertebral augmentation of the thoracic and lumbar spine.

For the purposes of reporting 22510, 22511, 22512, 22513, 22514, 22515, "vertebroplasty" is the process of injecting a material (cement) into the vertebral body to reinforce the structure of the body using image guidance. "Vertebral augmentation" is the process of cavity creation followed by the injection of the material (cement) under image guidance. For 0200T and 0201T, "sacral augmentation (sacroplasty)" refers to the creation of a cavity within a sacral vertebral body followed by injection of a material to fill that cavity.

The procedure codes are inclusive of bone biopsy, when performed, and imaging guidance necessary to perform the procedure. Use one primary procedure code and an add-on code for additional levels. When treating the sacrum, sacral procedures are reported only once per encounter.

22510 Percutaneous vertebroplasty (bone biopsy included when performed), 1 vertebral body, unilateral or bilateral injection, inclusive of all imaging guidance; cervicothoracic
➔ *CPT Changes: An Insider's View* 2015, 2017
➔ *CPT Assistant* Jan 15:8
➔ *Clinical Examples in Radiology* Fall 14:3, Summer 15:14

Percutaneous Vertebroplasty
22510

Augmentation of a vertebral fracture is achieved by percutaneous injections of polymethylmethacrylate under fluoroscopic guidance.

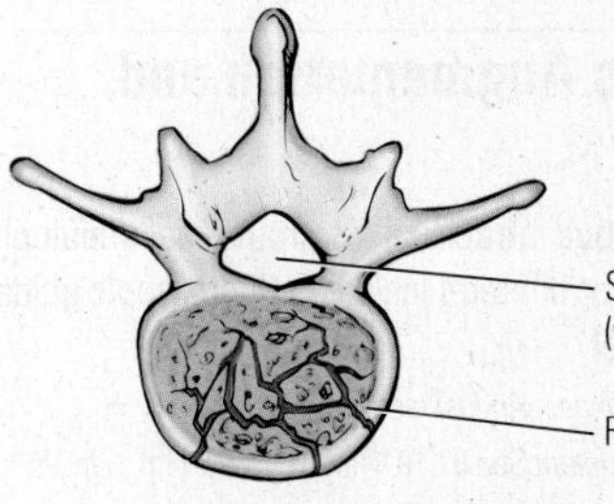

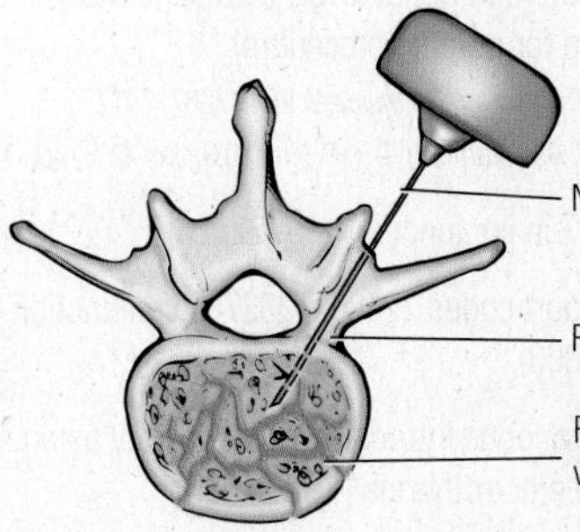

Musculoskeletal 20100-29999

22511 lumbosacral
➲ *CPT Changes: An Insider's View* 2015, 2017
➲ *CPT Assistant* Jan 15:8, Apr 15:8
➲ *Clinical Examples in Radiology* Fall 14:3, 4

+ 22512 each additional cervicothoracic or lumbosacral vertebral body (List separately in addition to code for primary procedure)
➲ *CPT Changes: An Insider's View* 2015, 2017
➲ *CPT Assistant* Jan 15:8
➲ *Clinical Examples in Radiology* Fall 14:3, 4, Summer 15:14

(Use 22512 in conjunction with 22510, 22511)

(Do not report 22510, 22511, 22512 in conjunction with 20225, 22310, 22315, 22325, 22327, when performed at the same level as 22510, 22511, 22512)

22513 Percutaneous vertebral augmentation, including cavity creation (fracture reduction and bone biopsy included when performed) using mechanical device (eg, kyphoplasty), 1 vertebral body, unilateral or bilateral cannulation, inclusive of all imaging guidance; thoracic
➲ *CPT Changes: An Insider's View* 2015, 2017
➲ *CPT Assistant* Jan 15:8
➲ *Clinical Examples in Radiology* Fall 14:3

22514 lumbar
➲ *CPT Changes: An Insider's View* 2015, 2017
➲ *CPT Assistant* Jan 15:8
➲ *Clinical Examples in Radiology* Fall 14:3, 4

+ 22515 each additional thoracic or lumbar vertebral body (List separately in addition to code for primary procedure)
➲ *CPT Changes: An Insider's View* 2015, 2017
➲ *CPT Assistant* Jan 15:8
➲ *Clinical Examples in Radiology* Fall 14:3

(Use 22515 in conjunction with 22513, 22514)

(Do not report 22513, 22514, 22515 in conjunction with 20225, 22310, 22315, 22325, 22327, when performed at the same level as 22513, 22514, 22515)

Percutaneous Augmentation and Annuloplasty

22526 Percutaneous intradiscal electrothermal annuloplasty, unilateral or bilateral including fluoroscopic guidance; single level
➲ *CPT Changes: An Insider's View* 2007, 2017
➲ *CPT Assistant* Sep 07:10, Nov 10:3, Jan 11:8, Jan 15:8

+ 22527 1 or more additional levels (List separately in addition to code for primary procedure)
➲ *CPT Changes: An Insider's View* 2007, 2017
➲ *CPT Assistant* Sep 07:10, Nov 10:3, Jan 11:8, Jan 15:8

(Use 22527 in conjunction with 22526)

(Do not report codes 22526, 22527 in conjunction with 77002, 77003)

(For percutaneous intradiscal annuloplasty using method other than electrothermal, use 22899)

Arthrodesis

Arthrodesis may be performed in the absence of other procedures and therefore when it is combined with another definitive procedure (eg, osteotomy, fracture care, vertebral corpectomy or laminectomy), modifier 51 is appropriate. However, arthrodesis codes 22585, 22614, and 22632 are considered add-on procedure codes and should not be used with modifier 51.

To report instrumentation procedures, see 22840-22855, 22859. (Codes 22840-22848, 22853, 22854, 22859 are reported in conjunction with code[s] for the definitive procedure[s]. When instrumentation reinsertion or removal is reported in conjunction with other definitive procedures, including arthrodesis, decompression, and exploration of fusion, append modifier 51 to 22849, 22850, 22852, and 22855.) To report exploration of fusion, use 22830. (When exploration is reported in conjunction with other definitive procedures, including arthrodesis and decompression, append modifier 51 to 22830.) Do not append modifier 62 to spinal instrumentation codes 22840-22848, 22850, 22852, 22853, 22854, 22859.

To report bone graft procedures, see 20930-20938. (Report in addition to code[s] for the definitive procedure[s].) Do not append modifier 62 to bone graft codes 20900-20938.

Lateral Extracavitary Approach Technique

22532 Arthrodesis, lateral extracavitary technique, including minimal discectomy to prepare interspace (other than for decompression); thoracic
➲ *CPT Changes: An Insider's View* 2004
➲ *CPT Assistant* Apr 12:16, Jul 13:3

22533 lumbar
➲ *CPT Changes: An Insider's View* 2004
➲ *CPT Assistant* Apr 12:16, Jul 13:3

+ 22534 thoracic or lumbar, each additional vertebral segment (List separately in addition to code for primary procedure)
➲ *CPT Changes: An Insider's View* 2004

(Use 22534 in conjunction with 22532 and 22533)

Anterior or Anterolateral Approach Technique

Procedure codes 22554-22558 are for SINGLE interspace; for additional interspaces, use 22585. A vertebral interspace is the non-bony compartment between two adjacent vertebral bodies, which contains the intervertebral disc, and includes the nucleus pulposus, annulus fibrosus, and two cartilaginous endplates.

For the following codes, when two surgeons work together as primary surgeons performing distinct part(s) of an anterior interbody arthrodesis, each surgeon should report his/her distinct operative work by appending modifier 62 to the procedure code. In this situation, modifier 62 may be appended to the procedure code(s) 22548-22558 and, as appropriate, to the associated additional interspace add-on code 22585 as long as both surgeons continue to work together as primary surgeons.

22548 Arthrodesis, anterior transoral or extraoral technique, clivus-C1-C2 (atlas-axis), with or without excision of odontoid process

➔ *CPT Assistant* Spring 93:36, Feb 96:7, Sep 97:8, Sep 00:10, Feb 02:4, Apr 12:16, Jul 13:3

(For intervertebral disc excision by laminotomy or laminectomy, see 63020-63042)

Arthrodesis (Anterior Transoral Technique)

22548

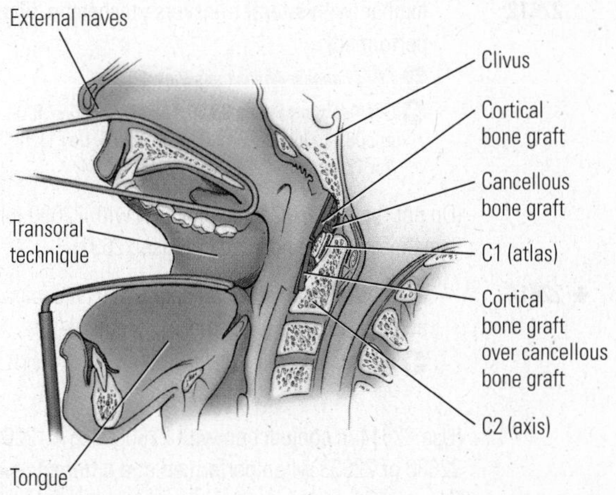

22551 Arthrodesis, anterior interbody, including disc space preparation, discectomy, osteophytectomy and decompression of spinal cord and/or nerve roots; cervical below C2

➔ *CPT Changes: An Insider's View* 2011

➔ *CPT Assistant* Apr 12:16, Jul 13:3, Jan 15:13, May 16:13

+ 22552 cervical below C2, each additional interspace (List separately in addition to code for primary procedure)

➔ *CPT Changes: An Insider's View* 2011

➔ *CPT Assistant* Apr 12:16, Jul 13:3

(Use 22552 in conjunction with 22551)

22554 Arthrodesis, anterior interbody technique, including minimal discectomy to prepare interspace (other than for decompression); cervical below C2

➔ *CPT Assistant* Spring 93:36, Sep 97:8, Sep 00:10, Jan 01:12, Feb 02:4, Apr 12:16, Jul 13:3, Apr 15:7

(Do not report 22554 in conjunction with 63075, even if performed by a separate individual. To report anterior cervical discectomy and interbody fusion at the same level during the same session, use 22551)

Anterior Approach for Cervical Fusion

22554

An example of an exposure technique used to reach anterior cervical vertebrae for spinal procedures (eg, discectomy, arthrodesis, spinal instrumentation)

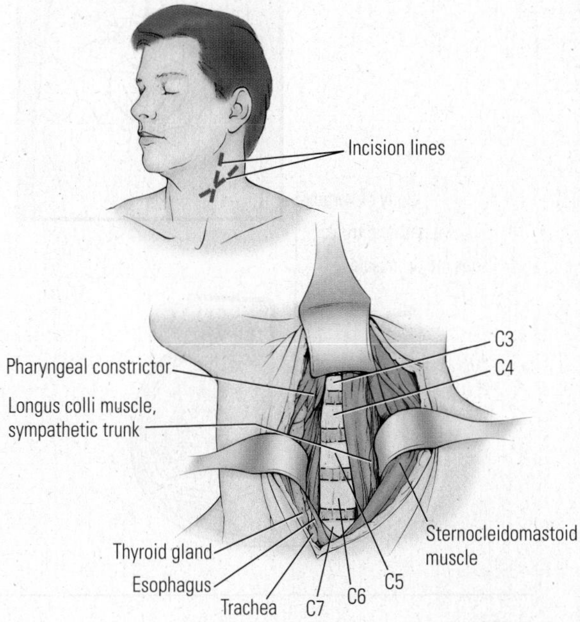

22556 thoracic

➔ *CPT Assistant* Spring 93:36, Jul 96:7, Sep 97:8, Sep 00:10, Feb 02:4, Apr 12:16, Jul 13:3

22558 lumbar

➔ *CPT Assistant* Spring 93:36, Mar 96:6, Jul 96:7, Sep 97:8, Sep 00:10, Feb 02:4, Oct 09:9, Apr 12:16, Jul 13:3, Mar 15:9

▶(For arthrodesis using pre-sacral interbody technique, use 22586)◀

+ 22585 each additional interspace (List separately in addition to code for primary procedure)

➔ *CPT Changes: An Insider's View* 2011

➔ *CPT Assistant* Spring 93:36, Feb 96:6, Mar 96:6, Sep 97:8, Sep 00:10, Feb 02:4, Apr 08:11

(Use 22585 in conjunction with 22554, 22556, 22558)

(Do not report 22585 in conjunction with 63075, even if performed by a separate individual. To report anterior cervical discectomy and interbody fusion at the same level during the same session, use 22552)

Anterior Approach for Lumbar Fusion (Anterior Retroperitoneal Exposure)

22558

An example of an exposure technique used to reach anterior lumbar vertebrae for spinal procedures (eg, discectomy, arthrodesis, spinal instrumentation)

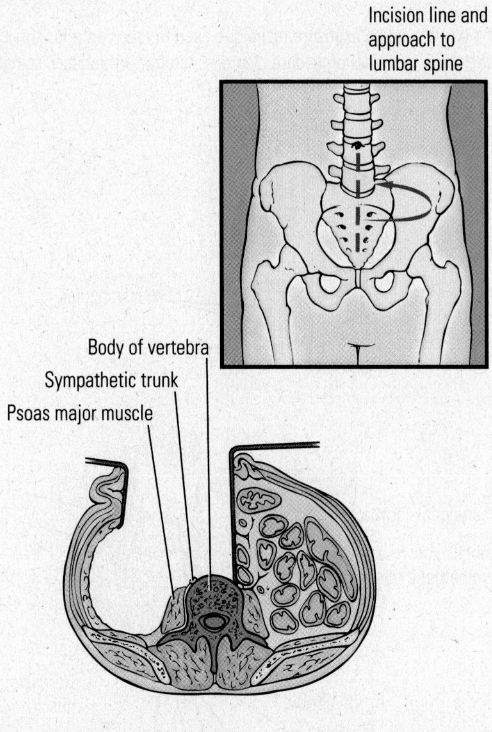

22586 Arthrodesis, pre-sacral interbody technique, including disc space preparation, discectomy, with posterior instrumentation, with image guidance, includes bone graft when performed, L5-S1 interspace

➲ *CPT Changes: An Insider's View* 2013

(Do not report 22586 in conjunction with 20930-20938, 22840, 22848, 72275, 77002, 77003, 77011, 77012)

Posterior, Posterolateral or Lateral Transverse Process Technique

To report instrumentation procedures, see 22840-22855, 22859. (Report in addition to code[s] for the definitive procedure[s].) Do not append modifier 62 to spinal instrumentation codes 22840-22848, 22850, 22852, 22853, 22854, 22859.

To report bone graft procedures, see 20930-20938. (Report in addition to code[s] for the definitive procedure[s].) Do not append modifier 62 to bone graft codes 20900-20938.

A vertebral segment describes the basic constituent part into which the spine may be divided. It represents a single complete vertebral bone with its associated articular processes and laminae. A vertebral interspace is the non-bony compartment between two adjacent vertebral bodies which contains the intervertebral disc, and includes the nucleus pulposus, annulus fibrosus, and two cartilaginous endplates.

22590 Arthrodesis, posterior technique, craniocervical (occiput-C2)

➲ *CPT Assistant* Spring 93:36, Sep 97:8, Apr 12:16, Jul 13:3

22595 Arthrodesis, posterior technique, atlas-axis (C1-C2)

➲ *CPT Assistant* Spring 93:36, Sep 97:8, Apr 12:12, Jul 13:3

22600 Arthrodesis, posterior or posterolateral technique, single level; cervical below C2 segment

➲ *CPT Assistant* Spring 93:36, Sep 97:8, Nov 10:8, Apr 12:16, Jun 12:11, Jul 13:3

22610 thoracic (with lateral transverse technique, when performed)

➲ *CPT Changes: An Insider's View* 2012

➲ *CPT Assistant* Spring 93:36, Sep 97:8, Nov 10:8, Apr 12:16, Jun 12:10, Jul 13:3

22612 lumbar (with lateral transverse technique, when performed)

➲ *CPT Changes: An Insider's View* 2012

➲ *CPT Assistant* Spring 93:36, Mar 96:7, Sep 97:8, 11, Apr 08:11, Jul 08:7, Oct 09:9, Nov 10:8, Dec 11:14, Jan 12:3, Apr 12:16, Jun 12:10, Jul 13:3, Dec 13:14

(Do not report 22612 in conjunction with 22630 for the same interspace and segment, use 22633)

+ 22614 each additional vertebral segment (List separately in addition to code for primary procedure)

➲ *CPT Assistant* Feb 96:6, Mar 96:7, Nov 10:8, Jun 12:11, Jul 13:3

(Use 22614 in conjunction with 22600, 22610, 22612, 22630 or 22633 when performed at a different level. When performing a posterior or posterolateral technique for fusion/arthrodesis at an additional level, use 22614. When performing a posterior interbody fusion arthrodesis at an additional level, use 22632. When performing a combined posterior or posterolateral technique with posterior interbody arthrodesis at an additional level, use 22634)

(For facet joint fusion, see 0219T-0222T)

(For placement of a posterior intrafacet implant, see 0219T-0222T)

22630 Arthrodesis, posterior interbody technique, including laminectomy and/or discectomy to prepare interspace (other than for decompression), single interspace; lumbar

➲ *CPT Changes: An Insider's View* 2000

➲ *CPT Assistant* Spring 93:36, Sep 97:8, Nov 99:11, Dec 99:2, Jan 01:12, Oct 09:9, Nov 11:10, Dec 11:14, Jan 12:3, Apr 12:16, Jun 12:11, Jul 13:3

(Do not report 22630 in conjunction with 22612 for the same interspace and segment, use 22633)

Musculoskeletal 20100-29999

+ 22632 each additional interspace (List separately in addition to code for primary procedure)

➲ *CPT Assistant* Feb 96:6, Sep 97:8, Dec 99:2, Jun 12:11, Jul 13:3

(Use 22632 in conjunction with 22612, 22630, or 22633 when performed at a different level. When performing a posterior interbody fusion arthrodesis at an additional level, use 22632. When performing a posterior or posterolateral technique for fusion/arthrodesis at an additional level, use 22614. When performing a combined posterior or posterolateral technique with posterior interbody arthrodesis at an additional level, use 22634)

22633 Arthrodesis, combined posterior or posterolateral technique with posterior interbody technique including laminectomy and/or discectomy sufficient to prepare interspace (other than for decompression), single interspace and segment; lumbar

➲ *CPT Changes: An Insider's View* 2012

➲ *CPT Assistant* Dec 11:14, Jan 12:3, Jun 12:10, Jul 13:3, Oct 16:11

(Do not report with 22612 or 22630 at the same level)

+ 22634 each additional interspace and segment (List separately in addition to code for primary procedure)

➲ *CPT Changes: An Insider's View* 2012

➲ *CPT Assistant* Dec 11:14, Jan 12:3, Jun 12:10, Jul 13:3

(Use 22634 in conjunction with 22633)

Spine Deformity (eg, Scoliosis, Kyphosis)

To report instrumentation procedures, see 22840-22855, 22859. (Report in addition to code[s] for the definitive procedure[s].) Do not append modifier 62 to spinal instrumentation codes 22840-22848, 22850, 22852, 22853, 22854, 22859.

To report bone graft procedures, see 20930-20938. (Report in addition to code[s] for the definitive procedure[s].) Do not append modifier 62 to bone graft codes 20900-20938.

A vertebral segment describes the basic constituent part into which the spine may be divided. It represents a single complete vertebral bone with its associated articular processes and laminae.

For the following codes, when two surgeons work together as primary surgeons performing distinct part(s) of an arthrodesis for spinal deformity, each surgeon should report his/her distinct operative work by appending modifier 62 to the procedure code. In this situation, modifier 62 may be appended to procedure code(s) 22800-22819 as long as both surgeons continue to work together as primary surgeons.

22800 Arthrodesis, posterior, for spinal deformity, with or without cast; up to 6 vertebral segments

➲ *CPT Assistant* Apr 12:16, Jul 13:3, Sep 17:14

22802 7 to 12 vertebral segments

➲ *CPT Assistant* Mar 96:10, Apr 12:16, Jul 13:3, Sep 17:14

22804 13 or more vertebral segments

➲ *CPT Assistant* Apr 12:16, Jul 13:3, Sep 17:14

22808 Arthrodesis, anterior, for spinal deformity, with or without cast; 2 to 3 vertebral segments

➲ *CPT Assistant* Feb 02:4, Apr 12:16, Jul 13:3, Sep 17:14

22810 4 to 7 vertebral segments

➲ *CPT Assistant* Mar 96:10, Sep 97:8, Feb 02:4, Apr 12:16, Jul 13:3, Sep 17:14

22812 8 or more vertebral segments

➲ *CPT Assistant* Feb 02:4, Apr 12:16, Jul 13:3, Sep 17:14

22818 Kyphectomy, circumferential exposure of spine and resection of vertebral segment(s) (including body and posterior elements); single or 2 segments

➲ *CPT Assistant* Nov 97:14, Sep 17:14

22819 3 or more segments

➲ *CPT Assistant* Nov 97:14, Sep 17:14

(To report arthrodesis, see 22800-22804 and add modifier 51)

Exploration

To report instrumentation procedures, see 22840-22855, 22859. (Codes 22840-22848, 22853, 22854, 22859 are reported in conjunction with code[s] for the definitive procedure[s]. When instrumentation reinsertion or removal is reported in conjunction with other definitive procedures, including arthrodesis, decompression, and exploration of fusion, append modifier 51 to 22849, 22850, 22852, and 22855.) Code 22849 should not be reported with 22850, 22852, and 22855 at the same spinal levels. To report exploration of fusion, see 22830. (When exploration is reported in conjunction with other definitive procedures, including arthrodesis and decompression, append modifier 51 to 22830.)

(To report bone graft procedures, see 20930-20938)

22830 Exploration of spinal fusion

➲ *CPT Assistant* Sep 97:11, Mar 10:9

Spinal Instrumentation

Segmental instrumentation is defined as fixation at each end of the construct and at least one additional interposed bony attachment.

Non-segmental instrumentation is defined as fixation at each end of the construct and may span several vertebral segments without attachment to the intervening segments.

Insertion of spinal instrumentation is reported separately and in addition to arthrodesis. Instrumentation procedure codes 22840-22848, 22853, 22854, 22859 are reported in addition to the definitive procedure(s). Do not append modifier 62 to spinal instrumentation codes 22840-22848, 22850, 22852, 22853, 22854, 22859.

To report bone graft procedures, see 20930-20938. (Report in addition to code[s] for definitive procedure[s].) Do not append modifier 62 to bone graft codes 20900-20938.

A vertebral segment describes the basic constituent part into which the spine may be divided. It represents a single complete vertebral bone with its associated articular processes and laminae. A vertebral interspace is the non-bony compartment between two adjacent vertebral bodies, which contains the intervertebral disc, and includes the nucleus pulposus, annulus fibrosus, and two cartilaginous endplates.

Codes 22849, 22850, 22852, and 22855 are subject to modifier 51 if reported with other definitive procedure(s), including arthrodesis, decompression, and exploration of fusion. Code 22849 should not be reported in conjunction with 22850, 22852, and 22855 at the same spinal levels. Only the appropriate insertion code (22840-22848) should be reported when previously placed spinal instrumentation is being removed or revised during the same session where new instrumentation is inserted at levels including all or part of the previously instrumented segments. Do not report the reinsertion (22849) or removal (22850, 22852, 22855) procedures in addition to the insertion of the new instrumentation (22840-22848).

+ 22840 Posterior non-segmental instrumentation (eg, Harrington rod technique, pedicle fixation across 1 interspace, atlantoaxial transarticular screw fixation, sublaminar wiring at C1, facet screw fixation) (List separately in addition to code for primary procedure)

➲ *CPT Changes: An Insider's View* 2000, 2008

➲ *CPT Assistant* Feb 96:6, Jul 96:10, Sep 97:8, Nov 99:12, Feb 02:6, Nov 10:8, Jan 11:9, Dec 11:15, Apr 12:12, Jun 12:11, Jul 13:3, Dec 13:17, Oct 14:15, Jun 17:10

(Use 22840 in conjunction with 22100-22102, 22110-22114, 22206, 22207, 22210-22214, 22220-22224, 22310-22327, 22532, 22533, 22548-22558, 22590-22612, 22630, 22633, 22634, 22800-22812, 63001-63030, 63040-63042, 63045-63047, 63050-63056, 63064, 63075, 63077, 63081, 63085, 63087, 63090, 63101, 63102, 63170-63290, 63300-63307)

+ 22841 Internal spinal fixation by wiring of spinous processes (List separately in addition to code for primary procedure)

➲ *CPT Changes: An Insider's View* 2008

➲ *CPT Assistant* Feb 96:6, Sep 97:8, Feb 02:6, Jun 12:11, Jul 13:3

(Use 22841 in conjunction with 22100-22102, 22110-22114, 22206, 22207, 22210-22214, 22220-22224, 22310-22327, 22532, 22533, 22548-22558, 22590-22612, 22630, 22633, 22634, 22800-22812, 63001-63030, 63040-63042, 63045-63047, 63050-63056, 63064, 63075, 63077, 63081, 63085, 63087, 63090, 63101, 63102, 63170-63290, 63300-63307)

Non-Segmental Spinal Instrumentation
22840

Fixation at each end of the construct

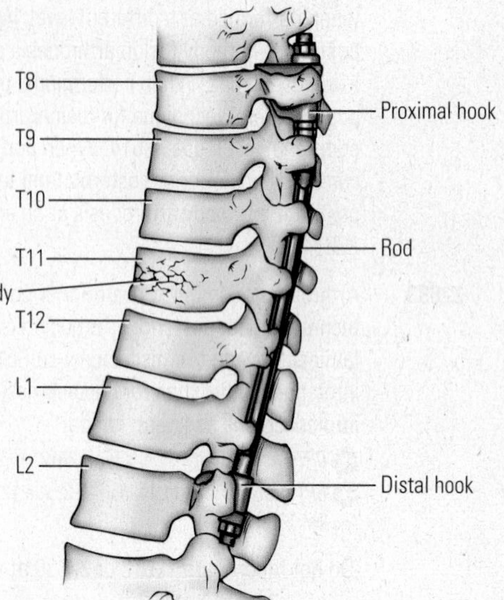

+ 22842 Posterior segmental instrumentation (eg, pedicle fixation, dual rods with multiple hooks and sublaminar wires); 3 to 6 vertebral segments (List separately in addition to code for primary procedure)

➲ *CPT Changes: An Insider's View* 2008

➲ *CPT Assistant* Feb 96:6, Mar 96:7, Sep 97:8, Feb 02:6, Dec 11:15, Jun 12:11, Jul 13:3

(Use 22842 in conjunction with 22100-22102, 22110-22114, 22206, 22207, 22210-22214, 22220-22224, 22310-22327, 22532, 22533, 22548-22558, 22590-22612, 22630, 22633, 22634, 22800-22812, 63001-63030, 63040-63042, 63045-63047, 63050-63056, 63064, 63075, 63077, 63081, 63085, 63087, 63090, 63101, 63102, 63170-63290, 63300-63307)

+ 22843 7 to 12 vertebral segments (List separately in addition to code for primary procedure)

➲ *CPT Changes: An Insider's View* 2008

➲ *CPT Assistant* Feb 96:6, Sep 97:8, Feb 02:6, Dec 11:15, Jun 12:11, Jul 13:3

(Use 22843 in conjunction with 22100-22102, 22110-22114, 22206, 22207, 22210-22214, 22220-22224, 22310-22327, 22532, 22533, 22548-22558, 22590-22612, 22630, 22633, 22634, 22800-22812, 63001-63030, 63040-63042, 63045-63047, 63050-63056, 63064, 63075, 63077, 63081, 63085, 63087, 63090, 63101, 63102, 63170-63290, 63300-63307)

+ 22844 13 or more vertebral segments (List separately in addition to code for primary procedure)

➲ *CPT Changes: An Insider's View* 2008

➲ *CPT Assistant* Feb 96:6, Sep 97:8, Feb 02:6, Dec 11:15, Jun 12:11, Jul 13:3

(Use 22844 in conjunction with 22100-22102, 22110-22114, 22206, 22207, 22210-22214, 22220-22224, 22310-22327, 22532, 22533, 22548-22558, 22590-22612, 22630, 22633, 22634, 22800-22812, 63001-63030, 63040-63042, 63045-63047, 63050-63056, 63064, 63075, 63077, 63081, 63085, 63087, 63090, 63101, 63102, 63170-63290, 63300-63307)

Segmental Spinal Instrumentation

22842-22844

Fixation at each end of the construct and at least one additional interposed bony attachment

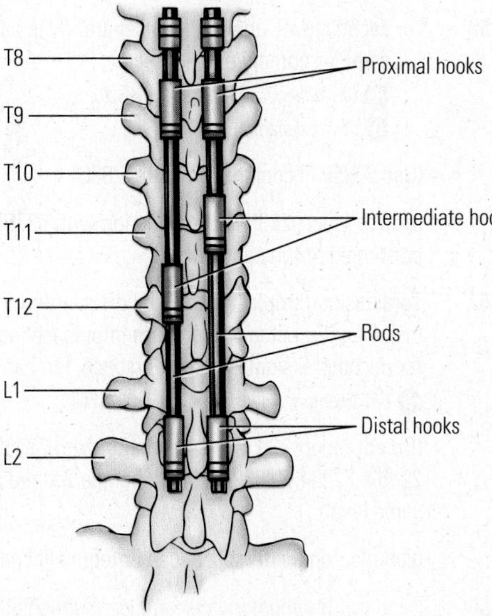

+ 22845 Anterior instrumentation; 2 to 3 vertebral segments (List separately in addition to code for primary procedure)

CPT Changes: An Insider's View 2008

CPT Assistant Feb 96:6, Mar 96:10, Jul 96:7, 10, Sep 97:8, Feb 02:6, Jun 12:11, Jul 13:3, Nov 14:14, Jan 15:13, Mar 15:9, Apr 15:7, May 16:13, Mar 17:7

(Use 22845 in conjunction with 22100-22102, 22110-22114, 22206, 22207, 22210-22214, 22220-22224, 22310-22327, 22532, 22533, 22548-22558, 22590-22612, 22630, 22633, 22634, 22800-22812, 63001-63030, 63040-63042, 63045-63047, 63050-63056, 63064, 63075, 63077, 63081, 63085, 63087, 63090, 63101, 63102, 63170-63290, 63300-63307)

+ 22846 4 to 7 vertebral segments (List separately in addition to code for primary procedure)

CPT Changes: An Insider's View 2008

CPT Assistant Feb 96:6, Sep 97:8, Feb 02:6, Jun 12:11, Jul 13:3, May 16:13

(Use 22846 in conjunction with 22100-22102, 22110-22114, 22206, 22207, 22210-22214, 22220-22224, 22310-22327, 22532, 22533, 22548-22558, 22590-22612, 22630, 22633, 22634, 22800-22812, 63001-63030, 63040-63042, 63045-63047, 63050-63056, 63064, 63075, 63077, 63081, 63085, 63087, 63090, 63101, 63102, 63170-63290, 63300-63307)

+ 22847 8 or more vertebral segments (List separately in addition to code for primary procedure)

CPT Changes: An Insider's View 2008

CPT Assistant Feb 96:6, Sep 97:8, Feb 02:6, Jun 12:11, Jul 13:3, May 16:13

(Use 22847 in conjunction with 22100-22102, 22110-22114, 22206, 22207, 22210-22214, 22220-22224, 22310-22327, 22532, 22533, 22548-22558, 22590-22612, 22630, 22633, 22634, 22800-22812, 63001-63030, 63040-63042, 63045-63047, 63050-63056, 63064, 63075, 63077, 63081, 63085, 63087, 63090, 63101, 63102, 63170-63290, 63300-63307)

+ 22848 Pelvic fixation (attachment of caudal end of instrumentation to pelvic bony structures) other than sacrum (List separately in addition to code for primary procedure)

CPT Changes: An Insider's View 2008

CPT Assistant Feb 96:6, Sep 97:8, Feb 02:6, Jun 12:11, Jul 13:3

(Use 22848 in conjunction with 22100-22102, 22110-22114, 22206, 22207, 22210-22214, 22220-22224, 22310-22327, 22532, 22533, 22548-22558, 22590-22612, 22630, 22633, 22634, 22800-22812, 63001-63030, 63040-63042, 63045-63047, 63050-63056, 63064, 63075, 63077, 63081, 63085, 63087, 63090, 63101, 63102, 63170-63290, 63300-63307)

22849 Reinsertion of spinal fixation device

CPT Assistant Feb 96:6, Sep 97:8, Feb 02:6, Nov 02:3, Oct 11:10, Jun 12:11, Jul 13:3, May 16:13, Jun 17:10

22850 Removal of posterior nonsegmental instrumentation (eg, Harrington rod)

CPT Assistant Feb 96:6, Sep 97:8, Feb 02:6, Jun 12:11, Jul 13:3, May 16:13, Jun 17:10

(22851 has been deleted. To report, see 22853, 22854, 22859)

22852 Removal of posterior segmental instrumentation

CPT Assistant Feb 96:6, Sep 97:8, Feb 02:6, May 06:16, Jun 12:11, Jun 17:10

+ 22853 Insertion of interbody biomechanical device(s) (eg, synthetic cage, mesh) with integral anterior instrumentation for device anchoring (eg, screws, flanges), when performed, to intervertebral disc space in conjunction with interbody arthrodesis, each interspace (List separately in addition to code for primary procedure)

CPT Changes: An Insider's View 2017

CPT Assistant Mar 17:7, Aug 17:9

(Use 22853 in conjunction with 22100-22102, 22110-22114, 22206, 22207, 22210-22214, 22220-22224, 22310-22327, 22532, 22533, 22548-22558, 22590-22612, 22630, 22633, 22634, 22800-22812, 63001-63030, 63040-63042, 63045-63047, 63050-63056, 63064, 63075, 63077, 63081, 63085, 63087, 63090, 63101, 63102, 63170-63290, 63300-63307)

(Report 22853 for each treated intervertebral disc space)

Musculoskeletal 20100-29999

Spinal Prosthetic Devices

22853, 22854, 22859

Application of prosthetic device

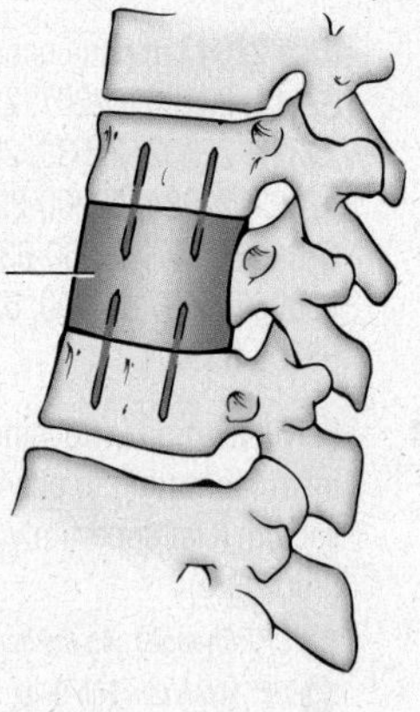

+ 22854 Insertion of intervertebral biomechanical device(s) (eg, synthetic cage, mesh) with integral anterior instrumentation for device anchoring (eg, screws, flanges), when performed, to vertebral corpectomy(ies) (vertebral body resection, partial or complete) defect, in conjunction with interbody arthrodesis, each contiguous defect (List separately in addition to code for primary procedure)

➔ *CPT Changes: An Insider's View* 2017

➔ *CPT Assistant* Mar 17:7

(Use 22854 in conjunction with 22100-22102, 22110-22114, 22206, 22207, 22210-22214, 22220-22224, 22310-22327, 22532, 22533, 22548-22558, 22590-22612, 22630, 22633, 22634, 22800-22812, 63001-63030, 63040-63042, 63045-63047, 63050-63056, 63064, 63075, 63077, 63081, 63085, 63087, 63090, 63101, 63102, 63170-63290, 63300-63307)

#+ 22859 Insertion of intervertebral biomechanical device(s) (eg, synthetic cage, mesh, methylmethacrylate) to intervertebral disc space or vertebral body defect without interbody arthrodesis, each contiguous defect (List separately in addition to code for primary procedure)

➔ *CPT Changes: An Insider's View* 2017

➔ *CPT Assistant* Mar 17:7

(Use 22859 in conjunction with 22100-22102, 22110-22114, 22206, 22207, 22210-22214, 22220-22224, 22310-22327, 22532, 22533, 22548-22558, 22590-22612, 22630, 22633, 22634, 22800-22812, 63001-63030, 63040-63042, 63045-63047, 63050-63056, 63064, 63075, 63077, 63081, 63085, 63087, 63090, 63101, 63102, 63170-63290, 63300-63307)

(22853, 22854, 22859 may be reported more than once for noncontiguous defects)

(For application of an intervertebral bone device/graft, see 20930, 20931, 20936, 20937, 20938)

22855 Removal of anterior instrumentation

➔ *CPT Assistant* Feb 96:6, Sep 97:8, Feb 02:6, Nov 02:2, Jun 12:11, Jun 17:10

22856 Total disc arthroplasty (artificial disc), anterior approach, including discectomy with end plate preparation (includes osteophytectomy for nerve root or spinal cord decompression and microdissection); single interspace, cervical

➔ *CPT Changes: An Insider's View* 2009, 2015

➔ *CPT Assistant* Apr 15:7

(Do not report 22856 in conjunction with 22554, 22845, 22853, 22854, 22859, 63075, 0375T when performed at the same level)

(Do not report 22856 in conjunction with 69990)

(For additional interspace cervical total disc arthroplasty, see 22858, 0375T)

#+ 22858 second level, cervical (List separately in addition to code for primary procedure)

➔ *CPT Changes: An Insider's View* 2015

➔ *CPT Assistant* Apr 15:7

(Use 22858 in conjunction with 22856)

(Do not report 22858 in conjunction with 0375T, when performed at the same level)

22857 Total disc arthroplasty (artificial disc), anterior approach, including discectomy to prepare interspace (other than for decompression), single interspace, lumbar

➔ *CPT Changes: An Insider's View* 2007, 2009

(Do not report 22857 in conjunction with 22558, 22845, 22853, 22854, 22859, 49010 when performed at the same level)

(For additional interspace, use Category III code 0163T)

22858 Code is out of numerical sequence. See 22853-22861

22859 Code is out of numerical sequence. See 22853-22861

22861 Revision including replacement of total disc arthroplasty (artificial disc), anterior approach, single interspace; cervical

➔ *CPT Changes: An Insider's View* 2009

(Do not report 22861 in conjunction with 22845, 22853, 22854, 22859, 22864, 63075 when performed at the same level)

(Do not report 22861 in conjunction with 69990)

(For additional interspace revision of cervical total disc arthroplasty, use 0098T)

22862 lumbar

➔ *CPT Changes: An Insider's View* 2007, 2009

➔ *CPT Assistant* Jun 07:1

(Do not report 22862 in conjunction with 22558, 22845, 22853, 22854, 22859, 22865, 49010 when performed at the same level)

(For additional interspace, use Category III code 0165T)

22864 Removal of total disc arthroplasty (artificial disc), anterior approach, single interspace; cervical

➔ *CPT Changes: An Insider's View* 2009

(Do not report 22864 in conjunction with 22861, 69990)

(For additional interspace removal of cervical total disc arthroplasty, use 0095T)

22865 lumbar

CPT Changes: An Insider's View 2007, 2009

CPT Assistant Jun 07:1

(Do not report 22865 in conjunction with 49010)

(For additional interspace, see Category III code 0164T)

(22856-22865 include fluoroscopy when performed)

(For decompression, see 63001-63048)

22867 Insertion of interlaminar/interspinous process stabilization/distraction device, without fusion, including image guidance when performed, with open decompression, lumbar; single level

CPT Changes: An Insider's View 2017

CPT Assistant Feb 17:9

+ 22868 second level (List separately in addition to code for primary procedure)

CPT Changes: An Insider's View 2017

CPT Assistant Feb 17:9

(Use 22868 in conjunction with 22867)

(Do not report 22867, 22868 in conjunction with 22532, 22533, 22534, 22558, 22612, 22614, 22630, 22632, 22633, 22634, 22800, 22802, 22804, 22840, 22841, 22842, 22869, 22870, 63005, 63012, 63017, 63030, 63035, 63042, 63044, 63047, 63048, 77003 for the same level)

(For insertion of interlaminar/interspinous process stabilization/distraction device, without open decompression or fusion, see 22869, 22870)

22869 Insertion of interlaminar/interspinous process stabilization/distraction device, without open decompression or fusion, including image guidance when performed, lumbar; single level

CPT Changes: An Insider's View 2017

CPT Assistant Feb 17:9

+ 22870 second level (List separately in addition to code for primary procedure)

CPT Changes: An Insider's View 2017

CPT Assistant Feb 17:9

(Use 22870 in conjunction with 22869)

(Do not report 22869, 22870 in conjunction with 22532, 22533, 22534, 22558, 22612, 22614, 22630, 22632, 22633, 22634, 22800, 22802, 22804, 22840, 22841, 22842, 63005, 63012, 63017, 63030, 63035, 63042, 63044, 63047, 63048, 77003)

Other Procedures

22899 Unlisted procedure, spine

CPT Assistant May 00:11, Sep 00:10, Jul 06:19, Feb 10:13, Nov 10:4, Jan 12:14, Sep 12:16, Dec 12:13, Dec 13:14, 17, Oct 14:15, Jan 15:8, Feb 17:9

Clinical Examples in Radiology Fall 14:3

Abdomen

Excision

22900 Excision, tumor, soft tissue of abdominal wall, subfascial (eg, intramuscular); less than 5 cm

CPT Changes: An Insider's View 2010

22901 5 cm or greater

CPT Changes: An Insider's View 2010

22902 Excision, tumor, soft tissue of abdominal wall, subcutaneous; less than 3 cm

CPT Changes: An Insider's View 2010

22903 3 cm or greater

CPT Changes: An Insider's View 2010

(For excision of benign lesions of cutaneous origin [eg, sebaceous cyst], see 11400-11406)

22904 Radical resection of tumor (eg, sarcoma), soft tissue of abdominal wall; less than 5 cm

CPT Changes: An Insider's View 2010, 2014

22905 5 cm or greater

CPT Changes: An Insider's View 2010, 2014

(For radical resection of tumor[s] of cutaneous origin [eg, melanoma], see 11600-11606)

Other Procedures

22999 Unlisted procedure, abdomen, musculoskeletal system

Shoulder

The area known as the shoulder is made up of the clavicle, scapula, humerus head and neck, sterno-clavicular joint, acromioclavicular joint, and shoulder joint.

Incision

23000 Removal of subdeltoid calcareous deposits, open

CPT Changes: An Insider's View 2002, 2003

(For arthroscopic removal of bursal deposits, use 29999)

23020 Capsular contracture release (eg, Sever type procedure)

(For incision and drainage procedures, superficial, see 10040-10160)

23030 Incision and drainage, shoulder area; deep abscess or hematoma

23031 infected bursa

23035 Incision, bone cortex (eg, osteomyelitis or bone abscess), shoulder area

23040 Arthrotomy, glenohumeral joint, including exploration, drainage, or removal of foreign body

CPT Assistant Nov 98:8

Musculoskeletal 20100-29999

23044 Arthrotomy, acromioclavicular, sternoclavicular joint, including exploration, drainage, or removal of foreign body
➔ *CPT Assistant* Nov 98:8

Excision

23065 Biopsy, soft tissue of shoulder area; superficial

23066 deep

(For needle biopsy of soft tissue, use 20206)

23071 Code is out of numerical sequence. See 23066-23078

23073 Code is out of numerical sequence. See 23066-23078

23075 Excision, tumor, soft tissue of shoulder area, subcutaneous; less than 3 cm
➔ *CPT Changes: An Insider's View* 2010
➔ *CPT Assistant* Summer 92:22, Nov 98:8

 # 23071 3 cm or greater
➔ *CPT Changes: An Insider's View* 2010

(For excision of benign lesions of cutaneous origin [eg, sebaceous cyst], see 11400-11406)

23076 Excision, tumor, soft tissue of shoulder area, subfascial (eg, intramuscular); less than 5 cm
➔ *CPT Changes: An Insider's View* 2010
➔ *CPT Assistant* Summer 92:22, Oct 09:7

 # 23073 5 cm or greater
➔ *CPT Changes: An Insider's View* 2010

23077 Radical resection of tumor (eg, sarcoma), soft tissue of shoulder area; less than 5 cm
➔ *CPT Changes: An Insider's View* 2010, 2014

23078 5 cm or greater
➔ *CPT Changes: An Insider's View* 2010, 2014

(For radical resection of tumor[s] of cutaneous origin [eg, melanoma], see 11600-11606)

23100 Arthrotomy, glenohumeral joint, including biopsy
➔ *CPT Assistant* Nov 98:8

23101 Arthrotomy, acromioclavicular joint or sternoclavicular joint, including biopsy and/or excision of torn cartilage
➔ *CPT Assistant* Nov 98:8

23105 Arthrotomy; glenohumeral joint, with synovectomy, with or without biopsy
➔ *CPT Assistant* Nov 98:8

23106 sternoclavicular joint, with synovectomy, with or without biopsy

23107 Arthrotomy, glenohumeral joint, with joint exploration, with or without removal of loose or foreign body

23120 Claviculectomy; partial
➔ *CPT Assistant* Sep 12:16

(For arthroscopic procedure, use 29824)

23125 total

23130 Acromioplasty or acromionectomy, partial, with or without coracoacromial ligament release
➔ *CPT Assistant* Aug 01:11, Feb 15:10, Mar 15:7

23140 Excision or curettage of bone cyst or benign tumor of clavicle or scapula;

23145 with autograft (includes obtaining graft)

23146 with allograft

23150 Excision or curettage of bone cyst or benign tumor of proximal humerus;

23155 with autograft (includes obtaining graft)

23156 with allograft

23170 Sequestrectomy (eg, for osteomyelitis or bone abscess), clavicle

23172 Sequestrectomy (eg, for osteomyelitis or bone abscess), scapula

23174 Sequestrectomy (eg, for osteomyelitis or bone abscess), humeral head to surgical neck

23180 Partial excision (craterization, saucerization, or diaphysectomy) bone (eg, osteomyelitis), clavicle
➔ *CPT Assistant* Nov 98:9

23182 Partial excision (craterization, saucerization, or diaphysectomy) bone (eg, osteomyelitis), scapula
➔ *CPT Assistant* Nov 98:9

23184 Partial excision (craterization, saucerization, or diaphysectomy) bone (eg, osteomyelitis), proximal humerus
➔ *CPT Assistant* Nov 98:9

23190 Ostectomy of scapula, partial (eg, superior medial angle)

23195 Resection, humeral head

(For replacement with implant, use 23470)

23200 Radical resection of tumor; clavicle
➔ *CPT Changes: An Insider's View* 2010

23210 scapula
➔ *CPT Changes: An Insider's View* 2010

23220 Radical resection of tumor, proximal humerus
➔ *CPT Changes: An Insider's View* 2010
➔ *CPT Assistant* Nov 98:8

(23221, 23222 have been deleted)

Introduction or Removal

(For arthrocentesis or needling of bursa, use 20610)

(For K-wire or pin insertion or removal, see 20650, 20670, 20680)

23330 Removal of foreign body, shoulder; subcutaneous
➔ *CPT Assistant* Aug 99:3, Mar 14:4

(To report removal of foreign body, see 23330, 23333)

23333 deep (subfascial or intramuscular)
➔ *CPT Changes: An Insider's View* 2014
➔ *CPT Assistant* Mar 14:4

23334 Removal of prosthesis, includes debridement and synovectomy when performed; humeral **or** glenoid component
➔ *CPT Changes: An Insider's View* 2014
➔ *CPT Assistant* Mar 14:4

23335 humeral **and** glenoid components (eg, total shoulder)
➔ *CPT Changes: An Insider's View* 2014
➔ *CPT Assistant* Mar 14:4

(Do not report 23334, 23335 in conjunction with 23473, 23474 if a prosthesis [ie, humeral and/or glenoid component(s)] is being removed and replaced in the same shoulder during the same surgical session)

(To report removal of hardware, other than humeral and/or glenoid prosthesis, use 20680)

23350 Injection procedure for shoulder arthrography or enhanced CT/MRI shoulder arthrography
➔ *CPT Changes: An Insider's View* 2002
➔ *CPT Assistant* Jul 01:3, Aug 15:6, May 16:13
➔ *Clinical Examples in Radiology* Spring 05:5, Spring 09:6, 7

(For radiographic arthrography, radiological supervision and interpretation, use 73040. Fluoroscopy [77002] is inclusive of radiographic arthrography)

(When fluoroscopic guided injection is performed for enhanced CT arthrography, use 23350, 77002, and 73201 or 73202)

(When fluoroscopic guided injection is performed for enhanced MR arthrography, use 23350, 77002, and 73222 or 73223)

(For enhanced CT or enhanced MRI arthrography, use 77002 and either 73201, 73202, 73222, or 73223)

(To report biopsy of the shoulder and joint, see 29805-29826)

Repair, Revision, and/or Reconstruction

23395 Muscle transfer, any type, shoulder or upper arm; single

23397 multiple

23400 Scapulopexy (eg, Sprengels deformity or for paralysis)

23405 Tenotomy, shoulder area; single tendon
➔ *CPT Assistant* Nov 98:8

23406 multiple tendons through same incision
➔ *CPT Assistant* Nov 98:8

23410 Repair of ruptured musculotendinous cuff (eg, rotator cuff) open; acute
➔ *CPT Changes: An Insider's View* 2003
➔ *CPT Assistant* Aug 01:11, Feb 02:11

23412 chronic
➔ *CPT Assistant* Feb 02:11, Sep 12:16, Feb 15:10, Jun 15:10

(For arthroscopic procedure, use 29827)

23415 Coracoacromial ligament release, with or without acromioplasty
➔ *CPT Assistant* Mar 15:7

(For arthroscopic procedure, use 29826)

23420 Reconstruction of complete shoulder (rotator) cuff avulsion, chronic (includes acromioplasty)
➔ *CPT Assistant* Feb 02:11, Oct 05:23

23430 Tenodesis of long tendon of biceps

(For arthroscopic biceps tenodesis, use 29828)

23440 Resection or transplantation of long tendon of biceps

23450 Capsulorrhaphy, anterior; Putti-Platt procedure or Magnuson type operation

(To report arthroscopic thermal capsulorrhaphy, use 29999)

23455 with labral repair (eg, Bankart procedure)
➔ *CPT Assistant* Nov 98:8

(For arthroscopic procedure, use 29806)

23460 Capsulorrhaphy, anterior, any type; with bone block

23462 with coracoid process transfer

(To report open thermal capsulorrhaphy, use 23929)

23465 Capsulorrhaphy, glenohumeral joint, posterior, with or without bone block
➔ *CPT Assistant* Nov 98:8

(For sternoclavicular and acromioclavicular reconstruction, see 23530, 23550)

23466 Capsulorrhaphy, glenohumeral joint, any type multi-directional instability
➔ *CPT Assistant* Nov 98:8

23470 Arthroplasty, glenohumeral joint; hemiarthroplasty
➔ *CPT Assistant* Nov 98:8, Mar 14:4

23472 total shoulder (glenoid and proximal humeral replacement (eg, total shoulder))
➔ *CPT Assistant* Jun 96:10, Nov 98:8, Mar 13:12, Mar 14:4

(For removal of total shoulder implants, see 23334, 23335)

(For osteotomy, proximal humerus, use 24400)

23473 Revision of total shoulder arthroplasty, including allograft when performed; humeral **or** glenoid component
➔ *CPT Changes: An Insider's View* 2013
➔ *CPT Assistant* Feb 13:11, Mar 13:12, Mar 14:4

23474 humeral **and** glenoid component
➔ *CPT Changes: An Insider's View* 2013
➔ *CPT Assistant* Feb 13:11, Mar 13:12, Mar 14:4

(Do not report 23473, 23474 in conjunction with 23334, 23335 if a prosthesis [ie, humeral and/or glenoid component(s)] is being removed and replaced in the same shoulder during the same surgical session)

23480 Osteotomy, clavicle, with or without internal fixation;

23485 with bone graft for nonunion or malunion (includes obtaining graft and/or necessary fixation)

23490 Prophylactic treatment (nailing, pinning, plating or wiring) with or without methylmethacrylate; clavicle

23491 proximal humerus
➲ *CPT Assistant* Nov 98:8

Fracture and/or Dislocation

Coding Tip

Reporting for Categories of Manipulation and/or Fracture

The codes for treatment of fractures and joint injuries (dislocations) are categorized by the type of manipulation (reduction) and stabilization (fixation or immobilization). These codes can apply to either open (compound) or closed fractures or joint injuries.

CPT Coding Guidelines, Musculoskeletal System

23500 Closed treatment of clavicular fracture; without manipulation

23505 with manipulation

23515 Open treatment of clavicular fracture, includes internal fixation, when performed
➲ *CPT Changes: An Insider's View* 2008
➲ *CPT Assistant* Jan 08:4

23520 Closed treatment of sternoclavicular dislocation; without manipulation

23525 with manipulation

23530 Open treatment of sternoclavicular dislocation, acute or chronic;

23532 with fascial graft (includes obtaining graft)

23540 Closed treatment of acromioclavicular dislocation; without manipulation

23545 with manipulation

23550 Open treatment of acromioclavicular dislocation, acute or chronic;

23552 with fascial graft (includes obtaining graft)

23570 Closed treatment of scapular fracture; without manipulation

23575 with manipulation, with or without skeletal traction (with or without shoulder joint involvement)

23585 Open treatment of scapular fracture (body, glenoid or acromion) includes internal fixation, when performed
➲ *CPT Changes: An Insider's View* 2009
➲ *CPT Assistant* Oct 04:10

23600 Closed treatment of proximal humeral (surgical or anatomical neck) fracture; without manipulation

23605 with manipulation, with or without skeletal traction

23615 Open treatment of proximal humeral (surgical or anatomical neck) fracture, includes internal fixation, when performed, includes repair of tuberosity(s), when performed;
➲ *CPT Changes: An Insider's View* 2008
➲ *CPT Assistant* Jan 08:4

23616 with proximal humeral prosthetic replacement
➲ *CPT Changes: An Insider's View* 2008

23620 Closed treatment of greater humeral tuberosity fracture; without manipulation
➲ *CPT Assistant* Nov 98:8

23625 with manipulation

23630 Open treatment of greater humeral tuberosity fracture, includes internal fixation, when performed
➲ *CPT Changes: An Insider's View* 2008
➲ *CPT Assistant* Nov 98:8

23650 Closed treatment of shoulder dislocation, with manipulation; without anesthesia

23655 requiring anesthesia

23660 Open treatment of acute shoulder dislocation
➲ *CPT Assistant* Feb 96:5

(Repairs for recurrent dislocations, see 23450-23466)

23665 Closed treatment of shoulder dislocation, with fracture of greater humeral tuberosity, with manipulation
➲ *CPT Assistant* Nov 98:8

23670 Open treatment of shoulder dislocation, with fracture of greater humeral tuberosity, includes internal fixation, when performed
➲ *CPT Changes: An Insider's View* 2008
➲ *CPT Assistant* Nov 98:8

23675 Closed treatment of shoulder dislocation, with surgical or anatomical neck fracture, with manipulation

23680 Open treatment of shoulder dislocation, with surgical or anatomical neck fracture, includes internal fixation, when performed
➲ *CPT Changes: An Insider's View* 2008

Manipulation

23700 Manipulation under anesthesia, shoulder joint, including application of fixation apparatus (dislocation excluded)
➲ *CPT Assistant* Jan 99:10, Apr 05:14, May 09:8, Jun 15:10

Arthrodesis

23800 Arthrodesis, glenohumeral joint;
➲ *CPT Assistant* Nov 98:8

23802 with autogenous graft (includes obtaining graft)

Amputation

23900 Interthoracoscapular amputation (forequarter)

23920 Disarticulation of shoulder;

23921 secondary closure or scar revision

Other Procedures

23929 Unlisted procedure, shoulder

Humerus (Upper Arm) and Elbow

The elbow area includes the head and neck of the radius and olecranon process.

Incision

(For incision and drainage procedures, superficial, see 10040-10160)

23930 Incision and drainage, upper arm or elbow area; deep abscess or hematoma

23931 bursa

➔ *CPT Assistant* Nov 98:8

23935 Incision, deep, with opening of bone cortex (eg, for osteomyelitis or bone abscess), humerus or elbow

24000 Arthrotomy, elbow, including exploration, drainage, or removal of foreign body

➔ *CPT Assistant* Nov 98:8-9

24006 Arthrotomy of the elbow, with capsular excision for capsular release (separate procedure)

Excision

24065 Biopsy, soft tissue of upper arm or elbow area; superficial

24066 deep (subfascial or intramuscular)

(For needle biopsy of soft tissue, use 20206)

24071 Code is out of numerical sequence. See 24066-24079

24073 Code is out of numerical sequence. See 24066-24079

24075 Excision, tumor, soft tissue of upper arm or elbow area, subcutaneous; less than 3 cm

➔ *CPT Changes: An Insider's View* 2002, 2010

 # 24071 3 cm or greater

➔ *CPT Changes: An Insider's View* 2010

(For excision of benign lesions of cutaneous origin [eg, sebaceous cyst], see 11400-11406)

24076 Excision, tumor, soft tissue of upper arm or elbow area, subfascial (eg, intramuscular); less than 5 cm

➔ *CPT Changes: An Insider's View* 2010

 # 24073 5 cm or greater

➔ *CPT Changes: An Insider's View* 2010

24077 Radical resection of tumor (eg, sarcoma), soft tissue of upper arm or elbow area; less than 5 cm

➔ *CPT Changes: An Insider's View* 2010, 2014

24079 5 cm or greater

➔ *CPT Changes: An Insider's View* 2010, 2014

(For radical resection of tumor[s] of cutaneous origin [eg, melanoma], see 11600-11606)

24100 Arthrotomy, elbow; with synovial biopsy only

24101 with joint exploration, with or without biopsy, with or without removal of loose or foreign body

24102 with synovectomy

24105 Excision, olecranon bursa

24110 Excision or curettage of bone cyst or benign tumor, humerus;

24115 with autograft (includes obtaining graft)

24116 with allograft

24120 Excision or curettage of bone cyst or benign tumor of head or neck of radius or olecranon process;

24125 with autograft (includes obtaining graft)

24126 with allograft

24130 Excision, radial head

(For replacement with implant, use 24366)

24134 Sequestrectomy (eg, for osteomyelitis or bone abscess), shaft or distal humerus

24136 Sequestrectomy (eg, for osteomyelitis or bone abscess), radial head or neck

24138 Sequestrectomy (eg, for osteomyelitis or bone abscess), olecranon process

24140 Partial excision (craterization, saucerization, or diaphysectomy) bone (eg, osteomyelitis), humerus

➔ *CPT Assistant* Nov 98:9

24145 Partial excision (craterization, saucerization, or diaphysectomy) bone (eg, osteomyelitis), radial head or neck

➔ *CPT Assistant* Nov 98:9

24147 Partial excision (craterization, saucerization, or diaphysectomy) bone (eg, osteomyelitis), olecranon process

➔ *CPT Assistant* Nov 98:9

24149 Radical resection of capsule, soft tissue, and heterotopic bone, elbow, with contracture release (separate procedure)

➔ *CPT Assistant* Nov 96:4

(For capsular and soft tissue release only, use 24006)

24150 Radical resection of tumor, shaft or distal humerus

➔ *CPT Changes: An Insider's View* 2010

24152 Radical resection of tumor, radial head or neck

➔ *CPT Changes: An Insider's View* 2010

24155 Resection of elbow joint (arthrectomy)

Musculoskeletal 20100-29999

Introduction or Removal

(For K-wire or pin insertion or removal, see 20650, 20670, 20680)

(For arthrocentesis or needling of bursa or joint, use 20605)

24160 Removal of prosthesis, includes debridement and synovectomy when performed; humeral **and** ulnar components
- *CPT Changes: An Insider's View* 2014
- *CPT Assistant* Feb 13:11, Mar 14:4

(To report removal of foreign body, elbow, see 24200, 24201)

(To report removal of hardware from the distal humerus or proximal ulna, other than humeral and ulnar prosthesis, use 20680)

(Do not report 24160 in conjunction with 24370 or 24371 if a prosthesis [ie, humeral and/or ulnar component(s)] is being removed and replaced in the same elbow during the same surgical session)

24164 radial head
- *CPT Changes: An Insider's View* 2014
- *CPT Assistant* Mar 14:4

(To report removal of foreign body, elbow, see 24200, 24201)

(To report removal of hardware from proximal radius, other than radial head prosthesis, use 20680)

24200 Removal of foreign body, upper arm or elbow area; subcutaneous
- *CPT Assistant* Mar 14:4

24201 deep (subfascial or intramuscular)
- *CPT Assistant* Nov 98:8, Mar 14:4

24220 Injection procedure for elbow arthrography
- *CPT Assistant* Aug 15:6, May 16:13

(For radiological supervision and interpretation, use 73085. Do not report 77002 in conjunction with 73085)

(For injection for tennis elbow, use 20550)

Repair, Revision, and/or Reconstruction

24300 Manipulation, elbow, under anesthesia
- *CPT Changes: An Insider's View* 2002

(For application of external fixation, see 20690 or 20692)

24301 Muscle or tendon transfer, any type, upper arm or elbow, single (excluding 24320-24331)

24305 Tendon lengthening, upper arm or elbow, each tendon
- *CPT Assistant* Nov 98:8

24310 Tenotomy, open, elbow to shoulder, each tendon
- *CPT Assistant* Nov 98:8

24320 Tenoplasty, with muscle transfer, with or without free graft, elbow to shoulder, single (Seddon-Brookes type procedure)

24330 Flexor-plasty, elbow (eg, Steindler type advancement);

24331 with extensor advancement

24332 Tenolysis, triceps
- *CPT Changes: An Insider's View* 2002

24340 Tenodesis of biceps tendon at elbow (separate procedure)

24341 Repair, tendon or muscle, upper arm or elbow, each tendon or muscle, primary or secondary (excludes rotator cuff)
- *CPT Assistant* Nov 96:4

24342 Reinsertion of ruptured biceps or triceps tendon, distal, with or without tendon graft
- *CPT Assistant* Nov 96:4, Apr 17:9

24343 Repair lateral collateral ligament, elbow, with local tissue
- *CPT Changes: An Insider's View* 2002

24344 Reconstruction lateral collateral ligament, elbow, with tendon graft (includes harvesting of graft)
- *CPT Changes: An Insider's View* 2002

24345 Repair medial collateral ligament, elbow, with local tissue
- *CPT Changes: An Insider's View* 2002

24346 Reconstruction medial collateral ligament, elbow, with tendon graft (includes harvesting of graft)
- *CPT Changes: An Insider's View* 2002

24357 Tenotomy, elbow, lateral or medial (eg, epicondylitis, tennis elbow, golfer's elbow); percutaneous
- *CPT Changes: An Insider's View* 2008
- *CPT Assistant* Jan 08:4

24358 debridement, soft tissue and/or bone, open
- *CPT Changes: An Insider's View* 2008
- *CPT Assistant* Jan 08:4

24359 debridement, soft tissue and/or bone, open with tendon repair or reattachment
- *CPT Changes: An Insider's View* 2008
- *CPT Assistant* Jan 08:4

(Do not report 24357-24359 in conjunction with 29837, 29838)

24360 Arthroplasty, elbow; with membrane (eg, fascial)
- *CPT Assistant* Nov 98:8

24361 with distal humeral prosthetic replacement

24362 with implant and fascia lata ligament reconstruction

24363 with distal humerus and proximal ulnar prosthetic replacement (eg, total elbow)
- *CPT Assistant* Feb 13:11

(For revision of total elbow implant, see 24370, 24371)

24365 Arthroplasty, radial head;

24366 with implant

24370 Revision of total elbow arthroplasty, including allograft when performed; humeral **or** ulnar component
- *CPT Changes: An Insider's View* 2013
- *CPT Assistant* Feb 13:11, Mar 14:4

24371 humeral **and** ulnar component
CPT Changes: An Insider's View 2013
CPT Assistant Feb 13:11, Mar 14:4

(Do not report 24370, 24371 in conjunction with 24160 if a prosthesis [ie, humeral and/or ulnar component(s)] is being removed and replaced in the same elbow)

24400 Osteotomy, humerus, with or without internal fixation
CPT Assistant Mar 14:4

24410 Multiple osteotomies with realignment on intramedullary rod, humeral shaft (Sofield type procedure)

24420 Osteoplasty, humerus (eg, shortening or lengthening) (excluding 64876)

24430 Repair of nonunion or malunion, humerus; without graft (eg, compression technique)

24435 with iliac or other autograft (includes obtaining graft)

(For proximal radius and/or ulna, see 25400-25420)

24470 Hemiepiphyseal arrest (eg, cubitus varus or valgus, distal humerus)

24495 Decompression fasciotomy, forearm, with brachial artery exploration

24498 Prophylactic treatment (nailing, pinning, plating or wiring), with or without methylmethacrylate, humeral shaft
CPT Assistant Nov 98:8

Fracture and/or Dislocation

Coding Tip

Reporting for Categories of Manipulation and/or Fracture

The codes for treatment of fractures and joint injuries (dislocations) are categorized by the type of manipulation (reduction) and stabilization (fixation or immobilization). These codes can apply to either open (compound) or closed fractures or joint injuries.

CPT Coding Guidelines, Musculoskeletal System

24500 Closed treatment of humeral shaft fracture; without manipulation

24505 with manipulation, with or without skeletal traction

24515 Open treatment of humeral shaft fracture with plate/screws, with or without cerclage

24516 Treatment of humeral shaft fracture, with insertion of intramedullary implant, with or without cerclage and/or locking screws
CPT Changes: An Insider's View 2003
CPT Assistant Feb 96:4, Jun 09:7, Jan 18:3

24530 Closed treatment of supracondylar or transcondylar humeral fracture, with or without intercondylar extension; without manipulation

24535 with manipulation, with or without skin or skeletal traction

24538 Percutaneous skeletal fixation of supracondylar or transcondylar humeral fracture, with or without intercondylar extension
CPT Assistant Winter 92:10

24545 Open treatment of humeral supracondylar or transcondylar fracture, includes internal fixation, when performed; without intercondylar extension
CPT Changes: An Insider's View 2008

24546 with intercondylar extension
CPT Changes: An Insider's View 2008

24560 Closed treatment of humeral epicondylar fracture, medial or lateral; without manipulation

24565 with manipulation

24566 Percutaneous skeletal fixation of humeral epicondylar fracture, medial or lateral, with manipulation

24575 Open treatment of humeral epicondylar fracture, medial or lateral, includes internal fixation, when performed
CPT Changes: An Insider's View 2008

24576 Closed treatment of humeral condylar fracture, medial or lateral; without manipulation

24577 with manipulation

24579 Open treatment of humeral condylar fracture, medial or lateral, includes internal fixation, when performed
CPT Changes: An Insider's View 2008

(To report closed treatment of fractures without manipulation, see 24530, 24560, 24576, 24650, 24670)

(To report closed treatment of fractures with manipulation, see 24535, 24565, 24577, 24675)

24582 Percutaneous skeletal fixation of humeral condylar fracture, medial or lateral, with manipulation

24586 Open treatment of periarticular fracture and/or dislocation of the elbow (fracture distal humerus and proximal ulna and/or proximal radius);

24587 with implant arthroplasty

(See also 24361)

24600 Treatment of closed elbow dislocation; without anesthesia

24605 requiring anesthesia

24615 Open treatment of acute or chronic elbow dislocation

24620 Closed treatment of Monteggia type of fracture dislocation at elbow (fracture proximal end of ulna with dislocation of radial head), with manipulation

24635 Open treatment of Monteggia type of fracture dislocation at elbow (fracture proximal end of ulna with dislocation of radial head), includes internal fixation, when performed
CPT Changes: An Insider's View 2008

24640 Closed treatment of radial head subluxation in child, nursemaid elbow, with manipulation

Musculoskeletal 20100-29999

24650 Closed treatment of radial head or neck fracture; without manipulation

24655 with manipulation

24665 Open treatment of radial head or neck fracture, includes internal fixation or radial head excision, when performed;
➔ *CPT Changes: An Insider's View* 2008

24666 with radial head prosthetic replacement
➔ *CPT Changes: An Insider's View* 2008

24670 Closed treatment of ulnar fracture, proximal end (eg, olecranon or coronoid process[es]); without manipulation
➔ *CPT Changes: An Insider's View* 2008

24675 with manipulation
➔ *CPT Changes: An Insider's View* 2008

24685 Open treatment of ulnar fracture, proximal end (eg, olecranon or coronoid process[es]), includes internal fixation, when performed
➔ *CPT Changes: An Insider's View* 2008
➔ *CPT Assistant* Jan 18:3

(Do not report 24685 in conjunction with 24100-24102)

Arthrodesis

24800 Arthrodesis, elbow joint; local

24802 with autogenous graft (includes obtaining graft)

Amputation

24900 Amputation, arm through humerus; with primary closure

24920 open, circular (guillotine)

24925 secondary closure or scar revision

24930 re-amputation

24931 with implant

24935 Stump elongation, upper extremity

24940 Cineplasty, upper extremity, complete procedure

Other Procedures

24999 Unlisted procedure, humerus or elbow

Forearm and Wrist

Radius, ulna, carpal bones, and joints.

Incision

25000 Incision, extensor tendon sheath, wrist (eg, de Quervains disease)
➔ *CPT Assistant* Nov 98:8

(For decompression median nerve or for carpal tunnel syndrome, use 64721)

25001 Incision, flexor tendon sheath, wrist (eg, flexor carpi radialis)
➔ *CPT Changes: An Insider's View* 2002

25020 Decompression fasciotomy, forearm and/or wrist, flexor OR extensor compartment; without debridement of nonviable muscle and/or nerve
➔ *CPT Changes: An Insider's View* 2002

25023 with debridement of nonviable muscle and/or nerve

(For decompression fasciotomy with brachial artery exploration, use 24495)

(For incision and drainage procedures, superficial, see 10060-10160)

(For debridement, see also 11000-11044)

25024 Decompression fasciotomy, forearm and/or wrist, flexor AND extensor compartment; without debridement of nonviable muscle and/or nerve
➔ *CPT Changes: An Insider's View* 2002

25025 with debridement of nonviable muscle and/or nerve
➔ *CPT Changes: An Insider's View* 2002

25028 Incision and drainage, forearm and/or wrist; deep abscess or hematoma

25031 bursa
➔ *CPT Assistant* Nov 98:9

25035 Incision, deep, bone cortex, forearm and/or wrist (eg, osteomyelitis or bone abscess)

25040 Arthrotomy, radiocarpal or midcarpal joint, with exploration, drainage, or removal of foreign body

Excision

25065 Biopsy, soft tissue of forearm and/or wrist; superficial

25066 deep (subfascial or intramuscular)
➔ *CPT Assistant* Nov 98:8, Apr 10:3

(For needle biopsy of soft tissue, use 20206)

25071 Code is out of numerical sequence. See 25066-25078

25073 Code is out of numerical sequence. See 25066-25078

25075 Excision, tumor, soft tissue of forearm and/or wrist area, subcutaneous; less than 3 cm
➔ *CPT Changes: An Insider's View* 2002, 2010

 # 25071 3 cm or greater
➔ *CPT Changes: An Insider's View* 2010

(For excision of benign lesions of cutaneous origin [eg, sebaceous cyst], see 11400-11406)

25076 Excision, tumor, soft tissue of forearm and/or wrist area, subfascial (eg, intramuscular); less than 3 cm
➔ *CPT Changes: An Insider's View* 2010

 # 25073 3 cm or greater
➔ *CPT Changes: An Insider's View* 2010

25077 Radical resection of tumor (eg, sarcoma), soft tissue of forearm and/or wrist area; less than 3 cm
CPT Changes: An Insider's View 2010, 2014

25078 3 cm or greater
CPT Changes: An Insider's View 2010, 2014

(For radical resection of tumor[s] of cutaneous origin [eg, melanoma], see 11600-11606)

25085 Capsulotomy, wrist (eg, contracture)

25100 Arthrotomy, wrist joint; with biopsy

25101 with joint exploration, with or without biopsy, with or without removal of loose or foreign body

25105 with synovectomy

25107 Arthrotomy, distal radioulnar joint including repair of triangular cartilage, complex

25109 Excision of tendon, forearm and/or wrist, flexor or extensor, each
CPT Changes: An Insider's View 2007

25110 Excision, lesion of tendon sheath, forearm and/or wrist

25111 Excision of ganglion, wrist (dorsal or volar); primary

25112 recurrent

(For hand or finger, use 26160)

25115 Radical excision of bursa, synovia of wrist, or forearm tendon sheaths (eg, tenosynovitis, fungus, Tbc, or other granulomas, rheumatoid arthritis); flexors
CPT Assistant Jun 12:15

25116 extensors, with or without transposition of dorsal retinaculum

(For finger synovectomies, use 26145)

25118 Synovectomy, extensor tendon sheath, wrist, single compartment;
CPT Assistant Apr 12:17, Jun 15:10

25119 with resection of distal ulna

25120 Excision or curettage of bone cyst or benign tumor of radius or ulna (excluding head or neck of radius and olecranon process);

(For head or neck of radius or olecranon process, see 24120-24126)

25125 with autograft (includes obtaining graft)

25126 with allograft

25130 Excision or curettage of bone cyst or benign tumor of carpal bones;

25135 with autograft (includes obtaining graft)

25136 with allograft

25145 Sequestrectomy (eg, for osteomyelitis or bone abscess), forearm and/or wrist

25150 Partial excision (craterization, saucerization, or diaphysectomy) of bone (eg, for osteomyelitis); ulna

25151 radius

(For head or neck of radius or olecranon process, see 24145, 24147)

25170 Radical resection of tumor, radius or ulna
CPT Changes: An Insider's View 2010

25210 Carpectomy; 1 bone

(For carpectomy with implant, see 25441-25445)

25215 all bones of proximal row

25230 Radial styloidectomy (separate procedure)

25240 Excision distal ulna partial or complete (eg, Darrach type or matched resection)

(For implant replacement, distal ulna, use 25442)

(For obtaining fascia for interposition, see 20920, 20922)

Introduction or Removal

(For K-wire, pin or rod insertion or removal, see 20650, 20670, 20680)

25246 Injection procedure for wrist arthrography
CPT Assistant Aug 15:6

(For radiological supervision and interpretation, use 73115. Do not report 77002 in conjunction with 73115)

(For foreign body removal, superficial use 20520)

25248 Exploration with removal of deep foreign body, forearm or wrist

25250 Removal of wrist prosthesis; (separate procedure)

25251 complicated, including total wrist

25259 Manipulation, wrist, under anesthesia
CPT Changes: An Insider's View 2002
CPT Assistant Jan 04:27, Jun 05:12

(For application of external fixation, see 20690 or 20692)

Repair, Revision, and/or Reconstruction

25260 Repair, tendon or muscle, flexor, forearm and/or wrist; primary, single, each tendon or muscle

25263 secondary, single, each tendon or muscle

25265 secondary, with free graft (includes obtaining graft), each tendon or muscle

25270 Repair, tendon or muscle, extensor, forearm and/or wrist; primary, single, each tendon or muscle

25272 secondary, single, each tendon or muscle

25274 secondary, with free graft (includes obtaining graft), each tendon or muscle
CPT Changes: An Insider's View 2002

25275 Repair, tendon sheath, extensor, forearm and/or wrist, with free graft (includes obtaining graft) (eg, for extensor carpi ulnaris subluxation)
CPT Changes: An Insider's View 2002

25280 Lengthening or shortening of flexor or extensor tendon, forearm and/or wrist, single, each tendon

25290 Tenotomy, open, flexor or extensor tendon, forearm and/or wrist, single, each tendon

25295 Tenolysis, flexor or extensor tendon, forearm and/or wrist, single, each tendon
➔ *CPT Assistant* Apr 97:11, Aug 98:10

25300 Tenodesis at wrist; flexors of fingers

25301 extensors of fingers

25310 Tendon transplantation or transfer, flexor or extensor, forearm and/or wrist, single; each tendon
➔ *CPT Assistant* Jun 02:11

25312 with tendon graft(s) (includes obtaining graft), each tendon

25315 Flexor origin slide (eg, for cerebral palsy, Volkmann contracture), forearm and/or wrist;

25316 with tendon(s) transfer

25320 Capsulorrhaphy or reconstruction, wrist, open (eg, capsulodesis, ligament repair, tendon transfer or graft) (includes synovectomy, capsulotomy and open reduction) for carpal instability
➔ *CPT Changes: An Insider's View* 2003

25332 Arthroplasty, wrist, with or without interposition, with or without external or internal fixation
➔ *CPT Assistant* Nov 96:5, Jan 05:8

(For obtaining fascia for interposition, see 20920, 20922)

(For prosthetic replacement arthroplasty, see 25441-25446)

25335 Centralization of wrist on ulna (eg, radial club hand)

25337 Reconstruction for stabilization of unstable distal ulna or distal radioulnar joint, secondary by soft tissue stabilization (eg, tendon transfer, tendon graft or weave, or tenodesis) with or without open reduction of distal radioulnar joint

(For harvesting of fascia lata graft, see 20920, 20922)

25350 Osteotomy, radius; distal third

25355 middle or proximal third

25360 Osteotomy; ulna

25365 radius AND ulna

25370 Multiple osteotomies, with realignment on intramedullary rod (Sofield type procedure); radius OR ulna

25375 radius AND ulna

25390 Osteoplasty, radius OR ulna; shortening

25391 lengthening with autograft

25392 Osteoplasty, radius AND ulna; shortening (excluding 64876)

25393 lengthening with autograft

25394 Osteoplasty, carpal bone, shortening
➔ *CPT Changes: An Insider's View* 2002

25400 Repair of nonunion or malunion, radius OR ulna; without graft (eg, compression technique)

25405 with autograft (includes obtaining graft)
➔ *CPT Changes: An Insider's View* 2002

25415 Repair of nonunion or malunion, radius AND ulna; without graft (eg, compression technique)

25420 with autograft (includes obtaining graft)
➔ *CPT Changes: An Insider's View* 2002

25425 Repair of defect with autograft; radius OR ulna

25426 radius AND ulna

25430 Insertion of vascular pedicle into carpal bone (eg, Hori procedure)
➔ *CPT Changes: An Insider's View* 2002

25431 Repair of nonunion of carpal bone (excluding carpal scaphoid (navicular)) (includes obtaining graft and necessary fixation), each bone
➔ *CPT Changes: An Insider's View* 2002

25440 Repair of nonunion, scaphoid carpal (navicular) bone, with or without radial styloidectomy (includes obtaining graft and necessary fixation)
➔ *CPT Changes: An Insider's View* 2002

25441 Arthroplasty with prosthetic replacement; distal radius
➔ *CPT Assistant* Jan 05:8-9, Aug 17:9

25442 distal ulna
➔ *CPT Assistant* Jan 05:8-9, Aug 17:9

25443 scaphoid carpal (navicular)
➔ *CPT Changes: An Insider's View* 2002
➔ *CPT Assistant* Jan 05:8-9

25444 lunate
➔ *CPT Assistant* Jan 05:8, 10

25445 trapezium
➔ *CPT Assistant* Jan 05:8, 10

25446 distal radius and partial or entire carpus (total wrist)
➔ *CPT Assistant* Jan 05:8, 11

25447 Arthroplasty, interposition, intercarpal or carpometacarpal joints
➔ *CPT Assistant* Nov 98:8, Jan 05:8, 11-12

(For wrist arthroplasty, use 25332)

25449 Revision of arthroplasty, including removal of implant, wrist joint

25450 Epiphyseal arrest by epiphysiodesis or stapling; distal radius OR ulna

25455 distal radius AND ulna

25490 Prophylactic treatment (nailing, pinning, plating or wiring) with or without methylmethacrylate; radius

25491 ulna

25492 radius AND ulna

Fracture and/or Dislocation

(For application of external fixation in addition to internal fixation, use 20690 and the appropriate internal fixation code)

25500 Closed treatment of radial shaft fracture; without manipulation

25505 with manipulation

25515 Open treatment of radial shaft fracture, includes internal fixation, when performed
➲ *CPT Changes: An Insider's View* 2008

25520 Closed treatment of radial shaft fracture and closed treatment of dislocation of distal radioulnar joint (Galeazzi fracture/dislocation)
➲ *CPT Changes: An Insider's View* 2002

25525 Open treatment of radial shaft fracture, includes internal fixation, when performed, and closed treatment of distal radioulnar joint dislocation (Galeazzi fracture/dislocation), includes percutaneous skeletal fixation, when performed
➲ *CPT Changes: An Insider's View* 2008

25526 Open treatment of radial shaft fracture, includes internal fixation, when performed, and open treatment of distal radioulnar joint dislocation (Galeazzi fracture/dislocation), includes internal fixation, when performed, includes repair of triangular fibrocartilage complex
➲ *CPT Changes: An Insider's View* 2002, 2008

25530 Closed treatment of ulnar shaft fracture; without manipulation
➲ *CPT Assistant* Apr 02:14

25535 with manipulation
➲ *CPT Assistant* Sep 10:7

25545 Open treatment of ulnar shaft fracture, includes internal fixation, when performed
➲ *CPT Changes: An Insider's View* 2008
➲ *CPT Assistant* Fall 93:23, Oct 99:5

25560 Closed treatment of radial and ulnar shaft fractures; without manipulation

25565 with manipulation

25574 Open treatment of radial AND ulnar shaft fractures, with internal fixation, when performed; of radius OR ulna
➲ *CPT Changes: An Insider's View* 2008
➲ *CPT Assistant* Fall 93:23, Oct 99:5

25575 of radius AND ulna
➲ *CPT Changes: An Insider's View* 2008

25600 Closed treatment of distal radial fracture (eg, Colles or Smith type) or epiphyseal separation, includes closed treatment of fracture of ulnar styloid, when performed; without manipulation
➲ *CPT Changes: An Insider's View* 2007
➲ *CPT Assistant* Oct 07:7, Apr 13:10

25605 with manipulation
➲ *CPT Assistant* Oct 07:7, Apr 13:10

(Do not report 25600, 25605 in conjunction with 25650)

25606 Percutaneous skeletal fixation of distal radial fracture or epiphyseal separation
➲ *CPT Changes: An Insider's View* 2007

(Do not report 25606 in conjunction with 25650)

(For percutaneous treatment of ulnar styloid fracture, use 25651)

(For open treatment of ulnar styloid fracture, use 25652)

25607 Open treatment of distal radial extra-articular fracture or epiphyseal separation, with internal fixation
➲ *CPT Changes: An Insider's View* 2007
➲ *CPT Assistant* Oct 07:7, Nov 12:13

(Do not report 25607 in conjunction with 25650)

(For percutaneous treatment of ulnar styloid fracture, use 25651)

(For open treatment of ulnar styloid fracture, use 25652)

25608 Open treatment of distal radial intra-articular fracture or epiphyseal separation; with internal fixation of 2 fragments
➲ *CPT Changes: An Insider's View* 2007
➲ *CPT Assistant* Oct 07:7

(Do not report 25608 in conjunction with 25609)

25609 with internal fixation of 3 or more fragments
➲ *CPT Changes: An Insider's View* 2007
➲ *CPT Assistant* Oct 07:7, Mar 13:13, Dec 13:14

(Do not report 25608, 25609 in conjunction with 25650)

(For percutaneous treatment of ulnar styloid fracture, use 25651)

(For open treatment of ulnar styloid fracture, use 25652)

25622 Closed treatment of carpal scaphoid (navicular) fracture; without manipulation

25624 with manipulation

25628 Open treatment of carpal scaphoid (navicular) fracture, includes internal fixation, when performed
➲ *CPT Changes: An Insider's View* 2008

25630 Closed treatment of carpal bone fracture (excluding carpal scaphoid [navicular]); without manipulation, each bone

25635 with manipulation, each bone

25645 Open treatment of carpal bone fracture (other than carpal scaphoid [navicular]), each bone
➲ *CPT Changes: An Insider's View* 2002

25650 Closed treatment of ulnar styloid fracture
➲ *CPT Assistant* Oct 07:7, Apr 13:10

(Do not report 25650 in conjunction with 25600, 25605, 25607-25609)

Musculoskeletal 20100-29999

25651 Percutaneous skeletal fixation of ulnar styloid fracture
➲ *CPT Changes: An Insider's View* 2002

25652 Open treatment of ulnar styloid fracture
➲ *CPT Changes: An Insider's View* 2002
➲ *CPT Assistant* Oct 07:7

25660 Closed treatment of radiocarpal or intercarpal dislocation, 1 or more bones, with manipulation

25670 Open treatment of radiocarpal or intercarpal dislocation, 1 or more bones

25671 Percutaneous skeletal fixation of distal radioulnar dislocation
➲ *CPT Changes: An Insider's View* 2002

25675 Closed treatment of distal radioulnar dislocation with manipulation

25676 Open treatment of distal radioulnar dislocation, acute or chronic

25680 Closed treatment of trans-scaphoperilunar type of fracture dislocation, with manipulation

25685 Open treatment of trans-scaphoperilunar type of fracture dislocation

25690 Closed treatment of lunate dislocation, with manipulation

25695 Open treatment of lunate dislocation

Arthrodesis

25800 Arthrodesis, wrist; complete, without bone graft (includes radiocarpal and/or intercarpal and/or carpometacarpal joints)
➲ *CPT Assistant* Nov 98:8

25805 with sliding graft

25810 with iliac or other autograft (includes obtaining graft)

25820 Arthrodesis, wrist; limited, without bone graft (eg, intercarpal or radiocarpal)
➲ *CPT Assistant* Nov 98:8

25825 with autograft (includes obtaining graft)
➲ *CPT Assistant* Jul 12:12

25830 Arthrodesis, distal radioulnar joint with segmental resection of ulna, with or without bone graft (eg, Sauve-Kapandji procedure)
➲ *CPT Assistant* Nov 98:8

Amputation

25900 Amputation, forearm, through radius and ulna;

25905 open, circular (guillotine)

25907 secondary closure or scar revision

25909 re-amputation

25915 Krukenberg procedure

25920 Disarticulation through wrist;

25922 secondary closure or scar revision

25924 re-amputation

25927 Transmetacarpal amputation;

25929 secondary closure or scar revision

25931 re-amputation

Other Procedures

25999 Unlisted procedure, forearm or wrist

Hand and Fingers

Incision

26010 Drainage of finger abscess; simple

26011 complicated (eg, felon)

26020 Drainage of tendon sheath, digit and/or palm, each

26025 Drainage of palmar bursa; single, bursa
➲ *CPT Assistant* Nov 98:8

26030 multiple bursa
➲ *CPT Assistant* Nov 98:8

26034 Incision, bone cortex, hand or finger (eg, osteomyelitis or bone abscess)
➲ *CPT Assistant* Nov 98:8

26035 Decompression fingers and/or hand, injection injury (eg, grease gun)

26037 Decompressive fasciotomy, hand (excludes 26035)

(For injection injury, use 26035)

26040 Fasciotomy, palmar (eg, Dupuytren's contracture); percutaneous
➲ *CPT Assistant* Nov 98:8, Apr 10:10, Oct 10:10

26045 open, partial

(For palmar fasciotomy by enzyme injection (eg, collagenase), see 20527, 26341)

(For fasciectomy, see 26121-26125)

26055 Tendon sheath incision (eg, for trigger finger)

26060 Tenotomy, percutaneous, single, each digit

26070 Arthrotomy, with exploration, drainage, or removal of loose or foreign body; carpometacarpal joint
➲ *CPT Assistant* Nov 98:10

26075 metacarpophalangeal joint, each
➲ *CPT Assistant* Sep 12:10

26080 interphalangeal joint, each
➲ *CPT Assistant* Sep 12:10

Excision

26100 Arthrotomy with biopsy; carpometacarpal joint, each

26105 metacarpophalangeal joint, each

26110 interphalangeal joint, each

26111 Code is out of numerical sequence. See 26110-26118

26113 Code is out of numerical sequence. See 26110-26118

26115 Excision, tumor or vascular malformation, soft tissue of hand or finger, subcutaneous; less than 1.5 cm
➔ *CPT Changes: An Insider's View* 2002, 2010

 # 26111 1.5 cm or greater
➔ *CPT Changes: An Insider's View* 2010

(For excision of benign lesions of cutaneous origin [eg, sebaceous cyst], see 11420-11426)

26116 Excision, tumor, soft tissue, or vascular malformation, of hand or finger, subfascial (eg, intramuscular); less than 1.5 cm
➔ *CPT Changes: An Insider's View* 2002, 2010
➔ *CPT Assistant* Apr 10:3

 # 26113 1.5 cm or greater
➔ *CPT Changes: An Insider's View* 2010
➔ *CPT Assistant* Apr 10:3

26117 Radical resection of tumor (eg, sarcoma), soft tissue of hand or finger; less than 3 cm
➔ *CPT Changes: An Insider's View* 2010, 2014

26118 3 cm or greater
➔ *CPT Changes: An Insider's View* 2010, 2014

(For radical resection of tumor[s] of cutaneous origin [eg, melanoma], see 11620-11626)

26121 Fasciectomy, palm only, with or without Z-plasty, other local tissue rearrangement, or skin grafting (includes obtaining graft)
➔ *CPT Assistant* Oct 10:10, Jun 11:13

26123 Fasciectomy, partial palmar with release of single digit including proximal interphalangeal joint, with or without Z-plasty, other local tissue rearrangement, or skin grafting (includes obtaining graft);
➔ *CPT Assistant* Jan 05:8, Oct 10:10, Jun 11:13

+ 26125 each additional digit (List separately in addition to code for primary procedure)
➔ *CPT Assistant* Jan 05:8, Oct 10:10, Jun 11:13

(Use 26125 in conjunction with 26123)

(For palmar fasciotomy by enzyme injection (eg, collagenase), see 20527, 26341)

(For fasciotomy, see 26040, 26045)

26130 Synovectomy, carpometacarpal joint

26135 Synovectomy, metacarpophalangeal joint including intrinsic release and extensor hood reconstruction, each digit

26140 Synovectomy, proximal interphalangeal joint, including extensor reconstruction, each interphalangeal joint

26145 Synovectomy, tendon sheath, radical (tenosynovectomy), flexor tendon, palm and/or finger, each tendon
➔ *CPT Assistant* Nov 98:8

(For tendon sheath synovectomies at wrist, see 25115, 25116)

26160 Excision of lesion of tendon sheath or joint capsule (eg, cyst, mucous cyst, or ganglion), hand or finger
➔ *CPT Changes: An Insider's View* 2002

(For wrist ganglion, see 25111, 25112)

(For trigger digit, use 26055)

26170 Excision of tendon, palm, flexor or extensor, single, each tendon
➔ *CPT Changes: An Insider's View* 2007
➔ *CPT Assistant* Jun 13:13

(Do not report 26170 in conjunction with 26390, 26415)

26180 Excision of tendon, finger, flexor or extensor, each tendon
➔ *CPT Changes: An Insider's View* 2007
➔ *CPT Assistant* Nov 98:8

(Do not report 26180 in conjunction with 26390, 26415)

26185 Sesamoidectomy, thumb or finger (separate procedure)

26200 Excision or curettage of bone cyst or benign tumor of metacarpal;

26205 with autograft (includes obtaining graft)

26210 Excision or curettage of bone cyst or benign tumor of proximal, middle, or distal phalanx of finger;

26215 with autograft (includes obtaining graft)

26230 Partial excision (craterization, saucerization, or diaphysectomy) bone (eg, osteomyelitis); metacarpal

26235 proximal or middle phalanx of finger

26236 distal phalanx of finger

26250 Radical resection of tumor, metacarpal
➔ *CPT Changes: An Insider's View* 2010
➔ *CPT Assistant* Nov 98:8

26260 Radical resection of tumor, proximal or middle phalanx of finger
➔ *CPT Changes: An Insider's View* 2010
➔ *CPT Assistant* Nov 98:8

26262 Radical resection of tumor, distal phalanx of finger
➔ *CPT Changes: An Insider's View* 2010
➔ *CPT Assistant* Nov 98:8

Introduction or Removal

26320 Removal of implant from finger or hand

(For removal of foreign body in hand or finger, see 20520, 20525)

Repair, Revision, and/or Reconstruction

26340 Manipulation, finger joint, under anesthesia, each joint
➔ *CPT Changes: An Insider's View* 2002
➔ *CPT Assistant* Nov 02:10

(For application of external fixation, see 20690 or 20692)

Musculoskeletal 20100-29999

26341 Manipulation, palmar fascial cord (ie, Dupuytren's cord), post enzyme injection (eg, collagenase), single cord
➲ *CPT Changes: An Insider's View* 2012
➲ *CPT Assistant* Jul 12:8, 14

(For enzyme injection (eg, collagenase), palmar fascial cord (eg, Dupuytren's contracture), use 20527)

(Report custom orthotic fabrication/application separately)

26350 Repair or advancement, flexor tendon, not in zone 2 digital flexor tendon sheath (eg, no man's land); primary or secondary without free graft, each tendon
➲ *CPT Changes: An Insider's View* 2002
➲ *CPT Assistant* Nov 98:8

26352 secondary with free graft (includes obtaining graft), each tendon

26356 Repair or advancement, flexor tendon, in zone 2 digital flexor tendon sheath (eg, no man's land); primary, without free graft, each tendon
➲ *CPT Changes: An Insider's View* 2002, 2004
➲ *CPT Assistant* Nov 98:8, Dec 98:9, Dec 08:6, Sep 14:13, Dec 17:15

26357 secondary, without free graft, each tendon
➲ *CPT Changes: An Insider's View* 2004

26358 secondary, with free graft (includes obtaining graft), each tendon

26370 Repair or advancement of profundus tendon, with intact superficialis tendon; primary, each tendon
➲ *CPT Assistant* Nov 98:8, Dec 08:6

26372 secondary with free graft (includes obtaining graft), each tendon
➲ *CPT Assistant* Nov 98:8

26373 secondary without free graft, each tendon
➲ *CPT Assistant* Nov 98:8

26390 Excision flexor tendon, with implantation of synthetic rod for delayed tendon graft, hand or finger, each rod
➲ *CPT Changes: An Insider's View* 2002
➲ *CPT Assistant* Nov 98:8

26392 Removal of synthetic rod and insertion of flexor tendon graft, hand or finger (includes obtaining graft), each rod
➲ *CPT Changes: An Insider's View* 2002
➲ *CPT Assistant* Nov 98:8

26410 Repair, extensor tendon, hand, primary or secondary; without free graft, each tendon
➲ *CPT Assistant* Nov 98:8

26412 with free graft (includes obtaining graft), each tendon
➲ *CPT Assistant* Nov 98:8

26415 Excision of extensor tendon, with implantation of synthetic rod for delayed tendon graft, hand or finger, each rod
➲ *CPT Changes: An Insider's View* 2002
➲ *CPT Assistant* Nov 98:8

26416 Removal of synthetic rod and insertion of extensor tendon graft (includes obtaining graft), hand or finger, each rod
➲ *CPT Changes: An Insider's View* 2000, 2002
➲ *CPT Assistant* Nov 99:12

26418 Repair, extensor tendon, finger, primary or secondary; without free graft, each tendon
➲ *CPT Assistant* Nov 98:8, Dec 99:10, Dec 00:14

26420 with free graft (includes obtaining graft) each tendon

26426 Repair of extensor tendon, central slip, secondary (eg, boutonniere deformity); using local tissue(s), including lateral band(s), each finger
➲ *CPT Changes: An Insider's View* 2002
➲ *CPT Assistant* Nov 98:8

26428 with free graft (includes obtaining graft), each finger
➲ *CPT Changes: An Insider's View* 2002

26432 Closed treatment of distal extensor tendon insertion, with or without percutaneous pinning (eg, mallet finger)
➲ *CPT Assistant* Nov 98:8

26433 Repair of extensor tendon, distal insertion, primary or secondary; without graft (eg, mallet finger)
➲ *CPT Assistant* Nov 98:8

26434 with free graft (includes obtaining graft)

(For tenovaginotomy for trigger finger, use 26055)

26437 Realignment of extensor tendon, hand, each tendon
➲ *CPT Assistant* Nov 98:8

26440 Tenolysis, flexor tendon; palm OR finger, each tendon
➲ *CPT Changes: An Insider's View* 2003
➲ *CPT Assistant* Apr 02:18, Jun 15:10

26442 palm AND finger, each tendon

26445 Tenolysis, extensor tendon, hand OR finger, each tendon
➲ *CPT Changes: An Insider's View* 2002
➲ *CPT Assistant* Nov 98:8, Dec 02:11, Mar 03:20

26449 Tenolysis, complex, extensor tendon, finger, including forearm, each tendon
➲ *CPT Assistant* Nov 98:8

26450 Tenotomy, flexor, palm, open, each tendon
➲ *CPT Assistant* Nov 98:8

26455 Tenotomy, flexor, finger, open, each tendon
➲ *CPT Assistant* Nov 98:8

26460 Tenotomy, extensor, hand or finger, open, each tendon
➲ *CPT Assistant* Nov 98:8

26471 Tenodesis; of proximal interphalangeal joint, each joint
➲ *CPT Assistant* Nov 98:8

26474 of distal joint, each joint
➲ *CPT Assistant* Nov 98:8

26476 Lengthening of tendon, extensor, hand or finger, each tendon
➲ *CPT Assistant* Nov 98:8

26477 Shortening of tendon, extensor, hand or finger, each tendon
➔ *CPT Assistant* Nov 98:8

26478 Lengthening of tendon, flexor, hand or finger, each tendon
➔ *CPT Assistant* Nov 98:8, Dec 13:16

26479 Shortening of tendon, flexor, hand or finger, each tendon
➔ *CPT Assistant* Nov 98:8

26480 Transfer or transplant of tendon, carpometacarpal area or dorsum of hand; without free graft, each tendon
➔ *CPT Assistant* Nov 98:8, Dec 13:16

26483 with free tendon graft (includes obtaining graft), each tendon

26485 Transfer or transplant of tendon, palmar; without free tendon graft, each tendon
➔ *CPT Assistant* Nov 98:8

26489 with free tendon graft (includes obtaining graft), each tendon

26490 Opponensplasty; superficialis tendon transfer type, each tendon

26492 tendon transfer with graft (includes obtaining graft), each tendon

26494 hypothenar muscle transfer

26496 other methods

(For thumb fusion in opposition, use 26820)

26497 Transfer of tendon to restore intrinsic function; ring and small finger
➔ *CPT Assistant* Nov 98:8

26498 all 4 fingers

26499 Correction claw finger, other methods

26500 Reconstruction of tendon pulley, each tendon; with local tissues (separate procedure)
➔ *CPT Assistant* Nov 98:8

26502 with tendon or fascial graft (includes obtaining graft) (separate procedure)

26508 Release of thenar muscle(s) (eg, thumb contracture)
➔ *CPT Assistant* Nov 98:8

26510 Cross intrinsic transfer, each tendon
➔ *CPT Changes: An Insider's View* 2002

26516 Capsulodesis, metacarpophalangeal joint; single digit
➔ *CPT Assistant* Nov 98:8

26517 2 digits

26518 3 or 4 digits

26520 Capsulectomy or capsulotomy; metacarpophalangeal joint, each joint
➔ *CPT Assistant* Nov 98:8

26525 interphalangeal joint, each joint
➔ *CPT Assistant* Nov 98:8, Apr 02:18, Mar 03:20, Jun 15:10

26530 Arthroplasty, metacarpophalangeal joint; each joint
➔ *CPT Assistant* Nov 98:8

(To report carpometacarpal joint arthroplasty, use 25447)

26531 with prosthetic implant, each joint
➔ *CPT Assistant* Nov 98:8, Sep 11:12

26535 Arthroplasty, interphalangeal joint; each joint
➔ *CPT Assistant* Nov 98:8

26536 with prosthetic implant, each joint
➔ *CPT Assistant* Nov 98:8

26540 Repair of collateral ligament, metacarpophalangeal or interphalangeal joint
➔ *CPT Assistant* Nov 96:6

26541 Reconstruction, collateral ligament, metacarpophalangeal joint, single; with tendon or fascial graft (includes obtaining graft)
➔ *CPT Assistant* Jan 97:3

26542 with local tissue (eg, adductor advancement)
➔ *CPT Assistant* Jan 97:3

26545 Reconstruction, collateral ligament, interphalangeal joint, single, including graft, each joint

26546 Repair non-union, metacarpal or phalanx (includes obtaining bone graft with or without external or internal fixation)
➔ *CPT Assistant* Nov 96:6

26548 Repair and reconstruction, finger, volar plate, interphalangeal joint

26550 Pollicization of a digit

26551 Transfer, toe-to-hand with microvascular anastomosis; great toe wrap-around with bone graft
➔ *CPT Assistant* Nov 96:6, Apr 97:7, Jun 97:9, Nov 98:8, 10-11

(For great toe with web space, use 20973)

26553 other than great toe, single
➔ *CPT Assistant* Nov 96:6, Apr 97:7, Jun 97:9, Nov 98:8, 10-11

26554 other than great toe, double
➔ *CPT Assistant* Nov 96:6, Apr 97:7, Jun 97:9, Nov 98:8, 10-11

(Do not report code 69990 in addition to codes 26551-26554)

26555 Transfer, finger to another position without microvascular anastomosis
➔ *CPT Assistant* Nov 98:8, 10-11

26556 Transfer, free toe joint, with microvascular anastomosis
➔ *CPT Assistant* Nov 96:6, Apr 97:7, Jun 97:9, Nov 98:8

(Do not report code 69990 in addition to code 26556)

(To report great toe-to-hand transfer, use 20973)

26560 Repair of syndactyly (web finger) each web space; with skin flaps

26561 with skin flaps and grafts

26562 complex (eg, involving bone, nails)

26565 Osteotomy; metacarpal, each
CPT Assistant Nov 98:9

26567 phalanx of finger, each
CPT Assistant Apr 12:17

26568 Osteoplasty, lengthening, metacarpal or phalanx

26580 Repair cleft hand

26587 Reconstruction of polydactylous digit, soft tissue and bone
CPT Changes: An Insider's View 2002
CPT Assistant Oct 01:10, Aug 03:14, May 04:16

(For excision of polydactylous digit, soft tissue only, use 11200)

26590 Repair macrodactylia, each digit
CPT Changes: An Insider's View 2002
CPT Assistant Oct 01:10, Aug 03:14, May 04:16

26591 Repair, intrinsic muscles of hand, each muscle
CPT Assistant May 98:11, Jul 98:11, Nov 98:8, 11

26593 Release, intrinsic muscles of hand, each muscle
CPT Assistant Nov 98:8, 11

26596 Excision of constricting ring of finger, with multiple Z-plasties

(To report release of scar contracture or graft repairs see 11042, 14040-14041, or 15120, 15240)

Fracture and/or Dislocation

Coding Tip

Reporting for Categories of Manipulation and/or Fracture

The codes for treatment of fractures and joint injuries (dislocations) are categorized by the type of manipulation (reduction) and stabilization (fixation or immobilization). These codes can apply to either open (compound) or closed fractures or joint injuries.

CPT Coding Guidelines, Musculoskeletal System

26600 Closed treatment of metacarpal fracture, single; without manipulation, each bone

26605 with manipulation, each bone

26607 Closed treatment of metacarpal fracture, with manipulation, with external fixation, each bone
CPT Changes: An Insider's View 2002

26608 Percutaneous skeletal fixation of metacarpal fracture, each bone

26615 Open treatment of metacarpal fracture, single, includes internal fixation, when performed, each bone
CPT Changes: An Insider's View 2008

26641 Closed treatment of carpometacarpal dislocation, thumb, with manipulation

26645 Closed treatment of carpometacarpal fracture dislocation, thumb (Bennett fracture), with manipulation

26650 Percutaneous skeletal fixation of carpometacarpal fracture dislocation, thumb (Bennett fracture), with manipulation
CPT Changes: An Insider's View 2008

26665 Open treatment of carpometacarpal fracture dislocation, thumb (Bennett fracture), includes internal fixation, when performed
CPT Changes: An Insider's View 2008

26670 Closed treatment of carpometacarpal dislocation, other than thumb, with manipulation, each joint; without anesthesia
CPT Changes: An Insider's View 2002

26675 requiring anesthesia

26676 Percutaneous skeletal fixation of carpometacarpal dislocation, other than thumb, with manipulation, each joint
CPT Changes: An Insider's View 2002

26685 Open treatment of carpometacarpal dislocation, other than thumb; includes internal fixation, when performed, each joint
CPT Changes: An Insider's View 2002, 2008

26686 complex, multiple, or delayed reduction

26700 Closed treatment of metacarpophalangeal dislocation, single, with manipulation; without anesthesia
CPT Assistant May 14:10

26705 requiring anesthesia

26706 Percutaneous skeletal fixation of metacarpophalangeal dislocation, single, with manipulation

26715 Open treatment of metacarpophalangeal dislocation, single, includes internal fixation, when performed
CPT Changes: An Insider's View 2008

26720 Closed treatment of phalangeal shaft fracture, proximal or middle phalanx, finger or thumb; without manipulation, each

26725 with manipulation, with or without skin or skeletal traction, each

26727 Percutaneous skeletal fixation of unstable phalangeal shaft fracture, proximal or middle phalanx, finger or thumb, with manipulation, each

26735 Open treatment of phalangeal shaft fracture, proximal or middle phalanx, finger or thumb, includes internal fixation, when performed, each
CPT Changes: An Insider's View 2008

26740 Closed treatment of articular fracture, involving metacarpophalangeal or interphalangeal joint; without manipulation, each

26742 with manipulation, each

26746 Open treatment of articular fracture, involving metacarpophalangeal or interphalangeal joint, includes internal fixation, when performed, each
➔ *CPT Changes: An Insider's View* 2008

26750 Closed treatment of distal phalangeal fracture, finger or thumb; without manipulation, each

26755 with manipulation, each

26756 Percutaneous skeletal fixation of distal phalangeal fracture, finger or thumb, each

26765 Open treatment of distal phalangeal fracture, finger or thumb, includes internal fixation, when performed, each
➔ *CPT Changes: An Insider's View* 2008

26770 Closed treatment of interphalangeal joint dislocation, single, with manipulation; without anesthesia

26775 requiring anesthesia

26776 Percutaneous skeletal fixation of interphalangeal joint dislocation, single, with manipulation

26785 Open treatment of interphalangeal joint dislocation, includes internal fixation, when performed, single
➔ *CPT Changes: An Insider's View* 2008

Arthrodesis

26820 Fusion in opposition, thumb, with autogenous graft (includes obtaining graft)

26841 Arthrodesis, carpometacarpal joint, thumb, with or without internal fixation;

26842 with autograft (includes obtaining graft)

26843 Arthrodesis, carpometacarpal joint, digit, other than thumb, each;
➔ *CPT Changes: An Insider's View* 2002

26844 with autograft (includes obtaining graft)

26850 Arthrodesis, metacarpophalangeal joint, with or without internal fixation;

26852 with autograft (includes obtaining graft)

26860 Arthrodesis, interphalangeal joint, with or without internal fixation;

+ 26861 each additional interphalangeal joint (List separately in addition to code for primary procedure)

(Use 26861 in conjunction with 26860)

26862 with autograft (includes obtaining graft)

+ 26863 with autograft (includes obtaining graft), each additional joint (List separately in addition to code for primary procedure)

(Use 26863 in conjunction with 26862)

Amputation

(For hand through metacarpal bones, use 25927)

26910 Amputation, metacarpal, with finger or thumb (ray amputation), single, with or without interosseous transfer

(For repositioning, see 26550, 26555)

26951 Amputation, finger or thumb, primary or secondary, any joint or phalanx, single, including neurectomies; with direct closure

26952 with local advancement flaps (V-Y, hood)

(For repair of soft tissue defect requiring split or full thickness graft or other pedicle flaps, see 15050-15758)

Other Procedures

26989 Unlisted procedure, hands or fingers

Pelvis and Hip Joint

Including head and neck of femur.

Incision

(For incision and drainage procedures, superficial, see 10040-10160)

26990 Incision and drainage, pelvis or hip joint area; deep abscess or hematoma

26991 infected bursa

26992 Incision, bone cortex, pelvis and/or hip joint (eg, osteomyelitis or bone abscess)
➔ *CPT Assistant* Jan 02:10, Oct 12:14

27000 Tenotomy, adductor of hip, percutaneous (separate procedure)

27001 Tenotomy, adductor of hip, open

(To report bilateral procedure, report 27001 with modifier 50)

27003 Tenotomy, adductor, subcutaneous, open, with obturator neurectomy

(To report bilateral procedure, report 27003 with modifier 50)

27005 Tenotomy, hip flexor(s), open (separate procedure)

27006 Tenotomy, abductors and/or extensor(s) of hip, open (separate procedure)

27025 Fasciotomy, hip or thigh, any type

(To report bilateral procedure, report 27025 with modifier 50)

27027 Decompression fasciotomy(ies), pelvic (buttock) compartment(s) (eg, gluteus medius-minimus, gluteus maximus, iliopsoas, and/or tensor fascia lata muscle), unilateral
➔ *CPT Changes: An Insider's View* 2009

(To report bilateral procedure, report 27027 with modifier 50)

27030 Arthrotomy, hip, with drainage (eg, infection)
CPT Assistant Nov 98:8

27033 Arthrotomy, hip, including exploration or removal of loose or foreign body
CPT Assistant Spring 92:11

27035 Denervation, hip joint, intrapelvic or extrapelvic intra-articular branches of sciatic, femoral, or obturator nerves
CPT Assistant Nov 98:8, Mar 14:13

(For obturator neurectomy, see 64763, 64766)

27036 Capsulectomy or capsulotomy, hip, with or without excision of heterotopic bone, with release of hip flexor muscles (ie, gluteus medius, gluteus minimus, tensor fascia latae, rectus femoris, sartorius, iliopsoas)
CPT Assistant Jan 05:8

Excision

27040 Biopsy, soft tissue of pelvis and hip area; superficial

27041 deep, subfascial or intramuscular
CPT Assistant Nov 98:8

(For needle biopsy of soft tissue, use 20206)

27043 Code is out of numerical sequence. See 27041-27052

27045 Code is out of numerical sequence. See 27041-27052

27047 Excision, tumor, soft tissue of pelvis and hip area, subcutaneous; less than 3 cm
CPT Changes: An Insider's View 2010
CPT Assistant Nov 98:8

 # 27043 3 cm or greater
CPT Changes: An Insider's View 2010

(For excision of benign lesions of cutaneous origin [eg, sebaceous cyst], see 11400-11406)

27048 Excision, tumor, soft tissue of pelvis and hip area, subfascial (eg, intramuscular); less than 5 cm
CPT Changes: An Insider's View 2010

 # 27045 5 cm or greater
CPT Changes: An Insider's View 2010

27049 Radical resection of tumor (eg, sarcoma), soft tissue of pelvis and hip area; less than 5 cm
CPT Changes: An Insider's View 2010, 2014
CPT Assistant Nov 98:8

 # 27059 5 cm or greater
CPT Changes: An Insider's View 2010, 2014

(For radical resection of tumor[s] of cutaneous origin [eg, melanoma], see 11600-11606)

27050 Arthrotomy, with biopsy; sacroiliac joint

27052 hip joint

27054 Arthrotomy with synovectomy, hip joint

27057 Decompression fasciotomy(ies), pelvic (buttock) compartment(s) (eg, gluteus medius-minimus, gluteus maximus, iliopsoas, and/or tensor fascia lata muscle) with debridement of nonviable muscle, unilateral
CPT Changes: An Insider's View 2009

(To report bilateral procedure, report 27057 with modifier 50)

27059 Code is out of numerical sequence. See 27041-27052

27060 Excision; ischial bursa

27062 trochanteric bursa or calcification

(For arthrocentesis or needling of bursa, use 20610)

27065 Excision of bone cyst or benign tumor, wing of ilium, symphysis pubis, or greater trochanter of femur; superficial, includes autograft, when performed
CPT Changes: An Insider's View 2011

27066 deep (subfascial), includes autograft, when performed
CPT Changes: An Insider's View 2011

27067 with autograft requiring separate incision
CPT Changes: An Insider's View 2011

27070 Partial excision, wing of ilium, symphysis pubis, or greater trochanter of femur, (craterization, saucerization) (eg, osteomyelitis or bone abscess); superficial
CPT Changes: An Insider's View 2011

27071 deep (subfascial or intramuscular)
CPT Changes: An Insider's View 2011

27075 Radical resection of tumor; wing of ilium, 1 pubic or ischial ramus or symphysis pubis
CPT Changes: An Insider's View 2010

27076 ilium, including acetabulum, both pubic rami, or ischium and acetabulum
CPT Changes: An Insider's View 2010

27077 innominate bone, total
CPT Changes: An Insider's View 2010

27078 ischial tuberosity and greater trochanter of femur
CPT Changes: An Insider's View 2010

27080 Coccygectomy, primary

(For pressure (decubitus) ulcer, see 15920, 15922 and 15931-15958)

Introduction or Removal

27086 Removal of foreign body, pelvis or hip; subcutaneous tissue
CPT Assistant Jul 98:8

27087 deep (subfascial or intramuscular)
CPT Assistant Nov 98:8

27090 Removal of hip prosthesis; (separate procedure)

27091 complicated, including total hip prosthesis, methylmethacrylate with or without insertion of spacer

27093 Injection procedure for hip arthrography; without anesthesia

➲ *CPT Assistant* Jun 12:14, Aug 15:6

➲ *Clinical Examples in Radiology* Fall 07:7, Spring 13:11

(For radiological supervision and interpretation, use 73525. Do not report 77002 in conjunction with 73525)

27095 with anesthesia

➲ *CPT Assistant* Jun 12:14, Aug 15:6, Jan 16:11

➲ *Clinical Examples in Radiology* Fall 07:7

(For radiological supervision and interpretation, use 73525. Do not report 77002 in conjunction with 73525)

27096 Injection procedure for sacroiliac joint, anesthetic/steroid, with image guidance (fluoroscopy or CT) including arthrography when performed

➲ *CPT Changes: An Insider's View* 2000, 2012

➲ *CPT Assistant* Nov 99:12, Apr 03:8, Apr 04:15, Jul 08:9, Jan 12:3, Aug 15:6

➲ *Clinical Examples in Radiology* Fall 11:10

(27096 is to be used only with CT or fluoroscopic imaging confirmation of intra-articular needle positioning)

(If CT or fluoroscopy imaging is not performed, use 20552)

(Code 27096 is a unilateral procedure. For bilateral procedure, use modifier 50)

Repair, Revision, and/or Reconstruction

27097 Release or recession, hamstring, proximal

➲ *CPT Assistant* Nov 98:8

27098 Transfer, adductor to ischium

➲ *CPT Assistant* Nov 98:8

27100 Transfer external oblique muscle to greater trochanter including fascial or tendon extension (graft)

27105 Transfer paraspinal muscle to hip (includes fascial or tendon extension graft)

27110 Transfer iliopsoas; to greater trochanter of femur

➲ *CPT Changes: An Insider's View* 2002

27111 to femoral neck

27120 Acetabuloplasty; (eg, Whitman, Colonna, Haygroves, or cup type)

27122 resection, femoral head (eg, Girdlestone procedure)

27125 Hemiarthroplasty, hip, partial (eg, femoral stem prosthesis, bipolar arthroplasty)

➲ *CPT Assistant* Spring 92:8, Feb 98:11, Nov 98:8

(For prosthetic replacement following fracture of the hip, use 27236)

27130 Arthroplasty, acetabular and proximal femoral prosthetic replacement (total hip arthroplasty), with or without autograft or allograft

➲ *CPT Changes: An Insider's View* 2002

➲ *CPT Assistant* Spring 92:8, Jan 07:1, Dec 11:14

Partial Hip Replacement With or Without Bipolar Prosthesis

27125

The femoral neck is excised so the physician can measure and then replace the femoral stem.

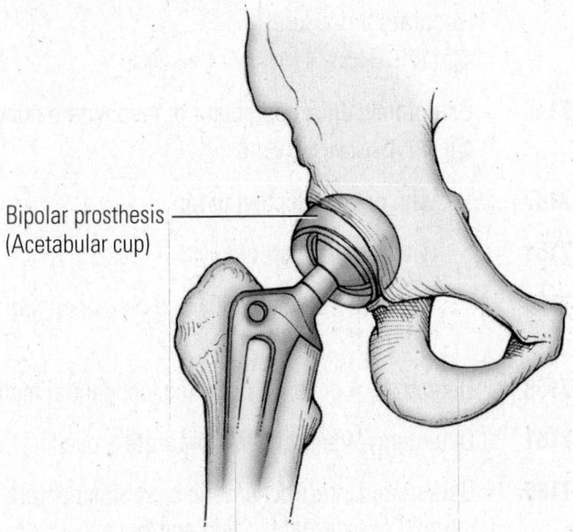

Total Hip Replacement

27130

The femoral head is excised, osteophytes are removed, and acetabulum is reamed out before replacement is inserted in the femoral shaft.

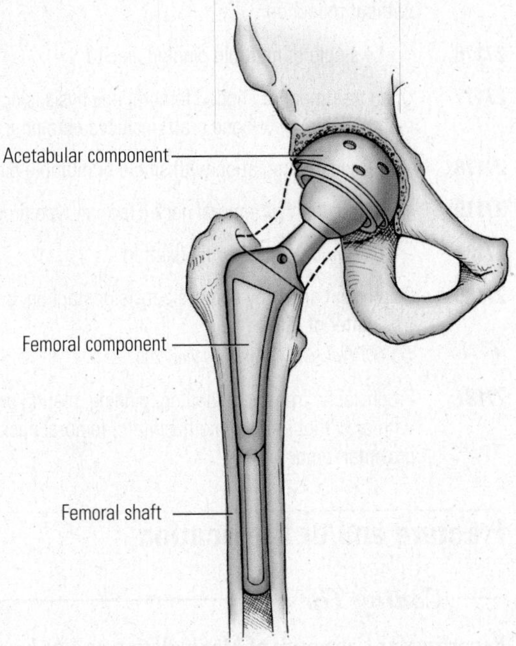

27132 Conversion of previous hip surgery to total hip arthroplasty, with or without autograft or allograft

➲ *CPT Changes: An Insider's View* 2002

➲ *CPT Assistant* Spring 92:11, Dec 08:3, May 17:10, Sep 17:14

27134 Revision of total hip arthroplasty; both components, with or without autograft or allograft

➲ *CPT Assistant* Spring 92:7, Dec 08:3

27137 acetabular component only, with or without autograft or allograft

➲ *CPT Assistant* Spring 92:7

27138 femoral component only, with or without allograft

➲ *CPT Assistant* Spring 92:7

27140 Osteotomy and transfer of greater trochanter of femur (separate procedure)

➲ *CPT Changes: An Insider's View* 2002

27146 Osteotomy, iliac, acetabular or innominate bone;

➲ *CPT Assistant* Feb 99:10

27147 with open reduction of hip

27151 with femoral osteotomy

27156 with femoral osteotomy and with open reduction of hip

27158 Osteotomy, pelvis, bilateral (eg, congenital malformation)

27161 Osteotomy, femoral neck (separate procedure)

27165 Osteotomy, intertrochanteric or subtrochanteric including internal or external fixation and/or cast

➲ *CPT Assistant* Spring 92:11

27170 Bone graft, femoral head, neck, intertrochanteric or subtrochanteric area (includes obtaining bone graft)

➲ *CPT Assistant* Spring 92:11

27175 Treatment of slipped femoral epiphysis; by traction, without reduction

27176 by single or multiple pinning, in situ

27177 Open treatment of slipped femoral epiphysis; single or multiple pinning or bone graft (includes obtaining graft)

27178 closed manipulation with single or multiple pinning

27179 osteoplasty of femoral neck (Heyman type procedure)

27181 osteotomy and internal fixation

27185 Epiphyseal arrest by epiphysiodesis or stapling, greater trochanter of femur

➲ *CPT Changes: An Insider's View* 2002

27187 Prophylactic treatment (nailing, pinning, plating or wiring) with or without methylmethacrylate, femoral neck and proximal femur

Fracture and/or Dislocation

Coding Tip

Reporting for Categories of Manipulation and/or Fracture

The codes for treatment of fractures and joint injuries (dislocations) are categorized by the type of manipulation (reduction) and stabilization (fixation or immobilization). These codes can apply to either open (compound) or closed fractures or joint injuries.

CPT Coding Guidelines, Musculoskeletal System

(27193, 27194 have been deleted. To report, see 27197, 27198)

27197 Closed treatment of posterior pelvic ring fracture(s), dislocation(s), diastasis or subluxation of the ilium, sacroiliac joint, and/or sacrum, with or without anterior pelvic ring fracture(s) and/or dislocation(s) of the pubic symphysis and/or superior/inferior rami, unilateral or bilateral; without manipulation

➲ *CPT Changes: An Insider's View* 2017

➲ *CPT Assistant* Jun 17:9

27198 with manipulation, requiring more than local anesthesia (ie, general anesthesia, moderate sedation, spinal/epidural)

➲ *CPT Changes: An Insider's View* 2017

➲ *CPT Assistant* Jun 17:9, Jan 18:3

(To report closed treatment of **only** anterior pelvic ring fracture(s) and/or dislocation(s) of the pubic symphysis and/or superior/inferior rami, unilateral or bilateral, use the appropriate evaluation and management services codes)

27200 Closed treatment of coccygeal fracture

27202 Open treatment of coccygeal fracture

27215 Open treatment of iliac spine(s), tuberosity avulsion, or iliac wing fracture(s), unilateral, for pelvic bone fracture patterns that do not disrupt the pelvic ring, includes internal fixation, when performed

➲ *CPT Changes: An Insider's View* 2009

(To report bilateral procedure, report 27215 with modifier 50)

27216 Percutaneous skeletal fixation of posterior pelvic bone fracture and/or dislocation, for fracture patterns that disrupt the pelvic ring, unilateral (includes ipsilateral ilium, sacroiliac joint and/or sacrum)

➲ *CPT Changes: An Insider's View* 2009

➲ *CPT Assistant* Sep 13:19, Mar 14:4

(To report bilateral procedure, report 27216 with modifier 50)

(For percutaneous/minimally invasive arthrodesis of the sacroiliac joint without fracture and/or dislocation, use 27279)

27217 Open treatment of anterior pelvic bone fracture and/or dislocation for fracture patterns that disrupt the pelvic ring, unilateral, includes internal fixation, when performed (includes pubic symphysis and/or ipsilateral superior/inferior rami)

➲ *CPT Changes: An Insider's View* 2009

(To report bilateral procedure, report 27217 with modifier 50)

27218 Open treatment of posterior pelvic bone fracture and/or dislocation, for fracture patterns that disrupt the pelvic ring, unilateral, includes internal fixation, when performed (includes ipsilateral ilium, sacroiliac joint and/or sacrum)

➲ *CPT Changes: An Insider's View* 2009

➲ *CPT Assistant* Mar 14:4

(To report bilateral procedure, report 27218 with modifier 50)

(For percutaneous/minimally invasive arthrodesis of the sacroiliac joint without fracture and/or dislocation, use 27279)

27220 Closed treatment of acetabulum (hip socket) fracture(s); without manipulation

27222 with manipulation, with or without skeletal traction

27226 Open treatment of posterior or anterior acetabular wall fracture, with internal fixation

27227 Open treatment of acetabular fracture(s) involving anterior or posterior (one) column, or a fracture running transversely across the acetabulum, with internal fixation

27228 Open treatment of acetabular fracture(s) involving anterior and posterior (two) columns, includes T-fracture and both column fracture with complete articular detachment, or single column or transverse fracture with associated acetabular wall fracture, with internal fixation

27230 Closed treatment of femoral fracture, proximal end, neck; without manipulation

27232 with manipulation, with or without skeletal traction

27235 Percutaneous skeletal fixation of femoral fracture, proximal end, neck

➔ *CPT Changes: An Insider's View* 2003

27236 Open treatment of femoral fracture, proximal end, neck, internal fixation or prosthetic replacement

➔ *CPT Changes: An Insider's View* 2000

➔ *CPT Assistant* Spring 92:10, Feb 98:11, Jan 07:1, Nov 16:9

27238 Closed treatment of intertrochanteric, peritrochanteric, or subtrochanteric femoral fracture; without manipulation

➔ *CPT Assistant* Summer 93:12

Percutaneous Treatment of Femoral Fracture

27235

Femoral fracture treatment without fracture exposure

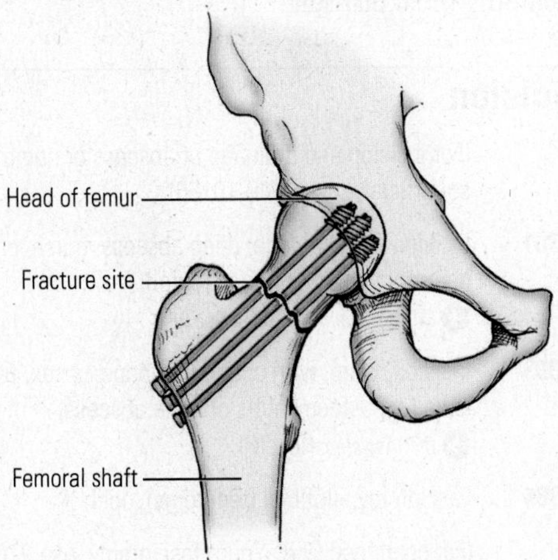

Open Treatment of Femoral Fracture

27236

A. Femoral fracture treatment by internal fixation device (with fracture exposure)

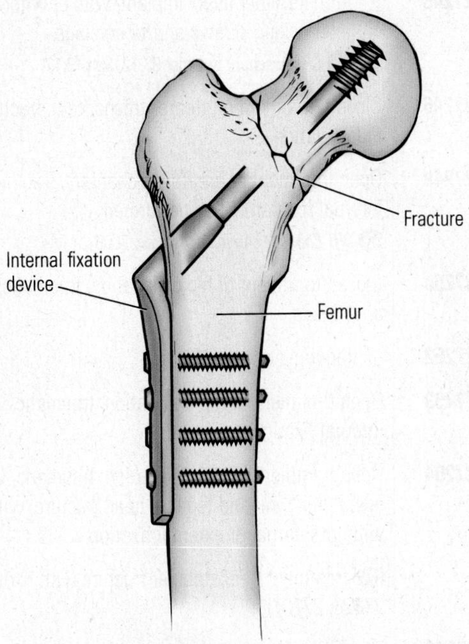

B. Femoral fracture treatment by prosthetic replacement

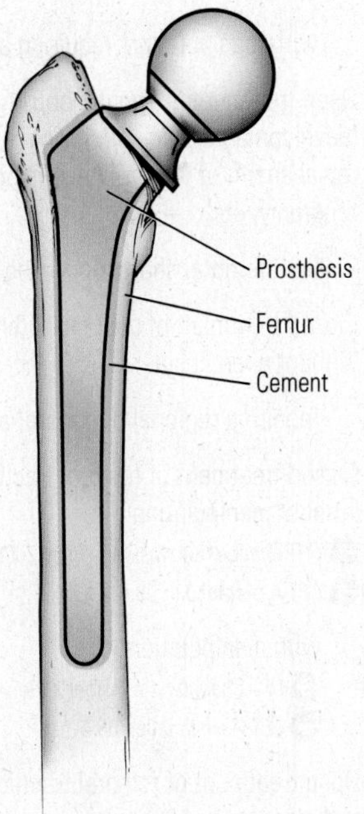

27240 with manipulation, with or without skin or skeletal traction

➔ *CPT Assistant* Summer 93:12

27244 Treatment of intertrochanteric, peritrochanteric, or subtrochanteric femoral fracture; with plate/screw type implant, with or without cerclage
➲ *CPT Changes: An Insider's View* 2003
➲ *CPT Assistant* Summer 93:12

27245 with intramedullary implant, with or without interlocking screws and/or cerclage
➲ *CPT Assistant* Summer 93:12, Sep 13:17

27246 Closed treatment of greater trochanteric fracture, without manipulation

27248 Open treatment of greater trochanteric fracture, includes internal fixation, when performed
➲ *CPT Changes: An Insider's View* 2008

27250 Closed treatment of hip dislocation, traumatic; without anesthesia

27252 requiring anesthesia

27253 Open treatment of hip dislocation, traumatic, without internal fixation

27254 Open treatment of hip dislocation, traumatic, with acetabular wall and femoral head fracture, with or without internal or external fixation

(For treatment of acetabular fracture with fixation, see 27226, 27227)

27256 Treatment of spontaneous hip dislocation (developmental, including congenital or pathological), by abduction, splint or traction; without anesthesia, without manipulation

27257 with manipulation, requiring anesthesia

27258 Open treatment of spontaneous hip dislocation (developmental, including congenital or pathological), replacement of femoral head in acetabulum (including tenotomy, etc);

27259 with femoral shaft shortening

27265 Closed treatment of post hip arthroplasty dislocation; without anesthesia

27266 requiring regional or general anesthesia

27267 Closed treatment of femoral fracture, proximal end, head; without manipulation
➲ *CPT Changes: An Insider's View* 2008
➲ *CPT Assistant* Jan 08:4

27268 with manipulation
➲ *CPT Changes: An Insider's View* 2008
➲ *CPT Assistant* Jan 08:4

27269 Open treatment of femoral fracture, proximal end, head, includes internal fixation, when performed
➲ *CPT Changes: An Insider's View* 2008
➲ *CPT Assistant* Jan 08:4, Dec 08:3

(Do not report 27269 in conjunction with 27033, 27253)

Manipulation

27275 Manipulation, hip joint, requiring general anesthesia
➲ *CPT Assistant* Jan 16:11, May 16:13

Arthrodesis

27279 Arthrodesis, sacroiliac joint, percutaneous or minimally invasive (indirect visualization), with image guidance, includes obtaining bone graft when performed, and placement of transfixing device
➲ *CPT Changes: An Insider's View* 2015

(For bilateral procedure, report 27279 with modifier 50)

27280 Arthrodesis, open, sacroiliac joint, including obtaining bone graft, including instrumentation, when performed
➲ *CPT Changes: An Insider's View* 2015
➲ *CPT Assistant* Sep 13:19, Mar 14:4

(To report bilateral procedure, report 27280 with modifier 50)

(For percutaneous/minimally invasive arthrodesis of the sacroiliac joint without fracture and/or dislocation, use 27279)

27282 Arthrodesis, symphysis pubis (including obtaining graft)

27284 Arthrodesis, hip joint (including obtaining graft);

27286 with subtrochanteric osteotomy

Amputation

27290 Interpelviabdominal amputation (hindquarter amputation)

27295 Disarticulation of hip

Other Procedures

27299 Unlisted procedure, pelvis or hip joint
➲ *CPT Assistant* Jan 02:10, Dec 05:9, Dec 08:3, Oct 12:14, Nov 12:13, Mar 14:13, Jun 16:8

Femur (Thigh Region) and Knee Joint

Including tibial plateaus.

Incision

(For incision and drainage of abscess or hematoma, superficial, see 10040-10160)

27301 Incision and drainage, deep abscess, bursa, or hematoma, thigh or knee region
➲ *CPT Assistant* Nov 98:9, Dec 08:3

27303 Incision, deep, with opening of bone cortex, femur or knee (eg, osteomyelitis or bone abscess)
➲ *CPT Assistant* Nov 98:8

27305 Fasciotomy, iliotibial (tenotomy), open

(For combined Ober-Yount fasciotomy, use 27025)

27306 Tenotomy, percutaneous, adductor or hamstring; single tendon (separate procedure)
➔ *CPT Assistant* Nov 98:8, Aug 17:9

27307 multiple tendons
➔ *CPT Assistant* Nov 98:8, Aug 17:9

27310 Arthrotomy, knee, with exploration, drainage, or removal of foreign body (eg, infection)
➔ *CPT Assistant* Nov 98:8, Dec 08:3

Excision

27323 Biopsy, soft tissue of thigh or knee area; superficial
➔ *CPT Assistant* Jun 97:12

27324 deep (subfascial or intramuscular)
➔ *CPT Assistant* Mar 97:4, Nov 98:8

(For needle biopsy of soft tissue, use 20206)

27325 Neurectomy, hamstring muscle
➔ *CPT Changes: An Insider's View* 2007

27326 Neurectomy, popliteal (gastrocnemius)
➔ *CPT Changes: An Insider's View* 2007

27327 Excision, tumor, soft tissue of thigh or knee area, subcutaneous; less than 3 cm
➔ *CPT Changes: An Insider's View* 2010

 # 27337 3 cm or greater
➔ *CPT Changes: An Insider's View* 2010

(For excision of benign lesions of cutaneous origin [eg, sebaceous cyst], see 11400-11406)

27328 Excision, tumor, soft tissue of thigh or knee area, subfascial (eg, intramuscular); less than 5 cm
➔ *CPT Changes: An Insider's View* 2010
➔ *CPT Assistant* Nov 16:9

27329 Code is out of numerical sequence. See 27358-27365

 # 27339 5 cm or greater
➔ *CPT Changes: An Insider's View* 2010

27330 Arthrotomy, knee; with synovial biopsy only
➔ *CPT Assistant* Mar 12:9

27331 including joint exploration, biopsy, or removal of loose or foreign bodies
➔ *CPT Assistant* May 96:6, Nov 98:8, Nov 12:13

27332 Arthrotomy, with excision of semilunar cartilage (meniscectomy) knee; medial OR lateral
➔ *CPT Assistant* Nov 98:8

27333 medial AND lateral
➔ *CPT Assistant* Mar 12:9

27334 Arthrotomy, with synovectomy, knee; anterior OR posterior
➔ *CPT Assistant* Nov 98:8

27335 anterior AND posterior including popliteal area

27337 Code is out of numerical sequence. See 27326-27331

27339 Code is out of numerical sequence. See 27326-27331

27340 Excision, prepatellar bursa

27345 Excision of synovial cyst of popliteal space (eg, Baker's cyst)

27347 Excision of lesion of meniscus or capsule (eg, cyst, ganglion), knee
➔ *CPT Assistant* Nov 98:11

27350 Patellectomy or hemipatellectomy

27355 Excision or curettage of bone cyst or benign tumor of femur;

27356 with allograft

27357 with autograft (includes obtaining graft)
➔ *CPT Assistant* Dec 02:11

+ 27358 with internal fixation (List in addition to code for primary procedure)

(Use 27358 in conjunction with 27355, 27356, or 27357)

27360 Partial excision (craterization, saucerization, or diaphysectomy) bone, femur, proximal tibia and/or fibula (eg, osteomyelitis or bone abscess)
➔ *CPT Assistant* Nov 98:8

 # 27329 Radical resection of tumor (eg, sarcoma), soft tissue of thigh or knee area; less than 5 cm
➔ *CPT Changes: An Insider's View* 2010, 2014

27364 5 cm or greater
➔ *CPT Changes: An Insider's View* 2010, 2014

(For radical resection of tumor[s] of cutaneous origin [eg, melanoma], see 11600-11606)

27365 Radical resection of tumor, femur or knee
➔ *CPT Changes: An Insider's View* 2010

(For radical resection of tumor, soft tissue of thigh or knee area, see 27329, 27364)

Introduction or Removal

● 27369 Injection procedure for contrast knee arthrography or contrast enhanced CT/MRI knee arthrography
➔ *CPT Changes: An Insider's View* 2019

►(Use 27369 in conjunction with 73580, 73701, 73702, 73722, 73723)◄

►(Do not report 27369 in conjunction with 20610, 20611, 29871)◄

►(For arthrocentesis of the knee or injection of any material other than contrast for subsequent arthrography, see 20610, 20611)◄

►(When fluoroscopic guided injection is performed for enhanced CT arthrography, use 27369, 77002, and 73701 or 73702)◄

►(When fluoroscopic guided injection is performed for enhanced MR arthrography, use 27369, 77002, and 73722 or 73723)◄

►(For arthroscopic lavage and drainage of the knee, use 29871)◄

►(For radiographic arthrography, radiological supervision and interpretation, use 73580)◄

►(27370 has been deleted)◄

►(For arthrocentesis of the knee or injection of any material other than contrast for subsequent arthrography, see 20610, 20611)◄

►(For injection procedure for contrast knee arthrography or contrast enhanced CT/MRI knee arthrography, use 27369)◄

27372 Removal of foreign body, deep, thigh region or knee area

(For removal of knee prosthesis including "total knee," use 27488)

(For surgical arthroscopic knee procedures, see 29870-29887)

Repair, Revision, and/or Reconstruction

27380 Suture of infrapatellar tendon; primary

27381 secondary reconstruction, including fascial or tendon graft

27385 Suture of quadriceps or hamstring muscle rupture; primary
➲ *CPT Assistant* Aug 17:9

27386 secondary reconstruction, including fascial or tendon graft

27390 Tenotomy, open, hamstring, knee to hip; single tendon
➲ *CPT Assistant* Nov 98:8

27391 multiple tendons, 1 leg
➲ *CPT Assistant* Nov 98:8

27392 multiple tendons, bilateral
➲ *CPT Assistant* Nov 98:8

27393 Lengthening of hamstring tendon; single tendon
➲ *CPT Assistant* Nov 98:8

27394 multiple tendons, 1 leg
➲ *CPT Assistant* Nov 98:8

27395 multiple tendons, bilateral
➲ *CPT Assistant* Nov 98:8

27396 Transplant or transfer (with muscle redirection or rerouting), thigh (eg, extensor to flexor); single tendon
➲ *CPT Changes: An Insider's View* 2009
➲ *CPT Assistant* Nov 98:8

27397 multiple tendons
➲ *CPT Changes: An Insider's View* 2009
➲ *CPT Assistant* Nov 98:8

27400 Transfer, tendon or muscle, hamstrings to femur (eg, Egger's type procedure)
➲ *CPT Assistant* Nov 98:8

27403 Arthrotomy with meniscus repair, knee
➲ *CPT Assistant* Nov 98:8

(For arthroscopic repair, use 29882)

27405 Repair, primary, torn ligament and/or capsule, knee; collateral
➲ *CPT Assistant* Dec 12:12

27407 cruciate

(For cruciate ligament reconstruction, use 27427)

27409 collateral and cruciate ligaments

(For ligament reconstruction, see 27427-27429)

27412 Autologous chondrocyte implantation, knee
➲ *CPT Changes: An Insider's View* 2005

(Do not report 27412 in conjunction with 20926, 27331, 27570)

(For harvesting of chondrocytes, use 29870)

27415 Osteochondral allograft, knee, open
➲ *CPT Changes: An Insider's View* 2005

(For arthroscopic implant of osteochondral allograft, use 29867)

(Do not report 27415 in conjunction with 27416)

27416 Osteochondral autograft(s), knee, open (eg, mosaicplasty) (includes harvesting of autograft[s])
➲ *CPT Changes: An Insider's View* 2008
➲ *CPT Assistant* Jan 08:4

(Do not report 27416 in conjunction with 27415, 29870, 29871, 29875, 29884 when performed at the same session and/or 29874, 29877, 29879, 29885-29887 when performed in the same compartment)

(For arthroscopic osteochondral autograft of knee, use 29866)

27418 Anterior tibial tubercleplasty (eg, Maquet type procedure)
➲ *CPT Assistant* Feb 10:13

27420 Reconstruction of dislocating patella; (eg, Hauser type procedure)
➲ *CPT Assistant* Nov 12:13

27422 with extensor realignment and/or muscle advancement or release (eg, Campbell, Goldwaite type procedure)
➲ *CPT Assistant* Mar 11:9

27424 with patellectomy

27425 Lateral retinacular release, open
➲ *CPT Changes: An Insider's View* 2002, 2003
➲ *CPT Assistant* Nov 00:11, Mar 11:9, Nov 15:7

(For arthroscopic lateral release, use 29873)

Posterolateral Corner of the Knee
27405, 27427

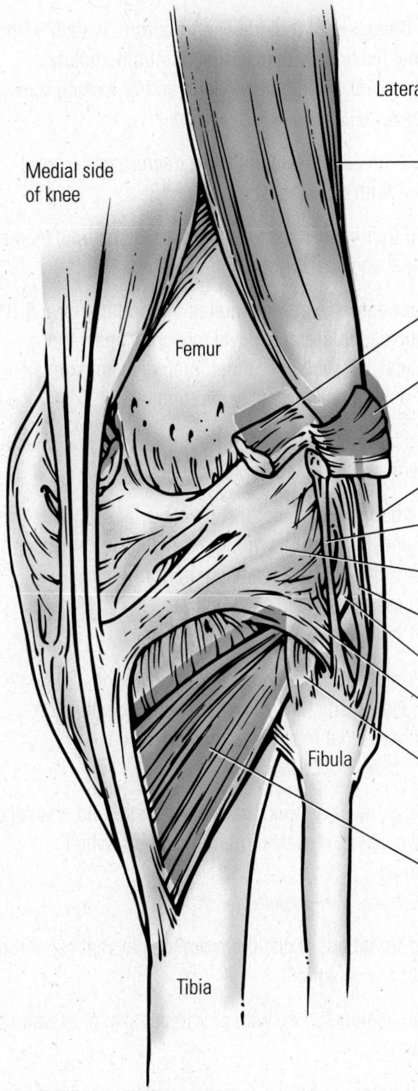

27427 Ligamentous reconstruction (augmentation), knee; extra-articular
➲ *CPT Changes: An Insider's View* 2000
➲ *CPT Assistant* Nov 99:13, Dec 12:12, May 17:10

27428 intra-articular (open)
➲ *CPT Changes: An Insider's View* 2000
➲ *CPT Assistant* Nov 99:13, Apr 09:8

27429 intra-articular (open) and extra-articular
➲ *CPT Changes: An Insider's View* 2000
➲ *CPT Assistant* Nov 99:13, Apr 09:8

(For primary repair of ligament(s) performed in conjunction with reconstruction, report 27405, 27407 or 27409 in conjunction with 27427, 27428 or 27429)

27430 Quadricepsplasty (eg, Bennett or Thompson type)

27435 Capsulotomy, posterior capsular release, knee
➲ *CPT Assistant* Nov 98:8

27437 Arthroplasty, patella; without prosthesis

27438 with prosthesis

27440 Arthroplasty, knee, tibial plateau;

27441 with debridement and partial synovectomy

27442 Arthroplasty, femoral condyles or tibial plateau(s), knee;
➲ *CPT Assistant* Nov 99:13, Jun 16:8

27443 with debridement and partial synovectomy

27445 Arthroplasty, knee, hinge prosthesis (eg, Walldius type)
➲ *CPT Assistant* Nov 98:8

27446 Arthroplasty, knee, condyle and plateau; medial OR lateral compartment
➲ *CPT Assistant* Dec 17:13

27447 medial AND lateral compartments with or without patella resurfacing (total knee arthroplasty)
➲ *CPT Changes: An Insider's View* 2002
➲ *CPT Assistant* Jan 07:1

(For revision of total knee arthroplasty, use 27487)

(For removal of total knee prosthesis, use 27488)

27448 Osteotomy, femur, shaft or supracondylar; without fixation

(To report bilateral procedure, report 27448 with modifier 50)

27450 with fixation

(To report bilateral procedure, report 27450 with modifier 50)

27454 Osteotomy, multiple, with realignment on intramedullary rod, femoral shaft (eg, Sofield type procedure)
➲ *CPT Assistant* Nov 98:8

27455 Osteotomy, proximal tibia, including fibular excision or osteotomy (includes correction of genu varus [bowleg] or genu valgus [knock-knee]); before epiphyseal closure

(To report bilateral procedure, report 27455 with modifier 50)

27457 after epiphyseal closure

(To report bilateral procedure, report 27457 with modifier 50)

27465 Osteoplasty, femur; shortening (excluding 64876)

27466 lengthening

27468 combined, lengthening and shortening with femoral segment transfer

27470 Repair, nonunion or malunion, femur, distal to head and neck; without graft (eg, compression technique)

27472 with iliac or other autogenous bone graft (includes obtaining graft)

Musculoskeletal 20100-29999

27475 Arrest, epiphyseal, any method (eg, epiphysiodesis); distal femur
CPT Assistant Nov 98:8

27477 tibia and fibula, proximal

27479 combined distal femur, proximal tibia and fibula

27485 Arrest, hemiepiphyseal, distal femur or proximal tibia or fibula (eg, genu varus or valgus)
CPT Assistant Nov 98:8

27486 Revision of total knee arthroplasty, with or without allograft; 1 component
CPT Assistant Dec 13:16, Jul 15:10, Apr 18:10

27487 femoral and entire tibial component
CPT Assistant Nov 98:8, Jul 13:6

27488 Removal of prosthesis, including total knee prosthesis, methylmethacrylate with or without insertion of spacer, knee
CPT Assistant Nov 98:8, Jul 13:6

27495 Prophylactic treatment (nailing, pinning, plating, or wiring) with or without methylmethacrylate, femur

27496 Decompression fasciotomy, thigh and/or knee, 1 compartment (flexor or extensor or adductor);

27497 with debridement of nonviable muscle and/or nerve

27498 Decompression fasciotomy, thigh and/or knee, multiple compartments;

27499 with debridement of nonviable muscle and/or nerve

Fracture and/or Dislocation

Coding Tip

Reporting for Categories of Manipulation and/or Fracture

The codes for treatment of fractures and joint injuries (dislocations) are categorized by the type of manipulation (reduction) and stabilization (fixation or immobilization). These codes can apply to either open (compound) or closed fractures or joint injuries.

CPT Coding Guidelines, Musculoskeletal System

(For arthroscopic treatment of intercondylar spine[s] and tuberosity fracture[s] of the knee, see 29850, 29851)

(For arthroscopic treatment of tibial fracture, see 29855, 29856)

27500 Closed treatment of femoral shaft fracture, without manipulation

27501 Closed treatment of supracondylar or transcondylar femoral fracture with or without intercondylar extension, without manipulation

27502 Closed treatment of femoral shaft fracture, with manipulation, with or without skin or skeletal traction
CPT Assistant Fall 93:22, Oct 99:5

27503 Closed treatment of supracondylar or transcondylar femoral fracture with or without intercondylar extension, with manipulation, with or without skin or skeletal traction

27506 Open treatment of femoral shaft fracture, with or without external fixation, with insertion of intramedullary implant, with or without cerclage and/or locking screws
CPT Assistant Winter 92:10, Jun 09:7

27507 Open treatment of femoral shaft fracture with plate/screws, with or without cerclage

27508 Closed treatment of femoral fracture, distal end, medial or lateral condyle, without manipulation

27509 Percutaneous skeletal fixation of femoral fracture, distal end, medial or lateral condyle, or supracondylar or transcondylar, with or without intercondylar extension, or distal femoral epiphyseal separation

27510 Closed treatment of femoral fracture, distal end, medial or lateral condyle, with manipulation

27511 Open treatment of femoral supracondylar or transcondylar fracture without intercondylar extension, includes internal fixation, when performed
CPT Changes: An Insider's View 2008
CPT Assistant May 96:6

27513 Open treatment of femoral supracondylar or transcondylar fracture with intercondylar extension, includes internal fixation, when performed
CPT Changes: An Insider's View 2008

27514 Open treatment of femoral fracture, distal end, medial or lateral condyle, includes internal fixation, when performed
CPT Changes: An Insider's View 2008

27516 Closed treatment of distal femoral epiphyseal separation; without manipulation

27517 with manipulation, with or without skin or skeletal traction

27519 Open treatment of distal femoral epiphyseal separation, includes internal fixation, when performed
CPT Changes: An Insider's View 2008

27520 Closed treatment of patellar fracture, without manipulation

27524 Open treatment of patellar fracture, with internal fixation and/or partial or complete patellectomy and soft tissue repair

27530 Closed treatment of tibial fracture, proximal (plateau); without manipulation

27532 with or without manipulation, with skeletal traction

(For arthroscopic treatment, see 29855, 29856)

27535 Open treatment of tibial fracture, proximal (plateau); unicondylar, includes internal fixation, when performed
CPT Changes: An Insider's View 2008

27536 bicondylar, with or without internal fixation

(For arthroscopic treatment, see 29855, 29856)

27538 Closed treatment of intercondylar spine(s) and/or tuberosity fracture(s) of knee, with or without manipulation

(For arthroscopic treatment, see 29850, 29851)

27540 Open treatment of intercondylar spine(s) and/or tuberosity fracture(s) of the knee, includes internal fixation, when performed

➔ *CPT Changes: An Insider's View* 2008

27550 Closed treatment of knee dislocation; without anesthesia

27552 requiring anesthesia

27556 Open treatment of knee dislocation, includes internal fixation, when performed; without primary ligamentous repair or augmentation/reconstruction

➔ *CPT Changes: An Insider's View* 2008

27557 with primary ligamentous repair

➔ *CPT Changes: An Insider's View* 2008

27558 with primary ligamentous repair, with augmentation/reconstruction

➔ *CPT Changes: An Insider's View* 2008

27560 Closed treatment of patellar dislocation; without anesthesia

➔ *CPT Assistant* Apr 02:15

(For recurrent dislocation, see 27420-27424)

27562 requiring anesthesia

27566 Open treatment of patellar dislocation, with or without partial or total patellectomy

Manipulation

27570 Manipulation of knee joint under general anesthesia (includes application of traction or other fixation devices)

➔ *CPT Assistant* Mar 11:9

Arthrodesis

27580 Arthrodesis, knee, any technique

Amputation

27590 Amputation, thigh, through femur, any level;

➔ *CPT Assistant* Dec 17:13

27591 immediate fitting technique including first cast

27592 open, circular (guillotine)

27594 secondary closure or scar revision

27596 re-amputation

27598 Disarticulation at knee

Other Procedures

27599 Unlisted procedure, femur or knee

➔ *CPT Assistant* Mar 08:14, Dec 12:13, Jan 14:9, Jan 15:13, Jun 16:8, Nov 16:9, Mar 17:10, Aug 17:9, Apr 18:10

Leg (Tibia and Fibula) and Ankle Joint

Incision

27600 Decompression fasciotomy, leg; anterior and/or lateral compartments only

27601 posterior compartment(s) only

27602 anterior and/or lateral, and posterior compartment(s)

(For incision and drainage procedures, superficial, see 10040-10160)

(For decompression fasciotomy with debridement, see 27892-27894)

27603 Incision and drainage, leg or ankle; deep abscess or hematoma

27604 infected bursa

27605 Tenotomy, percutaneous, Achilles tendon (separate procedure); local anesthesia

27606 general anesthesia

27607 Incision (eg, osteomyelitis or bone abscess), leg or ankle

27610 Arthrotomy, ankle, including exploration, drainage, or removal of foreign body

➔ *CPT Assistant* Nov 98:9

27612 Arthrotomy, posterior capsular release, ankle, with or without Achilles tendon lengthening

➔ *CPT Assistant* Nov 98:8

(See also 27685)

Excision

27613 Biopsy, soft tissue of leg or ankle area; superficial

27614 deep (subfascial or intramuscular)

➔ *CPT Assistant* Nov 98:8

(For needle biopsy of soft tissue, use 20206)

27615 Radical resection of tumor (eg, sarcoma), soft tissue of leg or ankle area; less than 5 cm

➔ *CPT Changes: An Insider's View* 2010, 2014

27616 5 cm or greater

➔ *CPT Changes: An Insider's View* 2010, 2014

(For radical resection of tumor[s] of cutaneous origin [eg, melanoma], see 11600-11606)

27618 Excision, tumor, soft tissue of leg or ankle area, subcutaneous; less than 3 cm

➔ *CPT Changes: An Insider's View* 2010

27632 3 cm or greater
CPT Changes: An Insider's View 2010
CPT Assistant Apr 10:3

(For excision of benign lesions of cutaneous origin [eg, sebaceous cyst], see 11400-11406)

27619 Excision, tumor, soft tissue of leg or ankle area, subfascial (eg, intramuscular); less than 5 cm
CPT Changes: An Insider's View 2010

27634 5 cm or greater
CPT Changes: An Insider's View 2010

27620 Arthrotomy, ankle, with joint exploration, with or without biopsy, with or without removal of loose or foreign body

27625 Arthrotomy, with synovectomy, ankle;
CPT Assistant Nov 98:8

27626 including tenosynovectomy

27630 Excision of lesion of tendon sheath or capsule (eg, cyst or ganglion), leg and/or ankle

27632 Code is out of numerical sequence. See 27616-27625

27634 Code is out of numerical sequence. See 27616-27625

27635 Excision or curettage of bone cyst or benign tumor, tibia or fibula;
CPT Assistant Apr 12:17

27637 with autograft (includes obtaining graft)

27638 with allograft

27640 Partial excision (craterization, saucerization, or diaphysectomy), bone (eg, osteomyelitis); tibia
CPT Changes: An Insider's View 2010
CPT Assistant Apr 12:17

(For exostosis excision, use 27635)

27641 fibula
CPT Changes: An Insider's View 2010

(For exostosis excision, use 27635)

27645 Radical resection of tumor; tibia
CPT Changes: An Insider's View 2010

27646 fibula
CPT Changes: An Insider's View 2010

27647 talus or calcaneus
CPT Changes: An Insider's View 2010

Introduction or Removal

27648 Injection procedure for ankle arthrography
CPT Assistant Aug 15:6

(For radiological supervision and interpretation, use 73615. Do not report 77002 in conjunction with 73615)

(For ankle arthroscopy, see 29894-29898)

Repair, Revision, and/or Reconstruction

27650 Repair, primary, open or percutaneous, ruptured Achilles tendon;
CPT Assistant Jul 14:5

27652 with graft (includes obtaining graft)
CPT Assistant Jul 14:5

27654 Repair, secondary, Achilles tendon, with or without graft
CPT Assistant Jul 14:5, Dec 16:16

27656 Repair, fascial defect of leg

27658 Repair, flexor tendon, leg; primary, without graft, each tendon
CPT Assistant Nov 98:8

27659 secondary, with or without graft, each tendon
CPT Assistant Jan 15:13

27664 Repair, extensor tendon, leg; primary, without graft, each tendon
CPT Assistant Nov 98:8, Jan 15:13

27665 secondary, with or without graft, each tendon
CPT Assistant Nov 98:8

27675 Repair, dislocating peroneal tendons; without fibular osteotomy

27676 with fibular osteotomy

27680 Tenolysis, flexor or extensor tendon, leg and/or ankle; single, each tendon
CPT Assistant Nov 98:8

27681 multiple tendons (through separate incision[s])
CPT Assistant Nov 98:8

27685 Lengthening or shortening of tendon, leg or ankle; single tendon (separate procedure)
CPT Assistant Nov 98:8, Sep 09:11

27686 multiple tendons (through same incision), each
CPT Assistant Nov 98:8, Sep 09:11

27687 Gastrocnemius recession (eg, Strayer procedure)

(Toe extensors are considered as a group to be a single tendon when transplanted into midfoot)

27690 Transfer or transplant of single tendon (with muscle redirection or rerouting); superficial (eg, anterior tibial extensors into midfoot)

27691 deep (eg, anterior tibial or posterior tibial through interosseous space, flexor digitorum longus, flexor hallucis longus, or peroneal tendon to midfoot or hindfoot)

+ 27692 each additional tendon (List separately in addition to code for primary procedure)

(Use 27692 in conjunction with 27690, 27691)

27695 Repair, primary, disrupted ligament, ankle; collateral
CPT Assistant Mar 14:14

27696 both collateral ligaments
CPT Assistant Mar 14:14

27698 Repair, secondary, disrupted ligament, ankle, collateral (eg, Watson-Jones procedure)
CPT Assistant Mar 14:14

27700 Arthroplasty, ankle;

27702 with implant (total ankle)

Musculoskeletal 20100-29999

27703 revision, total ankle

27704 Removal of ankle implant

27705 Osteotomy; tibia

27707 fibula

27709 tibia and fibula

27712 multiple, with realignment on intramedullary rod (eg, Sofield type procedure)

(For osteotomy to correct genu varus [bowleg] or genu valgus [knock-knee], see 27455-27457)

27715 Osteoplasty, tibia and fibula, lengthening or shortening

27720 Repair of nonunion or malunion, tibia; without graft, (eg, compression technique)

27722 with sliding graft

27724 with iliac or other autograft (includes obtaining graft)

➲ *CPT Assistant* May 12:11

27725 by synostosis, with fibula, any method

27726 Repair of fibula nonunion and/or malunion with internal fixation

➲ *CPT Changes: An Insider's View* 2008

➲ *CPT Assistant* Jan 08:4, Apr 09:9

(Do not report 27726 in conjunction with 27707)

27727 Repair of congenital pseudarthrosis, tibia

27730 Arrest, epiphyseal (epiphysiodesis), open; distal tibia

➲ *CPT Changes: An Insider's View* 2003

➲ *CPT Assistant* Nov 98:8

27732 distal fibula

27734 distal tibia and fibula

27740 Arrest, epiphyseal (epiphysiodesis), any method, combined, proximal and distal tibia and fibula;

➲ *CPT Assistant* Nov 98:8

27742 and distal femur

(For epiphyseal arrest of proximal tibia and fibula, use 27477)

27745 Prophylactic treatment (nailing, pinning, plating or wiring) with or without methylmethacrylate, tibia

Fracture and/or Dislocation

Coding Tip

Reporting for Categories of Manipulation and/or Fracture

The codes for treatment of fractures and joint injuries (dislocations) are categorized by the type of manipulation (reduction) and stabilization (fixation or immobilization). These codes can apply to either open (compound) or closed fractures or joint injuries.

CPT Coding Guidelines, Musculoskeletal System

27750 Closed treatment of tibial shaft fracture (with or without fibular fracture); without manipulation

➲ *CPT Assistant* Winter 92:10, Fall 93:21, Mar 96:10

27752 with manipulation, with or without skeletal traction

➲ *CPT Assistant* Winter 92:10, Fall 93:21, Feb 96:3, Mar 96:10, Jan 18:3

27756 Percutaneous skeletal fixation of tibial shaft fracture (with or without fibular fracture) (eg, pins or screws)

➲ *CPT Assistant* Winter 92:10

27758 Open treatment of tibial shaft fracture (with or without fibular fracture), with plate/screws, with or without cerclage

➲ *CPT Assistant* Winter 92:10, Mar 00:11

27759 Treatment of tibial shaft fracture (with or without fibular fracture) by intramedullary implant, with or without interlocking screws and/or cerclage

➲ *CPT Changes: An Insider's View* 2003

➲ *CPT Assistant* Winter 92:10

27760 Closed treatment of medial malleolus fracture; without manipulation

27762 with manipulation, with or without skin or skeletal traction

27766 Open treatment of medial malleolus fracture, includes internal fixation, when performed

➲ *CPT Changes: An Insider's View* 2008

27767 Closed treatment of posterior malleolus fracture; without manipulation

➲ *CPT Changes: An Insider's View* 2008

27768 with manipulation

➲ *CPT Changes: An Insider's View* 2008

27769 Open treatment of posterior malleolus fracture, includes internal fixation, when performed

➲ *CPT Changes: An Insider's View* 2008

(Do not report 27767-27769 in conjunction with 27808-27823)

27780 Closed treatment of proximal fibula or shaft fracture; without manipulation

➲ *CPT Assistant* Winter 92:11

27781 with manipulation

27784 Open treatment of proximal fibula or shaft fracture, includes internal fixation, when performed

➲ *CPT Changes: An Insider's View* 2008

➲ *CPT Assistant* Mar 00:11

27786 Closed treatment of distal fibular fracture (lateral malleolus); without manipulation

27788 with manipulation

27792 Open treatment of distal fibular fracture (lateral malleolus), includes internal fixation, when performed

➲ *CPT Changes: An Insider's View* 2008

(For treatment of tibia and fibula shaft fractures, see 27750-27759)

27808 Closed treatment of bimalleolar ankle fracture (eg, lateral and medial malleoli, or lateral and posterior malleoli or medial and posterior malleoli); without manipulation
➲ *CPT Changes: An Insider's View* 2008

27810 with manipulation
➲ *CPT Changes: An Insider's View* 2008

27814 Open treatment of bimalleolar ankle fracture (eg, lateral and medial malleoli, or lateral and posterior malleoli, or medial and posterior malleoli), includes internal fixation, when performed
➲ *CPT Changes: An Insider's View* 2008
➲ *CPT Assistant* Feb 16:13

27816 Closed treatment of trimalleolar ankle fracture; without manipulation

27818 with manipulation

27822 Open treatment of trimalleolar ankle fracture, includes internal fixation, when performed, medial and/or lateral malleolus; without fixation of posterior lip
➲ *CPT Changes: An Insider's View* 2008

27823 with fixation of posterior lip
➲ *CPT Changes: An Insider's View* 2008

27824 Closed treatment of fracture of weight bearing articular portion of distal tibia (eg, pilon or tibial plafond), with or without anesthesia; without manipulation

27825 with skeletal traction and/or requiring manipulation

27826 Open treatment of fracture of weight bearing articular surface/portion of distal tibia (eg, pilon or tibial plafond), with internal fixation, when performed; of fibula only
➲ *CPT Changes: An Insider's View* 2008

27827 of tibia only
➲ *CPT Changes: An Insider's View* 2008

27828 of both tibia and fibula
➲ *CPT Changes: An Insider's View* 2008
➲ *CPT Assistant* Apr 14:10

27829 Open treatment of distal tibiofibular joint (syndesmosis) disruption, includes internal fixation, when performed
➲ *CPT Changes: An Insider's View* 2008
➲ *CPT Assistant* Winter 92:11, Mar 09:10, Feb 16:13

27830 Closed treatment of proximal tibiofibular joint dislocation; without anesthesia

27831 requiring anesthesia

27832 Open treatment of proximal tibiofibular joint dislocation, includes internal fixation, when performed, or with excision of proximal fibula
➲ *CPT Changes: An Insider's View* 2008

27840 Closed treatment of ankle dislocation; without anesthesia

27842 requiring anesthesia, with or without percutaneous skeletal fixation

27846 Open treatment of ankle dislocation, with or without percutaneous skeletal fixation; without repair or internal fixation

27848 with repair or internal or external fixation

(For surgical or diagnostic arthroscopic procedures, see 29894-29898)

Manipulation

27860 Manipulation of ankle under general anesthesia (includes application of traction or other fixation apparatus)

Arthrodesis

27870 Arthrodesis, ankle, open
➲ *CPT Changes: An Insider's View* 2003

(For arthroscopic ankle arthrodesis, use 29899)

27871 Arthrodesis, tibiofibular joint, proximal or distal

Amputation

27880 Amputation, leg, through tibia and fibula;

27881 with immediate fitting technique including application of first cast

27882 open, circular (guillotine)

27884 secondary closure or scar revision

27886 re-amputation

27888 Amputation, ankle, through malleoli of tibia and fibula (eg, Syme, Pirogoff type procedures), with plastic closure and resection of nerves

27889 Ankle disarticulation

Other Procedures

27892 Decompression fasciotomy, leg; anterior and/or lateral compartments only, with debridement of nonviable muscle and/or nerve

(For decompression fasciotomy of the leg without debridement, use 27600)

27893 posterior compartment(s) only, with debridement of nonviable muscle and/or nerve

(For decompression fasciotomy of the leg without debridement, use 27601)

27894 anterior and/or lateral, and posterior compartment(s), with debridement of nonviable muscle and/or nerve

(For decompression fasciotomy of the leg without debridement, use 27602)

27899 Unlisted procedure, leg or ankle
➲ *CPT Assistant* Aug 00:11, Dec 16:16

Foot and Toes

Incision

(For incision and drainage procedures, superficial, see 10040-10160)

28001 Incision and drainage, bursa, foot
➔ *CPT Assistant* Nov 98:9

28002 Incision and drainage below fascia, with or without tendon sheath involvement, foot; single bursal space
➔ *CPT Assistant* Nov 98:8

28003 multiple areas
➔ *CPT Assistant* Nov 98:9

28005 Incision, bone cortex (eg, osteomyelitis or bone abscess), foot
➔ *CPT Assistant* Nov 98:9

28008 Fasciotomy, foot and/or toe

(See also 28060, 28062, 28250)

28010 Tenotomy, percutaneous, toe; single tendon
➔ *CPT Assistant* Nov 98:8

28011 multiple tendons
➔ *CPT Assistant* Nov 98:8

(For open tenotomy, see 28230-28234)

28020 Arthrotomy, including exploration, drainage, or removal of loose or foreign body; intertarsal or tarsometatarsal joint

28022 metatarsophalangeal joint

28024 interphalangeal joint

28035 Release, tarsal tunnel (posterior tibial nerve decompression)
➔ *CPT Assistant* Nov 98:8

(For other nerve entrapments, see 64704, 64722)

Excision

28039 Code is out of numerical sequence. See 28035-28047

28041 Code is out of numerical sequence. See 28035-28047

28043 Excision, tumor, soft tissue of foot or toe, subcutaneous; less than 1.5 cm
➔ *CPT Changes: An Insider's View* 2010

 # 28039 1.5 cm or greater
➔ *CPT Changes: An Insider's View* 2010

(For excision of benign lesions of cutaneous origin [eg, sebaceous cyst], see 11420-11426)

28045 Excision, tumor, soft tissue of foot or toe, subfascial (eg, intramuscular); less than 1.5 cm
➔ *CPT Changes: An Insider's View* 2010

 # 28041 1.5 cm or greater
➔ *CPT Changes: An Insider's View* 2010

28046 Radical resection of tumor (eg, sarcoma), soft tissue of foot or toe; less than 3 cm
➔ *CPT Changes: An Insider's View* 2010, 2014

28047 3 cm or greater
➔ *CPT Changes: An Insider's View* 2010, 2014

(For radical resection of tumor[s] of cutaneous origin [eg, melanoma], see 11620-11626)

28050 Arthrotomy with biopsy; intertarsal or tarsometatarsal joint

28052 metatarsophalangeal joint

28054 interphalangeal joint

28055 Neurectomy, intrinsic musculature of foot
➔ *CPT Changes: An Insider's View* 2007

28060 Fasciectomy, plantar fascia; partial (separate procedure)
➔ *CPT Assistant* Mar 08:14

28062 radical (separate procedure)

(For plantar fasciotomy, see 28008, 28250)

28070 Synovectomy; intertarsal or tarsometatarsal joint, each

28072 metatarsophalangeal joint, each

28080 Excision, interdigital (Morton) neuroma, single, each

28086 Synovectomy, tendon sheath, foot; flexor

28088 extensor

28090 Excision of lesion, tendon, tendon sheath, or capsule (including synovectomy) (eg, cyst or ganglion); foot
➔ *CPT Assistant* Nov 98:8

28092 toe(s), each

28100 Excision or curettage of bone cyst or benign tumor, talus or calcaneus;

28102 with iliac or other autograft (includes obtaining graft)

28103 with allograft

28104 Excision or curettage of bone cyst or benign tumor, tarsal or metatarsal, except talus or calcaneus;
➔ *CPT Changes: An Insider's View* 2002

28106 with iliac or other autograft (includes obtaining graft)

28107 with allograft

28108 Excision or curettage of bone cyst or benign tumor, phalanges of foot

(For partial excision of bossing or exostosis for phalanx in the foot, use 28124)

28110 Ostectomy, partial excision, fifth metatarsal head (bunionette) (separate procedure)
➔ *CPT Assistant* Oct 98:10, Sep 00:9, Dec 10:17

28111 Ostectomy, complete excision; first metatarsal head

28112 other metatarsal head (second, third or fourth)

28113 fifth metatarsal head

Musculoskeletal 20100-29999

28114 all metatarsal heads, with partial proximal phalangectomy, excluding first metatarsal (eg, Clayton type procedure)

28116 Ostectomy, excision of tarsal coalition

28118 Ostectomy, calcaneus;
➲ *CPT Assistant* May 11:9, Jan 15:13

28119 for spur, with or without plantar fascial release
➲ *CPT Assistant* May 11:9

28120 Partial excision (craterization, saucerization, sequestrectomy, or diaphysectomy) bone (eg, osteomyelitis or bossing); talus or calcaneus
➲ *CPT Assistant* May 11:9

28122 tarsal or metatarsal bone, except talus or calcaneus
➲ *CPT Assistant* Nov 98:11

(For partial excision of talus or calcaneus, use 28120)

(For cheilectomy for hallux rigidus, use 28289)

28124 phalanx of toe

28126 Resection, partial or complete, phalangeal base, each toe
➲ *CPT Assistant* Nov 98:8, Mar 15:9

28130 Talectomy (astragalectomy)

(For calcanectomy, use 28118)

28140 Metatarsectomy

28150 Phalangectomy, toe, each toe
➲ *CPT Assistant* Nov 98:8

28153 Resection, condyle(s), distal end of phalanx, each toe
➲ *CPT Assistant* Nov 98:8, Dec 11:15

28160 Hemiphalangectomy or interphalangeal joint excision, toe, proximal end of phalanx, each
➲ *CPT Assistant* Nov 98:8

28171 Radical resection of tumor; tarsal (except talus or calcaneus)
➲ *CPT Changes: An Insider's View* 2010

28173 metatarsal
➲ *CPT Changes: An Insider's View* 2010

28175 phalanx of toe
➲ *CPT Changes: An Insider's View* 2010

(For talus or calcaneus, use 27647)

Introduction or Removal

28190 Removal of foreign body, foot; subcutaneous
➲ *CPT Assistant* Dec 13:16

28192 deep
➲ *CPT Assistant* Dec 13:16

28193 complicated

Repair, Revision, and/or Reconstruction

28200 Repair, tendon, flexor, foot; primary or secondary, without free graft, each tendon
➲ *CPT Assistant* Nov 98:8, Jul 14:5, Feb 16:15

28202 secondary with free graft, each tendon (includes obtaining graft)

28208 Repair, tendon, extensor, foot; primary or secondary, each tendon
➲ *CPT Assistant* Nov 98:8

28210 secondary with free graft, each tendon (includes obtaining graft)

28220 Tenolysis, flexor, foot; single tendon
➲ *CPT Assistant* Nov 98:8

28222 multiple tendons
➲ *CPT Assistant* Nov 98:8

28225 Tenolysis, extensor, foot; single tendon
➲ *CPT Assistant* Nov 98:8

28226 multiple tendons
➲ *CPT Assistant* Nov 98:8

28230 Tenotomy, open, tendon flexor; foot, single or multiple tendon(s) (separate procedure)
➲ *CPT Assistant* Nov 98:8

28232 toe, single tendon (separate procedure)
➲ *CPT Assistant* Nov 98:8, Mar 15:9

28234 Tenotomy, open, extensor, foot or toe, each tendon
➲ *CPT Assistant* Nov 98:8, Sep 10:9

(For tendon transfer to midfoot or hindfoot, see 27690, 27691)

28238 Reconstruction (advancement), posterior tibial tendon with excision of accessory tarsal navicular bone (eg, Kidner type procedure)
➲ *CPT Changes: An Insider's View* 2002

(For subcutaneous tenotomy, see 28010, 28011)

(For transfer or transplant of tendon with muscle redirection or rerouting, see 27690-27692)

(For extensor hallucis longus transfer with great toe IP fusion (Jones procedure), use 28760)

28240 Tenotomy, lengthening, or release, abductor hallucis muscle

28250 Division of plantar fascia and muscle (eg, Steindler stripping) (separate procedure)

28260 Capsulotomy, midfoot; medial release only (separate procedure)

28261 with tendon lengthening

28262 extensive, including posterior talotibial capsulotomy and tendon(s) lengthening (eg, resistant clubfoot deformity)

28264 Capsulotomy, midtarsal (eg, Heyman type procedure)

28270 Capsulotomy; metatarsophalangeal joint, with or without tenorrhaphy, each joint (separate procedure)
➔ *CPT Assistant* Sep 10:9, Sep 11:11, Sep 14:13

28272 interphalangeal joint, each joint (separate procedure)
➔ *CPT Assistant* Dec 02:11

28280 Syndactylization, toes (eg, webbing or Kelikian type procedure)
➔ *CPT Assistant* Nov 98:8

28285 Correction, hammertoe (eg, interphalangeal fusion, partial or total phalangectomy)
➔ *CPT Assistant* Nov 98:8, May 06:18, Sep 10:9, Sep 11:11, Mar 15:9, Jun 16:8

28286 Correction, cock-up fifth toe, with plastic skin closure (eg, Ruiz-Mora type procedure)
➔ *CPT Assistant* Nov 98:8

28288 Ostectomy, partial, exostectomy or condylectomy, metatarsal head, each metatarsal head

28289 Hallux rigidus correction with cheilectomy, debridement and capsular release of the first metatarsophalangeal joint; without implant
➔ *CPT Changes: An Insider's View* 2017
➔ *CPT Assistant* Nov 98:11, May 11:3, Sep 15:12, Dec 16:7

(28290 has been deleted. To report, use 28292)

28291 with implant
➔ *CPT Changes: An Insider's View* 2017
➔ *CPT Assistant* Dec 16:7, Nov 17:10

Hallux Rigidus Correction
28289

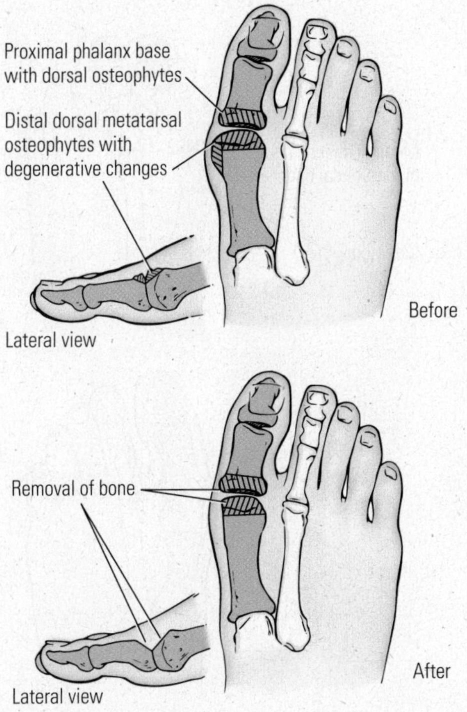

Hallux Rigidus Correction with Implant
28291

A single- or double-stem implant may be used

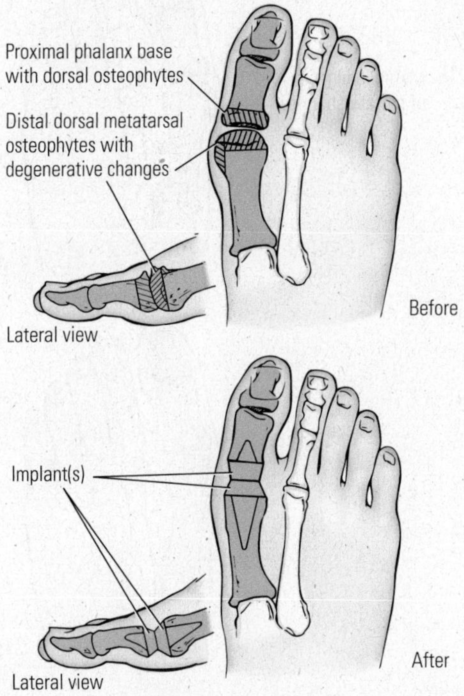

28292 Correction, hallux valgus (bunionectomy), with sesamoidectomy, when performed; with resection of proximal phalanx base, when performed, any method
➔ *CPT Changes: An Insider's View* 2017
➔ *CPT Assistant* Dec 96:5, Sep 00:9, Jan 07:31, May 10:9, Dec 10:12, Dec 16:3

(28293 has been deleted. To report, use 28291)

(28294 has been deleted. To report, use 28899)

28295 Code is out of numerical sequence. See 28292-28298

28296 with distal metatarsal osteotomy, any method
➔ *CPT Changes: An Insider's View* 2017
➔ *CPT Assistant* Dec 96:6, Jan 97:10, Jan 07:31, May 10:9, Sep 13:17, Dec 16:4

 # 28295 with proximal metatarsal osteotomy, any method
➔ *CPT Changes: An Insider's View* 2017
➔ *CPT Assistant* Dec 16:5

28297 with first metatarsal and medial cuneiform joint arthrodesis, any method
➔ *CPT Changes: An Insider's View* 2017
➔ *CPT Assistant* Dec 96:6, Jan 07:31, May 10:9, Dec 16:5

28298 with proximal phalanx osteotomy, any method
➔ *CPT Changes: An Insider's View* 2017
➔ *CPT Assistant* Dec 96:7, Jan 07:31, May 10:9, Oct 13:18, Dec 16:6

28299 with double osteotomy, any method
➔ *CPT Changes: An Insider's View* 2002, 2017
➔ *CPT Assistant* Dec 96:7, Jan 07:31, May 10:9, Sep 13:17, Oct 13:18, Apr 16:8, Dec 16:6

Hallux Valgus Correction
28292

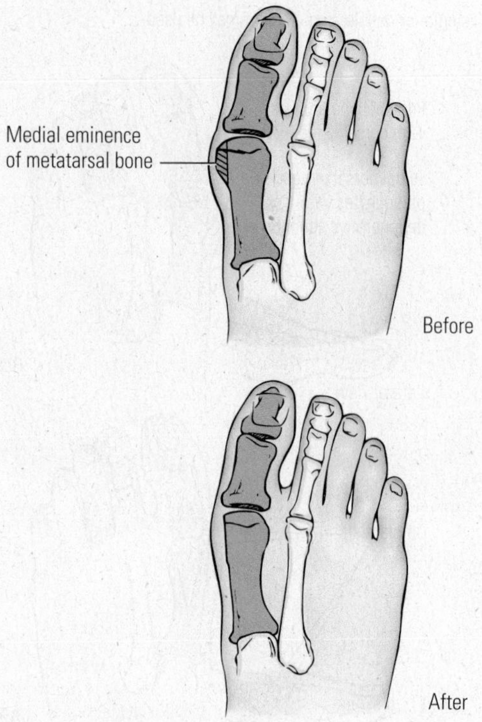

Hallux Valgus Correction with Proximal First Metatarsal Osteotomy
28295

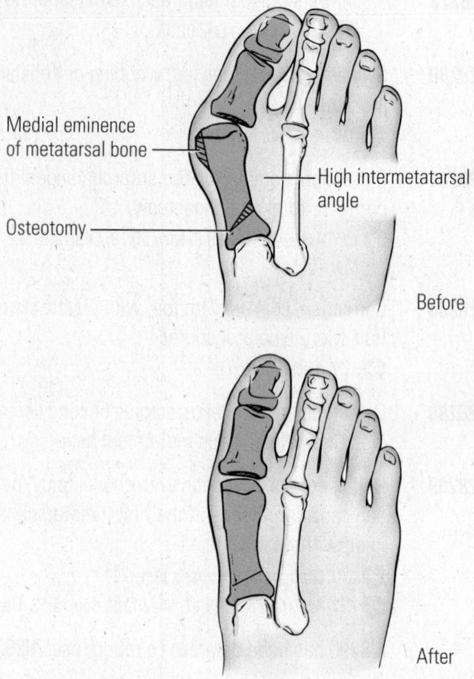

Hallux Valgus Correction with Proximal Phalanx Base Resection
28292

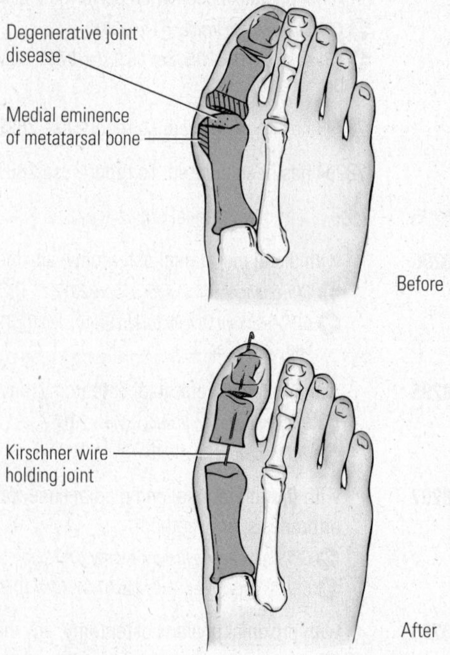

Hallux Valgus Correction with Distal First Metatarsal Osteotomy
28296

A single or multiple plane osteotomy originating through the distal aspect of the first metatarsal

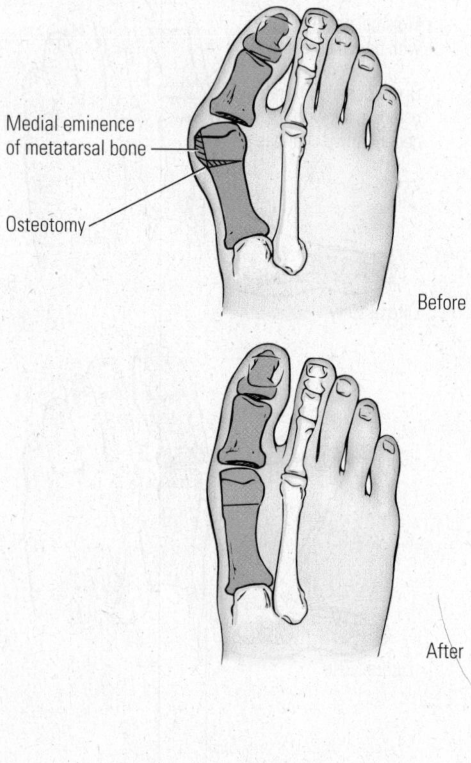

Hallux Valgus Correction with Metatarsal-Medial Cuneiform Joint Arthrodesis
28297

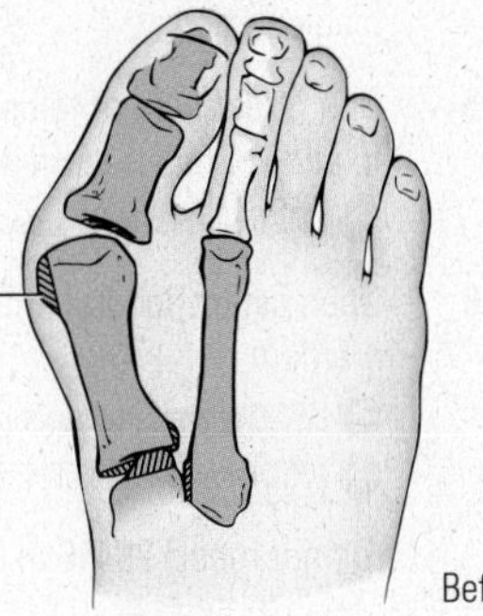

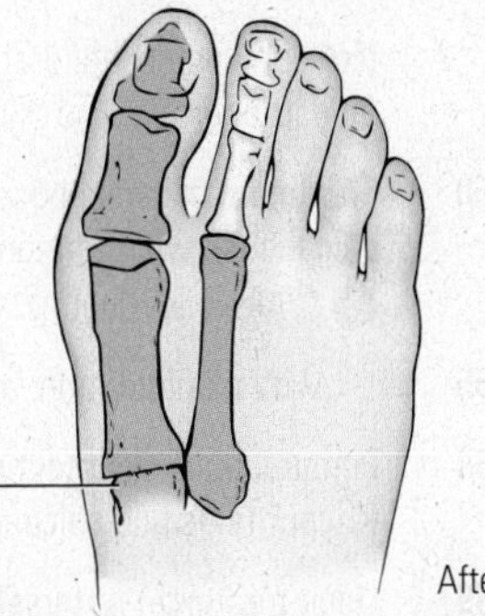

Hallux Valgus Correction with Proximal Phalanx Osteotomy
28298

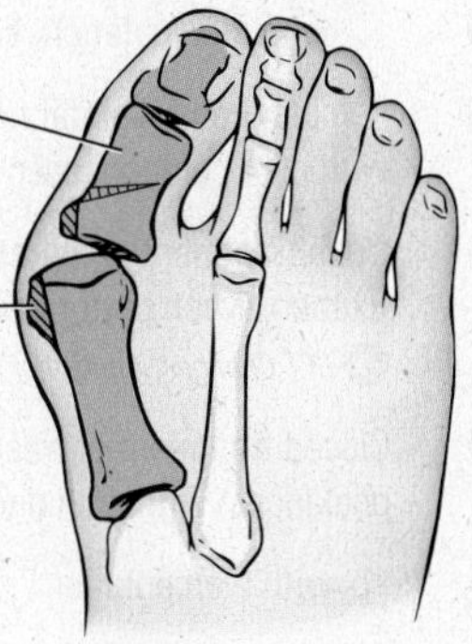

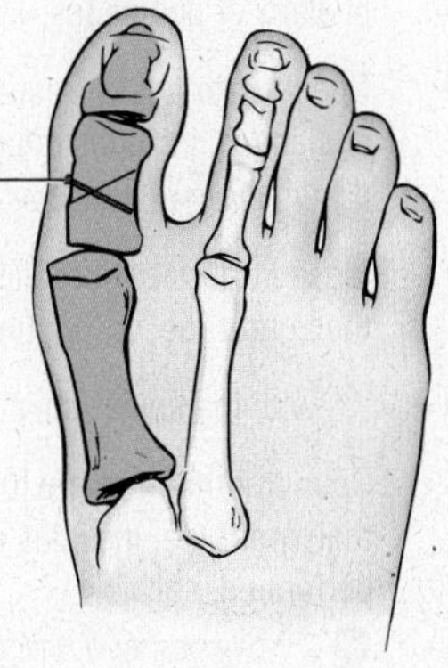

Hallux Valgus Correction with Double Osteotomy
28299

These illustrations depict medial resection of the first metatarsal along with several first ray double osteotomy options for hallux valgus and metatarsus primus adductus (high intermetatarsal angle) correction.

Surgical Option 1

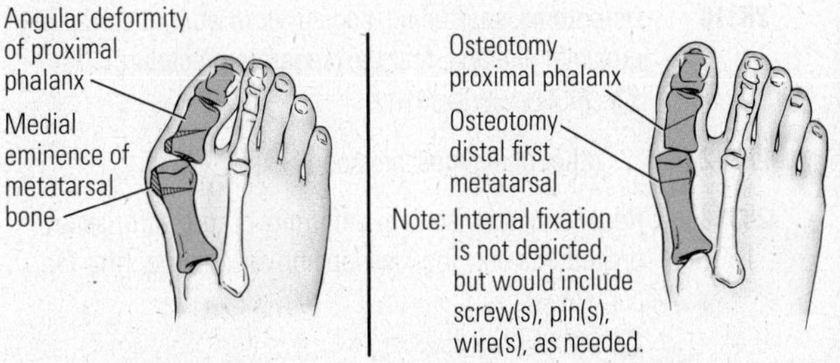

Surgical Option 2

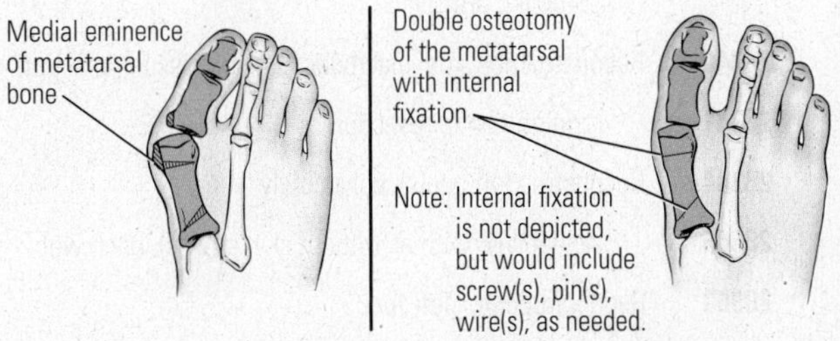

Surgical Option 3

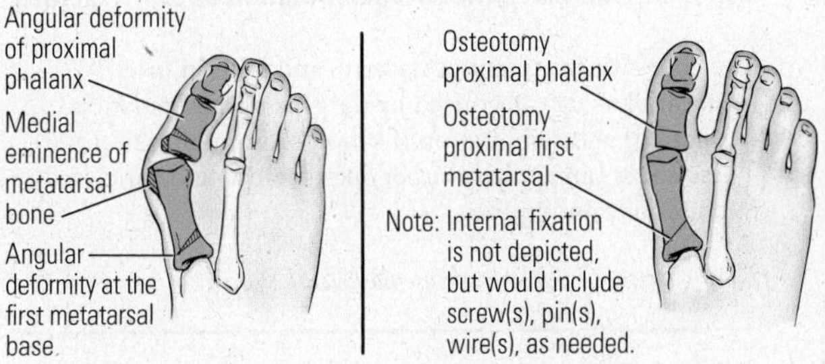

28300 Osteotomy; calcaneus (eg, Dwyer or Chambers type procedure), with or without internal fixation

28302 talus

28304 Osteotomy, tarsal bones, other than calcaneus or talus;

➔ *CPT Assistant* Nov 98:8

28305 with autograft (includes obtaining graft) (eg, Fowler type)

28306 Osteotomy, with or without lengthening, shortening or angular correction, metatarsal; first metatarsal
➔ *CPT Assistant* Nov 98:8, Dec 99:7, Dec 10:12

28307 first metatarsal with autograft (other than first toe)
➔ *CPT Assistant* Nov 98:9

28308 other than first metatarsal, each

28309 multiple (eg, Swanson type cavus foot procedure)
➔ *CPT Assistant* Nov 98:8, Dec 99:7

28310 Osteotomy, shortening, angular or rotational correction; proximal phalanx, first toe (separate procedure)
➔ *CPT Assistant* Sep 13:17

28312 other phalanges, any toe

28313 Reconstruction, angular deformity of toe, soft tissue procedures only (eg, overlapping second toe, fifth toe, curly toes)
➔ *CPT Assistant* Nov 98:8

28315 Sesamoidectomy, first toe (separate procedure)

28320 Repair, nonunion or malunion; tarsal bones
➔ *CPT Assistant* Nov 98:9

28322 metatarsal, with or without bone graft (includes obtaining graft)

28340 Reconstruction, toe, macrodactyly; soft tissue resection

28341 requiring bone resection

28344 Reconstruction, toe(s); polydactyly

28345 syndactyly, with or without skin graft(s), each web

28360 Reconstruction, cleft foot

Fracture and/or Dislocation

Coding Tip

Reporting for Categories of Manipulation and/or Fracture

The codes for treatment of fractures and joint injuries (dislocations) are categorized by the type of manipulation (reduction) and stabilization (fixation or immobilization). These codes can apply to either open (compound) or closed fractures or joint injuries.

CPT Coding Guidelines, Musculoskeletal System

28400 Closed treatment of calcaneal fracture; without manipulation

28405 with manipulation

28406 Percutaneous skeletal fixation of calcaneal fracture, with manipulation

28415 Open treatment of calcaneal fracture, includes internal fixation, when performed;
➔ *CPT Changes: An Insider's View* 2008

28420 with primary iliac or other autogenous bone graft (includes obtaining graft)
➔ *CPT Changes: An Insider's View* 2008

28430 Closed treatment of talus fracture; without manipulation

28435 with manipulation

28436 Percutaneous skeletal fixation of talus fracture, with manipulation

28445 Open treatment of talus fracture, includes internal fixation, when performed
➔ *CPT Changes: An Insider's View* 2008

28446 Open osteochondral autograft, talus (includes obtaining graft[s])
➔ *CPT Changes: An Insider's View* 2008
➔ *CPT Assistant* Jan 08:4, Dec 08:6

(Do not report 28446 in conjunction with 27705, 27707)

(For arthroscopic osteochondral talus graft, use 29892)

(For open osteochondral allograft or repairs with industrial grafts, use 28899)

28450 Treatment of tarsal bone fracture (except talus and calcaneus); without manipulation, each
➔ *CPT Assistant* Dec 01:7

28455 with manipulation, each

28456 Percutaneous skeletal fixation of tarsal bone fracture (except talus and calcaneus), with manipulation, each

28465 Open treatment of tarsal bone fracture (except talus and calcaneus), includes internal fixation, when performed, each
➔ *CPT Changes: An Insider's View* 2008

28470 Closed treatment of metatarsal fracture; without manipulation, each

28475 with manipulation, each

28476 Percutaneous skeletal fixation of metatarsal fracture, with manipulation, each

28485 Open treatment of metatarsal fracture, includes internal fixation, when performed, each
➔ *CPT Changes: An Insider's View* 2008

28490 Closed treatment of fracture great toe, phalanx or phalanges; without manipulation

28495 with manipulation

28496 Percutaneous skeletal fixation of fracture great toe, phalanx or phalanges, with manipulation

28505 Open treatment of fracture, great toe, phalanx or phalanges, includes internal fixation, when performed
➔ *CPT Changes: An Insider's View* 2008

28510 Closed treatment of fracture, phalanx or phalanges, other than great toe; without manipulation, each

28515 with manipulation, each

28525 Open treatment of fracture, phalanx or phalanges, other than great toe, includes internal fixation, when performed, each
➔ *CPT Changes: An Insider's View* 2008

28530 Closed treatment of sesamoid fracture

28531 Open treatment of sesamoid fracture, with or without internal fixation

28540 Closed treatment of tarsal bone dislocation, other than talotarsal; without anesthesia

28545 requiring anesthesia

28546 Percutaneous skeletal fixation of tarsal bone dislocation, other than talotarsal, with manipulation

28555 Open treatment of tarsal bone dislocation, includes internal fixation, when performed

➲ *CPT Changes: An Insider's View* 2008

28570 Closed treatment of talotarsal joint dislocation; without anesthesia

28575 requiring anesthesia

28576 Percutaneous skeletal fixation of talotarsal joint dislocation, with manipulation

28585 Open treatment of talotarsal joint dislocation, includes internal fixation, when performed

➲ *CPT Changes: An Insider's View* 2008

➲ *CPT Assistant* Sep 11:12

28600 Closed treatment of tarsometatarsal joint dislocation; without anesthesia

28605 requiring anesthesia

28606 Percutaneous skeletal fixation of tarsometatarsal joint dislocation, with manipulation

28615 Open treatment of tarsometatarsal joint dislocation, includes internal fixation, when performed

➲ *CPT Changes: An Insider's View* 2008

28630 Closed treatment of metatarsophalangeal joint dislocation; without anesthesia

28635 requiring anesthesia

28636 Percutaneous skeletal fixation of metatarsophalangeal joint dislocation, with manipulation

28645 Open treatment of metatarsophalangeal joint dislocation, includes internal fixation, when performed

➲ *CPT Changes: An Insider's View* 2008

➲ *CPT Assistant* Sep 14:13

28660 Closed treatment of interphalangeal joint dislocation; without anesthesia

28665 requiring anesthesia

28666 Percutaneous skeletal fixation of interphalangeal joint dislocation, with manipulation

28675 Open treatment of interphalangeal joint dislocation, includes internal fixation, when performed

➲ *CPT Changes: An Insider's View* 2008

Arthrodesis

28705 Arthrodesis; pantalar

28715 triple

28725 subtalar

➲ *CPT Assistant* Sep 11:11

28730 Arthrodesis, midtarsal or tarsometatarsal, multiple or transverse;

28735 with osteotomy (eg, flatfoot correction)

28737 Arthrodesis, with tendon lengthening and advancement, midtarsal, tarsal navicular-cuneiform (eg, Miller type procedure)

➲ *CPT Changes: An Insider's View* 2002

28740 Arthrodesis, midtarsal or tarsometatarsal, single joint

28750 Arthrodesis, great toe; metatarsophalangeal joint

➲ *CPT Assistant* Dec 96:7, Dec 16:8

28755 interphalangeal joint

28760 Arthrodesis, with extensor hallucis longus transfer to first metatarsal neck, great toe, interphalangeal joint (eg, Jones type procedure)

➲ *CPT Assistant* Nov 98:8

(For hammertoe operation or interphalangeal fusion, use 28285)

Amputation

28800 Amputation, foot; midtarsal (eg, Chopart type procedure)

28805 transmetatarsal

➲ *CPT Assistant* May 97:8

28810 Amputation, metatarsal, with toe, single

28820 Amputation, toe; metatarsophalangeal joint

➲ *CPT Assistant* May 97:8

28825 interphalangeal joint

Other Procedures

28890 Extracorporeal shock wave, high energy, performed by a physician or other qualified health care professional, requiring anesthesia other than local, including ultrasound guidance, involving the plantar fascia

➲ *CPT Changes: An Insider's View* 2006, 2013

➲ *CPT Assistant* Dec 05:10, Mar 06:1

(For extracorporeal shock wave therapy involving musculoskeletal system not otherwise specified, see 0101T, 0102T)

►(For extracorporeal shock wave therapy involving integumentary system not otherwise specified, see 0512T, 0513T)◄

►(Do not report 28890 in conjunction with 0512T, 0513T, when treating the same area)◄

28899 Unlisted procedure, foot or toes

➲ *CPT Assistant* Sep 11:12, Nov 15:10, Jun 16:8, Sep 17:14, Nov 17:10

Application of Casts and Strapping

The listed procedures apply when the cast application or strapping is a replacement procedure used during or after the period of follow-up care, or when the cast application or strapping is an initial service performed without a restorative treatment or procedure(s) to stabilize or protect a fracture, injury, or dislocation and/or to afford comfort to a patient. Restorative treatment or procedure(s) rendered by another individual following the application of the initial cast/splint/strap may be reported with a treatment of fracture and/or dislocation code.

An individual who applies the initial cast, strap, or splint and also assumes all of the subsequent fracture, dislocation, or injury care cannot use the application of casts and strapping codes as an initial service, since the first cast/splint or strap application is included in the treatment of fracture and/or dislocation codes. (See notes under Musculoskeletal System, page 116.) A temporary cast/splint/strap is not considered to be part of the preoperative care, and the use of the modifier 56 is not applicable. Additional evaluation and management services are reportable only if significant identifiable further services are provided at the time of the cast application or strapping.

If cast application or strapping is provided as an initial service (eg, casting of a sprained ankle or knee) in which no other procedure or treatment (eg, surgical repair, reduction of a fracture, or joint dislocation) is performed or is expected to be performed by an individual rendering the initial care only, use the casting, strapping, and/or supply code (99070) in addition to an evaluation and management code as appropriate.

Listed procedures include removal of cast or strapping.

(For orthotics management and training, see 97760, 97761, 97763)

Body and Upper Extremity

Casts

29000 Application of halo type body cast (see 20661-20663 for insertion)
➲ *CPT Assistant* Feb 96:3, 5, Apr 02:13, Jan 18:3

29010 Application of Risser jacket, localizer, body; only
➲ *CPT Assistant* Feb 96:3, Apr 02:13

29015 including head
➲ *CPT Assistant* Feb 96:3, Apr 02:13

29035 Application of body cast, shoulder to hips;
➲ *CPT Assistant* Feb 96:3, Apr 02:13

29040 including head, Minerva type
➲ *CPT Assistant* Feb 96:3, Apr 02:13

29044 including 1 thigh
➲ *CPT Assistant* Feb 96:3, Apr 02:13

29046 including both thighs
➲ *CPT Assistant* Feb 96:3, Apr 02:13

29049 Application, cast; figure-of-eight
➲ *CPT Changes: An Insider's View* 2002
➲ *CPT Assistant* Feb 96:3, Apr 02:13

29055 shoulder spica
➲ *CPT Assistant* Feb 96:3, Apr 02:13

29058 plaster Velpeau
➲ *CPT Assistant* Feb 96:3, Apr 02:13

29065 shoulder to hand (long arm)
➲ *CPT Assistant* Feb 96:3, Apr 02:13

29075 elbow to finger (short arm)
➲ *CPT Assistant* Feb 96:3-4, Apr 02:13

29085 hand and lower forearm (gauntlet)
➲ *CPT Assistant* Feb 96:3, Apr 02:13, Dec 02:11

29086 finger (eg, contracture)
➲ *CPT Changes: An Insider's View* 2002
➲ *CPT Assistant* Apr 02:13

Splints

29105 Application of long arm splint (shoulder to hand)
➲ *CPT Assistant* Feb 96:3, Apr 02:13, May 09:8, Jan 18:3

29125 Application of short arm splint (forearm to hand); static
➲ *CPT Assistant* Feb 96:3-4, Apr 02:13, Jan 18:3

29126 dynamic
➲ *CPT Assistant* Feb 96:3, Apr 02:13

29130 Application of finger splint; static
➲ *CPT Assistant* Feb 96:3, Apr 02:13

29131 dynamic
➲ *CPT Assistant* Feb 96:3, Apr 02:13

Strapping—Any Age

29200 Strapping; thorax
➲ *CPT Assistant* Feb 96:3, Apr 02:13

(To report low back strapping, use 29799)

29240 shoulder (eg, Velpeau)
➲ *CPT Assistant* Feb 96:3, Apr 02:13, Jun 10:8

29260 elbow or wrist
➲ *CPT Assistant* Feb 96:3, Apr 02:13

29280 hand or finger
➲ *CPT Assistant* Feb 96:3, Apr 02:13

Lower Extremity

Casts

29305 Application of hip spica cast; 1 leg
CPT Assistant Feb 96:3, Apr 02:13

29325 1 and one-half spica or both legs
CPT Assistant Feb 96:3, Apr 02:13

(For hip spica (body) cast, including thighs only, use 29046)

29345 Application of long leg cast (thigh to toes);
CPT Assistant Feb 96:3, Apr 02:13, Sep 11:11

29355 walker or ambulatory type
CPT Assistant Feb 96:3, Apr 02:13, Sep 11:11, Jan 18:3

29358 Application of long leg cast brace
CPT Assistant Feb 96:3, Apr 02:13, Sep 11:11

29365 Application of cylinder cast (thigh to ankle)
CPT Assistant Feb 96:3, Apr 02:13, Sep 11:11

29405 Application of short leg cast (below knee to toes);
CPT Assistant Feb 96:3, Apr 02:13, Mar 03:17, Sep 11:11, Jan 18:3

29425 walking or ambulatory type
CPT Assistant Feb 96:3, Apr 02:13, Sep 11:11

29435 Application of patellar tendon bearing (PTB) cast
CPT Assistant Feb 96:3, Apr 02:13, Sep 11:11

29440 Adding walker to previously applied cast
CPT Assistant Feb 96:3, Apr 02:13

29445 Application of rigid total contact leg cast
CPT Assistant Feb 96:3, Apr 02:13, Sep 11:11

29450 Application of clubfoot cast with molding or manipulation, long or short leg
CPT Assistant Feb 96:3, Apr 02:13

(To report bilateral procedure, use 29450 with modifier 50)

Splints

29505 Application of long leg splint (thigh to ankle or toes)
CPT Assistant Feb 96:3, Apr 02:13, May 09:8

29515 Application of short leg splint (calf to foot)
CPT Assistant Feb 96:3, Apr 02:13, Mar 03:18, Jan 18:3

Strapping—Any Age

29520 Strapping; hip
CPT Assistant Feb 96:3, Apr 02:13

29530 knee
CPT Assistant Feb 96:3, Apr 02:13, Jun 10:8, Aug 10:15

29540 ankle and/or foot
CPT Changes: An Insider's View 2003
CPT Assistant Feb 96:3, Apr 02:13, Mar 03:17, Jun 10:8, Aug 10:15, Mar 14:4

►(Do not report 29540 in conjunction with 29580, 29581, for the same extremity)◄

29550 toes
CPT Assistant Feb 96:3, Apr 02:13

29580 Unna boot
CPT Assistant Feb 96:3, Jul 99:10, Apr 02:13, Mar 14:4

►(Do not report 29580 in conjunction with 29540, 29581, for the same extremity)◄

29581 Application of multi-layer compression system; leg (below knee), including ankle and foot
CPT Changes: An Insider's View 2010, 2012
CPT Assistant May 11:11, Sep 12:16, Sep 13:17, Mar 14:4, Oct 14:6, Mar 15:10, Aug 16:3

►(Do not report 29581 in conjunction with 29540, 29580, for the same extremity)◄

►(Do not report 29520, 29530, 29540, 29550, 29580, 29581 in conjunction with 36465, 36466, 36468, 36470, 36471, 36473, 36474, 36475, 36476, 36478, 36479, 36482, 36483, for the same extremity)◄

(29582, 29583 have been deleted)

29584 upper arm, forearm, hand, and fingers
CPT Changes: An Insider's View 2012
CPT Assistant Mar 15:10, Aug 16:3

►(Do not report 29584 in conjunction with 36465, 36466, 36468, 36470, 36471, 36473, 36474, 36475, 36476, 36478, 36479, 36482, 36483, for the same extremity)◄

Removal or Repair

Codes for cast removals should be employed only for casts applied by another individual.

29700 Removal or bivalving; gauntlet, boot or body cast
CPT Assistant Apr 02:13

29705 full arm or full leg cast
CPT Assistant Apr 02:13

29710 shoulder or hip spica, Minerva, or Risser jacket, etc.
CPT Assistant Apr 02:13

29720 Repair of spica, body cast or jacket
CPT Assistant Apr 02:13

29730 Windowing of cast
CPT Assistant Apr 02:13

29740 Wedging of cast (except clubfoot casts)
CPT Assistant Apr 02:13

29750 Wedging of clubfoot cast
CPT Assistant Apr 02:13, Jan 18:3

(To report bilateral procedure, use 29750 with modifier 50)

Other Procedures

29799 Unlisted procedure, casting or strapping
CPT Assistant Sep 12:16, Aug 16:11, Jan 18:3

Endoscopy/Arthroscopy

Surgical endoscopy/arthroscopy always includes a diagnostic endoscopy/arthroscopy.

When arthroscopy is performed in conjunction with arthrotomy, add modifier 51.

29800 Arthroscopy, temporomandibular joint, diagnostic, with or without synovial biopsy (separate procedure)
CPT Assistant May 13:12

29804 Arthroscopy, temporomandibular joint, surgical
CPT Assistant May 13:12

(For open procedure, use 21010)

29805 Arthroscopy, shoulder, diagnostic, with or without synovial biopsy (separate procedure)
CPT Changes: An Insider's View 2002
CPT Assistant May 13:12, Jun 15:10

(For open procedure, see 23065-23066, 23100-23101)

29806 Arthroscopy, shoulder, surgical; capsulorrhaphy
CPT Changes: An Insider's View 2002
CPT Assistant May 13:12, Mar 15:7, Jul 15:10

(For open procedure, see 23450-23466)

(To report thermal capsulorrhaphy, use 29999)

29807 repair of SLAP lesion
CPT Changes: An Insider's View 2002
CPT Assistant May 13:12, Mar 15:7

29819 with removal of loose body or foreign body
CPT Changes: An Insider's View 2002
CPT Assistant May 13:12, Mar 15:7

(For open procedure, see 23040-23044, 23107)

29820 synovectomy, partial
CPT Assistant May 13:12, Jun 13:13, Mar 15:7

(For open procedure, see 23105)

29821 synovectomy, complete
CPT Assistant May 13:12, Jun 13:13, Mar 15:7

(For open procedure, see 23105)

29822 debridement, limited
CPT Assistant May 01:9, Apr 12:17, Sep 12:16, May 13:12, Mar 15:7, Jan 18:7

(For open procedure, see specific open shoulder procedure performed)

29823 debridement, extensive
CPT Assistant Apr 12:17, Sep 12:16, May 13:12, Mar 15:7, Dec 16:16, Jan 18:7

(For open procedure, see specific open shoulder procedure performed)

29824 distal claviculectomy including distal articular surface (Mumford procedure)
CPT Changes: An Insider's View 2002
CPT Assistant May 13:12, Mar 15:7

(For open procedure, use 23120)

Arthroscopy, Shoulder, Distal Claviculectomy (Mumford Procedure)
29824

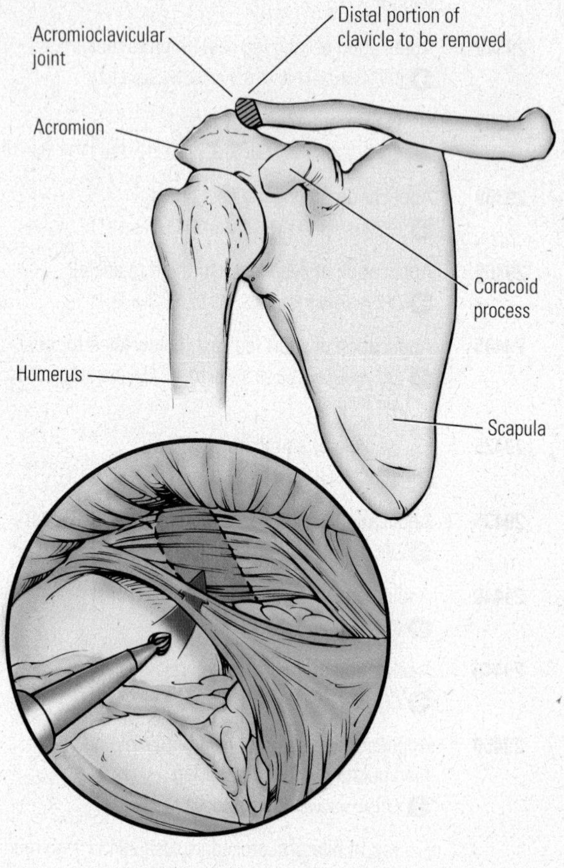

29825 with lysis and resection of adhesions, with or without manipulation
CPT Assistant May 13:12, Mar 15:7

(For open procedure, see specific open shoulder procedure performed)

+ 29826 decompression of subacromial space with partial acromioplasty, with coracoacromial ligament (ie, arch) release, when performed (List separately in addition to code for primary procedure)
CPT Changes: An Insider's View 2012
CPT Assistant May 01:9, Aug 02:10, May 13:12, Mar 15:7

(For open procedure, use 23130 or 23415)

(Use 29826 in conjunction with 29806-29825, 29827, 29828)

29827 with rotator cuff repair
➔ *CPT Changes: An Insider's View* 2003
➔ *CPT Assistant* Mar 08:14, May 13:12, Mar 15:7, Jul 16:8

(For open or mini-open rotator cuff repair, use 23412)

(When arthroscopic distal clavicle resection is performed at the same setting, use 29824 and append modifier 51)

29828 biceps tenodesis
➔ *CPT Changes: An Insider's View* 2008
➔ *CPT Assistant* Feb 08:9, May 13:12, Mar 15:7, Jul 16:8

(Do not report 29828 in conjunction with 29805, 29820, 29822)

(For open biceps tenodesis, use 23430)

29830 Arthroscopy, elbow, diagnostic, with or without synovial biopsy (separate procedure)
➔ *CPT Assistant* May 13:12

29834 Arthroscopy, elbow, surgical; with removal of loose body or foreign body
➔ *CPT Assistant* May 13:12

29835 synovectomy, partial
➔ *CPT Assistant* May 13:12

29836 synovectomy, complete
➔ *CPT Assistant* May 13:12

29837 debridement, limited
➔ *CPT Assistant* May 13:12

29838 debridement, extensive
➔ *CPT Assistant* May 13:12

29840 Arthroscopy, wrist, diagnostic, with or without synovial biopsy (separate procedure)
➔ *CPT Assistant* May 13:12

29843 Arthroscopy, wrist, surgical; for infection, lavage and drainage
➔ *CPT Assistant* May 13:12

29844 synovectomy, partial
➔ *CPT Assistant* May 13:12

29845 synovectomy, complete
➔ *CPT Assistant* Dec 03:11, May 13:12

29846 excision and/or repair of triangular fibrocartilage and/or joint debridement
➔ *CPT Assistant* Dec 03:11, May 13:12

29847 internal fixation for fracture or instability
➔ *CPT Assistant* May 13:12

29848 Endoscopy, wrist, surgical, with release of transverse carpal ligament
➔ *CPT Assistant* Dec 99:7, May 13:12, Jul 15:10, Jan 17:6, Apr 18:10

(For open procedure, use 64721)

29850 Arthroscopically aided treatment of intercondylar spine(s) and/or tuberosity fracture(s) of the knee, with or without manipulation; without internal or external fixation (includes arthroscopy)
➔ *CPT Assistant* May 13:12

29851 with internal or external fixation (includes arthroscopy)
➔ *CPT Assistant* May 13:12

(For bone graft, use 20900, 20902)

29855 Arthroscopically aided treatment of tibial fracture, proximal (plateau); unicondylar, includes internal fixation, when performed (includes arthroscopy)
➔ *CPT Changes: An Insider's View* 2008
➔ *CPT Assistant* May 13:12

29856 bicondylar, includes internal fixation, when performed (includes arthroscopy)
➔ *CPT Changes: An Insider's View* 2008
➔ *CPT Assistant* May 13:12

(For bone graft, use 20900, 20902)

29860 Arthroscopy, hip, diagnostic with or without synovial biopsy (separate procedure)
➔ *CPT Assistant* Nov 97:15, Jul 98:8, Sep 11:6, May 13:12

29861 Arthroscopy, hip, surgical; with removal of loose body or foreign body
➔ *CPT Assistant* Nov 97:15, Jul 98:8, Sep 11:5, May 13:12

29862 with debridement/shaving of articular cartilage (chondroplasty), abrasion arthroplasty, and/or resection of labrum
➔ *CPT Assistant* Nov 97:15, Jul 98:8, Sep 11:5, May 13:12

29863 with synovectomy
➔ *CPT Assistant* Nov 97:15, Jul 98:8, Sep 11:5, May 13:12

 # 29914 with femoroplasty (ie, treatment of cam lesion)
➔ *CPT Changes: An Insider's View* 2011
➔ *CPT Assistant* Sep 11:5

 # 29915 with acetabuloplasty (ie, treatment of pincer lesion)
➔ *CPT Changes: An Insider's View* 2011
➔ *CPT Assistant* Sep 11:5

(Do not report 29914, 29915 in conjunction with 29862, 29863)

 # 29916 with labral repair
➔ *CPT Changes: An Insider's View* 2011
➔ *CPT Assistant* Sep 11:5

(Do not report 29916 in conjunction with 29915, 29862, 29863)

29866 Arthroscopy, knee, surgical; osteochondral autograft(s) (eg, mosaicplasty) (includes harvesting of the autograft[s])
➔ *CPT Changes: An Insider's View* 2005, 2008
➔ *CPT Assistant* May 13:12

Arthroscopy of the Knee
29866-29887

Portal incisions are made on either side of the patellar tendon and compartments of the knee are examined using the arthroscope and a probe. Additional treatment is performed as needed.

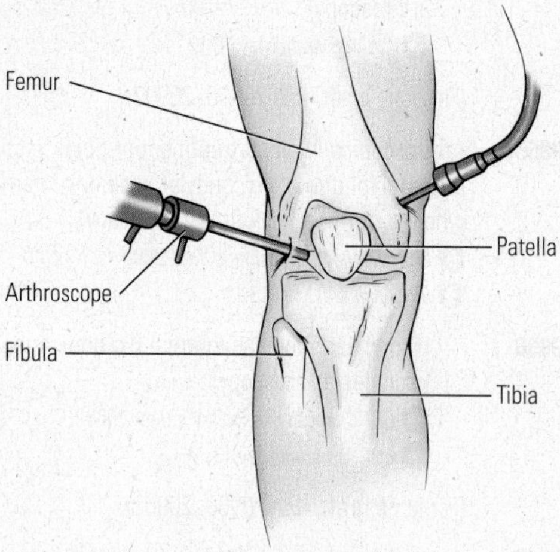

(Do not report 29866 in conjunction with 29870, 29871, 29875, 29884 when performed at the same session and/or 29874, 29877, 29879, 29885-29887 when performed in the same compartment)

(For open osteochondral autograft of knee, use 27416)

29867 osteochondral allograft (eg, mosaicplasty)
- *CPT Changes: An Insider's View* 2005
- *CPT Assistant* May 13:12

(Do not report 29867 in conjunction with 27570, 29870, 29871, 29875, 29884 when performed at the same session and/or 29874, 29877, 29879, 29885-29887 when performed in the same compartment)

(Do not report 29867 in conjunction with 27415)

29868 meniscal transplantation (includes arthrotomy for meniscal insertion), medial or lateral
- *CPT Changes: An Insider's View* 2005
- *CPT Assistant* May 13:12

(Do not report 29868 in conjunction with 29870, 29871, 29875, 29880, 29883, 29884 when performed at the same session or 29874, 29877, 29881, 29882 when performed in the same compartment)

29870 Arthroscopy, knee, diagnostic, with or without synovial biopsy (separate procedure)
- *CPT Assistant* Dec 07:10, Mar 11:9, May 13:12

(For open autologous chondrocyte implantation of the knee, use 27412)

29871 Arthroscopy, knee, surgical; for infection, lavage and drainage
- *CPT Assistant* Aug 01:6, May 13:12

►(Do not report 29871 in conjunction with 27369)◄

(For implantation of osteochondral graft for treatment of articular surface defect, see 27412, 27415, 29866, 29867)

29873 with lateral release
- *CPT Changes: An Insider's View* 2003
- *CPT Assistant* Dec 07:10, Aug 09:11, May 13:12, Nov 15:7

(For open lateral release, use 27425)

29874 for removal of loose body or foreign body (eg, osteochondritis dissecans fragmentation, chondral fragmentation)
- *CPT Assistant* Aug 01:6, Apr 03:12, May 13:12

29875 synovectomy, limited (eg, plica or shelf resection) (separate procedure)
- *CPT Assistant* Aug 01:6, May 13:12, May 14:10, Jan 16:11

29876 synovectomy, major, 2 or more compartments (eg, medial or lateral)
- *CPT Assistant* Aug 01:6, May 13:12

29877 debridement/shaving of articular cartilage (chondroplasty)
- *CPT Assistant* Feb 96:9, Jun 99:11, Aug 01:7, Apr 03:7, Apr 05:14, Dec 07:10, May 13:12

(When performed with arthroscopic meniscectomy, see 29880 or 29881)

29879 abrasion arthroplasty (includes chondroplasty where necessary) or multiple drilling or microfracture
- *CPT Changes: An Insider's View* 2000
- *CPT Assistant* Nov 99:13, Aug 01:7, May 13:12

29880 with meniscectomy (medial AND lateral, including any meniscal shaving) including debridement/shaving of articular cartilage (chondroplasty), same or separate compartment(s), when performed
- *CPT Changes: An Insider's View* 2012
- *CPT Assistant* Jun 99:11, Aug 01:7, Jan 12:3, May 13:12

29881 with meniscectomy (medial OR lateral, including any meniscal shaving) including debridement/shaving of articular cartilage (chondroplasty), same or separate compartment(s), when performed
- *CPT Changes: An Insider's View* 2012
- *CPT Assistant* Feb 96:9, Jun 99:11, Aug 01:7, Oct 03:11, Apr 05:14, Dec 07:10, Jan 12:3, May 13:12, May 14:10, Jan 16:11

29882 with meniscus repair (medial OR lateral)
- *CPT Assistant* Aug 01:7, Sep 04:12, Dec 07:10, Dec 11:15, May 13:12

29883 with meniscus repair (medial AND lateral)
- *CPT Assistant* Aug 01:7, Sep 04:12, Dec 07:10, Dec 11:15, May 13:12

(For meniscal transplantation, medial or lateral, knee, use 29868)

29884 with lysis of adhesions, with or without manipulation (separate procedure)
- *CPT Assistant* Aug 01:7, Mar 11:9, May 13:12

29885 drilling for osteochondritis dissecans with bone grafting, with or without internal fixation (including debridement of base of lesion)
➲ *CPT Assistant* Aug 01:7, May 13:12

29886 drilling for intact osteochondritis dissecans lesion
➲ *CPT Assistant* Aug 01:12, May 13:12

29887 drilling for intact osteochondritis dissecans lesion with internal fixation
➲ *CPT Assistant* Aug 01:12, May 13:12

29888 Arthroscopically aided anterior cruciate ligament repair/augmentation or reconstruction
➲ *CPT Assistant* Oct 03:11, Dec 07:10, May 13:12, Nov 16:9, May 17:10

29889 Arthroscopically aided posterior cruciate ligament repair/augmentation or reconstruction
➲ *CPT Assistant* Sep 96:9, Oct 98:11, Aug 01:8, Dec 07:10, May 13:12

29891 Arthroscopy, ankle, surgical, excision of osteochondral defect of talus and/or tibia, including drilling of the defect
➲ *CPT Assistant* Nov 97:15, May 13:12

29892 Arthroscopically aided repair of large osteochondritis dissecans lesion, talar dome fracture, or tibial plafond fracture, with or without internal fixation (includes arthroscopy)
➲ *CPT Assistant* Nov 97:15, Dec 08:6, May 13:12

29893 Endoscopic plantar fasciotomy
➲ *CPT Assistant* Nov 97:15, May 13:12

29894 Arthroscopy, ankle (tibiotalar and fibulotalar joints), surgical; with removal of loose body or foreign body
➲ *CPT Assistant* May 13:12

29895 synovectomy, partial
➲ *CPT Assistant* May 13:12

29897 debridement, limited
➲ *CPT Assistant* May 13:12

29898 debridement, extensive
➲ *CPT Assistant* May 13:12

29899 with ankle arthrodesis
➲ *CPT Changes: An Insider's View* 2003
➲ *CPT Assistant* May 13:12

(For open ankle arthrodesis, use 27870)

29900 Arthroscopy, metacarpophalangeal joint, diagnostic, includes synovial biopsy
➲ *CPT Changes: An Insider's View* 2002
➲ *CPT Assistant* May 13:12

(Do not report 29900 with 29901, 29902)

29901 Arthroscopy, metacarpophalangeal joint, surgical; with debridement
➲ *CPT Changes: An Insider's View* 2002
➲ *CPT Assistant* May 13:12

Arthroscopy of the Ankle
29894-29899

Incisions are made allowing the ankle to be examined using the arthroscope and a probe. Additional treatment is performed as needed.

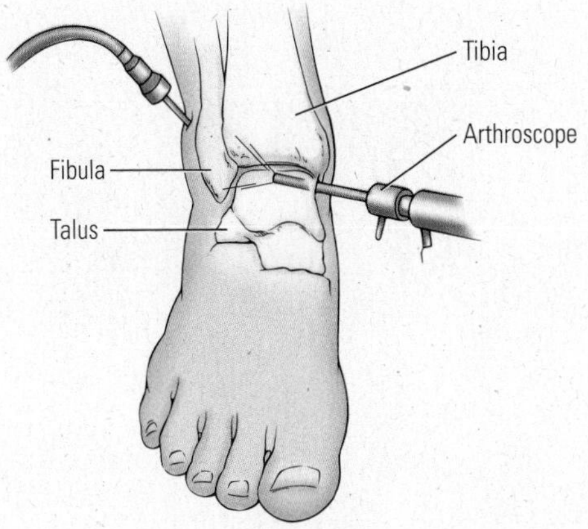

29902 with reduction of displaced ulnar collateral ligament (eg, Stener lesion)
➲ *CPT Changes: An Insider's View* 2002
➲ *CPT Assistant* May 13:12

29904 Arthroscopy, subtalar joint, surgical; with removal of loose body or foreign body
➲ *CPT Changes: An Insider's View* 2008
➲ *CPT Assistant* May 13:12

29905 with synovectomy
➲ *CPT Changes: An Insider's View* 2008
➲ *CPT Assistant* May 13:12

29906 with debridement
➲ *CPT Changes: An Insider's View* 2008
➲ *CPT Assistant* May 13:12

29907 with subtalar arthrodesis
➲ *CPT Changes: An Insider's View* 2008
➲ *CPT Assistant* May 13:12

29914 Code is out of numerical sequence. See 29862-29867

29915 Code is out of numerical sequence. See 29862-29867

29916 Code is out of numerical sequence. See 29862-29867

29999 Unlisted procedure, arthroscopy
➲ *CPT Changes: An Insider's View* 2002
➲ *CPT Assistant* Aug 02:10, Sep 04:12, Nov 08:10, Mar 09:10, Dec 11:15, Apr 12:17, May 13:12, Dec 15:18, Dec 16:16, Apr 17:9

Notes

Musculoskeletal

Surgery

Respiratory System (30000-32999) 187

The following is a listing of headings and subheadings that appear within the Respiratory System section of the CPT codebook. The subheadings or subsections denoted with asterisks (*) below have special instructions unique to that subsection. Where these are indicated, special notes or guidelines will be presented preceding those procedural terminology listings, referring to that subsection specifically.

Nose (30000-30999) 187
- Incision (30000-30020) 187
- Excision (30100-30160) 187
- Introduction (30200-30220) 187
- Removal of Foreign Body (30300-30320) 187
- Repair (30400-30630) 187
- Destruction (30801-30802) 188
- Other Procedures (30901-30999) 188

Accessory Sinuses (31000-31299) 188
- Incision (31000-31090) 188
- Excision (31200-31230) 189

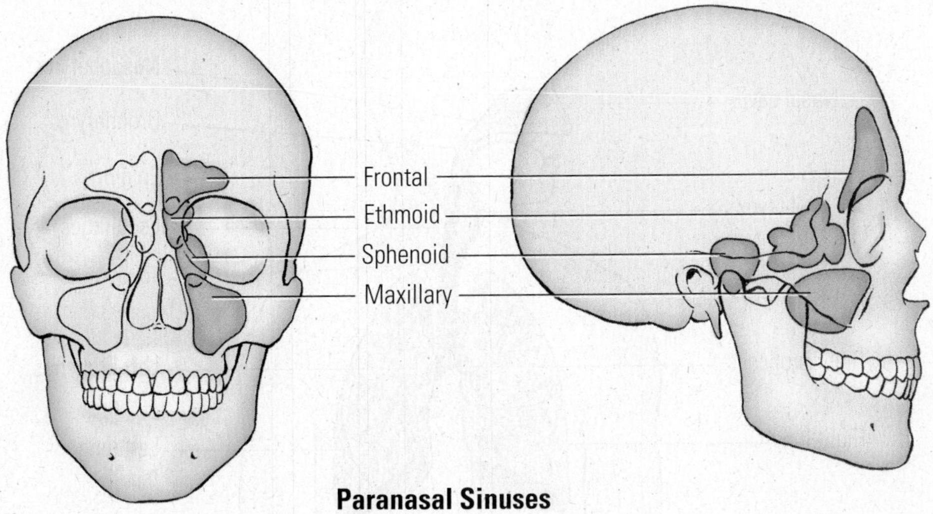

Paranasal Sinuses

- Endoscopy* (31231-31298) 189
- Other Procedures (31299) 192

Larynx (31300-31599) 192
- Excision (31300-31420) 192
- Introduction (31500-31502) 192
- Endoscopy* (31505-31579) 192
- Repair (31580-31592) 194
- Destruction 195
- Other Procedures (31599) 195

Trachea and Bronchi (31600-31899) 195
- Incision (31600-31614) 195
- Endoscopy* (31615-31654) 195

Bronchial Thermoplasty (31660-31661) 197
Introduction (31717-31730) 198
Excision, Repair (31750-31830) 198
Other Procedures (31899) 198

Lungs and Pleura* (32035-32999) 198
Incision (32035-32225) 199
Excision/Resection (32310-32405) 199
Removal (32440-32540) 199
Introduction and Removal (32550-32557) 200
Destruction* (32560-32562) 201
Thoracoscopy (Video-assisted thoracic surgery* [VATS]) (32601-32674) 201
Stereotactic Radiation Therapy* (32701) 204
Repair (32800-32820) 204
Lung Transplantation* (32850-32856) 204
Surgical Collapse Therapy; Thoracoplasty (32900-32960) 204
Other Procedures (32994-32999) 205

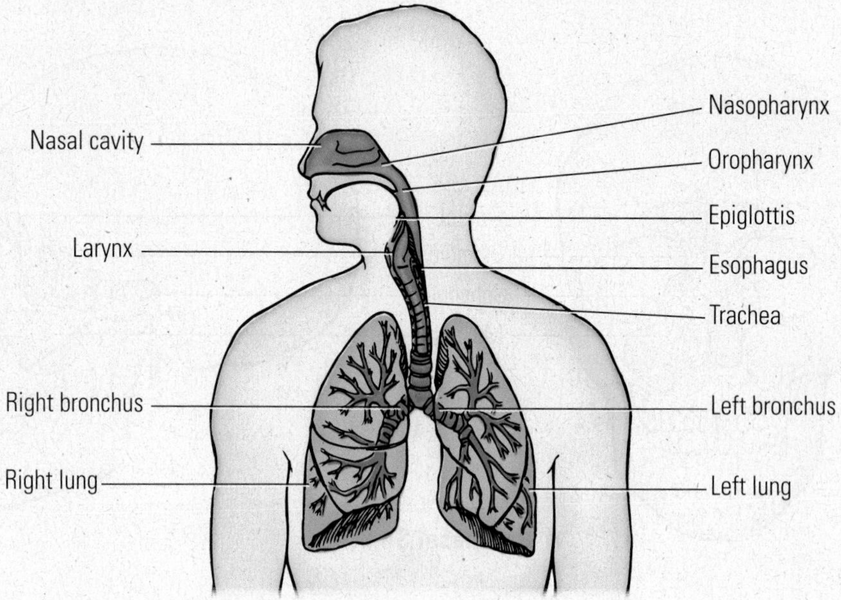

Respiratory System

Respiratory System

Nose

Incision

30000 Drainage abscess or hematoma, nasal, internal approach

(For external approach, see 10060, 10140)

30020 Drainage abscess or hematoma, nasal septum

(For lateral rhinotomy, see specific application [eg, 30118, 30320])

Excision

30100 Biopsy, intranasal

►(For biopsy skin of nose, see 11102, 11103, 11104, 11105, 11106, 11107)◄

30110 Excision, nasal polyp(s), simple

(30110 would normally be completed in an office setting)

(To report bilateral procedure, use 30110 with modifier 50)

30115 Excision, nasal polyp(s), extensive

(30115 would normally require the facilities available in a hospital setting)

(To report bilateral procedure, use 30115 with modifier 50)

30117 Excision or destruction (eg, laser), intranasal lesion; internal approach

➲ *CPT Changes: An Insider's View* 2002

30118 external approach (lateral rhinotomy)

➲ *CPT Changes: An Insider's View* 2002

30120 Excision or surgical planing of skin of nose for rhinophyma

➲ *CPT Assistant* May 07:9

30124 Excision dermoid cyst, nose; simple, skin, subcutaneous

30125 complex, under bone or cartilage

30130 Excision inferior turbinate, partial or complete, any method

➲ *CPT Changes: An Insider's View* 2006

➲ *CPT Assistant* Feb 98:11, Nov 98:11, Sep 01:10, May 03:5

(For excision of superior or middle turbinate, use 30999)

30140 Submucous resection inferior turbinate, partial or complete, any method

➲ *CPT Changes: An Insider's View* 2006

➲ *CPT Assistant* Nov 98:11, Dec 02:10, Apr 03:26, May 03:5, Dec 04:18, Mar 08:14

(Do not report 30130 or 30140 in conjunction with 30801, 30802, 30930)

(For submucous resection of superior or middle turbinate, use 30999)

(For endoscopic resection of concha bullosa of middle turbinate, use 31240)

(For submucous resection of nasal septum, use 30520)

30150 Rhinectomy; partial

30160 total

(For closure and/or reconstruction, primary or delayed, see **Integumentary System,** 13151-13160, 14060-14302, 15120, 15121, 15260, 15261, 15760, 20900-20912)

Introduction

30200 Injection into turbinate(s), therapeutic

➲ *CPT Assistant* Dec 04:19

30210 Displacement therapy (Proetz type)

30220 Insertion, nasal septal prosthesis (button)

Removal of Foreign Body

30300 Removal foreign body, intranasal; office type procedure

➲ *CPT Assistant* Jan 12:13

30310 requiring general anesthesia

30320 by lateral rhinotomy

Repair

(For obtaining tissues for graft, see 20900-20926, 21210)

30400 Rhinoplasty, primary; lateral and alar cartilages and/or elevation of nasal tip

(For columellar reconstruction, see 13151 et seq)

30410 complete, external parts including bony pyramid, lateral and alar cartilages, and/or elevation of nasal tip

30420 including major septal repair

➲ *CPT Assistant* Jul 16:8

30430 Rhinoplasty, secondary; minor revision (small amount of nasal tip work)

30435 intermediate revision (bony work with osteotomies)

30450 major revision (nasal tip work and osteotomies)

30460 Rhinoplasty for nasal deformity secondary to congenital cleft lip and/or palate, including columellar lengthening; tip only

➲ *CPT Assistant* Dec 14:18

30462 tip, septum, osteotomies

➲ *CPT Assistant* Dec 14:18

30465 Repair of nasal vestibular stenosis (eg, spreader grafting, lateral nasal wall reconstruction)

➲ *CPT Changes: An Insider's View* 2001

(30465 excludes obtaining graft. For graft procedure, see 20900-20926, 21210)

(30465 is used to report a bilateral procedure. For unilateral procedure, use modifier 52)

Surgical Repair of Vestibular Stenosis
30465

An incision is made in the upper lateral cartilage and continued as an osteotomy of the medial aspect of the nasal bones. The spreader graft is placed to widen the nasal vestibule.

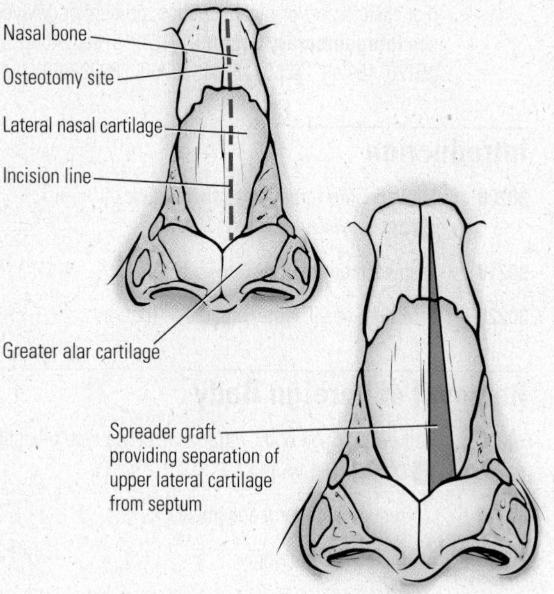

30520 Septoplasty or submucous resection, with or without cartilage scoring, contouring or replacement with graft
CPT Assistant Oct 97:11, Dec 02:10, Mar 12:9, Jul 15:10

(For submucous resection of turbinates, use 30140)

30540 Repair choanal atresia; intranasal

30545 transpalatine

(Do not report modifier 63 in conjunction with 30540, 30545)

30560 Lysis intranasal synechia

30580 Repair fistula; oromaxillary (combine with 31030 if antrotomy is included)

30600 oronasal

30620 Septal or other intranasal dermatoplasty (does not include obtaining graft)

30630 Repair nasal septal perforations
CPT Assistant Aug 12:13

Destruction

30801 Ablation, soft tissue of inferior turbinates, unilateral or bilateral, any method (eg, electrocautery, radiofrequency ablation, or tissue volume reduction); superficial
CPT Changes: An Insider's View 2002, 2006, 2010

(For ablation of superior or middle turbinates, use 30999)

30802 intramural (ie, submucosal)
CPT Changes: An Insider's View 2010
CPT Assistant Mar 08:14, Sep 10:10

(Do not report 30801 in conjunction with 30802)

(Do not report 30801, 30802, 30930 in conjunction with 30130 or 30140)

(For cautery performed for control of nasal hemorrhage, see 30901-30906)

Other Procedures

30901 Control nasal hemorrhage, anterior, simple (limited cautery and/or packing) any method

(To report bilateral procedure, use 30901 with modifier 50)

30903 Control nasal hemorrhage, anterior, complex (extensive cautery and/or packing) any method

(To report bilateral procedure, use 30903 with modifier 50)

30905 Control nasal hemorrhage, posterior, with posterior nasal packs and/or cautery, any method; initial
CPT Changes: An Insider's View 2002
CPT Assistant Sep 10:7

30906 subsequent

30915 Ligation arteries; ethmoidal

30920 internal maxillary artery, transantral

(For ligation external carotid artery, use 37600)

30930 Fracture nasal inferior turbinate(s), therapeutic
CPT Changes: An Insider's View 2006
CPT Assistant Jul 01:11, Dec 02:10, Jul 03:15, Aug 03:14, Dec 04:18, Sep 10:10, Jul 16:8

(Do not report 30801, 30802, 30930 in conjunction with 30130 or 30140)

(For fracture of superior or middle turbinate[s], use 30999)

30999 Unlisted procedure, nose
CPT Assistant Feb 13:13

Accessory Sinuses

Incision

31000 Lavage by cannulation; maxillary sinus (antrum puncture or natural ostium)
CPT Assistant Apr 14:10

(To report bilateral procedure, use 31000 with modifier 50)

31002 sphenoid sinus

31020 Sinusotomy, maxillary (antrotomy); intranasal

(To report bilateral procedure, use 31020 with modifier 50)

31030 radical (Caldwell-Luc) without removal of antrochoanal polyps

(To report bilateral procedure, use 31030 with modifier 50)

31032 radical (Caldwell-Luc) with removal of antrochoanal polyps

(To report bilateral procedure, use 31032 with modifier 50)

31040 Pterygomaxillary fossa surgery, any approach

(For transantral ligation of internal maxillary artery, use 30920)

31050 Sinusotomy, sphenoid, with or without biopsy;

31051 with mucosal stripping or removal of polyp(s)

31070 Sinusotomy frontal; external, simple (trephine operation)

(For frontal intranasal sinusotomy, use 31276)

Sinusotomy, Frontal
31070

A trephine is used to access the frontal sinus.

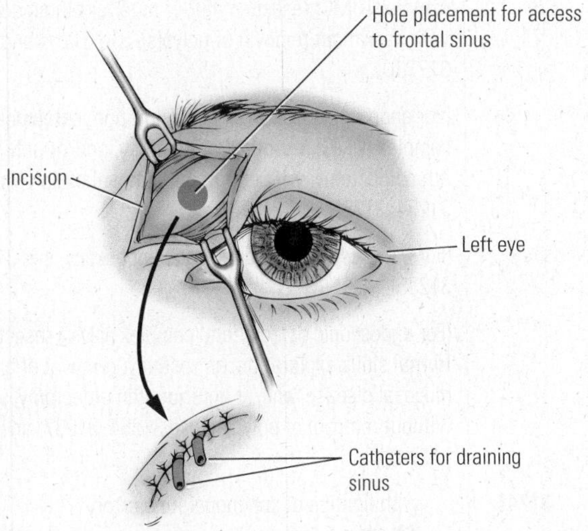

31075 transorbital, unilateral (for mucocele or osteoma, Lynch type)

31080 obliterative without osteoplastic flap, brow incision (includes ablation)

31081 obliterative, without osteoplastic flap, coronal incision (includes ablation)

31084 obliterative, with osteoplastic flap, brow incision

31085 obliterative, with osteoplastic flap, coronal incision

31086 nonobliterative, with osteoplastic flap, brow incision

31087 nonobliterative, with osteoplastic flap, coronal incision

31090 Sinusotomy, unilateral, 3 or more paranasal sinuses (frontal, maxillary, ethmoid, sphenoid)
➲ *CPT Assistant* Nov 97:15, Nov 98:11

Excision

31200 Ethmoidectomy; intranasal, anterior
➲ *CPT Assistant* Feb 16:10

31201 intranasal, total
➲ *CPT Assistant* Feb 16:10

31205 extranasal, total
➲ *CPT Assistant* Feb 16:10

31225 Maxillectomy; without orbital exenteration

31230 with orbital exenteration (en bloc)

(For orbital exenteration only, see 65110 et seq)

(For skin grafts, see 15120 et seq)

Endoscopy

A surgical sinus endoscopy includes a sinusotomy (when appropriate) and diagnostic endoscopy.

Codes 31295-31298 describe dilation of sinus ostia by displacement of tissue, any method, and include fluoroscopy if performed.

Stereotactic computer-assisted navigation may be used to facilitate the performance of endoscopic sinus surgery, and may be reported with 61782.

Codes 31233-31298 are used to report unilateral procedures unless otherwise specified.

Codes 31231-31235 for diagnostic evaluation refer to employing a nasal/sinus endoscope to inspect the interior of the nasal cavity and the middle and superior meatus, the turbinates, and the spheno-ethmoid recess. Any time a diagnostic evaluation is performed all these areas would be inspected and a separate code is not reported for each area. To report these services when all of the elements are not fully examined (eg, judged not clinically pertinent), or because the clinical situation precludes such exam (eg, technically unable, altered anatomy), append modifier 52 if repeat examination is not planned, or modifier 53 if repeat examination is planned.

Sinus Endoscopy
31231-31294

The physician uses an endoscope for visualizing and magnifying the internal structure of the sinuses.

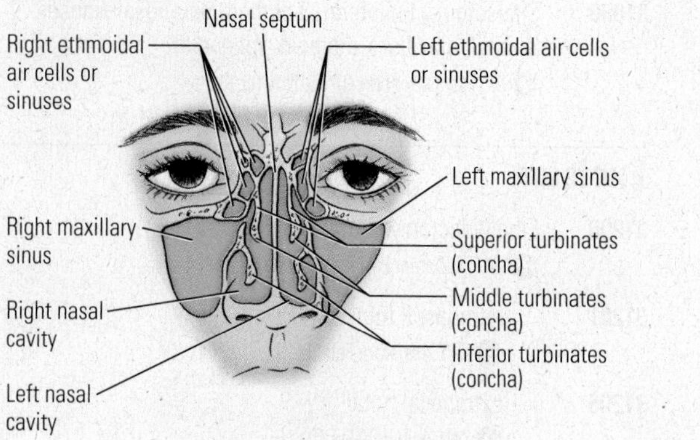

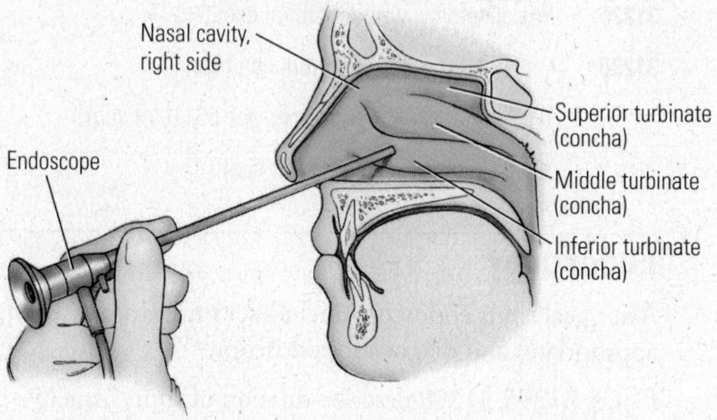

31231 Nasal endoscopy, diagnostic, unilateral or bilateral (separate procedure)
➔ *CPT Assistant* Winter 93:22, Jan 97:4, Feb 16:10, Jan 17:6, Apr 18:3

31233 Nasal/sinus endoscopy, diagnostic with maxillary sinusoscopy (via inferior meatus or canine fossa puncture)
➔ *CPT Assistant* Winter 93:22, Jan 97:4, Jun 11:11, Apr 18:3

(Do not report 31233 in conjunction with 31295 when performed on the same sinus)

31235 Nasal/sinus endoscopy, diagnostic with sphenoid sinusoscopy (via puncture of sphenoidal face or cannulation of ostium)
➔ *CPT Assistant* Winter 93:22, Jan 97:4, Apr 18:3

(Do not report 31235 in conjunction with 31297 when performed on the same sinus)

►(To report endoscopic placement of a drug-eluting implant in the ethmoid sinus without any other nasal/sinus endoscopic surgical service, use 31299. To report endoscopic placement of a drug-eluting implant in the ethmoid sinus in conjunction with biopsy, polypectomy, or debridement, use 31237)◄

31237 Nasal/sinus endoscopy, surgical; with biopsy, polypectomy or debridement (separate procedure)
➔ *CPT Assistant* Winter 93:23, Jan 97:4, Dec 01:6, May 03:5, Dec 11:13, Jan 15:13, Feb 16:10, Apr 18:3

31238 with control of nasal hemorrhage
➔ *CPT Changes: An Insider's View* 2002
➔ *CPT Assistant* Winter 93:23, Jan 97:4, Apr 18:3

(Do not report 31238 in conjunction with 31241, when performed on the ipsilateral side)

31239 with dacryocystorhinostomy
➔ *CPT Assistant* Winter 93:23, Jan 97:4, Apr 18:3

31240 with concha bullosa resection
➔ *CPT Assistant* Winter 93:23, Jan 97:4, May 03:5, Feb 16:10, Apr 18:3

(For endoscopic osteomeatal complex [OMC] resection with antrostomy and/or anterior ethmoidectomy, with or without removal of polyp[s], use 31254 and 31256)

(For endoscopic osteomeatal complex [OMC] resection with antrostomy, removal of antral mucosal disease, and/or anterior ethmoidectomy, with or without removal of polyp[s], use 31254 and 31267)

(For endoscopic frontal sinus exploration, osteomeatal complex [OMC] resection and/or anterior ethmoidectomy, with or without removal of polyp[s], use 31254 and 31276)

(For endoscopic frontal sinus exploration, osteomeatal complex [OMC] resection, antrostomy, and/or anterior ethmoidectomy, with or without removal of polyp[s], use 31254, 31256, and 31276)

(For endoscopic nasal diagnostic endoscopy, see 31231-31235)

(For endoscopic osteomeatal complex [OMC] resection, frontal sinus exploration, antrostomy, removal of antral mucosal disease, and/or anterior ethmoidectomy, with or without removal of polyp[s], use 31254, 31267, and 31276)

31241 with ligation of sphenopalatine artery
➔ *CPT Changes: An Insider's View* 2018
➔ *CPT Assistant* Apr 18:3

(Do not report 31241 in conjunction with 31238, when performed on the ipsilateral side)

31253 Code is out of numerical sequence. See 31254-31267

31254 Nasal/sinus endoscopy, surgical with ethmoidectomy; partial (anterior)
➔ *CPT Changes: An Insider's View* 2018
➔ *CPT Assistant* Winter 93:23, Jan 97:4, Sep 97:10, Oct 97:5, Dec 01:6, May 03:5, Jul 11:13, Feb 16:10, Apr 18:3

►(Do not report 31254 in conjunction with 31253, 31255, 31257, 31259, when performed on the ipsilateral side)◄

31255 total (anterior and posterior)

CPT Changes: An Insider's View 2018

CPT Assistant Winter 93:23, Jan 97:4, Dec 02:10, May 03:5, Jul 11:13, Feb 16:10, Apr 18:4

►(Do not report 31255 in conjunction with 31253, 31254, 31257, 31259, 31276, 31287, 31288, when performed on the ipsilateral side)◄

 # 31253 total (anterior and posterior), including frontal sinus exploration, with removal of tissue from frontal sinus, when performed

CPT Changes: An Insider's View 2018

CPT Assistant Apr 18:4

►(Do not report 31253 in conjunction with 31237, 31254, 31255, 31276, 31296, 31298, when performed on the ipsilateral side)◄

 # 31257 total (anterior and posterior), including sphenoidotomy

CPT Changes: An Insider's View 2018

CPT Assistant Apr 18:4

►(Do not report 31257 in conjunction with 31235, 31237, 31254, 31255, 31259, 31287, 31288, 31297, 31298, when performed on the ipsilateral side)◄

 # 31259 total (anterior and posterior), including sphenoidotomy, with removal of tissue from the sphenoid sinus

CPT Changes: An Insider's View 2018

CPT Assistant Apr 18:3

►(Do not report 31259 in conjunction with 31235, 31237, 31254, 31255, 31257, 31287, 31288, 31297, 31298, when performed on the ipsilateral side)◄

31256 Nasal/sinus endoscopy, surgical, with maxillary antrostomy;

CPT Assistant Winter 93:23, Jan 97:4, Jun 11:11, Jul 11:13, Jun 13:13, Apr 18:11

(For endoscopic anterior and posterior ethmoidectomy [APE] and antrostomy, with or without removal of polyp[s], use 31255 and 31256)

(For endoscopic anterior and posterior ethmoidectomy [APE], antrostomy and removal of antral mucosal disease, with or without removal of polyp[s], use 31255 and 31267)

(For endoscopic anterior and posterior ethmoidectomy [APE], and frontal sinus exploration, with or without removal of polyp[s], use 31255 and 31276)

31257 Code is out of numerical sequence. See 31254-31267

31259 Code is out of numerical sequence. See 31254-31267

31267 with removal of tissue from maxillary sinus

CPT Assistant Jan 97:4, Dec 01:6, Jun 11:11, Jul 11:13, Apr 18:3

(Do not report 31256, 31267 in conjunction with 31295 when performed on the same sinus)

(For endoscopic anterior and posterior ethmoidectomy [APE], and frontal sinus exploration and antrostomy, with or without removal of polyp[s], use 31255, 31256, and 31276)

(For endoscopic anterior and posterior ethmoidectomy [APE], frontal sinus exploration, antrostomy, and removal of antral mucosal disease, with or without removal of polyp[s], use 31255, 31267, and 31276)

31276 Nasal/sinus endoscopy, surgical, with frontal sinus exploration, including removal of tissue from frontal sinus, when performed

CPT Changes: An Insider's View 2018

CPT Assistant Winter 93:24, Jan 97:4, Jan 10:11, Jun 11:13, Apr 18:4

(Do not report 31276 in conjunction with 31253, 31255, 31296, 31298, when performed on the ipsilateral side)

(For endoscopic anterior and posterior ethmoidectomy and sphenoidotomy [APS], with or without removal of polyp[s], use 31255, 31287 or 31288)

(For endoscopic anterior and posterior ethmoidectomy and sphenoidotomy [APS], and antrostomy, with or without removal of polyp[s], use 31255, 31256, and 31287 or 31288)

(For endoscopic anterior and posterior ethmoidectomy and sphenoidotomy [APS], antrostomy and removal of antral mucosal disease, with or without removal of polyp[s], use 31255, 31267, and 31287 or 31288)

(For endoscopic anterior and posterior ethmoidectomy and sphenoidotomy [APS], and frontal sinus exploration with or without removal of polyp[s], use 31255, 31287 or 31288, and 31276)

(For endoscopic anterior and posterior ethmoidectomy and sphenoidotomy [APS], with or without removal of polyp[s], with frontal sinus exploration and antrostomy, use 31255, 31256, 31287 or 31288, and 31276)

(For unilateral endoscopy of 2 or more sinuses, see 31231-31235)

(For endoscopic anterior and posterior ethmoidectomy and sphenoidotomy [APS], frontal sinus exploration, antrostomy and removal of antral mucosal disease, with or without removal of polyp[s], see 31255, 31267, 31287 or 31288 and 31276)

31287 Nasal/sinus endoscopy, surgical, with sphenoidotomy;

CPT Assistant Winter 93:24, Jan 97:4, Jun 11:11, Apr 18:3

(Do not report 31287 in conjunction with 31235, 31255, 31257, 31259, 31288, 31297, 31298, when performed on the ipsilateral side)

31288 with removal of tissue from the sphenoid sinus

CPT Assistant Winter 93:24, Jan 97:4, Jun 11:11, Feb 16:10, Apr 18:3

(Do not report 31288 in conjunction with 31235, 31255, 31257, 31259, 31287, 31297, 31298, when performed on the ipsilateral side)

Respiratory 30000-32999

31290 Nasal/sinus endoscopy, surgical, with repair of cerebrospinal fluid leak; ethmoid region
➔ *CPT Assistant* Winter 93:24, Jan 97:4, Jul 11:13, Feb 16:10, Apr 18:3

31291 sphenoid region
➔ *CPT Assistant* Winter 93:24, Jan 97:4, Jul 11:13, Apr 18:3

31292 Nasal/sinus endoscopy, surgical; with medial or inferior orbital wall decompression
➔ *CPT Assistant* Winter 93:24, Jan 97:4, Jul 11:13, Apr 18:3

31293 with medial orbital wall and inferior orbital wall decompression
➔ *CPT Assistant* Winter 93:24, Jan 97:4, Jul 11:13, Apr 18:3

31294 with optic nerve decompression
➔ *CPT Assistant* Winter 93:24, Jan 97:4, Jul 11:13, Apr 18:3

31295 Nasal/sinus endoscopy, surgical; with dilation of maxillary sinus ostium (eg, balloon dilation), transnasal or via canine fossa
➔ *CPT Changes: An Insider's View* 2011
➔ *CPT Assistant* Jun 11:11, Apr 18:3

(Do not report 31295 in conjunction with 31233, 31256, 31267, when performed on the ipsilateral side)

31296 with dilation of frontal sinus ostium (eg, balloon dilation)
➔ *CPT Changes: An Insider's View* 2011
➔ *CPT Assistant* Jun 11:11, Apr 18:3

(Do not report 31296 in conjunction with 31253, 31276, 31297, 31298, when performed on the ipsilateral side)

31297 with dilation of sphenoid sinus ostium (eg, balloon dilation)
➔ *CPT Changes: An Insider's View* 2011
➔ *CPT Assistant* Jun 11:11, Apr 18:3

(Do not report 31297 in conjunction with 31235, 31257, 31259, 31287, 31288, 31296, 31298, when performed on the ipsilateral side)

31298 with dilation of frontal and sphenoid sinus ostia (eg, balloon dilation)
➔ *CPT Changes: An Insider's View* 2018
➔ *CPT Assistant* Apr 18:3

(Do not report 31298 in conjunction with 31235, 31237, 31253, 31257, 31259, 31276, 31287, 31288, 31296, 31297, when performed on the ipsilateral side)

Other Procedures

(For hypophysectomy, transantral or transeptal approach, use 61548)

(For transcranial hypophysectomy, use 61546)

31299 Unlisted procedure, accessory sinuses
➔ *CPT Assistant* Jan 10:11, Jun 11:11, Jun 13:13, Jul 15:10, Feb 16:10

Larynx

Excision

31300 Laryngotomy (thyrotomy, laryngofissure), with removal of tumor or laryngocele, cordectomy

(31320 has been deleted)

31360 Laryngectomy; total, without radical neck dissection
➔ *CPT Assistant* Aug 10:4

31365 total, with radical neck dissection
➔ *CPT Assistant* Oct 01:10, Aug 10:4

31367 subtotal supraglottic, without radical neck dissection
➔ *CPT Assistant* Aug 10:4

31368 subtotal supraglottic, with radical neck dissection

31370 Partial laryngectomy (hemilaryngectomy); horizontal

31375 laterovertical

31380 anterovertical

31382 antero-latero-vertical

31390 Pharyngolaryngectomy, with radical neck dissection; without reconstruction

31395 with reconstruction

31400 Arytenoidectomy or arytenoidopexy, external approach

(For endoscopic arytenoidectomy, use 31560)

31420 Epiglottidectomy

Introduction

⊘ **31500** Intubation, endotracheal, emergency procedure
➔ *CPT Assistant* Nov 99:32-33, Oct 03:2, Aug 04:8, Jul 06:4, Jul 07:1, Dec 09:10, May 16:3, Oct 16:8

31502 Tracheotomy tube change prior to establishment of fistula tract
➔ *CPT Assistant* Winter 90:6

Endoscopy

For endoscopic procedures, report appropriate endoscopy of each anatomic site examined. Laryngoscopy includes examination of the tongue base, larynx, and hypopharynx. The anatomic structures examined with this procedure include both midline (single anatomic sites) and paired structures. Midline, single anatomic sites include tongue base, vallecula, epiglottis, subglottis, and posterior pharyngeal wall. Paired structures include true vocal cords, arytenoids, false vocal cords, ventricles, pyriform sinuses, and aryepiglottic folds. For the purposes of reporting therapeutic interventions, all paired structures contained within one side of the larynx/pharynx are considered unilateral. If using operating microscope, telescope, or both, use the applicable code only once per operative session.

31505 Laryngoscopy, indirect; diagnostic (separate procedure)
➔ *CPT Changes: An Insider's View* 2000
➔ *CPT Assistant* Nov 99:13

31510 with biopsy
➔ *CPT Assistant* Nov 99:13

31511 with removal of foreign body
➔ *CPT Assistant* Nov 99:13

31512 with removal of lesion
➔ *CPT Assistant* Nov 99:13

31513 with vocal cord injection
➔ *CPT Assistant* Nov 99:13

31515 Laryngoscopy direct, with or without tracheoscopy; for aspiration

31520 diagnostic, newborn

(Do not report modifier 63 in conjunction with 31520)

31525 diagnostic, except newborn
➔ *CPT Assistant* Aug 10:3

31526 diagnostic, with operating microscope or telescope
➔ *CPT Changes: An Insider's View* 2006
➔ *CPT Assistant* Nov 98:11-12, Jun 17:10

(Do not report 31526 in conjunction with 69990)

31527 with insertion of obturator

31528 with dilation, initial
➔ *CPT Changes: An Insider's View* 2002

31529 with dilation, subsequent
➔ *CPT Changes: An Insider's View* 2002

31530 Laryngoscopy, direct, operative, with foreign body removal;

31531 with operating microscope or telescope
➔ *CPT Changes: An Insider's View* 2006
➔ *CPT Assistant* Nov 98:11-12, Jun 17:10

(Do not report code 69990 in addition to code 31531)

31535 Laryngoscopy, direct, operative, with biopsy;

31536 with operating microscope or telescope
➔ *CPT Changes: An Insider's View* 2006
➔ *CPT Assistant* Nov 98:11-12, Jun 17:10

(Do not report code 69990 in addition to code 31536)

31540 Laryngoscopy, direct, operative, with excision of tumor and/or stripping of vocal cords or epiglottis;

31541 with operating microscope or telescope
➔ *CPT Changes: An Insider's View* 2006
➔ *CPT Assistant* Nov 98:11-12, Jun 17:10

(Do not report code 69990 in addition to code 31541)

31545 Laryngoscopy, direct, operative, with operating microscope or telescope, with submucosal removal of non-neoplastic lesion(s) of vocal cord; reconstruction with local tissue flap(s)
➔ *CPT Changes: An Insider's View* 2005

31546 reconstruction with graft(s) (includes obtaining autograft)
➔ *CPT Changes: An Insider's View* 2005

(Do not report 31546 in addition to 20926 for graft harvest)

(For reconstruction of vocal cord with allograft, use 31599)

(Do not report 31545 or 31546 in conjunction with 31540, 31541, 69990)

31551 Code is out of numerical sequence. See 31579-31587

31552 Code is out of numerical sequence. See 31579-31587

31553 Code is out of numerical sequence. See 31579-31587

31554 Code is out of numerical sequence. See 31579-31587

31560 Laryngoscopy, direct, operative, with arytenoidectomy;

31561 with operating microscope or telescope
➔ *CPT Changes: An Insider's View* 2006
➔ *CPT Assistant* Nov 98:11-12, Jun 17:10

(Do not report code 69990 in addition to code 31561)

31570 Laryngoscopy, direct, with injection into vocal cord(s), therapeutic;
➔ *CPT Assistant* Jan 14:6, Jan 17:6

31571 with operating microscope or telescope
➔ *CPT Changes: An Insider's View* 2006
➔ *CPT Assistant* Nov 98:11-12, Nov 12:14, Jan 14:6, Jan 17:6, Jun 17:10

(Do not report 31571 in conjunction with 69990)

31572 Code is out of numerical sequence. See 31577-31580

31573 Code is out of numerical sequence. See 31577-31580

31574 Code is out of numerical sequence. See 31577-31580

31575 Laryngoscopy, flexible; diagnostic
➔ *CPT Changes: An Insider's View* 2017
➔ *CPT Assistant* Dec 16:13, Apr 17:8, Jul 17:7

(Do not report 31575 in conjunction with 31231, unless performed for a separate condition using a separate endoscope)

(Do not report 31575 in conjunction with 31572, 31573, 31574, 31576, 31577, 31578, 43197, 43198, 92511, 92612, 92614, 92616)

31576 with biopsy(ies)
➔ *CPT Changes: An Insider's View* 2017
➔ *CPT Assistant* Dec 16:13, Apr 17:8, Jul 17:7

(Do not report 31576 in conjunction with 31572, 31578)

31577 with removal of foreign body(s)
➔ *CPT Changes: An Insider's View* 2017
➔ *CPT Assistant* Dec 16:13, Apr 17:8, Jul 17:7

31578 with removal of lesion(s), non-laser
➔ *CPT Changes: An Insider's View* 2017
➔ *CPT Assistant* Dec 16:13, Apr 17:8, Jul 17:7

 # 31572 with ablation or destruction of lesion(s) with laser, unilateral
➲ *CPT Changes: An Insider's View* 2017
➲ *CPT Assistant* Dec 16:13, Apr 17:8, Jul 17:7

(Do not report 31572 in conjunction with 31576, 31578)

(To report flexible endoscopic evaluation of swallowing, see 92612-92613)

(To report flexible endoscopic evaluation with sensory testing, see 92614-92615)

(To report flexible endoscopic evaluation of swallowing with sensory testing, see 92616-92617)

(For flexible laryngoscopy as part of flexible endoscopic evaluation of swallowing and/or laryngeal sensory testing by cine or video recording, see 92612-92617)

 # 31573 with therapeutic injection(s) (eg, chemodenervation agent or corticosteroid, injected percutaneous, transoral, or via endoscope channel), unilateral
➲ *CPT Changes: An Insider's View* 2017
➲ *CPT Assistant* Dec 16:13, Apr 17:8, Jul 17:7

 # 31574 with injection(s) for augmentation (eg, percutaneous, transoral), unilateral
➲ *CPT Changes: An Insider's View* 2017
➲ *CPT Assistant* Dec 16:13, Apr 17:8, Jul 17:7

31579 Laryngoscopy, flexible or rigid telescopic, with stroboscopy
➲ *CPT Changes: An Insider's View* 2017
➲ *CPT Assistant* Dec 16:13, Apr 17:8, Jul 17:7

Repair

31580 Laryngoplasty; for laryngeal web, with indwelling keel or stent insertion
➲ *CPT Changes: An Insider's View* 2017
➲ *CPT Assistant* Mar 17:10, Apr 17:5

(Do not report 31580 in conjunction with 31551, 31552, 31553, 31554)

(To report tracheostomy, see 31600, 31601, 31603, 31605, 31610)

(To report removal of the keel or stent, use 31599)

(31582 has been deleted. To report, see 31551, 31552, 31553, 31554)

 # 31551 for laryngeal stenosis, with graft, without indwelling stent placement, younger than 12 years of age
➲ *CPT Changes: An Insider's View* 2017
➲ *CPT Assistant* Mar 17:10, Apr 17:5, Jul 17:7

(Do not report graft separately if harvested through the laryngoplasty incision [eg, thyroid cartilage graft])

(Do not report 31551 in conjunction with 31552, 31553, 31554, 31580)

(To report tracheostomy, see 31600, 31601, 31603, 31605, 31610)

 # 31552 for laryngeal stenosis, with graft, without indwelling stent placement, age 12 years or older
➲ *CPT Changes: An Insider's View* 2017
➲ *CPT Assistant* Mar 17:10, Apr 17:5, Jul 17:7

(Do not report graft separately if harvested through the laryngoplasty incision [eg, thyroid cartilage graft])

(Do not report 31552 in conjunction with 31551, 31553, 31554, 31580)

(To report tracheostomy, see 31600, 31601, 31603, 31605, 31610)

 # 31553 for laryngeal stenosis, with graft, with indwelling stent placement, younger than 12 years of age
➲ *CPT Changes: An Insider's View* 2017
➲ *CPT Assistant* Mar 17:10, Apr 17:5, Jul 17:7

(Do not report graft separately if harvested through the laryngoplasty incision [eg, thyroid cartilage graft])

(Do not report 31553 in conjunction with 31551, 31552, 31554, 31580)

(To report tracheostomy, see 31600, 31601, 31603, 31605, 31610)

(To report removal of the stent, use 31599)

 # 31554 for laryngeal stenosis, with graft, with indwelling stent placement, age 12 years or older
➲ *CPT Changes: An Insider's View* 2017
➲ *CPT Assistant* Mar 17:10, Apr 17:5, Jul 17:7

(Do not report graft separately if harvested through the laryngoplasty incision [eg, thyroid cartilage graft])

(Do not report 31554 in conjunction with 31551, 31552, 31553, 31580)

(To report tracheostomy, see 31600, 31601, 31603, 31605, 31610)

(To report removal of the stent, use 31599)

31584 with open reduction and fixation of (eg, plating) fracture, includes tracheostomy, if performed
➲ *CPT Changes: An Insider's View* 2017
➲ *CPT Assistant* Mar 17:10, Apr 17:5

(Do not report graft separately if harvested through the laryngoplasty incision [eg, thyroid cartilage graft])

31587 Laryngoplasty, cricoid split, without graft placement
➲ *CPT Changes: An Insider's View* 2017
➲ *CPT Assistant* Mar 17:10, Apr 17:5

(To report tracheostomy, see 31600, 31601, 31603, 31605, 31610)

(31588 has been deleted. To report laryngoplasty not otherwise specified, use 31599)

31590 Laryngeal reinnervation by neuromuscular pedicle
➲ *CPT Assistant* Mar 17:10

31591 Laryngoplasty, medialization, unilateral
➲ *CPT Changes: An Insider's View* 2017
➲ *CPT Assistant* Mar 17:10, Apr 17:5, Jul 17:7

31592 Cricotracheal resection
➲ *CPT Changes: An Insider's View* 2017
➲ *CPT Assistant* Feb 17:14, Mar 17:10, Apr 17:5, Jul 17:7

(Do not report graft separately if harvested through cricotracheal resection incision [eg, trachealis muscle])

(Do not report local advancement and rotational flaps separately if performed through the same incision)

(To report tracheostomy, see 31600, 31601, 31603, 31605, 31610)

(To report excision of tracheal stenosis and anastomosis, see 31780, 31781)

Destruction

►(31595 has been deleted)◄

Other Procedures

31599 Unlisted procedure, larynx
➲ *CPT Assistant* Nov 12:14, Jan 17:6

Trachea and Bronchi

Incision

31600 Tracheostomy, planned (separate procedure);
➲ *CPT Assistant* Aug 10:5

31601 younger than 2 years

31603 Tracheostomy, emergency procedure; transtracheal

31605 cricothyroid membrane

31610 Tracheostomy, fenestration procedure with skin flaps

(For endotracheal intubation, use 31500)

(For tracheal aspiration under direct vision, use 31515)

31611 Construction of tracheoesophageal fistula and subsequent insertion of an alaryngeal speech prosthesis (eg, voice button, Blom-Singer prosthesis)

31612 Tracheal puncture, percutaneous with transtracheal aspiration and/or injection

31613 Tracheostoma revision; simple, without flap rotation

31614 complex, with flap rotation

Endoscopy

For endoscopy procedures, code appropriate endoscopy of each anatomic site examined. Surgical bronchoscopy always includes diagnostic bronchoscopy when performed by the same physician. Codes 31622-31651, 31660, 31661 include fluoroscopic guidance, when performed.

Codes 31652 and 31653 are complete services used for sampling (eg, aspiration/biopsy) lymph node(s) or adjacent structure(s) utilizing endobronchial ultrasound (EBUS) and are reported separately. Code 31654 is an add-on code and should be reported for identifying one or more peripheral lesion(s) with transendoscopic ultrasound.

31615 Tracheobronchoscopy through established tracheostomy incision
➲ *CPT Changes: An Insider's View* 2017
➲ *CPT Assistant* Feb 10:6, Nov 12:14

(For tracheoscopy, see laryngoscopy codes 31515-31574)

(For bronchoscopy with endobronchial ultrasound [EBUS] guided transtracheal/transbronchial sampling of mediastinal and/or hilar lymph node stations or structures, see 31652, 31653. For transendoscopic ultrasound during bronchoscopic diagnostic or therapeutic intervention[s] for peripheral lesion[s], use 31654)

31622 Bronchoscopy, rigid or flexible, including fluoroscopic guidance, when performed; diagnostic, with cell washing, when performed (separate procedure)
➲ *CPT Changes: An Insider's View* 2004, 2010, 2017
➲ *CPT Assistant* Jul 96:11, Nov 98:12, Dec 98:8, Mar 99:3, Apr 00:10, Jun 01:10, Jan 02:10, Sep 04:8, 12, Aug 05:4, Dec 09:10, Feb 10:6, Apr 10:5, Feb 11:8

31623 with brushing or protected brushings
➲ *CPT Changes: An Insider's View* 2017
➲ *CPT Assistant* Nov 98:12, Mar 99:3, Nov 99:13, Jan 02:10, Sep 04:8, Aug 05:4, May 08:15, Apr 10:5, Mar 13:8

31624 with bronchial alveolar lavage
➲ *CPT Changes: An Insider's View* 2017
➲ *CPT Assistant* Nov 98:12, Feb 99:9, Mar 99:3, 11, Jan 02:10, Sep 04:8, Aug 05:4, May 08:15, Feb 10:6, Apr 10:5, Mar 13:8, Jun 17:10

31625 with bronchial or endobronchial biopsy(s), single or multiple sites
➲ *CPT Changes: An Insider's View* 2004, 2017
➲ *CPT Assistant* Spring 91:2, Jan 02:10, Jun 02:10, Sep 03:15, Sep 04:9, Aug 05:4, Feb 10:6, Apr 10:5, Mar 13:8

Bronchoscopy

31622-31661

A rigid or flexible bronchoscope is inserted through the oropharynx and vocal cords and beyond the trachea into the right or left bronchi.

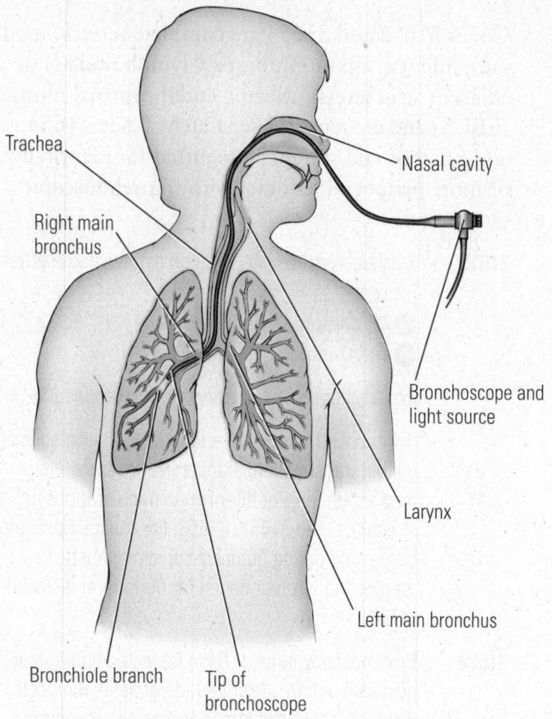

31626 with placement of fiducial markers, single or multiple
- *CPT Changes: An Insider's View* 2010, 2017
- *CPT Assistant* Feb 10:6, Apr 10:5, Jan 11:6, Mar 13:8, Jun 15:6, Jun 17:10

(Report supply of device separately)

+ 31627 with computer-assisted, image-guided navigation (List separately in addition to code for primary procedure[s])
- *CPT Changes: An Insider's View* 2010, 2017
- *CPT Assistant* Feb 10:6, Apr 10:5, Jan 11:6, Mar 13:8

(31627 includes 3D reconstruction. Do not report 31627 in conjunction with 76376, 76377)

(Use 31627 in conjunction with 31615, 31622-31626, 31628-31631, 31635, 31636, 31638-31643)

31628 with transbronchial lung biopsy(s), single lobe
- *CPT Changes: An Insider's View* 2004, 2017
- *CPT Assistant* Jun 01:10, Jan 02:10, Sep 04:9, Aug 05:4, May 08:15, Feb 10:6, Apr 10:5, Mar 13:8, Jun 17:10

(31628 should be reported only once regardless of how many transbronchial lung biopsies are performed in a lobe)

(To report transbronchial lung biopsies performed on additional lobe, use 31632)

31629 with transbronchial needle aspiration biopsy(s), trachea, main stem and/or lobar bronchus(i)
- *CPT Changes: An Insider's View* 2004, 2017
- *CPT Assistant* Apr 00:10, Jan 02:10, Sep 03:15, May 04:15, Jul 04:13, Aug 05:4, Nov 09:8, Feb 10:6, Apr 10:5, Apr 11:12, Mar 13:8

(31629 should be reported only once for upper airway biopsies regardless of how many transbronchial needle aspiration biopsies are performed in the upper airway or in a lobe)

(To report transbronchial needle aspiration biopsies performed on additional lobe[s], use 31633)

31630 with tracheal/bronchial dilation or closed reduction of fracture
- *CPT Changes: An Insider's View* 2005
- *CPT Assistant* Jan 02:10, Aug 05:4, Feb 10:6, Apr 10:5, Mar 13:8

31631 with placement of tracheal stent(s) (includes tracheal/bronchial dilation as required)
- *CPT Changes: An Insider's View* 2005
- *CPT Assistant* Jan 02:10, Aug 05:4, Feb 10:6, Apr 10:5, Mar 13:8

(For placement of bronchial stent, see 31636, 31637)

(For revision of tracheal/bronchial stent, use 31638)

+ 31632 with transbronchial lung biopsy(s), each additional lobe (List separately in addition to code for primary procedure)
- *CPT Changes: An Insider's View* 2004, 2016, 2017
- *CPT Assistant* Jan 02:10, Sep 04:9, Aug 05:4, Mar 13:8

(Use 31632 in conjunction with 31628)

(31632 should be reported only once regardless of how many transbronchial lung biopsies are performed in a lobe)

+ 31633 with transbronchial needle aspiration biopsy(s), each additional lobe (List separately in addition to code for primary procedure)
- *CPT Changes: An Insider's View* 2004, 2016, 2017
- *CPT Assistant* Jan 02:10, May 04:15, Jul 04:13, Sep 04:10, Aug 05:4, Nov 09:8, Apr 11:12, Mar 13:8

(Use 31633 in conjunction with 31629)

(31633 should be reported only once regardless of how many transbronchial needle aspiration biopsies are performed in the trachea or the additional lobe)

31634 with balloon occlusion, with assessment of air leak, with administration of occlusive substance (eg, fibrin glue), if performed
- *CPT Changes: An Insider's View* 2011, 2017
- *CPT Assistant* Jan 11:6, Mar 13:8

(Do not report 31634 in conjunction with 31647, 31651 at the same session)

31635 with removal of foreign body
- *CPT Changes: An Insider's View* 2017
- *CPT Assistant* Jan 02:10, Jun 02:10, Feb 10:6, Apr 10:5, Jan 11:6, Mar 13:8

(For removal of implanted bronchial valves, see 31648-31649)

31636 with placement of bronchial stent(s) (includes tracheal/bronchial dilation as required), initial bronchus

➔ *CPT Changes: An Insider's View* 2005

➔ *CPT Assistant* Aug 05:4, Apr 10:5, Mar 13:8

+ 31637 each additional major bronchus stented (List separately in addition to code for primary procedure)

➔ *CPT Changes: An Insider's View* 2005

➔ *CPT Assistant* Aug 05:4, Mar 13:8

(Use 31637 in conjunction with 31636)

31638 with revision of tracheal or bronchial stent inserted at previous session (includes tracheal/bronchial dilation as required)

➔ *CPT Changes: An Insider's View* 2005

➔ *CPT Assistant* Aug 05:4, Apr 10:5, Mar 13:8

31640 with excision of tumor

➔ *CPT Assistant* Jan 02:10, Aug 05:4, Apr 10:5, Mar 13:8

31641 with destruction of tumor or relief of stenosis by any method other than excision (eg, laser therapy, cryotherapy)

➔ *CPT Changes: An Insider's View* 2002, 2010

➔ *CPT Assistant* Nov 99:13, Sep 00:5, Jan 02:10, Aug 05:4, Apr 10:5, Oct 11:11, Mar 13:8, Apr 13:8

(For bronchoscopic photodynamic therapy, report 31641 in addition to 96570, 96571 as appropriate)

31643 with placement of catheter(s) for intracavitary radioelement application

➔ *CPT Changes: An Insider's View* 2010

➔ *CPT Assistant* Nov 98:12, Mar 99:3, Jan 02:10, Aug 05:4, Apr 09:3, Mar 13:8

(For intracavitary radioelement application, see 77761-77763, 77770, 77771, 77772)

31645 with therapeutic aspiration of tracheobronchial tree, initial

➔ *CPT Changes: An Insider's View* 2010, 2017, 2018

➔ *CPT Assistant* Jan 02:10, Aug 05:4, Mar 13:8

31646 with therapeutic aspiration of tracheobronchial tree, subsequent, same hospital stay

➔ *CPT Changes: An Insider's View* 2010, 2017, 2018

➔ *CPT Assistant* Jan 02:10, Aug 05:4, Mar 13:8

(For catheter aspiration of tracheobronchial tree with fiberscope at bedside, use 31725)

31647 with balloon occlusion, when performed, assessment of air leak, airway sizing, and insertion of bronchial valve(s), initial lobe

➔ *CPT Changes: An Insider's View* 2013, 2017

➔ *CPT Assistant* Mar 13:8

#+ 31651 with balloon occlusion, when performed, assessment of air leak, airway sizing, and insertion of bronchial valve(s), each additional lobe (List separately in addition to code for primary procedure[s])

➔ *CPT Changes: An Insider's View* 2013, 2017

➔ *CPT Assistant* Mar 13:8

(Use 31651 in conjunction with 31647)

31648 with removal of bronchial valve(s), initial lobe

➔ *CPT Changes: An Insider's View* 2013, 2017

➔ *CPT Assistant* Mar 13:8

(For removal and insertion of a bronchial valve at the same session, see 31647, 31648, and 31651)

+ 31649 with removal of bronchial valve(s), each additional lobe (List separately in addition to code for primary procedure)

➔ *CPT Changes: An Insider's View* 2013, 2017

➔ *CPT Assistant* Mar 13:8

(Use 31649 in conjunction with 31648)

31651 Code is out of numerical sequence. See 31646-31649

31652 with endobronchial ultrasound (EBUS) guided transtracheal and/or transbronchial sampling (eg, aspiration[s]/biopsy[ies]), one or two mediastinal and/or hilar lymph node stations or structures

➔ *CPT Changes: An Insider's View* 2016, 2017

➔ *CPT Assistant* Apr 16:5

31653 with endobronchial ultrasound (EBUS) guided transtracheal and/or transbronchial sampling (eg, aspiration[s]/biopsy[ies]), 3 or more mediastinal and/or hilar lymph node stations or structures

➔ *CPT Changes: An Insider's View* 2016, 2017

➔ *CPT Assistant* Apr 16:5

+ 31654 with transendoscopic endobronchial ultrasound (EBUS) during bronchoscopic diagnostic or therapeutic intervention(s) for peripheral lesion(s) (List separately in addition to code for primary procedure[s])

➔ *CPT Changes: An Insider's View* 2016, 2017

➔ *CPT Assistant* Apr 16:5

(Use 31654 in conjunction with 31622, 31623, 31624, 31625, 31626, 31628, 31629, 31640, 31643, 31645, 31646)

(For EBUS to access mediastinal or hilar lymph node station[s] or adjacent structure[s], see 31652, 31653)

(Report 31652, 31653, 31654 only once per session)

Bronchial Thermoplasty

31660 Bronchoscopy, rigid or flexible, including fluoroscopic guidance, when performed; with bronchial thermoplasty, 1 lobe

➔ *CPT Changes: An Insider's View* 2013, 2017

➔ *CPT Assistant* Mar 13:8

31661 with bronchial thermoplasty, 2 or more lobes
➔ *CPT Changes: An Insider's View* 2013, 2017
➔ *CPT Assistant* Mar 13:8

Introduction

(For endotracheal intubation, use 31500)

(For tracheal aspiration under direct vision, see 31515)

31717 Catheterization with bronchial brush biopsy
➔ *CPT Assistant* Feb 01:11

31720 Catheter aspiration (separate procedure); nasotracheal

31725 tracheobronchial with fiberscope, bedside
➔ *CPT Changes: An Insider's View* 2017

31730 Transtracheal (percutaneous) introduction of needle wire dilator/stent or indwelling tube for oxygen therapy

Excision, Repair

31750 Tracheoplasty; cervical
➔ *CPT Assistant* Jul 11:12

31755 tracheopharyngeal fistulization, each stage

31760 intrathoracic

31766 Carinal reconstruction

31770 Bronchoplasty; graft repair

31775 excision stenosis and anastomosis

(For lobectomy and bronchoplasty, use 32501)

31780 Excision tracheal stenosis and anastomosis; cervical
➔ *CPT Assistant* Feb 17:14

31781 cervicothoracic
➔ *CPT Assistant* Feb 17:14

31785 Excision of tracheal tumor or carcinoma; cervical

31786 thoracic

31800 Suture of tracheal wound or injury; cervical

31805 intrathoracic

31820 Surgical closure tracheostomy or fistula; without plastic repair

31825 with plastic repair

(For repair tracheoesophageal fistula, see 43305, 43312)

31830 Revision of tracheostomy scar

Other Procedures

31899 Unlisted procedure, trachea, bronchi
➔ *CPT Assistant* Jan 10:11, May 14:10

Lungs and Pleura

Pleural cavity or lung biopsy procedures may be accomplished using a percutaneous, thoracoscopic (Video-Assisted Thoracoscopic Surgery [VATS]), or thoracotomy approach. They involve the removal of differing amounts of tissue for diagnosis. A biopsy may be performed using different techniques such as incision or wedge. Lung resection procedures include diagnostic and therapeutic procedures, including the removal of blebs, bullae, cysts, and benign or malignant tumors or lesions. These procedures may involve the removal of small portions of the lung or even an entire lung. Additionally, lung resection procedures may require the removal of adjacent structures. Both diagnostic lung biopsies and therapeutic lung resections can be performed utilizing a wedge technique. However, a diagnostic biopsy of a lung nodule using a wedge technique requires only that a tissue sample be obtained without particular attention to resection margins. A therapeutic wedge resection requires attention to margins and complete resection even when the wedge resection is ultimately followed by a more extensive resection. In the case of a wedge resection in which intraoperative pathology consultation determines that a more extensive resection is required in the same anatomic location, it becomes classified as a diagnostic wedge resection (32507, 32668). When no more extensive resection is required, the same procedure is a therapeutic wedge resection (32505, 32666).

Pleural or lung biopsies or diagnostic wedge resections should be reported using codes 32096, 32097, 32098, 32400, 32405, 32507, 32607, 32608, 32609, or 32668. The open or thoracoscopic (VATS) therapeutic resection of lung mass or nodules via a wedge resection is reported using codes 32505, 32506, 32666, and 32667. More extensive anatomic lung resection procedures, which can be performed with either thoracotomy or thoracoscopic (VATS) approaches, include: segmentectomy, lobectomy, bilobectomy, and pneumonectomy.

When diagnostic biopsy(ies) of the lung are performed, regardless of the approach (ie, open or thoracoscopic [VATS]) or technique (eg, incisional resection, cautery resection, or stapled wedge), and the specimen is sent for intraoperative pathology consultation, and during that same operative session the surgeon uses these results to determine the extent of the necessary surgical resection that includes the anatomical location biopsied, only the most extensive procedure performed (eg, segmentectomy, lobectomy, thoracoscopic [VATS] lobectomy) should be reported.

The therapeutic wedge resection codes (32505, 32506, 32666, or 32667) should not be reported in addition to the more extensive lung procedure (eg, lobectomy) unless the therapeutic wedge resection was performed on a different lobe or on the contralateral lung, whether or not an intraoperative pathology consultation is used to determine the extent of lung resection. When a diagnostic wedge resection is followed by a more extensive procedure in the same anatomical location, report add-on codes 32507 or 32668 with the more extensive procedure(s). When a therapeutic wedge resection (32505, 32506, 32666, or 32667) is performed in a different lobe than the more extensive lung resection (eg, lobectomy), report the therapeutic wedge resection with modifier 59.

Incision

32035 Thoracostomy; with rib resection for empyema

32036 with open flap drainage for empyema

(To report wound exploration due to penetrating trauma without thoractomy, use 20101)

32096 Thoracotomy, with diagnostic biopsy(ies) of lung infiltrate(s) (eg, wedge, incisional), unilateral

➲ *CPT Changes: An Insider's View* 2012

➲ *CPT Assistant* Sep 12:3

(Do not report 32096 more than once per lung)

(Do not report 32096 in conjunction with 32440, 32442, 32445, 32488)

32097 Thoracotomy, with diagnostic biopsy(ies) of lung nodule(s) or mass(es) (eg, wedge, incisional), unilateral

➲ *CPT Changes: An Insider's View* 2012

➲ *CPT Assistant* Sep 12:3

(Do not report 32097 more than once per lung)

(Do not report 32097 in conjunction with 32440, 32442, 32445, 32488)

32098 Thoracotomy, with biopsy(ies) of pleura

➲ *CPT Changes: An Insider's View* 2012

➲ *CPT Assistant* Sep 12:3

32100 Thoracotomy; with exploration

➲ *CPT Changes: An Insider's View* 2012

➲ *CPT Assistant* Mar 07:1, Sep 12:3, Jan 13:6

(Do not report 32100 in conjunction with 19260, 19271, 19272, 32503, 32504, 33955, 33956, 33957, 33963, 33964)

32110 with control of traumatic hemorrhage and/or repair of lung tear

➲ *CPT Changes: An Insider's View* 2012

➲ *CPT Assistant* Sep 12:3

32120 for postoperative complications

➲ *CPT Changes: An Insider's View* 2012

32124 with open intrapleural pneumonolysis

➲ *CPT Changes: An Insider's View* 2012

➲ *CPT Assistant* Sep 12:3

32140 with cyst(s) removal, includes pleural procedure when performed

➲ *CPT Changes: An Insider's View* 2012

➲ *CPT Assistant* Sep 12:3

32141 with resection-plication of bullae, includes any pleural procedure when performed

➲ *CPT Changes: An Insider's View* 2012

➲ *CPT Assistant* Sep 12:3

(For lung volume reduction, use 32491)

32150 with removal of intrapleural foreign body or fibrin deposit

➲ *CPT Changes: An Insider's View* 2012

➲ *CPT Assistant* Sep 12:3

32151 with removal of intrapulmonary foreign body

➲ *CPT Changes: An Insider's View* 2012

32160 with cardiac massage

➲ *CPT Changes: An Insider's View* 2012

(For segmental or other resections of lung, see 32480-32504)

32200 Pneumonostomy, with open drainage of abscess or cyst

➲ *CPT Assistant* Nov 97:15

(For percutaneous image-guided drainage of abscess or cyst of lungs or mediastinum by catheter placement, use 49405)

32215 Pleural scarification for repeat pneumothorax

32220 Decortication, pulmonary (separate procedure); total

32225 partial

Excision/Resection

32310 Pleurectomy, parietal (separate procedure)

32320 Decortication and parietal pleurectomy

32400 Biopsy, pleura, percutaneous needle

➲ *CPT Assistant* Fall 94:1-2

➲ *Clinical Examples in Radiology* Summer 08:5, 6, Winter 17:5

(If imaging guidance is performed, see 76942, 77002, 77012, 77021)

►(For fine needle aspiration biopsy, see 10004, 10005, 10006, 10007, 10008, 10009, 10010, 10011, 10012, 10021)◄

32405 Biopsy, lung or mediastinum, percutaneous needle

➲ *CPT Changes: An Insider's View* 2012, 2017

➲ *CPT Assistant* Fall 94:1-2, Mar 97:4, Aug 02:10

➲ *Clinical Examples in Radiology* Summer 08:5, 6, Winter 17:5

(For open biopsy of lung, see 32096, 32097. For open biopsy of mediastinum, see 39000 or 39010. For thoracoscopic [VATS] biopsy of lung, pleura, pericardium, or mediastinal space structure, see 32604, 32606, 32607, 32608, 32609)

(For radiological supervision and interpretation, see 76942, 77002, 77012, 77021)

►(For fine needle aspiration biopsy, see 10005, 10006, 10007, 10008, 10009, 10010, 10011, 10012)◄

Removal

32440 Removal of lung, pneumonectomy;

➲ *CPT Changes: An Insider's View* 2012

➲ *CPT Assistant* Fall 94:1, Sep 12:3

32442 with resection of segment of trachea followed by broncho-tracheal anastomosis (sleeve pneumonectomy)
➔ *CPT Changes: An Insider's View* 2012
➔ *CPT Assistant* Fall 94:1, 3, Jun 17:10

32445 extrapleural
➔ *CPT Changes: An Insider's View* 2012
➔ *CPT Assistant* Fall 94:1, 3, Sep 12:3

(For extrapleural pneumonectomy, with empyemectomy, use 32445 and 32540)

(If lung resection is performed with chest wall tumor resection, report the appropriate chest wall tumor resection 19260-19272, in addition to lung resection 32440-32445)

32480 Removal of lung, other than pneumonectomy; single lobe (lobectomy)
➔ *CPT Changes: An Insider's View* 2012
➔ *CPT Assistant* Spring 91:5, Fall 94:1, 4, Sep 12:3

32482 2 lobes (bilobectomy)
➔ *CPT Changes: An Insider's View* 2012
➔ *CPT Assistant* Fall 94:1, 4, Jan 07:31, Sep 12:3

32484 single segment (segmentectomy)
➔ *CPT Changes: An Insider's View* 2012
➔ *CPT Assistant* Fall 94:1, 4, Sep 12:3

(For removal of lung with bronchoplasty, use 32501)

32486 with circumferential resection of segment of bronchus followed by broncho-bronchial anastomosis (sleeve lobectomy)
➔ *CPT Changes: An Insider's View* 2012
➔ *CPT Assistant* Fall 94:1, 4, Jun 17:10

32488 with all remaining lung following previous removal of a portion of lung (completion pneumonectomy)
➔ *CPT Changes: An Insider's View* 2012
➔ *CPT Assistant* Fall 94:1, 4, Sep 12:3

(For lobectomy or segmentectomy, with concomitant decortication, use 32320 and the appropriate removal of lung code)

32491 with resection-plication of emphysematous lung(s) (bullous or non-bullous) for lung volume reduction, sternal split or transthoracic approach, includes any pleural procedure, when performed
➔ *CPT Changes: An Insider's View* 2012
➔ *CPT Assistant* Nov 96:7, Sep 12:3

(If lung resection is performed with chest wall tumor resection, report the appropriate chest wall tumor resection 19260-19272, in addition to lung resection 32480, 32482, 32484, 32486, 32488, 32505, 32506, 32507)

+ 32501 Resection and repair of portion of bronchus (bronchoplasty) when performed at time of lobectomy or segmentectomy (List separately in addition to code for primary procedure)

(Use 32501 in conjunction with 32480, 32482, 32484)

(32501 is to be used when a portion of the bronchus to preserved lung is removed and requires plastic closure to preserve function of that preserved lung. It is not to be used for closure for the proximal end of a resected bronchus)

32503 Resection of apical lung tumor (eg, Pancoast tumor), including chest wall resection, rib(s) resection(s), neurovascular dissection, when performed; without chest wall reconstruction(s)
➔ *CPT Changes: An Insider's View* 2006

32504 with chest wall reconstruction
➔ *CPT Changes: An Insider's View* 2006

(Do not report 32503, 32504 in conjunction with 19260, 19271, 19272, 32100, 32551, 32554, 32555)

32505 Thoracotomy; with therapeutic wedge resection (eg, mass, nodule), initial
➔ *CPT Changes: An Insider's View* 2012
➔ *CPT Assistant* Sep 12:3

(Do not report 32505 in conjunction with 32440, 32442, 32445, 32488)

+ 32506 with therapeutic wedge resection (eg, mass or nodule), each additional resection, ipsilateral (List separately in addition to code for primary procedure)
➔ *CPT Changes: An Insider's View* 2012
➔ *CPT Assistant* Sep 12:3

(Report 32506 only in conjunction with 32505)

(If lung resection is performed with chest wall tumor resection, report the appropriate chest wall tumor resection 19260-19272, in addition to lung resection 32480, 32482, 32484, 32486, 32488, 32505, 32506, 32507)

+ 32507 with diagnostic wedge resection followed by anatomic lung resection (List separately in addition to code for primary procedure)
➔ *CPT Changes: An Insider's View* 2012
➔ *CPT Assistant* Sep 12:3

(Report 32507 in conjunction with 32440, 32442, 32445, 32480, 32482, 32484, 32486, 32488, 32503, 32504)

32540 Extrapleural enucleation of empyema (empyemectomy)

(For extrapleural enucleation of empyema [empyemectomy] with lobectomy, use 32540 and the appropriate removal of lung code)

Introduction and Removal

32550 Insertion of indwelling tunneled pleural catheter with cuff
➔ *CPT Changes: An Insider's View* 2008, 2017
➔ *CPT Assistant* Jul 10:10, Mar 14:14, May 14:3

(Do not report 32550 in conjunction with 32554, 32555, 32556, 32557 when performed on the same side of the chest)

(If imaging guidance is performed, use 75989)

32551 Tube thoracostomy, includes connection to drainage system (eg, water seal), when performed, open (separate procedure)

►(Do not report 32551 in conjunction with 33020, 33025, if pleural drain/chest tube is placed on the ipsilateral side)◄

➲ *CPT Changes: An Insider's View* 2008, 2013, 2017

➲ *CPT Assistant* Feb 09:7, Sep 10:6, Aug 11:4, Nov 12:3, May 14:3, Jun 17:10

➲ *Clinical Examples in Radiology* Fall 10:10, Winter 13:5

32552 Removal of indwelling tunneled pleural catheter with cuff

➲ *CPT Changes: An Insider's View* 2010

➲ *CPT Assistant* Feb 10:6

32553 Placement of interstitial device(s) for radiation therapy guidance (eg, fiducial markers, dosimeter), percutaneous, intra-thoracic, single or multiple

➲ *CPT Changes: An Insider's View* 2010, 2017

➲ *CPT Assistant* Feb 10:6, 7, Jun 15:6, Jun 16:3

(Report supply of device separately)

(For imaging guidance, see 76942, 77002, 77012, 77021)

(For percutaneous placement of interstitial device[s] for intra-abdominal, intrapelvic, and/or retroperitoneal radiation therapy guidance, use 49411)

32554 Thoracentesis, needle or catheter, aspiration of the pleural space; without imaging guidance

➲ *CPT Changes: An Insider's View* 2013

➲ *CPT Assistant* Nov 12:3, May 14:3

➲ *Clinical Examples in Radiology* Winter 13:5, 6, Summer 13:6

32555 with imaging guidance

➲ *CPT Changes: An Insider's View* 2013

➲ *CPT Assistant* Nov 12:3

➲ *Clinical Examples in Radiology* Winter 13:6, Summer 13:6

32556 Pleural drainage, percutaneous, with insertion of indwelling catheter; without imaging guidance

➲ *CPT Changes: An Insider's View* 2013

➲ *Clinical Examples in Radiology* Winter 13:6, Summer 13:6

32557 with imaging guidance

➲ *CPT Changes: An Insider's View* 2013

➲ *CPT Assistant* Nov 12:3, May 14:3

➲ *Clinical Examples in Radiology* Winter 13:5, 6, Summer 13:5, 6

(For insertion of indwelling tunneled pleural catheter with cuff, use 32550)

(For open procedure, use 32551)

(Do not report 32554-32557 in conjunction with 32550, 32551 when performed on the same side of the chest)

(Do not report 32554-32557 in conjunction with 75989, 76942, 77002, 77012, 77021)

Thoracentesis
32554, 32555

Accumulated fluid or air is removed from the pleural space by puncturing space between the ribs. In 32555, a tube is inserted and a syringe attached to the catheter for the removal of fluid and/or air.

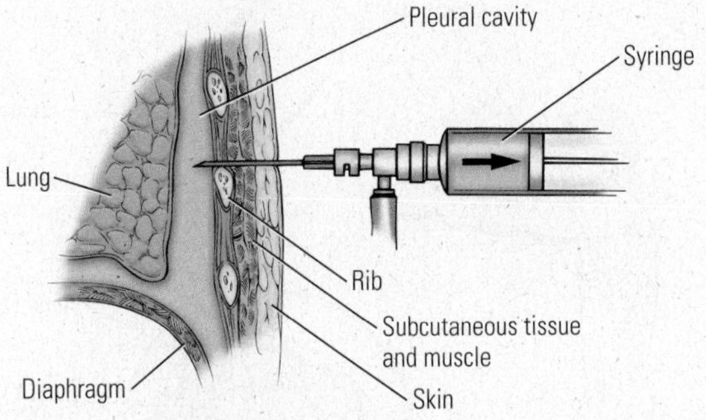

Destruction

The instillation of a fibrinolytic agent may be performed multiple times per day over the course of several days. Code 32561 should be reported only once on the initial day treatment. Code 32562 should be reported only once on each subsequent day of treatment.

32560 Instillation, via chest tube/catheter, agent for pleurodesis (eg, talc for recurrent or persistent pneumothorax)

➲ *CPT Changes: An Insider's View* 2008, 2010

➲ *CPT Assistant* Feb 10:6

(For chest tube insertion, use 32551)

32561 Instillation(s), via chest tube/catheter, agent for fibrinolysis (eg, fibrinolytic agent for break up of multiloculated effusion); initial day

➲ *CPT Changes: An Insider's View* 2010

➲ *CPT Assistant* Feb 10:6

(For chest tube insertion, use 32551)

32562 subsequent day

➲ *CPT Changes: An Insider's View* 2010

➲ *CPT Assistant* Feb 10:6

(For chest tube insertion, use 32551)

Thoracoscopy (Video-assisted thoracic surgery [VATS])

Surgical thoracoscopy (video-assisted thoracic surgery [VATS]) always includes diagnostic thoracoscopy.

32601 Thoracoscopy, diagnostic (separate procedure); lungs, pericardial sac, mediastinal or pleural space, without biopsy

➲ *CPT Changes: An Insider's View* 2012

➲ *CPT Assistant* Fall 94:1, 4, Sep 12:3, Aug 13:14

32604 pericardial sac, with biopsy

➲ *CPT Assistant* Fall 94:1, 4, Aug 13:14

(For open pericardial bipsy, use 39010)

Respiratory 30000-32999

Thoracoscopy
32601-32665

The inside of the chest cavity is examined through a fiberoptic endoscope.

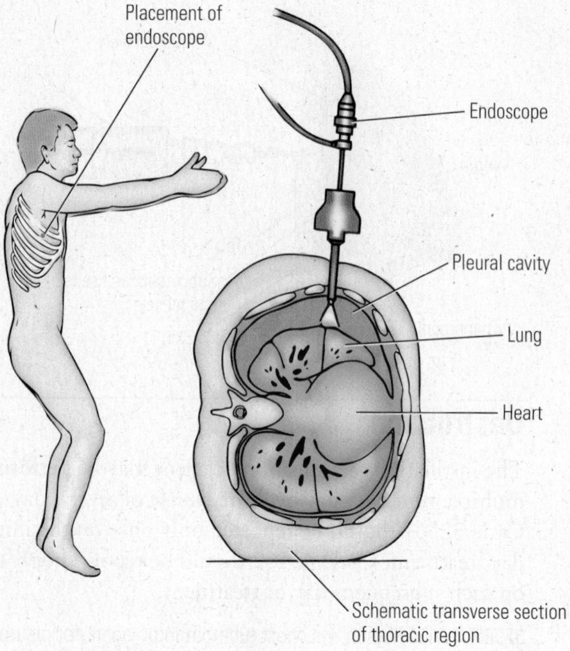

32606 mediastinal space, with biopsy
➲ *CPT Assistant* Fall 94:1, 5, Aug 13:14

32607 Thoracoscopy; with diagnostic biopsy(ies) of lung infiltrate(s) (eg, wedge, incisional), unilateral
➲ *CPT Changes: An Insider's View* 2012
➲ *CPT Assistant* Sep 12:3, Aug 13:14

(Do not report 32607 more than once per lung)

(Do not report 32607 in conjunction with 32440, 32442, 32445, 32488, 32671)

32608 with diagnostic biopsy(ies) of lung nodule(s) or mass(es) (eg, wedge, incisional), unilateral
➲ *CPT Changes: An Insider's View* 2012
➲ *CPT Assistant* Sep 12:3, Aug 13:14

(Do not report 32608 more than once per lung)

(Do not report 32608 in conjunction with 32440, 32442, 32445, 32488, 32671)

32609 with biopsy(ies) of pleura
➲ *CPT Changes: An Insider's View* 2012
➲ *CPT Assistant* Sep 12:3, Aug 13:14

32650 Thoracoscopy, surgical; with pleurodesis (eg, mechanical or chemical)
➲ *CPT Changes: An Insider's View* 2002
➲ *CPT Assistant* Fall 94:1, 6, Aug 13:14

32651 with partial pulmonary decortication
➲ *CPT Assistant* Fall 94:1, 6, Aug 13:14

32652 with total pulmonary decortication, including intrapleural pneumonolysis
➲ *CPT Assistant* Fall 94:1, 6, Aug 13:14

32653 with removal of intrapleural foreign body or fibrin deposit
➲ *CPT Assistant* Fall 94:1, 6, Aug 13:14

32654 with control of traumatic hemorrhage
➲ *CPT Assistant* Fall 94:1, 6, Aug 13:14

32655 with resection-plication of bullae, includes any pleural procedure when performed
➲ *CPT Changes: An Insider's View* 2012
➲ *CPT Assistant* Fall 94:1, 6, Aug 05:15, Aug 13:14

(For thoracoscopic [VATS] lung volume reduction surgery, use 32672)

32656 with parietal pleurectomy
➲ *CPT Assistant* Fall 94:1, 6, Aug 13:14

32658 with removal of clot or foreign body from pericardial sac
➲ *CPT Assistant* Fall 94:1, 6, Aug 13:14

32659 with creation of pericardial window or partial resection of pericardial sac for drainage
➲ *CPT Assistant* Fall 94:1, 6, Aug 13:14

32661 with excision of pericardial cyst, tumor, or mass
➲ *CPT Assistant* Fall 94:1, 6, Aug 13:14

32662 with excision of mediastinal cyst, tumor, or mass
➲ *CPT Assistant* Fall 94:1, 6, Aug 13:14

32663 with lobectomy (single lobe)
➲ *CPT Changes: An Insider's View* 2012
➲ *CPT Assistant* Fall 94:1, 6, Sep 12:3, Aug 13:14

(For thoracoscopic [VATS] segmentectomy, use 32669)

32664 with thoracic sympathectomy
➲ *CPT Assistant* Fall 94:1, Oct 99:10, Aug 13:14, Dec 15:16

32665 with esophagomyotomy (Heller type)
➲ *CPT Assistant* Fall 94:1, 6, Aug 13:14

(For exploratory thoracoscopy, and exploratory thoracoscopy with biopsy, see 32601-32609)

32666 with therapeutic wedge resection (eg, mass, nodule), initial unilateral
➲ *CPT Changes: An Insider's View* 2012
➲ *CPT Assistant* Sep 12:3, Aug 13:14

(To report bilateral procedure, report 32666 with modifier 50)

(Do not report 32666 in conjunction with 32440, 32442, 32445, 32488, 32671)

+ 32667 with therapeutic wedge resection (eg, mass or nodule), each additional resection, ipsilateral (List separately in addition to code for primary procedure)
➲ *CPT Changes: An Insider's View* 2012
➲ *CPT Assistant* Sep 12:3, Aug 13:14

(Report 32667 only in conjunction with 32666)

(Do not report 32667 in conjunction with 32440, 32442, 32445, 32488, 32671)

+ 32668 with diagnostic wedge resection followed by anatomic lung resection (List separately in addition to code for primary procedure)

➔ *CPT Changes: An Insider's View* 2012

➔ *CPT Assistant* Sep 12:3, Aug 13:14

(Report 32668 in conjunction with 32440, 32442, 32445, 32480, 32482, 32484, 32486, 32488, 32503, 32504, 32663, 32669, 32670, 32671)

32669 with removal of a single lung segment (segmentectomy)

➔ *CPT Changes: An Insider's View* 2012

➔ *CPT Assistant* Sep 12:3, Aug 13:14

32670 with removal of two lobes (bilobectomy)

➔ *CPT Changes: An Insider's View* 2012

➔ *CPT Assistant* Sep 12:3, Aug 13:14

32671 with removal of lung (pneumonectomy)

➔ *CPT Changes: An Insider's View* 2012

➔ *CPT Assistant* Sep 12:3, Aug 13:14

32672 with resection-plication for emphysematous lung (bullous or non-bullous) for lung volume reduction (LVRS), unilateral includes any pleural procedure, when performed

➔ *CPT Changes: An Insider's View* 2012

➔ *CPT Assistant* Sep 12:3, Aug 13:14

32673 with resection of thymus, unilateral or bilateral

➔ *CPT Changes: An Insider's View* 2012

➔ *CPT Assistant* Sep 12:3, Aug 13:14

(For open thymectomy see 60520, 60521, 60522)

(For open excision mediastinal cyst, see 39200; for open excision mediastinal tumor, use 39220)

(For exploratory thoracoscopy, and exploratory thoracoscopy with biopsy, see 32601-32609)

+ 32674 with mediastinal and regional lymphadenectomy (List separately in addition to code for primary procedure)

➔ *CPT Changes: An Insider's View* 2012

➔ *CPT Assistant* Sep 12:3, Aug 13:14, May 14:3

(On the right, mediastinal lymph nodes include the paratracheal, subcarinal, paraesophageal, and inferior pulmonary ligament)

(On the left, mediastinal lymph nodes include the aortopulmonary window, subcarinal, paraesophageal, and inferior pulmonary ligament)

(Report 32674 in conjunction with 19260, 31760, 31766, 31786, 32096-32200, 32220-32320, 32440-32491, 32503-32505, 32601-32663, 32666, 32669-32673, 32815, 33025, 33030, 33050-33130, 39200-39220, 39560, 39561, 43101, 43112, 43117, 43118, 43122, 43123, 43287, 43288, 43351, 60270, 60505)

(To report mediastinal and regional lymphadenectomy via thoracotomy, use 38746)

Mediastinal Lymph Nodes: Station Number and Descriptions

32674

Relevant mediastinal lymph nodes typically removed with procedures described by code 38746, and sampled removal described with code 39402.

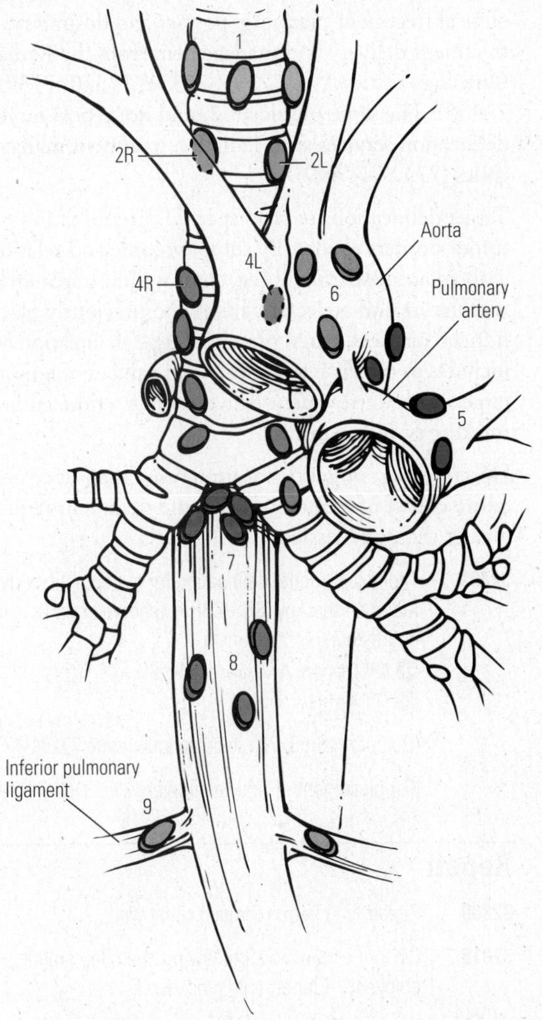

Station #	Lymph Node Descriptions
1	Low cervical, supraclavicular, and sternal notch
2	Upper paratracheal (R & L)
4	Lower paratracheal (R & L)
5	Subaortic or aortopulmonary window
6	Para-aortic
7	Subcarinal
8	Paraesophageal (below the carina)
9	Inferior pulmonary ligament

*Station #3 is not depicted as it is not applicable to the use of codes 32674, 38746, or 39402.

Respiratory 30000-32999

Stereotactic Radiation Therapy

Thoracic stereotactic body radiation therapy (SRS/SBRT) is a distinct procedure which may involve collaboration between a surgeon and radiation oncologist. The surgeon identifies and delineates the target for therapy. The radiation oncologist reports the appropriate code(s) for clinical treatment planning, physics and dosimetry, treatment delivery and management from the Radiation Oncology section (see 77295, 77331, 77370, 77373, 77435). The same physician should not report target delineation services with radiation treatment management codes (77427-77499).

Target delineation involves specific determination of tumor borders to identify tumor volume and relationship with adjacent structures (eg, chest wall, intraparenchymal vasculature and atelectatic lung) and previously placed fiducial markers, when present. Target delineation also includes availability to identify and validate the thoracic target prior to treatment delivery when a fiducial-less tracking system is utilized.

Do not report target delineation more than once per entire course of treatment when the treatment requires greater than one session.

32701 Thoracic target(s) delineation for stereotactic body radiation therapy (SRS/SBRT), (photon or particle beam), entire course of treatment

➔ *CPT Changes: An Insider's View* 2013

➔ *CPT Assistant* Jun 15:6

(Do not report 32701 in conjunction with 77261-77799)

(For placement of fiducial markers, see 31626, 32553)

Repair

32800 Repair lung hernia through chest wall

32810 Closure of chest wall following open flap drainage for empyema (Clagett type procedure)

32815 Open closure of major bronchial fistula

32820 Major reconstruction, chest wall (posttraumatic)

Lung Transplantation

Lung allotransplantation involves three distinct components of physician work:

1. ***Cadaver donor pneumonectomy(s)***, which include(s) harvesting the allograft and cold preservation of the allograft (perfusing with cold preservation solution and cold maintenance) (use 32850).
2. ***Backbench work***:

   Preparation of a cadaver donor single lung allograft prior to transplantation, including dissection of the allograft from surrounding soft tissues to prepare the pulmonary venous/atrial cuff, pulmonary artery, and bronchus unilaterally (use 32855).

   Preparation of a cadaver donor double lung allograft prior to transplantation, including dissection of the allograft from surrounding soft tissues to prepare the pulmonary venous/atrial cuff, pulmonary artery, and bronchus bilaterally (use 32856).
3. ***Recipient lung allotransplantation***, which includes transplantation of a single or double lung allograft and care of the recipient (see 32851-32854).

(For ex-vivo assessment of marginal donor lung transplant, see 0494T, 0495T, 0496T)

32850 Donor pneumonectomy(s) (including cold preservation), from cadaver donor

➔ *CPT Changes: An Insider's View* 2005

32851 Lung transplant, single; without cardiopulmonary bypass

32852 with cardiopulmonary bypass

32853 Lung transplant, double (bilateral sequential or en bloc); without cardiopulmonary bypass

32854 with cardiopulmonary bypass

32855 Backbench standard preparation of cadaver donor lung allograft prior to transplantation, including dissection of allograft from surrounding soft tissues to prepare pulmonary venous/atrial cuff, pulmonary artery, and bronchus; unilateral

➔ *CPT Changes: An Insider's View* 2005

32856 bilateral

➔ *CPT Changes: An Insider's View* 2005

(For repair or resection procedures on the donor lung, see 32491, 32505, 32506, 32507, 35216, 35276)

Surgical Collapse Therapy; Thoracoplasty

(See also 32503, 32504)

32900 Resection of ribs, extrapleural, all stages

32905 Thoracoplasty, Schede type or extrapleural (all stages);

32906 with closure of bronchopleural fistula

(For open closure of major bronchial fistula, use 32815)

(For resection of first rib for thoracic outlet compression, see 21615, 21616)

32940 Pneumonolysis, extraperiosteal, including filling or packing procedures

32960 Pneumothorax, therapeutic, intrapleural injection of air

Other Procedures

32994 Code is out of numerical sequence. See 32997-32999

32997 Total lung lavage (unilateral)
- *CPT Changes: An Insider's View* 2000, 2002
- *CPT Assistant* Nov 98:13, Nov 99:14

(For bronchoscopic bronchial alveolar lavage, use 31624)

32998 Ablation therapy for reduction or eradication of 1 or more pulmonary tumor(s) including pleura or chest wall when involved by tumor extension, percutaneous, including imaging guidance when performed, unilateral; radiofrequency
- *CPT Changes: An Insider's View* 2007, 2018
- *CPT Assistant* Nov 17:8
- *Clinical Examples in Radiology* Summer 12:11

 # 32994 cryoablation
- *CPT Changes: An Insider's View* 2018
- *CPT Assistant* Nov 17:8
- *Clinical Examples in Radiology* Fall 17:4

(For bilateral procedure, report 32994, 32998 with modifier 50)

32999 Unlisted procedure, lungs and pleura
- *CPT Assistant* Jan 02:11, Feb 02:11, Jul 08:10, Apr 10:10, Aug 11:9, Jun 15:6, Dec 15:16
- *Clinical Examples in Radiology* Spring 06:8,9

Cryoablation Therapy of Pulmonary Tumors
32994

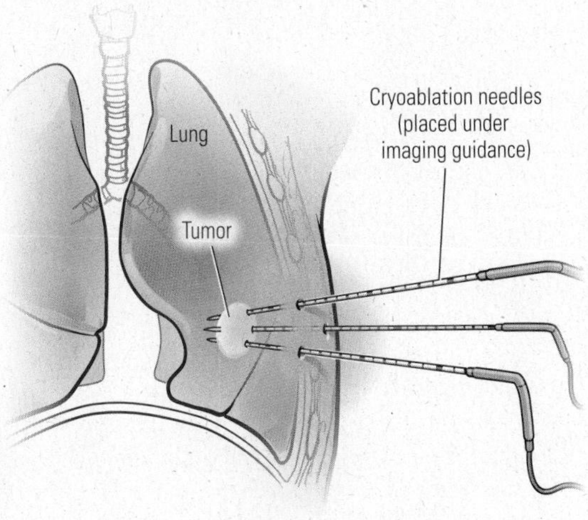

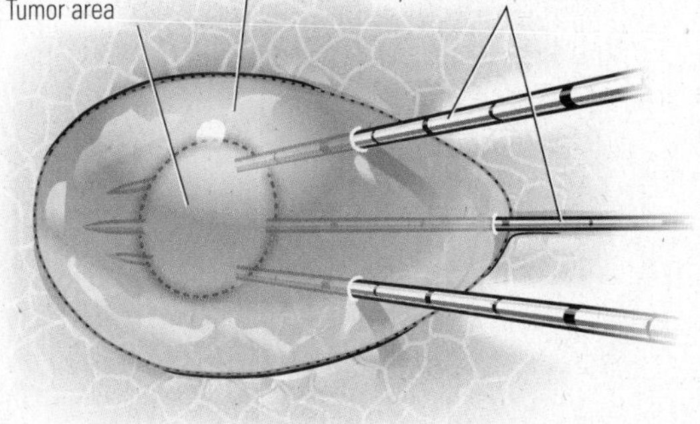

Respiratory 30000-32999

Notes

Surgery

Cardiovascular System* (33010-37799)....214

The following is a listing of headings and subheadings that appear within the Cardiovascular System section of the CPT codebook. The subheadings or subsections denoted with asterisks (*) below have special instructions unique to that subsection. Where these are indicated, special notes or guidelines will be presented preceding those procedural terminology listings, referring to that subsection specifically.

Heart and Pericardium (33010, 33999)....214

Pericardium (33010-33050)....214

Cardiac Tumor (33120-33130)....214

Transmyocardial Revascularization (33140, 33141)....214

Pacemaker or Implantable Defibrillator* (33202-33275)....214

Electrophysiologic Operative Procedures* (33250-33266)....221

Incision (33250-33261)....222

Endoscopy (33265, 33266)....223

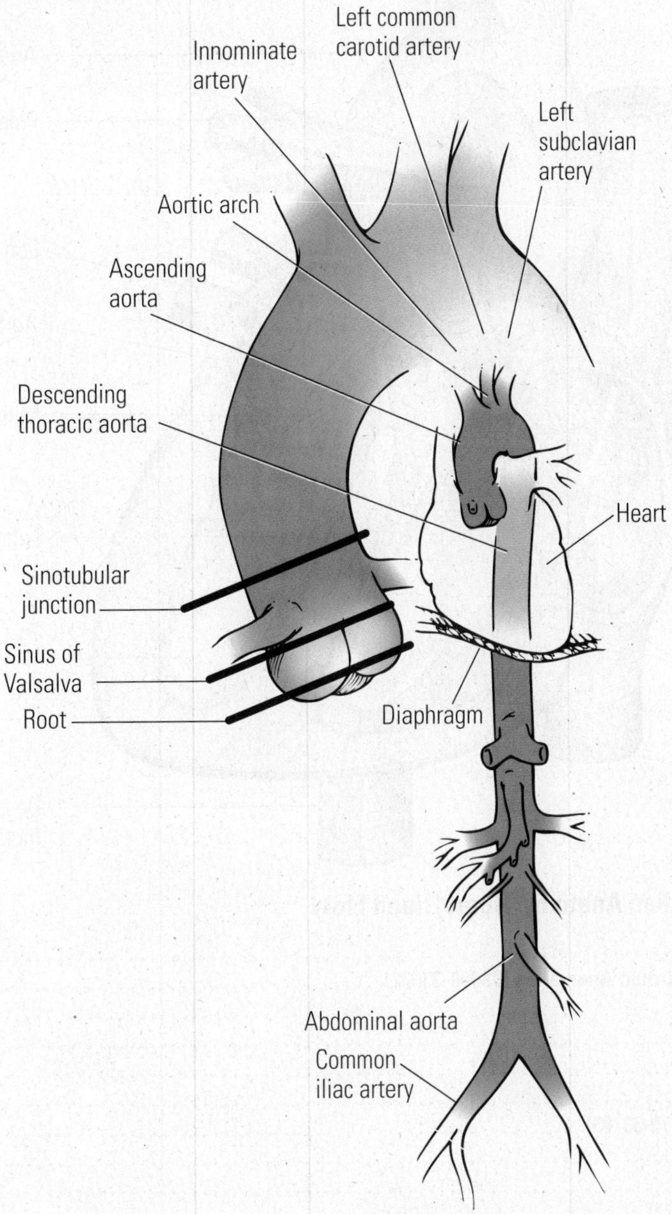

Aortic Anatomy

►Subcutaneous Cardiac Rhythm Monitor*◄ (33285-33286) 223
►Implantable Hemodynamic Monitors*◄ (33289) 223
Heart (Including Valves) and Great Vessels* (33300-33340) 223
Cardiac Valves (33361-33478) 224
Aortic Valve* (33361-33417, 33440) 224
Mitral Valve* (33418-33430) 226
Tricuspid Valve (33460-33468) 227
Pulmonary Valve* (33470-33478) 227
Other Valvular Procedures (33496) 228
Coronary Artery Anomalies* (33500-33507) 228
Endoscopy* (33508) 228
Venous Grafting Only for Coronary Artery Bypass* (33510-33516) 228
Combined Arterial-Venous Grafting for Coronary Bypass* (33517-33530) 229
Arterial Grafting for Coronary Artery Bypass* (33533-33548) 230

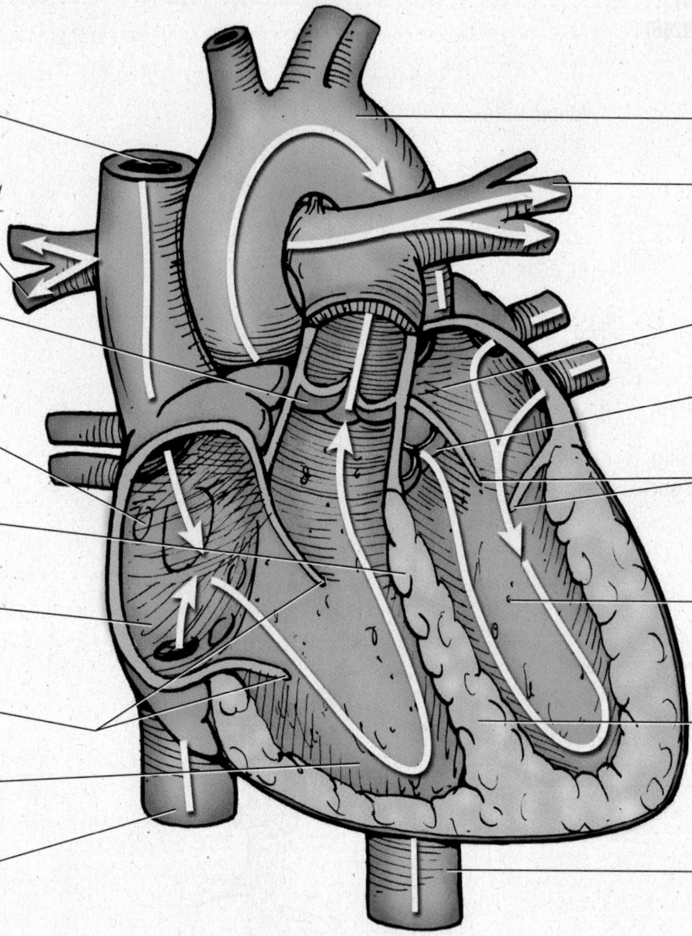

Cardiac Anatomy, Heart Blood Flow

Coronary Endarterectomy (33572) 231
Single Ventricle and Other Complex Cardiac Anomalies (33600-33622) 231
Septal Defect (33641-33697) 232
Sinus of Valsalva (33702-33722) 233
Venous Anomalies (33724-33732) 233
Shunting Procedures (33735-33768) 233
Transposition of the Great Vessels (33770-33783) 233
Truncus Arteriosus (33786-33788) 234
Aortic Anomalies (33800-33853) 234
Thoracic Aortic Aneurysm* (33860-33877) 234
Endovascular Repair of Descending Thoracic Aorta* (33880-33891) 235
Pulmonary Artery (33910-33926) 236
Heart/Lung Transplantation* (33927-33945) 237

Extracorporeal Membrane Oxygenation or Extracorporeal Life Support Services* (33946-33989) 238
Cardiac Assist* (33967-33993) 241
Other Procedures (33999) 243

Arteries and Veins* (34001-37799) 243
Embolectomy/Thrombectomy (34001-34490) 243
Arterial, With or Without Catheter (34001-34203) 243
Venous, Direct or With Catheter (34401-34490) 243
Venous Reconstruction (34501-34530) 243
Endovascular Repair of Abdominal Aorta and/or Iliac Arteries* (34701-34834) 243
Fenestrated Endovascular Repair of the Visceral and Infrarenal Aorta* (34839-34848) 249
Endovascular Repair of Iliac Aneurysm 251
Direct Repair of Aneurysm or Excision (Partial or Total) and Graft Insertion for Aneurysm, Pseudoaneurysm, Ruptured Aneurysm, and Associated Occlusive Disease* (35001-35152) 251
Repair Arteriovenous Fistula (35180-35190) 252
Repair Blood Vessel Other Than for Fistula, With or Without Patch Angioplasty (35201-35286) 252
Thromboendarterectomy (35301-35390) 252
Angioscopy (35400) 253
Transluminal Angioplasty 253
Open 253
Percutaneous 253
Bypass Graft (35500-35671) 253
Vein* (35500-35572) 253
In-Situ Vein (35583-35587) 255
Other Than Vein (35600-35671) 255
Composite Grafts* (35681-35683) 256
Adjuvant Techniques* (35685-35686) 256
Arterial Transposition (35691-35697) 257
Excision, Exploration, Repair, Revision (35700-35907) 257
Vascular Injection Procedures* (36000-36598) 258
Intravenous* (36000-36015) 258
Intra-Arterial—Intra-Aortic* (36100-36299) 259
Venous* (36400-36522) 262
Central Venous Access Procedures* (36555-36598) 266
Insertion of Central Venous Access Device (36555-36573) 266
Repair of Central Venous Access Device (36575-36576) 269
Partial Replacement of Central Venous Access Device (Catheter Only) (36578) 269
Complete Replacement of Central Venous Access Device Through Same Venous Access Site (36580-36585) 269
Removal of Central Venous Access Device (36589-36590) 271
Other Central Venous Access Procedures (36591-36598) 271
Arterial (36600-36660) 272
Intraosseous (36680) 272
Hemodialysis Access, Intervascular Cannulation for Extracorporeal Circulation, or Shunt Insertion (36800-36861) 272
Dialysis Circuit* (36901-36909) 273
Portal Decompression Procedures (37140-37183) 277
Transcatheter Procedures* (37184-37218) 277
Arterial Mechanical Thrombectomy (37184-37186) 278
Venous Mechanical Thrombectomy (37187-37188) 278
Other Procedures (37191-37218) 279
Endovascular Revascularization (Open or Percutaneous, Transcatheter)* (37220-37239, 37246-37249) 281
Vascular Embolization and Occlusion* (37241-37244) 286
Intravascular Ultrasound Services* (37252-37253) 288
Endoscopy* (37500-37501) 288
Ligation (37565-37785) 288
Other Procedures (37788-37799) 290

Hemic and Lymphatic Systems (38100-38999) 290
Spleen (38100-38200) 290
Excision (38100-38102) 290

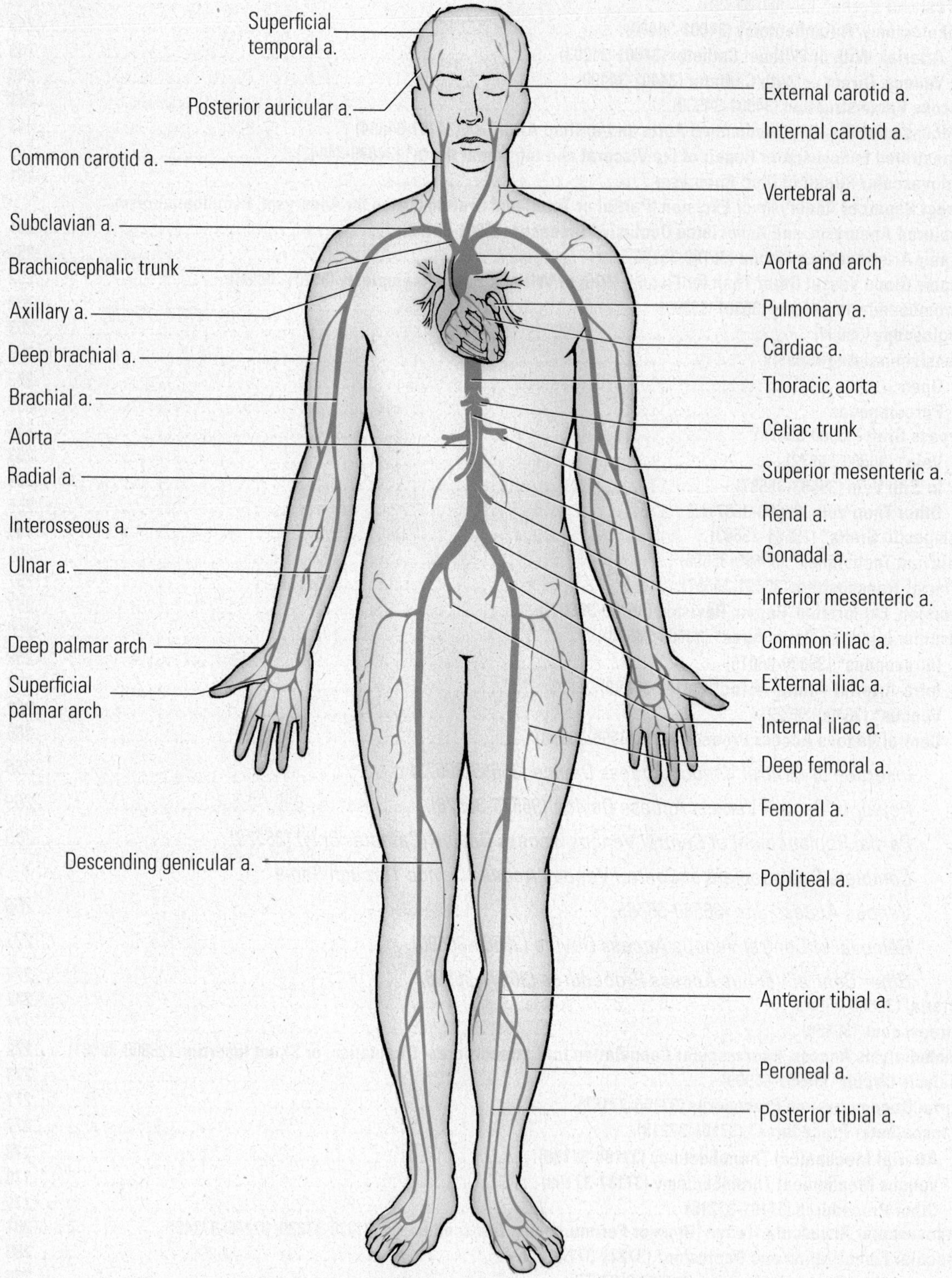

Circulatory System, Arteries

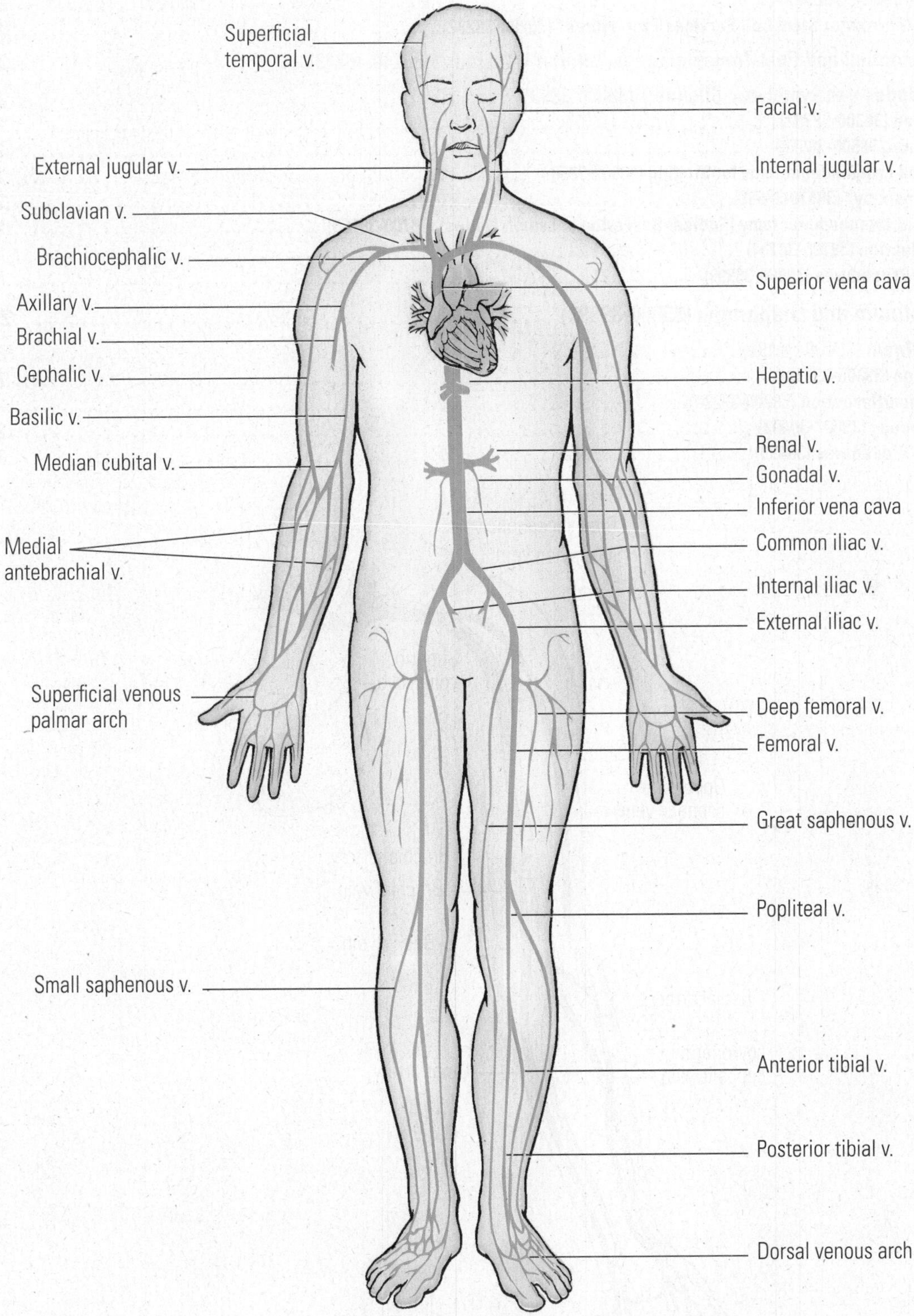

Circulatory System, Veins

Repair (38115) 290
Laparoscopy* (38120-38129) 290
Introduction (38200) 290

General (38204-38232) 290
Bone Marrow or Stem Cell Services/Procedures* (38204-38232) 290

Transplantation and Post-Transplantation Cellular Infusions* (38240-38243) 291

Lymph Nodes and Lymphatic Channels (38300-38999) 292
Incision (38300-38382) 292
Excision (38500-38555) 292
Limited Lymphadenectomy for Staging (38562-38564) 293
Laparoscopy* (38570-38589) 293
Radical Lymphadenectomy (Radical Resection of Lymph Nodes) (38700-38780) 293
Introduction (38790-38794) 294
Other Procedures (38900-38999) 294

Mediastinum and Diaphragm (39000-39599) 295

Mediastinum (39000-39499) 295
Incision (39000-39010) 295
Excision/Resection (39200-39220) 295
Endoscopy (39401-39402) 295
Other Procedures (39499) 295

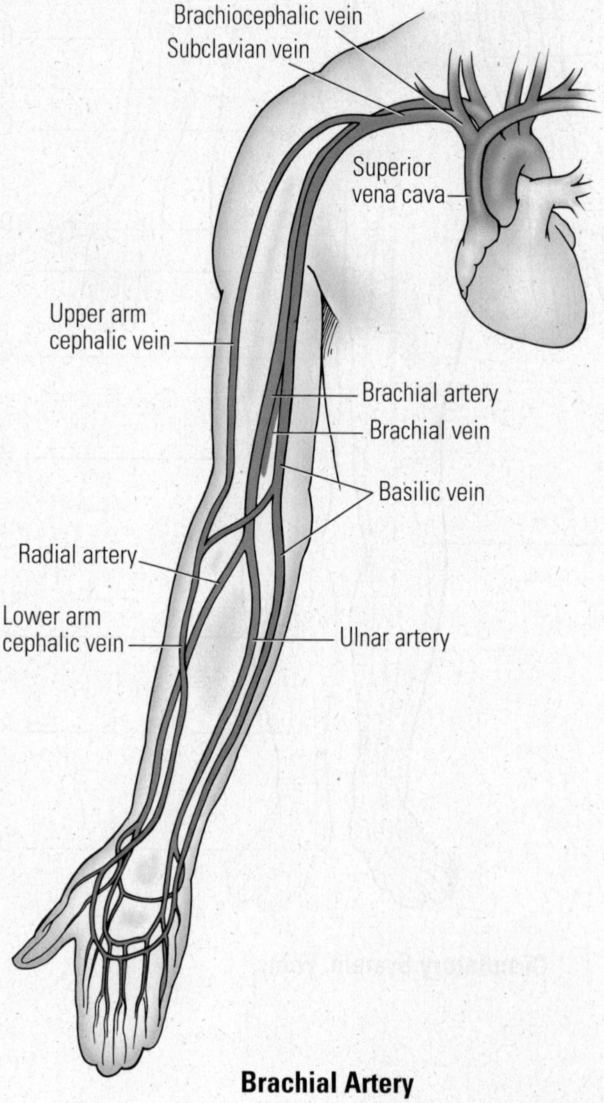

Brachial Artery

Diapraghm (39501-39599) 295
Repair (39501-39561) 295
Other Procedures (39599) 295

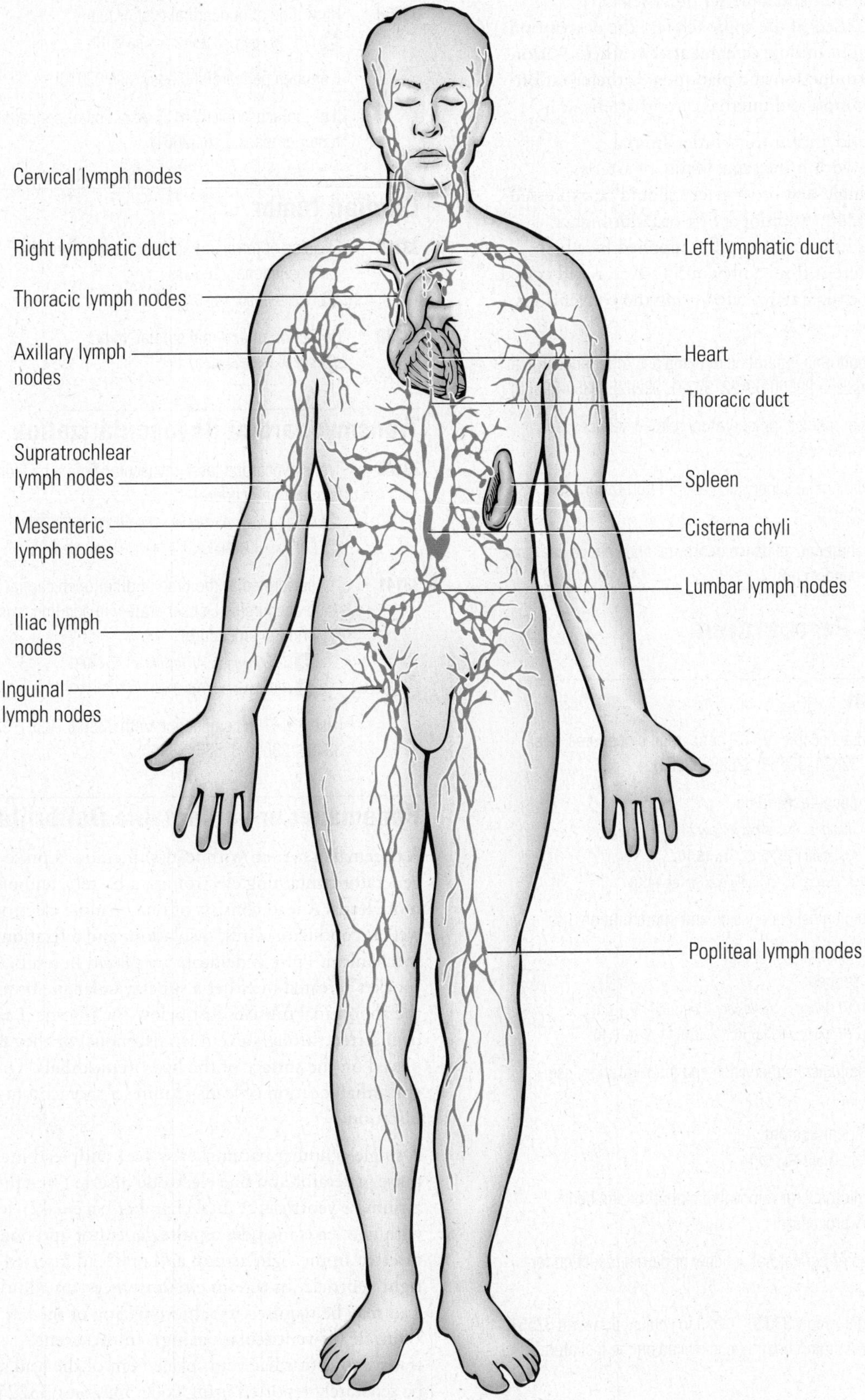

Lymphatic System

Cardiovascular System

Selective vascular catheterizations should be coded to include introduction and all lesser order selective catheterizations used in the approach (eg, the description for a selective right middle cerebral artery catheterization includes the introduction and placement catheterization of the right common and internal carotid arteries).

Additional second and/or third order arterial catheterizations within the same family of arteries supplied by a single first order artery should be expressed by 36218 or 36248. Additional first order or higher catheterizations in vascular families supplied by a first order vessel different from a previously selected and coded family should be separately coded using the conventions described above.

(For monitoring, operation of pump and other nonsurgical services, see 99190-99192, 99291, 99292, 99354-99360)

(For other medical or laboratory related services, see appropriate section)

(For radiological supervision and interpretation, see 75600-75970)

►(For anatomic guidance of arterial and venous anatomy, see Appendix L)◄

Heart and Pericardium

Pericardium

(For thoracoscopic (VATS) pericardial procedures, see 32601, 32604, 32658, 32659, 32661)

33010 Pericardiocentesis; initial
- *CPT Changes: An Insider's View* 2017
- *CPT Assistant* Feb 15:11, Sep 16:10
- *Clinical Examples in Radiology* Spring 14:10

(For radiological supervision and interpretation, use 76930)

33011 subsequent
- *CPT Changes: An Insider's View* 2017
- *CPT Assistant* Sep 10:7, Feb 15:11, Sep 16:10

(For radiological supervision and interpretation, use 76930)

33015 Tube pericardiostomy
- *CPT Assistant* Aug 14:14

33020 Pericardiotomy for removal of clot or foreign body (primary procedure)

33025 Creation of pericardial window or partial resection for drainage

►(Do not report 33020, 33025 in conjunction with 32551, if pleural drain/chest tube is placed on the ipsilateral side)◄

(For thoracoscopic (VATS) pericardial window, use 32659)

33030 Pericardiectomy, subtotal or complete; without cardiopulmonary bypass

33031 with cardiopulmonary bypass

33050 Resection of pericardial cyst or tumor
- *CPT Changes: An Insider's View* 2012

(For open pericardial biopsy, use 39010)

(For thoracoscopic (VATS) resection of pericardial cyst, tumor or mass, use 32661)

Cardiac Tumor

33120 Excision of intracardiac tumor, resection with cardiopulmonary bypass
- *CPT Assistant* Mar 07:1

33130 Resection of external cardiac tumor
- *CPT Assistant* Mar 07:1

Transmyocardial Revascularization

33140 Transmyocardial laser revascularization, by thoracotomy; (separate procedure)
- *CPT Changes: An Insider's View* 2000, 2001, 2002
- *CPT Assistant* Nov 99:14, Nov 00:5, Apr 01:7

+ 33141 performed at the time of other open cardiac procedure(s) (List separately in addition to code for primary procedure)
- *CPT Changes: An Insider's View* 2001
- *CPT Assistant* Apr 01:7

(Use 33141 in conjunction with 33390, 33391, 33404-33496, 33510-33536, 33542)

Pacemaker or Implantable Defibrillator

A pacemaker system with lead(s) includes a pulse generator containing electronics, a battery, and one or more leads. A lead consists of one or more electrodes, as well as conductor wires, insulation, and a fixation mechanism. Pulse generators are placed in a subcutaneous "pocket" created in either a subclavicular site or just above the abdominal muscles just below the ribcage. Leads may be inserted through a vein (transvenous) or they may be placed on the surface of the heart (epicardial). The epicardial location of leads requires a thoracotomy for insertion.

A single chamber pacemaker system with lead includes a pulse generator and one electrode inserted in either the atrium or ventricle. A dual chamber pacemaker system with two leads includes a pulse generator and one lead inserted in the right atrium and one lead inserted in the right ventricle. In certain circumstances, an additional lead may be required to achieve pacing of the left ventricle (bi-ventricular pacing). In this event, transvenous (cardiac vein) placement of the lead should be separately reported using code 33224 or 33225. Epicardial placement of the lead should be separately reported using 33202, 33203.

►A leadless cardiac pacemaker system includes a pulse generator with built-in battery and electrode for implantation in a cardiac chamber via a transcatheter approach. For implantation of a leadless pacemaker system, use 33274. Insertion, replacement, or removal of a leadless pacemaker system includes insertion of a catheter into the right ventricle.

Right heart catheterization (93451, 93453, 93456, 93457, 93460, 93461, 93530, 93531, 93532, 93533) may not be reported in conjunction with leadless pacemaker insertion and removal codes 33274, 33275 unless complete right heart catheterization is performed for an indication distinct from the leadless pacemaker procedure.◄

Like a pacemaker system, an implantable defibrillator system includes a pulse generator and electrodes. Two general categories of implantable defibrillators exist: transvenous implantable pacing cardioverter-defibrillator (ICD) and subcutaneous implantable defibrillator (S-ICD). Implantable pacing cardioverter-defibrillator devices use a combination of antitachycardia pacing, low-energy cardioversion or defibrillating shocks to treat ventricular tachycardia or ventricular fibrillation. The subcutaneous implantable defibrillator uses a single subcutaneous electrode to treat ventricular tachyarrhythmias. Subcutaneous implantable defibrillators differ from transvenous implantable pacing cardioverter-defibrillators in that subcutaneous defibrillators do not provide antitachycardia pacing or chronic pacing.

Implantable defibrillator pulse generators may be implanted in a subcutaneous infraclavicular, axillary, or abdominal pocket. Removal of an implantable defibrillator pulse generator requires opening of the existing subcutaneous pocket and disconnection of the pulse generator from its electrode(s). A thoracotomy (or laparotomy in the case of abdominally placed pulse generators) is not required to remove the pulse generator.

The electrodes (leads) of an implantable defibrillator system may be positioned within the atrial and/or ventricular chambers of the heart via the venous system (transvenously), or placed on the surface of the heart (epicardial), or positioned under the skin overlying the heart (subcutaneous). Electrode positioning on the epicardial surface of the heart requires a thoracotomy or thoracoscopic placement of the leads. Epicardial placement of electrode(s) may be separately reported using 33202, 33203. The electrode (lead) of a subcutaneous implantable defibrillator system is tunneled under the skin to the left parasternal margin. Subcutaneous placement of electrode may be reported using 33270 or 33271. In certain circumstances, an additional electrode may be required to achieve pacing of the left ventricle (bi-ventricular pacing). In this event, transvenous (cardiac vein) placement of the electrode may be separately reported using 33224 or 33225.

►Removal of a transvenous electrode(s) may first be attempted by transvenous extraction (33234, 33235, or 33244). However, if transvenous extraction is unsuccessful, a thoracotomy may be required to remove the electrodes (33238 or 33243). Use 33212, 33213, 33221, 33230, 33231, 33240 as appropriate, in addition to the thoracotomy or endoscopic epicardial lead placement codes (33202 or 33203) to report the insertion of the generator if done by the same physician during the same session. Removal of a subcutaneous implantable defibrillator electrode may be separately reported using 33272. For removal of a leadless pacemaker system without replacement, use 33275. For removal and replacement of a leadless pacemaker system during the same session, use 33274.◄

When the "battery" of a pacemaker system with lead(s) or implantable defibrillator is changed, it is actually the pulse generator that is changed. Removal of only the pacemaker or implantable defibrillator pulse generator is reported with 33233 or 33241. If only a pulse generator is inserted or replaced without any right atrial and/or right ventricular lead(s) inserted or replaced, report the appropriate code for only pulse generator insertion or replacement based on the number of final existing lead(s) (33227, 33228, 33229 and 33262, 33263, 33264). Do not report removal of a pulse generator (33233 or 33241) separately for this service. Insertion of a new pulse generator, when existing lead(s) are already in place and when no prior pulse generator is removed, is reported with 33212, 33213, 33221, 33230, 33231, 33240. When a pulse generator insertion involves the insertion or replacement of one or more right atrial and/or right ventricular lead(s) or subcutaneous lead(s), use system codes 33206, 33207, 33208 for pacemaker, 33249 for implantable pacing cardioverter-defibrillator, or 33270 for subcutaneous implantable defibrillator. When reporting the system insertion or replacement codes, removal of a pulse generator (33233 or 33241) may be reported separately, when performed. In addition, extraction of leads 33234, 33235 or 33244 for transvenous or 33272 for subcutaneous may be reported separately, when performed. An exception involves a pacemaker upgrade from single to dual system that includes removal of pulse generator, replacement of new pulse generator, and insertion of new lead, reported with 33214.

Revision of a skin pocket is included in 33206-33249, 33262, 33263, 33264, 33270, 33271, 33272, 33273. When revision of a skin pocket involves incision and drainage of a hematoma or complex wound infection, see 10140, 10180, 11042, 11043, 11044, 11045, 11046, 11047, as appropriate.

Relocation of a skin pocket for a pacemaker (33222) or implantable defibrillator (33223) is necessary for various clinical situations such as infection or erosion. Relocation of an existing pulse generator may be performed as a stand-alone procedure or at the time of a pulse generator or electrode insertion, replacement, or repositioning.

When skin pocket relocation is performed as part of an explant of an existing generator followed by replacement with a new generator, the pocket relocation is reported separately. Skin pocket relocation includes all work associated with the initial pocket (eg, opening the pocket, incision and drainage of hematoma or abscess if performed, and any closure performed), in addition to the creation of a new pocket for the new generator to be placed.

Repositioning of a pacemaker electrode, implantable defibrillator electrode(s), or a left ventricular pacing electrode is reported using 33215, 33226, or 33273, as appropriate.

Procedure	System	
	Pacemaker	Implantable Defibrillator
Insert transvenous single lead only without pulse generator	33216	33216
Insert transvenous dual leads without pulse generator	33217	33217
Insert transvenous multiple leads without pulse generator	33217 + 33224	33217 + 33224
Insert subcutaneous defibrillator electrode only without pulse generator	N/A	33271
Initial pulse generator insertion only with existing single lead, includes transvenous or subcutaneous defibrillator lead	33212	33240
Initial pulse generator insertion only with existing dual leads	33213	33230
Initial pulse generator insertion only with existing multiple leads	33221	33231
Initial pulse generator insertion or replacement plus insertion of transvenous single lead	33206 (atrial) or 33207 (ventricular)	33249
Initial pulse generator insertion or replacement plus insertion of transvenous dual leads	33208	33249
Initial pulse generator insertion or replacement plus insertion of transvenous multiple leads	33208 + 33225	33249 + 33225
Initial pulse generator insertion or replacement plus insertion of subcutaneous defibrillator electrode	N/A	33270
▶Insertion, replacement, or removal and replacement of permanent leadless pacemaker	33274	N/A◀
Upgrade single chamber system to dual chamber system	33214 (includes removal of existing pulse generator)	33241 + 33249
Removal pulse generator only (without replacement)	33233	33241
Removal pulse generator with replacement pulse generator only single lead system, includes transvenous or subcutaneous defibrillator lead	33227	33262
Removal pulse generator with replacement pulse generator only dual lead system (transvenous)	33228	33263
Removal pulse generator with replacement pulse generator only multiple lead system (transvenous)	33229	33264
Removal transvenous electrode only single lead system	33234	33244
Removal transvenous electrode only dual lead system	33235	33244
Removal subcutaneous defibrillator lead only	N/A	33272
Removal and replacement of pulse generator and transvenous electrodes	33233 + (33234 or 33235) + (33206, 33207, or 33208) and 33225, when appropriate	33241 + 33244 + 33249 and 33225, when appropriate
Removal and replacement of implantable defibrillator pulse generator and subcutaneous electrode	N/A	33272 + 33241 + 33270
▶Removal of permanent leadless pacemaker	33275	N/A◀
Conversion of existing system to bi-ventricular system (addition of LV lead and removal of current pulse generator with insertion of new pulse generator with bi-ventricular pacing capabilities)	33225 + 33228 or 33229	33225 + 33263 or 33264

►Device evaluation codes 93260, 93261, 93279-93299 for pacemaker system with lead(s) may not be reported in conjunction with pulse generator and lead insertion or revision codes 33206-33249, 33262, 33263, 33264, 33270, 33271, 33272, 33273. For leadless pacemaker systems, device evaluation codes 93279, 93286, 93288, 93294, 93296 may not be reported in conjunction with leadless pacemaker insertion and removal codes 33274, 33275. Defibrillator threshold testing (DFT) during transvenous implantable defibrillator insertion or replacement may be separately reported using 93640, 93641. DFT testing during subcutaneous implantable defibrillator system insertion is not separately reportable. DFT testing for transvenous or subcutaneous implantable defibrillator in follow-up or at the time of replacement may be separately reported using 93642 or 93644.

Radiological supervision and interpretation related to the pacemaker or implantable defibrillator procedure is included in 33206-33249, 33262, 33263, 33264, 33270, 33271, 33272, 33273, 33274, 33275. Fluoroscopy (76000, 77002), ultrasound guidance for vascular access (76937), right ventriculography (93566), and femoral venography (75820) are included in 33274, 33275, when performed). To report fluoroscopic guidance for diagnostic lead evaluation without lead insertion, replacement, or revision procedures, use 76000.◄

The following definitions apply to 33206-33249, 33262, 33263, 33264, 33270, 33271, 33272, 33273.

Single lead: a pacemaker or implantable defibrillator with pacing and sensing function in only one chamber of the heart or a subcutaneous electrode.

Dual lead: a pacemaker or implantable defibrillator with pacing and sensing function in only two chambers of the heart.

Multiple lead: a pacemaker or implantable defibrillator with pacing and sensing function in three or more chambers of the heart.

33202 Insertion of epicardial electrode(s); open incision (eg, thoracotomy, median sternotomy, subxiphoid approach)

➲ *CPT Changes: An Insider's View* 2007

➲ *CPT Assistant* Jun 12:5, Nov 14:5, May 15:3, Aug 16:5

33203 endoscopic approach (eg, thoracoscopy, pericardioscopy)

➲ *CPT Changes: An Insider's View* 2007

➲ *CPT Assistant* Jun 12:4, Nov 14:5, May 15:3, Aug 16:5

(When epicardial lead placement is performed with insertion of the generator, report 33202, 33203 in conjunction with 33212, 33213, 33221, 33230, 33231, 33240)

33206 Insertion of new or replacement of permanent pacemaker with transvenous electrode(s); atrial

➲ *CPT Changes: An Insider's View* 2012, 2017

➲ *CPT Assistant* Summer 94:10, 17, Oct 96:9, Nov 99:15, Jun 08:14, Jun 12:3, Apr 13:10, Nov 14:5, May 15:3, Aug 16:5

33207 ventricular

➲ *CPT Changes: An Insider's View* 2012, 2017

➲ *CPT Assistant* Summer 94:10, 17, Oct 96:9, Nov 99:15, Jun 08:14, Jun 12:3, Apr 13:10, May 15:3, Aug 16:5

33208 atrial and ventricular

➲ *CPT Changes: An Insider's View* 2012, 2017

➲ *CPT Assistant* Summer 94:10, 17, Jul 96:10, Nov 99:15, Jun 08:14, Jun 12:3, Apr 13:10, Nov 14:5, May 15:3, Aug 16:5

(Do not report 33206-33208 in conjunction with 33227-33229)

(Do not report 33206, 33207, 33208 in conjunction with 33216, 33217)

(Codes 33206-33208 include subcutaneous insertion of the pulse generator and transvenous placement of electrode[s])

(For removal and replacement of pacemaker pulse generator and transvenous electrode(s), use 33233 in conjunction with either 33234 or 33235 and 33206-33208)

33210 Insertion or replacement of temporary transvenous single chamber cardiac electrode or pacemaker catheter (separate procedure)

➲ *CPT Changes: An Insider's View* 2017

➲ *CPT Assistant* Summer 94:10, 17, Mar 07:1, Aug 11:4, Jun 12:3, Jan 13:6, May 15:3, Aug 16:5

Temporary Pacemaker
33210

The pacemaker pulse generator with the electrodes transvenously placed

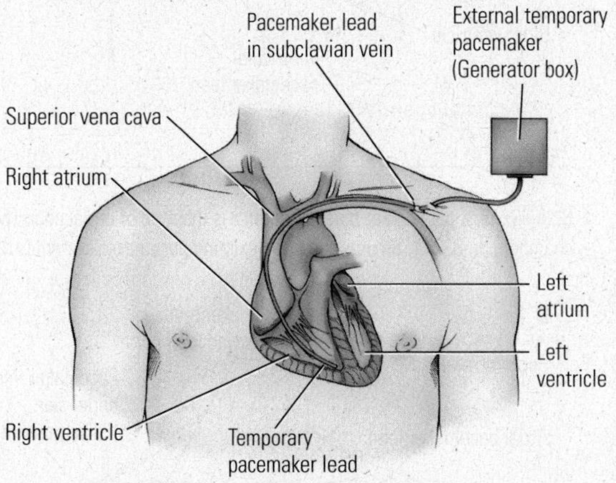

33211 Insertion or replacement of temporary transvenous dual chamber pacing electrodes (separate procedure)

➲ *CPT Changes: An Insider's View* 2017

➲ *CPT Assistant* Summer 94:10, 17, Mar 07:1, Aug 11:4, Jun 12:3, May 15:3, Aug 16:5

33212 Insertion of pacemaker pulse generator only; with existing single lead

➲ *CPT Changes: An Insider's View* 2012, 2017

➲ *CPT Assistant* Summer 94:10, 18, Fall 94:24, May 04:15, Jun 08:14, Jun 12:3, Nov 14:5, May 15:3, Aug 16:5

33213 with existing dual leads

➲ *CPT Changes: An Insider's View* 2012, 2017

➲ *CPT Assistant* Summer 94:10, 18, Oct 96:10, Feb 98:11, Jun 12:3, Nov 14:5, May 15:3, Aug 16:5

 # 33221 with existing multiple leads

➲ *CPT Changes: An Insider's View* 2012, 2017

➲ *CPT Assistant* Jun 12:3, Nov 14:5, May 15:3, Aug 16:5

(Do not report 33212, 33213, 33221 in conjunction with 33216, 33217)

Implanted Pacemaker
33212-33214

A. In 33212, a pacemaker pulse generator is inserted with an existing single lead.

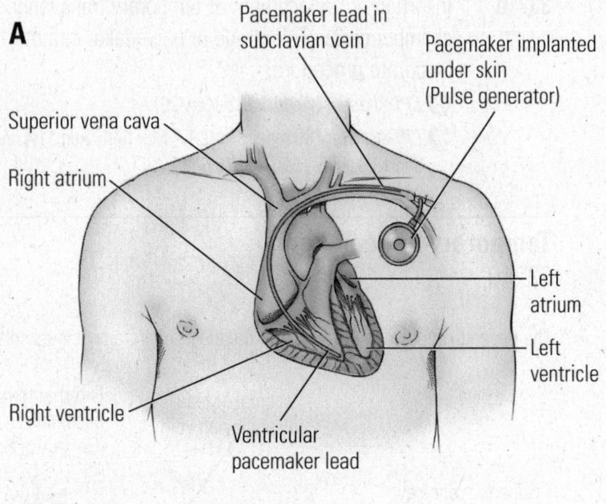

B. In 33213, a pacemaker pulse generator is inserted or replaced in two chambers. In 33214, an upgrade to an existing pacemaker system is done.

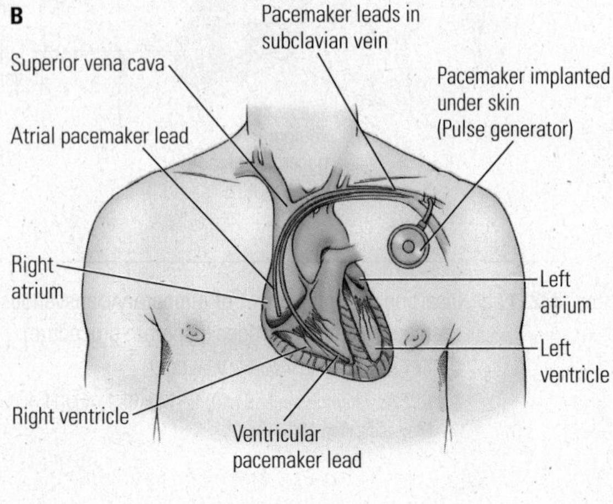

(Do not report 33212, 33213, 33221 in conjunction with 33233 for removal and replacement of the pacemaker pulse generator. Use 33227-33229, as appropriate, when pulse generator replacement is indicated)

(When epicardial lead placement is performed with insertion of generator, report 33202, 33203 in conjunction with 33212, 33213, 33221)

33214 Upgrade of implanted pacemaker system, conversion of single chamber system to dual chamber system (includes removal of previously placed pulse generator, testing of existing lead, insertion of new lead, insertion of new pulse generator)

➲ *CPT Changes: An Insider's View* 2017

➲ *CPT Assistant* Summer 94:10, 18, Fall 94:24, Jun 08:14, Jun 12:3, Nov 14:5, Aug 16:5

(Do not report 33214 in conjunction with 33216, 33217, 33227, 33228, 33229)

33215 Repositioning of previously implanted transvenous pacemaker or implantable defibrillator (right atrial or right ventricular) electrode

➲ *CPT Changes: An Insider's View* 2003, 2015

➲ *CPT Assistant* Jun 12:3, Nov 14:5, Aug 16:5

33216 Insertion of a single transvenous electrode, permanent pacemaker or implantable defibrillator

➲ *CPT Changes: An Insider's View* 2000, 2003, 2010, 2015, 2017

➲ *CPT Assistant* Summer 94:10, 18, Jul 96:10, Nov 99:15-16, Aug 16:5

(Do not report 33216 in conjunction with 33206, 33207, 33208, 33212, 33213, 33214, 33221, 33227, 33228, 33229, 33230, 33231, 33240, 33249, 33262, 33263, 33264)

33217 Insertion of 2 transvenous electrodes, permanent pacemaker or implantable defibrillator

➲ *CPT Changes: An Insider's View* 2000, 2010, 2015, 2017

➲ *CPT Assistant* Summer 94:10, 18, Jul 96:10, Nov 99:15-16, Jul 00:5, Apr 09:8, Jun 12:3, Aug 16:5

(Do not report 33217 in conjunction with 33206, 33207, 33208, 33212, 33213, 33214, 33221, 33227, 33228, 33229, 33230, 33231, 33240, 33249, 33262, 33263, 33264)

(For insertion or replacement of a cardiac venous system lead, see 33224, 33225)

33218 Repair of single transvenous electrode, permanent pacemaker or implantable defibrillator

➲ *CPT Changes: An Insider's View* 2000, 2012, 2015, 2017

➲ *CPT Assistant* Summer 94:10, 19, Oct 96:9, Nov 99:15-16, Jun 12:3, Aug 16:5

(For repair of single permanent pacemaker or implantable defibrillator electrode with replacement of pulse generator, see 33227, 33228, 33229 or 33262, 33263, 33264 and 33218)

33220 Repair of 2 transvenous electrodes for permanent pacemaker or implantable defibrillator

➲ *CPT Changes: An Insider's View* 2000, 2012, 2015, 2017

➲ *CPT Assistant* Summer 94:10, 19, Oct 96:9, Nov 99:15-16, Jun 08:14, Jun 12:3, Aug 16:5

(For repair of 2 transvenous electrodes for permanent pacemaker or implantable defibrillator with replacement of pulse generator, use 33220 in conjunction with 33228, 33229, 33263, 33264)

33221 Code is out of numerical sequence. See 33212-33215

33222 Relocation of skin pocket for pacemaker

➲ *CPT Changes: An Insider's View* 2000, 2014, 2017

➲ *CPT Assistant* Spring 94:30, Summer 94:10, Nov 99:15-16, Jun 08:14, Jun 12:3, Nov 14:5, May 15:3, Aug 16:5

(Do not report 33222 in conjunction with 10140, 10180, 11042, 11043, 11044, 11045, 11046, 11047, 13100, 13101, 13102)

33223 Relocation of skin pocket for implantable defibrillator

➲ *CPT Changes: An Insider's View* 2000, 2010, 2014, 2015, 2017

➲ *CPT Assistant* Summer 94:10, 19, Nov 99:15-16, Jun 08:14, Jun 12:3, Nov 14:5, Aug 16:5

(Do not report 33223 in conjunction with 10140, 10180, 11042, 11043, 11044, 11045, 11046, 11047, 13100, 13101, 13102)

33224 Insertion of pacing electrode, cardiac venous system, for left ventricular pacing, with attachment to previously placed pacemaker or implantable defibrillator pulse generator (including revision of pocket, removal, insertion, and/or replacement of existing generator)

➲ *CPT Changes: An Insider's View* 2003, 2012, 2015

➲ *CPT Assistant* Dec 07:16, Jun 12:3, Nov 14:5, May 15:3, Aug 16:5

(When epicardial electrode placement is performed, report 33224 in conjunction with 33202, 33203)

+ 33225 Insertion of pacing electrode, cardiac venous system, for left ventricular pacing, at time of insertion of implantable defibrillator or pacemaker pulse generator (eg, for upgrade to dual chamber system) (List separately in addition to code for primary procedure)

➲ *CPT Changes: An Insider's View* 2003, 2012, 2013, 2015

➲ *CPT Assistant* Dec 07:16, Jun 12:3, Nov 14:5, May 15:3, Aug 16:5

(Use 33225 in conjunction with 33206, 33207, 33208, 33212, 33213, 33214, 33216, 33217, 33221, 33223, 33228, 33229, 33230, 33231, 33233, 33234, 33235, 33240, 33249, 33263, 33264)

(Use 33225 in conjunction with 33222 only with pacemaker pulse generator pocket relocation and with 33223 only with implantable defibrillator [ICD] pocket relocation)

Biventricular Pacing
33224-33226

Insertion or repositioning of venous pacing electrode

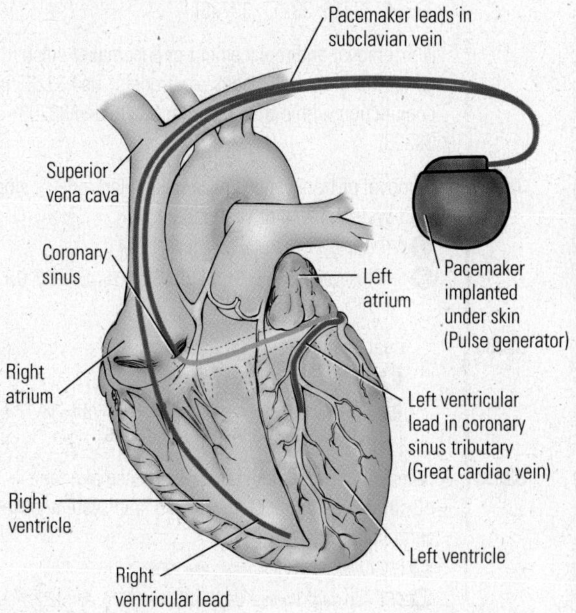

33226 Repositioning of previously implanted cardiac venous system (left ventricular) electrode (including removal, insertion and/or replacement of existing generator)

➲ *CPT Changes: An Insider's View* 2003, 2012

➲ *CPT Assistant* Jun 12:3, Nov 14:5, May 15:3, Aug 16:5

33227 Code is out of numerical sequence. See 33226-33244

33228 Code is out of numerical sequence. See 33226-33244

33229 Code is out of numerical sequence. See 33226-33244

33230 Code is out of numerical sequence. See 33226-33244

33231 Code is out of numerical sequence. See 33226-33244

33233 Removal of permanent pacemaker pulse generator only

➲ *CPT Changes: An Insider's View* 2000, 2012, 2017

➲ *CPT Assistant* Summer 94:10, 19, Fall 94:24, Oct 96:10, Jun 12:3, Nov 14:5, Aug 16:5

 # 33227 Removal of permanent pacemaker pulse generator with replacement of pacemaker pulse generator; single lead system

➲ *CPT Changes: An Insider's View* 2012, 2017

➲ *CPT Assistant* Jun 12:3, Apr 13:10, Nov 14:5, Aug 16:5

 # 33228 dual lead system

➲ *CPT Changes: An Insider's View* 2012, 2017

➲ *CPT Assistant* Jun 12:3, Apr 13:10, Aug 16:5

 # 33229 multiple lead system

CPT Changes: An Insider's View 2012, 2017

CPT Assistant Jun 12:3, Apr 13:10, Nov 14:5, Aug 16:5

(Do not report 33227, 33228, 33229 in conjunction with 33214, 33216, 33217, 33233)

(For removal and replacement of pacemaker pulse generator and transvenous electrode[s], use 33233 in conjunction with either 33234 or 33235 and 33206-33208)

33234 Removal of transvenous pacemaker electrode(s); single lead system, atrial or ventricular

CPT Changes: An Insider's View 2000, 2017

CPT Assistant Summer 94:10, 19, Nov 99:16, Jun 12:3, Oct 12:15, Nov 14:5, Aug 16:5

33235 dual lead system

CPT Changes: An Insider's View 2000, 2017

CPT Assistant Summer 94:10, 19, Nov 99:16, Jun 12:3, Oct 12:15, Dec 13:14, Nov 14:5, Aug 16:5

33236 Removal of permanent epicardial pacemaker and electrodes by thoracotomy; single lead system, atrial or ventricular

CPT Changes: An Insider's View 2000

CPT Assistant Summer 94:10, 19, Nov 99:16, Jun 12:3, Aug 16:5

33237 dual lead system

CPT Changes: An Insider's View 2000

CPT Assistant Summer 94:10, 19, Nov 99:16, Jun 12:3, Aug 16:5

33238 Removal of permanent transvenous electrode(s) by thoracotomy

CPT Changes: An Insider's View 2000

CPT Assistant Summer 94:10, 19, Nov 99:16, Jun 12:3, Nov 14:5, Aug 16:5

33240 Insertion of implantable defibrillator pulse generator only; with existing single lead

CPT Changes: An Insider's View 2000, 2012, 2015, 2017

CPT Assistant Summer 94:40, Jun 96:10, Nov 99:16-17, Jul 00:5, Apr 04:6, Jun 08:14, Jun 12:3, Nov 14:5, Aug 16:5

(Do not report 33240 in conjunction with 33271, 93260, 93261)

(Use 33240, as appropriate, in addition to the epicardial lead placement codes to report the insertion of the generator when done by the same physician during the same session)

 # 33230 with existing dual leads

CPT Changes: An Insider's View 2012, 2015, 2017

CPT Assistant Jun 12:3, Nov 14:5, Aug 16:5

 # 33231 with existing multiple leads

CPT Changes: An Insider's View 2012, 2015, 2017

CPT Assistant Jun 12:3, Nov 14:5, Aug 16:5

(Do not report 33230, 33231, 33240 in conjunction with 33216, 33217)

(Do not report 33230, 33231, 33240 in conjunction with 33241 for removal and replacement of the implantable defibrillator pulse generator. Use 33262, 33263, 33264, as appropriate, when pulse generator replacement is indicated)

(When epicardial lead placement is performed with insertion of generator, report 33202, 33203 in conjunction with 33230, 33231, 33240)

33241 Removal of implantable defibrillator pulse generator only

CPT Changes: An Insider's View 2000, 2012, 2015, 2017

CPT Assistant Summer 94:40, Nov 99:16-17, Jun 12:3, Nov 14:5, Aug 16:5

(Do not report 33241 in conjunction with 93260, 93261)

(Do not report 33241 in conjunction with 33230, 33231, 33240 for removal and replacement of the implantable defibrillator pulse generator. Use 33262, 33263, 33264, as appropriate, when pulse generator replacement is indicated)

(For removal and replacement of an implantable defibrillator pulse generator and electrode[s], use 33241 in conjunction with either 33243 or 33244 and 33249 for transvenous electrode[s] or 33270 and 33272 for subcutaneous electrode)

 # 33262 Removal of implantable defibrillator pulse generator with replacement of implantable defibrillator pulse generator; single lead system

CPT Changes: An Insider's View 2012, 2015, 2017

CPT Assistant Jun 12:3, Nov 14:5, Aug 16:5

(Do not report 33262 in conjunction with 33271, 93260, 93261)

 # 33263 dual lead system

CPT Changes: An Insider's View 2012, 2015, 2017

CPT Assistant Jun 12:3, Dec 13:17, Nov 14:5, Aug 16:5

 # 33264 multiple lead system

CPT Changes: An Insider's View 2012, 2015, 2017

CPT Assistant Jun 12:3, Dec 13:17, Nov 14:5, Aug 16:5

(Do not report 33262, 33263, 33264 in conjunction with 33216, 33217, 33241)

(For removal of electrode[s] by thoracotomy in conjunction with pulse generator removal or replacement, use 33243 in conjunction with 33241 or 33262, 33263, 33264)

(For removal of electrode[s] by transvenous extraction in conjunction with pulse generator removal or replacement, use 33244 in conjunction with 33241 or 33262, 33263, 33264)

(For repair of implantable defibrillator pulse generator and/or leads, see 33218, 33220)

(For removal of subcutaneous electrode in conjunction with implantable defibrillator pulse generator removal or replacement, use 33272 in conjunction with 33241 or 33262)

Coding Tip

Reporting for Electrode Removal and Lead Placement

Removal of electrode(s) may first be attempted by transvenous extraction (code 33244). However, if transvenous extraction is unsuccessful, a thoracotomy may be required to remove the electrodes (code 33243). Use codes 33212, 33213, 33240 as appropriate in addition to the thoracotomy or endoscopic epicardial lead placement codes to report the insertion of the generator if done by the same physician during the same session.

CPT Coding Guidelines, Pacemaker or Pacing Cardioverter-Defibrillator

33243 Removal of single or dual chamber implantable defibrillator electrode(s); by thoracotomy

➲ *CPT Changes: An Insider's View* 2000, 2015

➲ *CPT Assistant* Summer 94:40, Nov 99:16-17, Jun 12:3, Nov 14:5, Aug 16:5

33244 by transvenous extraction

➲ *CPT Changes: An Insider's View* 2000, 2012, 2015, 2017

➲ *CPT Assistant* Summer 94:40, Nov 99:16-17, Jul 00:5, Jun 12:3, Nov 14:5, Aug 16:5

33249 Insertion or replacement of permanent implantable defibrillator system, with transvenous lead(s), single or dual chamber

➲ *CPT Changes: An Insider's View* 2000, 2012, 2015, 2017

➲ *CPT Assistant* Summer 94:21, Nov 99:16-17, Apr 04:6, May 08:14, Jun 08:14, Jun 12:3, Nov 14:5, Aug 16:5

(Do not report 33249 in conjunction with 33216, 33217)

(For removal and replacement of an implantable defibrillator pulse generator and transvenous electrode[s], use 33241 in conjunction with either 33243 or 33244 and 33249)

(For insertion of transvenous implantable defibrillator lead(s), without thoracotomy, use 33216 or 33217)

 # 33270 Insertion or replacement of permanent subcutaneous implantable defibrillator system, with subcutaneous electrode, including defibrillation threshold evaluation, induction of arrhythmia, evaluation of sensing for arrhythmia termination, and programming or reprogramming of sensing or therapeutic parameters, when performed

➲ *CPT Changes: An Insider's View* 2015

➲ *CPT Assistant* Nov 14:5, Aug 16:5

(Do not report 33270 in conjunction with 33271, 93260, 93261, 93644)

(For removal and replacement of an implantable defibrillator pulse generator and subcutaneous electrode, use 33241 in conjunction with 33270 and 33272)

(For insertion of subcutaneous implantable defibrillator lead[s], use 33271)

 # 33271 Insertion of subcutaneous implantable defibrillator electrode

➲ *CPT Changes: An Insider's View* 2015

➲ *CPT Assistant* Nov 14:5, Aug 16:5

(Do not report 33271 in conjunction with 33240, 33262, 33270, 93260, 93261)

(For insertion or replacement of a cardiac venous system lead, see 33224, 33225)

 # 33272 Removal of subcutaneous implantable defibrillator electrode

➲ *CPT Changes: An Insider's View* 2015

➲ *CPT Assistant* Nov 14:5, Aug 16:5

 # 33273 Repositioning of previously implanted subcutaneous implantable defibrillator electrode

➲ *CPT Changes: An Insider's View* 2015

➲ *CPT Assistant* Nov 14:5, Aug 16:5

(Do not report 33272, 33273 in conjunction with 93260, 93261)

#● 33274 Transcatheter insertion or replacement of permanent leadless pacemaker, right ventricular, including imaging guidance (eg, fluoroscopy, venous ultrasound, ventriculography, femoral venography) and device evaluation (eg, interrogation or programming), when performed

➲ *CPT Changes: An Insider's View* 2019

#● 33275 Transcatheter removal of permanent leadless pacemaker, right ventricular

➲ *CPT Changes: An Insider's View* 2019

►(Do not report 33275 in conjunction with 33274)◄

►(Do not report 33274, 33275 in conjunction with femoral venography [75820], fluoroscopy [76000, 77002], ultrasound guidance for vascular access [76937], right ventriculography [93566])◄

►(Do not report 33274, 33275 in conjunction with 93451, 93453, 93456, 93457, 93460, 93461, 93530, 93531, 93532, 93533, unless complete right heart catheterization is performed for indications distinct from the leadless pacemaker procedure)◄

►(For subsequent leadless pacemaker device evaluation, see 93279, 93286, 93288, 93294, 93296)◄

►(For insertion, replacement, repositioning, and removal of pacemaker systems with leads, see 33202, 33203, 33206, 33207, 33208, 33212, 33213, 33214, 33215, 33216, 33217, 33218, 33220, 33221, 33227, 33228, 33229, 33233, 33234, 33235, 33236, 33237)◄

Electrophysiologic Operative Procedures

This family of codes describes the surgical treatment of supraventricular dysrhythmias. Tissue ablation, disruption, and reconstruction can be accomplished by many methods including surgical incision or through the use of a variety of energy sources (eg, radiofrequency, cryotherapy, microwave, ultrasound, laser). If excision or isolation of the left atrial appendage by any method, including stapling, oversewing, ligation, or plication, is performed in conjunction with any of the atrial tissue ablation and reconstruction (maze) procedures (33254-33259, 33265-33266), it is considered part of the procedure. Codes 33254-33256 are only to be reported when there is no concurrently performed procedure that requires median sternotomy or cardiopulmonary bypass. The appropriate atrial tissue ablation add-on code, 33257, 33258, 33259 should be reported in addition to an open cardiac procedure requiring sternotomy or cardiopulmonary bypass if performed concurrently.

Definitions

Limited operative ablation and reconstruction includes:

Surgical isolation of triggers of supraventricular dysrhythmias by operative ablation that isolates the pulmonary veins or other anatomically defined triggers in the left or right atrium.

Extensive operative ablation and reconstruction includes:

1. The services included in *"limited"*
2. Additional ablation of atrial tissue to eliminate sustained supraventricular dysrhythmias. This must include operative ablation that involves either the right atrium, the atrial septum, or left atrium in continuity with the atrioventricular annulus.

Incision

33250 Operative ablation of supraventricular arrhythmogenic focus or pathway (eg, Wolff-Parkinson-White, atrioventricular node re-entry), tract(s) and/or focus (foci); without cardiopulmonary bypass

➲ *CPT Changes: An Insider's View* 2000, 2002

➲ *CPT Assistant* Summer 94:16, Nov 99:17-18

(For intraoperative pacing and mapping by a separate provider, use 93631)

33251 with cardiopulmonary bypass

➲ *CPT Changes: An Insider's View* 2000

➲ *CPT Assistant* Summer 94:16, Nov 99:17-18

Coding Tip

Reporting Restriction for Operative Tissue Ablation

Codes 33254-33256 are only to be reported when there is no concurrently performed procedure that requires median sternotomy or cardiopulmonary bypass.

CPT Coding Guidelines, Electrophysiologic Operative Procedures

33254 Operative tissue ablation and reconstruction of atria, limited (eg, modified maze procedure)

➲ *CPT Changes: An Insider's View* 2007

➲ *CPT Assistant* Mar 07:1

33255 Operative tissue ablation and reconstruction of atria, extensive (eg, maze procedure); without cardiopulmonary bypass

➲ *CPT Changes: An Insider's View* 2007

➲ *CPT Assistant* Mar 07:1

33256 with cardiopulmonary bypass

➲ *CPT Changes: An Insider's View* 2007

➲ *CPT Assistant* Mar 07:1

(Do not report 33254-33256 in conjunction with 32100, 32551, 33120, 33130, 33210, 33211, 33390, 33391, 33404-33507, 33510-33523, 33533-33548, 33600-33853, 33860-33864, 33910-33920)

+ 33257 Operative tissue ablation and reconstruction of atria, performed at the time of other cardiac procedure(s), limited (eg, modified maze procedure) (List separately in addition to code for primary procedure)

➲ *CPT Changes: An Insider's View* 2008

(Use 33257 in conjunction with 33120-33130, 33250, 33251, 33261, 33300-33335, 33390, 33391, 33404-33496, 33500-33507, 33510-33516, 33533-33548, 33600-33619, 33641-33697, 33702-33732, 33735-33767, 33770-33814, 33840-33877, 33910-33922, 33925, 33926, 33935, 33945, 33975-33980)

+ 33258 Operative tissue ablation and reconstruction of atria, performed at the time of other cardiac procedure(s), extensive (eg, maze procedure), without cardiopulmonary bypass (List separately in addition to code for primary procedure)

➲ *CPT Changes: An Insider's View* 2008

(Use 33258 in conjunction with 33130, 33250, 33300, 33310, 33320, 33321, 33330, 33390, 33391, 33414-33417, 33420, 33470, 33471, 33501-33503, 33510-33516, 33533-33536, 33690, 33735, 33737, 33800-33813, 33840-33852, 33915, 33925, when the procedure is performed without cardiopulmonary bypass)

+ 33259 Operative tissue ablation and reconstruction of atria, performed at the time of other cardiac procedure(s), extensive (eg, maze procedure), with cardiopulmonary bypass (List separately in addition to code for primary procedure)

➲ *CPT Changes: An Insider's View* 2008

(Use 33259 in conjunction with 33120, 33251, 33261, 33305, 33315, 33322, 33335, 33390, 33391, 33404, 33405, 33406, 33410, 33411, 33412, 33413, 33422-33468, 33474-33478, 33496, 33500, 33504-33507, 33510-33516, 33533-33548, 33600-33688, 33692-33722, 33730, 33732, 33736, 33750-33767, 33770-33781, 33786-33788, 33814, 33853, 33860-33877, 33910, 33916-33922, 33926, 33935, 33945, 33975-33980, when the procedure is performed with cardiopulmonary bypass)

(Do not report 33257, 33258 and 33259 in conjunction with 32551, 33210, 33211, 33254-33256, 33265, 33266)

33261 Operative ablation of ventricular arrhythmogenic focus with cardiopulmonary bypass

➲ *CPT Assistant* Summer 94:16

33262 Code is out of numerical sequence. See 33226-33244

33263 Code is out of numerical sequence. See 33226-33244

33264 Code is out of numerical sequence. See 33226-33244

Cardiovascular 33010-39599

Endoscopy

33265 Endoscopy, surgical; operative tissue ablation and reconstruction of atria, limited (eg, modified maze procedure), without cardiopulmonary bypass
➔ *CPT Changes: An Insider's View* 2007
➔ *CPT Assistant* Mar 07:1

33266 operative tissue ablation and reconstruction of atria, extensive (eg, maze procedure), without cardiopulmonary bypass
➔ *CPT Changes: An Insider's View* 2007
➔ *CPT Assistant* Mar 07:1

(Do not report 33265-33266 in conjunction with 32551, 33210, 33211)

33270 Code is out of numerical sequence. See 33244-33251

33271 Code is out of numerical sequence. See 33244-33251

33272 Code is out of numerical sequence. See 33244-33251

33273 Code is out of numerical sequence. See 33244-33251

33274 Code is out of numerical sequence. See 33244-33251

33275 Code is out of numerical sequence. See 33244-33251

►Subcutaneous Cardiac Rhythm Monitor◄

►A subcutaneous cardiac rhythm monitor, also known as a cardiac event recorder or implantable/insertable loop recorder (ILR), is a subcutaneously placed device that continuously records the electrocardiographic rhythm, triggered automatically by rapid, irregular and/or slow heart rates or by the patient during a symptomatic episode. A subcutaneous cardiac rhythm monitor is placed using a small parasternal incision followed by insertion of the monitor into a small subcutaneous pre-pectoral pocket, followed by closure of the incision.◄

►(33282, 33284 have been deleted. To report, see 33285, 33286)◄

● **33285** Insertion, subcutaneous cardiac rhythm monitor, including programming
➔ *CPT Changes: An Insider's View* 2019

● **33286** Removal, subcutaneous cardiac rhythm monitor
➔ *CPT Changes: An Insider's View* 2019

►(Initial insertion includes programming. For subsequent electronic analysis and/or reprogramming, see 93285, 93291, 93298, 93299)◄

►Implantable Hemodynamic Monitors◄

►Transcatheter implantation of a wireless pulmonary artery pressure sensor (33289) establishes an intravascular device used for long-term remote monitoring of pulmonary artery pressures (93264). The hemodynamic data derived from this device is used to guide management of patients with heart failure. Code 33289 includes deployment and calibration of the sensor, right heart catheterization, selective pulmonary artery catheterization, radiological supervision and interpretation, and pulmonary artery angiography, when performed.◄

● **33289** Transcatheter implantation of wireless pulmonary artery pressure sensor for long-term hemodynamic monitoring, including deployment and calibration of the sensor, right heart catheterization, selective pulmonary catheterization, radiological supervision and interpretation, and pulmonary artery angiography, when performed
➔ *CPT Changes: An Insider's View* 2019

►(For remote monitoring of an implantable wireless pulmonary artery pressure sensor, use 93264)◄

►(Do not report 33289 in conjunction with 36013, 36014, 36015, 75741, 75743, 75746, 76000, 93451, 93453, 93456, 93457, 93460, 93461, 93530, 93531, 93532, 93533, 93568)◄

Heart (Including Valves) and Great Vessels

Patients receiving major cardiac procedures may require simultaneous cardiopulmonary bypass insertion of cannulae into the venous and arterial vasculatures with support of circulation and oxygenation by a heart-lung machine. Most services are described by codes in dyad arrangements to allow distinct reporting of procedures with or without cardiopulmonary bypass. Cardiopulmonary bypass is distinct from support of cardiac output using devices (eg, ventricular assist or intra-aortic balloon). For cardiac assist services, see 33946, 33947, 33948, 33949, 33967-33983, 33990, 33991, 33992, 33993.

33300 Repair of cardiac wound; without bypass

33305 with cardiopulmonary bypass

33310 Cardiotomy, exploratory (includes removal of foreign body, atrial or ventricular thrombus); without bypass
➔ *CPT Changes: An Insider's View* 2004

33315 with cardiopulmonary bypass
➔ *CPT Assistant* Oct 10:12, Dec 10:12

(Do not report removal of thrombus [33310-33315] in conjunction with other cardiac procedures unless a separate incision in the heart is required to remove the atrial or ventricular thrombus)

(If removal of thrombus with cardiopulmonary bypass [33315] is reported in conjunction with 33120, 33130, 33420-33430, 33460-33468, 33496, 33542, 33545, 33641-33647, 33670, 33681, 33975-33980 which requires a separate heart incision, report 33315 with modifier 59)

33320 Suture repair of aorta or great vessels; without shunt or cardiopulmonary bypass
➔ *CPT Assistant* Fall 91:7

33321 with shunt bypass
➔ *CPT Assistant* Fall 91:7

Cardiovascular 33010-39599

33322 with cardiopulmonary bypass
➲ *CPT Assistant* Fall 91:7

33330 Insertion of graft, aorta or great vessels; without shunt, or cardiopulmonary bypass

33335 with cardiopulmonary bypass

33340 Percutaneous transcatheter closure of the left atrial appendage with endocardial implant, including fluoroscopy, transseptal puncture, catheter placement(s), left atrial angiography, left atrial appendage angiography, when performed, and radiological supervision and interpretation
➲ *CPT Changes: An Insider's View* 2017
➲ *CPT Assistant* Jul 17:3

(Do not report 33340 in conjunction with 93462)

(Do not report 33340 in conjunction with 93452, 93453, 93458, 93459, 93460, 93461, 93531, 93532, 93533, unless catheterization of the left ventricle is performed by a non-transseptal approach for indications distinct from the left atrial appendage closure procedure)

(Do not report 33340 in conjunction with 93451, 93453, 93456, 93460, 93461, 93530, 93531, 93532, 93533, unless complete right heart catheterization is performed for indications distinct from the left atrial appendage closure procedure)

Cardiac Valves

(For multiple valve procedures, see 33390, 33391, 33404-33478 and add modifier 51 to the secondary valve procedure code)

Aortic Valve

Codes 33361, 33362, 33363, 33364, 33365, 33366 are used to report transcatheter aortic valve replacement (TAVR)/transcatheter aortic valve implantation (TAVI). TAVR/TAVI requires two physician operators and all components of the procedure are reported using modifier 62.

Codes 33361, 33362, 33363, 33364, 33365, 33366 include the work, when performed, of percutaneous access, placing the access sheath, balloon aortic valvuloplasty, advancing the valve delivery system into position, repositioning the valve as needed, deploying the valve, temporary pacemaker insertion for rapid pacing (33210), and closure of the arteriotomy when performed. Codes 33361, 33362, 33363, 33364, 33365, 33366 include open arterial or cardiac approach.

Angiography, radiological supervision, and interpretation performed to guide TAVR/TAVI (eg, guiding valve placement, documenting completion of the intervention, assessing the vascular access site for closure) are included in these codes.

Diagnostic left heart catheterization codes (93452, 93453, 93458-93461) and the supravalvular aortography code (93567) should **not** be used with TAVR/TAVI services (33361, 33362, 33363, 33364, 33365, 33366) to report:

1. Contrast injections, angiography, roadmapping, and/or fluoroscopic guidance for the TAVR/TAVI,
2. Aorta/left ventricular outflow tract measurement for the TAVR/TAVI, or
3. Post-TAVR/TAVI aortic or left ventricular angiography, as this work is captured in the TAVR/TAVI services codes (33361, 33362, 33363, 33364, 33365, 33366).

Diagnostic coronary angiography performed at the time of TAVR/TAVI may be separately reportable if:

1. No prior catheter-based coronary angiography study is available and a full diagnostic study is performed, or
2. A prior study is available, but as documented in the medical record:
   a. The patient's condition with respect to the clinical indication has changed since the prior study, or
   b. There is inadequate visualization of the anatomy and/or pathology, or
   c. There is a clinical change during the procedure that requires new evaluation.
   d. For same session/same day diagnostic coronary angiography services, report the appropriate diagnostic cardiac catheterization code(s) appended with modifier 59 indicating separate and distinct procedural service from TAVR/TAVI.

Diagnostic coronary angiography performed at a separate session from an interventional procedure may be separately reportable.

Other cardiac catheterization services may be reported separately when performed for diagnostic purposes not intrinsic to TAVR/TAVI.

Percutaneous coronary interventional procedures are reported separately, when performed.

When transcatheter ventricular support is required in conjunction with TAVR/TAVI, the appropriate code should be reported with the appropriate ventricular assist device (VAD) procedure code (33990-33993, 33975, 33976, 33999) or balloon pump insertion code (33967, 33970, 33973).

The TAVR/TAVI cardiovascular access and delivery procedures are reported with 33361, 33362, 33363, 33364, 33365, 33366. When cardiopulmonary bypass is performed in conjunction with TAVR/TAVI, codes 33361, 33362, 33363, 33364, 33365, 33366 should be reported with the appropriate add-on code for percutaneous peripheral bypass (33367), open peripheral bypass (33368), or central bypass (33369).

33361 Transcatheter aortic valve replacement (TAVR/TAVI) with prosthetic valve; percutaneous femoral artery approach
CPT Changes: An Insider's View 2013
CPT Assistant Jan 13:6, Jan 14:5, Jul 14:8, Mar 15:9

33362 open femoral artery approach
CPT Changes: An Insider's View 2013
CPT Assistant Jan 13:6, Jan 14:5, Mar 15:9

33363 open axillary artery approach
CPT Changes: An Insider's View 2013
CPT Assistant Jan 13:6, Jan 14:5, Mar 15:9

33364 open iliac artery approach
CPT Changes: An Insider's View 2013
CPT Assistant Jan 13:6, Jan 14:5, Mar 15:9

33365 transaortic approach (eg, median sternotomy, mediastinotomy)
CPT Changes: An Insider's View 2013
CPT Assistant Jan 13:6, Jan 14:5, Mar 15:9

33366 transapical exposure (eg, left thoracotomy)
CPT Changes: An Insider's View 2014
CPT Assistant Jan 14:5, Jul 14:8, Mar 15:9

+ 33367 cardiopulmonary bypass support with percutaneous peripheral arterial and venous cannulation (eg, femoral vessels) (List separately in addition to code for primary procedure)
CPT Changes: An Insider's View 2013
CPT Assistant Jan 13:6, Sep 15:3, Mar 16:5

(Use 33367 in conjunction with 33361, 33362, 33363, 33364, 33365, 33366, 33418, 33477, 0483T, 0484T)

(Do not report 33367 in conjunction with 33368, 33369)

+ 33368 cardiopulmonary bypass support with open peripheral arterial and venous cannulation (eg, femoral, iliac, axillary vessels) (List separately in addition to code for primary procedure)
CPT Changes: An Insider's View 2013
CPT Assistant Jan 13:6, Sep 15:3, Mar 16:5

(Use 33368 in conjunction with 33361, 33362, 33363, 33364, 33365, 33366, 33418, 33477, 0483T, 0484T)

(Do not report 33368 in conjunction with 33367, 33369)

+ 33369 cardiopulmonary bypass support with central arterial and venous cannulation (eg, aorta, right atrium, pulmonary artery) (List separately in addition to code for primary procedure)
CPT Changes: An Insider's View 2013
CPT Assistant Jan 13:6, Sep 15:3, Mar 16:5

(Use 33369 in conjunction with 33361, 33362, 33363, 33364, 33365, 33366, 33418, 33477, 0483T, 0484T)

(Do not report 33369 in conjunction with 33367, 33368)

33390 Valvuloplasty, aortic valve, open, with cardiopulmonary bypass; simple (ie, valvotomy, debridement, debulking, and/or simple commissural resuspension)
CPT Changes: An Insider's View 2017
CPT Assistant May 17:9

33391 complex (eg, leaflet extension, leaflet resection, leaflet reconstruction, or annuloplasty)
CPT Changes: An Insider's View 2017
CPT Assistant May 17:9

(Do not report 33391 in conjunction with 33390)

(33400, 33401, 33403 have been deleted. To report, see 33390, 33391)

33404 Construction of apical-aortic conduit
CPT Assistant Jan 04:28, Feb 05:14

33405 Replacement, aortic valve, open, with cardiopulmonary bypass; with prosthetic valve other than homograft or stentless valve
CPT Changes: An Insider's View 2000, 2017
CPT Assistant Nov 99:18, Feb 05:14, Aug 11:3, Jan 13:6, May 17:9

33406 with allograft valve (freehand)
CPT Changes: An Insider's View 2002, 2017
CPT Assistant Nov 99:18, Feb 05:14, Aug 11:3, May 17:9

33410 with stentless tissue valve
CPT Changes: An Insider's View 2000, 2017
CPT Assistant Nov 99:18, Feb 05:14, Aug 11:3, May 17:9

#● 33440 Replacement, aortic valve; by translocation of autologous pulmonary valve and transventricular aortic annulus enlargement of the left ventricular outflow tract with valved conduit replacement of pulmonary valve (Ross-Konno procedure)
CPT Changes: An Insider's View 2019

►(Do not report 33440 in conjunction with 33405, 33406, 33410, 33411, 33412, 33413, 33414, 33416, 33417, 33475, 33608, 33920)◄

33411 with aortic annulus enlargement, noncoronary sinus
CPT Changes: An Insider's View 2011
CPT Assistant Feb 05:14, Aug 11:3

33412 with transventricular aortic annulus enlargement (Konno procedure)
CPT Assistant Feb 05:14, Aug 11:3

►(Do not report 33412 in conjunction with 33413, 33440)◄

►(For replacement of aortic valve with transventricular aortic annulus enlargement [Konno procedure] in conjunction with translocation of autologous pulmonary valve with allograft replacement of pulmonary valve [Ross procedure], use 33440)◄

33413 by translocation of autologous pulmonary valve with allograft replacement of pulmonary valve (Ross procedure)
CPT Changes: An Insider's View 2002
CPT Assistant Feb 05:14, Aug 11:3

►(Do not report 33413 in conjunction with 33412, 33440)◄

►(For replacement of aortic valve with transventricular aortic annulus enlargement [Konno procedure] in conjunction with translocation of autologous pulmonary valve with allograft replacement of pulmonary valve [Ross procedure], use 33440)◄

33414 Repair of left ventricular outflow tract obstruction by patch enlargement of the outflow tract
➲ *CPT Assistant* Feb 05:14

33415 Resection or incision of subvalvular tissue for discrete subvalvular aortic stenosis
➲ *CPT Assistant* Feb 05:14

33416 Ventriculomyotomy (-myectomy) for idiopathic hypertrophic subaortic stenosis (eg, asymmetric septal hypertrophy)
➲ *CPT Assistant* Feb 05:14

(For percutaneous transcatheter septal reduction therapy, use 93583)

33417 Aortoplasty (gusset) for supravalvular stenosis
➲ *CPT Assistant* Feb 05:14

Mitral Valve

Codes 33418 and 33419 are used to report transcatheter mitral valve repair (TMVR). Code 33419 should only be reported once per session.

Codes 33418 and 33419 include the work, when performed, of percutaneous access, placing the access sheath, transseptal puncture, advancing the repair device delivery system into position, repositioning the device as needed, and deploying the device(s).

Angiography, radiological supervision, and interpretation performed to guide TMVR (eg, guiding device placement and documenting completion of the intervention) are included in these codes.

Diagnostic right and left heart catheterization codes (93451, 93452, 93453, 93456, 93457, 93458, 93459, 93460, 93461, 93530, 93531, 93532, 93533) should **not** be used with 33418, 33419 to report:

1. Contrast injections, angiography, road-mapping, and/or fluoroscopic guidance for the transcatheter mitral valve repair (TMVR),
2. Left ventricular angiography to assess mitral regurgitation for guidance of TMVR, or
3. Right and left heart catheterization for hemodynamic measurements before, during, and after TMVR for guidance of TMVR.

Diagnostic right and left heart catheterization codes (93451, 93452, 93453, 93456, 93457, 93458, 93459, 93460, 93461, 93530, 93531, 93532, 93533) and diagnostic coronary angiography codes (93454, 93455, 93456, 93457, 93458, 93459, 93460, 93461, 93563, 93564) may be reported with 33418, 33419, representing separate and distinct services from TMVR, if:

1. No prior study is available and a full diagnostic study is performed, or
2. A prior study is available, but as documented in the medical record:
   a. There is inadequate visualization of the anatomy and/or pathology, or
   b. The patient's condition with respect to the clinical indication has changed since the prior study, or
   c. There is a clinical change during the procedure that requires new evaluation.

Other cardiac catheterization services may be reported separately when performed for diagnostic purposes not intrinsic to TMVR.

For same session/same day diagnostic cardiac catheterization services, report the appropriate diagnostic cardiac catheterization code(s) appended with modifier 59 indicating separate and distinct procedural service from TMVR.

Diagnostic coronary angiography performed at a separate session from an interventional procedure may be separately reportable.

Percutaneous coronary interventional procedures may be reported separately, when performed.

When transcatheter ventricular support is required in conjunction with TMVR, the appropriate code may be reported with the appropriate ventricular assist device (VAD) procedure code (33990, 33991, 33992, 33993) or balloon pump insertion code (33967, 33970, 33973).

When cardiopulmonary bypass is performed in conjunction with TMVR, 33418, 33419 may be reported with the appropriate add-on code for percutaneous peripheral bypass (33367), open peripheral bypass (33368), or central bypass (33369).

33418 Transcatheter mitral valve repair, percutaneous approach, including transseptal puncture when performed; initial prosthesis
➲ *CPT Changes: An Insider's View* 2015
➲ *CPT Assistant* Sep 15:3

(Do not report 33418 in conjunction with 93462 unless transapical puncture is performed)

+ 33419 additional prosthesis(es) during same session (List separately in addition to code for primary procedure)
➲ *CPT Changes: An Insider's View* 2015
➲ *CPT Assistant* Sep 15:3

(Use 33419 in conjunction with 33418)

(For transcatheter mitral valve repair, percutaneous approach via the coronary sinus, use 0345T)

(For transcatheter mitral valve implantation/replacement [TMVI], see 0483T, 0484T)

33420 Valvotomy, mitral valve; closed heart
➲ *CPT Assistant* Feb 05:14

33422 open heart, with cardiopulmonary bypass
➔ *CPT Assistant* Feb 05:14

33425 Valvuloplasty, mitral valve, with cardiopulmonary bypass;
➔ *CPT Assistant* May 03:19, Feb 05:14

33426 with prosthetic ring
➔ *CPT Assistant* Feb 05:14

33427 radical reconstruction, with or without ring
➔ *CPT Assistant* Feb 05:14

33430 Replacement, mitral valve, with cardiopulmonary bypass
➔ *CPT Assistant* Feb 05:14

33440 Code is out of numerical sequence. See 33406-33412

Tricuspid Valve

33460 Valvectomy, tricuspid valve, with cardiopulmonary bypass
➔ *CPT Assistant* Feb 05:14

33463 Valvuloplasty, tricuspid valve; without ring insertion
➔ *CPT Assistant* Feb 05:14

33464 with ring insertion
➔ *CPT Assistant* Feb 05:14

33465 Replacement, tricuspid valve, with cardiopulmonary bypass
➔ *CPT Assistant* Feb 05:14

33468 Tricuspid valve repositioning and plication for Ebstein anomaly
➔ *CPT Assistant* Feb 05:14

Pulmonary Valve

Code 33477 is used to report transcatheter pulmonary valve implantation (TPVI). Code 33477 should only be reported once per session.

Code 33477 includes the work, when performed, of percutaneous access, placing the access sheath, advancing the repair device delivery system into position, repositioning the device as needed, and deploying the device(s). Angiography, radiological supervision, and interpretation performed to guide TPVI (eg, guiding device placement and documenting completion of the intervention) are included in the code.

►Code 33477 includes all cardiac catheterization(s), intraprocedural contrast injection(s), fluoroscopic radiological supervision and interpretation, and imaging guidance performed to complete the pulmonary valve procedure. Do not report 33477 in conjunction with 76000, 93451, 93453, 93454, 93455, 93456, 93457, 93458, 93459, 93460, 93461, 93530, 93531, 93532, 93533, 93563, 93566, 93567, 93568 for angiography intrinsic to the procedure.◄

Code 33477 includes percutaneous balloon angioplasty of the conduit/treatment zone, valvuloplasty of the pulmonary valve conduit, and stent deployment within the pulmonary conduit or an existing bioprosthetic pulmonary valve, when performed. Do not report 33477 in conjunction with 37236, 37237, 92997, 92998 for pulmonary artery angioplasty/valvuloplasty or stenting within the prosthetic valve delivery site.

Codes 92997, 92998 may be reported separately when pulmonary artery angioplasty is performed at a site separate from the prosthetic valve delivery site.Codes 37236, 37237 may be reported separately when pulmonary artery stenting is performed at a site separate from the prosthetic valve delivery site.

Diagnostic right heart catheterization and diagnostic coronary angiography codes (93451, 93453, 93454, 93455, 93456, 93457, 93458, 93459, 93460, 93461, 93530, 93531, 93532, 93533, 93563, 93566, 93567, 93568) should **not** be used with 33477 to report:

1. Contrast injections, angiography, roadmapping, and/or fluoroscopic guidance for the TPVI,
2. Pulmonary conduit angiography for guidance of TPVI, or
3. Right heart catheterization for hemodynamic measurements before, during, and after TPVI for guidance of TPVI.

Diagnostic right and left heart catheterization codes (93451, 93452, 93453, 93456, 93457, 93458, 93459, 93460, 93461, 93530, 93531, 93532, 93533), diagnostic coronary angiography codes (93454, 93455, 93456, 93457, 93458, 93459, 93460, 93461, 93563, 93564), and diagnostic pulmonary angiography code (93568) may be reported with 33477, representing separate and distinct services from TPVI, if:

1. No prior study is available and a full diagnostic study is performed, or
2. A prior study is available, but as documented in the medical record:
   a. There is inadequate visualization of the anatomy and/or pathology, or
   b. The patient's condition with respect to the clinical indication has changed since the prior study, or
   c. There is a clinical change during the procedure that requires new evaluation.

Other cardiac catheterization services may be reported separately when performed for diagnostic purposes not intrinsic to TPVI.

For same session/same day diagnostic cardiac catheterization services, report the appropriate diagnostic cardiac catheterization code(s) appended with modifier 59 to indicate separate and distinct procedural services from TPVI.

Diagnostic coronary angiography performed at a separate session from an interventional procedure may be separately reportable, when performed.

Percutaneous coronary interventional procedures may be reported separately, when performed.

Percutaneous pulmonary artery branch interventions may be reported separately, when performed.

When transcatheter ventricular support is required in conjunction with TPVI, the appropriate code may be reported with the appropriate percutaneous ventricular assist device (VAD) procedure codes (33990, 33991, 33992, 33993), extracorporeal membrane oxygenation (ECMO) or extracorporeal life support services (ECLS) procedure codes (33946-33989), or balloon pump insertion codes (33967, 33970, 33973).

When cardiopulmonary bypass is performed in conjunction with TPVI, code 33477 may be reported with the appropriate add-on code for percutaneous peripheral bypass (33367), open peripheral bypass (33368), or central bypass (33369).

33470 Valvotomy, pulmonary valve, closed heart; transventricular
➔ *CPT Assistant* Feb 05:14

(Do not report modifier 63 in conjunction with 33470)

33471 via pulmonary artery
➔ *CPT Assistant* Feb 05:14

(To report percutaneous valvuloplasty of pulmonary valve, use 92990)

33474 Valvotomy, pulmonary valve, open heart, with cardiopulmonary bypass
➔ *CPT Assistant* Feb 05:14

33475 Replacement, pulmonary valve
➔ *CPT Assistant* Feb 05:14

33476 Right ventricular resection for infundibular stenosis, with or without commissurotomy
➔ *CPT Assistant* Feb 05:14

33477 Transcatheter pulmonary valve implantation, percutaneous approach, including pre-stenting of the valve delivery site, when performed
➔ *CPT Changes: An Insider's View* 2016
➔ *CPT Assistant* Mar 16:5, Aug 16:10

33478 Outflow tract augmentation (gusset), with or without commissurotomy or infundibular resection
➔ *CPT Assistant* Feb 05:14

(Use 33478 in conjunction with 33768 when a cavopulmonary anastomosis to a second superior vena cava is performed)

Other Valvular Procedures

33496 Repair of non-structural prosthetic valve dysfunction with cardiopulmonary bypass (separate procedure)
➔ *CPT Assistant* Nov 97:16, Feb 05:14

(For reoperation, use 33530 in addition to 33496)

Coronary Artery Anomalies

Basic procedures include endarterectomy or angioplasty.

33500 Repair of coronary arteriovenous or arteriocardiac chamber fistula; with cardiopulmonary bypass

33501 without cardiopulmonary bypass

33502 Repair of anomalous coronary artery from pulmonary artery origin; by ligation
➔ *CPT Changes: An Insider's View* 2006

33503 by graft, without cardiopulmonary bypass

(Do not report modifier 63 in conjunction with 33502, 33503)

33504 by graft, with cardiopulmonary bypass

33505 with construction of intrapulmonary artery tunnel (Takeuchi procedure)

33506 by translocation from pulmonary artery to aorta

(Do not report modifier 63 in conjunction with 33505, 33506)

33507 Repair of anomalous (eg, intramural) aortic origin of coronary artery by unroofing or translocation
➔ *CPT Changes: An Insider's View* 2006
➔ *CPT Assistant* Mar 07:1

Endoscopy

Surgical vascular endoscopy always includes diagnostic endoscopy.

+ 33508 Endoscopy, surgical, including video-assisted harvest of vein(s) for coronary artery bypass procedure (List separately in addition to code for primary procedure)
➔ *CPT Changes: An Insider's View* 2003

(Use 33508 in conjunction with 33510-33523)

(For open harvest of upper extremity vein procedure, use 35500)

Venous Grafting Only for Coronary Artery Bypass

The following codes are used to report coronary artery bypass procedures using venous grafts only. These codes should NOT be used to report the performance of coronary artery bypass procedures using arterial grafts and venous grafts during the same procedure. See 33517-33523 and 33533-33536 for reporting combined arterial-venous grafts.

Procurement of the saphenous vein graft is included in the description of the work for 33510-33516 and should not be reported as a separate service or co-surgery. To report harvesting of an upper extremity vein, use 35500 in addition to the bypass procedure. To report harvesting of a femoropopliteal vein segment, report 35572 in addition to the bypass procedure. When surgical assistant performs graft procurement, add modifier 80 to 33510-33516. For percutaneous ventricular assist device insertion, removal, repositioning, see 33990-33993.

33510 Coronary artery bypass, vein only; single coronary venous graft

➲ *CPT Assistant* Fall 91:5, Winter 92:12, Jul 99:11, Apr 01:7, Feb 05:14, Jan 07:7, Mar 07:1, Aug 14:14

33511 2 coronary venous grafts

➲ *CPT Assistant* Fall 91:5, Winter 92:12, Jul 99:11, Apr 01:7, Feb 05:14, Jan 07:7, Mar 07:1

33512 3 coronary venous grafts

➲ *CPT Assistant* Fall 91:5, Winter 92:12, Apr 01:7, Feb 05:14, Jan 07:7, Mar 07:1

33513 4 coronary venous grafts

➲ *CPT Assistant* Fall 91:5, Winter 92:12, Apr 01:7, Feb 05:14, Jan 07:7, Mar 07:1

Coronary Artery Bypass-Venous Grafting Only

33510-33516

A. Use 33510 to report a single coronary venous graft.

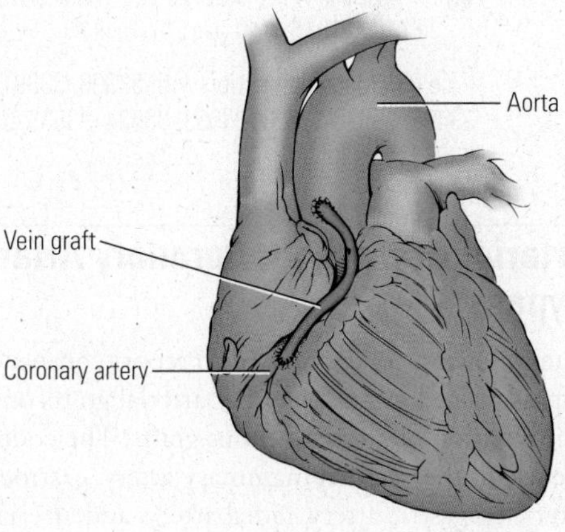

B. Report 33512 when 3 coronary venous grafts are performed.

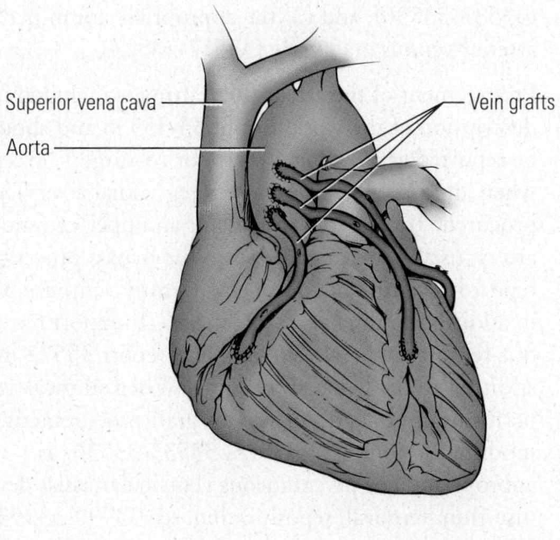

33514 5 coronary venous grafts

➲ *CPT Assistant* Fall 91:5, Winter 92:12, Apr 01:7, Feb 05:14, Jan 07:7, Mar 07:1

33516 6 or more coronary venous grafts

➲ *CPT Assistant* Fall 91:5, Winter 92:12, Jul 99:11, Apr 01:7, Feb 05:14, Jan 07:7, Mar 07:1, Aug 14:14

Combined Arterial-Venous Grafting for Coronary Bypass

The following codes are used to report coronary artery bypass procedures using venous grafts and arterial grafts during the same procedure. These codes may NOT be used alone.

To report combined arterial-venous grafts it is necessary to report two codes: (1) the appropriate combined arterial-venous graft code (33517-33523); and (2) the appropriate arterial graft code (33533-33536).

Procurement of the saphenous vein graft is included in the description of the work for 33517-33523 and should not be reported as a separate service or co-surgery. Procurement of the artery for grafting is included in the description of the work for 33533-33536 and should not be reported as a separate service or co-surgery, except when an upper extremity artery (eg, radial artery) is procured. To report harvesting of an upper extremity artery, use 35600 in addition to the bypass procedure. To report harvesting of an upper extremity vein, use 35500 in addition to the bypass procedure. To report harvesting of a femoropopliteal vein segment, report 35572 in addition to the bypass procedure. When surgical assistant performs arterial and/or venous graft procurement, add modifier 80 to 33517-33523, 33533-33536, as appropriate. For percutaneous ventricular assist device insertion, removal, repositioning, see 33990-33993.

+ 33517 Coronary artery bypass, using venous graft(s) and arterial graft(s); single vein graft (List separately in addition to code for primary procedure)

➲ *CPT Changes: An Insider's View* 2000, 2008

➲ *CPT Assistant* Fall 91:5, Winter 92:13, Nov 99:18, Apr 01:7, Feb 05:14

(Use 33517 in conjunction with 33533-33536)

+ 33518 2 venous grafts (List separately in addition to code for primary procedure)

➲ *CPT Changes: An Insider's View* 2008

➲ *CPT Assistant* Fall 91:5, Winter 92:13, Apr 01:7, Feb 05:14, Jan 07:7, Mar 07:1

(Use 33518 in conjunction with 33533-33536)

+ 33519 3 venous grafts (List separately in addition to code for primary procedure)

➲ *CPT Changes: An Insider's View* 2008

➲ *CPT Assistant* Fall 91:5, Winter 92:13, Apr 01:7, Feb 05:14, Jan 07:7, Mar 07:1

(Use 33519 in conjunction with 33533-33536)

Coronary Artery Bypass Combined Arterial-Venous Grafting

33517-33530

Both venous and arterial grafts are used in these bypass procedures. The appropriate arterial graft codes (33533-33536) must also be reported in conjunction with codes 33517-33530.

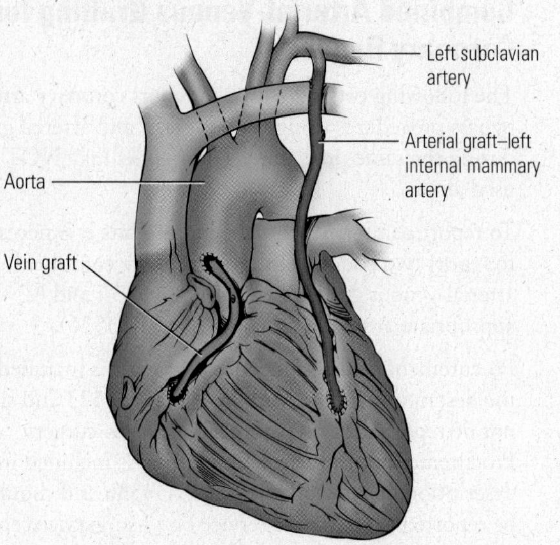

Coronary Artery Bypass-Sequential Combined Arterial-Venous Grafting

33517-33530

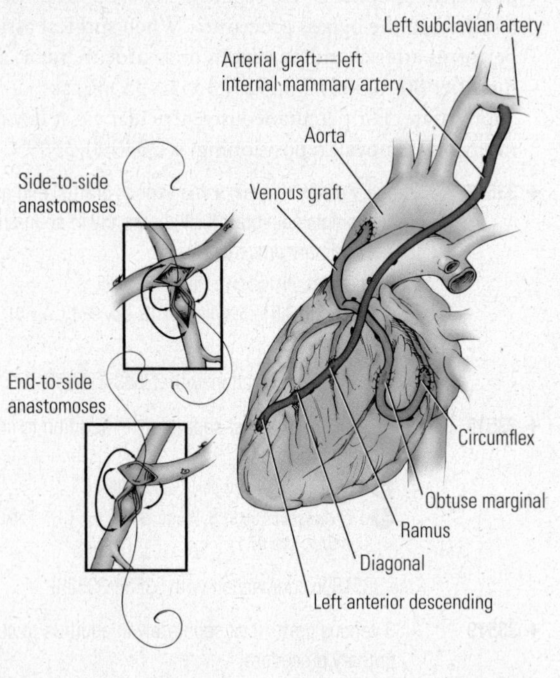

Note: To determine the number of bypass grafts in a coronary artery bypass (CABG), count the number of distal anastomoses (contact point[s]) where the bypass graft artery or vein is sutured to the diseased coronary artery(s).

+ 33521 4 venous grafts (List separately in addition to code for primary procedure)

➲ *CPT Changes: An Insider's View* 2008

➲ *CPT Assistant* Fall 91:5, Winter 92:13, Apr 01:7, Feb 05:14, Jan 07:7, Mar 07:1

(Use 33521 in conjunction with 33533-33536)

+ 33522 5 venous grafts (List separately in addition to code for primary procedure)

➲ *CPT Changes: An Insider's View* 2008

➲ *CPT Assistant* Fall 91:5, Winter 92:13, Apr 01:7, Feb 05:14, Jan 07:7, Mar 07:1

(Use 33522 in conjunction with 33533-33536)

+ 33523 6 or more venous grafts (List separately in addition to code for primary procedure)

➲ *CPT Changes: An Insider's View* 2008

➲ *CPT Assistant* Fall 91:5, Winter 92:13, Apr 01:7, Feb 05:14, Jan 07:7, Mar 07:1

(Use 33523 in conjunction with 33533-33536)

+ 33530 Reoperation, coronary artery bypass procedure or valve procedure, more than 1 month after original operation (List separately in addition to code for primary procedure)

➲ *CPT Assistant* Winter 90:6, Fall 91:5, Winter 92:13, Apr 01:7, Jul 01:11, Feb 05:13-14, Jan 07:7, Feb 11:8

(Use 33530 in conjunction with 33390, 33391, 33404-33496, 33510-33523, 33533, 33534, 33535, 33536, 33863)

Arterial Grafting for Coronary Artery Bypass

The following codes are used to report coronary artery bypass procedures using either arterial grafts only or a combination of arterial-venous grafts. The codes include the use of the internal mammary artery, gastroepiploic artery, epigastric artery, radial artery, and arterial conduits procured from other sites.

To report combined arterial-venous grafts it is necessary to report two codes: (1) the appropriate arterial graft code (33533-33536); and (2) the appropriate combined arterial-venous graft code (33517-33523).

Procurement of the artery for grafting is included in the description of the work for 33533-33536 and should not be reported as a separate service or co-surgery, except when an upper extremity artery (eg, radial artery) is procured. To report harvesting of an upper extremity artery, use 35600 in addition to the bypass procedure. To report harvesting of an upper extremity vein, use 35500 in addition to the bypass procedure. To report harvesting of a femoropopliteal vein segment, report 35572 in addition to the bypass procedure. When surgical assistant performs arterial and/or venous graft procurement, add modifier 80 to 33517-33523, 33533-33536, as appropriate. For percutaneous ventricular assist device insertion, removal, repositioning, see 33990-33993.

33533 Coronary artery bypass, using arterial graft(s); single arterial graft

➲ *CPT Changes: An Insider's View* 2000

➲ *CPT Assistant* Winter 92:12, Nov 99:18, Apr 01:7, Feb 05:14, Jan 07:7, Mar 07:1, Nov 14:14

33534 2 coronary arterial grafts

➲ *CPT Assistant* Winter 92:12, Apr 01:7, Feb 05:14, Jan 07:7, Mar 07:1

33535 3 coronary arterial grafts

➲ *CPT Assistant* Winter 92:12, Apr 01:7, Feb 05:14, Jan 07:7, Mar 07:1

33536 4 or more coronary arterial grafts

➲ *CPT Assistant* Winter 92:12, Apr 01:7, Feb 05:14, Jan 07:7, Mar 07:1, Nov 14:14

33542 Myocardial resection (eg, ventricular aneurysmectomy)

➲ *CPT Assistant* Winter 92:12, Mar 07:1

33545 Repair of postinfarction ventricular septal defect, with or without myocardial resection

➲ *CPT Assistant* Winter 92:12, Mar 07:1

33548 Surgical ventricular restoration procedure, includes prosthetic patch, when performed (eg, ventricular remodeling, SVR, SAVER, Dor procedures)

➲ *CPT Changes: An Insider's View* 2006

➲ *CPT Assistant* Nov 06:21, Dec 06:10, Mar 07:1

(Do not report 33548 in conjunction with 32551, 33210, 33211, 33310, 33315)

(For Batista procedure or pachopexy, use 33999)

Coronary Endarterectomy

+ 33572 Coronary endarterectomy, open, any method, of left anterior descending, circumflex, or right coronary artery performed in conjunction with coronary artery bypass graft procedure, each vessel (List separately in addition to primary procedure)

(Use 33572 in conjunction with 33510-33516, 33533-33536)

Single Ventricle and Other Complex Cardiac Anomalies

33600 Closure of atrioventricular valve (mitral or tricuspid) by suture or patch

➲ *CPT Assistant* Mar 07:1

33602 Closure of semilunar valve (aortic or pulmonary) by suture or patch

33606 Anastomosis of pulmonary artery to aorta (Damus-Kaye-Stansel procedure)

33608 Repair of complex cardiac anomaly other than pulmonary atresia with ventricular septal defect by construction or replacement of conduit from right or left ventricle to pulmonary artery

(For repair of pulmonary artery arborization anomalies by unifocalization, see 33925-33926)

33610 Repair of complex cardiac anomalies (eg, single ventricle with subaortic obstruction) by surgical enlargement of ventricular septal defect

➲ *CPT Changes: An Insider's View* 2002

(Do not report modifier 63 in conjunction with 33610)

33611 Repair of double outlet right ventricle with intraventricular tunnel repair;

(Do not report modifier 63 in conjunction with 33611)

33612 with repair of right ventricular outflow tract obstruction

33615 Repair of complex cardiac anomalies (eg, tricuspid atresia) by closure of atrial septal defect and anastomosis of atria or vena cava to pulmonary artery (simple Fontan procedure)

33617 Repair of complex cardiac anomalies (eg, single ventricle) by modified Fontan procedure

(Use 33617 in conjunction with 33768 when a cavopulmonary anastomosis to a second superior vena cava is performed)

33619 Repair of single ventricle with aortic outflow obstruction and aortic arch hypoplasia (hypoplastic left heart syndrome) (eg, Norwood procedure)

➲ *CPT Assistant* Mar 07:1, Apr 11:6, May 12:14, Jul 16:3

(Do not report modifier 63 in conjunction with 33619)

33620 Application of right and left pulmonary artery bands (eg, hybrid approach stage 1)

➲ *CPT Changes: An Insider's View* 2011

➲ *CPT Assistant* Apr 11:3, May 12:14, Jul 16:3

(For banding of the main pulmonary artery related to septal defect, use 33690)

33621 Transthoracic insertion of catheter for stent placement with catheter removal and closure (eg, hybrid approach stage 1)

➲ *CPT Changes: An Insider's View* 2011

➲ *CPT Assistant* Apr 11:3, Jul 16:3

(For placement of stent, use 37236)

(Report both 33620, 33621 if performed in same session)

Initial Hybrid Palliation
33621

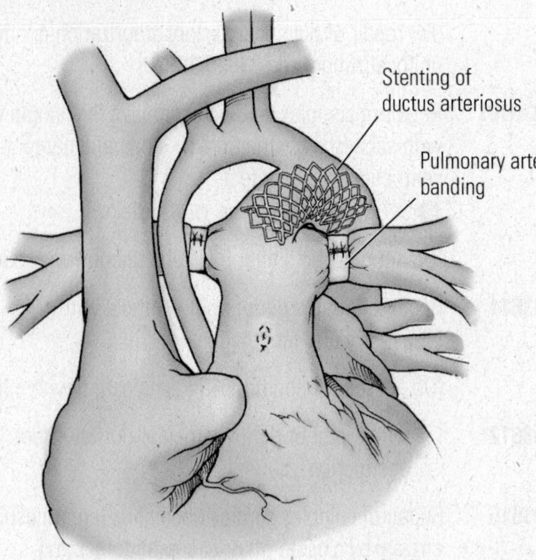

33622 Reconstruction of complex cardiac anomaly (eg, single ventricle or hypoplastic left heart) with palliation of single ventricle with aortic outflow obstruction and aortic arch hypoplasia, creation of cavopulmonary anastomosis, and removal of right and left pulmonary bands (eg, hybrid approach stage 2, Norwood, bidirectional Glenn, pulmonary artery debanding)
➲ *CPT Changes: An Insider's View* 2011
➲ *CPT Assistant* Apr 11:3, May 12:14, Jul 16:3

(Do not report 33622 in conjunction with 33619, 33767, 33822, 33840, 33845, 33851, 33853, 33917)

(For bilateral, bidirectional Glenn procedure, use 33622 in conjunction with 33768)

Hybrid Reconstruction
33622

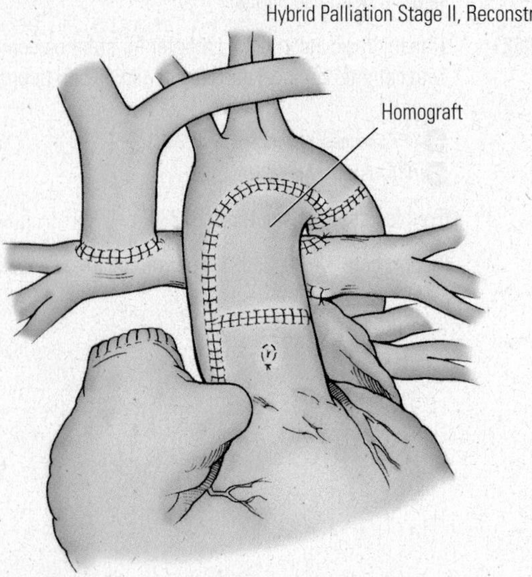

Septal Defect

33641 Repair atrial septal defect, secundum, with cardiopulmonary bypass, with or without patch
➲ *CPT Assistant* Mar 07:1, Dec 10:12

33645 Direct or patch closure, sinus venosus, with or without anomalous pulmonary venous drainage

(Do not report 33645 in conjunction with 33724, 33726)

33647 Repair of atrial septal defect and ventricular septal defect, with direct or patch closure

(Do not report modifier 63 in conjunction with 33647)

(For repair of tricuspid atresia (eg, Fontan, Gago procedures), use 33615)

33660 Repair of incomplete or partial atrioventricular canal (ostium primum atrial septal defect), with or without atrioventricular valve repair

33665 Repair of intermediate or transitional atrioventricular canal, with or without atrioventricular valve repair

33670 Repair of complete atrioventricular canal, with or without prosthetic valve

(Do not report modifier 63 in conjunction with 33670)

33675 Closure of multiple ventricular septal defects;
➲ *CPT Changes: An Insider's View* 2007
➲ *CPT Assistant* Mar 07:1

33676 with pulmonary valvotomy or infundibular resection (acyanotic)
➲ *CPT Changes: An Insider's View* 2007
➲ *CPT Assistant* Mar 07:1

33677 with removal of pulmonary artery band, with or without gusset
➲ *CPT Changes: An Insider's View* 2007
➲ *CPT Assistant* Mar 07:1

(Do not report 33675-33677 in conjunction with 32100, 32551, 32554, 32555, 33210, 33681, 33684, 33688)

(For percutaneous closure, use 93581)

33681 Closure of single ventricular septal defect, with or without patch;
➲ *CPT Changes: An Insider's View* 2007
➲ *CPT Assistant* Mar 07:1

33684 with pulmonary valvotomy or infundibular resection (acyanotic)

33688 with removal of pulmonary artery band, with or without gusset

(For pulmonary vein repair requiring creation of atrial septal defect, use 33724)

33690 Banding of pulmonary artery
➲ *CPT Assistant* Apr 11:4, May 12:14

(For right and left pulmonary artery banding in a single ventricle [eg, hybrid approach stage 1], use 33620)

(Do not report modifier 63 in conjunction with 33690)

33692 Complete repair tetralogy of Fallot without pulmonary atresia;

33694 with transannular patch

(Do not report modifier 63 in conjunction with 33694)

(For ligation and takedown of a systemic-to-pulmonary artery shunt, performed in conjunction with a congenital heart procedure; see 33924)

33697 Complete repair tetralogy of Fallot with pulmonary atresia including construction of conduit from right ventricle to pulmonary artery and closure of ventricular septal defect

➔ *CPT Assistant* Mar 07:1

(For ligation and takedown of a systemic-to-pulmonary artery shunt, performed in conjunction with a congenital heart procedure; see 33924)

Sinus of Valsalva

33702 Repair sinus of Valsalva fistula, with cardiopulmonary bypass;

➔ *CPT Assistant* Mar 07:1

33710 with repair of ventricular septal defect

33720 Repair sinus of Valsalva aneurysm, with cardiopulmonary bypass

33722 Closure of aortico-left ventricular tunnel

➔ *CPT Assistant* Mar 07:1

Venous Anomalies

33724 Repair of isolated partial anomalous pulmonary venous return (eg, Scimitar Syndrome)

➔ *CPT Changes: An Insider's View* 2007

➔ *CPT Assistant* Mar 07:1

(Do not report 33724 in conjunction with 32551, 33210, 33211)

33726 Repair of pulmonary venous stenosis

➔ *CPT Changes: An Insider's View* 2007

➔ *CPT Assistant* Mar 07:1

(Do not report 33726 in conjunction with 32551, 33210, 33211)

33730 Complete repair of anomalous pulmonary venous return (supracardiac, intracardiac, or infracardiac types)

➔ *CPT Assistant* Mar 07:1

(Do not report modifier 63 in conjunction with 33730)

(For partial anomalous pulmonary venous return, use 33724; for repair of pulmonary venous stenosis, use 33726)

33732 Repair of cor triatriatum or supravalvular mitral ring by resection of left atrial membrane

➔ *CPT Assistant* Mar 07:1

(Do not report modifier 63 in conjunction with 33732)

Shunting Procedures

33735 Atrial septectomy or septostomy; closed heart (Blalock-Hanlon type operation)

➔ *CPT Assistant* Mar 07:1

33736 open heart with cardiopulmonary bypass

(Do not report modifier 63 in conjunction with 33735, 33736)

33737 open heart, with inflow occlusion

(For transvenous method cardiac catheterization balloon atrial septectomy or septostomy (Rashkind type), use 92992)

(For blade method cardiac catheterization atrial septectomy or septostomy (Sang-Park septostomy), use 92993)

33750 Shunt; subclavian to pulmonary artery (Blalock-Taussig type operation)

33755 ascending aorta to pulmonary artery (Waterston type operation)

33762 descending aorta to pulmonary artery (Potts-Smith type operation)

(Do not report modifier 63 in conjunction with 33750, 33755, 33762)

33764 central, with prosthetic graft

33766 superior vena cava to pulmonary artery for flow to 1 lung (classical Glenn procedure)

33767 superior vena cava to pulmonary artery for flow to both lungs (bidirectional Glenn procedure)

➔ *CPT Assistant* Apr 11:6, Jul 16:3

+ 33768 Anastomosis, cavopulmonary, second superior vena cava (List separately in addition to primary procedure)

➔ *CPT Changes: An Insider's View* 2006

➔ *CPT Assistant* Mar 07:1, Apr 11:6, Jul 16:3

(Use 33768 in conjunction with 33478, 33617, 33622, 33767)

(Do not report 33768 in conjunction with 32551, 33210, 33211)

Transposition of the Great Vessels

33770 Repair of transposition of the great arteries with ventricular septal defect and subpulmonary stenosis; without surgical enlargement of ventricular septal defect

➔ *CPT Assistant* Mar 07:1

33771 with surgical enlargement of ventricular septal defect

33774 Repair of transposition of the great arteries, atrial baffle procedure (eg, Mustard or Senning type) with cardiopulmonary bypass;

33775 with removal of pulmonary band

33776 with closure of ventricular septal defect

33777 with repair of subpulmonic obstruction

33778 Repair of transposition of the great arteries, aortic pulmonary artery reconstruction (eg, Jatene type);

(Do not report modifier 63 in conjunction with 33778)

33779 with removal of pulmonary band

33780 with closure of ventricular septal defect

33781 with repair of subpulmonic obstruction
➲ *CPT Assistant* Mar 07:1

33782 Aortic root translocation with ventricular septal defect and pulmonary stenosis repair (ie, Nikaidoh procedure); without coronary ostium reimplantation
➲ *CPT Changes: An Insider's View* 2010

(Do not report 33782 in conjunction with 33412, 33413, 33608, 33681, 33770, 33771, 33778, 33780, 33920)

33783 with reimplantation of 1 or both coronary ostia
➲ *CPT Changes: An Insider's View* 2010

Truncus Arteriosus

33786 Total repair, truncus arteriosus (Rastelli type operation)
➲ *CPT Assistant* Mar 07:1

(Do not report modifier 63 in conjunction with 33786)

33788 Reimplantation of an anomalous pulmonary artery
➲ *CPT Assistant* Mar 07:1

(For pulmonary artery band, use 33690)

Aortic Anomalies

33800 Aortic suspension (aortopexy) for tracheal decompression (eg, for tracheomalacia) (separate procedure)
➲ *CPT Assistant* Mar 07:1

33802 Division of aberrant vessel (vascular ring);

33803 with reanastomosis

33813 Obliteration of aortopulmonary septal defect; without cardiopulmonary bypass

33814 with cardiopulmonary bypass

33820 Repair of patent ductus arteriosus; by ligation
➲ *CPT Assistant* Mar 07:1

33822 by division, younger than 18 years
➲ *CPT Assistant* Mar 07:1, Apr 11:6, Jul 16:3

Patent Ductus Arteriosus
33820

The tissues surrounding the ductus are dissected away and then several heavy ligatures are passed around the ductus and tied off on both ends.

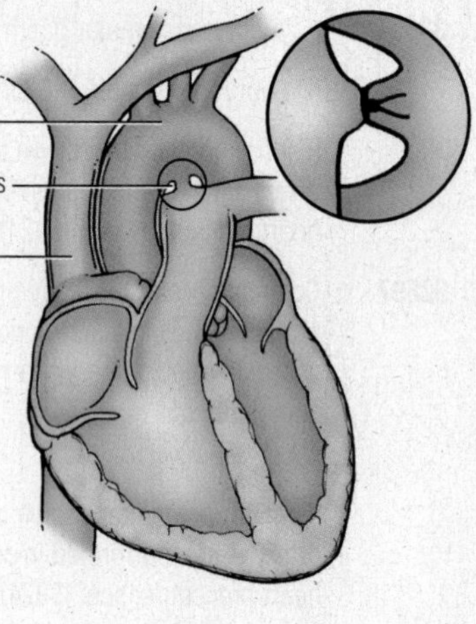

33824 by division, 18 years and older

(For percutaneous transcatheter closure of patent ductus arteriosus, use 93582)

33840 Excision of coarctation of aorta, with or without associated patent ductus arteriosus; with direct anastomosis
➲ *CPT Assistant* Apr 11:6, Jul 16:3

33845 with graft
➲ *CPT Assistant* Apr 11:6, Jul 16:3

33851 repair using either left subclavian artery or prosthetic material as gusset for enlargement
➲ *CPT Assistant* Apr 11:6, Jul 16:3

33852 Repair of hypoplastic or interrupted aortic arch using autogenous or prosthetic material; without cardiopulmonary bypass

33853 with cardiopulmonary bypass
➲ *CPT Assistant* Mar 07:1, Apr 11:6, Jul 16:3

(For repair of hypoplastic left heart syndrome (eg, Norwood type), via excision of coarctation of aorta, use 33619)

Thoracic Aortic Aneurysm

▶When ascending aortic disease involves the aortic arch, an aortic hemiarch graft may be necessary in conjunction with the ascending aortic graft and may be reported with add-on code 33866 in conjunction with the appropriate ascending aortic graft code (33860, 33863, 33864). Aortic hemiarch graft requires all of the following components:

1. Either total circulatory arrest or isolated cerebral perfusion (retrograde or antegrade);

2. Incision into the transverse arch extending under one or more of the arch vessels (eg, innominate, left common carotid, or left subclavian arteries); and
3. Extension of the ascending aortic graft under the aortic arch by construction of a beveled anastomosis to the distal ascending aorta and aortic arch without a cross-clamp (an open anastomosis).

An ascending aortic repair with a beveled anastomosis into the arch with a cross-clamp cannot be reported separately as a hemiarch graft using 33866. Use 33866 for aortic hemiarch graft when performed in conjunction with the ascending aortic graft codes 33860, 33863, 33864.◄

33860 Ascending aorta graft, with cardiopulmonary bypass, includes valve suspension, when performed

➲ *CPT Changes: An Insider's View* 2011

➲ *CPT Assistant* Mar 07:1, Aug 11:3

►(Do not report 33860 in conjunction with 33870)◄

33863 Ascending aorta graft, with cardiopulmonary bypass, with aortic root replacement using valved conduit and coronary reconstruction (eg, Bentall)

➲ *CPT Changes: An Insider's View* 2011

➲ *CPT Assistant* Feb 05:14, Mar 07:1, Aug 11:3

►(Do not report 33863 in conjunction with 33405, 33406, 33410, 33411, 33412, 33413, 33860, 33870)◄

33864 Ascending aorta graft, with cardiopulmonary bypass with valve suspension, with coronary reconstruction and valve-sparing aortic root remodeling (eg, David Procedure, Yacoub Procedure)

➲ *CPT Changes: An Insider's View* 2008, 2011

➲ *CPT Assistant* Aug 11:3

►(Do not report 33864 in conjunction with 33860, 33863, 33870)◄

+● **33866** Aortic hemiarch graft including isolation and control of the arch vessels, beveled open distal aortic anastomosis extending under one or more of the arch vessels, and total circulatory arrest or isolated cerebral perfusion (List separately in addition to code for primary procedure)

➲ *CPT Changes: An Insider's View* 2019

►(Use 33866 in conjunction with 33860, 33863, 33864)◄

►(Do not report 33866 in conjunction with 33870)◄

33870 Transverse arch graft, with cardiopulmonary bypass

►(Do not report 33870 in conjunction with 33860, 33863, 33864, 33866)◄

►(Use 33866 for aortic hemiarch graft when performed in conjunction with ascending aortic graft [33860, 33863, 33864])◄

33875 Descending thoracic aorta graft, with or without bypass

33877 Repair of thoracoabdominal aortic aneurysm with graft, with or without cardiopulmonary bypass

Aortic Root Remodeling: Coronary Arteries Reimplanted

33864

Valve-sparing aortic root replacement (code 33864)

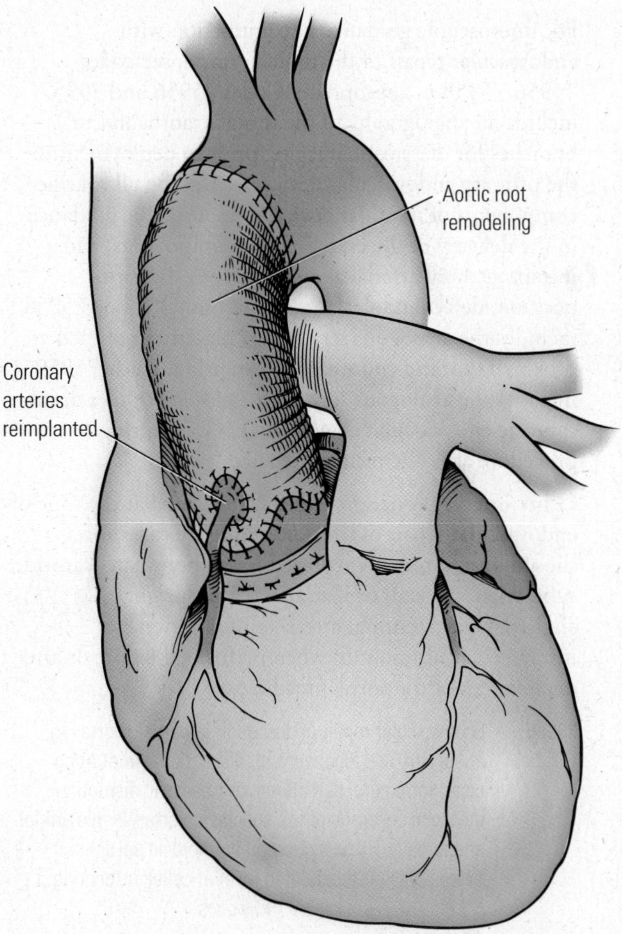

Endovascular Repair of Descending Thoracic Aorta

Codes 33880-33891 represent a family of procedures to report placement of an endovascular graft for repair of the descending thoracic aorta. These codes include all device introduction, manipulation, positioning, and deployment. All balloon angioplasty and/or stent deployment within the target treatment zone for the endoprosthesis, either before or after endograft deployment, are not separately reportable.

Open arterial exposure and associated closure of the arteriotomy sites (eg, 34714, 34715, 34716, 34812, 34820, 34833, 34834), introduction of guidewires and catheters (eg, 36140, 36200-36218), and extensive repair or replacement of an artery (eg, 35226, 35286) may be additionally reported. Transposition of subclavian artery to carotid, and carotid-carotid bypass performed in

Cardiovascular 33010-39599

conjunction with endovascular repair of the descending thoracic aorta (eg, 33889, 33891) may be separately reported. The primary codes, 33880 and 33881, include placement of all distal extensions, if required, in the distal thoracic aorta, while proximal extensions, if needed, may be reported separately.

For fluoroscopic guidance in conjunction with endovascular repair of the thoracic aorta, see codes 75956-75959 as appropriate. Codes 75956 and 75957 include all angiography of the thoracic aorta and its branches for diagnostic imaging prior to deployment of the primary endovascular devices (including all routine components of modular devices), fluoroscopic guidance in the delivery of the endovascular components, and intraprocedural arterial angiography (eg, confirm position, detect endoleak, evaluate runoff). Code 75958 includes the analogous services for placement of each proximal thoracic endovascular extension. Code 75959 includes the analogous services for placement of a distal thoracic endovascular extension(s) placed during a procedure after the primary repair.

Other interventional procedures performed at the time of endovascular repair of the descending thoracic aorta should be additionally reported (eg, innominate, carotid, subclavian, visceral, or iliac artery transluminal angioplasty or stenting, arterial embolization, intravascular ultrasound) when performed before or after deployment of the aortic prostheses.

33880 Endovascular repair of descending thoracic aorta (eg, aneurysm, pseudoaneurysm, dissection, penetrating ulcer, intramural hematoma, or traumatic disruption); involving coverage of left subclavian artery origin, initial endoprosthesis plus descending thoracic aortic extension(s), if required, to level of celiac artery origin

➔ *CPT Changes: An Insider's View* 2006
➔ *CPT Assistant* Dec 17:3
➔ *Clinical Examples in Radiology* Winter 06:14

(For radiological supervision and interpretation, use 75956 in conjunction with 33880)

33881 not involving coverage of left subclavian artery origin, initial endoprosthesis plus descending thoracic aortic extension(s), if required, to level of celiac artery origin

➔ *CPT Changes: An Insider's View* 2006
➔ *CPT Assistant* Dec 17:3
➔ *Clinical Examples in Radiology* Winter 06:14

(For radiological supervision and interpretation, use 75957 in conjunction with 33881)

33883 Placement of proximal extension prosthesis for endovascular repair of descending thoracic aorta (eg, aneurysm, pseudoaneurysm, dissection, penetrating ulcer, intramural hematoma, or traumatic disruption); initial extension

➔ *CPT Changes: An Insider's View* 2006
➔ *CPT Assistant* Dec 17:3
➔ *Clinical Examples in Radiology* Winter 06:14

(For radiological supervision and interpretation, use 75958 in conjunction with 33883)

(Do not report 33881, 33883 when extension placement converts repair to cover left subclavian origin. Use only 33880)

+ 33884 each additional proximal extension (List separately in addition to code for primary procedure)

➔ *CPT Changes: An Insider's View* 2006
➔ *CPT Assistant* Dec 17:3
➔ *Clinical Examples in Radiology* Winter 06:14

(Use 33884 in conjunction with 33883)

(For radiological supervision and interpretation, use 75958 in conjunction with 33884)

33886 Placement of distal extension prosthesis(s) delayed after endovascular repair of descending thoracic aorta

➔ *CPT Changes: An Insider's View* 2006
➔ *CPT Assistant* Dec 17:3
➔ *Clinical Examples in Radiology* Winter 06:14

(Do not report 33886 in conjunction with 33880, 33881)

(Report 33886 once, regardless of number of modules deployed)

(For radiological supervision and interpretation, use 75959 in conjunction with 33886)

33889 Open subclavian to carotid artery transposition performed in conjunction with endovascular repair of descending thoracic aorta, by neck incision, unilateral

➔ *CPT Changes: An Insider's View* 2006
➔ *Clinical Examples in Radiology* Winter 06:15

(Do not report 33889 in conjunction with 35694)

33891 Bypass graft, with other than vein, transcervical retropharyngeal carotid-carotid, performed in conjunction with endovascular repair of descending thoracic aorta, by neck incision

➔ *CPT Changes: An Insider's View* 2006
➔ *Clinical Examples in Radiology* Winter 06:15

(Do not report 33891 in conjunction with 35509, 35601)

Pulmonary Artery

33910 Pulmonary artery embolectomy; with cardiopulmonary bypass

➔ *CPT Assistant* Mar 07:1

33915 without cardiopulmonary bypass

➔ *CPT Assistant* Mar 07:1

33916 Pulmonary endarterectomy, with or without embolectomy, with cardiopulmonary bypass

➔ *CPT Assistant* Mar 07:1

33917 Repair of pulmonary artery stenosis by reconstruction with patch or graft

➔ *CPT Assistant* Mar 07:1, Apr 11:6, Jul 16:3

33920 Repair of pulmonary atresia with ventricular septal defect, by construction or replacement of conduit from right or left ventricle to pulmonary artery

➲ *CPT Assistant* Mar 07:1

(For repair of other complex cardiac anomalies by construction or replacement of right or left ventricle to pulmonary artery conduit, use 33608)

33922 Transection of pulmonary artery with cardiopulmonary bypass

(Do not report modifier 63 in conjunction with 33922)

+ 33924 Ligation and takedown of a systemic-to-pulmonary artery shunt, performed in conjunction with a congenital heart procedure (List separately in addition to code for primary procedure)

(Use 33924 in conjunction with 33470-33478, 33600-33617, 33622, 33684-33688, 33692-33697, 33735-33767, 33770-33783, 33786, 33917, 33920, 33922, 33925, 33926, 33935, 33945)

33925 Repair of pulmonary artery arborization anomalies by unifocalization; without cardiopulmonary bypass

➲ *CPT Changes: An Insider's View* 2006

33926 with cardiopulmonary bypass

➲ *CPT Changes: An Insider's View* 2006

Heart/Lung Transplantation

Heart with or without lung allotransplantation involves three distinct components of physician work:

1. ***Cadaver donor cardiectomy with or without pneumonectomy,*** which includes harvesting the allograft and cold preservation of the allograft (perfusing with cold preservation solution and cold maintenance) (see 33930, 33940).
2. ***Backbench work:***

   Preparation of a cadaver donor heart and lung allograft prior to transplantation, including dissection of the allograft from surrounding soft tissues to prepare the aorta, superior vena cava, inferior vena cava, and trachea for implantation (use 33933).

   Preparation of a cadaver donor heart allograft prior to transplantation, including dissection of the allograft from surrounding soft tissues to prepare aorta, superior vena cava, inferior vena cava, pulmonary artery, and left atrium for implantation (use 33944).
3. ***Recipient heart with or without lung allotransplantation,*** which includes transplantation of allograft and care of the recipient (see 33935, 33945).

(For implantation of a total replacement heart system [artificial heart] with recipient cardiectomy, use 33927)

33927 Implantation of a total replacement heart system (artificial heart) with recipient cardiectomy

➲ *CPT Changes: An Insider's View* 2018

(For implantation of ventricular assist device, see 33975, 33976, 33979, 33990, 33991)

Total Heart Implantation Device
33927, 33928, 33929

Total heart implantation device in place after cardiectomy

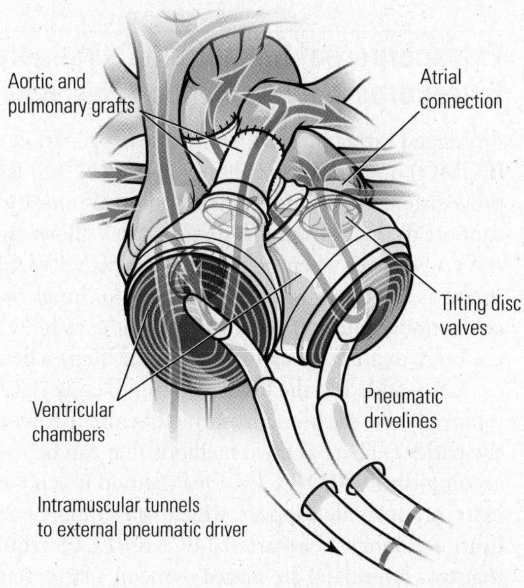

33928 Removal and replacement of total replacement heart system (artificial heart)

➲ *CPT Changes: An Insider's View* 2018

(For revision or replacement of components only of a replacement heart system [artificial heart], use 33999)

+ 33929 Removal of a total replacement heart system (artificial heart) for heart transplantation (List separately in addition to code for primary procedure)

➲ *CPT Changes: An Insider's View* 2018

(Use 33929 in conjunction with 33945)

33930 Donor cardiectomy-pneumonectomy (including cold preservation)

➲ *CPT Changes: An Insider's View* 2005

33933 Backbench standard preparation of cadaver donor heart/lung allograft prior to transplantation, including dissection of allograft from surrounding soft tissues to prepare aorta, superior vena cava, inferior vena cava, and trachea for implantation

➲ *CPT Changes: An Insider's View* 2005

33935 Heart-lung transplant with recipient cardiectomy-pneumonectomy

33940 Donor cardiectomy (including cold preservation)

➲ *CPT Changes: An Insider's View* 2005

➲ *CPT Assistant* Apr 05:10-11

33944 Backbench standard preparation of cadaver donor heart allograft prior to transplantation, including dissection of allograft from surrounding soft tissues to prepare aorta, superior vena cava, inferior vena cava, pulmonary artery, and left atrium for implantation

➔ *CPT Changes: An Insider's View* 2005

(For repair or resection procedures on the donor heart, see 33300, 33310, 33320, 33390, 33463, 33464, 33510, 33641, 35216, 35276, 35685)

33945 Heart transplant, with or without recipient cardiectomy

➔ *CPT Assistant* Fall 92:20

Extracorporeal Membrane Oxygenation or Extracorporeal Life Support Services

Prolonged extracorporeal membrane oxygenation (ECMO) or extracorporeal life support (ECLS) is a procedure that provides cardiac and/or respiratory support to the heart and/or lungs, which allows them to rest and recover when sick or injured. ECMO/ECLS supports the function of the heart and/or lungs by continuously pumping some of the patient's blood out of the body to an oxygenator (membrane lung) where oxygen is added to the blood, carbon dioxide (CO_2)is removed, and the blood is warmed before it is returned to the patient. There are two methods that can be used to accomplish ECMO/ECLS. One method is veno-arterial extracorporeal life support, which will support both the heart and lungs. Veno-arterial ECMO/ECLS requires that two cannula(e) are placed—one in a large vein and one in a large artery. The other method is veno-venous extracorporeal life support. Veno-venous ECMO/ECLS is used for lung support only and requires one or two cannula(e), which are placed in a vein.

Services directly related to the cannulation, initiation, management, and discontinuation of the ECMO/ECLS circuit and parameters (33946, 33947, 33948, 33949) are distinct from the daily overall management of the patient. The daily overall management of the patient is a factor that will vary greatly depending on the patient's age, disease process, and condition. Daily overall management of the patient may be separately reported using the relevant hospital observation services, hospital inpatient services, or critical care evaluation and management codes (99218, 99219, 99220, 99221, 99222, 99223, 99231, 99232, 99233, 99234, 99235, 99236, 99291, 99292, 99468, 99469, 99471, 99472, 99475, 99476, 99477, 99478, 99479, 99480).

Services directly related to the ECMO/ECLS involve the initial cannulation and repositioning, removing, or adding cannula(e) while the patient is being supported by the ECMO/ECLS. Initiation of the ECMO/ECLS circuit and setting parameters (33946, 33947) is performed by the physician and involves determining the necessary ECMO/ECLS device components, blood flow, gas exchange, and other necessary parameters to manage the circuit. The daily management of the ECMO/ECLS circuit and monitoring parameters (33948, 33949) requires physician oversight to ensure that specific features of the interaction of the circuit with the patient are met. Daily management of the circuit and parameters includes management of blood flow, oxygenation, CO_2 clearance by the membrane lung, systemic response, anticoagulation and treatment of bleeding, and cannula(e) positioning, alarms and safety. Once the patient's heart and/or lung function has sufficiently recovered, the physician will wean the patient from the ECMO/ECLS circuit and finally decannulate the patient. The basic management of the ECMO/ECLS circuit and parameters are similar, regardless of the patient's condition.

ECMO/ECLS commonly involves multiple physicians and supporting nonphysician personnel to manage each patient. Different physicians may insert the cannula(e) and initiate ECMO/ECLS, manage the ECMO/ECLS circuit, and decannulate the patient. In addition, it would be common for one physician to manage the ECMO/ECLS circuit and patient-related issues (eg, anticoagulation, complications related to the ECMO/ECLS devices), while another physician manages the overall patient medical condition and underlying disorders, all on a daily basis. The physicians involved in the patient's care are commonly of different specialties, and significant physician team interaction may be required. Depending on the type of circuit and the patient's condition, there is substantial nonphysician work by ECMO/ECLS specialists, cardiac perfusionists, respiratory therapists, and specially trained nurses who provide long periods of constant attention.

If the same physician provides any or all of the services for placing a patient on an ECMO/ECLS circuit, they may report the appropriate codes for the services they performed, which may include codes for the cannula(e) insertion (33951, 33952, 33953, 33954, 33955, 33956), ECMO/ECLS initiation (33946 or 33947), and overall patient management (99218, 99219, 99220, 99221, 99222, 99223, 99231, 99232, 99233, 99234, 99235, 99236, 99291, 99292, 99468, 99469, 99471, 99472, 99475, 99476, 99477, 99478, 99479, 99480).

ECMO/ECLS daily management (33948, 33949) and repositioning services (33957, 33958, 33959, 33962, 33963, 33964) may not be reported on the same day as initiation services (33946, 33947) by the same or different individuals.

If different physicians provide parts of the service, each physician may report the correct code(s) for the service(s) they provided, except as noted.

Repositioning of the ECMO/ECLS cannula(e) (33957, 33958, 33959, 33962, 33963, 33964) at the same session as insertion (33951, 33952, 33953, 33954, 33955, 33956) is not separately reportable. Replacement of ECMO/ECLS cannula(e) in the same vessel should only be reported using the insertion code (33951, 33952, 33953, 33954, 33955, 33956). If cannula(e) are removed from one vessel and new cannula(e) are placed in a different vessel, report the appropriate cannula(e) removal (33965, 33966, 33969, 33984, 33985, 33986) and insertion (33951, 33952, 33953, 33954, 33955, 33956) codes. Extensive repair or replacement of an artery may be additionally reported (eg, 35266, 35286, 35371, and 35665). Fluoroscopic guidance used for cannula(e) repositioning (33957, 33958, 33959, 33962, 33963, 33964) is included in the procedure when performed and should not be separately reported.

Daily management codes (33948 and 33949) should not be reported on the same day as initiation of ECMO (33946 or 33947).

Initiation codes (33946 or 33947) should not be reported on the same day as repositioning codes (33957, 33958, 33959, 33962, 33963, 33964). See the CPT codes for ECMO/ECLS Procedure Chart.

33946 Extracorporeal membrane oxygenation (ECMO)/extracorporeal life support (ECLS) provided by physician; initiation, veno-venous

➔ *CPT Changes: An Insider's View* 2015

➔ *CPT Assistant* Jul 15:3, Mar 16:5

(Do not report modifier 63 in conjunction with 33946, 33947, 33948, 33949)

(For insertion of cannula[e] for extracorporeal circulation, see 33951, 33952, 33953, 33954, 33955, 33956)

33947 initiation, veno-arterial

➔ *CPT Changes: An Insider's View* 2015

➔ *CPT Assistant* Jul 15:3, Mar 16:5

(Do not report modifier 63 in conjunction with 33946, 33947, 33948, 33949)

(Do not report 33946, 33947 in conjunction with 33948, 33949,33957, 33958, 33959, 33962, 33963, 33964)

33948 daily management, each day, veno-venous

➔ *CPT Changes: An Insider's View* 2015

➔ *CPT Assistant* Jul 15:3, Mar 16:5

(Do not report modifier 63 in conjunction with 33946, 33947, 33948, 33949)

33949 daily management, each day, veno-arterial

➔ *CPT Changes: An Insider's View* 2015

➔ *CPT Assistant* Jul 15:3, Mar 16:5

(Do not report modifier 63 in conjunction with 33946, 33947, 33948, 33949)

(Do not report 33948, 33949 in conjunction with 33946, 33947)

33951 insertion of peripheral (arterial and/or venous) cannula(e), percutaneous, birth through 5 years of age (includes fluoroscopic guidance, when performed)

➔ *CPT Changes: An Insider's View* 2015

➔ *CPT Assistant* Jul 15:3, Mar 16:5

(For initiation and daily management of extracorporeal circulation, see 33946, 33947, 33948, 33949)

33952 insertion of peripheral (arterial and/or venous) cannula(e), percutaneous, 6 years and older (includes fluoroscopic guidance, when performed)

➔ *CPT Changes: An Insider's View* 2015

➔ *CPT Assistant* Jul 15:3, Mar 16:5

(For maintenance of extracorporeal circulation, see 33946, 33947, 33948, 33949)

33953 insertion of peripheral (arterial and/or venous) cannula(e), open, birth through 5 years of age

➔ *CPT Changes: An Insider's View* 2015

➔ *CPT Assistant* Jul 15:3, Mar 16:5

(For maintenance of extracorporeal circulation, see 33946, 33947, 33948, 33949)

33954 insertion of peripheral (arterial and/or venous) cannula(e), open, 6 years and older

➔ *CPT Changes: An Insider's View* 2015

➔ *CPT Assistant* Jul 15:3, Mar 16:5

(Do not report 33953, 33954 in conjunction with 34714, 34715, 34716, 34812, 34820, 34833, 34834)

(For maintenance of extracorporeal circulation, see 33946, 33947, 33948, 33949)

33955 insertion of central cannula(e) by sternotomy or thoracotomy, birth through 5 years of age

➔ *CPT Changes: An Insider's View* 2015

➔ *CPT Assistant* Jul 15:3, Mar 16:5

(For maintenance of extracorporeal circulation, see 33946, 33947, 33948, 33949)

33956 insertion of central cannula(e) by sternotomy or thoracotomy, 6 years and older

➔ *CPT Changes: An Insider's View* 2015

➔ *CPT Assistant* Jul 15:3, Mar 16:5

(Do not report 33955, 33956 in conjunction with 32100, 39010)

(For maintenance of extracorporeal circulation, see 33946, 33947, 33948, 33949)

33957 reposition peripheral (arterial and/or venous) cannula(e), percutaneous, birth through 5 years of age (includes fluoroscopic guidance, when performed)

➔ *CPT Changes: An Insider's View* 2015

➔ *CPT Assistant* Jul 15:3, Mar 16:5

33958 reposition peripheral (arterial and/or venous) cannula(e), percutaneous, 6 years and older (includes fluoroscopic guidance, when performed)

➔ *CPT Changes: An Insider's View* 2015

➔ *CPT Assistant* Jul 15:3, Mar 16:5

(Do not report 33957, 33958 in conjunction with 34713)

CPT Codes For ECMO/ECLS Procedures

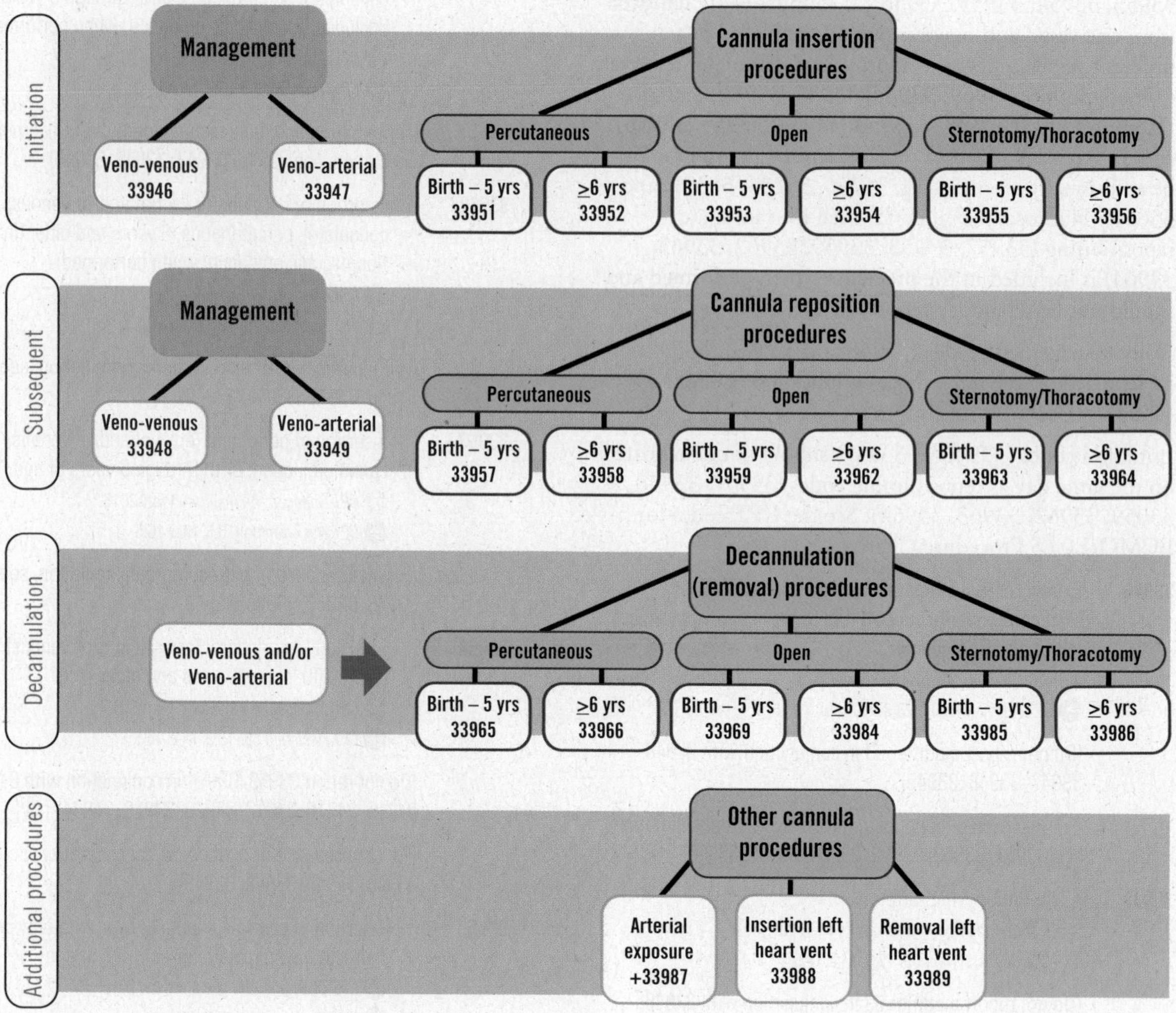

Abbreviations: Yrs indicates years; and ≥ indicates greater or equal to.

33959 reposition peripheral (arterial and/or venous) cannula(e), open, birth through 5 years of age (includes fluoroscopic guidance, when performed)

➲ *CPT Changes: An Insider's View* 2015

➲ *CPT Assistant* Jul 15:3, Mar 16:5

 # 33962 reposition peripheral (arterial and/or venous) cannula(e), open, 6 years and older (includes fluoroscopic guidance, when performed)

➲ *CPT Changes: An Insider's View* 2015

➲ *CPT Assistant* Jul 15:3, Mar 16:5

(Do not report 33959, 33962 in conjunction with 34714, 34715, 34716, 34812, 34820, 34834)

 # 33963 reposition of central cannula(e) by sternotomy or thoracotomy, birth through 5 years of age (includes fluoroscopic guidance, when performed)

➲ *CPT Changes: An Insider's View* 2015

➲ *CPT Assistant* Jul 15:3, Mar 16:5

 # 33964 reposition central cannula(e) by sternotomy or thoracotomy, 6 years and older (includes fluoroscopic guidance, when performed)

➲ *CPT Changes: An Insider's View* 2015

➲ *CPT Assistant* Jul 15:3, Mar 16:5

(Do not report 33963, 33964 in conjunction with 32100, 39010)

(Do not report 33957, 33958, 33959, 33962, 33963, 33964 in conjunction with 33946, 33947)

 # 33965 removal of peripheral (arterial and/or venous) cannula(e), percutaneous, birth through 5 years of age

➲ *CPT Changes: An Insider's View* 2015

➲ *CPT Assistant* Jul 15:3, Mar 16:5

 # 33966 removal of peripheral (arterial and/or venous) cannula(e), percutaneous, 6 years and older

➲ *CPT Changes: An Insider's View* 2015

➲ *CPT Assistant* Jul 15:3, Mar 16:5

 # 33969 removal of peripheral (arterial and/or venous) cannula(e), open, birth through 5 years of age

➲ *CPT Changes: An Insider's View* 2015

➲ *CPT Assistant* Jul 15:3, Mar 16:5

(Do not report 33969 in conjunction with 34714, 34715, 34716, 34812, 34820, 34834, 35201, 35206, 35211, 35226)

 # 33984 removal of peripheral (arterial and/or venous) cannula(e), open, 6 years and older

➲ *CPT Changes: An Insider's View* 2015

➲ *CPT Assistant* Jul 15:3, Mar 16:5

(Do not report 33984 in conjunction with 34714, 34715, 34716, 34812, 34820, 34834, 35201, 35206, 35211, 35226)

 # 33985 removal of central cannula(e) by sternotomy or thoracotomy, birth through 5 years of age

➲ *CPT Changes: An Insider's View* 2015

➲ *CPT Assistant* Jul 15:3, Mar 16:5

(Do not report 33985 in conjunction with 35211)

 # 33986 removal of central cannula(e) by sternotomy or thoracotomy, 6 years and older

➲ *CPT Changes: An Insider's View* 2015

➲ *CPT Assistant* Jul 15:3, Mar 16:5

(Do not report 33986 in conjunction with 35211)

#+ 33987 Arterial exposure with creation of graft conduit (eg, chimney graft) to facilitate arterial perfusion for ECMO/ECLS (List separately in addition to code for primary procedure)

➲ *CPT Changes: An Insider's View* 2015

➲ *CPT Assistant* Jul 15:3, Mar 16:5

(Use 33987 in conjunction with 33953, 33954, 33955, 33956)

(Do not report 33987 in conjunction with 34714, 34716, 34833)

 # 33988 Insertion of left heart vent by thoracic incision (eg, sternotomy, thoracotomy) for ECMO/ECLS

➲ *CPT Changes: An Insider's View* 2015

➲ *CPT Assistant* Jul 15:3, Mar 16:5

 # 33989 Removal of left heart vent by thoracic incision (eg, sternotomy, thoracotomy) for ECMO/ECLS

➲ *CPT Changes: An Insider's View* 2015

➲ *CPT Assistant* Jul 15:3, Mar 16:5

Cardiac Assist

The insertion of a ventricular assist device (VAD) can be performed via percutaneous (33990, 33991) or transthoracic (33975, 33976, 33979) approach. The location of the ventricular assist device may be intracorporeal or extracorporeal.

Open arterial exposure when necessary to facilitate percutaneous ventricular assist device insertion (33990, 33991), may be reported separately (34714, 34715, 34716, 34812, 34820, 34833, 34834). Extensive repair or replacement of an artery may be additionally reported (eg, 35226 or 35286).

Removal of a ventricular assist device (33977, 33978, 33980, 33992) includes removal of the entire device, including the cannulas. Removal of a percutaneous ventricular assist device at the same session as insertion is not separately reportable. For removal of a percutaneous ventricular assist device at a separate and distinct session, but on the same day as insertion, report 33992 appended with modifier 59 indicating a distinct procedural service.

Repositioning of a percutaneous ventricular assist device at the same session as insertion is not separately reportable. Repositioning of percutaneous ventricular assist device not necessitating imaging guidance is not a reportable service. For repositioning of a percutaneous ventricular assist device necessitating imaging guidance at a separate and distinct session, but on the same day as insertion, report 33993 with modifier 59 indicating a distinct procedural service.

Replacement of a ventricular assist device pump (ie, 33981-33983) includes the removal of the pump and insertion of a new pump, connection, de-airing, and initiation of the new pump.

Replacement of the entire implantable ventricular assist device system, ie, pump(s) and cannulas, is reported using the insertion codes (ie, 33975, 33976, 33979). Removal (ie, 33977, 33978, 33980) of the ventricular assist device system being replaced is not separately reported. Replacement of a percutaneous ventricular assist device is reported using implantation codes (ie, 33990, 33991). Removal (ie, 33992) is not reported separately.

33962 Code is out of numerical sequence. See 33958-33968

33963 Code is out of numerical sequence. See 33958-33968

33964 Code is out of numerical sequence. See 33958-33968

33965 Code is out of numerical sequence. See 33958-33968

33966 Code is out of numerical sequence. See 33958-33968

33967 Insertion of intra-aortic balloon assist device, percutaneous

➲ *CPT Changes: An Insider's View* 2002

➲ *CPT Assistant* Feb 02:2, Nov 11:8, Mar 13:10, Sep 15:3, Mar 16:5

33968 Removal of intra-aortic balloon assist device, percutaneous

➲ *CPT Changes: An Insider's View* 2000

➲ *CPT Assistant* Nov 99:19, Jan 00:10, Nov 11:8

(For removal of implantable aortic counterpulsation ventricular assist system, see 0455T, 0456T, 0457T, 0458T)

33969 Code is out of numerical sequence. See 33958-33968

33970 Insertion of intra-aortic balloon assist device through the femoral artery, open approach

➲ *CPT Changes: An Insider's View* 2000

➲ *CPT Assistant* Nov 99:19, Nov 11:8, Mar 13:10, Sep 15:3, Mar 16:5

(For insertion or replacement of implantable aortic counterpulsation ventricular assist system, see 0451T, 0452T, 0453T, 0454T)

33971 Removal of intra-aortic balloon assist device including repair of femoral artery, with or without graft

➲ *CPT Assistant* Nov 11:8

(For removal of implantable aortic counterpulsation ventricular assist system, see 0455T, 0456T, 0457T, 0458T)

33973 Insertion of intra-aortic balloon assist device through the ascending aorta

➲ *CPT Assistant* Nov 11:8, Mar 13:10, Sep 15:3, Mar 16:5

(For insertion or replacement of implantable aortic counterpulsation ventricular assist system, see 0451T, 0452T, 0453T, 0454T)

33974 Removal of intra-aortic balloon assist device from the ascending aorta, including repair of the ascending aorta, with or without graft

➲ *CPT Assistant* Nov 11:8

(For removal of implantable aortic counterpulsation ventricular assist system, see 0455T, 0456T, 0457T, 0458T)

33975 Insertion of ventricular assist device; extracorporeal, single ventricle

➲ *CPT Changes: An Insider's View* 2002

➲ *CPT Assistant* Feb 92:2, Jan 04:28, Nov 09:10, Jan 10:11, Apr 10:6, Mar 13:10

33976 extracorporeal, biventricular

➲ *CPT Changes: An Insider's View* 2002

➲ *CPT Assistant* Feb 02:2, Nov 09:10, Jan 10:11, Apr 10:6, Mar 13:10

33977 Removal of ventricular assist device; extracorporeal, single ventricle

➲ *CPT Changes: An Insider's View* 2002

➲ *CPT Assistant* Feb 02:2, Nov 09:10, Jan 10:11, Apr 10:6, Mar 13:10

33978 extracorporeal, biventricular

➲ *CPT Changes: An Insider's View* 2002

➲ *CPT Assistant* Feb 02:2, Nov 09:10, Jan 10:11, Apr 10:6, Mar 13:10

33979 Insertion of ventricular assist device, implantable intracorporeal, single ventricle

➲ *CPT Changes: An Insider's View* 2002

➲ *CPT Assistant* Feb 02:3, Jan 04:28, Nov 09:10, Jan 10:11, Apr 10:6, Mar 13:10

(For insertion or replacement of implantable aortic counterpulsation ventricular assist system, see 0451T, 0452T, 0453T, 0454T)

Insertion of Implantable Single Ventricle Assist Device
33979

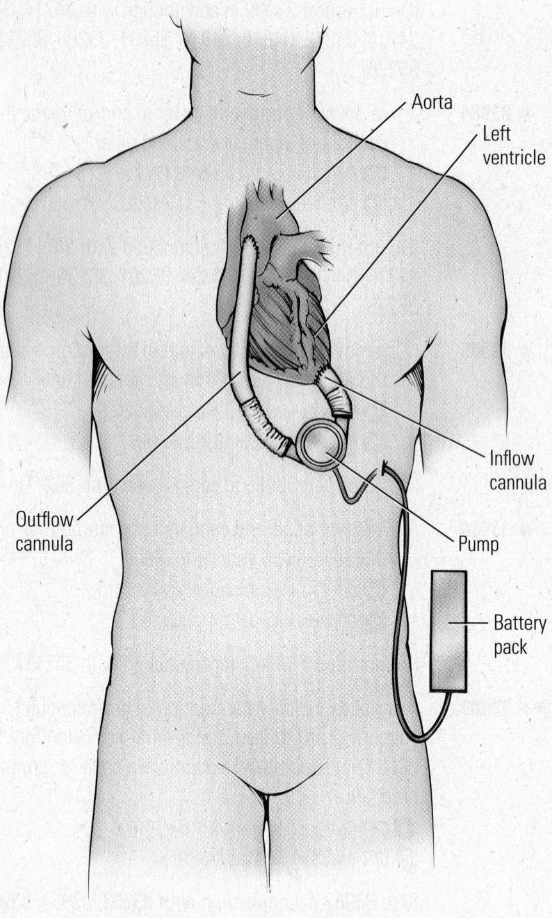

33980 Removal of ventricular assist device, implantable intracorporeal, single ventricle

➲ *CPT Changes: An Insider's View* 2002

➲ *CPT Assistant* Feb 02:3, Nov 09:10, Apr 10:6, Mar 13:10

(For removal of implantable aortic counterpulsation ventricular assist system, see 0455T, 0456T, 0457T, 0458T)

33981 Replacement of extracorporeal ventricular assist device, single or biventricular, pump(s), single or each pump

➲ *CPT Changes: An Insider's View* 2010

➲ *CPT Assistant* Apr 10:6

33982 Replacement of ventricular assist device pump(s); implantable intracorporeal, single ventricle, without cardiopulmonary bypass

➲ *CPT Changes: An Insider's View* 2010

➲ *CPT Assistant* Apr 10:6

33983 implantable intracorporeal, single ventricle, with cardiopulmonary bypass

➲ *CPT Changes: An Insider's View* 2010

➲ *CPT Assistant* Apr 10:6

(For insertion or replacement of implantable aortic counterpulsation ventricular assist system, see 0451T, 0452T, 0453T, 0454T)

33984 Code is out of numerical sequence. See 33958-33968

33985 Code is out of numerical sequence. See 33958-33968

33986 Code is out of numerical sequence. See 33958-33968

33987 Code is out of numerical sequence. See 33958-33968

33988 Code is out of numerical sequence. See 33958-33968

33989 Code is out of numerical sequence. See 33958-33968

33990 Insertion of ventricular assist device, percutaneous including radiological supervision and interpretation; arterial access only
➔ *CPT Changes: An Insider's View* 2013, 2017
➔ *CPT Assistant* Mar 13:10, Oct 14:15, Sep 15:3, Mar 16:5

33991 both arterial and venous access, with transseptal puncture
➔ *CPT Changes: An Insider's View* 2013, 2017
➔ *CPT Assistant* Mar 13:10, Sep 15:3, Mar 16:5

(For insertion or replacement of implantable aortic counterpulsation ventricular assist system, see 0451T, 0452T, 0453T, 0454T)

33992 Removal of percutaneous ventricular assist device at separate and distinct session from insertion
➔ *CPT Changes: An Insider's View* 2013, 2017
➔ *CPT Assistant* Mar 13:10, Sep 15:3, Mar 16:5

(For removal of implantable aortic counterpulsation ventricular assist system, see 0455T, 0456T, 0457T, 0458T)

33993 Repositioning of percutaneous ventricular assist device with imaging guidance at separate and distinct session from insertion
➔ *CPT Changes: An Insider's View* 2013, 2017
➔ *CPT Assistant* Mar 13:10, Sep 15:3, Mar 16:5

(For relocating and repositioning of implantable aortic counterpulsation ventricular assist system, see 0459T, 0460T, 0461T)

Other Procedures

33999 Unlisted procedure, cardiac surgery
➔ *CPT Assistant* Oct 99:11, Jan 04:7, Mar 07:1, Nov 09:10, Jan 10:11, Apr 10:6, Feb 13:13, Mar 13:10, Dec 13:14, Dec 14:17

Arteries and Veins

Primary vascular procedure listings include establishing both inflow and outflow by whatever procedures necessary. Also included is that portion of the operative arteriogram performed by the surgeon, as indicated. Sympathectomy, when done, is included in the listed aortic procedures. For unlisted vascular procedure, use 37799.

Embolectomy/Thrombectomy

Arterial, With or Without Catheter

34001 Embolectomy or thrombectomy, with or without catheter; carotid, subclavian or innominate artery, by neck incision

34051 innominate, subclavian artery, by thoracic incision

34101 axillary, brachial, innominate, subclavian artery, by arm incision

34111 radial or ulnar artery, by arm incision

34151 renal, celiac, mesentery, aortoiliac artery, by abdominal incision

34201 femoropopliteal, aortoiliac artery, by leg incision
➔ *CPT Assistant* Aug 11:9

34203 popliteal-tibio-peroneal artery, by leg incision

Venous, Direct or With Catheter

34401 Thrombectomy, direct or with catheter; vena cava, iliac vein, by abdominal incision

34421 vena cava, iliac, femoropopliteal vein, by leg incision
➔ *CPT Assistant* Spring 94:30

34451 vena cava, iliac, femoropopliteal vein, by abdominal and leg incision

34471 subclavian vein, by neck incision

34490 axillary and subclavian vein, by arm incision

Venous Reconstruction

34501 Valvuloplasty, femoral vein

34502 Reconstruction of vena cava, any method

34510 Venous valve transposition, any vein donor

34520 Cross-over vein graft to venous system

34530 Saphenopopliteal vein anastomosis

Endovascular Repair of Abdominal Aorta and/or Iliac Arteries

Codes 34701, 34702, 34703, 34704, 34705, 34706 describe introduction, positioning, and deployment of an endograft for treatment of abdominal aortic pathology (with or without rupture), such as aneurysm, pseudoaneurysm, dissection, penetrating ulcer, or traumatic disruption in the infrarenal abdominal aorta with or without extension into the iliac artery(ies). The terms, endovascular graft, endoprosthesis, endograft, and stentgraft, refer to a covered stent. The infrarenal aortic endograft may be an aortic tube device, a bifurcated unibody device, a modular bifurcated docking system with docking limb(s), or an aorto-uni-iliac device. Codes

Cardiovascular 33010-39599

34707 and 34708 describe introduction, positioning, and deployment of an ilio-iliac endograft for treatment of isolated arterial pathology (with or without rupture), such as aneurysm, pseudoaneurysm, arteriovenous malformation, or trauma involving the iliac artery. For treatment of atherosclerotic occlusive disease in the iliac artery(ies) with a covered stent(s), see 37221, 37223. For covered stent placement for atherosclerotic occlusive disease in the aorta, see 37236, 37237.

Report 34705 or 34706 for simultaneous bilateral iliac artery aneurysm repairs with aorto-bi-iliac endograft. For isolated bilateral iliac artery repair, report 34707 or 34708 with modifier 50 appended.

Decompressive laparotomy for abdominal compartment syndrome after ruptured abdominal aortic and/or iliac artery aneurysm repair may be separately reported with 49000 in addition to 34702, 34704, 34706, or 34708.

The treatment zone for endograft procedures is defined by those vessels that contain an endograft(s) (main body, docking limb[s], and/or extension[s]) deployed during that operative session. Adjunctive procedures outside the treatment zone may be separately reported (eg, angioplasty, endovascular stent placement, embolization). For example, when an endograft terminates in the common iliac artery, any additional treatment performed in the external and/or internal iliac artery may be separately reportable. Placement of a docking limb is inherent to a modular endograft(s), and, therefore, 34709 may not be reported separately if the docking limb extends into the external iliac artery. In addition, any interventions (eg, angioplasty, stenting, additional stent graft extension[s]) in the external iliac artery where the docking limb terminates may not be reported separately. Any catheterization or treatment of the internal iliac artery, such as embolization, may be separately reported. For 34701 and 34702, the abdominal aortic treatment zone is defined as the infrarenal aorta. For 34703 and 34704, the abdominal aortic treatment zone is typically defined as the infrarenal aorta and ipsilateral common iliac artery. For 34705 and 34706, the abdominal aortic treatment zone is typically defined as the infrarenal aorta and both common iliac arteries. For 34707 and 34708, the treatment zone is defined as the portion of the iliac artery(ies) (eg, common, internal, external iliac arteries) that contains the endograft. For a bifurcated iliac branch device, use 0254T.

Codes 34702, 34704, 34706, 34708 are reported when endovascular repair is performed on ruptured aneurysm in the aorta or iliac artery(ies). Rupture is defined as clinical and/or radiographic evidence of acute hemorrhage for purposes of reporting these codes. A chronic, contained rupture is considered a pseudoaneurysm, and endovascular treatment of a chronic, contained rupture is reported with 34701, 34703, 34705, or 34707.

Code 34709 is reported for placement of extension prosthesis(es) that terminate(s) either in the internal iliac, external iliac, or common femoral artery(ies) or in the abdominal aorta proximal to the renal artery(ies) in conjunction with 34701, 34702, 34703, 34704, 34705, 34706, 34707, 34708. Code 34709 may only be reported once per vessel treated (ie, multiple endograft extensions placed in a single vessel may only be reported once). Endograft extension(s) that terminate(s) in the common iliac arteries are included in 34703, 34704, 34705, 34706, 34707, 34708 and are not separately reported. Treatment zone angioplasty/stenting, when performed, is included in 34709. In addition, proximal infrarenal abdominal aortic extension prosthesis(es) that terminate(s) in the aorta below the renal artery(ies) are also included in 34701, 34702, 34703, 34704, 34705, 34706 and are not separately reportable.

Codes 34710, 34711 are reported for delayed placement of distal or proximal extension prosthesis(es) for endovascular repair of infrarenal abdominal aortic or iliac aneurysm, false aneurysm, dissection, endoleak, or endograft migration. Pre-procedure sizing and device selection, all nonselective catheterization(s), all associated radiological supervision and interpretation, and treatment zone angioplasty/stenting, when performed, are included in 34710 and 34711. Codes 34710 and 34711 may only be reported once per vessel treated (ie, multiple endograft extensions placed in a single vessel may only be reported once).

Nonselective catheterization is included in 34701, 34702, 34703, 34704, 34705, 34706, 34707, 34708 and is not separately reported. However, selective catheterization of the hypogastric artery(ies), renal artery(ies), and/or arterial families outside the treatment zone of the endograft may be separately reported. Intravascular ultrasound (37252, 37253) performed during endovascular aneurysm repair may be separately reported. Balloon angioplasty and/or stenting within the treatment zone of the endograft, either before or after endograft deployment, is not separately reported. Fluoroscopic guidance and radiological supervision and interpretation in conjunction with endograft repair is not separately reported, and includes all intraprocedural imaging (eg, angiography, rotational CT) of the aorta and its branches prior to deployment of the endovascular device, fluoroscopic guidance and roadmapping used in the delivery of the endovascular components, and intraprocedural and completion angiography (eg, confirm position, detect endoleak, evaluate runoff) performed at the time of the endovascular infrarenal aorta and/or iliac repair.

Codes 34709, 34710, 34711 include nonselective introduction of guidewires and catheters into the treatment zone from peripheral artery access(es). However, selective catheterization of the hypogastric artery(ies), renal artery(ies), and/or arterial families outside the treatment zone may be separately reported. Codes 34709, 34710, 34711 also include balloon angioplasty and/or stenting within the treatment zone of the endograft extension, either before or after deployment of the endograft, fluoroscopic guidance, and all associated radiological supervision and interpretation performed in conjunction with endovascular endograft extension (eg, angiographic diagnostic imaging of the aorta and its branches prior to deployment of the endovascular device, fluoroscopic guidance in the delivery of the endovascular components, and intraprocedural and completion angiography to confirm endograft position, detect endoleak, and evaluate runoff).

Code 34712 describes transcatheter delivery of accessory-enhanced fixation devices to the endograft (eg, anchor, screw, tack), including all associated radiological supervision and interpretation. Code 34712 may only be reported once per operative session.

Vascular access requiring use of closure devices for large sheaths (ie, 12 French or larger) or access requiring open surgical arterial exposure may be separately reported (eg, 34713, 34714, 34715, 34716, 34812, 34820, 34833, 34834). Code 34713 describes percutaneous access and closure of a femoral arteriotomy for delivery of endovascular prosthesis through a large arterial sheath (ie, 12 French or larger). Ultrasound guidance (ie, 76937), when performed, is included in 34713. (Percutaneous access using a sheath smaller than 12 French is included in 34701-34712 and is not separately reported.)

Code 34812 describes open repair and closure of the femoral artery. Extensive repair of an artery (eg, 35226, 35286, 35371) may also be reported separately. Iliac exposure for device delivery through a retroperitoneal incision, open brachial exposure, or axillary or subclavian exposure through an infraclavicular, or supraclavicular or sternotomy incision during endovascular aneurysm repair may be separately reported (eg, 34715, 34812, 34820, 34834). Endovascular device delivery or establishment of cardiopulmonary bypass that requires creation of a prosthetic conduit utilizing a femoral artery, iliac artery with a retroperitoneal incision, or axillary or subclavian artery exposure through an infraclavicular, supraclavicular, or sternotomy incision (34714, 34716, 34833) and oversewing of the conduit at the time of procedure completion may be separately reported during endovascular aneurysm repair or cardiac procedures requiring cardiopulmonary bypass. If a conduit is converted to a bypass, report the bypass (eg, 35665) and not the arterial exposure with conduit (34714, 34716, 34833). Arterial embolization(s) of renal, lumbar, inferior mesenteric, hypogastric or external iliac arteries to facilitate complete endovascular aneurysm exclusion may be separately reported (eg, 37242).

Balloon angioplasty and/or stenting at the sealing zone(s) of an endograft is an integral part of the procedure and is not separately reported. However, balloon angioplasty and/or stent deployment in vessels that do not contain endograft (outside the treatment zone for the endograft), either before or after endograft deployment, may be separately reported (eg, 37220, 37221, 37222, 37223).

Other interventional procedures performed at the time of endovascular abdominal aortic aneurysm repair may be additionally reported (eg, renal transluminal angioplasty, arterial embolization, intravascular ultrasound, balloon angioplasty or stenting of native artery[s] outside the endograft treatment zone, when done before or after deployment of endograft).

(For fenestrated endovascular repair of the visceral aorta, see 34841-34844. For fenestrated endovascular repair of the visceral aorta and concomitant infrarenal abdominal aorta, see 34845-34848)

34701 Endovascular repair of infrarenal aorta by deployment of an aorto-aortic tube endograft including pre-procedure sizing and device selection, all nonselective catheterization(s), all associated radiological supervision and interpretation, all endograft extension(s) placed in the aorta from the level of the renal arteries to the aortic bifurcation, and all angioplasty/stenting performed from the level of the renal arteries to the aortic bifurcation; for other than rupture (eg, for aneurysm, pseudoaneurysm, dissection, penetrating ulcer)

➲ *CPT Changes: An Insider's View* 2018

➲ *CPT Assistant* Dec 17:3

(For covered stent placement[s] for atherosclerotic occlusive disease isolated to the aorta, see 37236, 37237)

34702 for rupture including temporary aortic and/or iliac balloon occlusion, when performed (eg, for aneurysm, pseudoaneurysm, dissection, penetrating ulcer, traumatic disruption)

➲ *CPT Changes: An Insider's View* 2018

➲ *CPT Assistant* Dec 17:3

34703 Endovascular repair of infrarenal aorta and/or iliac artery(ies) by deployment of an aorto-uni-iliac endograft including pre-procedure sizing and device selection, all nonselective catheterization(s), all associated radiological supervision and interpretation, all endograft extension(s) placed in the aorta from the level of the renal arteries to the iliac bifurcation, and all angioplasty/stenting performed from the level of the renal arteries to the iliac bifurcation; for other than rupture (eg, for aneurysm, pseudoaneurysm, dissection, penetrating ulcer)

➲ *CPT Changes: An Insider's View* 2018

➲ *CPT Assistant* Dec 17:3

34704 for rupture including temporary aortic and/or iliac balloon occlusion, when performed (eg, for aneurysm, pseudoaneurysm, dissection, penetrating ulcer, traumatic disruption)

➲ *CPT Changes: An Insider's View* 2018

➲ *CPT Assistant* Dec 17:3

34705 Endovascular repair of infrarenal aorta and/or iliac artery(ies) by deployment of an aorto-bi-iliac endograft including pre-procedure sizing and device selection, all nonselective catheterization(s), all associated radiological supervision and interpretation, all endograft extension(s) placed in the aorta from the level of the renal arteries to the iliac bifurcation, and all angioplasty/stenting performed from the level of the renal arteries to the iliac bifurcation; for other than rupture (eg, for aneurysm, pseudoaneurysm, dissection, penetrating ulcer)

➔ *CPT Changes: An Insider's View* 2018

➔ *CPT Assistant* Dec 17:3

34706 for rupture including temporary aortic and/or iliac balloon occlusion, when performed (eg, for aneurysm, pseudoaneurysm, dissection, penetrating ulcer, traumatic disruption)

➔ *CPT Changes: An Insider's View* 2018

➔ *CPT Assistant* Dec 17:3

34707 Endovascular repair of iliac artery by deployment of an ilio-iliac tube endograft including pre-procedure sizing and device selection, all nonselective catheterization(s), all associated radiological supervision and interpretation, and all endograft extension(s) proximally to the aortic bifurcation and distally to the iliac bifurcation, and treatment zone angioplasty/stenting, when performed, unilateral; for other than rupture (eg, for aneurysm, pseudoaneurysm, dissection, arteriovenous malformation)

➔ *CPT Changes: An Insider's View* 2018

➔ *CPT Assistant* Dec 17:3

(For covered stent placement[s] for atherosclerotic occlusive disease of the abdominal aorta, see 37236, 37237)

(For covered stent placement[s] for atherosclerotic occlusive disease of the iliac artery, see 37221, 37223)

34708 for rupture including temporary aortic and/or iliac balloon occlusion, when performed (eg, for aneurysm, pseudoaneurysm, dissection, arteriovenous malformation, traumatic disruption)

➔ *CPT Changes: An Insider's View* 2018

➔ *CPT Assistant* Dec 17:3

+ 34709 Placement of extension prosthesis(es) distal to the common iliac artery(ies) or proximal to the renal artery(ies) for endovascular repair of infrarenal abdominal aortic or iliac aneurysm, false aneurysm, dissection, penetrating ulcer, including pre-procedure sizing and device selection, all nonselective catheterization(s), all associated radiological supervision and interpretation, and treatment zone angioplasty/stenting, when performed, per vessel treated (List separately in addition to code for primary procedure)

➔ *CPT Changes: An Insider's View* 2018

➔ *CPT Assistant* Dec 17:3

(Use 34709 in conjunction with 34701, 34702, 34703, 34704, 34705, 34706, 34707, 34708)

(34709 may only be reported once per vessel treated [ie, multiple endograft extensions placed in a single vessel may only be reported once])

Endovascular Repair

34705, 34706, 34709, 34710, 34711

Endovascular repair of abdominal aorta and/or iliac arteries

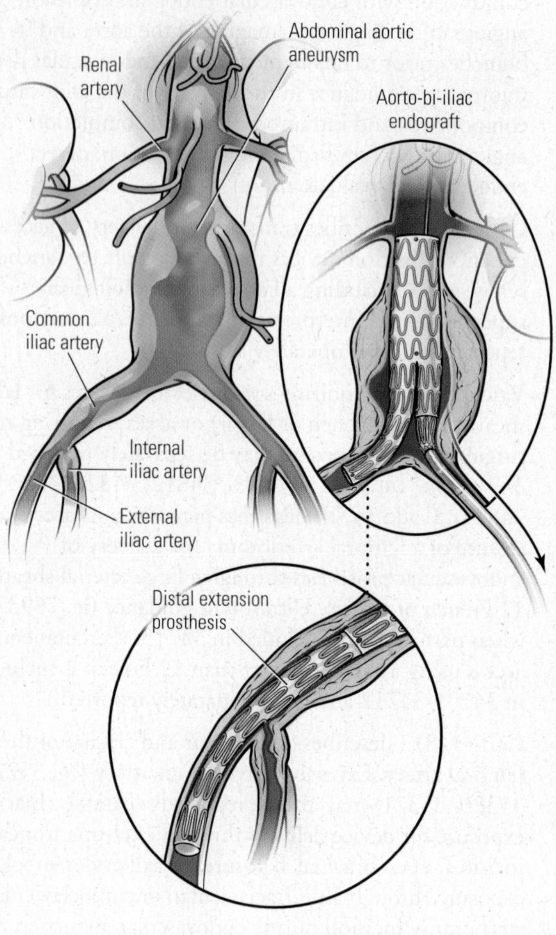

(Do not report 34709 for placement of a docking limb that extends into the external iliac artery)

(For endograft placement into a renal artery that is being covered by a proximal extension, see 37236, 37237)

34710 Delayed placement of distal or proximal extension prosthesis for endovascular repair of infrarenal abdominal aortic or iliac aneurysm, false aneurysm, dissection, endoleak, or endograft migration, including pre-procedure sizing and device selection, all nonselective catheterization(s), all associated radiological supervision and interpretation, and treatment zone angioplasty/stenting, when performed; initial vessel treated

➔ *CPT Changes: An Insider's View* 2018

➔ *CPT Assistant* Dec 17:3

+ 34711 each additional vessel treated (List separately in addition to code for primary procedure)

➔ *CPT Changes: An Insider's View* 2018

➔ *CPT Assistant* Dec 17:3

(Use 34711 in conjunction with 34710)

(34710, 34711 may each be reported only once per operative session [ie, multiple endograft extensions placed in a single vessel may only be reported with a single code])

(For decompressive laparotomy, use 49000 in conjunction with 34702, 34704, 34706, 34708, 34710)

(If the delayed revision is a transcatheter enhanced fixation device [eg, anchors, screws], report 34712)

(Do not report 34710, 34711 in conjunction with 34701, 34702, 34703, 34704, 34705, 34706, 34707, 34708, 34709)

(Do not report 34701-34711 in conjunction with 34841, 34842, 34843, 34844, 34845, 34846, 34847, 34848)

(For endovascular repair of iliac artery bifurcation [eg, aneurysm, pseudoaneurysm, arteriovenous malformation, trauma] using bifurcated endograft, use 0254T)

(Report 37252, 37253 for intravascular ultrasound when performed during endovascular aneurysm repair)

(For isolated bilateral iliac artery repair, report 34707 or 34708 with modifier 50)

(For open arterial exposure, report 34714, 34715, 34716, 34812, 34820, 34833, 34834 as appropriate, in conjunction with 34701, 34702, 34703, 34704, 34705, 34706, 34707, 34708, 34710)

(For percutaneous arterial closure, report 34713 as appropriate, in conjunction with 34701, 34702, 34703, 34704, 34705, 34706, 34707, 34708, 34710)

(For simultaneous bilateral iliac artery aneurysm repairs with aorto-biiliac endograft, see 34705, 34706, as appropriate)

34712 Transcatheter delivery of enhanced fixation device(s) to the endograft (eg, anchor, screw, tack) and all associated radiological supervision and interpretation

➔ *CPT Changes: An Insider's View* 2018

➔ *CPT Assistant* Dec 17:3

(Report 34712 only once per operative session)

+ 34713 Percutaneous access and closure of femoral artery for delivery of endograft through a large sheath (12 French or larger), including ultrasound guidance, when performed, unilateral (List separately in addition to code for primary procedure)

➔ *CPT Changes: An Insider's View* 2018

➔ *CPT Assistant* Dec 17:3

►(Use 34713 in conjunction with 33880, 33881, 33883, 33884, 33886, 34701, 34702, 34703, 34704, 34705, 34706, 34707, 34708, 34710, 34841, 34842, 34843, 34844, 34845, 34846, 34847, 34848, as appropriate. Do not report 34713 in conjunction with 33880, 33881, 33883, 33884, 33886, 34701, 34702, 34703, 34704, 34705, 34706, 34707, 34708, 34710, 34841, 34842, 34843, 34844, 34845, 34846, 34847, 34848, for percutaneous closure of femoral artery after delivery of endovascular prosthesis if a sheath smaller than 12 French was used)◄

(34713 may only be reported once per side. For bilateral procedure, report 34713 twice)

(Do not report ultrasound guidance [ie, 76937] for percutaneous vascular access in conjunction with 34713 for the same access)

(Do not report 34713 for percutaneous access and closure of the femoral artery in conjunction with 37221, 37223, 37236, 37237)

(Do not report 34713 in conjunction with 37221, 37223 for covered stent placement[s] for atherosclerotic occlusive disease of the iliac artery[ies])

#+ 34812 Open femoral artery exposure for delivery of endovascular prosthesis, by groin incision, unilateral (List separately in addition to code for primary procedure)

➔ *CPT Changes: An Insider's View* 2001, 2003, 2018

➔ *CPT Assistant* Dec 00:6, Sep 02:3, Feb 03:2, Mar 04:10, Jul 06:7, Mar 13:10, Dec 13:8, Dec 17:3

➔ *Clinical Examples in Radiology* Summer 14:2, 3

(Use 34812 in conjunction with 33880, 33881, 33883, 33884, 33886, 33990, 33991, 34701, 34702, 34703, 34704, 34705, 34706, 34707, 34708, 34841, 34842, 34843, 34844, 34845, 34846, 34847, 34848, 0254T)

(34812 may only be reported once per side. For bilateral procedure, report 34812 twice)

(Do not report 34812 in conjunction with 33953, 33954, 33959, 33962, 33969, 33984, 33987)

+ 34714 Open femoral artery exposure with creation of conduit for delivery of endovascular prosthesis or for establishment of cardiopulmonary bypass, by groin incision, unilateral (List separately in addition to code for primary procedure)

➔ *CPT Changes: An Insider's View* 2018

➔ *CPT Assistant* Dec 17:3

(Use 34714 in conjunction with 32852, 32854, 33031, 33120, 33251, 33256, 33259, 33261, 33305, 33315, 33322, 33335, 33390, 33391, 33404-33417, 33422, 33425, 33426, 33427, 33430, 33460, 33463, 33464, 33465, 33468, 33474, 33475, 33476, 33478, 33496, 33500, 33502, 33504, 33505, 33506, 33507, 33510, 33511, 33512, 33513, 33514, 33516, 33533, 33534, 33535, 33536, 33542, 33545, 33548, 33600-33688, 33692, 33694, 33697, 33702, 33710, 33720, 33722, 33724, 33726, 33730, 33732, 33736, 33750, 33755, 33762, 33764, 33766, 33767, 33770-33783, 33786, 33788, 33802, 33803, 33814, 33820, 33822, 33824, 33840, 33845, 33851, 33853, 33860, 33863, 33864, 33870, 33875, 33877, 33880, 33881, 33883, 33884, 33886, 33910, 33916, 33917, 33920, 33922, 33926, 33935, 33945, 33975, 33976, 33977, 33978, 33979, 33980, 33983, 33990, 33991, 34701, 34702, 34703, 34704, 34705, 34706, 34707, 34708, 34841, 34842, 34843, 34844, 34845, 34846, 34847, 34848, 0254T)

(34714 may only be reported once per side. For bilateral procedure, report 34714 twice)

(Do not report 34714 in conjunction with 33362, 33953, 33954, 33959, 33962, 33969, 33984, 34812 when performed on the same side)

#+ 34820 Open iliac artery exposure for delivery of endovascular prosthesis or iliac occlusion during endovascular therapy, by abdominal or retroperitoneal incision, unilateral (List separately in addition to code for primary procedure)

➲ *CPT Changes: An Insider's View* 2001, 2018

➲ *CPT Assistant* Dec 00:7-8, Sep 02:3, Feb 03:4, Aug 04:10, Jul 06:7, Dec 17:3

(Use 34820 in conjunction with 33880, 33881, 33883, 33884, 33886, 33990, 33991, 34701, 34702, 34703, 34704, 34705, 34706, 34707, 34708, 34841, 34842, 34843, 34844, 34845, 34846, 34847, 34848, 0254T)

(34820 may only be reported once per side. For bilateral procedure, report 34820 twice)

(Do not report 34820 in conjunction with 33953, 33954, 33959, 33962, 33969, 33984)

#+ 34833 Open iliac artery exposure with creation of conduit for delivery of endovascular prosthesis or for establishment of cardiopulmonary bypass, by abdominal or retroperitoneal incision, unilateral (List separately in addition to code for primary procedure)

➲ *CPT Changes: An Insider's View* 2003, 2006, 2018

➲ *CPT Assistant* Feb 03:4, Aug 04:10, Jul 06:7, Dec 17:3

➲ *Clinical Examples in Radiology* Winter 06:19

(Use 34833 in conjunction with 32852, 32854, 33031, 33120, 33251, 33256, 33259, 33261, 33305, 33315, 33322, 33335, 33390, 33391, 33404-33417, 33422, 33425, 33426, 33427, 33430, 33460, 33463, 33464, 33465, 33468, 33474, 33475, 33476, 33478, 33496, 33500, 33502, 33504, 33505, 33506, 33507, 33510, 33511, 33512, 33513, 33514, 33516, 33533, 33534, 33535, 33536, 33542, 33545, 33548, 33600-33688, 33692, 33694, 33697, 33702, 33710, 33720, 33722, 33724, 33726, 33730, 33732, 33736, 33750, 33755, 33762, 33764, 33766, 33767, 33770-33783, 33786, 33788, 33802, 33803, 33814, 33820, 33822, 33824, 33840, 33845, 33851, 33853, 33860, 33863, 33864, 33870, 33875, 33877, 33880, 33881, 33883, 33884, 33886, 33910, 33916, 33917, 33920, 33922, 33926, 33935, 33945, 33975, 33976, 33977, 33978, 33979, 33980, 33983, 33990, 33991, 34701, 34702, 34703, 34704, 34705, 34706, 34707, 34708, 34841, 34842, 34843, 34844, 34845, 34846, 34847, 34848, 0254T)

(34833 may only be reported once per side. For bilateral procedure, report 34833 twice)

(Do not report 34833 in conjunction with 33364, 33953, 33954, 33959, 33962, 33969, 33984, 34820 when performed on the same side)

#+ 34834 Open brachial artery exposure for delivery of endovascular prosthesis, unilateral (List separately in addition to code for primary procedure)

➲ *CPT Changes: An Insider's View* 2003, 2006, 2018

➲ *CPT Assistant* Feb 03:4, Jul 06:7, Dec 17:3

➲ *Clinical Examples in Radiology* Winter 06:19

(Use 34834 in conjunction with 33880, 33881, 33883, 33884, 33886, 33990, 33991, 34701, 34702, 34703, 34704, 34705, 34706, 34707, 34708, 34841, 34842, 34843, 34844, 34845, 34846, 34847, 34848, 0254T)

(34834 may only be reported once per side. For bilateral procedure, report 34834 twice)

(Do not report 34834 in conjunction with 33953, 33954, 33959, 33962, 33969, 33984)

+ 34715 Open axillary/subclavian artery exposure for delivery of endovascular prosthesis by infraclavicular or supraclavicular incision, unilateral (List separately in addition to code for primary procedure)

➲ *CPT Changes: An Insider's View* 2018

➲ *CPT Assistant* Dec 17:3

(Use 34715 in conjunction with 33880, 33881, 33883, 33884, 33886, 33990, 33991, 34701, 34702, 34703, 34704, 34705, 34706, 34707, 34708, 34841, 34842, 34843, 34844, 34845, 34846, 34847, 34848, 0254T)

(34715 may only be reported once per side. For bilateral procedure, report 34715 twice)

(Do not report 34715 in conjunction with 33363, 33953, 33954, 33959, 33962, 33969, 33984, 0451T, 0452T, 0455T, 0456T)

+ 34716 Open axillary/subclavian artery exposure with creation of conduit for delivery of endovascular prosthesis or for establishment of cardiopulmonary bypass, by infraclavicular or supraclavicular incision, unilateral (List separately in addition to code for primary procedure)

➲ *CPT Changes: An Insider's View* 2018

➲ *CPT Assistant* Dec 17:3

(Use 34716 in conjunction with 32852, 32854, 33031, 33120, 33251, 33256, 33259-33261, 33305, 33315, 33322, 33335, 33390, 33391, 33404-33417, 33422, 33425, 33426, 33427, 33430, 33460, 33463, 33464, 33465, 33468, 33474, 33475, 33476, 33478, 33496, 33500, 33502, 33504, 33505, 33506, 33507, 33510, 33511, 33512, 33513, 33514, 33516, 33533, 33534, 33535, 33536, 33542, 33545, 33548, 33600-33688, 33692, 33694, 33697, 33702-33722, 33724, 33726, 33730, 33732, 33736, 33750, 33755, 33762, 33764, 33766, 33767, 33770-33783, 33786, 33788, 33802, 33803, 33814, 33820, 33822, 33824, 33840, 33845, 33851, 33853, 33860, 33863, 33864, 33870, 33875, 33877, 33880, 33881, 33883, 33884, 33886, 33910, 33916, 33917, 33920, 33922, 33926, 33935, 33945, 33975, 33976, 33977, 33978, 33979, 33980, 33983, 33990, 33991, 34701, 34702, 34703, 34704, 34705, 34706, 34707, 34708, 34841, 34842, 34843, 34844, 34845, 34846, 34847, 34848, 0254T)

(34716 may only be reported once per side. For bilateral procedure, report 34716 twice)

(Do not report 34716 in conjunction with 33953, 33954, 33959, 33962, 33969, 33984, 0451T, 0452T, 0455T, 0456T)

(34800, 34802, 34803, 34804, 34805, 34806 have been deleted. To report, see 34701, 34702, 34703, 34704, 34705, 34706, 34707, 34708)

+ 34808 Endovascular placement of iliac artery occlusion device (List separately in addition to code for primary procedure)

➲ *CPT Changes: An Insider's View* 2001

➲ *CPT Assistant* Dec 00:6, Sep 02:3, Apr 12:3

(Use 34808 in conjunction with 34701, 34702, 34707, 34708, 34709, 34710, 34813, 34841, 34842, 34843, 34844)

34812 Code is out of numerical sequence. See 34712-34716

+ 34813 Placement of femoral-femoral prosthetic graft during endovascular aortic aneurysm repair (List separately in addition to code for primary procedure)

➲ *CPT Changes: An Insider's View* 2001

➲ *CPT Assistant* Dec 00:6, Sep 02:3, Apr 12:3

(Use 34813 in conjunction with 34812)

(For femoral artery grafting, see 35521, 35533, 35539, 35540, 35556, 35558, 35566, 35621, 35646, 35654-35661, 35666, 35700)

34820 Code is out of numerical sequence. See 34712-34716

(34825, 34826 have been deleted. To report, see 34709, 34710, 34711)

34830 Open repair of infrarenal aortic aneurysm or dissection, plus repair of associated arterial trauma, following unsuccessful endovascular repair; tube prosthesis

➲ *CPT Changes: An Insider's View* 2001

➲ *CPT Assistant* Dec 00:6, Sep 02:3, Oct 08:10

34831 aorto-bi-iliac prosthesis

➲ *CPT Changes: An Insider's View* 2001

➲ *CPT Assistant* Dec 00:6, Sep 02:3, Oct 08:10

34832 aorto-bifemoral prosthesis

➲ *CPT Changes: An Insider's View* 2001

➲ *CPT Assistant* Dec 00:6, Sep 02:3, Oct 08:10

34833 Code is out of numerical sequence. See 34712-34716

34834 Code is out of numerical sequence. See 34712-34716

Fenestrated Endovascular Repair of the Visceral and Infrarenal Aorta

The upper abdominal aorta that contains the celiac, superior mesenteric, and renal arteries is termed the visceral aorta. For reporting purposes, the thoracic aorta extends from the aortic valve to the aortic segment just proximal to the celiac artery.

Code 34839 is used to report the physician planning and sizing for a patient-specific fenestrated visceral aortic endograft. The planning includes review of high-resolution cross-sectional images (eg, CT, CTA, MRI) and utilization of 3D software for iterative modeling of the aorta and device in multiplanar views and center line of flow analysis. Code 34839 may only be reported when the physician spends a minimum of 90 total minutes performing patient-specific fenestrated endograft planning. Physician planning time does not need to be continuous and should be clearly documented in the patient record. Code 34839 is reported on the date that planning work is complete and may not include time spent on the day before or the day of the fenestrated endovascular repair procedure (34841, 34842, 34843, 34844, 34845, 34846, 34847, 34848) nor be reported on the day before or the day of the fenestrated endovascular repair procedure.

Codes 34841, 34842, 34843, 34844, 34845, 34846, 34847, 34848 are used to report placement of a fenestrated endovascular graft in the visceral aorta, either alone or in combination with the infrarenal aorta for aneurysm, pseudoaneurysm, dissection, penetrating ulcer, intramural hematoma, or traumatic disruption. The fenestrated main body endoprosthesis is deployed within the visceral aorta. Fenestrations within the fabric allow for selective catheterization of the visceral and/or renal arteries and subsequent placement of an endoprosthesis (ie, bare metal or covered stent) to maintain flow to the visceral artery. Patient variation in the location and relative orientation of the renal and visceral artery origins requires use of a patient-specific fenestrated endograft for endovascular repair that preserves flow to essential visceral arteries and allows proximal seal and fixation to be achieved above the renal level as well as in the distal aorta or iliac vessel(s).

Fenestrated aortic repair is reported based on the extent of aorta treated. Codes 34841, 34842, 34843, 34844 describe repair using proximal endoprostheses that span from the visceral aortic component to one, two, three, or four visceral artery origins and distal extent limited to the infrarenal aorta. These devices do not extend into the common iliac arteries. Codes 34845, 34846, 34847, 34848 are used to report deployment of a fenestrated endograft that spans from the visceral aorta (including one, two, three, or four visceral artery origins) through the infrarenal aorta into the common iliac arteries. The infrarenal component may be a bifurcated unibody device, a modular bifurcated docking system with docking limb(s), or an aorto-uniiliac device. Codes 34845, 34846, 34847, 34848 include placement of unilateral or bilateral docking limbs (depending on the device). Any additional endograft extensions that terminate in the common iliac arteries are included in 34845, 34846, 34847, 34848. Codes 34709, 34710, 34711 may not be separately reported for proximal abdominal aortic extension prosthesis(es) or for distal extension prosthesis(es) that terminate(s) in the aorta or the common iliac arteries. However, 34709, 34710, 34711 may be reported for distal extension prosthesis(es) that terminate(s) in the internal iliac, external iliac, or common femoral artery(ies).

Codes 34841-34844 and 34845-34848 define the total number of visceral and/or renal arteries (ie, celiac, superior mesenteric, and/or unilateral or bilateral renal artery[s]) requiring placement of an endoprosthesis (ie, bare metal or covered stent) through an aortic endograft fenestration.

Introduction of guide wires and catheters in the aorta and visceral and/or renal arteries is included in the work of 34841-34848 and is not separately reportable. However, catheterization of the hypogastric artery(s) and/or arterial families outside the treatment zone of the graft may be separately reported. Balloon angioplasty within the target treatment zone of the endograft, either before or after endograft deployment, is not separately reportable. Fluoroscopic guidance and radiological supervision and interpretation in conjunction with fenestrated endovascular aortic repair is not separately reportable and includes angiographic diagnostic imaging of the aorta and its branches prior to deployment of the fenestrated endovascular device, fluoroscopic guidance in the delivery of the fenestrated endovascular components, and intraprocedural arterial angiography (eg, confirm position, detect endoleak, evaluate runoff) done at the time of the endovascular aortic repair.

Exposure of the access vessels (eg, 34713, 34714, 34715, 34716, 34812, 34820, 34833, 34834) may be reported separately. Extensive repair of an artery (eg, 35226, 35286) may be reported separately. For concomitant endovascular treatment of the descending thoracic aorta, 33880-33886 and 75956-75959 may be reported with 34841, 34842, 34843, 34844, 34845, 34846, 34847, 34848. For isolated endovascular infrarenal abdominal aortic aneurysm repair that does not require placement of a fenestrated graft to preserve flow to the visceral branch(es), see 34701, 34702, 34703, 34704, 34705, 34706.

Other interventional procedures performed at the time of fenestrated endovascular abdominal aortic aneurysm repair may be reported separately (eg, arterial embolization, intravascular ultrasound, balloon angioplasty or stenting of native artery[s] outside the endoprosthesis target zone, when done before or after deployment of endoprosthesis).

34839 Physician planning of a patient-specific fenestrated visceral aortic endograft requiring a minimum of 90 minutes of physician time

➲ *CPT Changes: An Insider's View* 2015

(Do not report 34839 in conjunction with 76376, 76377)

(Do not report 34839 in conjunction with 34841, 34842, 34843, 34844, 34845, 34846, 34847, 34848, when performed on the day before or the day of the fenestrated endovascular repair procedure)

34841 Endovascular repair of visceral aorta (eg, aneurysm, pseudoaneurysm, dissection, penetrating ulcer, intramural hematoma, or traumatic disruption) by deployment of a fenestrated visceral aortic endograft and all associated radiological supervision and interpretation, including target zone angioplasty, when performed; including one visceral artery endoprosthesis (superior mesenteric, celiac or renal artery)

➲ *CPT Changes: An Insider's View* 2014

➲ *CPT Assistant* Dec 13:8, Dec 17:3

34842 including two visceral artery endoprostheses (superior mesenteric, celiac and/or renal artery[s])

➲ *CPT Changes: An Insider's View* 2014

➲ *CPT Assistant* Dec 13:8, Dec 17:3

34843 including three visceral artery endoprostheses (superior mesenteric, celiac and/or renal artery[s])

➲ *CPT Changes: An Insider's View* 2014

➲ *CPT Assistant* Dec 13:8, Dec 17:3

34844 including four or more visceral artery endoprostheses (superior mesenteric, celiac and/or renal artery[s])

➲ *CPT Changes: An Insider's View* 2014

➲ *CPT Assistant* Dec 13:8, Dec 17:3

(Do not report 34841, 34842, 34843, 34844 in conjunction with 34701, 34702, 34703, 34704, 34705, 34706, 34845, 34846, 34847, 34848)

(Do not report 34841, 34842, 34843, 34844 in conjunction with 34839, when planning services are performed on the day before or the day of the fenestrated endovascular repair procedure)

34845 Endovascular repair of visceral aorta and infrarenal abdominal aorta (eg, aneurysm, pseudoaneurysm, dissection, penetrating ulcer, intramural hematoma, or traumatic disruption) with a fenestrated visceral aortic endograft and concomitant unibody or modular infrarenal aortic endograft and all associated radiological supervision and interpretation, including target zone angioplasty, when performed; including one visceral artery endoprosthesis (superior mesenteric, celiac or renal artery)

➲ *CPT Changes: An Insider's View* 2014

➲ *CPT Assistant* Dec 13:8, Dec 17:3

34846 including two visceral artery endoprostheses (superior mesenteric, celiac and/or renal artery[s])

➲ *CPT Changes: An Insider's View* 2014

➲ *CPT Assistant* Dec 13:8, Dec 17:3

34847 including three visceral artery endoprostheses (superior mesenteric, celiac and/or renal artery[s])

➲ *CPT Changes: An Insider's View* 2014

➲ *CPT Assistant* Dec 13:8, Dec 17:3

34848 including four or more visceral artery endoprostheses (superior mesenteric, celiac and/or renal artery[s])
CPT Changes: An Insider's View 2014
CPT Assistant Dec 13:8, Jul 16:6, Aug 17:10, Dec 17:3

(Do not report 34845, 34846, 34847, 34848 in conjunction with 34701, 34702, 34703, 34704, 34705, 34706, 34841, 34842, 34843, 34844, 35081, 35102)

(Do not report 34845, 34846, 34847, 34848 in conjunction with 34839, when planning services are performed on the day before or the day of the fenestrated endovascular repair procedure)

(Do not report 34841-34848 in conjunction with 37236, 37237 for bare metal or covered stents placed into the visceral branches within the endoprosthesis target zone)

(For placement of distal extension prosthesis[es] terminating in the internal iliac, external iliac, or common femoral artery[s], see 34709, 34710, 34711, 0254T)

(Use 34845, 34846, 34847, 34848 in conjunction with 37220, 37221, 37222, 37223, only when 37220, 37221, 37222, 37223 are performed outside the target treatment zone of the endoprosthesis)

Endovascular Repair of Iliac Aneurysm

(34900 has been deleted. To report, see 34707, 34708)

Direct Repair of Aneurysm or Excision (Partial or Total) and Graft Insertion for Aneurysm, Pseudoaneurysm, Ruptured Aneurysm, and Associated Occlusive Disease

Procedures 35001-35152 include preparation of artery for anastomosis including endarterectomy.

(For direct repairs associated with occlusive disease only, see 35201-35286)

(For intracranial aneurysm, see 61700 et seq)

(For endovascular repair of abdominal aortic and/or iliac artery aneurysm, see 34701-34716)

(For thoracic aortic aneurysm, see 33860-33875)

(For endovascular repair of descending thoracic aorta, involving coverage of left subclavian artery origin, use 33880)

35001 Direct repair of aneurysm, pseudoaneurysm, or excision (partial or total) and graft insertion, with or without patch graft; for aneurysm and associated occlusive disease, carotid, subclavian artery, by neck incision
CPT Changes: An Insider's View 2002

35002 for ruptured aneurysm, carotid, subclavian artery, by neck incision

35005 for aneurysm, pseudoaneurysm, and associated occlusive disease, vertebral artery
CPT Changes: An Insider's View 2002

35011 for aneurysm and associated occlusive disease, axillary-brachial artery, by arm incision

35013 for ruptured aneurysm, axillary-brachial artery, by arm incision

35021 for aneurysm, pseudoaneurysm, and associated occlusive disease, innominate, subclavian artery, by thoracic incision
CPT Changes: An Insider's View 2002

35022 for ruptured aneurysm, innominate, subclavian artery, by thoracic incision

35045 for aneurysm, pseudoaneurysm, and associated occlusive disease, radial or ulnar artery
CPT Changes: An Insider's View 2002

35081 for aneurysm, pseudoaneurysm, and associated occlusive disease, abdominal aorta
CPT Changes: An Insider's View 2002
CPT Assistant Dec 00:2, Dec 01:7, Dec 13:8

35082 for ruptured aneurysm, abdominal aorta

35091 for aneurysm, pseudoaneurysm, and associated occlusive disease, abdominal aorta involving visceral vessels (mesenteric, celiac, renal)
CPT Changes: An Insider's View 2002
CPT Assistant Dec 00:2

35092 for ruptured aneurysm, abdominal aorta involving visceral vessels (mesenteric, celiac, renal)

35102 for aneurysm, pseudoaneurysm, and associated occlusive disease, abdominal aorta involving iliac vessels (common, hypogastric, external)
CPT Changes: An Insider's View 2002
CPT Assistant Dec 13:8

35103 for ruptured aneurysm, abdominal aorta involving iliac vessels (common, hypogastric, external)

35111 for aneurysm, pseudoaneurysm, and associated occlusive disease, splenic artery
CPT Changes: An Insider's View 2002

35112 for ruptured aneurysm, splenic artery

35121 for aneurysm, pseudoaneurysm, and associated occlusive disease, hepatic, celiac, renal, or mesenteric artery
CPT Changes: An Insider's View 2002

35122 for ruptured aneurysm, hepatic, celiac, renal, or mesenteric artery

35131 for aneurysm, pseudoaneurysm, and associated occlusive disease, iliac artery (common, hypogastric, external)
CPT Changes: An Insider's View 2002
CPT Assistant Feb 03:2

35132 for ruptured aneurysm, iliac artery (common, hypogastric, external)

35141 for aneurysm, pseudoaneurysm, and associated occlusive disease, common femoral artery (profunda femoris, superficial femoral)
➔ *CPT Changes: An Insider's View* 2002

35142 for ruptured aneurysm, common femoral artery (profunda femoris, superficial femoral)

35151 for aneurysm, pseudoaneurysm, and associated occlusive disease, popliteal artery
➔ *CPT Changes: An Insider's View* 2002

35152 for ruptured aneurysm, popliteal artery

Repair Arteriovenous Fistula

35180 Repair, congenital arteriovenous fistula; head and neck
➔ *CPT Assistant* Aug 11:9

35182 thorax and abdomen
➔ *CPT Assistant* Apr 11:9

35184 extremities
➔ *CPT Assistant* Apr 11:9

35188 Repair, acquired or traumatic arteriovenous fistula; head and neck
➔ *CPT Assistant* Apr 11:9

35189 thorax and abdomen
➔ *CPT Assistant* Apr 11:9

35190 extremities
➔ *CPT Assistant* Aug 11:9

Repair Blood Vessel Other Than for Fistula, With or Without Patch Angioplasty

(For AV fistula repair, see 35180-35190)

35201 Repair blood vessel, direct; neck
➔ *CPT Assistant* Mar 14:8, Apr 14:10

(Do not report 35201 in conjunction with 33969, 33984, 33985, 33986)

35206 upper extremity
➔ *CPT Assistant* Oct 00:3, Nov 03:5, Apr 12:4, Apr 14:10

(Do not report 35206 in conjunction with 33969, 33984, 33985, 33986)

35207 hand, finger

35211 intrathoracic, with bypass

(Do not report 35211 in conjunction with 33969, 33984, 33985, 33986)

35216 intrathoracic, without bypass
➔ *CPT Assistant* Apr 05:10-11

(Do not report 35216 in conjunction with 33969, 33984, 33985, 33986)

35221 intra-abdominal

35226 lower extremity
➔ *CPT Assistant* Apr 12:8, 9, Mar 13:10, Dec 13:8, Jul 17:5

(Do not report 35226 in conjunction with 33969, 33984, 33985, 33986)

35231 Repair blood vessel with vein graft; neck

35236 upper extremity
➔ *CPT Assistant* Oct 04:8

35241 intrathoracic, with bypass

35246 intrathoracic, without bypass

35251 intra-abdominal

35256 lower extremity

35261 Repair blood vessel with graft other than vein; neck

35266 upper extremity

35271 intrathoracic, with bypass

35276 intrathoracic, without bypass

35281 intra-abdominal

35286 lower extremity
➔ *CPT Assistant* Apr 12:8, 9, Mar 13:10, Dec 13:8, Apr 14:10, Jul 17:5

Thromboendarterectomy

(For coronary artery, see 33510-33536 and 33572)

(35301-35372 include harvest of saphenous or upper extremity vein when performed)

35301 Thromboendarterectomy, including patch graft, if performed; carotid, vertebral, subclavian, by neck incision
➔ *CPT Changes: An Insider's View* 2007
➔ *CPT Assistant* Jan 07:7, Sep 10:7

35302 superficial femoral artery
➔ *CPT Changes: An Insider's View* 2007
➔ *CPT Assistant* Jan 07:7, May 07:9

35303 popliteal artery
➔ *CPT Changes: An Insider's View* 2007
➔ *CPT Assistant* Jan 07:7, May 07:9

(Do not report 35302, 35303 in conjunction with 37225, 37227 when performed in the same vessel)

35304 tibioperoneal trunk artery
➔ *CPT Changes: An Insider's View* 2007
➔ *CPT Assistant* Jan 07:7, May 07:9

35305 tibial or peroneal artery, initial vessel
➔ *CPT Changes: An Insider's View* 2007
➔ *CPT Assistant* May 07:9

+ **35306** each additional tibial or peroneal artery (List separately in addition to code for primary procedure)
➔ *CPT Changes: An Insider's View* 2007
➔ *CPT Assistant* Jan 07:7, May 07:9

(Use 35306 in conjunction with 35305)

(Do not report 35304, 35305, 35306 in conjunction with 37229, 37231, 37233, 37235 when performed in the same vessel)

35311 subclavian, innominate, by thoracic incision

35321 axillary-brachial

35331 abdominal aorta

35341 mesenteric, celiac, or renal

35351 iliac

35355 iliofemoral

35361 combined aortoiliac

35363 combined aortoiliofemoral

35371 common femoral
CPT Assistant Jan 07:7, Jul 17:5

35372 deep (profunda) femoral
CPT Assistant Jan 07:7

Thromboendarterectomy
35371-35372

The common femoral artery (35371) or the deep (profunda) femoral artery (35372) is incised and the plaque and lining are removed, enlarging the diameter of the artery.

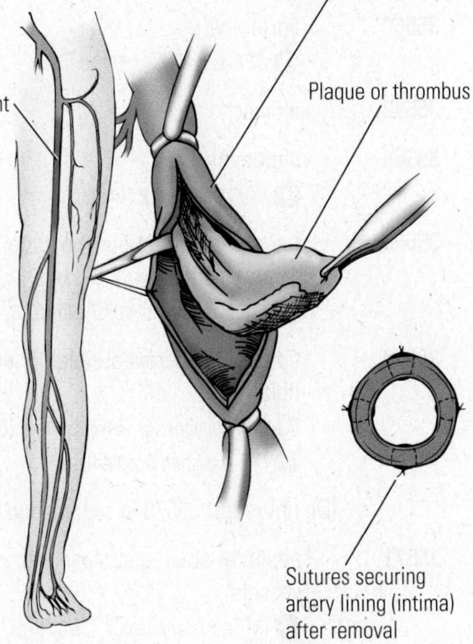

+ 35390 Reoperation, carotid, thromboendarterectomy, more than 1 month after original operation (List separately in addition to code for primary procedure)
CPT Assistant Nov 97:16

(Use 35390 in conjunction with 35301)

Angioscopy

+ 35400 Angioscopy (noncoronary vessels or grafts) during therapeutic intervention (List separately in addition to code for primary procedure)
CPT Assistant Nov 97:16

Transluminal Angioplasty

Open

(35450, 35452, 35458, 35460 have been deleted. To report, see 36902, 36905, 36907, 37246, 37247, 37248, 37249)

Percutaneous

(35471, 35472, 35475, 35476 have been deleted. To report, see 36902, 36905, 36907, 37246, 37247, 37248, 37249)

Bypass Graft

Vein

Procurement of the saphenous vein graft is included in the description of the work for 35501-35587 and should not be reported as a separate service or co-surgery. To report harvesting of an upper extremity vein, use 35500 in addition to the bypass procedure. To report harvesting of a femoropopliteal vein segment, use 35572 in addition to the bypass procedure. To report harvesting and construction of an autogenous composite graft of two segments from two distant locations, report 35682 in addition to the bypass procedure, for autogenous composite of three or more segments from distant sites, report 35683.

+ 35500 Harvest of upper extremity vein, 1 segment, for lower extremity or coronary artery bypass procedure (List separately in addition to code for primary procedure)
CPT Changes: An Insider's View 2000
CPT Assistant Nov 98:13, Mar 99:6, Nov 99:19, Jan 07:7, Apr 12:4

(Use 35500 in conjunction with 33510-33536, 35556, 35566, 35570, 35571, 35583-35587)

(For harvest of more than one vein segment, see 35682, 35683)

(For endoscopic procedure, use 33508)

35501 Bypass graft, with vein; common carotid-ipsilateral internal carotid
CPT Changes: An Insider's View 2007
CPT Assistant Apr 99:11

35506 carotid-subclavian or subclavian-carotid
CPT Changes: An Insider's View 2007
CPT Assistant Oct 04:6, Jan 07:7

35508 carotid-vertebral

35509 carotid-contralateral carotid
CPT Changes: An Insider's View 2007
CPT Assistant Jan 07:7, May 07:9

35510 carotid-brachial
➔ *CPT Changes: An Insider's View* 2004
➔ *CPT Assistant* Oct 04:6, Nov 07:8

35511 subclavian-subclavian

35512 subclavian-brachial
➔ *CPT Changes: An Insider's View* 2004
➔ *CPT Assistant* Oct 04:7

35515 subclavian-vertebral

35516 subclavian-axillary

35518 axillary-axillary
➔ *CPT Assistant* Oct 04:9

35521 axillary-femoral

(For bypass graft performed with synthetic graft, use 35621)

35522 axillary-brachial
➔ *CPT Changes: An Insider's View* 2004
➔ *CPT Assistant* Oct 04:9

35523 brachial-ulnar or -radial
➔ *CPT Changes: An Insider's View* 2008

(Do not report 35523 in conjunction with 35206, 35500, 35525, 36838)

(For bypass graft performed with synthetic conduit, use 37799)

35525 brachial-brachial
➔ *CPT Changes: An Insider's View* 2004
➔ *CPT Assistant* Oct 04:10

35526 aortosubclavian, aortoinnominate, or aortocarotid
➔ *CPT Changes: An Insider's View* 2011

(For bypass graft performed with synthetic graft, use 35626)

35531 aortoceliac or aortomesenteric

35533 axillary-femoral-femoral

(For bypass graft performed with synthetic graft, use 35654)

35535 hepatorenal
➔ *CPT Changes: An Insider's View* 2009

(Do not report 35535 in conjunction with 35221, 35251, 35281, 35500, 35536, 35560, 35631, 35636)

35536 splenorenal
➔ *CPT Assistant* Jun 99:10

35537 aortoiliac
➔ *CPT Changes: An Insider's View* 2007
➔ *CPT Assistant* Jan 07:7

(For bypass graft performed with synthetic graft, use 35637)

(Do not report 35537 in conjunction with 35538)

35538 aortobi-iliac
➔ *CPT Changes: An Insider's View* 2007
➔ *CPT Assistant* Jan 07:7

(For bypass graft performed with synthetic graft, use 35638)

(Do not report 35538 in conjunction with 35537)

35539 aortofemoral
➔ *CPT Changes: An Insider's View* 2007
➔ *CPT Assistant* Jan 07:7

(For bypass graft performed with synthetic graft, use 35647)

(Do not report 35539 in conjunction with 35540)

35540 aortobifemoral
➔ *CPT Changes: An Insider's View* 2007
➔ *CPT Assistant* Jan 07:7

(For bypass graft performed with synthetic graft, use 35646)

(Do not report 35540 in conjunction with 35539)

35556 femoral-popliteal
➔ *CPT Assistant* Fall 92:20, May 97:10, Jan 07:7, Nov 07:8

35558 femoral-femoral

35560 aortorenal
➔ *CPT Assistant* Jun 99:10

35563 ilioiliac

35565 iliofemoral
➔ *CPT Assistant* Oct 04:8

35566 femoral-anterior tibial, posterior tibial, peroneal artery or other distal vessels
➔ *CPT Assistant* Jan 07:7, Nov 07:8

35570 tibial-tibial, peroneal-tibial, or tibial/peroneal trunk-tibial
➔ *CPT Changes: An Insider's View* 2009
➔ *CPT Assistant* Apr 12:4

(Do not report 35570 in conjunction with 35256, 35286)

35571 popliteal-tibial, -peroneal artery or other distal vessels
➔ *CPT Assistant* Jan 07:7, Nov 07:8

+ 35572 Harvest of femoropopliteal vein, 1 segment, for vascular reconstruction procedure (eg, aortic, vena caval, coronary, peripheral artery) (List separately in addition to code for primary procedure)
➔ *CPT Changes: An Insider's View* 2003
➔ *CPT Assistant* Jan 07:28

(Use 35572 in conjunction with 33510-33516, 33517-33523, 33533-33536, 34502, 34520, 35001, 35002, 35011-35022, 35102, 35103, 35121-35152, 35231-35256, 35501-35571, 35583, 35585, 35587, 35879-35907)

(For bilateral procedure, use modifier 50)

Bypass Graft, Vein
35571

The physician creates a bypass around the popliteal artery, using a harvested vein that is sutured to the tibial artery.

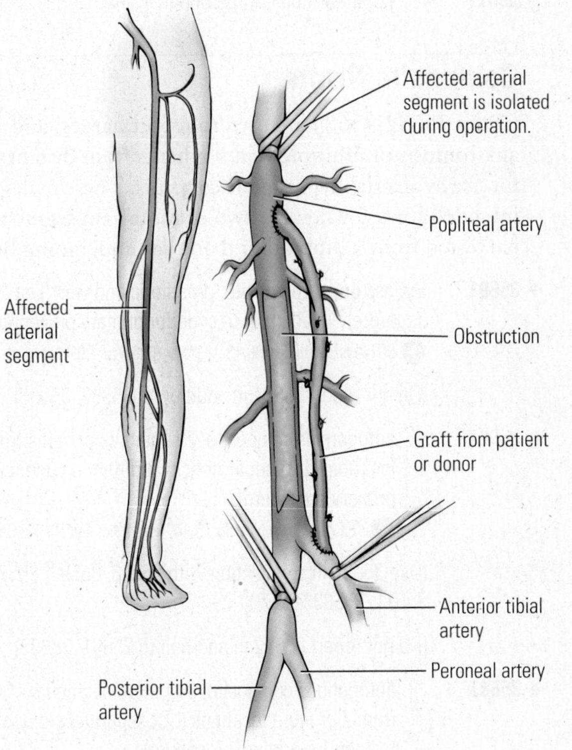

In-Situ Vein

(To report aortobifemoral bypass using synthetic conduit, and femoral-popliteal bypass with vein conduit in-situ, use 35646 and 35583. To report aorto[uni]femoral bypass with synthetic conduit, and femoral-popliteal bypass with vein conduit in-situ, use 35647 and 35583. To report aortofemoral bypass using vein conduit, and femoral-popliteal bypass with vein conduit in-situ, use 35539 and 35583)

35583 In-situ vein bypass; femoral-popliteal
➔ *CPT Assistant* Jan 07:7, Nov 07:8

35585 femoral-anterior tibial, posterior tibial, or peroneal artery
➔ *CPT Assistant* Jan 07:7, Nov 07:8

35587 popliteal-tibial, peroneal
➔ *CPT Assistant* Apr 99:11, Jan 07:7, Nov 07:8

Other Than Vein

(For arterial transposition and/or reimplantation, see 35691-35695)

+ 35600 Harvest of upper extremity artery, 1 segment, for coronary artery bypass procedure (List separately in addition to code for primary procedure)
➔ *CPT Changes: An Insider's View* 2001, 2008
➔ *CPT Assistant* Apr 07:12

(Use 35600 in conjunction with 33533–33536)

Harvest of Upper Extremity Artery
35600

Open procurement of a radial artery to secure conduit for construction of a coronary artery bypass graft

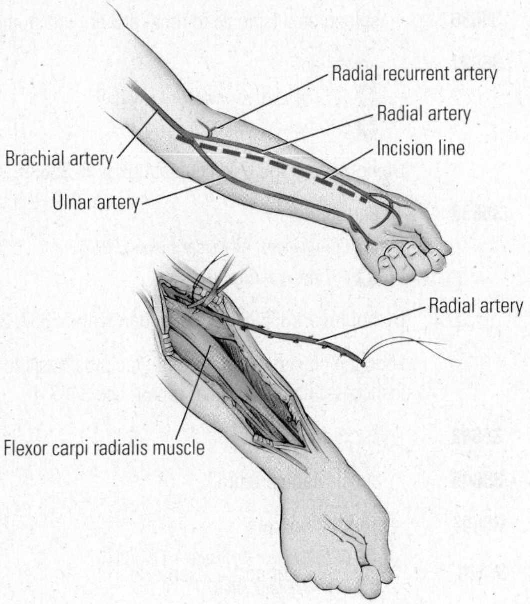

35601 Bypass graft, with other than vein; common carotid-ipsilateral internal carotid
➔ *CPT Changes: An Insider's View* 2007
➔ *CPT Assistant* Jul 06:7, Jan 07:7

35606 carotid-subclavian

(For open transcervical common carotid-common carotid bypass performed in conjunction with endovascular repair of descending thoracic aorta, use 33891)

(For open subclavian to carotid artery transposition performed in conjunction with endovascular thoracic aneurysm repair by neck incision, use 33889)

35612 subclavian-subclavian

35616 subclavian-axillary

35621 axillary-femoral
➔ *CPT Assistant* Jan 07:7

35623 axillary-popliteal or -tibial

35626 aortosubclavian, aortoinnominate, or aortocarotid
CPT Changes: An Insider's View 2011

35631 aortoceliac, aortomesenteric, aortorenal

35632 ilio-celiac
CPT Changes: An Insider's View 2009

(Do not report 35632 in conjunction with 35221, 35251, 35281, 35531, 35631)

35633 ilio-mesenteric
CPT Changes: An Insider's View 2009

(Do not report 35633 in conjunction with 35221, 35251, 35281, 35531, 35631)

35634 iliorenal
CPT Changes: An Insider's View 2009

(Do not report 35634 in conjunction with 35221, 35251, 35281, 35560, 35536, 35631)

35636 splenorenal (splenic to renal arterial anastomosis)

35637 aortoiliac
CPT Changes: An Insider's View 2007
CPT Assistant Jan 07:7

(Do not report 35637 in conjunction with 35638, 35646)

35638 aortobi-iliac
CPT Changes: An Insider's View 2007
CPT Assistant Jan 07:7

(Do not report 35638 in conjunction with 35637, 35646)

(For open placement of aortobi-iliac prosthesis following unsuccessful endovascular repair, use 34831)

35642 carotid-vertebral

35645 subclavian-vertebral

35646 aortobifemoral
CPT Changes: An Insider's View 2002
CPT Assistant Jan 07:7

(For bypass graft performed with vein graft, use 35540)

(For open placement of aortobifemoral prosthesis following unsuccessful endovascular repair, use 34832)

35647 aortofemoral
CPT Changes: An Insider's View 2002
CPT Assistant Jan 07:7

(For bypass graft performed with vein graft, use 35539)

35650 axillary-axillary

35654 axillary-femoral-femoral
CPT Assistant Jan 07:7

35656 femoral-popliteal
CPT Assistant Nov 07:8

35661 femoral-femoral
CPT Assistant Dec 04:6, Jan 07:7

35663 ilioiliac

35665 iliofemoral
CPT Assistant Jan 07:7

35666 femoral-anterior tibial, posterior tibial, or peroneal artery
CPT Assistant Nov 07:8

35671 popliteal-tibial or -peroneal artery

Composite Grafts

Codes 35682-35683 are used to report harvest and anastomosis of multiple vein segments from distant sites for use as arterial bypass graft conduits. These codes are intended for use when the two or more vein segments are harvested from a limb other than that undergoing bypass.

+ 35681 Bypass graft; composite, prosthetic and vein (List separately in addition to code for primary procedure)
CPT Assistant Nov 98:13-14, Mar 99:6, Apr 99:11

(Do not report 35681 in addition to 35682, 35683)

+ 35682 autogenous composite, 2 segments of veins from 2 locations (List separately in addition to code for primary procedure)
CPT Assistant Nov 98:13-14, Mar 99:6, Apr 99:11, Sep 02:4

(Use 35682 in conjunction with 35556, 35566, 35570, 35571, 35583-35587)

(Do not report 35682 in addition to 35681, 35683)

+ 35683 autogenous composite, 3 or more segments of vein from 2 or more locations (List separately in addition to code for primary procedure)
CPT Assistant Nov 98:13-14, Mar 99:6, Apr 99:11, Sep 02:4

(Use 35683 in conjunction with 35556, 35566, 35570, 35571, 35583-35587)

(Do not report 35683 in addition to 35681, 35682)

Adjuvant Techniques

Adjuvant (additional) technique(s) may be required at the time a bypass graft is created to improve patency of the lower extremity autogenous or synthetic bypass graft (eg, femoral-popliteal, femoral-tibial, or popliteal-tibial arteries). Code 35685 should be reported in addition to the primary synthetic bypass graft procedure, when an interposition of venous tissue (vein patch or cuff) is placed at the anastomosis between the synthetic bypass conduit and the involved artery (includes harvest).

Code 35686 should be reported in addition to the primary bypass graft procedure, when autogenous vein is used to create a fistula between the tibial or peroneal artery and vein at or beyond the distal bypass anastomosis site of the involved artery.

(For composite graft(s), see 35681-35683)

+ 35685 Placement of vein patch or cuff at distal anastomosis of bypass graft, synthetic conduit (List separately in addition to code for primary procedure)
➲ *CPT Changes: An Insider's View* 2002
➲ *CPT Assistant* Sep 02:3

(Use 35685 in conjunction with 35656, 35666, or 35671)

+ 35686 Creation of distal arteriovenous fistula during lower extremity bypass surgery (non-hemodialysis) (List separately in addition to code for primary procedure)
➲ *CPT Changes: An Insider's View* 2002
➲ *CPT Assistant* Sep 02:3, Apr 12:4

(Use 35686 in conjunction with 35556, 35566, 35570, 35571, 35583-35587, 35623, 35656, 35666, 35671)

Arterial Transposition

35691 Transposition and/or reimplantation; vertebral to carotid artery

35693 vertebral to subclavian artery

35694 subclavian to carotid artery

(For open subclavian to carotid artery transposition performed in conjunction with endovascular repair of descending thoracic aorta, use 33889)

35695 carotid to subclavian artery

+ 35697 Reimplantation, visceral artery to infrarenal aortic prosthesis, each artery (List separately in addition to code for primary procedure)
➲ *CPT Changes: An Insider's View* 2004

(Do not report 35697 in conjunction with 33877)

Excision, Exploration, Repair, Revision

+ 35700 Reoperation, femoral-popliteal or femoral (popliteal)-anterior tibial, posterior tibial, peroneal artery, or other distal vessels, more than 1 month after original operation (List separately in addition to code for primary procedure)
➲ *CPT Assistant* Apr 12:4

(Use 35700 in conjunction with 35556, 35566, 35570, 35571, 35583, 35585, 35587, 35656, 35666, 35671)

35701 Exploration (not followed by surgical repair), with or without lysis of artery; carotid artery

35721 femoral artery
➲ *CPT Assistant* Jun 96:8

35741 popliteal artery

35761 other vessels

35800 Exploration for postoperative hemorrhage, thrombosis or infection; neck

35820 chest

35840 abdomen
➲ *CPT Assistant* May 97:8

35860 extremity
➲ *CPT Assistant* Fall 92:21, Apr 14:10

35870 Repair of graft-enteric fistula

35875 Thrombectomy of arterial or venous graft (other than hemodialysis graft or fistula);
➲ *CPT Assistant* Nov 98:14, Feb 99:6, Mar 99:6, Apr 00:10

35876 with revision of arterial or venous graft
➲ *CPT Assistant* Nov 98:14

(For thrombectomy of hemodialysis graft or fistula, see 36831, 36833)

Codes 35879 and 35881 describe open revision of graft-threatening stenoses of lower extremity arterial bypass graft(s) (previously constructed with autogenous vein conduit) using vein patch angioplasty or segmental vein interposition techniques. For thrombectomy with revision of any noncoronary arterial or venous graft, including those of the lower extremity, (other than hemodialysis graft or fistula), use 35876. For direct repair (other than for fistula) of a lower extremity blood vessel (with or without patch angioplasty), use 35226. For repair (other than for fistula) of a lower extremity blood vessel using a vein graft, use 35256.

35879 Revision, lower extremity arterial bypass, without thrombectomy, open; with vein patch angioplasty
➲ *CPT Changes: An Insider's View* 2000
➲ *CPT Assistant* Nov 99:19

35881 with segmental vein interposition
➲ *CPT Changes: An Insider's View* 2000
➲ *CPT Assistant* Nov 99:19

(For revision of femoral anastomosis of synthetic arterial bypass graft, see 35883, 35884)

(For excision of infected graft, see 35901-35907 and appropriate revascularization code)

35883 Revision, femoral anastomosis of synthetic arterial bypass graft in groin, open; with nonautogenous patch graft (eg, Dacron, ePTFE, bovine pericardium)
➲ *CPT Changes: An Insider's View* 2007
➲ *CPT Assistant* Jan 07:7

(For bilateral procedure, use modifier 50)

(Do not report 35883 in conjunction with 35700, 35875, 35876, 35884)

35884 with autogenous vein patch graft
➲ *CPT Changes: An Insider's View* 2007
➲ *CPT Assistant* Jan 07:7

(For bilateral procedure, use modifier 50)

(Do not report 35884 in conjunction with 35700, 35875, 35876, 35883)

35901 Excision of infected graft; neck

35903 extremity

35905 thorax

35907 abdomen

Vascular Injection Procedures

Listed services for injection procedures include necessary local anesthesia, introduction of needles or catheter, injection of contrast media with or without automatic power injection, and/or necessary pre- and postinjection care specifically related to the injection procedure.

Selective vascular catheterization should be coded to include introduction and all lesser order selective catheterization used in the approach (eg, the description for a selective right middle cerebral artery catheterization includes the introduction and placement catheterization of the right common and internal carotid arteries).

Additional second and/or third order arterial catheterization within the same family of arteries or veins supplied by a single first order vessel should be expressed by 36012, 36218, or 36248.

Additional first order or higher catheterization in vascular families supplied by a first order vessel different from a previously selected and coded family should be separately coded using the conventions described above.

(For radiological supervision and interpretation, see **Radiology**)

(For injection procedures in conjunction with cardiac catheterization, see 93452-93461, 93563-93568)

(For chemotherapy of malignant disease, see 96401-96549)

Intravenous

An intracatheter is a sheathed combination of needle and short catheter.

36000 Introduction of needle or intracatheter, vein
- *CPT Assistant* Summer 95:2, Apr 98:1, 3, 7, Jul 98:1, Apr 03:26, Oct 03:2, Jul 06:4, Feb 07:10, Jul 07:1, Dec 08:7, May 14:4, Sep 14:13, Oct 14:6

36002 Injection procedures (eg, thrombin) for percutaneous treatment of extremity pseudoaneurysm
- *CPT Changes: An Insider's View* 2002
- *CPT Assistant* Nov 13:6, Oct 14:6

(For imaging guidance, see 76942, 77002, 77012, 77021)

(For ultrasound guided compression repair of pseudoaneurysms, use 76936)

(Do not report 36002 for vascular sealant of an arteriotomy site)

36005 Injection procedure for extremity venography (including introduction of needle or intracatheter)
- *CPT Changes: An Insider's View* 2002
- *CPT Assistant* Oct 14:6
- *Clinical Examples in Radiology* Spring 14:7

(For radiological supervision and interpretation, see 75820, 75822)

Injection Procedure (eg, Thrombin) for Percutaneous Treatment of Extremity Pseudoaneurysm
36002

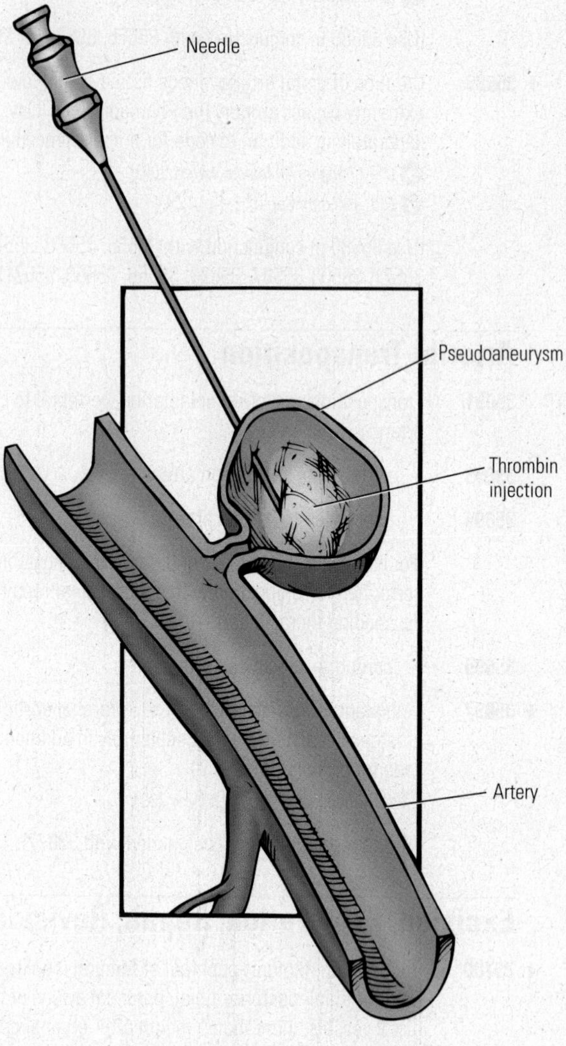

36010 Introduction of catheter, superior or inferior vena cava
- *CPT Changes: An Insider's View* 2013, 2017
- *CPT Assistant* Aug 96:2, Apr 98:7, Sep 00:11, May 01:10, Jul 03:12, Oct 08:11, Jan 09:7, Apr 12:4, Feb 17:14
- *Clinical Examples in Radiology* Winter 05:5-6, Spring 08:7-8, Winter 12:3, Spring 13:3, Winter 16:2

36011 Selective catheter placement, venous system; first order branch (eg, renal vein, jugular vein)
- *CPT Assistant* Aug 96:11, Apr 98:7, Jul 03:12, Dec 03:2, Apr 12:5
- *Clinical Examples in Radiology* Winter 12:3, Summer 16:3

36012 second order, or more selective, branch (eg, left adrenal vein, petrosal sinus)
- *CPT Assistant* Aug 96:11, Sep 98:7, Jul 03:12, Apr 12:5
- *Clinical Examples in Radiology* Winter 12:3

36013 Introduction of catheter, right heart or main pulmonary artery
- *CPT Assistant* Aug 96:11, Oct 08:11, Jan 09:7

36014 Selective catheter placement, left or right pulmonary artery
CPT Assistant Aug 96:11, Apr 98:7

36015 Selective catheter placement, segmental or subsegmental pulmonary artery
CPT Assistant Aug 96:11, Sep 00:11, Mar 12:10
Clinical Examples in Radiology Summer 12:1, 2, Spring 13:1, 2

(For insertion of flow directed catheter (eg, Swan-Ganz), use 93503)

(For venous catheterization for selective organ blood sampling, use 36500)

Intra-Arterial—Intra-Aortic

(For radiological supervision and interpretation, see Radiology)

36100 Introduction of needle or intracatheter, carotid or vertebral artery
CPT Assistant Aug 96:11

(For bilateral procedure, report 36100 with modifier 50)

(36120 has been deleted)

36140 Introduction of needle or intracatheter, upper or lower extremity artery
CPT Changes: An Insider's View 2013, 2017, 2018
CPT Assistant Fall 93:16, Aug 96:3, Nov 99:32-33, Oct 03:2, Jul 06:4, 7, Jul 07:1, Dec 07:10, 11, Jun 09:10, Jul 11:5

(For insertion of arteriovenous cannula, see 36810-36821)

(36147, 36148 have been deleted. To report, see 36901, 36902, 36903, 36904, 36905, 36906)

36160 Introduction of needle or intracatheter, aortic, translumbar
CPT Assistant Aug 96:3

Diagnostic Studies of Cervicocerebral Arteries: Codes 36221-36228 describe non-selective and selective arterial catheter placement and diagnostic imaging of the aortic arch, carotid, and vertebral arteries. Codes 36221-36226 include the work of accessing the vessel, placement of catheter(s), contrast injection(s), fluoroscopy, radiological supervision and interpretation, and closure of the arteriotomy by pressure, or application of an arterial closure device. Codes 36221-36228 describe arterial contrast injections with arterial, capillary, and venous phase imaging, when performed.

Code 36227 is an add-on code to report unilateral selective arterial catheter placement and diagnostic imaging of the ipsilateral external carotid circulation and includes all the work of accessing the additional vessel, placement of catheter(s), contrast injection(s), fluoroscopy, radiological supervision and interpretation. Code 36227 is reported in conjunction with 36222, 36223, or 36224.

Code 36228 is an add-on code to report unilateral selective arterial catheter placement and diagnostic imaging of the initial and each additional intracranial branch of the internal carotid or vertebral arteries. Code 36228 is reported in conjunction with 36223, 36224, 36225 or 36226. This includes any additional second or third order catheter selective placement in the same primary branch of the internal carotid, vertebral, or basilar artery and includes all the work of accessing the additional vessel, placement of catheter(s), contrast injection(s), fluoroscopy, radiological supervision and interpretation. It is not reported more than twice per side, regardless of the number of additional branches selectively catheterized.

Codes 36221-36226 are built on progressive hierarchies with more intensive services inclusive of less intensive services. The code inclusive of all of the services provided for that vessel should be reported (ie, use the code inclusive of the most intensive services provided). Only one code in the range 36222-36224 may be reported for each ipsilateral carotid territory. Only one code in the range 36225-36226 may be reported for each ipsilateral vertebral territory.

Code 36221 is reported for non-selective arterial catheter placement in the thoracic aorta and diagnostic imaging of the aortic arch and great vessel origins. Codes 36222-36228 are reported for unilateral artery catheterization. Do not report 36221 in conjunction with 36222-36226 as these selective codes include the work of 36221 when performed.

Do not report 36222, 36223, or 36224 together for ipsilateral angiography. Instead, select the code that represents the most comprehensive service using the following hierarchy of complexity (listed in descending order of complexity): 36224>36223>36222.

Do not report 36225 and 36226 together for ipsilateral angiography. Select the code that represents the more comprehensive service using the following hierarchy of complexity (listed in descending order of complexity): 36226>36225.

When bilateral carotid and/or vertebral arterial catheterization and imaging is performed, add modifier 50 to codes 36222-36228 if the same procedure is performed on both sides. For example, bilateral extracranial carotid angiography with selective catheterization of each common carotid artery would be reported with 36222 and modifier 50. However, when different territory(ies) is studied in the same session on both sides of the body, modifiers may be required to report the imaging performed. Use modifier 59 to denote that different carotid and/or vertebral arteries are being studied. For example, when selective right internal carotid artery catheterization accompanied by right extracranial and intracranial carotid angiography is followed by selective left common carotid artery catheterization with left extracranial carotid angiography, use 36224 to report the right side and 36222-59 to report the left side.

Diagnostic angiography of the cervicocerebral vessels may be followed by an interventional procedure at the same session. Interventional procedures may be separately reportable using standard coding conventions.

Do not report 36218 or 75774 as part of diagnostic angiography of the extracranial and intracranial cervicocerebral vessels. It may be appropriate to report 36218 and 75774 for diagnostic angiography of upper extremities and other vascular beds of the neck and/or shoulder girdle performed in the same session as vertebral angiography (eg, workup of a neck tumor that requires catheterization and angiography of the vertebral artery as well as other brachiocephalic arteries).

Report 76376 or 76377 for 3D rendering when performed in conjunction with 36221-36228.

Report 76937 for ultrasound guidance for vascular access, when performed in conjunction with 36221-36228.

36200 Introduction of catheter, aorta

➔ *CPT Changes: An Insider's View* 2012, 2017

➔ *CPT Assistant* Fall 93:16, Aug 96:3, Jul 06:7, Dec 07:10, 14, Apr 08:11, Dec 09:13, Jul 11:5, Oct 11:9, Apr 12:4, Feb 13:16, Mar 17:4

➔ *Clinical Examples in Radiology* Spring 12:6, Summer 14:2, 3, Winter 14:5-6

(For non-selective angiography of the extracranial carotid and/or cerebral vessels and cervicocerebral arch, when performed, use 36221)

36215 Selective catheter placement, arterial system; each first order thoracic or brachiocephalic branch, within a vascular family

➔ *CPT Assistant* Fall 93:15, Aug 96:3, Nov 97:16, Apr 98:9, Sep 00:11, Oct 00:4, Feb 03:3, Apr 12:4, Mar 17:4, May 17:8

➔ *Clinical Examples in Radiology* Spring 12:4, Spring 13:4, 5, 6, Winter 18:2

(For catheter placement for coronary angiography, see 93454-93461)

36216 initial second order thoracic or brachiocephalic branch, within a vascular family

➔ *CPT Assistant* Fall 93:15, Aug 96:3, Oct 00:4, Dec 07:10, Dec 11:12, Apr 12:4, Nov 13:14

➔ *Clinical Examples in Radiology* Spring 13:4, 5, 6, Winter 18:2

36217 initial third order or more selective thoracic or brachiocephalic branch, within a vascular family

➔ *CPT Assistant* Fall 93:15, Aug 96:3, Oct 00:4, Dec 07:10, Dec 11:12, Apr 12:5

➔ *Clinical Examples in Radiology* Summer 07:1, 2

+ 36218 additional second order, third order, and beyond, thoracic or brachiocephalic branch, within a vascular family (List in addition to code for initial second or third order vessel as appropriate)

➔ *CPT Assistant* Fall 93:15, Aug 96:3, Oct 00:4, Jul 06:7, Dec 07:10, Apr 12:5, May 13:3

➔ *Clinical Examples in Radiology* Winter 15:4, 5, 6, Winter 18:2

(Use 36218 in conjunction with 36216, 36217, 36225, 36226)

(For angiography, see 36222-36228, 75600-75774)

(For transluminal balloon angioplasty [except lower extremity artery[ies] for occlusive disease, intracranial, coronary, pulmonary, or dialysis circuit], see 37246, 37247)

(For transcatheter therapies, see 37200, 37211, 37213, 37214, 37236, 37237, 37238, 37239, 37241, 37242, 37243, 37244, 61624, 61626)

(When coronary artery, arterial conduit [eg, internal mammary, inferior epigastric or free radical artery] or venous bypass graft angiography is performed in conjunction with cardiac catheterization, see the appropriate cardiac catheterization, injection procedure, and imaging supervision code[s] [93455, 93457, 93459, 93461, 93530-93533, 93564] in the **Medicine** section. When internal mammary artery angiography only is performed without a concomitant cardiac catheterization, use 36216 or 36217 as appropriate)

36221 Non-selective catheter placement, thoracic aorta, with angiography of the extracranial carotid, vertebral, and/or intracranial vessels, unilateral or bilateral, and all associated radiological supervision and interpretation, includes angiography of the cervicocerebral arch, when performed

➔ *CPT Changes: An Insider's View* 2013, 2017

➔ *CPT Assistant* Feb 13:16, May 13:3, Jun 13:12, Oct 13:18, Mar 14:8, May 15:7

➔ *Clinical Examples in Radiology* Winter 15:6

(Do not report 36221 with 36222-36226)

36222 Selective catheter placement, common carotid or innominate artery, unilateral, any approach, with angiography of the ipsilateral extracranial carotid circulation and all associated radiological supervision and interpretation, includes angiography of the cervicocerebral arch, when performed

➔ *CPT Changes: An Insider's View* 2013, 2017

➔ *CPT Assistant* Feb 13:17, May 13:3, Jun 13:12, Oct 13:18, Nov 13:14, Mar 14:8, May 15:7, Nov 15:10

➔ *Clinical Examples in Radiology* Winter 15:6, Spring 16:6

(Do not report 36222 in conjunction with 37215, 37216, 37218 for the treated carotid artery)

36223 Selective catheter placement, common carotid or innominate artery, unilateral, any approach, with angiography of the ipsilateral intracranial carotid circulation and all associated radiological supervision and interpretation, includes angiography of the extracranial carotid and cervicocerebral arch, when performed

➔ *CPT Changes: An Insider's View* 2013, 2017

➔ *CPT Assistant* Feb 13:17, May 13:3, Jun 13:12, Oct 13:18, Mar 14:8

➔ *Clinical Examples in Radiology* Winter 15:6, Spring 16:6

(Do not report 36223 in conjunction with 37215, 37216, 37218 for the treated carotid artery)

36224 Selective catheter placement, internal carotid artery, unilateral, with angiography of the ipsilateral intracranial carotid circulation and all associated radiological supervision and interpretation, includes angiography of the extracranial carotid and cervicocerebral arch, when performed

- *CPT Changes: An Insider's View* 2013, 2017
- *CPT Assistant* Feb 13:17, May 13:3, Jun 13:12, Oct 13:18, Mar 14:8
- *Clinical Examples in Radiology* Winter 15:5, 6, Spring 16:5

(Do not report 36224 in conjunction with 37215, 37216, 37218 for the treated carotid artery)

36225 Selective catheter placement, subclavian or innominate artery, unilateral, with angiography of the ipsilateral vertebral circulation and all associated radiological supervision and interpretation, includes angiography of the cervicocerebral arch, when performed

- *CPT Changes: An Insider's View* 2013, 2017
- *CPT Assistant* May 13:3, Jun 13:12, Oct 13:18, Nov 13:14, Mar 14:8
- *Clinical Examples in Radiology* Spring 13:6, Winter 15:6

36226 Selective catheter placement, vertebral artery, unilateral, with angiography of the ipsilateral vertebral circulation and all associated radiological supervision and interpretation, includes angiography of the cervicocerebral arch, when performed

- *CPT Changes: An Insider's View* 2013, 2017
- *CPT Assistant* May 13:3, Jun 13:12, Oct 13:18, Mar 14:8
- *Clinical Examples in Radiology* Winter 15:4, 5, 6, Winter 18:2

+ 36227 Selective catheter placement, external carotid artery, unilateral, with angiography of the ipsilateral external carotid circulation and all associated radiological supervision and interpretation (List separately in addition to code for primary procedure)

- *CPT Changes: An Insider's View* 2013, 2017
- *CPT Assistant* Feb 13:17, May 13:3, Jun 13:12, Oct 13:18, Mar 14:8, Nov 15:10
- *Clinical Examples in Radiology* Winter 15:5, 6, Spring 16:5

(Use 36227 in conjunction with 36222, 36223, or 36224)

(Do not report 36221-36227 in conjunction with 37217 for ipsilateral services)

+ 36228 Selective catheter placement, each intracranial branch of the internal carotid or vertebral arteries, unilateral, with angiography of the selected vessel circulation and all associated radiological supervision and interpretation (eg, middle cerebral artery, posterior inferior cerebellar artery) (List separately in addition to code for primary procedure)

- *CPT Changes: An Insider's View* 2013, 2017
- *CPT Assistant* Feb 13:17, May 13:3, Jun 13:12, Oct 13:18

(Use 36228 in conjunction with 36223, 36224, 36225 or 36226)

(Do not report 36228 more than twice per side)

Angiography, Carotid Artery
36222-36228

A radiologic contrast study is performed on the carotid artery vascular family.

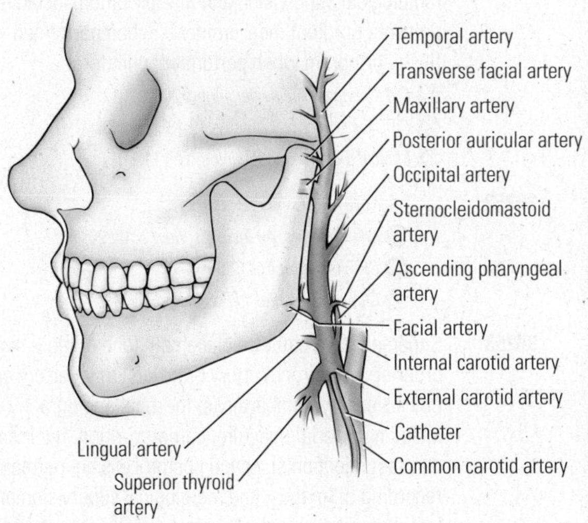

36245 Selective catheter placement, arterial system; each first order abdominal, pelvic, or lower extremity artery branch, within a vascular family

- *CPT Changes: An Insider's View* 2012, 2017
- *CPT Assistant* Fall 93:15, Aug 96:3, Jan 01:14, Jan 07:7, Dec 07:10, Jul 11:5, Oct 11:9, Apr 12:4, Nov 13:14
- *Clinical Examples in Radiology* Summer 08:1-3, Fall 11:3, Winter 14:2-3, Winter 18:2

36246 initial second order abdominal, pelvic, or lower extremity artery branch, within a vascular family

- *CPT Changes: An Insider's View* 2012, 2017
- *CPT Assistant* Fall 93:15, Aug 96:3, Jan 01:14, Jan 07:7, Dec 07:10, 11, Jul 11:5, Oct 11:9, Apr 12:4, Nov 13:14
- *Clinical Examples in Radiology* Winter 13:2, 3, Winter 14:1-3, Winter 18:11

36247 initial third order or more selective abdominal, pelvic, or lower extremity artery branch, within a vascular family

- *CPT Changes: An Insider's View* 2012, 2017
- *CPT Assistant* Fall 93:15, Aug 96:3, Jan 01:14, Jan 07:7, Dec 07:10, Jul 11:5, Apr 12:4, Fall 13:2, 3, 4, Nov 13:14
- *Clinical Examples in Radiology* Summer 08:1-3, Winter 08:1, Winter 13:1, 3, Summer 15:2, Winter 18:11

+ 36248 additional second order, third order, and beyond, abdominal, pelvic, or lower extremity artery branch, within a vascular family (List in addition to code for initial second or third order vessel as appropriate)

- *CPT Changes: An Insider's View* 2012, 2017
- *CPT Assistant* Fall 93:15, Aug 96:3, Apr 98:1, 7, Oct 00:4, Jan 01:14, Jan 07:7, Jul 11:5, Apr 12:4
- *Clinical Examples in Radiology* Winter 10:7

(Use 36248 in conjunction with 36246, 36247)

36251 Selective catheter placement (first-order), main renal artery and any accessory renal artery(s) for renal angiography, including arterial puncture and catheter placement(s), fluoroscopy, contrast injection(s), image postprocessing, permanent recording of images, and radiological supervision and interpretation, including pressure gradient measurements when performed, and flush aortogram when performed; unilateral

➔ *CPT Changes: An Insider's View* 2012, 2017

➔ *CPT Assistant* Apr 12:6, Aug 12:13, Nov 13:14

➔ *Clinical Examples in Radiology* Fall 11:2

36252 bilateral

➔ *CPT Changes: An Insider's View* 2012, 2017

➔ *CPT Assistant* Apr 12:6

➔ *Clinical Examples in Radiology* Fall 11:2

36253 Superselective catheter placement (one or more second order or higher renal artery branches) renal artery and any accessory renal artery(s) for renal angiography, including arterial puncture, catheterization, fluoroscopy, contrast injection(s), image postprocessing, permanent recording of images, and radiological supervision and interpretation, including pressure gradient measurements when performed, and flush aortogram when performed; unilateral

➔ *CPT Changes: An Insider's View* 2012, 2017

➔ *CPT Assistant* Apr 12:6, Aug 12:13, Nov 13:14

➔ *Clinical Examples in Radiology* Fall 11:2

(Do not report 36253 in conjunction with 36251 when performed for the same kidney)

36254 bilateral

➔ *CPT Changes: An Insider's View* 2012, 2017

➔ *CPT Assistant* Apr 12:6, Aug 12:13

➔ *Clinical Examples in Radiology* Fall 11:2

(Do not report 36254 in conjunction with 36252)

(Placement of closure device at the vascular access site is not separately reported with 36251-36254)

(Do not report 36251, 36252, 36253, 36254 in conjunction with 0338T, 0339T)

36260 Insertion of implantable intra-arterial infusion pump (eg, for chemotherapy of liver)

➔ *CPT Assistant* Fall 95:5

36261 Revision of implanted intra-arterial infusion pump

36262 Removal of implanted intra-arterial infusion pump

36299 Unlisted procedure, vascular injection

Venous

Venipuncture, needle or catheter for diagnostic study or intravenous therapy, percutaneous. These codes are also used to report the therapy as specified. For collection of a specimen from an established catheter, use 36592. For collection of a specimen from a completely implantable venous access device, use 36591.

36400 Venipuncture, younger than age 3 years, necessitating the skill of a physician or other qualified health care professional, not to be used for routine venipuncture; femoral or jugular vein

➔ *CPT Changes: An Insider's View* 2002, 2004, 2013

➔ *CPT Assistant* Jul 06:4, Jul 07:1, Dec 08:7, May 14:4

36405 scalp vein

➔ *CPT Changes: An Insider's View* 2013

➔ *CPT Assistant* Jul 06:4, Jul 07:1, Dec 08:7, May 14:4

36406 other vein

➔ *CPT Changes: An Insider's View* 2013

➔ *CPT Assistant* Jul 06:4, Jul 07:1, May 14:4

36410 Venipuncture, age 3 years or older, necessitating the skill of a physician or other qualified health care professional (separate procedure), for diagnostic or therapeutic purposes (not to be used for routine venipuncture)

➔ *CPT Changes: An Insider's View* 2004, 2013

➔ *CPT Assistant* Jun 96:10, May 01:11, Aug 02:2, Oct 03:10, Feb 07:10, Jul 07:1, Dec 08:7, Sep 13:18, Oct 14:6

➔ *Clinical Examples in Radiology* Spring 09:8

Coding Tip

Instructions for Use of the CPT Codebook

When advanced practice nurses and physician assistants are working with physicians they are considered as working in the exact same specialty and exact same subspecialties as the physician. A "physician or other qualified health care professional" is an individual who is qualified by education, training, licensure/regulation (when applicable), and facility privileging (when applicable) who performs a professional service within his or her scope of practice and independently reports that professional service. These professionals are distinct from "clinical staff." A clinical staff member is a person who works under the supervision of a physician or other qualified health care professional, and who is allowed by law, regulation, and facility policy to perform or assist in the performance of a specific professional service, but does not individually report that professional service. Other policies may also affect who may report specific services.

CPT Coding Guidelines, Introduction, Instructions for Use of the CPT Codebook

36415 Collection of venous blood by venipuncture

➔ *CPT Changes: An Insider's View* 2003

➔ *CPT Assistant* Jun 96:10, Mar 98:10, Oct 99:11, Aug 00:2, Feb 07:10, Jul 07:1, Dec 08:7, May 14:4

(Do not report modifier 63 in conjunction with 36415)

36416 Collection of capillary blood specimen (eg, finger, heel, ear stick)

➔ *CPT Changes: An Insider's View* 2003

36420 Venipuncture, cutdown; younger than age 1 year

➔ *CPT Assistant* Nov 99:32-33, Aug 00:2, Oct 03:2, Jul 06:4

(Do not report modifier 63 in conjunction with 36420)

36425 age 1 or over
➲ *CPT Assistant* Oct 14:6
➲ *Clinical Examples in Radiology* Summer 08:1

(Do not report 36425 in conjunction with 36475, 36476, 36478)

36430 Transfusion, blood or blood components
➲ *CPT Assistant* Aug 97:18, Nov 99:32-33, Aug 00:2, Mar 01:10, Oct 03:2, Jul 06:4, Jul 07:1, Jul 17:4

(When a partial exchange transfusion is performed in a newborn, use 36456)

36440 Push transfusion, blood, 2 years or younger
➲ *CPT Assistant* Aug 00:2, Oct 03:2, Jul 06:4, Jul 07:1, Jul 17:4

(When a partial exchange transfusion is performed in a newborn, use 36456)

36450 Exchange transfusion, blood; newborn
➲ *CPT Assistant* Jul 17:3

(When a partial exchange transfusion is performed in a newborn, use 36456)

(Do not report modifier 63 in conjunction with 36450)

36455 other than newborn

36456 Partial exchange transfusion, blood, plasma or crystalloid necessitating the skill of a physician or other qualified health care professional, newborn
➲ *CPT Changes: An Insider's View* 2017, 2018
➲ *CPT Assistant* Jul 17:3

(Do not report 36456 in conjunction with 36430, 36440, 36450)

(Do not report modifier 63 in conjunction with 36456)

36460 Transfusion, intrauterine, fetal

(Do not report modifier 63 in conjunction with 36460)

(For radiological supervision and interpretation, use 76941)

Codes 36468, 36470, 36471 describe injection(s) of a sclerosant for sclerotherapy of telangiectasia and/or incompetent vein(s). Code 36468 may only be reported once per extremity per session, regardless of the number of needle injections performed. Codes 36466, 36471 may only be reported once per extremity, regardless of the number of veins treated. Ultrasound guidance (76942), when performed, is not included in 36468, 36470, 36471 and may be reported separately.

Codes 36465, 36466 describe injection(s) of a non-compounded foam sclerosant into an extremity truncal vein (eg, great saphenous vein, accessory saphenous vein) using ultrasound-guided compression of the junction of the central vein (saphenofemoral junction or saphenopopliteal junction) to limit the dispersion of injectate. Do not report 36465, 36466 for injection of compounded foam sclerosant(s).

Compounding is a practice in which a qualified health care professional (eg, pharmacist, physician) combines, mixes, or alters ingredients of a drug to create a medication tailored to the needs of an individual patient.

When performed in the office setting, all required supplies and equipment are included in 36465, 36466, 36468, 36470, 36471 and may not be separately reported. In addition, application of compression dressing(s) (eg, compression bandages/stockings) is included in 36465, 36466, 36468, 36470, 36471, when performed, and may not be reported separately.

36465 Code is out of numerical sequence. See 36470-36474

36466 Code is out of numerical sequence. See 36470-36474

36468 Injection(s) of sclerosant for spider veins (telangiectasia), limb or trunk
➲ *CPT Changes: An Insider's View* 2018
➲ *CPT Assistant* Aug 14:14, Oct 14:6, Apr 15:10, Nov 16:3, Mar 18:3
➲ *Clinical Examples in Radiology* Summer 15:8, Spring 17:3

(For ultrasound imaging guidance performed in conjunction with 36468, use 76942)

►(Do not report 36468 in conjunction with 29520, 29530, 29540, 29550, 29580, 29581, 29584, for the same extremity)◄

(Do not report 36468 more than once per extremity)

(Do not report 36468 in conjunction with 37241 in the same surgical field)

36470 Injection of sclerosant; single incompetent vein (other than telangiectasia)
➲ *CPT Changes: An Insider's View* 2018
➲ *CPT Assistant* Oct 14:6, Apr 15:10, Nov 15:10, Nov 16:3, Mar 18:3
➲ *Clinical Examples in Radiology* Summer 15:8, Spring 17:3

36471 multiple incompetent veins (other than telangiectasia), same leg
➲ *CPT Changes: An Insider's View* 2018
➲ *CPT Assistant* Oct 14:6, Apr 15:10, Aug 15:8, Nov 15:10, Nov 16:3, Mar 18:3
➲ *Clinical Examples in Radiology* Summer 15:8, Spring 17:3

(For ultrasound imaging guidance performed in conjunction with 36470, 36471, use 76942)

►(Do not report 36470, 36471 in conjunction with 29520, 29530, 29540, 29550, 29580, 29581, 29584, for the same extremity)◄

(Do not report 36471 more than once per extremity)

(If the targeted vein is an extremity truncal vein and injection of non-compounded foam sclerosant with ultrasound guided compression maneuvers to guide dispersion of the injectate is performed, see 36465, 36466)

(Do not report 36470, 36471 in conjunction with 37241 in the same surgical field)

 # 36465 Injection of non-compounded foam sclerosant with ultrasound compression maneuvers to guide dispersion of the injectate, inclusive of all imaging guidance and monitoring; single incompetent extremity truncal vein (eg, great saphenous vein, accessory saphenous vein)

➲ *CPT Changes: An Insider's View* 2018

➲ *CPT Assistant* Mar 18:3

 # 36466 multiple incompetent truncal veins (eg, great saphenous vein, accessory saphenous vein), same leg

➲ *CPT Changes: An Insider's View* 2018

➲ *CPT Assistant* Mar 18:3

►(Do not report 36465, 36466 in conjunction with 29520, 29530, 29540, 29550, 29580, 29581, 29584, for the same extremity)◄

(Do not report 36465, 36466 in conjunction with 37241 in the same surgical field)

(For extremity truncal vein injection of compounded foam sclerosant[s], see 36470, 36471)

(For injection of a sclerosant into an incompetent vein without compression maneuvers to guide dispersion of the injectate, see 36470, 36471)

(For endovenous ablation therapy of incompetent vein[s] by transcatheter delivery of a chemical adhesive, see 36482, 36483)

(For vascular embolization and occlusion procedures, see 37241, 37242, 37243, 37244)

Codes 36473, 36474, 36475, 36476, 36478, 36479, 36482, 36483 describe endovascular ablation therapy of incompetent extremity vein(s), including all necessary imaging guidance and monitoring. Sclerosant injection(s) of vein(s) by needle or mini-catheter (36468, 36470, 36471) followed by a compression technique is not endovascular ablation therapy. Codes 36473, 36474, 36482, 36483 can be performed under local anesthesia without the need for tumescent (peri-saphenous) anesthesia. Codes 36475, 36476, 36478, 36479 are performed using adjunctive tumescent anesthesia.

Codes 36473, 36474 involve concomitant use of an intraluminal device that mechanically disrupts/abrades the venous intima and infusion of a physician-specified medication in the target vein(s).

Codes 36482, 36483 involve positioning an intravenous catheter the length of an incompetent vein, remote from the percutaneous access site, with subsequent delivery of a chemical adhesive to ablate the incompetent vein. This often includes ultrasound compression of the outflow vein to limit the dispersion of the injected solution.

Codes 36475, 36476 involve advancing a radiofrequency device the length of an incompetent vein, with subsequent delivery of radiofrequency energy to ablate the incompetent vein.

Codes 36478, 36479 involve advancing a laser device the length of an incompetent vein, with subsequent delivery of thermal energy to ablate the incompetent vein.

Codes 36474, 36476, 36479, 36483 for subsequent vein(s) treated in the same extremity may only be reported once per extremity, regardless of the number of additional vein(s) treated.

When performed in the office setting, all required supplies and equipment are included in 36473, 36474, 36475, 36476, 36478, 36479, 36482, 36483 and may not be separately reported. In addition, application of compression dressing(s) (eg, compression bandages/stockings) is included in 36473, 36474, 36475, 36476, 36478, 36479, 36482, 36483, when performed, and may not be reported separately.

36473 Endovenous ablation therapy of incompetent vein, extremity, inclusive of all imaging guidance and monitoring, percutaneous, mechanochemical; first vein treated

➲ *CPT Changes: An Insider's View* 2017

➲ *CPT Assistant* Nov 16:3, May 17:3, Mar 18:3

➲ *Clinical Examples in Radiology* Spring 17:2

+ 36474 subsequent vein(s) treated in a single extremity, each through separate access sites (List separately in addition to code for primary procedure)

➲ *CPT Changes: An Insider's View* 2017

➲ *CPT Assistant* Nov 16:3, May 17:3, Mar 18:3

➲ *Clinical Examples in Radiology* Spring 17:3

(Use 36474 in conjunction with 36473)

(Do not report 36474 more than once per extremity)

►(Do not report 36473, 36474 in conjunction with 29520, 29530, 29540, 29550, 29580, 29581, 29584, for the same extremity)◄

►(Do not report 36473, 36474 in conjunction with 36000, 36002, 36005, 36410, 36425, 36475, 36476, 36478, 36479, 37241, 75894, 76000, 76937, 76942, 76998, 77022, 93970, 93971, in the same surgical field)◄

36475 Endovenous ablation therapy of incompetent vein, extremity, inclusive of all imaging guidance and monitoring, percutaneous, radiofrequency; first vein treated

➲ *CPT Changes: An Insider's View* 2005

➲ *CPT Assistant* Jul 10:11, Mar 14:4, Oct 14:6, Apr 15:10, Nov 16:3, Mar 18:3

➲ *Clinical Examples in Radiology* Fall 08:10, Spring 17:3

+ 36476 subsequent vein(s) treated in a single extremity, each through separate access sites (List separately in addition to code for primary procedure)

➲ *CPT Changes: An Insider's View* 2005, 2017

➲ *CPT Assistant* Jul 10:11, Mar 14:4, Oct 14:6, Apr 15:10, Nov 16:3, Mar 18:3

➲ *Clinical Examples in Radiology* Spring 17:3

(Use 36476 in conjunction with 36475)

(Do not report 36476 more than once per extremity)

►(Do not report 36475, 36476 in conjunction with 29520, 29530, 29540, 29550, 29580, 29581, 29584, for the same extremity)◄

►(Do not report 36475, 36476 in conjunction with 36000, 36002, 36005, 36410, 36425, 36478, 36479, 36482, 36483, 37241-37244, 75894, 76000, 76937, 76942, 76998, 77022, 93970, 93971, in the same surgical field)◄

36478 Endovenous ablation therapy of incompetent vein, extremity, inclusive of all imaging guidance and monitoring, percutaneous, laser; first vein treated

➲ *CPT Changes: An Insider's View* 2005

➲ *CPT Assistant* Jul 12:12, Mar 14:4, Oct 14:6, Apr 15:10, Nov 16:3, Mar 18:3

➲ *Clinical Examples in Radiology* Spring 17:3

+ 36479 subsequent vein(s) treated in a single extremity, each through separate access sites (List separately in addition to code for primary procedure)

➲ *CPT Changes: An Insider's View* 2005, 2017

➲ *CPT Assistant* Jul 10:11, Jul 12:12, Mar 14:4, Aug 14:14, Oct 14:6, Apr 15:10, Nov 16:3, Mar 18:3

➲ *Clinical Examples in Radiology* Spring 17:3

(Use 36479 in conjunction with 36478)

(Do not report 36479 more than once per extremity)

►(Do not report 36478, 36479 in conjunction with 29520, 29530, 29540, 29550, 29580, 29581, 29584, for the same extremity)◄

►(Do not report 36478, 36479 in conjunction with 36000, 36002, 36005, 36410, 36425, 36475, 36476, 36482, 36483, 37241, 75894, 76000, 76937, 76942, 76998, 77022, 93970, 93971, in the same surgical field)◄

 # 36482 Endovenous ablation therapy of incompetent vein, extremity, by transcatheter delivery of a chemical adhesive (eg, cyanoacrylate) remote from the access site, inclusive of all imaging guidance and monitoring, percutaneous; first vein treated

➲ *CPT Changes: An Insider's View* 2018

➲ *CPT Assistant* Mar 18:3

#+ 36483 subsequent vein(s) treated in a single extremity, each through separate access sites (List separately in addition to code for primary procedure)

➲ *CPT Changes: An Insider's View* 2018

➲ *CPT Assistant* Mar 18:3

(Use 36483 in conjunction with 36482)

(Do not report 36483 more than once per extremity)

►(Do not report 36482, 36483 in conjunction with 29520, 29530, 29540, 29550, 29580, 29581, 29584, for the same extremity)◄

►(Do not report 36482, 36483 in conjunction with 36000, 36002, 36005, 36410, 36425, 36475, 36476, 36478, 36479, 37241, 75894, 76000, 76937, 76942, 76998, 77022, 93970, 93971, in the same surgical field)◄

36481 Percutaneous portal vein catheterization by any method

➲ *CPT Changes: An Insider's View* 2010, 2017

➲ *CPT Assistant* Oct 96:1, Mar 02:10, Dec 03:2

➲ *Clinical Examples in Radiology* Winter 18:11

36482 Code is out of numerical sequence. See 36478-36500

36483 Code is out of numerical sequence. See 36478-36500

(For radiological supervision and interpretation, see 75885, 75887)

36500 Venous catheterization for selective organ blood sampling

➲ *Clinical Examples in Radiology* Summer 16:2

(For catheterization in superior or inferior vena cava, use 36010)

(For radiological supervision and interpretation, use 75893)

36510 Catheterization of umbilical vein for diagnosis or therapy, newborn

➲ *CPT Assistant* Nov 99:5-6, Aug 00:2, Oct 03:2, Jul 06:4, Jul 07:1, May 16:3

(Do not report modifier 63 in conjunction with 36510)

36511 Therapeutic apheresis; for white blood cells

➲ *CPT Changes: An Insider's View* 2003

➲ *CPT Assistant* Oct 13:3

36512 for red blood cells

➲ *CPT Changes: An Insider's View* 2003

➲ *CPT Assistant* Oct 13:3

36513 for platelets

➲ *CPT Changes: An Insider's View* 2003

➲ *CPT Assistant* Oct 13:3

(Report 36513 only when platelets are removed by apheresis for treatment of the patient. Do not report 36513 for donor platelet collections)

36514 for plasma pheresis

➲ *CPT Changes: An Insider's View* 2003

➲ *CPT Assistant* Oct 13:3

(36515 has been deleted. For therapeutic apheresis with extracorporeal immunoadsorption and plasma reinfusion, use 36516)

36516 with extracorporeal immunoadsorption, selective adsorption or selective filtration and plasma reinfusion

➲ *CPT Changes: An Insider's View* 2003, 2018

➲ *CPT Assistant* Oct 13:3

(For professional evaluation, use modifier 26)

36522 Photopheresis, extracorporeal

➲ *CPT Assistant* Fall 93:25, Jun 09:3, Sep 09:3, Aug 10:12, Oct 13:3

(For dialysis services, see 90935-90999)

(For ultrafiltration, use 90999)

(For therapeutic apheresis for white blood cells, red blood cells, platelets and plasma pheresis, see 36511, 36512, 36513, 36514)

(For therapeutic apheresis extracorporeal adsorption procedures, use 36516)

Central Venous Access Procedures

►To qualify as a central venous access catheter or device, the tip of the catheter/device must terminate in the subclavian, brachiocephalic (innominate) or iliac veins, the superior or inferior vena cava, or the right atrium. The venous access device may be either centrally inserted (jugular, subclavian, femoral vein or inferior vena cava catheter entry site) or peripherally inserted (eg, basilic, cephalic, or saphenous vein entry site). The device may be accessed for use either via exposed catheter (external to the skin), via a subcutaneous port or via a subcutaneous pump.◄

The procedures involving these types of devices fall into five categories:

1. ***Insertion*** (placement of catheter through a newly established venous access)
2. ***Repair*** (fixing device without replacement of either catheter or port/pump, other than pharmacologic or mechanical correction of intracatheter or pericatheter occlusion [see 36595 or 36596])
3. ***Partial replacement*** of only the catheter component associated with a port/pump device, but not entire device
4. ***Complete replacement*** of entire device via same venous access site (complete exchange)
5. ***Removal*** of entire device.

There is no coding distinction between venous access achieved percutaneously versus by cutdown or based on catheter size.

For the repair, partial (catheter only) replacement, complete replacement, or removal of both catheters (placed from separate venous access sites) of a multi-catheter device, with or without subcutaneous ports/pumps, use the appropriate code describing the service with a frequency of two.

If an existing central venous access device is removed and a new one placed via a separate venous access site, appropriate codes for both procedures (removal of old, if code exists, and insertion of new device) should be reported.

►When imaging guidance is used for centrally inserted central venous catheters, for gaining access to the venous entry site and/or for manipulating the catheter into final central position, imaging guidance codes (eg, 76937, 77001) may be reported separately. Do not use 76937, 77001 in conjunction with 36568, 36569, 36572, 36573, 36584.◄

(For refilling and maintenance of an implantable pump or reservoir for intravenous or intra-arterial drug delivery, use 96522)

Insertion of Central Venous Access Device

36555 Insertion of non-tunneled centrally inserted central venous catheter; younger than 5 years of age

➲ *CPT Changes: An Insider's View* 2004, 2017

➲ *CPT Assistant* Dec 04:7, Jul 06:4, Jul 07:1, Jun 08:8

➲ *Clinical Examples in Radiology* Summer 06:8-9, Spring 09:10, Winter 09:9, Winter 17:8

(For peripherally inserted non-tunneled central venous catheter, younger than 5 years of age, use 36568)

Insertion of Non-Tunneled Centrally Inserted Central Venous Catheter
36555

During placement of a central venous catheter, a short tract is developed as the catheter is advanced from the skin entry site to the point of venous cannulation. The catheter tip must reside in the subclavian, innominate or iliac veins, the inferior or superior vena cava, or right atrium to be considered a "central venous" catheter.

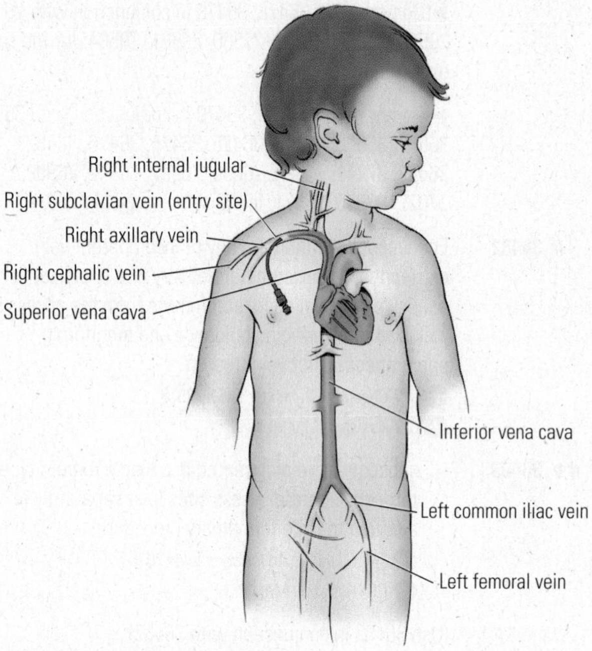

36556 age 5 years or older

➲ *CPT Changes: An Insider's View* 2004

➲ *CPT Assistant* Dec 04:7, Jun 08:8

➲ *Clinical Examples in Radiology* Summer 06:8-9, Spring 08:7, 8, Spring 09:10, Winter 09:8, 9, Winter 17:8

(For peripherally inserted non-tunneled central venous catheter, age 5 years or older, use 36569)

36557 Insertion of tunneled centrally inserted central venous catheter, without subcutaneous port or pump; younger than 5 years of age

➲ *CPT Changes: An Insider's View* 2004, 2017

➲ *CPT Assistant* Dec 04:7, Jun 08:8

➲ *Clinical Examples in Radiology* Spring 09:10, Winter 09:9, Winter 17:10

Insertion of Non-Tunneled Centrally Inserted Central Venous Catheter
36556

During placement of a central venous catheter, a short tract is developed as the catheter is advanced from the skin entry site to the point of venous cannulation. The catheter tip must reside in the subclavian, innominate or iliac veins, the inferior or superior vena cava, or right atrium, to be considered a "central venous" catheter.

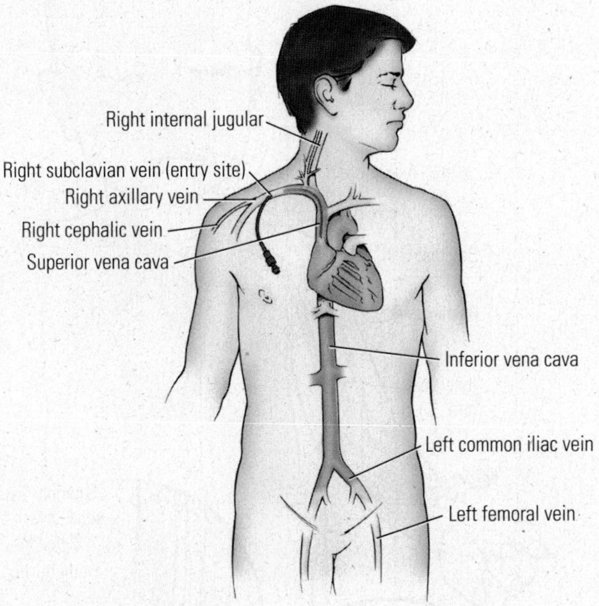

36558 age 5 years or older
- ➲ *CPT Changes: An Insider's View* 2004, 2017
- ➲ *CPT Assistant* Dec 04:7, Jun 08:8, Jan 15:13
- ➲ *Clinical Examples in Radiology* Spring 09:10, Winter 09:9, Winter 17:10

(For peripherally inserted central venous catheter with port, 5 years or older, use 36571)

36560 Insertion of tunneled centrally inserted central venous access device, with subcutaneous port; younger than 5 years of age
- ➲ *CPT Changes: An Insider's View* 2004, 2017
- ➲ *CPT Assistant* Dec 04:7, Jun 08:8, Dec 09:11
- ➲ *Clinical Examples in Radiology* Spring 09:10, Winter 09:9, Winter 17:10

(For peripherally inserted central venous access device with subcutaneous port, younger than 5 years of age, use 36570)

36561 age 5 years or older
- ➲ *CPT Changes: An Insider's View* 2004, 2017
- ➲ *CPT Assistant* Dec 04:7, Jun 08:8, Dec 09:11
- ➲ *Clinical Examples in Radiology* Spring 09:10, Winter 09:9, Winter 17:10

(For peripherally inserted central venous catheter with subcutaneous port, 5 years or older, use 36571)

Insertion of Tunneled Central Venous Catheter
36557-36558

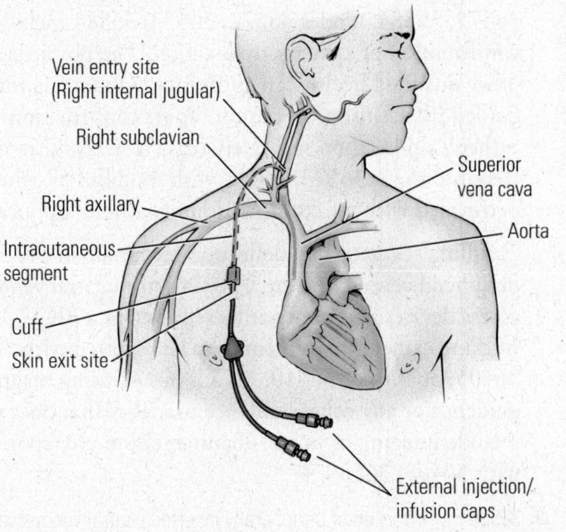

36563 Insertion of tunneled centrally inserted central venous access device with subcutaneous pump
- ➲ *CPT Changes: An Insider's View* 2004, 2017
- ➲ *CPT Assistant* Dec 04:8, Jun 08:8
- ➲ *Clinical Examples in Radiology* Spring 09:10, Winter 09:9, Winter 17:10

36565 Insertion of tunneled centrally inserted central venous access device, requiring 2 catheters via 2 separate venous access sites; without subcutaneous port or pump (eg, Tesio type catheter)
- ➲ *CPT Changes: An Insider's View* 2004, 2017
- ➲ *CPT Assistant* Dec 04:8, Jun 08:8
- ➲ *Clinical Examples in Radiology* Spring 09:10, Winter 09:9, Winter 17:10

36566 with subcutaneous port(s)
- ➲ *CPT Changes: An Insider's View* 2004, 2017
- ➲ *CPT Assistant* Dec 04:8, Jun 08:8
- ➲ *Clinical Examples in Radiology* Spring 09:10, Winter 09:9, Winter 17:10

▶Peripherally inserted central venous catheters (PICCs) may be placed or replaced with or without imaging guidance. When performed without imaging guidance, report using 36568 or 36569. When imaging guidance (eg, ultrasound, fluoroscopy) is used for PICC placement or repositioning, bundled service codes 36572, 36573, 36584 include all imaging necessary to complete the procedure, image documentation (representative images from all modalities used are stored to patient's permanent record), associated radiological supervision and interpretation, venography performed through the same venous puncture, and documentation of final central position of the catheter with imaging. Ultrasound guidance for PICC placement should include documentation of evaluation of the potential puncture sites, patency of the entry vein, and real-time ultrasound visualization of needle entry into the vein.

Codes 71045, 71046, 71047, 71048 should not be reported for the purpose of documenting the final catheter position on the same day of service as 36572, 36573, 36584. Codes 36572, 36573, 36584 include confirmation of catheter tip location. The physician or other qualified health care professional reporting image-guided PICC insertion cannot report confirmation of catheter tip location separately (eg, via X ray, ultrasound). Report 36572, 36573, 36584 with modifier 52 when performed without confirmation of catheter tip location.

"Midline" catheters by definition terminate in the peripheral venous system. They are **not** central venous access devices and may not be reported as a PICC service. Midline catheter placement may be reported with 36400, 36405, 36406, or 36410. PICCs placed using magnetic guidance or any other guidance modality that does not include imaging or image documentation are reported with 36568, 36569.◄

▲ **36568** Insertion of peripherally inserted central venous catheter (PICC), without subcutaneous port or pump, without imaging guidance; younger than 5 years of age

➲ *CPT Changes: An Insider's View* 2004, 2017, 2019

➲ *CPT Assistant* Oct 04:14, Dec 04:8, May 05:13, Jun 08:8, Nov 12:14

➲ *Clinical Examples in Radiology* Spring 09:10, Winter 09:9, Winter 17:10

(For placement of centrally inserted non-tunneled central venous catheter, without subcutaneous port or pump, younger than 5 years of age, use 36555)

►(For placement of peripherally inserted non-tunneled central venous catheter, without subcutaneous port or pump, with imaging guidance, younger than 5 years of age, use 36572)◄

▲ **36569** age 5 years or older

➲ *CPT Changes: An Insider's View* 2004, 2019

➲ *CPT Assistant* Oct 04:14, Dec 04:8, May 05:13, Jun 08:8, Nov 12:14, Sep 13:18, Sep 14:13

➲ *Clinical Examples in Radiology* 2004_Inaugural 04:1-2, Spring 08:7, Fall 08:5, 6, Spring 09:10, Winter 09:9, Winter 17:10

►(Do not report 36568, 36569 in conjunction with 76937, 77001)◄

(For placement of centrally inserted non-tunneled central venous catheter, without subcutaneous port or pump, age 5 years or older, use 36556)

►(For placement of peripherally inserted non-tunneled central venous catheter, without subcutaneous port or pump, with imaging guidance, age 5 years or older, use 36573)◄

#● **36572** Insertion of peripherally inserted central venous catheter (PICC), without subcutaneous port or pump, including all imaging guidance, image documentation, and all associated radiological supervision and interpretation required to perform the insertion; younger than 5 years of age

➲ *CPT Changes: An Insider's View* 2019

Peripherally Inserted Central Catheter

36572

A peripherally inserted central catheter, which is non-tunneled and without a subcutaneous port/pump, is placed in a child younger than 5 years of age.

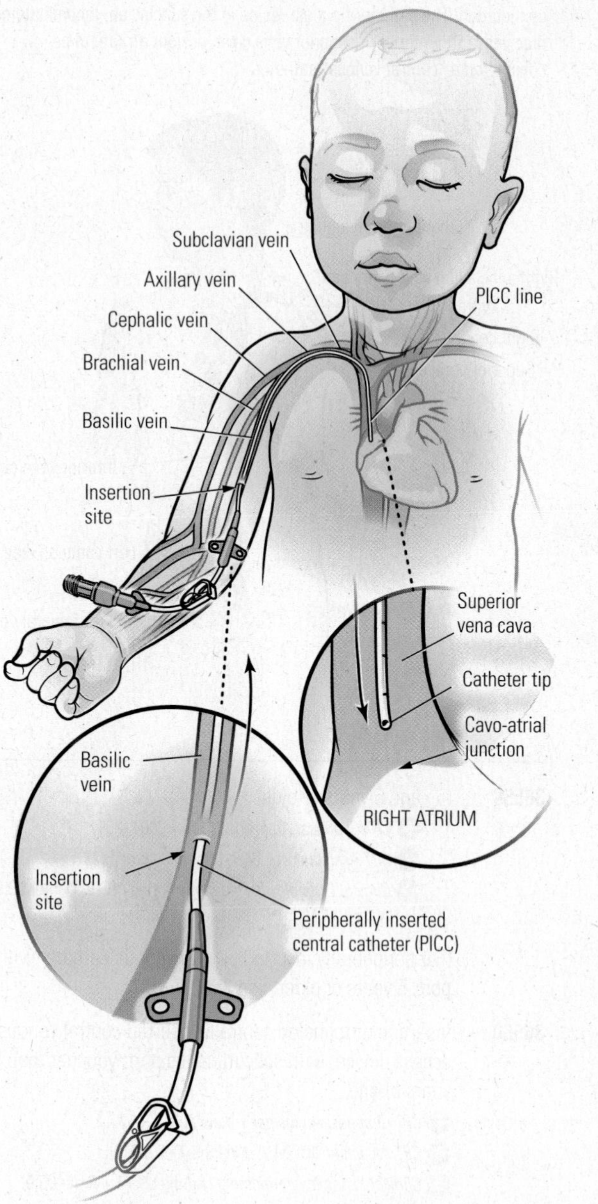

►(For placement of centrally inserted non-tunneled central venous catheter, without subcutaneous port or pump, younger than 5 years of age, use 36555)◄

►(For placement of peripherally inserted non-tunneled central venous catheter, without subcutaneous port or pump, without imaging guidance, younger than 5 years of age, use 36568)◄

#● **36573** age 5 years or older

➲ *CPT Changes: An Insider's View* 2019

►(For placement of centrally inserted non-tunneled central venous catheter, without subcutaneous port or pump, age 5 years or older, use 36556)◄

►(For placement of peripherally inserted non-tunneled central venous catheter, without subcutaneous port or pump, without imaging guidance, age 5 years or older, use 36569)◄

►(Do not report 36572, 36573 in conjunction with 76937, 77001)◄

36570 Insertion of peripherally inserted central venous access device, with subcutaneous port; younger than 5 years of age

➲ *CPT Changes: An Insider's View* 2004, 2017

➲ *CPT Assistant* Dec 04:8, Jun 08:8, Dec 09:11

➲ *Clinical Examples in Radiology* Spring 09:10, Winter 09:9, Winter 17:10

(For insertion of tunneled centrally inserted central venous access device with subcutaneous port, younger than 5 years of age, use 36560)

36571 age 5 years or older

➲ *CPT Changes: An Insider's View* 2004, 2017

➲ *CPT Assistant* Dec 04:9, Jun 08:8, Dec 09:11

➲ *Clinical Examples in Radiology* Spring 09:10, Winter 09:9, Winter 17:10

(For insertion of tunneled centrally inserted central venous access device with subcutaneous port, age 5 years or older, use 36561)

36572 Code is out of numerical sequence. See 36568-36571

36573 Code is out of numerical sequence. See 36568-36571

Implantable Venous Access Port
36570, 36571, 36576, 36578

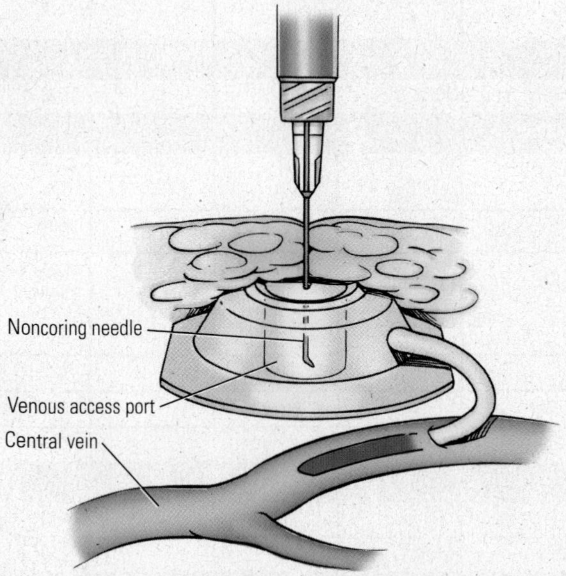

Repair of Central Venous Access Device

(For mechanical removal of pericatheter obstructive material, use 36595)

(For mechanical removal of intracatheter obstructive material, use 36596)

36575 Repair of tunneled or non-tunneled central venous access catheter, without subcutaneous port or pump, central or peripheral insertion site

➲ *CPT Changes: An Insider's View* 2004

➲ *Clinical Examples in Radiology* Spring 09:10, Summer 10:11

36576 Repair of central venous access device, with subcutaneous port or pump, central or peripheral insertion site

➲ *CPT Changes: An Insider's View* 2004, 2017

➲ *CPT Assistant* Dec 04:9, Jun 08:8

➲ *Clinical Examples in Radiology* Spring 09:10

Partial Replacement of Central Venous Access Device (Catheter Only)

36578 Replacement, catheter only, of central venous access device, with subcutaneous port or pump, central or peripheral insertion site

➲ *CPT Changes: An Insider's View* 2004, 2017

➲ *CPT Assistant* Dec 04:10, Jun 08:8

➲ *Clinical Examples in Radiology* Spring 09:10, Winter 09:9, Winter 17:10

(For complete replacement of entire device through same venous access, use 36582 or 36583)

Complete Replacement of Central Venous Access Device Through Same Venous Access Site

36580 Replacement, complete, of a non-tunneled centrally inserted central venous catheter, without subcutaneous port or pump, through same venous access

➲ *CPT Changes: An Insider's View* 2004

➲ *CPT Assistant* Dec 04:10, Jun 08:8

➲ *Clinical Examples in Radiology* Spring 09:10, Winter 09:9, Winter 17:10

36581 Replacement, complete, of a tunneled centrally inserted central venous catheter, without subcutaneous port or pump, through same venous access

➲ *CPT Changes: An Insider's View* 2004, 2017

➲ *CPT Assistant* Dec 04:10, Jun 08:8

➲ *Clinical Examples in Radiology* Spring 09:10, Winter 09:9, Winter 17:10

The Central Venous Access Procedures Table

	Non-tunneled	Tunneled Without Port or Pump (w/out port or pump)	Central Tunneled	Tunneled With Port (w/port)	Tunneled With Pump (w/pump)	Peripheral	<5 years	≥5 years	Any Age
Insertion									
Catheter (without imaging guidance)	36555						36555		
	36556							36556	
		36557	36557				36557		
		36558	36558					36558	
	36568 (w/o port or pump)					36568 (w/o port or pump)	36568 (w/o port or pump)		
	36569 (w/o port or pump)					36569 (w/o port or pump)		36569 (w/o port or pump)	
Catheter (with bundled imaging guidance)						36572 (w/o port or pump)	36572 (w/o port or pump)		
						36573 (w/o port or pump)		36573 (w/o port or pump)	
Device			36560	36560			36560		
			36561	36561				36561	
			36563		36563				36563
		36565	36565						36565
			36566	36566					
	36570 (w/port)			36570 (w/port)		36570 (w/port)	36570 (w/port)		
	36571 (w/port)			36571 (w/port)		36571 (w/port)		36571 (w/port)	
Repair									
Catheter	36575 (w/o port or pump)	36575 (w/o port or pump)	36575 (w/o port or pump)			36575 (w/o port or pump)			36575
Device	36576 (w/port or pump)					36576 (w/port or pump)			36576
Partial Replacement - Central Venous Access Device (Catheter only)									
			36578	36578	36578	36578			36578
Complete Replacement - Central Venous Access Device (Through Same Venous Access Site)									
Catheter (without imaging guidance)	36580 (w/o port or pump)								36580
		36581	36581						36581
Catheter (with bundled imaging guidance)	36584 (w/o port or pump)					36584 (w/o port or pump)			36584 (w/o port or pump)
Device			36582	36582					36582
			36583		36583				36583
				36585 (w/port)		36585 (w/port)			36585
Removal									
Catheter		36589							36589
Device			36590	36590	36590	36590			36590
Removal of Obstructive Material from Device									
	36595 (pericatheter)	36595 (pericatheter)	36595 (pericatheter)	36595 (pericatheter)	36595 (pericatheter)	36595 (pericatheter)			36595 (pericatheter)
	36596 (intraluminal)	36596 (intraluminal)	36596 (intraluminal)	36596 (intraluminal)	36596 (intraluminal)	36596 (intraluminal)			36596 (intraluminal)
Repositioning of Catheter									
	36597	36597	36597	36597	36597	36597	36597	36597	36597

36582 Replacement, complete, of a tunneled centrally inserted central venous access device, with subcutaneous port, through same venous access
- *CPT Changes: An Insider's View* 2004, 2017
- *CPT Assistant* Dec 04:10, Jun 08:8
- *Clinical Examples in Radiology* Spring 09:10, Winter 09:9, Winter 17:10

36583 Replacement, complete, of a tunneled centrally inserted central venous access device, with subcutaneous pump, through same venous access
- *CPT Changes: An Insider's View* 2004, 2017
- *CPT Assistant* Dec 04:10-11, Jun 08:8
- *Clinical Examples in Radiology* Spring 09:10, Winter 09:9, Winter 17:10

▲ **36584** Replacement, complete, of a peripherally inserted central venous catheter (PICC), without subcutaneous port or pump, through same venous access, including all imaging guidance, image documentation, and all associated radiological supervision and interpretation required to perform the replacement
- *CPT Changes: An Insider's View* 2004, 2019
- *CPT Assistant* Dec 04:11, Jun 08:8
- *Clinical Examples in Radiology* Spring 09:10, Winter 09:9, Winter 17:10

►(For replacement of a peripherally inserted central venous catheter [PICC] without subcutaneous port or pump, through same venous access, without imaging guidance, use 37799)◄

►(Do not report 36584 in conjunction with 76937, 77001)◄

36585 Replacement, complete, of a peripherally inserted central venous access device, with subcutaneous port, through same venous access
- *CPT Changes: An Insider's View* 2004, 2017
- *CPT Assistant* Dec 04:11, Jun 08:8
- *Clinical Examples in Radiology* Spring 09:10, Winter 09:9, Winter 17:10

Removal of Central Venous Access Device

36589 Removal of tunneled central venous catheter, without subcutaneous port or pump
- *CPT Changes: An Insider's View* 2004
- *CPT Assistant* Dec 04:11, Jun 08:8, Nov 15:10

36590 Removal of tunneled central venous access device, with subcutaneous port or pump, central or peripheral insertion
- *CPT Changes: An Insider's View* 2004, 2017
- *CPT Assistant* Dec 04:11, Jun 08:8, Jul 10:10
- *Clinical Examples in Radiology* Spring 08:7

(Do not report 36589 or 36590 for removal of non-tunneled central venous catheters)

Other Central Venous Access Procedures

36591 Collection of blood specimen from a completely implantable venous access device
- *CPT Changes: An Insider's View* 2008
- *CPT Assistant* Apr 08:9, Jul 11:16, May 14:4

(Do not report 36591 in conjunction with other services except a laboratory service)

(For collection of venous blood specimen by venipuncture, use 36415)

(For collection of capillary blood specimen, use 36416)

36592 Collection of blood specimen using established central or peripheral catheter, venous, not otherwise specified
- *CPT Changes: An Insider's View* 2008
- *CPT Assistant* Apr 08:9, Jul 11:16

(For blood collection from an established arterial catheter, use 37799)

(Do not report 36592 in conjunction with other services except a laboratory service)

36593 Declotting by thrombolytic agent of implanted vascular access device or catheter
- *CPT Changes: An Insider's View* 2008
- *CPT Assistant* Apr 08:9, Dec 09:11, Aug 11:9, Feb 13:3
- *Clinical Examples in Radiology* Summer 12:4, 5

36595 Mechanical removal of pericatheter obstructive material (eg, fibrin sheath) from central venous device via separate venous access
- *CPT Changes: An Insider's View* 2004
- *CPT Assistant* Dec 04:9, 12

(Do not report 36595 in conjunction with 36593)

(For venous catheterization, see 36010-36012)

(For radiological supervision and interpretation, use 75901)

36596 Mechanical removal of intraluminal (intracatheter) obstructive material from central venous device through device lumen
- *CPT Changes: An Insider's View* 2004
- *CPT Assistant* Dec 04:9, 12

(Do not report 36596 in conjunction with 36593)

(For venous catheterization, see 36010-36012)

(For radiological supervision and interpretation, use 75902)

36597 Repositioning of previously placed central venous catheter under fluoroscopic guidance
➔ *CPT Changes: An Insider's View* 2004
➔ *CPT Assistant* Dec 04:12, Sep 14:5

(For fluoroscopic guidance, use 76000)

36598 Contrast injection(s) for radiologic evaluation of existing central venous access device, including fluoroscopy, image documentation and report
➔ *CPT Changes: An Insider's View* 2006
➔ *Clinical Examples in Radiology* Winter 06:15, Spring 08:7, Summer 12:4

(Do not report 36598 in conjunction with 76000)

(Do not report 36598 in conjunction with 36595, 36596)

(For complete diagnostic studies, see 75820, 75825, 75827)

Arterial

36600 Arterial puncture, withdrawal of blood for diagnosis
➔ *CPT Assistant* Fall 95:7, Aug 00:2, Oct 03:2, Jul 05:11, Jul 06:4, Feb 07:10, Jul 07:1, May 14:4

⊘ **36620** Arterial catheterization or cannulation for sampling, monitoring or transfusion (separate procedure); percutaneous
➔ *CPT Assistant* Fall 95:7, Apr 98:3, Nov 99:32-33, Aug 00:2, Oct 03:2, Jul 06:4, Jul 07:1

36625 cutdown
➔ *CPT Assistant* Fall 95:7

36640 Arterial catheterization for prolonged infusion therapy (chemotherapy), cutdown
➔ *CPT Assistant* Fall 95:7

(See also 96420-96425)

(For arterial catheterization for occlusion therapy, see 75894)

36660 Catheterization, umbilical artery, newborn, for diagnosis or therapy
➔ *CPT Changes: An Insider's View* 2008
➔ *CPT Assistant* Fall 95:8, Oct 03:2, Jul 06:4, Jul 07:1

(Do not report modifier 63 in conjunction with 36660)

Intraosseous

36680 Placement of needle for intraosseous infusion

Hemodialysis Access, Intervascular Cannulation for Extracorporeal Circulation, or Shunt Insertion

36800 Insertion of cannula for hemodialysis, other purpose (separate procedure); vein to vein
➔ *CPT Assistant* Fall 93:3

36810 arteriovenous, external (Scribner type)
➔ *CPT Assistant* Fall 93:3, May 97:10

36815 arteriovenous, external revision, or closure
➔ *CPT Assistant* Fall 93:3

36818 Arteriovenous anastomosis, open; by upper arm cephalic vein transposition
➔ *CPT Changes: An Insider's View* 2005
➔ *CPT Assistant* Jul 05:9, Mar 16:10, Mar 17:5

(Do not report 36818 in conjunction with 36819, 36820, 36821, 36830 during a unilateral upper extremity procedure. For bilateral upper extremity open arteriovenous anastomoses performed at the same operative session, use modifier 50 or 59 as appropriate)

36819 by upper arm basilic vein transposition
➔ *CPT Changes: An Insider's View* 2000, 2002
➔ *CPT Assistant* Nov 99:20, Jul 05:9, Mar 17:5

(Do not report 36819 in conjunction with 36818, 36820, 36821, 36830 during a unilateral upper extremity procedure. For bilateral upper extremity open arteriovenous anastomoses performed at the same operative session, use modifier 50 or 59 as appropriate)

36820 by forearm vein transposition
➔ *CPT Changes: An Insider's View* 2002
➔ *CPT Assistant* Fall 93:4, Jul 05:9, Mar 17:5

36821 direct, any site (eg, Cimino type) (separate procedure)
➔ *CPT Changes: An Insider's View* 2000
➔ *CPT Assistant* Fall 93:3, Feb 97:2, Nov 99:20, Jul 05:9, Aug 15:8, Mar 17:5

Arteriovenous Anastomosis, Direct
36821

A section of artery and a neighboring vein are joined, allowing blood to flow down the artery and into the vein for the purpose of increasing blood flow, usually in hemodialysis.

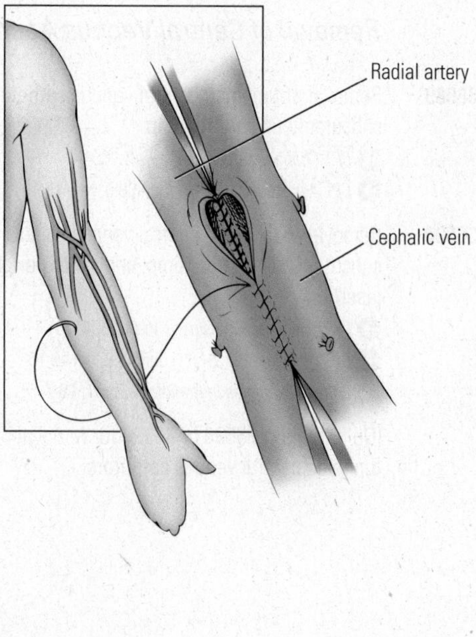

36823 Insertion of arterial and venous cannula(s) for isolated extracorporeal circulation including regional chemotherapy perfusion to an extremity, with or without hyperthermia, with removal of cannula(s) and repair of arteriotomy and venotomy sites

➔ *CPT Changes: An Insider's View* 2002

➔ *CPT Assistant* Nov 98:14-15, Mar 17:5

(36823 includes chemotherapy perfusion supported by a membrane oxygenator/perfusion pump. Do not report 96409-96425 in conjunction with 36823)

36825 Creation of arteriovenous fistula by other than direct arteriovenous anastomosis (separate procedure); autogenous graft

➔ *CPT Assistant* Fall 93:3, Feb 97:2, Jul 05:9, Mar 17:5

(For direct arteriovenous anastomosis, use 36821)

36830 nonautogenous graft (eg, biological collagen, thermoplastic graft)

➔ *CPT Changes: An Insider's View* 2003

➔ *CPT Assistant* Fall 93:3, Feb 97:2, Jul 05:9, Jan 15:13, Mar 17:5

(For direct arteriovenous anastomosis, use 36821)

36831 Thrombectomy, open, arteriovenous fistula without revision, autogenous or nonautogenous dialysis graft (separate procedure)

➔ *CPT Changes: An Insider's View* 2001

➔ *CPT Assistant* Nov 98:14-15, Feb 99:6, Mar 99:6, Apr 99:11, Mar 17:5

Arteriovenous Fistula
36825-36830

A donor's vein (36825) or a synthetic vein (36830) is used to connect an artery and vein.

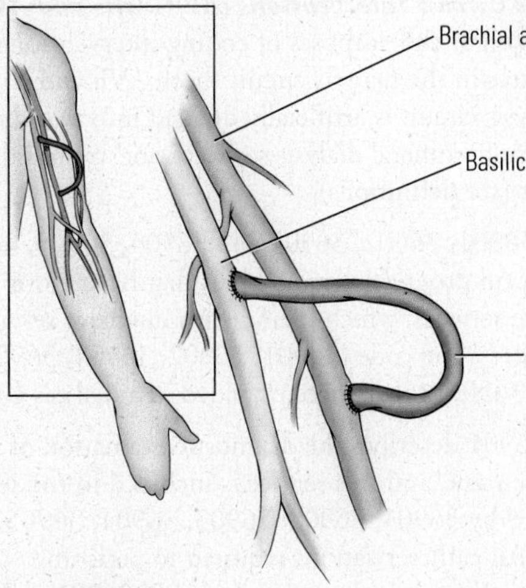

36832 Revision, open, arteriovenous fistula; without thrombectomy, autogenous or nonautogenous dialysis graft (separate procedure)

➔ *CPT Changes: An Insider's View* 2000, 2001

➔ *CPT Assistant* Fall 93:3, Feb 97:2, Nov 98:15, Feb 99:6, Mar 99:6, Apr 99:11, Nov 99:20-21, Mar 17:5

36833 with thrombectomy, autogenous or nonautogenous dialysis graft (separate procedure)

➔ *CPT Assistant* Nov 98:15, Feb 99:6, Apr 99:11, Mar 17:5

(For percutaneous thrombectomy within the dialysis circuit, see 36904, 36905, 36906)

(For central dialysis segment angioplasty in conjunction with 36818-36833, use 36907)

(For central dialysis segment stent placement in conjunction with 36818-36833, use 36908)

(Do not report 36832, 36833 in conjunction with 36901, 36902, 36903, 36904, 36905, 36906 for revision of the dialysis circuit)

36835 Insertion of Thomas shunt (separate procedure)

36838 Distal revascularization and interval ligation (DRIL), upper extremity hemodialysis access (steal syndrome)

➔ *CPT Changes: An Insider's View* 2004

(Do not report 36838 in conjunction with 35512, 35522, 35523, 36832, 37607, 37618)

36860 External cannula declotting (separate procedure); without balloon catheter

➔ *CPT Assistant* Fall 93:3, Feb 97:2, Nov 98:15, Feb 99:6, May 01:3

36861 with balloon catheter

➔ *CPT Assistant* Fall 93:3, Feb 97:2, May 01:3

(If imaging guidance is performed, use 76000)

(36870 has been deleted. To report percutaneous transluminal mechanical thrombectomy and/or infusion for thrombolysis within the dialysis circuit, see 36904, 36905, 36906)

Dialysis Circuit

Definitions

Dialysis circuit: The arteriovenous (AV) dialysis circuit is designed for easy and repetitive access to perform hemodialysis. It begins at the arterial anastomosis and extends to the right atrium. The circuit may be created using either an arterial-venous anastomosis, known as an arteriovenous fistula (AVF), or a prosthetic graft placed between an artery and vein, known as an arteriovenous graft (AVG). The dialysis circuit is comprised of two segments, termed the (1) peripheral dialysis segment and (2) central dialysis segment. Both are defined as follows.

Peripheral dialysis segment: The peripheral dialysis segment is the portion of the dialysis circuit that begins at the arterial anastomosis and extends to the central dialysis segment. In the upper extremity, the peripheral dialysis segment extends through the axillary vein (or entire cephalic vein in the case of cephalic venous outflow). In the lower extremity, the peripheral dialysis segment extends through the common femoral vein. The peripheral dialysis segment includes the historic "peri-anastomotic region" (defined below).

Central dialysis segment: The central dialysis segment includes all draining veins central to the peripheral dialysis segment. In the upper extremity, the central dialysis segment includes the veins central to the axillary and cephalic veins, including the subclavian and innominate veins through the superior vena cava. In the lower extremity, the central dialysis segment includes the veins central to the common femoral vein, including the external iliac and common iliac veins through the inferior vena cava.

Peri-anastomotic region: A historic term referring to the region of a dialysis circuit near the arterial anastomosis encompassing a short segment of the parent artery, the anastomosis, and a short segment of the dialysis circuit immediately adjacent to the anastomosis. The peri-anastomotic region is included within the peripheral segment of the dialysis circuit.

Performed through dialysis circuit: Any diagnostic study or therapeutic intervention within the dialysis circuit that is performed through a direct percutaneous access to the dialysis circuit.

Code 36901 includes direct access and imaging of the entire dialysis circuit. Antegrade and/or retrograde punctures of the dialysis circuit are typically used for imaging, and contrast may be injected directly through a needle or through a catheter placed into the dialysis circuit. All dialysis circuit punctures required to perform the procedure are included in 36901. Occasionally, the catheter needs to be advanced further into the circuit to adequately visualize the arterial anastomosis or the central veins, or selective catheterization of a venous branch may be required. All manipulation(s) of the catheter for diagnostic imaging of the dialysis circuit is included in 36901. Advancement of the catheter to the vena cava to adequately image that segment of the dialysis circuit is included in 36901 and is not separately reported. Code 36901 also includes catheterization of additional venous side branches communicating with the dialysis circuit, known as accessory veins. Advancement of the catheter tip through the arterial anastomosis to adequately visualize the anastomosis is also included in the service described by 36901 and is not separately reported.

Evaluation of the peri-anastomotic portion of the inflow is an integral part of the dialysis circuit angiogram and is included in 36901.

For the purposes of reporting dialysis access maintenance services, the arterial inflow to the dialysis circuit is considered a separate vessel. If a more proximal arterial inflow problem separate from the peripheral dialysis segment is suspected, additional catheter placement and imaging required for adequate evaluation of the artery may be separately reported. If a catheter is selectively advanced from the dialysis circuit puncture beyond the peri-anastomotic segment into the inflow artery, an additional catheterization code may be reported. For example, 36215 may be used to report image-guided retrograde catheter placement into the inflow artery and into the aorta, if necessary (36200 is not reported in addition to 36215 in this example). Note that 75710 may also be reported if contrast injection for diagnostic arteriography is performed through this catheter and radiological supervision and interpretation and imaging documentation is performed.

Ultrasound guidance for puncture of the dialysis circuit access is not typically performed and is not included in 36901, 36902, 36903, 36904, 36905, 36906. However, in the case of a new (immature) or failing AVF, ultrasound may be necessary to safely and effectively puncture the dialysis circuit for evaluation, and this may be reported separately with 76937, if all the appropriate elements for reporting 76937 are performed and documented.

For radiological supervision and interpretation of dialysis circuit angiography performed through existing access(es) or catheter-based arterial access, report 36901 with modifier 52.

Dialysis Circuit Interventions (AV Grafts and AV Fistulae): For the purposes of coding interventional procedures in the dialysis circuit (both AVF and AVG), the dialysis circuit is artificially divided into two distinct segments: peripheral dialysis segment and central dialysis segment (see definitions).

Codes 36901, 36902, 36903 and 36904, 36905, 36906 are built on progressive hierarchies that have more intensive services, which include less intensive services. Report only one code (36901, 36902, 36903, 36904, 36905, 36906) for services provided in a dialysis circuit.

Code 36901 describes the diagnostic evaluation of the dialysis circuit, and this service is included in the services described by 36901, 36902, 36903, 36904, 36905, 36906. All catheterizations required to perform diagnostic fistulography are included in 36901. All catheterizations required to perform additional interventional services are included in codes 36902, 36903, 36904, 36905, 36906, 36907, 36908, 36909 and not separately reported. All angiography, fluoroscopic image guidance, roadmapping, and radiological supervision and interpretation required to perform each service are included in each code. Closure of the puncture(s) by any method is included in the service of each individual code.

Code 36902 includes the services in 36901 plus transluminal balloon angioplasty in the peripheral segment of the dialysis circuit. Code 36902 would be reported only once per session to describe all angioplasty services performed in the peripheral segment of the dialysis circuit, regardless of the number of distinct lesions treated within that segment, the number of times the balloon is inflated, or the number of balloon catheters or sizes required to open all lesions, and includes angioplasty of the peri-anastomotic segment when performed. Code 36903 includes the services in 36902 plus transcatheter stent placement in the peripheral segment of the dialysis circuit. Code 36903 is reported only once per session to describe placing stent(s) within the peripheral segment, regardless of the number of stent(s) placed or the number of discrete lesion(s) treated within the peripheral segment. If both angioplasty and stenting are performed in the peripheral segment, including treatment of separate lesions, report 36903 only once.

Code 36904 describes percutaneous transluminal mechanical thrombectomy and/or infusion for thrombolysis in the dialysis circuit (all thrombus treated in both the peripheral and central dialysis circuit segments) and includes diagnostic angiography (36901), fluoroscopic image guidance, catheter placement(s), and all maneuvers required to remove thrombus from the peripheral and/or central segments, including all intraprocedural pharmacological thrombolytic injection(s)/infusion(s). It is never appropriate to report removal of the arterial plug during a declot/thrombectomy procedure as an angioplasty (36905). Removal of the arterial plug is included in a fistula thrombectomy, even if a balloon catheter is used to mechanically dislodge the resistant thrombus. Codes 36905 (angioplasty) and 36906 (stent) describe services in the peripheral circuit when performed in conjunction with thrombolysis/thrombectomy. Code 36905 includes the services in 36904 plus transluminal balloon angioplasty in the peripheral segment of the dialysis circuit. Code 36905 may be reported only once per session to describe all angioplasty performed in the peripheral segment of the dialysis circuit, regardless of the number of distinct lesions treated within that segment, the number of times the balloon is inflated, or the number of balloon catheters required to open all lesions. Code 36906 includes the services in 36905 plus transcatheter stent placement in the peripheral segment of the dialysis circuit. Code 36906 is reported only once per session to describe placing stent(s) within the peripheral segment, regardless of the number of stent(s) placed or the number of discrete lesion(s) treated within the peripheral segment.

Codes 36907 and 36908 describe procedures performed through puncture(s) in the dialysis circuit. Similar procedures performed from a different access (eg, common femoral vein) may be reported using 37248, 37249 or 37238, 37239. Code 36907 is an add-on code used in conjunction with 36901, 36902, 36903, 36904, 36905, 36906 to report angioplasty within the central dialysis segment when performed through puncture of the dialysis circuit, and is reported once per session independent of the number of discrete lesions treated, the number of balloon inflations, and number of balloon catheters or sizes required. These additional services should be clearly documented in the patient record, including the recorded images. Code 36907 may be reported only once per session with 36901, 36902, 36903, 36904, 36905, 36906, as appropriate. Report 36907 once for all angioplasty performed within the central dialysis segment.

Code 36908 is an add-on code used in conjunction with 36901, 36902, 36903, 36904, 36905, 36906 to report stenting lesion(s) in the central dialysis segment when performed through puncture of the dialysis circuit. It is reported once, regardless of the number of discrete lesions treated or the number of stents placed. Code 36908 includes the services in 36907; therefore, 36908 may not be reported with 36907 in the same session. Code 36908 may be reported only once per session with 36901, 36902, 36903, 36904, 36905, 36906, as appropriate.

Code 36909 is an add-on code used to report endovascular embolization or occlusion of the main vessel or side branches arising from (emptying into) the dialysis circuit. Code 36909 may only be reported once per therapeutic session, irrespective of the number of branches embolized or occluded. Embolization or occlusion of the main vessel or these side branches may not be reported with 37241.

If open dialysis circuit creation, revision, and/or thrombectomy (36818-36833) are performed, completion angiography is bundled, as is peripheral segment angioplasty and/or stent placement (36901, 36902, 36903) and, therefore, not separately reported. However, dialysis circuit central segment angioplasty and/or stent placement may be separately reported (36907, 36908).

36901 Introduction of needle(s) and/or catheter(s), dialysis circuit, with diagnostic angiography of the dialysis circuit, including all direct puncture(s) and catheter placement(s), injection(s) of contrast, all necessary imaging from the arterial anastomosis and adjacent artery through entire venous outflow including the inferior or superior vena cava, fluoroscopic guidance, radiological supervision and interpretation and image documentation and report

➔ *CPT Changes: An Insider's View* 2017

➔ *CPT Assistant* Mar 17:3, May 17:3

➔ *Clinical Examples in Radiology* Spring 18:8

(Do not report 36901 in conjunction with 36833, 36902, 36903, 36904, 36905, 36906)

36902 with transluminal balloon angioplasty, peripheral dialysis segment, including all imaging and radiological supervision and interpretation necessary to perform the angioplasty

➔ *CPT Changes: An Insider's View* 2017

➔ *CPT Assistant* Mar 17:3, May 17:3

➔ *Clinical Examples in Radiology* Spring 18:8

(Do not report 36902 in conjunction with 36903)

36903 with transcatheter placement of intravascular stent(s), peripheral dialysis segment, including all imaging and radiological supervision and interpretation necessary to perform the stenting, and all angioplasty within the peripheral dialysis segment

➔ *CPT Changes: An Insider's View* 2017

➔ *CPT Assistant* Mar 17:3, May 17:3

➔ *Clinical Examples in Radiology* Spring 18:9

(Do not report 36902, 36903 in conjunction with 36833, 36904, 36905, 36906)

(Do not report 36901, 36902, 36903 more than once per operative session)

(For transluminal balloon angioplasty within central vein(s) when performed through dialysis circuit, use 36907)

(For transcatheter placement of intravascular stent(s) within central vein(s) when performed through dialysis circuit, use 36908)

36904 Percutaneous transluminal mechanical thrombectomy and/or infusion for thrombolysis, dialysis circuit, any method, including all imaging and radiological supervision and interpretation, diagnostic angiography, fluoroscopic guidance, catheter placement(s), and intraprocedural pharmacological thrombolytic injection(s)

➔ *CPT Changes: An Insider's View* 2017

➔ *CPT Assistant* Mar 17:3, May 17:3

➔ *Clinical Examples in Radiology* Spring 18:9

(For open thrombectomy within the dialysis circuit, see 36831, 36833)

36905 with transluminal balloon angioplasty, peripheral dialysis segment, including all imaging and radiological supervision and interpretation necessary to perform the angioplasty

➔ *CPT Changes: An Insider's View* 2017

➔ *CPT Assistant* Mar 17:3, May 17:3

➔ *Clinical Examples in Radiology* Spring 18:9

(Do not report 36905 in conjunction with 36904)

36906 with transcatheter placement of intravascular stent(s), peripheral dialysis segment, including all imaging and radiological supervision and interpretation necessary to perform the stenting, and all angioplasty within the peripheral dialysis circuit

➔ *CPT Changes: An Insider's View* 2017

➔ *CPT Assistant* Mar 17:3, May 17:3

➔ *Clinical Examples in Radiology* Spring 18:9

(Do not report 36906 in conjunction with 36901, 36902, 36903, 36904, 36905)

(Do not report 36904, 36905, 36906 more than once per operative session)

(For transluminal balloon angioplasty within central vein(s) when performed through dialysis circuit, use 36907)

(For transcatheter placement of intravascular stent(s) within central vein(s) when performed through dialysis circuit, use 36908)

+ 36907 Transluminal balloon angioplasty, central dialysis segment, performed through dialysis circuit, including all imaging and radiological supervision and interpretation required to perform the angioplasty (List separately in addition to code for primary procedure)

➔ *CPT Changes: An Insider's View* 2017

➔ *CPT Assistant* Mar 17:3, May 17:3

➔ *Clinical Examples in Radiology* Spring 18:8

(Use 36907 in conjunction with 36818-36833, 36901, 36902, 36903, 36904, 36905, 36906)

(Do not report 36907 in conjunction with 36908)

(Report 36907 once for all angioplasty performed within the central dialysis segment)

+ 36908 Transcatheter placement of intravascular stent(s), central dialysis segment, performed through dialysis circuit, including all imaging and radiological supervision and interpretation required to perform the stenting, and all angioplasty in the central dialysis segment (List separately in addition to code for primary procedure)

➔ *CPT Changes: An Insider's View* 2017, 2018

➔ *CPT Assistant* Mar 17:3, May 17:3

(Use 36908 in conjunction with 36818-36833, 36901, 36902, 36903, 36904, 36905, 36906)

(Do not report 36908 in conjunction with 36907)

(Report 36908 once for all stenting performed within the central dialysis segment)

+ **36909** Dialysis circuit permanent vascular embolization or occlusion (including main circuit or any accessory veins), endovascular, including all imaging and radiological supervision and interpretation necessary to complete the intervention (List separately in addition to code for primary procedure)

➔ *CPT Changes: An Insider's View* 2017

➔ *CPT Assistant* Mar 17:3, May 17:3

(36909 includes all permanent vascular occlusions within the dialysis circuit and may only be reported once per encounter per day)

(Report 36909 in conjunction with 36901, 36902, 36903, 36904, 36905, 36906)

(For open ligation/occlusion in dialysis access, use 37607)

Portal Decompression Procedures

37140 Venous anastomosis, open; portocaval

➔ *CPT Changes: An Insider's View* 2003

(For peritoneal-venous shunt, use 49425)

37145 renoportal

37160 caval-mesenteric

37180 splenorenal, proximal

37181 splenorenal, distal (selective decompression of esophagogastric varices, any technique)

(For percutaneous procedure, use 37182)

37182 Insertion of transvenous intrahepatic portosystemic shunt(s) (TIPS) (includes venous access, hepatic and portal vein catheterization, portography with hemodynamic evaluation, intrahepatic tract formation/dilatation, stent placement and all associated imaging guidance and documentation)

➔ *CPT Changes: An Insider's View* 2003

➔ *CPT Assistant* Dec 03:2, Sep 13:17

➔ *Clinical Examples in Radiology* Summer 10:2

(Do not report 75885 or 75887 in conjunction with 37182)

(For open procedure, use 37140)

37183 Revision of transvenous intrahepatic portosystemic shunt(s) (TIPS) (includes venous access, hepatic and portal vein catheterization, portography with hemodynamic evaluation, intrahepatic tract recannulization/dilatation, stent placement and all associated imaging guidance and documentation)

➔ *CPT Changes: An Insider's View* 2003, 2010, 2017

➔ *CPT Assistant* Dec 03:2

➔ *Clinical Examples in Radiology* Fall 09:9, Summer 10:3

(Do not report 75885 or 75887 in conjunction with 37183)

(For repair of arteriovenous aneurysm, use 36832)

Transcatheter Procedures

Codes for catheter placement and the radiologic supervision and interpretation should also be reported, in addition to the code(s) for the therapeutic aspect of the procedure.

Mechanical Thrombectomy

Code(s) for catheter placement(s), diagnostic studies, and other percutaneous interventions (eg, transluminal balloon angioplasty, stent placement) provided are separately reportable.

Codes 37184-37188 specifically include intraprocedural fluoroscopic radiological supervision and interpretation services for guidance of the procedure.

Intraprocedural injection(s) of a thrombolytic agent is an included service and not separately reportable in conjunction with mechanical thrombectomy. However, subsequent or prior continuous infusion of a thrombolytic is not an included service and is separately reportable (see 37211-37214).

For coronary mechanical thrombectomy, use 92973.

For intracranial arterial mechanical thrombectomy, use 61645.

Transcatheter Thrombolytic Infusion

Codes 37211 or 37212 are used to report the initial day of transcatheter thrombolytic infusion(s) including follow-up arteriography/venography, and catheter position change or exchange, when performed. To report bilateral thrombolytic infusion through a separate access site(s), use modifier 50 in conjunction with 37211, 37212. Code 37213 is used to report continued transcatheter thrombolytic infusion(s) on subsequent day(s), other than initial day and final day of treatment. Code 37214 is used to report final day of transcatheter thrombolytic infusion(s). When initiation and completion of thrombolysis occur on the same day, report only 37211 or 37212.

Code(s) for catheter placement(s), diagnostic studies, and other percutaneous interventions (eg, transluminal balloon angioplasty, stent placement) provided may be separately reportable.

Codes 37211-37214 include fluoroscopic guidance and associated radiological supervision and interpretation.

Ongoing evaluation and management services on the day of the procedure related to thrombolysis are included in 37211-37214. If a significant, separately identifiable E/M service is performed by the same physician on the same day of the procedure, report the appropriate level of E/M service and append modifier 25.

Ultrasound guidance for vascular access is not included in 37211-37214. Code 76937 may be reported separately when performed if all the required elements are performed.

For intracranial arterial mechanical thrombectomy and/or infusion for thrombolysis, use 61645.

Arterial Mechanical Thrombectomy

►Arterial mechanical thrombectomy may be performed as a "primary" transcatheter procedure with pretreatment planning, performance of the procedure, and postprocedure evaluation focused on providing this service. Typically, the diagnosis of thrombus has been made prior to the procedure, and a mechanical thrombectomy is planned preoperatively. Primary mechanical thrombectomy is reported per vascular family using 37184 for the initial vessel treated and 37185 for second or all subsequent vessel(s) within the same vascular family. To report mechanical thrombectomy of an additional vascular family treated through a separate access site, use modifier 59 in conjunction with the primary service code (37184) for the mechanical transluminal thrombectomy.◄

Primary mechanical thrombectomy may precede or follow another percutaneous intervention. Most commonly primary mechanical thrombectomy will precede another percutaneous intervention with the decision regarding the need for other services not made until after mechanical thrombectomy has been performed. Occasionally, the performance of primary mechanical thrombectomy may follow another percutaneous intervention.

Do **NOT** report 37184-37185 for mechanical thrombectomy performed for the retrieval of short segments of thrombus or embolus evident during other percutaneous interventional procedures. See 37186 for these procedures.

Arterial mechanical thrombectomy is considered a "secondary" transcatheter procedure for removal or retrieval of short segments of thrombus or embolus when performed either before or after another percutaneous intervention (eg, percutaneous transluminal balloon angioplasty, stent placement). Secondary mechanical thrombectomy is reported using 37186. Do **NOT** report 37186 in conjunction with 37184-37185.

Venous Mechanical Thrombectomy

Use 37187 to report the initial application of venous mechanical thrombectomy. To report bilateral venous mechanical thrombectomy performed through a separate access site(s), use modifier 50 in conjunction with 37187. For repeat treatment on a subsequent day during a course of thrombolytic therapy, use 37188.

Arterial Mechanical Thrombectomy

37184 Primary percutaneous transluminal mechanical thrombectomy, noncoronary, non-intracranial, arterial or arterial bypass graft, including fluoroscopic guidance and intraprocedural pharmacological thrombolytic injection(s); initial vessel

➲ *CPT Changes: An Insider's View* 2006, 2016, 2017

➲ *CPT Assistant* Nov 11:11, Feb 13:3, Apr 15:10, Nov 15:3

➲ *Clinical Examples in Radiology* Winter 06:15, Summer 10:4, Winter 13:2, 3, 4, Spring 16:3

►(Do not report 37184 in conjunction with 61645, 76000, 96374)◄

+ 37185 second and all subsequent vessel(s) within the same vascular family (List separately in addition to code for primary mechanical thrombectomy procedure)

➲ *CPT Changes: An Insider's View* 2006, 2016, 2017

➲ *CPT Assistant* Nov 11:11, Feb 13:3, Apr 15:10, Nov 15:3

➲ *Clinical Examples in Radiology* Winter 06:15, Winter 13:2, 3, Spring 16:3

►(Do not report 37185 in conjunction with 76000, 96375)◄

(Do not report 37185 in conjunction with 61645 for treatment of the same vascular territory. See Nervous System Endovascular Therapy)

+ 37186 Secondary percutaneous transluminal thrombectomy (eg, nonprimary mechanical, snare basket, suction technique), noncoronary, non-intracranial, arterial or arterial bypass graft, including fluoroscopic guidance and intraprocedural pharmacological thrombolytic injections, provided in conjunction with another percutaneous intervention other than primary mechanical thrombectomy (List separately in addition to code for primary procedure)

➲ *CPT Changes: An Insider's View* 2006, 2016, 2017

➲ *CPT Assistant* Jul 11:11, Nov 11:9, Feb 13:3, Nov 15:3

➲ *Clinical Examples in Radiology* Winter 06:15, Winter 13:4, Spring 16:3

►(Do not report 37186 in conjunction with 76000, 96375)◄

(Do not report 37186 in conjunction with 61645 for treatment of the same vascular territory. See Nervous System Endovascular Therapy)

Venous Mechanical Thrombectomy

37187 Percutaneous transluminal mechanical thrombectomy, vein(s), including intraprocedural pharmacological thrombolytic injections and fluoroscopic guidance

➲ *CPT Changes: An Insider's View* 2006, 2017

➲ *CPT Assistant* Nov 11:11, Feb 13:3

➲ *Clinical Examples in Radiology* Winter 06:15, Winter 12:3, Summer 13:1, 2, 3, 4, Winter 13:4

►(Do not report 37187 in conjunction with 76000, 96375)◄

37188 Percutaneous transluminal mechanical thrombectomy, vein(s), including intraprocedural pharmacological thrombolytic injections and fluoroscopic guidance, repeat treatment on subsequent day during course of thrombolytic therapy

➲ *CPT Changes: An Insider's View* 2006, 2017

➲ *CPT Assistant* Nov 11:11, Feb 13:3

➲ *Clinical Examples in Radiology* Winter 06:15, Winter 12:3, Summer 13:4, Winter 13:4

►(Do not report 37188 in conjunction with 76000, 96375)◄

Other Procedures

37191 Insertion of intravascular vena cava filter, endovascular approach including vascular access, vessel selection, and radiological supervision and interpretation, intraprocedural roadmapping, and imaging guidance (ultrasound and fluoroscopy), when performed

➲ *CPT Changes: An Insider's View* 2012, 2017

➲ *CPT Assistant* Apr 12:8, Feb 13:3, May 16:11, Feb 17:14

➲ *Clinical Examples in Radiology* Winter 12:1, Winter 16:4

(For open surgical interruption of the inferior vena cava through a laparotomy or retroperitoneal exposure, use 37619)

37192 Repositioning of intravascular vena cava filter, endovascular approach including vascular access, vessel selection, and radiological supervision and interpretation, intraprocedural roadmapping, and imaging guidance (ultrasound and fluoroscopy), when performed

➲ *CPT Changes: An Insider's View* 2012, 2017

➲ *CPT Assistant* Apr 12:8, Feb 13:3, May 16:11

➲ *Clinical Examples in Radiology* Winter 12:2, Winter 16:4

(Do not report 37192 in conjunction with 37191)

37193 Retrieval (removal) of intravascular vena cava filter, endovascular approach including vascular access, vessel selection, and radiological supervision and interpretation, intraprocedural roadmapping, and imaging guidance (ultrasound and fluoroscopy), when performed

➲ *CPT Changes: An Insider's View* 2012, 2017

➲ *CPT Assistant* Apr 12:8, Feb 13:3, May 16:11

➲ *Clinical Examples in Radiology* Winter 12:2, Summer 16:12, Winter 16:4

(Do not report 37193 in conjunction with 37197)

37195 Thrombolysis, cerebral, by intravenous infusion

➲ *CPT Assistant* Nov 97:16

37197 Transcatheter retrieval, percutaneous, of intravascular foreign body (eg, fractured venous or arterial catheter), includes radiological supervision and interpretation, and imaging guidance (ultrasound or fluoroscopy), when performed

➲ *CPT Changes: An Insider's View* 2013, 2017

➲ *CPT Assistant* Feb 13:3, May 16:11, Feb 17:14

➲ *Clinical Examples in Radiology* Spring 13:2, 3, Winter 16:4

(For percutaneous retrieval of a vena cava filter, use 37193)

►(For transcatheter removal of permanent leadless pacemaker, use 33275)◄

Vena Cava Filter
37191

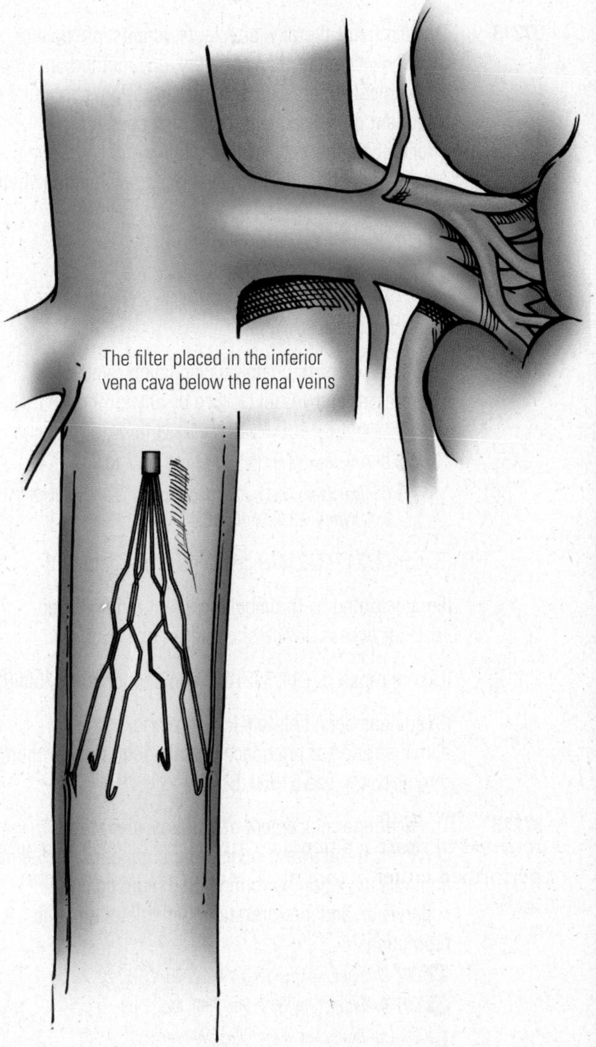

37200 Transcatheter biopsy

(For radiological supervision and interpretation, use 75970)

37211 Transcatheter therapy, arterial infusion for thrombolysis other than coronary or intracranial, any method, including radiological supervision and interpretation, initial treatment day

➲ *CPT Changes: An Insider's View* 2013, 2016, 2017

➲ *CPT Assistant* Feb 13:3, Nov 15:3, Mar 16:3

➲ *Clinical Examples in Radiology* Spring 13:11, Summer 13:3, 4, Winter 13:2, 3, 4, Spring 16:3

(For intracranial arterial mechanical thrombectomy and/or infusion for thrombolysis, use 61645)

37212 Transcatheter therapy, venous infusion for thrombolysis, any method, including radiological supervision and interpretation, initial treatment day

➲ *CPT Changes: An Insider's View* 2013, 2017

➲ *CPT Assistant* Feb 13:3, Nov 15:3, Mar 16:3

➲ *Clinical Examples in Radiology* Spring 13:11, Summer 13:4, Winter 13:4, Spring 16:4

37213 Transcatheter therapy, arterial or venous infusion for thrombolysis other than coronary, any method, including radiological supervision and interpretation, continued treatment on subsequent day during course of thrombolytic therapy, including follow-up catheter contrast injection, position change, or exchange, when performed;

➲ *CPT Changes: An Insider's View* 2013, 2017

➲ *CPT Assistant* Feb 13:3, Nov 15:3, Mar 16:3

➲ *Clinical Examples in Radiology* Spring 13:11, Summer 13:1, 2, 3, 4, Winter 13:4, Spring 16:4

37214 cessation of thrombolysis including removal of catheter and vessel closure by any method

➲ *CPT Changes: An Insider's View* 2013, 2017

➲ *CPT Assistant* Feb 13:3, Nov 15:3, Mar 16:3

➲ *Clinical Examples in Radiology* Spring 13:11, Summer 13:2, 3, 4, Winter 13:4, Spring 16:4

(Report 37211-37214 once per date of treatment)

(For declotting by thrombolytic agent of implanted vascular access device or catheter, use 36593)

(Do not report 37211-37214 in conjunction with 75898)

(37202 has been deleted. For intracranial arterial administration of pharmacological agent[s] other than for thrombolysis, see 61650, 61651)

37215 Transcatheter placement of intravascular stent(s), cervical carotid artery, open or percutaneous, including angioplasty, when performed, and radiological supervision and interpretation; with distal embolic protection

➲ *CPT Changes: An Insider's View* 2005, 2015, 2017

➲ *CPT Assistant* May 05:7, Feb 13:3, Mar 14:8

➲ *Clinical Examples in Radiology* Winter 15:2, 3

37216 without distal embolic protection

➲ *CPT Changes: An Insider's View* 2005, 2015, 2017

➲ *CPT Assistant* May 05:7, Feb 13:3, Mar 14:8

➲ *Clinical Examples in Radiology* Winter 15:3

(37215 and 37216 include all ipsilateral selective carotid catheterization, all diagnostic imaging for ipsilateral, cervical and cerebral carotid arteriography, and all related radiological supervision and interpretation. When ipsilateral carotid arteriogram (including imaging and selective catheterization) confirms the need for carotid stenting, 37215 and 37216 are inclusive of these services. If carotid stenting is not indicated, then the appropriate codes for carotid catheterization and imaging should be reported in lieu of 37215 and 37216)

(Do not report 37215, 37216 in conjunction with 36222-36224 for the treated carotid artery)

(For open or percutaneous transcatheter placement of extracranial vertebral artery stent[s], see Category III codes 0075T, 0076T)

37217 Transcatheter placement of intravascular stent(s), intrathoracic common carotid artery or innominate artery by retrograde treatment, open ipsilateral cervical carotid artery exposure, including angioplasty, when performed, and radiological supervision and interpretation

➲ *CPT Changes: An Insider's View* 2014, 2015

➲ *CPT Assistant* Mar 14:8, May 15:7

(37217 includes open vessel exposure and vascular access closure, all access and selective catheterization of the vessel, traversing the lesion, and any radiological supervision and interpretation directly related to the intervention when performed, standard closure of arteriotomy by suture, and imaging performed to document completion of the intervention in addition to the intervention[s] performed. Carotid artery revascularization services [eg, 33891, 35301, 35509, 35510, 35601, 35606] performed during the same session may be reported separately, when performed)

(Do not report 37217 in conjunction with 35201, 36221-36227, 37246, 37247 for ipsilateral services)

(For open or percutaneous transcatheter placement of intravascular cervical carotid artery stent[s], see 37215, 37216)

(For open or percutaneous antegrade transcatheter placement of innominate and/or intrathoracic carotid artery stent[s], use 37218)

(For open or percutaneous transcatheter placement of extracranial vertebral artery stent[s], see 0075T, 0076T)

(For transcatheter placement of intracranial stent[s], use 61635)

37218 Transcatheter placement of intravascular stent(s), intrathoracic common carotid artery or innominate artery, open or percutaneous antegrade approach, including angioplasty, when performed, and radiological supervision and interpretation

➲ *CPT Changes: An Insider's View* 2015, 2017

➲ *CPT Assistant* May 15:7

(37218 includes all ipsilateral extracranial intrathoracic selective innominate and carotid catheterization, all diagnostic imaging for ipsilateral extracranial intrathoracic innominate and/or carotid artery stenting, and all related radiologic supervision and interpretation. Report 37218 when the ipsilateral extracranial intrathoracic carotid arteriogram (including imaging and selective catheterization) confirms the need for stenting. If stenting is not indicated, report the appropriate codes for selective catheterization and imaging)

(Do not report 37218 in conjunction with 36222, 36223, 36224 for the treated carotid artery)

(For open or percutaneous transcatheter placement of intravascular cervical carotid artery stent[s], see 37215, 37216)

(For open or percutaneous transcatheter placement of extracranial vertebral artery stent[s], see 0075T, 0076T)

(For transcatheter placement of intracranial stent[s], use 61635)

Endovascular Revascularization (Open or Percutaneous, Transcatheter)

Codes 37220-37235 are to be used to describe lower extremity endovascular revascularization services performed for occlusive disease. These lower extremity codes are built on progressive hierarchies with more intensive services inclusive of lesser intensive services. The code inclusive of all of the services provided for that vessel should be reported (ie, use the code inclusive of the most intensive services provided). Only one code from this family (37220-37235) should be reported for each lower extremity vessel treated.

These lower extremity endovascular revascularization codes all include the work of accessing and selectively catheterizing the vessel, traversing the lesion, radiological supervision and interpretation directly related to the intervention(s) performed, embolic protection if used, closure of the arteriotomy by pressure and application of an arterial closure device or standard closure of the puncture by suture, and imaging performed to document completion of the intervention in addition to the intervention(s) performed. Extensive repair or replacement of an artery may be additionally reported (eg, 35226 or 35286). These codes describe endovascular procedures performed percutaneously and/or through an open surgical exposure. These codes include balloon angioplasty (eg, low-profile, cutting balloon, cryoplasty), atherectomy (eg, directional, rotational, laser), and stenting (eg, balloon-expandable, self-expanding, bare metal, covered, drug-eluting). Each code in this family (37220-37235) includes balloon angioplasty, when performed.

These codes describe revascularization therapies (ie, transluminal angioplasty, atherectomy, and stent placement) provided in three arterial vascular territories: iliac, femoral/popliteal, and tibial/peroneal.

When treating multiple vessels within a territory, report each additional vessel using an add-on code, as applicable. Select the base code that represents the most complex service using the following hierarchy of complexity (in descending order of complexity): atherectomy and stent> atherectomy>stent>angioplasty. When treating multiple lesions within the same vessel, report one service that reflects the combined procedures, whether done on one lesion or different lesions, using the same hierarchy.

1. ***Iliac Vascular Territory***—The iliac territory is divided into 3 vessels: common iliac, internal iliac, and external iliac.
2. ***Femoral/Popliteal Vascular Territory***—The entire femoral/popliteal territory in 1 lower extremity is considered a single vessel for CPT reporting specifically for the endovascular lower extremity revascularization codes 37224-37227.
3. ***Tibial/Peroneal Territory***—The tibial/peroneal territory is divided into 3 vessels: anterior tibial, posterior tibial, and peroneal arteries.

There are specific coding guidelines for each of the 3 vascular territories:

1. ***Iliac Vascular Territory***—A single primary code is used for the initial iliac artery treated in each leg (37220 or 37221). If other iliac vessels are also treated in that leg, these interventions are reported with the appropriate add-on code(s) (37222, 37223). Up to 2 add-on codes can be used in a unilateral iliac vascular territory since there are 3 vessels which could be treated. Add-on codes are used for different vessels, not distinct lesions within the same vessel.
2. ***Femoral/Popliteal Territory***—A single interventional code is used no matter what combination of angioplasty/stent/atherectomy is applied to all segments, including the common, deep and superficial femoral arteries as well as the popliteal artery (37224, 37225, 37226, or 37227). There are no add-on codes for additional vessels treated within the femoral/popliteal territory. Because only 1 service is reported when 2 lesions are treated in this territory, report the most complex service (eg, use 37227 if a stent is placed for 1 lesion and an atherectomy is performed on a second lesion).
3. ***Tibial/Peroneal Territory***—A single primary code is used for the initial tibial/peroneal artery treated in each leg (37228, 37229, 37230, or 37231). If other tibial/peroneal vessels are also treated in the same leg, these interventions are reported with the appropriate add-on code(s) (37232-37235). Up to 2 add-on codes could be used to describe services provided in a single leg since there are 3 tibial/peroneal vessels which could be treated. Add-on codes are used for different vessels, not distinct lesions within the same vessel. The common tibio-peroneal trunk is considered part of the tibial/peroneal territory, but is not considered a separate, fourth segment of vessel in the tibio-peroneal family for CPT reporting of endovascular lower extremity interventions. For instance, if lesions in the common tibio-peroneal trunk are treated in conjunction with lesions in the posterior tibial artery, a single code would be reported for treatment of this segment.

When treating multiple territories in the same leg, one primary lower extremity revascularization code is used for each territory treated. When second or third vessel(s) are treated in the iliac and/or tibial/peroneal territories, add-on code(s) are used to report the additional service(s). When more than one stent is placed in the same vessel, the code should be reported only once.

When multiple vessels in multiple territories in a single leg are treated at the same setting, the primary code for the treatment in the initial vessel in each vascular territory is reported. Add-on code(s) are reported when second and third iliac or tibial/peroneal arteries are treated in addition to the initial vessel in that vascular territory.

If a lesion extends across the margins of one vessel vascular territory into another, but can be opened with a single therapy, this intervention should be reported with a single code despite treating more than one vessel and/or vascular territory. For instance, if a stenosis extends from the common iliac artery into the proximal external iliac artery, and a single stent is placed to open the entire lesion, this therapy should be coded as a single stent placement in the iliac artery (37221). In this example, a code for an additional vessel treatment would not be used (do not report both 37221 and 37223).

For bifurcation lesions distal to the common iliac origins which require therapy of 2 distinct branches of the iliac or tibial/peroneal vascular territories, a primary code and an add-on code would be used to describe the intervention. In the femoral/popliteal territory, all branches are included in the primary code, so treatment of a bifurcation lesion would be reported as a single code.

When the same territory(ies) of both legs are treated in the same session, modifiers may be required to describe the interventions. Use modifier 59 to denote that different legs are being treated, even if the mode of therapy is different.

Mechanical thrombectomy and/or thrombolysis in the lower extremity vessels are sometimes necessary to aid in restoring flow to areas of occlusive disease, and are reported separately.

37220 Revascularization, endovascular, open or percutaneous, iliac artery, unilateral, initial vessel; with transluminal angioplasty

➲ *CPT Changes: An Insider's View* 2011, 2017

➲ *CPT Assistant* Jul 11:3, Oct 11:9, Dec 13:8, Jul 16:8

➲ *Clinical Examples in Radiology* Winter 11:3, Spring 14:9

37221 with transluminal stent placement(s), includes angioplasty within the same vessel, when performed

➲ *CPT Changes: An Insider's View* 2011, 2017

➲ *CPT Assistant* Jul 11:3, Oct 11:9, Jan 15:13, Jul 16:8

➲ *Clinical Examples in Radiology* Winter 11:2, Spring 16:13

(Use 37220, 37221 in conjunction with 34701-34711, 34845, 34846, 34847, 34848, 0254T only when 37220 or 37221 are performed outside the treatment zone of the endograft)

Transluminal Balloon Angioplasty

37220 and 37222

A balloon catheter is passed into the iliac artery and inflated to stretch the blood vessel to a larger diameter.

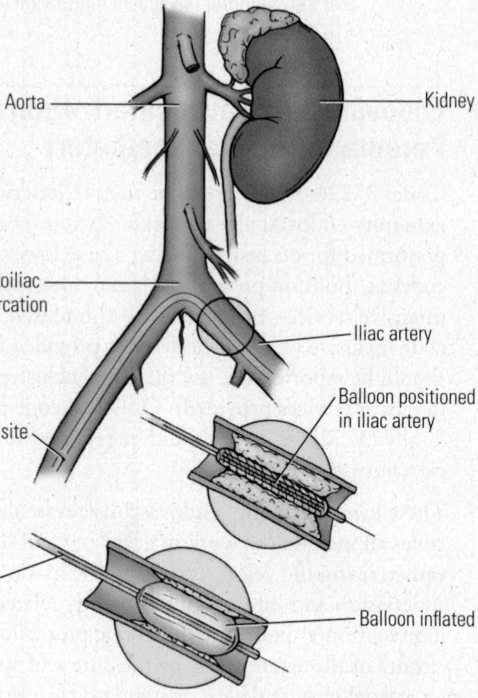

+ 37222 Revascularization, endovascular, open or percutaneous, iliac artery, each additional ipsilateral iliac vessel; with transluminal angioplasty (List separately in addition to code for primary procedure)

➲ *CPT Changes: An Insider's View* 2011, 2017

➲ *CPT Assistant* Jul 11:3, Oct 11:9, Jul 16:8

➲ *Clinical Examples in Radiology* Winter 11:2, Spring 16:13

(Use 37222 in conjunction with 37220, 37221)

+ 37223 with transluminal stent placement(s), includes angioplasty within the same vessel, when performed (List separately in addition to code for primary procedure)

➲ *CPT Changes: An Insider's View* 2011, 2017

➲ *CPT Assistant* Jul 11:3, Oct 11:9, Apr 12:8, Dec 13:8, Jul 16:8

➲ *Clinical Examples in Radiology* Winter 11:3, Spring 16:13

(Use 37223 in conjunction with 37221)

(Use 37222, 37223 in conjunction with 34701-34711, 34845, 34846, 34847, 34848, 0254T only when 37222 or 37223 are performed outside the treatment zone of the endograft)

37224 Revascularization, endovascular, open or percutaneous, femoral, popliteal artery(s), unilateral; with transluminal angioplasty
- *CPT Changes: An Insider's View* 2011, 2017
- *CPT Assistant* Jul 11:3, Oct 11:9, Dec 11:15, Jul 16:8
- *Clinical Examples in Radiology* Summer 11:10, Winter 11:3, Spring 16:13

37225 with atherectomy, includes angioplasty within the same vessel, when performed
- *CPT Changes: An Insider's View* 2011, 2017
- *CPT Assistant* Jul 11:3, Oct 11:9, Nov 11:9, Jul 16:8
- *Clinical Examples in Radiology* Spring 11:3, Winter 11:3, Spring 16:13

37226 with transluminal stent placement(s), includes angioplasty within the same vessel, when performed
- *CPT Changes: An Insider's View* 2011, 2017
- *CPT Assistant* Jul 11:3, Oct 11:9, Dec 11:15, Jul 16:8
- *Clinical Examples in Radiology* Winter 11:2, Spring 16:13

37227 with transluminal stent placement(s) and atherectomy, includes angioplasty within the same vessel, when performed
- *CPT Changes: An Insider's View* 2011, 2017
- *CPT Assistant* Jul 11:3, Oct 11:9, Nov 11:9, Jul 16:8
- *Clinical Examples in Radiology* Spring 11:2, Winter 11:3, Spring 16:13

►(Do not report 37224, 37225, 37226, 37227 in conjunction with 0505T, within the femoral-popliteal segment)◄

37228 Revascularization, endovascular, open or percutaneous, tibial, peroneal artery, unilateral, initial vessel; with transluminal angioplasty
- *CPT Changes: An Insider's View* 2011, 2017
- *CPT Assistant* Jul 11:3, Oct 11:9, Jul 16:8
- *Clinical Examples in Radiology* Spring 11:2, Winter 11:2, Spring 16:13

37229 with atherectomy, includes angioplasty within the same vessel, when performed
- *CPT Changes: An Insider's View* 2011, 2017
- *CPT Assistant* Jul 11:3, Oct 11:9, Nov 11:9, Jul 16:8
- *Clinical Examples in Radiology* Spring 11:3, Winter 11:3, Spring 16:13

37230 with transluminal stent placement(s), includes angioplasty within the same vessel, when performed
- *CPT Changes: An Insider's View* 2011, 2017
- *CPT Assistant* Jul 11:3, Oct 11:9, Jul 16:8
- *Clinical Examples in Radiology* Winter 11:3, Spring 16:13

37231 with transluminal stent placement(s) and atherectomy, includes angioplasty within the same vessel, when performed
- *CPT Changes: An Insider's View* 2011, 2017
- *CPT Assistant* Jul 11:3, Oct 11:9, Nov 11:9, Jul 16:8
- *Clinical Examples in Radiology* Spring 11:3, Winter 11:3, Spring 16:13

Iliac and Lower Extremity Arterial Anatomy Territory
37220-37235

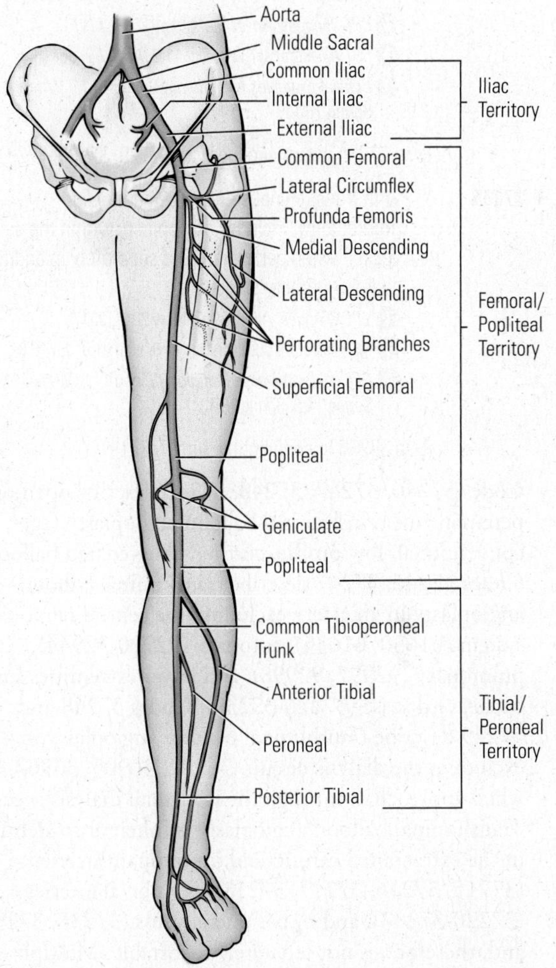

+ 37232 Revascularization, endovascular, open or percutaneous, tibial/peroneal artery, unilateral, each additional vessel; with transluminal angioplasty (List separately in addition to code for primary procedure)
- *CPT Changes: An Insider's View* 2011, 2017
- *CPT Assistant* Jul 11:3, Oct 11:9, Apr 12:8, Jul 16:8
- *Clinical Examples in Radiology* Winter 11:3, Spring 16:13

(Use 37232 in conjunction with 37228-37231)

+ 37233 with atherectomy, includes angioplasty within the same vessel, when performed (List separately in addition to code for primary procedure)
- *CPT Changes: An Insider's View* 2011, 2017
- *CPT Assistant* Jul 11:3, Oct 11:9, Nov 11:9, Apr 12:8, Jul 16:8
- *Clinical Examples in Radiology* Spring 11:3, Winter 11:3, Spring 16:13

(Use 37233 in conjunction with 37229, 37231)

Cardiovascular 33010-39599

+ 37234 with transluminal stent placement(s), includes angioplasty within the same vessel, when performed (List separately in addition to code for primary procedure)

CPT Changes: An Insider's View 2011, 2017

CPT Assistant Jul 11:3, Oct 11:9, Apr 12:9, Jul 16:8

Clinical Examples in Radiology Spring 11:11, Winter 11:3, Spring 16:13

(Use 37234 in conjunction with 37229, 37230, 37231)

+ 37235 with transluminal stent placement(s) and atherectomy, includes angioplasty within the same vessel, when performed (List separately in addition to code for primary procedure)

CPT Changes: An Insider's View 2011, 2017

CPT Assistant Jul 11:3, Oct 11:9, Nov 11:9, Jul 16:8

Clinical Examples in Radiology Spring 11:3, Winter 11:3, Spring 14:9, Spring 16:13

(Use 37235 in conjunction with 37231)

Codes 37246, 37247, 37248, 37249 describe open or percutaneous transluminal balloon angioplasty (eg, conventional, low profile, cutting, drug-coated balloon). Codes 37246, 37247 describe transluminal balloon angioplasty in an artery excluding the central nervous system (61630, 61635), coronary (92920-92944), pulmonary (92997, 92998), and lower extremities for occlusive disease (37220-37235). Codes 37248 and 37249 describe transluminal balloon angioplasty in a vein excluding the dialysis circuit (36902, 36905, 36907) when approached through the ipsilateral dialysis access. Transluminal balloon angioplasty is inherent to stenting in the extracranial carotid and innominate arteries (37215, 37216, 37217, 37218), peripheral arteries (37220-37237), and in peripheral veins (37238, 37239) and, therefore, is not separately reportable. Multiple angioplasties performed in a single vessel, including treatment of separate and distinct lesions within a single vessel, are reported with a single code. If a lesion extends across the margins of one vessel into another, but can be treated with a single therapy, the intervention should be reported only once. When additional, separate and distinct ipsilateral or contralateral vessels are treated in the same session, 37247 and/or 37249 may be reported as appropriate.

Non-selective and/or selective catheterization (eg, 36005, 36010, 36011, 36012, 36200, 36215, 36216, 36217, 36218, 36245, 36246, 36247, 36248) is reported separately. Codes 37246, 37247, 37248, 37249 include radiological supervision and interpretation directly related to the intervention performed and imaging performed to document completion of the intervention. Extensive repair or replacement of an artery may be reported separately (eg, 35226, 35286). Intravascular ultrasound may be reported separately (ie, 37252, 37253). Mechanical thrombectomy and/or thrombolytic therapy, when performed, may be reported separately (eg, 37184, 37185, 37186, 37187, 37188, 37211, 37212, 37213, 37214).

 # 37246 Transluminal balloon angioplasty (except lower extremity artery(ies) for occlusive disease, intracranial, coronary, pulmonary, or dialysis circuit), open or percutaneous, including all imaging and radiological supervision and interpretation necessary to perform the angioplasty within the same artery; initial artery

CPT Changes: An Insider's View 2017

CPT Assistant May 17:3, Jul 17:3

Transluminal Balloon Angioplasty
37246

A balloon catheter is inserted and advanced across the lesion into the narrowed portion of the vessel. The balloon is inflated to enlarge the diameter and restore normal blood flow.

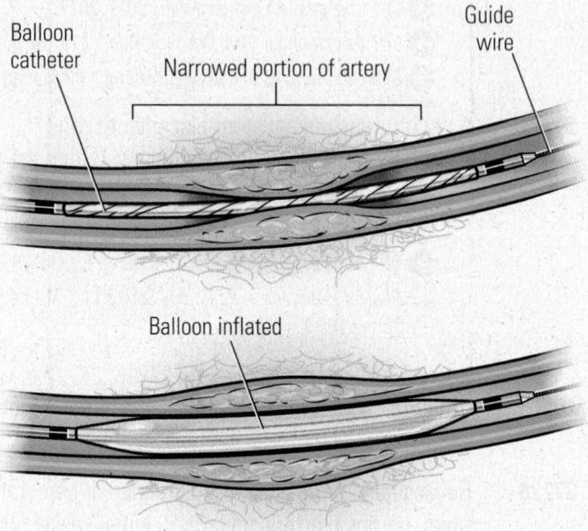

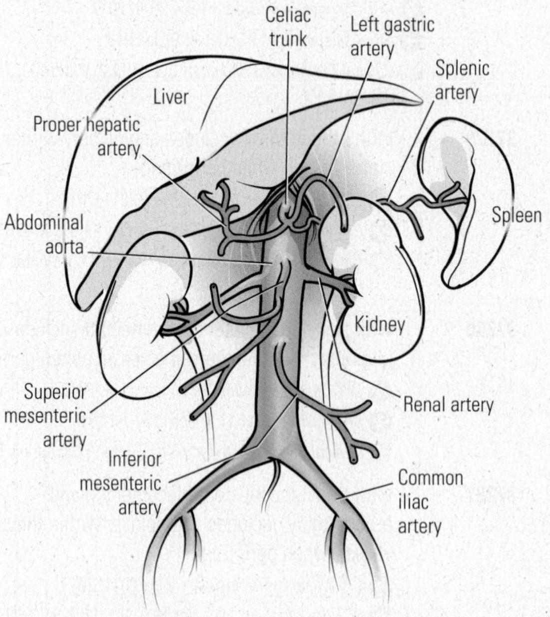

#+ 37247 each additional artery (List separately in addition to code for primary procedure)

CPT Changes: An Insider's View 2017

CPT Assistant May 17:3, Jul 17:3

(Use 37247 in conjunction with 37246)

(Do not report 37246, 37247 in conjunction with 37215, 37216, 37217, 37218, 37220-37237 when performed in the same artery during the same operative session)

(Do not report 37246, 37247 in conjunction with 34841, 34842, 34843, 34844, 34845, 34846, 34847, 34848 for angioplasty[ies] performed, when placing bare metal or covered stents into the visceral branches within the endoprosthesis target zone)

 # 37248 Transluminal balloon angioplasty (except dialysis circuit), open or percutaneous, including all imaging and radiological supervision and interpretation necessary to perform the angioplasty within the same vein; initial vein

➔ *CPT Changes: An Insider's View* 2017

➔ *CPT Assistant* Mar 17:4, May 17:3, Jul 17:3

#+ 37249 each additional vein (List separately in addition to code for primary procedure)

➔ *CPT Changes: An Insider's View* 2017

➔ *CPT Assistant* Mar 17:4, May 17:3, Jul 17:3

(Use 37249 in conjunction with 37248)

(Do not report 37248, 37249 in conjunction with 37238, 37239 when performed in the same vein during the same operative session)

►(Do not report 37248, 37249 in conjunction with 0505T, within the femoral-popliteal segment)◄

(For transluminal balloon angioplasty in aorta/visceral artery[ies] in conjunction with fenestrated endovascular repair, see 34841, 34842, 34843, 34844, 34845, 34846, 34847, 34848)

(For transluminal balloon angioplasty in iliac, femoral, popliteal, or tibial/peroneal artery[ies] for occlusive disease, see 37220-37235)

(For transluminal balloon angioplasty in a dialysis circuit performed through the circuit, see 36902, 36903, 36904, 36905, 36906, 36907, 36908)

(For transluminal balloon angioplasty in an intracranial artery, see 61630, 61635)

(For transluminal balloon angioplasty in a coronary artery, see 92920-92944)

(For transluminal balloon angioplasty in a pulmonary artery, see 92997, 92998)

Codes 37236-37239 are used to report endovascular revascularization for vessels other than lower extremity artery(ies) for occlusive disease (ie, 37221, 37223, 37226, 37227, 37230, 37231, 37234, 37235), cervical carotid (ie, 37215, 37216), intracranial (ie, 61635), intracoronary (ie, 92928, 92929, 92933, 92934, 92937, 92938, 92941, 92943, 92944), innominate and/or intrathoracic carotid artery through an antegrade approach (37218), extracranial vertebral (ie, 0075T, 0076T) performed percutaneously and/or through an open surgical exposure, open retrograde intrathoracic common carotid or innominate (37217), or dialysis circuit when performed through the dialysis circuit (36903, 36905, 36908).

Codes 37236, 37237 describe transluminal intravascular stent insertion in an artery while 37238, 37239 describe transluminal intravascular stent insertion in a vein. Multiple stents placed in a single vessel may only be reported with a single code. If a lesion extends across the margins of one vessel into another, but can be treated with a single therapy, the intervention should be reported only once. When additional, different vessels are treated in the same session, report 37237 and/or 37239 as appropriate. Each code in this family (37236-37239) includes any and all balloon angioplasty(s) performed in the treated vessel, including any pre-dilation (whether performed as a primary or secondary angioplasty), post-dilation following stent placement, treatment of a lesion outside the stented segment but in the same vessel, or use of larger/smaller balloon to achieve therapeutic result. Angioplasty in a separate and distinct vessel may be reported separately. Non-selective and/or selective catheterization(s) (eg, 36005, 36010-36015, 36200, 36215-36218, 36245-36248) is reported separately.

Codes 37236-37239 include radiological supervision and interpretation directly related to the intervention(s) performed, closure of the arteriotomy by pressure, application of an arterial closure device or standard closure of the puncture by suture, and imaging performed to document completion of the intervention in addition to the intervention(s) performed. Extensive repair or replacement of an artery may be reported separately (eg, 35226 or 35286). Report 76937 for ultrasound guidance for vascular access, when performed in conjunction with 37236-37239. Intravascular ultrasound may be reported separately (ie, 37252, 37253). For mechanical thrombectomy and/or thrombolytic therapy, when performed, see 37184-37188, 37211-37214.

Intravascular stents, both covered and uncovered, are a class of devices that may be used as part of an embolization procedure. As such, there is the potential for overlap among codes used for placement of vascular stents and those used for embolization. When a stent is placed for the purpose of providing a latticework for deployment of embolization coils, such as for embolization of an aneurysm, the embolization code is reported and not the stent code. If a covered stent is deployed as the sole management of an aneurysm, pseudoaneurysm, or vascular extravasation, then the stent deployment code should be reported and not the embolization code.

37236 Transcatheter placement of an intravascular stent(s) (except lower extremity artery(s) for occlusive disease, cervical carotid, extracranial vertebral or intrathoracic carotid, intracranial, or coronary), open or percutaneous, including radiological supervision and interpretation and including all angioplasty within the same vessel, when performed; initial artery

➔ *CPT Changes: An Insider's View* 2014, 2015, 2017

➔ *CPT Assistant* Dec 13:8, May 15:7, Mar 16:5, Jul 16:3

➔ *Clinical Examples in Radiology* Spring 14:9, Winter 14:5-6, Spring 16:13

+ 37237 each additional artery (List separately in addition to code for primary procedure)

➲ *CPT Changes: An Insider's View* 2014, 2015, 2017

➲ *CPT Assistant* Dec 13:8, Mar 16:5, Jul 16:6

➲ *Clinical Examples in Radiology* Winter 14:6, Spring 16:13

(Use 37237 in conjunction with 37236)

(Do not report 37236, 37237 in conjunction with 34841-34848 for bare metal or covered stents placed into the visceral branches within the endoprosthesis target zone)

(For stent placement(s) in iliac, femoral, popliteal, or tibial/peroneal artery(s) for occlusive disease, see 37221, 37223, 37226, 37227, 37230, 37231, 37234, 37235)

(For transcatheter placement of intravascular cervical carotid artery stent(s), see 37215, 37216)

(For transcatheter placement of intracranial stent(s), use 61635)

(For transcatheter placement of intracoronary stent(s), see 92928, 92929, 92933, 92934, 92937, 92938, 92941, 92943, 92944)

(For stenting of visceral arteries in conjunction with fenestrated endovascular repair, see 34841-34848)

(For open or percutaneous antegrade transcatheter placement of intrathoracic carotid/innominate artery stent(s), use 37218)

(For open or percutaneous transcatheter placement of extracranial vertebral artery stent(s), see Category III codes 0075T, 0076T)

(For open retrograde transcatheter placement of intrathoracic common carotid/innominate artery stent(s), use 37217)

(For placement of a stent at the arterial anastomosis of a dialysis circuit with or without transluminal mechanical thrombectomy and/or infusion for thrombolysis, see 36903, 36906)

37238 Transcatheter placement of an intravascular stent(s), open or percutaneous, including radiological supervision and interpretation and including angioplasty within the same vessel, when performed; initial vein

➲ *CPT Changes: An Insider's View* 2014, 2017

➲ *CPT Assistant* Jun 16:8, Jul 16:6, Mar 17:4

➲ *Clinical Examples in Radiology* Winter 14:6, Spring 16:13

+ 37239 each additional vein (List separately in addition to code for primary procedure)

➲ *CPT Changes: An Insider's View* 2014, 2017

➲ *CPT Assistant* Jul 16:6, Mar 17:4

➲ *Clinical Examples in Radiology* Spring 14:9, Winter 14:6, Spring 16:13

(Use 37239 in conjunction with 37238)

►(Do not report 37238, 37239 in conjunction with 0505T, within the femoral-popliteal segment)◄

(For placement of a stent[s] within the peripheral segment of the dialysis circuit, see 36903, 36906)

(For transcatheter placement of an intravascular stent[s] within central dialysis segment when performed through the dialysis circuit, use 36908)

Vascular Embolization and Occlusion

Codes 37241-37244 are used to describe vascular embolization and occlusion procedures, excluding the central nervous system and the head and neck, which are reported using 61624, 61626, 61710, and 75894, and excluding the ablation/sclerotherapy procedures for venous insufficiency/telangiectasia of the extremities/skin, which are reported using 36468, 36470, and 36471. Embolization and occlusion procedures are performed for a wide variety of clinical indications and in a range of vascular territories. Arteries, veins, and lymphatics may all be the target of embolization.

The embolization codes include all associated radiological supervision and interpretation, intra-procedural guidance and road-mapping, and imaging necessary to document completion of the procedure. They do not include diagnostic angiography and all necessary catheter placement(s). Code(s) for catheter placement(s) may be separately reported using selective catheter placement code(s), if used consistent with guidelines. Code(s) for diagnostic angiography may also be separately reported, when performed according to guidelines for diagnostic angiography during endovascular procedures, using the appropriate diagnostic angiography codes. Report these services with an appropriate modifier (eg, modifier 59). Please see the guidelines on the reporting of diagnostic angiography preceding 75600 in the **Vascular Procedures, Aorta and Arteries** section.

Code 37241 is used to report endovascular embolization or occlusion procedures performed for venous conditions other than hemorrhage or hemodialysis access. Examples include embolization of venous malformations, capillary hemangiomas, varicoceles, and visceral varices. (For endovascular embolization or occlusion of side branch[es] of an outflow vein[s] from a hemodialysis access, use 36909.)

Code 37242 is used to report vascular embolization or occlusion performed for arterial conditions other than hemorrhage or tumor such as arteriovenous malformations and arteriovenous fistulas whether congenital or acquired. Embolizations of aneurysms and pseudoaneurysms are also reported with 37242. Tumor embolization is reported with 37243. Note that injection to treat an extremity pseudoaneurysm is correctly reported with 36002. Sometimes, embolization and occlusion of an artery are performed prior to another planned interventional procedure; an example is embolization of the left gastric artery prior to planned implantation of a hepatic artery chemotherapy port. The artery embolization is reported with 37242.

Code 37243 is used to report embolization for the purpose of tissue ablation and organ infarction or ischemia. This can be performed in many clinical circumstances, including embolization of benign or malignant tumors of the liver, kidney, uterus, or other organs. When chemotherapy is given as part of an embolization procedure, additional codes (eg, 96420) may be separately reported. When a radioisotope (eg, Yttrium-90) is injected as part of an embolization, then additional codes (eg, 79445) may be separately reported. Uterine fibroid embolization is reported with 37243.

Code 37244 is used to report embolization for treatment of hemorrhage or vascular or lymphatic extravasation. Examples include embolization for management of gastrointestinal bleed, trauma-induced hemorrhage of the viscera or pelvis, embolization of the thoracic duct for chylous effusion and bronchial artery embolization for hemoptysis. Embolization of the uterine arteries for management of hemorrhage (eg, postpartum hemorrhage) is also reported with 37244.

Intravascular stents, both covered and uncovered, are a class of devices that may be used as part of an embolization procedure. As such, there is the potential for overlap among codes used for placement of vascular stents and those used for embolization. When a stent is placed for the purpose of providing a latticework for deployment of embolization coils, such as for embolization of an aneurysm, the embolization code is reported and not the stent code. If a stent is deployed as the sole management of an aneurysm, pseudoaneurysm, or vascular extravasation, then the stent deployment code should be reported and not the embolization code.

Only one embolization code should be reported for each surgical field (ie, the area immediately surrounding and directly involved in a treatment/procedure). Embolization procedures performed at a single setting and including multiple surgical fields (eg, a patient with multiple trauma and bleeding from the pelvis and the spleen) may be reported with multiple embolization codes with the appropriate modifier (eg, modifier 59).

There may be overlapping indications for an embolization procedure. The code for the immediate indication for the embolization should be used. For instance, if the immediate cause for embolization is bleeding in a patient with an aneurysm, report 37244.

37241 Vascular embolization or occlusion, inclusive of all radiological supervision and interpretation, intraprocedural roadmapping, and imaging guidance necessary to complete the intervention; venous, other than hemorrhage (eg, congenital or acquired venous malformations, venous and capillary hemangiomas, varices, varicoceles)

➔ *CPT Changes: An Insider's View* 2014, 2017

➔ *CPT Assistant* Nov 13:6, Aug 14:14, Oct 14:6, Apr 15:10, Aug 15:8, Nov 15:3, Mar 18:3

➔ *Clinical Examples in Radiology* Spring 14:7, Spring 16:4, Winter 18:10

(Do not report 37241 in conjunction with 36468, 36470, 36471, 36473, 36474, 36475-36479, 75894, 75898 in the same surgical field)

(For sclerosis of veins or endovenous ablation of incompetent extremity veins, see 36468-36479)

(For dialysis circuit permanent endovascular embolization or occlusion, use 36909)

37242 arterial, other than hemorrhage or tumor (eg, congenital or acquired arterial malformations, arteriovenous malformations, arteriovenous fistulas, aneurysms, pseudoaneurysms)

➔ *CPT Changes: An Insider's View* 2014, 2017

➔ *CPT Assistant* Nov 13:6, Oct 14:6, Nov 15:3

➔ *Clinical Examples in Radiology* Spring 14:8, Summer 15:8, Spring 16:4, Winter 18:10

(For percutaneous treatment of extremity pseudoaneurysm, use 36002)

37243 for tumors, organ ischemia, or infarction

➔ *CPT Changes: An Insider's View* 2014, 2017

➔ *CPT Assistant* Nov 13:7, Oct 14:6, Nov 15:3

➔ *Clinical Examples in Radiology* Winter 14:4, Summer 15:2, Spring 16:4, Winter 18:10

37244 for arterial or venous hemorrhage or lymphatic extravasation

➔ *CPT Changes: An Insider's View* 2014, 2017

➔ *CPT Assistant* Nov 13:7, Aug 14:14, Oct 14:6, Nov 15:3, Oct 17:9

➔ *Clinical Examples in Radiology* Spring 14:7, Winter 14:2-4, Summer 15:8, Spring 16:4, Winter 18:11

(Do not report 37242-37244 in conjunction with 75894, 75898 in the same surgical field)

(For embolization procedures of the central nervous system or head and neck, see 61624, 61626, 61710)

37246 Code is out of numerical sequence. See 37234-37237

37247 Code is out of numerical sequence. See 37234-37237

37248 Code is out of numerical sequence. See 37234-37237

37249 Code is out of numerical sequence. See 37234-37237

Intravascular Ultrasound Services

Intravascular ultrasound (IVUS) services include all transducer manipulations and repositioning within the specific vessel being examined during a diagnostic procedure or before, during, and/or after therapeutic intervention (eg, stent or stent graft placement, angioplasty, atherectomy, embolization, thrombolysis, transcatheter biopsy).

IVUS is included in the work described by codes 37191, 37192, 37193, 37197 (intravascular vena cava [IVC] filter placement, repositioning and removal, and intravascular foreign body retrieval) and should not be separately reported with those procedures. If a lesion extends across the margins of one vessel into another, this should be reported with a single code despite imaging more than one vessel.

Non-selective and/or selective vascular catheterization may be separately reportable (eg, 36005-36248).

+ 37252 Intravascular ultrasound (noncoronary vessel) during diagnostic evaluation and/or therapeutic intervention, including radiological supervision and interpretation; initial noncoronary vessel (List separately in addition to code for primary procedure)

➲ *CPT Changes: An Insider's View* 2016, 2017

➲ *CPT Assistant* May 16:11, Mar 17:4

➲ *Clinical Examples in Radiology* Winter 16:2

+ 37253 each additional noncoronary vessel (List separately in addition to code for primary procedure)

➲ *CPT Changes: An Insider's View* 2016, 2017

➲ *CPT Assistant* May 16:11, Mar 17:4

➲ *Clinical Examples in Radiology* Winter 16:2

(Use 37253 in conjunction with 37252)

(Report 37252, 37253 in conjunction with 33361, 33362, 33363, 33364, 33365, 33366, 33367, 33368, 33369, 33477, 33880, 33881, 33883, 33884, 33886, 34701, 34702, 34703, 34704, 34705, 34706, 34707, 34708, 34709, 34710, 34711, 34841, 34842, 34843, 34844, 34845, 34846, 34847, 34848, 36010, 36011, 36012, 36013, 36014, 36015, 36100, 36140, 36160, 36200, 36215, 36216, 36217, 36218, 36221, 36222, 36223, 36224, 36225, 36226, 36227, 36228, 36245, 36246, 36247, 36248, 36251, 36252, 36253, 36254, 36481, 36555-36571, 36578, 36580, 36581, 36582, 36583, 36584, 36585, 36595, 36901, 36902, 36903, 36904, 36905, 36906, 36907, 36908, 36909, 37184, 37185, 37186, 37187, 37188, 37200, 37211, 37212, 37213, 37214, 37215, 37216, 37218, 37220, 37221, 37222, 37223, 37224, 37225, 37226, 37227, 37228, 37229, 37230, 37231, 37232, 37233, 37234, 37235, 37236, 37237, 37238, 37239, 37241, 37242, 37243, 37244, 37246, 37247, 37248, 37249, 61623, 75600, 75605, 75625, 75630, 75635, 75705, 75710, 75716, 75726, 75731, 75733, 75736, 75741, 75743, 75746, 75756, 75774, 75805, 75807, 75810, 75820, 75822, 75825, 75827, 75831, 75833, 75860, 75870, 75872, 75885, 75887, 75889, 75891, 75893, 75894, 75898, 75901, 75902, 75956, 75957, 75958, 75959, 75970, 76000, 77001, 0075T, 0076T, 0234T, 0235T, 0236T, 0237T, 0238T, 0254T, 0338T)

(Do not report 37252, 37253 in conjunction with 37191, 37192, 37193, 37197)

Endoscopy

Surgical vascular endoscopy always includes diagnostic endoscopy.

37500 Vascular endoscopy, surgical, with ligation of perforator veins, subfascial (SEPS)

➲ *CPT Changes: An Insider's View* 2003

➲ *CPT Assistant* Jul 10:6

(For open procedure, use 37760)

37501 Unlisted vascular endoscopy procedure

➲ *CPT Changes: An Insider's View* 2003

Ligation

(For phleborrhaphy and arteriorrhaphy, see 35201-35286)

37565 Ligation, internal jugular vein

37600 Ligation; external carotid artery

37605 internal or common carotid artery

37606 internal or common carotid artery, with gradual occlusion, as with Selverstone or Crutchfield clamp

(For transcatheter permanent arterial occlusion or embolization, see 61624-61626)

(For endovascular temporary arterial balloon occlusion, use 61623)

(For ligation treatment of intracranial aneurysm, use 61703)

37607 Ligation or banding of angioaccess arteriovenous fistula

37609 Ligation or biopsy, temporal artery

37615 Ligation, major artery (eg, post-traumatic, rupture); neck

37616 chest

37617 abdomen

➲ *CPT Assistant* Aug 13:14

37618 extremity

37619 Ligation of inferior vena cava

➲ *CPT Changes: An Insider's View* 2012

➲ *CPT Assistant* Apr 12:8

(For endovascular delivery of an inferior vena cava filter, use 37191)

37650 Ligation of femoral vein

(For bilateral procedure, report 37650 with modifier 50)

37660 Ligation of common iliac vein

37700 Ligation and division of long saphenous vein at saphenofemoral junction, or distal interruptions

➔ *CPT Assistant* Aug 96:10, Nov 16:3, Mar 18:3

➔ *Clinical Examples in Radiology* Spring 17:3

(Do not report 37700 in conjunction with 37718, 37722)

(For bilateral procedure, report 37700 with modifier 50)

Ligation and Division of Long Saphenous Vein
37700

The physician ligates sections of the saphenous vein along the leg.

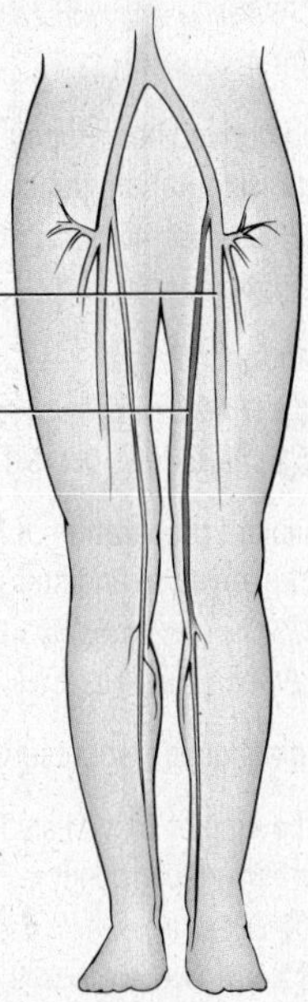

37718 Ligation, division, and stripping, short saphenous vein

➔ *CPT Changes: An Insider's View* 2006

➔ *CPT Assistant* Nov 16:3, Mar 18:3

➔ *Clinical Examples in Radiology* Spring 17:3

(For bilateral procedure, use modifier 50)

(Do not report 37718 in conjunction with 37735, 37780)

37722 Ligation, division, and stripping, long (greater) saphenous veins from saphenofemoral junction to knee or below

➔ *CPT Changes: An Insider's View* 2006

➔ *CPT Assistant* Nov 16:3, Mar 18:3

➔ *Clinical Examples in Radiology* Spring 17:3

(For ligation and stripping of the short saphenous vein, use 37718)

(For bilateral procedure, report 37722 with modifier 50)

(Do not report 37722 in conjunction with 37700, 37735)

(For ligation, division, and stripping of the greater saphenous vein, use 37722. For ligation, division, and stripping of the short saphenous vein, use 37718)

37735 Ligation and division and complete stripping of long or short saphenous veins with radical excision of ulcer and skin graft and/or interruption of communicating veins of lower leg, with excision of deep fascia

➔ *CPT Assistant* Nov 16:3, Mar 18:3

➔ *Clinical Examples in Radiology* Spring 17:3

(Do not report 37735 in conjunction with 37700, 37718, 37722, 37780)

(For bilateral procedure, report 37735 with modifier 50)

37760 Ligation of perforator veins, subfascial, radical (Linton type), including skin graft, when performed, open,1 leg

➔ *CPT Changes: An Insider's View* 2003, 2010

➔ *CPT Assistant* Jul 10:6, Nov 16:3, Mar 18:3

➔ *Clinical Examples in Radiology* Spring 17:3

(For endoscopic procedure, use 37500)

37761 Ligation of perforator vein(s), subfascial, open, including ultrasound guidance, when performed, 1 leg

➔ *CPT Changes: An Insider's View* 2010

➔ *CPT Assistant* Jul 10:6, Nov 16:3, Mar 18:3

➔ *Clinical Examples in Radiology* Spring 17:3

(For bilateral procedure, report 37761 with modifier 50)

(Do not report 37760, 37761 in conjunction with 76937, 76942, 76998, 93971)

(For endoscopic ligation of subfascial perforator veins, use 37500)

37765 Stab phlebectomy of varicose veins, 1 extremity; 10-20 stab incisions

➔ *CPT Changes: An Insider's View* 2004

➔ *CPT Assistant* Aug 04:6, Nov 10:9, Oct 14:6, Nov 16:3, Mar 18:3

➔ *Clinical Examples in Radiology* Spring 17:3

(For less than 10 incisions, use 37799)

(For more than 20 incisions, use 37766)

37766 more than 20 incisions

➔ *CPT Changes: An Insider's View* 2004

➔ *CPT Assistant* Aug 04:6, Sep 13:17, Oct 14:6, Nov 16:3, Mar 18:3

➔ *Clinical Examples in Radiology* Spring 17:3

37780 Ligation and division of short saphenous vein at saphenopopliteal junction (separate procedure)

➔ *CPT Assistant* Aug 96:10, Nov 16:3

➔ *Clinical Examples in Radiology* Spring 17:3

(For bilateral procedure, report 37780 with modifier 50)

37785 Ligation, division, and/or excision of varicose vein cluster(s), 1 leg

➔ *CPT Changes: An Insider's View* 2004

➔ *CPT Assistant* Aug 04:5, Nov 10:9, Nov 16:3

➔ *Clinical Examples in Radiology* Spring 17:3

(For bilateral procedure, report 37785 with modifier 50)

Other Procedures

37788 Penile revascularization, artery, with or without vein graft

37790 Penile venous occlusive procedure

37799 Unlisted procedure, vascular surgery

CPT Assistant Spring 93:12, Fall 93:3, Feb 97:10, Sep 97:10, May 01:11, Oct 04:16, Nov 10:9, Aug 11:9, Nov 13:14, Mar 14:8, Aug 14:14, Oct 14:6, Apr 15:10, Nov 16:3

Clinical Examples in Radiology Summer 15:7, Spring 17:3

Hemic and Lymphatic Systems

Spleen

Excision

38100 Splenectomy; total (separate procedure)

CPT Assistant Summer 93:10, July 93:9, Sep 12:11

38101 partial (separate procedure)

CPT Assistant Summer 93:10, Sep 12:11

+ 38102 total, en bloc for extensive disease, in conjunction with other procedure (List in addition to code for primary procedure)

CPT Assistant Summer 93:10, Sep 12:11

Repair

38115 Repair of ruptured spleen (splenorrhaphy) with or without partial splenectomy

CPT Assistant Summer 93:10, Sep 12:11

Laparoscopy

Surgical laparoscopy always includes diagnostic laparoscopy. To report a diagnostic laparoscopy (peritoneoscopy) (separate procedure), use 49320.

38120 Laparoscopy, surgical, splenectomy

CPT Changes: An Insider's View 2000

CPT Assistant Nov 99:20-21, Mar 00:8, Sep 12:11

38129 Unlisted laparoscopy procedure, spleen

CPT Changes: An Insider's View 2000

CPT Assistant Nov 99:20-21, Mar 00:8, Sep 12:11

Introduction

38200 Injection procedure for splenoportography

(For radiological supervision and interpretation, use 75810)

General

Bone Marrow or Stem Cell Services/ Procedures

Codes 38207-38215 describe various steps used to preserve, prepare and purify bone marrow/stem cells prior to transplantation or reinfusion. Each code may be reported only once per day regardless of the quantity of bone marrow/stem cells manipulated.

38204 Management of recipient hematopoietic progenitor cell donor search and cell acquisition

CPT Changes: An Insider's View 2003

CPT Assistant Oct 13:3

38205 Blood-derived hematopoietic progenitor cell harvesting for transplantation, per collection; allogeneic

CPT Changes: An Insider's View 2003, 2012

CPT Assistant Oct 13:3

38206 autologous

CPT Changes: An Insider's View 2003

CPT Assistant Oct 13:3

38207 Transplant preparation of hematopoietic progenitor cells; cryopreservation and storage

CPT Changes: An Insider's View 2003

CPT Assistant Jul 03:9, Jun 09:3, Oct 13:3

(For diagnostic cryopreservation and storage, use 88240)

38208 thawing of previously frozen harvest, without washing, per donor

CPT Changes: An Insider's View 2003, 2004, 2012

CPT Assistant Jul 03:9, Jun 09:3, Oct 13:3

(For diagnostic thawing and expansion of frozen cells, use 88241)

38209 thawing of previously frozen harvest, with washing, per donor

CPT Changes: An Insider's View 2003, 2004, 2012

CPT Assistant Oct 13:3

38210 specific cell depletion within harvest, T-cell depletion

CPT Changes: An Insider's View 2003

CPT Assistant Oct 13:3

38211 tumor cell depletion

CPT Changes: An Insider's View 2003

CPT Assistant Oct 13:3

38212 red blood cell removal

CPT Changes: An Insider's View 2003

CPT Assistant Oct 13:3

38213 platelet depletion

CPT Changes: An Insider's View 2003

CPT Assistant Oct 13:3

38214 plasma (volume) depletion

CPT Changes: An Insider's View 2003

CPT Assistant Oct 13:3

38215 cell concentration in plasma, mononuclear, or buffy coat layer

➲ *CPT Changes: An Insider's View* 2003

➲ *CPT Assistant* Oct 13:3

(Do not report 38207-38215 in conjunction with 88182, 88184-88189)

38220 Diagnostic bone marrow; aspiration(s)

➲ *CPT Changes: An Insider's View* 2002, 2003, 2018

➲ *CPT Assistant* Jan 04:26, Jun 07:10, Apr 12:15, May 12:11, Oct 13:3, Mar 15:9

➲ *Clinical Examples in Radiology* Spring 18:5

(Do not report 38220 in conjunction with 38221)

(For diagnostic bone marrow biopsy[ies] and aspiration[s] performed at the same session, use 38222)

(For aspiration of bone marrow for bone graft, spine surgery only, use 20939)

(For bone marrow aspiration[s] for platelet-rich stem cell injection, use 0232T)

38221 biopsy(ies)

➲ *CPT Changes: An Insider's View* 2002, 2003, 2018

➲ *CPT Assistant* Mar 15:9

➲ *Clinical Examples in Radiology* Winter 17:5, Spring 18:5

(Do not report 38221 in conjunction with 38220)

(For diagnostic bone marrow biopsy[ies] and aspiration[s] performed at the same session, use 38222)

38222 biopsy(ies) and aspiration(s)

➲ *CPT Changes: An Insider's View* 2018

➲ *Clinical Examples in Radiology* Spring 18:4

(Do not report 38222 in conjunction with 38220 and 38221)

(For bilateral procedure, report 38220, 38221, 38222 with modifier 50)

(For bone marrow biopsy interpretation, use 88305)

38230 Bone marrow harvesting for transplantation; allogeneic

➲ *CPT Changes: An Insider's View* 2012

➲ *CPT Assistant* Apr 96:1, Jun 09:3, May 12:11, Oct 13:3

38232 autologous

➲ *CPT Changes: An Insider's View* 2012

➲ *CPT Assistant* Oct 13:3

(For autologous and allogeneic blood-derived peripheral stem cell harvesting for transplantation, see 38205, 38206)

(For diagnostic bone marrow aspiration[s], see 38220, 38222)

(For aspiration of bone marrow for bone graft, spine surgery only, use 20939)

(For bone marrow aspiration[s] for platelet-rich stem cell injection, use 0232T)

Bone Marrow Harvesting for Transplantation
38230

A biopsy needle is inserted into the marrow cavity of the iliac crest and bone marrow is removed from the donor.

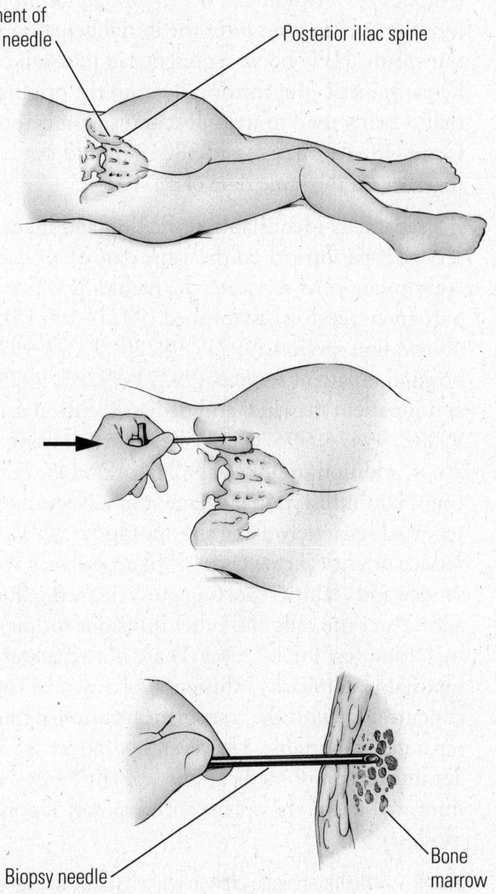

Transplantation and Post-Transplantation Cellular Infusions

Hematopoietic cell transplantation (HCT) refers to the infusion of hematopoietic progenitor cells (HPC) obtained from bone marrow, peripheral blood apheresis, and/or umbilical cord blood. These procedure codes (38240-38243) include physician monitoring of multiple physiologic parameters, physician verification of cell processing, evaluation of the patient during as well as immediately before and after the HPC/lymphocyte infusion, physician presence during the HPC/lymphocyte infusion with associated direct physician supervision of clinical staff, and management of uncomplicated adverse events (eg, nausea, urticaria) during the infusion, which is not separately reportable.

HCT may be autologous (when the HPC donor and recipient are the same person) or allogeneic (when the HPC donor and recipient are not the same person). Code 38241 is used to report any autologous transplant while 38240 is used to report an allogeneic transplant. In some cases allogeneic transplants involve more than one donor and cells from each donor are infused sequentially whereby one unit of 38240 is reported for each donor infused. Code 38242 is used to report a donor lymphocyte infusion. Code 38243 is used to report a HPC boost from the original allogeneic HPC donor. A lymphocyte infusion or HPC boost can occur days, months or even years after the initial hematopoietic cell transplant. HPC boost represents an infusion of hematopoietic progenitor cells from the original donor that is being used to treat post-transplant cytopenia(s). Codes 38240, 38242, and 38243 should not be reported together on the same date of service.

If a separately identifiable evaluation and management service is performed on the same date of service, the appropriate E/M service code, including office or other outpatient services, established (99211-99215), hospital observation services (99217-99220, 99224-99226), hospital inpatient services (99221-99223, 99231-99239), and inpatient neonatal and pediatric critical care (99471, 99472, 99475, 99476) may be reported, using modifier 25, in addition to 38240, 38242 or 38243. Post-transplant infusion management of adverse reactions is reported separately using the appropriate E/M, prolonged service or critical care code(s). In accordance with place of service and facility reporting guidelines, the fluid used to administer the cells and other infusions for incidental hydration (eg, 96360, 96361) are not separately reportable. Similarly, infusion(s) of any medication(s) concurrently with the transplant infusion are not separately reportable. However, hydration or administration of medications (eg, antibiotics, narcotics) unrelated to the transplant are separately reportable using modifier 59.

38240 Hematopoietic progenitor cell (HPC); allogeneic transplantation per donor
- ➲ *CPT Changes: An Insider's View* 2000, 2012, 2013
- ➲ *CPT Assistant* Apr 96:2, Nov 98:15, Nov 99:21, Jun 09:3, Oct 13:3

38241 autologous transplantation
- ➲ *CPT Changes: An Insider's View* 2000, 2013
- ➲ *CPT Assistant* Apr 96:2, Nov 98:15, Nov 99:21, Jun 09:3, Oct 13:3, Feb 15:10

 # 38243 HPC boost
- ➲ *CPT Changes: An Insider's View* 2013
- ➲ *CPT Assistant* Jun 13:13, Oct 13:3, Feb 15:10

38242 Allogeneic lymphocyte infusions
- ➲ *CPT Changes: An Insider's View* 2003, 2013
- ➲ *CPT Assistant* Jun 13:13, Oct 13:3

(For diagnostic bone marrow aspiration[s], see 38220, 38222)

(For aspiration of bone marrow for bone graft, spine surgery only, use 20939)

(For bone marrow aspiration[s] for platelet-rich stem cell injection, use 0232T)

(For modification, treatment, and processing of hematopoietic progenitor cell specimens for transplantation, see 38210-38215)

(For cryopreservation, freezing, and storage of hematopoietic progenitor cells for transplantation, use 38207)

(For thawing and expansion of hematopoietic progenitor cells for transplantation, see 38208, 38209)

(For compatibility studies, see 81379-81383, 86812, 86813, 86816, 86817, 86821)

38243 Code is out of numerical sequence. See 38240-38300

Lymph Nodes and Lymphatic Channels

Incision

38300 Drainage of lymph node abscess or lymphadenitis; simple

38305 extensive

38308 Lymphangiotomy or other operations on lymphatic channels

38380 Suture and/or ligation of thoracic duct; cervical approach

38381 thoracic approach

38382 abdominal approach

Excision

(For injection for sentinel node identification, use 38792)

38500 Biopsy or excision of lymph node(s); open, superficial
- ➲ *CPT Changes: An Insider's View* 2001
- ➲ *CPT Assistant* Jun 97:5, Jul 99:7, Oct 05:23, Dec 07:8, Sep 08:5, Jan 09:7, Jun 12:15

(Do not report 38500 with 38700-38780)

38505 by needle, superficial (eg, cervical, inguinal, axillary)
- ➲ *CPT Assistant* Jul 99:6, Jan 09:7
- ➲ *Clinical Examples in Radiology* Winter 17:5

(If imaging guidance is performed, see 76942, 77002, 77012, 77021)

►(For fine needle aspiration biopsy, see 10004, 10005, 10006, 10007, 10008, 10009, 10010, 10011, 10012, 10021)◄

(For evaluation of fine needle aspirate, see 88172, 88173)

38510 open, deep cervical node(s)
- ➲ *CPT Changes: An Insider's View* 2001
- ➲ *CPT Assistant* May 98:10, Jul 99:6, Jun 12:15

38520 open, deep cervical node(s) with excision scalene fat pad
- ➲ *CPT Changes: An Insider's View* 2001
- ➲ *CPT Assistant* May 98:10, Jul 99:6

38525 open, deep axillary node(s)
➲ *CPT Changes: An Insider's View* 2001
➲ *CPT Assistant* May 98:10, Jul 99:7, Oct 05:23, Dec 07:8, Sep 08:5, Apr 14:11, Mar 15:5

38530 open, internal mammary node(s)
➲ *CPT Changes: An Insider's View* 2001
➲ *CPT Assistant* May 98:10, Jul 99:6, Aug 10:6, Apr 14:11

(Do not report 38530 with 38720-38746)

►(For percutaneous needle biopsy, retroperitoneal lymph node or mass, use 49180)◄

►(For fine needle aspiration biopsy, retroperitoneal lymph node or mass, see 10005, 10006, 10007, 10008, 10009, 10010, 10011, 10012)◄

● **38531** open, inguinofemoral node(s)
➲ *CPT Changes: An Insider's View* 2019

►(For bilateral procedure, report 38531 with modifier 50)◄

38542 Dissection, deep jugular node(s)
➲ *CPT Assistant* Jul 99:7, Aug 10:6

(For radical cervical neck dissection, use 38720)

38550 Excision of cystic hygroma, axillary or cervical; without deep neurovascular dissection

38555 with deep neurovascular dissection

Limited Lymphadenectomy for Staging

38562 Limited lymphadenectomy for staging (separate procedure); pelvic and para-aortic
➲ *CPT Assistant* Mar 01:10

(When combined with prostatectomy, use 55812 or 55842)

(When combined with insertion of radioactive substance into prostate, use 55862)

38564 retroperitoneal (aortic and/or splenic)

Laparoscopy

Surgical laparoscopy always includes diagnostic laparoscopy. To report a diagnostic laparoscopy (peritoneoscopy) (separate procedure), use 49320.

38570 Laparoscopy, surgical; with retroperitoneal lymph node sampling (biopsy), single or multiple
➲ *CPT Changes: An Insider's View* 2000
➲ *CPT Assistant* Nov 99:21, Mar 00:8

38571 with bilateral total pelvic lymphadenectomy
➲ *CPT Changes: An Insider's View* 2000
➲ *CPT Assistant* Nov 99:21, Mar 00:8

38572 with bilateral total pelvic lymphadenectomy and peri-aortic lymph node sampling (biopsy), single or multiple
➲ *CPT Changes: An Insider's View* 2000
➲ *CPT Assistant* Nov 99:21, Jan 15:14

(For drainage of lymphocele to peritoneal cavity, use 49323)

38573 with bilateral total pelvic lymphadenectomy and peri-aortic lymph node sampling, peritoneal washings, peritoneal biopsy(ies), omentectomy, and diaphragmatic washings, including diaphragmatic and other serosal biopsy(ies), when performed
➲ *CPT Changes: An Insider's View* 2018
➲ *CPT Assistant* Apr 18:11

(Do not report 38573 in conjunction with 38562, 38564, 38570, 38571, 38572, 38589, 38770, 38780, 49255, 49320, 49326, 58541, 58542, 58543, 58544, 58548, 58550, 58552, 58553, 58554)

38589 Unlisted laparoscopy procedure, lymphatic system
➲ *CPT Changes: An Insider's View* 2000
➲ *CPT Assistant* Nov 99:21, Mar 00:8, Apr 18:11

Radical Lymphadenectomy (Radical Resection of Lymph Nodes)

(For limited pelvic and retroperitoneal lymphadenectomies, see 38562, 38564)

38700 Suprahyoid lymphadenectomy
➲ *CPT Assistant* Aug 02:8, Aug 10:3

(For bilateral procedure, report 38700 with modifier 50)

38720 Cervical lymphadenectomy (complete)
➲ *CPT Assistant* Oct 01:10, Aug 02:8, Aug 10:4

(For bilateral procedure, report 38720 with modifier 50)

38724 Cervical lymphadenectomy (modified radical neck dissection)
➲ *CPT Assistant* Jan 01:13, Aug 02:8, Aug 10:4, Dec 12:3

38740 Axillary lymphadenectomy; superficial
➲ *CPT Assistant* Apr 14:11

38745 complete

+ **38746** Thoracic lymphadenectomy by thoracotomy, mediastinal and regional lymphadenectomy (List separately in addition to code for primary procedure)
➲ *CPT Changes: An Insider's View* 2012
➲ *CPT Assistant* Sep 12:3, May 14:3

(On the right, mediastinal lymph nodes include the paratracheal, subcarinal, paraesophageal, and inferior pulmonary ligament)

(On the left, mediastinal lymph nodes include the aortopulmonary window, subcarinal, paraesophageal, and inferior pulmonary ligament)

(Report 38746 in conjunction with 19260, 31760, 31766, 31786, 32096-32200, 32220-32320, 32440-32491, 32503-32505, 33025, 33030, 33050-33130, 39200-39220, 39560, 39561, 43101, 43112, 43117, 43118, 43122, 43123, 43351, 60270, 60505)

(To report mediastinal and regional lymphadenectomy via thoracoscopy [VATS], see 32674)

Mediastinal Lymph Nodes: Station Number and Descriptions
38746

Relevant mediastinal lymph nodes typically removed with procedures described by code 38746, and sampled removal described with code 39402.

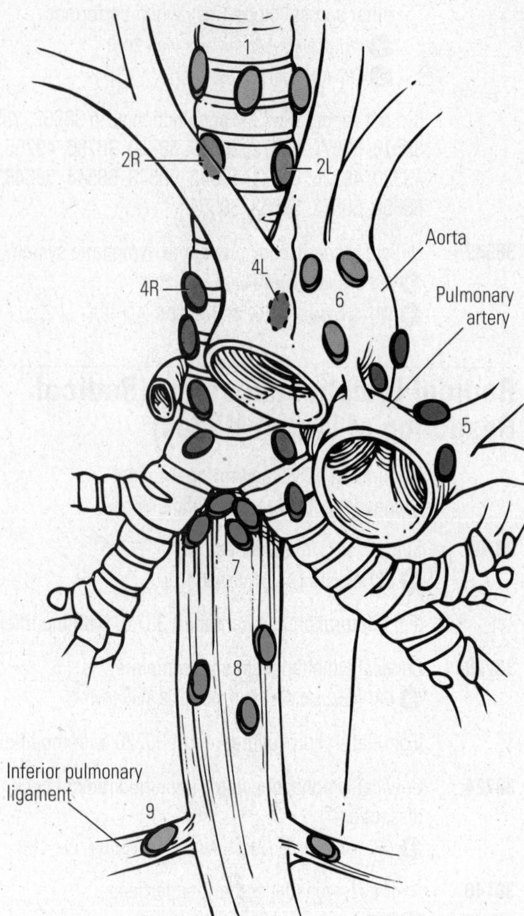

Station #	Lymph Node Descriptions
1	Low cervical, supraclavicular, and sternal notch
2	Upper paratracheal (R & L)
4	Lower paratracheal (R & L)
5	Subaortic or aortopulmonary window
6	Para-aortic
7	Subcarinal
8	Paraesophageal (below the carina)
9	Inferior pulmonary ligament

*Station #3 is not depicted as it is not applicable to the use of codes 32674, 38746, or 39402.

+ 38747 Abdominal lymphadenectomy, regional, including celiac, gastric, portal, peripancreatic, with or without para-aortic and vena caval nodes (List separately in addition to code for primary procedure)

➔ *CPT Assistant* Nov 98:15

38760 Inguinofemoral lymphadenectomy, superficial, including Cloquet's node (separate procedure)

(For bilateral procedure, report 38760 with modifier 50)

38765 Inguinofemoral lymphadenectomy, superficial, in continuity with pelvic lymphadenectomy, including external iliac, hypogastric, and obturator nodes (separate procedure)

(For bilateral procedure, report 38765 with modifier 50)

38770 Pelvic lymphadenectomy, including external iliac, hypogastric, and obturator nodes (separate procedure)

(For bilateral procedure, report 38770 with modifier 50)

38780 Retroperitoneal transabdominal lymphadenectomy, extensive, including pelvic, aortic, and renal nodes (separate procedure)

(For excision and repair of lymphedematous skin and subcutaneous tissue, see 15004-15005, 15570-15650)

Introduction

38790 Injection procedure; lymphangiography

➔ *CPT Assistant* Jul 99:6

➔ *Clinical Examples in Radiology* Summer 15:8

(For bilateral procedure, report 38790 with modifier 50)

(For radiological supervision and interpretation, see 75801-75807)

38792 radioactive tracer for identification of sentinel node

➔ *CPT Changes: An Insider's View* 2008, 2012

➔ *CPT Assistant* Nov 98:15, Jul 99:6, Dec 99:8, Sep 08:5, Mar 15:5

(For excision of sentinel node, see 38500-38542)

(For nuclear medicine lymphatics and lymph gland imaging, use 78195)

(For intraoperative identification (eg, mapping) of sentinel lymph node(s) including injection of non-radioactive dye, see 38900)

38794 Cannulation, thoracic duct

Other Procedures

+ 38900 Intraoperative identification (eg, mapping) of sentinel lymph node(s) includes injection of non-radioactive dye, when performed (List separately in addition to code for primary procedure)

➔ *CPT Changes: An Insider's View* 2011

➔ *CPT Assistant* Mar 15:5

►(Use 38900 in conjunction with 19302, 19307, 38500, 38510, 38520, 38525, 38530, 38531, 38542, 38562, 38564, 38570, 38571, 38572, 38740, 38745, 38760, 38765, 38770, 38780, 56630, 56631, 56632, 56633, 56634, 56637, 56640)◄

(For injection of radioactive tracer for identification of sentinel node, use 38792)

38999 Unlisted procedure, hemic or lymphatic system
➔ *CPT Assistant* May 98:10

Mediastinum and Diaphragm

Mediastinum

Incision

39000 Mediastinotomy with exploration, drainage, removal of foreign body, or biopsy; cervical approach

39010 transthoracic approach, including either transthoracic or median sternotomy
➔ *CPT Assistant* Jan 13:6, Jan 14:5

(Do not report 39010 in conjunction with 33955, 33956, 33963, 33964)

(For VATS pericardial biopsy, use 32604)

Excision/Resection

39200 Resection of mediastinal cyst
➔ *CPT Changes: An Insider's View* 2012

39220 Resection of mediastinal tumor
➔ *CPT Changes: An Insider's View* 2012

(For substernal thyroidectomy, use 60270)

(For thymectomy, use 60520)

(For thoracoscopic [VATS] resection of mediastinal cyst, tumor, or mass, use 32662)

Endoscopy

(39400 has been deleted. To report mediastinoscopy with biopsy, see 39401, 39402)

39401 Mediastinoscopy; includes biopsy(ies) of mediastinal mass (eg, lymphoma), when performed
➔ *CPT Changes: An Insider's View* 2016
➔ *CPT Assistant* Jun 16:4

39402 with lymph node biopsy(ies) (eg, lung cancer staging)
➔ *CPT Changes: An Insider's View* 2016
➔ *CPT Assistant* Jun 16:4

Other Procedures

39499 Unlisted procedure, mediastinum

Diaphragm

Repair

(For transabdominal repair of diaphragmatic [esophageal hiatal] hernia, use 43325)

(For laparoscopic repair of diaphragmatic [esophageal hiatal] hernias and fundoplication, see 43280, 43281, 43282)

39501 Repair, laceration of diaphragm, any approach
➔ *CPT Assistant* Nov 00:3, Dec 14:16

(For laparoscopic paraesophageal hernia repair, see 43281, 43282)

39503 Repair, neonatal diaphragmatic hernia, with or without chest tube insertion and with or without creation of ventral hernia
➔ *CPT Assistant* Feb 12:3

(Do not report modifier 63 in conjunction with 39503)

(For laparoscopic paraesophageal hernia repair, see 43281, 43282)

39540 Repair, diaphragmatic hernia (other than neonatal), traumatic; acute
➔ *CPT Assistant* Nov 00:9, Jun 08:3

39541 chronic

39545 Imbrication of diaphragm for eventration, transthoracic or transabdominal, paralytic or nonparalytic
➔ *CPT Assistant* Nov 00:3

39560 Resection, diaphragm; with simple repair (eg, primary suture)
➔ *CPT Changes: An Insider's View* 2000
➔ *CPT Assistant* Nov 99:21, Nov 00:3

39561 with complex repair (eg, prosthetic material, local muscle flap)
➔ *CPT Changes: An Insider's View* 2000
➔ *CPT Assistant* Nov 99:21, Nov 00:3

Other Procedures

39599 Unlisted procedure, diaphragm

Notes

Surgery

Digestive System (40490-49999) 300

The following is a listing of headings and subheadings that appear within the Digestive System section of the CPT codebook. The subheadings or subsections denoted with asterisks (*) below have special instructions unique to that subsection. Where these are indicated, special notes or guidelines will be presented preceding those procedural terminology listings, referring to that subsection specifically.

Lips (40490-40799) 300
- Excision (40490-40530) 300
- Repair (Cheiloplasty) (40650-40761) 300
- Other Procedures (40799) 300

Vestibule of Mouth* (40800-40899) 300
- Incision (40800-40806) 300
- Excision, Destruction (40808-40820) 300
- Repair (40830-40845) 300
- Other Procedures (40899) 300

Tongue and Floor of Mouth (41000-41599) 301
- Incision (41000-41019) 301
- Excision (41100-41155) 301
- Repair (41250-41252) 301
- Other Procedures (41510-41599) 301

Dentoalveolar Structures (41800-41899) 302
- Incision (41800-41806) 302
- Excision, Destruction (41820-41850) 302
- Other Procedures (41870-41899) 302

Palate and Uvula (42000-42299) 302
- Incision (42000) 302
- Excision, Destruction (42100-42160) 302
- Repair (42180-42281) 302
- Other Procedures (42299) 302

Salivary Gland and Ducts (42300-42699) 303
- Incision (42300-42340) 303
- Excision (42400-42450) 303
- Repair (42500-42510) 303
- Other Procedures (42550-42699) 303

Pharynx, Adenoids, and Tonsils (42700-42999) 303
- Incision (42700-42725) 303
- Excision, Destruction (42800-42894) 303
- Repair (42900-42953) 304
- Other Procedures (42955-42999) 304

Esophagus (43020-43499) 304
- Incision (43020-43045) 304
- Excision (43100-43135) 304
- Endoscopy* (43180-43278) 305
  - Esophagoscopy (43180-43233) 305
  - Esophagogastroduodenoscopy* (43210, 43233, 43235-43259, 43266, 43270) 308
  - Endoscopic Retrograde Cholangiopancreatography (ERCP)* (43260-43265, 43273-43278) 311
- Laparoscopy* (43279-43289) 313
- Repair (43300-43425) 315
- Manipulation (43450-43460) 316
- Other Procedures (43496-43499) 316

Stomach (43500-43999) 317
- Incision (43500-43520) 317
- Excision (43605-43641) 317
- Laparoscopy* (43644-43659) 317
- Introduction (43752-43763) 318
- Bariatric Surgery* (43770-43775) 319

Digestive System

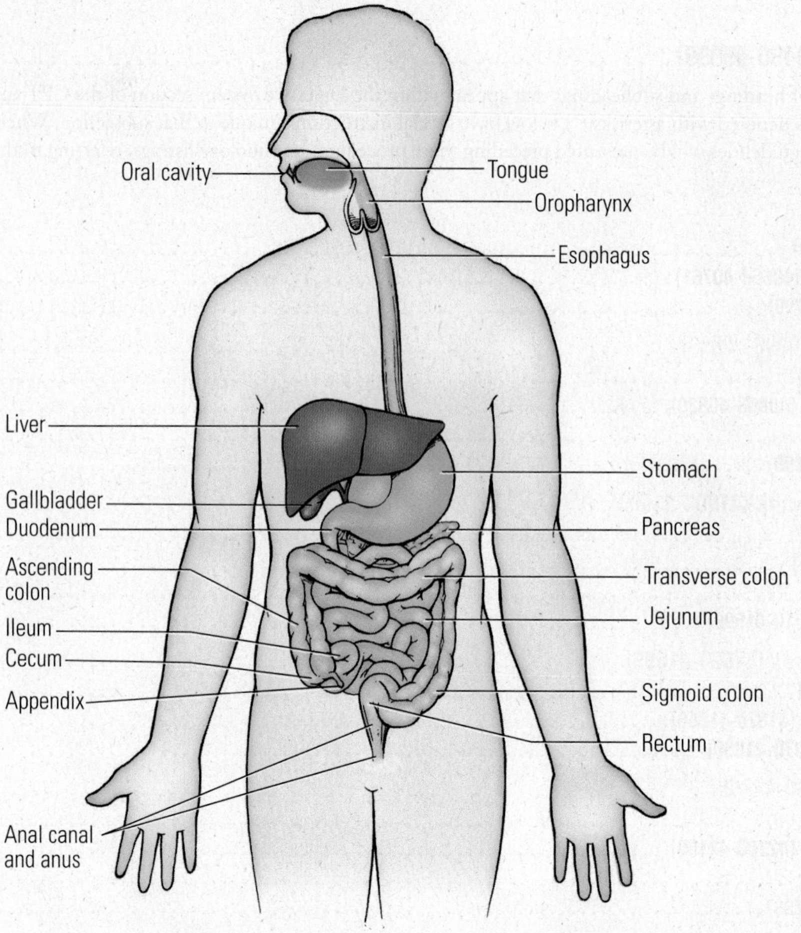

Laparoscopy* (43770-43775) 319
Other Procedures (43800-43999) 319

Intestines (Except Rectum) (44005-44799) 320
Incision (44005-44055) 320
Excision* (44100-44160) 321
Laparoscopy* (44180-44238) 322
Incision (44180) 323
Enterostomy—External Fistulization of Intestines (44186-44188) 323
Excision (44202-44213) 323
Repair (44227) 324
Other Procedures (44238) 324
Enterostomy—External Fistulization of Intestines (44300-44346) 324
Endoscopy, Small Intestine* (44360-44379) 324
Endoscopy, Stomal* (44380-44408) 325
Introduction (44500) 327
Repair (44602-44680) 327
Other Procedures (44700-44799) 328

Meckel's Diverticulum and the Mesentery (44800-44899) 328
Excision (44800-44820) 328
Suture (44850) 328
Other Procedures (44899) 328

Appendix (44900-44979) 328
Incision (44900).....328
Excision (44950-44960).....328
Laparoscopy* (44970-44979).....328
Colon and Rectum (45000-45999).....329
Incision (45000-45020).....329
Excision (45100-45172).....329
Destruction (45190).....330
Endoscopy* (45300-45393, 45398).....330
Laparoscopy* (45395-45499).....334
Excision (45395, 45397).....334
Repair (45400, 45499).....334
Repair (45500-45825).....334
Manipulation (45900-45915).....335
Other Procedures* (45399-45999).....335
Anus* (46020-46999).....335
Incision (46020-46083).....335
Excision (46200, 46220, 46221, 46230, 46250-46288, 46945, 46946).....336
Introduction (46500-46505).....336
Endoscopy* (46600-46615).....337
Repair (46700-46761, 46947).....337
Destruction (46900-46942).....338
Other Procedures (46999).....338
Liver (47000-47399).....338
Incision (47000-47015).....338
Excision (47100-47130).....338
Liver Transplantation* (47133-47147).....338
Repair (47300-47362).....339
Laparoscopy* (47370-47379).....339
Other Procedures (47380-47399).....339
Biliary Tract (47400-47999).....340
Incision (47400-47480).....340
Introduction* (47490-47544).....340
Endoscopy* (47550-47556).....343
Laparoscopy* (47562-47579).....343
Excision (47600-47715).....344
Repair (47720-47900).....344
Other Procedures (47999).....344
Pancreas (48000-48999).....344
Incision (48000-48020).....344
Excision (48100-48160).....344
Introduction (48400).....345
Repair (48500-48548).....345
Pancreas Transplantation* (48550-48556).....345
Other Procedures (48999).....345
Abdomen, Peritoneum, and Omentum (49000-49999).....345
Incision (49000-49084).....345
Excision, Destruction* (49180-49255).....346
Laparoscopy* (49320-49329).....347
Introduction, Revision, Removal (49400-49465).....348
Initial Placement* (49440-49442).....349
Conversion (49446).....350
Replacement* (49450-49452).....350
Mechanical Removal of Obstructive Material (49460).....350
Other (49465).....350
Repair (49491-49659).....350
Hernioplasty, Herniorrhaphy, Herniotomy* (49491-49659).....350
Laparoscopy (49650-49659)*.....*352*
Suture (49900).....352
Other Procedures (49904-49999).....352

Digestive 40490-49999

Digestive System

Lips

(For procedures on skin of lips, see 10040 et seq)

Excision

40490 Biopsy of lip

40500 Vermilionectomy (lip shave), with mucosal advancement

40510 Excision of lip; transverse wedge excision with primary closure

40520 V-excision with primary direct linear closure

(For excision of mucous lesions, see 40810-40816)

40525 full thickness, reconstruction with local flap (eg, Estlander or fan)

40527 full thickness, reconstruction with cross lip flap (Abbe-Estlander)

40530 Resection of lip, more than one-fourth, without reconstruction

(For reconstruction, see 13131 et seq)

Repair (Cheiloplasty)

40650 Repair lip, full thickness; vermilion only
➔ *CPT Assistant* Jul 00:10, Nov 16:7

40652 up to half vertical height
➔ *CPT Assistant* Jul 00:10, Nov 16:7

40654 over one-half vertical height, or complex
➔ *CPT Assistant* Nov 16:7

40700 Plastic repair of cleft lip/nasal deformity; primary, partial or complete, unilateral
➔ *CPT Assistant* Dec 14:18

40701 primary bilateral, 1-stage procedure

40702 primary bilateral, 1 of 2 stages

40720 secondary, by recreation of defect and reclosure
➔ *CPT Assistant* Dec 14:18

(For bilateral procedure, report 40720 with modifier 50)

(To report rhinoplasty only for nasal deformity secondary to congenital cleft lip, see 30460, 30462)

(For repair of cleft lip, with cross lip pedicle flap (Abbe-Estlander type), use 40527)

40761 with cross lip pedicle flap (Abbe-Estlander type), including sectioning and inserting of pedicle

(For repair cleft palate, see 42200 et seq)

(For other reconstructive procedures, see 14060, 14061, 15120-15261, 15574, 15576, 15630)

Other Procedures

40799 Unlisted procedure, lips

Vestibule of Mouth

The vestibule is the part of the oral cavity outside the dentoalveolar structures; it includes the mucosal and submucosal tissue of lips and cheeks.

Incision

40800 Drainage of abscess, cyst, hematoma, vestibule of mouth; simple

40801 complicated

40804 Removal of embedded foreign body, vestibule of mouth; simple

40805 complicated

40806 Incision of labial frenum (frenotomy)

Excision, Destruction

40808 Biopsy, vestibule of mouth

40810 Excision of lesion of mucosa and submucosa, vestibule of mouth; without repair

40812 with simple repair

40814 with complex repair

40816 complex, with excision of underlying muscle

40818 Excision of mucosa of vestibule of mouth as donor graft

40819 Excision of frenum, labial or buccal (frenumectomy, frenulectomy, frenectomy)

40820 Destruction of lesion or scar of vestibule of mouth by physical methods (eg, laser, thermal, cryo, chemical)

Repair

40830 Closure of laceration, vestibule of mouth; 2.5 cm or less

40831 over 2.5 cm or complex

40840 Vestibuloplasty; anterior

40842 posterior, unilateral

40843 posterior, bilateral

40844 entire arch

40845 complex (including ridge extension, muscle repositioning)

(For skin grafts, see 15002 et seq)

Other Procedures

40899 Unlisted procedure, vestibule of mouth

Tongue and Floor of Mouth

Incision

41000 Intraoral incision and drainage of abscess, cyst, or hematoma of tongue or floor of mouth; lingual

41005 sublingual, superficial

41006 sublingual, deep, supramylohyoid

41007 submental space

41008 submandibular space

41009 masticator space

41010 Incision of lingual frenum (frenotomy)
➔ *CPT Assistant* Sep 17:14, Nov 17:10

41015 Extraoral incision and drainage of abscess, cyst, or hematoma of floor of mouth; sublingual

41016 submental

41017 submandibular

41018 masticator space

(For frenoplasty, use 41520)

41019 Placement of needles, catheters, or other device(s) into the head and/or neck region (percutaneous, transoral, or transnasal) for subsequent interstitial radioelement application
➔ *CPT Changes: An Insider's View* 2008

(For imaging guidance, see 76942, 77002, 77012, 77021)

(For stereotactic insertion of intracranial brachytherapy radiation sources, use 61770)

(For interstitial radioelement application, see 77770, 77771, 77772, 77778)

Excision

41100 Biopsy of tongue; anterior two-thirds

41105 posterior one-third

41108 Biopsy of floor of mouth

41110 Excision of lesion of tongue without closure

41112 Excision of lesion of tongue with closure; anterior two-thirds

41113 posterior one-third

41114 with local tongue flap

(Do not report 41114 in conjunction with 41112 or 41113)

41115 Excision of lingual frenum (frenectomy)
➔ *CPT Assistant* Sep 17:14, Nov 17:10

41116 Excision, lesion of floor of mouth

41120 Glossectomy; less than one-half tongue
➔ *CPT Assistant* Aug 10:10

41130 hemiglossectomy
➔ *CPT Assistant* Aug 10:5

41135 partial, with unilateral radical neck dissection
➔ *CPT Assistant* Aug 10:5

41140 complete or total, with or without tracheostomy, without radical neck dissection
➔ *CPT Assistant* Aug 10:5

41145 complete or total, with or without tracheostomy, with unilateral radical neck dissection
➔ *CPT Assistant* Aug 10:5

41150 composite procedure with resection floor of mouth and mandibular resection, without radical neck dissection
➔ *CPT Assistant* Aug 10:5

41153 composite procedure with resection floor of mouth, with suprahyoid neck dissection
➔ *CPT Assistant* Aug 10:3

41155 composite procedure with resection floor of mouth, mandibular resection, and radical neck dissection (Commando type)
➔ *CPT Assistant* Jan 01:13, Aug 10:3

Repair

41250 Repair of laceration 2.5 cm or less; floor of mouth and/or anterior two-thirds of tongue

41251 posterior one-third of tongue

41252 Repair of laceration of tongue, floor of mouth, over 2.6 cm or complex

Other Procedures

►(41500 has been deleted)◄

41510 Suture of tongue to lip for micrognathia (Douglas type procedure)
➔ *CPT Assistant* Aug 10:11

41512 Tongue base suspension, permanent suture technique
➔ *CPT Changes: An Insider's View* 2009
➔ *CPT Assistant* Aug 10:11, Aug 12:13

(For suture of tongue to lip for micrognathia, use 41510)

41520 Frenoplasty (surgical revision of frenum, eg, with Z-plasty)
➔ *CPT Assistant* Sep 17:14, Nov 17:10

(For frenotomy, see 40806, 41010)

41530 Submucosal ablation of the tongue base, radiofrequency, 1 or more sites, per session
➔ *CPT Changes: An Insider's View* 2009
➔ *CPT Assistant* Aug 10:10

41599 Unlisted procedure, tongue, floor of mouth
➔ *CPT Assistant* Dec 00:14
➔ *Clinical Examples in Radiology* Fall 09:11

Dentoalveolar Structures

Incision

41800 Drainage of abscess, cyst, hematoma from dentoalveolar structures

41805 Removal of embedded foreign body from dentoalveolar structures; soft tissues

41806 bone

Excision, Destruction

41820 Gingivectomy, excision gingiva, each quadrant

41821 Operculectomy, excision pericoronal tissues

41822 Excision of fibrous tuberosities, dentoalveolar structures

41823 Excision of osseous tuberosities, dentoalveolar structures

41825 Excision of lesion or tumor (except listed above), dentoalveolar structures; without repair

41826 with simple repair

41827 with complex repair

(For nonexcisional destruction, use 41850)

41828 Excision of hyperplastic alveolar mucosa, each quadrant (specify)

41830 Alveolectomy, including curettage of osteitis or sequestrectomy

41850 Destruction of lesion (except excision), dentoalveolar structures

Other Procedures

41870 Periodontal mucosal grafting

41872 Gingivoplasty, each quadrant (specify)

41874 Alveoloplasty, each quadrant (specify)

(For closure of lacerations, see 40830, 40831)

(For segmental osteotomy, use 21206)

(For reduction of fractures, see 21421-21490)

41899 Unlisted procedure, dentoalveolar structures

Palate and Uvula

Incision

42000 Drainage of abscess of palate, uvula

Excision, Destruction

42100 Biopsy of palate, uvula

42104 Excision, lesion of palate, uvula; without closure

42106 with simple primary closure

42107 with local flap closure

(For skin graft, see 14040-14302)

(For mucosal graft, use 40818)

42120 Resection of palate or extensive resection of lesion

(For reconstruction of palate with extraoral tissue, see 14040-14302, 15050, 15120, 15240, 15576)

42140 Uvulectomy, excision of uvula

42145 Palatopharyngoplasty (eg, uvulopalatopharyngoplasty, uvulopharyngoplasty)
➔ *CPT Assistant* Dec 04:19

(For removal of exostosis of the bony palate, see 21031, 21032)

42160 Destruction of lesion, palate or uvula (thermal, cryo or chemical)
➔ *CPT Assistant* Apr 10:10

Repair

42180 Repair, laceration of palate; up to 2 cm

42182 over 2 cm or complex

42200 Palatoplasty for cleft palate, soft and/or hard palate only
➔ *CPT Assistant* Jul 14:8, Mar 15:9

42205 Palatoplasty for cleft palate, with closure of alveolar ridge; soft tissue only

42210 with bone graft to alveolar ridge (includes obtaining graft)

42215 Palatoplasty for cleft palate; major revision

42220 secondary lengthening procedure

42225 attachment pharyngeal flap

42226 Lengthening of palate, and pharyngeal flap

42227 Lengthening of palate, with island flap

42235 Repair of anterior palate, including vomer flap
➔ *CPT Assistant* Jul 14:8, Mar 15:9

(For repair of oronasal fistula, use 30600)

42260 Repair of nasolabial fistula

(For repair of cleft lip, see 40700 et seq)

42280 Maxillary impression for palatal prosthesis

42281 Insertion of pin-retained palatal prosthesis

Other Procedures

42299 Unlisted procedure, palate, uvula
➔ *CPT Assistant* Dec 04:19, Apr 10:10, Nov 10:9, Jul 14:8

Salivary Gland and Ducts

Incision

42300 Drainage of abscess; parotid, simple

42305 parotid, complicated

42310 Drainage of abscess; submaxillary or sublingual, intraoral

➔ *CPT Changes: An Insider's View* 2003

42320 submaxillary, external

42330 Sialolithotomy; submandibular (submaxillary), sublingual or parotid, uncomplicated, intraoral

42335 submandibular (submaxillary), complicated, intraoral

42340 parotid, extraoral or complicated intraoral

Excision

42400 Biopsy of salivary gland; needle

➔ *Clinical Examples in Radiology* Winter 17:5

►(For fine needle aspiration biopsy, see 10004, 10005, 10006, 10007, 10008, 10009, 10010, 10011, 10012, 10021)◄

(For evaluation of fine needle aspirate, see 88172, 88173)

(If imaging guidance is performed, see 76942, 77002, 77012, 77021)

42405 incisional

(If imaging guidance is performed, see 76942, 77002, 77012, 77021)

42408 Excision of sublingual salivary cyst (ranula)

42409 Marsupialization of sublingual salivary cyst (ranula)

42410 Excision of parotid tumor or parotid gland; lateral lobe, without nerve dissection

42415 lateral lobe, with dissection and preservation of facial nerve

42420 total, with dissection and preservation of facial nerve

➔ *CPT Assistant* Aug 10:4

42425 total, en bloc removal with sacrifice of facial nerve

42426 total, with unilateral radical neck dissection

(For suture or grafting of facial nerve, see 64864, 64865, 69740, 69745)

42440 Excision of submandibular (submaxillary) gland

42450 Excision of sublingual gland

Repair

42500 Plastic repair of salivary duct, sialodochoplasty; primary or simple

42505 secondary or complicated

42507 Parotid duct diversion, bilateral (Wilke type procedure);

42509 with excision of both submandibular glands

42510 with ligation of both submandibular (Wharton's) ducts

Other Procedures

42550 Injection procedure for sialography

➔ *Clinical Examples in Radiology* Fall 09:9

(For radiological supervision and interpretation, use 70390)

42600 Closure salivary fistula

42650 Dilation salivary duct

42660 Dilation and catheterization of salivary duct, with or without injection

42665 Ligation salivary duct, intraoral

42699 Unlisted procedure, salivary glands or ducts

Pharynx, Adenoids, and Tonsils

Incision

42700 Incision and drainage abscess; peritonsillar

42720 retropharyngeal or parapharyngeal, intraoral approach

42725 retropharyngeal or parapharyngeal, external approach

Excision, Destruction

42800 Biopsy; oropharynx

42804 nasopharynx, visible lesion, simple

42806 nasopharynx, survey for unknown primary lesion

(For laryngoscopic biopsy, see 31510, 31535, 31536)

42808 Excision or destruction of lesion of pharynx, any method

42809 Removal of foreign body from pharynx

42810 Excision branchial cleft cyst or vestige, confined to skin and subcutaneous tissues

42815 Excision branchial cleft cyst, vestige, or fistula, extending beneath subcutaneous tissues and/or into pharynx

42820 Tonsillectomy and adenoidectomy; younger than age 12

➔ *CPT Assistant* Feb 98:11, Mar 08:15, May 08:14

42821 age 12 or over

➔ *CPT Assistant* Aug 97:18, Feb 98:11, Mar 08:15, May 08:14

42825 Tonsillectomy, primary or secondary; younger than age 12

➔ *CPT Assistant* Aug 97:18, Feb 98:11, Mar 08:15

42826 age 12 or over

➔ *CPT Assistant* Aug 97:18, Feb 98:11, Mar 08:15, Apr 10:10

42830 Adenoidectomy, primary; younger than age 12

42831 age 12 or over

42835 Adenoidectomy, secondary; younger than age 12

42836 age 12 or over
➲ *CPT Assistant* Feb 98:11, Nov 10:9

42842 Radical resection of tonsil, tonsillar pillars, and/or retromolar trigone; without closure
➲ *CPT Assistant* Aug 10:6

42844 closure with local flap (eg, tongue, buccal)
➲ *CPT Assistant* Aug 10:6

42845 closure with other flap
➲ *CPT Assistant* Aug 10:6

(For closure with other flap(s), use appropriate number for flap(s))

(When combined with radical neck dissection, use also 38720)

42860 Excision of tonsil tags

42870 Excision or destruction lingual tonsil, any method (separate procedure)

(For resection of the nasopharynx [eg, juvenile angiofibroma] by bicoronal and/or transzygomatic approach, see 61586 and 61600)

42890 Limited pharyngectomy

42892 Resection of lateral pharyngeal wall or pyriform sinus, direct closure by advancement of lateral and posterior pharyngeal walls
➲ *CPT Assistant* Aug 10:6

(When combined with radical neck dissection, use also 38720)

42894 Resection of pharyngeal wall requiring closure with myocutaneous or fasciocutaneous flap or free muscle, skin, or fascial flap with microvascular anastomosis
➲ *CPT Changes: An Insider's View* 2010
➲ *CPT Assistant* Nov 07:8, Aug 10:6

(When combined with radical neck dissection, use also 38720)

(For limited pharyngectomy with radical neck dissection, use 38720 with 42890)

(For flap used for reconstruction, see 15730, 15733, 15734, 15756, 15757, 15758)

Repair

42900 Suture pharynx for wound or injury

42950 Pharyngoplasty (plastic or reconstructive operation on pharynx)
➲ *CPT Assistant* Apr 16:8

(For pharyngeal flap, use 42225)

42953 Pharyngoesophageal repair

(For closure with myocutaneous or other flap, use appropriate number in addition)

Other Procedures

42955 Pharyngostomy (fistulization of pharynx, external for feeding)

42960 Control oropharyngeal hemorrhage, primary or secondary (eg, post-tonsillectomy); simple

42961 complicated, requiring hospitalization

42962 with secondary surgical intervention

42970 Control of nasopharyngeal hemorrhage, primary or secondary (eg, postadenoidectomy); simple, with posterior nasal packs, with or without anterior packs and/or cautery
➲ *CPT Changes: An Insider's View* 2002

42971 complicated, requiring hospitalization

42972 with secondary surgical intervention

42999 Unlisted procedure, pharynx, adenoids, or tonsils
➲ *CPT Assistant* Feb 14:11

Esophagus

Incision

(For esophageal intubation with laparotomy, use 43510)

43020 Esophagotomy, cervical approach, with removal of foreign body

43030 Cricopharyngeal myotomy

43045 Esophagotomy, thoracic approach, with removal of foreign body

Excision

(For gastrointestinal reconstruction for previous esophagectomy, see 43360, 43361)

43100 Excision of lesion, esophagus, with primary repair; cervical approach

43101 thoracic or abdominal approach
➲ *CPT Assistant* Aug 10:4

(For wide excision of malignant lesion of cervical esophagus, with total laryngectomy without radical neck dissection, see 43107, 43116, 43124, and 31360)

(For wide excision of malignant lesion of cervical esophagus, with total laryngectomy with radical neck dissection, see 43107, 43116, 43124, and 31365)

43107 Total or near total esophagectomy, without thoracotomy; with pharyngogastrostomy or cervical esophagogastrostomy, with or without pyloroplasty (transhiatal)
➲ *CPT Assistant* Aug 10:4

43108 with colon interposition or small intestine reconstruction, including intestine mobilization, preparation and anastomosis(es)
➲ *CPT Changes: An Insider's View* 2002

43112 Total or near total esophagectomy, with thoracotomy; with pharyngogastrostomy or cervical esophagogastrostomy, with or without pyloroplasty (ie, McKeown esophagectomy or tri-incisional esophagectomy)

➔ *CPT Changes: An Insider's View* 2018

➔ *CPT Assistant* Aug 13:14

43113 with colon interposition or small intestine reconstruction, including intestine mobilization, preparation, and anastomosis(es)

➔ *CPT Changes: An Insider's View* 2002

43116 Partial esophagectomy, cervical, with free intestinal graft, including microvascular anastomosis, obtaining the graft and intestinal reconstruction

➔ *CPT Assistant* Nov 97:17, Nov 98:16, Aug 10:4

(Do not report 43116 in conjunction with 69990)

(Report 43116 with the modifier 52 appended if intestinal or free jejunal graft with microvascular anastomosis is performed by another physician)

(For free jejunal graft with microvascular anastomosis performed by another physician, use 43496)

43117 Partial esophagectomy, distal two-thirds, with thoracotomy and separate abdominal incision, with or without proximal gastrectomy; with thoracic esophagogastrostomy, with or without pyloroplasty (Ivor Lewis)

43118 with colon interposition or small intestine reconstruction, including intestine mobilization, preparation, and anastomosis(es)

➔ *CPT Changes: An Insider's View* 2002

(For total esophagectomy with gastropharyngostomy, see 43107, 43124)

(For esophagogastrectomy (lower third) and vagotomy, use 43122)

43121 Partial esophagectomy, distal two-thirds, with thoracotomy only, with or without proximal gastrectomy, with thoracic esophagogastrostomy, with or without pyloroplasty

43122 Partial esophagectomy, thoracoabdominal or abdominal approach, with or without proximal gastrectomy; with esophagogastrostomy, with or without pyloroplasty

43123 with colon interposition or small intestine reconstruction, including intestine mobilization, preparation, and anastomosis(es)

➔ *CPT Changes: An Insider's View* 2002

43124 Total or partial esophagectomy, without reconstruction (any approach), with cervical esophagostomy

43130 Diverticulectomy of hypopharynx or esophagus, with or without myotomy; cervical approach

➔ *CPT Assistant* Oct 10:12, Dec 10:12

43135 thoracic approach

➔ *CPT Assistant* Oct 10:12, Dec 10:12

(For endoscopic diverticulectomy of hypopharynx or cervical esophagus, use 43180)

Endoscopy

When bleeding occurs as a result of an endoscopic procedure, control of bleeding is not reported separately during the same operative session.

Esophagoscopy includes examination from the cricopharyngeus muscle (upper esophageal sphincter) to and including the gastroesophageal junction. It may also include examination of the proximal region of the stomach via retroflexion when performed.

Esophagoscopy

43180 Esophagoscopy, rigid, transoral with diverticulectomy of hypopharynx or cervical esophagus (eg, Zenker's diverticulum), with cricopharyngeal myotomy, includes use of telescope or operating microscope and repair, when performed

➔ *CPT Changes: An Insider's View* 2015

➔ *CPT Assistant* Nov 15:8

(Do not report 43180 in conjunction with 43210, 69990)

(For diverticulectomy of hypopharynx or esophagus [open], see 43130, 43135)

43191 Esophagoscopy, rigid, transoral; diagnostic, including collection of specimen(s) by brushing or washing when performed (separate procedure)

➔ *CPT Changes: An Insider's View* 2014

➔ *CPT Assistant* Dec 13:3, Feb 14:9, 11, Nov 15:8

(Do not report 43191 in conjunction with 43192, 43193, 43194, 43195, 43196, 43197, 43198, 43210)

(For diagnostic transnasal esophagoscopy, see 43197, 43198)

(For diagnostic flexible transoral esophagoscopy, use 43200)

43192 with directed submucosal injection(s), any substance

➔ *CPT Changes: An Insider's View* 2014

➔ *CPT Assistant* Dec 13:3

(Do not report 43192 in conjunction with 43191, 43197, 43198)

(For flexible transoral esophagoscopy with directed submucosal injection(s), use 43201)

(For flexible transoral esophagoscopy with injection sclerosis of esophageal varices, use 43204)

(For rigid transoral esophagoscopy with injection sclerosis of esophageal varices, use 43499)

43193 with biopsy, single or multiple

➔ *CPT Changes: An Insider's View* 2014

➔ *CPT Assistant* Dec 13:3

(Do not report 43193 in conjunction with 43191, 43197, 43198)

(For flexible transoral esophagoscopy with biopsy, use 43202)

43194 with removal of foreign body(s)

➔ *CPT Changes: An Insider's View* 2014, 2015

➔ *CPT Assistant* Dec 13:3

(Do not report 43194 in conjunction with 43191, 43197, 43198)

(If fluoroscopic guidance is performed, use 76000)

(For flexible transoral esophagoscopy with removal of foreign body(s), use 43215)

43195 with balloon dilation (less than 30 mm diameter)

➔ *CPT Changes: An Insider's View* 2014

➔ *CPT Assistant* Dec 13:3

(Do not report 43195 in conjunction with 43191, 43197, 43198)

(If fluoroscopic guidance is performed, use 74360)

(For esophageal dilation with balloon 30 mm diameter or larger, see 43214, 43233)

(For dilation without endoscopic visualization, see 43450, 43453)

(For flexible transoral esophagoscopy with balloon dilation [less than 30 mm diameter], use 43220)

43196 with insertion of guide wire followed by dilation over guide wire

➔ *CPT Changes: An Insider's View* 2014

➔ *CPT Assistant* Dec 13:3, Feb 14:9

(Do not report 43196 in conjunction with 43191, 43197, 43198)

(If fluoroscopic guidance is performed, use 74360)

(For flexible transoral esophagoscopy with insertion of guide wire followed by dilation over guide wire, use 43226)

43197 Esophagoscopy, flexible, transnasal; diagnostic, including collection of specimen(s) by brushing or washing, when performed (separate procedure)

➔ *CPT Changes: An Insider's View* 2014, 2015

➔ *CPT Assistant* Dec 13:3, Feb 14:9, Nov 15:8

(Do not report 43197 in conjunction with 31575, 43191, 43192, 43193, 43194, 43195, 43196, 43198, 43200-43232, 43235-43259, 43266, 43270, 92511)

(Do not report 43197 in conjunction with 31231 unless separate type of endoscope [eg, rigid endoscope] is used)

(For transoral esophagoscopy, see 43191, 43200)

43198 with biopsy, single or multiple

➔ *CPT Changes: An Insider's View* 2014

➔ *CPT Assistant* Dec 13:3, Feb 14:9

(Do not report 43198 in conjunction with 31575, 43191, 43192, 43193, 43194, 43195, 43196, 43197, 43200-43232, 43235-43259, 43266, 43270, 92511)

(Do not report 43198 in conjunction with 31231 unless separate type of endoscope [eg, rigid endoscope] is used)

(For transoral esophagoscopy with biopsy, see 43193, 43202)

43200 Esophagoscopy, flexible, transoral; diagnostic, including collection of specimen(s) by brushing or washing, when performed (separate procedure)

➔ *CPT Changes: An Insider's View* 2000, 2014, 2017

➔ *CPT Assistant* Spring 91:7, Spring 94:1, Jun 98:10, Nov 99:21, Sep 03:3, Oct 08:6, Jan 13:11, Feb 13:16, Dec 13:3, Feb 14:9, Nov 15:8

(Do not report 43200 in conjunction with 43197, 43198, 43201-43232)

(For diagnostic rigid transoral esophagoscopy, use 43191)

(For diagnostic flexible transnasal esophagoscopy, use 43197)

(For diagnostic flexible esophagogastroduodenoscopy, use 43235)

43201 with directed submucosal injection(s), any substance

➔ *CPT Changes: An Insider's View* 2003, 2014, 2017

➔ *CPT Assistant* Jun 10:4, Jan 13:11, Dec 13:3

(Do not report 43201 in conjunction with 43204, 43211, 43227 for the same lesion)

(Do not report 43201 in conjunction with 43197, 43198, 43200)

(For rigid transoral esophagoscopy with directed submucosal injection[s], use 43192)

(For flexible transoral esophagoscopy with injection sclerosis of esophageal varices, use 43204)

(For rigid transoral esophagoscopy with injection sclerosis of esophageal varices, use 43499)

43202 with biopsy, single or multiple

➔ *CPT Changes: An Insider's View* 2014, 2017

➔ *CPT Assistant* Spring 94:1, Oct 08:6, Jan 13:11, Dec 13:3

(Do not report 43202 in conjunction with 43211 for the same lesion)

(Do not report 43202 in conjunction with 43197, 43198, 43200)

(For rigid transoral esophagoscopy with biopsy, use 43193)

(For flexible transnasal esophagoscopy with biopsy, use 43198)

43204 with injection sclerosis of esophageal varices

➔ *CPT Changes: An Insider's View* 2014, 2017

➔ *CPT Assistant* Spring 94:1, Oct 08:6, Jun 10:5, Jan 13:11, Dec 13:3

(Do not report 43204 in conjunction with 43201, 43227 for the same lesion)

(Do not report 43204 in conjunction with 43197, 43198, 43200)

(For rigid transoral esophagoscopy with injection sclerosis of esophageal varices, use 43499)

43205 with band ligation of esophageal varices

➲ *CPT Changes: An Insider's View* 2014, 2017

➲ *CPT Assistant* Spring 94:1, Oct 08:6, Jan 13:11, Dec 13:3

(Do not report 43205 in conjunction with 43227 for the same lesion)

(Do not report 43205 in conjunction with 43197, 43198, 43200)

(To report control of nonvariceal bleeding with band ligation, use 43227)

43206 with optical endomicroscopy

➲ *CPT Changes: An Insider's View* 2013, 2014, 2017

➲ *CPT Assistant* Jan 13:11, Aug 13:5, Dec 13:3, Nov 17:10

(Report supply of contrast agent separately)

(Do not report 43206 in conjunction with 43197, 43198, 43200, 88375)

43210 Code is out of numerical sequence. See 43254-43261

43211 Code is out of numerical sequence. See 43216-43227

43212 Code is out of numerical sequence. See 43216-43227

43213 Code is out of numerical sequence. See 43216-43227

43214 Code is out of numerical sequence. See 43216-43227

43215 with removal of foreign body(s)

➲ *CPT Changes: An Insider's View* 2014, 2015, 2017

➲ *CPT Assistant* Spring 94:1, Oct 08:6, Dec 13:3

(Do not report 43215 in conjunction with 43197, 43198, 43200)

(If fluoroscopic guidance is performed, use 76000)

(For rigid transoral esophagoscopy with removal of foreign body(s), use 43194)

43216 with removal of tumor(s), polyp(s), or other lesion(s) by hot biopsy forceps

➲ *CPT Changes: An Insider's View* 2014, 2015, 2017

➲ *CPT Assistant* Spring 94:1, Oct 08:6, Jan 13:11, Dec 13:3

(Do not report 43216 in conjunction with 43197, 43198, 43200)

43217 with removal of tumor(s), polyp(s), or other lesion(s) by snare technique

➲ *CPT Changes: An Insider's View* 2014, 2017

➲ *CPT Assistant* Spring 94:1, Oct 08:6, Jan 13:11, Dec 13:3

(Do not report 43217 in conjunction with 43211 for the same lesion)

(Do not report 43217 in conjunction with 43197, 43198, 43200)

(For esophagogastroduodenoscopy with removal of tumor[s], polyp[s], or other lesion[s] by snare technique, use 43251)

(For endoscopic mucosal resection, use 43211)

 # 43211 with endoscopic mucosal resection

➲ *CPT Changes: An Insider's View* 2014, 2017

➲ *CPT Assistant* Dec 13:3, Nov 17:10

(Do not report 43211 in conjunction with 43201, 43202, 43217 for the same lesion)

(Do not report 43211 in conjunction with 43197, 43198, 43200)

 # 43212 with placement of endoscopic stent (includes pre- and post-dilation and guide wire passage, when performed)

➲ *CPT Changes: An Insider's View* 2014, 2017

➲ *CPT Assistant* Dec 13:3

(Do not report 43212 in conjunction with 43197, 43198, 43200, 43220, 43226, 43241)

(If fluoroscopic guidance is performed, use 74360)

43220 with transendoscopic balloon dilation (less than 30 mm diameter)

➲ *CPT Changes: An Insider's View* 2014, 2017

➲ *CPT Assistant* Spring 94:2, Jan 97:10, May 05:3, Oct 08:6, Jan 13:11, Dec 13:3

(Do not report 43220 in conjunction with 43197, 43198, 43200, 43212, 43226, 43229)

(If fluoroscopic guidance is performed, use 74360)

(For rigid transoral esophagoscopy with balloon dilation [less than 30 mm diameter], use 43195)

(For esophageal dilation with balloon 30 mm diameter or larger, use 43214)

(For dilation without endoscopic visualization, see 43450, 43453)

 # 43213 with dilation of esophagus, by balloon or dilator, retrograde (includes fluoroscopic guidance, when performed)

➲ *CPT Changes: An Insider's View* 2014, 2017

➲ *CPT Assistant* Dec 13:3

►(Do not report 43213 in conjunction with 43197, 43198, 43200, 74360, 76000)◄

(For transendoscopic balloon dilation of multiple strictures during the same session, report 43213 with modifier 59 for each additional stricture dilated)

 # 43214 with dilation of esophagus with balloon (30 mm diameter or larger) (includes fluoroscopic guidance, when performed)

➲ *CPT Changes: An Insider's View* 2014, 2017

➲ *CPT Assistant* Dec 13:3

►(Do not report 43214 in conjunction with 43197, 43198, 43200, 74360, 76000)◄

43226 with insertion of guide wire followed by passage of dilator(s) over guide wire

➲ *CPT Changes: An Insider's View* 2014, 2017

➲ *CPT Assistant* Spring 94:2, Jan 13:11, Dec 13:3

(Do not report 43226 in conjunction with 43229 for the same lesion)

(Do not report 43226 in conjunction with 43197, 43198, 43200, 43212, 43220)

(If fluoroscopic guidance is performed, use 74360)

Digestive 40490-49999

(For rigid transoral esophagoscopy with insertion of guide wire followed by dilation over guide wire, use 43196)

43227 with control of bleeding, any method

➔ *CPT Changes: An Insider's View* 2002, 2014, 2017

➔ *CPT Assistant* Spring 94:2, Oct 08:6, Jun 10:4, Jan 13:11, Dec 13:3, Feb 14:11

(Do not report 43227 in conjunction with 43201, 43204, 43205 for the same lesion)

(Do not report 43227 in conjunction with 43197, 43198, 43200)

43229 with ablation of tumor(s), polyp(s), or other lesion(s) (includes pre- and post-dilation and guide wire passage, when performed)

➔ *CPT Changes: An Insider's View* 2014, 2017

➔ *CPT Assistant* Dec 13:3

(Do not report 43229 in conjunction with 43220, 43226 for the same lesion)

(Do not report 43229 in conjunction with 43197, 43198, 43200)

(For esophagoscopic photodynamic therapy, report 43229 in conjunction with 96570, 96571 as appropriate)

43231 with endoscopic ultrasound examination

➔ *CPT Changes: An Insider's View* 2001, 2014, 2017

➔ *CPT Assistant* Oct 01:4, May 04:6, Oct 08:6, Mar 09:8, Jan 13:11, Dec 13:3

(Do not report 43231 in conjunction with 43197, 43198, 43200, 43232, 76975)

(Do not report 43231 more than once per session)

43232 with transendoscopic ultrasound-guided intramural or transmural fine needle aspiration/biopsy(s)

➔ *CPT Changes: An Insider's View* 2001, 2014, 2017

➔ *CPT Assistant* Oct 01:4, Mar 04:11, May 04:6, Oct 08:6, Mar 09:8, Jan 13:11, Dec 13:3, Feb 14:9

(Do not report 43232 in conjunction with 43197, 43198, 43200, 43231, 76942, 76975)

(Do not report 43232 more than once per session)

43233 Code is out of numerical sequence. See 43248-43251

Esophagogastroduodenoscopy

(For examination of the esophagus from the cricopharyngeus muscle [upper esophageal sphincter] to and including the gastroesophageal junction, including examination of the proximal region of the stomach via retroflexion when performed, see 43197, 43198, 43200, 43201, 43202, 43204, 43205, 43206, 43211, 43212, 43213, 43214, 43215, 43216, 43217, 43220, 43226, 43227, 43229, 43231, 43232)

(Use 43233, 43235-43259, 43266, 43270 for examination of a surgically altered stomach where the jejunum is examined distal to the anastomosis [eg, gastric bypass, gastroenterostomy {Billroth II}])

To report esophagogastroscopy where the duodenum is deliberately not examined (eg, judged clinically not pertinent), or because the clinical situation precludes such exam (eg, significant gastric retention precludes safe exam of duodenum), append modifier 52 if repeat examination is not planned, or modifier 53 if repeat examination is planned.

43235 Esophagogastroduodenoscopy, flexible, transoral; diagnostic, including collection of specimen(s) by brushing or washing, when performed (separate procedure)

➔ *CPT Changes: An Insider's View* 2014, 2017

➔ *CPT Assistant* Spring 94:4, Dec 97:11, Jun 03:11, Sep 03:3, Oct 08:6, May 09:8, Jan 13:11, Dec 13:3, Nov 15:8, Jul 17:10

(Do not report 43235 in conjunction with 43197, 43198, 43210, 43236-43259, 43266, 43270, 44360, 44361, 44363, 44364, 44365, 44366, 44369, 44370, 44372, 44373, 44376, 44377, 44378, 44379)

Esophagogastroduodenoscopy
43235

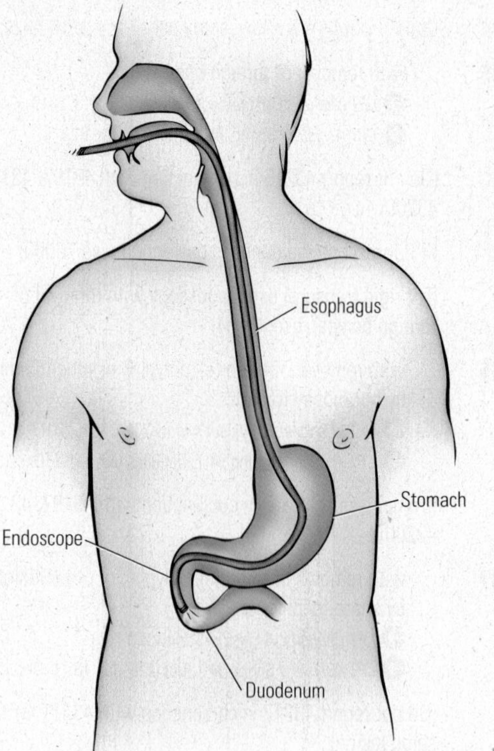

43236 with directed submucosal injection(s), any substance

➔ *CPT Changes: An Insider's View* 2003, 2014, 2017

➔ *CPT Assistant* Jun 10:4, Jan 13:11, Dec 13:3

(Do not report 43236 in conjunction with 43243, 43254, 43255 for the same lesion)

(Do not report 43236 in conjunction with 43197, 43198, 43235, 44360, 44361, 44363, 44364, 44365, 44366, 44369, 44370, 44372, 44373, 44376, 44377, 44378, 44379)

(For flexible, transoral esophagogastroduodenoscopy with injection sclerosis of esophageal and/or gastric varices, use 43243)

43237 with endoscopic ultrasound examination limited to the esophagus, stomach or duodenum, and adjacent structures

➲ *CPT Changes: An Insider's View* 2004, 2014, 2017

➲ *CPT Assistant* Jan 13:11, Dec 13:3, Jan 16:11

(Do not report 43237 in conjunction with 43197, 43198, 43235, 43238, 43242, 43253, 43259, 44360, 44361, 44363, 44364, 44365, 44366, 44369, 44370, 44372, 44373, 44376, 44377, 44378, 44379, 76975)

(Do not report 43237 more than once per session)

43238 with transendoscopic ultrasound-guided intramural or transmural fine needle aspiration/biopsy(s), (includes endoscopic ultrasound examination limited to the esophagus, stomach or duodenum, and adjacent structures)

➲ *CPT Changes: An Insider's View* 2004, 2014, 2017

➲ *CPT Assistant* Jan 13:11, Dec 13:3

(Do not report 43238 in conjunction with 43197, 43198, 43235, 43237, 43242, 44360, 44361, 44363, 44364, 44365, 44366, 44369, 44370, 44372, 44373, 44376, 44377, 44378, 44379, 76942, 76975)

(Do not report 43238 more than once per session)

43239 with biopsy, single or multiple

➲ *CPT Changes: An Insider's View* 2014, 2017

➲ *CPT Assistant* Spring 94:4, Apr 98:14, Feb 99:11, Oct 01:4, Nov 07:9, Jan 13:11, Dec 13:3

(Do not report 43239 in conjunction with 43254 for the same lesion)

(Do not report 43239 in conjunction with 43197, 43198, 43235, 44360, 44361, 44363, 44364, 44365, 44366, 44369, 44370, 44372, 44373, 44376, 44377, 44378, 44379)

43240 with transmural drainage of pseudocyst (includes placement of transmural drainage catheter[s]/stent[s], when performed, and endoscopic ultrasound, when performed)

➲ *CPT Changes: An Insider's View* 2001, 2014, 2017

➲ *CPT Assistant* Oct 01:4, Jan 13:11, Dec 13:3

(Do not report 43240 in conjunction with 43253 for the same lesion)

(Do not report 43240 in conjunction with 43197, 43198, 43235, 43242, 43259, 43266, 44360, 44361, 44363, 44364, 44365, 44366, 44369, 44370, 44372, 44373, 44376, 44377, 44378, 44379)

(Do not report 43240 more than once per session)

(For endoscopic pancreatic necrosectomy, use 48999)

43241 with insertion of intraluminal tube or catheter

➲ *CPT Changes: An Insider's View* 2001, 2014, 2017

➲ *CPT Assistant* Spring 94:4, Nov 01:7, Apr 09:3, Jan 13:11, Dec 13:3

(Do not report 43241 in conjunction with 43197, 43198, 43212, 43235, 43266, 44360, 44361, 44363, 44364, 44365, 44366, 44369, 44370, 44372, 44373, 44376, 44377, 44378, 44379)

(For naso- or oro-gastric tube placement requiring physician's or other qualified health care professional's skill and fluoroscopic guidance, use 43752)

(For nonendoscopic enteric tube placement, see 44500, 74340)

43242 with transendoscopic ultrasound-guided intramural or transmural fine needle aspiration/biopsy(s) (includes endoscopic ultrasound examination of the esophagus, stomach, and either the duodenum or a surgically altered stomach where the jejunum is examined distal to the anastomosis)

➲ *CPT Changes: An Insider's View* 2001, 2004, 2014, 2017

➲ *CPT Assistant* Oct 01:4, Mar 09:8, Jan 13:11, Dec 13:3

(Do not report 43242 in conjunction with 43197, 43198, 43235, 43237, 43238, 43240, 43259, 44360, 44361, 44363, 44364, 44365, 44366, 44369, 44370, 44372, 44373, 44376, 44377, 44378, 44379, 76942, 76975)

(Do not report 43242 more than once per session)

(For transendoscopic ultrasound-guided transmural fine needle aspiration/biopsy limited to the esophagus, stomach, duodenum, or adjacent structure, use 43238)

43243 with injection sclerosis of esophageal/gastric varices

➲ *CPT Changes: An Insider's View* 2014, 2017

➲ *CPT Assistant* Spring 94:4, Jun 10:5, Jan 13:11, Dec 13:3

(Do not report 43243 in conjunction with 43236, 43255 for the same lesion)

(Do not report 43243 in conjunction with 43197, 43198, 43235, 44360, 44361, 44363, 44364, 44365, 44366, 44369, 44370, 44372, 44373, 44376, 44377, 44378, 44379)

43244 with band ligation of esophageal/gastric varices

➲ *CPT Changes: An Insider's View* 2014, 2017

➲ *CPT Assistant* Spring 94:4, Jun 11:13, Jan 13:11, Dec 13:3

(Do not report 43244 in conjunction with 43197, 43198, 43235, 43255, 44360, 44361, 44363, 44364, 44365, 44366, 44369, 44370, 44372, 44373, 44376, 44377, 44378, 44379)

(To report control of nonvariceal bleeding with band ligation, use 43255)

43245 with dilation of gastric/duodenal stricture(s) (eg, balloon, bougie)

➲ *CPT Changes: An Insider's View* 2002, 2003, 2014, 2017

➲ *CPT Assistant* Spring 94:4, Oct 01:4, Jan 04:26, Jan 13:11, Dec 13:3

(Do not report 43245 in conjunction with 43197, 43198, 43235, 43266, 44360, 44361, 44363, 44364, 44365, 44366, 44369, 44370, 44372, 44373, 44376, 44377, 44378, 44379)

(If fluoroscopic guidance is performed, use 74360)

43246 with directed placement of percutaneous gastrostomy tube

➲ *CPT Changes: An Insider's View* 2014, 2017

➲ *CPT Assistant* Spring 94:4, Feb 97:10, Mar 10:10, Jan 13:11, May 13:12, Dec 13:3

(Do not report 43246 in conjunction with 43197, 43198, 43235, 44360, 44361, 44363, 44364, 44365, 44366, 44369, 44370, 44372, 44376, 44377, 44378, 44379)

►(For percutaneous insertion of gastrostomy tube under fluoroscopic guidance, use 49440)◄

►(For percutaneous replacement of gastrostomy tube without imaging or endoscopy, see 43762, 43763)◄

43247 with removal of foreign body(s)

➲ *CPT Changes: An Insider's View* 2014, 2015, 2017

➲ *CPT Assistant* Spring 94:4, Jan 13:11, Dec 13:3

(Do not report 43247 in conjunction with 43197, 43198, 43235, 44360, 44361, 44363, 44364, 44365, 44366, 44369, 44370, 44372, 44373, 44376, 44377, 44378, 44379)

(If fluoroscopic guidance is performed, use 76000)

43248 with insertion of guide wire followed by passage of dilator(s) through esophagus over guide wire

➲ *CPT Changes: An Insider's View* 2014, 2017

➲ *CPT Assistant* Spring 94:4, Dec 97:11, Oct 08:6, Jan 13:11, Dec 13:3, Jul 17:10

(Do not report 43248 in conjunction with 43197, 43198, 43235, 43266, 43270, 44360, 44361, 44363, 44364, 44365, 44366, 44369, 44370, 44372, 44373, 44376, 44377, 44378, 44379)

(If fluoroscopic guidance is performed, use 74360)

43249 with transendoscopic balloon dilation of esophagus (less than 30 mm diameter)

➲ *CPT Changes: An Insider's View* 2014, 2017

➲ *CPT Assistant* May 05:3, Jan 13:11, Dec 13:3

(Do not report 43249 in conjunction with 43197, 43198, 43235, 43266, 43270, 44360, 44361, 44363, 44364, 44365, 44366, 44369, 44370, 44372, 44373, 44376, 44377, 44378, 44379)

(If fluoroscopic guidance is performed, use 74360)

 # 43233 with dilation of esophagus with balloon (30 mm diameter or larger) (includes fluoroscopic guidance, when performed)

➲ *CPT Changes: An Insider's View* 2014, 2017

➲ *CPT Assistant* Dec 13:3

►(Do not report 43233 in conjunction with 43197, 43198, 43235, 44360, 44361, 44363, 44364, 44365, 44366, 44369, 44370, 44372, 44373, 44376, 44377, 44378, 44379, 74360, 76000)◄

43250 with removal of tumor(s), polyp(s), or other lesion(s) by hot biopsy forceps

➲ *CPT Changes: An Insider's View* 2014, 2015, 2017

➲ *CPT Assistant* Spring 94:4, Feb 99:11, Nov 07:9, Jan 13:11, Dec 13:3

(Do not report 43250 in conjunction with 43197, 43198, 43235, 44360, 44361, 44363, 44364, 44365, 44366, 44369, 44370, 44372, 44373, 44376, 44377, 44378, 44379)

43251 with removal of tumor(s), polyp(s), or other lesion(s) by snare technique

➲ *CPT Changes: An Insider's View* 2014, 2017

➲ *CPT Assistant* Spring 94:4, Oct 04:12, Nov 07:9, Jun 11:13, Jan 13:11, Dec 13:3

(Do not report 43251 in conjunction with 43254 for the same lesion)

(Do not report 43251 in conjunction with 43197, 43198, 43235, 44360, 44361, 44363, 44364, 44365, 44366, 44369, 44370, 44372, 44373, 44376, 44377, 44378, 44379)

(For endoscopic mucosal resection, use 43254)

43252 with optical endomicroscopy

➲ *CPT Changes: An Insider's View* 2013, 2014, 2017

➲ *CPT Assistant* Jan 13:11, Aug 13:5, Dec 13:3

(Report supply of contrast agent separately)

(Do not report 43252 in conjunction with 43197, 43198, 43235, 44360, 44361, 44363, 44364, 44365, 44366, 44369, 44370, 44372, 44373, 44376, 44377, 44378, 44379, 88375)

43253 with transendoscopic ultrasound-guided transmural injection of diagnostic or therapeutic substance(s) (eg, anesthetic, neurolytic agent) or fiducial marker(s) (includes endoscopic ultrasound examination of the esophagus, stomach, and either the duodenum or a surgically altered stomach where the jejunum is examined distal to the anastomosis)

➲ *CPT Changes: An Insider's View* 2014, 2017

➲ *CPT Assistant* Dec 13:3, Apr 18:11

(Do not report 43253 in conjunction with 43240 for the same lesion)

(Do not report 43253 in conjunction with 43197, 43198, 43235, 43237, 43259, 44360, 44361, 44363, 44364, 44365, 44366, 44369, 44370, 44372, 44373, 44376, 44377, 44378, 44379, 76942, 76975)

(Do not report 43253 more than once per session)

(For transendoscopic ultrasound-guided transmural fine needle aspiration/biopsy, see 43238, 43242)

43254 with endoscopic mucosal resection

➲ *CPT Changes: An Insider's View* 2014, 2017

➲ *CPT Assistant* Dec 13:3

(Do not report 43254 in conjunction with 43236, 43239, 43251 for the same lesion)

(Do not report 43254 in conjunction with 43197, 43198, 43235, 44360, 44361, 44363, 44364, 44365, 44366, 44369, 44370, 44372, 44373, 44376, 44377, 44378, 44379)

43255 with control of bleeding, any method

➔ *CPT Changes: An Insider's View* 2014, 2017

➔ *CPT Assistant* Spring 94:4, Jun 10:4, Dec 13:3

(Do not report 43255 in conjunction with 43236, 43243, 43244 for the same lesion)

(Do not report 43255 in conjunction with 43197, 43198, 43235, 44360, 44361, 44363, 44364, 44365, 44366, 44369, 44370, 44372, 44373, 44376, 44377, 44378, 44379)

 # 43266 with placement of endoscopic stent (includes pre- and post-dilation and guide wire passage, when performed)

➔ *CPT Changes: An Insider's View* 2014, 2017

➔ *CPT Assistant* Dec 13:3

(Do not report 43266 in conjunction with 43197, 43198, 43235, 43240, 43241, 43245, 43248, 43249, 44360, 44361, 44363, 44364, 44365, 44366, 44369, 44370, 44372, 44373, 44376, 44377, 44378, 44379)

(If fluoroscopic guidance is performed, use 74360)

43257 with delivery of thermal energy to the muscle of lower esophageal sphincter and/or gastric cardia, for treatment of gastroesophageal reflux disease

➔ *CPT Changes: An Insider's View* 2005, 2014, 2017

➔ *CPT Assistant* May 05:3, Jan 13:11, Dec 13:3

(Do not report 43257 in conjunction with 43197, 43198, 43235, 44360, 44361, 44363, 44364, 44365, 44366, 44369, 44370, 44372, 44373, 44376, 44377, 44378, 44379)

(For ablation of metaplastic/dysplastic esophageal lesion [eg, Barrett's esophagus], see 43229, 43270)

 # 43270 with ablation of tumor(s), polyp(s), or other lesion(s) (includes pre- and post-dilation and guide wire passage, when performed)

➔ *CPT Changes: An Insider's View* 2014, 2017

➔ *CPT Assistant* Dec 13:3

(Do not report 43270 in conjunction with 43248, 43249 for the same lesion)

(Do not report 43270 in conjunction with 43197, 43198, 43235, 44360, 44361, 44363, 44364, 44365, 44366, 44369, 44370, 44372, 44373, 44376, 44377, 44378, 44379)

(For esophagoscopic photodynamic therapy, use 43270 in conjunction with 96570, 96571 as appropriate)

43259 with endoscopic ultrasound examination, including the esophagus, stomach, and either the duodenum or a surgically altered stomach where the jejunum is examined distal to the anastomosis

➔ *CPT Changes: An Insider's View* 2004, 2014, 2017

➔ *CPT Assistant* Spring 94:4, May 04:7, Mar 09:8, Jan 13:11, Dec 13:3, Jan 16:11

(Do not report 43259 in conjunction with 43197, 43198, 43235, 43237, 43240, 43242, 43253, 44360, 44361, 44363, 44364, 44365, 44366, 44369, 44370, 44372, 44373, 44376, 44377, 44378, 44379, 76975)

(Do not report 43259 more than once per session)

 # 43210 with esophagogastric fundoplasty, partial or complete, includes duodenoscopy when performed

➔ *CPT Changes: An Insider's View* 2016

➔ *CPT Assistant* Nov 15:8

(Do not report 43210 in conjunction with 43180, 43191, 43197, 43200, 43235)

Endoscopic Retrograde Cholangiopancreatography (ERCP)

Report the appropriate code(s) for each service performed. Therapeutic ERCP (43261, 43262, 43263, 43264, 43265, 43274, 43275, 43276, 43277, 43278) includes diagnostic ERCP (43260). ERCP includes guide wire passage when performed. An ERCP is considered complete if one or more of the ductal system(s), (pancreatic/biliary) is visualized. To report ERCP attempted but with unsuccessful cannulation of any ductal system, see 43235-43259, 43266, 43270.

(For percutaneous biliary catheter procedures, see 47490-47544)

Codes 43274, 43275, 43276, and 43277 describe ERCP with stent placement, removal or replacement (exchange) of stent(s), and balloon dilation within the pancreatico-biliary system. For reporting purposes, ducts that may be reported as stented or subject to stent replacement (exchange) or to balloon dilation include:

Pancreas: major and minor ducts

Biliary tree: common bile duct, right hepatic duct, left hepatic duct, cystic duct/gallbladder

ERCP with stent placement includes any balloon dilation performed in that duct. ERCP with more than one stent placement (eg, different ducts or side by side in the same duct) performed during the same day/session may be reported with 43274 more than once with modifier 59 appended to the subsequent procedure(s). For ERCP with more than one stent exchanged during the same day/session, 43276 may be reported for the initial stent exchange, and 43276 with modifier 59 for each additional stent exchange. ERCP with balloon dilation of more than one duct during the same day/session may be reported with modifier 59 appended to the subsequent procedure(s). Sphincteroplasty, which is balloon dilation of the ampulla (sphincter of Oddi), is reported with 43277, and includes sphincterotomy (43262) when performed.

To report ERCP via altered postoperative anatomy, see 43260, 43262, 43263, 43264, 43265, 43273, 43274, 43275, 43276, 43277, 43278, for Billroth II gastroenterostomy. See 47999 (Unlisted procedure, biliary tract) or 48999 (Unlisted procedure, pancreas) for ERCP via gastrostomy (laparoscopic or open) or via Roux-en-Y anatomy (eg, post-bariatric gastric bypass, post-total gastrectomy).

To report optical endomicroscopy of the biliary tract and pancreas, use 0397T. Do not report optical endomicroscopy more than once per session.

Stone destruction includes any stone removal in the same ductal system (biliary/pancreatic). Code 43277 may be separately reported if sphincteroplasty or dilation of a ductal stricture is required before proceeding to remove stones/debris from the duct during the same session. Dilation that is incidental to the passage of an instrument to clear stones or debris is not separately reported.

(Do not report 43277 for use of a balloon catheter to clear stones/debris from a duct. Any dilation of the duct that may occur during this maneuver is considered inherent to the work of 43264 and 43265)

(If imaging of the ductal systems is performed, including images saved to the permanent record and report of the imaging, see 74328, 74329, 74330)

43260 Endoscopic retrograde cholangiopancreatography (ERCP); diagnostic, including collection of specimen(s) by brushing or washing, when performed (separate procedure)

➲ *CPT Changes: An Insider's View* 2014, 2017

➲ *CPT Assistant* Spring 94:5, Oct 04:13, May 08:14, Aug 08:12, Jan 12:12, Jan 13:11, Dec 13:3

(Do not report 43260 in conjunction with 43261, 43262, 43263, 43264, 43265, 43274, 43275, 43276, 43277, 43278)

43261 with biopsy, single or multiple

➲ *CPT Changes: An Insider's View* 2017

➲ *CPT Assistant* Spring 94:5, Aug 08:12, Jun 11:13, Jan 13:11

(Do not report 43261 in conjunction with 43260)

(For percutaneous endoluminal biopsy of biliary tree, use 47543)

43262 with sphincterotomy/papillotomy

➲ *CPT Changes: An Insider's View* 2017

➲ *CPT Assistant* Spring 94:5, Oct 04:13, Jul 09:10, Jan 13:11

(43262 may be reported when sphincterotomy is performed in addition to 43261, 43263, 43264, 43265, 43275, 43278)

(Do not report 43262 in conjunction with 43274 for stent placement or with 43276 for stent replacement [exchange] in the same location)

(Do not report 43262 in conjunction with 43260, 43277)

Endoscopic Retrograde Cholangiopancreatography (ERCP)

43260

Examination of the hepatobiliary system (pancreatic ducts, hepatic ducts, common bile ducts, duodenal papilla [ampulla of Vater] and gallbladder [if present]) is performed through a side-viewing flexible fiberoptic endoscope.

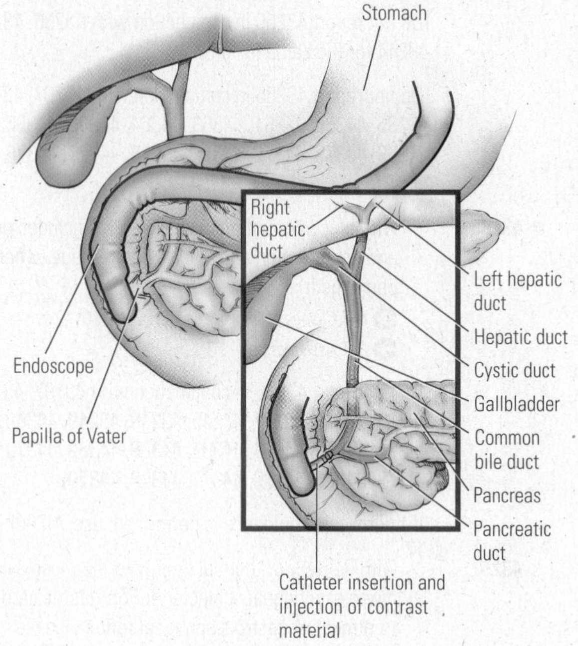

(For percutaneous balloon dilation of biliary duct(s) or of ampulla, use 47542)

43263 with pressure measurement of sphincter of Oddi

➲ *CPT Changes: An Insider's View* 2014, 2017

➲ *CPT Assistant* Spring 94:5, Oct 04:13, Jan 13:11, Dec 13:3

(Do not report 43263 in conjunction with 43260)

(Do not report 43263 more than once per session)

43264 with removal of calculi/debris from biliary/pancreatic duct(s)

➲ *CPT Changes: An Insider's View* 2002, 2014, 2017

➲ *CPT Assistant* Spring 94:5, Jan 13:11, Dec 13:3

(Do not report 43264 if no calculi or debris are found, even if balloon catheter is deployed)

(Do not report 43264 in conjunction with 43260, 43265)

(For percutaneous removal of calculi/debris, use 47544)

43265 with destruction of calculi, any method (eg, mechanical, electrohydraulic, lithotripsy)

➲ *CPT Changes: An Insider's View* 2002, 2014, 2017

➲ *CPT Assistant* Spring 94:5, Jan 13:11, Dec 13:3

(Do not report 43265 in conjunction with 43260, 43264)

(For percutaneous removal of calculi/debris, use 47544)

43266 Code is out of numerical sequence. See 43254-43261

43270 Code is out of numerical sequence. See 43254-43261

 # 43274 with placement of endoscopic stent into biliary or pancreatic duct, including pre- and post-dilation and guide wire passage, when performed, including sphincterotomy, when performed, each stent

➲ *CPT Changes: An Insider's View* 2014, 2017

➲ *CPT Assistant* Dec 13:3

(Do not report 43274 in conjunction with 43262, 43275, 43276, 43277 for stent placement or replacement [exchange] in the same duct)

(For stent placement in both the pancreatic duct and the common bile duct during the same operative session, placement of separate stents in both the right and left hepatic ducts, or placement of two side-by-side stents in the same duct, 43274 may be reported for each additional stent placed, using modifier 59 with the subsequent procedure[s])

(To report naso-biliary or naso-pancreatic drainage tube placement, use 43274)

(For percutaneous placement of biliary stent(s), see 47538, 47539, 47540)

 # 43275 with removal of foreign body(s) or stent(s) from biliary/pancreatic duct(s)

➲ *CPT Changes: An Insider's View* 2014, 2017

➲ *CPT Assistant* Dec 13:3

(Do not report 43275 in conjunction with 43260, 43274, 43276)

(For removal of stent from biliary or pancreatic duct without ERCP, use 43247)

(Report 43275 only once for removal of one or more stents or foreign bodies from biliary/pancreatic duct[s] during the same session)

(For percutaneous removal of calculi/debris, use 47544)

 # 43276 with removal and exchange of stent(s), biliary or pancreatic duct, including pre- and post-dilation and guide wire passage, when performed, including sphincterotomy, when performed, each stent exchanged

➲ *CPT Changes: An Insider's View* 2014, 2017

➲ *CPT Assistant* Dec 13:3

(43276 includes removal and replacement [exchange] of one stent. For replacement [exchange] of additional stent[s] during the same session, report 43276 with modifier 59 for each additional replacement [exchange])

(Do not report 43276 in conjunction with 43260, 43275)

(Do not report 43276 in conjunction with 43262, 43274 for stent placement or exchange in the same duct)

 # 43277 with trans-endoscopic balloon dilation of biliary/pancreatic duct(s) or of ampulla (sphincteroplasty), including sphincterotomy, when performed, each duct

➲ *CPT Changes: An Insider's View* 2014, 2017

➲ *CPT Assistant* Dec 13:3

(Do not report 43277 in conjunction with 43278 for the same lesion)

(Do not report 43277 in conjunction with 43260, 43262)

(Do not report 43277 for incidental dilation using balloon for stone/debris removal performed with 43264, 43265)

(If sphincterotomy without sphincteroplasty is performed on a separate pancreatic duct orifice during the same session [ie, pancreas divisum], report 43262 with modifier 59)

(Do not report 43277 in conjunction with 43274, 43276 for dilation and stent placement/replacement [exchange] in the same duct)

(For transendoscopic balloon dilation of multiple strictures during the same session, use 43277 with modifier 59 for each additional stricture dilated)

(For bilateral balloon dilation [both right and left hepatic ducts], 43277 may be reported twice with modifier 59 appended to the second procedure)

(For percutaneous balloon dilation of biliary duct(s) or of ampulla (sphincteroplasty), use 47542)

 # 43278 with ablation of tumor(s), polyp(s), or other lesion(s), including pre- and post-dilation and guide wire passage, when performed

➲ *CPT Changes: An Insider's View* 2014, 2017

➲ *CPT Assistant* Dec 13:3

(Do not report 43278 in conjunction with 43277 for the same lesion)

(Do not report 43278 in conjunction with 43260)

(For ampullectomy, use 43254)

+ 43273 Endoscopic cannulation of papilla with direct visualization of pancreatic/common bile duct(s) (List separately in addition to code(s) for primary procedure)

➲ *CPT Changes: An Insider's View* 2009, 2014, 2017

➲ *CPT Assistant* Jan 13:11, Dec 13:3

(Report 43273 once per procedure)

(Use 43273 in conjunction with 43260, 43261, 43262, 43263, 43264, 43265, 43274, 43275, 43276, 43277, 43278)

43274 Code is out of numerical sequence. See 43264-43279

43275 Code is out of numerical sequence. See 43264-43279

43276 Code is out of numerical sequence. See 43264-43279

43277 Code is out of numerical sequence. See 43264-43279

43278 Code is out of numerical sequence. See 43264-43279

Laparoscopy

Surgical laparoscopy always includes diagnostic laparoscopy. To report a diagnostic laparoscopy (peritoneoscopy) (separate procedure), use 49320.

43279 Laparoscopy, surgical, esophagomyotomy (Heller type), with fundoplasty, when performed

➲ *CPT Changes: An Insider's View* 2009

➲ *CPT Assistant* Feb 12:3

(For open approach, see 43330, 43331)

(Do not report 43279 in conjunction with 43280)

43280 Laparoscopy, surgical, esophagogastric fundoplasty (eg, Nissen, Toupet procedures)

➔ *CPT Changes: An Insider's View* 2000

➔ *CPT Assistant* Nov 99:22, Mar 00:8, Dec 02:2, Jun 11:8, Feb 12:3, Dec 14:16, Nov 15:8

(Do not report 43280 in conjunction with 43279, 43281, 43282)

(For open esophagogastric fundoplasty, see 43327, 43328)

(For laparoscopy, surgical, esophageal sphincter augmentation procedure, placement of sphincter augmentation device, see43284, 43285)

(For esophagogastroduodenoscopy fundoplasty, partial or complete, transoral approach, use 43210)

Laparoscopic Fundoplasty

43280

With the esophagus and fundus held aside, sutures are placed in both crus diaphragmatis muscles below the esophagus to bring them together to close the hiatal hernia, and the anterior and posterior walls of the fundus are wrapped and stitched around the esophagus to complete the laparoscopic fundoplasty.

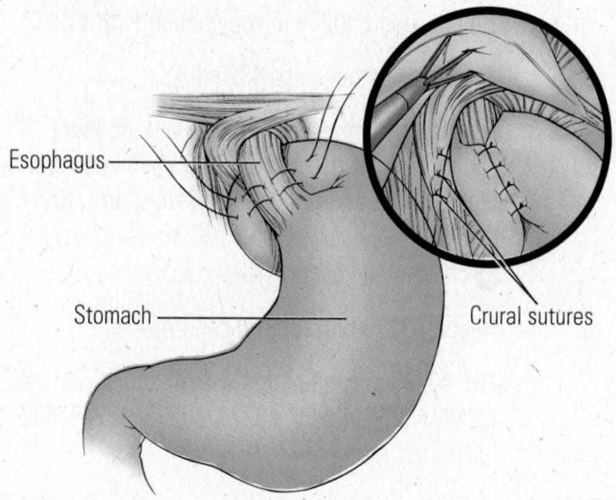

43281 Laparoscopy, surgical, repair of paraesophageal hernia, includes fundoplasty, when performed; without implantation of mesh

➔ *CPT Changes: An Insider's View* 2010

➔ *CPT Assistant* Jun 11:9, Feb 12:3, Dec 14:16

43282 with implantation of mesh

➔ *CPT Changes: An Insider's View* 2010

➔ *CPT Assistant* Jun 11:9, Feb 12:3, Dec 14:16, Aug 16:9

(To report transabdominal paraesophageal hiatal hernia repair, see 43332, 43333)

(To report transthoracic diaphragmatic hernia repair, see 43334, 43335)

(Do not report 43281, 43282 in conjunction with 43280, 43450, 43453)

+ 43283 Laparoscopy, surgical, esophageal lengthening procedure (eg, Collis gastroplasty or wedge gastroplasty) (List separately in addition to code for primary procedure)

➔ *CPT Changes: An Insider's View* 2011

➔ *CPT Assistant* Jun 11:9, Feb 12:3

(Use 43283 in conjunction with 43280, 43281, 43282)

43284 Laparoscopy, surgical, esophageal sphincter augmentation procedure, placement of sphincter augmentation device (ie, magnetic band), including cruroplasty when performed

➔ *CPT Changes: An Insider's View* 2017

➔ *CPT Assistant* Aug 17:6

(Do not report 43284 in conjunction with 43279, 43280, 43281, 43282)

Laparoscopic Esophageal Sphincter Augmentation

43284

Implanted magnetic sphincter augmentation device

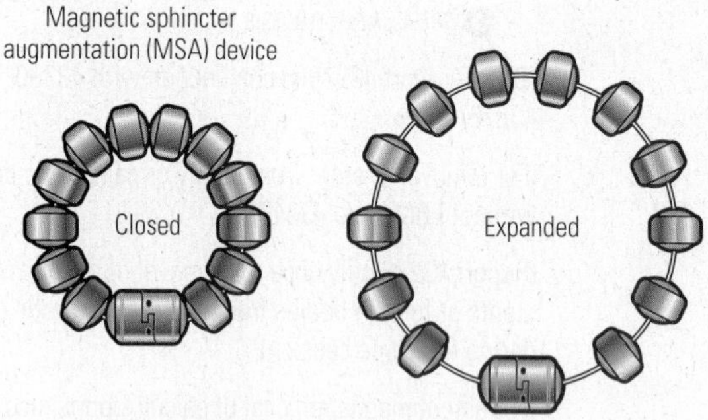

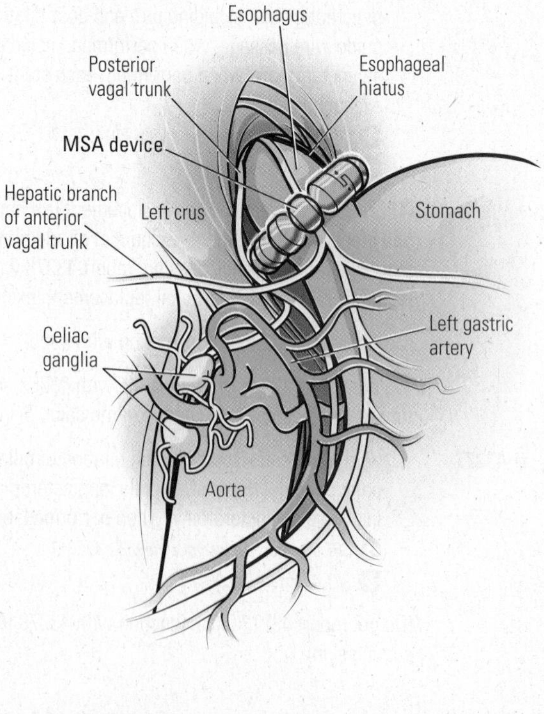

43285 Removal of esophageal sphincter augmentation device
➔ *CPT Changes: An Insider's View* 2017
➔ *CPT Assistant* Aug 17:6

43286 Esophagectomy, total or near total, with laparoscopic mobilization of the abdominal and mediastinal esophagus and proximal gastrectomy, with laparoscopic pyloric drainage procedure if performed, with open cervical pharyngogastrostomy or esophagogastrostomy (ie, laparoscopic transhiatal esophagectomy)
➔ *CPT Changes: An Insider's View* 2018

43287 Esophagectomy, distal two-thirds, with laparoscopic mobilization of the abdominal and lower mediastinal esophagus and proximal gastrectomy, with laparoscopic pyloric drainage procedure if performed, with separate thoracoscopic mobilization of the middle and upper mediastinal esophagus and thoracic esophagogastrostomy (ie, laparoscopic thoracoscopic esophagectomy, Ivor Lewis esophagectomy)
➔ *CPT Changes: An Insider's View* 2018

(Do not report 43287 in conjunction with 32551 for right tube thoracostomy)

43288 Esophagectomy, total or near total, with thoracoscopic mobilization of the upper, middle, and lower mediastinal esophagus, with separate laparoscopic proximal gastrectomy, with laparoscopic pyloric drainage procedure if performed, with open cervical pharyngogastrostomy or esophagogastrostomy (ie, thoracoscopic, laparoscopic and cervical incision esophagectomy, McKeown esophagectomy, tri-incisional esophagectomy)
➔ *CPT Changes: An Insider's View* 2018

(Do not report 43288 in conjunction with 32551 for right tube thoracostomy)

43289 Unlisted laparoscopy procedure, esophagus
➔ *CPT Changes: An Insider's View* 2000
➔ *CPT Assistant* Nov 99:22, Mar 00:8, Dec 14:16

Repair

43300 Esophagoplasty (plastic repair or reconstruction), cervical approach; without repair of tracheoesophageal fistula

43305 with repair of tracheoesophageal fistula

43310 Esophagoplasty (plastic repair or reconstruction), thoracic approach; without repair of tracheoesophageal fistula

43312 with repair of tracheoesophageal fistula

43313 Esophagoplasty for congenital defect (plastic repair or reconstruction), thoracic approach; without repair of congenital tracheoesophageal fistula
➔ *CPT Changes: An Insider's View* 2002

43314 with repair of congenital tracheoesophageal fistula
➔ *CPT Changes: An Insider's View* 2002

(Do not report modifier 63 in conjunction with 43313, 43314)

43320 Esophagogastrostomy (cardioplasty), with or without vagotomy and pyloroplasty, transabdominal or transthoracic approach

(For laparoscopic procedure, use 43280)

43325 Esophagogastric fundoplasty, with fundic patch (Thal-Nissen procedure)
➔ *CPT Assistant* Winter 90:6

(For cricopharyngeal myotomy, use 43030)

43327 Esophagogastric fundoplasty partial or complete; laparotomy
➔ *CPT Changes: An Insider's View* 2011
➔ *CPT Assistant* Jun 11:8, Feb 12:3, Nov 15:8

43328 thoracotomy
➔ *CPT Changes: An Insider's View* 2011
➔ *CPT Assistant* Jun 11:8, Feb 12:3, Nov 15:8

(For esophagogastroduodenoscopy fundoplasty, partial or complete, transoral approach, use 43210)

Nissen Fundoplasty
43327, 43328

The lower esophagus is accessed through an upper abdominal or lower thoracic incision. The fundus of the stomach is mobilized and wrapped around the lower esophageal sphincter, and the wrap is sutured into place.

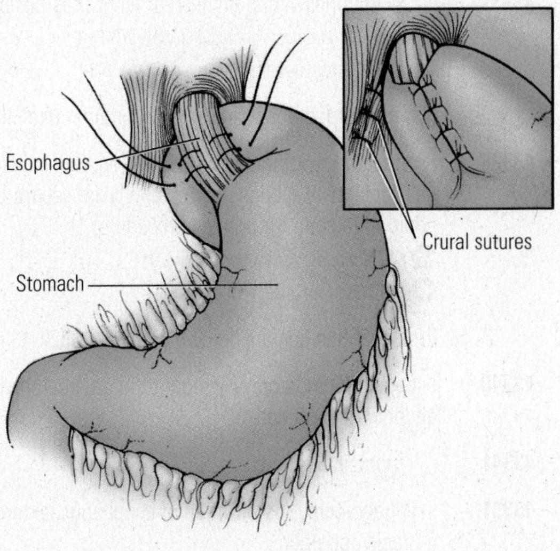

43330 Esophagomyotomy (Heller type); abdominal approach
➔ *CPT Changes: An Insider's View* 2000
➔ *CPT Assistant* Nov 99:22

(For laparoscopic esophagomyotomy procedure, use 43279)

43331 thoracic approach
➔ *CPT Changes: An Insider's View* 2000
➔ *CPT Assistant* Nov 99:22

(For thoracoscopic esophagomyotomy, use 32665)

Digestive 40490-49999

43332 Repair, paraesophageal hiatal hernia (including fundoplication), via laparotomy, except neonatal; without implantation of mesh or other prosthesis
➔ *CPT Changes: An Insider's View* 2011
➔ *CPT Assistant* Feb 12:3

43333 with implantation of mesh or other prosthesis
➔ *CPT Changes: An Insider's View* 2011
➔ *CPT Assistant* Feb 12:3

(For neonatal diaphragmatic hernia repair, use 39503)

43334 Repair, paraesophageal hiatal hernia (including fundoplication), via thoracotomy, except neonatal; without implantation of mesh or other prosthesis
➔ *CPT Changes: An Insider's View* 2011
➔ *CPT Assistant* Feb 12:3

43335 with implantation of mesh or other prosthesis
➔ *CPT Changes: An Insider's View* 2011
➔ *CPT Assistant* Feb 12:3

(For neonatal diaphragmatic hernia repair, use 39503)

43336 Repair, paraesophageal hiatal hernia, (including fundoplication), via thoracoabdominal incision, except neonatal; without implantation of mesh or other prosthesis
➔ *CPT Changes: An Insider's View* 2011
➔ *CPT Assistant* Feb 12:3

43337 with implantation of mesh or other prosthesis
➔ *CPT Changes: An Insider's View* 2011
➔ *CPT Assistant* Feb 12:3

(For neonatal diaphragmatic hernia repair, use 39503)

+ 43338 Esophageal lengthening procedure (eg, Collis gastroplasty or wedge gastroplasty) (List separately in addition to code for primary procedure)
➔ *CPT Changes: An Insider's View* 2011
➔ *CPT Assistant* Jun 11:10, Feb 12:3

(Use 43338 in conjunction with 43280, 43327-43337)

43340 Esophagojejunostomy (without total gastrectomy); abdominal approach

43341 thoracic approach

43351 Esophagostomy, fistulization of esophagus, external; thoracic approach
➔ *CPT Changes: An Insider's View* 2015

43352 cervical approach
➔ *CPT Changes: An Insider's View* 2015

43360 Gastrointestinal reconstruction for previous esophagectomy, for obstructing esophageal lesion or fistula, or for previous esophageal exclusion; with stomach, with or without pyloroplasty

43361 with colon interposition or small intestine reconstruction, including intestine mobilization, preparation, and anastomosis(es)
➔ *CPT Changes: An Insider's View* 2002

43400 Ligation, direct, esophageal varices

43401 Transection of esophagus with repair, for esophageal varices

43405 Ligation or stapling at gastroesophageal junction for pre-existing esophageal perforation

43410 Suture of esophageal wound or injury; cervical approach
➔ *CPT Assistant* Jun 96:7

43415 transthoracic or transabdominal approach

43420 Closure of esophagostomy or fistula; cervical approach

43425 transthoracic or transabdominal approach

(To report transabdominal paraesophageal hiatal hernia repair, see 43332, 43333. To report transthoracic diaphragmatic hernia repair, see 43334, 43335)

Manipulation

(For associated esophagogram, use 74220)

43450 Dilation of esophagus, by unguided sound or bougie, single or multiple passes
➔ *CPT Changes: An Insider's View* 2014
➔ *CPT Assistant* Spring 94:1, Jan 97:10, Apr 98:14, Jun 98:10, Dec 13:3, Jul 17:10

(For radiological supervision and interpretation, use 74360)

43453 Dilation of esophagus, over guide wire
➔ *CPT Changes: An Insider's View* 2017
➔ *CPT Assistant* Spring 94:1, Jan 97:10, Dec 97:11

(For dilation with endoscopic visualization, see 43195, 43226)

(For dilation of esophagus, by balloon or dilator, see 43214, 43220, 43233, 43249)

(For radiological supervision and interpretation, use 74360)

(For endoscopic dilation of esophagus with balloon less than 30 mm diameter, see 43195, 43220, 43249)

(For endoscopic dilation of esophagus with balloon 30 mm diameter or larger, see 43214, 43233)

43460 Esophagogastric tamponade, with balloon (Sengstaken type)
➔ *CPT Changes: An Insider's View* 2009

(For removal of esophageal foreign body by balloon catheter, see 43499, 74235)

Other Procedures

43496 Free jejunum transfer with microvascular anastomosis
➔ *CPT Assistant* Nov 96:8, Apr 97:4, Jun 97:10, Nov 97:17, Nov 98:16

(Do not report code 69990 in addition to code 43496)

43499 Unlisted procedure, esophagus
➔ *CPT Assistant* May 07:10, Oct 10:12, Dec 10:12, May 11:9, Dec 11:19, Mar 13:13, Nov 15:8, 11

Stomach

Incision

43500 Gastrotomy; with exploration or foreign body removal

43501 with suture repair of bleeding ulcer

43502 with suture repair of pre-existing esophagogastric laceration (eg, Mallory-Weiss)

43510 with esophageal dilation and insertion of permanent intraluminal tube (eg, Celestin or Mousseaux-Barbin)

43520 Pyloromyotomy, cutting of pyloric muscle (Fredet-Ramstedt type operation)

(Do not report modifier 63 in conjunction with 43520)

Excision

43605 Biopsy of stomach, by laparotomy
CPT Changes: An Insider's View 2011

43610 Excision, local; ulcer or benign tumor of stomach

43611 malignant tumor of stomach

43620 Gastrectomy, total; with esophagoenterostomy

43621 with Roux-en-Y reconstruction

43622 with formation of intestinal pouch, any type

43631 Gastrectomy, partial, distal; with gastroduodenostomy

43632 with gastrojejunostomy

43633 with Roux-en-Y reconstruction

43634 with formation of intestinal pouch

+ 43635 Vagotomy when performed with partial distal gastrectomy (List separately in addition to code[s] for primary procedure)
CPT Assistant Nov 97:17

(Use 43635 in conjunction with 43631, 43632, 43633, 43634)

43640 Vagotomy including pyloroplasty, with or without gastrostomy; truncal or selective

(For pyloroplasty, use 43800)

(For vagotomy, see 64755, 64760)

43641 parietal cell (highly selective)

(For upper gastrointestinal endoscopy, see 43235-43259)

Laparoscopy

Surgical laparoscopy always includes diagnostic laparoscopy. To report a diagnostic laparoscopy (peritoneoscopy) (separate procedure), use 49320.

(For upper gastrointestinal endoscopy including esophagus, stomach, and either the duodenum and/or jejunum, see 43235-43259)

43644 Laparoscopy, surgical, gastric restrictive procedure; with gastric bypass and Roux-en-Y gastroenterostomy (roux limb 150 cm or less)
CPT Changes: An Insider's View 2005
CPT Assistant May 05:3

(Do not report 43644 in conjunction with 43846, 49320)

(Esophagogastroduodenoscopy [EGD] performed for a separate condition should be reported with modifier 59)

(For greater than 150 cm, use 43645)

(For open procedure, use 43846)

43645 with gastric bypass and small intestine reconstruction to limit absorption
CPT Changes: An Insider's View 2005
CPT Assistant May 05:3

(Do not report 43645 in conjunction with 49320, 43847)

43647 Laparoscopy, surgical; implantation or replacement of gastric neurostimulator electrodes, antrum
CPT Changes: An Insider's View 2007
CPT Assistant Mar 07:4

43648 revision or removal of gastric neurostimulator electrodes, antrum
CPT Changes: An Insider's View 2007
CPT Assistant Mar 07:4

(For open approach, see 43881, 43882)

(For insertion of gastric neurostimulator pulse generator, use 64590)

(For revision or removal of gastric neurostimulator pulse generator, use 64595)

(For electronic analysis and programming of gastric neurostimulator pulse generator, see 95980-95982)

(For laparoscopic implantation, revision, or removal of gastric neurostimulator electrodes, lesser curvature [morbid obesity], use 43659)

(For laparoscopic implantation, revision, replacement, or removal of vagus nerve blocking neurostimulator electrode array and/or pulse generator at the esophagogastric junction, see 0312T-0317T)

43651 Laparoscopy, surgical; transection of vagus nerves, truncal
CPT Changes: An Insider's View 2000
CPT Assistant Nov 99:22, Mar 00:8

43652 transection of vagus nerves, selective or highly selective
CPT Changes: An Insider's View 2000
CPT Assistant Nov 99:22, Mar 00:8

43653 gastrostomy, without construction of gastric tube (eg, Stamm procedure) (separate procedure)
CPT Changes: An Insider's View 2000
CPT Assistant Nov 99:22, Mar 00:8

43659 Unlisted laparoscopy procedure, stomach
➲ *CPT Changes: An Insider's View* 2000
➲ *CPT Assistant* Nov 99:22, Mar 00:8, Apr 06:19, Jun 06:16, Dec 07:12, Jun 11:8, Dec 11:19, Feb 13:13, Jun 13:13

Introduction

43752 Naso- or oro-gastric tube placement, requiring physician's skill and fluoroscopic guidance (includes fluoroscopy, image documentation and report)
➲ *CPT Changes: An Insider's View* 2001, 2004
➲ *CPT Assistant* Jan 02:11, Apr 03:7, Oct 03:2, Jul 06:4, Feb 07:10, Jul 07:1, Aug 08:7, Sep 11:4, May 14:4, Mar 18:11

(Do not report 43752 in conjunction with critical care codes 99291-99292, neonatal critical care codes 99468, 99469, pediatric critical care codes 99471, 99472 or low birth weight intensive care service codes 99478, 99479)

(For percutaneous placement of gastrostomy tube, use 49440)

(For enteric tube placement, see 44500, 74340)

43753 Gastric intubation and aspiration(s) therapeutic, necessitating physician's skill (eg, for gastrointestinal hemorrhage), including lavage if performed
➲ *CPT Changes: An Insider's View* 2011
➲ *CPT Assistant* Sep 11:3, May 14:4

Gastric Intubation
43753

A large-bore gastric lavage tube is inserted orally through the esophagus into the stomach for expedient lavage and evacuation of stomach contents (eg, poisonings, hemorrhage).

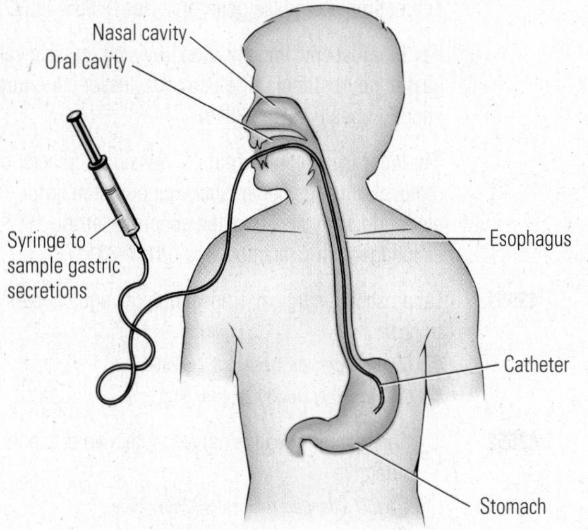

43754 Gastric intubation and aspiration, diagnostic; single specimen (eg, acid analysis)
➲ *CPT Changes: An Insider's View* 2011
➲ *CPT Assistant* Dec 10:10, Sep 11:3

43755 collection of multiple fractional specimens with gastric stimulation, single or double lumen tube (gastric secretory study) (eg, histamine, insulin, pentagastrin, calcium, secretin), includes drug administration
➲ *CPT Changes: An Insider's View* 2011
➲ *CPT Assistant* Dec 10:10, Sep 11:3

(For gastric acid analysis, use 82930)

(For naso- or oro-gastric tube placement by physician with fluoroscopic guidance, use 43752)

(Report the drug[s] or substance[s] administered. The fluid used to administer the drug[s] is not separately reported)

43756 Duodenal intubation and aspiration, diagnostic, includes image guidance; single specimen (eg, bile study for crystals or afferent loop culture)
➲ *CPT Changes: An Insider's View* 2011
➲ *CPT Assistant* Dec 10:10, Sep 11:3

43757 collection of multiple fractional specimens with pancreatic or gallbladder stimulation, single or double lumen tube, includes drug administration
➲ *CPT Changes: An Insider's View* 2011
➲ *CPT Assistant* Dec 10:10, Sep 11:3

(For appropriate chemical analysis procedures, see 89049-89240)

(Report the substances[s] or drug[s] administered. The fluid used to administer the drug[s] is not separately reported)

►(43760 has been deleted. To report replacement of gastrostomy tube without imaging or endoscopy, see 43762, 43763)◄

(To report fluoroscopically guided replacement of gastrostomy tube, use 49450)

(For endoscopic placement of gastrostomy tube, use 43246)

43761 Repositioning of a naso- or oro-gastric feeding tube, through the duodenum for enteric nutrition
➲ *CPT Changes: An Insider's View* 2000, 2008, 2010
➲ *CPT Assistant* Oct 96:9, Nov 99:22, Jun 08:8, Aug 08:7

(Do not report 43761 in conjunction with 44500, 49446)

(If imaging guidance is performed, use 76000)

(For endoscopic conversion of a gastrostomy tube to jejunostomy tube, use 44373)

(For placement of a long gastrointestinal tube into the duodenum, use 44500)

● **43762** Replacement of gastrostomy tube, percutaneous, includes removal, when performed, without imaging or endoscopic guidance; not requiring revision of gastrostomy tract
➲ *CPT Changes: An Insider's View* 2019

● **43763** requiring revision of gastrostomy tract

CPT Changes: An Insider's View 2019

►(For percutaneous replacement of gastrostomy tube under fluoroscopic guidance, use 49450)◄

►(For endoscopically directed placement of gastrostomy tube, use 43246)◄

Bariatric Surgery

Bariatric surgical procedures may involve the stomach, duodenum, jejunum, and/or the ileum.

Laparoscopy

Surgical laparoscopy always includes diagnostic laparoscopy. To report a diagnostic laparoscopy (separate procedure), use 49320.

Typical postoperative follow-up care (see Surgery Guidelines, CPT Surgical Package Definition) after gastric restriction using the adjustable gastric restrictive device includes subsequent restrictive device adjustment(s) through the postoperative period for the typical patient. Adjustment consists of changing the gastric restrictive device component diameter by injection or aspiration of fluid through the subcutaneous port component.

43770 Laparoscopy, surgical, gastric restrictive procedure; placement of adjustable gastric restrictive device (eg, gastric band and subcutaneous port components)

CPT Changes: An Insider's View 2006, 2008

CPT Assistant Dec 10:13

(For individual component placement, report 43770 with modifier 52)

43771 revision of adjustable gastric restrictive device component only

CPT Changes: An Insider's View 2006, 2008

43772 removal of adjustable gastric restrictive device component only

CPT Changes: An Insider's View 2006, 2008

43773 removal and replacement of adjustable gastric restrictive device component only

CPT Changes: An Insider's View 2006, 2008

(Do not report 43773 in conjunction with 43772)

43774 removal of adjustable gastric restrictive device and subcutaneous port components

CPT Changes: An Insider's View 2006, 2008

(For removal and replacement of both gastric band and subcutaneous port components, use 43659)

43775 longitudinal gastrectomy (ie, sleeve gastrectomy)

CPT Changes: An Insider's View 2010

(For open gastric restrictive procedure, without gastric bypass, for morbid obesity, other than vertical-banded gastroplasty, use 43843)

(For laparoscopic implantation, revision, replacement, removal or reprogramming of vagus nerve blocking neurostimulator electrode array and/or pulse generator at the esophagogastric junction, see 0312T-0317T)

Other Procedures

43800 Pyloroplasty

(For pyloroplasty and vagotomy, use 43640)

43810 Gastroduodenostomy

43820 Gastrojejunostomy; without vagotomy

43825 with vagotomy, any type

43830 Gastrostomy, open; without construction of gastric tube (eg, Stamm procedure) (separate procedure)

CPT Changes: An Insider's View 2000

CPT Assistant Nov 99:22

43831 neonatal, for feeding

CPT Changes: An Insider's View 2000

CPT Assistant Nov 99:22

►(For percutaneous replacement of gastrostomy tube with removal when performed without imaging or endoscopy, see 43762, 43763)◄

►(For percutaneous replacement of gastrostomy tube under fluoroscopic guidance, use 49450)◄

(Do not report modifier 63 in conjunction with 43831)

43832 with construction of gastric tube (eg, Janeway procedure)

CPT Changes: An Insider's View 2000

CPT Assistant Nov 99:22

(For percutaneous endoscopic gastrostomy, use 43246)

43840 Gastrorrhaphy, suture of perforated duodenal or gastric ulcer, wound, or injury

43842 Gastric restrictive procedure, without gastric bypass, for morbid obesity; vertical-banded gastroplasty

CPT Assistant May 98:5

43843 other than vertical-banded gastroplasty

CPT Assistant May 98:5

(For laparoscopic longitudinal gastrectomy [ie, sleeve gastrectomy], use 43775)

43845 Gastric restrictive procedure with partial gastrectomy, pylorus-preserving duodenoileostomy and ileoileostomy (50 to 100 cm common channel) to limit absorption (biliopancreatic diversion with duodenal switch)

CPT Changes: An Insider's View 2005

CPT Assistant May 05:3

(Do not report 43845 in conjunction with 43633, 43847, 44130, 49000)

43846 Gastric restrictive procedure, with gastric bypass for morbid obesity; with short limb (150 cm or less) Roux-en-Y gastroenterostomy
- ➲ *CPT Changes: An Insider's View* 2005
- ➲ *CPT Assistant* May 98:5, May 05:3

(For greater than 150 cm, use 43847)

(For laparoscopic procedure, use 43644)

Gastric Bypass for Morbid Obesity
43846

The stomach is partitioned with a staple line on the lesser curvature (no band, no gastric transection). A short limb of small bowel (less than 100 cm) is divided and anastomosed to the small upper stomach pouch.

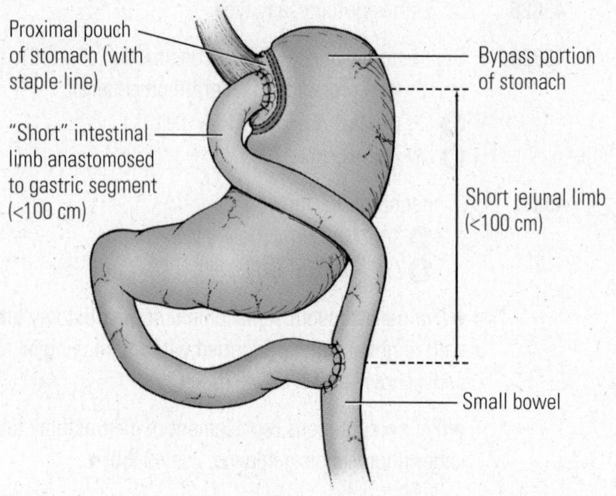

43847 with small intestine reconstruction to limit absorption
- ➲ *CPT Changes: An Insider's View* 2015
- ➲ *CPT Assistant* May 98:5, May 02:7

43848 Revision, open, of gastric restrictive procedure for morbid obesity, other than adjustable gastric restrictive device (separate procedure)
- ➲ *CPT Changes: An Insider's View* 2006, 2008
- ➲ *CPT Assistant* May 98:5, Apr 06:1

(For laparoscopic adjustable gastric restrictive procedures, see 43770-43774)

(For gastric restrictive port procedures, see 43886-43888)

43850 Revision of gastroduodenal anastomosis (gastroduodenostomy) with reconstruction; without vagotomy

43855 with vagotomy

43860 Revision of gastrojejunal anastomosis (gastrojejunostomy) with reconstruction, with or without partial gastrectomy or intestine resection; without vagotomy
- ➲ *CPT Changes: An Insider's View* 2002

43865 with vagotomy

43870 Closure of gastrostomy, surgical

43880 Closure of gastrocolic fistula

43881 Implantation or replacement of gastric neurostimulator electrodes, antrum, open
- ➲ *CPT Changes: An Insider's View* 2007
- ➲ *CPT Assistant* Mar 07:4

43882 Revision or removal of gastric neurostimulator electrodes, antrum, open
- ➲ *CPT Changes: An Insider's View* 2007
- ➲ *CPT Assistant* Mar 07:4

(For laparoscopic approach, see 43647, 43648)

(For insertion of gastric neurostimulator pulse generator, use 64590)

(For revision or removal of gastric neurostimulator pulse generator, use 64595)

(For electronic analysis and programming of gastric neurostimulator pulse generator, see 95980-95982)

(For open implantation, revision, or removal of gastric neurostimulator electrodes, lesser curvature [morbid obesity], use 43999)

(For laparoscopic implantation, revision, replacement, removal or reprogramming of vagus nerve blocking neurostimulator electrode array and/or pulse generator at the esophagogastric junction, see 0312T-0317T)

(For open implantation, revision, or removal of gastric lesser curvature or vagal trunk (EGJ) neurostimulator electrodes, [morbid obesity], use 43999)

43886 Gastric restrictive procedure, open; revision of subcutaneous port component only
- ➲ *CPT Changes: An Insider's View* 2006

43887 removal of subcutaneous port component only
- ➲ *CPT Changes: An Insider's View* 2006

43888 removal and replacement of subcutaneous port component only
- ➲ *CPT Changes: An Insider's View* 2006

(Do not report 43888 in conjunction with 43774, 43887)

(For laparoscopic removal of both gastric restrictive device and subcutaneous port components, use 43774)

(For removal and replacement of both gastric restrictive device and subcutaneous port components, use 43659)

43999 Unlisted procedure, stomach
- ➲ *CPT Assistant* Mar 10:10, Jun 11:13, Feb 13:13

Intestines (Except Rectum)

Incision

44005 Enterolysis (freeing of intestinal adhesion) (separate procedure)
- ➲ *CPT Changes: An Insider's View* 2000
- ➲ *CPT Assistant* Winter 90:6, Nov 97:17, Nov 99:23, Jan 00:11, Apr 00:10, Feb 18:11

(Do not report 44005 in addition to 45136)

(For laparoscopic approach, use 44180)

44010 Duodenotomy, for exploration, biopsy(s), or foreign body removal

+ 44015 Tube or needle catheter jejunostomy for enteral alimentation, intraoperative, any method (List separately in addition to primary procedure)

➔ *CPT Assistant* Mar 02:10, Jul 10:10

44020 Enterotomy, small intestine, other than duodenum; for exploration, biopsy(s), or foreign body removal

➔ *CPT Changes: An Insider's View* 2002

44021 for decompression (eg, Baker tube)

44025 Colotomy, for exploration, biopsy(s), or foreign body removal

(For exteriorization of intestine (Mikulicz resection with crushing of spur), see 44602-44605)

44050 Reduction of volvulus, intussusception, internal hernia, by laparotomy

44055 Correction of malrotation by lysis of duodenal bands and/or reduction of midgut volvulus (eg, Ladd procedure)

(Do not report modifier 63 in conjunction with 44055)

Excision

Intestinal allotransplantation involves three distinct components of physician work:

1. ***Cadaver donor enterectomy,*** which includes harvesting the intestine graft and cold preservation of the graft (perfusing with cold preservation solution and cold maintenance) (use 44132). ***Living donor enterectomy,*** which includes harvesting the intestine graft, cold preservation of the graft (perfusing with cold preservation solution and cold maintenance), and care of the donor (use 44133).
2. ***Backbench work:***

   Standard preparation of an intestine allograft prior to transplantation includes mobilization and fashioning of the superior mesenteric artery and vein (see 44715).

   Additional reconstruction of an intestine allograft prior to transplantation may include venous and/or arterial anastomosis(es) (see 44720-44721).
3. ***Recipient intestinal allotransplantation with or without recipient enterectomy,*** which includes transplantation of allograft and care of the recipient (see 44135, 44136).

44100 Biopsy of intestine by capsule, tube, peroral (1 or more specimens)

44110 Excision of 1 or more lesions of small or large intestine not requiring anastomosis, exteriorization, or fistulization; single enterotomy

➔ *CPT Changes: An Insider's View* 2002

44111 multiple enterotomies

44120 Enterectomy, resection of small intestine; single resection and anastomosis

➔ *CPT Assistant* Mar 04:3, Aug 08:7

+ 44121 each additional resection and anastomosis (List separately in addition to code for primary procedure)

(Use 44121 in conjunction with 44120)

44125 with enterostomy

44126 Enterectomy, resection of small intestine for congenital atresia, single resection and anastomosis of proximal segment of intestine; without tapering

➔ *CPT Changes: An Insider's View* 2002

44127 with tapering

➔ *CPT Changes: An Insider's View* 2002

Enterectomy, Resection for Congenital Atresia
44127

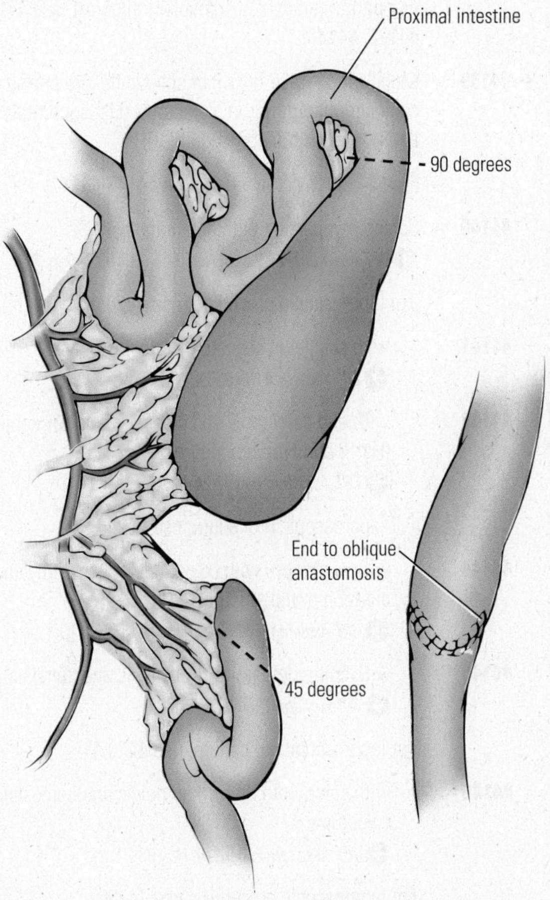

+ 44128 each additional resection and anastomosis (List separately in addition to code for primary procedure)

➔ *CPT Changes: An Insider's View* 2002

(Use 44128 in conjunction with 44126, 44127)

(Do not report modifier 63 in conjunction with 44126, 44127, 44128)

44130 Enteroenterostomy, anastomosis of intestine, with or without cutaneous enterostomy (separate procedure)

44132 Donor enterectomy (including cold preservation), open; from cadaver donor
➲ *CPT Changes: An Insider's View* 2001, 2005

44133 partial, from living donor
➲ *CPT Changes: An Insider's View* 2001

(For backbench intestinal graft preparation or reconstruction, see 44715, 44720, 44721)

44135 Intestinal allotransplantation; from cadaver donor
➲ *CPT Changes: An Insider's View* 2001

44136 from living donor
➲ *CPT Changes: An Insider's View* 2001

44137 Removal of transplanted intestinal allograft, complete
➲ *CPT Changes: An Insider's View* 2005

(For partial removal of transplant allograft, see 44120, 44121, 44140)

+ 44139 Mobilization (take-down) of splenic flexure performed in conjunction with partial colectomy (List separately in addition to primary procedure)

(Use 44139 in conjunction with 44140-44147)

44140 Colectomy, partial; with anastomosis
➲ *CPT Assistant* Fall 92:23, Aug 08:7, Nov 08:7, Sep 10:7

(For laparoscopic procedure, use 44204)

44141 with skin level cecostomy or colostomy
➲ *CPT Assistant* Fall 92:24, Nov 08:7

44143 with end colostomy and closure of distal segment (Hartmann type procedure)
➲ *CPT Assistant* Fall 92:24, Nov 08:7

(For laparoscopic procedure, use 44206)

44144 with resection, with colostomy or ileostomy and creation of mucofistula
➲ *CPT Assistant* Fall 92:24, Nov 08:7

44145 with coloproctostomy (low pelvic anastomosis)
➲ *CPT Assistant* Fall 92:24

(For laparoscopic procedure, use 44207)

44146 with coloproctostomy (low pelvic anastomosis), with colostomy
➲ *CPT Assistant* Fall 92:24, Nov 08:7

(For laparoscopic procedure, use 44208)

44147 abdominal and transanal approach
➲ *CPT Assistant* Fall 92:24, Nov 08:7

44150 Colectomy, total, abdominal, without proctectomy; with ileostomy or ileoproctostomy

(For laparoscopic procedure, use 44210)

Colectomy, Partial
44140

A segment of the colon is resected and an anastomosis is performed between the remaining ends of the colon.

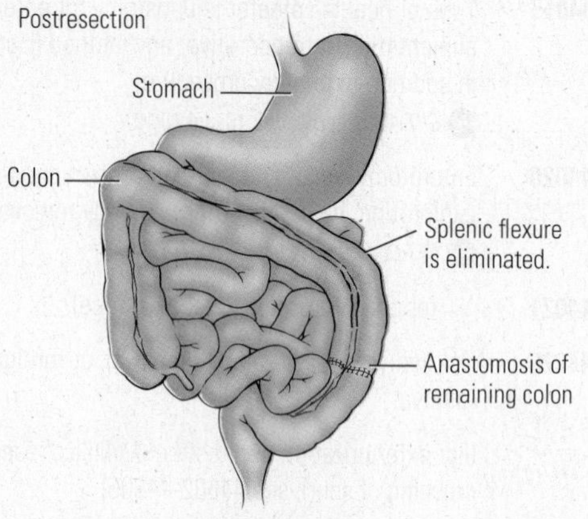

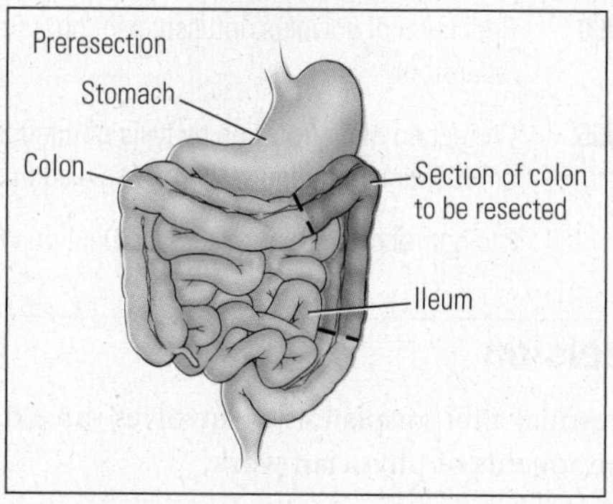

44151 with continent ileostomy

44155 Colectomy, total, abdominal, with proctectomy; with ileostomy

(For laparoscopic procedure, use 44212)

44156 with continent ileostomy

44157 with ileoanal anastomosis, includes loop ileostomy, and rectal mucosectomy, when performed
➲ *CPT Changes: An Insider's View* 2007

44158 with ileoanal anastomosis, creation of ileal reservoir (S or J), includes loop ileostomy, and rectal mucosectomy, when performed
➲ *CPT Changes: An Insider's View* 2007

(For laparoscopic procedure, use 44211)

44160 Colectomy, partial, with removal of terminal ileum with ileocolostomy
➲ *CPT Changes: An Insider's View* 2002

(For laparoscopic procedure, use 44205)

Laparoscopy

Surgical laparoscopy always includes diagnostic laparoscopy. To report a diagnostic laparoscopy (peritoneoscopy) (separate procedure), use 49320.

Colectomy With Removal of Terminal Ileum and Ileocolostomy
44160

A segment of the colon and terminal ileum is removed and an anastomosis is performed between the remaining ileum and colon.

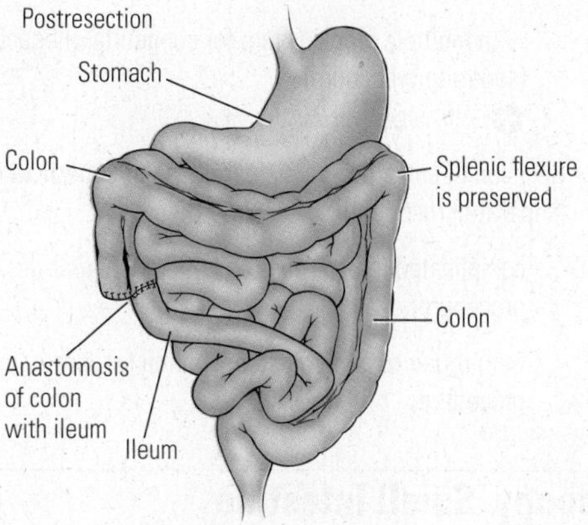

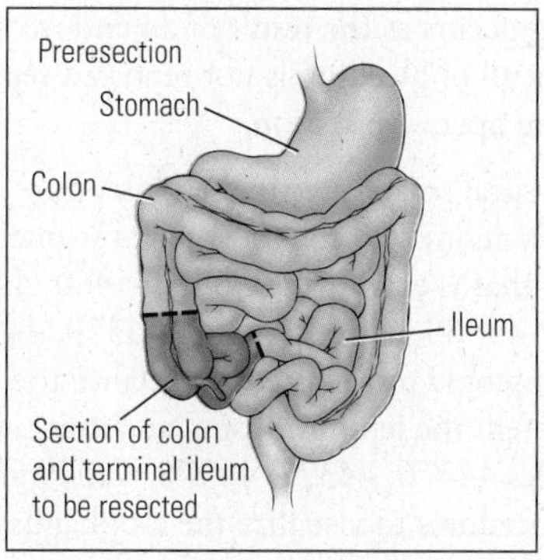

Incision

44180 Laparoscopy, surgical, enterolysis (freeing of intestinal adhesion) (separate procedure)
➔ *CPT Changes: An Insider's View* 2006
➔ *CPT Assistant* Feb 18:11

(For laparoscopy with salpingolysis, ovariolysis, use 58660)

Enterostomy—External Fistulization of Intestines

44186 Laparoscopy, surgical; jejunostomy (eg, for decompression or feeding)
➔ *CPT Changes: An Insider's View* 2006

44187 ileostomy or jejunostomy, non-tube
➔ *CPT Changes: An Insider's View* 2006

(For open procedure, use 44310)

44188 Laparoscopy, surgical, colostomy or skin level cecostomy
➔ *CPT Changes: An Insider's View* 2006

(For open procedure, use 44320)

(Do not report 44188 in conjunction with 44970)

Excision

44202 Laparoscopy, surgical; enterectomy, resection of small intestine, single resection and anastomosis
➔ *CPT Changes: An Insider's View* 2000, 2002, 2006
➔ *CPT Assistant* Nov 99:23, Mar 00:9, May 03:2, Apr 06:1

+ 44203 each additional small intestine resection and anastomosis (List separately in addition to code for primary procedure)
➔ *CPT Changes: An Insider's View* 2002
➔ *CPT Assistant* May 03:2

(Use 44203 in conjunction with 44202)

(For open procedure, see 44120, 44121)

44204 colectomy, partial, with anastomosis
➔ *CPT Changes: An Insider's View* 2002
➔ *CPT Assistant* May 03:3, Apr 06:1, 19, Dec 17:14

(For open procedure, use 44140)

44205 colectomy, partial, with removal of terminal ileum with ileocolostomy
➔ *CPT Changes: An Insider's View* 2002
➔ *CPT Assistant* May 03:3, Apr 06:1

(For open procedure, use 44160)

44206 colectomy, partial, with end colostomy and closure of distal segment (Hartmann type procedure)
➔ *CPT Changes: An Insider's View* 2003
➔ *CPT Assistant* May 03:3, Apr 06:1

(For open procedure, use 44143)

44207 colectomy, partial, with anastomosis, with coloproctostomy (low pelvic anastomosis)
➔ *CPT Changes: An Insider's View* 2003
➔ *CPT Assistant* May 03:3, Apr 06:1

(For open procedure, use 44145)

44208 colectomy, partial, with anastomosis, with coloproctostomy (low pelvic anastomosis) with colostomy
➔ *CPT Changes: An Insider's View* 2003
➔ *CPT Assistant* May 03:3, Apr 06:1

(For open procedure, use 44146)

44210 colectomy, total, abdominal, without proctectomy, with ileostomy or ileoproctostomy
➔ *CPT Changes: An Insider's View* 2003
➔ *CPT Assistant* May 03:3

(For open procedure, use 44150)

44211 colectomy, total, abdominal, with proctectomy, with ileoanal anastomosis, creation of ileal reservoir (S or J), with loop ileostomy, includes rectal mucosectomy, when performed
➔ *CPT Changes: An Insider's View* 2003, 2007
➔ *CPT Assistant* May 03:3

(For open procedure, see 44157, 44158)

44212 colectomy, total, abdominal, with proctectomy, with ileostomy
➲ *CPT Changes: An Insider's View* 2003
➲ *CPT Assistant* May 03:3

(For open procedure, use 44155)

+ 44213 Laparoscopy, surgical, mobilization (take-down) of splenic flexure performed in conjunction with partial colectomy (List separately in addition to primary procedure)
➲ *CPT Changes: An Insider's View* 2006

(Use 44213 in conjunction with 44204-44208)

(For open procedure, use 44139)

Repair

44227 Laparoscopy, surgical, closure of enterostomy, large or small intestine, with resection and anastomosis
➲ *CPT Changes: An Insider's View* 2006

(For open procedure, see 44625, 44626)

Other Procedures

44238 Unlisted laparoscopy procedure, intestine (except rectum)
➲ *CPT Changes: An Insider's View* 2003
➲ *CPT Assistant* May 03:4, Jul 17:10

Enterostomy—External Fistulization of Intestines

44300 Placement, enterostomy or cecostomy, tube open (eg, for feeding or decompression) (separate procedure)
➲ *CPT Changes: An Insider's View* 2008
➲ *CPT Assistant* Mar 02:10, Aug 08:7

(Do not report 44300 in conjunction with 44701 for cannulation of the colon for intraoperative colonic lavage)

(For percutaneous placement of duodenostomy, jejunostomy, gastro-jejunostomy or cecostomy [or other colonic] tube including fluoroscopic imaging guidance, see 49441-49442)

44310 Ileostomy or jejunostomy, non-tube
➲ *CPT Changes: An Insider's View* 2006
➲ *CPT Assistant* Mar 02:10, Apr 06:1

(For laparoscopic procedure, use 44187)

(Do not report 44310 in conjunction with 44144, 44150-44151, 44155, 44156, 45113, 45119, 45136)

44312 Revision of ileostomy; simple (release of superficial scar) (separate procedure)
➲ *CPT Assistant* Spring 93:35

44314 complicated (reconstruction in-depth) (separate procedure)

44316 Continent ileostomy (Kock procedure) (separate procedure)

(For fiberoptic evaluation, use 44385)

44320 Colostomy or skin level cecostomy;
➲ *CPT Changes: An Insider's View* 2006

(For laparoscopic procedure, use 44188)

(Do not report 44320 in conjunction with 44141, 44144, 44146, 44605, 45110, 45119, 45126, 45563, 45805, 45825, 50810, 51597, 57307, or 58240)

44322 with multiple biopsies (eg, for congenital megacolon) (separate procedure)
➲ *CPT Changes: An Insider's View* 2002

44340 Revision of colostomy; simple (release of superficial scar) (separate procedure)

44345 complicated (reconstruction in-depth) (separate procedure)

44346 with repair of paracolostomy hernia (separate procedure)

Endoscopy, Small Intestine

When bleeding occurs as the result of an endoscopic procedure, control of bleeding is not reported separately during the same operative session.

Antegrade transoral small intestinal endoscopy (enteroscopy) is defined by the most distal segment of small intestine that is examined. Codes 44360, 44361, 44363, 44364, 44365, 44366, 44369, 44370, 44372, 44373 are endoscopic procedures to visualize the esophagus through the jejunum using an antegrade approach. Codes 44376, 44377, 44378, 44379 are endoscopic procedures to visualize the esophagus through the ileum using an antegrade approach. If an endoscope cannot be advanced at least 50 cm beyond the pylorus, see 43233, 43235-43259, 43266, 43270; if an endoscope can be passed at least 50 cm beyond pylorus but only into jejunum, see 44360, 44361, 44363, 44364, 44365, 44366, 44369, 44370, 44372, 44373.

To report retrograde examination of small intestine via anus or colon stoma, use 44799, unlisted procedure, intestine.

(Do not report 44360, 44361, 44363, 44364, 44365, 44366, 44369, 44370, 44372, 44373 in conjunction with 43233, 43235-43259, 43266, 43270, 44376, 44377, 44378, 44379)

(Do not report 44376, 44377, 44378, 44379 in conjunction with 43233, 43235-43259, 43266, 43270, 44360, 44361, 44363, 44364, 44365, 44366, 44369, 44370, 44372, 44373)

(For esophagogastroduodenoscopy, see 43233, 43235-43259, 43266, 43270)

44360 Small intestinal endoscopy, enteroscopy beyond second portion of duodenum, not including ileum; diagnostic, including collection of specimen(s) by brushing or washing, when performed (separate procedure)
➲ *CPT Changes: An Insider's View* 2015, 2017
➲ *CPT Assistant* Spring 94:7, Mar 11:10, Dec 13:3, Nov 14:3

44361 with biopsy, single or multiple

➲ *CPT Changes: An Insider's View* 2017

44363 with removal of foreign body(s)

➲ *CPT Changes: An Insider's View* 2015, 2017

44364 with removal of tumor(s), polyp(s), or other lesion(s) by snare technique

➲ *CPT Changes: An Insider's View* 2017

44365 with removal of tumor(s), polyp(s), or other lesion(s) by hot biopsy forceps or bipolar cautery

➲ *CPT Changes: An Insider's View* 2017

44366 with control of bleeding (eg, injection, bipolar cautery, unipolar cautery, laser, heater probe, stapler, plasma coagulator)

➲ *CPT Changes: An Insider's View* 2002, 2017

➲ *CPT Assistant* Jun 10:4

44369 with ablation of tumor(s), polyp(s), or other lesion(s) not amenable to removal by hot biopsy forceps, bipolar cautery or snare technique

➲ *CPT Changes: An Insider's View* 2017

44370 with transendoscopic stent placement (includes predilation)

➲ *CPT Changes: An Insider's View* 2001, 2017

➲ *CPT Assistant* Nov 01:7

44372 with placement of percutaneous jejunostomy tube

➲ *CPT Changes: An Insider's View* 2017

➲ *CPT Assistant* Spring 94:7

44373 with conversion of percutaneous gastrostomy tube to percutaneous jejunostomy tube

➲ *CPT Changes: An Insider's View* 2017

➲ *CPT Assistant* Spring 94:7, Dec 13:3

(For fiberoptic jejunostomy through stoma, use 43235)

44376 Small intestinal endoscopy, enteroscopy beyond second portion of duodenum, including ileum; diagnostic, with or without collection of specimen(s) by brushing or washing (separate procedure)

➲ *CPT Changes: An Insider's View* 2017

➲ *CPT Assistant* Spring 94:7, Mar 11:10, Dec 13:3

(Do not report 44376 in conjunction with 44360, 44361, 44363, 44364, 44365, 44366, 44369, 44370, 44372, 44373)

44377 with biopsy, single or multiple

➲ *CPT Changes: An Insider's View* 2017

➲ *CPT Assistant* Spring 94:7

(Do not report 44377 in conjunction with 44360, 44361, 44363, 44364, 44365, 44366, 44369, 44370, 44372, 44373)

44378 with control of bleeding (eg, injection, bipolar cautery, unipolar cautery, laser, heater probe, stapler, plasma coagulator)

➲ *CPT Changes: An Insider's View* 2002, 2017

➲ *CPT Assistant* Spring 94:7, Jun 10:4, Apr 12:17, Dec 13:3

(Do not report 44378 in conjunction with 44360, 44361, 44363, 44364, 44365, 44366, 44369, 44370, 44372, 44373)

44379 with transendoscopic stent placement (includes predilation)

➲ *CPT Changes: An Insider's View* 2001, 2017

➲ *CPT Assistant* Nov 01:7, Nov 14:3

(Do not report 44379 in conjunction with 44360, 44361, 44363, 44364, 44365, 44366, 44369, 44370, 44372, 44373)

Endoscopy, Stomal

Definitions

Proctosigmoidoscopy is the examination of the rectum and may include examination of a portion of the sigmoid colon.

Sigmoidoscopy is the examination of the entire rectum, sigmoid colon and may include examination of a portion of the descending colon.

Colonoscopy is the examination of the entire colon, from the rectum to the cecum, and may include examination of the terminal ileum or small intestine proximal to an anastomosis.

Colonoscopy through stoma is the examination of the colon, from the colostomy stoma to the cecum or colon-small intestine anastomosis, and may include examination of the terminal ileum or small intestine proximal to an anastomosis.

When performing a diagnostic or screening endoscopic procedure on a patient who is scheduled and prepared for a total colonoscopy, if the physician is unable to advance the colonoscope to the cecum or colon-small intestine anastomosis due to unforeseen circumstances, report 45378 (colonoscopy) or 44388 (colonoscopy through stoma) with modifier 53 and provide appropriate documentation.

If a therapeutic colonoscopy (44389-44407, 45379, 45380, 45381, 45382, 45384, 45388, 45398) is performed and does not reach the cecum or colon-small intestine anastomosis, report the appropriate therapeutic colonoscopy code with modifier 52 and provide appropriate documentation.

Report ileoscopy through stoma (44380, 44381, 44382, 44384) for endoscopic examination of a patient who has an ileostomy.

Report colonoscopy through stoma (44388-44408) for endoscopic examination of a patient who has undergone segmental resection of the colon (eg, hemicolectomy, sigmoid colectomy, low anterior resection) and has a colostomy.

Coding Tip

For definitions of proctosigmoidoscopy, sigmoidoscopy, colonoscopy, and guidelines for colonoscopies that do not reach the cecum or colon-small intestine anastomosis, see Colon and Rectum/Endoscopy.

For colonoscopy per rectum, see 45378, 45390, 45392, 45393, 45398.

Report proctosigmoidoscopy (45300-45327), flexible sigmoidoscopy (45330-45347), or anoscopy (46600, 46604, 46606, 46608, 46610, 46611, 46612, 46614, 46615), as appropriate for endoscopic examination of the defunctionalized rectum or distal colon in a patient who has undergone colectomy, in addition to colonoscopy through stoma (44388-44408) or ileoscopy through stoma (44380, 44381, 44382, 44384) if appropriate.

When bleeding occurs as the result of an endoscopic procedure, control of bleeding is not reported separately during the same operative session.

For computed tomographic colonography, see 74261, 74262, 74263.

44380 Ileoscopy, through stoma; diagnostic, including collection of specimen(s) by brushing or washing, when performed (separate procedure)

CPT Changes: An Insider's View 2015, 2017

CPT Assistant Dec 13:3, Nov 14:3, Dec 14:3

44381 Code is out of numerical sequence. See 44380-44385

(Do not report 44380 in conjunction with 44381, 44382, 44384)

44382 with biopsy, single or multiple

CPT Changes: An Insider's View 2017

CPT Assistant Dec 13:3

(Do not report 44382 in conjunction with 44380)

 # 44381 with transendoscopic balloon dilation

CPT Changes: An Insider's View 2015, 2017

CPT Assistant Nov 14:3

(Do not report 44381 in conjunction with 44380, 44384)

(If fluoroscopic guidance is performed, use 74360)

(For transendoscopic balloon dilation of multiple strictures during the same session, report 44381 with modifier 59 for each additional stricture dilated)

44384 with placement of endoscopic stent (includes pre- and post-dilation and guide wire passage, when performed)

CPT Changes: An Insider's View 2015, 2017

CPT Assistant Nov 14:3

(Do not report 44384 in conjunction with 44380, 44381)

(If fluoroscopic guidance is performed, use 74360)

44385 Endoscopic evaluation of small intestinal pouch (eg, Kock pouch, ileal reservoir [S or J]); diagnostic, including collection of specimen(s) by brushing or washing, when performed (separate procedure)

CPT Changes: An Insider's View 2015, 2017

(Do not report 44385 in conjunction with 44386)

44386 with biopsy, single or multiple

CPT Changes: An Insider's View 2015, 2017

CPT Assistant Dec 13:3

(Do not report 44386 in conjunction with 44385)

Coding Tip

Definition of Colonoscopy through Stoma

Colonoscopy through stoma is the examination of the colon, from the stoma to the cecum, and may include the examination of the terminal ileum or small intestine proximal to an anastomosis. When performing an endoscopic procedure on a patient who is scheduled and prepared for a colonoscopy through stoma, if the physician is unable to advance the colonoscope to the cecum or colon-small intestine anastomosis due to unforeseen circumstances, report 44388 with modifier 53 and provide appropriate documentation.

44388 Colonoscopy through stoma; diagnostic, including collection of specimen(s) by brushing or washing, when performed (separate procedure)

CPT Changes: An Insider's View 2015, 2017

CPT Assistant Nov 07:8, Dec 13:3, Nov 14:3

(Do not report 44388 in conjunction with 44389-44408)

44389 with biopsy, single or multiple

CPT Changes: An Insider's View 2017

CPT Assistant Dec 14:3

(Do not report 44389 in conjunction with 44403 for the same lesion)

(Do not report 44389 in conjunction with 44388)

44390 with removal of foreign body(s)

CPT Changes: An Insider's View 2015, 2017

(Do not report 44390 in conjunction with 44388)

(If fluoroscopic guidance is performed, use 76000)

44391 with control of bleeding, any method

CPT Changes: An Insider's View 2002, 2015, 2017

CPT Assistant Jun 10:4

(Do not report 44391 in conjunction with 44404 for the same lesion)

(Do not report 44391 in conjunction with 44388)

44392 with removal of tumor(s), polyp(s), or other lesion(s) by hot biopsy forceps

CPT Changes: An Insider's View 2015, 2017

(Do not report 44392 in conjunction with 44388)

 # 44401 with ablation of tumor(s), polyp(s), or other lesion(s) (includes pre-and post-dilation and guide wire passage, when performed)

➔ *CPT Changes: An Insider's View* 2015, 2017

➔ *CPT Assistant* Nov 14:3

(Do not report 44401 in conjunction with 44405 for the same lesion)

(Do not report 44401 in conjunction with 44388)

44394 with removal of tumor(s), polyp(s), or other lesion(s) by snare technique

➔ *CPT Changes: An Insider's View* 2017

(Do not report 44394 in conjunction with 44403 for the same lesion)

(Do not report 44394 in conjunction with 44388)

(For endoscopic mucosal resection, use 44403)

44401 Code is out of numerical sequence. See 44391-44402

44402 with endoscopic stent placement (including pre- and post-dilation and guide wire passage, when performed)

➔ *CPT Changes: An Insider's View* 2015, 2017

➔ *CPT Assistant* Nov 14:3

(Do not report 44402 in conjunction with 44388, 44405)

(If fluoroscopic guidance is performed, use 74360)

44403 with endoscopic mucosal resection

➔ *CPT Changes: An Insider's View* 2015, 2017

➔ *CPT Assistant* Nov 14:3

(Do not report 44403 in conjunction with 44389, 44394, 44404 for the same lesion)

(Do not report 44403 in conjunction with 44388)

44404 with directed submucosal injection(s), any substance

➔ *CPT Changes: An Insider's View* 2015, 2017

➔ *CPT Assistant* Nov 14:3

(Do not report 44404 in conjunction with 44391, 44403 for the same lesion)

(Do not report 44404 in conjunction with 44388)

44405 with transendoscopic balloon dilation

➔ *CPT Changes: An Insider's View* 2015, 2017

➔ *CPT Assistant* Nov 14:3

(Do not report 44405 in conjunction with 44388, 44401, 44402)

(If fluoroscopic guidance is performed, use 74360)

(For transendoscopic balloon dilation of multiple strictures during the same session, report 44405 with modifier 59 for each additional stricture dilated)

44406 with endoscopic ultrasound examination, limited to the sigmoid, descending, transverse, or ascending colon and cecum and adjacent structures

➔ *CPT Changes: An Insider's View* 2015, 2017

➔ *CPT Assistant* Nov 14:3

(Do not report 44406 in conjunction with 44388, 44407, 76975)

(Do not report 44406 more than once per session)

44407 with transendoscopic ultrasound guided intramural or transmural fine needle aspiration/biopsy(s), includes endoscopic ultrasound examination limited to the sigmoid, descending, transverse, or ascending colon and cecum and adjacent structures

➔ *CPT Changes: An Insider's View* 2015, 2017

➔ *CPT Assistant* Nov 14:3, Dec 14:3

(Do not report 44407 in conjunction with 44388, 44406, 76942, 76975)

(Do not report 44407 more than once per session)

44408 with decompression (for pathologic distention) (eg, volvulus, megacolon), including placement of decompression tube, when performed

➔ *CPT Changes: An Insider's View* 2015, 2017

➔ *CPT Assistant* Nov 14:3, Dec 14:3

(Do not report 44408 in conjunction with 44388)

(Do not report 44408 more than once per session)

Introduction

⊘ **44500** Introduction of long gastrointestinal tube (eg, Miller-Abbott) (separate procedure)

➔ *CPT Changes: An Insider's View* 2017

➔ *CPT Assistant* Sep 16:9

(For radiological supervision and interpretation, use 74340)

(For naso- or oro-gastric tube placement, use 43752)

Repair

44602 Suture of small intestine (enterorrhaphy) for perforated ulcer, diverticulum, wound, injury or rupture; single perforation

44603 multiple perforations

44604 Suture of large intestine (colorrhaphy) for perforated ulcer, diverticulum, wound, injury or rupture (single or multiple perforations); without colostomy

44605 with colostomy

44615 Intestinal stricturoplasty (enterotomy and enterorrhaphy) with or without dilation, for intestinal obstruction

44620 Closure of enterostomy, large or small intestine;

➔ *CPT Assistant* Nov 97:17, May 02:7

44625 with resection and anastomosis other than colorectal

➔ *CPT Assistant* Nov 97:17

44626 with resection and colorectal anastomosis (eg, closure of Hartmann type procedure)

➔ *CPT Assistant* Nov 97:17

(For laparoscopic procedure, use 44227)

44640 Closure of intestinal cutaneous fistula

44650 Closure of enteroenteric or enterocolic fistula

44660 Closure of enterovesical fistula; without intestinal or bladder resection

44661 with intestine and/or bladder resection
➲ *CPT Changes: An Insider's View* 2002

(For closure of renocolic fistula, see 50525, 50526)

(For closure of gastrocolic fistula, use 43880)

(For closure of rectovesical fistula, see 45800, 45805)

44680 Intestinal plication (separate procedure)

Other Procedures

44700 Exclusion of small intestine from pelvis by mesh or other prosthesis, or native tissue (eg, bladder or omentum)
➲ *CPT Changes: An Insider's View* 2002
➲ *CPT Assistant* Nov 97:18

(For therapeutic radiation clinical treatment, see **Radiation Oncology** section)

+ 44701 Intraoperative colonic lavage (List separately in addition to code for primary procedure)
➲ *CPT Changes: An Insider's View* 2003

(Use 44701 in conjunction with 44140, 44145, 44150, or 44604 as appropriate)

(Do not report 44701 in conjunction with 44950-44960)

44705 Preparation of fecal microbiota for instillation, including assessment of donor specimen
➲ *CPT Changes: An Insider's View* 2013
➲ *CPT Assistant* Jan 13:11, May 13:12

(Do not report 44705 in conjunction with 74283)

(For fecal instillation by oro-nasogastric tube or enema, use 44799)

44715 Backbench standard preparation of cadaver or living donor intestine allograft prior to transplantation, including mobilization and fashioning of the superior mesenteric artery and vein
➲ *CPT Changes: An Insider's View* 2005

44720 Backbench reconstruction of cadaver or living donor intestine allograft prior to transplantation; venous anastomosis, each
➲ *CPT Changes: An Insider's View* 2005

44721 arterial anastomosis, each
➲ *CPT Changes: An Insider's View* 2005
➲ *CPT Assistant* Apr 05:10-11

44799 Unlisted procedure, small intestine
➲ *CPT Changes: An Insider's View* 2015
➲ *CPT Assistant* Dec 00:14, May 08:15, Nov 08:11, Mar 10:10, Jul 10:10, Mar 11:10, May 11:9, May 13:12, Nov 14:3

(For unlisted laparoscopic procedure, intestine except rectum, use 44238)

(For unlisted procedure, colon, use 45399)

Meckel's Diverticulum and the Mesentery

Excision

44800 Excision of Meckel's diverticulum (diverticulectomy) or omphalomesenteric duct

44820 Excision of lesion of mesentery (separate procedure)

(With intestine resection, see 44120 or 44140 et seq)

Suture

44850 Suture of mesentery (separate procedure)

(For reduction and repair of internal hernia, use 44050)

Other Procedures

44899 Unlisted procedure, Meckel's diverticulum and the mesentery

Appendix

Incision

44900 Incision and drainage of appendiceal abscess, open
➲ *CPT Assistant* Nov 97:18

(For percutaneous image-guided drainage by catheter of appendiceal abscess, use 49406)

Excision

44950 Appendectomy;
➲ *CPT Assistant* Feb 92:22, Sep 96:4, Aug 02:2, Nov 08:7

(Incidental appendectomy during intra-abdominal surgery does not usually warrant a separate identification. If necessary to report, add modifier 52)

+ 44955 when done for indicated purpose at time of other major procedure (not as separate procedure) (List separately in addition to code for primary procedure)
➲ *CPT Assistant* Fall 92:22, Sep 96:4, Apr 97:3, Nov 08:7, Jan 12:13

44960 for ruptured appendix with abscess or generalized peritonitis
➲ *CPT Assistant* Fall 92:22, Nov 08:7

Laparoscopy

Surgical laparoscopy always includes diagnostic laparoscopy. To report a diagnostic laparoscopy (peritoneoscopy) (separate procedure), use 49320.

44970 Laparoscopy, surgical, appendectomy
➲ *CPT Changes: An Insider's View* 2000
➲ *CPT Assistant* Nov 99:23, Mar 00:9, Apr 06:1, 20, Mar 15:3

44979 Unlisted laparoscopy procedure, appendix
➔ *CPT Changes: An Insider's View* 2000
➔ *CPT Assistant* Nov 99:23, Mar 00:9, Jan 12:13

Colon and Rectum

Incision

45000 Transrectal drainage of pelvic abscess

(For transrectal image-guided fluid collection drainage by catheter of pelvic abscess, use 49407)

45005 Incision and drainage of submucosal abscess, rectum

45020 Incision and drainage of deep supralevator, pelvirectal, or retrorectal abscess

(See also 46050, 46060)

Excision

45100 Biopsy of anorectal wall, anal approach (eg, congenital megacolon)

(For endoscopic biopsy, use 45305)

45108 Anorectal myomectomy

45110 Proctectomy; complete, combined abdominoperineal, with colostomy

(For laparoscopic procedure, use 45395)

45111 partial resection of rectum, transabdominal approach

45112 Proctectomy, combined abdominoperineal, pull-through procedure (eg, colo-anal anastomosis)
➔ *CPT Assistant* Nov 97:18

(For colo-anal anastomosis with colonic reservoir or pouch, use 45119)

45113 Proctectomy, partial, with rectal mucosectomy, ileoanal anastomosis, creation of ileal reservoir (S or J), with or without loop ileostomy

45114 Proctectomy, partial, with anastomosis; abdominal and transsacral approach

45116 transsacral approach only (Kraske type)

45119 Proctectomy, combined abdominoperineal pull-through procedure (eg, colo-anal anastomosis), with creation of colonic reservoir (eg, J-pouch), with diverting enterostomy when performed
➔ *CPT Changes: An Insider's View* 2006
➔ *CPT Assistant* Nov 97:18, Apr 06:1

(For laparoscopic procedure, use 45397)

45120 Proctectomy, complete (for congenital megacolon), abdominal and perineal approach; with pull-through procedure and anastomosis (eg, Swenson, Duhamel, or Soave type operation)

45121 with subtotal or total colectomy, with multiple biopsies

45123 Proctectomy, partial, without anastomosis, perineal approach

45126 Pelvic exenteration for colorectal malignancy, with proctectomy (with or without colostomy), with removal of bladder and ureteral transplantations, and/or hysterectomy, or cervicectomy, with or without removal of tube(s), with or without removal of ovary(s), or any combination thereof
➔ *CPT Assistant* Nov 98:16

45130 Excision of rectal procidentia, with anastomosis; perineal approach

45135 abdominal and perineal approach

45136 Excision of ileoanal reservoir with ileostomy
➔ *CPT Changes: An Insider's View* 2002

(Do not report 45136 in conjunction with 44005, 44310)

45150 Division of stricture of rectum

45160 Excision of rectal tumor by proctotomy, transsacral or transcoccygeal approach

45171 Excision of rectal tumor, transanal approach; not including muscularis propria (ie, partial thickness)
➔ *CPT Changes: An Insider's View* 2010
➔ *CPT Assistant* Jun 10:3

45172 including muscularis propria (ie, full thickness)
➔ *CPT Changes: An Insider's View* 2010
➔ *CPT Assistant* Jun 10:3, Feb 18:11

Rectal Tumor Excision
45171-45172

A rectal tumor is excised via transanal approach.

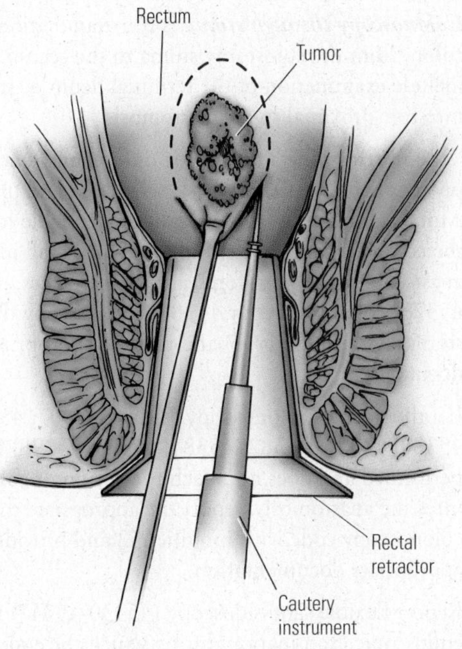

Digestive 40490-49999

(For destruction of rectal tumor, transanal approach, use 45190)

(For transanal endoscopic microsurgical [ie, TEMS] excision of rectal tumor, including muscularis propria [ie, full thickness], use 0184T)

Destruction

45190 Destruction of rectal tumor (eg, electrodesiccation, electrosurgery, laser ablation, laser resection, cryosurgery) transanal approach

➔ *CPT Changes: An Insider's View* 2002

➔ *CPT Assistant* Jun 10:3

(For excision of rectal tumor, transanal approach, see 45171, 45172)

(For transanal endoscopic microsurgical [ie, TEMS] excision of rectal tumor, including muscularis propria [ie, full thickness], use 0184T)

Endoscopy

Definitions

Proctosigmoidoscopy is the examination of the rectum and may include examination of a portion of the sigmoid colon.

Sigmoidoscopy is the examination of the entire rectum, sigmoid colon and may include examination of a portion of the descending colon.

Colonoscopy is the examination of the entire colon, from the rectum to the cecum, and may include examination of the terminal ileum or small intestine proximal to an anastomosis.

Colonoscopy through stoma is the examination of the colon, from the colostomy stoma to the cecum, and may include examination of the terminal ileum or small intestine proximal to an anastomosis.

When performing a diagnostic or screening endoscopic procedure on a patient who is scheduled and prepared for a total colonoscopy, if the physician is unable to advance the colonoscope to the cecum or colon-small intestine anastomosis due to unforeseen circumstances, report 45378 (colonoscopy) or 44388 (colonoscopy through stoma) with modifier 53 and provide appropriate documentation.

If a therapeutic colonoscopy (44389-44407, 45379, 45380, 45381, 45382, 45384, 45388, 45398) is performed and does not reach the cecum or colon-small intestine anastomosis, report the appropriate therapeutic colonoscopy code with modifier 52 and provide appropriate documentation.

Report flexible sigmoidoscopy (45330-45347) for endoscopic examination during which the endoscope is not advanced beyond the splenic flexure.

Report flexible sigmoidoscopy (45330-45347) for endoscopic examination of a patient who has undergone resection of the colon proximal to the sigmoid (eg, subtotal colectomy) and has an ileo-sigmoid or ileo-rectal anastomosis. Report pouch endoscopy codes (44385, 44386) for endoscopic examination of a patient who has undergone resection of colon with ileo-anal anastomosis (eg, J-pouch).

Report colonoscopy (45378-45398) for endoscopic examination of a patient who has undergone segmental resection of the colon (eg, hemicolectomy, sigmoid colectomy, low anterior resection).

For colonoscopy through stoma, see 44388-44408.

Report proctosigmoidoscopy (45300-45327), flexible sigmoidoscopy (45330-45347), or anoscopy (46600, 46604, 46606, 46608, 46610, 46611, 46612, 46614, 46615), as appropriate for endoscopic examination of the defunctionalized rectum or distal colon in a patient who has undergone colectomy, in addition to colonoscopy through stoma (44388-44408) or ileoscopy through stoma (44380, 44381, 44382, 44384) if appropriate.

When bleeding occurs as a result of an endoscopic procedure, control of bleeding is not reported separately during the same operative session.

For computed tomographic colonography, see 74261-74263.

45300 Proctosigmoidoscopy, rigid; diagnostic, with or without collection of specimen(s) by brushing or washing (separate procedure)

➔ *CPT Assistant* Spring 94:8, Oct 97:6, Apr 06:1

45303 with dilation (eg, balloon, guide wire, bougie)

➔ *CPT Changes: An Insider's View* 2002, 2017

➔ *CPT Assistant* Spring 94:8, Oct 97:6, Apr 06:1

(For radiological supervision and interpretation, use 74360)

45305 with biopsy, single or multiple

➔ *CPT Changes: An Insider's View* 2017

➔ *CPT Assistant* Spring 94:8, Oct 97:6, Apr 06:1

45307 with removal of foreign body

➔ *CPT Changes: An Insider's View* 2017

➔ *CPT Assistant* Spring 94:8, Oct 97:6, Apr 06:1

45308 with removal of single tumor, polyp, or other lesion by hot biopsy forceps or bipolar cautery

➔ *CPT Changes: An Insider's View* 2017

➔ *CPT Assistant* Spring 94:8, Oct 97:6, Apr 06:1

45309 with removal of single tumor, polyp, or other lesion by snare technique

➔ *CPT Changes: An Insider's View* 2017

➔ *CPT Assistant* Spring 94:8, Oct 97:6, Apr 06:1

45315 with removal of multiple tumors, polyps, or other lesions by hot biopsy forceps, bipolar cautery or snare technique

➔ *CPT Changes: An Insider's View* 2017

➔ *CPT Assistant* Spring 94:8, Oct 97:6, Apr 06:1

45317 with control of bleeding (eg, injection, bipolar cautery, unipolar cautery, laser, heater probe, stapler, plasma coagulator)

➔ *CPT Changes: An Insider's View* 2002, 2017

➔ *CPT Assistant* Spring 94:8, Oct 97:6, Apr 06:1

45320 with ablation of tumor(s), polyp(s), or other lesion(s) not amenable to removal by hot biopsy forceps, bipolar cautery or snare technique (eg, laser)

➔ *CPT Changes: An Insider's View* 2017

➔ *CPT Assistant* Spring 94:8, Oct 97:6, Apr 06:1

45321 with decompression of volvulus

➔ *CPT Changes: An Insider's View* 2017

➔ *CPT Assistant* Spring 94:8, Oct 97:6, Apr 06:1

45327 with transendoscopic stent placement (includes predilation)

➔ *CPT Changes: An Insider's View* 2001, 2017

➔ *CPT Assistant* Nov 01:7, Apr 06:1

Coding Tip

Definition of Sigmoidoscopy

Sigmoidoscopy is the examination of the entire rectum, sigmoid colon and may include examination of a portion of the descending colon.

CPT Coding Guidelines, Endoscopy

45330 Sigmoidoscopy, flexible; diagnostic, including collection of specimen(s) by brushing or washing, when performed (separate procedure)

➔ *CPT Changes: An Insider's View* 2015

➔ *CPT Assistant* Spring 94:9, May 05:3, May 07:10, Nov 07:8, Dec 13:3, Dec 14:3, 19, Sep 15:12, Feb 16:13

(Do not report 45330 in conjunction with 45331-45342, 45346, 45347, 45349, 45350)

45331 with biopsy, single or multiple

➔ *CPT Assistant* Spring 94:9, Sep 96:6, Jan 07:28

(Do not report 45331 in conjunction with 45349 for the same lesion)

45332 with removal of foreign body(s)

➔ *CPT Changes: An Insider's View* 2015, 2017

➔ *CPT Assistant* Winter 90:3, Spring 94:9, Dec 14:3

(Do not report 45332 in conjunction with 45330)

(If fluoroscopic guidance is performed, use 76000)

45333 with removal of tumor(s), polyp(s), or other lesion(s) by hot biopsy forceps

➔ *CPT Changes: An Insider's View* 2015, 2017

➔ *CPT Assistant* Winter 90:3, Spring 94:9, Dec 14:3

(Do not report 45333 in conjunction with 45330)

45334 with control of bleeding, any method

➔ *CPT Changes: An Insider's View* 2002, 2015, 2017

➔ *CPT Assistant* Spring 94:9, Sep 96:6, Jan 07:28, Jun 10:5, Dec 14:3

(Do not report 45334 in conjunction with 45335, 45350 for the same lesion)

(Do not report 45334 in conjunction with 45330)

45335 with directed submucosal injection(s), any substance

➔ *CPT Changes: An Insider's View* 2003, 2017

➔ *CPT Assistant* Mar 03:22, Jun 10:5

(Do not report 45335 in conjunction with 45334, 45349 for the same lesion)

(Do not report 45335 in conjunction with 45330)

45337 with decompression (for pathologic distention) (eg, volvulus, megacolon), including placement of decompression tube, when performed

➔ *CPT Changes: An Insider's View* 2015, 2017

➔ *CPT Assistant* Spring 94:9, Dec 14:3

(Do not report 45337 in conjunction with 45330)

(Do not report 45337 more than once per session)

45338 with removal of tumor(s), polyp(s), or other lesion(s) by snare technique

➔ *CPT Changes: An Insider's View* 2017

➔ *CPT Assistant* Spring 94:9

(Do not report 45338 in conjunction with 45349 for the same lesion)

(Do not report 45338 in conjunction with 45330)

(For endoscopic mucosal resection, use 45349)

 # 45346 with ablation of tumor(s), polyp(s), or other lesion(s) (includes pre- and post-dilation and guide wire passage, when performed)

➔ *CPT Changes: An Insider's View* 2015, 2017

➔ *CPT Assistant* Dec 14:3

(Do not report 45346 in conjunction with 45330)

(Do not report 45346 in conjunction with 45340 for the same lesion)

45340 with transendoscopic balloon dilation

➔ *CPT Changes: An Insider's View* 2003, 2015, 2017

➔ *CPT Assistant* Dec 14:3

(Do not report 45340 in conjunction with 45330, 45346, 45347)

(If fluoroscopic guidance is performed, use 74360)

(For transendoscopic balloon dilation of multiple strictures during the same session, use 45340 with modifier 59 for each additional stricture dilated)

45341 with endoscopic ultrasound examination

➔ *CPT Changes: An Insider's View* 2001, 2017

➔ *CPT Assistant* Oct 01:4, May 05:3, Dec 13:3

Colonoscopy Decision Tree

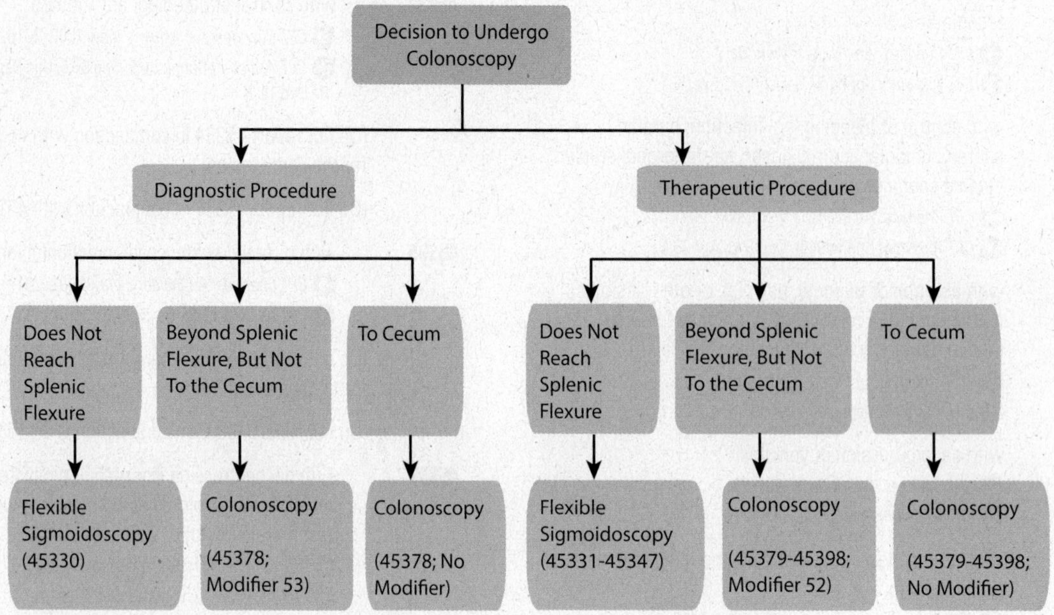

(Do not report 45341 in conjunction with 45330, 45342, 76872, 76975)

(Do not report 45341 more than once per session)

45342 with transendoscopic ultrasound guided intramural or transmural fine needle aspiration/biopsy(s)

➲ *CPT Changes: An Insider's View* 2001, 2017

➲ *CPT Assistant* Oct 01:4, May 05:3, Dec 13:3

(Do not report 45342 in conjunction with 45330, 45341, 76872, 76942, 76975)

(Do not report 45342 more than once per session)

45346 Code is out of numerical sequence. See 45337-45341

45347 with placement of endoscopic stent (includes pre- and post-dilation and guide wire passage, when performed)

➲ *CPT Changes: An Insider's View* 2015, 2017

➲ *CPT Assistant* Dec 14:3, Feb 16:13

(Do not report 45347 in conjunction with 45330, 45340)

(If fluoroscopic guidance is performed, use 74360)

45349 with endoscopic mucosal resection

➲ *CPT Changes: An Insider's View* 2015, 2017

➲ *CPT Assistant* Dec 14:3

(Do not report 45349 in conjunction with 45331, 45335, 45338, 45350 for the same lesion)

(Do not report 45349 in conjunction with 45330)

45350 with band ligation(s) (eg, hemorrhoids)

➲ *CPT Changes: An Insider's View* 2015, 2017

➲ *CPT Assistant* Dec 14:3

(Do not report 45350 in conjunction with 45334 for the same lesion)

(Do not report 45350 in conjunction with 45330, 45349, 46221)

(Do not report 45350 more than once per session)

(To report control of active bleeding with band ligation[s], use 45334)

Coding Tip

Definition of Colonoscopy

Colonoscopy is the examination of the entire colon, from the rectum to the cecum, and may include the examination of the terminal ileum or small intestine proximal to an anastomosis. When performing a diagnostic or screening endoscopic procedure on a patient who is scheduled and prepared for a total colonoscopy, if the physician is unable to advance the colonoscope to the cecum or colon-small intestine anastomosis due to unforeseen circumstances, report 45378 (colonoscopy) or 44388 (colonoscopy through stoma) with modifier 53 and provide appropriate documentation.

CPT Coding Guidelines, Endoscopy

45378 Colonoscopy, flexible; diagnostic, including collection of specimen(s) by brushing or washing, when performed (separate procedure)

➲ *CPT Changes: An Insider's View* 2015, 2017

➲ *CPT Assistant* Spring 94:9, Aug 99:3, Jan 02:12, Jan 04:4, May 05:3, Dec 10:3, Apr 11:12, Jan 13:11, Nov 14:3, Dec 14:3, Sep 15:12, Sep 17:14, Jan 18:7

(Do not report 45378 in conjunction with 45379-45393, 45398)

(For colonoscopy with decompression [pathologic distention], use 45393)

Colonoscopy
45378

A colonoscope is inserted in the anus and moved through the colon to the cecum in order to visualize the lumen of the rectum and colon.

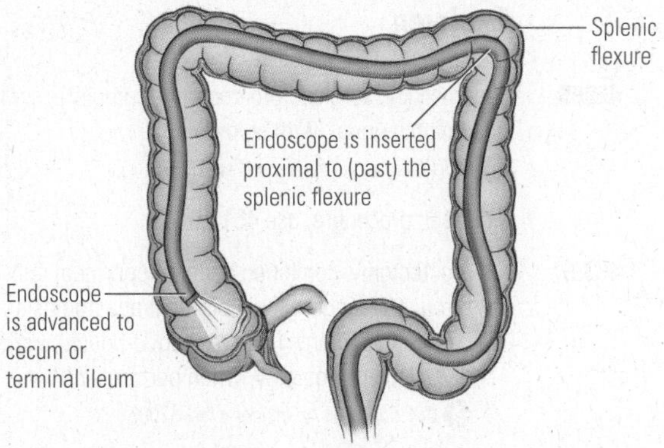

45379 with removal of foreign body(s)
➔ *CPT Changes: An Insider's View* 2015, 2017
➔ *CPT Assistant* Spring 94:9, Aug 99:3, Dec 14:3

(Do not report 45379 in conjunction with 45378)

(If fluoroscopic guidance is performed, use 76000)

45380 with biopsy, single or multiple
➔ *CPT Changes: An Insider's View* 2015, 2017
➔ *CPT Assistant* Spring 94:9, Jan 96:7, Feb 99:11, Aug 99:3, Jan 04:7, Jul 04:15, Dec 14:3

(Do not report 45380 in conjunction with 45390 for the same lesion)

(Do not report 45380 in conjunction with 45378)

45381 with directed submucosal injection(s), any substance
➔ *CPT Changes: An Insider's View* 2003, 2015, 2017
➔ *CPT Assistant* Mar 03:22, Jan 04:7, Jun 10:5, Jan 17:6

(Do not report 45381 in conjunction with 45382, 45390 for the same lesion)

(Do not report 45381 in conjunction with 45378)

45382 with control of bleeding, any method
➔ *CPT Changes: An Insider's View* 2002, 2015, 2017
➔ *CPT Assistant* Spring 94:9, Aug 99:3, Jun 10:5, Dec 14:3

(Do not report 45382 in conjunction with 45381, 45398 for the same lesion)

(Do not report 45382 in conjunction with 45378)

 # 45388 with ablation of tumor(s), polyp(s), or other lesion(s) (includes pre- and post-dilation and guide wire passage, when performed)
➔ *CPT Changes: An Insider's View* 2015, 2017
➔ *CPT Assistant* Dec 14:3

(Do not report 45388 in conjunction with 45386 for the same lesion)

(Do not report 45388 in conjunction with 45378)

45384 with removal of tumor(s), polyp(s), or other lesion(s) by hot biopsy forceps
➔ *CPT Changes: An Insider's View* 2015, 2017
➔ *CPT Assistant* Spring 94:9, Jul 98:10, Feb 99:11, Aug 99:3, Jan 04:6, Jul 04:15, Apr 11:12, Dec 14:3, Jun 15:10

(Do not report 45384 in conjunction with 45378)

45385 with removal of tumor(s), polyp(s), or other lesion(s) by snare technique
➔ *CPT Changes: An Insider's View* 2015, 2017
➔ *CPT Assistant* Spring 94:9, Jan 96:7, Jul 98:10, Aug 99:3, Jan 04:5, Jul 04:15, Jun 10:5, Jan 17:6

(Do not report 45385 in conjunction with 45390 for the same lesion)

(Do not report 45385 in conjunction with 45378)

(For endoscopic mucosal resection, use 45390)

45386 with transendoscopic balloon dilation
➔ *CPT Changes: An Insider's View* 2003, 2015, 2017
➔ *CPT Assistant* Dec 14:3

(Do not report 45386 in conjunction with 45378, 45388, 45389)

(If fluoroscopic guidance is performed, use 74360)

(For transendoscopic balloon dilation of multiple strictures during the same session, report 45386 with modifier 59 for each additional stricture dilated)

45388 Code is out of numerical sequence. See 45381-45385

Colonoscopy With Lesion Ablation or Removal
45385, 45388

Insertion and advancement of a colonoscope through the colon and to the cecum for ablation (45388) or removal (45385) of tumors, polyps, or other lesions

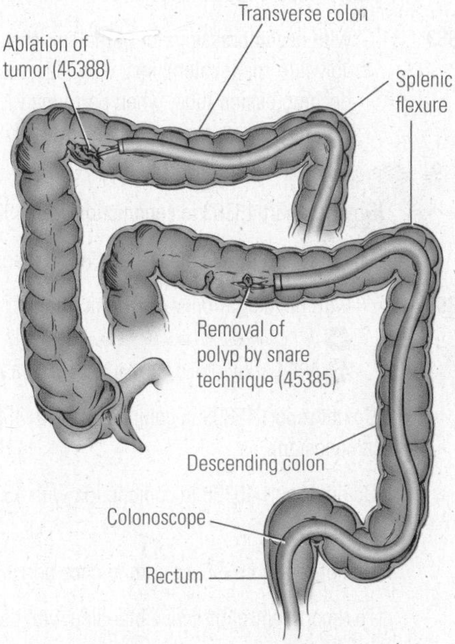

45389 with endoscopic stent placement (includes pre- and post-dilation and guide wire passage, when performed)
➲ *CPT Changes: An Insider's View* 2015, 2017
➲ *CPT Assistant* Dec 14:3

(Do not report 45389 in conjunction with 45378, 45386)

(If fluoroscopic guidance is performed, use 74360)

45390 Code is out of numerical sequence. See 45391-45397

45391 with endoscopic ultrasound examination limited to the rectum, sigmoid, descending, transverse, or ascending colon and cecum, and adjacent structures
➲ *CPT Changes: An Insider's View* 2005, 2015, 2017
➲ *CPT Assistant* May 05:3, Dec 13:3, Dec 14:3

(Do not report 45391 in conjunction with 45378, 45392, 76872, 76975)

(Do not report 45391 more than once per session)

45392 with transendoscopic ultrasound guided intramural or transmural fine needle aspiration/biopsy(s), includes endoscopic ultrasound examination limited to the rectum, sigmoid, descending, transverse, or ascending colon and cecum, and adjacent structures
➲ *CPT Changes: An Insider's View* 2005, 2015, 2017
➲ *CPT Assistant* May 05:3, Dec 13:3, Dec 14:3

(Do not report 45392 in conjunction with 45378, 45391, 76872, 76942, 76975)

(Do not report 45392 more than once per session)

 # 45390 with endoscopic mucosal resection
➲ *CPT Changes: An Insider's View* 2015, 2017
➲ *CPT Assistant* Dec 14:3, Jan 17:6

(Do not report 45390 in conjunction with 45380, 45381, 45385, 45398 for the same lesion)

(Do not report 45390 in conjunction with 45378)

45393 with decompression (for pathologic distention) (eg, volvulus, megacolon), including placement of decompression tube, when performed
➲ *CPT Changes: An Insider's View* 2015, 2017
➲ *CPT Assistant* Dec 14:4

(Do not report 45393 in conjunction with 45378)

(Do not report 45393 more than once per session)

 # 45398 with band ligation(s) (eg, hemorrhoids)
➲ *CPT Changes: An Insider's View* 2015, 2017
➲ *CPT Assistant* Dec 14:3, Sep 17:14, Jan 18:7

(Do not report 45398 in conjunction with 45382 for the same lesion)

(Do not report 45398 in conjunction with 45378, 45390, 46221)

(Do not report 45398 more than once per session)

(To report control of active bleeding with band ligation[s], use 45382)

Laparoscopy

Surgical laparoscopy always includes diagnostic laparoscopy. To report a diagnostic laparoscopy (peritoneoscopy) (separate procedure), use 49320.

Excision

45395 Laparoscopy, surgical; proctectomy, complete, combined abdominoperineal, with colostomy
➲ *CPT Changes: An Insider's View* 2006

(For open procedure, use 45110)

45397 proctectomy, combined abdominoperineal pull-through procedure (eg, colo-anal anastomosis), with creation of colonic reservoir (eg, J-pouch), with diverting enterostomy, when performed
➲ *CPT Changes: An Insider's View* 2006

(For open procedure, use 45119)

45398 Code is out of numerical sequence. See 45391-45397

45399 Code is out of numerical sequence. See 45910-45999

Repair

45400 Laparoscopy, surgical; proctopexy (for prolapse)
➲ *CPT Changes: An Insider's View* 2006

(For open procedure, use 45540, 45541)

45402 proctopexy (for prolapse), with sigmoid resection
➲ *CPT Changes: An Insider's View* 2006

(For open procedure, use 45550)

45499 Unlisted laparoscopy procedure, rectum
➲ *CPT Changes: An Insider's View* 2006

Repair

45500 Proctoplasty; for stenosis

45505 for prolapse of mucous membrane
➲ *CPT Assistant* Oct 13:19, Mar 15:10

45520 Perirectal injection of sclerosing solution for prolapse
➲ *CPT Assistant* Jul 01:11, Aug 01:10

45540 Proctopexy (eg, for prolapse); abdominal approach
➲ *CPT Changes: An Insider's View* 2006

(For laparoscopic procedure, use 45400)

45541 perineal approach

45550 with sigmoid resection, abdominal approach
➲ *CPT Changes: An Insider's View* 2006

(For laparoscopic procedure, use 45402)

45560 Repair of rectocele (separate procedure)

(For repair of rectocele with posterior colporrhaphy, use 57250)

45562 Exploration, repair, and presacral drainage for rectal injury;

45563 with colostomy

45800 Closure of rectovesical fistula;

45805 with colostomy

45820 Closure of rectourethral fistula;

45825 with colostomy

(For rectovaginal fistula closure, see 57300-57308)

Manipulation

45900 Reduction of procidentia (separate procedure) under anesthesia

45905 Dilation of anal sphincter (separate procedure) under anesthesia other than local

45910 Dilation of rectal stricture (separate procedure) under anesthesia other than local

45915 Removal of fecal impaction or foreign body (separate procedure) under anesthesia
➔ *CPT Changes: An Insider's View* 2003

Other Procedures

Surgical diagnostic anorectal exam (45990) includes the following elements: external perineal exam, digital rectal exam, pelvic exam (when performed), diagnostic anoscopy, and diagnostic rigid proctoscopy.

\# **45399** Unlisted procedure, colon
➔ *CPT Changes: An Insider's View* 2015
➔ *CPT Assistant* Nov 14:3, Dec 14:4

45990 Anorectal exam, surgical, requiring anesthesia (general, spinal, or epidural), diagnostic
➔ *CPT Changes: An Insider's View* 2006

(Do not report 45990 in conjunction with 45300-45327, 46600, 57410, 99170)

45999 Unlisted procedure, rectum

(For unlisted laparoscopic procedure, rectum, use 45499)

Anus

For incision of thrombosed external hemorrhoid, use 46083. For ligation of internal hemorrhoid(s), see 46221, 46945, 46946. For excision of internal and/or external hemorrhoid(s), see 46250-46262, 46320. For injection of hemorrhoid(s), use 46500. For destruction of internal hemorrhoid(s) by thermal energy, use 46930. For destruction of hemorrhoid(s) by cryosurgery, use 46999. For hemorrhoidopexy, use 46947. Do not report 46600 in conjunction with 46020-46942, 0184T, 0249T, 0377T during the same operative session.

Incision

(For subcutaneous fistulotomy, use 46270)

46020 Placement of seton
➔ *CPT Changes: An Insider's View* 2002

(Do not report 46020 in addition to 46060, 46280, 46600, 0249T)

Placement of Seton
46020

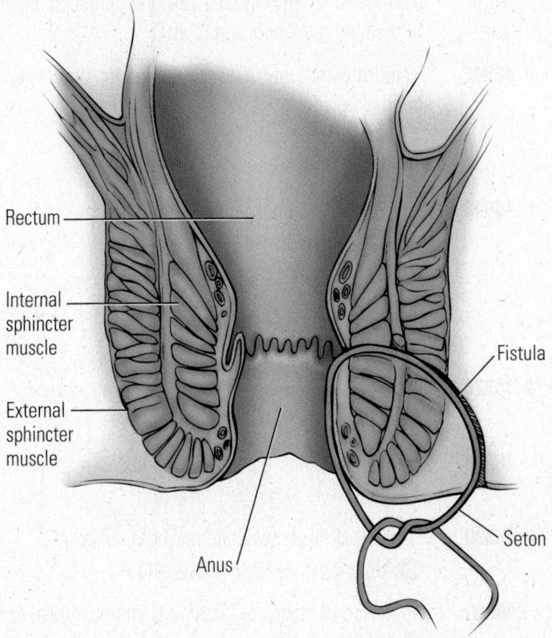

46030 Removal of anal seton, other marker

46040 Incision and drainage of ischiorectal and/or perirectal abscess (separate procedure)

46045 Incision and drainage of intramural, intramuscular, or submucosal abscess, transanal, under anesthesia

46050 Incision and drainage, perianal abscess, superficial

(See also 45020, 46060)

46060 Incision and drainage of ischiorectal or intramural abscess, with fistulectomy or fistulotomy, submuscular, with or without placement of seton

(Do not report 46060 in addition to 46020)

(See also 45020)

46070 Incision, anal septum (infant)

(For anoplasty, see 46700-46705)

(Do not report modifier 63 in conjunction with 46070)

46080 Sphincterotomy, anal, division of sphincter (separate procedure)

46083 Incision of thrombosed hemorrhoid, external
➔ *CPT Assistant* Jun 97:10

Excision

46200 Fissurectomy, including sphincterotomy, when performed
➲ *CPT Changes: An Insider's View* 2010

(46210, 46211 have been deleted. To report, use 46999)

46220 Code is out of numerical sequence. See 46200-46255

46221 Hemorrhoidectomy, internal, by rubber band ligation(s)
➲ *CPT Changes: An Insider's View* 2010
➲ *CPT Assistant* Oct 97:8, Dec 14:3, Apr 15:10, Sep 17:14, Jan 18:7

(Do not report 46221 in conjunction with 45350, 45398)

(For ligation, hemorrhoidal vascular bundle(s), including ultrasound guidance, use 0249T)

 # 46945 Hemorrhoidectomy, internal, by ligation other than rubber band; single hemorrhoid column/group
➲ *CPT Changes: An Insider's View* 2010
➲ *CPT Assistant* Apr 15:10

 # 46946 2 or more hemorrhoid columns/groups
➲ *CPT Changes: An Insider's View* 2010
➲ *CPT Assistant* Apr 15:10

(Do not report 46221, 46945, and 46946 in conjunction with 0249T)

 # 46220 Excision of single external papilla or tag, anus
➲ *CPT Changes: An Insider's View* 2010

46230 Excision of multiple external papillae or tags, anus
➲ *CPT Changes: An Insider's View* 2010

 # 46320 Excision of thrombosed hemorrhoid, external
➲ *CPT Changes: An Insider's View* 2010

46250 Hemorrhoidectomy, external, 2 or more columns/groups
➲ *CPT Changes: An Insider's View* 2010

(For hemorrhoidectomy, external, single column/group, use 46999)

46255 Hemorrhoidectomy, internal and external, single column/group;
➲ *CPT Changes: An Insider's View* 2010
➲ *CPT Assistant* Oct 14:15

46257 with fissurectomy

46258 with fistulectomy, including fissurectomy, when performed
➲ *CPT Changes: An Insider's View* 2010

46260 Hemorrhoidectomy, internal and external, 2 or more columns/groups;
➲ *CPT Changes: An Insider's View* 2010

46261 with fissurectomy

46262 with fistulectomy, including fissurectomy, when performed
➲ *CPT Changes: An Insider's View* 2010
➲ *CPT Assistant* May 05:3

(Do not report 46250-46262 in conjunction with 0249T)

Hemorrhoidectomy of Internal Prolapsed Hemorrhoid Columns
46250-46262

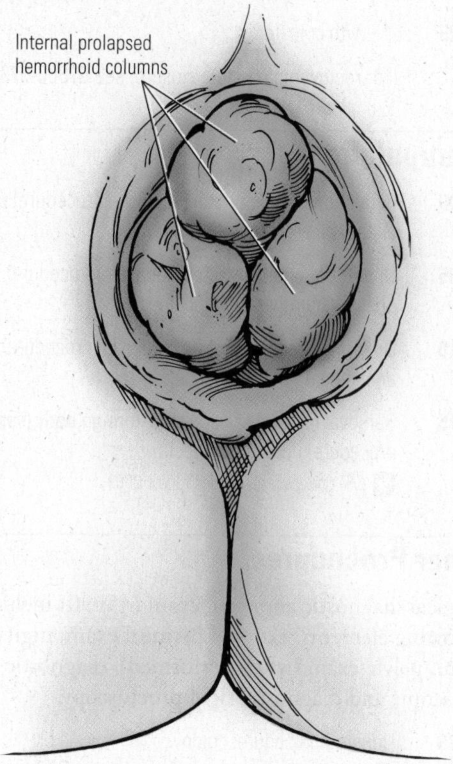

Anal column is considered to be an internal hemorrhoid with 3 major areas in the anal canal: right posterior (1 o'clock), right anterior (5 o'clock), and left lateral (9 o'clock) positions of the anus.

46270 Surgical treatment of anal fistula (fistulectomy/fistulotomy); subcutaneous

46275 intersphincteric
➲ *CPT Changes: An Insider's View* 2010

46280 transsphincteric, suprasphincteric, extrasphincteric or multiple, including placement of seton, when performed
➲ *CPT Changes: An Insider's View* 2010

(Do not report 46280 in conjunction with 46020)

46285 second stage

46288 Closure of anal fistula with rectal advancement flap

46320 Code is out of numerical sequence. See 46200-46255

Introduction

46500 Injection of sclerosing solution, hemorrhoids
➲ *CPT Assistant* May 05:3

(For anoscopy with directed submucosal injection of bulking agent for fecal incontinence, use 0377T)

46505 Chemodenervation of internal anal sphincter

➔ *CPT Changes: An Insider's View* 2006

(For chemodenervation of other muscles, see 64612, 64616, 64617, 64642, 64643, 64644, 64645, 64646, 64647. For destruction of nerve by neurolytic agent, use 64630)

(Report the specific service in conjunction with the specific substance(s) or drug(s) provided)

Endoscopy

Surgical endoscopy always includes diagnostic endoscopy.

(For anoscopy with directed submucosal injection of bulking agent for fecal incontinence, use 0377T)

46600 Anoscopy; diagnostic, including collection of specimen(s) by brushing or washing, when performed (separate procedure)

➔ *CPT Changes: An Insider's View* 2015

➔ *CPT Assistant* Spring 94:9, Oct 97:6, Apr 06:1, Jun 10:3, Aug 11:9, Jan 18:7

(Do not report 46600 in conjunction with 46020-46947, 0184T, 0249T, 0377T during the same operative session)

(For diagnostic high-resolution anoscopy [HRA], use 46601)

46601 diagnostic, with high-resolution magnification (HRA) (eg, colposcope, operating microscope) and chemical agent enhancement, including collection of specimen(s) by brushing or washing, when performed

➔ *CPT Changes: An Insider's View* 2015

(Do not report 46601 in conjunction with 69990)

46604 with dilation (eg, balloon, guide wire, bougie)

➔ *CPT Changes: An Insider's View* 2002

➔ *CPT Assistant* Spring 94:9, Oct 97:6

46606 with biopsy, single or multiple

➔ *CPT Assistant* Spring 94:9, Oct 97:6

(For high-resolution anoscopy [HRA] with biopsy, use 46607)

46607 with high-resolution magnification (HRA) (eg, colposcope, operating microscope) and chemical agent enhancement, with biopsy, single or multiple

➔ *CPT Changes: An Insider's View* 2015

(Do not report 46607 in conjunction with 69990)

46608 with removal of foreign body

➔ *CPT Assistant* Spring 94:9, Oct 97:6

46610 with removal of single tumor, polyp, or other lesion by hot biopsy forceps or bipolar cautery

➔ *CPT Assistant* Spring 94:10, Oct 97:6

46611 with removal of single tumor, polyp, or other lesion by snare technique

➔ *CPT Assistant* Spring 94:10, Oct 97:6

46612 with removal of multiple tumors, polyps, or other lesions by hot biopsy forceps, bipolar cautery or snare technique

➔ *CPT Assistant* Spring 94:10, Oct 97:6

46614 with control of bleeding (eg, injection, bipolar cautery, unipolar cautery, laser, heater probe, stapler, plasma coagulator)

➔ *CPT Changes: An Insider's View* 2002

➔ *CPT Assistant* Spring 94:10, Oct 97:6

46615 with ablation of tumor(s), polyp(s), or other lesion(s) not amenable to removal by hot biopsy forceps, bipolar cautery or snare technique

➔ *CPT Assistant* Spring 94:10, Oct 97:6

Repair

46700 Anoplasty, plastic operation for stricture; adult

46705 infant

(Do not report modifier 63 in conjunction with 46705)

(For simple incision of anal septum, use 46070)

46706 Repair of anal fistula with fibrin glue

➔ *CPT Changes: An Insider's View* 2003

46707 Repair of anorectal fistula with plug (eg, porcine small intestine submucosa [SIS])

➔ *CPT Changes: An Insider's View* 2010

➔ *CPT Assistant* Jan 12:10, Oct 13:15

46710 Repair of ileoanal pouch fistula/sinus (eg, perineal or vaginal), pouch advancement; transperineal approach

➔ *CPT Changes: An Insider's View* 2006

46712 combined transperineal and transabdominal approach

➔ *CPT Changes: An Insider's View* 2006

46715 Repair of low imperforate anus; with anoperineal fistula (cut-back procedure)

46716 with transposition of anoperineal or anovestibular fistula

(Do not report modifier 63 in conjunction with 46715, 46716)

46730 Repair of high imperforate anus without fistula; perineal or sacroperineal approach

46735 combined transabdominal and sacroperineal approaches

(Do not report modifier 63 in conjunction with 46730, 46735)

46740 Repair of high imperforate anus with rectourethral or rectovaginal fistula; perineal or sacroperineal approach

46742 combined transabdominal and sacroperineal approaches

(Do not report modifier 63 in conjunction with 46740, 46742)

46744 Repair of cloacal anomaly by anorectovaginoplasty and urethroplasty, sacroperineal approach

(Do not report modifier 63 in conjunction with 46744)

46746 Repair of cloacal anomaly by anorectovaginoplasty and urethroplasty, combined abdominal and sacroperineal approach;

46748 with vaginal lengthening by intestinal graft or pedicle flaps

46750 Sphincteroplasty, anal, for incontinence or prolapse; adult

46751 child

46753 Graft (Thiersch operation) for rectal incontinence and/or prolapse

46754 Removal of Thiersch wire or suture, anal canal

46760 Sphincteroplasty, anal, for incontinence, adult; muscle transplant

46761 levator muscle imbrication (Park posterior anal repair)

►(46762 has been deleted)◄

(For anoscopy with directed submucosal injection of bulking agent for fecal incontinence, use 0377T)

 # 46947 Hemorrhoidopexy (eg, for prolapsing internal hemorrhoids) by stapling
➔ *CPT Changes: An Insider's View* 2005
➔ *CPT Assistant* May 05:3, 14

Destruction

46900 Destruction of lesion(s), anus (eg, condyloma, papilloma, molluscum contagiosum, herpetic vesicle), simple; chemical

46910 electrodesiccation

46916 cryosurgery

46917 laser surgery

46922 surgical excision

46924 Destruction of lesion(s), anus (eg, condyloma, papilloma, molluscum contagiosum, herpetic vesicle), extensive (eg, laser surgery, electrosurgery, cryosurgery, chemosurgery)
➔ *CPT Changes: An Insider's View* 2002

46930 Destruction of internal hemorrhoid(s) by thermal energy (eg, infrared coagulation, cautery, radiofrequency)
➔ *CPT Changes: An Insider's View* 2009
➔ *CPT Assistant* Apr 15:10, Jul 16:8

(46934-46936 have been deleted)

(46937, 46938 have been deleted. To report, use 45190)

46940 Curettage or cautery of anal fissure, including dilation of anal sphincter (separate procedure); initial
➔ *CPT Changes: An Insider's View* 2002

46942 subsequent

46945 Code is out of numerical sequence. See 46200-46255

46946 Code is out of numerical sequence. See 46200-46255

46947 Code is out of numerical sequence. See 46760-46910

Other Procedures

46999 Unlisted procedure, anus
➔ *CPT Assistant* Oct 97:8, Apr 15:10

Liver

Incision

47000 Biopsy of liver, needle; percutaneous
➔ *CPT Changes: An Insider's View* 2012, 2017
➔ *CPT Assistant* Fall 93:12
➔ *Clinical Examples in Radiology* Winter 17:4

(If imaging guidance is performed, see 76942, 77002, 77012, 77021)

+ 47001 when done for indicated purpose at time of other major procedure (List separately in addition to code for primary procedure)
➔ *CPT Assistant* Jun 07:10

(If imaging guidance is performed, see 76942, 77002)

►(For fine needle aspiration biopsy in conjunction with 47000, 47001, see 10004, 10005, 10006, 10007, 10008, 10009, 10010, 10011, 10012, 10021)◄

(For evaluation of fine needle aspirate in conjunction with 47000, 47001, see 88172, 88173)

47010 Hepatotomy, for open drainage of abscess or cyst, 1 or 2 stages
➔ *CPT Assistant* Nov 97:18

(For percutaneous image-guided fluid collection drainage by catheter of hepatic abscess or cyst, use 49405)

47015 Laparotomy, with aspiration and/or injection of hepatic parasitic (eg, amoebic or echinococcal) cyst(s) or abscess(es)

Excision

47100 Biopsy of liver, wedge

47120 Hepatectomy, resection of liver; partial lobectomy
➔ *CPT Assistant* May 98:10, Sep 14:14, Oct 16:11

47122 trisegmentectomy

47125 total left lobectomy

47130 total right lobectomy

Liver Transplantation

Liver allotransplantation involves three distinct components of physician work:

1. ***Cadaver donor hepatectomy,*** which includes harvesting the graft and cold preservation of the graft (perfusing with cold preservation solution and cold

maintenance) (use 47133). ***Living donor hepatectomy,*** which includes harvesting the graft, cold preservation of the graft (perfusing with cold preservation solution and cold maintenance), and care of the donor (see 47140-47142).

2. ***Backbench work:***

   Standard preparation of the whole liver graft will include one of the following:

   Preparation of whole liver graft (including cholecystectomy, if necessary, and dissection and removal of surrounding soft tissues to prepare vena cava, portal vein, hepatic artery, and common bile duct for implantation) (use 47143).

   Preparation as described for whole liver graft, plus trisegment split into two partial grafts (use 47144).

   Preparation as described for whole liver graft, plus lobe split into two partial grafts (use 47145).

   Additional reconstruction of the liver graft may include venous and/or arterial anastomosis(es) (see 47146, 47147).

3. ***Recipient liver allotransplantation,*** which includes recipient hepatectomy (partial or whole), transplantation of the allograft (partial or whole), and care of the recipient (use 47135).

47133 Donor hepatectomy (including cold preservation), from cadaver donor
➔ *CPT Changes: An Insider's View* 2005

47135 Liver allotransplantation, orthotopic, partial or whole, from cadaver or living donor, any age
➔ *CPT Assistant* Dec 11:16

(47136 has been deleted. To report, use 47399)

47140 Donor hepatectomy (including cold preservation), from living donor; left lateral segment only (segments II and III)
➔ *CPT Changes: An Insider's View* 2004, 2005
➔ *CPT Assistant* Aug 11:9

47141 total left lobectomy (segments II, III and IV)
➔ *CPT Changes: An Insider's View* 2004

47142 total right lobectomy (segments V, VI, VII and VIII)
➔ *CPT Changes: An Insider's View* 2004

47143 Backbench standard preparation of cadaver donor whole liver graft prior to allotransplantation, including cholecystectomy, if necessary, and dissection and removal of surrounding soft tissues to prepare the vena cava, portal vein, hepatic artery, and common bile duct for implantation; without trisegment or lobe split
➔ *CPT Changes: An Insider's View* 2005
➔ *CPT Assistant* Apr 05:10, 12

47144 with trisegment split of whole liver graft into 2 partial liver grafts (ie, left lateral segment [segments II and III] and right trisegment [segments I and IV through VIII])
➔ *CPT Changes: An Insider's View* 2005, 2009

47145 with lobe split of whole liver graft into 2 partial liver grafts (ie, left lobe [segments II, III, and IV] and right lobe [segments I and V through VIII])
➔ *CPT Changes: An Insider's View* 2005

47146 Backbench reconstruction of cadaver or living donor liver graft prior to allotransplantation; venous anastomosis, each
➔ *CPT Changes: An Insider's View* 2005

47147 arterial anastomosis, each
➔ *CPT Changes: An Insider's View* 2005

(Do not report 47143-47147 in conjunction with 47120-47125, 47600, 47610)

Repair

47300 Marsupialization of cyst or abscess of liver

47350 Management of liver hemorrhage; simple suture of liver wound or injury

47360 complex suture of liver wound or injury, with or without hepatic artery ligation

47361 exploration of hepatic wound, extensive debridement, coagulation and/or suture, with or without packing of liver

47362 re-exploration of hepatic wound for removal of packing

Laparoscopy

Surgical laparoscopy always includes diagnostic laparoscopy. To report a diagnostic laparoscopy (peritoneoscopy) (separate procedure), use 49320.

47370 Laparoscopy, surgical, ablation of 1 or more liver tumor(s); radiofrequency
➔ *CPT Changes: An Insider's View* 2002
➔ *CPT Assistant* Oct 02:2

(For imaging guidance, use 76940)

47371 cryosurgical
➔ *CPT Changes: An Insider's View* 2002

(For imaging guidance, use 76940)

47379 Unlisted laparoscopic procedure, liver
➔ *CPT Changes: An Insider's View* 2001
➔ *CPT Assistant* Aug 06:10, Dec 07:12, Dec 14:18

Other Procedures

47380 Ablation, open, of 1 or more liver tumor(s); radiofrequency
➔ *CPT Changes: An Insider's View* 2002
➔ *CPT Assistant* Oct 02:1
➔ *Clinical Examples in Radiology* Summer 08:3

(For imaging guidance, use 76940)

47381 cryosurgical
➲ *CPT Changes: An Insider's View* 2002

(For imaging guidance, use 76940)

47382 Ablation, 1 or more liver tumor(s), percutaneous, radiofrequency
➲ *CPT Changes: An Insider's View* 2002, 2010, 2017
➲ *CPT Assistant* Oct 02:1
➲ *Clinical Examples in Radiology* Spring 08:1, 2, Summer 08:3, Summer 12:11

(For imaging guidance and monitoring, see 76940, 77013, 77022)

47383 Ablation, 1 or more liver tumor(s), percutaneous, cryoablation
➲ *CPT Changes: An Insider's View* 2015, 2017
➲ *CPT Assistant* Dec 14:18

(For imaging guidance and monitoring, see 76940, 77013, 77022)

47399 Unlisted procedure, liver
➲ *CPT Assistant* Dec 14:18, Mar 17:10

Biliary Tract

Incision

47400 Hepaticotomy or hepaticostomy with exploration, drainage, or removal of calculus

47420 Choledochotomy or choledochostomy with exploration, drainage, or removal of calculus, with or without cholecystotomy; without transduodenal sphincterotomy or sphincteroplasty

47425 with transduodenal sphincterotomy or sphincteroplasty

47460 Transduodenal sphincterotomy or sphincteroplasty, with or without transduodenal extraction of calculus (separate procedure)

47480 Cholecystotomy or cholecystostomy, open, with exploration, drainage, or removal of calculus (separate procedure)
➲ *CPT Changes: An Insider's View* 2011
➲ *CPT Assistant* Apr 11:12
➲ *Clinical Examples in Radiology* Summer 11:3

(For percutaneous cholecystostomy, use 47490)

Introduction

Percutaneous biliary procedures (eg, transhepatic, transcholecystic) are described by 47490 and 47531-47544, and are performed with imaging guidance. They are differentiated from endoscopic procedures that utilize an access to the biliary tree from a hollow viscus for diagnosis and therapy. Diagnostic cholangiography is typically performed with percutaneous biliary procedures, and is included in 47490, 47533, 47534, 47535, 47536, 47537, 47538, 47539, 47540, and 47541.

Codes 47531 and 47532 describe percutaneous diagnostic cholangiography that includes injection(s) of contrast material, all associated radiological supervision and interpretation, and procedural imaging guidance (eg, ultrasound and/or fluoroscopy). Code 47532 also includes accessing the biliary system with a needle or catheter. Codes 47531 and 47532 may not be reported with codes 47533, 47534, 47535, 47536, 47537, 47538, 47539, 47540, and 47541.

An external biliary drainage catheter is a catheter placed into a bile duct that does not terminate in bowel, and that drains bile externally only. An internal-external biliary drainage catheter is a single, externally accessible catheter that terminates in the small intestine, and may drain bile into the small intestine and/or externally. A "stent," as used in this code set, is a percutaneously placed device (eg, self-expanding metallic mesh stent, plastic tube) that is positioned within the biliary tree and is completely internal, with no portion extending outside the patient.

Codes 47533, 47534, 47535, 47536, 47537, 47538, 47539, and 47540 describe percutaneous therapeutic biliary procedures that include catheter or stent placement, catheter removal and replacement (exchange), and/or catheter removal. These codes include the elements of access, drainage catheter manipulations, diagnostic cholangiography, imaging guidance (eg, ultrasonography and/or fluoroscopy), and all associated radiological supervision and interpretation. Codes 47533, 47534, 47538, 47539, 47540 may be reported once for each catheter or stent placed (eg, bilobar placement, multi-segmental placement). Codes 47535, 47536, and 47537 may be reported once for each catheter conversion, exchange, or removal (eg, bilobar, bisegmental).

Codes 47538, 47539, 47540 may be reported only once per session to describe one or more overlapping or serial stent(s) placed within a single bile duct, or bridging more than one ductal segment (eg, left hepatic duct and common bile duct) through a single percutaneous access. Codes 47538, 47539, 47540 may be reported more than once in the same session using modifier 59 for the additional procedures in the following circumstances: (i) placement of side-by-side (double-barrel) stents within a single bile duct; (ii) placement of two or more stents into separate bile ducts through a single percutaneous access; or (iii) placement of stents through two or more percutaneous access sites (eg, placement of one stent through the interstices of another stent). Code 47538 describes biliary stent placement through an existing access. Therefore, 47538 should not be reported together with 47536 if a biliary drainage catheter (eg, external or internal-external) is replaced after the biliary stent is placed. Code 47540 describes biliary stent placement with the additional service of placing a biliary drainage catheter (eg, external or internal-external). Therefore, 47540 should not be reported with 47533, 47534 for the same ductal system.

Code 47541 describes a procedure to assist with endoscopic procedures performed in conjunction with other physician specialists. Access placed may include wire and/or catheter. Code 47541 may not be reported if a wire is placed through existing percutaneous access.

Codes 47542, 47543, and 47544 describe procedures that may be performed in conjunction with other codes in this family, are add-on codes and do not include access, catheter placement, or diagnostic imaging. Do not report 47542 with 47538, 47539, 47540 because balloon dilation is included in 47538, 47539, and 47540. Code 47544 should not be reported with 47531-47543 for incidental removal of debris. Code 47542 should not be reported with 47544, if a balloon is used for removal of calculi or debris rather than for dilation.

47490 Cholecystostomy, percutaneous, complete procedure, including imaging guidance, catheter placement, cholecystogram when performed, and radiological supervision and interpretation

➔ *CPT Changes: An Insider's View* 2011
➔ *CPT Assistant* Apr 11:12, Dec 15:3
➔ *Clinical Examples in Radiology* Summer 11:1-3, Winter 11:10

(Do not report 47490 in conjunction with 47531, 47532, 75989, 76942, 77002, 77012, 77021)

47531 Injection procedure for cholangiography, percutaneous, complete diagnostic procedure including imaging guidance (eg, ultrasound and/or fluoroscopy) and all associated radiological supervision and interpretation; existing access

➔ *CPT Changes: An Insider's View* 2016
➔ *CPT Assistant* Dec 15:3
➔ *Clinical Examples in Radiology* Fall 15:5

47532 new access (eg, percutaneous transhepatic cholangiogram)

➔ *CPT Changes: An Insider's View* 2016, 2017
➔ *CPT Assistant* Dec 15:3
➔ *Clinical Examples in Radiology* Fall 15:5

(Do not report 47531, 47532 in conjunction with 47490, 47533, 47534, 47535, 47536, 47537, 47538, 47539, 47540, 47541 for procedures performed through the same percutaneous access)

(For intraoperative cholangiography, see 74300, 74301)

47533 Placement of biliary drainage catheter, percutaneous, including diagnostic cholangiography when performed, imaging guidance (eg, ultrasound and/or fluoroscopy), and all associated radiological supervision and interpretation; external

➔ *CPT Changes: An Insider's View* 2016, 2017
➔ *CPT Assistant* Dec 15:3
➔ *Clinical Examples in Radiology* Fall 15:5

47534 internal-external

➔ *CPT Changes: An Insider's View* 2016, 2017
➔ *CPT Assistant* Dec 15:3
➔ *Clinical Examples in Radiology* Fall 15:4

47535 Conversion of external biliary drainage catheter to internal-external biliary drainage catheter, percutaneous, including diagnostic cholangiography when performed, imaging guidance (eg, fluoroscopy), and all associated radiological supervision and interpretation

➔ *CPT Changes: An Insider's View* 2016, 2017
➔ *CPT Assistant* Dec 15:3
➔ *Clinical Examples in Radiology* Fall 15:5

47536 Exchange of biliary drainage catheter (eg, external, internal-external, or conversion of internal-external to external only), percutaneous, including diagnostic cholangiography when performed, imaging guidance (eg, fluoroscopy), and all associated radiological supervision and interpretation

➔ *CPT Changes: An Insider's View* 2016, 2017
➔ *CPT Assistant* Dec 15:3
➔ *Clinical Examples in Radiology* Fall 15:5

(Do not report 47536 in conjunction with 47538 for the same access)

(47536 includes exchange of one catheter. For exchange of additional catheter[s] during the same session, report 47536 with modifier 59 for each additional exchange)

47537 Removal of biliary drainage catheter, percutaneous, requiring fluoroscopic guidance (eg, with concurrent indwelling biliary stents), including diagnostic cholangiography when performed, imaging guidance (eg, fluoroscopy), and all associated radiological supervision and interpretation

➔ *CPT Changes: An Insider's View* 2016
➔ *CPT Assistant* Dec 15:3
➔ *Clinical Examples in Radiology* Fall 15:5

Exchanges/Conversions

(Existing Access)

Do Not Report Exchange with Stent for Same Percutaneous Access		**To:** **Internal-External**	**External**	**Stent**
From	External Drain	47535 Conversion	47536 Exchange	47538 Stent
	Internal-External Drain	47536 Exchange	47536 Exchange	47538 Stent

Percutaneous Biliary Stent(s) and Drain Placement
47533, 47534, 47538, 47539, 47540

Biliary catheters (eg, external 47533, internal-external 47534) and multiple stents (eg, 47538, 47539, 47540)

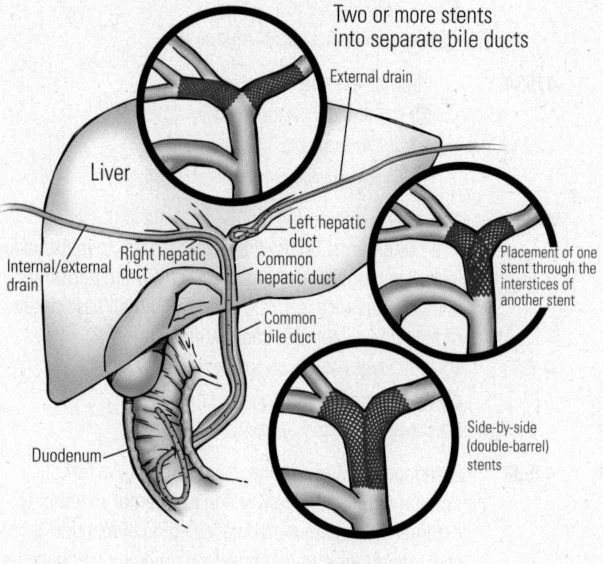

(Do not report 47537 in conjunction with 47538 for the same access)

(For removal of biliary drainage catheter not requiring fluoroscopic guidance, see E/M services and report the appropriate level of service provided [eg 99201-99215, 99217, 99218, 99219, 99220, 99221, 99222, 99223, 99224, 99225, 99226, 99231, 99232, 99233])

47538 Placement of stent(s) into a bile duct, percutaneous, including diagnostic cholangiography, imaging guidance (eg, fluoroscopy and/or ultrasound), balloon dilation, catheter exchange(s) and catheter removal(s) when performed, and all associated radiological supervision and interpretation; existing access

➲ *CPT Changes: An Insider's View* 2016, 2017
➲ *CPT Assistant* Dec 15:3, Mar 16:10
➲ *Clinical Examples in Radiology* Fall 15:5

(Do not report 47538 in conjunction with 47536, 47537 for the same percutaneous access)

47539 new access, without placement of separate biliary drainage catheter

➲ *CPT Changes: An Insider's View* 2016, 2017
➲ *CPT Assistant* Dec 15:3, Mar 16:10
➲ *Clinical Examples in Radiology* Fall 15:5

47540 new access, with placement of separate biliary drainage catheter (eg, external or internal-external)

➲ *CPT Changes: An Insider's View* 2016, 2017
➲ *CPT Assistant* Dec 15:3, Mar 16:10
➲ *Clinical Examples in Radiology* Fall 15:5

(Do not report 47538, 47539, 47540 in conjunction with 43277, 47542, 47555, 47556 for the same lesion in the same session)

(Do not report 47540 in conjunction with 47533, 47534 for the same percutaneous access)

(47538, 47539, 47540 may be reported more than once per session, when specific conditions described in the **Introduction** within the **Biliary Tract** subsection guidelines are met)

47541 Placement of access through the biliary tree and into small bowel to assist with an endoscopic biliary procedure (eg, rendezvous procedure), percutaneous, including diagnostic cholangiography when performed, imaging guidance (eg, ultrasound and/or fluoroscopy), and all associated radiological supervision and interpretation, new access

➲ *CPT Changes: An Insider's View* 2016, 2017
➲ *CPT Assistant* Dec 15:3
➲ *Clinical Examples in Radiology* Fall 15:6

(Do not report 47541 in conjunction with 47531, 47532, 47533, 47534, 47535, 47536, 47537, 47538, 47539, 47540)

(Do not report 47541 when there is existing catheter access)

(For use of existing access through the biliary tree into small bowel to assist with an endoscopic biliary procedure, see 47535, 47536, 47537)

+ 47542 Balloon dilation of biliary duct(s) or of ampulla (sphincteroplasty), percutaneous, including imaging guidance (eg, fluoroscopy), and all associated radiological supervision and interpretation, each duct (List separately in addition to code for primary procedure)

➲ *CPT Changes: An Insider's View* 2016, 2017
➲ *CPT Assistant* Dec 15:3
➲ *Clinical Examples in Radiology* Fall 15:6

(Use 47542 in conjunction with 47531, 47532, 47533, 47534, 47535, 47536, 47537, 47541)

(Do not report 47542 in conjunction with 43262, 43277, 47538, 47539, 47540, 47555, 47556)

(Do not report 47542 in conjunction with 47544 if a balloon is used for removal of calculi, debris, and/or sludge rather than for dilation)

(For percutaneous balloon dilation of multiple ducts during the same session, report an additional dilation once with 47542 and modifier 59, regardless of the number of additional ducts dilated)

(For endoscopic balloon dilation, see 43277, 47555, 47556)

+ 47543 Endoluminal biopsy(ies) of biliary tree, percutaneous, any method(s) (eg, brush, forceps, and/or needle), including imaging guidance (eg, fluoroscopy), and all associated radiological supervision and interpretation, single or multiple (List separately in addition to code for primary procedure)

➲ *CPT Changes: An Insider's View* 2016, 2017
➲ *CPT Assistant* Dec 15:3
➲ *Clinical Examples in Radiology* Fall 15:6

(Use 47543 in conjunction with 47531, 47532, 47533, 47534, 47535, 47536, 47537, 47538, 47539, 47540)

(Report 47543 once per session)

(For endoscopic brushings, see 43260, 47552)

(For endoscopic biopsy, see 43261, 47553)

+ 47544 Removal of calculi/debris from biliary duct(s) and/or gallbladder, percutaneous, including destruction of calculi by any method (eg, mechanical, electrohydraulic, lithotripsy) when performed, imaging guidance (eg, fluoroscopy), and all associated radiological supervision and interpretation (List separately in addition to code for primary procedure)

➲ *CPT Changes: An Insider's View* 2016, 2017
➲ *CPT Assistant* Dec 15:3
➲ *Clinical Examples in Radiology* Fall 15:6

(Use 47544 in conjunction with 47531, 47532, 47533, 47534, 47535, 47536, 47537, 47538, 47539, 47540)

(Do not report 47544 if no calculi or debris are found, even if removal device is deployed)

(Do not report 47544 in conjunction with 43264, 47554)

(Do not report 47544 in conjunction with 47531-47543 for incidental removal of debris)

(For endoscopic removal of calculi, see 43264, 47554)

(For endoscopic destruction of calculi, use 43265)

Endoscopy

Surgical endoscopy always includes diagnostic endoscopy.

+ 47550 Biliary endoscopy, intraoperative (choledochoscopy) (List separately in addition to code for primary procedure)

47552 Biliary endoscopy, percutaneous via T-tube or other tract; diagnostic, with collection of specimen(s) by brushing and/or washing, when performed (separate procedure)

➲ *CPT Changes: An Insider's View* 2014

47553 with biopsy, single or multiple

47554 with removal of calculus/calculi

➲ *CPT Changes: An Insider's View* 2002

47555 with dilation of biliary duct stricture(s) without stent

47556 with dilation of biliary duct stricture(s) with stent

(For ERCP, see 43260-43278, 74328, 74329, 74330, 74363)

(If imaging guidance is performed, use 74363)

Laparoscopy

Surgical laparoscopy always includes diagnostic laparoscopy. To report a diagnostic laparoscopy (peritoneoscopy) (separate procedure), use 49320.

(For percutaneous cholangiography, see 47531 or 47532)

47562 Laparoscopy, surgical; cholecystectomy

➲ *CPT Changes: An Insider's View* 2000
➲ *CPT Assistant* Nov 99:23, Mar 00:9, Sep 03:3, Dec 07:12

47563 cholecystectomy with cholangiography

➲ *CPT Changes: An Insider's View* 2000
➲ *CPT Assistant* Nov 99:23, Mar 00:9, Dec 00:14, Dec 07:12

(For intraoperative cholangiography radiological supervision and interpretation, see 74300, 74301)

(For percutaneous cholangiography, see 47531, 47532)

47564 cholecystectomy with exploration of common duct

➲ *CPT Changes: An Insider's View* 2000
➲ *CPT Assistant* Nov 99:23, Mar 00:9

47570 cholecystoenterostomy

➲ *CPT Changes: An Insider's View* 2000
➲ *CPT Assistant* Nov 99:23, Mar 00:9

Laparoscopic Cholecystectomy
47562

The gallbladder is dissected and removed from the liver bed under laparoscopic guidance.

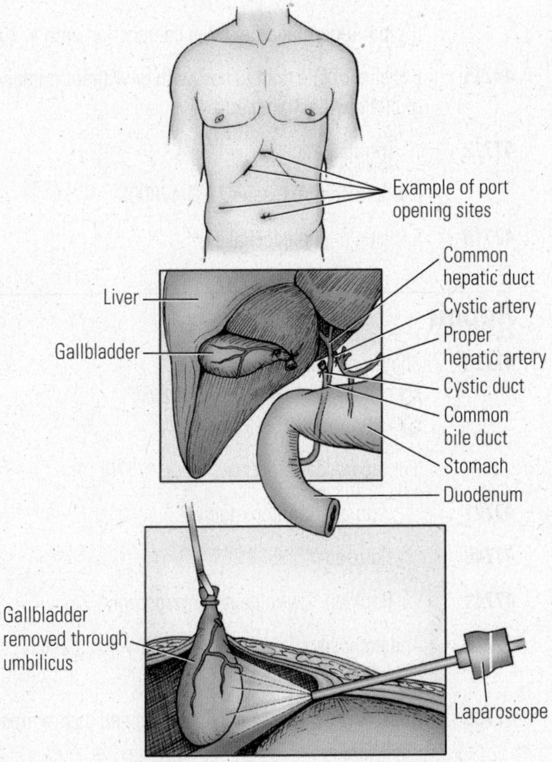

Digestive 40490-49999

47579 Unlisted laparoscopy procedure, biliary tract
➔ *CPT Changes: An Insider's View* 2000
➔ *CPT Assistant* Nov 99:23, Mar 00:9

Excision

47600 Cholecystectomy;
➔ *CPT Changes: An Insider's View* 2000
➔ *CPT Assistant* Fall 92:19, Nov 99:24

47605 with cholangiography
➔ *CPT Changes: An Insider's View* 2000
➔ *CPT Assistant* Nov 99:24, Apr 02:19

(For laparoscopic approach, see 47562-47564)

47610 Cholecystectomy with exploration of common duct;
➔ *CPT Assistant* Apr 02:19

(For cholecystectomy with exploration of common duct with biliary endoscopy, use 47610 with 47550)

47612 with choledochoenterostomy

47620 with transduodenal sphincterotomy or sphincteroplasty, with or without cholangiography

(47630 has been deleted. For percutaneous biliary duct stone extraction, use 47544)

47700 Exploration for congenital atresia of bile ducts, without repair, with or without liver biopsy, with or without cholangiography

(Do not report modifier 63 in conjunction with 47700)

47701 Portoenterostomy (eg, Kasai procedure)

(Do not report modifier 63 in conjunction with 47701)

47711 Excision of bile duct tumor, with or without primary repair of bile duct; extrahepatic

47712 intrahepatic

(For anastomosis, see 47760-47800)

47715 Excision of choledochal cyst

Repair

47720 Cholecystoenterostomy; direct
➔ *CPT Changes: An Insider's View* 2000
➔ *CPT Assistant* Nov 99:24

(For laparoscopic approach, use 47570)

47721 with gastroenterostomy

47740 Roux-en-Y

47741 Roux-en-Y with gastroenterostomy

47760 Anastomosis, of extrahepatic biliary ducts and gastrointestinal tract

47765 Anastomosis, of intrahepatic ducts and gastrointestinal tract

47780 Anastomosis, Roux-en-Y, of extrahepatic biliary ducts and gastrointestinal tract

47785 Anastomosis, Roux-en-Y, of intrahepatic biliary ducts and gastrointestinal tract

47800 Reconstruction, plastic, of extrahepatic biliary ducts with end-to-end anastomosis

47801 Placement of choledochal stent
➔ *CPT Assistant* Dec 10:13

47802 U-tube hepaticoenterostomy

47900 Suture of extrahepatic biliary duct for pre-existing injury (separate procedure)

Other Procedures

47999 Unlisted procedure, biliary tract
➔ *CPT Assistant* May 11:9

Pancreas

(For peroral pancreatic endoscopic procedures, see 43260-43265, 43274-43278)

Incision

48000 Placement of drains, peripancreatic, for acute pancreatitis;

48001 with cholecystostomy, gastrostomy, and jejunostomy

48020 Removal of pancreatic calculus
➔ *CPT Assistant* Spring 91:7

Excision

48100 Biopsy of pancreas, open (eg, fine needle aspiration, needle core biopsy, wedge biopsy)
➔ *CPT Changes: An Insider's View* 2002

48102 Biopsy of pancreas, percutaneous needle
➔ *Clinical Examples in Radiology* Winter 17:5

(For radiological supervision and interpretation, see 76942, 77002, 77012, 77021)

►(For fine needle aspiration biopsy, see 10005, 10006, 10007, 10008, 10009, 10010, 10011, 10012)◄

(For evaluation of fine needle aspirate, see 88172, 88173)

48105 Resection or debridement of pancreas and peripancreatic tissue for acute necrotizing pancreatitis
➔ *CPT Changes: An Insider's View* 2007

48120 Excision of lesion of pancreas (eg, cyst, adenoma)

48140 Pancreatectomy, distal subtotal, with or without splenectomy; without pancreaticojejunostomy
➔ *CPT Assistant* Jul 17:10

48145 with pancreaticojejunostomy

48146 Pancreatectomy, distal, near-total with preservation of duodenum (Child-type procedure)

48148 Excision of ampulla of Vater

48150 Pancreatectomy, proximal subtotal with total duodenectomy, partial gastrectomy, choledochoenterostomy and gastrojejunostomy (Whipple-type procedure); with pancreatojejunostomy
➲ *CPT Assistant* Dec 15:18

48152 without pancreatojejunostomy

48153 Pancreatectomy, proximal subtotal with near-total duodenectomy, choledochoenterostomy and duodenojejunostomy (pylorus-sparing, Whipple-type procedure); with pancreatojejunostomy

48154 without pancreatojejunostomy

48155 Pancreatectomy, total

48160 Pancreatectomy, total or subtotal, with autologous transplantation of pancreas or pancreatic islet cells
➲ *CPT Changes: An Insider's View* 2002

Introduction

+ 48400 Injection procedure for intraoperative pancreatography (List separately in addition to code for primary procedure)
➲ *CPT Assistant* Dec 07:12

(For radiological supervision and interpretation, see 74300, 74301)

(For intraoperative pancreatography radiological supervision and interpretation, see 74300, 74301)

Repair

48500 Marsupialization of pancreatic cyst
➲ *CPT Changes: An Insider's View* 2002

48510 External drainage, pseudocyst of pancreas, open
➲ *CPT Assistant* Nov 97:18

(For percutaneous image-guided fluid collection drainage by catheter of pancreatic pseudocyst, use 49405)

48520 Internal anastomosis of pancreatic cyst to gastrointestinal tract; direct

48540 Roux-en-Y

48545 Pancreatorrhaphy for injury
➲ *CPT Changes: An Insider's View* 2002

48547 Duodenal exclusion with gastrojejunostomy for pancreatic injury
➲ *CPT Changes: An Insider's View* 2002

48548 Pancreaticojejunostomy, side-to-side anastomosis (Puestow-type operation)
➲ *CPT Changes: An Insider's View* 2007

Pancreas Transplantation

Pancreas allotransplantation involves three distinct components of physician work:

1. ***Cadaver donor pancreatectomy,*** which includes harvesting the pancreas graft, with or without duodenal segment, and cold preservation of the graft (perfusing with cold preservation solution and cold maintenance) (use 48550).

2. ***Backbench work:***

   Standard preparation of a cadaver donor pancreas allograft prior to transplantation includes dissection of the allograft from surrounding soft tissues, splenectomy, duodenotomy, ligation of bile duct, ligation of mesenteric vessels, and Y-graft arterial anastomoses from the iliac artery to the superior mesenteric artery and to the splenic artery (use 48551).

   Additional reconstruction of a cadaver donor pancreas allograft prior to transplantation may include venous anastomosis(es) (use 48552).

3. ***Recipient pancreas allotransplantation,*** which includes transplantation of allograft, and care of the recipient (use 48554).

48550 Donor pancreatectomy (including cold preservation), with or without duodenal segment for transplantation
➲ *CPT Changes: An Insider's View* 2005
➲ *CPT Assistant* Apr 05:10, 12

48551 Backbench standard preparation of cadaver donor pancreas allograft prior to transplantation, including dissection of allograft from surrounding soft tissues, splenectomy, duodenotomy, ligation of bile duct, ligation of mesenteric vessels, and Y-graft arterial anastomoses from iliac artery to superior mesenteric artery and to splenic artery
➲ *CPT Changes: An Insider's View* 2005

48552 Backbench reconstruction of cadaver donor pancreas allograft prior to transplantation, venous anastomosis, each
➲ *CPT Changes: An Insider's View* 2005

(Do not report 48551 and 48552 in conjunction with 35531, 35563, 35685, 38100-38102, 44010, 44820, 44850, 47460, 47550-47556, 48100-48120, 48545)

48554 Transplantation of pancreatic allograft

48556 Removal of transplanted pancreatic allograft

Other Procedures

48999 Unlisted procedure, pancreas
➲ *CPT Assistant* Dec 07:12, May 11:9, Feb 13:13

Abdomen, Peritoneum, and Omentum

Incision

49000 Exploratory laparotomy, exploratory celiotomy with or without biopsy(s) (separate procedure)
➲ *CPT Assistant* Fall 92:23, Mar 01:10, Nov 08:7, Sep 12:11

(To report wound exploration due to penetrating trauma without laparotomy, use 20102)

49002 Reopening of recent laparotomy

➲ *CPT Assistant* Fall 92:23, Nov 08:7

(To report re-exploration of hepatic wound for removal of packing, use 47362)

49010 Exploration, retroperitoneal area with or without biopsy(s) (separate procedure)

(To report wound exploration due to penetrating trauma without laparotomy, use 20102)

49020 Drainage of peritoneal abscess or localized peritonitis, exclusive of appendiceal abscess, open

(For appendiceal abscess, use 44900)

(For percutaneous image-guided drainage of peritoneal abscess or localized peritonitis by catheter, use 49406)

(For transrectal or transvaginal image-guided drainage of peritoneal abscess by catheter, use 49407)

49040 Drainage of subdiaphragmatic or subphrenic abscess, open

➲ *CPT Assistant* Nov 97:18

(For percutaneous image-guided drainage of subdiaphragmatic or subphrenic abscess by catheter, use 49406)

49060 Drainage of retroperitoneal abscess, open

➲ *CPT Changes: An Insider's View* 2000

➲ *CPT Assistant* Nov 97:18, Nov 99:24, Jul 01:11, Aug 01:10

(For percutaneous image-guided drainage of retroperitoneal abscess by catheter, use 49406)

(For transrectal or transvaginal image-guided drainage of retroperitoneal abscess by catheter, use 49407)

49062 Drainage of extraperitoneal lymphocele to peritoneal cavity, open

➲ *CPT Assistant* Nov 97:19, Jul 01:11, Aug 01:10

(For laparoscopic drainage of lymphocele to peritoneal cavity, use 49323)

(For percutaneous image-guided drainage of peritoneal or retroperitoneal lymphocele by catheter, use 49406)

49082 Abdominal paracentesis (diagnostic or therapeutic); without imaging guidance

➲ *CPT Changes: An Insider's View* 2012

➲ *CPT Assistant* Dec 12:9

➲ *Clinical Examples in Radiology* Fall 11:11, Spring 12:10, Winter 12:9

49083 with imaging guidance

➲ *CPT Changes: An Insider's View* 2012

➲ *CPT Assistant* Dec 12:9, Mar 14:14

➲ *Clinical Examples in Radiology* Fall 11:11, Spring 12:10, Winter 12:9

(Do not report 49083 in conjunction with 76942, 77002, 77012, 77021)

(For percutaneous image-guided drainage of retroperitoneal abscess by catheter, use 49406)

49084 Peritoneal lavage, including imaging guidance, when performed

➲ *CPT Changes: An Insider's View* 2012

➲ *CPT Assistant* Dec 12:9

➲ *Clinical Examples in Radiology* Fall 11:11, Winter 12:9

(Do not report 49084 in conjunction with 76942, 77002, 77012, 77021)

(For percutaneous image-guided drainage of retroperitoneal abscess by catheter, use 49406)

Excision, Destruction

Code 49185 describes sclerotherapy of a fluid collection (eg, lymphocele, cyst, or seroma) through a percutaneous access. It includes contrast injection(s), sclerosant injection(s), sclerosant dwell time, diagnostic study, imaging guidance (eg, ultrasound, fluoroscopy), and radiological supervision and interpretation, when performed. Code 49185 may be reported once per day for each lesion treated through a separate catheter. Do not report 49185 more than once if treating multiple lesions through the same catheter. Codes for access to and drainage of the collection may be separately reportable according to location (eg, 10030, 10160, 49405, 49406, 49407, 50390).

(For lysis of intestinal adhesions, use 44005)

49180 Biopsy, abdominal or retroperitoneal mass, percutaneous needle

➲ *CPT Assistant* Fall 93:11

➲ *Clinical Examples in Radiology* Fall 10:7, Winter 17:5

(If imaging guidance is performed, see 76942, 77002, 77012, 77021)

►(For fine needle aspiration biopsy, see 10004, 10005, 10006, 10007, 10008, 10009, 10010, 10011, 10012, 10021)◄

(For evaluation of fine needle aspirate, see 88172, 88173)

49185 Sclerotherapy of a fluid collection (eg, lymphocele, cyst, or seroma), percutaneous, including contrast injection(s), sclerosant injection(s), diagnostic study, imaging guidance (eg, ultrasound, fluoroscopy) and radiological supervision and interpretation when performed

➲ *CPT Changes: An Insider's View* 2016

➲ *CPT Assistant* Mar 16:10

(For treatment of multiple lesions in a single day requiring separate access, use modifier 59 for each additional treated lesion)

(For treatment of multiple interconnected lesions treated through a single access, report 49185 once)

(For access/drainage with needle, see 10160, 50390)

(For access/drainage with catheter, see 10030, 49405, 49406, 49407, 50390)

(For exchange of existing catheter, before or after injection of sclerosant, see 49423, 75984)

(For sclerotherapy of a lymphatic/vascular malformation, use 37241)

(For sclerosis of veins or endovenous ablation of incompetent extremity veins, see 36468, 36470, 36471, 36475, 36476, 36478, 36479)

(For pleurodesis, use 32560)

(Do not report 49185 in conjunction with 49424, 76080)

49203 Excision or destruction, open, intra-abdominal tumors, cysts or endometriomas, 1 or more peritoneal, mesenteric, or retroperitoneal primary or secondary tumors; largest tumor 5 cm diameter or less
➔ *CPT Changes: An Insider's View* 2008
➔ *CPT Assistant* Aug 08:7, Dec 10:16

49204 largest tumor 5.1-10.0 cm diameter
➔ *CPT Changes: An Insider's View* 2008
➔ *CPT Assistant* Aug 08:7, Dec 10:16

49205 largest tumor greater than 10.0 cm diameter
➔ *CPT Changes: An Insider's View* 2008
➔ *CPT Assistant* Aug 08:7, Dec 10:16

(Do not report 49203-49205 in conjunction with 38770, 38780, 49000, 49010, 49215, 50010, 50205, 50225, 50236, 50250, 50290, 58920, 58925, 58940, 58943, 58951, 58952, 58953, 58954, 58956, 58957, 58958, 58960)

(For partial or total nephrectomy, use 50220 or 50240 in conjunction with 49203-49205)

(For colectomy, use 44140 in conjunction with 49203-49205)

(For small bowel resection, use 44120 in conjunction with 49203-49205)

(For vena caval resection with reconstruction, use 49203-49205 in conjunction with 37799)

(For resection of recurrent ovarian, tubal, primary peritoneal, or uterine malignancy, see 58957, 58958)

(For cryoablation of renal tumors, see 50250, 50593)

49215 Excision of presacral or sacrococcygeal tumor

(Do not report modifier 63 in conjunction with 49215)

49220 Staging laparotomy for Hodgkins disease or lymphoma (includes splenectomy, needle or open biopsies of both liver lobes, possibly also removal of abdominal nodes, abdominal node and/or bone marrow biopsies, ovarian repositioning)
➔ *CPT Changes: An Insider's View* 2002

49250 Umbilectomy, omphalectomy, excision of umbilicus (separate procedure)

49255 Omentectomy, epiploectomy, resection of omentum (separate procedure)
➔ *CPT Changes: An Insider's View* 2000
➔ *CPT Assistant* Nov 99:24, Mar 18:11

Laparoscopy

Surgical laparoscopy always includes diagnostic laparoscopy. To report a diagnostic laparoscopy (peritoneoscopy), (separate procedure), use 49320.

For laparoscopic fulguration or excision of lesions of the ovary, pelvic viscera, or peritoneal surface use 58662.

49320 Laparoscopy, abdomen, peritoneum, and omentum, diagnostic, with or without collection of specimen(s) by brushing or washing (separate procedure)
➔ *CPT Changes: An Insider's View* 2000, 2001
➔ *CPT Assistant* Nov 99:24, Mar 00:9, Apr 06:19, Mar 07:4, Nov 07:1, Dec 08:7, Jun 10:7, Dec 15:18, Apr 17:7

Laparoscopy
49320

The physician inserts a fiberoptic laparoscope to observe the necessary organs in these procedures.

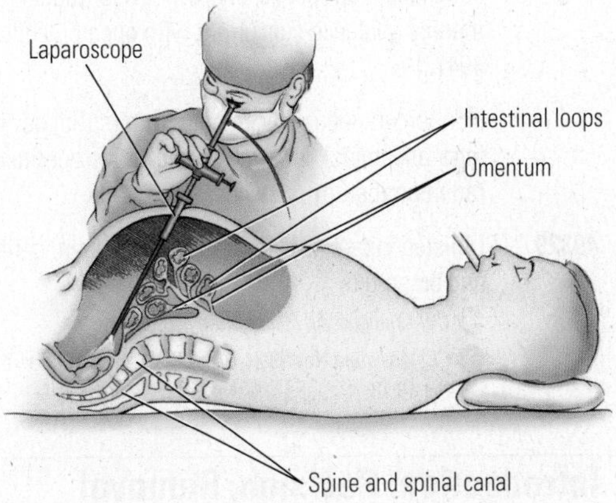

49321 Laparoscopy, surgical; with biopsy (single or multiple)
➔ *CPT Changes: An Insider's View* 2000, 2001
➔ *CPT Assistant* Nov 99:24, Mar 00:9

49322 with aspiration of cavity or cyst (eg, ovarian cyst) (single or multiple)
➔ *CPT Changes: An Insider's View* 2000
➔ *CPT Assistant* Nov 99:24, Mar 00:9

49323 with drainage of lymphocele to peritoneal cavity
➔ *CPT Changes: An Insider's View* 2000
➔ *CPT Assistant* Nov 99:24, Mar 00:9, May 00:4, Jul 01:11, Aug 01:10

(For open drainage of lymphocele to peritoneal cavity, use 49062)

49324 with insertion of tunneled intraperitoneal catheter
➔ *CPT Changes: An Insider's View* 2007, 2011

(For subcutaneous extension of intraperitoneal catheter with remote chest exit site, use 49435 in conjunction with 49324)

(For open insertion of tunneled intraperitoneal catheter, use 49421)

49325 with revision of previously placed intraperitoneal cannula or catheter, with removal of intraluminal obstructive material if performed

➲ *CPT Changes: An Insider's View* 2007

+ 49326 with omentopexy (omental tacking procedure) (List separately in addition to code for primary procedure)

➲ *CPT Changes: An Insider's View* 2007

(Use 49326 in conjunction with 49324, 49325)

+ 49327 with placement of interstitial device(s) for radiation therapy guidance (eg, fiducial markers, dosimeter), intra-abdominal, intrapelvic, and/or retroperitoneum, including imaging guidance, if performed, single or multiple (List separately in addition to code for primary procedure)

➲ *CPT Changes: An Insider's View* 2011

(Use 49327 in conjunction with laparoscopic abdominal, pelvic, or retroperitoneal procedure[s] performed concurrently)

(For placement of interstitial device[s] for intra-abdominal, intrapelvic, and/or retroperitoneal radiation therapy guidance concurrent with open procedure, use 49412)

(For percutaneous placement of interstitial device[s] for intra-abdominal, intrapelvic, and/or retroperitoneal radiation therapy guidance, use 49411)

49329 Unlisted laparoscopy procedure, abdomen, peritoneum and omentum

➲ *CPT Changes: An Insider's View* 2000

➲ *CPT Assistant* Nov 99:24, Mar 00:9, Feb 06:16, Dec 11:16, Oct 13:18

Introduction, Revision, Removal

49400 Injection of air or contrast into peritoneal cavity (separate procedure)

➲ *CPT Assistant* Dec 10:13

➲ *Clinical Examples in Radiology* Fall 07:1, 2

(For radiological supervision and interpretation, use 74190)

49402 Removal of peritoneal foreign body from peritoneal cavity

➲ *CPT Changes: An Insider's View* 2007

(For lysis of intestinal adhesions, use 44005)

(For open or percutaneous peritoneal drainage or lavage, see 49406, 49020, 49040, 49082-49084, as appropriate)

(For percutaneous insertion of a tunneled intraperitoneal catheter without subcutaneous port, use 49418)

49405 Image-guided fluid collection drainage by catheter (eg, abscess, hematoma, seroma, lymphocele, cyst); visceral (eg, kidney, liver, spleen, lung/mediastinum), percutaneous

➲ *CPT Changes: An Insider's View* 2014, 2017

➲ *CPT Assistant* May 14:9

➲ *Clinical Examples in Radiology* Fall 13:6, Spring 15:8, Winter 16:10

(Do not report 49405 in conjunction with 75989, 76942, 77002, 77003, 77012, 77021)

(For percutaneous cholecystostomy, use 47490)

(For pneumonostomy, use 32200)

(For thoracentesis, see 32554, 32555)

(For percutaneous pleural drainage, see 32556, 32557)

(For open visceral drainage, see 32200 [lung abscess or cyst], 47010 [liver abscess or cyst], 48510 [pseudocyst of pancreas], 50020 [perirenal or renal abscess])

49406 peritoneal or retroperitoneal, percutaneous

➲ *CPT Changes: An Insider's View* 2014, 2017

➲ *CPT Assistant* May 14:9

➲ *Clinical Examples in Radiology* Fall 13:6, Spring 15:8, Winter 16:10

(Do not report 49406 in conjunction with 75989, 76942, 77002, 77003, 77012, 77021)

(For abdominal paracentesis [diagnostic or therapeutic], see 49082, 49083)

(For transrectal or transvaginal image-guided peritoneal or retroperitoneal fluid collection drainage by catheter, use 49407)

(For open transrectal drainage of pelvic abscess, use 45000)

(For open peritoneal or retroperitoneal drainage, see 44900 [appendiceal abscess], 49020 [peritoneal abscess or localized peritonitis], 49040 [subdiaphragmatic or subphrenic abscess], 49060 [retroperitoneal abscess], 49062 [extraperitoneal lymphocele], 49084 [peritoneal lavage], 50020 [perirenal or renal abscess], 58805 [ovarian cyst], 58822 [ovarian abscess])

(For percutaneous paracentesis, see 49082, 49083)

(For percutaneous insertion of a tunneled intraperitoneal catheter without subcutaneous port, use 49418)

49407 peritoneal or retroperitoneal, transvaginal or transrectal

➲ *CPT Changes: An Insider's View* 2014, 2017

➲ *CPT Assistant* May 14:9

➲ *Clinical Examples in Radiology* Fall 13:6, Spring 15:8, Winter 16:10

(Do not report 49407 in conjunction with 75989, 76942, 77002, 77003, 77012, 77021)

(Report 49405, 49406, 49407 separately for each individual collection drained with a separate catheter)

(For open transrectal or transvaginal drainage, see 45000 [pelvic abscess], 58800 [ovarian cyst], 58820 [ovarian abscess])

(For percutaneous image-guided fluid collection drainage by catheter [eg, abscess, hematoma, seroma, lymphocele, cyst] for soft tissue [eg, extremity, abdominal wall, neck], use 10030)

49411 Placement of interstitial device(s) for radiation therapy guidance (eg, fiducial markers, dosimeter), percutaneous, intra-abdominal, intra-pelvic (except prostate), and/or retroperitoneum, single or multiple

➔ *CPT Changes: An Insider's View* 2010, 2017

➔ *CPT Assistant* Feb 10:7, Jun 16:3

(Report supply of device separately)

(For imaging guidance, see 76942, 77002, 77012, 77021)

(For percutaneous placement of interstitial device[s] for intra-thoracic radiation therapy guidance, use 32553)

+ 49412 Placement of interstitial device(s) for radiation therapy guidance (eg, fiducial markers, dosimeter), open, intra-abdominal, intrapelvic, and/or retroperitoneum, including image guidance, if performed, single or multiple (List separately in addition to code for primary procedure)

➔ *CPT Changes: An Insider's View* 2011

(Use 49412 in conjunction with open abdominal, pelvic, or retroperitoneal procedure[s] performed concurrently)

(For placement of interstitial device[s] for intra-abdominal, intrapelvic, and/or retroperitoneal radiation therapy guidance concurrent with laparoscopic procedure, use 49327)

(For percutaneous placement of interstitial device[s] for intra-abdominal, intrapelvic, and/or retroperitoneal radiation therapy guidance, use 49411)

49418 Insertion of tunneled intraperitoneal catheter (eg, dialysis, intraperitoneal chemotherapy instillation, management of ascites), complete procedure, including imaging guidance, catheter placement, contrast injection when performed, and radiological supervision and interpretation, percutaneous

➔ *CPT Changes: An Insider's View* 2011, 2017

49419 Insertion of tunneled intraperitoneal catheter, with subcutaneous port (ie, totally implantable)

➔ *CPT Changes: An Insider's View* 2003, 2011

(For removal, use 49422)

49421 Insertion of tunneled intraperitoneal catheter for dialysis, open

➔ *CPT Changes: An Insider's View* 2011

➔ *CPT Assistant* Fall 93:2, Jul 06:19

(For laparoscopic insertion of tunneled intraperitoneal catheter, use 49324)

(For subcutaneous extension of intraperitoneal catheter with remote chest exit site, use 49435 in conjunction with 49421)

49422 Removal of tunneled intraperitoneal catheter

➔ *CPT Changes: An Insider's View* 2011

(For removal of a non-tunneled catheter, use appropriate E/M code)

49423 Exchange of previously placed abscess or cyst drainage catheter under radiological guidance (separate procedure)

➔ *CPT Assistant* Nov 97:19, Mar 98:8

➔ *Clinical Examples in Radiology* Summer 13:6

(For radiological supervision and interpretation, use 75984)

49424 Contrast injection for assessment of abscess or cyst via previously placed drainage catheter or tube (separate procedure)

➔ *CPT Changes: An Insider's View* 2002

➔ *CPT Assistant* Nov 97:19, Mar 98:8, Nov 03:14

➔ *Clinical Examples in Radiology* Fall 09:9

(For radiological supervision and interpretation, use 76080)

49425 Insertion of peritoneal-venous shunt

49426 Revision of peritoneal-venous shunt

(For shunt patency test, use 78291)

49427 Injection procedure (eg, contrast media) for evaluation of previously placed peritoneal-venous shunt

(For radiological supervision and interpretation, see 75809, 78291)

49428 Ligation of peritoneal-venous shunt

49429 Removal of peritoneal-venous shunt

+ 49435 Insertion of subcutaneous extension to intraperitoneal cannula or catheter with remote chest exit site (List separately in addition to code for primary procedure)

➔ *CPT Changes: An Insider's View* 2007

(Use 49435 in conjunction with 49324, 49421)

49436 Delayed creation of exit site from embedded subcutaneous segment of intraperitoneal cannula or catheter

➔ *CPT Changes: An Insider's View* 2007

Initial Placement

Do not additionally report 43752 for placement of a nasogastric (NG) or orogastric (OG) tube to insufflate the stomach prior to percutaneous gastrointestinal tube placement. NG or OG tube placement is considered part of the procedure in this family of codes.

49440 Insertion of gastrostomy tube, percutaneous, under fluoroscopic guidance including contrast injection(s), image documentation and report

➔ *CPT Changes: An Insider's View* 2008, 2017

➔ *CPT Assistant* Jan 08:8, Jun 08:8, Aug 08:7, Sep 10:9, Sep 14:5, Dec 14:18

(For conversion to a gastro-jejunostomy tube at the time of initial gastrostomy tube placement, use 49440 in conjunction with 49446)

49441 Insertion of duodenostomy or jejunostomy tube, percutaneous, under fluoroscopic guidance including contrast injection(s), image documentation and report

➲ *CPT Changes: An Insider's View* 2008, 2017

➲ *CPT Assistant* Jan 08:8, Jun 08:8, Aug 08:7, Dec 14:18

(For conversion of gastrostomy tube to gastro-jejunostomy tube, use 49446)

49442 Insertion of cecostomy or other colonic tube, percutaneous, under fluoroscopic guidance including contrast injection(s), image documentation and report

➲ *CPT Changes: An Insider's View* 2008, 2017

➲ *CPT Assistant* Jan 08:8, Jun 08:8, Aug 08:7, Dec 14:18

Conversion

49446 Conversion of gastrostomy tube to gastro-jejunostomy tube, percutaneous, under fluoroscopic guidance including contrast injection(s), image documentation and report

➲ *CPT Changes: An Insider's View* 2008, 2017

(For conversion to a gastro-jejunostomy tube at the time of initial gastrostomy tube placement, use 49446 in conjunction with 49440)

Replacement

If an existing gastrostomy, duodenostomy, jejunostomy, gastro-jejunostomy, or cecostomy (or other colonic) tube is removed and a new tube is placed via a separate percutaneous access site, the placement of the new tube is not considered a replacement and would be reported using the appropriate initial placement codes 49440-49442.

49450 Replacement of gastrostomy or cecostomy (or other colonic) tube, percutaneous, under fluoroscopic guidance including contrast injection(s), image documentation and report

➲ *CPT Changes: An Insider's View* 2008

➲ *CPT Assistant* Sep 10:9, Dec 13:17

►(For percutaneous replacement of gastrostomy tube with removal when performed without imaging or endoscopy, see 43762, 43763)◄

49451 Replacement of duodenostomy or jejunostomy tube, percutaneous, under fluoroscopic guidance including contrast injection(s), image documentation and report

➲ *CPT Changes: An Insider's View* 2008

➲ *CPT Assistant* Jan 08:8, Jun 08:8, Aug 08:7, Jul 10:10, Dec 14:18

49452 Replacement of gastro-jejunostomy tube, percutaneous, under fluoroscopic guidance including contrast injection(s), image documentation and report

➲ *CPT Changes: An Insider's View* 2008

➲ *CPT Assistant* Mar 10:10

Mechanical Removal of Obstructive Material

49460 Mechanical removal of obstructive material from gastrostomy, duodenostomy, jejunostomy, gastro-jejunostomy, or cecostomy (or other colonic) tube, any method, under fluoroscopic guidance including contrast injection(s), if performed, image documentation and report

➲ *CPT Changes: An Insider's View* 2008

(Do not report 49460 in conjunction with 49450-49452, 49465)

Other

49465 Contrast injection(s) for radiological evaluation of existing gastrostomy, duodenostomy, jejunostomy, gastro-jejunostomy, or cecostomy (or other colonic) tube, from a percutaneous approach including image documentation and report

➲ *CPT Changes: An Insider's View* 2008

➲ *CPT Assistant* Sep 14:5

(Do not report 49465 in conjunction with 49450-49460)

Repair

Hernioplasty, Herniorrhaphy, Herniotomy

The hernia repair codes in this section are categorized primarily by the type of hernia (inguinal, femoral, incisional, etc).

Some types of hernias are further categorized as "initial" or "recurrent" based on whether or not the hernia has required previous repair(s).

Additional variables accounted for by some of the codes include patient age and clinical presentation (reducible vs. incarcerated or strangulated).

With the exception of the incisional hernia repairs (see 49560-49566) the use of mesh or other prostheses is not separately reported.

The excision/repair of strangulated organs or structures such as testicle(s), intestine, ovaries are reported by using the appropriate code for the excision/repair (eg, 44120, 54520, and 58940) in addition to the appropriate code for the repair of the strangulated hernia.

(For reduction and repair of intra-abdominal hernia, use 44050)

(For debridement of abdominal wall, see 11042, 11043)

(Codes 49491-49651 are unilateral procedures. To report bilateral procedure, report modifier 50 with the appropriate procedure code)

49491 Repair, initial inguinal hernia, preterm infant (younger than 37 weeks gestation at birth), performed from birth up to 50 weeks postconception age, with or without hydrocelectomy; reducible
➲ *CPT Changes: An Insider's View* 2002
➲ *CPT Assistant* Mar 04:2, Jun 08:3

49492 incarcerated or strangulated
➲ *CPT Changes: An Insider's View* 2002
➲ *CPT Assistant* Mar 04:2, Jun 08:3

(Do not report modifier 63 in conjunction with 49491, 49492)

(Postconception age equals gestational age at birth plus age of infant in weeks at the time of the hernia repair. Initial inguinal hernia repairs that are performed on preterm infants who are older than 50 weeks postconception age and younger than age 6 months at the time of surgery, should be reported using codes 49495, 49496)

49495 Repair, initial inguinal hernia, full term infant younger than age 6 months, or preterm infant older than 50 weeks postconception age and younger than age 6 months at the time of surgery, with or without hydrocelectomy; reducible
➲ *CPT Changes: An Insider's View* 2002
➲ *CPT Assistant* Winter 93:6, Winter 94:13, Jan 04:27, Mar 04:10, May 04:14, Nov 07:9, Jun 08:3

49496 incarcerated or strangulated
➲ *CPT Assistant* Winter 93:6, Winter 94:13, Jan 04:27, Mar 04:10, May 04:14, Jun 08:3

(Do not report modifier 63 in conjunction with 49495, 49496)

(Postconception age equals gestational age at birth plus age in weeks at the time of the hernia repair. Initial inguinal hernia repairs that are performed on preterm infants who are younger than or up to 50 weeks postconception age but younger than 6 months of age since birth, should be reported using codes 49491, 49492. Inguinal hernia repairs on infants age 6 months to younger than 5 years should be reported using codes 49500-49501)

49500 Repair initial inguinal hernia, age 6 months to younger than 5 years, with or without hydrocelectomy; reducible
➲ *CPT Changes: An Insider's View* 2002
➲ *CPT Assistant* Winter 94:13, Jan 04:27, Mar 04:10, Nov 07:9, Jun 08:3, Nov 14:14

49501 incarcerated or strangulated
➲ *CPT Changes: An Insider's View* 2002
➲ *CPT Assistant* Winter 94:13, Jan 04:27, Mar 04:12, Jun 08:3

49505 Repair initial inguinal hernia, age 5 years or older; reducible
➲ *CPT Assistant* Winter 94:13, Sep 00:10, Jan 04:27, Mar 04:12, Jun 08:3

49507 incarcerated or strangulated
➲ *CPT Assistant* Winter 94:13, Jan 04:27, Mar 04:10, Jun 08:3

(For inguinal hernia repair, with simple orchiectomy, see 49505 or 49507 and 54520)

(For inguinal hernia repair, with excision of hydrocele or spermatocele, see 49505 or 49507 and 54840 or 55040)

49520 Repair recurrent inguinal hernia, any age; reducible
➲ *CPT Assistant* Winter 94:13, Sep 03:3, Jan 04:27, Mar 04:3, Jun 08:3

49521 incarcerated or strangulated
➲ *CPT Assistant* Winter 94:13, Jan 04:27, Mar 04:10, Jun 08:3

49525 Repair inguinal hernia, sliding, any age
➲ *CPT Assistant* Winter 94:14, Jan 04:27, Mar 04:10, Nov 07:9, Jun 08:3

(For incarcerated or strangulated inguinal hernia repair, see 49496, 49501, 49507, 49521)

49540 Repair lumbar hernia
➲ *CPT Assistant* Winter 94:14, Jun 08:3

49550 Repair initial femoral hernia, any age; reducible
➲ *CPT Assistant* Winter 94:14, Jun 08:3

49553 incarcerated or strangulated
➲ *CPT Assistant* Winter 94:14, Jun 08:3

49555 Repair recurrent femoral hernia; reducible
➲ *CPT Assistant* Winter 94:14, Jun 08:3

49557 incarcerated or strangulated
➲ *CPT Assistant* Winter 94:14, Jun 08:3

49560 Repair initial incisional or ventral hernia; reducible
➲ *CPT Assistant* Winter 93:6, Winter 94:14, Nov 97:19, Jun 08:3, Jan 12:10, Oct 13:15

49561 incarcerated or strangulated
➲ *CPT Assistant* Winter 94:14, Jun 08:3, Jan 12:10, Oct 13:15, Mar 18:11

49565 Repair recurrent incisional or ventral hernia; reducible
➲ *CPT Assistant* Winter 94:14, Nov 97:19, Jun 08:3, Jan 12:10, Oct 13:15

49566 incarcerated or strangulated
➲ *CPT Assistant* Winter 94:14, Jun 08:3, Jan 12:10, Oct 13:15

Coding Tip

Restrictions for Reporting Insertion of Mesh and Other Prostheses with Hernia Repairs

With the exception of the incisional hernia repairs (see 49560-49566) the use of mesh or other prostheses is not separately reported.

CPT Coding Guidelines, Hernioplasty, Herniorrhaphy, Herniotomy

+ **49568** Implantation of mesh or other prosthesis for open incisional or ventral hernia repair or mesh for closure of debridement for necrotizing soft tissue infection (List separately in addition to code for the incisional or ventral hernia repair)
➔ *CPT Changes: An Insider's View* 2008, 2009
➔ *CPT Assistant* Winter 94:14, Nov 97:19, Sep 01:11, Nov 05:15, Nov 07:9, Jun 08:3, Jan 12:10, Oct 13:15

(Use 49568 in conjunction with 11004-11006, 49560-49566)

49570 Repair epigastric hernia (eg, preperitoneal fat); reducible (separate procedure)
➔ *CPT Assistant* Winter 94:15, Jun 08:3

49572 incarcerated or strangulated
➔ *CPT Assistant* Winter 94:15, Jun 08:3

49580 Repair umbilical hernia, younger than age 5 years; reducible
➔ *CPT Assistant* Winter 94:15, Jun 08:3

49582 incarcerated or strangulated
➔ *CPT Assistant* Winter 94:15, Jun 08:3

49585 Repair umbilical hernia, age 5 years or older; reducible
➔ *CPT Assistant* Winter 94:15

49587 incarcerated or strangulated
➔ *CPT Assistant* Winter 94:15

49590 Repair spigelian hernia
➔ *CPT Assistant* Winter 94:15

49600 Repair of small omphalocele, with primary closure
➔ *CPT Assistant* Winter 94:15

(Do not report modifier 63 in conjunction with 49600)

49605 Repair of large omphalocele or gastroschisis; with or without prosthesis
➔ *CPT Assistant* Winter 94:15

49606 with removal of prosthesis, final reduction and closure, in operating room
➔ *CPT Assistant* Winter 94:15

(Do not report modifier 63 in conjunction with 49605, 49606)

49610 Repair of omphalocele (Gross type operation); first stage
➔ *CPT Assistant* Winter 94:15

49611 second stage
➔ *CPT Assistant* Winter 94:15

(Do not report modifier 63 in conjunction with 49610, 49611)

(For diaphragmatic or hiatal hernia repair, see 39503, 43332)

(For surgical repair of omentum, use 49999)

Laparoscopy

Surgical laparoscopy always includes diagnostic laparoscopy. To report a diagnostic laparoscopy (peritoneoscopy) (separate procedure), use 49320.

49650 Laparoscopy, surgical; repair initial inguinal hernia
➔ *CPT Changes: An Insider's View* 2000
➔ *CPT Assistant* Nov 99:24, Mar 00:9, Jul 14:5

49651 repair recurrent inguinal hernia
➔ *CPT Changes: An Insider's View* 2000
➔ *CPT Assistant* Nov 99:24, Mar 00:9

49652 Laparoscopy, surgical, repair, ventral, umbilical, spigelian or epigastric hernia (includes mesh insertion, when performed); reducible
➔ *CPT Changes: An Insider's View* 2009

(Do not report 49652 in conjunction with 44180, 49568)

49653 incarcerated or strangulated
➔ *CPT Changes: An Insider's View* 2009

(Do not report 49653 in conjunction with 44180, 49568)

49654 Laparoscopy, surgical, repair, incisional hernia (includes mesh insertion, when performed); reducible
➔ *CPT Changes: An Insider's View* 2009
➔ *CPT Assistant* Jan 18:7

(Do not report 49654 in conjunction with 44180, 49568)

49655 incarcerated or strangulated
➔ *CPT Changes: An Insider's View* 2009
➔ *CPT Assistant* Jan 18:7

(Do not report 49655 in conjunction with 44180, 49568)

49656 Laparoscopy, surgical, repair, recurrent incisional hernia (includes mesh insertion, when performed); reducible
➔ *CPT Changes: An Insider's View* 2009

(Do not report 49656 in conjunction with 44180, 49568)

49657 incarcerated or strangulated
➔ *CPT Changes: An Insider's View* 2009

(Do not report 49657 in conjunction with 44180, 49568)

49659 Unlisted laparoscopy procedure, hernioplasty, herniorrhaphy, herniotomy
➔ *CPT Changes: An Insider's View* 2000
➔ *CPT Assistant* Nov 99:25, Mar 00:9, Sep 01:11, Nov 05:15, Feb 06:16, Jan 09:7, Jul 14:5, Dec 14:16, Jul 17:10

Suture

49900 Suture, secondary, of abdominal wall for evisceration or dehiscence
➔ *CPT Assistant* Sep 10:7

(For suture of ruptured diaphragm, see 39540, 39541)

(For debridement of abdominal wall, see 11042, 11043)

Other Procedures

49904 Omental flap, extra-abdominal (eg, for reconstruction of sternal and chest wall defects)
➔ *CPT Changes: An Insider's View* 2003

(Code 49904 includes harvest and transfer. If a second surgeon harvests the omental flap, then the 2 surgeons should code 49904 as co-surgeons, using modifier 62)

+ 49905 Omental flap, intra-abdominal (List separately in addition to code for primary procedure)

➔ *CPT Changes: An Insider's View* 2003

➔ *CPT Assistant* Nov 00:11

(Do not report 49905 in conjunction with 44700)

49906 Free omental flap with microvascular anastomosis

➔ *CPT Assistant* Nov 96:8, Apr 97:8, Nov 98:16

(Do not report code 69990 in addition to 49906)

49999 Unlisted procedure, abdomen, peritoneum and omentum

➔ *CPT Assistant* Jul 06:19, Sep 07:10, Nov 07:9, Aug 08:7, Apr 10:10, Dec 10:13, Jun 11:13, Jan 14:9

➔ *Clinical Examples in Radiology* Fall 07:1, 2

Digestive

Notes

Surgery

Urinary System (50010-53899) 357

The following is a listing of headings and subheadings that appear within the Urinary System section of the CPT codebook. The subheadings or subsections denoted with asterisks (*) below have special instructions unique to that subsection. Where these are indicated, special notes or guidelines will be presented preceding those procedural terminology listings referring to that subsection specifically.

Kidney (50010-50593) 357
- **Incision (50010-50135)** 357
- **Excision (50200-50290)** 358
- **Renal Transplantation* (50300-50380)** 358
- **Introduction (50382-50396, 50430-50437)** 359
  - **Renal Pelvis Catheter Procedures (50382-50389)** 359
    - *Internally Dwelling (50382-50386)* *359*
    - *Externally Accessible (50387-50389)* *359*
  - **Other Introduction (Injection/Change/Removal) Procedures* (50390-50396, 50430-50437)** 360
- **Repair (50400-50405, 50500-50540)** 361
- **Laparoscopy* (50541-50549)** 362
- **Endoscopy (50551-50580)** 363
- **Other Procedures (50590-50593)** 363

Ureter (50600-50980) 364
- **Incision/Biopsy* (50600-50630)** 364
- **Excision (50650-50660)** 365
- **Introduction (50684-50695)** 365
  - **Other Introduction (Injection/Change/Removal) Procedures* (50684-50695)** 365
- **Repair* (50700-50940)** 365
- **Laparoscopy* (50945-50949)** 367
- **Endoscopy (50951-50980)** 367

Bladder (51020-52700) 368
- **Incision (51020-51080)** 368
- **Removal (51100-51102)** 368
- **Excision (51500-51597)** 368
- **Introduction (51600-51720)** 368
- **Urodynamics* (51725-51798)** 369
- **Repair (51800-51980)** 370
- **Laparoscopy* (51990-51999)** 370
- **Endoscopy—Cystoscopy, Urethroscopy, Cystourethroscopy* (52000-52010)** 371
- **Transurethral Surgery (52204-52356)** 371
  - **Urethra and Bladder (52204-52318)** 371
  - **Ureter and Pelvis* (52320-52356)** 373
- **Vesical Neck and Prostate (52400-52700)** 374

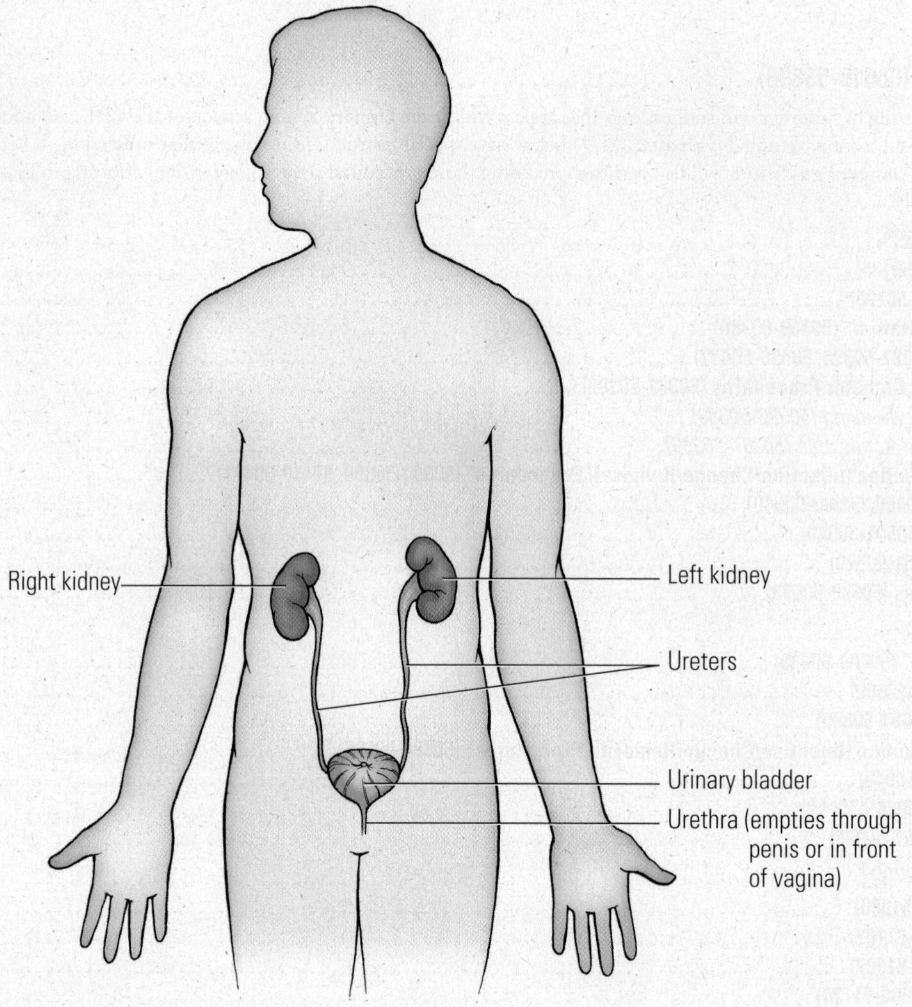

Urinary System

Urethra (53000-53899) 375
Incision (53000-53085) 375
Excision (53200-53275) 375
Repair (53400-53520) 376
Manipulation (53600-53665) 376
Other Procedures (53850-53899) 377

Urinary System

(For provision of chemotherapeutic agents, report both the specific service in addition to code(s) for the specific substance(s) or drug(s) provided)

Kidney

Incision

(For retroperitoneal exploration, abscess, tumor, or cyst, see 49010, 49060, 49203-49205)

50010 Renal exploration, not necessitating other specific procedures

(For laparoscopic ablation of renal mass lesion(s), use 50542)

50020 Drainage of perirenal or renal abscess, open

➔ *CPT Assistant* Nov 97:19, Oct 01:8, May 14:9

Drainage of Renal Abscess
50020

An incision is made to the abscess cavity and the site is irrigated and drained.

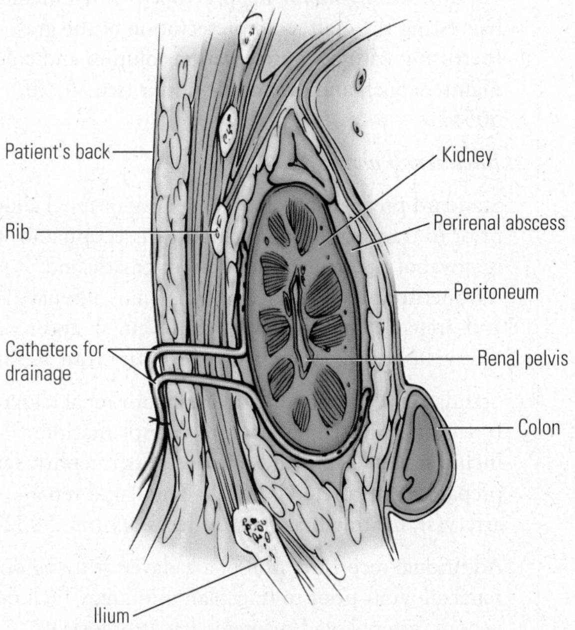

(For percutaneous image-guided fluid collection drainage by catheter of perirenal/renal abscess, use 49405)

50040 Nephrostomy, nephrotomy with drainage

➔ *CPT Assistant* Spring 93:35, Oct 01:8

50045 Nephrotomy, with exploration

➔ *CPT Assistant* Oct 01:8

(For renal endoscopy performed in conjunction with this procedure, see 50570-50580)

50060 Nephrolithotomy; removal of calculus

➔ *CPT Assistant* Oct 01:8

Nephrolithotomy With Calculus Removal
50060-50075

A kidney stone (calculus) is removed by an incision in the kidney. Use 50070 if complicated by a congenital kidney abnormality.

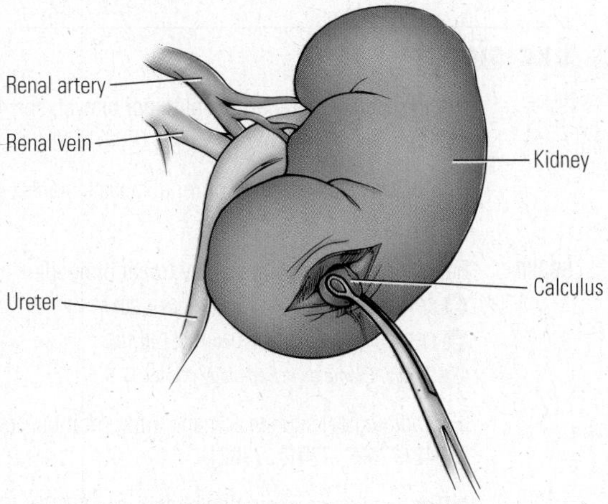

50065 secondary surgical operation for calculus

➔ *CPT Assistant* Oct 01:8

50070 complicated by congenital kidney abnormality

➔ *CPT Assistant* Oct 01:8

50075 removal of large staghorn calculus filling renal pelvis and calyces (including anatrophic pyelolithotomy)

➔ *CPT Assistant* Oct 01:8

50080 Percutaneous nephrostolithotomy or pyelostolithotomy, with or without dilation, endoscopy, lithotripsy, stenting, or basket extraction; up to 2 cm

➔ *CPT Assistant* Oct 01:8, Dec 08:7, Jun 09:10

50081 over 2 cm

➔ *CPT Assistant* Oct 01:8, Dec 08:7, Jun 09:10

►(For establishment of nephrostomy without nephrostolithotomy, see 50040, 50432, 50433, 52334)◄

►(For fluoroscopic guidance, use 76000)◄

►(Do not report 50080, 50081 in conjunction with 50436, 50437, when performed by the same physician or other qualified health care professional)◄

50100 Transection or repositioning of aberrant renal vessels (separate procedure)

➔ *CPT Assistant* Oct 01:8

50120 Pyelotomy; with exploration

➔ *CPT Assistant* Oct 01:8

(For renal endoscopy performed in conjunction with this procedure, see 50570-50580)

50125 with drainage, pyelostomy

➔ *CPT Assistant* Oct 01:8

50130 with removal of calculus (pyelolithotomy, pelviolithotomy, including coagulum pyelolithotomy)
➲ *CPT Assistant* Oct 01:8

50135 complicated (eg, secondary operation, congenital kidney abnormality)
➲ *CPT Assistant* Oct 01:8

(For supply of anticarcinogenic agents, use 99070 in addition to code for primary procedure)

Excision

(For excision of retroperitoneal tumor or cyst, see 49203-49205)

(For laparoscopic ablation of renal mass lesion(s), use 50542)

50200 Renal biopsy; percutaneous, by trocar or needle
➲ *CPT Changes: An Insider's View* 2010, 2017
➲ *CPT Assistant* Fall 93:13, Oct 01:8, Feb 10:7
➲ *Clinical Examples in Radiology* Winter 17:5

(For radiological supervision and interpretation, see 76942, 77002, 77012, 77021)

►(For fine needle aspiration biopsy, see 10005, 10006, 10007, 10008, 10009, 10010, 10011, 10012)◄

(For evaluation of fine needle aspirate, see 88172, 88173)

50205 by surgical exposure of kidney
➲ *CPT Assistant* Oct 01:8

50220 Nephrectomy, including partial ureterectomy, any open approach including rib resection;
➲ *CPT Changes: An Insider's View* 2002
➲ *CPT Assistant* Oct 01:8, Nov 02:3, Aug 08:7

50225 complicated because of previous surgery on same kidney
➲ *CPT Assistant* Oct 01:8, Nov 02:3

50230 radical, with regional lymphadenectomy and/or vena caval thrombectomy
➲ *CPT Assistant* Oct 01:8, Nov 02:3

(When vena caval resection with reconstruction is necessary, use 37799)

50234 Nephrectomy with total ureterectomy and bladder cuff; through same incision
➲ *CPT Assistant* Oct 01:8, Nov 02:3

50236 through separate incision
➲ *CPT Assistant* Oct 01:8, Nov 02:3

50240 Nephrectomy, partial
➲ *CPT Assistant* Oct 01:8, Nov 02:3, Jan 03:20, Apr 05:10, 12, Aug 08:7

(For laparoscopic partial nephrectomy, use 50543)

50250 Ablation, open, 1 or more renal mass lesion(s), cryosurgical, including intraoperative ultrasound guidance and monitoring, if performed
➲ *CPT Changes: An Insider's View* 2006, 2011
➲ *CPT Assistant* May 06:17

(For laparoscopic ablation of renal mass lesions, use 50542)

(For percutaneous ablation of renal tumors, see 50592, 50593)

50280 Excision or unroofing of cyst(s) of kidney
➲ *CPT Changes: An Insider's View* 2000
➲ *CPT Assistant* Nov 99:25, Oct 01:8

(For laparoscopic ablation of renal cysts, use 50541)

50290 Excision of perinephric cyst
➲ *CPT Assistant* Oct 01:8

Renal Transplantation

Renal *auto*transplantation includes reimplantation of the autograft as the primary procedure, along with secondary extra-corporeal procedure(s) (eg, partial nephrectomy, nephrolithotomy) reported with modifier 51 (see 50380 and applicable secondary procedure(s)).

Renal *allo*transplantation involves three distinct components of physician work:

1. ***Cadaver donor nephrectomy, unilateral or bilateral,*** which includes harvesting the graft(s) and cold preservation of the graft(s) (perfusing with cold preservation solution and cold maintenance) (use 50300). ***Living donor nephrectomy,*** which includes harvesting the graft, cold preservation of the graft (perfusing with cold preservation solution and cold maintenance), and care of the donor (see 50320, 50547).

2. ***Backbench work:***

   Standard preparation of a cadaver donor renal allograft prior to transplantation including dissection and removal of perinephric fat, diaphragmatic and retroperitoneal attachments; excision of adrenal gland; and preparation of ureter(s), renal vein(s), and renal artery(s), ligating branches, as necessary (use 50323).

   Standard preparation of a living donor renal allograft (open or laparoscopic) prior to transplantation including dissection and removal of perinephric fat and preparation of ureter(s), renal vein(s), and renal artery(s), ligating branches, as necessary (use 50325).

   Additional reconstruction of a cadaver or living donor renal allograft prior to transplantation may include venous, arterial, and/or ureteral anastomosis(es) necessary for implantation (see 50327-50329).

3. ***Recipient renal allotransplantation,*** which includes transplantation of the allograft (with or without recipient nephrectomy) and care of the recipient (see 50360, 50365).

(For dialysis, see 90935-90999)

(For laparoscopic donor nephrectomy, use 50547)

(For laparoscopic drainage of lymphocele to peritoneal cavity, use 49323)

50300 Donor nephrectomy (including cold preservation); from cadaver donor, unilateral or bilateral
CPT Changes: An Insider's View 2000, 2005
CPT Assistant Nov 99:25, Apr 05:10-12

50320 open, from living donor
CPT Changes: An Insider's View 2000, 2005
CPT Assistant Nov 99:25, May 00:4

50323 Backbench standard preparation of cadaver donor renal allograft prior to transplantation, including dissection and removal of perinephric fat, diaphragmatic and retroperitoneal attachments, excision of adrenal gland; and preparation of ureter(s), renal vein(s), and renal artery(s), ligating branches, as necessary
CPT Changes: An Insider's View 2005
CPT Assistant Apr 05:10-11

(Do not report 50323 in conjunction with 60540, 60545)

50325 Backbench standard preparation of living donor renal allograft (open or laparoscopic) prior to transplantation, including dissection and removal of perinephric fat and preparation of ureter(s), renal vein(s), and renal artery(s), ligating branches, as necessary
CPT Changes: An Insider's View 2005

50327 Backbench reconstruction of cadaver or living donor renal allograft prior to transplantation; venous anastomosis, each
CPT Changes: An Insider's View 2005

50328 arterial anastomosis, each
CPT Changes: An Insider's View 2005

50329 ureteral anastomosis, each
CPT Changes: An Insider's View 2005

50340 Recipient nephrectomy (separate procedure)

(For bilateral procedure, report 50340 with modifier 50)

50360 Renal allotransplantation, implantation of graft; without recipient nephrectomy
CPT Changes: An Insider's View 2005

50365 with recipient nephrectomy
CPT Assistant Apr 05:10-11

(For bilateral procedure, report 50365 with modifier 50)

50370 Removal of transplanted renal allograft

50380 Renal autotransplantation, reimplantation of kidney
CPT Assistant Apr 05:10, 12

(For renal autotransplantation extra-corporeal [bench] surgery, use autotransplantation as the primary procedure and report secondary procedure[s] [eg, partial nephrectomy, nephrolithotomy] with modifier 51)

Introduction

Renal Pelvis Catheter Procedures

Internally Dwelling

50382 Removal (via snare/capture) and replacement of internally dwelling ureteral stent via percutaneous approach, including radiological supervision and interpretation
CPT Changes: An Insider's View 2006, 2017
CPT Assistant Sep 06:1, 16, Oct 08:8, Dec 09:4, Jan 16:3
Clinical Examples in Radiology Winter 06:15, Spring 08:5

(For bilateral procedure, use modifier 50)

(For removal and replacement of an internally dwelling ureteral stent via a transurethral approach, use 50385)

50384 Removal (via snare/capture) of internally dwelling ureteral stent via percutaneous approach, including radiological supervision and interpretation
CPT Changes: An Insider's View 2006, 2017
CPT Assistant Sep 06:2, 16, Oct 08:8, Jan 16:3
Clinical Examples in Radiology Winter 06:16, Spring 08:5

(For bilateral procedure, use modifier 50)

►(Do not report 50382, 50384 in conjunction with 50436, 50437)◄

(For removal of an internally dwelling ureteral stent via a transurethral approach, use 50386)

50385 Removal (via snare/capture) and replacement of internally dwelling ureteral stent via transurethral approach, without use of cystoscopy, including radiological supervision and interpretation
CPT Changes: An Insider's View 2008, 2017
CPT Assistant Oct 08:8, Dec 09:4, Jan 16:3
Clinical Examples in Radiology Spring 08:5

50386 Removal (via snare/capture) of internally dwelling ureteral stent via transurethral approach, without use of cystoscopy, including radiological supervision and interpretation
CPT Changes: An Insider's View 2008, 2017
CPT Assistant Oct 08:8, Jan 16:3
Clinical Examples in Radiology Spring 08:4

Externally Accessible

50387 Removal and replacement of externally accessible nephroureteral catheter (eg, external/internal stent) requiring fluoroscopic guidance, including radiological supervision and interpretation
CPT Changes: An Insider's View 2006, 2016, 2017
CPT Assistant Sep 06:2, 4, 16, Dec 09:4, Mar 12:3, Jan 16:3, Mar 16:10
Clinical Examples in Radiology Winter 06:16, Spring 08:5, Fall 15:4

(For bilateral procedure, use modifier 50)

(For removal and replacement of externally accessible ureteral stent via ureterostomy or ileal conduit, use 50688)

(For removal without replacement of an externally accessible ureteral stent not requiring fluoroscopic guidance, see Evaluation and Management services codes)

50389 Removal of nephrostomy tube, requiring fluoroscopic guidance (eg, with concurrent indwelling ureteral stent)

➲ *CPT Changes: An Insider's View* 2006

➲ *CPT Assistant* Sep 06:1, 2, 4, Jan 16:3

➲ *Clinical Examples in Radiology* Winter 06:16

(Removal of nephrostomy tube not requiring fluoroscopic guidance is considered inherent to E/M services. Report the appropriate level of E/M service provided)

Other Introduction (Injection/Change/Removal) Procedures

►Percutaneous genitourinary procedures are performed with imaging guidance (eg, fluoroscopy and/or ultrasound). Diagnostic nephrostogram and/or ureterogram are typically performed with percutaneous genitourinary procedures and are included in 50432, 50433, 50434, 50435, 50436, 50437, 50693, 50694, 50695.

Code 50436 describes enlargement of an existing percutaneous tract to the renal collecting system to accommodate large instruments used in an endourologic procedure. Code 50436 includes predilation urinary tract imaging, postprocedure nephrostomy tube placement, when performed, and includes all radiological supervision and interpretation and imaging guidance (eg, ultrasound, fluoroscopy). Code 50436 may not be reported with 50432, 50433, 52334 for basic dilation of a percutaneous tract during initial placement of a catheter or device.

Code 50437 includes all elements of 50436, but also includes new access into the renal collecting system performed in the same session when a pre-existing tract is not present.◄

Codes 50430 and 50431 are diagnostic procedure codes that include injection(s) of contrast material, all associated radiological supervision and interpretation, and procedural imaging guidance (eg, ultrasound and/or fluoroscopy). Code 50430 also includes accessing the collecting system and/or associated ureter with a needle and/or catheter. Codes 50430 or 50431 may not be reported together with 50432, 50433, 50434, 50435, 50693, 50694, 50695.

Codes 50432, 50433, 50434, 50435 represent therapeutic procedures describing catheter placement or exchange, and include the elements of access, drainage catheter manipulations, and imaging guidance (eg, ultra sonography and/or fluoroscopy), as well as diagnostic imaging supervision and interpretation, when performed.

Code 50433 describes percutaneous nephrostomy with the additional accessing of the ureter/bladder to ultimately place a nephroureteral catheter (a single transnephric catheter with nephrostomy and ureteral components that allows drainage internally, externally, or both).

For codes 50430, 50431, 50432, 50433, 50434, 50435, 50606, 50693, 50694, 50695, 50705, and 50706, the renal pelvis and its associated ureter are considered a single entity for reporting purposes. Codes 50430, 50431, 50432, 50433, 50434, 50435, 50606, 50693, 50694, 50695, 50705, and 50706 may be reported once for each renal collecting system/ureter accessed (eg, two separate codes would be reported for bilateral nephrostomy tube placement or for unilateral duplicated collecting system/ureter requiring two separate procedures.

50390 Aspiration and/or injection of renal cyst or pelvis by needle, percutaneous

➲ *CPT Assistant* Fall 93:14, Dec 97:7, Oct 01:8, Oct 05:18, Oct 08:8

(For radiological supervision and interpretation, see 74425, 74470, 76942, 77002, 77012, 77021)

(For antegrade nephrostogram and/or antegrade pyelogram, see 50430, 50431)

50391 Instillation(s) of therapeutic agent into renal pelvis and/or ureter through established nephrostomy, pyelostomy or ureterostomy tube (eg, anticarcinogenic or antifungal agent)

➲ *CPT Changes: An Insider's View* 2005

➲ *CPT Assistant* Oct 05:18

(50392 has been deleted. To report nephrostomy tube placement, use 50432)

(50393 has been deleted. To report ureteral catheter placement, see 50693, 50694, 50695)

(50394 has been deleted. To report injection procedures for antegrade nephrostogram and/or antegrade pyelogram, see 50430, 50431)

►(50395 has been deleted. To report, see 50436, 50437)◄

#● **50436** Dilation of existing tract, percutaneous, for an endourologic procedure including imaging guidance (eg, ultrasound and/or fluoroscopy) and all associated radiological supervision and interpretation, with postprocedure tube placement, when performed;

➲ *CPT Changes: An Insider's View* 2019

#● **50437** including new access into the renal collecting system

➲ *CPT Changes: An Insider's View* 2019

(For nephrostolithotomy, see 50080, 50081)

(For retrograde percutaneous nephrostomy, use 52334)

(For endoscopic surgery, see 50551-50561)

►(Do not report 50436, 50437 in conjunction with 50080, 50081, 50382, 50384, 50430, 50431, 50432, 50433, 52334, 74485)◄

50396 Manometric studies through nephrostomy or pyelostomy tube, or indwelling ureteral catheter
➲ *CPT Assistant* Fall 93:16, Dec 97:7, Oct 01:8

(For radiological supervision and interpretation, use 74425)

(50398 has been deleted. To report exchange of a percutaneous nephrostomy catheter, use 50435)

 # 50430 Injection procedure for antegrade nephrostogram and/or ureterogram, complete diagnostic procedure including imaging guidance (eg, ultrasound and fluoroscopy) and all associated radiological supervision and interpretation; new access
➲ *CPT Changes: An Insider's View* 2016, 2017
➲ *CPT Assistant* Oct 15:5, Jan 16:3
➲ *Clinical Examples in Radiology* Fall 15:3, Spring 16:12

 # 50431 existing access
➲ *CPT Changes: An Insider's View* 2016
➲ *CPT Assistant* Oct 15:5, Jan 16:3
➲ *Clinical Examples in Radiology* Fall 15:3, Spring 16:12

(Do not report 50430, 50431 in conjunction with 50432, 50433, 50434, 50435, 50693, 50694, 50695, 74425 for the same renal collecting system and/or associated ureter)

Introduction of Catheter Into Renal Pelvis
50432

The physician inserts a catheter into the renal pelvis in order to drain urine.

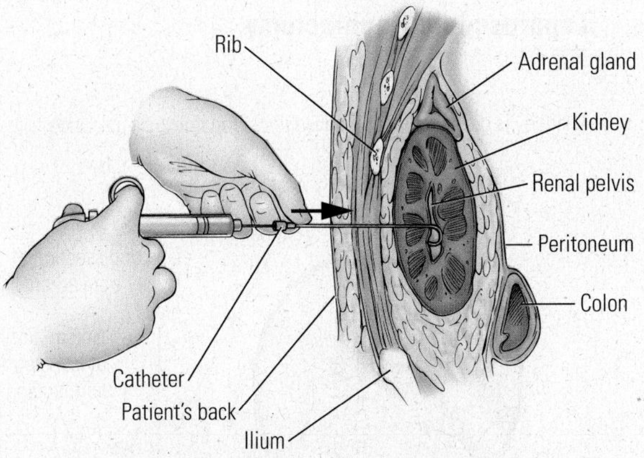

 # 50432 Placement of nephrostomy catheter, percutaneous, including diagnostic nephrostogram and/or ureterogram when performed, imaging guidance (eg, ultrasound and/or fluoroscopy) and all associated radiological supervision and interpretation
➲ *CPT Changes: An Insider's View* 2016, 2017
➲ *CPT Assistant* Oct 15:5, Jan 16:3, Mar 18:11
➲ *Clinical Examples in Radiology* Fall 15:2, Spring 16:12

►(Do not report 50432 in conjunction with 50430, 50431, 50433, 50436, 50437, 50694, 50695, 74425, for the same renal collecting system and/or associated ureter)◄

►(Do not report 50432 in conjunction with 50436, 50437, for dilation of the nephrostomy tube tract)◄

 # 50433 Placement of nephroureteral catheter, percutaneous, including diagnostic nephrostogram and/or ureterogram when performed, imaging guidance (eg, ultrasound and/or fluoroscopy) and all associated radiological supervision and interpretation, new access
➲ *CPT Changes: An Insider's View* 2016, 2017
➲ *CPT Assistant* Oct 15:5, Jan 16:3, Mar 18:11
➲ *Clinical Examples in Radiology* Fall 15:3, Spring 16:12

(Do not report 50433 in conjunction with 50430, 50431, 50432, 50693, 50694, 50695, 74425 for the same renal collecting system and/or associated ureter)

►(Do not report 50433 in conjunction with 50436, 50437, for dilation of the nephroureteral catheter tract)◄

(For nephroureteral catheter removal and replacement, use 50387)

 # 50434 Convert nephrostomy catheter to nephroureteral catheter, percutaneous, including diagnostic nephrostogram and/or ureterogram when performed, imaging guidance (eg, ultrasound and/or fluoroscopy) and all associated radiological supervision and interpretation, via pre-existing nephrostomy tract
➲ *CPT Changes: An Insider's View* 2016, 2017
➲ *CPT Assistant* Oct 15:5, Jan 16:3
➲ *Clinical Examples in Radiology* Fall 15:3, Spring 16:12

(Do not report 50434 in conjunction with 50430, 50431, 50435, 50684, 50693, 74425 for the same renal collecting system and/or associated ureter)

 # 50435 Exchange nephrostomy catheter, percutaneous, including diagnostic nephrostogram and/or ureterogram when performed, imaging guidance (eg, ultrasound and/or fluoroscopy) and all associated radiological supervision and interpretation
➲ *CPT Changes: An Insider's View* 2016
➲ *CPT Assistant* Oct 15:5, Jan 16:3, Mar 18:11
➲ *Clinical Examples in Radiology* Fall 15:3, Spring 16:12

(Do not report 50435 in conjunction with 50430, 50431, 50434, 50693, 74425 for the same renal collecting system and/or associated ureter)

(For removal of nephrostomy catheter requiring fluoroscopic guidance, use 50389)

Repair

50400 Pyeloplasty (Foley Y-pyeloplasty), plastic operation on renal pelvis, with or without plastic operation on ureter, nephropexy, nephrostomy, pyelostomy, or ureteral splinting; simple
➲ *CPT Changes: An Insider's View* 2000
➲ *CPT Assistant* Nov 99:25, May 00:4, Oct 01:8

50405 complicated (congenital kidney abnormality, secondary pyeloplasty, solitary kidney, calycoplasty)
➲ *CPT Changes: An Insider's View* 2000
➲ *CPT Assistant* Nov 99:25, May 00:4, Oct 01:8

(For laparoscopic approach, use 50544)

50430 Code is out of numerical sequence. See 50390-50405

50431 Code is out of numerical sequence. See 50390-50405

50432 Code is out of numerical sequence. See 50390-50405

50433 Code is out of numerical sequence. See 50390-50405

50434 Code is out of numerical sequence. See 50390-50405

50435 Code is out of numerical sequence. See 50390-50405

50436 Code is out of numerical sequence. See 50390-50405

50437 Code is out of numerical sequence. See 50390-50405

50500 Nephrorrhaphy, suture of kidney wound or injury

50520 Closure of nephrocutaneous or pyelocutaneous fistula

50525 Closure of nephrovisceral fistula (eg, renocolic), including visceral repair; abdominal approach

50526 thoracic approach

50540 Symphysiotomy for horseshoe kidney with or without pyeloplasty and/or other plastic procedure, unilateral or bilateral (1 operation)

Laparoscopy

Surgical laparoscopy always includes diagnostic laparoscopy. To report a diagnostic laparoscopy (peritoneoscopy) (separate procedure), use 49320.

50541 Laparoscopy, surgical; ablation of renal cysts
➲ *CPT Changes: An Insider's View* 2000
➲ *CPT Assistant* Nov 99:25, May 00:4, Oct 01:8, Nov 02:3, Jan 03:20

50542 ablation of renal mass lesion(s), including intraoperative ultrasound guidance and monitoring, when performed
➲ *CPT Changes: An Insider's View* 2003, 2011
➲ *CPT Assistant* Nov 02:3, Jan 03:21, Aug 04:12

(For open procedure, use 50250)

(For percutaneous ablation of renal tumors, see 50592, 50593)

50543 partial nephrectomy
➲ *CPT Changes: An Insider's View* 2003
➲ *CPT Assistant* Nov 02:3, Jan 03:21

(For open procedure, use 50240)

50544 pyeloplasty
➲ *CPT Changes: An Insider's View* 2000
➲ *CPT Assistant* Nov 99:25, May 00:4, Oct 01:8

50545 radical nephrectomy (includes removal of Gerota's fascia and surrounding fatty tissue, removal of regional lymph nodes, and adrenalectomy)
➲ *CPT Changes: An Insider's View* 2001
➲ *CPT Assistant* Oct 01:8

(For open procedure, use 50230)

50546 nephrectomy, including partial ureterectomy
➲ *CPT Changes: An Insider's View* 2000, 2001
➲ *CPT Assistant* Nov 99:25, May 00:4, Oct 01:8

Laparoscopic Radical Nephrectomy
50545

Radical nephrectomy (includes removal of Gerota's fascia and surrounding fatty tissue, removal of regional lymph nodes, and adrenalectomy)

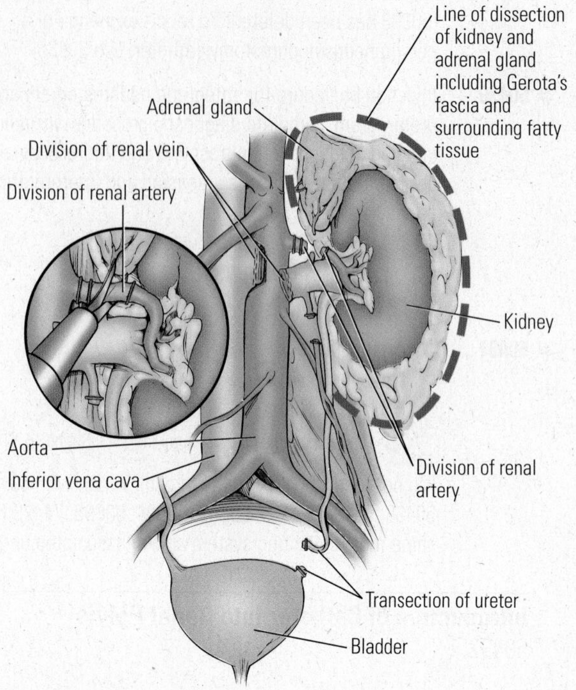

Laparoscopic Nephrectomy
50546

A kidney is dissected and removed under laparoscopic guidance.

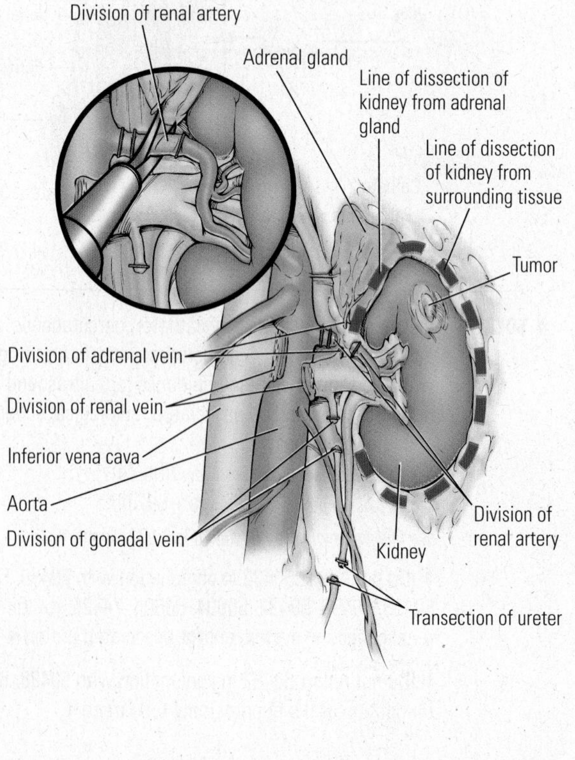

50547 donor nephrectomy (including cold preservation), from living donor
➔ *CPT Changes: An Insider's View* 2000, 2005
➔ *CPT Assistant* Nov 99:25, May 00:4, Oct 01:8

(For open procedure, use 50320)

(For backbench renal allograft standard preparation prior to transplantation, use 50325)

(For backbench renal allograft reconstruction prior to transplantation, see 50327-50329)

50548 nephrectomy with total ureterectomy
➔ *CPT Changes: An Insider's View* 2000, 2001
➔ *CPT Assistant* Nov 99:25, May 00:4, Oct 01:8

(For open procedure, see 50234, 50236)

50549 Unlisted laparoscopy procedure, renal
➔ *CPT Changes: An Insider's View* 2000
➔ *CPT Assistant* Nov 99:25, Mar 00:9, May 00:4, Feb 06:16

(For laparoscopic drainage of lymphocele to peritoneal cavity, use 49323)

Endoscopy

(For supplies and materials, use 99070)

50551 Renal endoscopy through established nephrostomy or pyelostomy, with or without irrigation, instillation, or ureteropyelography, exclusive of radiologic service;
➔ *CPT Assistant* Oct 01:8, Jan 03:21

50553 with ureteral catheterization, with or without dilation of ureter
➔ *CPT Assistant* Oct 01:8

(For image-guided dilation of ureter without endoscopic guidance, use 50706)

50555 with biopsy
➔ *CPT Assistant* Oct 01:8

(For image-guided biopsy of ureter and/or renal pelvis without endoscopic guidance, use 50606)

50557 with fulguration and/or incision, with or without biopsy
➔ *CPT Assistant* Oct 01:8

50561 with removal of foreign body or calculus
➔ *CPT Assistant* Oct 01:8, Jan 03:21

50562 with resection of tumor
➔ *CPT Changes: An Insider's View* 2003
➔ *CPT Assistant* Jan 03:21

(When procedures 50570-50580 provide a significant identifiable service, they may be added to 50045 and 50120)

50570 Renal endoscopy through nephrotomy or pyelotomy, with or without irrigation, instillation, or ureteropyelography, exclusive of radiologic service;
➔ *CPT Assistant* Oct 01:8

(For nephrotomy, use 50045)

(For pyelotomy, use 50120)

50572 with ureteral catheterization, with or without dilation of ureter
➔ *CPT Assistant* Oct 01:8

(For image-guided dilation of ureter without endoscopic guidance, use 50706)

50574 with biopsy
➔ *CPT Assistant* Oct 01:8

(For image-guided biopsy of ureter and/or renal pelvis without endoscopic guidance, use 50606)

50575 with endopyelotomy (includes cystoscopy, ureteroscopy, dilation of ureter and ureteral pelvic junction, incision of ureteral pelvic junction and insertion of endopyelotomy stent)
➔ *CPT Assistant* Oct 01:8, Aug 02:11

50576 with fulguration and/or incision, with or without biopsy
➔ *CPT Assistant* Oct 01:8

50580 with removal of foreign body or calculus
➔ *CPT Assistant* Oct 01:8

Other Procedures

50590 Lithotripsy, extracorporeal shock wave
➔ *CPT Assistant* Jul 01:11, Aug 01:10, Oct 01:8, Jul 03:16, Aug 03:14

Lithotripsy
50590

The physician breaks up a kidney stone (calculus) by directing shock waves through a liquid surrounding the patient.

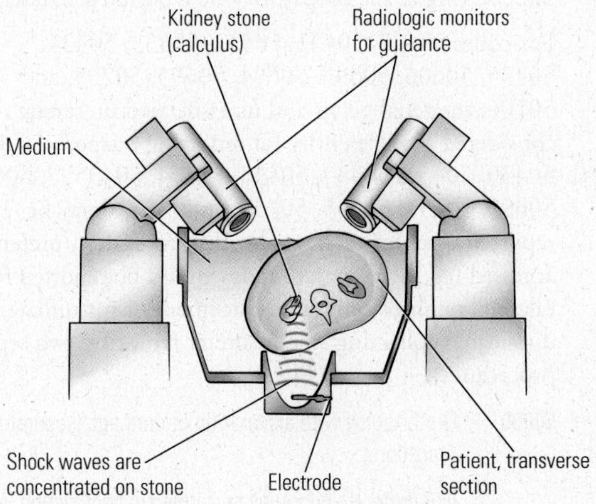

Urinary 50010-53899

50592 Ablation, 1 or more renal tumor(s), percutaneous, unilateral, radiofrequency

➲ *CPT Changes: An Insider's View* 2006, 2017

➲ *Clinical Examples in Radiology* Winter 06:16, Summer 12:11

(50592 is a unilateral procedure. For bilateral procedure, report 50592 with modifier 50)

(For imaging guidance and monitoring, see 76940, 77013, 77022)

50593 Ablation, renal tumor(s), unilateral, percutaneous, cryotherapy

➲ *CPT Changes: An Insider's View* 2008, 2017

➲ *CPT Assistant* May 17:3

(50593 is a unilateral procedure. For bilateral procedure, report 50593 with modifier 50)

(For imaging guidance and monitoring, see codes 76940, 77013, 77022)

Ureter

Incision/Biopsy

Code 50606 is an add-on code describing endoluminal biopsy (eg, brush) using non-endoscopic imaging guidance, which may be reported once per ureter per day. This code includes the work of the biopsy and the imaging guidance and radiological supervision and interpretation required to accomplish the biopsy. The biopsy may be performed through *de novo* transrenal access, an existing renal/ureteral access, transurethral access, an ileal conduit, or ureterostomy. The service of gaining access may be reported separately. Diagnostic pyelography/ureterography is not included in the work of 50606 and may be reported separately. Other interventions or catheter placements performed at the same setting as the biopsy may be reported separately.

For codes 50430, 50431, 50432, 50433, 50434, 50435, 50606, 50693, 50694, 50695, 50705, and 50706, the renal pelvis and its associated ureter are considered a single entity for reporting purposes. Codes 50430, 50431, 50432, 50433, 50434, 50435, 50606, 50693, 50694, 50695, 50705, and 50706 may be reported once for each renal collecting system/ureter accessed (eg, two separate codes would be reported for bilateral nephrostomy tube placement or for unilateral duplicated collecting system/ureter requiring two separate procedures).

50600 Ureterotomy with exploration or drainage (separate procedure)

(For ureteral endoscopy performed in conjunction with this procedure, see 50970-50980)

50605 Ureterotomy for insertion of indwelling stent, all types

➲ *CPT Assistant* Oct 01:8, Dec 09:4, Apr 12:18

Indwelling Ureteral Stent
50605

The physician makes an incision in the ureter (ureterotomy) and inserts a stent. For placement using cystourethroscopic technique, use 52332.

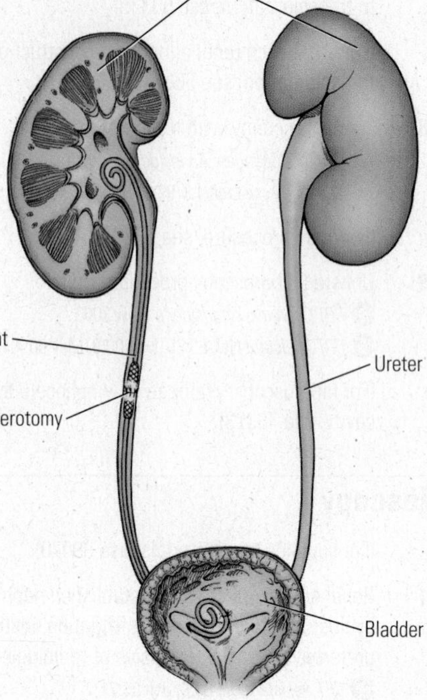

+ 50606 Endoluminal biopsy of ureter and/or renal pelvis, non-endoscopic, including imaging guidance (eg, ultrasound and/or fluoroscopy) and all associated radiological supervision and interpretation (List separately in addition to code for primary procedure)

➲ *CPT Changes: An Insider's View* 2016, 2017

➲ *CPT Assistant* Jan 16:3

➲ *Clinical Examples in Radiology* Fall 15:3, Spring 16:12

(Use 50606 in conjunction with 50382, 50384, 50385, 50386, 50387, 50389, 50430, 50431, 50432, 50433, 50434, 50435, 50684, 50688, 50690, 50693, 50694, 50695, 51610)

(Do not report 50606 in conjunction with 50555, 50574, 50955, 50974, 52007, 74425 for the same renal collecting system and/or associated ureter)

50610 Ureterolithotomy; upper one-third of ureter

➲ *CPT Changes: An Insider's View* 2000

➲ *CPT Assistant* Nov 99:26, Oct 01:8

50620 middle one-third of ureter

➲ *CPT Changes: An Insider's View* 2000

➲ *CPT Assistant* Nov 99:26, Oct 01:8

50630 lower one-third of ureter

➲ *CPT Changes: An Insider's View* 2000

➲ *CPT Assistant* Nov 99:26, Oct 01:8, May 14:3

(For laparoscopic approach, use 50945)

(For transvesical ureterolithotomy, use 51060)

(For cystotomy with stone basket extraction of ureteral calculus, use 51065)

(For endoscopic extraction or manipulation of ureteral calculus, see 50080, 50081, 50561, 50961, 50980, 52320-52330, 52352, 52353, 52356)

Excision

(For ureterocele, see 51535, 52300)

50650 Ureterectomy, with bladder cuff (separate procedure)

50660 Ureterectomy, total, ectopic ureter, combination abdominal, vaginal and/or perineal approach

Introduction

Other Introduction (Injection/Change/Removal) Procedures

Codes 50693, 50694, 50695 are therapeutic procedure codes describing percutaneous placement of ureteral stents. These codes include access, drainage, catheter manipulations, diagnostic nephrostogram and/or ureterogram, when performed, imaging guidance (eg, ultrasonography and/or fluoroscopy), and all associated radiological supervision and interpretation. When a separate ureteral stent and a nephrostomy catheter are placed into a ureter and its associated renal pelvis during the same session through a new percutaneous renal access, use 50695 to report the procedure.

50684 Injection procedure for ureterography or ureteropyelography through ureterostomy or indwelling ureteral catheter

➲ *CPT Assistant* Jan 16:3

(Do not report 50684 in conjunction with 50433, 50434, 50693, 50694, 50695)

(For radiological supervision and interpretation, use 74425)

50686 Manometric studies through ureterostomy or indwelling ureteral catheter

50688 Change of ureterostomy tube or externally accessible ureteral stent via ileal conduit

➲ *CPT Changes: An Insider's View* 2006

➲ *CPT Assistant* Jan 16:3

➲ *Clinical Examples in Radiology* Winter 06:20

(If imaging guidance is performed, use 75984)

50690 Injection procedure for visualization of ileal conduit and/or ureteropyelography, exclusive of radiologic service

➲ *CPT Assistant* Jan 16:3

(For radiological supervision and interpretation, use 74425)

50693 Placement of ureteral stent, percutaneous, including diagnostic nephrostogram and/or ureterogram when performed, imaging guidance (eg, ultrasound and/or fluoroscopy), and all associated radiological supervision and interpretation; pre-existing nephrostomy tract

➲ *CPT Changes: An Insider's View* 2016, 2017

➲ *CPT Assistant* Oct 15:5, Jan 16:3

➲ *Clinical Examples in Radiology* Fall 15:3, Spring 16:12

50694 new access, without separate nephrostomy catheter

➲ *CPT Changes: An Insider's View* 2016, 2017

➲ *CPT Assistant* Oct 15:5, Jan 16:3

➲ *Clinical Examples in Radiology* Fall 15:3, Spring 16:12

50695 new access, with separate nephrostomy catheter

➲ *CPT Changes: An Insider's View* 2016, 2017

➲ *CPT Assistant* Oct 15:5, Jan 16:3

➲ *Clinical Examples in Radiology* Fall 15:3, Spring 16:12

(Do not report 50693, 50694, 50695 in conjunction with 50430, 50431, 50432, 50433, 50434, 50435, 50684, 74425 for the same renal collecting system and/or associated ureter)

Repair

Codes 50705, 50706 are add-on codes describing embolization and balloon dilation of the ureter using non-endoscopic imaging guidance, and each may be reported once per ureter per day. These codes include embolization or dilation plus imaging guidance and radiological supervision and interpretation required to accomplish the embolization or dilation. These procedures may be performed through *de novo* transrenal access, an existing renal/ureteral access, transurethral access, an ileal conduit, or ureterostomy. The service of gaining access may be reported separately. Diagnostic pyelography/ureterography is not included in 50705 and 50706 and may be reported separately. Other interventions or catheter placements performed at the same setting as the embolization/dilation may be reported separately.

50700 Ureteroplasty, plastic operation on ureter (eg, stricture)

+ 50705 Ureteral embolization or occlusion, including imaging guidance (eg, ultrasound and/or fluoroscopy) and all associated radiological supervision and interpretation (List separately in addition to code for primary procedure)

➲ *CPT Changes: An Insider's View* 2016, 2017

➲ *CPT Assistant* Jan 16:3

➲ *Clinical Examples in Radiology* Fall 15:3, Spring 16:12

(Use 50705 in conjunction with 50382, 50384, 50385, 50386, 50387, 50389, 50430, 50431, 50432, 50433, 50434, 50435, 50684, 50688, 50690, 50693, 50694, 50695, 51610)

+ 50706 Balloon dilation, ureteral stricture, including imaging guidance (eg, ultrasound and/or fluoroscopy) and all associated radiological supervision and interpretation (List separately in addition to code for primary procedure)
➲ *CPT Changes: An Insider's View* 2016, 2017
➲ *CPT Assistant* Jan 16:3
➲ *Clinical Examples in Radiology* Fall 15:3, Spring 16:12

(Use 50706 in conjunction with 50382, 50384, 50385, 50386, 50387, 50389, 50430, 50431, 50432, 50433, 50434, 50435, 50684, 50688, 50690, 50693, 50694, 50695, 51610)

(Do not report 50706 in conjunction with 50553, 50572, 50953, 50972, 52341, 52344, 52345, 74485)

(For percutaneous nephrostomy, nephroureteral catheter, and/or ureteral catheter placement use 50385, 50387, 50432, 50433, 50434, 50435, 50693, 50694, 50695)

50715 Ureterolysis, with or without repositioning of ureter for retroperitoneal fibrosis

(For bilateral procedure, report 50715 with modifier 50)

50722 Ureterolysis for ovarian vein syndrome

50725 Ureterolysis for retrocaval ureter, with reanastomosis of upper urinary tract or vena cava

50727 Revision of urinary-cutaneous anastomosis (any type urostomy);

50728 with repair of fascial defect and hernia

50740 Ureteropyelostomy, anastomosis of ureter and renal pelvis
➲ *CPT Assistant* Oct 01:8

50750 Ureterocalycostomy, anastomosis of ureter to renal calyx
➲ *CPT Assistant* Oct 01:8

50760 Ureteroureterostomy
➲ *CPT Assistant* Oct 01:8

50770 Transureteroureterostomy, anastomosis of ureter to contralateral ureter

(Codes 50780-50785 include minor procedures to prevent vesicoureteral reflux)

50780 Ureteroneocystostomy; anastomosis of single ureter to bladder
➲ *CPT Assistant* Oct 01:8, Feb 18:11

(For bilateral procedure, report 50780 with modifier 50)

(When combined with cystourethroplasty or vesical neck revision, use 51820)

50782 anastomosis of duplicated ureter to bladder
➲ *CPT Assistant* Oct 01:8

50783 with extensive ureteral tailoring
➲ *CPT Assistant* Oct 01:8

50785 with vesico-psoas hitch or bladder flap
➲ *CPT Assistant* Oct 01:8

(For bilateral procedure, report 50785 with modifier 50)

50800 Ureteroenterostomy, direct anastomosis of ureter to intestine
➲ *CPT Assistant* Oct 01:8

(For bilateral procedure, report 50800 with modifier 50)

50810 Ureterosigmoidostomy, with creation of sigmoid bladder and establishment of abdominal or perineal colostomy, including intestine anastomosis
➲ *CPT Changes: An Insider's View* 2002
➲ *CPT Assistant* Oct 01:8

50815 Ureterocolon conduit, including intestine anastomosis
➲ *CPT Assistant* Oct 01:8

(For bilateral procedure, report 50815 with modifier 50)

50820 Ureteroileal conduit (ileal bladder), including intestine anastomosis (Bricker operation)
➲ *CPT Changes: An Insider's View* 2002
➲ *CPT Assistant* Oct 01:8

(For bilateral procedure, report 50820 with modifier 50)

(For combination of 50800-50820 with cystectomy, see 51580-51595)

50825 Continent diversion, including intestine anastomosis using any segment of small and/or large intestine (Kock pouch or Camey enterocystoplasty)
➲ *CPT Changes: An Insider's View* 2002
➲ *CPT Assistant* Oct 01:8

Ureteroileal Conduit
50820

The ureters are connected to a segment of intestine to divert urine flow through an opening in the skin.

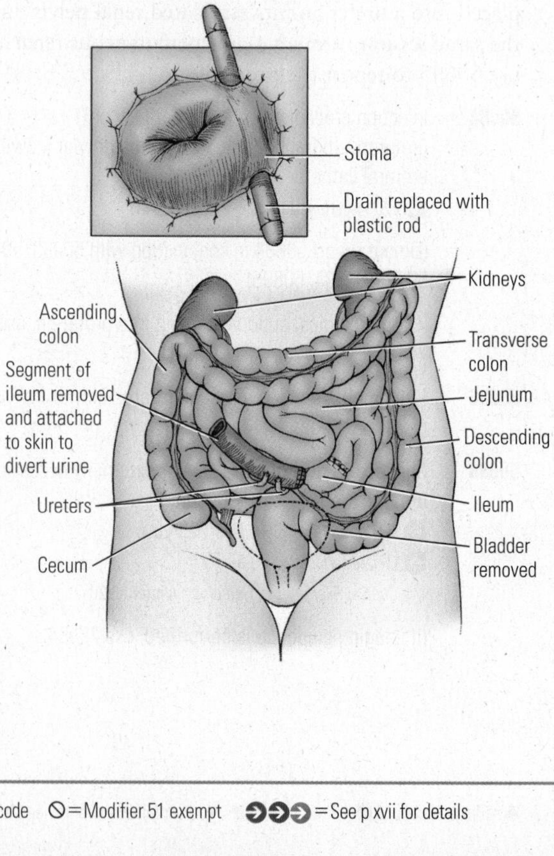

50830 Urinary undiversion (eg, taking down of ureteroileal conduit, ureterosigmoidostomy or ureteroenterostomy with ureteroureterostomy or ureteroneocystostomy)
➔ *CPT Assistant* Oct 01:8

50840 Replacement of all or part of ureter by intestine segment, including intestine anastomosis
➔ *CPT Changes: An Insider's View* 2002
➔ *CPT Assistant* Oct 01:8

(For bilateral procedure, report 50840 with modifier 50)

50845 Cutaneous appendico-vesicostomy

50860 Ureterostomy, transplantation of ureter to skin

(For bilateral procedure, report 50860 with modifier 50)

50900 Ureterorrhaphy, suture of ureter (separate procedure)

50920 Closure of ureterocutaneous fistula

50930 Closure of ureterovisceral fistula (including visceral repair)

50940 Deligation of ureter

(For ureteroplasty, ureterolysis, see 50700-50860)

Laparoscopy

Surgical laparoscopy always includes diagnostic laparoscopy. To report a diagnostic laparoscopy (peritoneoscopy) (separate procedure), use 49320.

50945 Laparoscopy, surgical; ureterolithotomy
➔ *CPT Changes: An Insider's View* 2000
➔ *CPT Assistant* Nov 99:26, May 00:4, Oct 01:8, Sep 06:13

50947 ureteroneocystostomy with cystoscopy and ureteral stent placement
➔ *CPT Changes: An Insider's View* 2001
➔ *CPT Assistant* Oct 01:8

50948 ureteroneocystostomy without cystoscopy and ureteral stent placement
➔ *CPT Changes: An Insider's View* 2001
➔ *CPT Assistant* Oct 01:8

(For open ureteroneocystostomy, see 50780-50785)

50949 Unlisted laparoscopy procedure, ureter
➔ *CPT Changes: An Insider's View* 2001
➔ *CPT Assistant* Oct 01:8

Endoscopy

50951 Ureteral endoscopy through established ureterostomy, with or without irrigation, instillation, or ureteropyelography, exclusive of radiologic service;
➔ *CPT Assistant* Oct 01:8

Laparoscopic Ureteroneocystostomy
50947

Ureteroneocystostomy with cystoscopy and ureteral stent placement

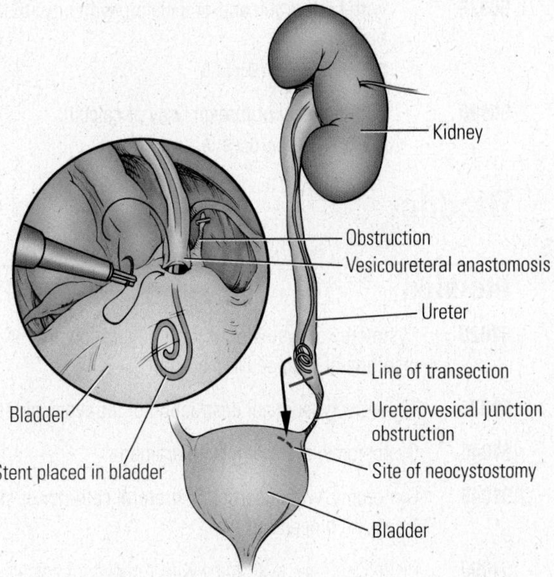

50953 with ureteral catheterization, with or without dilation of ureter
➔ *CPT Assistant* Oct 01:8

(For image-guided dilation of ureter without endoscopic guidance, use 50706)

50955 with biopsy
➔ *CPT Assistant* Oct 01:8

(For image-guided biopsy of ureter and/or renal pelvis without endoscopic guidance, use 50606)

50957 with fulguration and/or incision, with or without biopsy
➔ *CPT Assistant* Oct 01:8

50961 with removal of foreign body or calculus
➔ *CPT Assistant* Oct 01:8, Mar 07:10, Apr 07:12

50970 Ureteral endoscopy through ureterotomy, with or without irrigation, instillation, or ureteropyelography, exclusive of radiologic service;
➔ *CPT Assistant* Oct 01:8

(For ureterotomy, use 50600)

50972 with ureteral catheterization, with or without dilation of ureter
➔ *CPT Assistant* Oct 01:8

(For image-guided dilation of ureter without endoscopic guidance, use 50706)

50974 with biopsy
➔ *CPT Assistant* Oct 01:8

(For image-guided biopsy of ureter and/or renal pelvis without endoscopic guidance, use 50606)

50976 with fulguration and/or incision, with or without biopsy
➔ *CPT Assistant* Oct 01:8

50980 with removal of foreign body or calculus
➔ *CPT Assistant* Oct 01:8

Bladder

Incision

51020 Cystotomy or cystostomy; with fulguration and/or insertion of radioactive material

51030 with cryosurgical destruction of intravesical lesion

51040 Cystostomy, cystotomy with drainage

51045 Cystotomy, with insertion of ureteral catheter or stent (separate procedure)

51050 Cystolithotomy, cystotomy with removal of calculus, without vesical neck resection

51060 Transvesical ureterolithotomy

51065 Cystotomy, with calculus basket extraction and/or ultrasonic or electrohydraulic fragmentation of ureteral calculus
➔ *CPT Changes: An Insider's View* 2002

51080 Drainage of perivesical or prevesical space abscess

(For percutaneous image-guided fluid collection drainage by catheter of perivesicular or prevesicular space abscess, use 49406)

Removal

51100 Aspiration of bladder; by needle
➔ *CPT Changes: An Insider's View* 2008
➔ *CPT Assistant* Jun 08:11

51101 by trocar or intracatheter
➔ *CPT Changes: An Insider's View* 2008
➔ *CPT Assistant* Jun 08:11

51102 with insertion of suprapubic catheter
➔ *CPT Changes: An Insider's View* 2008
➔ *CPT Assistant* Jun 08:11

(For imaging guidance, see 76942, 77002, 77012)

Excision

51500 Excision of urachal cyst or sinus, with or without umbilical hernia repair

51520 Cystotomy; for simple excision of vesical neck (separate procedure)

51525 for excision of bladder diverticulum, single or multiple (separate procedure)

51530 for excision of bladder tumor

(For transurethral resection, see 52234-52240, 52305)

51535 Cystotomy for excision, incision, or repair of ureterocele

(For bilateral procedure, report 51535 with modifier 50)

(For transurethral excision, use 52300)

51550 Cystectomy, partial; simple

51555 complicated (eg, postradiation, previous surgery, difficult location)

51565 Cystectomy, partial, with reimplantation of ureter(s) into bladder (ureteroneocystostomy)

51570 Cystectomy, complete; (separate procedure)
➔ *CPT Assistant* Spring 93:35

51575 with bilateral pelvic lymphadenectomy, including external iliac, hypogastric, and obturator nodes
➔ *CPT Assistant* Spring 93:35

51580 Cystectomy, complete, with ureterosigmoidostomy or ureterocutaneous transplantations;

51585 with bilateral pelvic lymphadenectomy, including external iliac, hypogastric, and obturator nodes

51590 Cystectomy, complete, with ureteroileal conduit or sigmoid bladder, including intestine anastomosis;
➔ *CPT Changes: An Insider's View* 2002

51595 with bilateral pelvic lymphadenectomy, including external iliac, hypogastric, and obturator nodes

51596 Cystectomy, complete, with continent diversion, any open technique, using any segment of small and/or large intestine to construct neobladder
➔ *CPT Changes: An Insider's View* 2002

51597 Pelvic exenteration, complete, for vesical, prostatic or urethral malignancy, with removal of bladder and ureteral transplantations, with or without hysterectomy and/or abdominoperineal resection of rectum and colon and colostomy, or any combination thereof

(For pelvic exenteration for gynecologic malignancy, use 58240)

Introduction

51600 Injection procedure for cystography or voiding urethrocystography

(For radiological supervision and interpretation, see 74430, 74455)

51605 Injection procedure and placement of chain for contrast and/or chain urethrocystography

(For radiological supervision and interpretation, use 74430)

51610 Injection procedure for retrograde urethrocystography
➔ *CPT Assistant* Jan 16:3

(For radiological supervision and interpretation, use 74450)

51700 Bladder irrigation, simple, lavage and/or instillation

(Codes 51701-51702 are reported only when performed independently. Do not report 51701-51702 when catheter insertion is an inclusive component of another procedure.)

51701 Insertion of non-indwelling bladder catheter (eg, straight catheterization for residual urine)
➔ *CPT Changes: An Insider's View* 2003
➔ *CPT Assistant* Jul 06:4, Jan 07:31, Jul 07:1

51702 Insertion of temporary indwelling bladder catheter; simple (eg, Foley)
➔ *CPT Changes: An Insider's View* 2003
➔ *CPT Assistant* Oct 03:10, Jul 06:4, Jan 07:31, Jul 07:1, May 14:3
➔ *Clinical Examples in Radiology* Spring 12:1

(Do not report 51702 in conjunction with 0071T, 0072T)

51703 complicated (eg, altered anatomy, fractured catheter/balloon)
➔ *CPT Changes: An Insider's View* 2003
➔ *CPT Assistant* Jan 07:31

51705 Change of cystostomy tube; simple
➔ *CPT Assistant* Dec 07:13

51710 complicated
➔ *CPT Assistant* Dec 07:13

(If imaging guidance is performed, use 75984)

51715 Endoscopic injection of implant material into the submucosal tissues of the urethra and/or bladder neck

(For anoscopy with directed submucosal injection of bulking agent for fecal incontinence, use 0377T)

51720 Bladder instillation of anticarcinogenic agent (including retention time)
➔ *CPT Changes: An Insider's View* 2007
➔ *CPT Assistant* Nov 02:11

Urodynamics

The following section (51725-51798) lists procedures that may be used separately or in many and varied combinations.

When multiple procedures are performed in the same investigative session, modifier 51 should be employed.

All procedures in this section imply that these services are performed by, or are under the direct supervision of, a physician or other qualified health care professional and that all instruments, equipment, fluids, gases, probes, catheters, technician's fees, medications, gloves, trays, tubing, and other sterile supplies be provided by that individual. When the individual only interprets the results and/or operates the equipment, a professional component, modifier 26, should be used to identify these services.

51725 Simple cystometrogram (CMG) (eg, spinal manometer)
➔ *CPT Assistant* Sep 02:6, Feb 10:7

51726 Complex cystometrogram (ie, calibrated electronic equipment);
➔ *CPT Changes: An Insider's View* 2010
➔ *CPT Assistant* Sep 02:6, Feb 10:7

51727 with urethral pressure profile studies (ie, urethral closure pressure profile), any technique
➔ *CPT Changes: An Insider's View* 2010
➔ *CPT Assistant* Feb 10:7

51728 with voiding pressure studies (ie, bladder voiding pressure), any technique
➔ *CPT Changes: An Insider's View* 2010
➔ *CPT Assistant* Feb 10:7

51729 with voiding pressure studies (ie, bladder voiding pressure) and urethral pressure profile studies (ie, urethral closure pressure profile), any technique
➔ *CPT Changes: An Insider's View* 2010
➔ *CPT Assistant* Feb 10:7

#+ 51797 Voiding pressure studies, intra-abdominal (ie, rectal, gastric, intraperitoneal) (List separately in addition to code for primary procedure)
➔ *CPT Changes: An Insider's View* 2008, 2010
➔ *CPT Assistant* Dec 01:7, Sep 02:6, Oct 09:7, Feb 10:7

(Use 51797 in conjunction with 51728, 51729)

51736 Simple uroflowmetry (UFR) (eg, stop-watch flow rate, mechanical uroflowmeter)
➔ *CPT Assistant* Sep 02:6, Feb 10:7

51741 Complex uroflowmetry (eg, calibrated electronic equipment)
➔ *CPT Assistant* Sep 02:6, Feb 10:7, Sep 14:14

51784 Electromyography studies (EMG) of anal or urethral sphincter, other than needle, any technique
➔ *CPT Assistant* Sep 02:6, Feb 10:7, Feb 14:11, Sep 14:14

(Do not report 51784 in conjunction with 51792)

51785 Needle electromyography studies (EMG) of anal or urethral sphincter, any technique
➔ *CPT Assistant* Apr 02:6, Sep 02:6, Jul 04:13, Feb 10:7

51792 Stimulus evoked response (eg, measurement of bulbocavernosus reflex latency time)
➔ *CPT Assistant* Apr 02:6, Sep 02:6, Feb 10:7, Feb 14:11

(Do not report 51792 in conjunction with 51784)

51797 Code is out of numerical sequence. See 51728-51741

51798 Measurement of post-voiding residual urine and/or bladder capacity by ultrasound, non-imaging
➲ *CPT Changes: An Insider's View* 2003
➲ *CPT Assistant* Dec 05:3, Feb 10:7

Measurement of Postvoiding
51798

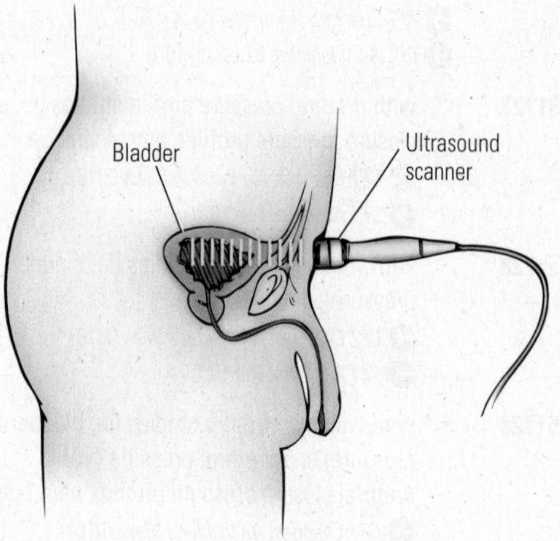

Repair

51800 Cystoplasty or cystourethroplasty, plastic operation on bladder and/or vesical neck (anterior Y-plasty, vesical fundus resection), any procedure, with or without wedge resection of posterior vesical neck

51820 Cystourethroplasty with unilateral or bilateral ureteroneocystostomy

51840 Anterior vesicourethropexy, or urethropexy (eg, Marshall-Marchetti-Krantz, Burch); simple
➲ *CPT Assistant* Jan 97:1, Nov 97:19, Apr 98:15, Jun 02:7, May 06:17, Jun 10:6, Aug 12:13

51841 complicated (eg, secondary repair)
➲ *CPT Assistant* Jan 97:1, Jun 02:7, Jun 10:6, Aug 12:13

(For urethropexy (Pereyra type), use 57289)

51845 Abdomino-vaginal vesical neck suspension, with or without endoscopic control (eg, Stamey, Raz, modified Pereyra)
➲ *CPT Assistant* Jan 97:3

51860 Cystorrhaphy, suture of bladder wound, injury or rupture; simple

51865 complicated

51880 Closure of cystostomy (separate procedure)

51900 Closure of vesicovaginal fistula, abdominal approach

(For vaginal approach, see 57320-57330)

51920 Closure of vesicouterine fistula;

51925 with hysterectomy

(For closure of vesicoenteric fistula, see 44660, 44661)

(For closure of rectovesical fistula, see 45800-45805)

51940 Closure, exstrophy of bladder
➲ *CPT Changes: An Insider's View* 2002

(See also 54390)

51960 Enterocystoplasty, including intestinal anastomosis
➲ *CPT Changes: An Insider's View* 2002

51980 Cutaneous vesicostomy

Laparoscopy

Surgical laparoscopy always includes diagnostic laparoscopy. To report a diagnostic laparoscopy (peritoneoscopy) (separate procedure), use 49320.

51990 Laparoscopy, surgical; urethral suspension for stress incontinence
➲ *CPT Changes: An Insider's View* 2000
➲ *CPT Assistant* Nov 99:26, May 00:4, Jun 10:6, Mar 12:10, Aug 12:13

51992 sling operation for stress incontinence (eg, fascia or synthetic)
➲ *CPT Changes: An Insider's View* 2000
➲ *CPT Assistant* Nov 99:26, May 00:4, Mar 12:10, Aug 12:13

(For open sling operation for stress incontinence, use 57288)

(For reversal or removal of sling operation for stress incontinence, use 57287)

Laparoscopic Sling Suspension Urinary Incontinence
51990

Nonabsorbable sutures are placed laparoscopically into the endopelvic fascia at the bladder neck region on each side and secured to the ipsilateral pectineal ligament. The sutures are tied using extra vaginal-urethral knots so as to create a hammock type suspension of the bladder neck, without urethral occlusion.

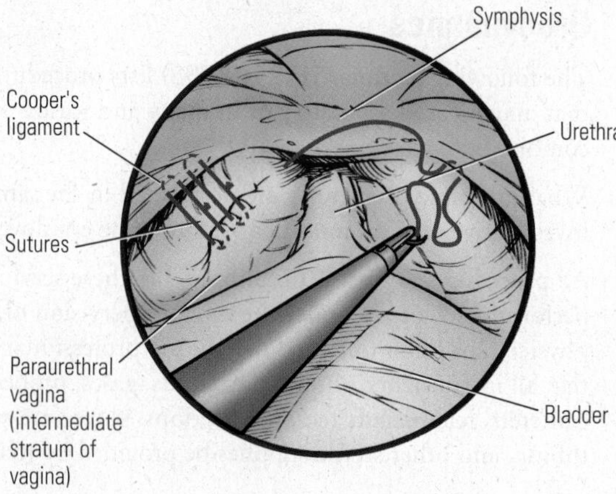

51999 Unlisted laparoscopy procedure, bladder
➔ *CPT Changes: An Insider's View* 2006
➔ *CPT Assistant* Dec 17:14

Endoscopy—Cystoscopy, Urethroscopy, Cystourethroscopy

Endoscopic descriptions are listed so that the main procedure can be identified without having to list all the minor related functions performed at the same time. For example: meatotomy, urethral calibration and/or dilation, urethroscopy, and cystoscopy prior to a transurethral resection of prostate; ureteral catheterization following extraction of ureteral calculus; internal urethrotomy and bladder neck fulguration when performing a cystourethroscopy for the female urethral syndrome. When the secondary procedure requires significant additional time and effort, it may be identified by the addition of modifier 22.

For example: urethrotomy performed for a documented pre-existing stricture or bladder neck contracture.

Because cutaneous urinary diversions utilizing ileum or colon serve as functional replacements of a native bladder, endoscopy of such bowel segments, as well as performance of secondary procedures can be captured by using the cystourethroscopy codes. For example, endoscopy of an ileal loop with removal of ureteral calculus would be coded as cystourethroscopy (including ureteral catheterization); with removal of ureteral calculus (52320).

52000 Cystourethroscopy (separate procedure)
➔ *CPT Assistant* Oct 00:7, May 01:5, Sep 04:11, Oct 05:23, Nov 07:9, Mar 13:14, May 14:3, Oct 17:9

(Do not report 52000 in conjunction with 52001, 52320, 52325, 52327, 52330, 52332, 52334, 52341, 52342, 52343, 52356)

(Do not report 52000 in conjunction with 57240, 57260, 57265)

52001 Cystourethroscopy with irrigation and evacuation of multiple obstructing clots
➔ *CPT Changes: An Insider's View* 2002, 2003

(Do not report 52001 in conjunction with 52000)

Coding Tip

Restrictions for Reporting Temporary Catheter Insertion and Removal with Cystourethroscopy

The insertion and removal of a temporary ureteral catheter (52005) during diagnostic or therapeutic cystourethroscopy with ureteroscopy and/or pyeloscopy is included in 52320-52356 and should not be reported separately.

CPT Coding Guidelines, Urinary System, Bladder Transurethral Surgery, Ureter and Pelvis

52005 Cystourethroscopy, with ureteral catheterization, with or without irrigation, instillation, or ureteropyelography, exclusive of radiologic service;
➔ *CPT Assistant* Sep 00:11, Jan 01:13, May 01:5, Oct 01:8, Dec 10:15

Cystourethroscopy With Ureteral Catheterization
52005

A cystourethroscope is passed through the urethra and bladder in order to view the urinary collecting system.

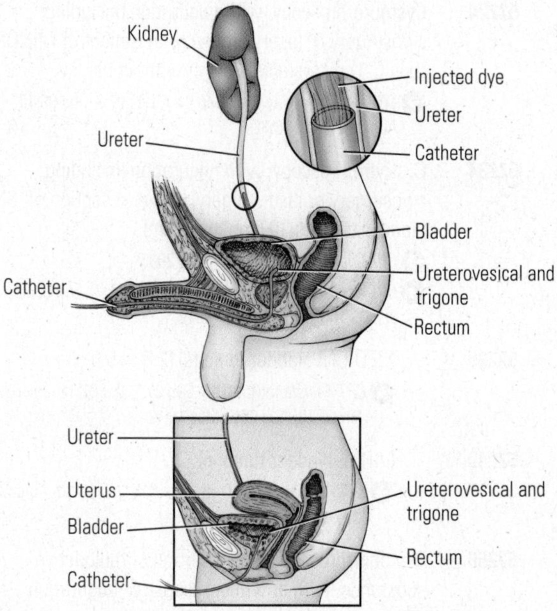

52007 with brush biopsy of ureter and/or renal pelvis
➔ *CPT Assistant* May 01:5, Oct 01:8

(For image-guided biopsy of ureter and/or renal pelvis without endoscopic guidance, use 50606)

52010 Cystourethroscopy, with ejaculatory duct catheterization, with or without irrigation, instillation, or duct radiography, exclusive of radiologic service
➔ *CPT Assistant* May 01:5

(For radiological supervision and interpretation, use 74440)

Transurethral Surgery

Urethra and Bladder

52204 Cystourethroscopy, with biopsy(s)
➔ *CPT Changes: An Insider's View* 2007
➔ *CPT Assistant* May 01:5, Sep 01:1, Sep 03:16, Aug 09:6, May 16:12

52214 Cystourethroscopy, with fulguration (including cryosurgery or laser surgery) of trigone, bladder neck, prostatic fossa, urethra, or periurethral glands
➔ *CPT Assistant* May 01:5, Sep 01:1, Aug 09:6, May 16:12

(For transurethral fulguration of prostate tissue performed within the postoperative period of 52601 or 52630 performed by the same physician, append modifier 78)

(For transurethral fulguration of prostate tissue performed within the postoperative period of a related procedure performed by the same physician, append modifier 78)

(For transurethral fulguration of prostate for postoperative bleeding performed by the same physician, append modifier 78)

52224 Cystourethroscopy, with fulguration (including cryosurgery or laser surgery) or treatment of MINOR (less than 0.5 cm) lesion(s) with or without biopsy

CPT Assistant May 01:5, Sep 01:1, Dec 07:7, Jun 09:10, Aug 09:6, May 16:12

52234 Cystourethroscopy, with fulguration (including cryosurgery or laser surgery) and/or resection of; SMALL bladder tumor(s) (0.5 up to 2.0 cm)

CPT Changes: An Insider's View 2005

CPT Assistant May 01:5, Sep 01:1, Oct 02:12, Jan 03:21, Jun 09:10, Aug 09:6, May 16:12

52235 MEDIUM bladder tumor(s) (2.0 to 5.0 cm)

CPT Assistant May 01:5, Sep 01:1, Oct 02:12, Jan 03:21, Jun 09:10, Aug 09:6, May 16:12

52240 LARGE bladder tumor(s)

CPT Assistant May 01:5, Sep 01:1, Jun 09:10, Aug 09:6, May 16:12

52250 Cystourethroscopy with insertion of radioactive substance, with or without biopsy or fulguration

CPT Assistant May 01:5, Sep 01:1

52260 Cystourethroscopy, with dilation of bladder for interstitial cystitis; general or conduction (spinal) anesthesia

CPT Assistant May 01:5, Sep 01:1, Oct 05:23

52265 local anesthesia

CPT Assistant May 01:5, Sep 01:1

52270 Cystourethroscopy, with internal urethrotomy; female

CPT Assistant May 01:5, Sep 01:1

52275 male

CPT Assistant May 01:5, Sep 01:1

52276 Cystourethroscopy with direct vision internal urethrotomy

CPT Assistant May 01:5, Sep 01:1, May 09:8, Feb 10:7

52277 Cystourethroscopy, with resection of external sphincter (sphincterotomy)

CPT Assistant May 01:5, Sep 01:1

52281 Cystourethroscopy, with calibration and/or dilation of urethral stricture or stenosis, with or without meatotomy, with or without injection procedure for cystography, male or female

CPT Assistant Nov 97:20, May 01:5, Sep 01:1, Jun 07:10, Oct 17:9

(To report cystourethroscopy with urethral therapeutic drug delivery, use 0499T)

52282 Cystourethroscopy, with insertion of permanent urethral stent

CPT Changes: An Insider's View 2010

CPT Assistant Nov 97:20, May 01:5, Sep 01:1, Feb 10:7, Jun 15:5

(For placement of temporary prostatic urethral stent, use 53855)

52283 Cystourethroscopy, with steroid injection into stricture

CPT Assistant May 01:5, Sep 01:1, Mar 15:9

52285 Cystourethroscopy for treatment of the female urethral syndrome with any or all of the following: urethral meatotomy, urethral dilation, internal urethrotomy, lysis of urethrovaginal septal fibrosis, lateral incisions of the bladder neck, and fulguration of polyp(s) of urethra, bladder neck, and/or trigone

CPT Assistant May 01:5, Sep 01:1

52287 Cystourethroscopy, with injection(s) for chemodenervation of the bladder

CPT Changes: An Insider's View 2013

(The supply of the chemodenervation agent is reported separately)

52290 Cystourethroscopy; with ureteral meatotomy, unilateral or bilateral

CPT Assistant May 01:5, Sep 01:1

52300 with resection or fulguration of orthotopic ureterocele(s), unilateral or bilateral

CPT Assistant May 01:5, Sep 01:1

52301 with resection or fulguration of ectopic ureterocele(s), unilateral or bilateral

CPT Assistant May 01:5, Sep 01:1

52305 with incision or resection of orifice of bladder diverticulum, single or multiple

CPT Assistant May 01:5, Sep 01:1

Coding Tip

Instructions for Reporting Stent Removal

To report cystourethroscopic removal of a self-retaining, indwelling ureteral stent, see 52310, 52315, and append modifier 58, if appropriate.

CPT Coding Guidelines, Urinary System, Bladder Transurethral Surgery, Ureter and Pelvis

---

52310 Cystourethroscopy, with removal of foreign body, calculus, or ureteral stent from urethra or bladder (separate procedure); simple

CPT Assistant May 01:5, Sep 01:1

52315 complicated

CPT Assistant May 01:5, Sep 01:1

52317 Litholapaxy: crushing or fragmentation of calculus by any means in bladder and removal of fragments; simple or small (less than 2.5 cm)

CPT Assistant May 01:5, Sep 01:1, Feb 12:11

52318 complicated or large (over 2.5 cm)

➲ *CPT Assistant* May 01:5, Sep 01:1, Feb 12:11

Ureter and Pelvis

Therapeutic cystourethroscopy always includes diagnostic cystourethroscopy. To report a diagnostic cystourethroscopy, use 52000. Therapeutic cystourethroscopy with ureteroscopy and/or pyeloscopy always includes diagnostic cystourethroscopy with ureteroscopy and/or pyeloscopy. To report a diagnostic cystourethroscopy with ureteroscopy and/or pyeloscopy, use 52351.

Do not report 52000 in conjunction with 52320-52343, 52356.

Do not report 52351 in conjunction with 52344-52346, 52352-52356.

The insertion and removal of a temporary ureteral catheter (52005) during diagnostic or therapeutic cystourethroscopy with ureteroscopy and/or pyeloscopy is included in 52320-52356 and should not be reported separately.

To report insertion of a self-retaining, indwelling stent performed during diagnostic or therapeutic cystourethroscopy with ureteroscopy and/or pyeloscopy, report 52332, in addition to primary procedure(s) performed (52320-52330, 52334-52352, 52354, 52355), and append modifier 51. Code 52332 is used to report a unilateral procedure unless otherwise specified.

For bilateral insertion of self-retaining, indwelling ureteral stents, use code 52332, and append modifier 50.

To report cystourethroscopic removal of a self-retaining, indwelling ureteral stent, see 52310, 52315, and append modifier 58, if appropriate.

52320 Cystourethroscopy (including ureteral catheterization); with removal of ureteral calculus

➲ *CPT Assistant* Mar 96:1, May 96:11, Jan 01:13, May 01:5, Sep 01:1, Oct 01:8, May 14:3

52325 with fragmentation of ureteral calculus (eg, ultrasonic or electro-hydraulic technique)

➲ *CPT Assistant* Mar 96:1, May 96:11, May 01:5, Sep 01:1, Oct 01:8, Dec 07:13

52327 with subureteric injection of implant material

➲ *CPT Assistant* Mar 96:1, May 96:11, May 01:5, Sep 01:1, Oct 01:8

52330 with manipulation, without removal of ureteral calculus

➲ *CPT Assistant* Mar 96:1, May 96:11, Sep 00:11, May 01:5, Sep 01:1, Oct 01:8, May 14:3

(Do not report 52320, 52325, 52327, 52330 in conjunction with 52000)

52332 Cystourethroscopy, with insertion of indwelling ureteral stent (eg, Gibbons or double-J type)

➲ *CPT Assistant* Mar 96:1, May 96:11, Nov 96:8, Jan 01:13, May 01:5, Sep 01:1, Oct 01:8, Oct 05:18, Dec 09:4, 12, May 14:3

(Do not report 52332 in conjunction with 52000, 52353, 52356 when performed together on the same side)

52334 Cystourethroscopy with insertion of ureteral guide wire through kidney to establish a percutaneous nephrostomy, retrograde

➲ *CPT Assistant* Mar 96:11, May 96:11, May 01:5, Sep 01:1, Oct 01:8, May 14:3

►(For percutaneous nephrostolithotomy, see 50080, 50081; for establishment of percutaneous nephrostomy, see 50432, 50433)◄

(For cystourethroscopy, with ureteroscopy and/or pyeloscopy, see 52351-52356)

(For cystourethroscopy with incision, fulguration, or resection of congenital posterior urethral valves or obstructive hypertrophic mucosal folds, use 52400)

►(Do not report 52334 in conjunction with 50437, 52000, 52351)◄

52341 Cystourethroscopy; with treatment of ureteral stricture (eg, balloon dilation, laser, electrocautery, and incision)

➲ *CPT Changes: An Insider's View* 2001

➲ *CPT Assistant* Nov 96:9, Apr 01:4, May 01:5, Sep 01:1, Oct 01:8

52342 with treatment of ureteropelvic junction stricture (eg, balloon dilation, laser, electrocautery, and incision)

➲ *CPT Changes: An Insider's View* 2001

➲ *CPT Assistant* Apr 01:4, May 01:5, Sep 01:1, Oct 01:8, Aug 02:11

52343 with treatment of intra-renal stricture (eg, balloon dilation, laser, electrocautery, and incision)

➲ *CPT Changes: An Insider's View* 2001

➲ *CPT Assistant* Apr 01:4, May 01:5, Sep 01:1, Oct 01:8, May 14:3

(Do not report 52341, 52342, 52343 in conjunction with 52000, 52351)

(For image-guided dilation of ureter, ureteropelvic junction stricture without endoscopic guidance, use 50706)

(For radiological supervision and interpretation, use 74485)

52344 Cystourethroscopy with ureteroscopy; with treatment of ureteral stricture (eg, balloon dilation, laser, electrocautery, and incision)

➲ *CPT Changes: An Insider's View* 2001

➲ *CPT Assistant* Apr 01:4, May 01:5, Sep 01:1, Oct 01:8

52345 with treatment of ureteropelvic junction stricture (eg, balloon dilation, laser, electrocautery, and incision)

➲ *CPT Changes: An Insider's View* 2001

➲ *CPT Assistant* Apr 01:4, May 01:5, Sep 01:1, Oct 01:8

52346 with treatment of intra-renal stricture (eg, balloon dilation, laser, electrocautery, and incision)

➲ *CPT Changes: An Insider's View* 2001

➲ *CPT Assistant* Apr 01:4, May 01:5, Sep 01:1, Oct 01:8, May 14:3

(For transurethral resection or incision of ejaculatory ducts, use 52402)

(Do not report 52344, 52345, 52346 in conjunction with 52351)

(For image-guided dilation of ureter, ureteropelvic junction stricture without endoscopic guidance, use 50706)

(For radiological supervision and interpretation, use 74485)

52351 Cystourethroscopy, with ureteroscopy and/or pyeloscopy; diagnostic
CPT Changes: An Insider's View 2001
CPT Assistant Apr 01:4, May 01:5, Sep 01:1, Oct 01:8, May 14:3

(Do not report 52351 in conjunction with 52341, 52342, 52343, 52344, 52345, 52346, 52352-52356)

52352 with removal or manipulation of calculus (ureteral catheterization is included)
CPT Changes: An Insider's View 2001
CPT Assistant Apr 01:4, May 01:5, Sep 01:1, Oct 01:8, Jun 07:10, Feb 10:13, May 14:3

52353 with lithotripsy (ureteral catheterization is included)
CPT Changes: An Insider's View 2001
CPT Assistant Apr 01:4, May 01:5, Sep 01:1, Oct 01:8, Dec 07:13, Apr 09:8, May 14:3

(Do not report 52353 in conjunction with 52332, 52356 when performed together on the same side)

 # 52356 with lithotripsy including insertion of indwelling ureteral stent (eg, Gibbons or double-J type)
CPT Changes: An Insider's View 2014
CPT Assistant May 14:3

(Do not report 52356 in conjunction with 52332, 52353 when performed together on the same side)

52354 with biopsy and/or fulguration of ureteral or renal pelvic lesion
CPT Changes: An Insider's View 2001, 2003
CPT Assistant Apr 01:4, May 01:5, Sep 01:1, Oct 01:8, May 14:3

(For image-guided biopsy of ureter and/or renal pelvis without endoscopic guidance, use 50606)

52355 with resection of ureteral or renal pelvic tumor
CPT Changes: An Insider's View 2001, 2003
CPT Assistant Apr 01:4, May 01:5, Sep 01:1, Oct 01:8, Jan 03:21, May 14:3

52356 Code is out of numerical sequence. See 52352-52355

Vesical Neck and Prostate

52400 Cystourethroscopy with incision, fulguration, or resection of congenital posterior urethral valves, or congenital obstructive hypertrophic mucosal folds
CPT Changes: An Insider's View 2001
CPT Assistant Apr 01:4

52402 Cystourethroscopy with transurethral resection or incision of ejaculatory ducts
CPT Changes: An Insider's View 2005

52441 Cystourethroscopy, with insertion of permanent adjustable transprostatic implant; single implant
CPT Changes: An Insider's View 2015
CPT Assistant Jun 15:5

+ 52442 each additional permanent adjustable transprostatic implant (List separately in addition to code for primary procedure)
CPT Changes: An Insider's View 2015
CPT Assistant Jun 15:5

(Use 52442 in conjunction with 52441)

(To report removal of implant[s], use 52310)

(For insertion of a permanent urethral stent, use 52282. For insertion of a temporary prostatic urethral stent, use 53855)

52450 Transurethral incision of prostate
CPT Assistant Apr 01:4, Jul 05:15, Jun 15:5

52500 Transurethral resection of bladder neck (separate procedure)
CPT Assistant Apr 01:4, Jan 04:27, Jul 05:15, May 09:8

52601 Transurethral electrosurgical resection of prostate, including control of postoperative bleeding, complete (vasectomy, meatotomy, cystourethroscopy, urethral calibration and/or dilation, and internal urethrotomy are included)
CPT Assistant Nov 97:20, Apr 01:4, Jun 03:6, Oct 11:10, Jun 15:5

(For transurethral waterjet ablation of prostate, use 0421T)

(For other approaches, see 55801-55845)

Transurethral Resection of Prostate, Complete
52601

The physician removes the prostate gland using an electrocautery knife.

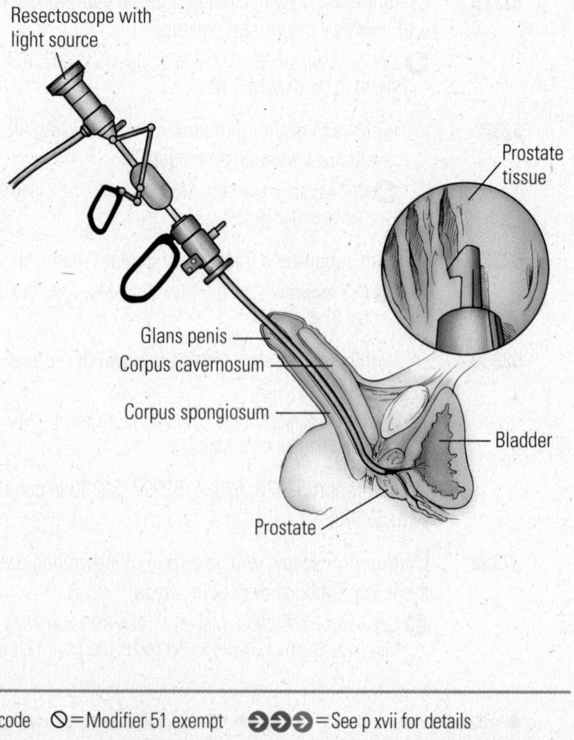

(52612, 52614, 52620 have been deleted. For first stage transurethral partial resection of prostate, use 52601. For second stage partial resection of prostate, use 52601 with modifier 58. For transurethral resection of residual or regrowth of obstructive prostate tissue, use 52630)

52630 Transurethral resection; residual or regrowth of obstructive prostate tissue including control of postoperative bleeding, complete (vasectomy, meatotomy, cystourethroscopy, urethral calibration and/or dilation, and internal urethrotomy are included)

➔ *CPT Changes: An Insider's View* 2009

➔ *CPT Assistant* Apr 01:4

(For resection of residual prostate tissue performed within the postoperative period of a related procedure performed by the same physician, append modifier 78)

(For transurethral waterjet ablation of prostate, use 0421T)

52640 of postoperative bladder neck contracture

➔ *CPT Assistant* Apr 01:4

52647 Laser coagulation of prostate, including control of postoperative bleeding, complete (vasectomy, meatotomy, cystourethroscopy, urethral calibration and/or dilation, and internal urethrotomy are included if performed)

➔ *CPT Changes: An Insider's View* 2006

➔ *CPT Assistant* Nov 97:20, Mar 98:11, Apr 01:4, Nov 06:21

52648 Laser vaporization of prostate, including control of postoperative bleeding, complete (vasectomy, meatotomy, cystourethroscopy, urethral calibration and/or dilation, internal urethrotomy and transurethral resection of prostate are included if performed)

➔ *CPT Changes: An Insider's View* 2006

➔ *CPT Assistant* Mar 98:11, Apr 01:5, Jul 05:15, Nov 06:21, Jun 15:5

52649 Laser enucleation of the prostate with morcellation, including control of postoperative bleeding, complete (vasectomy, meatotomy, cystourethroscopy, urethral calibration and/or dilation, internal urethrotomy and transurethral resection of prostate are included if performed)

➔ *CPT Changes: An Insider's View* 2008

➔ *CPT Assistant* Jun 15:5

(Do not report 52649 in conjunction with 52000, 52276, 52281, 52601, 52647, 52648, 53020, 55250)

52700 Transurethral drainage of prostatic abscess

➔ *CPT Assistant* Apr 01:4

(For litholapaxy, use 52317, 52318)

Urethra

(For endoscopy, see cystoscopy, urethroscopy, cystourethroscopy, 52000-52700)

(For injection procedure for urethrocystography, see 51600-51610)

Contact Laser Vaporization of Prostate
52648

A laser is used to vaporize the prostate.

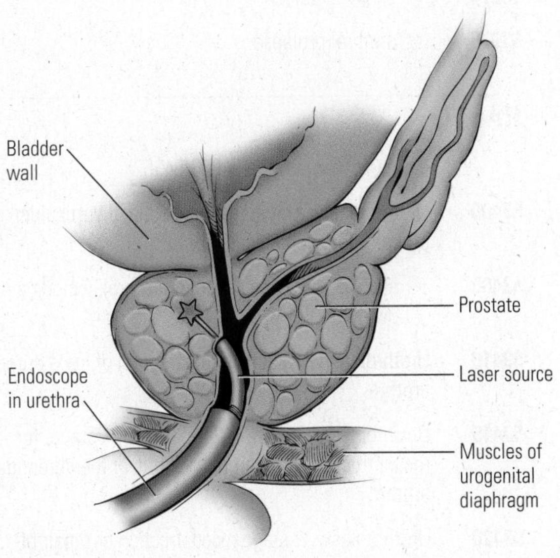

Incision

53000 Urethrotomy or urethrostomy, external (separate procedure); pendulous urethra

53010 perineal urethra, external

53020 Meatotomy, cutting of meatus (separate procedure); except infant

53025 infant

(Do not report modifier 63 in conjunction with 53025)

53040 Drainage of deep periurethral abscess

(For subcutaneous abscess, see 10060, 10061)

53060 Drainage of Skene's gland abscess or cyst

53080 Drainage of perineal urinary extravasation; uncomplicated (separate procedure)

53085 complicated

Excision

53200 Biopsy of urethra

53210 Urethrectomy, total, including cystostomy; female

53215 male

53220 Excision or fulguration of carcinoma of urethra

53230 Excision of urethral diverticulum (separate procedure); female

53235 male

53240 Marsupialization of urethral diverticulum, male or female

53250 Excision of bulbourethral gland (Cowper's gland)

53260 Excision or fulguration; urethral polyp(s), distal urethra

(For endoscopic approach, see 52214, 52224)

53265 urethral caruncle

53270 Skene's glands

53275 urethral prolapse

Repair

(For hypospadias, see 54300-54352)

53400 Urethroplasty; first stage, for fistula, diverticulum, or stricture (eg, Johannsen type)

53405 second stage (formation of urethra), including urinary diversion

53410 Urethroplasty, 1-stage reconstruction of male anterior urethra

53415 Urethroplasty, transpubic or perineal, 1-stage, for reconstruction or repair of prostatic or membranous urethra

53420 Urethroplasty, 2-stage reconstruction or repair of prostatic or membranous urethra; first stage

53425 second stage

53430 Urethroplasty, reconstruction of female urethra

53431 Urethroplasty with tubularization of posterior urethra and/or lower bladder for incontinence (eg, Tenago, Leadbetter procedure)

➲ *CPT Changes: An Insider's View* 2002

53440 Sling operation for correction of male urinary incontinence (eg, fascia or synthetic)

➲ *CPT Changes: An Insider's View* 2003

53442 Removal or revision of sling for male urinary incontinence (eg, fascia or synthetic)

➲ *CPT Changes: An Insider's View* 2003

53444 Insertion of tandem cuff (dual cuff)

➲ *CPT Changes: An Insider's View* 2002

53445 Insertion of inflatable urethral/bladder neck sphincter, including placement of pump, reservoir, and cuff

➲ *CPT Changes: An Insider's View* 2002

53446 Removal of inflatable urethral/bladder neck sphincter, including pump, reservoir, and cuff

➲ *CPT Changes: An Insider's View* 2002

53447 Removal and replacement of inflatable urethral/bladder neck sphincter including pump, reservoir, and cuff at the same operative session

➲ *CPT Changes: An Insider's View* 2002

53448 Removal and replacement of inflatable urethral/bladder neck sphincter including pump, reservoir, and cuff through an infected field at the same operative session including irrigation and debridement of infected tissue

➲ *CPT Changes: An Insider's View* 2002

(Do not report 11042, 11043 in addition to 53448)

53449 Repair of inflatable urethral/bladder neck sphincter, including pump, reservoir, and cuff

➲ *CPT Changes: An Insider's View* 2002

53450 Urethromeatoplasty, with mucosal advancement

➲ *CPT Assistant* Sep 12:16

(For meatotomy, see 53020, 53025)

53460 Urethromeatoplasty, with partial excision of distal urethral segment (Richardson type procedure)

53500 Urethrolysis, transvaginal, secondary, open, including cystourethroscopy (eg, postsurgical obstruction, scarring)

➲ *CPT Changes: An Insider's View* 2004

➲ *CPT Assistant* Sep 04:11

(For urethrolysis by retropubic approach, use 53899)

(Do not report 53500 in conjunction with 52000)

53502 Urethrorrhaphy, suture of urethral wound or injury, female

53505 Urethrorrhaphy, suture of urethral wound or injury; penile

53510 perineal

53515 prostatomembranous

53520 Closure of urethrostomy or urethrocutaneous fistula, male (separate procedure)

(For closure of urethrovaginal fistula, use 57310)

(For closure of urethrorectal fistula, see 45820, 45825)

Manipulation

(For radiological supervision and interpretation, use 74485)

53600 Dilation of urethral stricture by passage of sound or urethral dilator, male; initial

53601 subsequent

53605 Dilation of urethral stricture or vesical neck by passage of sound or urethral dilator, male, general or conduction (spinal) anesthesia

(For dilation of urethral stricture, male, performed under local anesthesia, see 53600, 53601, 53620, 53621)

53620 Dilation of urethral stricture by passage of filiform and follower, male; initial

53621 subsequent

53660 Dilation of female urethra including suppository and/or instillation; initial

53661 subsequent

53665 Dilation of female urethra, general or conduction (spinal) anesthesia

(For urethral catheterization, see 51701-51703)

(For dilation of urethra performed under local anesthesia, female, see 53660, 53661)

Other Procedures

(For 2 or 3 glass urinalysis, use 81020)

53850 Transurethral destruction of prostate tissue; by microwave thermotherapy
➔ *CPT Assistant* Nov 97:20, Apr 01:6, Feb 10:7, Jun 15:5

53852 by radiofrequency thermotherapy
➔ *CPT Assistant* Nov 97:20, Apr 01:6, Jun 15:5

● **53854** by radiofrequency generated water vapor thermotherapy
➔ *CPT Changes: An Insider's View* 2019

53855 Insertion of a temporary prostatic urethral stent, including urethral measurement
➔ *CPT Changes: An Insider's View* 2010
➔ *CPT Assistant* Feb 10:7

(For insertion of permanent urethral stent, use 52282)

Temporary Prostatic Urethral Stent Insertion
53855

A temporary prostatic urethral stent is inserted.

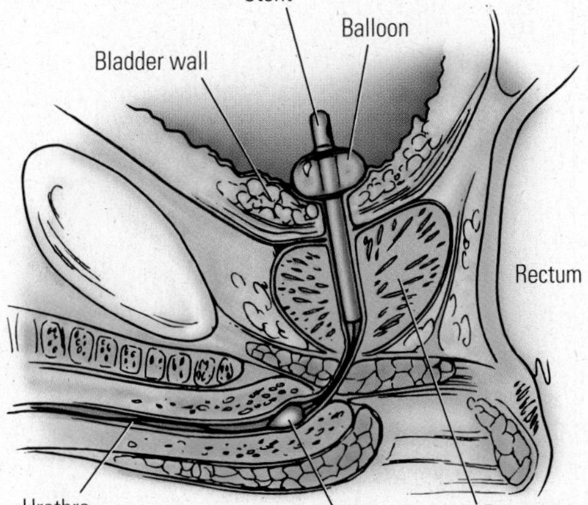

53860 Transurethral radiofrequency micro-remodeling of the female bladder neck and proximal urethra for stress urinary incontinence
➔ *CPT Changes: An Insider's View* 2011

53899 Unlisted procedure, urinary system
➔ *CPT Assistant* Aug 04:12, Sep 04:11, Oct 05:18, 23-24, Feb 06:14, May 10:10, Mar 15:9, Jun 15:5
➔ *Clinical Examples in Radiology* Summer 06:1-3

Urinary 50010-53899

Notes

Surgery

Male Genital System (54000-55899)....381

The following is a listing of headings and subheadings that appear within the Male Genital System section of the CPT codebook. The subheadings or subsections denoted with asterisks (*) below have special instructions unique to that subsection. Where these are indicated, special notes or guidelines will be presented preceding those procedural terminology listings, referring to that subsection specifically.

Penis (54000-54450)....381
- Incision (54000-54015)....381
- Destruction (54050-54065)....381
- Excision (54100-54164)....381
- Introduction (54200-54250)....381
- Repair (54300-54440)....382
- Manipulation (54450)....383

Testis (54500-54699)....383
- Excision (54500-54535)....383
- Exploration (54550-54560)....383
- Repair (54600-54680)....383
- Laparoscopy* (54690-54699)....383

Epididymis (54700-54901)....384
- Incision (54700)....384
- Excision (54800-54861)....384
- Exploration (54865)....384
- Repair (54900, 54901)....384

Tunica Vaginalis (55000-55060)....384
- Incision (55000)....384
- Excision (55040, 55041)....384
- Repair (55060)....384

Scrotum (55100-55180)....384
- Incision (55100-55120)....384
- Excision (55150)....384
- Repair (55175-55180)....385

Vas Deferens (55200-55400)....385
- Incision (55200)....385
- Excision (55250)....385
- Introduction (55300)....385
- Repair (55400)....385
- Suture....385

Spermatic Cord (55500-55559)....385
- Excision (55500-55540)....385
- Laparoscopy* (55550-55559)....385

Seminal Vesicles (55600-55680)....385
- Incision (55600-55605)....385
- Excision (55650-55680)....385

Prostate (55700-55899) 385
Incision (55700-55725) 385
Excision (55801-55865) 386
Laparoscopy* (55866) 386
Other Procedures (55870-55899) 386

Reproductive System Procedures (55920) 387

Intersex Surgery (55970-55980) 387

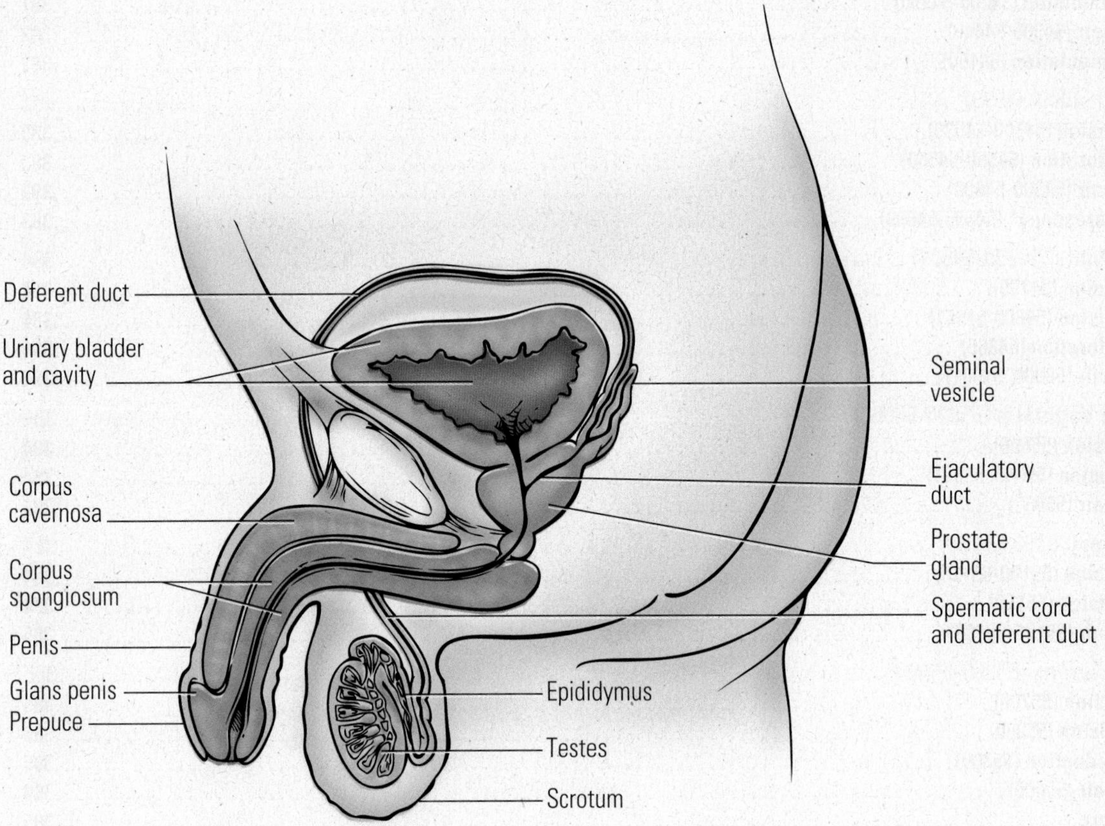

Male Genital System

Male Genital System

Penis

Incision

(For abdominal perineal gangrene debridement, see 11004-11006)

54000 Slitting of prepuce, dorsal or lateral (separate procedure); newborn

(Do not report modifier 63 in conjunction with 54000)

54001 except newborn

54015 Incision and drainage of penis, deep

(For skin and subcutaneous abscess, see 10060-10160)

Destruction

54050 Destruction of lesion(s), penis (eg, condyloma, papilloma, molluscum contagiosum, herpetic vesicle), simple; chemical

54055 electrodesiccation

54056 cryosurgery

54057 laser surgery

54060 surgical excision

54065 Destruction of lesion(s), penis (eg, condyloma, papilloma, molluscum contagiosum, herpetic vesicle), extensive (eg, laser surgery, electrosurgery, cryosurgery, chemosurgery)

➔ *CPT Changes: An Insider's View* 2002

(For destruction or excision of other lesions, see **Integumentary System**)

Excision

54100 Biopsy of penis; (separate procedure)

➔ *CPT Changes: An Insider's View* 2000

➔ *CPT Assistant* Nov 99:26

54105 deep structures

54110 Excision of penile plaque (Peyronie disease);

54111 with graft to 5 cm in length

➔ *CPT Assistant* Aug 99:5

54112 with graft greater than 5 cm in length

54115 Removal foreign body from deep penile tissue (eg, plastic implant)

54120 Amputation of penis; partial

54125 complete

54130 Amputation of penis, radical; with bilateral inguinofemoral lymphadenectomy

54135 in continuity with bilateral pelvic lymphadenectomy, including external iliac, hypogastric and obturator nodes

(For lymphadenectomy [separate procedure], see 38760-38770)

54150 Circumcision, using clamp or other device with regional dorsal penile or ring block

➔ *CPT Changes: An Insider's View* 2007

➔ *CPT Assistant* Sep 96:11, May 98:11, Apr 03:27, Aug 03:6, May 07:10, Jul 07:5

(Do not report modifier 63 in conjunction with 54150)

(Report 54150 with modifier 52 when performed without dorsal penile or ring block)

54160 Circumcision, surgical excision other than clamp, device, or dorsal slit; neonate (28 days of age or less)

➔ *CPT Changes: An Insider's View* 2007

➔ *CPT Assistant* Sep 96:11, May 98:11, May 07:10, Jul 07:5

(Do not report modifier 63 in conjunction with 54160)

54161 older than 28 days of age

➔ *CPT Changes: An Insider's View* 2007

➔ *CPT Assistant* Sep 96:11, Dec 96:10, May 98:11, Jul 07:5

54162 Lysis or excision of penile post-circumcision adhesions

➔ *CPT Changes: An Insider's View* 2002

54163 Repair incomplete circumcision

➔ *CPT Changes: An Insider's View* 2002

54164 Frenulotomy of penis

➔ *CPT Changes: An Insider's View* 2002

(Do not report 54164 with circumcision codes 54150-54161, 54162, 54163)

Introduction

54200 Injection procedure for Peyronie disease;

54205 with surgical exposure of plaque

54220 Irrigation of corpora cavernosa for priapism

54230 Injection procedure for corpora cavernosography

(For radiological supervision and interpretation, use 74445)

54231 Dynamic cavernosometry, including intracavernosal injection of vasoactive drugs (eg, papaverine, phentolamine)

54235 Injection of corpora cavernosa with pharmacologic agent(s) (eg, papaverine, phentolamine)

➔ *CPT Assistant* Sep 96:10

54240 Penile plethysmography

54250 Nocturnal penile tumescence and/or rigidity test

Repair

(For other urethroplasties, see 53400-53430)

(For penile revascularization, use 37788)

54300 Plastic operation of penis for straightening of chordee (eg, hypospadias), with or without mobilization of urethra

➲ *CPT Assistant* Dec 14:16

54304 Plastic operation on penis for correction of chordee or for first stage hypospadias repair with or without transplantation of prepuce and/or skin flaps

54308 Urethroplasty for second stage hypospadias repair (including urinary diversion); less than 3 cm

54312 greater than 3 cm

54316 Urethroplasty for second stage hypospadias repair (including urinary diversion) with free skin graft obtained from site other than genitalia

54318 Urethroplasty for third stage hypospadias repair to release penis from scrotum (eg, third stage Cecil repair)

54322 1-stage distal hypospadias repair (with or without chordee or circumcision); with simple meatal advancement (eg, Magpi, V-flap)

54324 with urethroplasty by local skin flaps (eg, flip-flap, prepucial flap)

54326 with urethroplasty by local skin flaps and mobilization of urethra

54328 with extensive dissection to correct chordee and urethroplasty with local skin flaps, skin graft patch, and/or island flap

➲ *CPT Assistant* Oct 04:15

(For urethroplasty and straightening of chordee, use 54308)

54332 1-stage proximal penile or penoscrotal hypospadias repair requiring extensive dissection to correct chordee and urethroplasty by use of skin graft tube and/or island flap

➲ *CPT Assistant* Mar 04:11, Sep 04:12

54336 1-stage perineal hypospadias repair requiring extensive dissection to correct chordee and urethroplasty by use of skin graft tube and/or island flap

➲ *CPT Assistant* Oct 04:15

54340 Repair of hypospadias complications (ie, fistula, stricture, diverticula); by closure, incision, or excision, simple

54344 requiring mobilization of skin flaps and urethroplasty with flap or patch graft

54348 requiring extensive dissection and urethroplasty with flap, patch or tubed graft (includes urinary diversion)

54352 Repair of hypospadias cripple requiring extensive dissection and excision of previously constructed structures including re-release of chordee and reconstruction of urethra and penis by use of local skin as grafts and island flaps and skin brought in as flaps or grafts

54360 Plastic operation on penis to correct angulation

54380 Plastic operation on penis for epispadias distal to external sphincter;

54385 with incontinence

54390 with exstrophy of bladder

54400 Insertion of penile prosthesis; non-inflatable (semi-rigid)

54401 inflatable (self-contained)

(For removal or replacement of penile prosthesis, see 54415, 54416)

54405 Insertion of multi-component, inflatable penile prosthesis, including placement of pump, cylinders, and reservoir

➲ *CPT Changes: An Insider's View* 2002

(For reduced services, report 54405 with modifier 52)

54406 Removal of all components of a multi-component, inflatable penile prosthesis without replacement of prosthesis

➲ *CPT Changes: An Insider's View* 2002

(For reduced services, report 54406 with modifier 52)

54408 Repair of component(s) of a multi-component, inflatable penile prosthesis

➲ *CPT Changes: An Insider's View* 2002

54410 Removal and replacement of all component(s) of a multi-component, inflatable penile prosthesis at the same operative session

➲ *CPT Changes: An Insider's View* 2002

54411 Removal and replacement of all components of a multi-component inflatable penile prosthesis through an infected field at the same operative session, including irrigation and debridement of infected tissue

➲ *CPT Changes: An Insider's View* 2002

(For reduced services, report 54411 with modifier 52)

(Do not report 11042, 11043 in addition to 54411)

54415 Removal of non-inflatable (semi-rigid) or inflatable (self-contained) penile prosthesis, without replacement of prosthesis

➲ *CPT Changes: An Insider's View* 2002

54416 Removal and replacement of non-inflatable (semi-rigid) or inflatable (self-contained) penile prosthesis at the same operative session

➲ *CPT Changes: An Insider's View* 2002

54417 Removal and replacement of non-inflatable (semi-rigid) or inflatable (self-contained) penile prosthesis through an infected field at the same operative session, including irrigation and debridement of infected tissue

➲ *CPT Changes: An Insider's View* 2002

(Do not report 11042, 11043 in addition to 54417)

54420 Corpora cavernosa-saphenous vein shunt (priapism operation), unilateral or bilateral

54430 Corpora cavernosa-corpus spongiosum shunt (priapism operation), unilateral or bilateral

54435 Corpora cavernosa-glans penis fistulization (eg, biopsy needle, Winter procedure, rongeur, or punch) for priapism

54437 Repair of traumatic corporeal tear(s)
➔ *CPT Changes: An Insider's View* 2016

(For repair of urethra, see 53410, 53415)

54438 Replantation, penis, complete amputation including urethral repair
➔ *CPT Changes: An Insider's View* 2016

(To report replantation of incomplete penile amputation, see 54437 for repair of corporeal tear[s], and 53410, 53415 for repair of the urethra)

54440 Plastic operation of penis for injury

Manipulation

54450 Foreskin manipulation including lysis of preputial adhesions and stretching

Testis

Excision

(For abdominal perineal gangrene debridement, see 11004-11006)

54500 Biopsy of testis, needle (separate procedure)
➔ *Clinical Examples in Radiology* Winter 17:5

►(For fine needle aspiration biopsy, see 10004, 10005, 10006, 10007, 10008, 10009, 10010, 10011, 10012, 10021)◄

(For evaluation of fine needle aspirate, see 88172, 88173)

54505 Biopsy of testis, incisional (separate procedure)
➔ *CPT Assistant* Oct 01:8

(For bilateral procedure, report 54505 with modifier 50)

(When combined with vasogram, seminal vesiculogram, or epididymogram, use 55300)

54512 Excision of extraparenchymal lesion of testis
➔ *CPT Changes: An Insider's View* 2001
➔ *CPT Assistant* Oct 01:8, Aug 05:13

54520 Orchiectomy, simple (including subcapsular), with or without testicular prosthesis, scrotal or inguinal approach
➔ *CPT Assistant* Winter 94:13, Oct 01:8, Mar 04:3

(For bilateral procedure, report 54520 with modifier 50)

54522 Orchiectomy, partial
➔ *CPT Changes: An Insider's View* 2001
➔ *CPT Assistant* Oct 01:8

54530 Orchiectomy, radical, for tumor; inguinal approach
➔ *CPT Assistant* Oct 01:8

54535 with abdominal exploration
➔ *CPT Assistant* Oct 01:8

(For orchiectomy with repair of hernia, see 49505 or 49507 and 54520)

(For radical retroperitoneal lymphadenectomy, use 38780)

Exploration

54550 Exploration for undescended testis (inguinal or scrotal area)
➔ *CPT Assistant* Oct 01:8, Mar 17:10

(For bilateral procedure, report 54550 with modifier 50)

54560 Exploration for undescended testis with abdominal exploration
➔ *CPT Assistant* Oct 01:8

(For bilateral procedure, report 54560 with modifier 50)

Repair

54600 Reduction of torsion of testis, surgical, with or without fixation of contralateral testis
➔ *CPT Assistant* Aug 05:13

54620 Fixation of contralateral testis (separate procedure)

54640 Orchiopexy, inguinal approach, with or without hernia repair
➔ *CPT Assistant* Oct 01:8, Jan 04:27, Mar 04:10, Jun 08:4, Mar 17:11

(For bilateral procedure, report 54640 with modifier 50)

(For inguinal hernia repair performed in conjunction with inguinal orchiopexy, see 49495-49525)

54650 Orchiopexy, abdominal approach, for intra-abdominal testis (eg, Fowler-Stephens)
➔ *CPT Changes: An Insider's View* 2000
➔ *CPT Assistant* Nov 99:26, May 00:4, Oct 01:8

(For laparoscopic approach, use 54692)

54660 Insertion of testicular prosthesis (separate procedure)
➔ *CPT Assistant* Oct 01:8

(For bilateral procedure, report 54660 with modifier 50)

54670 Suture or repair of testicular injury
➔ *CPT Assistant* Oct 01:8

54680 Transplantation of testis(es) to thigh (because of scrotal destruction)
➔ *CPT Assistant* Oct 01:8

Laparoscopy

Surgical laparoscopy always includes diagnostic laparoscopy. To report a diagnostic laparoscopy (peritoneoscopy) (separate procedure), use 49320.

54690 Laparoscopy, surgical; orchiectomy
➔ *CPT Changes: An Insider's View* 2000
➔ *CPT Assistant* Nov 99:26, Mar 00:5, Oct 01:8

54692 orchiopexy for intra-abdominal testis
➲ *CPT Changes: An Insider's View* 2000
➲ *CPT Assistant* Nov 99:27, May 00:4, Oct 01:8

Laparoscopic Orchiopexy
54692

Surgical fixation of an undescended testis in the scrotum under laparoscopic guidance

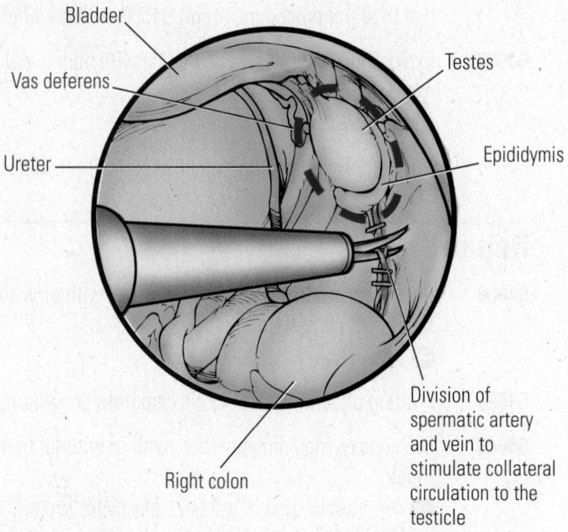

54699 Unlisted laparoscopy procedure, testis
➲ *CPT Changes: An Insider's View* 2000
➲ *CPT Assistant* Nov 99:27, Mar 00:9

Epididymis

Incision

54700 Incision and drainage of epididymis, testis and/or scrotal space (eg, abscess or hematoma)
➲ *CPT Assistant* Oct 01:8

(For debridement of necrotizing soft tissue infection of external genitalia, see 11004-11006)

Excision

54800 Biopsy of epididymis, needle
➲ *CPT Assistant* Oct 01:8
➲ *Clinical Examples in Radiology* Winter 17:5

►(For fine needle aspiration biopsy, see 10004, 10005, 10006, 10007, 10008, 10009, 10010, 10011, 10012, 10021)◄

(For evaluation of fine needle aspirate, see 88172, 88173)

54830 Excision of local lesion of epididymis
➲ *CPT Assistant* Oct 01:8

54840 Excision of spermatocele, with or without epididymectomy
➲ *CPT Assistant* Oct 01:8

54860 Epididymectomy; unilateral

54861 bilateral

Exploration

54865 Exploration of epididymis, with or without biopsy
➲ *CPT Changes: An Insider's View* 2007

Repair

54900 Epididymovasostomy, anastomosis of epididymis to vas deferens; unilateral
➲ *CPT Assistant* Nov 98:16, Jun 04:11

54901 bilateral
➲ *CPT Assistant* Nov 98:16, Jun 04:11

(For operating microscope, use 69990)

Tunica Vaginalis

Incision

55000 Puncture aspiration of hydrocele, tunica vaginalis, with or without injection of medication

Excision

55040 Excision of hydrocele; unilateral
➲ *CPT Assistant* Jun 08:4, Nov 17:10

55041 bilateral

(With hernia repair, see 49495-49501)

Repair

55060 Repair of tunica vaginalis hydrocele (Bottle type)
➲ *CPT Assistant* Nov 14:14

Scrotum

Incision

55100 Drainage of scrotal wall abscess

(See also 54700)

(For debridement of necrotizing soft tissue infection of external genitalia, see 11004-11006)

55110 Scrotal exploration

55120 Removal of foreign body in scrotum

Excision

(For excision of local lesion of skin of scrotum, see **Integumentary System**)

55150 Resection of scrotum

Repair

55175 Scroplasty; simple
➔ *CPT Assistant* Dec 14:16

55180 complicated

Vas Deferens

Incision

55200 Vasotomy, cannulization with or without incision of vas, unilateral or bilateral (separate procedure)

Excision

55250 Vasectomy, unilateral or bilateral (separate procedure), including postoperative semen examination(s)
➔ *CPT Assistant* Jun 98:10, Jul 98:10

Introduction

55300 Vasotomy for vasograms, seminal vesiculograms, or epididymograms, unilateral or bilateral

(For radiological supervision and interpretation, use 74440)

(When combined with biopsy of testis, see 54505 and use modifier 51)

Repair

55400 Vasovasostomy, vasovasorrhaphy
➔ *CPT Assistant* Nov 98:16, Oct 01:8, Jun 04:11

(For bilateral procedure, report 55400 with modifier 50)

(For operating microscope, use 69990)

Suture

(55450 has been deleted. To report, use 55250)

Spermatic Cord

Excision

55500 Excision of hydrocele of spermatic cord, unilateral (separate procedure)
➔ *CPT Assistant* Oct 01:8

55520 Excision of lesion of spermatic cord (separate procedure)
➔ *CPT Assistant* Sep 00:10, Oct 01:8

55530 Excision of varicocele or ligation of spermatic veins for varicocele; (separate procedure)
➔ *CPT Assistant* Oct 01:8

55535 abdominal approach
➔ *CPT Assistant* Oct 01:8

55540 with hernia repair
➔ *CPT Assistant* Oct 01:8

Laparoscopy

Surgical laparoscopy always includes diagnostic laparoscopy. To report a diagnostic laparoscopy (peritoneoscopy) (separate procedure), use 49320.

55550 Laparoscopy, surgical, with ligation of spermatic veins for varicocele
➔ *CPT Changes: An Insider's View* 2000
➔ *CPT Assistant* Nov 99:27, Mar 00:9, Oct 01:8

55559 Unlisted laparoscopy procedure, spermatic cord
➔ *CPT Changes: An Insider's View* 2000
➔ *CPT Assistant* Nov 99:27, Mar 00:9

Seminal Vesicles

Incision

55600 Vesiculotomy;

(For bilateral procedure, report 55600 with modifier 50)

55605 complicated

Excision

55650 Vesiculectomy, any approach

(For bilateral procedure, report 55650 with modifier 50)

55680 Excision of Mullerian duct cyst

(For injection procedure, see 52010, 55300)

Prostate

Incision

55700 Biopsy, prostate; needle or punch, single or multiple, any approach
➔ *CPT Assistant* May 96:3, Nov 10:5
➔ *Clinical Examples in Radiology* Spring 15:10, Winter 17:5

(If imaging guidance is performed, see 76942, 77002, 77012, 77021)

►(For fine needle aspiration biopsy, see 10004, 10005, 10006, 10007, 10008, 10009, 10010, 10011, 10012, 10021)◄

(For evaluation of fine needle aspirate, see 88172, 88173)

(For transperineal stereotactic template guided saturation prostate biopsies, use 55706)

55705 incisional, any approach

55706 Biopsies, prostate, needle, transperineal, stereotactic template guided saturation sampling, including imaging guidance
➔ *CPT Changes: An Insider's View* 2009
➔ *CPT Assistant* Nov 10:5

(Do not report 55706 in conjunction with 55700)

Male Genital 54000-55980

55720 Prostatotomy, external drainage of prostatic abscess, any approach; simple

55725 complicated

(For transurethral drainage, use 52700)

Excision

(For transurethral removal of prostate, see 52601-52640)

(For transurethral destruction of prostate, see 53850-53852)

(For limited pelvic lymphadenectomy for staging [separate procedure], use 38562)

(For independent node dissection, see 38770-38780)

55801 Prostatectomy, perineal, subtotal (including control of postoperative bleeding, vasectomy, meatotomy, urethral calibration and/or dilation, and internal urethrotomy)
➔ *CPT Assistant* Jun 03:6-7

55810 Prostatectomy, perineal radical;
➔ *CPT Assistant* Jun 03:7

55812 with lymph node biopsy(s) (limited pelvic lymphadenectomy)

55815 with bilateral pelvic lymphadenectomy, including external iliac, hypogastric and obturator nodes

(If 55815 is carried out on separate days, use 38770 with modifier 50 and 55810)

55821 Prostatectomy (including control of postoperative bleeding, vasectomy, meatotomy, urethral calibration and/or dilation, and internal urethrotomy); suprapubic, subtotal, 1 or 2 stages
➔ *CPT Assistant* Jun 03:6

55831 retropubic, subtotal
➔ *CPT Assistant* Jun 03:7

55840 Prostatectomy, retropubic radical, with or without nerve sparing;
➔ *CPT Assistant* Jun 03:8

55842 with lymph node biopsy(s) (limited pelvic lymphadenectomy)
➔ *CPT Assistant* Jun 03:8

55845 with bilateral pelvic lymphadenectomy, including external iliac, hypogastric, and obturator nodes
➔ *CPT Assistant* Jun 03:8

(If 55845 is carried out on separate days, use 38770 with modifier 50 and 55840)

(For laparoscopic retropubic radical prostatectomy, use 55866)

55860 Exposure of prostate, any approach, for insertion of radioactive substance;

(For application of interstitial radioelement, see 77770, 77771, 77772, 77778)

55862 with lymph node biopsy(s) (limited pelvic lymphadenectomy)

55865 with bilateral pelvic lymphadenectomy, including external iliac, hypogastric and obturator nodes

Laparoscopy

Surgical laparoscopy always includes diagnostic laparoscopy. To report a diagnostic laparoscopy (peritoneoscopy) (separate procedure), use 49320.

55866 Laparoscopy, surgical prostatectomy, retropubic radical, including nerve sparing, includes robotic assistance, when performed
➔ *CPT Changes: An Insider's View* 2003, 2011
➔ *CPT Assistant* Jun 03:8, Mar 12:10

(For open procedure, use 55840)

Other Procedures

(For artificial insemination, see 58321, 58322)

55870 Electroejaculation

55873 Cryosurgical ablation of the prostate (includes ultrasonic guidance and monitoring)
➔ *CPT Changes: An Insider's View* 2001, 2010
➔ *CPT Assistant* Apr 01:4, Sep 02:9, Jun 03:8, Feb 10:7, Sep 15:12

55874 Transperineal placement of biodegradable material, peri-prostatic, single or multiple injection(s), including image guidance, when performed
➔ *CPT Changes: An Insider's View* 2018

(Do not report 55874 in conjunction with 76942)

55875 Transperineal placement of needles or catheters into prostate for interstitial radioelement application, with or without cystoscopy
➔ *CPT Changes: An Insider's View* 2007
➔ *CPT Assistant* May 07:1, Apr 09:3

(For placement of needles or catheters into pelvic organs and/or genitalia [except prostate] for interstitial radioelement application, use 55920)

(For interstitial radioelement application, see 77770, 77771, 77772, 77778)

(For ultrasonic guidance for interstitial radioelement application, use 76965)

55876 Placement of interstitial device(s) for radiation therapy guidance (eg, fiducial markers, dosimeter), prostate (via needle, any approach), single or multiple
➔ *CPT Changes: An Insider's View* 2007, 2010, 2011
➔ *CPT Assistant* May 07:1, Oct 07:1, Feb 10:7, 12, Jun 16:3

(Report supply of device separately)

(For imaging guidance, see 76942, 77002, 77012, 77021)

55899 Unlisted procedure, male genital system
➔ *CPT Assistant* Jun 03:8, May 07:11, Jun 15:5, Jan 17:6
➔ *Clinical Examples in Radiology* Spring 06:8-9

Reproductive System Procedures

55920 Placement of needles or catheters into pelvic organs and/or genitalia (except prostate) for subsequent interstitial radioelement application

➔ *CPT Changes: An Insider's View* 2008

➔ *CPT Assistant* Apr 09:10

(For placement of needles or catheters into prostate, use 55875)

(For insertion of uterine tandems and/or vaginal ovoids for clinical brachytherapy, use 57155)

(For insertion of Heyman capsules for clinical brachytherapy, use 58346)

Intersex Surgery

55970 Intersex surgery; male to female

55980 female to male

Male Genital 54000-55980

Notes

Surgery

Female Genital System (56405-58999) 391

The following is a listing of headings and subheadings that appear within the Female Genital System section of the CPT codebook. The subheadings or subsections denoted with asterisks (*) below have special instructions unique to that subsection. Where these are indicated, special notes or guidelines will be presented preceding those procedural terminology listings, referring to that subsection specifically.

Female Genital System

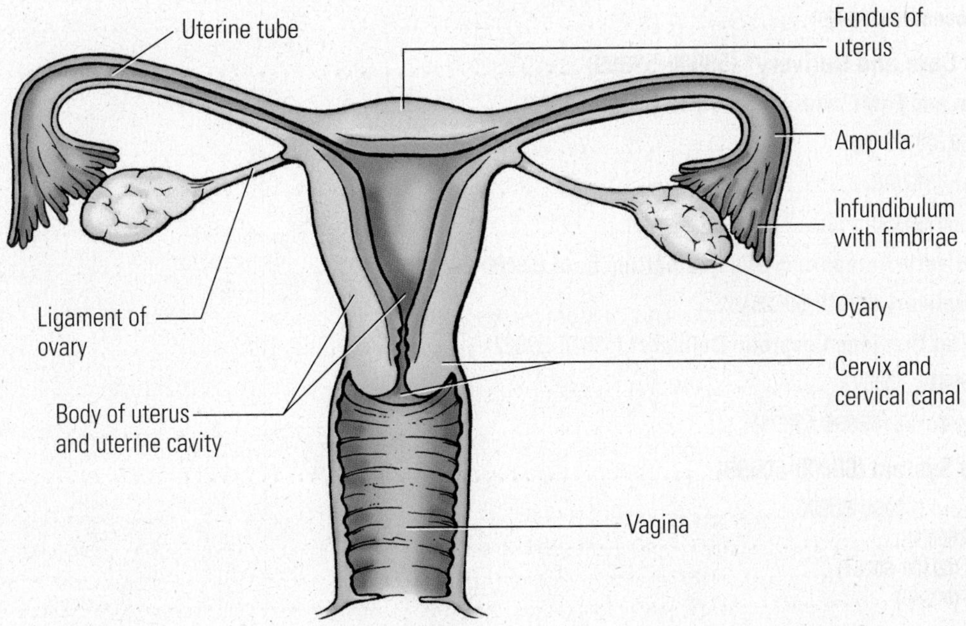

Vulva, Perineum, and Introitus* (56405-56821) 391
- **Incision (56405-56442)** 391
- **Destruction (56501-56515)** 391
- **Excision (56605-56740)** 391
- **Repair (56800-56810)** 391
- **Endoscopy (56820, 56821)** 392

Vagina (57000-57426) 392
- **Incision (57000-57023)** 392
- **Destruction (57061-57065)** 392
- **Excision (57100-57135)** 392
- **Introduction (57150-57180)** 392
- **Repair (57200-57335)** 393
- **Manipulation (57400-57415)** 394
- **Endoscopy/Laparoscopy (57420-57426)** 394

Cervix Uteri (57452-57800) 394
- **Endoscopy (57452-57461)** 394
- **Excision (57500-57558)** 395
- **Repair (57700-57720)** 395
- **Manipulation (57800)** 395

Corpus Uteri (58100-58579) 395
Excision (58100-58294) 395
Hysterectomy Procedures (58150-58294) 396
Introduction (58300-58356) 396
Repair (58400-58540) 397
Laparoscopy/Hysteroscopy* (58541-58579, 58674) 397
Oviduct/Ovary (58600-58770) 399
Incision (58600-58615) 399
Laparoscopy* (58660-58673, 58679) 399
Excision (58700-58720) 399
Repair (58740-58770) 399
Ovary (58800-58960) 400
Incision (58800-58825) 400
Excision (58900-58960) 400
In Vitro Fertilization (58970-58999) 400
Other Procedures (58999) 401
Maternity Care and Delivery* (59000-59899) 401
Antepartum and Fetal Invasive Services (59000-59076) 401
Excision (59100-59160) 402
Introduction (59200) 402
Repair (59300-59350) 402
Vaginal Delivery, Antepartum and Postpartum Care (59400-59430) 402
Cesarean Delivery (59510-59525) 403
Delivery After Previous Cesarean Delivery* (59610-59622) 404
Abortion (59812-59857) 404
Other Procedures (59866-59899) 404
Endocrine System (60000-60699) 404
Thyroid Gland (60000-60300) 404
Incision (60000) 404
Excision (60100-60281) 404
Removal (60300) 405
Parathyroid, Thymus, Adrenal Glands, Pancreas, and Carotid Body (60500-60699) 405
Excision (60500-60605) 405
Laparoscopy* (60650-60659) 406
Other Procedures (60699) 406

Female Genital System

(For pelvic laparotomy, use 49000)

(For excision or destruction of endometriomas, open method, see 49203-49205, 58957, 58958)

(For paracentesis, see 49082, 49083, 49084)

(For secondary closure of abdominal wall evisceration or disruption, use 49900)

(For fulguration or excision of lesions, laparoscopic approach, use 58662)

(For chemotherapy, see 96401-96549)

Vulva, Perineum, and Introitus

Definitions

The following definitions apply to the vulvectomy codes (56620-56640):

A ***simple*** procedure is the removal of skin and superficial subcutaneous tissues.

A ***radical*** procedure is the removal of skin and deep subcutaneous tissue.

A ***partial*** procedure is the removal of less than 80% of the vulvar area.

A ***complete*** procedure is the removal of greater than 80% of the vulvar area.

Incision

(For incision and drainage of sebaceous cyst, furuncle, or abscess, see 10040, 10060, 10061)

56405 Incision and drainage of vulva or perineal abscess

56420 Incision and drainage of Bartholin's gland abscess

(For incision and drainage of Skene's gland abscess or cyst, use 53060)

56440 Marsupialization of Bartholin's gland cyst

56441 Lysis of labial adhesions

➔ *CPT Assistant* Winter 90:7

56442 Hymenotomy, simple incision

➔ *CPT Changes: An Insider's View* 2007

Destruction

56501 Destruction of lesion(s), vulva; simple (eg, laser surgery, electrosurgery, cryosurgery, chemosurgery)

➔ *CPT Changes: An Insider's View* 2002

56515 extensive (eg, laser surgery, electrosurgery, cryosurgery, chemosurgery)

➔ *CPT Changes: An Insider's View* 2002

(For destruction of Skene's gland cyst or abscess, use 53270)

(For cautery destruction of urethral caruncle, use 53265)

Excision

56605 Biopsy of vulva or perineum (separate procedure); 1 lesion

➔ *CPT Assistant* Sep 00:9, Jun 08:6

+ 56606 each separate additional lesion (List separately in addition to code for primary procedure)

(Use 56606 in conjunction with 56605)

(For excision of local lesion, see 11420-11426, 11620-11626)

56620 Vulvectomy simple; partial

➔ *CPT Assistant* Dec 13:14

56625 complete

(For skin graft, see 15002 et seq)

56630 Vulvectomy, radical, partial;

(For skin graft, if used, see 15004-15005, 15120, 15121, 15240, 15241)

56631 with unilateral inguinofemoral lymphadenectomy

56632 with bilateral inguinofemoral lymphadenectomy

►(For partial radical vulvectomy with inguinofemoral lymph node biopsy without complete inguinofemoral lymphadenectomy, use 56630 in conjunction with 38531)◄

56633 Vulvectomy, radical, complete;

56634 with unilateral inguinofemoral lymphadenectomy

56637 with bilateral inguinofemoral lymphadenectomy

►(For complete radical vulvectomy with inguinofemoral lymph node biopsy without complete inguinofemoral lymphadenectomy, use 56633 in conjunction with 38531)◄

56640 Vulvectomy, radical, complete, with inguinofemoral, iliac, and pelvic lymphadenectomy

(For bilateral procedure, report 56640 with modifier 50)

(For lymphadenectomy, see 38760-38780)

56700 Partial hymenectomy or revision of hymenal ring

56740 Excision of Bartholin's gland or cyst

(For excision of Skene's gland, use 53270)

(For excision of urethral caruncle, use 53265)

(For excision or fulguration of urethral carcinoma, use 53220)

(For excision or marsupialization of urethral diverticulum, see 53230, 53240)

Repair

(For repair of urethra for mucosal prolapse, use 53275)

56800 Plastic repair of introitus

56805 Clitoroplasty for intersex state

56810 Perineoplasty, repair of perineum, nonobstetrical (separate procedure)

(See also 56800)

(For repair of wounds to genitalia, see 12001-12007, 12041-12047, 13131-13133)

(For repair of recent injury of vagina and perineum, nonobstetrical, use 57210)

(For anal sphincteroplasty, see 46750, 46751)

(For episiorrhaphy, episioperineorrhaphy for recent injury of vulva and/or perineum, nonobstetrical, use 57210)

Endoscopy

56820 Colposcopy of the vulva;
➲ *CPT Changes: An Insider's View* 2003
➲ *CPT Assistant* Feb 03:5

56821 with biopsy(s)
➲ *CPT Changes: An Insider's View* 2003
➲ *CPT Assistant* Feb 03:5, Jun 03:11

(For colposcopic examinations/procedures involving the vagina, see 57420, 57421; cervix, see 57452-57461)

Vagina

Incision

57000 Colpotomy; with exploration
➲ *CPT Assistant* Nov 07:1

57010 with drainage of pelvic abscess

57020 Colpocentesis (separate procedure)

57022 Incision and drainage of vaginal hematoma; obstetrical/postpartum
➲ *CPT Changes: An Insider's View* 2001, 2002

57023 non-obstetrical (eg, post-trauma, spontaneous bleeding)
➲ *CPT Changes: An Insider's View* 2001

Destruction

57061 Destruction of vaginal lesion(s); simple (eg, laser surgery, electrosurgery, cryosurgery, chemosurgery)
➲ *CPT Changes: An Insider's View* 2002
➲ *CPT Assistant* Apr 96:11

57065 extensive (eg, laser surgery, electrosurgery, cryosurgery, chemosurgery)
➲ *CPT Changes: An Insider's View* 2002
➲ *CPT Assistant* Apr 96:11

Excision

57100 Biopsy of vaginal mucosa; simple (separate procedure)

57105 extensive, requiring suture (including cysts)

57106 Vaginectomy, partial removal of vaginal wall;
➲ *CPT Assistant* Nov 98:17, Oct 99:5

Vaginectomy, Partial Removal of Vaginal Wall
57106

A specific portion of the upper or lower vaginal wall is excised.

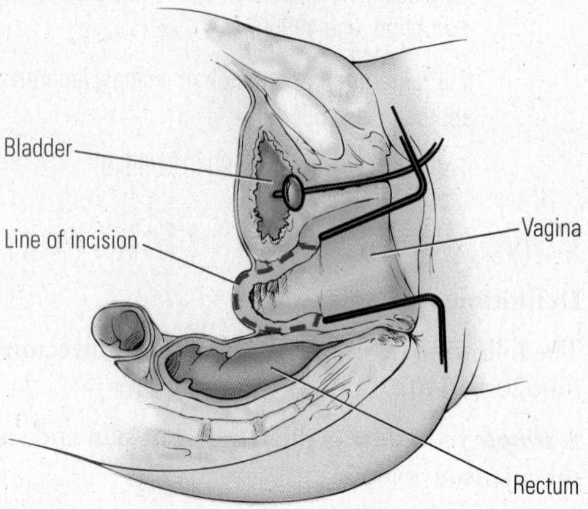

57107 with removal of paravaginal tissue (radical vaginectomy)
➲ *CPT Assistant* Nov 98:17, Oct 99:5

57109 with removal of paravaginal tissue (radical vaginectomy) with bilateral total pelvic lymphadenectomy and para-aortic lymph node sampling (biopsy)
➲ *CPT Assistant* Nov 98:17, Oct 99:5

57110 Vaginectomy, complete removal of vaginal wall;
➲ *CPT Assistant* Nov 98:17, Oct 99:5

57111 with removal of paravaginal tissue (radical vaginectomy)
➲ *CPT Assistant* Nov 98:17, Oct 99:5

57112 with removal of paravaginal tissue (radical vaginectomy) with bilateral total pelvic lymphadenectomy and para-aortic lymph node sampling (biopsy)
➲ *CPT Assistant* Nov 98:17, Oct 99:5

57120 Colpocleisis (Le Fort type)

57130 Excision of vaginal septum

57135 Excision of vaginal cyst or tumor

Introduction

57150 Irrigation of vagina and/or application of medicament for treatment of bacterial, parasitic, or fungoid disease

57155 Insertion of uterine tandem and/or vaginal ovoids for clinical brachytherapy
➲ *CPT Changes: An Insider's View* 2002, 2011, 2017
➲ *CPT Assistant* Feb 02:8, Apr 09:3

Vaginectomy, Complete Removal of Vaginal Wall (Radical Vaginectomy)
57111

Removal of all of the vaginal wall and removal of paravaginal tissue (the highly vascular supporting connective tissue next to the vagina)

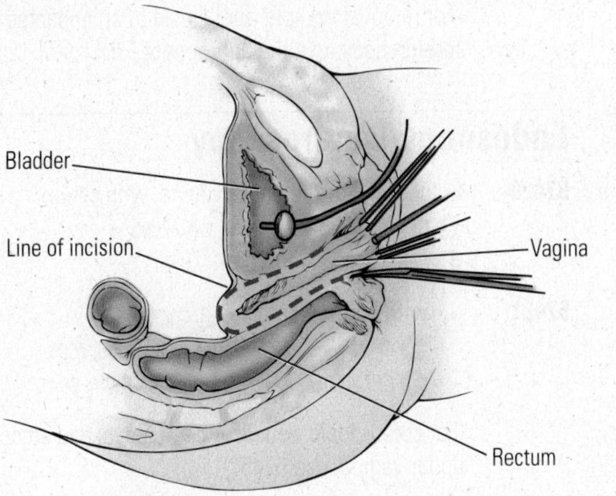

(For placement of needles or catheters into pelvic organs and/or genitalia [except prostate] for interstitial radioelement application, use 55920)

(For insertion of radioelement sources or ribbons, see 77761-77763, 77770, 77771, 77772)

57156 Insertion of a vaginal radiation afterloading apparatus for clinical brachytherapy
CPT Changes: An Insider's View 2011

57160 Fitting and insertion of pessary or other intravaginal support device
CPT Assistant Nov 96:9, Oct 98:11, Jun 00:11, May 10:10

57170 Diaphragm or cervical cap fitting with instructions

57180 Introduction of any hemostatic agent or pack for spontaneous or traumatic nonobstetrical vaginal hemorrhage (separate procedure)
CPT Assistant Nov 07:1

Repair

(For urethral suspension, Marshall-Marchetti-Krantz type, abdominal approach, see 51840, 51841)

(For laparoscopic suspension, use 51990)

57200 Colporrhaphy, suture of injury of vagina (nonobstetrical)

57210 Colpoperineorrhaphy, suture of injury of vagina and/or perineum (nonobstetrical)

57220 Plastic operation on urethral sphincter, vaginal approach (eg, Kelly urethral plication)
CPT Assistant Winter 90:7

57230 Plastic repair of urethrocele
CPT Assistant Winter 90:7

57240 Anterior colporrhaphy, repair of cystocele with or without repair of urethrocele, including cystourethroscopy, when performed
CPT Changes: An Insider's View 2018
CPT Assistant Winter 90:7, Jan 97:3, Jun 02:5, Jun 10:6

(Do not report 57240 in conjunction with 52000)

57250 Posterior colporrhaphy, repair of rectocele with or without perineorrhaphy
CPT Assistant Winter 90:7, Jun 02:4, May 11:9

(For repair of rectocele [separate procedure] without posterior colporrhaphy, use 45560)

57260 Combined anteroposterior colporrhaphy, including cystourethroscopy, when performed
CPT Changes: An Insider's View 2018
CPT Assistant Jun 02:5, Jun 10:6

(Do not report 57260 in conjunction with 52000)

57265 with enterocele repair
CPT Changes: An Insider's View 2018
CPT Assistant Jun 02:6, Jun 10:6

(Do not report 57265 in conjunction with 52000)

+ 57267 Insertion of mesh or other prosthesis for repair of pelvic floor defect, each site (anterior, posterior compartment), vaginal approach (List separately in addition to code for primary procedure)
CPT Changes: An Insider's View 2005
CPT Assistant Jul 05:16, May 11:9, Jan 12:10, Oct 13:15

(Use 57267 in conjunction with 45560, 57240-57265, 57285)

57268 Repair of enterocele, vaginal approach (separate procedure)
CPT Assistant Jun 02:6

57270 Repair of enterocele, abdominal approach (separate procedure)
CPT Assistant Jun 02:6

57280 Colpopexy, abdominal approach
CPT Assistant Jan 97:3, Jun 02:6

57282 Colpopexy, vaginal; extra-peritoneal approach (sacrospinous, iliococcygeus)
CPT Changes: An Insider's View 2005
CPT Assistant Jan 97:3, Jun 02:6

57283 intra-peritoneal approach (uterosacral, levator myorrhaphy)
CPT Changes: An Insider's View 2005
CPT Assistant May 11:9

(Do not report 57283 in conjunction with 57556, 58263, 58270, 58280, 58292, 58294)

57284 Paravaginal defect repair (including repair of cystocele, if performed); open abdominal approach
CPT Changes: An Insider's View 2008
CPT Assistant Jan 97:1, Jun 02:7, Jul 05:16, Jun 10:6

(Do not report 57284 in conjunction with 51840, 51841, 51990, 57240, 57260, 57265, 58152, 58267)

57285 vaginal approach
➲ *CPT Changes: An Insider's View* 2008
➲ *CPT Assistant* Jun 10:6

(Do not report 57285 in conjunction with 51990, 57240, 57260, 57265, 58267)

57287 Removal or revision of sling for stress incontinence (eg, fascia or synthetic)
➲ *CPT Changes: An Insider's View* 2001
➲ *CPT Assistant* Jun 02:7, Nov 07:9

57288 Sling operation for stress incontinence (eg, fascia or synthetic)
➲ *CPT Changes: An Insider's View* 2000
➲ *CPT Assistant* Nov 99:28, May 00:4, Oct 00:7, Apr 02:18, Jun 02:7

(For laparoscopic approach, use 51992)

57289 Pereyra procedure, including anterior colporrhaphy
➲ *CPT Assistant* Jan 97:3, Jun 02:7

57291 Construction of artificial vagina; without graft

57292 with graft

57295 Revision (including removal) of prosthetic vaginal graft; vaginal approach
➲ *CPT Changes: An Insider's View* 2006

57296 open abdominal approach
➲ *CPT Changes: An Insider's View* 2007

(For laparoscopic approach, use 57426)

57300 Closure of rectovaginal fistula; vaginal or transanal approach
➲ *CPT Assistant* Nov 97:21

57305 abdominal approach
➲ *CPT Assistant* Nov 97:21

57307 abdominal approach, with concomitant colostomy
➲ *CPT Assistant* Nov 97:21

57308 transperineal approach, with perineal body reconstruction, with or without levator plication
➲ *CPT Assistant* Nov 97:21

57310 Closure of urethrovaginal fistula;

57311 with bulbocavernosus transplant

57320 Closure of vesicovaginal fistula; vaginal approach

(For concomitant cystostomy, see 51020-51040, 51101, 51102)

57330 transvesical and vaginal approach

(For abdominal approach, use 51900)

57335 Vaginoplasty for intersex state

Manipulation

57400 Dilation of vagina under anesthesia (other than local)
➲ *CPT Changes: An Insider's View* 2009

57410 Pelvic examination under anesthesia (other than local)
➲ *CPT Changes: An Insider's View* 2009
➲ *CPT Assistant* Spring 93:34, Apr 06:1, Nov 07:1

57415 Removal of impacted vaginal foreign body (separate procedure) under anesthesia (other than local)
➲ *CPT Changes: An Insider's View* 2009

(For removal without anesthesia of an impacted vaginal foreign body, use the appropriate E/M code)

Endoscopy/Laparoscopy

57420 Colposcopy of the entire vagina, with cervix if present;
➲ *CPT Changes: An Insider's View* 2003
➲ *CPT Assistant* Feb 03:5

57421 with biopsy(s) of vagina/cervix
➲ *CPT Changes: An Insider's View* 2003, 2006
➲ *CPT Assistant* Feb 03:5, Jun 03:11, Jun 06:16

(For colposcopic visualization of cervix and adjacent upper vagina, use 57452)

(When reporting colposcopies of multiple sites, use modifier 51 as appropriate. For colposcopic examinations/procedures involving the vulva, see 56820, 56821; cervix, see 57452-57461)

(For endometrial sampling [biopsy] performed in conjunction with colposcopy, use 58110)

57423 Paravaginal defect repair (including repair of cystocele, if performed), laparoscopic approach
➲ *CPT Changes: An Insider's View* 2008
➲ *CPT Assistant* Jun 10:6

(Do not report 57423 in conjunction with 49320, 51840, 51841, 51990, 57240, 57260, 58152, 58267)

57425 Laparoscopy, surgical, colpopexy (suspension of vaginal apex)
➲ *CPT Changes: An Insider's View* 2004

57426 Revision (including removal) of prosthetic vaginal graft, laparoscopic approach
➲ *CPT Changes: An Insider's View* 2010

(For vaginal approach, see 57295. For open abdominal approach, see 57296)

Cervix Uteri

Endoscopy

(For colposcopic examinations/procedures involving the vulva, see 56820, 56821; vagina, see 57420, 57421)

57452 Colposcopy of the cervix including upper/adjacent vagina;
➲ *CPT Changes: An Insider's View* 2003
➲ *CPT Assistant* Apr 00:5, Feb 03:5, Jun 03:10

(Do not report 57452 in addition to 57454-57461)

Female Genital 56405-60699

Laparoscopic Revision of Prosthetic Vaginal Graft
57426

Location of prosthetic vaginal graft

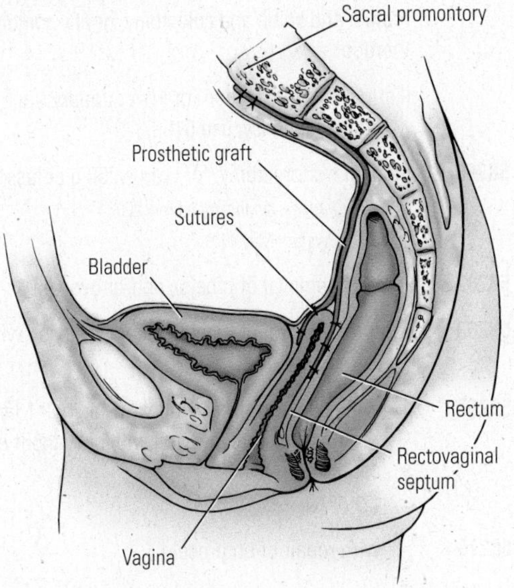

57454 with biopsy(s) of the cervix and endocervical curettage
➲ *CPT Changes: An Insider's View* 2003
➲ *CPT Assistant* Apr 00:5, Feb 03:5, Jun 03:10, Aug 11:9

57455 with biopsy(s) of the cervix
➲ *CPT Changes: An Insider's View* 2003
➲ *CPT Assistant* Apr 00:5, Feb 03:5, Jun 03:10

57456 with endocervical curettage
➲ *CPT Changes: An Insider's View* 2003
➲ *CPT Assistant* Apr 00:5, Jan 03:23, Feb 03:5, Jun 03:10

57460 with loop electrode biopsy(s) of the cervix
➲ *CPT Changes: An Insider's View* 2003
➲ *CPT Assistant* Apr 00:5, Jan 03:23, Feb 03:5, Jun 03:10, Jul 05:15

57461 with loop electrode conization of the cervix
➲ *CPT Changes: An Insider's View* 2003
➲ *CPT Assistant* Jan 03:23, Feb 03:5, Jun 03:10, Dec 06:15

(Do not report 57461 in addition to 57456)

(For endometrial sampling [biopsy] performed in conjunction with colposcopy, use 58110)

Excision

(For radical surgical procedures, see 58200-58240)

57500 Biopsy of cervix, single or multiple, or local excision of lesion, with or without fulguration (separate procedure)
➲ *CPT Changes: An Insider's View* 2008

57505 Endocervical curettage (not done as part of a dilation and curettage)
➲ *CPT Assistant* Jul 05:15

57510 Cautery of cervix; electro or thermal
➲ *CPT Changes: An Insider's View* 2002

57511 cryocautery, initial or repeat

57513 laser ablation

57520 Conization of cervix, with or without fulguration, with or without dilation and curettage, with or without repair; cold knife or laser
➲ *CPT Assistant* Apr 00:5

(See also 58120)

57522 loop electrode excision
➲ *CPT Assistant* Apr 00:5, Mar 03:22, Jul 03:15

57530 Trachelectomy (cervicectomy), amputation of cervix (separate procedure)

57531 Radical trachelectomy, with bilateral total pelvic lymphadenectomy and para-aortic lymph node sampling biopsy, with or without removal of tube(s), with or without removal of ovary(s)
➲ *CPT Assistant* Nov 97:21

(For radical abdominal hysterectomy, use 58210)

57540 Excision of cervical stump, abdominal approach;

57545 with pelvic floor repair

57550 Excision of cervical stump, vaginal approach;

57555 with anterior and/or posterior repair

57556 with repair of enterocele

(For insertion of intrauterine device, use 58300)

(For insertion of any hemostatic agent or pack for control of spontaneous non-obstetrical hemorrhage, see 57180)

57558 Dilation and curettage of cervical stump
➲ *CPT Changes: An Insider's View* 2007

Repair

57700 Cerclage of uterine cervix, nonobstetrical

57720 Trachelorrhaphy, plastic repair of uterine cervix, vaginal approach

Manipulation

57800 Dilation of cervical canal, instrumental (separate procedure)

Corpus Uteri

Excision

58100 Endometrial sampling (biopsy) with or without endocervical sampling (biopsy), without cervical dilation, any method (separate procedure)

(For endocervical curettage only, use 57505)

(For endometrial sampling [biopsy] performed in conjunction with colposcopy [57420, 57421, 57452-57461], use 58110)

+ 58110 Endometrial sampling (biopsy) performed in conjunction with colposcopy (List separately in addition to code for primary procedure)

➔ *CPT Changes: An Insider's View* 2006

➔ *CPT Assistant* Jun 06:17

(Use 58110 in conjunction with 57420, 57421, 57452-57461)

58120 Dilation and curettage, diagnostic and/or therapeutic (nonobstetrical)

➔ *CPT Assistant* Fall 95:16, Nov 97:21, May 03:19

(For postpartum hemorrhage, use 59160)

58140 Myomectomy, excision of fibroid tumor(s) of uterus, 1 to 4 intramural myoma(s) with total weight of 250 g or less and/or removal of surface myomas; abdominal approach

➔ *CPT Changes: An Insider's View* 2002, 2003

➔ *CPT Assistant* Feb 03:15, Jun 03:5

58145 vaginal approach

58146 Myomectomy, excision of fibroid tumor(s) of uterus, 5 or more intramural myomas and/or intramural myomas with total weight greater than 250 g, abdominal approach

➔ *CPT Changes: An Insider's View* 2003

➔ *CPT Assistant* Feb 03:15, Jun 03:5

(Do not report 58146 in addition to 58140-58145, 58150-58240)

Hysterectomy Procedures

58150 Total abdominal hysterectomy (corpus and cervix), with or without removal of tube(s), with or without removal of ovary(s);

➔ *CPT Assistant* Dec 96:10, Apr 97:3, Nov 97:21, Sep 00:9, Aug 01:11

58152 with colpo-urethrocystopexy (eg, Marshall-Marchetti-Krantz, Burch)

➔ *CPT Assistant* Jan 97:1, Nov 97:22, Jun 10:6

(For urethrocystopexy without hysterectomy, see 51840, 51841)

58180 Supracervical abdominal hysterectomy (subtotal hysterectomy), with or without removal of tube(s), with or without removal of ovary(s)

58200 Total abdominal hysterectomy, including partial vaginectomy, with para-aortic and pelvic lymph node sampling, with or without removal of tube(s), with or without removal of ovary(s)

58210 Radical abdominal hysterectomy, with bilateral total pelvic lymphadenectomy and para-aortic lymph node sampling (biopsy), with or without removal of tube(s), with or without removal of ovary(s)

➔ *CPT Assistant* Fall 92:21, May 12:14

(For radical hysterectomy with ovarian transposition, use also 58825)

58240 Pelvic exenteration for gynecologic malignancy, with total abdominal hysterectomy or cervicectomy, with or without removal of tube(s), with or without removal of ovary(s), with removal of bladder and ureteral transplantations, and/or abdominoperineal resection of rectum and colon and colostomy, or any combination thereof

(For pelvic exenteration for lower urinary tract or male genital malignancy, use 51597)

58260 Vaginal hysterectomy, for uterus 250 g or less;

➔ *CPT Changes: An Insider's View* 2003

➔ *CPT Assistant* May 11:9

58262 with removal of tube(s), and/or ovary(s)

58263 with removal of tube(s), and/or ovary(s), with repair of enterocele

58267 with colpo-urethrocystopexy (Marshall-Marchetti-Krantz type, Pereyra type) with or without endoscopic control

➔ *CPT Assistant* Jun 10:6

58270 with repair of enterocele

(For repair of enterocele with removal of tubes and/or ovaries, use 58263)

58275 Vaginal hysterectomy, with total or partial vaginectomy;

➔ *CPT Changes: An Insider's View* 2002

58280 with repair of enterocele

58285 Vaginal hysterectomy, radical (Schauta type operation)

➔ *CPT Assistant* Nov 07:1

58290 Vaginal hysterectomy, for uterus greater than 250 g;

➔ *CPT Changes: An Insider's View* 2003

58291 with removal of tube(s) and/or ovary(s)

➔ *CPT Changes: An Insider's View* 2003

58292 with removal of tube(s) and/or ovary(s), with repair of enterocele

➔ *CPT Changes: An Insider's View* 2003

58293 with colpo-urethrocystopexy (Marshall-Marchetti-Krantz type, Pereyra type) with or without endoscopic control

➔ *CPT Changes: An Insider's View* 2003

58294 with repair of enterocele

➔ *CPT Changes: An Insider's View* 2003

Introduction

(To report insertion of non-biodegradable drug delivery implant for contraception, use 11981. To report removal of implantable contraceptive capsules with subsequent insertion of non-biodegradable drug delivery implant, use 11976 and 11981)

58300 Insertion of intrauterine device (IUD)

➔ *CPT Assistant* Apr 98:14

58301 Removal of intrauterine device (IUD)

➔ *CPT Assistant* Apr 98:14

58321 Artificial insemination; intra-cervical

58322 intra-uterine

58323 Sperm washing for artificial insemination
➲ *CPT Assistant* Jan 98:6

58340 Catheterization and introduction of saline or contrast material for saline infusion sonohysterography (SIS) or hysterosalpingography
➲ *CPT Changes: An Insider's View* 2004
➲ *CPT Assistant* Nov 97:22, Jul 99:8, Mar 09:11

(For radiological supervision and interpretation of saline infusion sonohysterography, use 76831)

(For radiological supervision and interpretation of hysterosalpingography, use 74740)

58345 Transcervical introduction of fallopian tube catheter for diagnosis and/or re-establishing patency (any method), with or without hysterosalpingography
➲ *CPT Assistant* Nov 97:22, Mar 09:11

(For radiological supervision and interpretation, use 74742)

58346 Insertion of Heyman capsules for clinical brachytherapy
➲ *CPT Changes: An Insider's View* 2002
➲ *CPT Assistant* Feb 02:8, Apr 09:3

(For placement of needles or catheters into pelvic organs and/or genitalia [except prostate] for interstitial radioelement application, use 55920)

(For insertion of radioelement sources or ribbons, see 77761-77763, 77770, 77771, 77772)

58350 Chromotubation of oviduct, including materials
➲ *CPT Assistant* May 02:19, Dec 08:7

(To report the supply of any materials, use 99070)

58353 Endometrial ablation, thermal, without hysteroscopic guidance
➲ *CPT Changes: An Insider's View* 2001
➲ *CPT Assistant* Mar 02:11, Apr 02:19

(For hysteroscopic procedure, use 58563)

58356 Endometrial cryoablation with ultrasonic guidance, including endometrial curettage, when performed
➲ *CPT Changes: An Insider's View* 2005

(Do not report 58356 in conjunction with 58100, 58120, 58340, 76700, 76856)

Repair

58400 Uterine suspension, with or without shortening of round ligaments, with or without shortening of sacrouterine ligaments; (separate procedure)

58410 with presacral sympathectomy
➲ *CPT Assistant* Mar 07:9

(For anastomosis of tubes to uterus, use 58752)

58520 Hysterorrhaphy, repair of ruptured uterus (nonobstetrical)

58540 Hysteroplasty, repair of uterine anomaly (Strassman type)

(For closure of vesicouterine fistula, use 51920)

Laparoscopy/Hysteroscopy

Surgical laparoscopy always includes diagnostic laparoscopy. To report a diagnostic laparoscopy (peritoneoscopy) (separate procedure), use 49320. To report a diagnostic hysteroscopy (separate procedure), use 58555.

58674 Laparoscopy, surgical, ablation of uterine fibroid(s) including intraoperative ultrasound guidance and monitoring, radiofrequency
➲ *CPT Changes: An Insider's View* 2017
➲ *CPT Assistant* Feb 17:14, Apr 17:7

(Do not report 58674 in conjunction with 49320, 58541-58554, 58570, 58571, 58572, 58573, 76998)

58541 Laparoscopy, surgical, supracervical hysterectomy, for uterus 250 g or less;
➲ *CPT Changes: An Insider's View* 2007
➲ *CPT Assistant* Nov 07:1, Apr 17:7

58542 with removal of tube(s) and/or ovary(s)
➲ *CPT Changes: An Insider's View* 2007
➲ *CPT Assistant* Nov 07:1, Apr 17:7

(Do not report 58541, 58542 in conjunction with 49320, 57000, 57180, 57410, 58140-58146, 58545, 58546, 58561, 58661, 58670, 58671)

58543 Laparoscopy, surgical, supracervical hysterectomy, for uterus greater than 250 g;
➲ *CPT Changes: An Insider's View* 2007
➲ *CPT Assistant* Nov 07:1, Apr 17:7

58544 with removal of tube(s) and/or ovary(s)
➲ *CPT Changes: An Insider's View* 2007
➲ *CPT Assistant* Nov 07:1

(Do not report 58543-58544 in conjunction with 49320, 57000, 57180, 57410, 58140-58146, 58545, 58546, 58561, 58661, 58670, 58671)

58545 Laparoscopy, surgical, myomectomy, excision; 1 to 4 intramural myomas with total weight of 250 g or less and/or removal of surface myomas
➲ *CPT Changes: An Insider's View* 2003
➲ *CPT Assistant* Jun 03:5, 12

58546 5 or more intramural myomas and/or intramural myomas with total weight greater than 250 g
➲ *CPT Changes: An Insider's View* 2003
➲ *CPT Assistant* Jun 03:12, Jan 04:26, Apr 17:7

58548 Laparoscopy, surgical, with radical hysterectomy, with bilateral total pelvic lymphadenectomy and para-aortic lymph node sampling (biopsy), with removal of tube(s) and ovary(s), if performed
➲ *CPT Changes: An Insider's View* 2007
➲ *CPT Assistant* Nov 07:1, Sep 15:12, Apr 17:7

(Do not report 58548 in conjunction with 38570-38572, 58210, 58285, 58550-58554)

58550 Laparoscopy, surgical, with vaginal hysterectomy, for uterus 250 g or less;
- *CPT Changes: An Insider's View* 2000, 2003
- *CPT Assistant* Nov 99:28, Mar 00:9, Apr 17:7

58552 with removal of tube(s) and/or ovary(s)
- *CPT Changes: An Insider's View* 2003
- *CPT Assistant* Nov 07:1, Apr 17:7

(Do not report 58550-58552 in conjunction with 49320, 57000, 57180, 57410, 58140-58146, 58545, 58546, 58561, 58661, 58670, 58671)

58553 Laparoscopy, surgical, with vaginal hysterectomy, for uterus greater than 250 g;
- *CPT Changes: An Insider's View* 2003
- *CPT Assistant* Apr 17:7

58554 with removal of tube(s) and/or ovary(s)
- *CPT Changes: An Insider's View* 2003
- *CPT Assistant* Apr 17:7

(Do not report 58553-58554 in conjunction with 49320, 57000, 57180, 57410, 58140-58146, 58545, 58546, 58561, 58661, 58670, 58671)

58555 Hysteroscopy, diagnostic (separate procedure)
- *CPT Changes: An Insider's View* 2000
- *CPT Assistant* Nov 99:28, Mar 00:10

58558 Hysteroscopy, surgical; with sampling (biopsy) of endometrium and/or polypectomy, with or without D & C
- *CPT Changes: An Insider's View* 2000
- *CPT Assistant* Nov 99:28, Mar 00:10, Sep 02:10, Jan 03:7, May 03:19

58559 with lysis of intrauterine adhesions (any method)
- *CPT Changes: An Insider's View* 2000
- *CPT Assistant* Nov 99:28, Mar 00:10

58560 with division or resection of intrauterine septum (any method)
- *CPT Changes: An Insider's View* 2000
- *CPT Assistant* Nov 99:28, Mar 00:10

58561 with removal of leiomyomata
- *CPT Changes: An Insider's View* 2000
- *CPT Assistant* Nov 99:28, Mar 00:10, Jan 03:7

58562 with removal of impacted foreign body
- *CPT Changes: An Insider's View* 2000
- *CPT Assistant* Nov 99:28, Mar 00:10

58563 with endometrial ablation (eg, endometrial resection, electrosurgical ablation, thermoablation)
- *CPT Changes: An Insider's View* 2000, 2002
- *CPT Assistant* Nov 99:28, Mar 00:10, Mar 02:11, Apr 02:19, Jan 03:7, Feb 12:11, Jan 15:14

58565 with bilateral fallopian tube cannulation to induce occlusion by placement of permanent implants
- *CPT Changes: An Insider's View* 2005
- *CPT Assistant* Jan 11:9, Feb 12:11

Hysteroscopy
58563

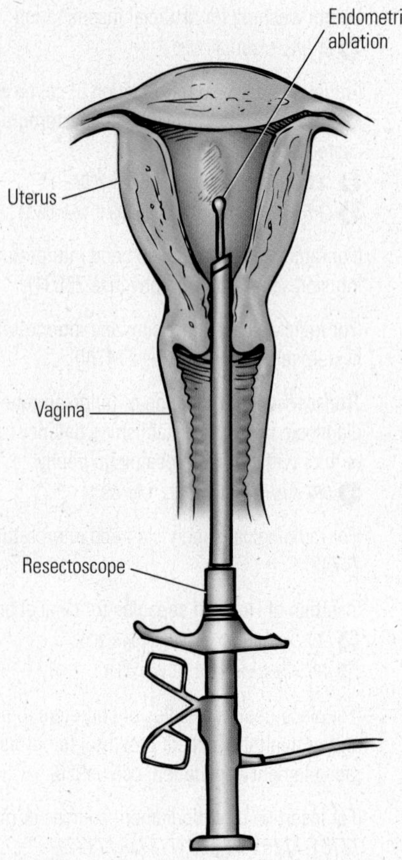

(Do not report 58565 in conjunction with 58555 or 57800)

(For unilateral procedure, use modifier 52)

58570 Laparoscopy, surgical, with total hysterectomy, for uterus 250 g or less;
- *CPT Changes: An Insider's View* 2008
- *CPT Assistant* Apr 17:7

58571 with removal of tube(s) and/or ovary(s)
- *CPT Changes: An Insider's View* 2008
- *CPT Assistant* May 12:14, Aug 12:13, Apr 17:7, Feb 18:11

58572 Laparoscopy, surgical, with total hysterectomy, for uterus greater than 250 g;
- *CPT Changes: An Insider's View* 2008
- *CPT Assistant* Apr 17:7

58573 with removal of tube(s) and/or ovary(s)
- *CPT Changes: An Insider's View* 2008
- *CPT Assistant* May 12:14, Aug 12:13, Apr 17:7, Feb 18:11, Apr 18:11

(Do not report 58570-58573 in conjunction with 49320, 57000, 57180, 57410, 58140-58146, 58150, 58545, 58546, 58561, 58661, 58670, 58671)

58575 Laparoscopy, surgical, total hysterectomy for resection of malignancy (tumor debulking), with omentectomy including salpingo-oophorectomy, unilateral or bilateral, when performed
➲ *CPT Changes: An Insider's View* 2018

(Do not report 58575 in conjunction with 49255, 49320, 49321, 58570, 58571, 58572, 58573, 58661)

58578 Unlisted laparoscopy procedure, uterus
➲ *CPT Changes: An Insider's View* 2000
➲ *CPT Assistant* Nov 99:28, Mar 00:10, Mar 07:9

58579 Unlisted hysteroscopy procedure, uterus
➲ *CPT Changes: An Insider's View* 2000
➲ *CPT Assistant* Nov 99:28, Mar 00:10

Oviduct/Ovary

Incision

58600 Ligation or transection of fallopian tube(s), abdominal or vaginal approach, unilateral or bilateral
➲ *CPT Changes: An Insider's View* 2000
➲ *CPT Assistant* Nov 99:28

58605 Ligation or transection of fallopian tube(s), abdominal or vaginal approach, postpartum, unilateral or bilateral, during same hospitalization (separate procedure)
➲ *CPT Changes: An Insider's View* 2000
➲ *CPT Assistant* Nov 99:28

(For laparoscopic procedures, use 58670, 58671)

+ 58611 Ligation or transection of fallopian tube(s) when done at the time of cesarean delivery or intra-abdominal surgery (not a separate procedure) (List separately in addition to code for primary procedure)
➲ *CPT Changes: An Insider's View* 2002

58615 Occlusion of fallopian tube(s) by device (eg, band, clip, Falope ring) vaginal or suprapubic approach
➲ *CPT Changes: An Insider's View* 2000
➲ *CPT Assistant* Nov 99:28

(For laparoscopic approach, use 58671)

(For lysis of adnexal adhesions, use 58740)

Laparoscopy

Surgical laparoscopy always includes diagnostic laparoscopy. To report a diagnostic laparoscopy (peritoneoscopy) (separate procedure), use 49320.

58660 Laparoscopy, surgical; with lysis of adhesions (salpingolysis, ovariolysis) (separate procedure)
➲ *CPT Changes: An Insider's View* 2000
➲ *CPT Assistant* Nov 99:28, Mar 00:10, Mar 03:22, Dec 11:16

58661 with removal of adnexal structures (partial or total oophorectomy and/or salpingectomy)
➲ *CPT Changes: An Insider's View* 2000
➲ *CPT Assistant* Nov 99:28, Mar 00:10, Jan 02:11, Nov 07:1, May 10:10

58662 with fulguration or excision of lesions of the ovary, pelvic viscera, or peritoneal surface by any method
➲ *CPT Changes: An Insider's View* 2000
➲ *CPT Assistant* Nov 99:28, Mar 00:10, Dec 17:14

58670 with fulguration of oviducts (with or without transection)
➲ *CPT Changes: An Insider's View* 2000
➲ *CPT Assistant* Nov 99:29, Mar 00:10, Nov 07:2

58671 with occlusion of oviducts by device (eg, band, clip, or Falope ring)
➲ *CPT Changes: An Insider's View* 2000
➲ *CPT Assistant* Nov 99:29, Mar 00:10

58672 with fimbrioplasty
➲ *CPT Changes: An Insider's View* 2000
➲ *CPT Assistant* Nov 99:29, Mar 00:10

58673 with salpingostomy (salpingoneostomy)
➲ *CPT Changes: An Insider's View* 2000
➲ *CPT Assistant* Nov 99:29, Mar 00:10, May 02:19

(Codes 58672 and 58673 are used to report unilateral procedures. For bilateral procedure, use modifier 50)

58674 Code is out of numerical sequence. See 58520-58542

58679 Unlisted laparoscopy procedure, oviduct, ovary
➲ *CPT Changes: An Insider's View* 2000
➲ *CPT Assistant* Nov 99:29, Mar 00:10

(For laparoscopic aspiration of ovarian cyst, use 49322)

(For laparoscopic biopsy of the ovary or fallopian tube, use 49321)

Excision

58700 Salpingectomy, complete or partial, unilateral or bilateral (separate procedure)

58720 Salpingo-oophorectomy, complete or partial, unilateral or bilateral (separate procedure)
➲ *CPT Assistant* Sep 00:9, Jul 06:19

Repair

58740 Lysis of adhesions (salpingolysis, ovariolysis)
➲ *CPT Changes: An Insider's View* 2000
➲ *CPT Assistant* Sep 96:9, Nov 99:29

(For laparoscopic approach, use 58660)

(For excision or destruction of endometriomas, open method, see 49203-49205, 58957, 58958)

(For fulguration or excision of lesions, laparoscopic approach, use 58662)

58750 Tubotubal anastomosis

58752 Tubouterine implantation

58760 Fimbrioplasty
➲ *CPT Changes: An Insider's View* 2000
➲ *CPT Assistant* Nov 99:29

(For laparoscopic approach, use 58672)

58770 Salpingostomy (salpingoneostomy)
➲ *CPT Changes: An Insider's View* 2000
➲ *CPT Assistant* Nov 99:29

(For laparoscopic approach, use 58673)

Ovary

Incision

58800 Drainage of ovarian cyst(s), unilateral or bilateral (separate procedure); vaginal approach

58805 abdominal approach

58820 Drainage of ovarian abscess; vaginal approach, open
➲ *CPT Assistant* Nov 97:22

58822 abdominal approach
➲ *CPT Assistant* Nov 97:22

(For transrectal image-guided fluid collection drainage by catheter of pelvic abscess, use 49407)

58825 Transposition, ovary(s)

Excision

58900 Biopsy of ovary, unilateral or bilateral (separate procedure)
➲ *CPT Changes: An Insider's View* 2000
➲ *CPT Assistant* Nov 99:29

(For laparoscopic biopsy of the ovary or fallopian tube, use 49321)

58920 Wedge resection or bisection of ovary, unilateral or bilateral

58925 Ovarian cystectomy, unilateral or bilateral

58940 Oophorectomy, partial or total, unilateral or bilateral;
➲ *CPT Assistant* Mar 04:3

(For oophorectomy with concomitant debulking for ovarian malignancy, use 58952)

58943 for ovarian, tubal or primary peritoneal malignancy, with para-aortic and pelvic lymph node biopsies, peritoneal washings, peritoneal biopsies, diaphragmatic assessments, with or without salpingectomy(s), with or without omentectomy
➲ *CPT Changes: An Insider's View* 2001
➲ *CPT Assistant* Oct 10:16, Dec 10:16

58950 Resection (initial) of ovarian, tubal or primary peritoneal malignancy with bilateral salpingo-oophorectomy and omentectomy;
➲ *CPT Changes: An Insider's View* 2001, 2007
➲ *CPT Assistant* Oct 10:16, Dec 10:16

58951 with total abdominal hysterectomy, pelvic and limited para-aortic lymphadenectomy
➲ *CPT Assistant* Aug 01:11, Oct 10:16, Dec 10:16

58952 with radical dissection for debulking (ie, radical excision or destruction, intra-abdominal or retroperitoneal tumors)
➲ *CPT Changes: An Insider's View* 2001
➲ *CPT Assistant* Dec 96:10, Aug 01:11, Oct 10:16, Dec 10:16

(For resection of recurrent ovarian, tubal, primary peritoneal, or uterine malignancy, see 58957, 58958)

58953 Bilateral salpingo-oophorectomy with omentectomy, total abdominal hysterectomy and radical dissection for debulking;
➲ *CPT Changes: An Insider's View* 2002
➲ *CPT Assistant* Feb 02:8, Oct 10:16, Dec 10:16, May 14:10

58954 with pelvic lymphadenectomy and limited para-aortic lymphadenectomy
➲ *CPT Changes: An Insider's View* 2002
➲ *CPT Assistant* Feb 02:9, Oct 10:16, Dec 10:16

58956 Bilateral salpingo-oophorectomy with total omentectomy, total abdominal hysterectomy for malignancy
➲ *CPT Changes: An Insider's View* 2005
➲ *CPT Assistant* May 14:10

(Do not report 58956 in conjunction with 49255, 58150, 58180, 58262, 58263, 58550, 58661, 58700, 58720, 58900, 58925, 58940, 58957, 58958)

58957 Resection (tumor debulking) of recurrent ovarian, tubal, primary peritoneal, uterine malignancy (intra-abdominal, retroperitoneal tumors), with omentectomy, if performed;
➲ *CPT Changes: An Insider's View* 2007

58958 with pelvic lymphadenectomy and limited para-aortic lymphadenectomy
➲ *CPT Changes: An Insider's View* 2007

(Do not report 58957, 58958 in conjunction with 38770, 38780, 44005, 49000, 49203-49215, 49255, 58900-58960)

58960 Laparotomy, for staging or restaging of ovarian, tubal, or primary peritoneal malignancy (second look), with or without omentectomy, peritoneal washing, biopsy of abdominal and pelvic peritoneum, diaphragmatic assessment with pelvic and limited para-aortic lymphadenectomy
➲ *CPT Changes: An Insider's View* 2001

(Do not report 58960 in conjunction with 58957, 58958)

In Vitro Fertilization

58970 Follicle puncture for oocyte retrieval, any method

(For radiological supervision and interpretation, use 76948)

58974 Embryo transfer, intrauterine

58976 Gamete, zygote, or embryo intrafallopian transfer, any method
➲ *CPT Changes: An Insider's View* 2000
➲ *CPT Assistant* Nov 99:29

(For laparoscopic adnexal procedures, see 58660-58673)

Other Procedures

58999 Unlisted procedure, female genital system (nonobstetrical)
➔ *CPT Assistant* Apr 09:9, 10

Maternity Care and Delivery

The services normally provided in uncomplicated maternity cases include antepartum care, delivery, and postpartum care. Pregnancy confirmation during a problem oriented or preventive visit is not considered a part of antepartum care and should be reported using the appropriate E/M service codes 99201, 99202, 99203, 99204, 99205, 99211, 99212, 99213, 99214, 99215, 99241, 99242, 99243, 99244, 99245, 99281, 99282, 99283, 99284, 99285, 99384, 99385, 99386, 99394, 99395, 99396 for that visit.

Antepartum care includes the initial prenatal history and physical examination; subsequent prenatal history and physical examinations; recording of weight, blood pressures, fetal heart tones, routine chemical urinalysis, and monthly visits up to 28 weeks gestation; biweekly visits to 36 weeks gestation; and weekly visits until delivery. Any other visits or services within this time period should be coded separately.

Delivery services include admission to the hospital, the admission history and physical examination, management of uncomplicated labor, vaginal delivery (with or without episiotomy, with or without forceps), or cesarean delivery. When reporting delivery only services (59409, 59514, 59612, 59620), report inpatient postdelivery management and discharge services using Evaluation and Management Services codes (99217-99239). Delivery and postpartum services (59410, 59515, 59614, 59622) include delivery services and all inpatient and outpatient postpartum services. Medical complications of pregnancy (eg, cardiac problems, neurological problems, diabetes, hypertension, toxemia, hyperemesis, preterm labor, premature rupture of membranes, trauma) and medical problems complicating labor and delivery management may require additional resources and may be reported separately.

Postpartum care only services (59430) include office or other outpatient visits following vaginal or cesarean section delivery.

For surgical complications of pregnancy (eg, appendectomy, hernia, ovarian cyst, Bartholin cyst), see services in the **Surgery** section.

If all or part of the antepartum and/or postpartum patient care is provided except delivery due to termination of pregnancy by abortion or referral to another physician or other qualified health care professional for delivery, see the antepartum and postpartum care codes 59425, 59426, and 59430.

(For circumcision of newborn, see 54150, 54160)

Antepartum and Fetal Invasive Services

(For fetal intrauterine transfusion, use 36460)

(For unlisted fetal invasive procedure, use 59897)

59000 Amniocentesis; diagnostic
➔ *CPT Changes: An Insider's View* 2002
➔ *CPT Assistant* Apr 97:2, Feb 02:7, Aug 02:2, May 04:2

(For radiological supervision and interpretation, use 76946)

59001 therapeutic amniotic fluid reduction (includes ultrasound guidance)
➔ *CPT Changes: An Insider's View* 2002
➔ *CPT Assistant* Feb 02:7, Aug 02:2

Amniocentesis, Therapeutic Amniotic Fluid Reduction
59001

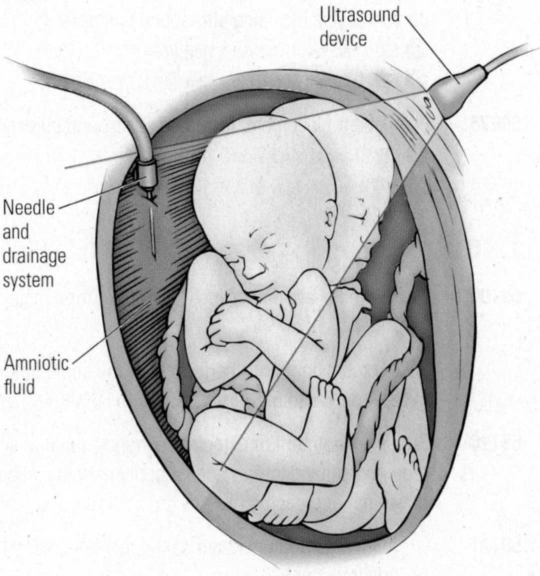

59012 Cordocentesis (intrauterine), any method
➔ *CPT Assistant* Aug 02:2

(For radiological supervision and interpretation, use 76941)

59015 Chorionic villus sampling, any method
➔ *CPT Assistant* Apr 97:2, Aug 02:2

(For radiological supervision and interpretation, use 76945)

59020 Fetal contraction stress test
➔ *CPT Assistant* Apr 97:2, Aug 02:2

59025 Fetal non-stress test
➔ *CPT Assistant* Apr 97:2, May 98:10, Oct 04:10, Dec 08:8

59030 Fetal scalp blood sampling
➲ *CPT Assistant* Aug 02:3

(For repeat fetal scalp blood sampling, use 59030 and see modifiers 76 and 77)

59050 Fetal monitoring during labor by consulting physician (ie, non-attending physician) with written report; supervision and interpretation
➲ *CPT Assistant* Nov 97:22

59051 interpretation only
➲ *CPT Assistant* Nov 97:22

59070 Transabdominal amnioinfusion, including ultrasound guidance
➲ *CPT Changes: An Insider's View* 2004
➲ *CPT Assistant* May 04:2, Jun 04:11

59072 Fetal umbilical cord occlusion, including ultrasound guidance
➲ *CPT Changes: An Insider's View* 2004
➲ *CPT Assistant* May 04:2, Jun 04:11

59074 Fetal fluid drainage (eg, vesicocentesis, thoracocentesis, paracentesis), including ultrasound guidance
➲ *CPT Changes: An Insider's View* 2004
➲ *CPT Assistant* May 04:2, 4, Jun 04:11, Dec 04:19

59076 Fetal shunt placement, including ultrasound guidance
➲ *CPT Changes: An Insider's View* 2004
➲ *CPT Assistant* May 04:2, 4, Jun 04:11, Dec 04:19

Excision

59100 Hysterotomy, abdominal (eg, for hydatidiform mole, abortion)

(When tubal ligation is performed at the same time as hysterotomy, use 58611 in addition to 59100)

59120 Surgical treatment of ectopic pregnancy; tubal or ovarian, requiring salpingectomy and/or oophorectomy, abdominal or vaginal approach

59121 tubal or ovarian, without salpingectomy and/or oophorectomy

59130 abdominal pregnancy

59135 interstitial, uterine pregnancy requiring total hysterectomy

59136 interstitial, uterine pregnancy with partial resection of uterus

59140 cervical, with evacuation

59150 Laparoscopic treatment of ectopic pregnancy; without salpingectomy and/or oophorectomy
➲ *CPT Assistant* Sep 96:9

59151 with salpingectomy and/or oophorectomy

59160 Curettage, postpartum
➲ *CPT Assistant* Nov 97:22, Sep 02:11

Laparoscopic Treatment of Ectopic Pregnancy
59150

The site of gestation is located with a laparoscope, and a small incision is made above the site. The ectopic pregnancy is then removed.

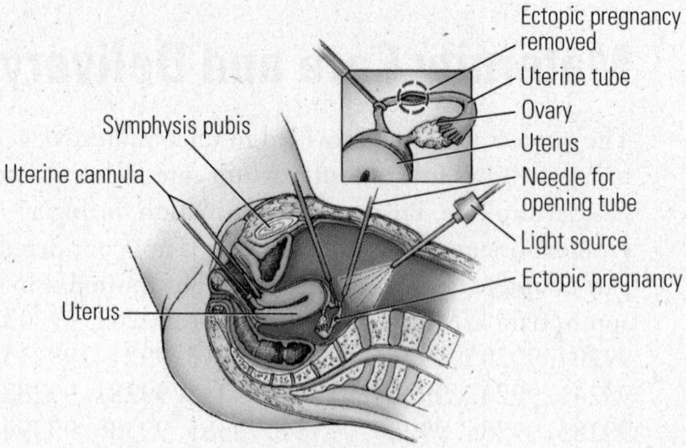

Introduction

(For intrauterine fetal transfusion, use 36460)

(For introduction of hypertonic solution and/or prostaglandins to initiate labor, see 59850-59857)

59200 Insertion of cervical dilator (eg, laminaria, prostaglandin) (separate procedure)
➲ *CPT Assistant* Fall 93:9, Apr 97:3, Jul 05:15, Dec 17:14

Repair

(For tracheloplasty, use 57700)

59300 Episiotomy or vaginal repair, by other than attending
➲ *CPT Changes: An Insider's View* 2013

59320 Cerclage of cervix, during pregnancy; vaginal
➲ *CPT Assistant* Aug 02:2, Nov 06:21, Feb 07:10

59325 abdominal
➲ *CPT Assistant* Aug 02:2, Nov 06:21, Feb 07:10

59350 Hysterorrhaphy of ruptured uterus
➲ *CPT Assistant* Aug 02:2

Vaginal Delivery, Antepartum and Postpartum Care

Coding Tip

Instructions for Reporting Antepartum and Postpartum Care

The services normally provided in uncomplicated maternity cases include antepartum care, delivery, and postpartum care.

CPT Coding Guidelines, Maternity Care and Delivery

59400 Routine obstetric care including antepartum care, vaginal delivery (with or without episiotomy, and/or forceps) and postpartum care
➔ *CPT Assistant* Feb 96:1, Mar 96:11, Feb 97:11, Apr 97:3, Apr 98:15, Jun 98:10, Aug 02:3, Feb 03:15

Vaginal Delivery
59400-59410

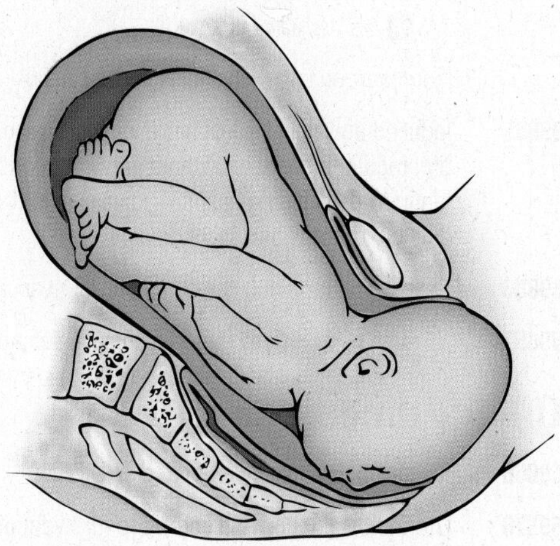

59409 Vaginal delivery only (with or without episiotomy and/or forceps);
➔ *CPT Assistant* Feb 96:1, Mar 96:11, Jul 96:11, Sep 96:4, Feb 97:11, Apr 97:1, Aug 02:3, Dec 07:13, Jun 09:10

59410 including postpartum care

59412 External cephalic version, with or without tocolysis
➔ *CPT Assistant* Fall 94:21, Feb 96:1, Aug 02:2-3

(Use 59412 in addition to code[s] for delivery)

59414 Delivery of placenta (separate procedure)
➔ *CPT Assistant* Jun 96:10, Jun 98:10, Aug 02:3

(For antepartum care only, see 59425, 59426 or appropriate E/M code[s])

(For 1-3 antepartum care visits, see appropriate E/M code[s])

59425 Antepartum care only; 4-6 visits
➔ *CPT Assistant* Fall 94:21, Apr 97:11, Aug 02:3

59426 7 or more visits
➔ *CPT Assistant* Fall 94:21, Apr 97:11, Aug 02:3

59430 Postpartum care only (separate procedure)
➔ *CPT Assistant* Jun 96:10, Aug 02:3

Cesarean Delivery

(For standby attendance for infant, use 99360)

(For low cervical cesarean section, see 59510, 59515, 59525)

Coding Tip

Instructions for Reporting Cesarean Delivery

Patients who have had a previous cesarean delivery and now present with the expectation of a vaginal delivery are coded using codes 59610-59622. If the patient has a successful vaginal delivery after a previous cesarean delivery (VBAC), use codes 59610-59614. If the attempt is unsuccessful and another cesarean delivery is carried out, use codes 59618-59622. To report elective cesarean deliveries, use code 59510, 59514 or 59515.

CPT Coding Guidelines, Maternity Care and Delivery, Delivery After Previous Cesarean Delivery

59510 Routine obstetric care including antepartum care, cesarean delivery, and postpartum care
➔ *CPT Assistant* Jul 96:11, Sep 96:4, Oct 96:10, Feb 97:11, Apr 97:2, Aug 02:3, Mar 13:13

59514 Cesarean delivery only;
➔ *CPT Assistant* Oct 96:10, Feb 97:11, Mar 13:13

59515 including postpartum care
➔ *CPT Assistant* Mar 13:13

(For classic cesarean section, see 59510, 59515, 59525)

+ 59525 Subtotal or total hysterectomy after cesarean delivery (List separately in addition to code for primary procedure)

(Use 59525 in conjunction with 59510, 59514, 59515, 59618, 59620, 59622)

Cesarean Delivery
59510-59515

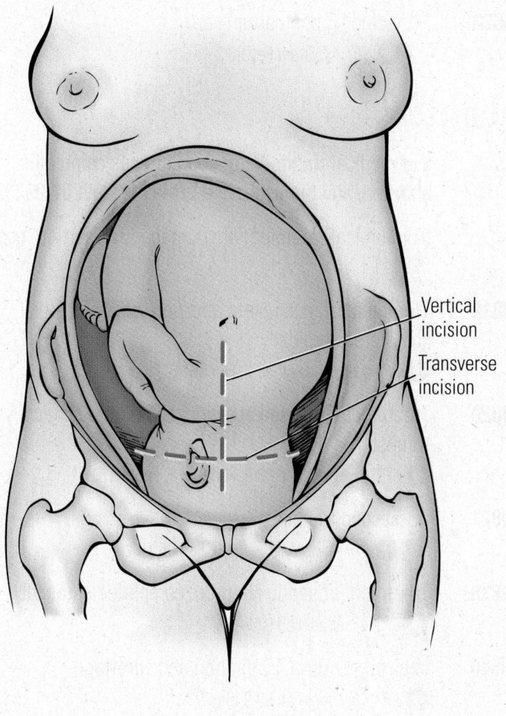

(For extraperitoneal cesarean section, or cesarean section with subtotal or total hysterectomy, see 59510, 59515, 59525)

Delivery After Previous Cesarean Delivery

Patients who have had a previous cesarean delivery and now present with the expectation of a vaginal delivery are coded using codes 59610-59622. If the patient has a successful vaginal delivery after a previous cesarean delivery (VBAC), use codes 59610-59614. If the attempt is unsuccessful and another cesarean delivery is carried out, use codes 59618-59622. To report elective cesarean deliveries use code 59510, 59514 or 59515.

59610 Routine obstetric care including antepartum care, vaginal delivery (with or without episiotomy, and/or forceps) and postpartum care, after previous cesarean delivery
➲ *CPT Assistant* Feb 96:2, Apr 97:3, Aug 02:3

59612 Vaginal delivery only, after previous cesarean delivery (with or without episiotomy and/or forceps);
➲ *CPT Assistant* Feb 96:2, Aug 02:3

59614 including postpartum care
➲ *CPT Assistant* Feb 96:2

59618 Routine obstetric care including antepartum care, cesarean delivery, and postpartum care, following attempted vaginal delivery after previous cesarean delivery
➲ *CPT Assistant* Feb 96:2, Aug 02:4

59620 Cesarean delivery only, following attempted vaginal delivery after previous cesarean delivery;
➲ *CPT Assistant* Feb 96:2

59622 including postpartum care
➲ *CPT Assistant* Feb 96:2

Abortion

(For medical treatment of spontaneous complete abortion, any trimester, use E/M codes 99201-99233)

(For surgical treatment of spontaneous abortion, use 59812)

59812 Treatment of incomplete abortion, any trimester, completed surgically
➲ *CPT Assistant* Fall 93:9, Fall 95:16

59820 Treatment of missed abortion, completed surgically; first trimester
➲ *CPT Assistant* Fall 93:9, Fall 95:16, Feb 99:10

59821 second trimester
➲ *CPT Assistant* Fall 93:9, Fall 95:16

59830 Treatment of septic abortion, completed surgically
➲ *CPT Assistant* Fall 93:9

59840 Induced abortion, by dilation and curettage
➲ *CPT Assistant* Fall 93:9, Sep 03:16

59841 Induced abortion, by dilation and evacuation
➲ *CPT Assistant* Fall 93:9

59850 Induced abortion, by 1 or more intra-amniotic injections (amniocentesis-injections), including hospital admission and visits, delivery of fetus and secundines;
➲ *CPT Assistant* Fall 93:10

59851 with dilation and curettage and/or evacuation
➲ *CPT Assistant* Fall 93:10

59852 with hysterotomy (failed intra-amniotic injection)
➲ *CPT Assistant* Fall 93:10

(For insertion of cervical dilator, use 59200)

59855 Induced abortion, by 1 or more vaginal suppositories (eg, prostaglandin) with or without cervical dilation (eg, laminaria), including hospital admission and visits, delivery of fetus and secundines;

59856 with dilation and curettage and/or evacuation

59857 with hysterotomy (failed medical evacuation)

Other Procedures

59866 Multifetal pregnancy reduction(s) (MPR)

59870 Uterine evacuation and curettage for hydatidiform mole
➲ *CPT Assistant* Feb 99:10

59871 Removal of cerclage suture under anesthesia (other than local)
➲ *CPT Assistant* Nov 97:22, Nov 06:21, Feb 07:10

59897 Unlisted fetal invasive procedure, including ultrasound guidance, when performed
➲ *CPT Changes: An Insider's View* 2004, 2010
➲ *CPT Assistant* May 04:5

59898 Unlisted laparoscopy procedure, maternity care and delivery
➲ *CPT Changes: An Insider's View* 2000
➲ *CPT Assistant* Nov 99:29, Mar 00:10

59899 Unlisted procedure, maternity care and delivery
➲ *CPT Assistant* Jun 97:10, May 04:2, Oct 13:3

Endocrine System

(For pituitary and pineal surgery, see **Nervous System**)

Thyroid Gland

Incision

60000 Incision and drainage of thyroglossal duct cyst, infected
➲ *CPT Changes: An Insider's View* 2002

Excision

60100 Biopsy thyroid, percutaneous core needle
➲ *CPT Assistant* Jun 97:5, Jun 07:10
➲ *Clinical Examples in Radiology* Winter 17:5

(If imaging guidance is performed, see 76942, 77002, 77012, 77021)

►(For fine needle aspiration biopsy, see 10004, 10005, 10006, 10007, 10008, 10009, 10010, 10011, 10012, 10021)◄

(For evaluation of fine needle aspirate, see 88172, 88173)

60200 Excision of cyst or adenoma of thyroid, or transection of isthmus
CPT Assistant Aug 11:10, Dec 12:3

60210 Partial thyroid lobectomy, unilateral; with or without isthmusectomy
CPT Assistant Winter 94:7, Aug 11:9, Dec 12:3

60212 with contralateral subtotal lobectomy, including isthmusectomy
CPT Assistant Dec 12:3

60220 Total thyroid lobectomy, unilateral; with or without isthmusectomy
CPT Assistant Oct 10:13, Dec 10:13, Aug 11:10, Dec 12:3

Thyroid Lobectomy
60220

The thyroid is exposed via a transverse cervical incision. The superior and inferior thyroid vessels serving the lobe are ligated, the isthmus is severed, and the entire thyroid lobe is resected.

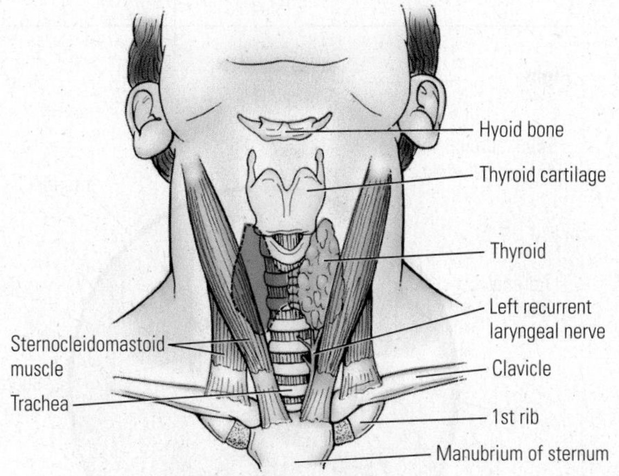

60225 with contralateral subtotal lobectomy, including isthmusectomy
CPT Assistant Dec 12:3

60240 Thyroidectomy, total or complete
CPT Assistant Dec 12:3

(For thyroidectomy, subtotal or partial, use 60271)

60252 Thyroidectomy, total or subtotal for malignancy; with limited neck dissection
CPT Assistant Nov 00:10, Dec 12:3

60254 with radical neck dissection
CPT Assistant Nov 00:10, Dec 12:3

60260 Thyroidectomy, removal of all remaining thyroid tissue following previous removal of a portion of thyroid
CPT Assistant Oct 10:13, Dec 10:13, Dec 12:3

(For bilateral procedure, report 60260 with modifier 50)

60270 Thyroidectomy, including substernal thyroid; sternal split or transthoracic approach
CPT Changes: An Insider's View 2002
CPT Assistant Dec 12:3

60271 cervical approach
CPT Assistant Dec 12:3

60280 Excision of thyroglossal duct cyst or sinus;

60281 recurrent

(For thyroid ultrasonography, use 76536)

Removal

60300 Aspiration and/or injection, thyroid cyst
CPT Changes: An Insider's View 2008

►(For fine needle aspiration biopsy, see 10004, 10005, 10006, 10007, 10008, 10009, 10010, 10011, 10012, 10021)◄

(If imaging guidance is performed, see 76942, 77012)

Parathyroid, Thymus, Adrenal Glands, Pancreas, and Carotid Body

Excision

(For pituitary and pineal surgery, see **Nervous System**)

60500 Parathyroidectomy or exploration of parathyroid(s);
CPT Assistant Dec 12:3

60502 re-exploration
CPT Assistant Dec 12:3

60505 with mediastinal exploration, sternal split or transthoracic approach
CPT Assistant Dec 12:3

+ **60512** Parathyroid autotransplantation (List separately in addition to code for primary procedure)
CPT Assistant Aug 11:9, Dec 12:3, Jan 17:7

(Use 60512 in conjunction with 60500, 60502, 60505, 60212, 60225, 60240, 60252, 60254, 60260, 60270, 60271)

60520 Thymectomy, partial or total; transcervical approach (separate procedure)

60521 sternal split or transthoracic approach, without radical mediastinal dissection (separate procedure)
CPT Assistant Dec 07:12

60522 sternal split or transthoracic approach, with radical mediastinal dissection (separate procedure)

(For thoracoscopic [VATS] thymectomy, see 32673)

Female Genital 56405-60699

Posterior View of the Pharynx
60512

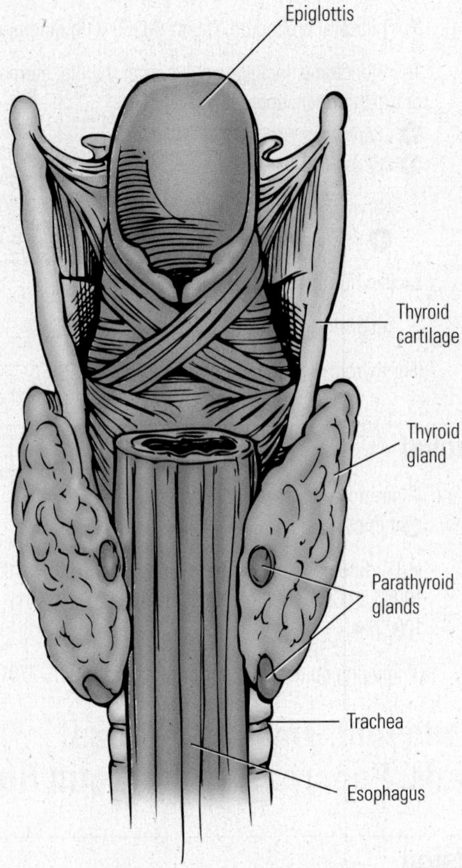

60540 Adrenalectomy, partial or complete, or exploration of adrenal gland with or without biopsy, transabdominal, lumbar or dorsal (separate procedure);
CPT Assistant Nov 98:17

60545 with excision of adjacent retroperitoneal tumor
CPT Assistant Nov 98:17

(Do not report 60540, 60545 in conjunction with 50323)

(For bilateral procedure, report 60540 with modifier 50)

(For excision of remote or disseminated pheochromocytoma, see 49203-49205)

(For laparoscopic approach, use 60650)

60600 Excision of carotid body tumor; without excision of carotid artery

60605 with excision of carotid artery

Laparoscopy

Surgical laparoscopy always includes diagnostic laparoscopy. To report a diagnostic laparoscopy (peritoneoscopy) (separate procedure), use 49320.

60650 Laparoscopy, surgical, with adrenalectomy, partial or complete, or exploration of adrenal gland with or without biopsy, transabdominal, lumbar or dorsal
CPT Changes: An Insider's View 2000
CPT Assistant Nov 99:30, Mar 00:10, Nov 01:8

Laparoscopic Adrenalectomy
60650

An adrenal gland is dissected and removed under laparoscopic guidance. Multiple small blood vessels from the vena cava and the aorta do not follow standard anatomic pattern, requiring intricate dissection.

Left

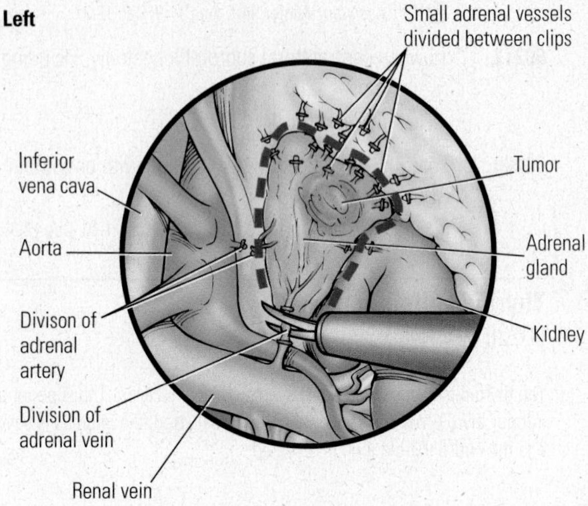

Right

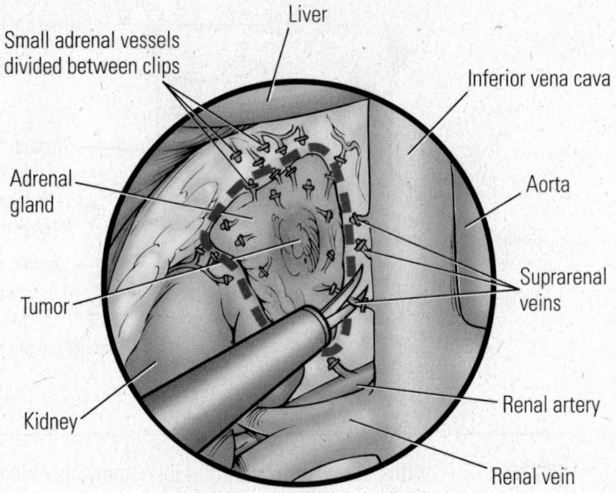

60659 Unlisted laparoscopy procedure, endocrine system
CPT Changes: An Insider's View 2000
CPT Assistant Nov 99:30, Mar 00:10

Other Procedures

60699 Unlisted procedure, endocrine system
CPT Assistant Feb 06:16, Dec 07:12

Notes

Notes

Surgery

Nervous System (61000-64999) 412

The following is a listing of headings and subheadings that appear within the Nervous System section of the CPT codebook. The subheadings or subsections denoted with asterisks (*) below have special instructions unique to that subsection. Where these are indicated, special notes or guidelines will be presented preceding those procedural terminology listings, referring to that subsection specifically.

Skull, Meninges, and Brain (61000-62258) 412
Injection, Drainage, or Aspiration (61000-61070) 412
Twist Drill, Burr Hole(s), or Trephine (61105-61253) 412
Craniectomy or Craniotomy (61304-61576) 412
Surgery of Skull Base* (61580-61619) 414
Approach Procedures (61580-61598) 415
Anterior Cranial Fossa (61580-61586) 415
Middle Cranial Fossa (61590-61592) 415
Posterior Cranial Fossa (61595-61598) 415
Definitive Procedures (61600-61616) 415
Base of Anterior Cranial Fossa (61600-61601) 415
Base of Middle Cranial Fossa (61605-61613) 415
Base of Posterior Cranial Fossa (61615-61616) 416
Repair and/or Reconstruction of Surgical Defects of Skull Base (61618-61619) 416
Endovascular Therapy (61623-61651) 416
Surgery for Aneurysm, Arteriovenous Malformation, or Vascular Disease* (61680-61711) 418
Stereotaxis (61720-61791) 418
Stereotactic Radiosurgery (Cranial)* (61796-61800) 419
Neurostimulators (Intracranial)* (61850-61888) 420
Repair (62000-62148) 421
Neuroendoscopy* (62160-62165) 421
Cerebrospinal Fluid (CSF) Shunt (62180-62258) 421

Spine and Spinal Cord (62263-63746) 422
Injection, Drainage, or Aspiration* (62263-62327) 422
Catheter Implantation (62350-62355) 425
Reservoir/Pump Implantation (62360-62370) 426
Endoscopic Decompression of Neural Elements and/or Excision of Herniated Intervertebral Discs* (62380) 426
Posterior Extradural Laminotomy or Laminectomy for Exploration/ Decompression of Neural Elements or Excision of Herniated Intervertebral Discs* (63001-63051) 427
Transpedicular or Costovertebral Approach for Posterolateral Extradural Exploration/Decompression (63055-63066) 428
Anterior or Anterolateral Approach for Extradural Exploration/Decompression* (63075-63091) 429
Lateral Extracavitary Approach for Extradural Exploration/Decompression* (63101-63103) 430
Incision (63170-63200) 430
Excision by Laminectomy of Lesion Other Than Herniated Disc (63250-63295) 430
Excision, Anterior or Anterolateral Approach, Intraspinal Lesion* (63300-63308) 431
Stereotaxis (63600-63610) 431
Stereotactic Radiosurgery (Spinal)* (63620-63621) 431
Neurostimulators (Spinal)* (63650-63688) 432
Repair (63700-63710) 433
Shunt, Spinal CSF (63740-63746) 433

Extracranial Nerves, Peripheral Nerves, and Autonomic Nervous System (64400-64999) 434
Introduction/Injection of Anesthetic Agent (Nerve Block), Diagnostic or Therapeutic (64400-64530) 434
Somatic Nerves (64400-64489) 434
Paravertebral Spinal Nerves and Branches (64490-64495) 435
Autonomic Nerves (64505-64530) 436
Neurostimulators (Peripheral Nerve)* (64553-64595) 436
Destruction by Neurolytic Agent (eg, Chemical, Thermal, Electrical or Radiofrequency), Chemodenervation* (64600-64681) 438

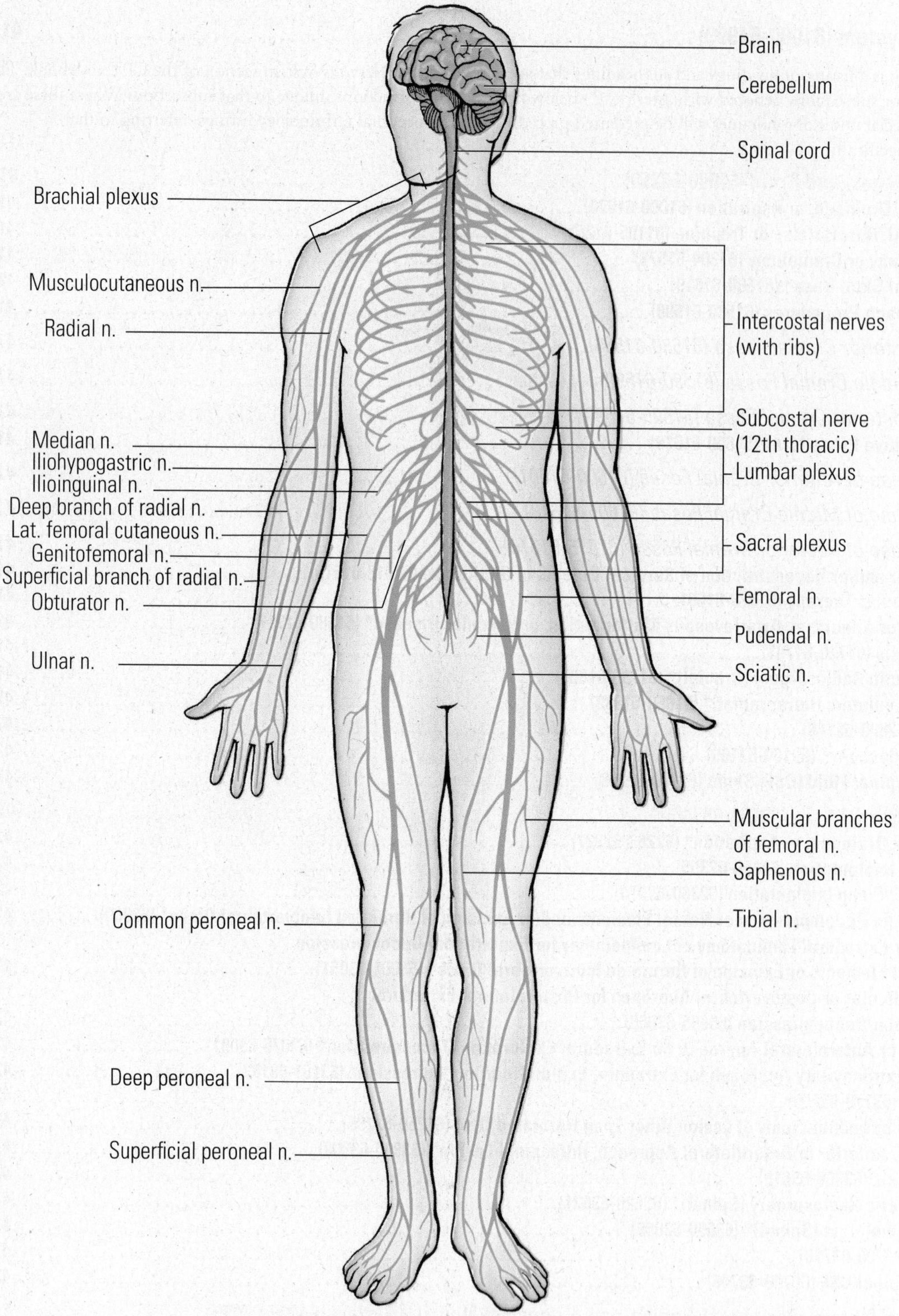

Nervous System

Somatic Nerves (64600-64647)....................438
Sympathetic Nerves (64650-64681)....................440
Neuroplasty (Exploration, Neurolysis or Nerve Decompression)* (64702-64727)....................440
Transection or Avulsion (64732-64772)....................441
Excision (64774-64823)....................441
Somatic Nerves (64774-64795)....................441
Sympathetic Nerves (64802-64823)....................442
Neurorrhaphy (64831-64876)....................442
Neurorrhaphy With Nerve Graft, Vein Graft, or Conduit (64885-64913)....................442
Other Procedures (64999)....................443

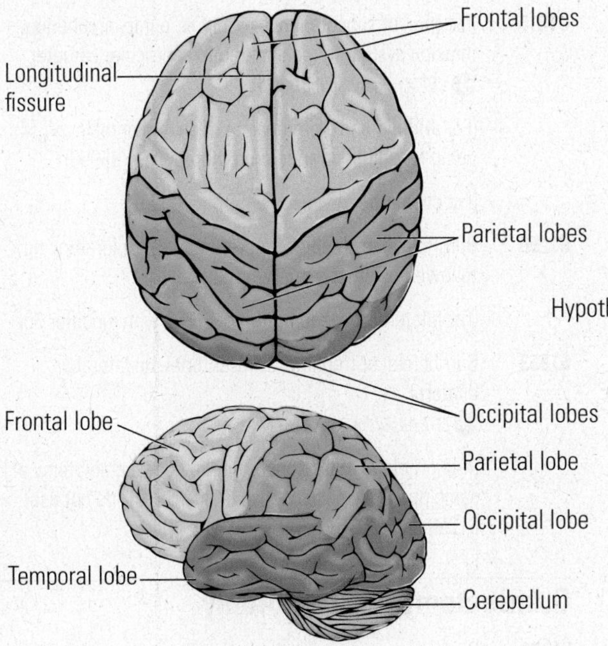

Brain Anatomy

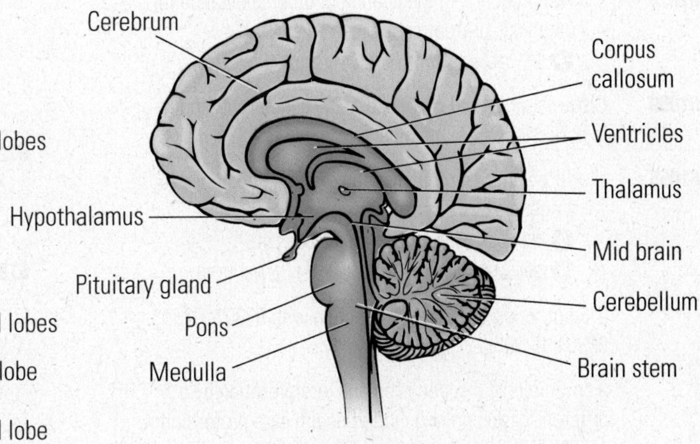

Sagittal Section of Brain and Brain Stem

Nervous System

Skull, Meninges, and Brain

(For injection procedure for cerebral angiography, see 36100-36218)

(For injection procedure for ventriculography, see 61026, 61120)

(For injection procedure for pneumoencephalography, use 61055)

Injection, Drainage, or Aspiration

61000 Subdural tap through fontanelle, or suture, infant, unilateral or bilateral; initial

61001 subsequent taps

61020 Ventricular puncture through previous burr hole, fontanelle, suture, or implanted ventricular catheter/reservoir; without injection

61026 with injection of medication or other substance for diagnosis or treatment
➲ *CPT Changes: An Insider's View* 2002

61050 Cisternal or lateral cervical (C1-C2) puncture; without injection (separate procedure)

61055 with injection of medication or other substance for diagnosis or treatment
➲ *CPT Changes: An Insider's View* 2002, 2015
➲ *Clinical Examples in Radiology* Fall 14:7, Fall 15:10

(Do not report 61055 in conjunction with 62302, 62303, 62304, 62305)

(For radiological supervision and interpretation by a different physician or qualified health care professional, see **Radiology**)

61070 Puncture of shunt tubing or reservoir for aspiration or injection procedure

(For radiological supervision and interpretation, use 75809)

Twist Drill, Burr Hole(s), or Trephine

61105 Twist drill hole for subdural or ventricular puncture

⊘ **61107** Twist drill hole(s) for subdural, intracerebral, or ventricular puncture; for implanting ventricular catheter, pressure recording device, or other intracerebral monitoring device
➲ *CPT Changes: An Insider's View* 2007

(For intracranial neuroendoscopic ventricular catheter placement, use 62160)

61108 for evacuation and/or drainage of subdural hematoma

61120 Burr hole(s) for ventricular puncture (including injection of gas, contrast media, dye, or radioactive material)

61140 Burr hole(s) or trephine; with biopsy of brain or intracranial lesion

61150 with drainage of brain abscess or cyst

61151 with subsequent tapping (aspiration) of intracranial abscess or cyst

61154 Burr hole(s) with evacuation and/or drainage of hematoma, extradural or subdural

(For bilateral procedure, report 61154 with modifier 50)

61156 Burr hole(s); with aspiration of hematoma or cyst, intracerebral

61210 for implanting ventricular catheter, reservoir, EEG electrode(s), pressure recording device, or other cerebral monitoring device (separate procedure)
➲ *CPT Changes: An Insider's View* 2007, 2008

(For intracranial neuroendoscopic ventricular catheter placement, use 62160)

61215 Insertion of subcutaneous reservoir, pump or continuous infusion system for connection to ventricular catheter
➲ *CPT Assistant* Spring 93:13

(For refilling and maintenance of an implantable infusion pump for spinal or brain drug therapy, use 95990)

(For chemotherapy, use 96450)

61250 Burr hole(s) or trephine, supratentorial, exploratory, not followed by other surgery

(For bilateral procedure, report 61250 with modifier 50)

61253 Burr hole(s) or trephine, infratentorial, unilateral or bilateral
➲ *CPT Assistant* Sep 02:10

(If burr hole[s] or trephine are followed by craniotomy at same operative session, use 61304-61321; do not use 61250 or 61253)

Craniectomy or Craniotomy

61304 Craniectomy or craniotomy, exploratory; supratentorial

61305 infratentorial (posterior fossa)

61312 Craniectomy or craniotomy for evacuation of hematoma, supratentorial; extradural or subdural

61313 intracerebral

61314 Craniectomy or craniotomy for evacuation of hematoma, infratentorial; extradural or subdural

61315 intracerebellar

+ **61316** Incision and subcutaneous placement of cranial bone graft (List separately in addition to code for primary procedure)
➲ *CPT Changes: An Insider's View* 2003

(Use 61316 in conjunction with 61304, 61312, 61313, 61322, 61323, 61340, 61570, 61571, 61680-61705)

61320 Craniectomy or craniotomy, drainage of intracranial abscess; supratentorial

61321 infratentorial

61322 Craniectomy or craniotomy, decompressive, with or without duraplasty, for treatment of intracranial hypertension, without evacuation of associated intraparenchymal hematoma; without lobectomy

➲ *CPT Changes: An Insider's View* 2003

(Do not report 61313 in addition to 61322)

(For subtemporal decompression, use 61340)

61323 with lobectomy

➲ *CPT Changes: An Insider's View* 2003

(Do not report 61313 in addition to 61323)

(For subtemporal decompression, use 61340)

61330 Decompression of orbit only, transcranial approach

(For bilateral procedure, report 61330 with modifier 50)

►(61332 has been deleted)◄

61333 Exploration of orbit (transcranial approach) with removal of lesion

61340 Subtemporal cranial decompression (pseudotumor cerebri, slit ventricle syndrome)

➲ *CPT Changes: An Insider's View* 2003

(For bilateral procedure, report 61340 with modifier 50)

(For decompressive craniotomy or craniectomy for intracranial hypertension, without hematoma evacuation, see 61322, 61323)

61343 Craniectomy, suboccipital with cervical laminectomy for decompression of medulla and spinal cord, with or without dural graft (eg, Arnold-Chiari malformation)

61345 Other cranial decompression, posterior fossa

(For orbital decompression by lateral wall approach, Kroenlein type, use 67445)

61450 Craniectomy, subtemporal, for section, compression, or decompression of sensory root of gasserian ganglion

61458 Craniectomy, suboccipital; for exploration or decompression of cranial nerves

61460 for section of 1 or more cranial nerves

►(61480 has been deleted)◄

61500 Craniectomy; with excision of tumor or other bone lesion of skull

➲ *CPT Assistant* Jan 14:9

61501 for osteomyelitis

➲ *CPT Assistant* Jan 14:9

61510 Craniectomy, trephination, bone flap craniotomy; for excision of brain tumor, supratentorial, except meningioma

61512 for excision of meningioma, supratentorial

61514 for excision of brain abscess, supratentorial

61516 for excision or fenestration of cyst, supratentorial

(For excision of pituitary tumor or craniopharyngioma, see 61545, 61546, 61548)

+ 61517 Implantation of brain intracavitary chemotherapy agent (List separately in addition to code for primary procedure)

➲ *CPT Changes: An Insider's View* 2003

(Use 61517 only in conjunction with 61510 or 61518)

(Do not report 61517 for brachytherapy insertion. For intracavitary insertion of radioelement sources or ribbons, see 77770, 77771, 77772)

61518 Craniectomy for excision of brain tumor, infratentorial or posterior fossa; except meningioma, cerebellopontine angle tumor, or midline tumor at base of skull

61519 meningioma

61520 cerebellopontine angle tumor

61521 midline tumor at base of skull

61522 Craniectomy, infratentorial or posterior fossa; for excision of brain abscess

61524 for excision or fenestration of cyst

61526 Craniectomy, bone flap craniotomy, transtemporal (mastoid) for excision of cerebellopontine angle tumor;

➲ *CPT Assistant* Summer 91:8, Mar 18:11

61530 combined with middle/posterior fossa craniotomy/craniectomy

61531 Subdural implantation of strip electrodes through 1 or more burr or trephine hole(s) for long-term seizure monitoring

(For stereotactic implantation of electrodes, use 61760)

(For craniotomy for excision of intracranial arteriovenous malformation, see 61680-61692)

61533 Craniotomy with elevation of bone flap; for subdural implantation of an electrode array, for long-term seizure monitoring

(For continuous EEG monitoring, see 95950-95954)

61534 for excision of epileptogenic focus without electrocorticography during surgery

61535 for removal of epidural or subdural electrode array, without excision of cerebral tissue (separate procedure)

61536 for excision of cerebral epileptogenic focus, with electrocorticography during surgery (includes removal of electrode array)

61537 for lobectomy, temporal lobe, without electrocorticography during surgery

➲ *CPT Changes: An Insider's View* 2004

61538 for lobectomy, temporal lobe, with electrocorticography during surgery

➲ *CPT Changes: An Insider's View* 2004

61539 for lobectomy, other than temporal lobe, partial or total, with electrocorticography during surgery
➲ *CPT Changes: An Insider's View* 2004

61540 for lobectomy, other than temporal lobe, partial or total, without electrocorticography during surgery
➲ *CPT Changes: An Insider's View* 2004

61541 for transection of corpus callosum

61543 for partial or subtotal (functional) hemispherectomy
➲ *CPT Changes: An Insider's View* 2004

61544 for excision or coagulation of choroid plexus

61545 for excision of craniopharyngioma

(For craniotomy for selective amygdalohippocampectomy, use 61566)

(For craniotomy for multiple subpial transections during surgery, use 61567)

61546 Craniotomy for hypophysectomy or excision of pituitary tumor, intracranial approach

61548 Hypophysectomy or excision of pituitary tumor, transnasal or transseptal approach, nonstereotactic
➲ *CPT Assistant* Nov 98:17, Jul 11:13

(Do not report code 69990 in addition to code 61548)

61550 Craniectomy for craniosynostosis; single cranial suture
➲ *CPT Assistant* Feb 12:11

61552 multiple cranial sutures
➲ *CPT Assistant* Feb 12:11

(For cranial reconstruction for orbital hypertelorism, see 21260-21263)

(For reconstruction, see 21172-21180)

61556 Craniotomy for craniosynostosis; frontal or parietal bone flap

61557 bifrontal bone flap
➲ *CPT Assistant* Feb 12:11

61558 Extensive craniectomy for multiple cranial suture craniosynostosis (eg, cloverleaf skull); not requiring bone grafts
➲ *CPT Assistant* Feb 12:11

61559 recontouring with multiple osteotomies and bone autografts (eg, barrel-stave procedure) (includes obtaining grafts)
➲ *CPT Assistant* Feb 12:11

(For reconstruction, see 21172-21180)

61563 Excision, intra and extracranial, benign tumor of cranial bone (eg, fibrous dysplasia); without optic nerve decompression

61564 with optic nerve decompression

(For reconstruction, see 21181-21183)

61566 Craniotomy with elevation of bone flap; for selective amygdalohippocampectomy
➲ *CPT Changes: An Insider's View* 2004

61567 for multiple subpial transections, with electrocorticography during surgery
➲ *CPT Changes: An Insider's View* 2004

61570 Craniectomy or craniotomy; with excision of foreign body from brain

61571 with treatment of penetrating wound of brain

(For sequestrectomy for osteomyelitis, use 61501)

61575 Transoral approach to skull base, brain stem or upper spinal cord for biopsy, decompression or excision of lesion;

61576 requiring splitting of tongue and/or mandible (including tracheostomy)

(For arthrodesis, use 22548)

Surgery of Skull Base

The surgical management of lesions involving the skull base (base of anterior, middle, and posterior cranial fossae) often requires the skills of several surgeons of different surgical specialties working together or in tandem during the operative session. These operations are usually not staged because of the need for definitive closure of dura, subcutaneous tissues, and skin to avoid serious infections such as osteomyelitis and/or meningitis.

The procedures are categorized according to:

(1) ***approach procedure*** necessary to obtain adequate exposure to the lesion (pathologic entity), (2) ***definitive procedure(s)*** necessary to biopsy, excise or otherwise treat the lesion, and (3) ***repair/reconstruction*** of the defect present following the definitive procedure(s).

The ***approach procedure*** is described according to anatomical area involved, ie, anterior cranial fossa, middle cranial fossa, posterior cranial fossa, and brain stem or upper spinal cord.

The ***definitive procedure(s)*** describes the repair, biopsy, resection, or excision of various lesions of the skull base and, when appropriate, primary closure of the dura, mucous membranes, and skin.

The ***repair/reconstruction procedure(s)*** is reported separately if extensive dural grafting, cranioplasty, local or regional myocutaneous pedicle flaps, or extensive skin grafts are required.

For primary closure, see the appropriate codes (ie, 15730, 15733, 15756, 15757, 15758).

When one surgeon performs the approach procedure, another surgeon performs the definitive procedure, and another surgeon performs the repair/reconstruction procedure, each surgeon reports only the code for the specific procedure performed.

Nervous 61000-64999

If one surgeon performs more than one procedure (ie, approach procedure and definitive procedure), then both codes are reported, adding modifier 51 to the secondary, additional procedure(s).

Approach Procedures

Anterior Cranial Fossa

61580 Craniofacial approach to anterior cranial fossa; extradural, including lateral rhinotomy, ethmoidectomy, sphenoidectomy, without maxillectomy or orbital exenteration

➲ *CPT Assistant* Winter 93:17, Spring 94:11

61581 extradural, including lateral rhinotomy, orbital exenteration, ethmoidectomy, sphenoidectomy and/or maxillectomy

➲ *CPT Assistant* Winter 93:17, Spring 94:11

61582 extradural, including unilateral or bifrontal craniotomy, elevation of frontal lobe(s), osteotomy of base of anterior cranial fossa

➲ *CPT Assistant* Winter 93:17, Spring 94:11

61583 intradural, including unilateral or bifrontal craniotomy, elevation or resection of frontal lobe, osteotomy of base of anterior cranial fossa

➲ *CPT Assistant* Winter 93:17, Spring 94:11, Dec 17:13

61584 Orbitocranial approach to anterior cranial fossa, extradural, including supraorbital ridge osteotomy and elevation of frontal and/or temporal lobe(s); without orbital exenteration

➲ *CPT Assistant* Winter 93:18

61585 with orbital exenteration

➲ *CPT Assistant* Winter 93:18

61586 Bicoronal, transzygomatic and/or LeFort I osteotomy approach to anterior cranial fossa with or without internal fixation, without bone graft

➲ *CPT Assistant* Winter 93:18, Nov 96:12

Middle Cranial Fossa

61590 Infratemporal pre-auricular approach to middle cranial fossa (parapharyngeal space, infratemporal and midline skull base, nasopharynx), with or without disarticulation of the mandible, including parotidectomy, craniotomy, decompression and/or mobilization of the facial nerve and/or petrous carotid artery

➲ *CPT Assistant* Winter 93:18

61591 Infratemporal post-auricular approach to middle cranial fossa (internal auditory meatus, petrous apex, tentorium, cavernous sinus, parasellar area, infratemporal fossa) including mastoidectomy, resection of sigmoid sinus, with or without decompression and/or mobilization of contents of auditory canal or petrous carotid artery

➲ *CPT Assistant* Winter 93:18

61592 Orbitocranial zygomatic approach to middle cranial fossa (cavernous sinus and carotid artery, clivus, basilar artery or petrous apex) including osteotomy of zygoma, craniotomy, extra- or intradural elevation of temporal lobe

➲ *CPT Assistant* Winter 93:18

Posterior Cranial Fossa

61595 Transtemporal approach to posterior cranial fossa, jugular foramen or midline skull base, including mastoidectomy, decompression of sigmoid sinus and/or facial nerve, with or without mobilization

➲ *CPT Assistant* Winter 93:18, Mar 18:11

61596 Transcochlear approach to posterior cranial fossa, jugular foramen or midline skull base, including labyrinthectomy, decompression, with or without mobilization of facial nerve and/or petrous carotid artery

➲ *CPT Assistant* Winter 93:18

61597 Transcondylar (far lateral) approach to posterior cranial fossa, jugular foramen or midline skull base, including occipital condylectomy, mastoidectomy, resection of C1-C3 vertebral body(s), decompression of vertebral artery, with or without mobilization

➲ *CPT Assistant* Winter 93:18

61598 Transpetrosal approach to posterior cranial fossa, clivus or foramen magnum, including ligation of superior petrosal sinus and/or sigmoid sinus

➲ *CPT Assistant* Winter 93:18

Definitive Procedures

Base of Anterior Cranial Fossa

61600 Resection or excision of neoplastic, vascular or infectious lesion of base of anterior cranial fossa; extradural

➲ *CPT Assistant* Winter 93:19, Spring 94:12, Nov 96:12

61601 intradural, including dural repair, with or without graft

➲ *CPT Assistant* Winter 93:19, Spring 94:12

Base of Middle Cranial Fossa

61605 Resection or excision of neoplastic, vascular or infectious lesion of infratemporal fossa, parapharyngeal space, petrous apex; extradural

➲ *CPT Assistant* Winter 93:19

61606 intradural, including dural repair, with or without graft

➲ *CPT Assistant* Winter 93:20

61607 Resection or excision of neoplastic, vascular or infectious lesion of parasellar area, cavernous sinus, clivus or midline skull base; extradural

➲ *CPT Assistant* Winter 93:20

61608 intradural, including dural repair, with or without graft

➔ *CPT Assistant* Winter 93:20

►Code 61611 is reported in addition to code(s) for primary procedure(s) 61605-61608. Report only one transection or ligation of carotid artery code per operative session.◄

►(61610 has been deleted)◄

+ 61611 Transection or ligation, carotid artery in petrous canal; without repair (List separately in addition to code for primary procedure)

➔ *CPT Assistant* Winter 93:20

►(61612 has been deleted)◄

61613 Obliteration of carotid aneurysm, arteriovenous malformation, or carotid-cavernous fistula by dissection within cavernous sinus

➔ *CPT Assistant* Winter 93:20

Base of Posterior Cranial Fossa

61615 Resection or excision of neoplastic, vascular or infectious lesion of base of posterior cranial fossa, jugular foramen, foramen magnum, or C1-C3 vertebral bodies; extradural

➔ *CPT Assistant* Winter 93:20

61616 intradural, including dural repair, with or without graft

➔ *CPT Assistant* Mar 18:11

Repair and/or Reconstruction of Surgical Defects of Skull Base

61618 Secondary repair of dura for cerebrospinal fluid leak, anterior, middle or posterior cranial fossa following surgery of the skull base; by free tissue graft (eg, pericranium, fascia, tensor fascia lata, adipose tissue, homologous or synthetic grafts)

➔ *CPT Assistant* Winter 93:20, Spring 94:19, Mar 00:11

61619 by local or regionalized vascularized pedicle flap or myocutaneous flap (including galea, temporalis, frontalis or occipitalis muscle)

➔ *CPT Assistant* Winter 93:20, Spring 94:19, Mar 00:11

Endovascular Therapy

61623 Endovascular temporary balloon arterial occlusion, head or neck (extracranial/intracranial) including selective catheterization of vessel to be occluded, positioning and inflation of occlusion balloon, concomitant neurological monitoring, and radiologic supervision and interpretation of all angiography required for balloon occlusion and to exclude vascular injury post occlusion

➔ *CPT Changes: An Insider's View* 2003

(If selective catheterization and angiography of arteries other than artery to be occluded is performed, use appropriate catheterization and radiologic supervision and interpretation codes)

(If complete diagnostic angiography of the artery to be occluded is performed immediately prior to temporary occlusion, use appropriate radiologic supervision and interpretation codes only)

61624 Transcatheter permanent occlusion or embolization (eg, for tumor destruction, to achieve hemostasis, to occlude a vascular malformation), percutaneous, any method; central nervous system (intracranial, spinal cord)

➔ *CPT Changes: An Insider's View* 2003

➔ *CPT Assistant* Jun 99:10, Nov 06:8, Nov 13:6

➔ *Clinical Examples in Radiology* Summer 07:2, Summer 16:13, Winter 18:2

(For non-central nervous system and non-head or neck embolization, see 37241-37244)

(For radiological supervision and interpretation, use 75894)

61626 non-central nervous system, head or neck (extracranial, brachiocephalic branch)

➔ *CPT Assistant* Nov 13:6

➔ *Clinical Examples in Radiology* Spring 16:5

(For non-central nervous system and non-head or neck embolization, see 37241-37244)

(For radiological supervision and interpretation, use 75894)

61630 Balloon angioplasty, intracranial (eg, atherosclerotic stenosis), percutaneous

➔ *CPT Changes: An Insider's View* 2006

➔ *CPT Assistant* Apr 17:10

➔ *Clinical Examples in Radiology* Winter 06:16

61635 Transcatheter placement of intravascular stent(s), intracranial (eg, atherosclerotic stenosis), including balloon angioplasty, if performed

➔ *CPT Changes: An Insider's View* 2006

➔ *CPT Assistant* Mar 14:8

➔ *Clinical Examples in Radiology* Winter 06:16

►(61630 and 61635 include all selective vascular catheterization of the target vascular territory, all diagnostic imaging for arteriography of the target vascular territory, and all related radiological supervision and interpretation. When diagnostic arteriogram (including imaging and selective catheterization) confirms the need for angioplasty or stent placement, 61630 and 61635 are inclusive of these services. If angioplasty or stenting are not indicated, then the appropriate codes for selective catheterization and imaging should be reported in lieu of 61630 and 61635)◄

(Do not report 61630 or 61635 in conjunction with 61645 for the same vascular territory)

(For definition of vascular territory, see the Nervous System Endovascular Therapy guidelines)

61640 Balloon dilatation of intracranial vasospasm, percutaneous; initial vessel
- *CPT Changes: An Insider's View* 2006
- *CPT Assistant* May 14:10
- *Clinical Examples in Radiology* Winter 06:16

+▲ 61641 each additional vessel in same vascular territory (List separately in addition to code for primary procedure)
- *CPT Changes: An Insider's View* 2006, 2019
- *CPT Assistant* May 14:10
- *Clinical Examples in Radiology* Winter 06:16

+▲ 61642 each additional vessel in different vascular territory (List separately in addition to code for primary procedure)
- *CPT Changes: An Insider's View* 2006, 2019
- *CPT Assistant* May 14:10
- *Clinical Examples in Radiology* Winter 06:16

(Use 61641 and 61642 in conjunction with 61640)

(61640, 61641, 61642 include all selective vascular catheterization of the target vessel, contrast injection[s], vessel measurement, roadmapping, postdilatation angiography, and fluoroscopic guidance for the balloon dilatation)

(Do not report 61640, 61642 in conjunction with 61650 or 61651 for the same vascular territory)

(For definition of vascular territory, see the Nervous System Endovascular Therapy guidelines)

Codes 61645, 61650, 61651 describe cerebral endovascular therapeutic interventions in any intracranial artery. They include selective catheterization, diagnostic angiography, and all subsequent angiography including associated radiological supervision and interpretation within the treated vascular territory, fluoroscopic guidance, neurologic and hemodynamic monitoring of the patient, and closure of the arteriotomy by manual pressure, an arterial closure device, or suture.

For purposes of reporting services described by 61645, 61650, 61651, the intracranial arteries are divided into three vascular territories: 1) right carotid circulation; 2) left carotid circulation; 3) vertebro-basilar circulation. Code 61645 may be reported once for each intracranial vascular territory treated. Code 61650 is reported once for the first intracranial vascular territory treated with intra-arterial prolonged administration of pharmacologic agent(s). If additional intracranial vascular territory(ies) is also treated with intra-arterial prolonged administration of pharmacologic agent(s) during the same session, the treatment of each additional vascular territory(ies) is reported using 61651 (may be reported maximally two times per day).

Code 61645 describes endovascular revascularization of thrombotic/embolic occlusion of intracranial arterial vessel(s) via any method, including mechanical thrombectomy (eg, mechanical retrieval device, aspiration catheter) and/or the administration of any agent(s) for the purpose of revascularization, such as thrombolytics or IIB/IIIA inhibitors.

Codes 61650, 61651 describe the cerebral endovascular continuous or intermittent therapeutic prolonged administration of any non-thrombolytic agent(s) (eg, spasmolytics or chemotherapy) into an artery to treat non-iatrogenic central nervous system diseases or sequelae thereof. These codes should not be used to report administration of agents (eg, heparin, nitroglycerin, saline) usually administered during endovascular interventions. These codes are used for prolonged administrations, ie, of at least 10 minutes continuous or intermittent duration.

Do not report 61645, 61650, or 61651 in conjunction with 36221, 36226, 36228, 37184, or 37186 for the treated vascular territory. Do not report 61645 in conjunction with 61650 or 61651 for the same vascular distribution. Diagnostic angiography of a non-treated vascular territory may be reported separately. For example, angiography of the left carotid and/or the vertebral circulations may be reported if the intervention is performed in the right carotid circulation.

61645 Percutaneous arterial transluminal mechanical thrombectomy and/or infusion for thrombolysis, intracranial, any method, including diagnostic angiography, fluoroscopic guidance, catheter placement, and intraprocedural pharmacological thrombolytic injection(s)
- *CPT Changes: An Insider's View* 2016
- *CPT Assistant* Nov 15:3, Dec 15:17, Mar 16:3
- *Clinical Examples in Radiology* Spring 16:2

(Do not report 61645 in conjunction with 36221, 36222, 36223, 36224, 36225, 36226, 37184, 61630, 61635, 61650, 61651 for the same vascular territory)

(To report venous mechanical thrombectomy and/or thrombolysis, see 37187, 37188, 37212, 37214)

61650 Endovascular intracranial prolonged administration of pharmacologic agent(s) other than for thrombolysis, arterial, including catheter placement, diagnostic angiography, and imaging guidance; initial vascular territory
- *CPT Changes: An Insider's View* 2016
- *CPT Assistant* Nov 15:3, Mar 16:3
- *Clinical Examples in Radiology* Spring 16:3

+ 61651 each additional vascular territory (List separately in addition to code for primary procedure)
- *CPT Changes: An Insider's View* 2016
- *CPT Assistant* Nov 15:3, Mar 16:3
- *Clinical Examples in Radiology* Spring 16:3

(Use 61651 in conjunction with 61650)

(Do not report 61650 or 61651 in conjunction with 36221, 36222, 36223, 36224, 36225, 36226, 61640, 61641, 61642, 61645 for the same vascular territory)

(Do not report 61650 or 61651 in conjunction with 96420, 96422, 96423, 96425 for the same vascular territory)

Surgery for Aneurysm, Arteriovenous Malformation, or Vascular Disease

Includes craniotomy when appropriate for procedure.

61680 Surgery of intracranial arteriovenous malformation; supratentorial, simple

61682 supratentorial, complex

➲ *CPT Assistant* Jun 13:14

61684 infratentorial, simple

61686 infratentorial, complex

➲ *CPT Assistant* Jun 13:14

61690 dural, simple

61692 dural, complex

➲ *CPT Assistant* Jun 13:14

61697 Surgery of complex intracranial aneurysm, intracranial approach; carotid circulation

➲ *CPT Changes: An Insider's View* 2001

➲ *CPT Assistant* Dec 17:13

61698 vertebrobasilar circulation

➲ *CPT Changes: An Insider's View* 2001

(61697, 61698 involve aneurysms that are larger than 15 mm or with calcification of the aneurysm neck, or with incorporation of normal vessels into the aneurysm neck, or a procedure requiring temporary vessel occlusion, trapping, or cardiopulmonary bypass to successfully treat the aneurysm)

61700 Surgery of simple intracranial aneurysm, intracranial approach; carotid circulation

➲ *CPT Changes: An Insider's View* 2001

➲ *CPT Assistant* Jun 99:11, Jul 99:10, Dec 17:13

61702 vertebrobasilar circulation

➲ *CPT Changes: An Insider's View* 2001

61703 Surgery of intracranial aneurysm, cervical approach by application of occluding clamp to cervical carotid artery (Selverstone-Crutchfield type)

(For cervical approach for direct ligation of carotid artery, see 37600-37606)

61705 Surgery of aneurysm, vascular malformation or carotid-cavernous fistula; by intracranial and cervical occlusion of carotid artery

61708 by intracranial electrothrombosis

(For ligation or gradual occlusion of internal/common carotid artery, see 37605, 37606)

61710 by intra-arterial embolization, injection procedure, or balloon catheter

➲ *CPT Assistant* Nov 13:6

Intracranial Aneurysm, Intracranial Approach
61700

Placement of ligating clip across the neck of an intracranial aneurysm

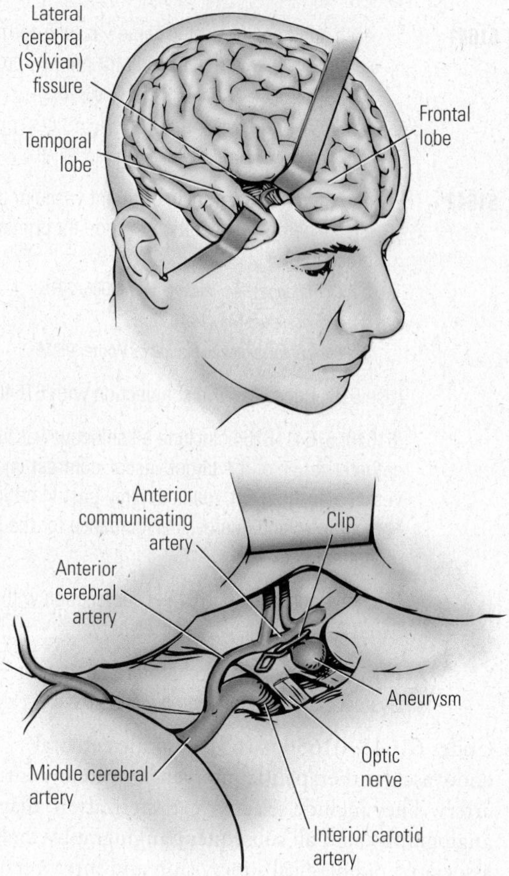

61711 Anastomosis, arterial, extracranial-intracranial (eg, middle cerebral/cortical) arteries

(For carotid or vertebral thromboendarterectomy, use 35301)

(Use 69990 when the surgical microscope is employed for the microsurgical procedure. Do not use 69990 for visualization with magnifying loupes or corrected vision)

Stereotaxis

61720 Creation of lesion by stereotactic method, including burr hole(s) and localizing and recording techniques, single or multiple stages; globus pallidus or thalamus

➲ *CPT Assistant* Jul 11:12, Jul 14:9

61735 subcortical structure(s) other than globus pallidus or thalamus

➲ *CPT Assistant* Jul 11:12

61750 Stereotactic biopsy, aspiration, or excision, including burr hole(s), for intracranial lesion;

➲ *CPT Changes: An Insider's View* 2000

➲ *CPT Assistant* Nov 99:30

61751 with computed tomography and/or magnetic resonance guidance
➲ *CPT Changes: An Insider's View* 2000, 2003
➲ *CPT Assistant* Jun 96:10, Nov 99:30, Dec 04:20, Jul 11:12

(For radiological supervision and interpretation of computerized tomography, see 70450, 70460, or 70470 as appropriate)

(For radiological supervision and interpretation of magnetic resonance imaging, see 70551, 70552, or 70553 as appropriate)

61760 Stereotactic implantation of depth electrodes into the cerebrum for long-term seizure monitoring
➲ *CPT Assistant* Jul 11:12

61770 Stereotactic localization, including burr hole(s), with insertion of catheter(s) or probe(s) for placement of radiation source
➲ *CPT Changes: An Insider's View* 2001
➲ *CPT Assistant* Jul 11:12

+ 61781 Stereotactic computer-assisted (navigational) procedure; cranial, intradural (List separately in addition to code for primary procedure)
➲ *CPT Changes: An Insider's View* 2011
➲ *CPT Assistant* Jul 11:12, Jul 14:9, Sep 14:14

(Do not report 61781 in conjunction with 61720-61791, 61796-61799, 61863-61868, 62201, 77371-77373, 77432)

+ 61782 cranial, extradural (List separately in addition to code for primary procedure)
➲ *CPT Changes: An Insider's View* 2011
➲ *CPT Assistant* Jul 11:12

(Do not report 61781, 61782 by the same individual during the same surgical session)

+ 61783 spinal (List separately in addition to code for primary procedure)
➲ *CPT Changes: An Insider's View* 2011
➲ *CPT Assistant* Jul 11:12

(Do not report 61783 in conjunction with 63620, 63621)

61790 Creation of lesion by stereotactic method, percutaneous, by neurolytic agent (eg, alcohol, thermal, electrical, radiofrequency); gasserian ganglion
➲ *CPT Assistant* Jul 11:12

61791 trigeminal medullary tract
➲ *CPT Assistant* Jul 11:12, Jul 14:9

Stereotactic Radiosurgery (Cranial)

Cranial stereotactic radiosurgery is a distinct procedure that utilizes externally generated ionizing radiation to inactivate or eradicate defined target(s) in the head without the need to make an incision. The target is defined by and the treatment is delivered using high-resolution stereotactic imaging. Stereotactic radiosurgery codes and headframe application procedures are reported by the neurosurgeon. The radiation oncologist reports the appropriate code(s) for clinical treatment planning, physics and dosimetry, treatment delivery, and management from the **Radiation Oncology** section (77261-77790). Any necessary planning, dosimetry, targeting, positioning, or blocking by the neurosurgeon is included in the stereotactic radiation surgery services. The same individual should not report stereotactic radiosurgery services with radiation treatment management codes (77427-77435).

Cranial stereotactic radiosurgery is typically performed in a single planning and treatment session, using a rigidly attached stereotactic guiding device, other immobilization technology and/or a stereotactic image-guidance system, but can be performed with more than one planning session and in a limited number of treatment sessions, up to a maximum of five sessions. Do not report stereotactic radiosurgery more than once per lesion per course of treatment when the treatment requires more than one session.

Codes 61796 and 61797 involve stereotactic radiosurgery for simple cranial lesions. Simple cranial lesions are lesions less than 3.5 cm in maximum dimension that do not meet the definition of a complex lesion provided below. Report code 61796 when all lesions are simple.

Codes 61798 and 61799 involve stereotactic radiosurgery for complex cranial lesions and procedures that create therapeutic lesions (eg, thalamotomy or pallidotomy). All lesions 3.5 cm in maximum dimension or greater are complex. When performing therapeutic lesion creation procedures, report code 61798 only once regardless of the number of lesions created. Schwannomas, arterio-venous malformations, pituitary tumors, glomus tumors, pineal region tumors and cavernous sinus/parasellar/petroclival tumors are complex. Any lesion that is adjacent (5mm or less) to the optic nerve/optic chasm/optic tract or within the brainstem is complex. If treating multiple lesions, and any single lesion treated is complex, use 61798.

Do not report codes 61796-61800 in conjunction with code 20660.

Codes 61796-61799 include computer-assisted planning. Do not report codes 61796-61799 in conjunction with 61781-61783.

(For intensity modulated beam delivery plan and treatment, see 77301, 77385, 77386. For stereotactic body radiation therapy, see 77373, 77435)

61796 Stereotactic radiosurgery (particle beam, gamma ray, or linear accelerator); 1 simple cranial lesion
➲ *CPT Changes: An Insider's View* 2009
➲ *CPT Assistant* Jul 11:12, Apr 12:11, Jul 14:9, Jun 15:6

(Do not report 61796 more than once per course of treatment)

(Do not report 61796 in conjunction with 61798)

+ 61797 each additional cranial lesion, simple (List separately in addition to code for primary procedure)
➲ *CPT Changes: An Insider's View* 2009
➲ *CPT Assistant* Jul 11:12, Apr 12:11, Jun 15:6

Nervous 61000-64999

(Use 61797 in conjunction with 61796, 61798)

(For each course of treatment, 61797 and 61799 may be reported no more than once per lesion. Do not report any combination of 61797 and 61799 more than 4 times for entire course of treatment regardless of number of lesions treated)

61798 1 complex cranial lesion

➔ *CPT Changes: An Insider's View* 2009

➔ *CPT Assistant* Jul 11:12, Apr 12:11, Jun 15:6

(Do not report 61798 more than once per course of treatment)

(Do not report 61798 in conjunction with 61796)

+ 61799 each additional cranial lesion, complex (List separately in addition to code for primary procedure)

➔ *CPT Changes: An Insider's View* 2009

➔ *CPT Assistant* Jul 11:12, Apr 12:11, Jul 14:9, Jun 15:6

(Use 61799 in conjunction with 61798)

(For each course of treatment, 61797 and 61799 may be reported no more than once per lesion. Do not report any combination of 61797 and 61799 more than 4 times for entire course of treatment regardless of number of lesions treated)

+ 61800 Application of stereotactic headframe for stereotactic radiosurgery (List separately in addition to code for primary procedure)

➔ *CPT Changes: An Insider's View* 2009

➔ *CPT Assistant* Apr 12:11, Jun 15:6

(Use 61800 in conjunction with 61796, 61798)

Neurostimulators (Intracranial)

►For electronic analysis with programming, when performed, of cranial nerve and brain neurostimulator pulse generator/transmitters, see codes 95970, 95976, 95977, 95983, 95984. Test stimulation to confirm correct target site placement of the electrode array(s) and/or to confirm the functional status of the system is inherent to placement and is not separately reported as electronic analysis or programming of the neurostimulator system. Electronic analysis (95970) at the time of implantation is not separately reported.◄

Microelectrode recording, when performed by the operating surgeon in association with implantation of neurostimulator electrode arrays, is an inclusive service and should not be reported separately. If another individual participates in neurophysiological mapping during a deep brain stimulator implantation procedure, this service may be reported by the second individual with codes 95961-95962.

61850 Twist drill or burr hole(s) for implantation of neurostimulator electrodes, cortical

➔ *CPT Changes: An Insider's View* 2000

➔ *CPT Assistant* Sep 99:5, Nov 99:30

61860 Craniectomy or craniotomy for implantation of neurostimulator electrodes, cerebral, cortical

➔ *CPT Changes: An Insider's View* 2000

➔ *CPT Assistant* Sep 99:5, Nov 99:30

61863 Twist drill, burr hole, craniotomy, or craniectomy with stereotactic implantation of neurostimulator electrode array in subcortical site (eg, thalamus, globus pallidus, subthalamic nucleus, periventricular, periaqueductal gray), without use of intraoperative microelectrode recording; first array

➔ *CPT Changes: An Insider's View* 2004

➔ *CPT Assistant* Sep 99:5, Oct 10:10, Jul 11:12, Jul 14:9

+ 61864 each additional array (List separately in addition to primary procedure)

➔ *CPT Changes: An Insider's View* 2004

➔ *CPT Assistant* Sep 99:5, Jul 11:12

(Use 61864 in conjunction with 61863)

61867 Twist drill, burr hole, craniotomy, or craniectomy with stereotactic implantation of neurostimulator electrode array in subcortical site (eg, thalamus, globus pallidus, subthalamic nucleus, periventricular, periaqueductal gray), with use of intraoperative microelectrode recording; first array

➔ *CPT Changes: An Insider's View* 2004

➔ *CPT Assistant* Jul 11:12

+ 61868 each additional array (List separately in addition to primary procedure)

➔ *CPT Changes: An Insider's View* 2004

➔ *CPT Assistant* Jul 11:12, Jul 14:9

(Use 61868 in conjunction with 61867)

Placement of Cranial Neurostimulator
61867-61868, 61885

Placement of subcortical (eg, thalamic) neurostimulator electrode via burr hole (61867-61868) with connection of the electrode to an implanted programmable pulse generator (61885) in the infraclavicular area

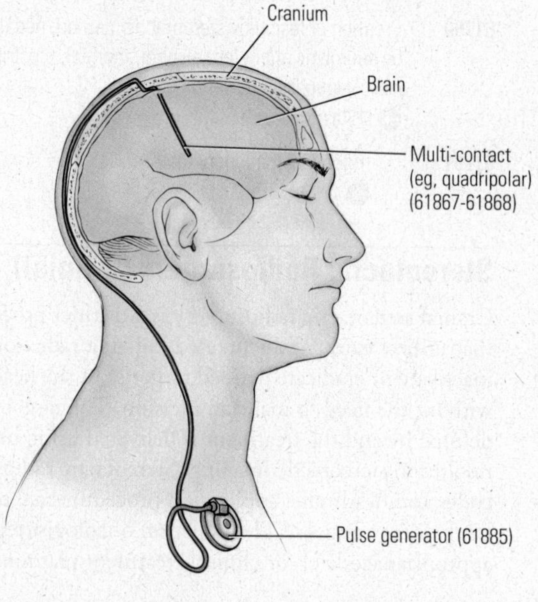

61870 Craniectomy for implantation of neurostimulator electrodes, cerebellar, cortical

61880 Revision or removal of intracranial neurostimulator electrodes

61885 Insertion or replacement of cranial neurostimulator pulse generator or receiver, direct or inductive coupling; with connection to a single electrode array

➲ *CPT Changes: An Insider's View* 2000, 2005

➲ *CPT Assistant* Sep 99:5, Nov 99:30, Jun 00:3, Apr 01:8, Sep 03:3, Dec 10:14, Feb 11:5, Sep 11:8

61886 with connection to 2 or more electrode arrays

➲ *CPT Changes: An Insider's View* 2000

➲ *CPT Assistant* Nov 99:30, Jun 00:3, Apr 01:8, Feb 11:5, Sep 11:8

(For percutaneous placement of cranial nerve (eg, vagus, trigeminal) neurostimulator electrode(s), use 64553)

(For revision or removal of cranial nerve (eg, vagus, trigeminal) neurostimulator electrode array, use 64569)

61888 Revision or removal of cranial neurostimulator pulse generator or receiver

➲ *CPT Assistant* Sep 11:8

(Do not report 61888 in conjunction with 61885 or 61886 for the same pulse generator)

Repair

62000 Elevation of depressed skull fracture; simple, extradural

62005 compound or comminuted, extradural

62010 with repair of dura and/or debridement of brain

62100 Craniotomy for repair of dural/cerebrospinal fluid leak, including surgery for rhinorrhea/otorrhea

➲ *CPT Changes: An Insider's View* 2002

(For repair of spinal dural/CSF leak, see 63707, 63709)

62115 Reduction of craniomegalic skull (eg, treated hydrocephalus); not requiring bone grafts or cranioplasty

62117 requiring craniotomy and reconstruction with or without bone graft (includes obtaining grafts)

62120 Repair of encephalocele, skull vault, including cranioplasty

62121 Craniotomy for repair of encephalocele, skull base

62140 Cranioplasty for skull defect; up to 5 cm diameter

➲ *CPT Assistant* Jan 14:9

62141 larger than 5 cm diameter

➲ *CPT Assistant* Jan 14:9

62142 Removal of bone flap or prosthetic plate of skull

➲ *CPT Assistant* Jan 14:9

62143 Replacement of bone flap or prosthetic plate of skull

➲ *CPT Assistant* Jan 14:9

62145 Cranioplasty for skull defect with reparative brain surgery

➲ *CPT Assistant* Jan 14:9

62146 Cranioplasty with autograft (includes obtaining bone grafts); up to 5 cm diameter

➲ *CPT Assistant* Jan 14:9

62147 larger than 5 cm diameter

➲ *CPT Assistant* Jan 14:9

+ 62148 Incision and retrieval of subcutaneous cranial bone graft for cranioplasty (List separately in addition to code for primary procedure)

➲ *CPT Changes: An Insider's View* 2003

(Use 62148 in conjunction with 62140-62147)

Neuroendoscopy

Surgical endoscopy always includes diagnostic endoscopy.

+ 62160 Neuroendoscopy, intracranial, for placement or replacement of ventricular catheter and attachment to shunt system or external drainage (List separately in addition to code for primary procedure)

➲ *CPT Changes: An Insider's View* 2003

➲ *CPT Assistant* Jun 07:11, Dec 12:14

(Use 62160 only in conjunction with 61107, 61210, 62220-62230, 62258)

62161 Neuroendoscopy, intracranial; with dissection of adhesions, fenestration of septum pellucidum or intraventricular cysts (including placement, replacement, or removal of ventricular catheter)

➲ *CPT Changes: An Insider's View* 2003

62162 with fenestration or excision of colloid cyst, including placement of external ventricular catheter for drainage

➲ *CPT Changes: An Insider's View* 2003

62163 with retrieval of foreign body

➲ *CPT Changes: An Insider's View* 2003

62164 with excision of brain tumor, including placement of external ventricular catheter for drainage

➲ *CPT Changes: An Insider's View* 2003

62165 with excision of pituitary tumor, transnasal or trans-sphenoidal approach

➲ *CPT Changes: An Insider's View* 2003

➲ *CPT Assistant* Dec 17:14

Cerebrospinal Fluid (CSF) Shunt

62180 Ventriculocisternostomy (Torkildsen type operation)

62190 Creation of shunt; subarachnoid/subdural-atrial, -jugular, -auricular

62192 subarachnoid/subdural-peritoneal, -pleural, other terminus

62194 Replacement or irrigation, subarachnoid/subdural catheter

➲ *CPT Assistant* Dec 11:6

62200 Ventriculocisternostomy, third ventricle;
➔ *CPT Changes: An Insider's View* 2003

62201 stereotactic, neuroendoscopic method
➔ *CPT Changes: An Insider's View* 2003
➔ *CPT Assistant* Aug 07:15, Jul 11:12, Jul 14:9

(For intracranial neuroendoscopic procedures, see 62161-62165)

62220 Creation of shunt; ventriculo-atrial, -jugular, -auricular
➔ *CPT Changes: An Insider's View* 2003

(For intracranial neuroendoscopic ventricular catheter placement, use 62160)

62223 ventriculo-peritoneal, -pleural, other terminus
➔ *CPT Changes: An Insider's View* 2003

(For intracranial neuroendoscopic ventricular catheter placement, use 62160)

Cerebrospinal Fluid (CSF) Shunt (Ventricular Peritoneal)
62223

A ventriculostomy is performed to drain CSF into the peritoneal cavity.

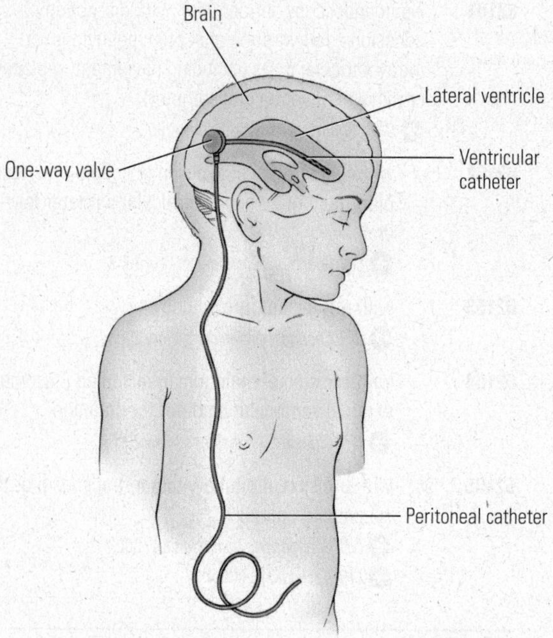

62225 Replacement or irrigation, ventricular catheter
➔ *CPT Changes: An Insider's View* 2003
➔ *CPT Assistant* Dec 11:6

(For intracranial neuroendoscopic ventricular catheter placement, use 62160)

62230 Replacement or revision of cerebrospinal fluid shunt, obstructed valve, or distal catheter in shunt system
➔ *CPT Changes: An Insider's View* 2002, 2003
➔ *CPT Assistant* Dec 11:6, Dec 12:14

(For intracranial neuroendoscopic ventricular catheter placement, use 62160)

(For replacement of **only** the valve and proximal catheter, use 62230 in conjunction with 62225)

62252 Reprogramming of programmable cerebrospinal shunt
➔ *CPT Changes: An Insider's View* 2001, 2002

62256 Removal of complete cerebrospinal fluid shunt system; without replacement
➔ *CPT Changes: An Insider's View* 2002

62258 with replacement by similar or other shunt at same operation
➔ *CPT Assistant* Dec 11:6

(For percutaneous irrigation or aspiration of shunt reservoir, use 61070)

(For reprogramming of programmable CSF shunt, use 62252)

(For intracranial neuroendoscopic ventricular catheter placement, use 62160)

Spine and Spinal Cord

(For application of caliper or tongs, use 20660)

(For treatment of fracture or dislocation of spine, see 22310-22327)

Injection, Drainage, or Aspiration

Injection of contrast during fluoroscopic guidance and localization is an inclusive component of 62263, 62264, 62267, 62270, 62272, 62273, 62280, 62281, 62282, 62302, 62303, 62304, 62305, 62321, 62323, 62325, 62327. Fluoroscopic guidance and localization is reported with 77003, unless a formal contrast study (myelography, epidurography, or arthrography) is performed, in which case the use of fluoroscopy is included in the supervision and interpretation codes or the myelography via lumbar injection code. Image guidance and the injection of contrast are inclusive components and are required for the performance of myelography, as described by codes 62302, 62303, 62304, 62305.

For radiologic supervision and interpretation of epidurography, use 72275. Code 72275 is only to be used when an epidurogram is performed, images documented, and a formal radiologic report is issued.

Code 62263 describes a catheter-based treatment involving targeted injection of various substances (eg, hypertonic saline, steroid, anesthetic) via an indwelling epidural catheter. Code 62263 includes percutaneous insertion and removal of an epidural catheter (remaining in place over a several-day period), for the administration of multiple injections of a neurolytic agent(s) performed during serial treatment sessions (ie, spanning two or more treatment days). If required, adhesions or scarring may also be lysed by mechanical means. Code 62263 is **not** reported for each adhesiolysis treatment, but should be reported **once** to describe the entire series of injections/infusions spanning two or more treatment days.

Code 62264 describes multiple adhesiolysis treatment sessions performed on the same day. Adhesions or scarring may be lysed by injections of neurolytic agent(s). If required, adhesions or scarring may also be lysed mechanically using a percutaneously-deployed catheter.

Codes 62263 and 62264 include the procedure of injections of contrast for epidurography (72275) and fluoroscopic guidance and localization (77003) during initial or subsequent sessions.

Fluoroscopy or CT and any injection of contrast are inclusive components of 62321, 62323, 62325, 62327. For epidurography, use 72275.

The placement and use of a catheter to administer one or more epidural or subarachnoid injections on a single calendar day should be reported in the same manner as if a needle had been used, ie, as a single injection using either 62320, 62321, 62322, or 62323. Such injections should not be reported with 62324, 62325, 62326, or 62327.

Threading a catheter into the epidural space, injecting substances at one or more levels and then removing the catheter should be treated as a single injection (62320, 62321, 62322, 62323). If the catheter is left in place to deliver substance(s) over a prolonged period (ie, more than a single calendar day) either continuously or via intermittent bolus, use 62324, 62325, 62326, 62327 as appropriate.

When reporting 62320, 62321, 62322, 62323, 62324, 62325, 62326, 62327 code choice is based on the region at which the needle or catheter entered the body (eg, lumbar). Codes 62320, 62321, 62322, 62323, 62324, 62325, 62326, 62327 should be reported only once, when the substance injected spreads or catheter tip insertion moves into another spinal region (eg, 62322 is reported only once for injection or catheter insertion at L3-4 with spread of the substance or placement of the catheter tip to the thoracic region).

Percutaneous spinal procedures are done with indirect visualization (eg, image guidance) (eg, 62287). Endoscopic assistance during an open procedure with continuous and direct visualization (light-based) is reported using excision codes (eg, 63020-63035).

(For transforaminal epidural injection, see 64479-64484)

(Report 01996 for daily hospital management of continuous epidural or subarachnoid drug administration performed in conjunction with 62324, 62325, 62326, 62327)

Definitions

For purposes of CPT coding, the following definitions of approach and visualization apply. The primary approach and visualization define the service, whether another method is incidentally applied. Surgical services are presumed open, unless otherwise specified.

Percutaneous: Image-guided procedures (eg, computer tomography [CT] or fluoroscopy) performed with indirect visualization of the spine without the use of any device that allows visualization through a surgical incision.

Endoscopic: Spinal procedures performed with continuous direct visualization of the spine through an endoscope.

Open: Spinal procedures performed with continuous direct visualization of the spine through a surgical opening.

Indirect visualization: Image-guided (eg, CT or fluoroscopy), not light-based visualization.

Direct visualization: Light-based visualization; can be performed by eye, or with surgical loupes, microscope, or endoscope.

(For the techniques of microsurgery and/or use of microscope, use 69990)

62263 Percutaneous lysis of epidural adhesions using solution injection (eg, hypertonic saline, enzyme) or mechanical means (eg, catheter) including radiologic localization (includes contrast when administered), multiple adhesiolysis sessions; 2 or more days

➲ *CPT Changes: An Insider's View* 2000, 2003

➲ *CPT Assistant* Nov 99:33, Dec 99:11, Mar 02:11, Dec 02:10, Nov 05:14, Jul 08:9, Oct 09:12, Nov 10:3, Jan 11:8, Jun 12:12

➲ *Clinical Examples in Radiology* Spring 11:10, Summer 16:4

(62263 includes codes 72275 and 77003)

62264 1 day

➲ *CPT Changes: An Insider's View* 2003

➲ *CPT Assistant* Nov 05:14, Jul 08:9, Oct 09:12, Nov 10:3, Jan 11:8, Jun 12:12

➲ *Clinical Examples in Radiology* Spring 11:10, Summer 16:4

(Do not report 62264 with 62263)

(62264 includes codes 72275 and 77003)

62267 Percutaneous aspiration within the nucleus pulposus, intervertebral disc, or paravertebral tissue for diagnostic purposes

➲ *CPT Changes: An Insider's View* 2009

➲ *CPT Assistant* Nov 10:3, Jan 11:8, Jul 12:3

➲ *Clinical Examples in Radiology* Fall 10:8, Spring 11:10, Winter 14:10, Summer 16:4

(For imaging, use 77003)

►(Do not report 62267 in conjunction with 10005, 10006, 10007, 10008, 10009, 10010, 10011, 10012, 20225, 62287, 62290, 62291)◄

62268 Percutaneous aspiration, spinal cord cyst or syrinx

➲ *CPT Assistant* Dec 17:13

(For radiological supervision and interpretation, see 76942, 77002, 77012)

62269 Biopsy of spinal cord, percutaneous needle

➲ *Clinical Examples in Radiology* Fall 10:7, Winter 17:5

(For radiological supervision and interpretation, see 76942, 77002, 77012)

►(For fine needle aspiration biopsy, see 10004, 10005, 10006, 10007, 10008, 10009, 10010, 10011, 10012, 10021)◄

(For evaluation of fine needle aspirate, see 88172, 88173)

62270 Spinal puncture, lumbar, diagnostic

➲ *CPT Changes: An Insider's View* 2000, 2002

➲ *CPT Assistant* Nov 99:32-33, Oct 03:2, Jul 06:4, Jul 07:1, Oct 09:12, Nov 10:3, Jan 11:8, Mar 12:3

➲ *Clinical Examples in Radiology* Spring 11:9, Winter 14:9-10, Summer 16:4

62272 Spinal puncture, therapeutic, for drainage of cerebrospinal fluid (by needle or catheter)

➲ *CPT Changes: An Insider's View* 2000

➲ *CPT Assistant* Nov 99:32-33, Nov 10:3, Dec 13:14

➲ *Clinical Examples in Radiology* Spring 11:10, Winter 14:9-10, Summer 16:4

62273 Injection, epidural, of blood or clot patch

➲ *CPT Changes: An Insider's View* 2000

➲ *CPT Assistant* Nov 99:32-34, Oct 09:12, Nov 10:3

➲ *Clinical Examples in Radiology* Spring 11:10, Winter 14:10, Summer 16:4

(For injection of diagnostic or therapeutic substance[s], see 62320, 62321, 62322, 62323, 62324, 62325, 62326, 62327)

62280 Injection/infusion of neurolytic substance (eg, alcohol, phenol, iced saline solutions), with or without other therapeutic substance; subarachnoid

➲ *CPT Changes: An Insider's View* 2000

➲ *CPT Assistant* Nov 99:32-34, Jan 00:2, Jul 08:9, Oct 09:12, Feb 10:11, Nov 10:3, Jan 11:8, Jun 12:12

➲ *Clinical Examples in Radiology* Spring 11:10, Winter 14:10, Summer 16:4

62281 epidural, cervical or thoracic

➲ *CPT Changes: An Insider's View* 2000

➲ *CPT Assistant* Apr 96:11, Nov 99:32-34, Jan 00:2, Jul 08:9, Oct 09:12, Feb 10:11, May 10:10, Nov 10:3, Jan 11:8, Jun 12:12

➲ *Clinical Examples in Radiology* Spring 11:10, Winter 14:10, Summer 16:4

62282 epidural, lumbar, sacral (caudal)

➲ *CPT Changes: An Insider's View* 2000

➲ *CPT Assistant* Apr 96:11, Nov 99:32-34, Jan 00:2, Jul 08:9, Oct 09:12, Feb 10:11, Nov 10:3, Jan 11:8, Jun 12:12

➲ *Clinical Examples in Radiology* Spring 11:10, Winter 14:10, Summer 16:4

62284 Injection procedure for myelography and/or computed tomography, lumbar

➲ *CPT Changes: An Insider's View* 2003, 2008, 2015

➲ *CPT Assistant* Fall 93:13, Sep 04:13

➲ *Clinical Examples in Radiology* Fall 06:5-6, 11-12, Spring 11:9, Fall 14:6, 7, 11

(Do not report 62284 in conjunction with 62302, 62303, 62304, 62305, 72240, 72255, 72265, 72270)

(When both 62284 and 72240, 72255, 72265, 72270 are performed by the same physician or other qualified health care professional for myelography, see 62302, 62303, 62304, 62305)

(For injection procedure at C1-C2, use 61055)

(For radiological supervision and interpretation, see **Radiology**)

62287 Decompression procedure, percutaneous, of nucleus pulposus of intervertebral disc, any method utilizing needle based technique to remove disc material under fluoroscopic imaging or other form of indirect visualization, with discography and/or epidural injection(s) at the treated level(s), when performed, single or multiple levels, lumbar

➲ *CPT Changes: An Insider's View* 2000, 2009, 2012, 2017

➲ *CPT Assistant* Nov 99:34, Mar 02:11, Oct 10:9, Jul 12:3, Oct 12:14, Apr 14:11, Mar 15:10, Feb 17:12

(Do not report 62287 in conjunction with 62267, 62290, 62322, 77003, 77012, 72295, when performed at same level)

(For non-needle based technique for percutaneous decompression of nucleus pulposus of intervertebral disc, see 0274T, 0275T)

62290 Injection procedure for discography, each level; lumbar

➲ *CPT Changes: An Insider's View* 2000

➲ *CPT Assistant* Nov 99:35, Apr 03:27, Mar 11:7, Jul 12:3

➲ *Clinical Examples in Radiology* Fall 10:10

62291 cervical or thoracic

➲ *CPT Changes: An Insider's View* 2000

➲ *CPT Assistant* Nov 99:35, Mar 11:7

➲ *Clinical Examples in Radiology* Fall 10:10

(For radiological supervision and interpretation, see 72285, 72295)

62292 Injection procedure for chemonucleolysis, including discography, intervertebral disc, single or multiple levels, lumbar

➲ *CPT Assistant* Oct 99:10

62294 Injection procedure, arterial, for occlusion of arteriovenous malformation, spinal

62302 Myelography via lumbar injection, including radiological supervision and interpretation; cervical

➲ *CPT Changes: An Insider's View* 2015

➲ *Clinical Examples in Radiology* Fall 14:6, Fall 15:10, Summer 16:4

(Do not report 62302 in conjunction with 62284, 62303, 62304, 62305, 72240, 72255, 72265, 72270)

62303 thoracic

➲ *CPT Changes: An Insider's View* 2015

➲ *Clinical Examples in Radiology* Fall 14:6, Fall 15:10, Summer 16:4

(Do not report 62303 in conjunction with 62284, 62302, 62304, 62305, 72240, 72255, 72265, 72270)

62304 lumbosacral

➔ *CPT Changes: An Insider's View* 2015

➔ *Clinical Examples in Radiology* Fall 14:3, 6, Fall 15:10, Summer 16:4

(Do not report 62304 in conjunction with 62284, 62302, 62303, 62305, 72240, 72255, 72265, 72270)

62305 2 or more regions (eg, lumbar/thoracic, cervical/thoracic, lumbar/cervical, lumbar/thoracic/cervical)

➔ *CPT Changes: An Insider's View* 2015

➔ *Clinical Examples in Radiology* Fall 14:6, 7, Fall 15:10, Summer 16:4

(Do not report 62305 in conjunction with 62284, 62302, 62303, 62304, 72240, 72255, 72265, 72270)

(For myelography lumbar injection and imaging performed by different physicians or other qualified health care professionals, see 62284 or 72240, 72255, 72265, 72270)

(For injection procedure at C1-C2, use 61055)

(62310 has been deleted. To report, use 62320)

(62311 has been deleted. To report, use 62322)

(62318 has been deleted. To report, use 62324)

(62319 has been deleted. To report, use 62326)

62320 Injection(s), of diagnostic or therapeutic substance(s) (eg, anesthetic, antispasmodic, opioid, steroid, other solution), not including neurolytic substances, including needle or catheter placement, interlaminar epidural or subarachnoid, cervical or thoracic; without imaging guidance

➔ *CPT Changes: An Insider's View* 2017

➔ *CPT Assistant* Sep 17:6

62321 with imaging guidance (ie, fluoroscopy or CT)

➔ *CPT Changes: An Insider's View* 2017

➔ *CPT Assistant* Sep 17:6

(Do not report 62321 in conjunction with 77003, 77012, 76942)

62322 Injection(s), of diagnostic or therapeutic substance(s) (eg, anesthetic, antispasmodic, opioid, steroid, other solution), not including neurolytic substances, including needle or catheter placement, interlaminar epidural or subarachnoid, lumbar or sacral (caudal); without imaging guidance

➔ *CPT Changes: An Insider's View* 2017

➔ *CPT Assistant* Sep 17:6

62323 with imaging guidance (ie, fluoroscopy or CT)

➔ *CPT Changes: An Insider's View* 2017

➔ *CPT Assistant* Sep 17:6

(Do not report 62323 in conjunction with 77003, 77012, 76942)

62324 Injection(s), including indwelling catheter placement, continuous infusion or intermittent bolus, of diagnostic or therapeutic substance(s) (eg, anesthetic, antispasmodic, opioid, steroid, other solution), not including neurolytic substances, interlaminar epidural or subarachnoid, cervical or thoracic; without imaging guidance

➔ *CPT Changes: An Insider's View* 2017

➔ *CPT Assistant* May 17:10, Sep 17:6

62325 with imaging guidance (ie, fluoroscopy or CT)

➔ *CPT Changes: An Insider's View* 2017

➔ *CPT Assistant* May 17:10, Sep 17:6

(Do not report 62325 in conjunction with 77003, 77012, 76942)

62326 Injection(s), including indwelling catheter placement, continuous infusion or intermittent bolus, of diagnostic or therapeutic substance(s) (eg, anesthetic, antispasmodic, opioid, steroid, other solution), not including neurolytic substances, interlaminar epidural or subarachnoid, lumbar or sacral (caudal); without imaging guidance

➔ *CPT Changes: An Insider's View* 2017

➔ *CPT Assistant* May 17:10, Sep 17:7

62327 with imaging guidance (ie, fluoroscopy or CT)

➔ *CPT Changes: An Insider's View* 2017

➔ *CPT Assistant* May 17:10, Sep 17:7

(Do not report 62327 in conjunction with 77003, 77012, 76942)

(Report 01996 for daily hospital management of continuous epidural or subarachnoid drug administration performed in conjunction with 62324, 62325, 62326, 62327)

Catheter Implantation

(For percutaneous placement of intrathecal or epidural catheter, see 62270, 62272, 62273, 62280, 62281, 62282, 62284, 62320, 62321, 62322, 62323, 62324, 62325, 62326, 62327)

62350 Implantation, revision or repositioning of tunneled intrathecal or epidural catheter, for long-term medication administration via an external pump or implantable reservoir/infusion pump; without laminectomy

➔ *CPT Changes: An Insider's View* 2000, 2001

➔ *CPT Assistant* Nov 99:36

62351 with laminectomy

➔ *CPT Changes: An Insider's View* 2000

➔ *CPT Assistant* Nov 99:36

(For refilling and maintenance of an implantable infusion pump for spinal or brain drug therapy, see 95990, 95991)

62355 Removal of previously implanted intrathecal or epidural catheter

Reservoir/Pump Implantation

62360 Implantation or replacement of device for intrathecal or epidural drug infusion; subcutaneous reservoir

62361 nonprogrammable pump

62362 programmable pump, including preparation of pump, with or without programming

➔ *CPT Assistant* Mar 97:11

Intrathecal or Epidural Drug Infusion Pump Implantation

62362

The reservoir is placed in the subcutaneous tissues and attached to a previously placed catheter for intrathecal or epidural drug infusion.

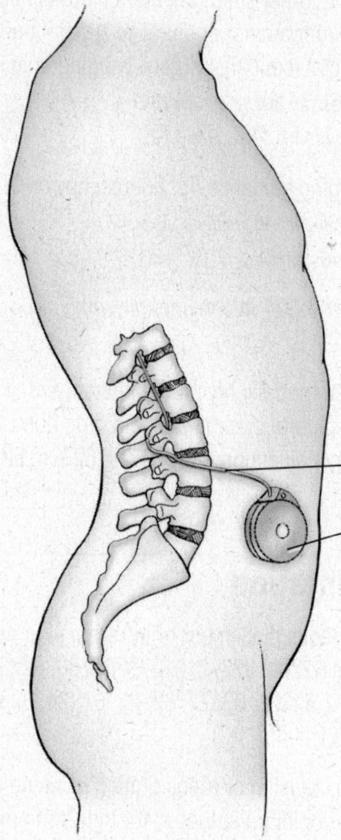

62365 Removal of subcutaneous reservoir or pump, previously implanted for intrathecal or epidural infusion

62367 Electronic analysis of programmable, implanted pump for intrathecal or epidural drug infusion (includes evaluation of reservoir status, alarm status, drug prescription status); without reprogramming or refill

➔ *CPT Changes: An Insider's View* 2012

➔ *CPT Assistant* Jul 12:5, 6, Aug 12:10, 11, 12, 15

62368 with reprogramming

➔ *CPT Assistant* Nov 02:10, Jul 06:1, Jul 12:5, 6, Aug 12:10, 11, 12, 15

(For refilling and maintenance of an implantable infusion pump for spinal or brain drug therapy, see 95990-95991)

62369 with reprogramming and refill

➔ *CPT Changes: An Insider's View* 2012

➔ *CPT Assistant* Jul 12:5, 6, Aug 12:10, 11, 12, 15

62370 with reprogramming and refill (requiring skill of a physician or other qualified health care professional)

➔ *CPT Changes: An Insider's View* 2012, 2013

➔ *CPT Assistant* Jul 12:5, 6, Aug 12:10, 11, 12, 15

(Do not report 62367-62370 in conjunction with 95990, 95991. For refilling and maintenance of a reservoir or an implantable infusion pump for spinal or brain drug delivery without reprogramming, see 95990, 95991)

Coding Tip

Instructions for Use of the CPT Codebook

When advanced practice nurses and physician assistants are working with physicians they are considered as working in the exact same specialty and exact same subspecialties as the physician. A "physician or other qualified health care professional" is an individual who is qualified by education, training, licensure/regulation (when applicable), and facility privileging (when applicable) who performs a professional service within his or her scope of practice and independently reports that professional service. These professionals are distinct from "clinical staff." A clinical staff member is a person who works under the supervision of a physician or other qualified health care professional, and who is allowed by law, regulation, and facility policy to perform or assist in the performance of a specific professional service, but does not individually report that professional service. Other policies may also affect who may report specific services.

CPT Coding Guidelines, Introduction, Instructions for Use of the CPT Codebook

Endoscopic Decompression of Neural Elements and/or Excision of Herniated Intervertebral Discs

Definitions

For purposes of CPT coding, the following definitions of approach and visualization apply. The primary approach and visualization define the service, whether another method is incidentally applied. Surgical services are presumed open, unless otherwise specified.

Percutaneous: Image-guided procedures (eg, computer tomography [CT] or fluoroscopy) performed with indirect visualization of the spine without the use of any device that allows visualization through a surgical incision.

Endoscopic: Spinal procedures performed with continuous direct visualization of the spine through an endoscope.

Open: Spinal procedures performed with continuous direct visualization of the spine through a surgical opening.

Indirect visualization: Image-guided (eg, CT or fluoroscopy), not light-based visualization.

Direct visualization: Light-based visualization; can be performed by eye, or with surgical loupes, microscope, or endoscope.

(For the techniques of microsurgery and/or use of microscope, use 69990)

(For percutaneous decompression, see 62287, 0274T, 0275T)

62380 Endoscopic decompression of spinal cord, nerve root(s), including laminotomy, partial facetectomy, foraminotomy, discectomy and/or excision of herniated intervertebral disc, 1 interspace, lumbar

➲ *CPT Changes: An Insider's View* 2017

➲ *CPT Assistant* Feb 17:12

(For open procedures, see 63030, 63056)

(For bilateral procedure, report 62380 with modifier 50)

Posterior Extradural Laminotomy or Laminectomy for Exploration/ Decompression of Neural Elements or Excision of Herniated Intervertebral Discs

Definitions

For purposes of CPT coding, the following definitions of approach and visualization apply. The primary approach and visualization define the service, whether another method is incidentally applied. Surgical services are presumed open, unless otherwise specified.

Percutaneous: Image-guided procedures (eg, computer tomography [CT] or fluoroscopy) performed with indirect visualization of the spine without the use of any device that allows visualization through a surgical incision.

Endoscopic: Spinal procedures performed with continuous direct visualization of the spine through an endoscope.

Open: Spinal procedures performed with continuous direct visualization of the spine through a surgical opening.

Indirect visualization: Image-guided (eg, CT or fluoroscopy), not light-based visualization.

Direct visualization: Light-based visualization; can be performed by eye, or with surgical loupes, microscope, or endoscope.

(When 63001-63048 are followed by arthrodesis, see 22590-22614)

(For the techniques of microsurgery and/or use of microscope, use 69990)

(For percutaneous decompression, see 62287, 0274T, 0275T)

63001 Laminectomy with exploration and/or decompression of spinal cord and/or cauda equina, without facetectomy, foraminotomy or discectomy (eg, spinal stenosis), 1 or 2 vertebral segments; cervical

➲ *CPT Assistant* Jan 01:12, Jun 07:1, Jul 11:13, Jul 12:3, Jul 13:3

63003 thoracic

➲ *CPT Assistant* Jan 01:12, Jul 12:3, Jul 13:3

63005 lumbar, except for spondylolisthesis

➲ *CPT Assistant* Jan 01:12, Jul 12:3, Jul 13:3, Dec 13:17

Lumbar Laminectomy
63005

With the patient prone and under general anesthesia, the laminae and underlying ligamentum flavum are removed.

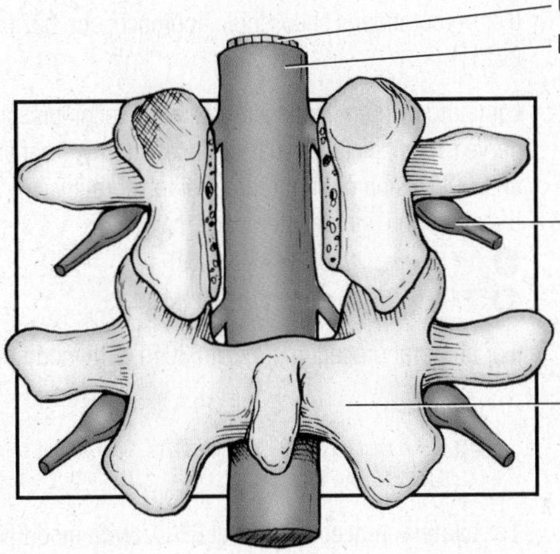

63011 sacral

➲ *CPT Assistant* Jan 01:12, Jul 13:3

63012 Laminectomy with removal of abnormal facets and/or pars inter-articularis with decompression of cauda equina and nerve roots for spondylolisthesis, lumbar (Gill type procedure)

➲ *CPT Assistant* Jan 01:12, Jul 13:3

63015 Laminectomy with exploration and/or decompression of spinal cord and/or cauda equina, without facetectomy, foraminotomy or discectomy (eg, spinal stenosis), more than 2 vertebral segments; cervical

➲ *CPT Assistant* Jan 01:12, Jul 13:3

63016 thoracic

➲ *CPT Assistant* Jan 01:12, Jul 13:3

63017 lumbar

➲ *CPT Assistant* Jan 01:12, Jul 13:3

63020 Laminotomy (hemilaminectomy), with decompression of nerve root(s), including partial facetectomy, foraminotomy and/or excision of herniated intervertebral disc; 1 interspace, cervical

➲ *CPT Changes: An Insider's View* 2000, 2009, 2012

➲ *CPT Assistant* Nov 99:36, Jan 01:12, Jul 12:4, Dec 12:13, Jul 13:3

Nervous 61000-64999

(For bilateral procedure, report 63020 with modifier 50)

63030 1 interspace, lumbar

CPT Changes: An Insider's View 2000, 2009, 2012

CPT Assistant Mar 96:7, Nov 99:36, Jan 01:12, Feb 01:10, Sep 02:10, Oct 04:12, Oct 08:10, Oct 09:9, Nov 10:4, Mar 11:7, Jul 11:13, Jul 12:3, 4, Dec 12:13, Jul 13:3, Dec 13:17, May 16:13, Feb 17:13

(For bilateral procedure, report 63030 with modifier 50)

+ 63035 each additional interspace, cervical or lumbar (List separately in addition to code for primary procedure)

CPT Changes: An Insider's View 2000, 2009, 2012

CPT Assistant Fall 91:8, Mar 96:7, Nov 99:36, Jan 01:12, Feb 01:10, Jul 12:4

(Use 63035 in conjunction with 63020-63030)

(For bilateral procedure, report 63035 with modifier 50)

(For percutaneous endoscopic approach, see 0274T, 0275T)

63040 Laminotomy (hemilaminectomy), with decompression of nerve root(s), including partial facetectomy, foraminotomy and/or excision of herniated intervertebral disc, reexploration, single interspace; cervical

CPT Changes: An Insider's View 2001

CPT Assistant Jan 99:11, Jan 01:12, Jul 13:3

(For bilateral procedure, report 63040 with modifier 50)

63042 lumbar

CPT Assistant Jan 99:11, Jan 01:12, Oct 08:10, Oct 09:9, Jul 11:13, Jul 13:3

(For bilateral procedure, report 63042 with modifier 50)

+ 63043 each additional cervical interspace (List separately in addition to code for primary procedure)

CPT Changes: An Insider's View 2001

(Use 63043 in conjunction with 63040)

(For bilateral procedure, report 63043 with modifier 50)

+ 63044 each additional lumbar interspace (List separately in addition to code for primary procedure)

CPT Changes: An Insider's View 2001

(Use 63044 in conjunction with 63042)

(For bilateral procedure, report 63044 with modifier 50)

63045 Laminectomy, facetectomy and foraminotomy (unilateral or bilateral with decompression of spinal cord, cauda equina and/or nerve root[s], [eg, spinal or lateral recess stenosis]), single vertebral segment; cervical

CPT Assistant Jan 01:12, Dec 12:13, Jul 13:3

63046 thoracic

CPT Assistant Jan 99:11, Jan 01:12, Dec 12:13, Jul 13:3

63047 lumbar

CPT Assistant Jan 99:11, Jan 01:12, Feb 01:10, Nov 02:11, Apr 08:11, Jul 08:7, Oct 08:10, Oct 09:9, Nov 10:4, Jul 11:13, Dec 12:13, Jul 13:3, Dec 13:17, Dec 14:16, Oct 16:11, Feb 17:13

+ 63048 each additional segment, cervical, thoracic, or lumbar (List separately in addition to code for primary procedure)

CPT Assistant Fall 91:8, Jan 99:11, Jan 01:12, Dec 12:13

(Use 63048 in conjunction with 63045-63047)

63050 Laminoplasty, cervical, with decompression of the spinal cord, 2 or more vertebral segments;

CPT Changes: An Insider's View 2005

CPT Assistant Jul 13:3

63051 with reconstruction of the posterior bony elements (including the application of bridging bone graft and non-segmental fixation devices [eg, wire, suture, mini-plates], when performed)

CPT Changes: An Insider's View 2005

CPT Assistant Jul 11:13, Jul 13:3

(Do not report 63050 or 63051 in conjunction with 22600, 22614, 22840-22842, 63001, 63015, 63045, 63048, 63295 for the same vertebral segment(s))

Transpedicular or Costovertebral Approach for Posterolateral Extradural Exploration/Decompression

63055 Transpedicular approach with decompression of spinal cord, equina and/or nerve root(s) (eg, herniated intervertebral disc), single segment; thoracic

CPT Changes: An Insider's View 2000

CPT Assistant Nov 99:36, Jul 13:3

63056 lumbar (including transfacet, or lateral extraforaminal approach) (eg, far lateral herniated intervertebral disc)

CPT Changes: An Insider's View 2000

CPT Assistant Nov 99:36, Oct 09:9, Nov 11:10, Jul 12:3, Jul 13:3, Jan 14:9

+ 63057 each additional segment, thoracic or lumbar (List separately in addition to code for primary procedure)

CPT Changes: An Insider's View 2000

CPT Assistant Nov 99:36

(Use 63057 in conjunction with 63055, 63056)

63064 Costovertebral approach with decompression of spinal cord or nerve root(s) (eg, herniated intervertebral disc), thoracic; single segment

CPT Assistant Fall 92:19, Jul 13:3

+ 63066 each additional segment (List separately in addition to code for primary procedure)

(Use 63066 in conjunction with 63064)

(For excision of thoracic intraspinal lesions by laminectomy, see 63266, 63271, 63276, 63281, 63286)

Anterior or Anterolateral Approach for Extradural Exploration/Decompression

For the following codes, when two surgeons work together as primary surgeons performing distinct part(s) of spinal cord exploration/decompression operation, each surgeon should report his/her distinct operative work by appending modifier 62 to the procedure code (and any associated add-on codes for that procedure code as long as both surgeons continue to work together as primary surgeons). In this situation, modifier 62 may be appended to the definitive procedure code(s) 63075, 63077, 63081, 63085, 63087, 63090 and, as appropriate, to associated additional interspace add-on code(s) 63076, 63078 or additional segment add-on code(s) 63082, 63086, 63088, 63091 as long as both surgeons continue to work together as primary surgeons.

For vertebral corpectomy, the term **partial** is used to describe removal of a substantial portion of the body of the vertebra. In the cervical spine, the amount of bone removed is defined as at least one-half of the vertebral body. In the thoracic and lumbar spine, the amount of bone removed is defined as at least one-third of the vertebral body.

63075 Discectomy, anterior, with decompression of spinal cord and/or nerve root(s), including osteophytectomy; cervical, single interspace

➲ *CPT Changes: An Insider's View* 2002

➲ *CPT Assistant* Nov 98:18, Jan 01:12, Feb 02:4, Jul 13:3, Apr 15:7

(Do not report 63075 in conjunction with 22554, even if performed by separate individuals. To report anterior cervical discectomy and interbody fusion at the same level during the same session, use 22551)

+ 63076 cervical, each additional interspace (List separately in addition to code for primary procedure)

➲ *CPT Changes: An Insider's View* 2002

➲ *CPT Assistant* Nov 98:18, Jan 01:12, Feb 02:4

(Do not report 63076 in conjunction with 22554, even if performed by separate individuals. To report anterior cervical discectomy and interbody fusion at the same level during the same session, use 22552)

(Use 63076 in conjunction with 63075)

63077 thoracic, single interspace

➲ *CPT Changes: An Insider's View* 2002

➲ *CPT Assistant* Nov 98:18, Jan 01:12, Feb 02:4, Jul 13:3

+ 63078 thoracic, each additional interspace (List separately in addition to code for primary procedure)

➲ *CPT Changes: An Insider's View* 2002

➲ *CPT Assistant* Nov 98:18, Jan 01:12, Feb 02:4

(Use 63078 in conjunction with 63077)

(Do not report code 69990 in addition to codes 63075-63078)

63081 Vertebral corpectomy (vertebral body resection), partial or complete, anterior approach with decompression of spinal cord and/or nerve root(s); cervical, single segment

➲ *CPT Changes: An Insider's View* 2002

➲ *CPT Assistant* Spring 93:37, Feb 02:4, Jul 13:3, Jun 15:10, Apr 16:8

+ 63082 cervical, each additional segment (List separately in addition to code for primary procedure)

➲ *CPT Changes: An Insider's View* 2002

➲ *CPT Assistant* Spring 93:37, Feb 02:4, Apr 16:8

(Use 63082 in conjunction with 63081)

(For transoral approach, see 61575, 61576)

63085 Vertebral corpectomy (vertebral body resection), partial or complete, transthoracic approach with decompression of spinal cord and/or nerve root(s); thoracic, single segment

➲ *CPT Changes: An Insider's View* 2002

➲ *CPT Assistant* Spring 93:37, Feb 02:4, Jul 13:3, Apr 16:8

+ 63086 thoracic, each additional segment (List separately in addition to code for primary procedure)

➲ *CPT Changes: An Insider's View* 2002

➲ *CPT Assistant* Spring 93:37, Feb 02:4, Apr 16:8

(Use 63086 in conjunction with 63085)

63087 Vertebral corpectomy (vertebral body resection), partial or complete, combined thoracolumbar approach with decompression of spinal cord, cauda equina or nerve root(s), lower thoracic or lumbar; single segment

➲ *CPT Changes: An Insider's View* 2002

➲ *CPT Assistant* Spring 93:37, Feb 02:4, Jul 13:3, Apr 16:8

+ 63088 each additional segment (List separately in addition to code for primary procedure)

➲ *CPT Changes: An Insider's View* 2002

➲ *CPT Assistant* Spring 93:37, Feb 02:4, Apr 16:8

(Use 63088 in conjunction with 63087)

63090 Vertebral corpectomy (vertebral body resection), partial or complete, transperitoneal or retroperitoneal approach with decompression of spinal cord, cauda equina or nerve root(s), lower thoracic, lumbar, or sacral; single segment

➲ *CPT Changes: An Insider's View* 2002

➲ *CPT Assistant* Spring 93:37, Mar 96:6, Feb 02:4, Jul 13:3, Apr 16:8

+ 63091 each additional segment (List separately in addition to code for primary procedure)

➲ *CPT Changes: An Insider's View* 2002

➲ *CPT Assistant* Spring 93:37, Mar 96:6, Feb 02:4, Apr 16:8

(Use 63091 in conjunction with 63090)

(Procedures 63081-63091 include discectomy above and/or below vertebral segment)

(If followed by arthrodesis, see 22548-22812)

(For reconstruction of spine, use appropriate vertebral corpectomy codes 63081-63091, bone graft codes 20930-20938, arthrodesis codes 22548-22812, and spinal instrumentation codes 22840-22855, 22859)

Lateral Extracavitary Approach for Extradural Exploration/Decompression

For vertebral corpectomy, the term **partial** is used to describe removal of a substantial portion of the body of the vertebra. In the cervical spine, the amount of bone removed is defined as at least one-half of the vertebral body. In the thoracic and lumbar spine, the amount of bone removed is defined as at least one-third of the vertebral body.

63101 Vertebral corpectomy (vertebral body resection), partial or complete, lateral extracavitary approach with decompression of spinal cord and/or nerve root(s) (eg, for tumor or retropulsed bone fragments); thoracic, single segment
➔ *CPT Changes: An Insider's View* 2004
➔ *CPT Assistant* Jul 13:3

63102 lumbar, single segment
➔ *CPT Changes: An Insider's View* 2004
➔ *CPT Assistant* Jul 13:3

+ 63103 thoracic or lumbar, each additional segment (List separately in addition to code for primary procedure)
➔ *CPT Changes: An Insider's View* 2004

(Use 63103 in conjunction with 63101 and 63102)

Incision

63170 Laminectomy with myelotomy (eg, Bischof or DREZ type), cervical, thoracic, or thoracolumbar
➔ *CPT Assistant* Jul 13:3

63172 Laminectomy with drainage of intramedullary cyst/syrinx; to subarachnoid space
➔ *CPT Assistant* Jul 13:3

63173 to peritoneal or pleural space
➔ *CPT Changes: An Insider's View* 2004
➔ *CPT Assistant* Jul 13:3

63180 Laminectomy and section of dentate ligaments, with or without dural graft, cervical; 1 or 2 segments
➔ *CPT Assistant* Jul 13:3

63182 more than 2 segments
➔ *CPT Assistant* Jul 13:3

63185 Laminectomy with rhizotomy; 1 or 2 segments
➔ *CPT Assistant* Jul 13:3

63190 more than 2 segments
➔ *CPT Assistant* Jul 13:3

63191 Laminectomy with section of spinal accessory nerve
➔ *CPT Assistant* Jul 13:3

(For bilateral procedure, report 63191 with modifier 50)

(For resection of sternocleidomastoid muscle, use 21720)

63194 Laminectomy with cordotomy, with section of 1 spinothalamic tract, 1 stage; cervical
➔ *CPT Assistant* Jul 13:3

63195 thoracic
➔ *CPT Assistant* Jul 13:3

63196 Laminectomy with cordotomy, with section of both spinothalamic tracts, 1 stage; cervical
➔ *CPT Assistant* Jul 13:3

63197 thoracic
➔ *CPT Assistant* Jul 13:3

63198 Laminectomy with cordotomy with section of both spinothalamic tracts, 2 stages within 14 days; cervical
➔ *CPT Assistant* Jul 13:3

63199 thoracic
➔ *CPT Assistant* Jul 13:3

63200 Laminectomy, with release of tethered spinal cord, lumbar
➔ *CPT Assistant* Jul 13:3

Excision by Laminectomy of Lesion Other Than Herniated Disc

63250 Laminectomy for excision or occlusion of arteriovenous malformation of spinal cord; cervical
➔ *CPT Assistant* Jul 13:3

63251 thoracic
➔ *CPT Assistant* Jul 13:3

63252 thoracolumbar
➔ *CPT Assistant* Jul 13:3

63265 Laminectomy for excision or evacuation of intraspinal lesion other than neoplasm, extradural; cervical
➔ *CPT Assistant* Jul 13:3

63266 thoracic

63267 lumbar
➔ *CPT Assistant* Jul 13:3

63268 sacral
➔ *CPT Assistant* Jul 13:3

63270 Laminectomy for excision of intraspinal lesion other than neoplasm, intradural; cervical
➔ *CPT Assistant* Jul 13:3

63271 thoracic
➔ *CPT Assistant* Jul 13:3

63272 lumbar
➔ *CPT Assistant* Jul 13:3

63273 sacral
➔ *CPT Assistant* Jul 13:3

63275 Laminectomy for biopsy/excision of intraspinal neoplasm; extradural, cervical
➔ *CPT Assistant* Jul 13:3

63276 extradural, thoracic
➔ *CPT Assistant* Jul 13:3

63277 extradural, lumbar
➔ *CPT Assistant* Jul 13:3

63278 extradural, sacral
➔ *CPT Assistant* Jul 13:3

63280 intradural, extramedullary, cervical
➔ *CPT Assistant* Jul 13:3

63281 intradural, extramedullary, thoracic
➔ *CPT Assistant* Jul 13:3

63282 intradural, extramedullary, lumbar
➔ *CPT Assistant* Jul 13:3

63283 intradural, sacral
➔ *CPT Assistant* Jul 13:3

63285 intradural, intramedullary, cervical
➔ *CPT Assistant* Jul 13:3

63286 intradural, intramedullary, thoracic
➔ *CPT Assistant* Jul 13:3

63287 intradural, intramedullary, thoracolumbar
➔ *CPT Assistant* Jul 13:3

63290 combined extradural-intradural lesion, any level
➔ *CPT Assistant* Jul 13:3

(For drainage of intramedullary cyst/syrinx, use 63172, 63173)

+ 63295 Osteoplastic reconstruction of dorsal spinal elements, following primary intraspinal procedure (List separately in addition to code for primary procedure)
➔ *CPT Changes: An Insider's View* 2005

(Use 63295 in conjunction with 63172, 63173, 63185, 63190, 63200-63290)

(Do not report 63295 in conjunction with 22590-22614, 22840-22844, 63050, 63051 for the same vertebral segment(s))

Excision, Anterior or Anterolateral Approach, Intraspinal Lesion

For the following codes, when two surgeons work together as primary surgeons performing distinct part(s) of an anterior approach for an intraspinal excision, each surgeon should report his/her distinct operative work by appending modifier 62 to the single definitive procedure code. In this situation, modifier 62 may be appended to the definitive procedure code(s) 63300-63307 and, as appropriate, to the associated additional segment add-on code 63308 as long as both surgeons continue to work together as primary surgeons.

For vertebral corpectomy, the term **partial** is used to describe removal of a substantial portion of the body of the vertebra. In the cervical spine, the amount of bone removed is defined as at least one-half of the vertebral body. In the thoracic and lumbar spine, the amount of bone removed is defined as at least one-third of the vertebral body.

(For arthrodesis, see 22548-22585)

(For reconstruction of spine, see 20930-20938)

63300 Vertebral corpectomy (vertebral body resection), partial or complete, for excision of intraspinal lesion, single segment; extradural, cervical
➔ *CPT Assistant* Feb 02:4, Jul 13:3

63301 extradural, thoracic by transthoracic approach
➔ *CPT Assistant* Feb 02:4, Jul 13:3

63302 extradural, thoracic by thoracolumbar approach
➔ *CPT Assistant* Feb 02:4, Jul 13:3

63303 extradural, lumbar or sacral by transperitoneal or retroperitoneal approach
➔ *CPT Assistant* Feb 02:4, Jul 13:3

63304 intradural, cervical
➔ *CPT Assistant* Feb 02:4, Jul 13:3

63305 intradural, thoracic by transthoracic approach
➔ *CPT Assistant* Feb 02:4, Jul 13:3

63306 intradural, thoracic by thoracolumbar approach
➔ *CPT Assistant* Feb 02:4, Jul 13:3

63307 intradural, lumbar or sacral by transperitoneal or retroperitoneal approach
➔ *CPT Assistant* Feb 02:4, Jul 13:3

+ 63308 each additional segment (List separately in addition to codes for single segment)
➔ *CPT Assistant* Feb 02:4

(Use 63308 in conjunction with 63300-63307)

Stereotaxis

63600 Creation of lesion of spinal cord by stereotactic method, percutaneous, any modality (including stimulation and/or recording)

63610 Stereotactic stimulation of spinal cord, percutaneous, separate procedure not followed by other surgery

►(63615 has been deleted)◄

Stereotactic Radiosurgery (Spinal)

Spinal stereotactic radiosurgery is a distinct procedure that utilizes externally generated ionizing radiation to inactivate or eradicate defined target(s) in the spine without the need to make an incision. The target is defined by and the treatment is delivered using high-resolution stereotactic imaging. These codes are reported by the surgeon. The radiation oncologist reports the appropriate code(s) for clinical treatment planning, physics and dosimetry, treatment delivery and management from the **Radiation Oncology** section (77261-77790). Any necessary planning, dosimetry, targeting, positioning, or blocking by the neurosurgeon is included in the stereotactic radiation surgery services. The same individual should not report stereotactic radiosurgery services with radiation treatment management codes (77427-77432).

Spinal stereotactic radiosurgery is typically performed in a single planning and treatment session using a stereotactic image-guidance system, but can be performed with a planning session and in a limited number of treatment sessions, up to a maximum of five sessions. Do not report stereotactic radiosurgery more than once per lesion per course of treatment when the treatment requires greater than one session.

Stereotactic spinal surgery is only used when the tumor being treated affects spinal neural tissue or abuts the dura mater. Arteriovenous malformations must be subdural. For other radiation services of the spine, see **Radiation Oncology** services.

Codes 63620, 63621 include computer-assisted planning. Do not report 63620, 63621 in conjunction with 61781-61783.

(For intensity modulated beam delivery plan and treatment, see 77301, 77385, 77386. For stereotactic body radiation therapy, see 77373, 77435)

63620 Stereotactic radiosurgery (particle beam, gamma ray, or linear accelerator); 1 spinal lesion

➔ *CPT Changes: An Insider's View* 2009

➔ *CPT Assistant* Oct 10:3, Jul 11:12, Jun 15:6

(Do not report 63620 more than once per course of treatment)

+ 63621 each additional spinal lesion (List separately in addition to code for primary procedure)

➔ *CPT Changes: An Insider's View* 2009

➔ *CPT Assistant* Oct 10:3, Jul 11:12, Jun 15:6

(Report 63621 in conjunction with 63620)

(For each course of treatment, 63621 may be reported no more than once per lesion. Do not report 63621 more than 2 times for entire course of treatment regardless of number of lesions treated)

Neurostimulators (Spinal)

►For electronic analysis with programming, when performed, of spinal cord neurostimulator pulse generator/transmitters, see codes 95970, 95971, 95972. Test stimulation to confirm correct target site placement of the electrode array(s) and/or to confirm the functional status of the system is inherent to placement, and is not separately reported as electronic analysis or programming of the neurostimulator system. Electronic analysis (95970) at the time of implantation is not separately reported.◄

Codes 63650, 63655, and 63661-63664 describe the operative placement, revision, replacement, or removal of the spinal neurostimulator system components to provide spinal electrical stimulation. A neurostimulator system includes an implanted neurostimulator, external controller, extension, and collection of contacts. Multiple contacts or electrodes (4 or more) provide the actual electrical stimulation in the epidural space.

For percutaneously placed neurostimulator systems (63650, 63661, 63663), the contacts are on a catheter-like lead. An array defines the collection of contacts that are on one catheter.

For systems placed via an open surgical exposure (63655, 63662, 63664), the contacts are on a plate or paddle-shaped surface.

Do not report 63661 or 63663 when removing or replacing a temporary percutaneously placed array for an external generator.

63650 Percutaneous implantation of neurostimulator electrode array, epidural

➔ *CPT Changes: An Insider's View* 2010

➔ *CPT Assistant* Jun 98:3-4, Nov 98:18, Mar 99:11, Apr 99:10, Sep 99:3, Dec 08:8, Feb 10:9, Aug 10:8, Dec 10:14, Apr 11:10, Oct 13:19, Dec 15:17, Jan 16:12, Dec 17:16

Percutaneous Implantation of Neurostimulator Electrodes
63650

Single catheter electrode array is inserted percutaneously into the epidural space. A simple or complex receiver is subcutaneously implanted.

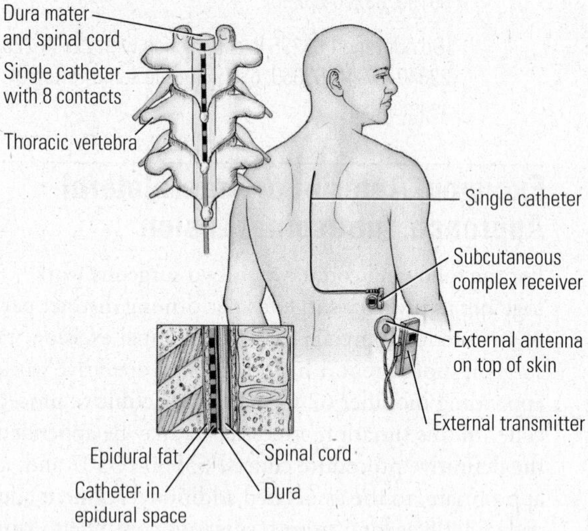

63655 Laminectomy for implantation of neurostimulator electrodes, plate/paddle, epidural

➔ *CPT Assistant* Jun 98:3-4, Nov 98:18, Sep 99:3-4, Dec 08:8, Aug 10:8, Dec 10:14, Apr 11:10

Placement of Neurostimulator Electrodes Through Laminectomy
63655

The electrode plate or paddle is placed in the epidural space via open exposure through large laminotomy or small laminectomy. The simple or complex receiver is subcutaneously implanted.

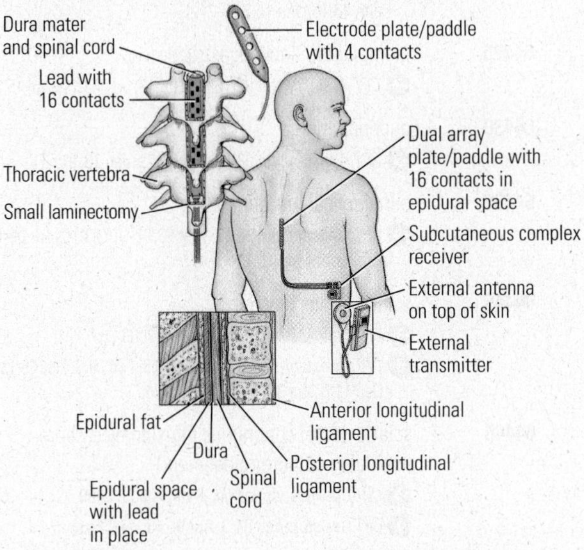

63661 Removal of spinal neurostimulator electrode percutaneous array(s), including fluoroscopy, when performed
➲ *CPT Changes: An Insider's View* 2010
➲ *CPT Assistant* Feb 10:9, Aug 10:8, Jan 11:8, Apr 11:10
➲ *Clinical Examples in Radiology* Spring 11:10

63662 Removal of spinal neurostimulator electrode plate/paddle(s) placed via laminotomy or laminectomy, including fluoroscopy, when performed
➲ *CPT Changes: An Insider's View* 2010
➲ *CPT Assistant* Feb 10:9, Aug 10:8, Apr 11:10
➲ *Clinical Examples in Radiology* Spring 11:10

63663 Revision including replacement, when performed, of spinal neurostimulator electrode percutaneous array(s), including fluoroscopy, when performed
➲ *CPT Changes: An Insider's View* 2010
➲ *CPT Assistant* Feb 10:9, Aug 10:8, Apr 11:10
➲ *Clinical Examples in Radiology* Spring 11:10

(Do not report 63663 in conjunction with 63661, 63662 for the same spinal level)

63664 Revision including replacement, when performed, of spinal neurostimulator electrode plate/paddle(s) placed via laminotomy or laminectomy, including fluoroscopy, when performed
➲ *CPT Changes: An Insider's View* 2010
➲ *CPT Assistant* Feb 10:9, Aug 10:8, Apr 11:10
➲ *Clinical Examples in Radiology* Spring 11:10

(Do not report 63664 in conjunction with 63661, 63662 for the same spinal level)

63685 Insertion or replacement of spinal neurostimulator pulse generator or receiver, direct or inductive coupling
➲ *CPT Changes: An Insider's View* 2005
➲ *CPT Assistant* Jun 98:3-4, Sep 99:5, Feb 10:9, Oct 10:14, Dec 10:14, Apr 11:10, Dec 17:16

(Do not report 63685 in conjunction with 63688 for the same pulse generator or receiver)

63688 Revision or removal of implanted spinal neurostimulator pulse generator or receiver
➲ *CPT Assistant* Jun 98:3-4, Sep 99:5, Feb 10:9, Apr 11:11

►(For electronic analysis with programming, when performed, of implanted spinal cord neurostimulator pulse generator/transmitter, see 95970, 95971, 95972)◄

Repair

63700 Repair of meningocele; less than 5 cm diameter

63702 larger than 5 cm diameter

(Do not use modifier 63 in conjunction with 63700, 63702)

63704 Repair of myelomeningocele; less than 5 cm diameter

63706 larger than 5 cm diameter

(Do not use modifier 63 in conjunction with 63704, 63706)

(For complex skin closure, see **Integumentary System**)

63707 Repair of dural/cerebrospinal fluid leak, not requiring laminectomy
➲ *CPT Changes: An Insider's View* 2002

63709 Repair of dural/cerebrospinal fluid leak or pseudomeningocele, with laminectomy
➲ *CPT Changes: An Insider's View* 2002

63710 Dural graft, spinal

(For laminectomy and section of dentate ligaments, with or without dural graft, cervical, see 63180, 63182)

Shunt, Spinal CSF

63740 Creation of shunt, lumbar, subarachnoid-peritoneal, -pleural, or other; including laminectomy
➲ *CPT Assistant* Winter 90:8

63741 percutaneous, not requiring laminectomy
➲ *CPT Assistant* Winter 90:8

63744 Replacement, irrigation or revision of lumbosubarachnoid shunt

63746 Removal of entire lumbosubarachnoid shunt system without replacement

(For insertion of subarachnoid catheter with reservoir and/or pump for intermittent or continuous infusion of drug including laminectomy, see 62351 and 62360, 62361 or 62362)

(For insertion or replacement of subarachnoid or epidural catheter, with reservoir and/or pump for drug infusion without laminectomy, see 62350 and 62360, 62361 or 62362)

Extracranial Nerves, Peripheral Nerves, and Autonomic Nervous System

(For intracranial surgery on cranial nerves, see 61450, 61460, 61790)

Introduction/Injection of Anesthetic Agent (Nerve Block), Diagnostic or Therapeutic

(For destruction by neurolytic agent or chemodenervation, see 62280-62282, 64600-64681)

(For epidural or subarachnoid injection, see 62320, 62321, 62322, 62323, 62324, 62325, 62326, 62327)

(64479-64487, 64490-64495 are unilateral procedures. For bilateral procedures, use modifier 50)

Somatic Nerves

64400 Injection, anesthetic agent; trigeminal nerve, any division or branch
- *CPT Changes: An Insider's View* 2000
- *CPT Assistant* Jul 98:10, May 99:8, Nov 99:36, Apr 05:13, Feb 10:9, Jan 13:13
- *Clinical Examples in Radiology* Summer 14:6

64402 facial nerve
- *CPT Assistant* Jul 98:10, Apr 05:13, Jan 13:13

64405 greater occipital nerve
- *CPT Assistant* Jul 98:10, Apr 05:13, Jan 13:13, Oct 16:11

64408 vagus nerve
- *CPT Assistant* Jul 98:10, Apr 05:13, Jan 13:13

64410 phrenic nerve
- *CPT Assistant* Jul 98:10, Apr 05:13, Jan 13:13

(64412 has been deleted. To report, use 64999)

64413 cervical plexus
- *CPT Assistant* Jul 98:10, Apr 05:13, Jan 13:13

64415 brachial plexus, single
- *CPT Changes: An Insider's View* 2003
- *CPT Assistant* Fall 92:17, Jul 98:10, May 99:8, Oct 01:9, Feb 04:7, Apr 05:13, Nov 06:23, Jan 13:13

64416 brachial plexus, continuous infusion by catheter (including catheter placement)
- *CPT Changes: An Insider's View* 2003, 2009
- *CPT Assistant* Feb 04:7, Apr 05:13, Jan 13:13

(Do not report 64416 in conjunction with 01996)

64417 axillary nerve
- *CPT Assistant* Jul 98:10, Apr 05:13, Jan 13:13

64418 suprascapular nerve
- *CPT Assistant* Jul 98:10, Apr 05:13, Aug 07:15, Jan 13:13

64420 intercostal nerve, single
- *CPT Assistant* Jul 98:10, Apr 05:13, Aug 10:12, Nov 10:9, Jan 13:13, Jun 15:3

64421 intercostal nerves, multiple, regional block
- *CPT Assistant* Jul 98:10, Apr 05:13, Aug 10:12, Nov 10:9, Jan 13:13, Jun 15:3

64425 ilioinguinal, iliohypogastric nerves
- *CPT Assistant* Jul 98:10, Apr 05:13, Jan 13:13, Jun 15:3

64430 pudendal nerve
- *CPT Assistant* Jul 98:10, Apr 05:13, Jan 13:13

64435 paracervical (uterine) nerve
- *CPT Assistant* Jul 98:10, Mar 03:22, Jul 03:15, Apr 05:13, Feb 12:11, Jan 13:13

64445 sciatic nerve, single
- *CPT Changes: An Insider's View* 2003
- *CPT Assistant* Jul 98:10, May 99:8, Feb 04:8, Apr 05:13, Dec 11:8, Apr 12:19, Jan 13:13

64446 sciatic nerve, continuous infusion by catheter (including catheter placement)
- *CPT Changes: An Insider's View* 2003, 2009
- *CPT Assistant* Feb 04:9, Apr 05:13, Jan 13:13

(Do not report 64446 in conjunction with 01996)

64447 femoral nerve, single
- *CPT Changes: An Insider's View* 2003
- *CPT Assistant* Feb 04:9, Apr 05:13, Jan 13:13, Nov 14:14, Dec 14:16, Sep 15:12

(Do not report 64447 in conjunction with 01996)

64448 femoral nerve, continuous infusion by catheter (including catheter placement)
- *CPT Changes: An Insider's View* 2003, 2009
- *CPT Assistant* Feb 04:10, Apr 05:13, Jan 13:13, Nov 14:14, Dec 14:16, Sep 15:12

(Do not report 64448 in conjunction with 01996)

64449 lumbar plexus, posterior approach, continuous infusion by catheter (including catheter placement)
- *CPT Changes: An Insider's View* 2004, 2009
- *CPT Assistant* Apr 05:13, Jan 13:13

(Do not report 64449 in conjunction with 01996)

64450 other peripheral nerve or branch
- *CPT Changes: An Insider's View* 2000
- *CPT Assistant* Jul 98:10, Nov 99:37, Dec 99:7, Oct 01:9, Aug 03:6, Apr 05:13, Jan 09:6, Jan 13:13, Sep 15:12, Nov 15:11, Oct 16:11
- *Clinical Examples in Radiology* Summer 14:6

64455 Injection(s), anesthetic agent and/or steroid, plantar common digital nerve(s) (eg, Morton's neuroma)
- *CPT Changes: An Insider's View* 2009
- *CPT Assistant* Jan 13:13

(Do not report 64455 in conjunction with 64632)

(Imaging guidance [fluoroscopy or CT] and any injection of contrast are inclusive components of 64479-64484. Imaging guidance and localization are required for the performance of 64479-64484)

(64470-64476 have been deleted. To report, see 64490-64495)

64461 Code is out of numerical sequence. See 64483-64487

64462 Code is out of numerical sequence. See 64483-64487

64463 Code is out of numerical sequence. See 64483-64487

64479 Injection(s), anesthetic agent and/or steroid, transforaminal epidural, with imaging guidance (fluoroscopy or CT); cervical or thoracic, single level

- *CPT Changes: An Insider's View* 2000, 2011
- *CPT Assistant* Nov 99:33, 37, Feb 00:4, Jul 08:9, Nov 08:11, Feb 10:9, Jan 11:8, Feb 11:4, Jul 11:16, Jul 12:5, Jan 16:9
- *Clinical Examples in Radiology* Summer 08:9, Spring 11:10, Winter 18:7

(For transforaminal epidural injection under ultrasound guidance, use 0228T)

+ 64480 cervical or thoracic, each additional level (List separately in addition to code for primary procedure)

- *CPT Changes: An Insider's View* 2000, 2011
- *CPT Assistant* Nov 99:33, 37, Feb 00:4, Feb 05:14, Jul 08:9, Feb 10:9, Jan 11:8, Feb 11:4, Jul 11:16, Jul 12:5
- *Clinical Examples in Radiology* Summer 08:9, Spring 11:10, Winter 18:7

(Use 64480 in conjunction with 64479)

(For transforaminal epidural injection under ultrasound guidance, use 0229T)

(For transforaminal epidural injection at the T12-L1 level, use 64479)

64483 lumbar or sacral, single level

- *CPT Changes: An Insider's View* 2000, 2011
- *CPT Assistant* Nov 99:33, 37, Feb 00:4, Jul 08:9, Feb 10:9, Jan 11:8, Feb 11:4, Jul 11:16, May 12:14, Jul 12:5, Oct 16:11
- *Clinical Examples in Radiology* Spring 11:10, Winter 18:7

(For transforaminal epidural injection under ultrasound guidance, use 0230T)

+ 64484 lumbar or sacral, each additional level (List separately in addition to code for primary procedure)

- *CPT Changes: An Insider's View* 2000, 2011
- *CPT Assistant* Nov 99:33, 37, Feb 00:4, Feb 05:14, Jul 08:9, Nov 08:11, Feb 10:9, Feb 11:4, Jul 11:16, Jul 12:5, Jan 16:9
- *Clinical Examples in Radiology* Spring 11:10, Winter 18:7

(Use 64484 in conjunction with 64483)

(For transforaminal epidural injection under ultrasound guidance, use 0231T)

(64479-64484 are unilateral procedures. For bilateral procedures, use modifier 50)

 # 64461 Paravertebral block (PVB) (paraspinous block), thoracic; single injection site (includes imaging guidance, when performed)

- *CPT Changes: An Insider's View* 2016
- *CPT Assistant* Jan 16:9

#+ 64462 second and any additional injection site(s) (includes imaging guidance, when performed) (List separately in addition to code for primary procedure)

- *CPT Changes: An Insider's View* 2016
- *CPT Assistant* Jan 16:9

(Use 64462 in conjunction with 64461)

(Do not report 64462 more than once per day)

 # 64463 continuous infusion by catheter (includes imaging guidance, when performed)

- *CPT Changes: An Insider's View* 2016
- *CPT Assistant* Jan 16:9

(Do not report 64461, 64462, 64463 in conjunction with 62320, 62324, 64420, 64421, 64479, 64480, 64490, 64491, 64492, 76942, 77002, 77003)

64486 Transversus abdominis plane (TAP) block (abdominal plane block, rectus sheath block) unilateral; by injection(s) (includes imaging guidance, when performed)

- *CPT Changes: An Insider's View* 2015
- *CPT Assistant* Jun 15:3
- *Clinical Examples in Radiology* Winter 18:8

64487 by continuous infusion(s) (includes imaging guidance, when performed)

- *CPT Changes: An Insider's View* 2015
- *CPT Assistant* Jun 15:3
- *Clinical Examples in Radiology* Winter 18:8

64488 Transversus abdominis plane (TAP) block (abdominal plane block, rectus sheath block) bilateral; by injections (includes imaging guidance, when performed)

- *CPT Changes: An Insider's View* 2015
- *CPT Assistant* Jun 15:3
- *Clinical Examples in Radiology* Winter 18:8

64489 by continuous infusions (includes imaging guidance, when performed)

- *CPT Changes: An Insider's View* 2015
- *CPT Assistant* Jun 15:3
- *Clinical Examples in Radiology* Winter 18:8

Paravertebral Spinal Nerves and Branches

(Image guidance [fluoroscopy or CT] and any injection of contrast are inclusive components of 64490-64495. Imaging guidance and localization are required for the performance of paravertebral facet joint injections described by codes 64490-64495. If imaging is not used, report 20552-20553. If ultrasound guidance is used, report 0213T-0218T)

(For bilateral paravertebral facet injection procedures, use modifier 50)

(For paravertebral facet injection of the T12-L1 joint, or nerves innervating that joint, use 64490)

64490 Injection(s), diagnostic or therapeutic agent, paravertebral facet (zygapophyseal) joint (or nerves innervating that joint) with image guidance (fluoroscopy or CT), cervical or thoracic; single level

➔ *CPT Changes: An Insider's View* 2010

➔ *CPT Assistant* Feb 10:9, Aug 10:12, Dec 10:13, Jan 11:8, Feb 11:4, Jun 12:10, Oct 12:15

➔ *Clinical Examples in Radiology* Winter 10:15, Spring 11:10, Winter 18:8

+ 64491 second level (List separately in addition to code for primary procedure)

➔ *CPT Changes: An Insider's View* 2010

➔ *CPT Assistant* Aug 10:12, Jun 12:10, Oct 12:15

➔ *Clinical Examples in Radiology* Winter 10:15

(Use 64491 in conjunction with 64490)

+ 64492 third and any additional level(s) (List separately in addition to code for primary procedure)

➔ *CPT Changes: An Insider's View* 2010

➔ *CPT Assistant* Feb 10:9, Aug 10:12, Jan 11:8, Feb 11:4, Jun 12:10, Oct 12:15

➔ *Clinical Examples in Radiology* Winter 10:14, Spring 11:10, Winter 18:8

(Do not report 64492 more than once per day)

(Use 64492 in conjunction with 64490, 64491)

64493 Injection(s), diagnostic or therapeutic agent, paravertebral facet (zygapophyseal) joint (or nerves innervating that joint) with image guidance (fluoroscopy or CT), lumbar or sacral; single level

➔ *CPT Changes: An Insider's View* 2010

➔ *CPT Assistant* Feb 10:9, Aug 10:12, Jan 11:8, Feb 11:4, Jun 12:10, Oct 12:15

➔ *Clinical Examples in Radiology* Winter 10:14, Spring 11:10, Winter 18:8

+ 64494 second level (List separately in addition to code for primary procedure)

➔ *CPT Changes: An Insider's View* 2010

➔ *CPT Assistant* Feb 10:9, Aug 10:12, Jan 11:8, Feb 11:4, Jun 12:10

➔ *Clinical Examples in Radiology* Winter 10:14, Spring 11:10, Winter 18:8

(Use 64494 in conjunction with 64493)

+ 64495 third and any additional level(s) (List separately in addition to code for primary procedure)

➔ *CPT Changes: An Insider's View* 2010

➔ *CPT Assistant* Feb 10:9, Aug 10:12, Jan 11:8, Feb 11:4, Jun 12:10, Oct 12:15

➔ *Clinical Examples in Radiology* Winter 10:14, Spring 11:10, Winter 18:8

(Do not report 64495 more than once per day)

(Use 64495 in conjunction with 64493, 64494)

Autonomic Nerves

64505 Injection, anesthetic agent; sphenopalatine ganglion

➔ *CPT Assistant* Jul 98:10, Apr 05:13, Jan 13:13, Jun 13:13, Jul 14:8

➔ *Clinical Examples in Radiology* Summer 14:6

►(64508 has been deleted)◄

64510 stellate ganglion (cervical sympathetic)

➔ *CPT Assistant* Jul 98:10, Apr 05:13, Jan 13:13

64517 superior hypogastric plexus

➔ *CPT Changes: An Insider's View* 2004

➔ *CPT Assistant* Oct 04:11, Apr 05:13, Jan 13:13

64520 lumbar or thoracic (paravertebral sympathetic)

➔ *CPT Assistant* Jul 98:10, Apr 05:13, Dec 10:14, Jan 13:13

64530 celiac plexus, with or without radiologic monitoring

➔ *CPT Assistant* Jul 98:10, Apr 05:13, Jan 13:13

➔ *Clinical Examples in Radiology* Summer 14:5, 6

(For transendoscopic ultrasound-guided transmural injection, anesthetic, celiac plexus, use 43253)

Neurostimulators (Peripheral Nerve)

►For electronic analysis with programming, when performed, of peripheral nerve neurostimulator pulse generator/transmitters, see codes 95970, 95971, 95972. An electrode array is a catheter or other device with more than one contact. The function of each contact may be capable of being adjusted during programming services. Test stimulation to confirm correct target site placement of the electrode array(s) and/or to confirm the functional status of the system is inherent to placement, and is not separately reported as electronic analysis or programming of the neurostimulator system. Electronic analysis (95970) at the time of implantation is not separately reported.

Codes 64553, 64555, and 64561 may be used to report both temporary and permanent placement of percutaneous electrode arrays.◄

►(64550 has been deleted)◄

►(For transcutaneous nerve stimulation [TENS], use 97014 for electrical stimulation requiring supervision only or use 97032 for electrical stimulation requiring constant attendance)◄

64553 Percutaneous implantation of neurostimulator electrode array; cranial nerve

➔ *CPT Changes: An Insider's View* 2000, 2012

➔ *CPT Assistant* Nov 99:38, Apr 01:9

(For percutaneous electrical stimulation of a cranial nerve using needle[s] or needle electrode[s] [eg, PENS, PNT], use 64999)

(For open placement of cranial nerve (eg, vagus, trigeminal) neurostimulator pulse generator or receiver, see 61885, 61886, as appropriate)

64555 peripheral nerve (excludes sacral nerve)
➔ *CPT Changes: An Insider's View* 2002, 2012
➔ *CPT Assistant* Jan 15:14, Feb 16:13, Dec 17:16

(Do not report 64555 in conjunction with 64566)

(For percutaneous electrical stimulation of a peripheral nerve using needle[s] or needle electrode[s] [eg, PENS, PNT], use 64999)

64561 sacral nerve (transforaminal placement) including image guidance, if performed
➔ *CPT Changes: An Insider's View* 2002, 2012, 2013
➔ *CPT Assistant* Dec 12:14, Sep 14:5

(64565 has been deleted)

(For percutaneous electrical neuromuscular stimulation or neuromodulation using needle[s] or needle electrode[s] [eg, PENS, PNT], use 64999)

64566 Posterior tibial neurostimulation, percutaneous needle electrode, single treatment, includes programming
➔ *CPT Changes: An Insider's View* 2011
➔ *CPT Assistant* Feb 11:5, Sep 11:8

(Do not report 64566 in conjunction with 64555, 95970-95972)

64568 Incision for implantation of cranial nerve (eg, vagus nerve) neurostimulator electrode array and pulse generator
➔ *CPT Changes: An Insider's View* 2011
➔ *CPT Assistant* Feb 11:5, Sep 11:8, 10, 12, Nov 16:6, Mar 18:9

(Do not report 64568 in conjunction with 61885, 61886, 64570)

(For insertion of chest wall respiratory sensor electrode or electrode array, including connection to pulse generator, use 0466T)

64569 Revision or replacement of cranial nerve (eg, vagus nerve) neurostimulator electrode array, including connection to existing pulse generator
➔ *CPT Changes: An Insider's View* 2011
➔ *CPT Assistant* Feb 11:5, Sep 11:8, Nov 16:6, Mar 18:9

(Do not report 64569 in conjunction with 64570 or 61888)

(For replacement of pulse generator, use 61885)

(For revision or replacement of chest wall respiratory sensor electrode or electrode array, including connection to existing pulse generator, use 0467T)

64570 Removal of cranial nerve (eg, vagus nerve) neurostimulator electrode array and pulse generator
➔ *CPT Changes: An Insider's View* 2011
➔ *CPT Assistant* Feb 11:5, Sep 11:10, Nov 16:6, Mar 18:9

(Do not report 64570 in conjunction with 61888)

(For laparoscopic implantation, revision, replacement, or removal of vagus nerve blocking neurostimulator electrode array and/or pulse generator at the esophagogastric junction, see 0312T-0317T)

(For removal of chest wall respiratory sensor electrode or electrode array, use 0468T)

Implantation Neurostimulator Electrodes, Cranial Nerve (Vagus Nerve Stimulation)
64568-64570

Implantation of a cranial nerve (eg, vagus nerve) neurostimulator electrode with connection of the electrode to an implanted programmable pulse generator in the infraclavicular area (64568). Revision or replacement of the cranial nerve electrode (64569). Replacement of the cranial nerve pulse generator (61885).

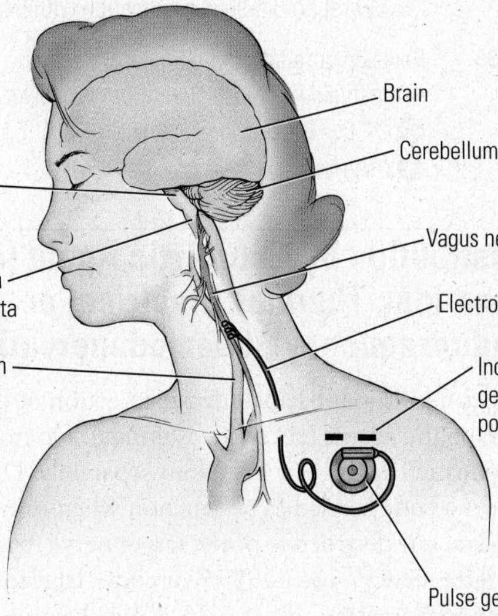

64575 Incision for implantation of neurostimulator electrode array; peripheral nerve (excludes sacral nerve)
➔ *CPT Changes: An Insider's View* 2002, 2011, 2012

64580 neuromuscular
➔ *CPT Changes: An Insider's View* 2012

64581 sacral nerve (transforaminal placement)
➔ *CPT Changes: An Insider's View* 2002, 2012
➔ *CPT Assistant* Dec 12:14, Sep 14:5

Incisional Implantation of Sacral Nerve Neurostimulator
64581

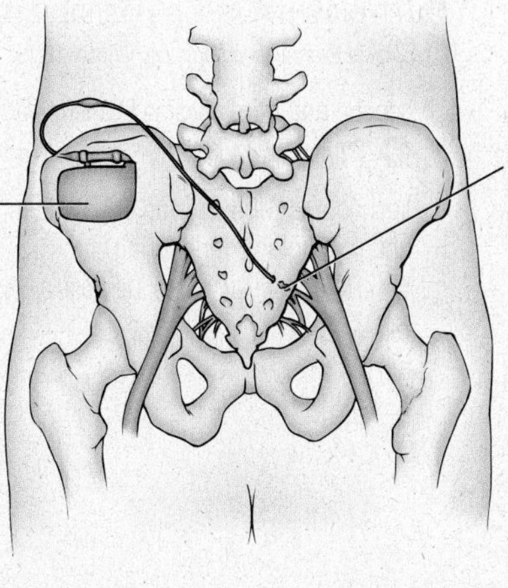

Nervous 61000-64999

64585 Revision or removal of peripheral neurostimulator electrode array
➲ *CPT Changes: An Insider's View* 2012

64590 Insertion or replacement of peripheral or gastric neurostimulator pulse generator or receiver, direct or inductive coupling
➲ *CPT Changes: An Insider's View* 2002, 2005, 2007
➲ *CPT Assistant* Sep 99:4, Apr 01:8, Mar 07:4, Apr 07:7, Sep 11:9, Dec 12:14, Jan 15:14, Dec 17:16

(Do not report 64590 in conjunction with 64595)

64595 Revision or removal of peripheral or gastric neurostimulator pulse generator or receiver
➲ *CPT Changes: An Insider's View* 2007
➲ *CPT Assistant* Sep 99:3, Mar 07:4, Jan 08:8

Destruction by Neurolytic Agent (eg, Chemical, Thermal, Electrical or Radiofrequency), Chemodenervation

Codes 64600-64681 include the injection of other therapeutic agents (eg, corticosteroids). Do not report diagnostic/therapeutic injections separately. Do not report a code labeled as destruction when using therapies that are not destructive of the target nerve (eg, pulsed radiofrequency), use 64999. For codes labeled as chemodenervation, the supply of the chemodenervation agent is reported separately.

(For chemodenervation of internal anal sphincter, use 46505)

(For chemodenervation of the bladder, use 52287)

(For chemodenervation for strabismus involving the extraocular muscles, use 67345)

(For chemodenervation guided by needle electromyography or muscle electrical stimulation, see 95873, 95874)

Somatic Nerves

64600 Destruction by neurolytic agent, trigeminal nerve; supraorbital, infraorbital, mental, or inferior alveolar branch
➲ *CPT Assistant* Aug 05:13, Feb 10:9, Sep 12:14
➲ *Clinical Examples in Radiology* Winter 18:19

64605 second and third division branches at foramen ovale
➲ *CPT Assistant* Aug 05:13, Feb 10:9, Sep 12:14

64610 second and third division branches at foramen ovale under radiologic monitoring
➲ *CPT Assistant* Aug 05:13, Feb 10:9, Sep 12:14, Apr 17:10

64611 Chemodenervation of parotid and submandibular salivary glands, bilateral
➲ *CPT Changes: An Insider's View* 2011
➲ *CPT Assistant* Feb 11:10, Sep 12:14

(Report 64611 with modifier 52 if fewer than four salivary glands are injected)

64612 Chemodenervation of muscle(s); muscle(s) innervated by facial nerve, unilateral (eg, for blepharospasm, hemifacial spasm)
➲ *CPT Changes: An Insider's View* 2000, 2001, 2013
➲ *CPT Assistant* Oct 98:10, Apr 01:2, Aug 05:13, Sep 06:5, Dec 08:9, Jan 09:8, Feb 10:9, 13, Dec 11:19, Sep 12:14, Apr 13:5, Dec 13:10, Jan 14:6, May 14:5

(For bilateral procedure, report 64612 with modifier 50)

64615 muscle(s) innervated by facial, trigeminal, cervical spinal and accessory nerves, bilateral (eg, for chronic migraine)
➲ *CPT Changes: An Insider's View* 2013
➲ *CPT Assistant* Apr 13:5, Jan 14:6

(Report 64615 only once per session)

(Do not report 64615 in conjunction with 64612, 64616, 64617, 64642, 64643, 64644, 64645, 64646, 64647)

(For guidance see 95873, 95874. Do not report more than one guidance code for 64615)

64616 neck muscle(s), excluding muscles of the larynx, unilateral (eg, for cervical dystonia, spasmodic torticollis)
➲ *CPT Changes: An Insider's View* 2014
➲ *CPT Assistant* Jan 14:6, May 14:5

(For bilateral procedure, report 64616 with modifier 50)

(For chemodenervation guided by needle electromyography or muscle electrical stimulation, see 95873, 95874. Do not report more than one guidance code for any unit of 64616)

64617 larynx, unilateral, percutaneous (eg, for spasmodic dysphonia), includes guidance by needle electromyography, when performed
➲ *CPT Changes: An Insider's View* 2014
➲ *CPT Assistant* Jan 14:6

(For bilateral procedure, report 64617 with modifier 50)

(Do not report 64617 in conjunction with 95873, 95874)

(For diagnostic needle electromyography of the larynx, use 95865)

(For chemodenervation of the larynx performed with direct laryngoscopy, see 31570, 31571)

64620 Destruction by neurolytic agent, intercostal nerve
➲ *CPT Changes: An Insider's View* 2000
➲ *CPT Assistant* Nov 99:38, Aug 05:13, Sep 12:14, Jan 14:6

(Imaging guidance [fluoroscopy or CT] are inclusive components of 64633-64636)

(Image guidance [fluoroscopy or CT] and any injection of contrast are inclusive components of 64633-64636. Image guidance and localization are required for the performance of paravertebral facet joint nerve destruction by neurolytic agent described by 64633-64636. If CT or fluoroscopic imaging is not used, report 64999)

Report 64633, 64634, 64635, 64636 per joint, not per nerve. Although two nerves innervate each facet joint, only one code may be reported for each joint denervated, regardless of the number of nerves treated. Use 64634 or 64636 to report each additional facet joint at a different vertebral level in the same spinal region.

For neurolytic destruction of the nerves innervating the T12-L1 paravertebral facet joint, use 64633.

Do not report 64633, 64634, 64635, 64636 for non-thermal facet joint denervation including chemical, low-grade thermal energy (<80 degrees Celsius), or any form of pulsed radiofrequency. To appropriately report any of these modalities, use 64999.

 # 64633 Destruction by neurolytic agent, paravertebral facet joint nerve(s), with imaging guidance (fluoroscopy or CT); cervical or thoracic, single facet joint

➲ *CPT Changes: An Insider's View* 2012

➲ *CPT Assistant* Jun 12:10, Jul 12:6, Sep 12:14, Apr 13:10, Feb 15:9

(For bilateral procedure, report 64633 with modifier 50)

#+ 64634 cervical or thoracic, each additional facet joint (List separately in addition to code for primary procedure)

➲ *CPT Changes: An Insider's View* 2012

➲ *CPT Assistant* Jun 12:10, Jul 12:6, Sep 12:14, Apr 13:10, Feb 15:9

(Use 64634 in conjunction with 64633)

(For bilateral procedure, report 64634 with modifier 50)

 # 64635 lumbar or sacral, single facet joint

➲ *CPT Changes: An Insider's View* 2012

➲ *CPT Assistant* Jun 12:10, Jul 12:6, 14, Sep 12:14, Apr 13:10, Feb 15:9

(For bilateral procedure, report 64635 with modifier 50)

#+ 64636 lumbar or sacral, each additional facet joint (List separately in addition to code for primary procedure)

➲ *CPT Changes: An Insider's View* 2012

➲ *CPT Assistant* Jun 12:10, Jul 12:6, 14, Sep 12:14, Apr 13:10, Feb 15:9

(Use 64636 in conjunction with 64635)

(For bilateral procedure, report 64636 with modifier 50)

(Do not report 64633-64636 in conjunction with 77003, 77012)

(For destruction by neurolytic agent, individual nerves, sacroiliac joint, use 64640)

64630 Destruction by neurolytic agent; pudendal nerve

➲ *CPT Changes: An Insider's View* 2001

➲ *CPT Assistant* Aug 05:13, Feb 10:9, Sep 12:14, Oct 17:9

64632 plantar common digital nerve

➲ *CPT Changes: An Insider's View* 2009

➲ *CPT Assistant* Jan 09:6, Sep 12:14, Jan 13:13, Jul 15:11, Oct 17:9

(Do not report 64632 in conjunction with 64455)

64633 Code is out of numerical sequence. See 64617-64632

64634 Code is out of numerical sequence. See 64617-64632

64635 Code is out of numerical sequence. See 64617-64632

64636 Code is out of numerical sequence. See 64617-64632

64640 other peripheral nerve or branch

➲ *CPT Assistant* Aug 05:13, Dec 09:11, Feb 10:9, Jun 12:15, Sep 12:14, May 17:10, Oct 17:9, Jan 18:7

Report 64642, 64643, 64644, 64645 once per extremity. Codes 64642, 64643, 64644, 64645 can be reported together up to a combined total of four units of service per patient when all four extremities are injected. Report only one base code (64642 or 64644) per session. Report one unit of additional extremity code(s) (64643 or 64645) for each additional extremity injected.

Report 64646 or 64647 for chemodenervation of muscles of the trunk.

Trunk muscles include the erector spinae and paraspinal muscles, rectus abdominus and obliques. All other somatic muscles are extremity muscles, head muscles, or neck muscles.

(For chemodenervation guided by needle electromyography or muscle electrical stimulation, see 95873, 95874. Do not report more than one guidance code for each corresponding chemodenervation of extremity or trunk code)

(Do not report modifier 50 in conjunction with 64642, 64643, 64644, 64645, 64646, 64647)

Chemodenervation of Extremity
64642

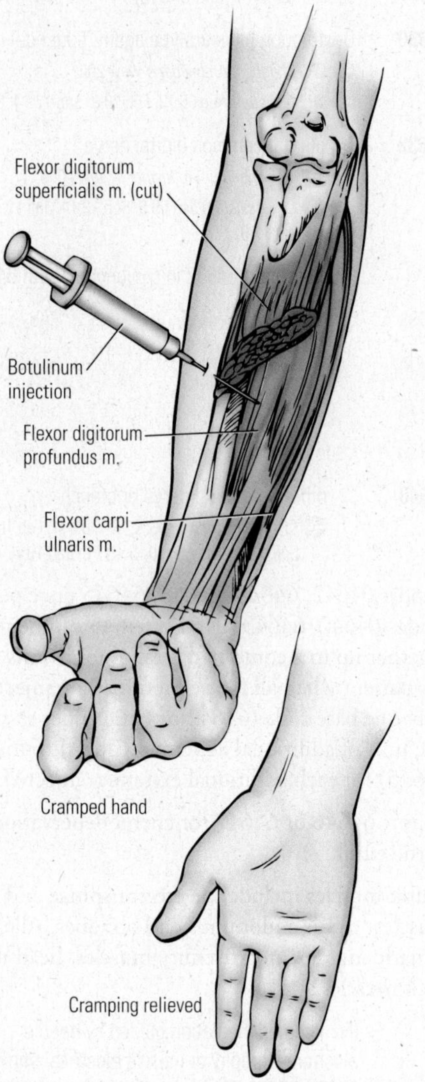

64642 Chemodenervation of one extremity; 1-4 muscle(s)
➔ *CPT Changes: An Insider's View* 2014
➔ *CPT Assistant* Jan 14:6, Oct 14:15

+ 64643 each additional extremity, 1-4 muscle(s) (List separately in addition to code for primary procedure)
➔ *CPT Changes: An Insider's View* 2014
➔ *CPT Assistant* Jan 14:6, Oct 14:15

(Use 64643 in conjunction with 64642, 64644)

64644 Chemodenervation of one extremity; 5 or more muscles
➔ *CPT Changes: An Insider's View* 2014
➔ *CPT Assistant* Jan 14:6, Oct 14:15

+ 64645 each additional extremity, 5 or more muscles (List separately in addition to code for primary procedure)
➔ *CPT Changes: An Insider's View* 2014
➔ *CPT Assistant* Jan 14:6, Oct 14:15

(Use 64645 in conjunction with 64644)

64646 Chemodenervation of trunk muscle(s); 1-5 muscle(s)
➔ *CPT Changes: An Insider's View* 2014
➔ *CPT Assistant* Jan 14:6

64647 6 or more muscles
➔ *CPT Changes: An Insider's View* 2014
➔ *CPT Assistant* Jan 14:6

(Report either 64646 or 64647 only once per session)

Sympathetic Nerves

64650 Chemodenervation of eccrine glands; both axillae
➔ *CPT Changes: An Insider's View* 2006
➔ *CPT Assistant* Jun 08:9, Feb 10:11, Sep 12:14

64653 other area(s) (eg, scalp, face, neck), per day
➔ *CPT Changes: An Insider's View* 2006
➔ *CPT Assistant* Jun 08:9, Sep 12:14

(Report the specific service in conjunction with code(s) for the specific substance(s) or drug(s) provided)

(For chemodenervation of extremities (eg, hands or feet), use 64999)

(For chemodenervation of bladder, use 52287)

64680 Destruction by neurolytic agent, with or without radiologic monitoring; celiac plexus
➔ *CPT Changes: An Insider's View* 2004
➔ *CPT Assistant* Feb 99:10, Aug 05:13, Jun 08:9, Sep 12:14
➔ *Clinical Examples in Radiology* Winter 18:19

(For transendoscopic ultrasound-guided transmural injection, neurolytic agent, celiac plexus, use 43253)

64681 superior hypogastric plexus
➔ *CPT Changes: An Insider's View* 2004
➔ *CPT Assistant* Aug 05:13, Dec 07:13, Sep 12:14
➔ *Clinical Examples in Radiology* Winter 18:19

Neuroplasty (Exploration, Neurolysis or Nerve Decompression)

Neuroplasty is the surgical decompression or freeing of intact nerve from scar tissue, including external neurolysis and/or transposition to repair or restore the nerve.

(For percutaneous neurolysis, see 62263, 62264, 62280-62282)

(For internal neurolysis requiring use of operating microscope, use 64727)

(For facial nerve decompression, use 69720)

(For neuroplasty with nerve wrapping, see 64702-64727, 64999)

64702 Neuroplasty; digital, 1 or both, same digit
➔ *CPT Assistant* Jun 01:11

64704 nerve of hand or foot
➔ *CPT Assistant* Jun 01:11

64708 Neuroplasty, major peripheral nerve, arm or leg, open; other than specified
➲ *CPT Changes: An Insider's View* 2011
➲ *CPT Assistant* Jun 01:11, Jun 12:12, Nov 17:10

64712 sciatic nerve
➲ *CPT Changes: An Insider's View* 2011
➲ *CPT Assistant* Jun 01:11, Jun 12:12

64713 brachial plexus
➲ *CPT Changes: An Insider's View* 2011
➲ *CPT Assistant* Jun 01:11, Jun 12:12, May 13:12

64714 lumbar plexus
➲ *CPT Changes: An Insider's View* 2011
➲ *CPT Assistant* Jun 97:11, Sep 98:16, Jun 01:11, Jun 12:12, Dec 13:17

64716 Neuroplasty and/or transposition; cranial nerve (specify)
➲ *CPT Assistant* Jun 01:11

64718 ulnar nerve at elbow
➲ *CPT Assistant* Jun 01:11, Mar 09:10

64719 ulnar nerve at wrist
➲ *CPT Assistant* Jun 01:11, Mar 09:10

64721 median nerve at carpal tunnel
➲ *CPT Assistant* Fall 92:17, Sep 97:10, Jun 01:11, Nov 06:23, Aug 09:11, Jun 12:15, Sep 12:16, Dec 13:14, Jul 15:10

(For arthroscopic procedure, use 29848)

64722 Decompression; unspecified nerve(s) (specify)
➲ *CPT Assistant* Sep 98:16, May 99:11, Jun 01:11, Oct 04:12

64726 plantar digital nerve
➲ *CPT Assistant* Jun 01:11

+ 64727 Internal neurolysis, requiring use of operating microscope (List separately in addition to code for neuroplasty) (Neuroplasty includes external neurolysis)
➲ *CPT Assistant* Nov 98:19, Jun 01:11, Jun 12:13

(Do not report code 69990 in addition to code 64727)

Transection or Avulsion

(For stereotactic lesion of gasserian ganglion, use 61790)

64732 Transection or avulsion of; supraorbital nerve
➲ *CPT Changes: An Insider's View* 2000
➲ *CPT Assistant* Nov 99:39

64734 infraorbital nerve

64736 mental nerve

64738 inferior alveolar nerve by osteotomy

64740 lingual nerve

64742 facial nerve, differential or complete

64744 greater occipital nerve

64746 phrenic nerve

64755 vagus nerves limited to proximal stomach (selective proximal vagotomy, proximal gastric vagotomy, parietal cell vagotomy, supra- or highly selective vagotomy)
➲ *CPT Changes: An Insider's View* 2000, 2002
➲ *CPT Assistant* Nov 99:39

(For laparoscopic approach, use 43652)

64760 vagus nerve (vagotomy), abdominal
➲ *CPT Changes: An Insider's View* 2000
➲ *CPT Assistant* Nov 99:39

(For laparoscopic approach, use 43651)

64763 Transection or avulsion of obturator nerve, extrapelvic, with or without adductor tenotomy

(For bilateral procedure, report 64763 with modifier 50)

64766 Transection or avulsion of obturator nerve, intrapelvic, with or without adductor tenotomy

(For bilateral procedure, report 64766 with modifier 50)

64771 Transection or avulsion of other cranial nerve, extradural

64772 Transection or avulsion of other spinal nerve, extradural
➲ *CPT Assistant* Apr 15:10

(For excision of tender scar, skin and subcutaneous tissue, with or without tiny neuroma, see 11400-11446, 13100-13153)

Excision

Somatic Nerves

(For Morton neurectomy, use 28080)

64774 Excision of neuroma; cutaneous nerve, surgically identifiable

64776 digital nerve, 1 or both, same digit

+ 64778 digital nerve, each additional digit (List separately in addition to code for primary procedure)

(Use 64778 in conjunction with 64776)

64782 hand or foot, except digital nerve

+ 64783 hand or foot, each additional nerve, except same digit (List separately in addition to code for primary procedure)

(Use 64783 in conjunction with 64782)

64784 major peripheral nerve, except sciatic

64786 sciatic nerve

+ 64787 Implantation of nerve end into bone or muscle (List separately in addition to neuroma excision)

(Use 64787 in conjunction with 64774-64786)

64788 Excision of neurofibroma or neurolemmoma; cutaneous nerve
➲ *CPT Assistant* Apr 16:3

64790 major peripheral nerve
CPT Assistant Apr 16:3

64792 extensive (including malignant type)
CPT Assistant Apr 16:3

(For destruction of extensive cutaneous neurofibroma, see 0419T, 0420T)

64795 Biopsy of nerve

Sympathetic Nerves

64802 Sympathectomy, cervical

(For bilateral procedure, report 64802 with modifier 50)

64804 Sympathectomy, cervicothoracic

(For bilateral procedure, report 64804 with modifier 50)

64809 Sympathectomy, thoracolumbar

(For bilateral procedure, report 64809 with modifier 50)

64818 Sympathectomy, lumbar

(For bilateral procedure, report 64818 with modifier 50)

64820 Sympathectomy; digital arteries, each digit
CPT Changes: An Insider's View 2002
CPT Assistant Jan 04:27

(Do not report 69990 in addition to code 64820)

64821 radial artery
CPT Changes: An Insider's View 2002

(Do not report 69990 in addition to code 64821)

64822 ulnar artery
CPT Changes: An Insider's View 2002

(Do not report 69990 in addition to code 64822)

64823 superficial palmar arch
CPT Changes: An Insider's View 2002

(Do not report 69990 in addition to code 64823)

Neurorrhaphy

64831 Suture of digital nerve, hand or foot; 1 nerve
CPT Assistant Apr 00:6, Sep 14:13

+ 64832 each additional digital nerve (List separately in addition to code for primary procedure)
CPT Assistant Apr 00:6

(Use 64832 in conjunction with 64831)

64834 Suture of 1 nerve; hand or foot, common sensory nerve
CPT Changes: An Insider's View 2008

64835 median motor thenar
CPT Changes: An Insider's View 2008

64836 ulnar motor
CPT Changes: An Insider's View 2008

+ 64837 Suture of each additional nerve, hand or foot (List separately in addition to code for primary procedure)

(Use 64837 in conjunction with 64834-64836)

64840 Suture of posterior tibial nerve

64856 Suture of major peripheral nerve, arm or leg, except sciatic; including transposition

64857 without transposition

64858 Suture of sciatic nerve

+ 64859 Suture of each additional major peripheral nerve (List separately in addition to code for primary procedure)

(Use 64859 in conjunction with 64856, 64857)

64861 Suture of; brachial plexus

64862 lumbar plexus

64864 Suture of facial nerve; extracranial

64865 infratemporal, with or without grafting

64866 Anastomosis; facial-spinal accessory

64868 facial-hypoglossal

+ 64872 Suture of nerve; requiring secondary or delayed suture (List separately in addition to code for primary neurorrhaphy)

(Use 64872 in conjunction with 64831-64865)

+ 64874 requiring extensive mobilization, or transposition of nerve (List separately in addition to code for nerve suture)

(Use 64874 in conjunction with 64831-64865)

+ 64876 requiring shortening of bone of extremity (List separately in addition to code for nerve suture)

(Use 64876 in conjunction with 64831-64865)

Neurorrhaphy With Nerve Graft, Vein Graft, or Conduit

64885 Nerve graft (includes obtaining graft), head or neck; up to 4 cm in length
CPT Assistant Nov 00:11, Dec 17:12

64886 more than 4 cm length
CPT Assistant Nov 00:11, Dec 17:12

64890 Nerve graft (includes obtaining graft), single strand, hand or foot; up to 4 cm length
CPT Assistant Apr 15:10, Aug 15:8, Dec 17:12

64891 more than 4 cm length
CPT Assistant Dec 17:12

64892 Nerve graft (includes obtaining graft), single strand, arm or leg; up to 4 cm length
CPT Assistant Dec 17:12

64893 more than 4 cm length
CPT Assistant Dec 17:12

64895 Nerve graft (includes obtaining graft), multiple strands (cable), hand or foot; up to 4 cm length
➔ *CPT Assistant* Nov 00:11, Dec 17:12

64896 more than 4 cm length
➔ *CPT Assistant* Nov 00:11, Dec 17:12

64897 Nerve graft (includes obtaining graft), multiple strands (cable), arm or leg; up to 4 cm length
➔ *CPT Assistant* Nov 00:11, Dec 17:12

64898 more than 4 cm length
➔ *CPT Assistant* Nov 00:11, Dec 17:12

+ 64901 Nerve graft, each additional nerve; single strand (List separately in addition to code for primary procedure)
➔ *CPT Assistant* Nov 00:11, Dec 17:12

(Use 64901 in conjunction with 64885-64893)

+ 64902 multiple strands (cable) (List separately in addition to code for primary procedure)
➔ *CPT Assistant* Nov 00:11, Dec 17:12

(Use 64902 in conjunction with 64885, 64886, 64895-64898)

64905 Nerve pedicle transfer; first stage
➔ *CPT Assistant* Dec 17:12

64907 second stage
➔ *CPT Assistant* Dec 17:12

64910 Nerve repair; with synthetic conduit or vein allograft (eg, nerve tube), each nerve
➔ *CPT Changes: An Insider's View* 2007
➔ *CPT Assistant* Nov 07:4, Apr 15:10, Aug 15:8, Dec 17:12

64911 with autogenous vein graft (includes harvest of vein graft), each nerve
➔ *CPT Changes: An Insider's View* 2007
➔ *CPT Assistant* Nov 07:4, Dec 17:12

(Do not report 69990 in addition to 64910, 64911)

64912 with nerve allograft, each nerve, first strand (cable)
➔ *CPT Changes: An Insider's View* 2018
➔ *CPT Assistant* Dec 17:12

+ 64913 with nerve allograft, each additional strand (List separately in addition to code for primary procedure)
➔ *CPT Changes: An Insider's View* 2018
➔ *CPT Assistant* Dec 17:12

(Use 64913 in conjunction with 64912)

(Do not report 64912, 64913 in conjunction with 69990)

Other Procedures

64999 Unlisted procedure, nervous system
➔ *CPT Assistant* Apr 96:11, Sep 98:16, Oct 98:10, Jan 00:10, Aug 00:7, Sep 00:10, Feb 02:10, Nov 03:5, Oct 04:11, Apr 05:13, Aug 05:13, Sep 05:9, Sep 07:10, Nov 07:4, Dec 07:8, Jul 08:9, Sep 08:11, Aug 09:8, Dec 09:11, Jun 10:8, Sep 10:10, Nov 10:4, Apr 11:12, Jul 11:12, 16-17, Sep 11:12, Jan 12:14, Feb 12:11, May 12:14, Sep 12:16, Oct 12:14, Dec 12:13, Apr 13:5, 10, Jun 13:13, Nov 13:14, Dec 13:14, Jan 14:8, 9, Feb 14:11, Jul 14:8, Feb 15:9, Apr 15:10, Jul 15:11, Aug 15:8, Oct 15:9, Feb 16:13, Oct 16:11, Nov 16:6, May 17:10, Dec 17:13, Jan 18:7, Mar 18:9
➔ *Clinical Examples in Radiology* Winter 17:3

Notes

Surgery

Eye and Ocular Adnexa (65091-68899) 447

The following is a listing of headings and subheadings that appear within the Eye and Ocular Adnexa section of the CPT codebook. The subheadings or subsections denoted with asterisks (*) below have special instructions unique to that subsection. Where these are indicated, special notes or guidelines will be presented preceding those procedural terminology listings, referring to that subsection specifically.

Eyeball (65091-65290) 447
Removal of Eye (65091-65114) 447
Secondary Implant(s) Procedures* (65125-65175) 447
Removal of Foreign Body (65205-65265) 447
Repair of Laceration (65270-65290) 447

Anterior Segment (65400-66999) 448
Cornea (65400-65785) 448
Excision (65400-65426) 448
Removal or Destruction (65430-65600) 448
Keratoplasty* (65710-65757) 448
Other Procedures* (65760-65785) 449
Anterior Chamber (65800-66030) 449
Incision (65800-65880) 449
Removal (65900-65930) 449
Introduction (66020-66030) 450
Anterior Sclera (66130-66250) 450
Excision (66130-66175) 450
Aqueous Shunt (66179-66185) 450
Repair or Revision (66225-66250) 450
Iris, Ciliary Body (66500-66770) 450
Incision (66500-66505) 450
Excision (66600-66635) 450
Repair (66680-66682) 451
Destruction (66700-66770) 451
Lens (66820-66940) 451
Incision (66820-66825) 451
Removal* (66830-66940) 451
Intraocular Lens Procedures (66982-66986) 451
Other Procedures (66990-66999) 452

Posterior Segment (67005-67299) 452
Vitreous (67005-67043) 452
Retina or Choroid (67101-67229) 453
Repair (67101-67121) 453
Prophylaxis* (67141-67145) 453
Destruction* (67208-67229) 454
Posterior Sclera (67250-67255) 454
Repair (67250-67255) 454
Other Procedures (67299) 454

Ocular Adnexa (67311-67999) 454
Extraocular Muscles (67311-67399) 454
Other Procedures (67399) 456
Orbit (67400-67599) 456
Exploration, Excision, Decompression (67400-67450) 456
Other Procedures (67500-67599) 456
Eyelids (67700-67999) 457
Incision (67700-67810) 457
Excision, Destruction* (67800-67850) 457
Tarsorrhaphy (67875-67882) 457
Repair (Brow Ptosis, Blepharoptosis, Lid Retraction, Ectropion, Entropion) (67900-67924) 457
Reconstruction* (67930-67975) 458
Other Procedures (67999) 458
Conjunctiva (68020-68899) 459
Incision and Drainage (68020-68040) 459
Excision and/or Destruction (68100-68135) 459
Injection (68200) 459
Conjunctivoplasty (68320-68340) 459
Other Procedures (68360-68399) 459
Lacrimal System (68400-68899) 459
Incision (68400-68440) 459
Excision (68500-68550) 459
Repair (68700-68770) 459
Probing and/or Related Procedures (68801-68850) 460
Other Procedures (68899) 460

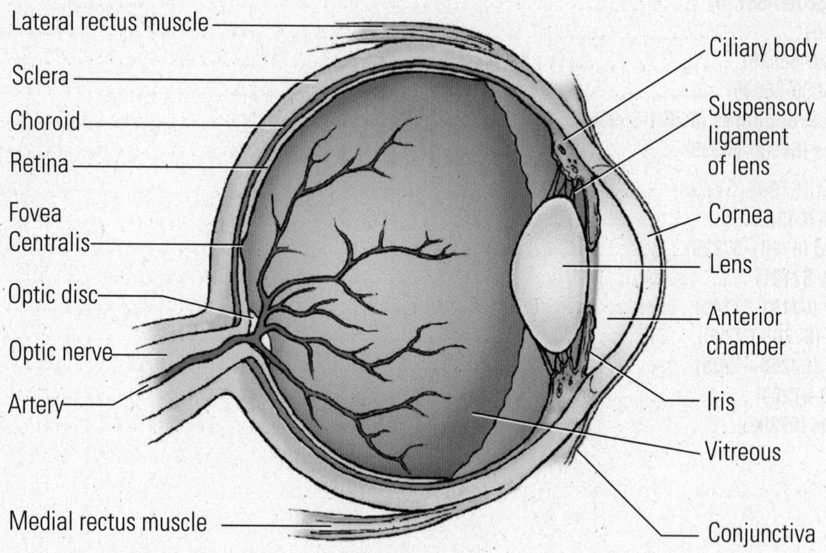

Eye Anatomy

Eye and Ocular Adnexa

(For diagnostic and treatment ophthalmological services, see **Medicine, Ophthalmology,** and 92002 et seq)

(Do not report code 69990 in addition to codes 65091-68850)

Eyeball

Removal of Eye

65091 Evisceration of ocular contents; without implant

65093 with implant

65101 Enucleation of eye; without implant

65103 with implant, muscles not attached to implant

65105 with implant, muscles attached to implant

(For conjunctivoplasty after enucleation, see 68320 et seq)

65110 Exenteration of orbit (does not include skin graft), removal of orbital contents; only

65112 with therapeutic removal of bone

65114 with muscle or myocutaneous flap

(For skin graft to orbit (split skin), see 15120, 15121; free, full thickness, see 15260, 15261)

(For eyelid repair involving more than skin, see 67930 et seq)

Secondary Implant(s) Procedures

An ocular implant is an implant inside muscular cone; an orbital implant is an implant outside muscular cone.

65125 Modification of ocular implant with placement or replacement of pegs (eg, drilling receptacle for prosthesis appendage) (separate procedure)

65130 Insertion of ocular implant secondary; after evisceration, in scleral shell

65135 after enucleation, muscles not attached to implant

65140 after enucleation, muscles attached to implant

65150 Reinsertion of ocular implant; with or without conjunctival graft

65155 with use of foreign material for reinforcement and/or attachment of muscles to implant

65175 Removal of ocular implant

(For orbital implant (implant outside muscle cone) insertion, use 67550; removal, use 67560)

Removal of Foreign Body

(For removal of implanted material: ocular implant, use 65175; anterior segment implant, use 65920; posterior segment implant, use 67120; orbital implant, use 67560)

(For diagnostic x-ray for foreign body, use 70030)

(For diagnostic echography for foreign body, use 76529)

(For removal of foreign body from orbit: frontal approach, use 67413; lateral approach, use 67430)

(For removal of foreign body from eyelid, embedded, use 67938)

(For removal of foreign body from lacrimal system, use 68530)

65205 Removal of foreign body, external eye; conjunctival superficial

➔ *CPT Assistant* Mar 05:17, Oct 13:19

65210 conjunctival embedded (includes concretions), subconjunctival, or scleral nonperforating

65220 corneal, without slit lamp

65222 corneal, with slit lamp

(For repair of corneal laceration with foreign body, use 65275)

65235 Removal of foreign body, intraocular; from anterior chamber of eye or lens

➔ *CPT Changes: An Insider's View* 2002

(For removal of implanted material from anterior segment, use 65920)

65260 from posterior segment, magnetic extraction, anterior or posterior route

65265 from posterior segment, nonmagnetic extraction

(For removal of implanted material from posterior segment, use 67120)

Repair of Laceration

(For fracture of orbit, see 21385 et seq)

(For repair of wound of eyelid, skin, linear, simple, see 12011-12018; intermediate, layered closure, see 12051-12057; linear, complex, see 13151-13160; other, see 67930, 67935)

(For repair of wound of lacrimal system, use 68700)

(For repair of operative wound, use 66250)

65270 Repair of laceration; conjunctiva, with or without nonperforating laceration sclera, direct closure

➔ *CPT Assistant* Aug 12:9

65272 conjunctiva, by mobilization and rearrangement, without hospitalization

65273 conjunctiva, by mobilization and rearrangement, with hospitalization

65275 cornea, nonperforating, with or without removal foreign body

65280 cornea and/or sclera, perforating, not involving uveal tissue
➲ *CPT Assistant* Aug 12:9

65285 cornea and/or sclera, perforating, with reposition or resection of uveal tissue
➲ *CPT Assistant* Aug 12:9

(65280 and 65285 are not used for repair of a surgical wound)

65286 application of tissue glue, wounds of cornea and/or sclera
➲ *CPT Assistant* May 99:11, Apr 09:5

(Repair of laceration includes use of conjunctival flap and restoration of anterior chamber, by air or saline injection when indicated)

(For repair of iris or ciliary body, use 66680)

65290 Repair of wound, extraocular muscle, tendon and/or Tenon's capsule

Anterior Segment

Cornea

Excision

65400 Excision of lesion, cornea (keratectomy, lamellar, partial), except pterygium

65410 Biopsy of cornea

65420 Excision or transposition of pterygium; without graft
➲ *CPT Assistant* Dec 07:13

65426 with graft

Removal or Destruction

65430 Scraping of cornea, diagnostic, for smear and/or culture

65435 Removal of corneal epithelium; with or without chemocauterization (abrasion, curettage)
➲ *CPT Assistant* Feb 16:12

(Do not report 65435 in conjunction with 0402T)

65436 with application of chelating agent (eg, EDTA)

65450 Destruction of lesion of cornea by cryotherapy, photocoagulation or thermocauterization

Cryotherapy of Lesion on Cornea
65450

A freezing probe is applied directly to the corneal defect to destroy it.

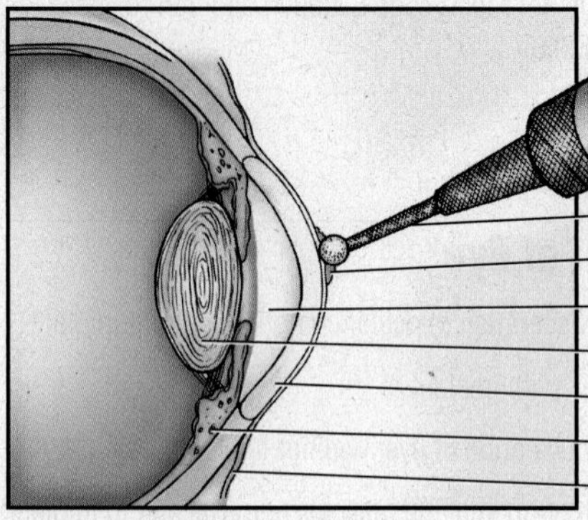

65600 Multiple punctures of anterior cornea (eg, for corneal erosion, tattoo)

Keratoplasty

Corneal transplant includes use of fresh or preserved grafts. The preparation of donor material is included for penetrating or anterior lamellar keratoplasty, but reported separately for endothelial keratoplasty. Do not report 65710-65757 in conjunction with 92025.

(Keratoplasty excludes refractive keratoplasty procedures, 65760, 65765, and 65767)

65710 Keratoplasty (corneal transplant); anterior lamellar
➲ *CPT Changes: An Insider's View* 2009
➲ *CPT Assistant* Oct 02:8, Apr 09:5, Dec 09:13, Aug 12:15

65730 penetrating (except in aphakia or pseudophakia)
➲ *CPT Changes: An Insider's View* 2009
➲ *CPT Assistant* Oct 02:8, Feb 06:1, Apr 09:5, Dec 09:13, Aug 12:15

65750 penetrating (in aphakia)
➲ *CPT Assistant* Oct 02:8, Apr 09:5, Dec 09:13, Aug 12:15

65755 penetrating (in pseudophakia)
➲ *CPT Assistant* Winter 90:8, Oct 02:9, Apr 09:5, Dec 09:13, Aug 12:15

65756 endothelial
➲ *CPT Changes: An Insider's View* 2009

+ 65757 Backbench preparation of corneal endothelial allograft prior to transplantation (List separately in addition to code for primary procedure)
➲ *CPT Changes: An Insider's View* 2009
➲ *CPT Assistant* Aug 14:15

(Use 65757 in conjunction with 65756)

Other Procedures

Do not report 65760-65771 in conjunction with 92025.

65760 Keratomileusis
➔ *CPT Assistant* Oct 02:9

65765 Keratophakia
➔ *CPT Assistant* Oct 02:10

65767 Epikeratoplasty
➔ *CPT Assistant* Winter 90:8, Oct 02:10

65770 Keratoprosthesis
➔ *CPT Assistant* Oct 02:10

65771 Radial keratotomy
➔ *CPT Assistant* Winter 90:8, Oct 02:10

65772 Corneal relaxing incision for correction of surgically induced astigmatism
➔ *CPT Assistant* Oct 02:10, 12

65775 Corneal wedge resection for correction of surgically induced astigmatism
➔ *CPT Assistant* Oct 02:10, 12, Aug 12:9

(For fitting of contact lens for treatment of disease, see 92071, 92072)

(For unlisted procedures on cornea, use 66999)

65778 Placement of amniotic membrane on the ocular surface; without sutures
➔ *CPT Changes: An Insider's View* 2011, 2014
➔ *CPT Assistant* May 14:5, Feb 18:11

65779 single layer, sutured
➔ *CPT Changes: An Insider's View* 2011, 2014
➔ *CPT Assistant* May 14:5, Feb 18:11

(Do not report 65778, 65779 in conjunction with 65430, 65435, 65780)

(For placement of amniotic membrane using tissue glue, use 66999)

65780 Ocular surface reconstruction; amniotic membrane transplantation, multiple layers
➔ *CPT Changes: An Insider's View* 2004, 2011
➔ *CPT Assistant* May 04:10, Jun 09:9, May 14:5, Feb 18:11

(For placement of amniotic membrane without reconstruction using no sutures or single layer suture technique, see 65778, 65779)

65781 limbal stem cell allograft (eg, cadaveric or living donor)
➔ *CPT Changes: An Insider's View* 2004
➔ *CPT Assistant* May 04:10

65782 limbal conjunctival autograft (includes obtaining graft)
➔ *CPT Changes: An Insider's View* 2004
➔ *CPT Assistant* Feb 04:11, May 04:10, Feb 05:15-16

(For harvesting conjunctival allograft, living donor, use 68371)

65785 Implantation of intrastromal corneal ring segments
➔ *CPT Changes: An Insider's View* 2016

Anterior Chamber

Incision

65800 Paracentesis of anterior chamber of eye (separate procedure); with removal of aqueous
➔ *CPT Changes: An Insider's View* 2013
➔ *CPT Assistant* Nov 12:10

65810 with removal of vitreous and/or discission of anterior hyaloid membrane, with or without air injection
➔ *CPT Assistant* Nov 12:10

65815 with removal of blood, with or without irrigation and/or air injection
➔ *CPT Assistant* Nov 12:10

(For injection, see 66020-66030)

(For removal of blood clot, use 65930)

65820 Goniotomy
➔ *CPT Assistant* Sep 05:12

(Do not report modifier 63 in conjunction with 65820)

(For use of ophthalmic endoscope with 65820, use 66990)

65850 Trabeculotomy ab externo

65855 Trabeculoplasty by laser surgery
➔ *CPT Changes: An Insider's View* 2016
➔ *CPT Assistant* Mar 98:7, Mar 03:23

(Do not report 65855 in conjunction with 65860, 65865, 65870, 65875, 65880)

(For trabeculectomy, use 66170)

65860 Severing adhesions of anterior segment, laser technique (separate procedure)

65865 Severing adhesions of anterior segment of eye, incisional technique (with or without injection of air or liquid) (separate procedure); goniosynechiae

(For trabeculoplasty by laser surgery, use 65855)

65870 anterior synechiae, except goniosynechiae

65875 posterior synechiae
➔ *CPT Assistant* Sep 05:12

(For use of ophthalmic endoscope with 65875, use 66990)

65880 corneovitreal adhesions

(For laser surgery, use 66821)

Removal

65900 Removal of epithelial downgrowth, anterior chamber of eye
➔ *CPT Changes: An Insider's View* 2002

Eye / Ocular Adnexa 65091-68899

65920 Removal of implanted material, anterior segment of eye
➔ *CPT Changes: An Insider's View* 2002
➔ *CPT Assistant* Sep 05:12

(For use of ophthalmic endoscope with 65920, use 66990)

65930 Removal of blood clot, anterior segment of eye
➔ *CPT Changes: An Insider's View* 2002

Introduction

66020 Injection, anterior chamber of eye (separate procedure); air or liquid
➔ *CPT Changes: An Insider's View* 2002
➔ *CPT Assistant* Nov 12:10

66030 medication
➔ *CPT Assistant* Nov 12:10

(For unlisted procedures on anterior segment, use 66999)

Anterior Sclera

Excision

(For removal of intraocular foreign body, use 65235)

(For operations on posterior sclera, use 67250, 67255)

66130 Excision of lesion, sclera

66150 Fistulization of sclera for glaucoma; trephination with iridectomy

66155 thermocauterization with iridectomy

66160 sclerectomy with punch or scissors, with iridectomy

66170 trabeculectomy ab externo in absence of previous surgery
➔ *CPT Assistant* Jul 03:4, Nov 03:10, Dec 12:14

(For trabeculotomy ab externo, use 65850)

(For repair of operative wound, use 66250)

66172 trabeculectomy ab externo with scarring from previous ocular surgery or trauma (includes injection of antifibrotic agents)
➔ *CPT Assistant* Jul 03:4, Nov 03:10, Dec 12:14

66174 Transluminal dilation of aqueous outflow canal; without retention of device or stent
➔ *CPT Changes: An Insider's View* 2011

66175 with retention of device or stent
➔ *CPT Changes: An Insider's View* 2011

Aqueous Shunt

66179 Aqueous shunt to extraocular equatorial plate reservoir, external approach; without graft
➔ *CPT Changes: An Insider's View* 2015
➔ *CPT Assistant* Jan 15:10

66180 with graft
➔ *CPT Changes: An Insider's View* 2015
➔ *CPT Assistant* Winter 90:8, Aug 03:9, Sep 03:2, Jun 12:15, Jan 15:10

(Do not report 66180 in conjunction with 67255)

66183 Insertion of anterior segment aqueous drainage device, without extraocular reservoir, external approach
➔ *CPT Changes: An Insider's View* 2014
➔ *CPT Assistant* May 14:5

66184 Revision of aqueous shunt to extraocular equatorial plate reservoir; without graft
➔ *CPT Changes: An Insider's View* 2015
➔ *CPT Assistant* Jan 15:10

66185 with graft
➔ *CPT Changes: An Insider's View* 2015
➔ *CPT Assistant* Winter 90:8, Jan 15:10

(Do not report 66185 in conjunction with 67255)

(For removal of implanted shunt, use 67120)

Repair or Revision

(For scleral procedures in retinal surgery, see 67101 et seq)

►(66220 has been deleted)◄

66225 Repair of scleral staphyloma with graft

(For scleral reinforcement, see 67250, 67255)

66250 Revision or repair of operative wound of anterior segment, any type, early or late, major or minor procedure
➔ *CPT Assistant* Oct 10:15, Dec 10:15

(For unlisted procedures on anterior sclera, use 66999)

Iris, Ciliary Body

Incision

66500 Iridotomy by stab incision (separate procedure); except transfixion

66505 with transfixion as for iris bombe

(For iridotomy by photocoagulation, use 66761)

Excision

66600 Iridectomy, with corneoscleral or corneal section; for removal of lesion

66605 with cyclectomy

66625 peripheral for glaucoma (separate procedure)

66630 sector for glaucoma (separate procedure)

66635 optical (separate procedure)

(For coreoplasty by photocoagulation, use 66762)

Repair

66680 Repair of iris, ciliary body (as for iridodialysis)

(For reposition or resection of uveal tissue with perforating wound of cornea or sclera, use 65285)

66682 Suture of iris, ciliary body (separate procedure) with retrieval of suture through small incision (eg, McCannel suture)

Destruction

66700 Ciliary body destruction; diathermy

66710 cyclophotocoagulation, transscleral

➔ *CPT Changes: An Insider's View* 2005

➔ *CPT Assistant* Mar 05:20, Sep 05:5

66711 cyclophotocoagulation, endoscopic

➔ *CPT Changes: An Insider's View* 2005

➔ *CPT Assistant* Mar 05:20, Sep 05:5, 12

(Do not report 66711 in conjunction with 66990)

66720 cryotherapy

➔ *CPT Changes: An Insider's View* 2017

66740 cyclodialysis

66761 Iridotomy/iridectomy by laser surgery (eg, for glaucoma) (per session)

➔ *CPT Changes: An Insider's View* 2011

➔ *CPT Assistant* Mar 98:7

66762 Iridoplasty by photocoagulation (1 or more sessions) (eg, for improvement of vision, for widening of anterior chamber angle)

➔ *CPT Assistant* Mar 98:7

66770 Destruction of cyst or lesion iris or ciliary body (nonexcisional procedure)

(For excision lesion iris, ciliary body, see 66600, 66605; for removal of epithelial downgrowth, use 65900)

(For unlisted procedures on iris, ciliary body, use 66999)

Lens

Incision

66820 Discission of secondary membranous cataract (opacified posterior lens capsule and/or anterior hyaloid); stab incision technique (Ziegler or Wheeler knife)

66821 laser surgery (eg, YAG laser) (1 or more stages)

66825 Repositioning of intraocular lens prosthesis, requiring an incision (separate procedure)

Removal

Lateral canthotomy, iridectomy, iridotomy, anterior capsulotomy, posterior capsulotomy, the use of viscoelastic agents, enzymatic zonulysis, use of other pharmacologic agents, and subconjunctival or sub-tenon injections are included as part of the code for the extraction of lens.

66830 Removal of secondary membranous cataract (opacified posterior lens capsule and/or anterior hyaloid) with corneo-scleral section, with or without iridectomy (iridocapsulotomy, iridocapsulectomy)

66840 Removal of lens material; aspiration technique, 1 or more stages

➔ *CPT Assistant* Fall 92:4, Jan 09:7, Apr 09:9, Sep 09:5, Apr 16:8, Jun 16:6, Sep 16:9

66850 phacofragmentation technique (mechanical or ultrasonic) (eg, phacoemulsification), with aspiration

➔ *CPT Assistant* Fall 92:6, Jan 09:7, Apr 09:9, Sep 09:5, Jun 16:6

66852 pars plana approach, with or without vitrectomy

➔ *CPT Assistant* Fall 92:8, Jan 09:7, Apr 09:9, Sep 09:5, Jun 16:6

66920 intracapsular

➔ *CPT Assistant* Fall 92:8, Sep 09:5

66930 intracapsular, for dislocated lens

➔ *CPT Assistant* Fall 92:8, Sep 09:5

66940 extracapsular (other than 66840, 66850, 66852)

➔ *CPT Assistant* Fall 92:4, Jan 09:7, Apr 09:9, Sep 09:5, Jun 16:6

(For removal of intralenticular foreign body without lens extraction, use 65235)

(For repair of operative wound, use 66250)

Intraocular Lens Procedures

66982 Extracapsular cataract removal with insertion of intraocular lens prosthesis (1-stage procedure), manual or mechanical technique (eg, irrigation and aspiration or phacoemulsification), complex, requiring devices or techniques not generally used in routine cataract surgery (eg, iris expansion device, suture support for intraocular lens, or primary posterior capsulorrhexis) or performed on patients in the amblyogenic developmental stage

➔ *CPT Changes: An Insider's View* 2001, 2002

➔ *CPT Assistant* Feb 01:7, Nov 03:10, Sep 09:5, Mar 13:6, Mar 16:10, Dec 17:14

(For insertion of ocular telescope prosthesis including removal of crystalline lens, use 0308T)

66983 Intracapsular cataract extraction with insertion of intraocular lens prosthesis (1 stage procedure)

➔ *CPT Assistant* Fall 92:5, 8, Nov 03:10, Sep 09:5, Mar 13:6

(Do not report 66983 in conjunction with 0308T)

66984 Extracapsular cataract removal with insertion of intraocular lens prosthesis (1 stage procedure), manual or mechanical technique (eg, irrigation and aspiration or phacoemulsification)

➔ *CPT Assistant* Fall 92:5, 8, Feb 01:7, Nov 03:10, Mar 05:11, Sep 09:5, Mar 13:6

(For complex extracapsular cataract removal, use 66982)

(For insertion of ocular telescope prosthesis including removal of crystalline lens, use 0308T)

66985 Insertion of intraocular lens prosthesis (secondary implant), not associated with concurrent cataract removal

➔ *CPT Assistant* Sep 05:12, Sep 09:5, Dec 11:16, Mar 13:6

(To code implant at time of concurrent cataract surgery, see 66982, 66983, 66984)

(To report supply of intraocular lens prosthesis, use 99070)

(For ultrasonic determination of intraocular lens power, use 76519)

(For removal of implanted material from anterior segment, use 65920)

(For secondary fixation (separate procedure), use 66682)

(For use of ophthalmic endoscope with 66985, use 66990)

66986 Exchange of intraocular lens

➔ *CPT Assistant* Sep 05:12

(For use of ophthalmic endoscope with 66986, use 66990)

Other Procedures

+ 66990 Use of ophthalmic endoscope (List separately in addition to code for primary procedure)

➔ *CPT Changes: An Insider's View* 2003

➔ *CPT Assistant* Sep 05:12, Oct 08:3

(66990 may be used only with codes 65820, 65875, 65920, 66985, 66986, 67036, 67039, 67040, 67041, 67042, 67043, 67113)

66999 Unlisted procedure, anterior segment of eye

➔ *CPT Assistant* Apr 16:8

Posterior Segment

Vitreous

67005 Removal of vitreous, anterior approach (open sky technique or limbal incision); partial removal

➔ *CPT Assistant* Fall 92:4

67010 subtotal removal with mechanical vitrectomy

➔ *CPT Assistant* Fall 92:4

(For removal of vitreous by paracentesis of anterior chamber, use 65810)

(For removal of corneovitreal adhesions, use 65880)

67015 Aspiration or release of vitreous, subretinal or choroidal fluid, pars plana approach (posterior sclerotomy)

67025 Injection of vitreous substitute, pars plana or limbal approach (fluid-gas exchange), with or without aspiration (separate procedure)

➔ *CPT Assistant* Feb 18:3

67027 Implantation of intravitreal drug delivery system (eg, ganciclovir implant), includes concomitant removal of vitreous

➔ *CPT Assistant* Nov 97:23, Nov 98:1, Feb 18:3

(For removal, use 67121)

Intravitreal Drug Delivery System

67027

A drug delivery system that releases medication into the vitreous is implanted into the vitreous by pars plana incision.

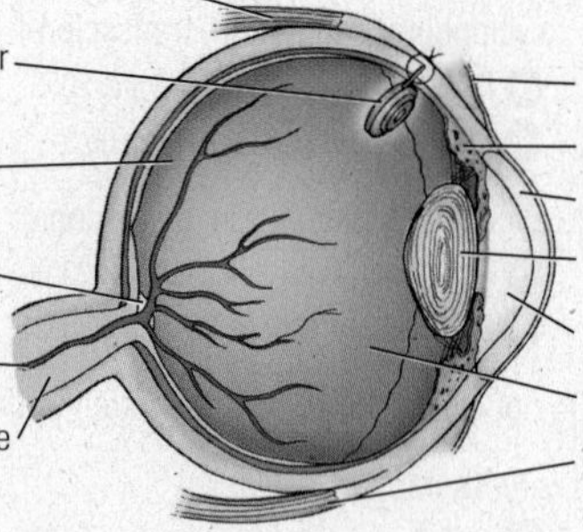

67028 Intravitreal injection of a pharmacologic agent (separate procedure)

➔ *CPT Assistant* Winter 90:9, Oct 12:15, Feb 18:3

67030 Discission of vitreous strands (without removal), pars plana approach

67031 Severing of vitreous strands, vitreous face adhesions, sheets, membranes or opacities, laser surgery (1 or more stages)

67036 Vitrectomy, mechanical, pars plana approach;

➔ *CPT Assistant* Fall 92:6, Oct 08:3

67039 with focal endolaser photocoagulation

➔ *CPT Assistant* Winter 90:9, Sep 05:12

67040 with endolaser panretinal photocoagulation

➔ *CPT Assistant* Winter 90:9, Sep 05:12, Jul 07:12

67041 with removal of preretinal cellular membrane (eg, macular pucker)

➔ *CPT Changes: An Insider's View* 2008

67042 with removal of internal limiting membrane of retina (eg, for repair of macular hole, diabetic macular edema), includes, if performed, intraocular tamponade (ie, air, gas or silicone oil)

➔ *CPT Changes: An Insider's View* 2008

67043 with removal of subretinal membrane (eg, choroidal neovascularization), includes, if performed, intraocular tamponade (ie, air, gas or silicone oil) and laser photocoagulation

➔ *CPT Changes: An Insider's View* 2008

(For use of ophthalmic endoscope with 67036, 67039, 67040-67043, use 66990)

(For associated lensectomy, use 66850)

(For use of vitrectomy in retinal detachment surgery, see 67108, 67113)

(For associated removal of foreign body, see 65260, 65265)

(For unlisted procedures on vitreous, use 67299)

Retina or Choroid

Repair

(If diathermy, cryotherapy and/or photocoagulation are combined, report under principal modality used)

67101 Repair of retinal detachment, including drainage of subretinal fluid when performed; cryotherapy

➲ *CPT Changes: An Insider's View* 2016, 2017

➲ *CPT Assistant* Mar 98:7, Jun 16:6, Sep 16:5, Feb 17:14

67105 photocoagulation

➲ *CPT Changes: An Insider's View* 2016, 2017

➲ *CPT Assistant* Mar 98:7, Jun 16:6, Sep 16:5, Feb 17:14

67107 Repair of retinal detachment; scleral buckling (such as lamellar scleral dissection, imbrication or encircling procedure), including, when performed, implant, cryotherapy, photocoagulation, and drainage of subretinal fluid

➲ *CPT Changes: An Insider's View* 2016

➲ *CPT Assistant* Jun 16:6, Sep 16:5

Repair of Retinal Detachment
67107

The retinal tear is treated externally by placing a hot or cold probe over the sclera and then depressing it. The burn seals the choroid to the retina at the site of the tear. The healing scar is supported by the encircling band, which buckles the eye.

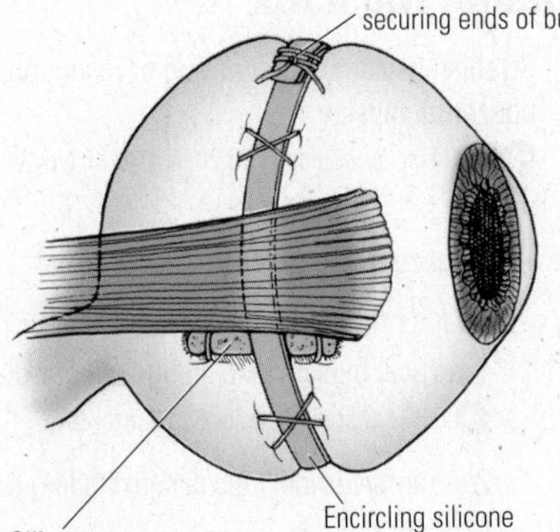

67108 with vitrectomy, any method, including, when performed, air or gas tamponade, focal endolaser photocoagulation, cryotherapy, drainage of subretinal fluid, scleral buckling, and/or removal of lens by same technique

➲ *CPT Changes: An Insider's View* 2016

➲ *CPT Assistant* Winter 90:9, Mar 12:9, Jun 16:6, Sep 16:5

67110 by injection of air or other gas (eg, pneumatic retinopexy)

➲ *CPT Assistant* Winter 90:9, Sep 16:5

(67112 has been deleted. To report, see 67107, 67108, 67110, 67113)

(For aspiration or drainage of subretinal or subchoroidal fluid, use 67015)

67113 Repair of complex retinal detachment (eg, proliferative vitreoretinopathy, stage C-1 or greater, diabetic traction retinal detachment, retinopathy of prematurity, retinal tear of greater than 90 degrees), with vitrectomy and membrane peeling, including, when performed, air, gas, or silicone oil tamponade, cryotherapy, endolaser photocoagulation, drainage of subretinal fluid, scleral buckling, and/or removal of lens

➲ *CPT Changes: An Insider's View* 2008, 2016

➲ *CPT Assistant* Jun 16:6, Sep 16:5

(To report vitrectomy, pars plana approach, other than in retinal detachment surgery, see 67036-67043)

(For use of ophthalmic endoscope with 67113, use 66990)

67115 Release of encircling material (posterior segment)

67120 Removal of implanted material, posterior segment; extraocular

67121 intraocular

➲ *CPT Assistant* Nov 97:23, Nov 98:19

(For removal from anterior segment, use 65920)

(For removal of foreign body, see 65260, 65265)

Prophylaxis

Codes 67141, 67145 include treatment at one or more sessions that may occur at different encounters. These codes should be reported once during a defined treatment period.

Repetitive services. The services listed below are often performed in multiple sessions or groups of sessions. The methods of reporting vary.

The following descriptors are intended to include all sessions in a defined treatment period.

67141 Prophylaxis of retinal detachment (eg, retinal break, lattice degeneration) without drainage, 1 or more sessions; cryotherapy, diathermy

➲ *CPT Assistant* Mar 98:7, Oct 08:3, Sep 16:5

67145 photocoagulation (laser or xenon arc)

➲ *CPT Assistant* Fall 92:4, Mar 98:7, Sep 16:5

Destruction

Codes 67208, 67210, 67218, 67220, 67229 include treatment at one or more sessions that may occur at different encounters. These codes should be reported once during a defined treatment period.

67208 Destruction of localized lesion of retina (eg, macular edema, tumors), 1 or more sessions; cryotherapy, diathermy
➔ *CPT Assistant* Mar 98:7, Nov 98:19, Oct 08:3

67210 photocoagulation
➔ *CPT Assistant* Mar 98:7, Nov 98:19, Oct 08:3, Jan 12:3

67218 radiation by implantation of source (includes removal of source)
➔ *CPT Assistant* Mar 98:7, Oct 08:3

67220 Destruction of localized lesion of choroid (eg, choroidal neovascularization); photocoagulation (eg, laser), 1 or more sessions
➔ *CPT Changes: An Insider's View* 2000, 2001
➔ *CPT Assistant* Nov 98:19, Nov 99:39, Feb 01:8, Oct 08:3, Jan 12:3

67221 photodynamic therapy (includes intravenous infusion)
➔ *CPT Changes: An Insider's View* 2001
➔ *CPT Assistant* Feb 01:8, Sep 01:10, Jun 02:10, Feb 18:10

+ 67225 photodynamic therapy, second eye, at single session (List separately in addition to code for primary eye treatment)
➔ *CPT Changes: An Insider's View* 2002
➔ *CPT Assistant* Jun 02:10

(Use 67225 in conjunction with 67221)

67227 Destruction of extensive or progressive retinopathy (eg, diabetic retinopathy), cryotherapy, diathermy
➔ *CPT Changes: An Insider's View* 2008, 2016
➔ *CPT Assistant* Mar 98:7, Oct 08:3

67228 Treatment of extensive or progressive retinopathy (eg, diabetic retinopathy), photocoagulation
➔ *CPT Changes: An Insider's View* 2008, 2016
➔ *CPT Assistant* Mar 98:7, Oct 08:3

67229 Treatment of extensive or progressive retinopathy, 1 or more sessions, preterm infant (less than 37 weeks gestation at birth), performed from birth up to 1 year of age (eg, retinopathy of prematurity), photocoagulation or cryotherapy
➔ *CPT Changes: An Insider's View* 2008

(For bilateral procedure, use modifier 50 with 67208, 67210, 67218, 67220, 67227, 67228, 67229)

(For unlisted procedures on retina, use 67299)

Posterior Sclera

Repair

(For excision lesion sclera, use 66130)

67250 Scleral reinforcement (separate procedure); without graft

67255 with graft
➔ *CPT Assistant* Jun 12:15, Jan 15:10

(Do not report 67255 in conjunction with 66180, 66185)

►(For repair scleral staphyloma, use 66225)◄

Other Procedures

67299 Unlisted procedure, posterior segment

Ocular Adnexa

Extraocular Muscles of Right Eye

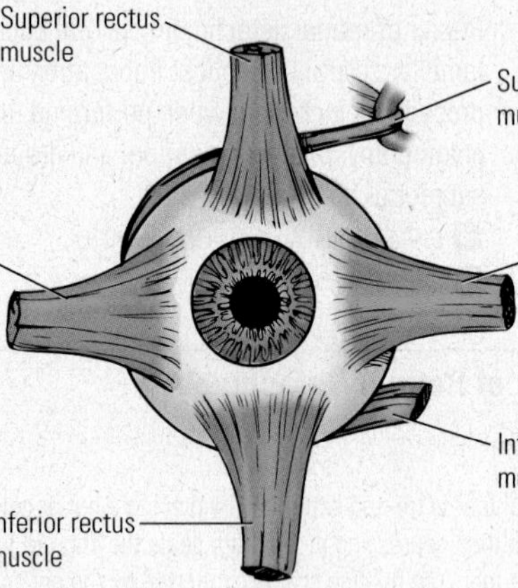

Extraocular Muscles

67311 Strabismus surgery, recession or resection procedure; 1 horizontal muscle
➔ *CPT Assistant* Summer 93:20, Mar 97:5, Nov 98:19, Sep 02:10, Jan 17:7

67312 2 horizontal muscles
➔ *CPT Assistant* Summer 93:20, Mar 97:5

67314 1 vertical muscle (excluding superior oblique)
➔ *CPT Assistant* Summer 93:20, Mar 97:5

67316 2 or more vertical muscles (excluding superior oblique)
➔ *CPT Assistant* Summer 93:20, Mar 97:5

(For adjustable sutures, use 67335 in addition to codes 67311-67334 for primary procedure reflecting number of muscles operated on)

Strabismus Surgery—Horizontal Muscles
67311-67312

In Figure A, the medial or lateral rectus muscle is made weaker by recession (retroplacement of the muscle attachment). In Figure B, it is made stronger by resection (removal of a segment). Use 67311 for one horizontal muscle and 67312 for two muscles of the same eye.

A

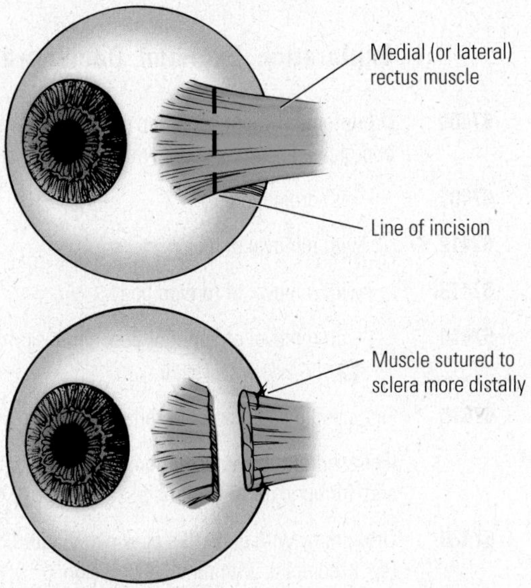

B

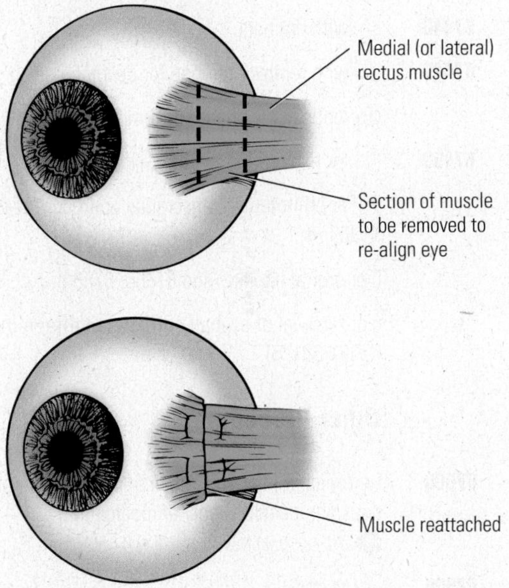

67318 Strabismus surgery, any procedure, superior oblique muscle

➔ *CPT Assistant* Summer 93:20, Mar 97:5, Nov 98:19

+ 67320 Transposition procedure (eg, for paretic extraocular muscle), any extraocular muscle (specify) (List separately in addition to code for primary procedure)

➔ *CPT Assistant* Summer 93:20, Mar 97:5

(Use 67320 in conjunction with 67311-67318)

Strabismus Surgery—Vertical Muscles
67314-67316

Either the superior or inferior rectus muscle is strengthened or weakened. Use 67316 for two muscles of the same eye.

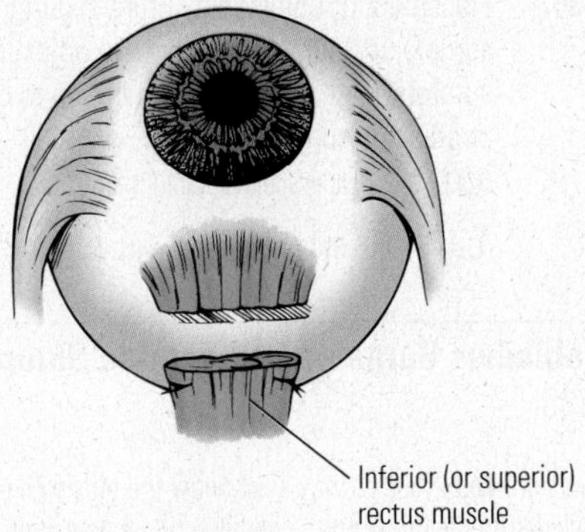

Transposition Procedure
67320

The extraocular muscles are transposed.

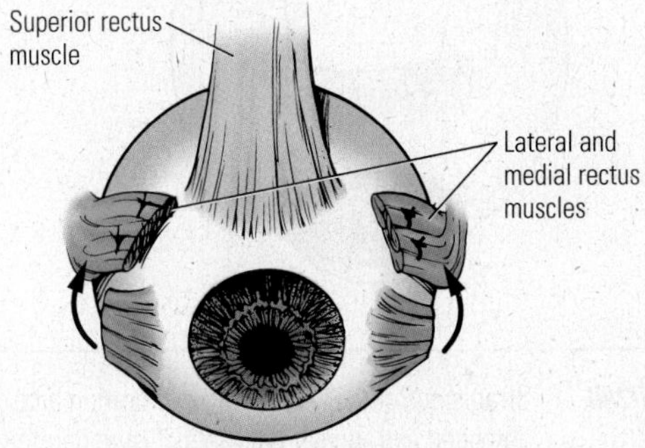

+ 67331 Strabismus surgery on patient with previous eye surgery or injury that did not involve the extraocular muscles (List separately in addition to code for primary procedure)

➔ *CPT Assistant* Summer 93:20, Mar 97:5

(Use 67331 in conjunction with 67311-67318)

+ 67332 Strabismus surgery on patient with scarring of extraocular muscles (eg, prior ocular injury, strabismus or retinal detachment surgery) or restrictive myopathy (eg, dysthyroid ophthalmopathy) (List separately in addition to code for primary procedure)

➔ *CPT Assistant* Summer 93:20, Mar 97:5

(Use 67332 in conjunction with 67311-67318)

+ 67334 Strabismus surgery by posterior fixation suture technique, with or without muscle recession (List separately in addition to code for primary procedure)
➔ *CPT Assistant* Summer 93:20, Mar 97:5

(Use 67334 in conjunction with 67311-67318)

+ 67335 Placement of adjustable suture(s) during strabismus surgery, including postoperative adjustment(s) of suture(s) (List separately in addition to code for specific strabismus surgery)
➔ *CPT Assistant* Summer 93:20, Mar 97:5

(Use 67335 in conjunction with 67311-67334)

Strabismus Surgery—Adjustable Sutures
67335

Sutures are tied in such a way as to allow the tension on the muscle to be adjusted after the anesthetic is not affecting the position of the globe.

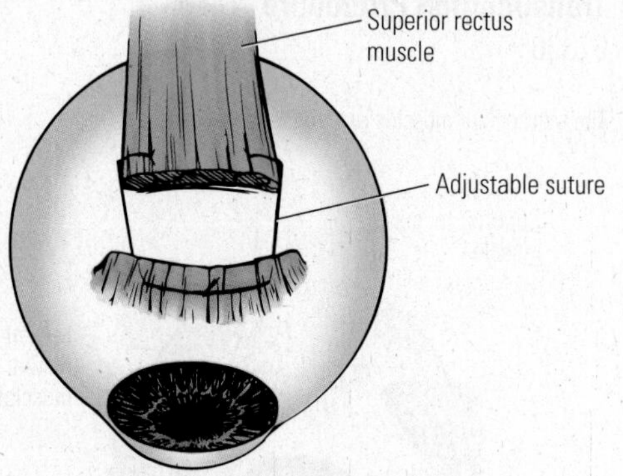

+ 67340 Strabismus surgery involving exploration and/or repair of detached extraocular muscle(s) (List separately in addition to code for primary procedure)
➔ *CPT Assistant* Summer 93:20, Mar 97:5

(Use 67340 in conjunction with 67311-67334)

67343 Release of extensive scar tissue without detaching extraocular muscle (separate procedure)
➔ *CPT Assistant* Summer 93:20, Mar 97:5

(Use 67343 in conjunction with 67311-67340, when such procedures are performed other than on the affected muscle)

67345 Chemodenervation of extraocular muscle
➔ *CPT Assistant* Summer 93:20, Mar 97:5, Apr 00:2, Feb 10:13, Dec 13:10, May 14:5

(For chemodenervation for blepharospasm and other neurological disorders, see 64612 and 64616)

67346 Biopsy of extraocular muscle
➔ *CPT Changes: An Insider's View* 2007

(For repair of wound, extraocular muscle, tendon or Tenon's capsule, use 65290)

Other Procedures

67399 Unlisted procedure, extraocular muscle
➔ *CPT Changes: An Insider's View* 2015
➔ *CPT Assistant* Jul 17:10

Orbit

Exploration, Excision, Decompression

67400 Orbitotomy without bone flap (frontal or transconjunctival approach); for exploration, with or without biopsy

67405 with drainage only

67412 with removal of lesion

67413 with removal of foreign body

67414 with removal of bone for decompression
➔ *CPT Assistant* Jul 99:10

67415 Fine needle aspiration of orbital contents

(For exenteration, enucleation, and repair, see 65101 et seq; for optic nerve decompression, use 67570)

67420 Orbitotomy with bone flap or window, lateral approach (eg, Kroenlein); with removal of lesion

67430 with removal of foreign body

67440 with drainage

67445 with removal of bone for decompression

(For optic nerve sheath decompression, use 67570)

67450 for exploration, with or without biopsy

►(For orbitotomy, transcranial approach, see 61330, 61333)◄

(For orbital implant, see 67550, 67560)

(For removal of eyeball or for repair after removal, see 65091-65175)

Other Procedures

67500 Retrobulbar injection; medication (separate procedure, does not include supply of medication)
➔ *CPT Assistant* Nov 12:10

67505 alcohol

67515 Injection of medication or other substance into Tenon's capsule
➔ *CPT Changes: An Insider's View* 2002
➔ *CPT Assistant* Nov 12:10

(For subconjunctival injection, use 68200)

67550 Orbital implant (implant outside muscle cone); insertion

67560 removal or revision

(For ocular implant (implant inside muscle cone), see 65093-65105, 65130-65175)

(For treatment of fractures of malar area, orbit, see 21355 et seq)

67570 Optic nerve decompression (eg, incision or fenestration of optic nerve sheath)

67599 Unlisted procedure, orbit

Eyelids

Incision

67700 Blepharotomy, drainage of abscess, eyelid
➲ *CPT Assistant* Mar 13:6

67710 Severing of tarsorrhaphy
➲ *CPT Assistant* Mar 13:6

67715 Canthotomy (separate procedure)
➲ *CPT Assistant* Mar 13:6

(For canthoplasty, use 67950)

(For division of symblepharon, use 68340)

 # 67810 Incisional biopsy of eyelid skin including lid margin
➲ *CPT Changes: An Insider's View* 2013
➲ *CPT Assistant* Dec 04:19, Feb 13:16, Mar 13:6

►(For biopsy of skin of the eyelid, see 11102, 11103, 11104, 11105, 11106, 11107)◄

Excision, Destruction

Codes for removal of lesion include more than skin (ie, involving lid margin, tarsus, and/or palpebral conjunctiva).

(For removal of lesion, involving mainly skin of eyelid, see 11310-11313; 11440-11446, 11640-11646; 17000-17004)

(For repair of wounds, blepharoplasty, grafts, reconstructive surgery, see 67930-67975)

67800 Excision of chalazion; single
➲ *CPT Assistant* Sep 99:10

67801 multiple, same lid

67805 multiple, different lids
➲ *CPT Assistant* Sep 99:10

67808 under general anesthesia and/or requiring hospitalization, single or multiple

67810 Code is out of numerical sequence. See 67710-67801

67820 Correction of trichiasis; epilation, by forceps only
➲ *CPT Assistant* Jul 98:10

Trichiasis
67820-67825

When the eyelashes are ingrown or misdirected (trichiasis), the physician uses a biomicroscope and forceps to remove the offending eyelashes. Report 67825 when cryosurgery or electrosurgery is used to destroy the follicles.

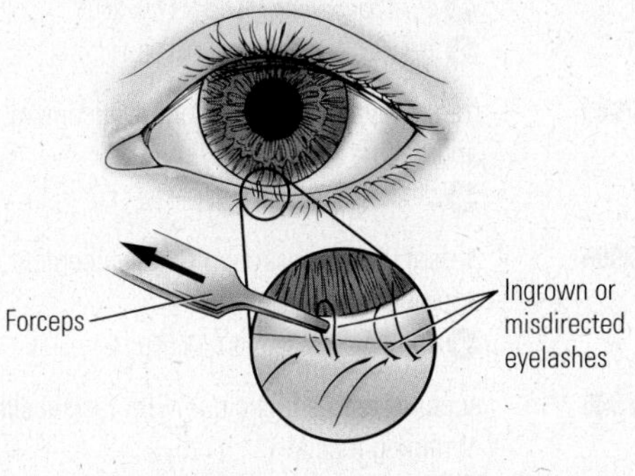

67825 epilation by other than forceps (eg, by electrosurgery, cryotherapy, laser surgery)
➲ *CPT Assistant* Jul 98:10

67830 incision of lid margin

67835 incision of lid margin, with free mucous membrane graft

67840 Excision of lesion of eyelid (except chalazion) without closure or with simple direct closure

(For excision and repair of eyelid by reconstructive surgery, see 67961, 67966)

67850 Destruction of lesion of lid margin (up to 1 cm)

(For Mohs micrographic surgery, see 17311-17315)

(For initiation or follow-up care of topical chemotherapy (eg, 5-FU or similar agents), see appropriate office visits)

Tarsorrhaphy

67875 Temporary closure of eyelids by suture (eg, Frost suture)
➲ *CPT Assistant* Winter 90:9

67880 Construction of intermarginal adhesions, median tarsorrhaphy, or canthorrhaphy;

67882 with transposition of tarsal plate

(For severing of tarsorrhaphy, use 67710)

(For canthoplasty, reconstruction canthus, use 67950)

(For canthotomy, use 67715)

Repair (Brow Ptosis, Blepharoptosis, Lid Retraction, Ectropion, Entropion)

67900 Repair of brow ptosis (supraciliary, mid-forehead or coronal approach)

(For forehead rhytidectomy, use 15824)

67901 Repair of blepharoptosis; frontalis muscle technique with suture or other material (eg, banked fascia)
CPT Changes: An Insider's View 2006
CPT Assistant Sep 00:7, Oct 06:11, Jul 17:10

67902 frontalis muscle technique with autologous fascial sling (includes obtaining fascia)
CPT Changes: An Insider's View 2006
CPT Assistant Sep 00:7, Oct 06:11

67903 (tarso) levator resection or advancement, internal approach
CPT Assistant Sep 00:7, Oct 06:11

67904 (tarso) levator resection or advancement, external approach
CPT Assistant Sep 00:7, Oct 06:11, Aug 11:8

67906 superior rectus technique with fascial sling (includes obtaining fascia)
CPT Assistant Sep 00:7, Oct 06:11

67908 conjunctivo-tarso-Muller's muscle-levator resection (eg, Fasanella-Servat type)
CPT Assistant Sep 00:7, Oct 06:11

67909 Reduction of overcorrection of ptosis

67911 Correction of lid retraction

(For obtaining autogenous graft materials, see 20920, 20922 or 20926)

(For correction of trichiasis by mucous membrane graft, use 67835)

67912 Correction of lagophthalmos, with implantation of upper eyelid lid load (eg, gold weight)
CPT Changes: An Insider's View 2004
CPT Assistant May 04:12, Aug 04:10, Oct 06:11

67914 Repair of ectropion; suture

67915 thermocauterization

67916 excision tarsal wedge
CPT Changes: An Insider's View 2004
CPT Assistant Feb 04:11, May 04:12, Feb 05:16, Oct 06:11

67917 extensive (eg, tarsal strip operations)
CPT Changes: An Insider's View 2004
CPT Assistant Feb 04:11, May 04:12, Oct 06:11

(For correction of everted punctum, use 68705)

67921 Repair of entropion; suture

67922 thermocauterization

67923 excision tarsal wedge
CPT Changes: An Insider's View 2004
CPT Assistant May 04:12, Oct 06:11

67924 extensive (eg, tarsal strip or capsulopalpebral fascia repairs operation)
CPT Changes: An Insider's View 2004
CPT Assistant May 04:12, Oct 06:11

(For repair of cicatricial ectropion or entropion requiring scar excision or skin graft, see also 67961 et seq)

Reconstruction

Codes for blepharoplasty involve more than skin (ie, involving lid margin, tarsus, and/or palpebral conjunctiva).

67930 Suture of recent wound, eyelid, involving lid margin, tarsus, and/or palpebral conjunctiva direct closure; partial thickness

67935 full thickness

67938 Removal of embedded foreign body, eyelid
CPT Assistant May 14:5

(For repair of skin of eyelid, see 12011-12018, 12051-12057, 13151-13153)

(For tarsorrhaphy, canthorrhaphy, see 67880, 67882)

(For repair of blepharoptosis and lid retraction, see 67901-67911)

(For blepharoplasty for entropion, ectropion, see 67916, 67917, 67923, 67924)

(For correction of blepharochalasis (blepharorhytidectomy), see 15820-15823)

(For repair of skin of eyelid, adjacent tissue transfer, see 14060, 14061; preparation for graft, use 15004; free graft, see 15120, 15121, 15260, 15261)

(For excision of lesion of eyelid, use 67800 et seq)

(For repair of lacrimal canaliculi, use 68700)

67950 Canthoplasty (reconstruction of canthus)

67961 Excision and repair of eyelid, involving lid margin, tarsus, conjunctiva, canthus, or full thickness, may include preparation for skin graft or pedicle flap with adjacent tissue transfer or rearrangement; up to one-fourth of lid margin

67966 over one-fourth of lid margin
CPT Assistant Nov 12:13

(For canthoplasty, use 67950)

(For free skin grafts, see 15120, 15121, 15260, 15261)

(For tubed pedicle flap preparation, use 15576; for delay, use 15630; for attachment, use 15650)

67971 Reconstruction of eyelid, full thickness by transfer of tarsoconjunctival flap from opposing eyelid; up to two-thirds of eyelid, 1 stage or first stage

67973 total eyelid, lower, 1 stage or first stage

67974 total eyelid, upper, 1 stage or first stage

67975 second stage

Other Procedures

67999 Unlisted procedure, eyelids
CPT Assistant Jul 17:10

Conjunctiva

(For removal of foreign body, see 65205 et seq)

Incision and Drainage

68020 Incision of conjunctiva, drainage of cyst

68040 Expression of conjunctival follicles (eg, for trachoma)
➔ *CPT Assistant* May 14:5

(To report automated evacuation of Meibomian glands, use 0207T)

Excision and/or Destruction

68100 Biopsy of conjunctiva

68110 Excision of lesion, conjunctiva; up to 1 cm
➔ *CPT Assistant* Jan 17:7, Feb 18:11

68115 over 1 cm
➔ *CPT Assistant* Feb 18:11

68130 with adjacent sclera

68135 Destruction of lesion, conjunctiva

Injection

(For injection into Tenon's capsule or retrobulbar injection, see 67500-67515)

68200 Subconjunctival injection
➔ *CPT Assistant* Aug 03:15, Nov 12:10

Conjunctivoplasty

(For wound repair, see 65270-65273)

68320 Conjunctivoplasty; with conjunctival graft or extensive rearrangement
➔ *CPT Assistant* Feb 04:11

68325 with buccal mucous membrane graft (includes obtaining graft)

68326 Conjunctivoplasty, reconstruction cul-de-sac; with conjunctival graft or extensive rearrangement

68328 with buccal mucous membrane graft (includes obtaining graft)

68330 Repair of symblepharon; conjunctivoplasty, without graft

68335 with free graft conjunctiva or buccal mucous membrane (includes obtaining graft)

68340 division of symblepharon, with or without insertion of conformer or contact lens

Other Procedures

68360 Conjunctival flap; bridge or partial (separate procedure)

68362 total (such as Gunderson thin flap or purse string flap)

(For conjunctival flap for perforating injury, see 65280, 65285)

(For repair of operative wound, use 66250)

(For removal of conjunctival foreign body, see 65205, 65210)

68371 Harvesting conjunctival allograft, living donor
➔ *CPT Changes: An Insider's View* 2004
➔ *CPT Assistant* May 04:10

68399 Unlisted procedure, conjunctiva

Lacrimal System

Incision

68400 Incision, drainage of lacrimal gland

68420 Incision, drainage of lacrimal sac (dacryocystotomy or dacryocystostomy)

68440 Snip incision of lacrimal punctum

Excision

68500 Excision of lacrimal gland (dacryoadenectomy), except for tumor; total

68505 partial

68510 Biopsy of lacrimal gland

68520 Excision of lacrimal sac (dacryocystectomy)

68525 Biopsy of lacrimal sac

68530 Removal of foreign body or dacryolith, lacrimal passages

68540 Excision of lacrimal gland tumor; frontal approach

68550 involving osteotomy

Repair

68700 Plastic repair of canaliculi

68705 Correction of everted punctum, cautery

68720 Dacryocystorhinostomy (fistulization of lacrimal sac to nasal cavity)
➔ *CPT Assistant* Sep 01:10, Jul 03:15, Aug 03:14, Aug 09:11

68745 Conjunctivorhinostomy (fistulization of conjunctiva to nasal cavity); without tube

68750 with insertion of tube or stent

68760 Closure of the lacrimal punctum; by thermocauterization, ligation, or laser surgery

68761 by plug, each

➔ *CPT Assistant* Jun 96:10, Jan 07:28

(For insertion and removal of drug-eluting implant into lacrimal canaliculus for intra-ocular pressure, use 0356T)

(For placement of drug-eluting insert under the eyelid[s], see 0444T, 0445T)

Closure of Lacrimal Punctum by Plug
68761

The physician inserts a lacrimal duct implant into a lacrimal punctum.

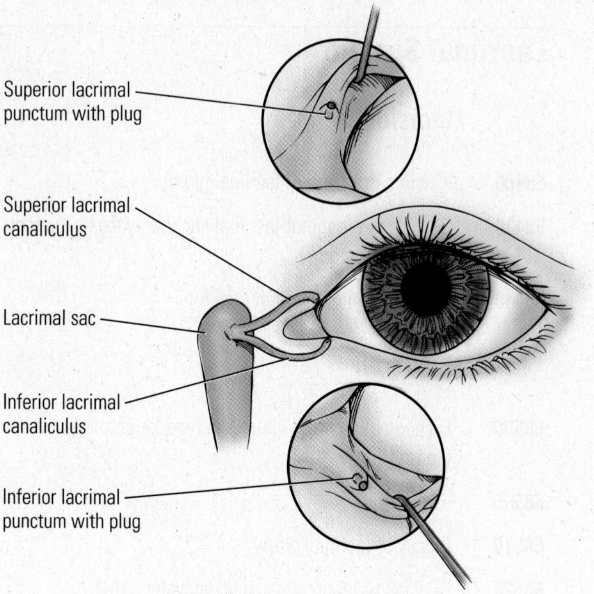

68770 Closure of lacrimal fistula (separate procedure)

Probing and/or Related Procedures

68801 Dilation of lacrimal punctum, with or without irrigation

(To report a bilateral procedure, use 68801 with modifier 50)

68810 Probing of nasolacrimal duct, with or without irrigation;

➔ *CPT Assistant* Nov 02:11, Oct 08:3

(For bilateral procedure, report 68810 with modifier 50)

68811 requiring general anesthesia

➔ *CPT Assistant* Nov 02:11, Oct 08:3

(For bilateral procedure, report 68811 with modifier 50)

68815 with insertion of tube or stent

➔ *CPT Assistant* Nov 02:11, Oct 08:3, Aug 09:11, Nov 10:9

(See also 92018)

(For bilateral procedure, report 68815 with modifier 50)

(For insertion and removal of drug-eluting implant into lacrimal canaliculus for intra-ocular pressure, use 0356T)

(For placement of drug-eluting insert under the eyelid[s], see 0444T, 0445T)

68816 with transluminal balloon catheter dilation

➔ *CPT Changes: An Insider's View* 2008

Probing of Nasolacrimal Duct
68816

A balloon catheter is in the nasolacrimal duct.

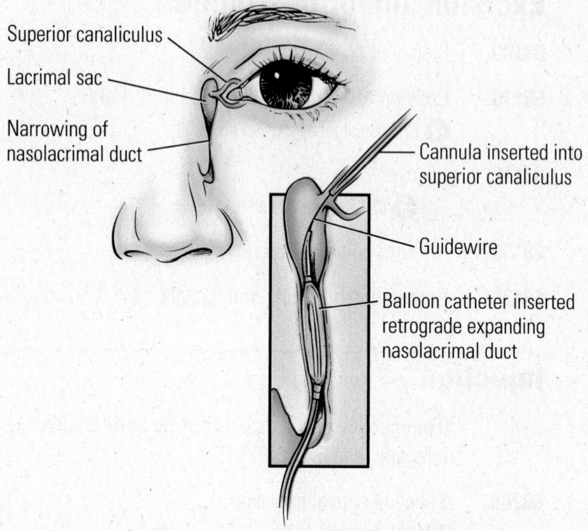

(Do not report 68816 in conjunction with 68810, 68811, 68815)

(For bilateral procedure, report 68816 with modifier 50)

68840 Probing of lacrimal canaliculi, with or without irrigation

68850 Injection of contrast medium for dacryocystography

➔ *CPT Assistant* Feb 01:9

(For radiological supervision and interpretation, see 70170, 78660)

Other Procedures

68899 Unlisted procedure, lacrimal system

Notes

Notes

Surgery

Auditory System (69000-69979) 464

The following is a listing of headings and subheadings that appear within the Auditory System and Operating Microscope sections of the CPT codebook. The subheadings or subsections denoted with asterisks (*) below have special instructions unique to that subsection. Where these are indicated, special notes or guidelines will be presented preceding those procedural terminology listings, referring to that subsection specifically.

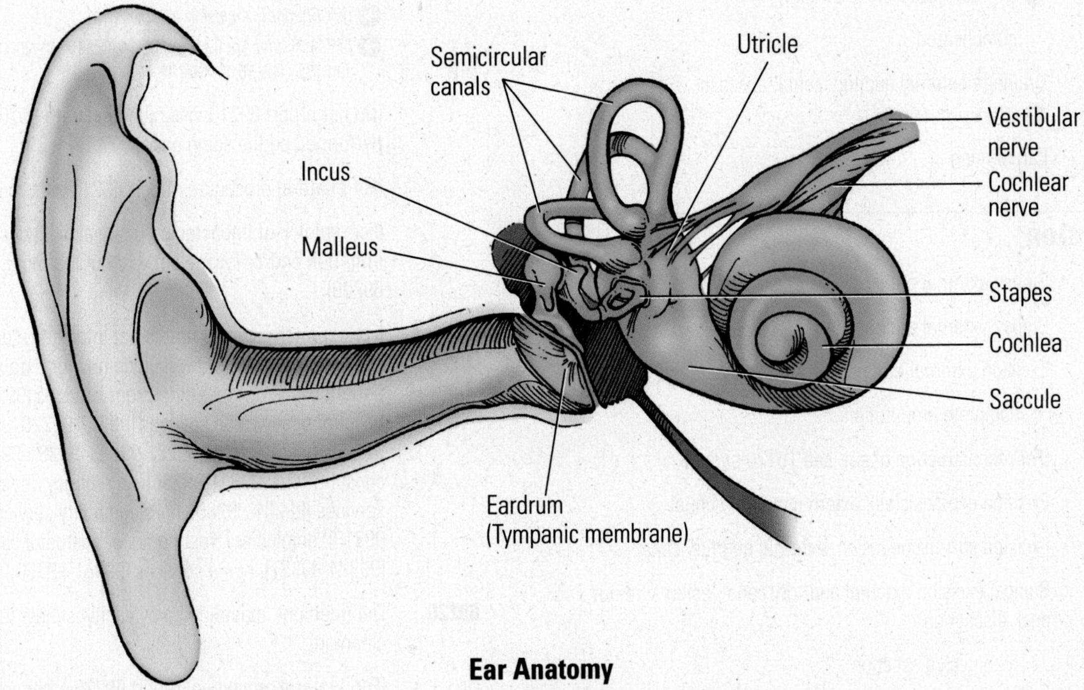

Ear Anatomy

External Ear (69000-69399) 464
- Incision (69000-69090) 464
- Excision (69100-69155) 464
- Removal (69200-69222) 464
- Repair (69300-69320) 464
- Other Procedures (69399) 465

Middle Ear (69420-69799) 465
- Incision (69420-69450) 465
- Excision (69501-69554) 465
- Repair (69601-69676) 466
- Other Procedures (69700-69799) 466

Inner Ear (69801-69949) 467
- Incision and/or Destruction (69801-69806) 467
- Excision (69905-69915) 467
- Introduction (69930) 467
- Other Procedures (69949) 467

Temporal Bone, Middle Fossa Approach (69950-69979) 467
- Other Procedures (69979) 467

Operating Microscope* (69990) 468

Auditory System

(For diagnostic services (eg, audiometry, vestibular tests), see 92502 et seq)

External Ear

Incision

69000 Drainage external ear, abscess or hematoma; simple
➔ *CPT Assistant* Oct 97:11, Oct 99:10

69005 complicated

69020 Drainage external auditory canal, abscess
➔ *CPT Assistant* Oct 97:11

69090 Ear piercing

Excision

69100 Biopsy external ear

69105 Biopsy external auditory canal

69110 Excision external ear; partial, simple repair

69120 complete amputation

(For reconstruction of ear, see 15120 et seq)

69140 Excision exostosis(es), external auditory canal

69145 Excision soft tissue lesion, external auditory canal

69150 Radical excision external auditory canal lesion; without neck dissection

69155 with neck dissection

(For resection of temporal bone, use 69535)

(For skin grafting, see 15004-15261)

Removal

69200 Removal foreign body from external auditory canal; without general anesthesia

69205 with general anesthesia
➔ *CPT Assistant* Apr 13:10

69209 Removal impacted cerumen using irrigation/lavage, unilateral
➔ *CPT Changes: An Insider's View* 2016
➔ *CPT Assistant* Jan 16:7, Feb 16:14, Mar 16:11

(Do not report 69209 in conjunction with 69210 when performed on the same ear)

(For bilateral procedure, report 69209 with modifier 50)

(For removal of impacted cerumen requiring instrumentation, use 69210)

(For cerumen removal that is not impacted, see E/M service code, which may include new or established patient office or other outpatient services [99201-99215], hospital observation services [99217-99220, 99224-99226], hospital care [99221-99223, 99231-99233], consultations [99241-99255], emergency department services [99281-99285], nursing facility services [99304-99318], domiciliary, rest home, or custodial care services [99324-99337], home services [99341-99350])

69210 Removal impacted cerumen requiring instrumentation, unilateral
➔ *CPT Changes: An Insider's View* 2014
➔ *CPT Assistant* Apr 03:9, Jul 05:14, Oct 13:14, Nov 14:14, Jan 16:7, Feb 16:14, Mar 16:11

(Do not report 69210 in conjunction with 69209 when performed on the same ear)

(For bilateral procedure, report 69210 with modifier 50)

(For removal of impacted cerumen achieved with irrigation and/or lavage but without instrumentation, use 69209)

(For cerumen removal that is not impacted, see E/M service code, which may include new or established patient office or other outpatient services [99201-99215], hospital observation services [99217-99220, 99224-99226], hospital care [99221-99223, 99231-99233], consultations [99241-99255], emergency department services [99281-99285], nursing facility services [99304-99318], domiciliary, rest home, or custodial care services [99324-99337], home services [99341-99350])

69220 Debridement, mastoidectomy cavity, simple (eg, routine cleaning)

(For bilateral procedure, report 69220 with modifier 50)

69222 Debridement, mastoidectomy cavity, complex (eg, with anesthesia or more than routine cleaning)

(For bilateral procedure, report 69222 with modifier 50)

Repair

(For suture of wound or injury of external ear, see 12011-14302)

69300 Otoplasty, protruding ear, with or without size reduction
➔ *CPT Changes: An Insider's View* 2017

(For bilateral procedure, report 69300 with modifier 50)

69310 Reconstruction of external auditory canal (meatoplasty) (eg, for stenosis due to injury, infection) (separate procedure)

➔ *CPT Changes: An Insider's View* 2002

➔ *CPT Assistant* Jan 14:9, Jul 14:9

69320 Reconstruction external auditory canal for congenital atresia, single stage

(For combination with middle ear reconstruction, see 69631, 69641)

(For other reconstructive procedures with grafts (eg, skin, cartilage, bone), see 13151-15760, 21230-21235)

Other Procedures

(For otoscopy under general anesthesia, use 92502)

69399 Unlisted procedure, external ear

Middle Ear

Incision

69420 Myringotomy including aspiration and/or eustachian tube inflation

➔ *CPT Assistant* May 11:8

69421 Myringotomy including aspiration and/or eustachian tube inflation requiring general anesthesia

➔ *CPT Assistant* May 11:8

69424 Ventilating tube removal requiring general anesthesia

➔ *CPT Changes: An Insider's View* 2003

➔ *CPT Assistant* Mar 05:17, Jun 10:11, Nov 10:9

(For bilateral procedure, report 69424 with modifier 50)

(Do not report code 69424 in conjunction with 69205, 69210, 69420, 69421, 69433-69676, 69710-69745, 69801-69930)

69433 Tympanostomy (requiring insertion of ventilating tube), local or topical anesthesia

➔ *CPT Assistant* May 11:8, Feb 18:11

(For bilateral procedure, report 69433 with modifier 50)

Tympanostomy
69433-69436

A ventilating tube is inserted into the opening of the tympanum.

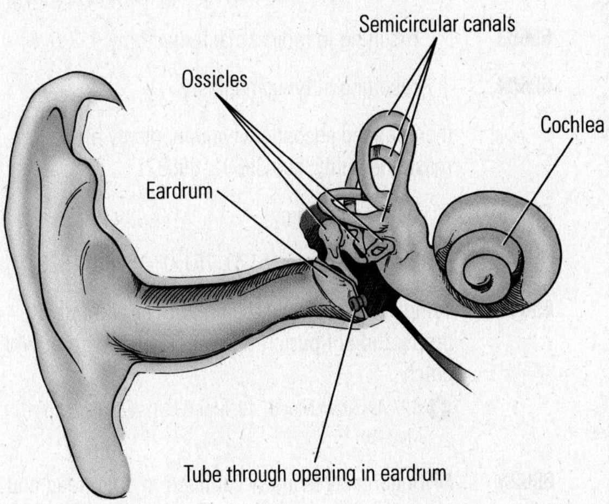

69436 Tympanostomy (requiring insertion of ventilating tube), general anesthesia

➔ *CPT Assistant* May 11:8, May 12:14, Feb 18:11

(For bilateral procedure, report 69436 with modifier 50)

69440 Middle ear exploration through postauricular or ear canal incision

(For atticotomy, see 69601 et seq)

69450 Tympanolysis, transcanal

Excision

69501 Transmastoid antrotomy (simple mastoidectomy)

69502 Mastoidectomy; complete

69505 modified radical

69511 radical

(For skin graft, see 15004 et seq)

(For mastoidectomy cavity debridement, see 69220, 69222)

69530 Petrous apicectomy including radical mastoidectomy

69535 Resection temporal bone, external approach

(For middle fossa approach, see 69950-69970)

69540 Excision aural polyp

69550 Excision aural glomus tumor; transcanal

69552 transmastoid

69554 extended (extratemporal)

Auditory 69000-69979

Repair

69601 Revision mastoidectomy; resulting in complete mastoidectomy

69602 resulting in modified radical mastoidectomy

69603 resulting in radical mastoidectomy

69604 resulting in tympanoplasty

(For planned secondary tympanoplasty after mastoidectomy, see 69631, 69632)

69605 with apicectomy

(For skin graft, see 15120, 15121, 15260, 15261)

69610 Tympanic membrane repair, with or without site preparation of perforation for closure, with or without patch

➔ *CPT Assistant* Mar 01:10, Mar 03:21, Aug 08:4, Apr 15:11, May 15:11

69620 Myringoplasty (surgery confined to drumhead and donor area)

➔ *CPT Assistant* Mar 01:10, Aug 08:4, Apr 15:11, May 15:11

69631 Tympanoplasty without mastoidectomy (including canalplasty, atticotomy and/or middle ear surgery), initial or revision; without ossicular chain reconstruction

➔ *CPT Assistant* Jul 98:11, Mar 01:10, Mar 07:9, Aug 08:4, Dec 12:11

69632 with ossicular chain reconstruction (eg, postfenestration)

69633 with ossicular chain reconstruction and synthetic prosthesis (eg, partial ossicular replacement prosthesis [PORP], total ossicular replacement prosthesis [TORP])

69635 Tympanoplasty with antrotomy or mastoidotomy (including canalplasty, atticotomy, middle ear surgery, and/or tympanic membrane repair); without ossicular chain reconstruction

69636 with ossicular chain reconstruction

69637 with ossicular chain reconstruction and synthetic prosthesis (eg, partial ossicular replacement prosthesis [PORP], total ossicular replacement prosthesis [TORP])

69641 Tympanoplasty with mastoidectomy (including canalplasty, middle ear surgery, tympanic membrane repair); without ossicular chain reconstruction

69642 with ossicular chain reconstruction

69643 with intact or reconstructed wall, without ossicular chain reconstruction

69644 with intact or reconstructed canal wall, with ossicular chain reconstruction

69645 radical or complete, without ossicular chain reconstruction

Tympanoplasty
69635-69646

A graft is used to repair the tympanic membrane perforation.

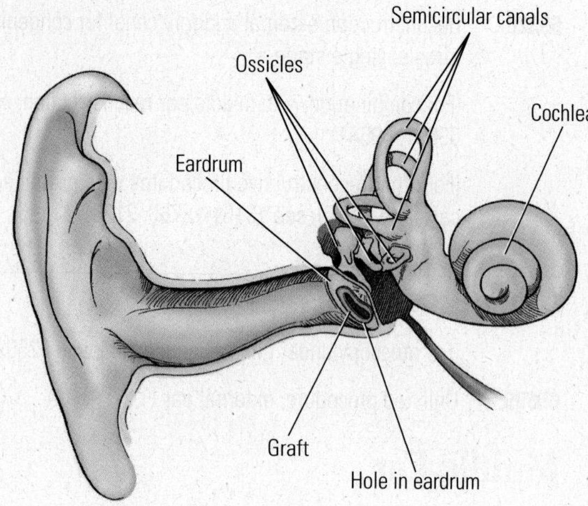

69646 radical or complete, with ossicular chain reconstruction

69650 Stapes mobilization

69660 Stapedectomy or stapedotomy with reestablishment of ossicular continuity, with or without use of foreign material;

69661 with footplate drill out

69662 Revision of stapedectomy or stapedotomy

69666 Repair oval window fistula

69667 Repair round window fistula

69670 Mastoid obliteration (separate procedure)

69676 Tympanic neurectomy

(For bilateral procedure, report 69676 with modifier 50)

Other Procedures

69700 Closure postauricular fistula, mastoid (separate procedure)

69710 Implantation or replacement of electromagnetic bone conduction hearing device in temporal bone

(Replacement procedure includes removal of old device)

69711 Removal or repair of electromagnetic bone conduction hearing device in temporal bone

69714 Implantation, osseointegrated implant, temporal bone, with percutaneous attachment to external speech processor/cochlear stimulator; without mastoidectomy

➔ *CPT Changes: An Insider's View* 2001

➔ *CPT Assistant* Oct 13:19

69715 with mastoidectomy

➔ *CPT Changes: An Insider's View* 2001

69717 Replacement (including removal of existing device), osseointegrated implant, temporal bone, with percutaneous attachment to external speech processor/cochlear stimulator; without mastoidectomy

➔ *CPT Changes: An Insider's View* 2001

69718 with mastoidectomy

➔ *CPT Changes: An Insider's View* 2001

69720 Decompression facial nerve, intratemporal; lateral to geniculate ganglion

69725 including medial to geniculate ganglion

69740 Suture facial nerve, intratemporal, with or without graft or decompression; lateral to geniculate ganglion

69745 including medial to geniculate ganglion

(For extracranial suture of facial nerve, use 64864)

69799 Unlisted procedure, middle ear

➔ *CPT Assistant* Oct 99:10

Inner Ear

Incision and/or Destruction

69801 Labyrinthotomy, with perfusion of vestibuloactive drug(s), transcanal

➔ *CPT Changes: An Insider's View* 2011

➔ *CPT Assistant* Nov 96:12, May 11:8

(Do not report 69801 more than once per day)

(Do not report 69801 in conjunction with 69420, 69421, 69433, 69436 when performed on the same ear)

69805 Endolymphatic sac operation; without shunt

69806 with shunt

➔ *CPT Assistant* Nov 96:12

(69820, 69840 have been deleted)

Excision

69905 Labyrinthectomy; transcanal

69910 with mastoidectomy

69915 Vestibular nerve section, translabyrinthine approach

(For transcranial approach, use 69950)

Introduction

69930 Cochlear device implantation, with or without mastoidectomy

Cochlear Device Implantation
69930

An internal coil is attached to the temporal bone and the ground wire attached to the internal coil is connected to the temporalis muscle.

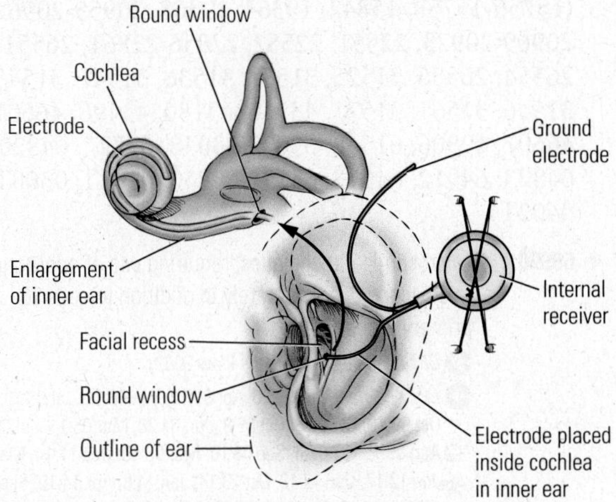

Other Procedures

69949 Unlisted procedure, inner ear

Temporal Bone, Middle Fossa Approach

(For external approach, use 69535)

69950 Vestibular nerve section, transcranial approach

69955 Total facial nerve decompression and/or repair (may include graft)

69960 Decompression internal auditory canal

69970 Removal of tumor, temporal bone

Other Procedures

69979 Unlisted procedure, temporal bone, middle fossa approach

➔ *CPT Assistant* Jan 07:30, Sep 14:14

Auditory 69000-69979

Operating Microscope

The surgical microscope is employed when the surgical services are performed using the techniques of microsurgery. Code 69990 should be reported (without modifier 51 appended) in addition to the code for the primary procedure performed. Do not use 69990 for visualization with magnifying loupes or corrected vision. Do not report 69990 in addition to procedures where use of the operating microscope is an inclusive component (15756-15758, 15842, 19364, 19368, 20955-20962, 20969-20973, 22551, 22552, 22856-22861, 26551-26554, 26556, 31526, 31531, 31536, 31541, 31545, 31546, 31561, 31571, 43116, 43180, 43496, 46601, 46607, 49906, 61548, 63075-63078, 64727, 64820-64823, 64912, 64913, 65091-68850, 0184T, 0308T, 0402T).

+ 69990 Microsurgical techniques, requiring use of operating microscope (List separately in addition to code for primary procedure)

➔ *CPT Changes: An Insider's View* 2002

➔ *CPT Assistant* Nov 98:20, Apr 99:11, Jun 99:11, Jul 99:10, Oct 99:10, Oct 00:3, Oct 02:8, Jan 04:28, Mar 05:11, Jul 05:14, Aug 05:1, Nov 07:4, Sep 08:10, Mar 09:10, Dec 11:14, Mar 12:9, Jun 12:17, Dec 12:13, Oct 13:14, Jan 14:8, Apr 14:10, Sep 14:13-14, Feb 16:12, Dec 17:13, Feb 18:11

Operating Microscope
69990

A surgical operating microscope is used to obtain good visualization of the fine structures in the operating field. The lens system may be operated by hand or foot controls to adjust to working distance, with interchangeable oculars providing magnification as needed.

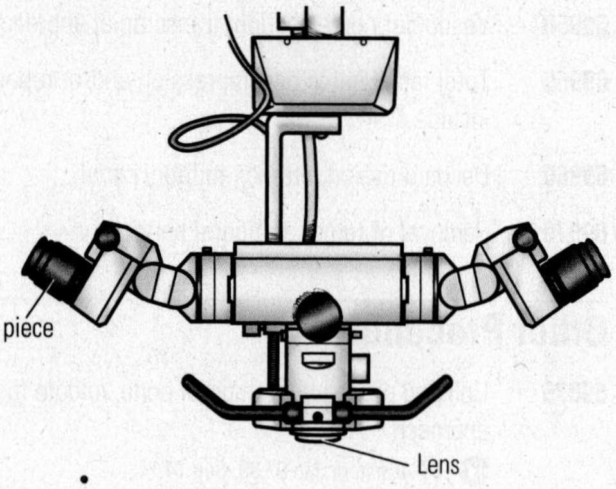

Notes

Operating Microscope 69990

Radiology Guidelines (Including Nuclear Medicine and Diagnostic Ultrasound)

Subject Listings ... 472
Separate Procedures ... 472
Unlisted Service or Procedure ... 472
Special Report ... 473
►Supervision and Interpretation, Imaging Guidance◄ ... 473
Administration of Contrast Material(s) ... 473
Written Report(s) ... 473

Radiology

The following is a listing of headings and subheadings that appear within the Radiology section of the CPT codebook. The subheadings or subsections denoted with asterisks (*) below have special instructions unique to that subsection. Where these are indicated, special notes or guidelines will be presented preceding those procedural terminology listings, referring to that subsection specifically.

Diagnostic Radiology (Diagnostic Imaging) (70010-76499) ... 474
Head and Neck (70010-70559) ... 474
Chest (71045-71555) ... 476
Spine and Pelvis (72020-72295) ... 477
Upper Extremities (73000-73225) ... 480
Lower Extremities (73501-73725) ... 481
Abdomen (74018-74190) ... 482
Gastrointestinal Tract (74210-74363) ... 483
Urinary Tract (74400-74485) ... 485
Gynecological and Obstetrical (74710-74775) ... 485
Heart (75557-75574) ... 485
Vascular Procedures (75600-75989) ... 486
Aorta and Arteries* (75600-75774) ... 486
Veins and Lymphatics* (75801-75893) ... 488
Transcatheter Procedures* (75894-75989) ... 490
Other Procedures (76000-76499) ... 492
Diagnostic Ultrasound* (76506-76999) ... 493
Head and Neck (76506-76536) ... 493
Chest* (76604-76642) ... 494
Abdomen and Retroperitoneum* (76700-76776) ... 494
Spinal Canal (76800) ... 495

Pelvis (76801-76857) 495
Obstetrical* (76801-76828) 495
Nonobstetrical* (76830-76857) 496
Genitalia (76870-76873) 497
Extremities* (76881-76886) 497
Ultrasonic Guidance Procedures (76930-76965) 498
Other Procedures (76970-76999) 498

Radiologic Guidance (77001-77022) 499
Fluoroscopic Guidance (77001-77003) 499
Computed Tomography Guidance (77011-77014) 500
►Magnetic Resonance Imaging Guidance◄ (77021-77022) 500

Breast, Mammography (77046-77067) 500

Bone/Joint Studies (77071-77086) 502

Radiation Oncology* (77261-77799) 502
Consultation: Clinical Management* 502
Clinical Treatment Planning (External and Internal Sources)* (77261-77293, 77299) 502
Medical Radiation Physics, Dosimetry, Treatment Devices, and Special Services (77295-77370) 503
Stereotactic Radiation Treatment Delivery (77371-77373) 504
Other Procedures (77399) 505
Radiation Treatment Delivery* (77385-77387, 77401-77417, 77424-77425) 505
Neutron Beam Treatment Delivery (77423) 506
Radiation Treatment Management* (77427-77499) 506
Proton Beam Treatment Delivery* (77520-77525) 508
Hyperthermia* (77600-77615) 508
Clinical Intracavitary Hyperthermia (77620) 509
Clinical Brachytherapy* (77750-77799) 509

Nuclear Medicine* (78012-79999) 510
Diagnostic (78012-78999) 510
Endocrine System (78012-78099) 510
Hematopoietic, Reticuloendothelial and Lymphatic System (78102-78199) 510
Gastrointestinal System (78201-78299) 511
Musculoskeletal System* (78300-78399) 511
Cardiovascular System* (78414-78499) 512
Respiratory System (78579-78599) 513

Nervous System (78600-78699) 513
Genitourinary System (78700-78799).....514
Other Procedures (78800-78999) 514
Therapeutic* (79005-79999) 515

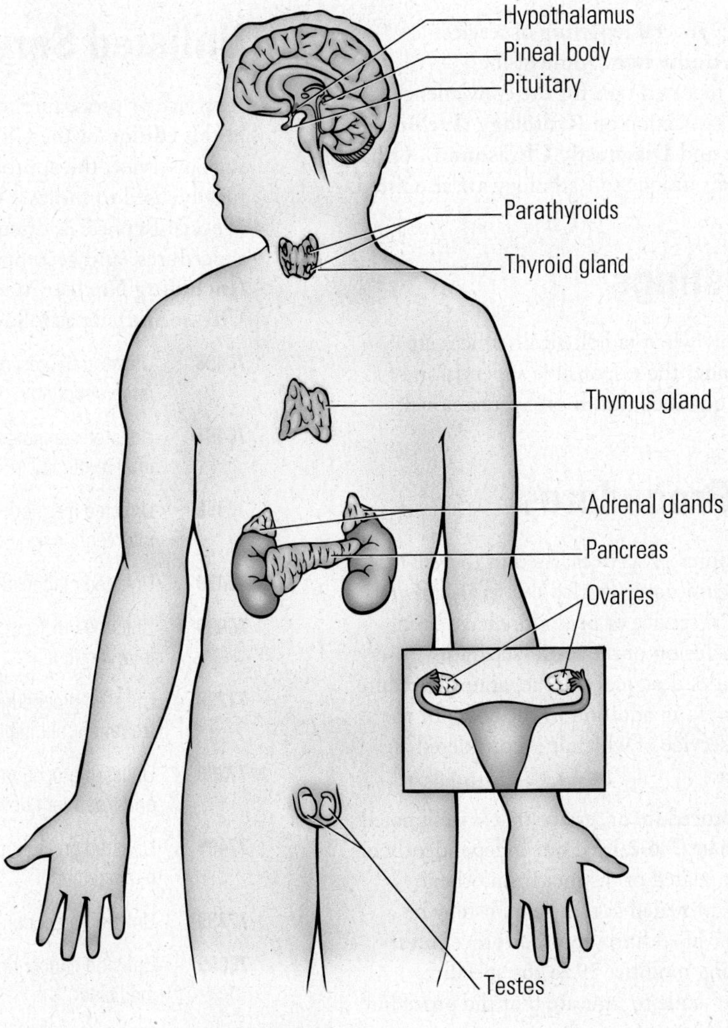

Endocrine System

Radiology Guidelines (Including Nuclear Medicine and Diagnostic Ultrasound)

Guidelines to direct general reporting of services are presented in the **Introduction.** Some of the commonalities are repeated here for the convenience of those referring to this section on **Radiology (Including Nuclear Medicine and Diagnostic Ultrasound).** Other definitions and items unique to Radiology are also listed.

Subject Listings

Subject listings apply when radiological services are performed by or under the responsible supervision of a physician or other qualified health care professional.

Separate Procedures

Some of the procedures or services listed in the CPT codebook that are commonly carried out as an integral component of a total service or procedure have been identified by the inclusion of the term "separate procedure." The codes designated as "separate procedure" should not be reported in addition to the code for the total procedure or service of which it is considered an integral component.

However, when a procedure or service that is designated as a "separate procedure" is carried out independently or considered to be unrelated or distinct from other procedures/services provided at that time, it may be reported by itself, or in addition to other procedures/services by appending modifier 59 to the specific "separate procedure" code to indicate that the procedure is not considered to be a component of another procedure, but is a distinct, independent procedure. This may represent a different session or patient encounter, different procedure or surgery, different site or organ system, separate incision/excision, separate lesion, separate injury, or area of injury in extensive injuries.

Unlisted Service or Procedure

A service or procedure may be provided that is not listed in this edition of the CPT codebook. When reporting such a service, the appropriate "Unlisted Procedure" code may be used to indicate the service, identifying it by "Special Report" as discussed below. The "Unlisted Procedures" and accompanying codes for **Radiology (Including Nuclear Medicine and Diagnostic Ultrasound)** are as follows:

76496 Unlisted fluoroscopic procedure (eg, diagnostic, interventional)

76497 Unlisted computed tomography procedure (eg, diagnostic, interventional)

76498 Unlisted magnetic resonance procedure (eg, diagnostic, interventional)

76499 Unlisted diagnostic radiographic procedure

76999 Unlisted ultrasound procedure (eg, diagnostic, interventional)

77299 Unlisted procedure, therapeutic radiology clinical treatment planning

77399 Unlisted procedure, medical radiation physics, dosimetry and treatment devices, and special services

77499 Unlisted procedure, therapeutic radiology treatment management

77799 Unlisted procedure, clinical brachytherapy

78099 Unlisted endocrine procedure, diagnostic nuclear medicine

78199 Unlisted hematopoietic, reticuloendothelial and lymphatic procedure, diagnostic nuclear medicine

78299 Unlisted gastrointestinal procedure, diagnostic nuclear medicine

78399 Unlisted musculoskeletal procedure, diagnostic nuclear medicine

78499 Unlisted cardiovascular procedure, diagnostic nuclear medicine

78599 Unlisted respiratory procedure, diagnostic nuclear medicine

78699 Unlisted nervous system procedure, diagnostic nuclear medicine

78799 Unlisted genitourinary procedure, diagnostic nuclear medicine

78999 Unlisted miscellaneous procedure, diagnostic nuclear medicine

79999 Radiopharmaceutical therapy, unlisted procedure

Special Report

A service that is rarely provided, unusual, variable, or new may require a special report. Pertinent information should include an adequate definition or description of the nature, extent, and need for the procedure; and the time, effort, and equipment necessary to provide the service.

▸Supervision and Interpretation, Imaging Guidance◂

▶Imaging may be required during the performance of certain procedures or certain imaging procedures may require surgical procedures to access the imaged area. Many services include image guidance, and imaging guidance is not separately reportable when it is included in the base service. The CPT code set typically defines in descriptors and/or guidelines when imaging guidance is included. When imaging is not included in a surgical procedure or procedure from the **Medicine** section, image guidance codes or codes labeled "radiological supervision and interpretation" (RS&I) may be reported for the portion of the service that requires imaging. All imaging guidance codes require: (1) image documentation in the patient record and (2) description of imaging guidance in the procedure report. All RS&I codes require: (1) image documentation in the patient's permanent record and (2) a procedure report or separate imaging report that includes written documentation of interpretive findings of information contained in the images and radiologic supervision of the service.

(The RS&I codes are not applicable to the Radiation Oncology subsection.)◀

Administration of Contrast Material(s)

The phrase "with contrast" used in the codes for procedures performed using contrast for imaging enhancement represents contrast material administered intravascularly, intra-articularly, or intrathecally.

For intra-articular injection, use the appropriate joint injection code. If radiographic arthrography is performed, also use the arthrography supervision and interpretation code for the appropriate joint (which includes fluoroscopy). If computed tomography (CT) or magnetic resonance (MR) arthrography are performed without radiographic arthrography, use the appropriate joint injection code, the appropriate CT or MR code ("with contrast" or "without followed by contrast"), and the appropriate imaging guidance code for needle placement for contrast injection.

For spine examinations using computed tomography, magnetic resonance imaging, magnetic resonance angiography, "with contrast" includes intrathecal or intravascular injection. For intrathecal injection, use also 61055 or 62284.

Injection of intravascular contrast material is part of the "with contrast" CT, computed tomographic angiography (CTA), magnetic resonance imaging (MRI), and magnetic resonance angiography (MRA) procedures.

Oral and/or rectal contrast administration alone does not qualify as a study "with contrast."

Written Report(s)

A written report (eg, handwritten or electronic) signed by the interpreting individual should be considered an integral part of a radiologic procedure or interpretation.

▶With regard to CPT descriptors for imaging services, "images" must contain anatomic information unique to the patient for which the imaging service is provided. "Images" refer to those acquired in either an analog (ie, film) or digital (ie, electronic) manner.◀

Radiology

Diagnostic Radiology (Diagnostic Imaging)

Head and Neck

70010 Myelography, posterior fossa, radiological supervision and interpretation
➔ *CPT Assistant* Mar 05:11, Dec 07:16

70015 Cisternography, positive contrast, radiological supervision and interpretation

70030 Radiologic examination, eye, for detection of foreign body

70100 Radiologic examination, mandible; partial, less than 4 views

70110 complete, minimum of 4 views

70120 Radiologic examination, mastoids; less than 3 views per side

70130 complete, minimum of 3 views per side

70134 Radiologic examination, internal auditory meati, complete

70140 Radiologic examination, facial bones; less than 3 views

70150 complete, minimum of 3 views

70160 Radiologic examination, nasal bones, complete, minimum of 3 views

70170 Dacryocystography, nasolacrimal duct, radiological supervision and interpretation

70190 Radiologic examination; optic foramina

70200 orbits, complete, minimum of 4 views

70210 Radiologic examination, sinuses, paranasal, less than 3 views

70220 Radiologic examination, sinuses, paranasal, complete, minimum of 3 views

70240 Radiologic examination, sella turcica

70250 Radiologic examination, skull; less than 4 views
➔ *CPT Changes: An Insider's View* 2004

70260 complete, minimum of 4 views
➔ *CPT Changes: An Insider's View* 2004

70300 Radiologic examination, teeth; single view

70310 partial examination, less than full mouth

70320 complete, full mouth

70328 Radiologic examination, temporomandibular joint, open and closed mouth; unilateral

70330 bilateral
➔ *CPT Assistant* May 11:10

70332 Temporomandibular joint arthrography, radiological supervision and interpretation
➔ *CPT Assistant* Feb 07:11

(Do not report 70332 in conjunction with 77002)

70336 Magnetic resonance (eg, proton) imaging, temporomandibular joint(s)
➔ *CPT Changes: An Insider's View* 2001
➔ *CPT Assistant* Jul 99:11, Jul 01:7, Aug 15:6

70350 Cephalogram, orthodontic
➔ *CPT Assistant* Aug 12:14

70355 Orthopantogram (eg, panoramic x-ray)
➔ *CPT Changes: An Insider's View* 2012
➔ *Clinical Examples in Radiology* Fall 11:11

70360 Radiologic examination; neck, soft tissue

70370 pharynx or larynx, including fluoroscopy and/or magnification technique

70371 Complex dynamic pharyngeal and speech evaluation by cine or video recording
➔ *CPT Assistant* Dec 04:17, Jul 14:5
➔ *Clinical Examples in Radiology* Spring 18:15

(70373 has been deleted. For contrast laryngography, use 76499)

(For laryngeal computed tomography, see 70490, 70491, 70492)

70380 Radiologic examination, salivary gland for calculus

70390 Sialography, radiological supervision and interpretation
➔ *Clinical Examples in Radiology* Fall 09:9

70450 Computed tomography, head or brain; without contrast material
➔ *CPT Changes: An Insider's View* 2003
➔ *CPT Assistant* Apr 96:11
➔ *Clinical Examples in Radiology* Winter 08:6, Fall 14:8

70460 with contrast material(s)
➔ *CPT Assistant* Apr 96:11
➔ *Clinical Examples in Radiology* Winter 10:11, Fall 14:8

70470 without contrast material, followed by contrast material(s) and further sections
➔ *CPT Assistant* Apr 96:11
➔ *Clinical Examples in Radiology* Fall 14:8

(To report 3D rendering, see 76376, 76377)

70480 Computed tomography, orbit, sella, or posterior fossa or outer, middle, or inner ear; without contrast material
➔ *CPT Changes: An Insider's View* 2003

70481 with contrast material(s)
➔ *CPT Assistant* Apr 08:11

70482 without contrast material, followed by contrast material(s) and further sections

(To report 3D rendering, see 76376, 76377)

70486 Computed tomography, maxillofacial area; without contrast material
➔ *CPT Changes: An Insider's View* 2003
➔ *CPT Assistant* Mar 02:11
➔ *Clinical Examples in Radiology* Spring 07:4, Winter 07:4-5, Fall 09:9

70487 with contrast material(s)

70488 without contrast material, followed by contrast material(s) and further sections

(To report 3D rendering, see 76376, 76377)

70490 Computed tomography, soft tissue neck; without contrast material
➔ *CPT Changes: An Insider's View* 2003

70491 with contrast material(s)

70492 without contrast material followed by contrast material(s) and further sections

(To report 3D rendering, see 76376, 76377)

(For cervical spine, see 72125, 72126)

70496 Computed tomographic angiography, head, with contrast material(s), including noncontrast images, if performed, and image postprocessing
➔ *CPT Changes: An Insider's View* 2001, 2008
➔ *CPT Assistant* Jul 01:4, Dec 05:7, Jan 07:31

70498 Computed tomographic angiography, neck, with contrast material(s), including noncontrast images, if performed, and image postprocessing
➔ *CPT Changes: An Insider's View* 2001, 2008
➔ *CPT Assistant* Jul 01:4, Dec 05:7, Jan 07:31
➔ *Clinical Examples in Radiology* Winter 09:2

70540 Magnetic resonance (eg, proton) imaging, orbit, face, and/or neck; without contrast material(s)
➔ *CPT Changes: An Insider's View* 2001, 2007
➔ *CPT Assistant* Jul 01:6, Mar 07:7, Sep 10:10
➔ *Clinical Examples in Radiology* Spring 05:3, Summer 07:7, Summer 13:9

(For head or neck magnetic resonance angiography studies, see 70544-70546, 70547-70549)

70542 with contrast material(s)
➔ *CPT Changes: An Insider's View* 2001
➔ *CPT Assistant* Jul 01:6, Sep 10:10
➔ *Clinical Examples in Radiology* Spring 05:3, Summer 07:7, Summer 13:9

70543 without contrast material(s), followed by contrast material(s) and further sequences
➔ *CPT Changes: An Insider's View* 2001
➔ *CPT Assistant* Jul 01:6, Sep 10:10
➔ *Clinical Examples in Radiology* Spring 05:2-3, Summer 07:7, Winter 07:7, 11, Summer 13:9

(Report 70540-70543 once per imaging session)

70544 Magnetic resonance angiography, head; without contrast material(s)
➔ *CPT Changes: An Insider's View* 2001
➔ *CPT Assistant* Sep 01:5, Dec 05:7, Jan 07:31

70545 with contrast material(s)
➔ *CPT Changes: An Insider's View* 2001
➔ *CPT Assistant* Jul 01:5, Dec 05:7

70546 without contrast material(s), followed by contrast material(s) and further sequences
➔ *CPT Changes: An Insider's View* 2001
➔ *CPT Assistant* Jul 01:5, Dec 05:7, Jan 07:31

70547 Magnetic resonance angiography, neck; without contrast material(s)
➔ *CPT Changes: An Insider's View* 2001
➔ *CPT Assistant* Sep 01:5, Dec 05:7, Jan 07:31
➔ *Clinical Examples in Radiology* Winter 09:2

70548 with contrast material(s)
➔ *CPT Changes: An Insider's View* 2001
➔ *CPT Assistant* Sep 01:6, Dec 05:7, Jan 07:31
➔ *Clinical Examples in Radiology* Winter 09:2

70549 without contrast material(s), followed by contrast material(s) and further sequences
➔ *CPT Changes: An Insider's View* 2001
➔ *CPT Assistant* Sep 01:6, Dec 05:7, Jan 07:31
➔ *Clinical Examples in Radiology* Winter 09:2

70551 Magnetic resonance (eg, proton) imaging, brain (including brain stem); without contrast material
➔ *CPT Assistant* May 98:10, Mar 05:20, Feb 07:6
➔ *Clinical Examples in Radiology* Spring 15:9

70552 with contrast material(s)
➔ *CPT Assistant* Jul 01:6, Mar 05:20, Feb 07:6
➔ *Clinical Examples in Radiology* Spring 15:9

70553 without contrast material, followed by contrast material(s) and further sequences
➔ *CPT Assistant* Nov 97:24, Jul 01:6, Mar 05:20, Feb 07:6
➔ *Clinical Examples in Radiology* Spring 05:2, Spring 06:4-5, Spring 15:9, Summer 15:13

(For magnetic spectroscopy, use 76390)

Functional MRI involves identification and mapping of stimulation of brain function. When neurofunctional tests are administered by a technologist or other non-physician or non-psychologist, use 70554. When neurofunctional tests are entirely administered by a physician or psychologist, use 70555.

70554 Magnetic resonance imaging, brain, functional MRI; including test selection and administration of repetitive body part movement and/or visual stimulation, not requiring physician or psychologist administration
➔ *CPT Changes: An Insider's View* 2007
➔ *CPT Assistant* Feb 07:6, Mar 07:7, Aug 08:13

(Do not report 70554 in conjunction with 96020)

70555 requiring physician or psychologist administration of entire neurofunctional testing
- *CPT Changes: An Insider's View* 2007
- *CPT Assistant* Feb 07:6, Mar 07:7

(Do not report 70555 unless 96020 is performed)

(Do not report 70554, 70555 in conjunction with 70551-70553 unless a separate diagnostic MRI is performed)

70557 Magnetic resonance (eg, proton) imaging, brain (including brain stem and skull base), during open intracranial procedure (eg, to assess for residual tumor or residual vascular malformation); without contrast material
- *CPT Changes: An Insider's View* 2004

70558 with contrast material(s)
- *CPT Changes: An Insider's View* 2004

70559 without contrast material(s), followed by contrast material(s) and further sequences
- *CPT Changes: An Insider's View* 2004

(For stereotactic biopsy of intracranial lesion with magnetic resonance guidance, use 61751,70557, 70558, or 70559 may be reported only if a separate report is generated. Report only 1 of the above codes once per operative session. Do not use these codes in conjunction with 61751, 77021, 77022)

Chest

(For fluoroscopic or ultrasonic guidance for needle placement procedures (eg, biopsy, aspiration, injection, localization device) of the thorax, see 76942, 77002)

(71010 has been deleted. To report, use 71045)

(71015 has been deleted. To report, use 71045)

(71020 has been deleted. To report, use 71046)

(71021 has been deleted. To report, use 71047)

(71022 has been deleted. To report, see 71047, 71048)

►(71023 has been deleted. To report, see 71046, 76000)◄

(71030 has been deleted. To report, use 71048)

►(71034 has been deleted. To report, see 71048, 76000)◄

(71035 has been deleted. To report, see 71046, 71047, 71048)

71045 Radiologic examination, chest; single view
- *CPT Changes: An Insider's View* 2018
- *CPT Assistant* Apr 18:7

71046 2 views
- *CPT Changes: An Insider's View* 2018
- *CPT Assistant* Apr 18:7

71047 3 views
- *CPT Changes: An Insider's View* 2018
- *CPT Assistant* Apr 18:7

71048 4 or more views
- *CPT Changes: An Insider's View* 2018
- *CPT Assistant* Apr 18:7

(For acute abdomen series that includes a single view of the chest and one or more views of the abdomen, use 74022)

(For concurrent computer-aided detection [CAD] performed in addition to 71045, 71046, 71047, 71048, use 0174T)

(Do not report 71045, 71046, 71047, 71048 in conjunction with 0175T for computer-aided detection [CAD] performed remotely from the primary interpretation)

71100 Radiologic examination, ribs, unilateral; 2 views
- *Clinical Examples in Radiology* Spring 14:6

71101 including posteroanterior chest, minimum of 3 views

71110 Radiologic examination, ribs, bilateral; 3 views
- *Clinical Examples in Radiology* Spring 14:6

71111 including posteroanterior chest, minimum of 4 views
- *Clinical Examples in Radiology* Spring 14:6

71120 Radiologic examination; sternum, minimum of 2 views

71130 sternoclavicular joint or joints, minimum of 3 views

71250 Computed tomography, thorax; without contrast material
- *CPT Changes: An Insider's View* 2003
- *CPT Assistant* Jul 07:13, Aug 11:10, Fall 13:9, 10
- *Clinical Examples in Radiology* Fall 08:7, Winter 18:17

71260 with contrast material(s)
- *CPT Assistant* Jul 01:4, Jun 09:9, Fall 13:9, 10
- *Clinical Examples in Radiology* Summer 05:4, Fall 08:7, 11, 12

71270 without contrast material, followed by contrast material(s) and further sections
- *CPT Assistant* Jun 01:10, Jul 07:13
- *Clinical Examples in Radiology* Fall 08:7, Fall 13:9, 10

(For cardiac computed tomography of the heart, see 75571-75574)

(To report 3D rendering, see 76376, 76377)

71275 Computed tomographic angiography, chest (noncoronary), with contrast material(s), including noncontrast images, if performed, and image postprocessing
- *CPT Changes: An Insider's View* 2001, 2007, 2008
- *CPT Assistant* Jul 01:4, Jun 05:11, Dec 05:7, Jan 07:31, Mar 07:7, Jun 09:9, Aug 11:10
- *Clinical Examples in Radiology* Spring 05:7, Fall 08:11, 12, Spring 09:11, Fall 09:10, Winter 10:2, Fall 13:9, 10, Spring 16:13

(For coronary artery computed tomographic angiography including calcification score and/or cardiac morphology, use 75574)

71550 Magnetic resonance (eg, proton) imaging, chest (eg, for evaluation of hilar and mediastinal lymphadenopathy); without contrast material(s)
- *CPT Changes: An Insider's View* 2001
- *CPT Assistant* Jul 01:7, Apr 10:10, Sep 10:10
- *Clinical Examples in Radiology* Summer 13:9

71551 with contrast material(s)
CPT Changes: An Insider's View 2001
CPT Assistant Jul 01:7, Sep 10:10
Clinical Examples in Radiology Summer 13:9

71552 without contrast material(s), followed by contrast material(s) and further sequences
CPT Changes: An Insider's View 2001
CPT Assistant Jul 01:7, Apr 10:10, Sep 10:10
Clinical Examples in Radiology Summer 13:9

►(For breast MRI, see 77046, 77047, 77048, 77049)◄

71555 Magnetic resonance angiography, chest (excluding myocardium), with or without contrast material(s)
CPT Assistant Fall 95:2, Dec 05:7, Jan 07:31
Clinical Examples in Radiology Spring 16:13, Spring 17:14

Spine and Pelvis

(72010 has been deleted. To report, use 72082)

72020 Radiologic examination, spine, single view, specify level
CPT Assistant Jul 13:10, Oct 15:9
Clinical Examples in Radiology Spring 13:8, 9, Winter 18:15

(For a single view that includes the entire thoracic and lumbar spine, use 72081)

72040 Radiologic examination, spine, cervical; 2 or 3 views
CPT Changes: An Insider's View 2001, 2013, 2014
CPT Assistant Sep 01:7, Jul 13:10
Clinical Examples in Radiology Fall 09:10, Summer 11:8, Fall 11:9, Spring 13:8, 9, Winter 18:15

72050 4 or 5 views
CPT Changes: An Insider's View 2013
Clinical Examples in Radiology Summer 11:8, Fall 11:9, Spring 13:9, Winter 18:15

72052 6 or more views
CPT Changes: An Insider's View 2013
Clinical Examples in Radiology Summer 11:8, Fall 11:9, Spring 13:9, Winter 18:15

(72069 has been deleted. To report, see 72081, 72082, 72083, 72084)

72070 Radiologic examination, spine; thoracic, 2 views
CPT Changes: An Insider's View 2001
CPT Assistant Sep 01:7
Clinical Examples in Radiology Fall 11:9, Spring 13:9, Winter 18:15

72072 thoracic, 3 views
CPT Changes: An Insider's View 2001
CPT Assistant Sep 01:7
Clinical Examples in Radiology Fall 11:9, Spring 13:9, Winter 18:15

72074 thoracic, minimum of 4 views
CPT Changes: An Insider's View 2001
CPT Assistant Sep 01:7
Clinical Examples in Radiology Fall 11:9, Spring 13:9, Winter 18:15

72080 thoracolumbar junction, minimum of 2 views
CPT Changes: An Insider's View 2001, 2016
CPT Assistant Sep 01:7, Oct 15:9, Sep 16:4
Clinical Examples in Radiology Fall 11:9, Spring 13:8, 9, Fall 15:7, Winter 18:15

(For a single view examination of the thoracolumbar junction, use 72020)

72081 Radiologic examination, spine, entire thoracic and lumbar, including skull, cervical and sacral spine if performed (eg, scoliosis evaluation); one view
CPT Changes: An Insider's View 2016
CPT Assistant Sep 16:4
Clinical Examples in Radiology Fall 15:7, Winter 18:15

72082 2 or 3 views
CPT Changes: An Insider's View 2016
CPT Assistant Sep 16:4
Clinical Examples in Radiology Fall 15:7, Winter 18:15

72083 4 or 5 views
CPT Changes: An Insider's View 2016
CPT Assistant Sep 16:4
Clinical Examples in Radiology Fall 15:7, Winter 18:15

72084 minimum of 6 views
CPT Changes: An Insider's View 2016
CPT Assistant Sep 16:4
Clinical Examples in Radiology Fall 15:7, Winter 18:15

(72090 has been deleted. To report, see 72081, 72082, 72083, 72084)

72100 Radiologic examination, spine, lumbosacral; 2 or 3 views
CPT Changes: An Insider's View 2001
CPT Assistant Sep 01:7
Clinical Examples in Radiology Fall 11:9, 10, Spring 13:8, 9, Spring 14:10, Winter 18:15

72110 minimum of 4 views
CPT Changes: An Insider's View 2001
CPT Assistant Sep 01:7
Clinical Examples in Radiology Fall 11:10, Spring 13:9, Winter 18:15

72114 complete, including bending views, minimum of 6 views
CPT Changes: An Insider's View 2012
Clinical Examples in Radiology Summer 12:11, Spring 13:9, Winter 18:15

72120 bending views only, 2 or 3 views
CPT Changes: An Insider's View 2012
CPT Assistant Aug 16:7
Clinical Examples in Radiology Fall 11:9, 10, Spring 13:8, 9, Spring 14:10, Winter 18:15

(Contrast material in CT of spine is either by intrathecal or intravenous injection. For intrathecal injection, use also 61055 or 62284. IV injection of contrast material is part of the CT procedure)

72125 Computed tomography, cervical spine; without contrast material
CPT Changes: An Insider's View 2003
Clinical Examples in Radiology Fall 14:7, 11

72126 with contrast material

➔ *CPT Assistant* Sep 14:3

➔ *Clinical Examples in Radiology* Fall 15:10

72127 without contrast material, followed by contrast material(s) and further sections

(For intrathecal injection procedure, see 61055, 62284)

72128 Computed tomography, thoracic spine; without contrast material

➔ *CPT Changes: An Insider's View* 2003

72129 with contrast material

➔ *CPT Assistant* Sep 14:3

➔ *Clinical Examples in Radiology* Fall 15:10

(For intrathecal injection procedure, see 61055, 62284)

72130 without contrast material, followed by contrast material(s) and further sections

(For intrathecal injection procedure, see 61055, 62284)

72131 Computed tomography, lumbar spine; without contrast material

➔ *CPT Changes: An Insider's View* 2003

➔ *Clinical Examples in Radiology* Summer 07:11, Spring 12:10

72132 with contrast material

➔ *CPT Assistant* Fall 93:13, Sep 14:3

➔ *Clinical Examples in Radiology* Fall 06:5-6, 11-12, Fall 14:6, Fall 15:10

72133 without contrast material, followed by contrast material(s) and further sections

➔ *Clinical Examples in Radiology* Fall 14:7, 11

(For intrathecal injection procedure, see 61055, 62284)

(To report 3D rendering, see 76376, 76377)

72141 Magnetic resonance (eg, proton) imaging, spinal canal and contents, cervical; without contrast material

➔ *CPT Assistant* Apr 10:10, Jun 14:14

72142 with contrast material(s)

➔ *CPT Assistant* Apr 10:10

(For cervical spinal canal imaging without contrast material followed by contrast material, use 72156)

72146 Magnetic resonance (eg, proton) imaging, spinal canal and contents, thoracic; without contrast material

➔ *CPT Assistant* May 99:10, Apr 10:10, Jun 14:14

72147 with contrast material(s)

➔ *CPT Assistant* May 99:10, Apr 10:10

(For thoracic spinal canal imaging without contrast material followed by contrast material, use 72157)

72148 Magnetic resonance (eg, proton) imaging, spinal canal and contents, lumbar; without contrast material

➔ *CPT Assistant* Nov 05:15, Jun 14:14

➔ *Clinical Examples in Radiology* Spring 06:6, 11

72149 with contrast material(s)

(For lumbar spinal canal imaging without contrast material followed by contrast material, use 72158)

72156 Magnetic resonance (eg, proton) imaging, spinal canal and contents, without contrast material, followed by contrast material(s) and further sequences; cervical

72157 thoracic

72158 lumbar

72159 Magnetic resonance angiography, spinal canal and contents, with or without contrast material(s)

➔ *CPT Assistant* Dec 05:7, Jan 07:31

72170 Radiologic examination, pelvis; 1 or 2 views

➔ *CPT Changes: An Insider's View* 2001

➔ *CPT Assistant* Sep 01:7, Mar 03:23, Aug 16:7

➔ *Clinical Examples in Radiology* Spring 05:12, Fall 15:8, Summer 16:8, Winter 16:13

72190 complete, minimum of 3 views

➔ *Clinical Examples in Radiology* Fall 15:9, Summer 16:8, Winter 16:13

(For pelvimetry, use 74710)

(For a combined computed tomography [CT] or computed tomographic angiography abdomen and pelvis study, see 74174, 74176-74178)

72191 Computed tomographic angiography, pelvis, with contrast material(s), including noncontrast images, if performed, and image postprocessing

➔ *CPT Changes: An Insider's View* 2001, 2008

➔ *CPT Assistant* Jul 01:4, 6, Dec 05:7, Jan 07:31

➔ *Clinical Examples in Radiology* Summer 08:8, Fall 09:10, Fall 11:9

(Do not report 72191 in conjunction with 73706 or 75635. For CTA aorto-iliofemoral runoff, use 75635)

(Do not report 72191 in conjunction with 74175. For a combined computed tomographic angiography abdomen and pelvis study, use 74174)

72192 Computed tomography, pelvis; without contrast material

➔ *CPT Changes: An Insider's View* 2003

➔ *CPT Assistant* Mar 05:1, 4, Mar 07:10, Apr 10:9, Nov 11:6, Oct 12:12

➔ *Clinical Examples in Radiology* Winter 06:11, Spring 07:3, 11, Summer 07:11, Fall 09:9, Fall 11:8, Winter 11:8-10, Spring 16:9

72193 with contrast material(s)

➔ *CPT Assistant* Mar 05:1, 4, Mar 07:10, Apr 10:9, Nov 11:6, Oct 12:12

➔ *Clinical Examples in Radiology* Winter 05:1, 7, Spring 07:3, 11, Fall 11:8, Winter 11:8-10, Spring 16:9

72194 without contrast material, followed by contrast material(s) and further sections

➔ *CPT Assistant* Mar 05:1, 4, Mar 07:10, Apr 10:9, Nov 11:6, Oct 12:12

➔ *Clinical Examples in Radiology* Spring 07:3, 11, Fall 11:8, Winter 11:8-10, Spring 16:9

(For a combined CT abdomen and pelvis study, see 74176-74178)

(To report 3D rendering, see 76376, 76377)

(For computed tomographic colonography, diagnostic, see 74261-74262. For computed tomographic colonography, screening, use 74263)

(Do not report 72192-72194 in conjunction with 74261-74263)

72195 Magnetic resonance (eg, proton) imaging, pelvis; without contrast material(s)

- *CPT Changes: An Insider's View* 2001
- *CPT Assistant* Jul 01:7, Jun 06:17, Jun 14:14, Jun 16:5
- *Clinical Examples in Radiology* Spring 06:8-9, Fall 06:7-8, Summer 07:4, 5, Winter 16:12, Spring 18:12

72196 with contrast material(s)

- *CPT Changes: An Insider's View* 2001
- *CPT Assistant* Jul 01:7, Jun 06:17, Jun 16:5
- *Clinical Examples in Radiology* Spring 06:8-9, Fall 06:7-8, Winter 16:12, Spring 18:12

72197 without contrast material(s), followed by contrast material(s) and further sequences

- *CPT Changes: An Insider's View* 2001
- *CPT Assistant* Jul 01:7, Jun 16:5
- *Clinical Examples in Radiology* Spring 06:8-9, Fall 06:2-3, 7-8, Spring 15:10, Winter 16:12, Spring 18:12

(Do not report 72195, 72196, 72197 in conjunction with 74712, 74713)

(For magnetic resonance imaging of a fetus[es], see 74712, 74713)

72198 Magnetic resonance angiography, pelvis, with or without contrast material(s)

- *CPT Assistant* Dec 05:7, Jan 07:31

72200 Radiologic examination, sacroiliac joints; less than 3 views

72202 3 or more views

72220 Radiologic examination, sacrum and coccyx, minimum of 2 views

72240 Myelography, cervical, radiological supervision and interpretation

- *CPT Assistant* Fall 93:13, Sep 14:3
- *Clinical Examples in Radiology* Fall 06:5-6, 11-12, Fall 14:6, 7, 11, Fall 15:10

(Do not report 72240 in conjunction with 62284, 62302, 62303, 62304, 62305)

(When both 62284 and 72240 are performed by the same physician or other qualified health care professional for cervical myelography, use 62302)

(For complete cervical myelography via injection procedure at C1-C2, see 61055, 72240)

72255 Myelography, thoracic, radiological supervision and interpretation

- *CPT Assistant* Sep 14:3
- *Clinical Examples in Radiology* Fall 14:7, 11, Fall 15:10

(Do not report 72255 in conjunction with 62284, 62302, 62303, 62304, 62305)

(When both 62284 and 72255 are performed by the same physician or other qualified health care professional for thoracic myelography, use 62303)

(For complete thoracic myelography via injection procedure at C1-C2, see 61055, 72255)

72265 Myelography, lumbosacral, radiological supervision and interpretation

- *CPT Assistant* Fall 93:13, Aug 00:7, Sep 14:3
- *Clinical Examples in Radiology* Fall 14:7, 11, Fall 15:10

(Do not report 72265 in conjunction with 62284, 62302, 62303, 62304, 62305)

(When both 62284 and 72265 are performed by the same physician or other qualified health care professional for lumbosacral myelography, use 62304)

(For complete lumbosacral myelography via injection procedure at C1-C2, see 61055, 72265)

72270 Myelography, 2 or more regions (eg, lumbar/thoracic, cervical/thoracic, lumbar/cervical, lumbar/thoracic/cervical), radiological supervision and interpretation

- *CPT Changes: An Insider's View* 2004
- *CPT Assistant* Sep 14:3
- *Clinical Examples in Radiology* Fall 14:6, 7, 11, Fall 15:10

(Do not report 72270 in conjunction with 62284, 62302, 62303, 62304, 62305)

(When both 62284 and 72270 are performed by the same physician or other qualified health care professional for myelography of 2 or more regions, use 62305)

(For complete myelography of 2 or more regions via injection procedure at C1-C2, see 61055, 72270)

72275 Epidurography, radiological supervision and interpretation

- *CPT Changes: An Insider's View* 2000
- *CPT Assistant* Nov 99:40, Jan 00:2, Aug 00:7, Jul 08:9, Oct 09:12, Feb 10:12, May 10:10, Jun 12:12, Jul 12:5, May 17:3
- *Clinical Examples in Radiology* Summer 13:12

(72275 includes 77003)

(For injection procedure, see 62280, 62281, 62282, 62320, 62321, 62322, 62323, 62324, 62325, 62326, 62327, 64479, 64480, 64483, 64484)

(Use 72275 only when an epidurogram is performed, images documented, and a formal radiologic report is issued)

►(Do not report 72275 in conjunction with 22586)◄

72285 Discography, cervical or thoracic, radiological supervision and interpretation

- *CPT Changes: An Insider's View* 2000
- *CPT Assistant* Nov 99:35, 40, Mar 11:7
- *Clinical Examples in Radiology* Fall 10:10

Radiology 70010-79999

Epidurography
72275

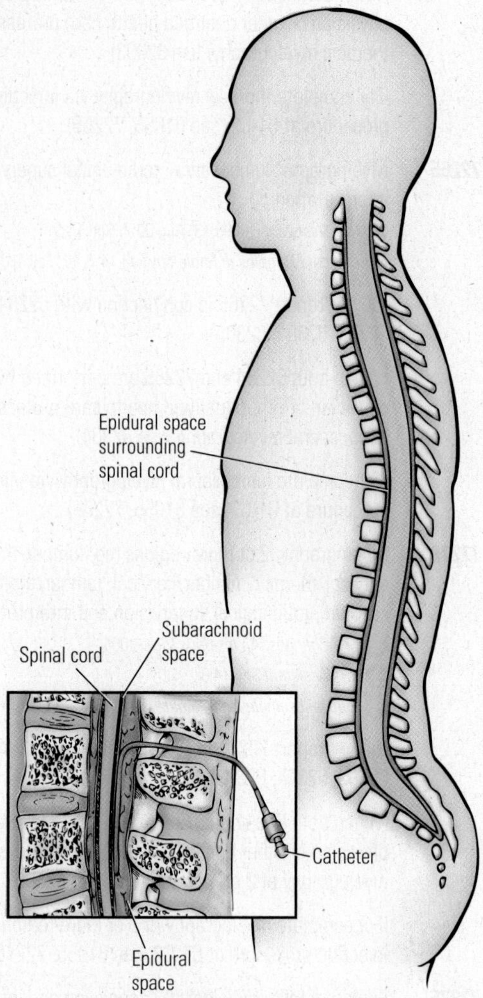

72295 Discography, lumbar, radiological supervision and interpretation
➔ *CPT Assistant* Apr 03:27, Mar 11:7, Jul 12:3
➔ *Clinical Examples in Radiology* Fall 10:10

Upper Extremities

(For stress views, any joint, use 77071)

73000 Radiologic examination; clavicle, complete

73010 scapula, complete

73020 Radiologic examination, shoulder; 1 view

73030 complete, minimum of 2 views

73040 Radiologic examination, shoulder, arthrography, radiological supervision and interpretation
➔ *CPT Assistant* Jul 01:7, Feb 07:11
➔ *Clinical Examples in Radiology* Spring 05:6, Spring 09:6, 7

(Do not report 77002 in conjunction with 73040)

73050 Radiologic examination; acromioclavicular joints, bilateral, with or without weighted distraction

73060 humerus, minimum of 2 views

73070 Radiologic examination, elbow; 2 views
➔ *CPT Changes: An Insider's View* 2001
➔ *CPT Assistant* Winter 90:9, Sep 01:8

73080 complete, minimum of 3 views

73085 Radiologic examination, elbow, arthrography, radiological supervision and interpretation
➔ *CPT Assistant* Feb 07:11
➔ *Clinical Examples in Radiology* Spring 05:6

(Do not report 77002 in conjunction with 73085)

73090 Radiologic examination; forearm, 2 views
➔ *CPT Changes: An Insider's View* 2001
➔ *CPT Assistant* Sep 01:8, Apr 02:14

73092 upper extremity, infant, minimum of 2 views

73100 Radiologic examination, wrist; 2 views
➔ *CPT Changes: An Insider's View* 2001
➔ *CPT Assistant* Winter 90:9, Sep 01:8

73110 complete, minimum of 3 views
➔ *CPT Assistant* Mar 97:10, Nov 06:22

73115 Radiologic examination, wrist, arthrography, radiological supervision and interpretation
➔ *CPT Assistant* Feb 07:11
➔ *Clinical Examples in Radiology* Spring 05:6

(Do not report 77002 in conjunction with 73115)

73120 Radiologic examination, hand; 2 views
➔ *CPT Assistant* Winter 90:9

73130 minimum of 3 views
➔ *Clinical Examples in Radiology* Winter 05:9, Spring 11:8

73140 Radiologic examination, finger(s), minimum of 2 views
➔ *CPT Assistant* Jan 07:29
➔ *Clinical Examples in Radiology* Spring 11:8

73200 Computed tomography, upper extremity; without contrast material
➔ *CPT Changes: An Insider's View* 2003
➔ *CPT Assistant* Jul 11:17

73201 with contrast material(s)
➔ *CPT Assistant* Jul 11:17, Aug 15:6
➔ *Clinical Examples in Radiology* Spring 09:6, 7

73202 without contrast material, followed by contrast material(s) and further sections

(To report 3D rendering, see 76376, 76377)

73206 Computed tomographic angiography, upper extremity, with contrast material(s), including noncontrast images, if performed, and image postprocessing
➔ *CPT Changes: An Insider's View* 2001, 2008
➔ *CPT Assistant* Jul 01:5, Dec 05:7, Jan 07:31

73218 Magnetic resonance (eg, proton) imaging, upper extremity, other than joint; without contrast material(s)
CPT Changes: An Insider's View 2001
CPT Assistant Jul 01:7, Sep 10:10, Feb 11:9
Clinical Examples in Radiology Summer 13:9

73219 with contrast material(s)
CPT Changes: An Insider's View 2001
CPT Assistant Jul 01:7, Sep 10:10
Clinical Examples in Radiology Summer 13:9

73220 without contrast material(s), followed by contrast material(s) and further sequences
CPT Changes: An Insider's View 2001
CPT Assistant Jul 01:7, Sep 10:10
Clinical Examples in Radiology Summer 13:9

73221 Magnetic resonance (eg, proton) imaging, any joint of upper extremity; without contrast material(s)
CPT Changes: An Insider's View 2001
CPT Assistant Jul 01:7, Sep 10:10, Feb 11:9
Clinical Examples in Radiology Summer 13:9

73222 with contrast material(s)
CPT Changes: An Insider's View 2001
CPT Assistant Jul 01:7, Sep 10:10, Aug 15:6
Clinical Examples in Radiology Spring 05:5, Summer 13:9

73223 without contrast material(s), followed by contrast material(s) and further sequences
CPT Changes: An Insider's View 2001
CPT Assistant Jul 01:7, Sep 10:10
Clinical Examples in Radiology Spring 09:6, Summer 13:9

73225 Magnetic resonance angiography, upper extremity, with or without contrast material(s)
CPT Assistant Dec 05:7, Jan 07:31
Clinical Examples in Radiology Summer 13:9, 10

Lower Extremities

(For stress views, any joint, use 77071)

(73500 has been deleted. To report, use 73501)

73501 Radiologic examination, hip, unilateral, with pelvis when performed; 1 view
CPT Changes: An Insider's View 2016
CPT Assistant Oct 15:9, Jun 16:9, Aug 16:7, Nov 16:10
Clinical Examples in Radiology Fall 15:9, Spring 16:14, Summer 16:9, 13

73502 2-3 views
CPT Changes: An Insider's View 2016
CPT Assistant Oct 15:9, Jun 16:9, Aug 16:7, Nov 16:10
Clinical Examples in Radiology Fall 15:9, Spring 16:14, Summer 16:8, 13

73503 minimum of 4 views
CPT Changes: An Insider's View 2016
CPT Assistant Oct 15:9, Jun 16:9, Aug 16:7, Nov 16:10
Clinical Examples in Radiology Fall 15:9, Summer 16:9, 13

(73510 has been deleted. To report, see 73502, 73503)

(73520 has been deleted. To report, see 73521, 73522, 73523)

73521 Radiologic examination, hips, bilateral, with pelvis when performed; 2 views
CPT Changes: An Insider's View 2016
CPT Assistant Oct 15:9, Jun 16:9, Aug 16:7, Nov 16:10
Clinical Examples in Radiology Fall 15:9, Summer 16:9, 13, Winter 16:13

73522 3-4 views
CPT Changes: An Insider's View 2016
CPT Assistant Oct 15:9, Jun 16:9, Aug 16:7, Nov 16:10
Clinical Examples in Radiology Fall 15:8, Summer 16:9, 13, Winter 16:13

73523 minimum of 5 views
CPT Changes: An Insider's View 2016
CPT Assistant Oct 15:9, Jun 16:9, Aug 16:7, Nov 16:10
Clinical Examples in Radiology Fall 15:9, Summer 16:9, 13, Winter 16:13

73525 Radiologic examination, hip, arthrography, radiological supervision and interpretation
CPT Assistant Feb 07:11, Jun 12:14, Nov 16:10
Clinical Examples in Radiology Spring 05:6

(Do not report 73525 in conjunction with 77002)

(73550 has been deleted. To report, see 73551, 73552)

73551 Radiologic examination, femur; 1 view
CPT Changes: An Insider's View 2016
CPT Assistant Aug 16:7, Nov 16:10
Clinical Examples in Radiology Fall 15:9, Summer 16:8

73552 minimum 2 views
CPT Changes: An Insider's View 2016
CPT Assistant Aug 16:7, Nov 16:10, Nov 17:10
Clinical Examples in Radiology Fall 15:9

73560 Radiologic examination, knee; 1 or 2 views
CPT Assistant Feb 15:10, May 15:10
Clinical Examples in Radiology Winter 15:11

73562 3 views
CPT Assistant Apr 02:15
Clinical Examples in Radiology Fall 06:4

73564 complete, 4 or more views
CPT Assistant Jun 98:11, Nov 98:21, Feb 15:10, May 15:10
Clinical Examples in Radiology Fall 06:4, Winter 15:11

73565 both knees, standing, anteroposterior
CPT Assistant Winter 90:9, Feb 15:10, May 15:10
Clinical Examples in Radiology Fall 06:4, Winter 15:11

73580 Radiologic examination, knee, arthrography, radiological supervision and interpretation
CPT Assistant Feb 07:11, Aug 15:6
Clinical Examples in Radiology Spring 05:6

(Do not report 73580 in conjunction with 77002)

73590 Radiologic examination; tibia and fibula, 2 views
CPT Changes: An Insider's View 2001
CPT Assistant Sep 01:8, Nov 17:10

73592 lower extremity, infant, minimum of 2 views
CPT Assistant Nov 17:10

73600 Radiologic examination, ankle; 2 views
➲ *CPT Changes: An Insider's View* 2001
➲ *CPT Assistant* Sep 01:8, Apr 02:15, Mar 03:9
➲ *Clinical Examples in Radiology* Winter 13:11

73610 complete, minimum of 3 views
➲ *CPT Assistant* Apr 02:15, Mar 03:9

73615 Radiologic examination, ankle, arthrography, radiological supervision and interpretation
➲ *CPT Assistant* Feb 07:11

(Do not report 73615 in conjunction with 77002)

73620 Radiologic examination, foot; 2 views
➲ *CPT Changes: An Insider's View* 2001
➲ *CPT Assistant* Sep 01:8, Apr 02:15, Mar 03:9

73630 complete, minimum of 3 views
➲ *Clinical Examples in Radiology* Summer 07:12

73650 Radiologic examination; calcaneus, minimum of 2 views

73660 toe(s), minimum of 2 views

73700 Computed tomography, lower extremity; without contrast material
➲ *CPT Changes: An Insider's View* 2003
➲ *CPT Assistant* Mar 07:10, Jul 11:17
➲ *Clinical Examples in Radiology* Fall 08:10, Fall 10:6

73701 with contrast material(s)
➲ *CPT Assistant* Mar 07:10, Jul 11:17
➲ *Clinical Examples in Radiology* Summer 10:10

73702 without contrast material, followed by contrast material(s) and further sections
➲ *CPT Assistant* Mar 07:10, Jul 11:17

(To report 3D rendering, see 76376, 76377)

73706 Computed tomographic angiography, lower extremity, with contrast material(s), including noncontrast images, if performed, and image postprocessing
➲ *CPT Changes: An Insider's View* 2001, 2008
➲ *CPT Assistant* Jul 01:5-6, Dec 05:7, Jan 07:31, Apr 08:11, Apr 11:13
➲ *Clinical Examples in Radiology* Summer 08:8

(For CTA aorto-iliofemoral runoff, use 75635)

73718 Magnetic resonance (eg, proton) imaging, lower extremity other than joint; without contrast material(s)
➲ *CPT Changes: An Insider's View* 2001
➲ *CPT Assistant* Jul 01:3
➲ *Clinical Examples in Radiology* Spring 07:7-9, 12, Summer 07:4, 5

73719 with contrast material(s)
➲ *CPT Changes: An Insider's View* 2001
➲ *CPT Assistant* Jul 01:3
➲ *Clinical Examples in Radiology* Spring 07:7-9, 12, Summer 07:4, 5

73720 without contrast material(s), followed by contrast material(s) and further sequences
➲ *CPT Changes: An Insider's View* 2001
➲ *CPT Assistant* Jul 01:3
➲ *Clinical Examples in Radiology* Spring 07:7-9, 12, Summer 07:4, 5

73721 Magnetic resonance (eg, proton) imaging, any joint of lower extremity; without contrast material
➲ *CPT Changes: An Insider's View* 2001
➲ *CPT Assistant* Jul 01:3, Jun 06:17
➲ *Clinical Examples in Radiology* Spring 07:7-9, 12, Summer 07:4, 5

73722 with contrast material(s)
➲ *CPT Changes: An Insider's View* 2001
➲ *CPT Assistant* Jul 01:3, Jun 06:17, Aug 15:6
➲ *Clinical Examples in Radiology* Spring 07:7-9, 12, Summer 07:4, 5, Spring 13:11

73723 without contrast material(s), followed by contrast material(s) and further sequences
➲ *CPT Changes: An Insider's View* 2001
➲ *CPT Assistant* Jul 01:3
➲ *Clinical Examples in Radiology* Spring 07:7-9, 12, Summer 07:4, 5

73725 Magnetic resonance angiography, lower extremity, with or without contrast material(s)
➲ *CPT Assistant* Dec 05:7, Jan 07:31
➲ *Clinical Examples in Radiology* Spring 06:1-3

Abdomen

(74000 has been deleted. To report, use 74018)

(74010 has been deleted. To report, see 74019, 74021)

(74020 has been deleted. To report, see 74019, 74021)

74018 Radiologic examination, abdomen; 1 view
➲ *CPT Changes: An Insider's View* 2018
➲ *CPT Assistant* Apr 18:7

74019 2 views
➲ *CPT Changes: An Insider's View* 2018
➲ *CPT Assistant* Apr 18:7

74021 3 or more views
➲ *CPT Changes: An Insider's View* 2018
➲ *CPT Assistant* Apr 18:7

74022 Radiologic examination, abdomen; complete acute abdomen series, including supine, erect, and/or decubitus views, single view chest
➲ *CPT Changes: An Insider's View* 2003

74150 Computed tomography, abdomen; without contrast material
➲ *CPT Changes: An Insider's View* 2003
➲ *CPT Assistant* Oct 02:12, Mar 05:1, 4, Apr 10:9, Nov 11:6, Oct 12:12
➲ *Clinical Examples in Radiology* Spring 07:3, 11, Fall 08:7, Fall 09:9, Fall 11:8, Winter 11:8, 9, Spring 16:9

74160 with contrast material(s)
➲ *CPT Assistant* Mar 05:1, 4, Apr 10:9, Nov 11:6, Oct 12:12
➲ *Clinical Examples in Radiology* Spring 07:3, 11, Fall 08:7, Summer 10:10, Fall 11:8, Winter 11:8, 9, Spring 16:9

74170 without contrast material, followed by contrast material(s) and further sections
➲ *CPT Assistant* Mar 05:4, Apr 10:9, Nov 11:6, Oct 12:12
➲ *Clinical Examples in Radiology* Winter 05:1, 7-8, 12, Spring 07:3, 11, Fall 08:7, Fall 11:8, Winter 11:8, 9, Spring 16:10

(For a combined CT abdomen and pelvis study, see 74176-74178)

(To report 3D rendering, see 76376, 76377)

(For computed tomographic colonography, diagnostic, see 74261-74262. For computed tomographic colonography, screening, use 74263)

(Do not report 74150-74170 in conjunction with 74261-74263)

74174 Computed tomographic angiography, abdomen and pelvis, with contrast material(s), including noncontrast images, if performed, and image postprocessing

➔ *CPT Changes: An Insider's View* 2012

➔ *Clinical Examples in Radiology* Fall 11:8, Spring 17:7

(Do not report 74174 in conjunction with 72191, 73706, 74175, 75635, 76376, 76377)

(For CTA aorto-iliofemoral runoff, use 75635)

74175 Computed tomographic angiography, abdomen, with contrast material(s), including noncontrast images, if performed, and image postprocessing

➔ *CPT Changes: An Insider's View* 2001, 2008

➔ *CPT Assistant* Jul 01:6, Dec 05:7, Jan 07:31, Apr 11:13

➔ *Clinical Examples in Radiology* Summer 08:8, Fall 09:10, Fall 11:8

(Do not report 74175 in conjunction with 73706 or 75635. For CTA aorto-iliofemoral runoff, use 75635)

(Do not report 74175 in conjunction with 72191. For a combined computed tomographic angiography abdomen and pelvis study, use 74174)

For combinations of CT of the abdomen with CT of the pelvis performed at the same session, use the following table. Do not report more than one CT of the abdomen or CT of the pelvis for any session.

Stand Alone Code	**74150 CT Abdomen WO Contrast**	**74160 CT Abdomen W Contrast**	**74170 CT Abdomen WO/W Contrast**
72192 CT Pelvis WO Contrast	74176	74178	74178
72193 CT Pelvis W Contrast	74178	74177	74178
72194 CT Pelvis WO/W Contrast	74178	74178	74178

74176 Computed tomography, abdomen and pelvis; without contrast material

➔ *CPT Changes: An Insider's View* 2011

➔ *CPT Assistant* Nov 11:6

➔ *Clinical Examples in Radiology* Fall 11:8, Winter 11:9, Spring 16:10, Spring 17:7

74177 with contrast material(s)

➔ *CPT Changes: An Insider's View* 2011

➔ *CPT Assistant* Nov 11:6

➔ *Clinical Examples in Radiology* Fall 11:8, Winter 11:9, Spring 16:10, Spring 17:7

74178 without contrast material in one or both body regions, followed by contrast material(s) and further sections in one or both body regions

➔ *CPT Changes: An Insider's View* 2011

➔ *CPT Assistant* Nov 11:6

➔ *Clinical Examples in Radiology* Fall 11:8, Winter 11:8, Spring 16:10, Spring 17:7

(Do not report 74176-74178 in conjunction with 72192-72194, 74150-74170)

(Report 74176, 74177, or 74178 only once per CT abdomen and pelvis examination)

74181 Magnetic resonance (eg, proton) imaging, abdomen; without contrast material(s)

➔ *CPT Changes: An Insider's View* 2001

➔ *CPT Assistant* Jul 01:3, Nov 07:9, May 09:9, Jul 09:10, Mar 18:11

➔ *Clinical Examples in Radiology* Fall 07:3, Spring 09:4

74182 with contrast material(s)

➔ *CPT Changes: An Insider's View* 2001

➔ *CPT Assistant* Jul 01:3, May 09:9, Jul 09:10, Mar 18:11

74183 without contrast material(s), followed by with contrast material(s) and further sequences

➔ *CPT Changes: An Insider's View* 2001

➔ *CPT Assistant* Jul 01:3, May 09:9, Jul 09:10, Mar 18:11

74185 Magnetic resonance angiography, abdomen, with or without contrast material(s)

➔ *CPT Assistant* Dec 05:7, Jan 07:31

➔ *Clinical Examples in Radiology* Spring 06:1-3

74190 Peritoneogram (eg, after injection of air or contrast), radiological supervision and interpretation

➔ *CPT Assistant* Dec 10:13

➔ *Clinical Examples in Radiology* Fall 07:1, 2

(For procedure, use 49400)

(For computed tomography, see 72192 or 74150)

Gastrointestinal Tract

(For percutaneous placement of gastrostomy tube, use 43246)

74210 Radiologic examination; pharynx and/or cervical esophagus

74220 esophagus

➔ *Clinical Examples in Radiology* Spring 18:15

74230 Swallowing function, with cineradiography/videoradiography

➔ *CPT Changes: An Insider's View* 2002

➔ *CPT Assistant* Dec 04:17, Jul 14:5

➔ *Clinical Examples in Radiology* Summer 06:4-5, Spring 18:14

74235 Removal of foreign body(s), esophageal, with use of balloon catheter, radiological supervision and interpretation

(For procedure, use 43499)

74240 Radiologic examination, gastrointestinal tract, upper; with or without delayed images, without KUB
➲ *CPT Changes: An Insider's View* 2016
➲ *CPT Assistant* Sep 16:7

74241 with or without delayed images, with KUB
➲ *CPT Changes: An Insider's View* 2016
➲ *CPT Assistant* Sep 16:7

74245 with small intestine, includes multiple serial images
➲ *CPT Changes: An Insider's View* 2002, 2016
➲ *CPT Assistant* Sep 16:7

74246 Radiological examination, gastrointestinal tract, upper, air contrast, with specific high density barium, effervescent agent, with or without glucagon; with or without delayed images, without KUB
➲ *CPT Changes: An Insider's View* 2016
➲ *CPT Assistant* Sep 16:7

74247 with or without delayed images, with KUB
➲ *CPT Changes: An Insider's View* 2016
➲ *CPT Assistant* Sep 16:7

74249 with small intestine follow-through
➲ *CPT Changes: An Insider's View* 2002

74250 Radiologic examination, small intestine, includes multiple serial images
➲ *CPT Changes: An Insider's View* 2002, 2016
➲ *CPT Assistant* Sep 16:7

74251 via enteroclysis tube
➲ *CPT Changes: An Insider's View* 2016
➲ *CPT Assistant* Sep 16:7

74260 Duodenography, hypotonic

74261 Computed tomographic (CT) colonography, diagnostic, including image postprocessing; without contrast material
➲ *CPT Changes: An Insider's View* 2010
➲ *CPT Assistant* Apr 10:9
➲ *Clinical Examples in Radiology* Winter 10:6

74262 with contrast material(s) including non-contrast images, if performed
➲ *CPT Changes: An Insider's View* 2010
➲ *CPT Assistant* Apr 10:9
➲ *Clinical Examples in Radiology* Winter 10:4-6

(Do not report 74261, 74262 in conjunction with 72192-72194, 74150-74170, 74263, 76376, 76377)

74263 Computed tomographic (CT) colonography, screening, including image postprocessing
➲ *CPT Changes: An Insider's View* 2010
➲ *CPT Assistant* Apr 10:9
➲ *Clinical Examples in Radiology* Winter 10:6

(Do not report 74263 in conjunction with 72192-72194, 74150-74170, 74261, 74262, 76376, 76377)

74270 Radiologic examination, colon; contrast (eg, barium) enema, with or without KUB
➲ *CPT Changes: An Insider's View* 2009
➲ *CPT Assistant* May 03:19

74280 air contrast with specific high density barium, with or without glucagon

74283 Therapeutic enema, contrast or air, for reduction of intussusception or other intraluminal obstruction (eg, meconium ileus)
➲ *CPT Assistant* Nov 97:24
➲ *Clinical Examples in Radiology* Spring 13:9

74290 Cholecystography, oral contrast

74300 Cholangiography and/or pancreatography; intraoperative, radiological supervision and interpretation
➲ *CPT Changes: An Insider's View* 2000
➲ *CPT Assistant* Nov 99:41, Dec 00:14

+ 74301 additional set intraoperative, radiological supervision and interpretation (List separately in addition to code for primary procedure)

(Use 74301 in conjunction with 74300)

(74305 has been deleted. To report, use 47531)

(74320 has been deleted. To report, use 47532)

(74327 has been deleted. For percutaneous biliary stone extraction, use 47544)

74328 Endoscopic catheterization of the biliary ductal system, radiological supervision and interpretation

(For procedure, see 43260-43278 as appropriate)

74329 Endoscopic catheterization of the pancreatic ductal system, radiological supervision and interpretation

(For procedure, see 43260-43278 as appropriate)

74330 Combined endoscopic catheterization of the biliary and pancreatic ductal systems, radiological supervision and interpretation

(For procedure, see 43260-43278 as appropriate)

74340 Introduction of long gastrointestinal tube (eg, Miller-Abbott), including multiple fluoroscopies and images, radiological supervision and interpretation
➲ *CPT Changes: An Insider's View* 2016
➲ *CPT Assistant* Sep 16:9

(For tube placement, use 44500)

74355 Percutaneous placement of enteroclysis tube, radiological supervision and interpretation
➲ *CPT Assistant* Feb 07:11, Nov 10:3, Jan 11:8

74360 Intraluminal dilation of strictures and/or obstructions (eg, esophagus), radiological supervision and interpretation
➲ *CPT Assistant* Spring 94:3, Oct 08:6

(Do not report 74360 in conjunction with 43213, 43214, 43233)

74363 Percutaneous transhepatic dilation of biliary duct stricture with or without placement of stent, radiological supervision and interpretation

➲ *CPT Changes: An Insider's View* 2002

(For procedure, see 47555, 47556)

Urinary Tract

74400 Urography (pyelography), intravenous, with or without KUB, with or without tomography

74410 Urography, infusion, drip technique and/or bolus technique;

74415 with nephrotomography

74420 Urography, retrograde, with or without KUB

➲ *CPT Assistant* Sep 00:11, Dec 10:15

74425 Urography, antegrade (pyelostogram, nephrostogram, loopogram), radiological supervision and interpretation

➲ *CPT Assistant* Fall 93:14, Dec 97:7, Oct 05:18

➲ *Clinical Examples in Radiology* Summer 06:1-3, Fall 15:2, Spring 16:12

(Do not report 74425 in conjunction with 50430, 50431, 50432, 50433, 50434, 50435, 50693, 50694, 50695)

74430 Cystography, minimum of 3 views, radiological supervision and interpretation

74440 Vasography, vesiculography, or epididymography, radiological supervision and interpretation

74445 Corpora cavernosography, radiological supervision and interpretation

➲ *CPT Assistant* Feb 07:11, Nov 10:3, Jan 11:8

74450 Urethrocystography, retrograde, radiological supervision and interpretation

74455 Urethrocystography, voiding, radiological supervision and interpretation

74470 Radiologic examination, renal cyst study, translumbar, contrast visualization, radiological supervision and interpretation

➲ *CPT Assistant* Oct 05:18, Feb 07:11, Nov 10:3, Jan 11:8

▲ **74485** Dilation of ureter(s) or urethra, radiological supervision and interpretation

➲ *CPT Changes: An Insider's View* 2019

➲ *CPT Assistant* Oct 05:18, Dec 08:7, Jan 09:7, Oct 15:5

➲ *Clinical Examples in Radiology* Summer 06:1-3

►(Do not report 74485 in conjunction with 50436, 50437)◄

(For dilation of ureter without radiologic guidance, use 52341, 52344)

(For change of nephrostomy or pyelostomy tube, use 50435)

►(For dilation of a nephrostomy tract for endourologic procedure, see 50436, 50437)◄

Gynecological and Obstetrical

(For abdomen and pelvis, see 72170-72190, 74018, 74019, 74021, 74022, 74150, 74160, 74170)

74710 Pelvimetry, with or without placental localization

74712 Magnetic resonance (eg, proton) imaging, fetal, including placental and maternal pelvic imaging when performed; single or first gestation

➲ *CPT Changes: An Insider's View* 2016

➲ *CPT Assistant* Jun 16:5

➲ *Clinical Examples in Radiology* Winter 16:12

+ **74713** each additional gestation (List separately in addition to code for primary procedure)

➲ *CPT Changes: An Insider's View* 2016

➲ *CPT Assistant* Jun 16:5

➲ *Clinical Examples in Radiology* Winter 16:12

(Use 74713 in conjunction with 74712)

(Do not report 74712, 74713 in conjunction with 72195, 72196, 72197)

(If only placenta or maternal pelvis is imaged without fetal imaging, see 72195, 72196, 72197)

74740 Hysterosalpingography, radiological supervision and interpretation

➲ *CPT Assistant* Nov 97:24, Jul 99:8, Mar 09:11

(For introduction of saline or contrast for hysterosalpingography, see 58340)

74742 Transcervical catheterization of fallopian tube, radiological supervision and interpretation

(For procedure, use 58345)

74775 Perineogram (eg, vaginogram, for sex determination or extent of anomalies)

Heart

Cardiac magnetic imaging differs from traditional magnetic resonance imaging (MRI) in its ability to provide a physiologic evaluation of cardiac function. Traditional MRI relies on static images to obtain clinical diagnoses based upon anatomic information. Improvement in spatial and temporal resolution has expanded the application from an anatomic test and includes physiologic evaluation of cardiac function. Flow and velocity assessment for valves and intracardiac shunts is performed in addition to a function and morphologic evaluation. Use 75559 with 75565 to report flow with pharmacologic wall motion stress evaluation without contrast. Use 75563 with 75565 to report flow with pharmacologic perfusion stress with contrast.

Cardiac MRI for velocity flow mapping can be reported in conjunction with 75557, 75559, 75561, or 75563.

Listed procedures may be performed independently or in the course of overall medical care. If the individual providing these services is also responsible for diagnostic workup and/or follow-up care of the patient, also see appropriate sections. Only one procedure in the series 75557-75563 is appropriately reported per session. Only one add-on code for flow velocity can be reported per session.

Cardiac MRI studies may be performed at rest and/or during pharmacologic stress. Therefore, the appropriate stress testing code from the 93015-93018 series should be reported in addition to 75559 or 75563.

Cardiac computed tomography (CT) and coronary computed tomographic angiography (CTA) include the axial source images of the pre-contrast, arterial phase sequence, and venous phase sequence (if performed), as well as the two-dimensional and three-dimensional reformatted images resulting from the study, including cine review. Contrast enhanced cardiac CT and coronary CTA codes 75571-75574 include any quantitative assessment when performed as part of the same encounter. Report only one computed tomography heart service per encounter.

(For separate injection procedures for vascular radiology, see **Surgery** section, 36000-36299)

(For cardiac catheterization procedures, see 93451-93572)

(75552-75556 have been deleted. To report, see 75557, 75559, 75561, 75563, 75565)

75557 Cardiac magnetic resonance imaging for morphology and function without contrast material;
- *CPT Changes: An Insider's View* 2008
- *CPT Assistant* Jul 10:7
- *Clinical Examples in Radiology* Spring 09:2

75559 with stress imaging
- *CPT Changes: An Insider's View* 2008
- *Clinical Examples in Radiology* Spring 09:2

75561 Cardiac magnetic resonance imaging for morphology and function without contrast material(s), followed by contrast material(s) and further sequences;
- *CPT Changes: An Insider's View* 2008
- *CPT Assistant* Jul 10:7
- *Clinical Examples in Radiology* Spring 09:2, Spring 16:13, Spring 17:14

75563 with stress imaging
- *CPT Changes: An Insider's View* 2008
- *CPT Assistant* Jul 10:7
- *Clinical Examples in Radiology* Spring 09:2

(75558, 75560, 75562, 75564 have been deleted. To report flow velocity, use 75565)

+ 75565 Cardiac magnetic resonance imaging for velocity flow mapping (List separately in addition to code for primary procedure)
- *CPT Changes: An Insider's View* 2010
- *CPT Assistant* Jul 10:7

(Use 75565 in conjunction with 75557, 75559, 75561, 75563)

(Do not report 75557, 75559, 75561, 75563, 75565 in conjunction with 76376, 76377)

75571 Computed tomography, heart, without contrast material, with quantitative evaluation of coronary calcium
- *CPT Changes: An Insider's View* 2010
- *CPT Assistant* Jul 10:7
- *Clinical Examples in Radiology* Winter 10:2, 3

75572 Computed tomography, heart, with contrast material, for evaluation of cardiac structure and morphology (including 3D image postprocessing, assessment of cardiac function, and evaluation of venous structures, if performed)
- *CPT Changes: An Insider's View* 2010
- *CPT Assistant* Jul 10:7
- *Clinical Examples in Radiology* Winter 10:2, 3, Spring 16:13

75573 Computed tomography, heart, with contrast material, for evaluation of cardiac structure and morphology in the setting of congenital heart disease (including 3D image postprocessing, assessment of LV cardiac function, RV structure and function and evaluation of venous structures, if performed)
- *CPT Changes: An Insider's View* 2010
- *CPT Assistant* Jul 10:7
- *Clinical Examples in Radiology* Winter 10:2, 3

75574 Computed tomographic angiography, heart, coronary arteries and bypass grafts (when present), with contrast material, including 3D image postprocessing (including evaluation of cardiac structure and morphology, assessment of cardiac function, and evaluation of venous structures, if performed)
- *CPT Changes: An Insider's View* 2010
- *CPT Assistant* Jul 10:7
- *Clinical Examples in Radiology* Winter 10:1-3

Vascular Procedures

Aorta and Arteries

Selective vascular catheterizations should be coded to include introduction and all lesser order selective catheterizations used in the approach (eg, the description for a selective right middle cerebral artery catheterization includes the introduction and placement catheterization of the right common and internal carotid arteries).

Additional second and/or third order arterial catheterizations within the same family of arteries supplied by a single first order artery should be expressed by 36218 or 36248. Additional first order or higher catheterizations in vascular families supplied by a first order vessel different from a previously selected and coded family should be separately coded using the conventions described above.

The lower extremity endovascular revascularization codes describing services performed for occlusive disease (37220-37235) include catheterization (36200, 36140, 36245-36248) in the work described by the codes. Catheterization codes are not additionally reported for diagnostic lower extremity angiography when performed through the same access site as the therapy (37220-37235) performed in the same session. However, catheterization for the diagnostic lower extremity angiogram may be reported separately if a different arterial puncture site is necessary.

For angiography performed in conjunction with therapeutic transcatheter radiological supervision and interpretation services, see the **Radiology Transcatheter Procedures** guidelines.

Diagnostic angiography (radiological supervision and interpretation) codes should NOT be used with interventional procedures for:

1. Contrast injections, angiography, roadmapping, and/or fluoroscopic guidance for the intervention,
2. Vessel measurement, and
3. Post-angioplasty/stent/atherectomy angiography, as this work is captured in the radiological supervision and interpretation code(s). In those therapeutic codes that include radiological supervision and interpretation, this work is captured in the therapeutic code.

Diagnostic angiography performed at the time of an interventional procedure is separately reportable if:

1. No prior catheter-based angiographic study is available and a full diagnostic study is performed, and the decision to intervene is based on the diagnostic study, OR
2. A prior study is available, but as documented in the medical record:
   a. The patient's condition with respect to the clinical indication has changed since the prior study, OR
   b. There is inadequate visualization of the anatomy and/or pathology, OR
   c. There is a clinical change during the procedure that requires new evaluation outside the target area of intervention.

Diagnostic angiography performed at a separate sessions from an interventional procedure is separately reported.

If diagnostic angiography is necessary, is performed at the same session as the interventional procedure and meets the above criteria, modifier 59 must be appended to the diagnostic radiological supervision and interpretation code(s) to denote that diagnostic work has been done following these guidelines.

Diagnostic angiography performed at the time of an interventional procedure is NOT separately reportable if it is specifically included in the interventional code descriptor.

(For intravenous procedure, see 36000, 36005-36015, and for intra-arterial procedure, see 36100-36248)

(For radiological supervision and interpretation, see 75600-75893)

75600 Aortography, thoracic, without serialography, radiological supervision and interpretation

(For supravalvular aortography performed at the time of cardiac catheterization, use 93567, which includes imaging supervision, interpretation, and report)

75605 Aortography, thoracic, by serialography, radiological supervision and interpretation

➔ *CPT Assistant* Spring 94:29, Dec 98:9, Jan 13:6

➔ *Clinical Examples in Radiology* Spring 13:4, 5, 6

(For supravalvular aortography performed at the time of cardiac catheterization, use 93567, which includes imaging supervision, interpretation, and report)

Aortography
75600-75630

A radiographic contrast study is performed on the abdominal or thoracic aorta.

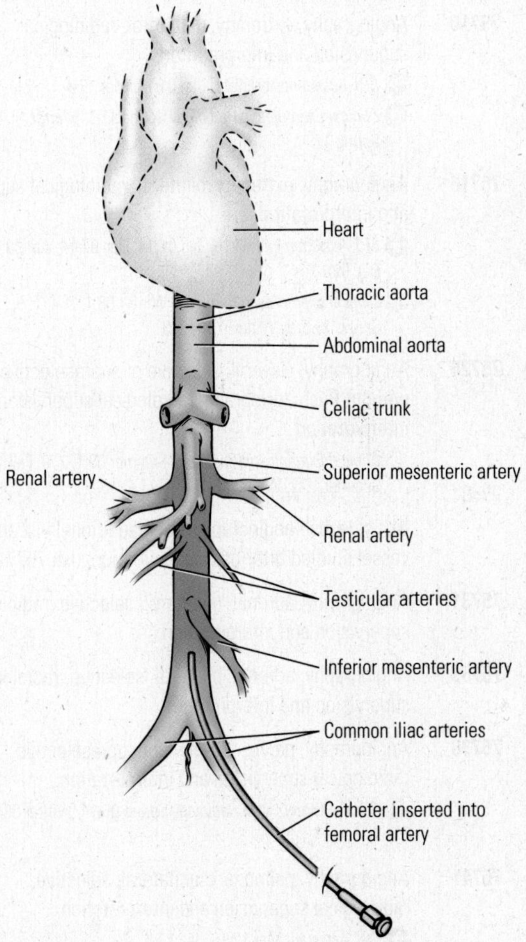

75625 Aortography, abdominal, by serialography, radiological supervision and interpretation

➔ *CPT Assistant* Fall 93:16, Jan 01:14, Dec 07:14, Apr 08:11, Dec 09:13, Jan 13:6, Feb 13:16

➔ *Clinical Examples in Radiology* Winter 08:1, 2, 4, 5, 9, Spring 13:11

Radiology 70010-79999

75630 Aortography, abdominal plus bilateral iliofemoral lower extremity, catheter, by serialography, radiological supervision and interpretation

➔ *CPT Assistant* Fall 93:16, Jan 01:14, Apr 08:11, Dec 09:13

➔ *Clinical Examples in Radiology* Winter 14:5, 7

75635 Computed tomographic angiography, abdominal aorta and bilateral iliofemoral lower extremity runoff, with contrast material(s), including noncontrast images, if performed, and image postprocessing

➔ *CPT Changes: An Insider's View* 2001, 2008

➔ *CPT Assistant* Jul 01:4-5, Dec 05:7, Jan 07:31, Apr 11:13

➔ *Clinical Examples in Radiology* Spring 06:1-3, Summer 08:7, 8, Summer 10:10

(Do not report 75635 in conjunction with 72191, 73706, 74174 or 74175)

(75658 has been deleted. To report, use 75710)

75705 Angiography, spinal, selective, radiological supervision and interpretation

➔ *Clinical Examples in Radiology* Winter 18:2

75710 Angiography, extremity, unilateral, radiological supervision and interpretation

➔ *CPT Assistant* Apr 99:11, Jan 01:14, Mar 17:4

➔ *Clinical Examples in Radiology* Spring 11:1, Winter 11:1, Spring 12:4

75716 Angiography, extremity, bilateral, radiological supervision and interpretation

➔ *CPT Assistant* Fall 93:16, Jan 01:14, Dec 07:14, Apr 08:11, Dec 09:13

➔ *Clinical Examples in Radiology* Winter 08:1, 2, 4, 5, 9, Spring 13:5, 6, Winter 13:1, 2, 3

75726 Angiography, visceral, selective or supraselective (with or without flush aortogram), radiological supervision and interpretation

➔ *Clinical Examples in Radiology* Summer 08:1, 2, 3, Fall 13:2, 3, 5, Summer 15:2, Winter 18:11

(For selective angiography, each additional visceral vessel studied after basic examination, use 75774)

75731 Angiography, adrenal, unilateral, selective, radiological supervision and interpretation

75733 Angiography, adrenal, bilateral, selective, radiological supervision and interpretation

75736 Angiography, pelvic, selective or supraselective, radiological supervision and interpretation

➔ *Clinical Examples in Radiology* Spring 05:14, Winter 08:4, 5, Winter 14:1-3

75741 Angiography, pulmonary, unilateral, selective, radiological supervision and interpretation

➔ *CPT Assistant* Mar 12:10, Jan 13:6

➔ *Clinical Examples in Radiology* Spring 13:1, 2

75743 Angiography, pulmonary, bilateral, selective, radiological supervision and interpretation

➔ *CPT Assistant* Spring 94:29, Apr 98:7, Jan 13:6

➔ *Clinical Examples in Radiology* Summer 12:1, 2

75746 Angiography, pulmonary, by nonselective catheter or venous injection, radiological supervision and interpretation

(For pulmonary angiography by nonselective catheter or venous injection performed at the time of cardiac catheterization, use 93568, which includes imaging supervision, interpretation, and report)

75756 Angiography, internal mammary, radiological supervision and interpretation

(For internal mammary angiography performed at the time of cardiac catheterization, see 93455, 93457, 93459, 93461, 93564, which include imaging supervision, interpretation, and report)

+ 75774 Angiography, selective, each additional vessel studied after basic examination, radiological supervision and interpretation (List separately in addition to code for primary procedure)

➔ *CPT Assistant* Fall 93:17, Spring 94:29, Apr 11:13, Fall 13:2, 3, 5, Feb 13:17, Jun 13:12, Oct 13:18, May 17:3

➔ *Clinical Examples in Radiology* Summer 08:1-3, Winter 08:1, 2, 4, 5, Spring 13:6, Winter 13:1-3, Winter 15:4-6, Winter 18:2

(Use 75774 in addition to code for specific initial vessel studied)

(Do not report 75774 as part of diagnostic angiography of the extracranial and intracranial cervicocerebral vessels. It may be appropriate to report 75774 for diagnostic angiography of upper extremities and other vascular beds performed in the same session)

(For angiography, see 75600-75756)

(For catheterizations, see codes 36215-36248)

(For cardiac catheterization procedures, see 93452-93462, 93531-93533, 93563-93568)

(75791 has been deleted. To report, see 36901, 36902, 36903, 36904, 36905, 36906)

(For radiological supervision and interpretation of dialysis circuit angiography performed through existing access[es] or catheter-based arterial access, use 36901 with modifier 52)

Veins and Lymphatics

For venography performed in conjunction with therapeutic transcatheter radiological supervision and interpretation services, see the **Radiology Transcatheter Procedures** guidelines.

Diagnostic venography (radiological supervision and interpretation) codes should NOT be used with interventional procedures for:

1. Contrast injections, venography, roadmapping, and/or fluoroscopic guidance for the intervention,
2. Vessel measurement, and
3. Post-angioplasty/stent venography, as this work is captured in the radiological supervision and interpretation code(s).

Diagnostic venography performed at the time of an interventional procedure is separately reportable if:

1. No prior catheter-based venographic study is available and a full diagnostic study is performed, and decision to intervene is based on the diagnostic study, OR
2. A prior study is available, but as documented in the medical record:
   a. The patient's condition with respect to the clinical indication has changed since the prior study, OR
   b. There is inadequate visualization of the anatomy and/or pathology, OR
   c. There is a clinical change during the procedure that requires new evaluation outside the target area of intervention.

Diagnostic venography performed at a separate setting from an interventional procedure is separately reported.

Diagnostic venography performed at the time of an interventional procedure is NOT separately reportable if it is specifically included in the interventional code descriptor.

(For injection procedure for venous system, see 36000-36015, 36400-36510)

(For injection procedure for lymphatic system, use 38790)

75801 Lymphangiography, extremity only, unilateral, radiological supervision and interpretation

➔ *Clinical Examples in Radiology* Summer 15:8

75803 Lymphangiography, extremity only, bilateral, radiological supervision and interpretation

➔ *Clinical Examples in Radiology* Summer 15:8

75805 Lymphangiography, pelvic/abdominal, unilateral, radiological supervision and interpretation

➔ *Clinical Examples in Radiology* Summer 15:8

75807 Lymphangiography, pelvic/abdominal, bilateral, radiological supervision and interpretation

➔ *Clinical Examples in Radiology* Summer 15:8

75809 Shuntogram for investigation of previously placed indwelling nonvascular shunt (eg, LeVeen shunt, ventriculoperitoneal shunt, indwelling infusion pump), radiological supervision and interpretation

➔ *CPT Changes: An Insider's View* 2001

➔ *CPT Assistant* Feb 07:11, Jul 08:13, Aug 08:13, Sep 08:10, Nov 10:3, Jan 11:8

(For procedure, see 49427 or 61070)

75810 Splenoportography, radiological supervision and interpretation

➔ *CPT Assistant* Feb 07:11, Nov 10:3, Jan 11:8

75820 Venography, extremity, unilateral, radiological supervision and interpretation

➔ *CPT Assistant* Oct 97:10, May 08:14, May 15:3, May 16:5

➔ *Clinical Examples in Radiology* Summer 06:8-9, Spring 08:12, Spring 14:7, Winter 16:2

Venography
75820-75822

A radiographic contrast study is performed on the veins of the lower extremities.

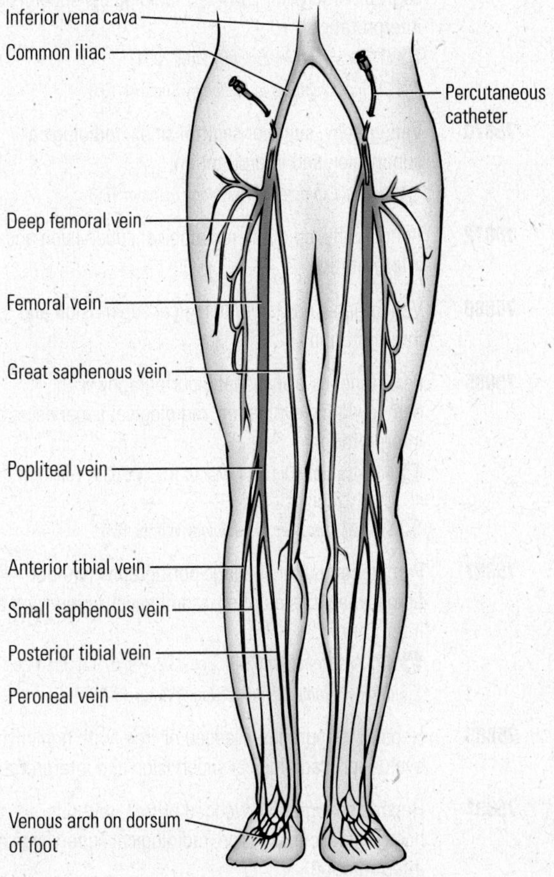

75822 Venography, extremity, bilateral, radiological supervision and interpretation

75825 Venography, caval, inferior, with serialography, radiological supervision and interpretation

➔ *CPT Assistant* Feb 17:14

➔ *Clinical Examples in Radiology* Winter 05:5-6, Winter 12:3, Winter 16:2

75827 Venography, caval, superior, with serialography, radiological supervision and interpretation

➔ *CPT Assistant* Apr 98:12

➔ *Clinical Examples in Radiology* Winter 12:3

75831 Venography, renal, unilateral, selective, radiological supervision and interpretation

➔ *CPT Assistant* Sep 98:7

➔ *Clinical Examples in Radiology* Winter 12:3

75833 Venography, renal, bilateral, selective, radiological supervision and interpretation

➔ *CPT Assistant* Sep 98:7

➔ *Clinical Examples in Radiology* Winter 12:3

75840 Venography, adrenal, unilateral, selective, radiological supervision and interpretation

75842 Venography, adrenal, bilateral, selective, radiological supervision and interpretation

75860 Venography, venous sinus (eg, petrosal and inferior sagittal) or jugular, catheter, radiological supervision and interpretation

➲ *CPT Changes: An Insider's View* 2004

➲ *Clinical Examples in Radiology* Summer 16:3

75870 Venography, superior sagittal sinus, radiological supervision and interpretation

➲ *Clinical Examples in Radiology* Summer 16:3

75872 Venography, epidural, radiological supervision and interpretation

75880 Venography, orbital, radiological supervision and interpretation

75885 Percutaneous transhepatic portography with hemodynamic evaluation, radiological supervision and interpretation

➲ *CPT Assistant* Oct 96:4, Mar 02:10, Dec 03:2, Feb 07:11, Nov 10:3, Jan 11:8

➲ *Clinical Examples in Radiology* Winter 18:11

75887 Percutaneous transhepatic portography without hemodynamic evaluation, radiological supervision and interpretation

➲ *CPT Assistant* Mar 02:10, Dec 03:2, Feb 07:11, Jan 11:8

➲ *Clinical Examples in Radiology* Winter 18:11

75889 Hepatic venography, wedged or free, with hemodynamic evaluation, radiological supervision and interpretation

75891 Hepatic venography, wedged or free, without hemodynamic evaluation, radiological supervision and interpretation

75893 Venous sampling through catheter, with or without angiography (eg, for parathyroid hormone, renin), radiological supervision and interpretation

➲ *Clinical Examples in Radiology* Summer 16:2

(For procedure, use 36500)

Transcatheter Procedures

Therapeutic transcatheter radiological supervision and interpretation code(s) include the following services associated with that intervention:

1. Contrast injections, angiography/venography, roadmapping, and fluoroscopic guidance for the intervention,
2. Vessel measurement, and
3. Completion angiography/venography (except for those uses permitted by 75898).

Unless specifically included in the code descriptor, diagnostic angiography/venography performed at the time of transcatheter therapeutic radiological and interpretation service(s) is separately reportable (eg, no prior catheter-based diagnostic angiography/venography study of the target vessel is available, prior diagnostic study is inadequate, patient's condition with respect to the clinical indication has changed since the prior study or during the intervention). See 75600-75893.

Codes 75956 and 75957 include all angiography of the thoracic aorta and its branches for diagnostic imaging prior to deployment of the primary endovascular devices (including all routine components of modular devices), fluoroscopic guidance in the delivery of the endovascular components, and intraprocedural arterial angiography (eg, confirm position, detect endoleak, evaluate runoff).

Code 75958 includes the analogous services for placement of each proximal thoracic endovascular extension. Code 75959 includes the analogous services for placement of a distal thoracic endovascular extension(s) placed during a procedure after the primary repair.

75894 Transcatheter therapy, embolization, any method, radiological supervision and interpretation

➲ *CPT Assistant* Sep 98:7, Feb 08:5, Apr 12:5, Fall 13:2, 3, 4, Nov 13:6, 7, 15, Oct 14:6

➲ *Clinical Examples in Radiology* Summer 07:2, Winter 07:1-3, Summer 08:1, 2, 3, Winter 08:4, 5, Fall 11:3, Spring 14:8, Spring 16:5, Summer 16:13, Winter 18:2

(Do not report 75894 in conjunction with 36475, 36476, 36478, 36479, 37241-37244)

(75896 has been deleted. For radiological supervision and interpretation for thrombolysis other than coronary, see 37211, 37212, 37213, 37214. For radiological supervision and interpretation for intracranial arterial administration of pharmacological agent(s) other than for thrombolysis, see 61650, 61651)

75898 Angiography through existing catheter for follow-up study for transcatheter therapy, embolization or infusion, other than for thrombolysis

➲ *CPT Changes: An Insider's View* 2002, 2013

➲ *CPT Assistant* Dec 07:11, Nov 11:11, Fall 13:2, 3, 4, Nov 13:6, 15, Oct 14:6, Nov 15:3

➲ *Clinical Examples in Radiology* Summer 07:2, Summer 08:1, 2, 3, Winter 08:4, 5, Summer 12:3, Spring 16:4, Winter 18:2

(For thrombolysis infusion management other than coronary, see 37211-37214, 61645)

(For non-thrombolysis infusion management other than coronary, see 61650, 61651)

(Do not report 75898 in conjunction with 37211-37214, 37241-37244, 61645, 61650, 61651)

75901 Mechanical removal of pericatheter obstructive material (eg, fibrin sheath) from central venous device via separate venous access, radiologic supervision and interpretation

➲ *CPT Changes: An Insider's View* 2003

➲ *CPT Assistant* Jul 03:13, Dec 04:12

(For procedure, use 36595)

(For venous catheterization, see 36010-36012)

75902 Mechanical removal of intraluminal (intracatheter) obstructive material from central venous device through device lumen, radiologic supervision and interpretation

➔ *CPT Changes: An Insider's View* 2003

➔ *CPT Assistant* Jul 03:13, Dec 04:12

(For procedure, use 36596)

(For venous catheterization, see 36010-36012)

(75952, 75953, 75954 have been deleted. To report, see 34701-34711, 0254T)

75956 Endovascular repair of descending thoracic aorta (eg, aneurysm, pseudoaneurysm, dissection, penetrating ulcer, intramural hematoma, or traumatic disruption); involving coverage of left subclavian artery origin, initial endoprosthesis plus descending thoracic aortic extension(s), if required, to level of celiac artery origin, radiological supervision and interpretation

➔ *CPT Changes: An Insider's View* 2006

➔ *Clinical Examples in Radiology* Winter 06:17

(For implantation of endovascular graft, use 33880)

75957 not involving coverage of left subclavian artery origin, initial endoprosthesis plus descending thoracic aortic extension(s), if required, to level of celiac artery origin, radiological supervision and interpretation

➔ *CPT Changes: An Insider's View* 2006

➔ *Clinical Examples in Radiology* Winter 06:17

(For implantation of endovascular graft, use 33881)

75958 Placement of proximal extension prosthesis for endovascular repair of descending thoracic aorta (eg, aneurysm, pseudoaneurysm, dissection, penetrating ulcer, intramural hematoma, or traumatic disruption), radiological supervision and interpretation

➔ *CPT Changes: An Insider's View* 2006

➔ *Clinical Examples in Radiology* Winter 06:17

(Report 75958 for each proximal extension)

(For implantation of proximal endovascular extension, see 33883, 33884)

75959 Placement of distal extension prosthesis(s) (delayed) after endovascular repair of descending thoracic aorta, as needed, to level of celiac origin, radiological supervision and interpretation

➔ *CPT Changes: An Insider's View* 2006

➔ *Clinical Examples in Radiology* Winter 06:17

(Do not report 75959 in conjunction with 75956, 75957)

(Report 75959 once, regardless of number of modules deployed)

(For implantation of distal endovascular extension, use 33886)

(Radiologic supervision for transcatheter placement of stent[s] is included in the therapeutic service codes)

(For removal of a vena cava filter, use 37193)

(75962, 75964, 75966, 75968 have been deleted. To report, see 36902, 36905, 37246, 37247)

75970 Transcatheter biopsy, radiological supervision and interpretation

➔ *CPT Assistant* May 17:3

(For injection procedure only for transcatheter therapy or biopsy, see 36100-36299)

(For transcatheter renal and ureteral biopsy, use 52007)

(For percutaneous needle biopsy of pancreas, use 48102; of retroperitoneal lymph node or mass, use 49180)

(75978 has been deleted. To report, see 36902, 36905, 36907, 37248, 37249)

(For radiological supervision and interpretation of transluminal balloon angioplasty within the peripheral and/or central segments of a dialysis circuit performed through the dialysis circuit, see 36902, 36905, 36907)

(75980 has been deleted. To report, see 47533, 47534, 47535, 47536, 47537)

(75982 has been deleted. To report, see 47533, 47534, 47535, 47536, 47537, 47538, 47539, 47540)

75984 Change of percutaneous tube or drainage catheter with contrast monitoring (eg, genitourinary system, abscess), radiological supervision and interpretation

➔ *CPT Changes: An Insider's View* 2008

➔ *CPT Assistant* Nov 97:24

➔ *Clinical Examples in Radiology* Summer 10:11, Fall 15:2, Spring 16:12

(For percutaneous replacement of gastrostomy, duodenostomy, jejunostomy, gastro-jejunostomy, or cecostomy [or other colonic] tube including fluoroscopic imaging guidance, see 49450-49452)

(To report exchange of a percutaneous nephrostomy catheter, use 50435)

(For percutaneous cholecystostomy, use 47490)

(For percutaneous biliary procedures, including radiological supervision and interpretation, see 47531-47544)

(For percutaneous nephrostolithotomy or pyelostolithotomy, see 50080, 50081)

(For removal and/or replacement of an internally dwelling ureteral stent via a transurethral approach, see 50385-50386)

75989 Radiological guidance (ie, fluoroscopy, ultrasound, or computed tomography), for percutaneous drainage (eg, abscess, specimen collection), with placement of catheter, radiological supervision and interpretation

➔ *CPT Changes: An Insider's View* 2001, 2002

➔ *CPT Assistant* Nov 97:24, Mar 98:8, Feb 07:11, Nov 10:3, Apr 11:12, Nov 12:3, Fall 13:5, 6, Nov 13:9, May 14:9

➔ *Clinical Examples in Radiology* Summer 10:3, Summer 11:3, Winter 11:10, Winter 13:5, Spring 14:10, Spring 15:8, Winter 16:10

(Do not report 75989 in conjunction with 10030, 32554, 32555, 32556, 32557, 47490, 49405, 49406, 49407)

Other Procedures

(For computed tomography cerebral perfusion analysis, see Category III code 0042T)

(For arthrography of shoulder, use 73040; elbow, use 73085; wrist, use 73115; hip, use 73525; knee, use 73580; ankle, use 73615)

76000 Fluoroscopy (separate procedure), up to 1 hour physician or other qualified health care professional time

➔ *CPT Changes: An Insider's View* 2000, 2013, 2018

➔ *CPT Assistant* Apr 96:11, Nov 99:32, Dec 00:14, Apr 03:7, Jul 03:16, Aug 03:14, Jul 08:9, Aug 08:7, Dec 08:7, 9, Aug 10:8, Oct 10:14, Nov 10:3, Dec 10:14, Jul 11:5, Nov 11:11, Feb 13:3, Mar 13:10, Sep 13:17, Sep 14:5, Oct 14:6, May 15:3, Sep 15:3, Jan 16:12, Mar 16:5, May 16:5, Aug 16:5

➔ *Clinical Examples in Radiology* Spring 18:14

►(Do not report 76000 in conjunction with 33274, 33275, 33957, 33958, 33959, 33962, 33963, 33964, 0515T, 0516T, 0517T, 0518T, 0519T, 0520T)◄

►(76001 has been deleted)◄

76010 Radiologic examination from nose to rectum for foreign body, single view, child

➔ *CPT Changes: An Insider's View* 2001

➔ *CPT Assistant* Feb 10:12

➔ *Clinical Examples in Radiology* Summer 09:11

76080 Radiologic examination, abscess, fistula or sinus tract study, radiological supervision and interpretation

➔ *CPT Assistant* Nov 97:24, Mar 98:8, Nov 03:14, Dec 06:10, Jan 09:8

➔ *Clinical Examples in Radiology* Fall 09:9, Summer 15:8

(For contrast injection[s] and radiological assessment of gastrostomy, duodenostomy, jejunostomy, gastro-jejunostomy, or cecostomy [or other colonic] tube including fluoroscopic imaging guidance, use 49465)

76098 Radiological examination, surgical specimen

➔ *Clinical Examples in Radiology* Fall 10:1, Summer 12:10, Fall 13:10, 11, Spring 14:10

(Do not report 76098 in conjunction with 19081-19086)

76100 Radiologic examination, single plane body section (eg, tomography), other than with urography

76101 Radiologic examination, complex motion (ie, hypercycloidal) body section (eg, mastoid polytomography), other than with urography; unilateral

76102 bilateral

(Do not report 76101, 76102 more than once per day)

(For panoramic X-ray, use 70355)

(For nephrotomography, use 74415)

76120 Cineradiography/videoradiography, except where specifically included

➔ *CPT Changes: An Insider's View* 2002

➔ *CPT Assistant* Sep 00:4, Apr 04:15, Apr 11:13

+ 76125 Cineradiography/videoradiography to complement routine examination (List separately in addition to code for primary procedure)

➔ *CPT Changes: An Insider's View* 2002

➔ *CPT Assistant* Oct 97:1, Sep 00:4

76140 Consultation on X-ray examination made elsewhere, written report

➔ *CPT Assistant* Summer 91:13, Oct 97:1

(2D reformatting is no longer separately reported. To report 3D rendering, see 76376, 76377)

76376 3D rendering with interpretation and reporting of computed tomography, magnetic resonance imaging, ultrasound, or other tomographic modality with image postprocessing under concurrent supervision; not requiring image postprocessing on an independent workstation

➔ *CPT Changes: An Insider's View* 2006, 2013

➔ *CPT Assistant* Dec 05:1, 7, Jan 07:31, Jul 08:3, May 09:9, Jun 09:9, Jul 09:10, Apr 10:5, Jul 10:7, May 13:3, Jun 13:12, Apr 16:9, May 17:11

➔ *Clinical Examples in Radiology* Spring 06:8-9, Fall 06:9-10, Winter 06:17, Winter 07:4-5, Summer 08:8, Fall 08:12, Spring 09:4, Summer 09:14, Fall 09:9, Spring 10:2, Summer 10:10, Fall 10:6, Winter 10:6, Winter 13:10, Fall 14:8, 11, Spring 17:7, Winter 17:14

(Use 76376 in conjunction with code[s] for base imaging procedure[s])

►(Do not report 76376 in conjunction with 31627, 34839, 70496, 70498, 70544, 70545, 70546, 70547, 70548, 70549, 71275, 71555, 72159, 72191, 72198, 73206, 73225, 73706, 73725, 74174, 74175, 74185, 74261, 74262, 74263, 75557, 75559, 75561, 75563, 75565, 75571, 75572, 75573, 75574, 75635, 76377, 77046, 77047, 77048, 77049, 77061, 77062, 77063, 78012-78999, 93355, 0523T)◄

76377 requiring image postprocessing on an independent workstation

➔ *CPT Changes: An Insider's View* 2006, 2013

➔ *CPT Assistant* Dec 05:1, Jan 07:31, Jul 08:3, May 09:9, Jun 09:9, Jul 09:10, Dec 09:13, Feb 10:6, Apr 10:5, 9, Jul 10:7, May 13:3, Jun 13:12, Apr 16:9, May 17:11

➔ *Clinical Examples in Radiology* Spring 06:8-9, Fall 06:9-10, Winter 06:17, Summer 07:1, 2, Winter 07:4-5, Summer 08:8, Fall 08:12, Spring 09:5, Summer 09:14, Fall 09:9, Spring 10:2, Summer 10:10, Fall 10:6, Winter 10:6, Winter 13:10, Spring 17:7, Winter 17:14

(Use 76377 in conjunction with code[s] for base imaging procedure[s])

►(Do not report 76377 in conjunction with 34839, 70496, 70498, 70544, 70545, 70546, 70547, 70548, 70549, 71275, 71555, 72159, 72191, 72198, 73206, 73225, 73706, 73725, 74174, 74175, 74185, 74261, 74262, 74263, 75557, 75559, 75561, 75563, 75565, 75571, 75572, 75573, 75574, 75635, 76376, 77046, 77047, 77048, 77049, 77061, 77062, 77063, 78012-78999, 93355, 0523T)◄

(76376, 76377 require concurrent supervision of image postprocessing 3D manipulation of volumetric data set and image rendering)

76380 Computed tomography, limited or localized follow-up study

➔ *CPT Changes: An Insider's View* 2002, 2003

➔ *CPT Assistant* Jul 07:13

➔ *Clinical Examples in Radiology* Summer 16:4

76390 Magnetic resonance spectroscopy

➔ *CPT Assistant* Nov 97:25

(For magnetic resonance imaging, use appropriate MRI body site code)

● **76391** Magnetic resonance (eg, vibration) elastography

➔ *CPT Changes: An Insider's View* 2019

76496 Unlisted fluoroscopic procedure (eg, diagnostic, interventional)

➔ *CPT Changes: An Insider's View* 2003

➔ *Clinical Examples in Radiology* Fall 07:3

76497 Unlisted computed tomography procedure (eg, diagnostic, interventional)

➔ *CPT Changes: An Insider's View* 2003

➔ *CPT Assistant* Jun 05:11

➔ *Clinical Examples in Radiology* Spring 05:1, 7

76498 Unlisted magnetic resonance procedure (eg, diagnostic, interventional)

➔ *CPT Changes: An Insider's View* 2003

➔ *CPT Assistant* Dec 11:17

➔ *Clinical Examples in Radiology* Fall 08:11, Spring 09:11, Winter 13:11, Spring 18:12

76499 Unlisted diagnostic radiographic procedure

➔ *CPT Changes: An Insider's View* 2003

➔ *CPT Assistant* Jul 99:10, Sep 00:4, Apr 04:15, Nov 06:22, Mar 08:15, Dec 11:17, Dec 13:17, Jul 16:8

➔ *Clinical Examples in Radiology* Spring 11:8, Fall 14:10, Summer 15:8

Diagnostic Ultrasound

All diagnostic ultrasound examinations require permanently recorded images with measurements, when such measurements are clinically indicated. For those codes whose sole diagnostic goal is a biometric measure (ie, 76514, 76516, and 76519), permanently recorded images are not required. A final, written report should be issued for inclusion in the patient's medical record. The prescription form for the intraocular lens satisfies the written report requirement for 76519. For those anatomic regions that have "complete" and "limited" ultrasound codes, note the elements that comprise a "complete" exam. The report should contain a description of these elements or the reason that an element could not be visualized (eg, obscured by bowel gas, surgically absent).

If less than the required elements for a "complete" exam are reported (eg, limited number of organs or limited portion of region evaluated), the "limited" code for that anatomic region should be used once per patient exam session. A "limited" exam of an anatomic region should not be reported for the same exam session as a "complete" exam of that same region.

Evaluation of vascular structures using both color and spectral Doppler is separately reportable. To report, see **Noninvasive Vascular Diagnostic Studies** (93880-93990). However, color Doppler alone, when performed for anatomic structure identification in conjunction with a real-time ultrasound examination, is not reported separately.

Ultrasound guidance procedures also require permanently recorded images of the site to be localized, as well as a documented description of the localization process, either separately or within the report of the procedure for which the guidance is utilized.

Use of ultrasound, without thorough evaluation of organ(s) or anatomic region, image documentation, and final, written report, is not separately reportable.

Definitions

A-mode implies a one-dimensional ultrasonic measurement procedure.

M-mode implies a one-dimensional ultrasonic measurement procedure with movement of the trace to record amplitude and velocity of moving echo-producing structures.

B-scan implies a two-dimensional ultrasonic scanning procedure with a two-dimensional display.

Real-time scan implies a two-dimensional ultrasonic scanning procedure with display of both two-dimensional structure and motion with time.

(To report diagnostic vascular ultrasound studies, see 93880-93990)

(For focused ultrasound ablation treatment of uterine leiomyomata, see Category III codes 0071T, 0072T)

Head and Neck

76506 Echoencephalography, real time with image documentation (gray scale) (for determination of ventricular size, delineation of cerebral contents, and detection of fluid masses or other intracranial abnormalities), including A-mode encephalography as secondary component where indicated

➔ *CPT Changes: An Insider's View* 2007, 2008

➔ *CPT Assistant* Mar 07:7

76510 Ophthalmic ultrasound, diagnostic; B-scan and quantitative A-scan performed during the same patient encounter

➔ *CPT Changes: An Insider's View* 2005

➔ *CPT Assistant* Dec 05:3

76511 quantitative A-scan only
CPT Changes: An Insider's View 2005
CPT Assistant Winter 93:12, Oct 96:9, Nov 99:42, Jul 04:12, Dec 05:3

76512 B-scan (with or without superimposed non-quantitative A-scan)
CPT Changes: An Insider's View 2005
CPT Assistant Winter 93:12, Oct 96:9, Dec 05:3

76513 anterior segment ultrasound, immersion (water bath) B-scan or high resolution biomicroscopy
CPT Changes: An Insider's View 2000
CPT Assistant Winter 93:12, Nov 99:42, Nov 09:9, Apr 13:7

(For scanning computerized ophthalmic diagnostic imaging of the anterior and posterior segments using technology other than ultrasound, see 92132, 92133, 92134)

76514 corneal pachymetry, unilateral or bilateral (determination of corneal thickness)
CPT Changes: An Insider's View 2004
CPT Assistant Jul 04:12, 15, Feb 05:13, Jun 05:11, Dec 05:3, Feb 16:12

(Do not report 76514 in conjunction with 0402T)

76516 Ophthalmic biometry by ultrasound echography, A-scan;
CPT Assistant Oct 03:10, Dec 05:3

76519 with intraocular lens power calculation
CPT Assistant Winter 93:12, Oct 03:10, Dec 05:3, Sep 09:5

(For partial coherence interferometry, use 92136)

76529 Ophthalmic ultrasonic foreign body localization
CPT Assistant Winter 93:12

76536 Ultrasound, soft tissues of head and neck (eg, thyroid, parathyroid, parotid), real time with image documentation
CPT Changes: An Insider's View 2002, 2007
CPT Assistant Mar 07:7, May 09:7, Oct 17:10
Clinical Examples in Radiology Winter 13:8, Spring 15:4, Spring 18:13

Chest

Code 76641 represents a complete ultrasound examination of the breast. Code 76641 consists of an ultrasound examination of all four quadrants of the breast and the retroareolar region. It also includes ultrasound examination of the axilla, if performed.

Code 76642 consists of a focused ultrasound examination of the breast limited to the assessment of one or more, but not all of the elements listed in code 76641. It also includes ultrasound examination of the axilla, if performed.

Use of ultrasound, without thorough evaluation of organ(s) or anatomic region, image documentation, and final written report, is not separately reportable.

76604 Ultrasound, chest (includes mediastinum), real time with image documentation
CPT Changes: An Insider's View 2002, 2007
CPT Assistant Nov 12:3, Oct 17:10
Clinical Examples in Radiology Spring 15:4, Summer 15:14, Winter 16:13

76641 Ultrasound, breast, unilateral, real time with image documentation, including axilla when performed; complete
CPT Changes: An Insider's View 2015
CPT Assistant Aug 15:11, Oct 17:10
Clinical Examples in Radiology Spring 15:4, Winter 15:10

76642 limited
CPT Changes: An Insider's View 2015
CPT Assistant Oct 17:10
Clinical Examples in Radiology Spring 15:4, Winter 15:10, Winter 16:13, Spring 18:13

(Report 76641, 76642 only once per breast, per session)

(For axillary ultrasound only, use 76882)

Abdomen and Retroperitoneum

A complete ultrasound examination of the abdomen (76700) consists of real time scans of the liver, gall bladder, common bile duct, pancreas, spleen, kidneys, and the upper abdominal aorta and inferior vena cava including any demonstrated abdominal abnormality.

A complete ultrasound examination of the retroperitoneum (76770) consists of real time scans of the kidneys, abdominal aorta, common iliac artery origins, and inferior vena cava, including any demonstrated retroperitoneal abnormality. Alternatively, if clinical history suggests urinary tract pathology, complete evaluation of the kidneys and urinary bladder also comprises a complete retroperitoneal ultrasound.

Use of ultrasound, without thorough evaluation of organ(s) or anatomic region, image documentation and final, written report, is not separately reportable.

76700 Ultrasound, abdominal, real time with image documentation; complete
CPT Changes: An Insider's View 2002, 2007
CPT Assistant Fall 93:13, Oct 01:3, Dec 05:3, Mar 07:7, Oct 17:10
Clinical Examples in Radiology Winter 05:9, 11, Fall 07:4, Spring 08:10, Summer 14:9, Spring 15:4, Winter 17:14

76705 limited (eg, single organ, quadrant, follow-up)
CPT Assistant Fall 93:13, Oct 01:3, Apr 03:27, Dec 05:3, Feb 09:22, May 09:7, Mar 12:10, Dec 12:9, Oct 17:10
Clinical Examples in Radiology Winter 05:9, 11, Fall 07:4, Summer 11:11, Spring 12:10, Winter 12:10, Summer 14:8, 9, Spring 15:4, Summer 15:13, Summer 16:10, Winter 17:14, Spring 18:13

76706 Ultrasound, abdominal aorta, real time with image documentation, screening study for abdominal aortic aneurysm (AAA)
CPT Changes: An Insider's View 2017
CPT Assistant May 17:3, Sep 17:12
Clinical Examples in Radiology Spring 17:5

(For ultrasound or duplex ultrasound of the abdominal aorta other than screening, see 76770, 76775, 93978, 93979)

76770 Ultrasound, retroperitoneal (eg, renal, aorta, nodes), real time with image documentation; complete

➔ *CPT Changes: An Insider's View* 2002, 2007

➔ *CPT Assistant* May 99:10, Jun 99:10, Mar 15:10, May 17:8, Oct 17:10

➔ *Clinical Examples in Radiology* Winter 05:9, 11, Fall 07:4, Winter 08:12, Summer 09:12, Summer 12:10, Summer 13:10, Spring 15:4, Spring 17:5

76775 limited

➔ *CPT Assistant* May 99:10, Jun 99:10, Dec 05:3, Feb 09:22, Mar 15:10, May 17:8, Oct 17:10

➔ *Clinical Examples in Radiology* Winter 05:9, 11, Spring 07:5-6, Fall 07:4, Winter 07:8-10, Summer 09:12, Summer 12:10, Summer 13:10, Spring 15:4, Summer 16:11, Spring 17:5

76776 Ultrasound, transplanted kidney, real time and duplex Doppler with image documentation

➔ *CPT Changes: An Insider's View* 2007

➔ *CPT Assistant* Mar 07:7

➔ *Clinical Examples in Radiology* Summer 12:10

(For ultrasound of transplanted kidney without duplex Doppler, use 76775)

(For ultrasound and duplex Doppler of a transplanted kidney, do not report 76776 in conjunction with 93975, 93976)

Spinal Canal

76800 Ultrasound, spinal canal and contents

➔ *CPT Changes: An Insider's View* 2002

➔ *CPT Assistant* Apr 98:15

Pelvis

Obstetrical

Codes 76801 and 76802 include determination of the number of gestational sacs and fetuses, gestational sac/fetal measurements appropriate for gestation (younger than 14 weeks 0 days), survey of visible fetal and placental anatomic structure, qualitative assessment of amniotic fluid volume/gestational sac shape and examination of the maternal uterus and adnexa.

Codes 76805 and 76810 include determination of number of fetuses and amniotic/chorionic sacs, measurements appropriate for gestational age (older than or equal to 14 weeks 0 days), survey of intracranial/spinal/abdominal anatomy, 4 chambered heart, umbilical cord insertion site, placenta location and amniotic fluid assessment and, when visible, examination of maternal adnexa.

Codes 76811 and 76812 include all elements of codes 76805 and 76810 plus detailed anatomic evaluation of the fetal brain/ventricles, face, heart/outflow tracts and chest anatomy, abdominal organ specific anatomy, number/length/architecture of limbs and detailed evaluation of the umbilical cord and placenta and other fetal anatomy as clinically indicated.

Report should document the results of the evaluation of each element described above or the reason for non-visualization.

Code 76815 represents a focused "quick look" exam limited to the assessment of one or more of the elements listed in code 76815.

Code 76816 describes an examination designed to reassess fetal size and interval growth or reevaluate one or more anatomic abnormalities of a fetus previously demonstrated on ultrasound, and should be coded once for each fetus requiring reevaluation using modifier 59 for each fetus after the first.

Code 76817 describes a transvaginal obstetric ultrasound performed separately or in addition to one of the transabdominal examinations described above. For transvaginal examinations performed for non-obstetrical purposes, use code 76830.

76801 Ultrasound, pregnant uterus, real time with image documentation, fetal and maternal evaluation, first trimester (< 14 weeks 0 days), transabdominal approach; single or first gestation

➔ *CPT Changes: An Insider's View* 2003

➔ *CPT Assistant* Mar 03:7, Nov 05:15

➔ *Clinical Examples in Radiology* Winter 07:6-7, Summer 10:8

(To report first trimester fetal nuchal translucency measurement, use 76813)

+ 76802 each additional gestation (List separately in addition to code for primary procedure)

➔ *CPT Changes: An Insider's View* 2003

➔ *CPT Assistant* Mar 03:7, Nov 05:15

➔ *Clinical Examples in Radiology* Winter 07:6-7, Summer 11:10

(Use 76802 in conjunction with 76801)

(To report first trimester fetal nuchal translucency measurement, use 76814)

76805 Ultrasound, pregnant uterus, real time with image documentation, fetal and maternal evaluation, after first trimester (> or = 14 weeks 0 days), transabdominal approach; single or first gestation

➔ *CPT Changes: An Insider's View* 2002, 2003

➔ *CPT Assistant* Apr 97:2, Nov 97:25, Oct 01:3, Aug 02:2, Mar 03:7

➔ *Clinical Examples in Radiology* Winter 05:3-4, Summer 12:11, Winter 14:11

+ 76810 each additional gestation (List separately in addition to code for primary procedure)

➔ *CPT Changes: An Insider's View* 2003

➔ *CPT Assistant* Apr 97:2, Oct 01:3, Aug 02:2, Mar 03:7

➔ *Clinical Examples in Radiology* Winter 05:4, Summer 11:10, Winter 14:11

(Use 76810 in conjunction with 76805)

Radiology 70010-79999

76811 Ultrasound, pregnant uterus, real time with image documentation, fetal and maternal evaluation plus detailed fetal anatomic examination, transabdominal approach; single or first gestation

➲ *CPT Changes: An Insider's View* 2003

➲ *CPT Assistant* Mar 03:7

➲ *Clinical Examples in Radiology* Winter 05:4, Winter 14:11

+ 76812 each additional gestation (List separately in addition to code for primary procedure)

➲ *CPT Changes: An Insider's View* 2003

➲ *CPT Assistant* Mar 03:7

➲ *Clinical Examples in Radiology* Summer 11:10, Winter 14:11

(Use 76812 in conjunction with 76811)

76813 Ultrasound, pregnant uterus, real time with image documentation, first trimester fetal nuchal translucency measurement, transabdominal or transvaginal approach; single or first gestation

➲ *CPT Changes: An Insider's View* 2007

➲ *CPT Assistant* Mar 07:7

➲ *Clinical Examples in Radiology* Winter 07:6

+ 76814 each additional gestation (List separately in addition to code for primary procedure)

➲ *CPT Changes: An Insider's View* 2007

➲ *CPT Assistant* Mar 07:7

➲ *Clinical Examples in Radiology* Winter 07:6, Summer 11:10

(Use 76814 in conjunction with 76813)

76815 Ultrasound, pregnant uterus, real time with image documentation, limited (eg, fetal heart beat, placental location, fetal position and/or qualitative amniotic fluid volume), 1 or more fetuses

➲ *CPT Changes: An Insider's View* 2003

➲ *CPT Assistant* Apr 97:2, Nov 97:25, Oct 01:3, Dec 01:6, Aug 02:2, Mar 03:7, Nov 03:14, May 10:9

➲ *Clinical Examples in Radiology* Winter 07:6-7, Summer 10:8, 9, Summer 12:11, Summer 14:7, 8, Summer 16:12

(Use 76815 only once per exam and not per element)

(To report first trimester fetal nuchal translucency measurement, see 76813, 76814)

76816 Ultrasound, pregnant uterus, real time with image documentation, follow-up (eg, re-evaluation of fetal size by measuring standard growth parameters and amniotic fluid volume, re-evaluation of organ system(s) suspected or confirmed to be abnormal on a previous scan), transabdominal approach, per fetus

➲ *CPT Changes: An Insider's View* 2003

➲ *CPT Assistant* Apr 97:2, Oct 01:3, Aug 02:2, Mar 03:7, May 10:9, Nov 11:10

➲ *Clinical Examples in Radiology* Summer 10:9, Summer 12:11, Summer 14:7, 8, Spring 16:13

(Report 76816 with modifier 59 for each additional fetus examined in a multiple pregnancy)

76817 Ultrasound, pregnant uterus, real time with image documentation, transvaginal

➲ *CPT Changes: An Insider's View* 2003

➲ *CPT Assistant* Mar 03:7, Nov 11:10

➲ *Clinical Examples in Radiology* Summer 10:8, Summer 11:10, Winter 14:11, Winter 16:13

(For non-obstetrical transvaginal ultrasound, use 76830)

(If transvaginal examination is done in addition to transabdominal obstetrical ultrasound exam, use 76817 in addition to appropriate transabdominal exam code)

76818 Fetal biophysical profile; with non-stress testing

➲ *CPT Changes: An Insider's View* 2001

➲ *CPT Assistant* Apr 97:2, May 98:10, Sep 01:4, Oct 01:3, Dec 01:6, Nov 04:10

➲ *Clinical Examples in Radiology* Summer 14:7, 8

76819 without non-stress testing

➲ *CPT Changes: An Insider's View* 2001, 2002

➲ *CPT Assistant* Sep 01:8, Dec 01:6

➲ *Clinical Examples in Radiology* Summer 14:7, 8

(Fetal biophysical profile assessments for the second and any additional fetuses, should be reported separately by code 76818 or 76819 with the modifier 59 appended)

(For amniotic fluid index without non-stress test, use 76815)

76820 Doppler velocimetry, fetal; umbilical artery

➲ *CPT Changes: An Insider's View* 2005

➲ *CPT Assistant* Dec 05:3, Jul 16:9

76821 middle cerebral artery

➲ *CPT Changes: An Insider's View* 2005

➲ *CPT Assistant* Dec 05:3

76825 Echocardiography, fetal, cardiovascular system, real time with image documentation (2D), with or without M-mode recording;

➲ *CPT Assistant* Apr 97:2, Aug 02:2, Sep 17:15

76826 follow-up or repeat study

➲ *CPT Assistant* Apr 97:2, Aug 02:2, Sep 17:15

76827 Doppler echocardiography, fetal, pulsed wave and/or continuous wave with spectral display; complete

➲ *CPT Changes: An Insider's View* 2005

➲ *CPT Assistant* Apr 97:2, Aug 02:2, Dec 05:3

76828 follow-up or repeat study

➲ *CPT Assistant* Apr 97:2, Aug 02:2, Dec 05:3

(To report the use of color mapping, use 93325)

Nonobstetrical

Code 76856 includes the complete evaluation of the female pelvic anatomy. Elements of this examination include a description and measurements of the uterus and adnexal structures, measurement of the endometrium, measurement of the bladder (when applicable), and a description of any pelvic pathology (eg, ovarian cysts, uterine leiomyomata, free pelvic fluid).

Code 76856 is also applicable to a complete evaluation of the male pelvis. Elements of the examination include evaluation and measurement (when applicable) of the urinary bladder, evaluation of the prostate and seminal vesicles to the extent that they are visualized transabdominally, and any pelvic pathology (eg, bladder tumor, enlarged prostate, free pelvic fluid, pelvic abscess).

Code 76857 represents a focused examination limited to the assessment of one or more elements listed in code 76856 and/or the reevaluation of one or more pelvic abnormalities previously demonstrated on ultrasound. Code 76857, rather than 76770, should be utilized if the urinary bladder alone (ie, not including the kidneys) is imaged, whereas code 51798 should be utilized if a bladder volume or post-void residual measurement is obtained without imaging the bladder.

Use of ultrasound, without thorough evaluation of organ(s) or anatomic region, image documentation, and final, written report, is not separately reportable.

76830 Ultrasound, transvaginal

➔ *CPT Changes: An Insider's View* 2002

➔ *CPT Assistant* Aug 96:10, Jul 99:8, Aug 02:2, Mar 03:7, Dec 05:3, Feb 09:22, Nov 11:10, Oct 17:10

➔ *Clinical Examples in Radiology* 2004_Inaugural 04:6-7, Spring 08:9, Summer 10:8, 9, Summer 12:7, Spring 15:4, Summer 15:10, Winter 16:13

(For obstetrical transvaginal ultrasound, use 76817)

(If transvaginal examination is done in addition to transabdominal non-obstetrical ultrasound exam, use 76830 in addition to appropriate transabdominal exam code)

76831 Saline infusion sonohysterography (SIS), including color flow Doppler, when performed

➔ *CPT Changes: An Insider's View* 2004

➔ *CPT Assistant* Nov 97:25, Jul 99:8, Dec 05:3, Mar 09:11

(For introduction of saline for saline infusion sonohysterography, use 58340)

76856 Ultrasound, pelvic (nonobstetric), real time with image documentation; complete

➔ *CPT Changes: An Insider's View* 2002, 2007

➔ *CPT Assistant* Oct 01:3, Dec 05:3, Jan 06:47, Mar 07:7, Feb 09:22, Aug 16:10, Oct 17:10

➔ *Clinical Examples in Radiology* 2004_Inaugural 04:6-7, Spring 08:9, Summer 10:8, Summer 12:7, Summer 14:9, Spring 15:4, Summer 15:10, Winter 18:15

76857 limited or follow-up (eg, for follicles)

➔ *CPT Assistant* Jun 97:10, Oct 01:3, Dec 05:3, Sep 07:10, May 09:7, Oct 17:10

➔ *Clinical Examples in Radiology* Spring 08:9, Summer 10:8, Summer 12:7, Summer 13:11, Summer 14:8, 9, Spring 15:4, Summer 15:10, Spring 18:13, Winter 18:15

Genitalia

76870 Ultrasound, scrotum and contents

➔ *CPT Changes: An Insider's View* 2002

➔ *CPT Assistant* May 05:3, Oct 17:10

➔ *Clinical Examples in Radiology* Spring 15:4, Winter 18:15

76872 Ultrasound, transrectal;

➔ *CPT Changes: An Insider's View* 2000, 2004

➔ *CPT Assistant* May 96:3, Nov 99:42, Oct 17:10

➔ *Clinical Examples in Radiology* Spring 15:4

(Do not report 76872 in conjunction with 45341, 45342, 45391, 45392, 0249T, 0421T)

76873 prostate volume study for brachytherapy treatment planning (separate procedure)

➔ *CPT Changes: An Insider's View* 2000

➔ *CPT Assistant* Nov 99:42

Extremities

Code 76881 represents a complete evaluation of a specific joint in an extremity. Code 76881 requires ultrasound examination of all of the following joint elements: joint space (eg, effusion), peri-articular soft-tissue structures that surround the joint (ie, muscles, tendons, other soft-tissue structures), and any identifiable abnormality. In some circumstances, additional evaluations such as dynamic imaging or stress maneuvers may be performed as part of the complete evaluation. Code 76881 also requires permanently recorded images and a written report containing a description of each of the required elements or reason that an element(s) could not be visualized (eg, absent secondary to surgery or trauma).

When fewer than all of the required elements for a "complete" exam (76881) are performed, report the "limited" code (76882).

Code 76882 represents a limited evaluation of a joint or an evaluation of a structure(s) in an extremity other than a joint (eg, soft-tissue mass, fluid collection, or nerve[s]). Limited evaluation of a joint includes assessment of a specific anatomic structure(s) (eg, joint space only [effusion] or tendon, muscle, and/or other soft-tissue structure[s] that surround the joint) that does not assess all of the required elements included in 76881. Code 76882 also requires permanently recorded images and a written report containing a description of each of the elements evaluated.

For spectral and color Doppler evaluation of the extremities, use 93925, 93926, 93930, 93931, 93970, or 93971 as appropriate.

76881 Ultrasound, complete joint (ie, joint space and peri-articular soft-tissue structures), real-time with image documentation

➔ *CPT Changes: An Insider's View* 2011, 2018

➔ *CPT Assistant* Sep 16:9, Oct 17:10

➔ *Clinical Examples in Radiology* Winter 11:7, 11, Summer 14:8, Spring 15:4, Winter 15:8, 9, Spring 17:12, Spring 18:12

76882 Ultrasound, limited, joint or other nonvascular extremity structure(s) (eg, joint space, peri-articular tendon[s], muscle[s], nerve[s], other soft-tissue structure[s], or soft-tissue mass[es]), real-time with image documentation

➲ *CPT Changes: An Insider's View* 2011, 2018

➲ *CPT Assistant* Sep 16:9, Oct 17:10

➲ *Clinical Examples in Radiology* Summer 11:11, Winter 11:7, Summer 14:8, 9, Spring 15:4, Summer 15:13, Winter 15:8-10, Spring 17:12

76885 Ultrasound, infant hips, real time with imaging documentation; dynamic (requiring physician or other qualified health care professional manipulation)

➲ *CPT Changes: An Insider's View* 2002, 2013

➲ *CPT Assistant* Nov 97:25

76886 limited, static (not requiring physician or other qualified health care professional manipulation)

➲ *CPT Changes: An Insider's View* 2002, 2013

➲ *CPT Assistant* Nov 97:25

Ultrasonic Guidance Procedures

76930 Ultrasonic guidance for pericardiocentesis, imaging supervision and interpretation

➲ *CPT Changes: An Insider's View* 2001

➲ *CPT Assistant* Sep 16:10

➲ *Clinical Examples in Radiology* Spring 14:10

76932 Ultrasonic guidance for endomyocardial biopsy, imaging supervision and interpretation

➲ *CPT Changes: An Insider's View* 2001

76936 Ultrasound guided compression repair of arterial pseudoaneurysm or arteriovenous fistulae (includes diagnostic ultrasound evaluation, compression of lesion and imaging)

+ 76937 Ultrasound guidance for vascular access requiring ultrasound evaluation of potential access sites, documentation of selected vessel patency, concurrent realtime ultrasound visualization of vascular needle entry, with permanent recording and reporting (List separately in addition to code for primary procedure)

➲ *CPT Changes: An Insider's View* 2004

➲ *CPT Assistant* Dec 04:13, Jan 09:7, Jul 10:6, Nov 10:3, Jan 11:8, Apr 12:6, Feb 13:3, May 13:3, Jun 13:12, Sep 13:18, Oct 14:6, Jul 15:10, Mar 17:4, Jul 17:5

➲ *Clinical Examples in Radiology* 2004_Inaugural 04:1-2, Winter 05:5-6, Summer 06:8-9, Spring 08:7, 8, Fall 08:5, 6, Spring 09:10, Winter 09:8, 9, Summer 10:1, 3, 4, Spring 12:4, Summer 12:3, Winter 12:3, Summer 13:4, Fall 13:1, 2, 3, 4, Winter 13:1, 2, 3, Summer 14:10, Winter 14:1-5, 7, Summer 15:2, Winter 15:2, 3, 4, 5, 6, Winter 16:2, Winter 17:8, Spring 18:8

►(Do not report 76937 in conjunction with 33274, 33275, 36568, 36569, 36572, 36573, 36584, 37191, 37192, 37193, 37760, 37761, 76942)◄

►(Do not report 76937 in conjunction with 0505T for ultrasound guidance for vascular access)◄

(If extremity venous non-invasive vascular diagnostic study is performed separate from venous access guidance, see 93970, 93971)

76940 Ultrasound guidance for, and monitoring of, parenchymal tissue ablation

➲ *CPT Changes: An Insider's View* 2004, 2007

➲ *CPT Assistant* Oct 02:2, Mar 07:7, Jul 15:8, May 17:3, Nov 17:8

➲ *Clinical Examples in Radiology* Spring 08:1, 2, Summer 12:11, Spring 15:3, Fall 17:3

(Do not report 76940 in conjunction with 20982, 20983, 32994, 32998, 50250, 50542, 76942, 76998)

(For ablation, see 47370-47382, 47383, 50592, 50593)

76941 Ultrasonic guidance for intrauterine fetal transfusion or cordocentesis, imaging supervision and interpretation

➲ *CPT Changes: An Insider's View* 2001

(For procedure, see 36460, 59012)

76942 Ultrasonic guidance for needle placement (eg, biopsy, aspiration, injection, localization device), imaging supervision and interpretation

➲ *CPT Changes: An Insider's View* 2001

➲ *CPT Assistant* Fall 93:12, Fall 94:2, May 96:3, Jun 97:5, Oct 01:2, May 04:7, Dec 04:12, Apr 05:15-16, Aug 08:7, Mar 09:8, Feb 10:6, Mar 10:9, Jul 10:6, Feb 11:4, Mar 11:10, Apr 11:12, Nov 12:3, Dec 12:9, Nov 13:9, Oct 14:6, Feb 15:6, Aug 15:8, Nov 15:10, Jan 16:9, Jun 16:3, Jun 17:10, Dec 17:16, Mar 18:3

➲ *Clinical Examples in Radiology* Summer 05:1, 2, 6, Fall 05:1, Summer 08:5, 6, Fall 08:2, 3, Fall 09:8, Winter 09:9, Summer 10:1, 3, 4, Fall 10:3, Summer 11:3, Spring 14:2-4, 7, Summer 14:9, Spring 15:10, Summer 15:7, Winter 16:6, Winter 17:3, Spring 18:3, Winter 18:8

►(Do not report 76942 in conjunction with 10004, 10005, 10006, 10021, 10030, 19083, 19285, 20604, 20606, 20611, 27096, 32554, 32555, 32556, 32557, 37760, 37761, 43232, 43237, 43242, 45341, 45342, 55874, 64479, 64480, 64483, 64484, 64490, 64491, 64493, 64494, 64495, 76975, 0213T, 0214T, 0215T, 0216T, 0217T, 0218T, 0228T, 0229T, 0230T, 0231T, 0232T, 0249T, 0481T)◄

(For harvesting, preparation, and injection[s] of platelet rich plasma, use 0232T)

76945 Ultrasonic guidance for chorionic villus sampling, imaging supervision and interpretation

➲ *CPT Changes: An Insider's View* 2001

(For procedure, use 59015)

76946 Ultrasonic guidance for amniocentesis, imaging supervision and interpretation

➲ *CPT Changes: An Insider's View* 2001

76948 Ultrasonic guidance for aspiration of ova, imaging supervision and interpretation

➲ *CPT Changes: An Insider's View* 2001

(For placement of interstitial device[s] for radiation therapy guidance, see 31627, 32553, 49411, 55876)

76965 Ultrasonic guidance for interstitial radioelement application

Other Procedures

76970 Ultrasound study follow-up (specify)

Radiology 70010-79999

76975 Gastrointestinal endoscopic ultrasound, supervision and interpretation

➲ *CPT Changes: An Insider's View* 2001

➲ *CPT Assistant* Spring 94:5, May 04:7, Mar 09:8

(Do not report 76975 in conjunction with 43231, 43232, 43237, 43238, 43240, 43242, 43259, 44406, 44407, 45341, 45342, 45391, 45392, 76942)

76977 Ultrasound bone density measurement and interpretation, peripheral site(s), any method

➲ *CPT Assistant* Nov 98:21

● **76978** Ultrasound, targeted dynamic microbubble sonographic contrast characterization (non-cardiac); initial lesion

➲ *CPT Changes: An Insider's View* 2019

+● **76979** each additional lesion with separate injection (List separately in addition to code for primary procedure)

➲ *CPT Changes: An Insider's View* 2019

►(Use 76979 in conjunction with 76978)◄

►(Do not report 76978, 76979 in conjunction with 96374)◄

● **76981** Ultrasound, elastography; parenchyma (eg, organ)

➲ *CPT Changes: An Insider's View* 2019

● **76982** first target lesion

➲ *CPT Changes: An Insider's View* 2019

+● **76983** each additional target lesion (List separately in addition to code for primary procedure)

➲ *CPT Changes: An Insider's View* 2019

►(Use 76983 in conjunction with 76982)◄

►(Report 76981 only once per session for evaluation of the same parenchymal organ)◄

►(To report shear wave liver elastography without imaging, use 91200)◄

►(For evaluation of a parenchymal organ and lesion[s] in the same parenchymal organ at the same session, report only 76981)◄

►(Do not report 76983 more than two times per organ)◄

76998 Ultrasonic guidance, intraoperative

➲ *CPT Changes: An Insider's View* 2007

➲ *CPT Assistant* Mar 07:7, Jul 10:6, Jan 13:6, Jan 14:5, Oct 14:6, Aug 15:8, Apr 17:7

➲ *Clinical Examples in Radiology* Winter 12:11

►(Do not report 76998 in conjunction with 36475, 36479, 37760, 37761, 47370, 47371, 47380, 47381, 47382, 0249T, 0515T, 0516T, 0517T, 0518T, 0519T, 0520T)◄

(For ultrasound guidance for open and laparoscopic radiofrequency tissue ablation, use 76940)

76999 Unlisted ultrasound procedure (eg, diagnostic, interventional)

➲ *CPT Changes: An Insider's View* 2003

➲ *Clinical Examples in Radiology* Summer 12:10, Spring 15:10, Winter 15:8, 9

Radiologic Guidance

Fluoroscopic Guidance

(Do not report guidance codes 77001, 77002, 77003 for services in which fluoroscopic guidance is included in the descriptor)

+ **77001** Fluoroscopic guidance for central venous access device placement, replacement (catheter only or complete), or removal (includes fluoroscopic guidance for vascular access and catheter manipulation, any necessary contrast injections through access site or catheter with related venography radiologic supervision and interpretation, and radiographic documentation of final catheter position) (List separately in addition to code for primary procedure)

➲ *CPT Changes: An Insider's View* 2007

➲ *CPT Assistant* Mar 07:7, Jul 08:9, Nov 10:3, Jan 11:8

➲ *Clinical Examples in Radiology* Spring 08:7, 8, Fall 08:5, 6, Winter 09:8, 9, Summer 10:11, Winter 17:8

►(Do not report 77001 in conjunction with 33957, 33958, 33959, 33962, 33963, 33964, 36568, 36569, 36572, 36573, 36584, 77002)◄

(If formal extremity venography is performed from separate venous access and separately interpreted, use 36005 and 75820, 75822, 75825, or 75827)

+ **77002** Fluoroscopic guidance for needle placement (eg, biopsy, aspiration, injection, localization device) (List separately in addition to code for primary procedure)

➲ *CPT Changes: An Insider's View* 2007, 2017

➲ *CPT Assistant* Feb 07:11, Mar 07:7, May 07:1, Jun 07:10, Jul 08:9, Aug 08:7, Dec 08:9, Dec 09:12, Feb 10:6, Nov 10:3, Jan 11:8, Apr 11:12, Feb 12:11, Apr 12:19, Jun 12:14, Nov 12:3, Dec 12:9, Nov 13:9, Jul 15:8, Aug 15:6, Jan 16:9, Jun 16:3, Sep 16:10, May 17:3, Jun 17:10, Nov 17:8

➲ *Clinical Examples in Radiology* Summer 08:5, 6, Spring 09:6, 7, Fall 09:7, Winter 09:9, Fall 10:10, Summer 11:3, Spring 13:11, Spring 14:4, 10, Winter 14:9-10, Spring 15:3, Winter 16:6, Winter 17:5, Spring 18:3

(See appropriate surgical code for procedure and anatomic location)

►(Use 77002 in conjunction with 10160, 20206, 20220, 20225, 20520, 20525, 20526, 20550, 20551, 20552, 20553, 20555, 20600, 20605, 20610, 20612, 20615, 21116, 21550, 23350, 24220, 25246, 27093, 27095, 27369, 27648, 32400, 32405, 32553, 36002, 38220, 38221, 38222, 38505, 38794, 41019, 42400, 42405, 47000, 47001, 48102, 49180, 49411, 50200, 50390, 51100, 51101, 51102, 55700, 55876, 60100, 62268, 62269, 64505, 64600, 64605)◄

(77002 is included in all arthrography radiological supervision and interpretation codes. See **Administration of Contrast Material[s]** introductory guidelines for reporting of arthrography procedures)

+ **77003** Fluoroscopic guidance and localization of needle or catheter tip for spine or paraspinous diagnostic or therapeutic injection procedures (epidural or subarachnoid) (List separately in addition to code for primary procedure)

➲ *CPT Changes: An Insider's View* 2007, 2010, 2011, 2012, 2017

➲ *CPT Assistant* Mar 07:7, Jul 08:9, Feb 10:12, May 10:10, Aug 10:8, Oct 10:14, Nov 10:3, Dec 10:14, Jan 11:8, Feb 11:4, Mar 11:7, Jul 11:17, Jun 12:12, Jul 12:3, 5, 6, Sep 12:14, Nov 13:9, Dec 13:14, Jan 16:9, 12, May 17:3, Dec 17:13

➲ *Clinical Examples in Radiology* Summer 08:9, 13, Winter 09:9, Spring 11:9, Spring 14:4, Winter 14:9-10, Fall 15:10, Summer 16:4, Winter 18:8

(Use 77003 in conjunction with 61050, 61055, 62267, 62270, 62272, 62273, 62280, 62281, 62282, 62284, 64510, 64517, 64520, 64610, 96450)

(Do not report 77003 in conjunction with 62320, 62321, 62322, 62323, 62324, 62325, 62326, 62327)

Computed Tomography Guidance

77011 Computed tomography guidance for stereotactic localization

➲ *CPT Changes: An Insider's View* 2007

➲ *CPT Assistant* Mar 07:7

77012 Computed tomography guidance for needle placement (eg, biopsy, aspiration, injection, localization device), radiological supervision and interpretation

➲ *CPT Changes: An Insider's View* 2007

➲ *CPT Assistant* Mar 07:7, May 07:1, Jun 07:10, Aug 08:7, Feb 10:6, Feb 11:4, Apr 11:12, Jul 12:3, 6, Sep 12:14, Nov 12:3, Dec 12:9, Nov 13:9, Feb 15:6, Jun 16:3

➲ *Clinical Examples in Radiology* Summer 08:5, 6, Fall 08:3, Fall 09:6, Fall 10:3, Summer 11:3, Spring 14:4, Spring 15:7, Summer 16:4, Winter 16:6, Winter 17:5, Spring 18:3, Winter 18:8

►(Do not report 77011, 77012 in conjunction with 22586)◄

►(Do not report 77012 in conjunction with 10009, 10010,10030, 27096, 32554, 32555, 32556, 32557, 64479, 64480, 64483, 64484, 64490, 64491, 64492, 64493, 64494, 64495, 64633, 64634, 64635, 64636, 0232T, 0481T)◄

(For harvesting, preparation, and injection[s] of platelet-rich plasma, use 0232T)

77013 Computed tomography guidance for, and monitoring of, parenchymal tissue ablation

➲ *CPT Changes: An Insider's View* 2007

➲ *CPT Assistant* Mar 07:7, Jul 15:8, May 17:3, Nov 17:8

➲ *Clinical Examples in Radiology* Summer 12:11, Spring 15:3, Fall 17:3

(Do not report 77013 in conjunction with 20982, 20983, 32994, 32998)

(For percutaneous ablation, see 47382, 47383, 50592, 50593)

77014 Computed tomography guidance for placement of radiation therapy fields

➲ *CPT Changes: An Insider's View* 2007

➲ *CPT Assistant* Mar 07:7, Apr 15:11, Feb 16:3

➲ *Clinical Examples in Radiology* Summer 09:2, 4, Spring 12:10, Winter 13:11

(For placement of interstitial device[s] for radiation therapy guidance, see 31627, 32553, 49411, 55876)

►Magnetic Resonance Imaging Guidance◄

▲ **77021** Magnetic resonance imaging guidance for needle placement (eg, for biopsy, needle aspiration, injection, or placement of localization device) radiological supervision and interpretation

➲ *CPT Changes: An Insider's View* 2007, 2019

➲ *CPT Assistant* Mar 07:7, May 07:1, Jun 07:10, Aug 08:7, Feb 10:6, Apr 11:12, Nov 12:3, Dec 12:9, Nov 13:9, Feb 15:6, Jun 16:3, Jun 17:10

➲ *Clinical Examples in Radiology* Summer 08:5, 6, 13, Fall 08:3, Fall 10:3, Summer 11:3, Spring 14:4, Spring 15:7, Winter 16:6, Winter 17:5, Spring 18:3

(For procedure, see appropriate organ or site)

►(Do not report 77021 in conjunction with 10011, 10012, 10030, 19085, 19287, 32554, 32555, 32556, 32557, 0232T, 0481T)◄

(For harvesting, preparation, and injection[s] of platelet-rich plasma, use 0232T)

▲ **77022** Magnetic resonance imaging guidance for, and monitoring of, parenchymal tissue ablation

➲ *CPT Changes: An Insider's View* 2007, 2019

➲ *CPT Assistant* Mar 07:7, Oct 14:6, Jul 15:8, May 17:3

➲ *Clinical Examples in Radiology* Summer 12:11, Spring 15:3, Fall 17:3

(Do not report 77022 in conjunction with 20982, 20983, 32994, 32998, 0071T, 0072T)

(For percutaneous ablation, see 47382, 47383, 50592, 50593)

(For focused ultrasound ablation treatment of uterine leiomyomata, see Category III codes 0071T, 0072T)

(To report stereotactic localization guidance for breast biopsy or for placement of breast localization device[s], see 19081, 19283)

(To report mammographic guidance for placement of breast localization device[s], use 19281)

Breast, Mammography

● **77046** Magnetic resonance imaging, breast, without contrast material; unilateral

➲ *CPT Changes: An Insider's View* 2019

● **77047** bilateral
➔ *CPT Changes: An Insider's View* 2019

● **77048** Magnetic resonance imaging, breast, without and with contrast material(s), including computer-aided detection (CAD real-time lesion detection, characterization and pharmacokinetic analysis), when performed; unilateral
➔ *CPT Changes: An Insider's View* 2019

● **77049** bilateral
➔ *CPT Changes: An Insider's View* 2019

(77051 has been deleted. To report, see 77065, 77066)

(77052 has been deleted. To report, use 77067)

77053 Mammary ductogram or galactogram, single duct, radiological supervision and interpretation
➔ *CPT Changes: An Insider's View* 2007
➔ *CPT Assistant* Mar 07:7

(For mammary ductogram or galactogram injection, use 19030)

77054 Mammary ductogram or galactogram, multiple ducts, radiological supervision and interpretation
➔ *CPT Changes: An Insider's View* 2007
➔ *CPT Assistant* Mar 07:7

(77055 has been deleted. To report, use 77065)

(77056 has been deleted. To report, use 77066)

(77057 has been deleted. To report, use 77067)

►(77058 has been deleted. To report, see 77046, 77048)◄

►(77059 has been deleted. To report, see 77047, 77049)◄

77061 Digital breast tomosynthesis; unilateral
➔ *CPT Changes: An Insider's View* 2015
➔ *CPT Assistant* May 17:3
➔ *Clinical Examples in Radiology* Fall 14:10

77062 bilateral
➔ *CPT Changes: An Insider's View* 2015
➔ *CPT Assistant* Dec 16:15, May 17:3
➔ *Clinical Examples in Radiology* Fall 14:10

(Do not report 77061, 77062 in conjunction with 76376, 76377, 77067)

+ **77063** Screening digital breast tomosynthesis, bilateral (List separately in addition to code for primary procedure)
➔ *CPT Changes: An Insider's View* 2015
➔ *CPT Assistant* Dec 16:15, May 17:3
➔ *Clinical Examples in Radiology* Fall 14:10

(Do not report 77063 in conjunction with 76376, 76377, 77065, 77066)

(Use 77063 in conjunction with 77067)

Screening Mammography
77067

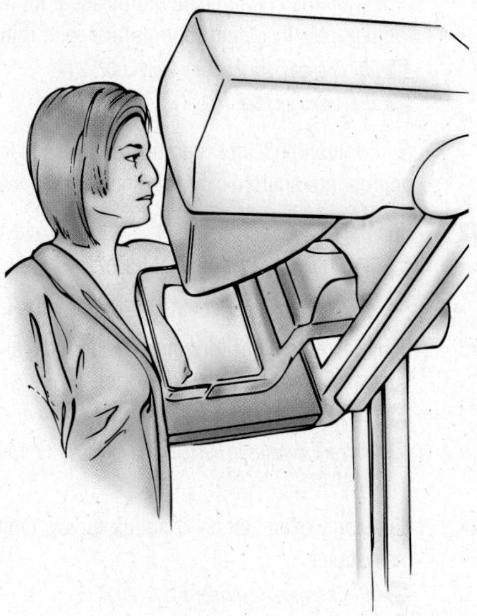

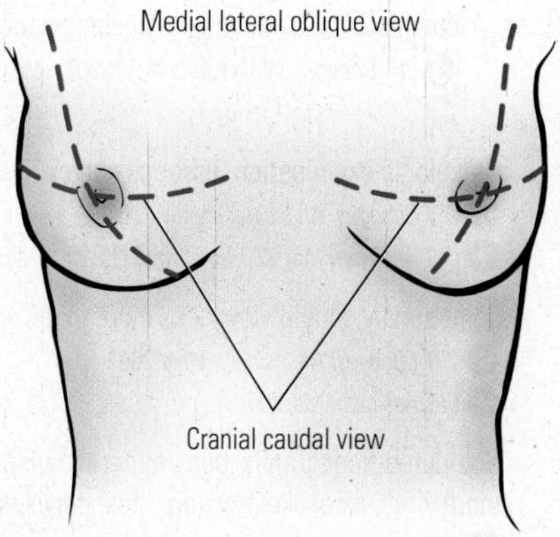

77065 Diagnostic mammography, including computer-aided detection (CAD) when performed; unilateral
➔ *CPT Changes: An Insider's View* 2017
➔ *CPT Assistant* Dec 16:15, May 17:3
➔ *Clinical Examples in Radiology* Winter 17:15, Spring 18:3

77066 bilateral
➔ *CPT Changes: An Insider's View* 2017
➔ *CPT Assistant* Dec 16:15, May 17:3
➔ *Clinical Examples in Radiology* Winter 17:15, Spring 18:12

77067 Screening mammography, bilateral (2-view study of each breast), including computer-aided detection (CAD) when performed
➔ *CPT Changes: An Insider's View* 2017
➔ *CPT Assistant* Dec 16:15, May 17:3
➔ *Clinical Examples in Radiology* Winter 17:15, Spring 18:12

(For electrical impedance breast scan, use 76499)

Bone/Joint Studies

77071 Manual application of stress performed by physician or other qualified health care professional for joint radiography, including contralateral joint if indicated

➔ *CPT Changes: An Insider's View* 2007, 2013

➔ *CPT Assistant* Mar 07:7

(For radiographic interpretation of stressed images, see appropriate anatomic site and number of views)

77072 Bone age studies

➔ *CPT Changes: An Insider's View* 2007

➔ *CPT Assistant* Mar 07:7

77073 Bone length studies (orthoroentgenogram, scanogram)

➔ *CPT Changes: An Insider's View* 2007

➔ *CPT Assistant* Mar 07:7

➔ *Clinical Examples in Radiology* Summer 07:12, Fall 08:10, Fall 10:6

77074 Radiologic examination, osseous survey; limited (eg, for metastases)

➔ *CPT Changes: An Insider's View* 2007

➔ *CPT Assistant* Mar 07:7

77075 complete (axial and appendicular skeleton)

➔ *CPT Changes: An Insider's View* 2007

➔ *CPT Assistant* Mar 07:7

77076 Radiologic examination, osseous survey, infant

➔ *CPT Changes: An Insider's View* 2007

➔ *CPT Assistant* Mar 07:7

77077 Joint survey, single view, 2 or more joints (specify)

➔ *CPT Changes: An Insider's View* 2007

➔ *CPT Assistant* Mar 07:7

77078 Computed tomography, bone mineral density study, 1 or more sites, axial skeleton (eg, hips, pelvis, spine)

➔ *CPT Changes: An Insider's View* 2007

➔ *CPT Assistant* Mar 07:7

77080 Dual-energy X-ray absorptiometry (DXA), bone density study, 1 or more sites; axial skeleton (eg, hips, pelvis, spine)

➔ *CPT Changes: An Insider's View* 2007

➔ *CPT Assistant* Mar 07:7

➔ *Clinical Examples in Radiology* Fall 07:11, Summer 10:6, Summer 15:12

(Do not report 77080 in conjunction with 77085, 77086)

77081 appendicular skeleton (peripheral) (eg, radius, wrist, heel)

➔ *CPT Changes: An Insider's View* 2007

➔ *CPT Assistant* Mar 07:7

(For dual energy x-ray absorptiometry [DXA] body composition study, use 76499)

 # 77085 axial skeleton (eg, hips, pelvis, spine), including vertebral fracture assessment

➔ *CPT Changes: An Insider's View* 2015

➔ *Clinical Examples in Radiology* Summer 15:12

(Do not report 77085 in conjunction with 77080, 77086)

 # 77086 Vertebral fracture assessment via dual-energy X-ray absorptiometry (DXA)

➔ *CPT Changes: An Insider's View* 2015

➔ *Clinical Examples in Radiology* Summer 15:12

(Do not report 77086 in conjunction with 77080, 77085)

77084 Magnetic resonance (eg, proton) imaging, bone marrow blood supply

➔ *CPT Changes: An Insider's View* 2007

➔ *CPT Assistant* Mar 07:7

77085 Code is out of numerical sequence. See 77080-77261

77086 Code is out of numerical sequence. See 77080-77261

Radiation Oncology

Listings for Radiation Oncology provide for teletherapy and brachytherapy to include initial consultation, clinical treatment planning, simulation, medical radiation physics, dosimetry, treatment devices, special services, and clinical treatment management procedures. They include normal follow-up care during course of treatment and for three months following its completion.

When a service or procedure is provided that is not listed in this edition of the CPT codebook it should be identified by a Special Report (see page 473) and one of the following unlisted procedure codes:

77299 Unlisted procedure, therapeutic radiology clinical treatment planning

77399 Unlisted procedure, medical radiation physics, dosimetry and treatment devices, and special services

77499 Unlisted procedure, therapeutic radiology treatment management

77799 Unlisted procedure, clinical brachytherapy

For treatment by injectable or ingestible isotopes, see subsection Nuclear Medicine.

Consultation: Clinical Management

Preliminary consultation, evaluation of patient prior to decision to treat, or full medical care (in addition to treatment management) when provided by the therapeutic radiologist may be identified by the appropriate procedure codes from **Evaluation and Management, Medicine,** or **Surgery** sections.

Clinical Treatment Planning (External and Internal Sources)

The clinical treatment planning process is a complex service including interpretation of special testing, tumor localization, treatment volume determination, treatment time/dosage determination, choice of treatment modality, determination of number and size of treatment ports, selection of appropriate treatment devices, and other procedures.

Definitions

Simple planning requires a single treatment area of interest encompassed in a single port or simple parallel opposed ports with simple or no blocking.

Intermediate planning requires 3 or more converging ports, 2 separate treatment areas, multiple blocks, or special time dose constraints.

Complex planning requires highly complex blocking, custom shielding blocks, tangential ports, special wedges or compensators, three or more separate treatment areas, rotational or special beam considerations, combination of therapeutic modalities.

77261 Therapeutic radiology treatment planning; simple
- *CPT Assistant* Fall 91:12, 15, Oct 97:2, Oct 10:3, Feb 16:3
- *Clinical Examples in Radiology* Summer 09:2, 4

77262 intermediate
- *CPT Assistant* Fall 91:12, 15, Oct 97:2, Apr 09:3, Nov 09:6, Oct 10:3, Feb 16:3
- *Clinical Examples in Radiology* Summer 09:2, 4

77263 complex
- *CPT Assistant* Fall 91:15, Oct 97:2, Apr 09:3, Nov 09:6, Oct 10:3, Feb 16:3
- *Clinical Examples in Radiology* Summer 09:2, 4, Summer 15:5

Simulation is the process of defining relevant normal and abnormal target anatomy, and acquiring the images and data necessary to develop the optimal radiation treatment process for the patient. A simulation is defined as complex if any of these criteria are met: particle, rotation or arc therapy, complex or custom blocking, brachytherapy simulation, hyperthermia probe verification, or any use of contrast material. If a simulation does not meet any of these criteria, the complexity is defined by the number of treatment areas: one treatment area is simple, two treatment areas are intermediate, and three or more treatment areas are complex.

A treatment area is a contiguous anatomic location that will be treated with radiation therapy. Generally, this includes the primary tumor organ or the resection bed and the draining lymph node chains, if indicated. An example is a breast cancer patient for whom a single treatment area could be the breast alone or the breast, adjacent supraclavicular fossa, and internal mammary nodes. In some cases, a patient might receive radiation therapy to more than one discontinuous anatomic location. An example would be a patient with multiple bone metastases in separate sites (eg, femur and cervical spine); in this case, each distinct and separate anatomic site to be irradiated is a separate treatment area.

Definitions

Simple: simulation of a single treatment area.

Intermediate: two separate treatment areas.

Complex: three or more treatment areas, or any number of treatment areas if any of the following are involved: particle, rotation or arc therapy, complex blocking, custom shielding blocks, brachytherapy simulation, hyperthermia probe verification, any use of contrast materials.

77280 Therapeutic radiology simulation-aided field setting; simple
- *CPT Assistant* Fall 91:15, Oct 97:2, Nov 97:26, Apr 09:10, Nov 09:6, Oct 10:3, Nov 13:11, Apr 15:11
- *Clinical Examples in Radiology* Summer 08:12, Summer 09:2, 4, 5

77285 intermediate
- *CPT Assistant* Fall 91:15, Oct 97:3, Nov 09:6, Oct 10:3, Apr 15:11
- *Clinical Examples in Radiology* Summer 08:12, Summer 09:4

77290 complex
- *CPT Assistant* Fall 91:12, 15, Oct 97:3, Apr 09:3, 10, Nov 09:6, Oct 10:3, Nov 13:11, Apr 15:11, Sep 16:10
- *Clinical Examples in Radiology* Summer 08:12, Summer 09:4

+ 77293 Respiratory motion management simulation (List separately in addition to code for primary procedure)
- *CPT Changes: An Insider's View* 2014
- *CPT Assistant* Nov 13:11, Dec 15:16

(Use 77293 in conjunction with 77295, 77301)

77295 Code is out of numerical sequence. See 77293-77301

77299 Unlisted procedure, therapeutic radiology clinical treatment planning
- *CPT Assistant* Oct 10:3

Medical Radiation Physics, Dosimetry, Treatment Devices, and Special Services

 # 77295 3-dimensional radiotherapy plan, including dose-volume histograms
- *CPT Changes: An Insider's View* 2014
- *CPT Assistant* Fall 91:15, Oct 97:3, Nov 97:26, May 05:7, Oct 07:1, Nov 09:3, Oct 10:3, Nov 13:11, Jun 15:6, Dec 15:16
- *Clinical Examples in Radiology* Summer 08:12, Summer 09:2, 5

77300 Basic radiation dosimetry calculation, central axis depth dose calculation, TDF, NSD, gap calculation, off axis factor, tissue inhomogeneity factors, calculation of non-ionizing radiation surface and depth dose, as required during course of treatment, only when prescribed by the treating physician
- *CPT Changes: An Insider's View* 2002
- *CPT Assistant* Fall 91:14, Oct 97:3, Dec 08:9, Nov 09:3, Oct 10:3
- *Clinical Examples in Radiology* Summer 08:12, Summer 09:2, 5, 6, Summer 15:5

(Do not report 77300 in conjunction with 77306, 77307, 77316, 77317, 77318, 77321, 77767, 77768, 77770, 77771, 77772, 0394T, 0395T)

77301 Intensity modulated radiotherapy plan, including dose-volume histograms for target and critical structure partial tolerance specifications
- *CPT Changes: An Insider's View* 2002
- *CPT Assistant* Mar 05:1, 6, May 05:7, Oct 07:1, Nov 09:3, Oct 10:3, Nov 13:11

Radiology 70010-79999

(Dose plan is optimized using inverse or forward planning technique for modulated beam delivery [eg, binary, dynamic MLC] to create highly conformal dose distribution. Computer plan distribution must be verified for positional accuracy based on dosimetric verification of the intensity map with verification of treatment set-up and interpretation of verification methodology)

77306 Teletherapy isodose plan; simple (1 or 2 unmodified ports directed to a single area of interest), includes basic dosimetry calculation(s)
- *CPT Changes: An Insider's View* 2015
- *CPT Assistant* Feb 16:3

77307 complex (multiple treatment areas, tangential ports, the use of wedges, blocking, rotational beam, or special beam considerations), includes basic dosimetry calculation(s)
- *CPT Changes: An Insider's View* 2015
- *CPT Assistant* Feb 16:3

(Only 1 teletherapy isodose plan may be reported for a given course of therapy to a specific treatment area)

(Do not report 77306, 77307 in conjunction with 77300)

77316 Brachytherapy isodose plan; simple (calculation[s] made from 1 to 4 sources, or remote afterloading brachytherapy, 1 channel), includes basic dosimetry calculation(s)
- *CPT Changes: An Insider's View* 2015
- *CPT Assistant* Feb 16:3

(For definition of source, see clinical brachytherapy introductory guidelines)

77317 intermediate (calculation[s] made from 5 to 10 sources, or remote afterloading brachytherapy, 2-12 channels), includes basic dosimetry calculation(s)
- *CPT Changes: An Insider's View* 2015
- *CPT Assistant* Feb 16:3

77318 complex (calculation[s] made from over 10 sources, or remote afterloading brachytherapy, over 12 channels), includes basic dosimetry calculation(s)
- *CPT Changes: An Insider's View* 2015
- *CPT Assistant* Feb 16:3

(Do not report 77316, 77317, 77318 in conjunction with 77300)

77321 Special teletherapy port plan, particles, hemibody, total body
- *CPT Assistant* Fall 91:14, Oct 97:4, Oct 10:3
- *Clinical Examples in Radiology* Summer 09:5, 6

77331 Special dosimetry (eg, TLD, microdosimetry) (specify), only when prescribed by the treating physician
- *CPT Assistant* Fall 91:13, Oct 97:4, Jun 15:6
- *Clinical Examples in Radiology* Summer 09:5, 6

77332 Treatment devices, design and construction; simple (simple block, simple bolus)
- *CPT Assistant* Oct 97:4, Oct 10:3, Feb 16:3
- *Clinical Examples in Radiology* Summer 07:10, Summer 08:12, Summer 09:6

77333 intermediate (multiple blocks, stents, bite blocks, special bolus)
- *CPT Assistant* Oct 97:3, Oct 10:3, Feb 16:3
- *Clinical Examples in Radiology* Summer 07:10, Summer 08:12, Summer 09:6

77334 complex (irregular blocks, special shields, compensators, wedges, molds or casts)
- *CPT Assistant* Fall 91:14, Oct 97:4, Dec 08:9, Nov 09:3, Oct 10:3, Dec 10:15, Dec 15:16, Feb 16:3, Sep 16:10
- *Clinical Examples in Radiology* Summer 07:9, 10, Summer 08:12, Summer 09:2, 6

77336 Continuing medical physics consultation, including assessment of treatment parameters, quality assurance of dose delivery, and review of patient treatment documentation in support of the radiation oncologist, reported per week of therapy
- *CPT Assistant* Fall 91:15, Oct 97:4, Nov 98:21, Oct 10:3, Feb 16:3
- *Clinical Examples in Radiology* Summer 08:12, Summer 09:2, 6

77338 Multi-leaf collimator (MLC) device(s) for intensity modulated radiation therapy (IMRT), design and construction per IMRT plan
- *CPT Changes: An Insider's View* 2010
- *CPT Assistant* Oct 10:3, Dec 10:15

(Do not report 77338 in conjunction with 77385 for compensator based IMRT)

(Do not report 77338 more than once per IMRT plan)

(For immobilization in IMRT treatment, see 77332-77334)

77370 Special medical radiation physics consultation
- *CPT Assistant* Fall 91:14, Oct 97:4, May 09:8, Oct 10:3, Jun 15:6, Feb 16:3
- *Clinical Examples in Radiology* Summer 08:12, Summer 09:6, 9

Stereotactic Radiation Treatment Delivery

77371 Radiation treatment delivery, stereotactic radiosurgery (SRS), complete course of treatment of cranial lesion(s) consisting of 1 session; multi-source Cobalt 60 based
- *CPT Changes: An Insider's View* 2007, 2008, 2010, 2017
- *CPT Assistant* Mar 07:7, Oct 07:1, Oct 10:3, Jul 11:12, Jul 14:9
- *Clinical Examples in Radiology* Summer 09:7

77372 linear accelerator based
- *CPT Changes: An Insider's View* 2007, 2008
- *CPT Assistant* Mar 07:7, Oct 07:1, Oct 10:3, Jul 11:12
- *Clinical Examples in Radiology* Summer 09:7

(For radiation treatment management, use 77432)

77373 Stereotactic body radiation therapy, treatment delivery, per fraction to 1 or more lesions, including image guidance, entire course not to exceed 5 fractions
- *CPT Changes: An Insider's View* 2007
- *CPT Assistant* Mar 07:7, Oct 07:1, Oct 10:3, Jul 11:12, Jul 14:9, Jun 15:6
- *Clinical Examples in Radiology* Summer 09:7

(Do not report 77373 in conjunction with 77385, 77386, 77401, 77402, 77407, 77412)

(For single fraction cranial lesion[s], see 77371, 77372)

77385 Code is out of numerical sequence. See 77412-77427

77386 Code is out of numerical sequence. See 77412-77427

77387 Code is out of numerical sequence. See 77412-77427

Other Procedures

77399 Unlisted procedure, medical radiation physics, dosimetry and treatment devices, and special services

➲ *CPT Assistant* Nov 98:21, Oct 10:3

Radiation Treatment Delivery

Following dosimetry calculations, there are a number of alternative methods to deliver external radiation treatments, which are described with specific CPT codes:

- X-ray (photon), including conventional and intensity modulated radiation therapy (IMRT) beams;
- Electron beams;
- Neutron beams;
- Proton beams.

All treatment delivery codes are reported once per treatment session. The treatment delivery codes recognize technical-only services and contain no physician work (the professional component). In contrast, the treatment management codes contain only the professional component.

Radiation treatment delivery with conventional X-ray or electron beams is assigned levels of complexity based on the number of treatment sites and complexity of the treatment fields, blocking, wedges, and physical or virtual tissue compensators. A simple block is straight-edged or an approximation of a straight edge created by a multileaf collimator (MLC). Energy of the megavoltage (≥ 1 MeV) beam does not contribute to complexity. Techniques such as treating a field-in-field to ensure dose homogeneity reflect added complexity.

Energies below the megavoltage range may be used in the treatment of skin lesions. Superficial radiation energies (up to 200 kV) may be generated by a variety of technologies and should not be reported with megavoltage (77402, 77407, 77412) for surface application. Do not report clinical treatment planning (77261, 77262, 77263), treatment devices (77332, 77333, 77334), isodose planning (77306, 77307, 77316, 77317, 77318), physics consultation (77336), or radiation treatment management (77427, 77431, 77432, 77435, 77469, 77470, 77499) with 77401, 0394T, or 0395T. When reporting 77401 alone, evaluation and management, when performed, may be reported with the appropriate E/M codes.

Intensity modulated radiation therapy (IMRT) uses computer-based optimization techniques with non-uniform radiation beam intensities to create highly conformal dose distributions that can be delivered by a radiotherapy treatment machine. A number of technologies, including spatially and temporally modulated beams, cylindrical beamlets, dynamic MLC, single or multiple fields or arcs, or compensators, may be used to generate IMRT. The complexity of IMRT may vary depending on the area being treated or the technique being used.

Image guided radiation therapy (IGRT) may be used to direct the radiation beam and to reflect motion during treatment. A variety of techniques may be used to perform this guidance including imaging (eg, ultrasound, CT, MRI, stereoscopic imaging) and non-imaging (eg, electromagnetic or infrared) techniques. Guidance may be used with any radiation treatment delivery technique and is typically used with IMRT delivery. IMRT delivery codes include the technical component of guidance or tracking, if performed. Because only the technical portion of IGRT is bundled into IMRT, the physician involvement in guidance or tracking may be reported separately. When guidance is required with conventional radiation treatment delivery, both the professional and technical components are reported because neither component of guidance is bundled into conventional radiation treatment delivery services.

The technical and professional components of guidance are handled differently with each radiation delivery code depending on the type of radiation being administered. The **Radiation Management and Treatment Table** is provided for clarity.

Definitions

Radiation Treatment Delivery, megavoltage (≥ 1 MeV), any energy

Simple: All of the following criteria are met (and none of the complex or intermediate criteria are met): single treatment area, one or two ports, and two or fewer simple blocks.

Intermediate: Any of the following criteria are met (and none of the complex criteria are met): 2 separate treatment areas, 3 or more ports on a single treatment area, or 3 or more simple blocks.

Complex: Any of the following criteria are met: 3 or more separate treatment areas, custom blocking, tangential ports, wedges, rotational beam, field-in-field or other tissue compensation that does not meet IMRT guidelines, or electron beam.

Intensity Modulated Radiation Therapy (IMRT), any energy, includes the technical services for guidance

Simple: Any of the following: prostate, breast, and all sites using physical compensator based IMRT.

Complex: Includes all other sites if not using physical compensator based IMRT.

77401 Radiation treatment delivery, superficial and/or ortho voltage, per day

CPT Changes: An Insider's View 2015

CPT Assistant Apr 03:14, Aug 03:10, Oct 07:1, Oct 10:3, Dec 15:14, Feb 16:3

Clinical Examples in Radiology Summer 08:12, Summer 09:7

(Do not report 77401 in conjunction with 77373)

77402 Radiation treatment delivery, >1 MeV; simple

CPT Changes: An Insider's View 2015

CPT Assistant Apr 03:14, Aug 03:10, Oct 07:1, Oct 10:3, Dec 15:14, Feb 16:3, Mar 16:7

Clinical Examples in Radiology Spring 07:7-9, 12, Summer 08:12, Summer 09:7

(Do not report 77402 in conjunction with 77373)

77407 intermediate

CPT Changes: An Insider's View 2015

CPT Assistant Apr 03:14, Aug 03:10, Oct 07:1, Dec 15:14, Feb 16:3, Mar 16:7

Clinical Examples in Radiology Spring 07:7-9, 12, Summer 08:12, Summer 09:7

(Do not report 77407 in conjunction with 77373)

77412 complex

CPT Changes: An Insider's View 2006, 2015

CPT Assistant Apr 03:14, Aug 03:10, Oct 07:1, Dec 15:14, Feb 16:3, Mar 16:7

Clinical Examples in Radiology Winter 06:20, Spring 07:7-9, 12, Summer 08:12, Summer 09:7

(Do not report 77412 in conjunction with 77373)

77417 Therapeutic radiology port image(s)

CPT Changes: An Insider's View 2016

CPT Assistant Fall 91:14, Dec 97:11, Feb 06:14, Oct 07:1, Dec 15:14, Dec 17:15

Clinical Examples in Radiology Summer 09:2, 7

(For intensity modulated treatment planning, use 77301)

 # 77385 Intensity modulated radiation treatment delivery (IMRT), includes guidance and tracking, when performed; simple

CPT Changes: An Insider's View 2015

CPT Assistant Feb 16:3

(To report professional component [PC] of guidance and tracking, use 77387 with modifier 26)

 # 77386 complex

CPT Changes: An Insider's View 2015

CPT Assistant Feb 16:3

(To report professional component [PC] of guidance and tracking, use 77387 with modifier 26)

(Do not report 77385, 77386 in conjunction with 77371, 77372, 77373)

#▲ 77387 Guidance for localization of target volume for delivery of radiation treatment, includes intrafraction tracking, when performed

CPT Changes: An Insider's View 2015, 2019

CPT Assistant Dec 15:14, 17, Feb 16:3

(Do not report technical component [TC] with 77385, 77386, 77371, 77372, 77373)

(For placement of interstitial device[s] for radiation therapy guidance, see 31627, 32553, 49411, 55876)

 # 77424 Intraoperative radiation treatment delivery, x-ray, single treatment session

CPT Changes: An Insider's View 2012

CPT Assistant Dec 15:14

Clinical Examples in Radiology Fall 11:11

 # 77425 Intraoperative radiation treatment delivery, electrons, single treatment session

CPT Changes: An Insider's View 2012

CPT Assistant Dec 15:14

Clinical Examples in Radiology Fall 11:11

Neutron Beam Treatment Delivery

(77422 has been deleted)

77423 High energy neutron radiation treatment delivery, 1 or more isocenter(s) with coplanar or non-coplanar geometry with blocking and/or wedge, and/or compensator(s)

CPT Changes: An Insider's View 2006, 2018

CPT Assistant Dec 15:14

Clinical Examples in Radiology Winter 06:18

77424 Code is out of numerical sequence. See 77412-77427

77425 Code is out of numerical sequence. See 77412-77427

Radiation Treatment Management

Radiation treatment management is reported in units of five fractions or treatment sessions, regardless of the actual time period in which the services are furnished. The services need not be furnished on consecutive days. Multiple fractions representing two or more treatment sessions furnished on the same day may be counted separately as long as there has been a distinct break in therapy sessions, and the fractions are of the character usually furnished on different days. Code 77427 is also reported if there are three or four fractions beyond a multiple of five at the end of a course of treatment; one or two fractions beyond a multiple of five at the end of a course of treatment are not reported separately.

Radiation treatment management requires **and includes** a minimum of one examination of the patient by the physician for medical evaluation and management (eg, assessment of the patient's response to treatment, coordination of care and treatment, review of imaging and/or lab test results with documentation) for each reporting of the radiation treatment management service. Code 77469 represents only the intraoperative session management and does not include medical evaluation and management outside of that session. The professional services furnished during treatment management typically include:

Radiation Management and Treatment Table

Category	Code	Descriptor	IGRT TC (77387-TC) Bundled into Code?	IGRT PC (77387-PC) Bundled into Code?	Code Type (Technical / Professional)
SRS: Stereotactic radiosurgery IMRT: Intensity modulated radiation therapy TC: Technical component			SBRT: Stereotactic body radiation therapy IGRT: Image guided radiation therapy PC: Professional component (modifier 26)		
Radiation Treatment Management	77427	Treatment Management, 1-5 Treatments	N	N	Professional
	77431	Treatment Management, 1-2 Fractions	N	N	Professional
	77432	SRS Management, Cranial Lesion(s)	N	Y	Professional
	77435	SBRT Management	N	Y	Professional
SRS Treatment Delivery	77371	SRS Multisource 60 Based	Y	N	Technical
	77372	SRS Linear Based	Y	N	Technical
SBRT Treatment Delivery	77373	SBRT, 1 or More Lesions, 1-5 Fractions	Y	N	Technical
Radiation Treatment Delivery	77401	Superficial and/or Ortho Voltage	N	N	Technical
	77402	Radiation Treatment Delivery, Simple	N	N	Technical
	77407	Radiation Treatment Delivery, Intermediate	N	N	Technical
	77412	Radiation Treatment Delivery, Complex	N	N	Technical
IMRT Treatment Delivery	77385	IMRT Treatment Delivery, Simple	Y	N	Technical
	77386	IMRT Treatment Delivery, Complex	Y	N	Technical
Neutron Beam Treatment Delivery	77423	Neutron Beam Treatment, Complex	N	N	Technical
Proton Treatment Delivery	77520	Proton Treatment, Simple	N	N	Technical
	77522	Proton Treatment, Simple	N	N	Technical
	77523	Proton Treatment, Intermediate	N	N	Technical
	77525	Proton Treatment, Complex	N	N	Technical

- Review of port images;
- Review of dosimetry, dose delivery, and treatment parameters;
- Review of patient treatment set-up.

Stereotactic radiosurgery (SRS-[77432]) and stereotactic body radiation treatment (SBRT-[77435]) management also include the professional component of guidance for localization of target volume for the delivery of radiation therapy (77387). ***See also the Radiation Management and Treatment Table.***

77427 Radiation treatment management, 5 treatments

CPT Changes: An Insider's View 2000

CPT Assistant Nov 99:42, Feb 00:7, Oct 07:1, Nov 09:6, Jun 15:6, Feb 16:3

Clinical Examples in Radiology Summer 08:12, Summer 09:2, 7, 8

77431 Radiation therapy management with complete course of therapy consisting of 1 or 2 fractions only

CPT Assistant Winter 90:10, Oct 97:4, Nov 09:6, Feb 16:3

Clinical Examples in Radiology Summer 08:12, Summer 09:7, 8

(77431 is not to be used to fill in the last week of a long course of therapy)

77432 Stereotactic radiation treatment management of cranial lesion(s) (complete course of treatment consisting of 1 session)

- *CPT Changes: An Insider's View* 2008
- *CPT Assistant* Oct 97:4, Nov 09:6, Jul 11:12, Jul 14:9, Dec 15:14, 17, Feb 16:3
- *Clinical Examples in Radiology* Summer 09:7, 8

(The same physician should not report both stereotactic radiosurgery services [61796-61800] and radiation treatment management [77432 or 77435] for cranial lesions)

(For stereotactic body radiation therapy treatment, use 77435)

(To report the technical component of guidance for localization of target volume, use 77387 with a technical component modifier [TC])

77435 Stereotactic body radiation therapy, treatment management, per treatment course, to 1 or more lesions, including image guidance, entire course not to exceed 5 fractions

- *CPT Changes: An Insider's View* 2007
- *CPT Assistant* Mar 07:7, Oct 07:1, Nov 09:6, Jun 15:6, Dec 15:14, Feb 16:3
- *Clinical Examples in Radiology* Summer 09:7, 8

(Do not report 77435 in conjunction with 77427-77432)

(The same physician should not report both stereotactic radiosurgery services [32701, 63620, 63621] and radiation treatment management [77435])

(To report the technical component of guidance for localization of target volume, use 77387 with a technical component modifier [TC])

77469 Intraoperative radiation treatment management

- *CPT Changes: An Insider's View* 2012
- *CPT Assistant* Feb 16:3
- *Clinical Examples in Radiology* Summer 09:7, Fall 11:11

77470 Special treatment procedure (eg, total body irradiation, hemibody radiation, per oral or endocavitary irradiation)

- *CPT Changes: An Insider's View* 2001, 2012
- *CPT Assistant* Winter 91:22, Oct 97:1, Apr 09:3, Feb 16:3
- *Clinical Examples in Radiology* Summer 08:12, Summer 09:7, 8, Spring 12:11

(77470 assumes that the procedure is performed 1 or more times during the course of therapy, in addition to daily or weekly patient management)

(For intraoperative radiation treatment delivery and management, see 77424, 77425, 77469)

77499 Unlisted procedure, therapeutic radiology treatment management

- *CPT Changes: An Insider's View* 2000
- *CPT Assistant* Nov 99:42, Feb 00:7, Nov 09:6, Jun 15:6, Feb 16:3
- *Clinical Examples in Radiology* Summer 09:7, 8

Proton Beam Treatment Delivery

Definitions

Simple proton treatment delivery to a single treatment area utilizing a single non-tangential/oblique port, custom block with compensation (77522) and without compensation (77520).

Intermediate proton treatment delivery to one or more treatment areas utilizing two or more ports or one or more tangential/oblique ports, with custom blocks and compensators.

Complex proton treatment delivery to one or more treatment areas utilizing two or more ports per treatment area with matching or patching fields and/or multiple isocenters, with custom blocks and compensators.

77520 Proton treatment delivery; simple, without compensation

- *CPT Changes: An Insider's View* 2000, 2001
- *CPT Assistant* Nov 99:43

77522 simple, with compensation

- *CPT Changes: An Insider's View* 2001

77523 intermediate

- *CPT Changes: An Insider's View* 2000, 2001
- *CPT Assistant* Nov 99:43

77525 complex

- *CPT Changes: An Insider's View* 2001

Hyperthermia

Hyperthermia treatments as listed in this section include external (superficial and deep), interstitial, and intracavitary.

Radiation therapy when given concurrently is listed separately.

Hyperthermia is used only as an adjunct to radiation therapy or chemotherapy. It may be induced by a variety of sources (eg, microwave, ultrasound, low energy radio-frequency conduction, or by probes).

The listed treatments include management during the course of therapy and follow-up care for three months after completion.

Preliminary consultation is not included (see **Evaluation and Management** 99241-99255).

Physics planning and interstitial insertion of temperature sensors, and use of external or interstitial heat generating sources are included.

The following descriptors are included in the treatment schedule:

77600 Hyperthermia, externally generated; superficial (ie, heating to a depth of 4 cm or less)

- *CPT Changes: An Insider's View* 2017
- *CPT Assistant* Winter 91:22, Dec 13:17

77605 deep (ie, heating to depths greater than 4 cm)
➔ *CPT Changes: An Insider's View* 2017
➔ *CPT Assistant* Winter 91:22, Dec 13:17

77610 Hyperthermia generated by interstitial probe(s); 5 or fewer interstitial applicators
➔ *CPT Changes: An Insider's View* 2017
➔ *CPT Assistant* Winter 91:22
➔ *Clinical Examples in Radiology* Spring 14:11

77615 more than 5 interstitial applicators
➔ *CPT Changes: An Insider's View* 2017
➔ *CPT Assistant* Winter 91:22

Clinical Intracavitary Hyperthermia

77620 Hyperthermia generated by intracavitary probe(s)
➔ *CPT Assistant* Winter 91:22, Dec 13:17

Clinical Brachytherapy

Clinical brachytherapy requires the use of either natural or man-made radioelements applied into or around a treatment field of interest. The supervision of radioelements and dose interpretation are performed solely by the therapeutic radiologist.

Services 77750-77799 include admission to the hospital and daily visits.

For insertion of ovoids and tandems, use 57155.

For insertion of Heyman capsules, use 58346.

Definitions

(Sources refer to intracavitary placement or permanent interstitial placement; ribbons refer to temporary interstitial placement)

A simple application has one to four sources/ribbons.

An intermediate application has five to 10 sources/ribbons.

A complex application has greater than 10 sources/ribbons.

High dose-rate brachytherapy involves treatment with radiation sources that cannot safely be handled manually. These systems are remotely controlled and place a radionuclide source (radioelement or radioisotope) within an applicator placed in or near the target. These applicators may be placed in the body or on the skin surface.

Small electronic X-ray sources placed into an applicator within or close to the target may also be used to generate radiation at high-dose rates. This is referred to as high dose-rate electronic brachytherapy.

To report high dose-rate electronic brachytherapy, see 0394T, 0395T.

77750 Infusion or instillation of radioelement solution (includes 3-month follow-up care)
➔ *CPT Changes: An Insider's View* 2005
➔ *CPT Assistant* Sep 05:1

(For administration of radiolabeled monoclonal antibodies, use 79403)

(For non-antibody radiopharmaceutical therapy by intravenous administration only, not including 3-month follow-up care, use 79101)

77761 Intracavitary radiation source application; simple
➔ *CPT Changes: An Insider's View* 2001
➔ *CPT Assistant* Winter 91:23, Jan 96:7, Mar 99:3, Feb 02:7, Sep 05:1

77762 intermediate
➔ *CPT Assistant* Winter 91:23, Feb 02:7, Sep 05:1

77763 complex
➔ *CPT Assistant* Winter 91:23, Mar 99:3, Feb 02:7, Sep 05:1

(Do not report 77761-77763 in conjunction with Category III code 0394T, 0395T)

77767 Remote afterloading high dose rate radionuclide skin surface brachytherapy, includes basic dosimetry, when performed; lesion diameter up to 2.0 cm or 1 channel
➔ *CPT Changes: An Insider's View* 2016

77768 lesion diameter over 2.0 cm and 2 or more channels, or multiple lesions
➔ *CPT Changes: An Insider's View* 2016

77770 Remote afterloading high dose rate radionuclide interstitial or intracavitary brachytherapy, includes basic dosimetry, when performed; 1 channel
➔ *CPT Changes: An Insider's View* 2016

77771 2-12 channels
➔ *CPT Changes: An Insider's View* 2016

77772 over 12 channels
➔ *CPT Changes: An Insider's View* 2016

(Do not report 77767, 77768, 77770, 77771, 77772 in conjunction with 77300, 0394T, 0395T)

(For non-brachytherapy superficial [eg, ≤200 kV] radiation treatment delivery, use 77401)

(77776, 77777 have been deleted. To report, use 77799)

77778 Interstitial radiation source application, complex, includes supervision, handling, loading of radiation source, when performed
➔ *CPT Changes: An Insider's View* 2016
➔ *CPT Assistant* Winter 91:23, Apr 04:6, Sep 05:1, May 07:1
➔ *Clinical Examples in Radiology* Summer 15:5

(Do not report 77778 in conjunction with Category III codes 0394T, 0395T)

(Do not report 77778 in conjunction with 77790)

(77782-77784 have been deleted. To report, see 77767, 77768, 77770, 77771, 77772)

77789 Surface application of low dose rate radionuclide source
➔ *CPT Changes: An Insider's View* 2001, 2016
➔ *CPT Assistant* Sep 05:1

(Do not report 77789 in conjunction with 77401, 77767, 77768, 0394T, 0395T)

77790 Supervision, handling, loading of radiation source
➔ *CPT Changes: An Insider's View* 2001
➔ *CPT Assistant* Sep 05:1
➔ *Clinical Examples in Radiology* Summer 15:5

(Do not report 77790 in conjunction with 77778)

77799 Unlisted procedure, clinical brachytherapy
➔ *CPT Assistant* Sep 05:1

Nuclear Medicine

Listed procedures may be performed independently or in the course of overall medical care. If the individual providing these services is also responsible for diagnostic workup and/or follow-up care of patient, see appropriate sections also.

Radioimmunoassay tests are found in the **Clinical Pathology** section (codes 82009-84999). These codes can be appropriately used by any specialist performing such tests in a laboratory licensed and/or certified for radioimmunoassays. The reporting of these tests is not confined to clinical pathology laboratories alone.

The services listed do not include the radiopharmaceutical or drug. To separately report supply of diagnostic and therapeutic radiopharmaceuticals and drugs, use the appropriate supply code(s), in addition to the procedure code.

Diagnostic

Endocrine System

78012 Thyroid uptake, single or multiple quantitative measurement(s) (including stimulation, suppression, or discharge, when performed)
➔ *CPT Changes: An Insider's View* 2013
➔ *CPT Assistant* Jun 13:9
➔ *Clinical Examples in Radiology* Winter 13:9

78013 Thyroid imaging (including vascular flow, when performed);
➔ *CPT Changes: An Insider's View* 2013
➔ *CPT Assistant* Jun 13:9
➔ *Clinical Examples in Radiology* Winter 13:9

78014 with single or multiple uptake(s) quantitative measurement(s) (including stimulation, suppression, or discharge, when performed)
➔ *CPT Changes: An Insider's View* 2013
➔ *CPT Assistant* Jun 13:9
➔ *Clinical Examples in Radiology* Winter 13:9

78015 Thyroid carcinoma metastases imaging; limited area (eg, neck and chest only)
➔ *CPT Assistant* Nov 98:21, Jan 07:31

78016 with additional studies (eg, urinary recovery)
➔ *CPT Assistant* Jan 07:31

78018 whole body
➔ *CPT Assistant* Apr 99:4, Jan 07:31
➔ *Clinical Examples in Radiology* Fall 09:3-5

+ 78020 Thyroid carcinoma metastases uptake (List separately in addition to code for primary procedure)
➔ *CPT Assistant* Nov 98:21, Apr 99:4, Jan 07:31
➔ *Clinical Examples in Radiology* Fall 09:3-5

(Use 78020 in conjunction with 78018 only)

78070 Parathyroid planar imaging (including subtraction, when performed);
➔ *CPT Changes: An Insider's View* 2013
➔ *CPT Assistant* Jan 07:31, Dec 16:10
➔ *Clinical Examples in Radiology* Summer 11:4, 5

78071 with tomographic (SPECT)
➔ *CPT Changes: An Insider's View* 2013
➔ *CPT Assistant* Dec 16:10

78072 with tomographic (SPECT), and concurrently acquired computed tomography (CT) for anatomical localization
➔ *CPT Changes: An Insider's View* 2013
➔ *CPT Assistant* Dec 16:10

78075 Adrenal imaging, cortex and/or medulla
➔ *CPT Assistant* Jan 07:31, Feb 12:9
➔ *Clinical Examples in Radiology* Summer 12:9

78099 Unlisted endocrine procedure, diagnostic nuclear medicine
➔ *CPT Assistant* Dec 05:7, Jan 07:31, Dec 16:10

(For chemical analysis, see **Chemistry** section)

Hematopoietic, Reticuloendothelial and Lymphatic System

78102 Bone marrow imaging; limited area
➔ *CPT Assistant* Dec 05:7, Feb 12:9

78103 multiple areas

78104 whole body

78110 Plasma volume, radiopharmaceutical volume-dilution technique (separate procedure); single sampling

78111 multiple samplings

78120 Red cell volume determination (separate procedure); single sampling

78121 multiple samplings

78122 Whole blood volume determination, including separate measurement of plasma volume and red cell volume (radiopharmaceutical volume-dilution technique)

78130 Red cell survival study;

78135 differential organ/tissue kinetics (eg, splenic and/or hepatic sequestration)

78140 Labeled red cell sequestration, differential organ/tissue (eg, splenic and/or hepatic)

78185 Spleen imaging only, with or without vascular flow

(If combined with liver study, use procedures 78215 and 78216)

(78190 has been deleted)

78191 Platelet survival study

78195 Lymphatics and lymph nodes imaging

➔ *CPT Changes: An Insider's View* 2000, 2002

➔ *CPT Assistant* Nov 98:22, Jul 99:6, Nov 99:43, Dec 99:8, Sep 08:5, Feb 12:9

(For sentinel node identification without scintigraphy imaging, use 38792)

(For sentinel node excision, see 38500-38542)

78199 Unlisted hematopoietic, reticuloendothelial and lymphatic procedure, diagnostic nuclear medicine

➔ *CPT Assistant* Dec 05:7

(For chemical analysis, see **Chemistry** section)

Gastrointestinal System

78201 Liver imaging; static only

➔ *CPT Assistant* Dec 05:7, Feb 12:9

78202 with vascular flow

➔ *CPT Assistant* Feb 12:9

(For spleen imaging only, use 78185)

78205 Liver imaging (SPECT);

➔ *CPT Assistant* Nov 98:22

➔ *Clinical Examples in Radiology* Summer 15:6

78206 with vascular flow

➔ *CPT Assistant* Nov 98:22

78215 Liver and spleen imaging; static only

78216 with vascular flow

78226 Hepatobiliary system imaging, including gallbladder when present;

➔ *CPT Changes: An Insider's View* 2012

➔ *Clinical Examples in Radiology* Winter 12:6

78227 with pharmacologic intervention, including quantitative measurement(s) when performed

➔ *CPT Changes: An Insider's View* 2012

➔ *Clinical Examples in Radiology* Winter 12:5

78230 Salivary gland imaging;

78231 with serial images

78232 Salivary gland function study

78258 Esophageal motility

78261 Gastric mucosa imaging

78262 Gastroesophageal reflux study

➔ *CPT Assistant* Dec 15:10

78264 Gastric emptying imaging study (eg, solid, liquid, or both)

➔ *CPT Changes: An Insider's View* 2016

➔ *CPT Assistant* Dec 15:10

78265 with small bowel transit

➔ *CPT Changes: An Insider's View* 2016

➔ *CPT Assistant* Dec 15:10

➔ *Clinical Examples in Radiology* Winter 17:12

78266 with small bowel and colon transit, multiple days

➔ *CPT Changes: An Insider's View* 2016

➔ *CPT Assistant* Dec 15:10

➔ *Clinical Examples in Radiology* Winter 17:6

(Report 78264, 78265, 78266 only once per imaging study)

78267 Urea breath test, C-14 (isotopic); acquisition for analysis

➔ *CPT Changes: An Insider's View* 2000, 2005

➔ *CPT Assistant* Nov 99:43

➔ *Clinical Examples in Radiology* Fall 07:9

78268 analysis

➔ *CPT Changes: An Insider's View* 2000

➔ *CPT Assistant* Nov 99:43

➔ *Clinical Examples in Radiology* Fall 07:9

(For breath hydrogen or methane testing and analysis, use 91065)

►(78270, 78271, 78272 have been deleted)◄

78278 Acute gastrointestinal blood loss imaging

78282 Gastrointestinal protein loss

78290 Intestine imaging (eg, ectopic gastric mucosa, Meckel's localization, volvulus)

➔ *CPT Changes: An Insider's View* 2002

78291 Peritoneal-venous shunt patency test (eg, for LeVeen, Denver shunt)

➔ *CPT Assistant* Feb 12:9

(For injection procedure, use 49427)

78299 Unlisted gastrointestinal procedure, diagnostic nuclear medicine

➔ *CPT Assistant* Dec 05:7

Musculoskeletal System

Bone and joint imaging can be used in the diagnosis of a variety of inflammatory processes (eg, osteomyelitis), as well as for localization of primary and/or metastatic neoplasms.

78300 Bone and/or joint imaging; limited area

➔ *CPT Assistant* Mar 97:11, Dec 05:7, Feb 12:9

➔ *Clinical Examples in Radiology* Winter 09:5, Spring 10:9

78305 multiple areas

➔ *CPT Assistant* Mar 97:11

➔ *Clinical Examples in Radiology* Winter 09:5, Spring 10:9

78306 whole body
➔ *CPT Assistant* Mar 97:11, Jan 02:10, Jun 03:11, Feb 12:10
➔ *Clinical Examples in Radiology* Summer 06:7, 12, Winter 09:3, 4, 5, Spring 10:9, Spring 13:10

78315 3 phase study
➔ *CPT Assistant* Jan 02:10
➔ *Clinical Examples in Radiology* Summer 06:7, 12, Winter 09:4, 5, Spring 10:9

78320 tomographic (SPECT)
➔ *CPT Assistant* Mar 97:11, Jun 03:11, Jan 08:9
➔ *Clinical Examples in Radiology* Winter 09:4, 5, Spring 10:9, Spring 13:10

78350 Bone density (bone mineral content) study, 1 or more sites; single photon absorptiometry
➔ *CPT Assistant* Nov 97:26

78351 dual photon absorptiometry, 1 or more sites
➔ *CPT Assistant* Nov 97:26, Feb 12:9

78399 Unlisted musculoskeletal procedure, diagnostic nuclear medicine
➔ *CPT Assistant* Dec 05:7

Cardiovascular System

Myocardial perfusion and cardiac blood pool imaging studies may be performed at rest and/or during stress. When performed during exercise and/or pharmacologic stress, the appropriate stress testing code from the 93015-93018 series should be reported in addition to 78451-78454, 78472-78492.

78414 Determination of central c-v hemodynamics (non-imaging) (eg, ejection fraction with probe technique) with or without pharmacologic intervention or exercise, single or multiple determinations
➔ *CPT Assistant* Dec 05:7, May 10:6, Feb 12:9

78428 Cardiac shunt detection
➔ *CPT Assistant* May 10:6

78445 Non-cardiac vascular flow imaging (ie, angiography, venography)
➔ *CPT Assistant* May 10:6
➔ *Clinical Examples in Radiology* Spring 10:9

78451 Myocardial perfusion imaging, tomographic (SPECT) (including attenuation correction, qualitative or quantitative wall motion, ejection fraction by first pass or gated technique, additional quantification, when performed); single study, at rest or stress (exercise or pharmacologic)
➔ *CPT Changes: An Insider's View* 2010
➔ *CPT Assistant* May 10:5, Feb 11:9, Feb 12:10
➔ *Clinical Examples in Radiology* Spring 10:9, Winter 10:11

78452 multiple studies, at rest and/or stress (exercise or pharmacologic) and/or redistribution and/or rest reinjection
➔ *CPT Changes: An Insider's View* 2010
➔ *CPT Assistant* May 10:5, Feb 11:9, Feb 12:9
➔ *Clinical Examples in Radiology* Spring 10:9, Winter 10:10, 11

78453 Myocardial perfusion imaging, planar (including qualitative or quantitative wall motion, ejection fraction by first pass or gated technique, additional quantification, when performed); single study, at rest or stress (exercise or pharmacologic)
➔ *CPT Changes: An Insider's View* 2010
➔ *CPT Assistant* May 10:5
➔ *Clinical Examples in Radiology* Winter 10:11

78454 multiple studies, at rest and/or stress (exercise or pharmacologic) and/or redistribution and/or rest reinjection
➔ *CPT Changes: An Insider's View* 2010
➔ *CPT Assistant* May 10:5
➔ *Clinical Examples in Radiology* Winter 10:11

78456 Acute venous thrombosis imaging, peptide
➔ *CPT Changes: An Insider's View* 2000
➔ *CPT Assistant* Nov 99:43, May 10:6

78457 Venous thrombosis imaging, venogram; unilateral
➔ *CPT Changes: An Insider's View* 2000
➔ *CPT Assistant* Nov 99:43

78458 bilateral
➔ *CPT Changes: An Insider's View* 2000
➔ *CPT Assistant* Nov 99:43, May 10:6

78459 Myocardial imaging, positron emission tomography (PET), metabolic evaluation
➔ *CPT Assistant* Jun 96:5, Nov 97:26, May 10:6
➔ *Clinical Examples in Radiology* Summer 10:11

(For myocardial perfusion study, see 78491-78492)

(78460-78465 have been deleted. To report, see 78451-78454)

78466 Myocardial imaging, infarct avid, planar; qualitative or quantitative
➔ *CPT Assistant* May 10:6

78468 with ejection fraction by first pass technique
➔ *CPT Assistant* May 10:6

78469 tomographic SPECT with or without quantification
➔ *CPT Assistant* May 10:6

(For myocardial sympathetic innervation imaging, see 0331T, 0332T)

78472 Cardiac blood pool imaging, gated equilibrium; planar, single study at rest or stress (exercise and/or pharmacologic), wall motion study plus ejection fraction, with or without additional quantitative processing
➔ *CPT Changes: An Insider's View* 2000
➔ *CPT Assistant* Nov 98:22, Nov 99:44, May 10:6

(For assessment of right ventricular ejection fraction by first pass technique, use 78496)

78473 multiple studies, wall motion study plus ejection fraction, at rest and stress (exercise and/or pharmacologic), with or without additional quantification
➔ *CPT Assistant* May 10:6

(Do not report 78472, 78473 in conjunction with 78451-78454, 78481, 78483, 78494)

(78478, 78480 have been deleted. To report, see 78451-78454)

78481 Cardiac blood pool imaging (planar), first pass technique; single study, at rest or with stress (exercise and/or pharmacologic), wall motion study plus ejection fraction, with or without quantification
➔ *CPT Assistant* May 10:6

78483 multiple studies, at rest and with stress (exercise and/or pharmacologic), wall motion study plus ejection fraction, with or without quantification
➔ *CPT Assistant* May 10:6

(For cerebral blood flow study, use 78610)

(Do not report 78481-78483 in conjunction with 78451-78454)

78491 Myocardial imaging, positron emission tomography (PET), perfusion; single study at rest or stress
➔ *CPT Assistant* Nov 97:27, May 10:6
➔ *Clinical Examples in Radiology* Summer 10:11

78492 multiple studies at rest and/or stress
➔ *CPT Assistant* Nov 97:27, May 10:6
➔ *Clinical Examples in Radiology* Summer 10:11

78494 Cardiac blood pool imaging, gated equilibrium, SPECT, at rest, wall motion study plus ejection fraction, with or without quantitative processing
➔ *CPT Assistant* Nov 98:22, Jun 99:3, May 10:6

+ 78496 Cardiac blood pool imaging, gated equilibrium, single study, at rest, with right ventricular ejection fraction by first pass technique (List separately in addition to code for primary procedure)
➔ *CPT Assistant* Nov 98:22, Jun 99:3, 11, May 10:6, Feb 12:9

(Use 78496 in conjunction with 78472)

78499 Unlisted cardiovascular procedure, diagnostic nuclear medicine
➔ *CPT Assistant* Dec 05:7, May 10:6
➔ *Clinical Examples in Radiology* Summer 08:12

Respiratory System

78579 Pulmonary ventilation imaging (eg, aerosol or gas)
➔ *CPT Changes: An Insider's View* 2012
➔ *CPT Assistant* Feb 12:9
➔ *Clinical Examples in Radiology* Fall 11:5

78580 Pulmonary perfusion imaging (eg, particulate)
➔ *CPT Changes: An Insider's View* 2012
➔ *CPT Assistant* Mar 99:4, Dec 05:7, May 10:6

78582 Pulmonary ventilation (eg, aerosol or gas) and perfusion imaging
➔ *CPT Changes: An Insider's View* 2012
➔ *Clinical Examples in Radiology* Fall 11:4, 5

78597 Quantitative differential pulmonary perfusion, including imaging when performed
➔ *CPT Changes: An Insider's View* 2012
➔ *Clinical Examples in Radiology* Fall 11:5, 6

78598 Quantitative differential pulmonary perfusion and ventilation (eg, aerosol or gas), including imaging when performed
➔ *CPT Changes: An Insider's View* 2012
➔ *CPT Assistant* Feb 12:9
➔ *Clinical Examples in Radiology* Fall 11:5

(Report 78579, 78580, 78582-78598 only once per imaging session)

(Do not report 78580, 78582-78598 in conjunction with 78451-78454)

78599 Unlisted respiratory procedure, diagnostic nuclear medicine
➔ *CPT Assistant* Dec 05:7

Nervous System

78600 Brain imaging, less than 4 static views;
➔ *CPT Changes: An Insider's View* 2008
➔ *CPT Assistant* Dec 05:7, Feb 12:9

78601 with vascular flow
➔ *CPT Changes: An Insider's View* 2008

78605 Brain imaging, minimum 4 static views;
➔ *CPT Changes: An Insider's View* 2008

78606 with vascular flow
➔ *CPT Changes: An Insider's View* 2008

78607 Brain imaging, tomographic (SPECT)
➔ *CPT Changes: An Insider's View* 2008
➔ *Clinical Examples in Radiology* Spring 12:9

78608 Brain imaging, positron emission tomography (PET); metabolic evaluation
➔ *Clinical Examples in Radiology* Spring 10:1, 2

78609 perfusion evaluation

78610 Brain imaging, vascular flow only

78630 Cerebrospinal fluid flow, imaging (not including introduction of material); cisternography
➔ *CPT Assistant* May 17:3

(For injection procedure, see 61000-61070, 62270-62327)

78635 ventriculography

(For injection procedure, see 61000-61070, 62270-62294)

78645 shunt evaluation

(For injection procedure, see 61000-61070, 62270-62294)

78647 tomographic (SPECT)

78650 Cerebrospinal fluid leakage detection and localization
➔ *CPT Changes: An Insider's View* 2002

(For injection procedure, see 61000-61070, 62270-62294)

78660 Radiopharmaceutical dacryocystography
➔ *CPT Assistant* Feb 12:9

78699 Unlisted nervous system procedure, diagnostic nuclear medicine
➔ *CPT Assistant* Dec 05:7

Genitourinary System

78700 Kidney imaging morphology;
CPT Changes: An Insider's View 2007
CPT Assistant Dec 05:7, Mar 07:7, Feb 12:9
Clinical Examples in Radiology Fall 09:2

78701 with vascular flow
Clinical Examples in Radiology Fall 09:2

78707 with vascular flow and function, single study without pharmacological intervention
CPT Changes: An Insider's View 2007
CPT Assistant Nov 97:27, Mar 07:7

78708 with vascular flow and function, single study, with pharmacological intervention (eg, angiotensin converting enzyme inhibitor and/or diuretic)
CPT Changes: An Insider's View 2007
CPT Assistant Nov 97:27, Mar 07:7
Clinical Examples in Radiology Fall 09:2

78709 with vascular flow and function, multiple studies, with and without pharmacological intervention (eg, angiotensin converting enzyme inhibitor and/or diuretic)
CPT Changes: An Insider's View 2007
CPT Assistant Nov 97:27, Mar 07:7
Clinical Examples in Radiology Fall 09:2

(For introduction of radioactive substance in association with renal endoscopy, use 77778)

78710 tomographic (SPECT)
CPT Changes: An Insider's View 2007
CPT Assistant Nov 97:27, Mar 07:7

78725 Kidney function study, non-imaging radioisotopic study
CPT Assistant Nov 98:22
Clinical Examples in Radiology Fall 09:2

+ 78730 Urinary bladder residual study (List separately in addition to code for primary procedure)
CPT Changes: An Insider's View 2007
CPT Assistant Mar 07:7
Clinical Examples in Radiology Spring 12:2

(Use 78730 in conjunction with 78740)

(For measurement of postvoid residual urine and/or bladder capacity by ultrasound, nonimaging, use 51798)

(For ultrasound imaging of the bladder only, with measurement of postvoid residual urine when performed, use 76857)

78740 Ureteral reflux study (radiopharmaceutical voiding cystogram)
Clinical Examples in Radiology Spring 12:1

(Use 78740 in conjunction with 78730 for urinary bladder residual study)

(For catheterization, see 51701, 51702, 51703)

78761 Testicular imaging with vascular flow
CPT Changes: An Insider's View 2007
CPT Assistant Mar 07:7, Feb 12:9

78799 Unlisted genitourinary procedure, diagnostic nuclear medicine
CPT Assistant Dec 05:7

(For chemical analysis, see **Chemistry** section)

Other Procedures

(For specific organ, see appropriate heading)

(For radiophosphorus tumor identification, ocular, see 78800)

78800 Radiopharmaceutical localization of tumor or distribution of radiopharmaceutical agent(s); limited area
CPT Changes: An Insider's View 2004
CPT Assistant Dec 05:7, Dec 11:17, Feb 12:9
Clinical Examples in Radiology Summer 06:6, 10-11, Spring 10:4, 8, Fall 10:11

(For specific organ, see appropriate heading)

78801 multiple areas
CPT Assistant Dec 11:17, Feb 12:9

78802 whole body, single day imaging
CPT Changes: An Insider's View 2004
CPT Assistant Jun 03:11, Feb 12:9
Clinical Examples in Radiology Summer 06:6, 10-11

78803 tomographic (SPECT)
CPT Assistant Jun 03:11, Feb 12:9, Oct 15:9, Dec 16:10
Clinical Examples in Radiology Summer 06:6, 10-11, Summer 12:8, Spring 15:10

78804 whole body, requiring 2 or more days imaging
CPT Changes: An Insider's View 2004
CPT Assistant Feb 12:9
Clinical Examples in Radiology Summer 12:8

78805 Radiopharmaceutical localization of inflammatory process; limited area
CPT Changes: An Insider's View 2001
CPT Assistant Nov 99:44, Feb 12:9

78806 whole body
CPT Changes: An Insider's View 2000
CPT Assistant Nov 99:44, Jun 03:11, Feb 12:9

78807 tomographic (SPECT)
CPT Assistant Jun 03:11, Feb 12:9

(For imaging bone infectious or inflammatory disease with a bone imaging radiopharmaceutical, see 78300, 78305, 78306)

78808 Injection procedure for radiopharmaceutical localization by non-imaging probe study, intravenous (eg, parathyroid adenoma)
CPT Changes: An Insider's View 2009
CPT Assistant Feb 12:9, Dec 16:10

(For sentinel lymph node identification, use 38792)

(For PET of brain, see 78608, 78609)

(For PET myocardial imaging, see 78459, 78491, 78492)

78811 Positron emission tomography (PET) imaging; limited area (eg, chest, head/neck)
- *CPT Changes: An Insider's View* 2005, 2008
- *CPT Assistant* Dec 05:7, Feb 12:9
- *Clinical Examples in Radiology* Spring 05:13, 15, Spring 10:2, 7, Spring 13:10

78812 skull base to mid-thigh
- *CPT Changes: An Insider's View* 2005, 2008
- *CPT Assistant* Dec 05:7, Feb 12:9, Feb 13:16
- *Clinical Examples in Radiology* Spring 05:13, 15, Spring 10:1, 2

78813 whole body
- *CPT Changes: An Insider's View* 2005, 2008
- *CPT Assistant* Dec 05:7, Feb 12:9, Feb 13:16
- *Clinical Examples in Radiology* Spring 05:13, 15, Spring 10:2

78814 Positron emission tomography (PET) with concurrently acquired computed tomography (CT) for attenuation correction and anatomical localization imaging; limited area (eg, chest, head/neck)
- *CPT Changes: An Insider's View* 2005, 2008
- *CPT Assistant* Feb 05:13, Jun 05:10, Dec 05:7, Feb 12:9, Feb 13:16
- *Clinical Examples in Radiology* Spring 05:13, 15, Spring 10:2, 4, Spring 13:10

78815 skull base to mid-thigh
- *CPT Changes: An Insider's View* 2005, 2008
- *CPT Assistant* Feb 05:13, Jun 05:10, Dec 05:7, Feb 12:9, Feb 13:16
- *Clinical Examples in Radiology* Spring 05:13, 15, Spring 10:2, 4, Spring 13:10

78816 whole body
- *CPT Changes: An Insider's View* 2005, 2008
- *CPT Assistant* Feb 05:13, Jun 05:10, Dec 05:7, Feb 12:9, Feb 13:16
- *Clinical Examples in Radiology* Spring 05:13, 15, Spring 10:2, Spring 13:10

(Report 78811-78816 only once per imaging session)

(Computed tomography [CT] performed for other than attenuation correction and anatomical localization is reported using the appropriate site specific CT code with modifier 59)

(78890, 78891 have been deleted)

78999 Unlisted miscellaneous procedure, diagnostic nuclear medicine
- *CPT Assistant* Dec 05:7, Feb 12:9, Oct 15:9, Dec 16:16
- *Clinical Examples in Radiology* Summer 08:12, Spring 10:2, 11, Spring 15:9

Therapeutic

The oral and intravenous administration codes in this section are inclusive of the mode of administration. For intra-arterial, intra-cavitary, and intra-articular administration, also use the appropriate injection and/or procedure codes, as well as imaging guidance and radiological supervision and interpretation codes, when appropriate.

79005 Radiopharmaceutical therapy, by oral administration
- *CPT Changes: An Insider's View* 2005
- *CPT Assistant* Sep 05:1, Feb 12:9
- *Clinical Examples in Radiology* Spring 05:14, Fall 09:5, Winter 12:8

(For monoclonal antibody therapy, use 79403)

79101 Radiopharmaceutical therapy, by intravenous administration
- *CPT Changes: An Insider's View* 2005
- *CPT Assistant* Sep 05:1, Feb 12:9
- *Clinical Examples in Radiology* Spring 10:8, Winter 12:8

(Do not report 79101 in conjunction with 36400, 36410, 79403, 96360, 96374 or 96375, 96409)

(For radiolabeled monoclonal antibody by intravenous infusion, use 79403)

(For infusion or instillation of non-antibody radioelement solution that includes 3 months follow-up care, use 77750)

79200 Radiopharmaceutical therapy, by intracavitary administration
- *CPT Changes: An Insider's View* 2005
- *CPT Assistant* Sep 05:1, Feb 12:9

79300 Radiopharmaceutical therapy, by interstitial radioactive colloid administration
- *CPT Changes: An Insider's View* 2005
- *CPT Assistant* Sep 05:1, Feb 12:9

79403 Radiopharmaceutical therapy, radiolabeled monoclonal antibody by intravenous infusion
- *CPT Changes: An Insider's View* 2004
- *CPT Assistant* Sep 05:1, Feb 12:9

(For pre-treatment imaging, see 78802, 78804)

(Do not report 79403 in conjunction with 79101)

79440 Radiopharmaceutical therapy, by intra-articular administration
- *CPT Changes: An Insider's View* 2005
- *CPT Assistant* Sep 05:1, Feb 12:9

79445 Radiopharmaceutical therapy, by intra-arterial particulate administration
- *CPT Changes: An Insider's View* 2005
- *CPT Assistant* Sep 05:1, Dec 06:10, Feb 12:9, Nov 13:6
- *Clinical Examples in Radiology* Summer 15:3, Winter 18:12

(Do not report 79445 in conjunction with 96373, 96420)

(Use appropriate procedural and radiological supervision and interpretation codes for the angiographic and interventional procedures provided prerequisite to intra-arterial radiopharmaceutical therapy)

79999 Radiopharmaceutical therapy, unlisted procedure
- *CPT Changes: An Insider's View* 2005
- *CPT Assistant* Mar 05:11, Sep 05:1, Jan 07:30, Feb 12:9
- *Clinical Examples in Radiology* Winter 12:8

Notes

Pathology and Laboratory Guidelines

Services in Pathology and Laboratory 536
Separate or Multiple Procedures 536
Unlisted Service or Procedure 536
Special Report 536

Pathology and Laboratory

The following is a listing of headings and subheadings that appear within the Pathology and Laboratory section of the CPT code set. The subheadings or subsections denoted with asterisks (*) below have special instructions unique to that subsection. Where these are indicated, special notes or guidelines will be presented preceding those procedural terminology listings, referring to that subsection specifically.

Organ or Disease-Oriented Panels* (80047-80081) 537
Drug Assay* (80305-80377) 539
Presumptive Drug Class Screening* (80305-80307) 542
Definitive Drug Testing* (80320-80377) 543
Definitive Drug Classes Listing* (80320-80373, 83992) 544
Therapeutic Drug Assays* (80150-80299) 546
Evocative/Suppression Testing* (80400-80439) 548
Consultations (Clinical Pathology)* (80500-80502) 550
Urinalysis* (81000-81099) 550
Molecular Pathology* (81105-81408, 81479) 551
Tier 1 Molecular Pathology Procedures* (81105-81383) 553
Tier 2 Molecular Pathology Procedures* (81400-81408) 563
Genomic Sequencing Procedures and Other Molecular Multianalyte Assays* (81410-81471) 578
Multianalyte Assays with Algorithmic Analyses* (81490-81599) 581
Chemistry* (82009-84999) 583
Hematology and Coagulation (85002-85999) 594
Immunology (86000-86849) 597
Tissue Typing (86805-86849) 602
Transfusion Medicine (86850-86999) 603
Microbiology* (87003-87999) 604
Anatomic Pathology (88000-88099) 612
Postmortem Examination* (88000-88099) 612
Cytopathology (88104-88199) 612
Cytogenetic Studies* (88230-88299) 614
Surgical Pathology* (88300-88399) 615
In Vivo (eg, Transcutaneous) Laboratory Procedures (88720-88749) 620
Other Procedures (89049-89240) 621
Reproductive Medicine Procedures (89250-89398) 621
Proprietary Laboratory Analyses* (0001U-0061U) 623

Molecular Pathology Gene Table

Claim Designation	Abbreviated Gene Name	Full Gene Name	Commonly Associated Proteins/Diseases (Not a complete list)	CPT Code(s)
ABCA4	ABCA4	ATP-binding cassette, sub-family A (ABC1), member 4	Stargardt disease, age-related macular degeneration, hereditary retinal disorders	81408, 81434
ABCC8	ABCC8	ATP-binding cassette, sub-family C (CFTR/MRP), member 8	Familial hyperinsulinism	81401, 81407
ABCD1	ABCD1	ATP-binding cassette, sub-family D (ALD), member 1	Adrenoleukodystrophy	81405
ABL1	ABL1	ABL proto-oncogene 1 non-receptor tyrosine kinase	Acquired imatinib resistance	81401
	ABL1	ABL proto-oncogene 1, non-receptor tyrosine kinase	Acquired imatinib tyrosine kinase inhibitor resistance	81170
ACADM	ACADM	Acyl-CoA dehydrogenase, C-4 to C-12 straight chain, MCAD	Medium chain acyl dehydrogenase deficiency, severe inherited conditions	81400, 81401, 81443
ACADS	ACADS	Acyl-CoA dehydrogenase, C-2 to C-3 short chain	Short chain acyl-CoA dehydrogenase deficiency	81404, 81405
ACADVL	ACADVL	Acyl-CoA dehydrogenase, very long chain	Very long chain acyl-coenzyme A dehydrogenase deficiency	81406
ACE	ACE	Angiotensin converting enzyme	Hereditary blood pressure regulation	81400
ACTA2	ACTA2	Actin, alpha 2, smooth muscle, aorta	Thoracic aortic aneurysms and aortic dissections, aortic dysfunction or dilation	81405, 81410
ACTC1	ACTC1	Actin, alpha, cardiac muscle 1	Familial hypertrophic cardiomyopathy	81405
ACTN4	ACTN4	Actinin, alpha 4	Focal segmental glomerulosclerosis	81406
ADRB2	ADRB2	Adrenergic beta-2 receptor surface	Drug metabolism	81401
AFF2	AFF2	AF4/FMR2 family, member 2 (FMR2)	Fragile X mental retardation 2 (FRAXE)	81171, 81172,
AFG3L2	AFG3L2	AFG3 ATPase family gene 3-like 2 (S. cerevisiae)	Spinocerebellar ataxia	81406
AGL	AGL	Amylo-alpha-1, 6-glucosidase, 4-alpha-glucanotransferase	Glycogen storage disease type III	81407
AGTR1	AGTR1	Angiotensin II receptor, type 1	Essential hypertension	81400
AHI1	AHI1	Abelson helper integration site 1	Joubert syndrome	81407
AIRE	AIRE	Autoimmune regulator	Autoimmune polyendocrinopathy syndrome type 1	81406
ALDH7A1	ALDH7A1	Aldehyde dehydrogenase 7 family, member A1	Pyridoxine-dependent epilepsy	81406
ALK	ALK	Anaplastic lymphoma receptor tyrosine kinase	Solid organ neoplasm or hematolymphoid neoplasm	81445, 81455
ANG	ANG	Angiogenin, ribonuclease, RNase A family, 5	Amyotrophic lateral sclerosis	81403
ANK2	ANK2	Ankyrin-2	Cardiac ion channelopathies	81413
ANKRD1	ANKRD1	Ankyrin repeat domain 1	Dilated cardiomyopathy	81405
ANO5	ANO5	Anoctamin 5	Limb-girdle muscular dystrophy	81406
ANOS1	ANOS1	Anosmin- 1	Kallman syndrome 1	81406
	APC	Adenomatous polyposis coli	Familial adenomatosis polyposis (FAP), attenuated FAP, hereditary colon cancer disorders	81201, 81202, 81203, 81435
APOB	APOB	Apolipoprotein B	Familial hypercholesterolemia type B	81401
APOE	APOE	Apolipoprotein E	Hyperlipoproteinemia type III, cardiovascular disease, Alzheimer disease	81401
APP	APP	Amyloid beta (A4) precursor protein	Alzheimer disease	81406
APTX	APTX	Aprataxin	Ataxia with oculomotor apraxia 1	81405
AQP2	AQP2	Aquaporin 2 (collecting duct)	Nephrogenic diabetes insipidus	81404
AR	AR	Androgen receptor	Spinal and bulbar muscular atrophy, Kennedy disease, X chromosome inactivation, androgen insensitivity syndrome	81173, 81174, 81204
ARSA	ARSA	Arylsulfatase A	Arylsulfatase A deficiency, severe inherited conditions	81405, 81443
ARX	ARX	Aristaless related homeobox	X-linked lissencephaly with ambiguous genitalia, X-linked mental retardation, X-linked intellectual disability (XLID)	81403, 81404, 81470, 81471
	ASPA	Aspartoacylase	Canavan disease, Ashkenazi Jewish-associated disorders, severe inherited conditions	81200, 81412, 81443
ASPM	ASPM	Asp (abnormal spindle) homolog, microcephaly associated (Drosophila)	Primary microcephaly	81407
ASS1	ASS1	Argininosuccinate synthase 1	Citrullinemia type I	81406
ASXL1	ASXL1	Additional sex combs like 1, transcriptional regulator	Myelodysplastic syndrome, myeloproliferative neoplasms, chronic myelomonocytic leukemia	81175, 81176

Molecular Pathology Gene Table, *continued*

Claim Designation	Abbreviated Gene Name	Full Gene Name	Commonly Associated Proteins/Diseases (Not a complete list)	CPT Code(s)
ATL1	ATL1	Atlastin GTPase 1	Spastic paraplegia	81406
ATM	ATM	Ataxia telangiectasia mutated	Ataxia telangiectasia	81408
ATN1	ATN1	Atrophin 1	Dentatorubral-pallidoluysian atrophy	81177
ATP1A2	ATP1A2	ATPase, Na+/K+ transporting, alpha 2 polypeptide	Familial hemiplegic migraine	81406
ATP7B	ATP7B	ATPase, Cu++ transporting, beta polypeptide	Wilson disease, severe inherited conditions	81406, 81443
ATRX	ATRX	Alpha thalassemia/mental retardation syndrome X-linked	X-linked intellectual disability (XLID)	81470, 81471
ATXN1	ATXN1	Ataxin 1	Spinocerebellar ataxia	81178
ATXN2	ATXN2	Ataxin 2	Spinocerebellar ataxia	81179
ATXN3	ATXN3	Ataxin 3	Spinocerebellar ataxia, Machado-Joseph disease	81180
ATXN7	ATXN7	Ataxin 7	Spinocerebellar ataxia	81181
ATXN8OS	ATXN8OS	ATXN8 opposite strand (non-protein coding)	Spinocerebellar ataxia	81182
ATXN10	ATXN10	Ataxin 10	Spinocerebellar ataxia	81183
AVPR2	AVPR2	Arginine vasopressin receptor 2	Nephrogenic diabetes insipidus	81404
BBS1	BBS1	Bardet-Biedl syndrome 1	Bardet-Biedl syndrome	81406
BBS2	BBS2	Bardet-Biedl syndrome 2	Bardet-Biedl syndrome	81406
BBS10	BBS10	Bardet-Biedl syndrome 10	Bardet-Biedl syndrome	81404
BCKDHA	BCKDHA	Branched-chain keto acid dehydrogenase E1, alpha polypeptide	Maple syrup urine disease type 1A, severe inherited conditions	81400, 81405, 81443
BCKDHB	BCKDHB	Branched-chain keto acid dehydrogenase E1, beta polypeptide	Maple syrup urine disease, maple syrup urine disease type 1B, severe inherited conditions	81205, 81406, 81443
	BCR/ABL1	t(9;22)	Chronic myelogenous leukemia	81206, 81207, 81208
BCS1L	BCS1L	BCS1-like (S. cerevisiae)	Leigh syndrome, mitochondrial complex III deficiency, GRACILE syndrome, mitochondrial disorders	81405, 81440
BEST1	BEST1	Bestrophin 1	Vitelliform macular dystrophy	81406
	BLM	Bloom syndrome, RecQ helicase-like	Bloom syndrome, Ashkenazi Jewish-associated disorders, severe inherited conditions	81209, 81412, 81443
BMPR1A	BMPR1A	Bone morphogenetic protein receptor, type IA	Hereditary colon cancer disorders	81435
BMPR2	BMPR2	Bone morphogenetic protein receptor, type II (serine/threonine kinase)	Heritable pulmonary arterial hypertension	81405, 81406
	BRAF	V-raf murine sarcoma viral oncogene homolog B1	Colon cancer	81210
BRAF	BRAF	B-Raf proto-oncogene, serine/threonine kinase	Noonan syndrome, Noonan spectrum disorders, solid organ neoplasm, hematolymphoid neoplasm or disorder	81406, 81442, 81445, 81450, 81455
	BRCA1	BRCA1, DNA repair associated	Hereditary breast and ovarian cancer, hereditary breast cancer-related disorders	81165, 81166, 81215, 81432, 81433
	BRCA2	BRCA2, DNA repair associated	Hereditary breast and ovarian cancer, hereditary breast cancer-related disorders	81167, 81216, 81217, 81432, 81433
	BRCA1 and BRCA2	BRCA1, DNA repair associated BRCA2, DNA repair associated	Hereditary breast and ovarian cancer	81162, 81163, 81164, 81212
BSCL2	BSCL2	Berardinelli-Seip congenital lipodystrophy 2 (seipin)	Berardinelli-Seip congenital lipodystrophy, hereditary peripheral neuropathies	81406, 81448
BTD	BTD	Biotinidase	Biotinidase deficiency	81404
BTK	BTK	Bruton agammaglobulinemia tyrosine kinase	X-linked agammaglobulinemia, chronic lymphocytic leukemia	81406, 81233
C10ORF2	C10orf2	Chromosome 10 open reading frame 2	Mitochondrial DNA depletion syndrome, mitochondrial disorders	81404, 81440
C1P19Q	Chromosome 1p-/19q- deletion analysis	N/A	Glial tumors	81402
CACNA1A	CACNA1A	Calcium channel, voltage-dependent, P/Q type, alpha 1A subunit	Spinocerebellar ataxia	81184, 81185, 81186

Molecular Pathology Gene Table, *continued*

Claim Designation	Abbreviated Gene Name	Full Gene Name	Commonly Associated Proteins/Diseases (Not a complete list)	CPT Code(s)
CACNB2	CACNB2	Calcium channel, voltage-dependent, beta 2 subunit	Brugada syndrome	81406
	CALR	Calreticulin	Myeloproliferative disorders	81219
CAPN3	CAPN3	Calpain 3	Limb-girdle muscular dystrophy (LGMD) type 2A, calpainopathy	81406
CASQ2	CASQ2	Calsequestrin 2 (cardiac muscle)	Catecholaminergic polymorphic ventricular tachycardia, cardiac ion channelopathies	81405, 81413
CASR	CASR	Calcium-sensing receptor	Hypocalcemia	81405
CAV3	CAV3	Caveolin 3	CAV3-related distal myopathy, limb-girdle muscular dystrophy type 1C, cardiac ion channelopathies	81404, 81413
CBFBMYH11	CBFB/MYH11	Inv(16)	Acute myeloid leukemia	81401
CBL	CBL	Cbl proto-oncogene, E3 ubiquitin protein ligase	Noonan spectrum disorders	81442
CBS	CBS	Cystathionine-beta-synthase	Homocystinuria, cystathionine beta-synthase deficiency	81401, 81406
CCND1IGH	CCND1/IGH	BCL1/IgH, t(11;14)	Mantle cell lymphoma	81401
CCR5	CCR5	Chemokine C-C motif receptor 5	HIV resistance	81400
CD40LG	CD40LG	CD40 ligand	X-linked hyper IgM syndrome	81404
CDH1	CDH1	Cadherin 1, type 1, E-cadherin (epithelial)	Hereditary diffuse gastric cancer, hereditary breast cancer-related disorders, hereditary colon cancer disorders	81406, 81432, 81435
CDH23	CDH23	Cadherin-related 23	Usher syndrome, type 1, hearing loss	81408, 81430
CDKL5	CDKL5	Cyclin-dependent kinase-like 5	Early infantile epileptic encephalopathy, X-linked intellectual disability (XLID)	81405, 81406, 81470, 81471
CDKN2A	CDKN2A	Cyclin-dependent kinase inhibitor 2A	CDKN2A-related cutaneous malignant melanoma, solid organ neoplasm or hematolymphoid neoplasm	81404, 81445, 81455
	CEBPA	CCAAT/enhancer binding protein (C/EBP), alpha	Acute myeloid leukemia, hematolymphoid neoplasm or disorder, solid organ neoplasm	81218, 81450, 81455
CEL	CEL	Carboxyl ester lipase (bile salt-stimulated lipase)	Maturity-onset diabetes of the young (MODY)	81403
CEP290	CEP290	Centrosomal protein 290kDa	Joubert syndrome	81408
CFHARMS2	CFH/ARMS2	Complement factor H/age-related maculopathy susceptibility 2	Macular degeneration	81401
	CFTR	Cystic fibrosis transmembrane conductance regulator	Cystic fibrosis, Ashkenazi Jewish-associated disorders, severe inherited conditions	81220, 81221, 81222, 81223, 81224, 81412, 81443
CGHSNP	Cytogenomic microarray analysis, neoplasia	N/A	N/A	81406
Ch22Q13	Cytogenomic constitutional targeted microarray analysis of chromosome 22q13 by interrogation of genomic regions for copy number and single nucleotide polymorphism variants	N/A	N/A	81405
CHD7	CHD7	Chromodomain helicase DNA binding protein 7	CHARGE syndrome	81407
	Chimerism engraftment analysis	N/A	Post transplantation specimen (eg, hematopoietic stem cell)	81267, 81268
CHRNA4	CHRNA4	Cholinergic receptor, nicotinic, alpha 4	Nocturnal frontal lobe epilepsy	81405
CHRNB2	CHRNB2	Cholinergic receptor, nicotinic, beta 2 (neuronal)	Nocturnal frontal lobe epilepsy	81405
CHROM18Q	Chromosome 18q-		Colon cancer	81402
CLCN1	CLCN1	Chloride channel 1, skeletal muscle	Myotonia congenita	81406
CLCNKB	CLCNKB	Chloride channel, voltage-sensitive Kb	Bartter syndrome 3 and 4b	81406
CLRN1	CLRN1	Clarin 1	Usher syndrome, type 3, hearing loss	81400, 81404, 81430

Molecular Pathology Gene Table, *continued*

Claim Designation	Abbreviated Gene Name	Full Gene Name	Commonly Associated Proteins/Diseases (Not a complete list)	CPT Code(s)
CNBP	CNBP	CCHC-type zinc finger, nucleic acid binding protein	Myotonic dystrophy type 2	81187
CNGA1	CNGA1	Cyclic nucleotide gated channel alpha 1	Hereditary retinal disorders	81434
CNTNAP2	CNTNAP2	Contactin associated protein-like 2	Pitt-Hopkins-like syndrome 1	81406
COL1A1	COL1A1	Collagen, type I, alpha 1	Osteogenesis imperfecta, type I	81408
COL1A1PDGFB	COL1A1/PDGFB	t(17;22)	Dermatofibrosarcoma protuberans	81402
COL1A2	COL1A2	Collagen, type I, alpha 2	Osteogenesis imperfecta, type I	81408
COL3A1	COL3A1	Collagen, type III, alpha 1	Aortic dysfunction or dilation	81410, 81411
COL4A1	COL4A1	Collagen, type IV, alpha 1	Brain small-vessel disease with hemorrhage	81408
COL4A3	COL4A3	Collagen, type IV, alpha 3 (Goodpasture antigen)	Alport syndrome	81408
COL4A4	COL4A4	Collagen, type IV, alpha 4	Alport syndrome	81407
COL4A5	COL4A5	Collagen, type IV, alpha 5	Alport syndrome	81407, 81408
COL6A1	COL6A1	Collagen, type VI, alpha 1	Collagen type VI-related disorders	81407
COL6A2	COL6A2	Collagen, type VI, alpha 2	Collagen type VI-related disorders	81406, 81407
COL6A3	COL6A3	Collagen, type VI, alpha 3	Collagen type VI-related disorders	81407
COQ2	COQ2	Coenzyme Q2, polyprenyltransferase	Mitochondrial disorders	81440
COX10	COX10	COX10 homolog, cytochrome c oxidase assembly protein	Mitochondrial respiratory chain complex IV deficiency, mitochondrial disorders	81405, 81440
COX15	COX15	COX15 homolog, cytochrome c oxidase assembly protein	Mitochondrial respiratory chain complex IV deficiency	81405
COX6B1	COX6B1	Cytochrome c oxidase subunit VIb polypeptide 1	Mitochondrial respiratory chain complex IV deficiency	81404
CPOX	CPOX	Coproporphyrinogen oxidase	Hereditary coproporphyria	81405
CPT1A	CPT1A	Carnitine palmitoyltransferase 1A (liver)	Carnitine palmitoyltransferase 1A (CPT1A) deficiency	81406
CPT2	CPT2	Carnitine palmitoyltransferase 2	Carnitine palmitoyltransferase II deficiency	81404
CRB1	CRB1	Crumbs homolog 1 (Drosophila)	Leber congenital amaurosis, hereditary retinal disorders	81406, 81434
CREBBP	CREBBP	CREB binding protein	Rubinstein-Taybi syndrome	81406, 81407
CRX	CRX	Cone-rod homeobox	Cone-rod dystrophy 2, Leber congenital amaurosis	81404
CSTB	CSTB	Cystatin B (stefin B)	Unverricht-Lundborg disease	81188, 81189, 81190
CTNNB1	CTNNB1	Catenin (cadherin-associated protein), beta 1, 88kDa	Desmoid tumors	81403
CTRC	CTRC	Chymotrypsin C	Hereditary pancreatitis	81405
CYP11B1	CYP11B1	Cytochrome P450, family 11, subfamily B, polypeptide 1	Congenital adrenal hyperplasia	81405
CYP17A1	CYP17A1	Cytochrome P450, family 17, subfamily A, polypeptide 1	Congenital adrenal hyperplasia	81405
CYP1B1	CYP1B1	Cytochrome P450, family 1, subfamily B, polypeptide 1	Primary congenital glaucoma	81404
CYP21A2	CYP21A2	Cytochrome P450, family 21, subfamily A, polypeptide 2	Congenital adrenal hyperplasia, 21-hydroxylase deficiency, steroid 21-hydroxylase isoform	81402, 81405
	CYP2C9	Cytochrome P450, family 2, subfamily C, polypeptide 9	Drug metabolism	81227
	CYP2C19	Cytochrome P450, family 2, subfamily C, polypeptide 19	Drug metabolism	81225
	CYP2D6	Cytochrome P450, family 2, subfamily D, polypeptide 6	Drug metabolism	81226
CYP3A4	CYP3A4	Cytochrome P450 family 3 subfamily A member 4	Drug metabolism	81230
CYP3A5	CYP3A5	Cytochrome P450 family 3 subfamily A member 5	Drug metabolism	81231
	Cytogenomic constitutional (genome-wide) microarray analysis	N/A	N/A	81228, 81229
DAZSRY	DAZ/SRY	Deleted in azoospermia and sex determining region Y	Male infertility	81403
DBT	DBT	Dihydrolipoamide branched chain transacylase E2	Maple syrup urine disease, type 2	81405, 81406
DCX	DCX	Doublecortin	X-linked lissencephaly	81405
DEKNUP214	DEK/NUP214	t(6;9)	Acute myeloid leukemia	81401

Molecular Pathology Gene Table, *continued*

Claim Designation	Abbreviated Gene Name	Full Gene Name	Commonly Associated Proteins/Diseases (Not a complete list)	CPT Code(s)
DES	DES	Desmin	Myofibrillar myopathy	81405
DFNB1	DFNB1	N/A	Hearing loss	81431
DFNB59	DFNB59	Deafness, autosomal recessive 59	Autosomal recessive nonsyndromic hearing impairment	81405
DGUOK	DGUOK	Deoxyguanosine kinase	Hepatocerebral mitochondrial DNA depletion syndrome, mitochondrial disorders	81405, 81440
DHCR7	DHCR7	7-dehydrocholesterol reductase	Smith-Lemli-Opitz syndrome, severe inherited conditions	81405, 81443
DLAT	DLAT	Dihydrolipoamide S-acetyltransferase	Pyruvate dehydrogenase E2 deficiency	81406
DLD	DLD	Dihydrolipoamide dehydrogenase	Maple syrup urine disease, type III	81406
	DMD	Dystrophin	Duchenne/Becker muscular dystrophy	81161
DMD	DMD	Dystrophin	Duchenne/Becker muscular dystrophy	81408
DMPK	DMPK	Dystrophia myotonica-protein kinase	Myotonic dystrophy, type 1	81234, 81239
DNMT3A	DNMT3A	DNA (cytosine-5-)-methyltransferase 3 alpha	Acute myeloid leukemia, hematolymphoid neoplasm or disorder, solid organ neoplasm	81403, 81450, 81455
DPYD	DPYD	Dihydropyrimidine dehydrogenase	5-fluorouracil/5-FU and capecitabine drug metabolism	81232
DSC2	DSC2	Desmocollin	Arrhythmogenic right ventricular dysplasia/cardiomyopathy 11	81406
DSG2	DSG2	Desmoglein 2	Arrhythmogenic right ventricular dysplasia/cardiomyopathy 10, hereditary cardiomyopathy	81406, 81439
DSP	DSP	Desmoplakin	Arrhythmogenic right ventricular dysplasia/cardiomyopathy 8	81406
DYSF	DYSF	Dysferlin, limb-girdle muscular dystrophy 2B (autosomal recessive)	Limb-girdle muscular dystrophy	81408
E2APBX1	E2A/PBX1	t(1;19)	Acute lymphocytic leukemia	81401
EFHC1	EFHC1	EF-hand domain (C-terminal) containing 1	Juvenile myoclonic epilepsy	81406
	EGFR	Epidermal growth factor receptor	Non-small cell lung cancer, solid organ neoplasm or hematolymphoid neoplasm	81235, 81445, 81455
EGR2	EGR2	Early growth response 2	Charcot-Marie-Tooth disease	81404
EIF2B2	EIF2B2	Eukaryotic translation initiation factor 2B, subunit 2 beta, 39kDa	Leukoencephalopathy with vanishing white matter	81405
EIF2B3	EIF2B3	Eukaryotic translation initiation factor 2B, subunit 3 gamma, 58kDa	Leukoencephalopathy with vanishing white matter	81406
EIF2B4	EIF2B4	Eukaryotic translation initiation factor 2B, subunit 4 delta, 67kDa	Leukoencephalopathy with vanishing white matter	81406
EIF2B5	EIF2B5	Eukaryotic translation initiation factor 2B, subunit 5 epsilon, 82kDa	Childhood ataxia with central nervous system hypomyelination/vanishing white matter	81406
EMD	EMD	Emerin	Emery-Dreifuss muscular dystrophy	81404, 81405
EML4ALK	EML4/ALK	Inv(2)	Non-small cell lung cancer	81401
ENG	ENG	Endoglin	Hereditary hemorrhagic telangiectasia, type 1	81405, 81406
EPCAM	EPCAM	Epithelial cell adhesion molecule	Lynch syndrome, hereditary colon cancer disorders	81403, 81436
EPM2A	EPM2A	Epilepsy, progressive myoclonus type 2A, Lafora disease (laforin)	Progressive myoclonus epilepsy	81404
ERBB2	ERBB2	V-Erb-B2 avian erythroblastic leukemia viral oncogene homolog 2	Solid organ neoplasm or hematolymphoid neoplasm	81445, 81455
ESR1PGR	ESR1/PGR	Receptor 1/progesterone receptor	Breast cancer	81402
ETV6NTRK3	ETV6/NTRK3	t(12;15)	Congenital/infantile fibrosarcoma	81401
ETV6RUNX1	ETV6/RUNX1	t(12;21)	Acute lymphocytic leukemia	81401
EWSR1ATF1	EWSR1/ATF1	t(12;22)	Clear cell sarcoma	81401
EWSR1ERG	EWSR1/ERG	t(21;22)	Ewing sarcoma/peripheral neuroectodermal tumor	81401
EWSR1FLI1	EWSR1/FLI1	t(11;22)	Ewing sarcoma/peripheral neuroectodermal tumor	81401
EWSR1WT1	EWSR1/WT1	t(11;22)	Desmoplastic small round cell tumor	81401
EYA1	EYA1	Eyes absent homolog 1 (Drosophila)	Branchio-oto-renal (BOR) spectrum disorders	81405, 81406
EYS	EYS	Eyes shut homolog (Drosophila)	Hereditary retinal disorders	81434

Molecular Pathology Gene Table, *continued*

Claim Designation	Abbreviated Gene Name	Full Gene Name	Commonly Associated Proteins/Diseases (Not a complete list)	CPT Code(s)
EZH2	EZH2	Enhancer of zeste 2 polycomb repressive complex 2 subunit	Myelodysplastic syndrome, myeloproliferative neoplasms, diffuse large B-cell lymphoma	81236, 81237, 81450, 81455
	F2	Prothrombin, coagulation factor II	Hereditary hypercoagulability	81240
F2	F2	Prothrombin, coagulation factor II	Hereditary hypercoagulability	81400
	F5	Coagulation factor V	Hereditary hypercoagulability	81241
F5	F5	Coagulation factor V	Hereditary hypercoagulability	81400
F7	F7	Coagulation factor VII (serum prothrombin conversion accelerator)	Hereditary hypercoagulability	81400
F8	F8	Coagulation factor VIII	Hemophilia A	81403, 81406, 81407
F9	F9	Coagulation factor IX	Hemophilia B	81238
F11	F11	Coagulation factor XI	Coagulation disorder	81401
F12	F12	Coagulation factor XII (Hageman factor)	Angioedema, hereditary, type III; factor XII deficiency	81403
F13B	F13B	Coagulation factor XIII, B polypeptide	Hereditary hypercoagulability	81400
FAH	FAH	Fumarylacetoacetate hydrolase (fumarylacetoacetase)	Tyrosinemia, type 1	81406
	FANCC	Fanconi anemia, complementation group C	Fanconi anemia, type C, Ashkenazi Jewish-associated disorders, severe inherited conditions	81242, 81412, 81443
FASTKD2	FASTKD2	FAST kinase domains 2	Mitochondrial respiratory chain complex IV deficiency	81406
FBN1	FBN1	Bibrillin 1	Marfan syndrome, aortic dysfunction or dilation	81408, 81410
FGB	FGB	Fibrinogen beta chain	Hereditary ischemic heart disease	81400
FGD1	FGD1	FYVE, RhoGEF and PH domain containing 1	X-linked intellectual disability (XLID)	81470, 81471
FGF23	FGF23	Fibroblast growth factor 23	Hypophosphatemic rickets	81404
FGFR1	FGFR1	Fibroblast growth factor receptor 1	Pfeiffer syndrome type 1, craniosynostosis, Kallmann syndrome	81400, 81405
FGFR2	FGFR2	Fibroblast growth factor receptor 2	Craniosynostosis, Apert syndrome, Crouzon syndrome	81404
FGFR3	FGFR3	Fibroblast growth factor receptor 3	Muenke syndrome, achondroplasia, hypochondroplasia, isolated craniosynostosis	81400, 81401, 81403, 81404
FH	FH	Fumarate hydratase	Fumarate Hydratase Deficiency, Hereditary Leiomyomatosis with renal cell cancer	81405
FHL1	FHL1	Four and a half LIM domains 1	Emery-Dreifuss muscular dystrophy	81404
FIG4	FIG4	FIG4 homolog, SAC1 lipid phosphatase domain containing (S. cerevisiae)	Charcot-Marie-Tooth disease	81406
FIP1L1PDGFRA	FIP1L1/PDGFRA	Del(4q12)	Imatinib-sensitive chronic eosinophilic leukemia	81401
FKRP	FKRP	Fukutin related protein	Congenital muscular dystrophy type 1C (MDC1C), limb-girdle muscular dystrophy (LGMD) type 2I	81404
FKTN	FKTN	Fukutin	Fukuyama congenital muscular dystrophy, limb-girdle muscular dystrophy (LGMD) type 2M or 2L	81400, 81405
FLG	FLG	Filaggrin	Ichthyosis vulgaris	81401
	FLT3	Fms-related tyrosine kinase 3	Acute myeloid leukemia, hematolymphoid neoplasm or disorder, solid organ neoplasm	81245, 81246, 81450, 81455
	FMR1	Fragile X mental retardation 1	Fragile X mental retardation, X-linked intellectual disability (XLID)	81243, 81244, 81470, 81471
FOXG1	FOXG1	Forkhead box G1	Rett syndrome	81404
FOXO1PAX3	FOXO1/PAX3	t(2;13)	Ewing sarcoma/peripheral neuroectodermal tumor, alveolar rhabdomyosarcoma	81401
FOXO1PAX7	FOXO1/PAX7	t(1;13)	Ewing sarcoma/peripheral neuroectodermal tumor, alveolar rhabdomyosarcoma	81401
FSHMD1A	FSHMD1A	Facioscapulohumeral muscular dystrophy 1A	Facioscapulohumeral muscular dystrophy	81404
FTSJ1	FTSJ1	FtsJ RNA methyltransferase homolog 1 (E. coli)	X-linked mental retardation 9	81405, 81406
FUS	FUS	Fused in sarcoma	Amyotrophic lateral sclerosis	81406
FUSDDIT3	FUS/DDIT3	t(12;16)	Myxoid Liposarcoma	81401
FXN	FXN	Frataxin	Friedreich ataxia	81284, 81285, 81286, 81289

Molecular Pathology Gene Table, *continued*

Claim Designation	Abbreviated Gene Name	Full Gene Name	Commonly Associated Proteins/Diseases (Not a complete list)	CPT Code(s)
G6PC	G6PC	Glucose-6-phosphatase, catalytic subunit	Glycogen storage disease, Type 1a, von Gierke disease, severe inherited conditions	81250, 81443
G6PD	G6PD	Glucose-6-phosphate dehydrogenase	Hemolytic anemia, jaundice	81247, 81248, 81249
GAA	GAA	Glucosidase, alpha; acid	Glycogen storage disease type II (Pompe disease), severe inherited conditions	81406, 81443
GABRG2	GABRG2	Gamma-aminobutyric acid (GABA) A receptor, gamma 2	Generalized epilepsy with febrile seizures	81405
GALC	GALC	Galactosylceramidase	Krabbe disease	81401, 81406
GALT	GALT	Galactose-1-phosphate uridylyltransferase	Galactosemia, severe inherited conditions	81401, 81406, 81443
GARS	GARS	Glycyl-tRNA synthetase	Charcot-Marie-Tooth disease	81406
	GBA	Glucosidase, beta, acid	Gaucher disease, Ashkenazi Jewish-associated disorders, severe inherited conditions	81251, 81412, 81443
GBE1		1,4-alpha-glucan branching enzyme 1	Severe inherited conditions	81443
GCDH	GCDH	Glutaryl-CoA dehydrogenase	Glutaricacidemia type 1	81406
GCH1	GCH1	GTP cyclohydrolase 1	Autosomal dominant dopa-responsive dystonia	81405
GCK	GCK	Glucokinase (hexokinase 4)	Maturity-onset diabetes of the young (MODY)	81406
GDAP1	GDAP1	Ganglioside-induced differentiation-associated protein 1	Charcot-Marie-Tooth disease	81405
GFAP	GFAP	Glial fibrillary acidic protein	Alexander disease	81405
GH1	GH1	Growth hormone 1	Growth hormone deficiency	81404
GHR	GHR	Growth hormone receptor	Laron syndrome	81405
GHRHR	GHRHR	Growth hormone releasing hormone receptor	Growth hormone deficiency	81405
GJB1	GJB1	Gap junction protein, beta 1	Charcot-Marie-Tooth X-linked, hereditary peripheral neuropathies	81403, 81448
	GJB2	Gap junction protein, beta 2, 26kDa, connexin 26	Nonsyndromic hearing loss	81252, 81253, 81430, 81431
	GJB6	Gap junction protein, beta 6, 30kDa, connexin 30	Nonsyndromic hearing loss	81254, 81431
GLA	GLA	Galactosidase, alpha	Fabry disease	81405
GLUD1	GLUD1	Glutamate dehydrogenase 1	Familial hyperinsulinism	81406
GNAQ	GNAQ	Guanine nucleotide-binding protein G(q) subunit alpha	Uveal melanoma	81403
GNE	GNE	Glucosamine (UDP-N-acetyl)-2-epimerase/N-acetyl-mannosamine kinase	Inclusion body myopathy 2 (IBM2), Nonaka myopathy	81400, 81406
GP1BB	GP1BB	Glycoprotein Ib (platelet), beta polypeptide	Bernard-Soulier syndrome type B	81404
GPR98	GPR98	G-protein coupled receptor 98	Hearing loss	81430
GRN	GRN	Granulin	Frontotemporal dementia	81406
H19	H19	Imprinted maternally expressed transcript (non-protein coding)	Beckwith-Wiedemann syndrome	81401
HADHA	HADHA	Hydroxyacyl-CoA dehydrogenase/3-ketoacyl-CoA thiolase/enoyl-CoA hydratase (trifunctional protein) alpha subunit	Long chain acyl-coenzyme A dehydrogenase deficiency	81406
HADHB	HADHB	Hydroxyacyl-CoA dehydrogenase/3-ketoacyl-CoA thiolase/enoyl-CoA hydratase (trifunctional protein), beta subunit	Trifunctional protein deficiency	81406
HBA1/HBA2	HBA1/HBA2	Alpha globin 1 and alpha globin 2	Alpha thalassemia, thalassemia, Hb Bart hydrops fetalis syndrome, HbH disease	81257, 81258, 81259, 81269
HBB	HBB	Hemoglobin, subunit beta	Sickle cell anemia, beta thalassemia, hemoglobinopathy, severe inherited conditions	81361, 81362, 81363, 81364, 81443
HEA	HEA	Human erythrocyte antigen	Sickle-cell disease, thalassemia, hemolytic transfusion reactions, hemolytic disease of the fetus or newborn	81403
	HEXA	Hexosaminidase A (alpha polypeptide)	Tay-Sachs disease, Ashkenazi Jewish-associated disorders, severe inherited conditions	81255, 81406, 81412, 81443

Molecular Pathology Gene Table, *continued*

Claim Designation	Abbreviated Gene Name	Full Gene Name	Commonly Associated Proteins/Diseases (Not a complete list)	CPT Code(s)
	HFE	Hemochromatosis	Hereditary hemochromatosis	81256
	HLA	Human leukocyte antigen genes	Pretransplant and drug therapy testing	81370-81383
HLCS	HLCS	HLCS holocarboxylase synthetase	Holocarboxylase synthetase deficiency	81406
HMBS	HMBS	hydroxymethylbilane synthase	Acute intermittent porphyria	81406
HNF1A	HNF1A	HNF1 homeobox A	Maturity-onset diabetes of the young (MODY)	81405
HNF1B	HNF1B	HNF1 homeobox B	Maturity-onset diabetes of the young (MODY)	81404, 81405
HNF4A	HNF4A	Hepatocyte nuclear factor 4, alpha	Maturity-onset diabetes of the young (MODY)	81406
HPA1	Human Platelet Antigen 1 genotyping (HPA-1), ITGB3	Integrin, beta 3 (platelet glycoprotein IIIa), antigen CD61 (GPIIIa)	Neonatal alloimmune thrombocytopenia (NAIT), post-transfusion purpura	81105
HPA2	Human Platelet Antigen 2 genotyping (HPA-2), GP1BA	Glycoprotein Ib (platelet), alpha polypeptide (GPIba)	Neonatal alloimmune thrombocytopenia (NAIT), post-transfusion purpura	81106
HPA3	Human Platelet Antigen 3 genotyping (HPA-3), ITGA2B	Integrin, alpha 2b (platelet glycoprotein IIb of IIb/IIIa complex), antigen CD41 (GPIIb)	Neonatal alloimmune thrombocytopenia (NAIT), post-transfusion purpura	81107
HPA4	Human Platelet Antigen 4 genotyping (HPA-4), ITGB3	Integrin, beta 3 (platelet glycoprotein IIIa), antigen CD61 (GPIIIa)	Neonatal alloimmune thrombocytopenia (NAIT), post-transfusion purpura	81108
HPA5	Human Platelet Antigen 5 genotyping (HPA-5), ITGA2	Integrin, alpha 2 (CD49B, alpha 2 subunit of VLA-2 receptor) (GPIa)	Neonatal alloimmune thrombocytopenia (NAIT), post-transfusion purpura	81109
HPA6	Human Platelet Antigen 6 genotyping (HPA-6w), ITGB3	Integrin, beta 3 (platelet glycoprotein IIIa, antigen CD61) (GPIIIa)	Neonatal alloimmune thrombocytopenia (NAIT), post-transfusion purpura	81110
HPA9	Human Platelet Antigen 9 genotyping (HPA-9w), ITGA2B	Integrin, alpha 2b (platelet glycoprotein IIb of IIb/IIIa complex, antigen CD41) (GPIIb)	Neonatal alloimmune thrombocytopenia (NAIT), post-transfusion purpura	81111
HPA15	Human Platelet Antigen 15 genotyping (HPA-15), CD109	CD109 molecule	Neonatal alloimmune thrombocytopenia (NAIT), post-transfusion purpura	81112
HRAS	HRAS	V-Ha-ras Harvey rat sarcoma viral oncogene homolog	Costello syndrome, Noonan spectrum disorders	81403, 81404, 81442
HSD3B2	HSD3B2	Hydroxy-delta-5-steroid dehydrogenase, 3 beta- and steroid delta-isomerase 2	3-beta-hydroxysteroid dehydrogenase type II deficiency	81404
HSD11B2	HSD11B2	Hydroxysteroid (11-beta) dehydrogenase 2	Mineralocorticoid excess syndrome	81404
HSPB1	HSPB1	Heat shock 27kDa protein 1	Charcot-Marie-Tooth disease	81404
HTRA1	HTRA1	HtrA serine peptidase 1	Macular degeneration	81405
HTT	HTT	Huntingtin	Huntington disease	81271, 81274
HUWE1	HUWE1	HECT, UBA and WWE domain containing 1, E3 ubiquitin protein ligase	X-linked intellectual disability (XLID)	81470, 81471
IDH1	IDH1	Isocitrate dehydrogenase 1 (NADP+), soluble	Glioma, hematolymphoid neoplasm or disorder, solid organ neoplasm	81120, 81450, 81455
IDH2	IDH2	Isocitrate dehydrogenase 2 (NADP+), mitochondrial	Glioma, hematolymphoid neoplasm or disorder, solid organ neoplasm	81121, 81450, 81455
IDS	IDS	Iduronate 2-sulfatase	Mucopolysaccharidosis, type II	81405
IDUA	IDUA	Iduronidase, alpha-L-	Mucopolysaccharidosis type I	81406
IFNL3	IFNL3	Interferon, lambda 3	Drug response	81283
	IGH@	Immunoglobulin heavy chain locus	Leukemias and lymphomas, B-cell	81261, 81262, 81263

Molecular Pathology Gene Table, *continued*

Claim Designation	Abbreviated Gene Name	Full Gene Name	Commonly Associated Proteins/Diseases (Not a complete list)	CPT Code(s)
IGHBCL2	IGH@/BCL2	t(14;18)	Follicular lymphoma	81401, 81402
	IGK@	Immunoglobulin kappa light chain locus	Leukemia and lymphoma, B-cell	81264
	IKBKAP	Inhibitor of kappa light polypeptide gene enhancer in B-cells, kinase complex-associated protein	Familial dysautonomia, Ashkenazi Jewish-associated disorders, severe inherited conditions	81260, 81412, 81443
IL1RAPL	IL1RAPL	Interleukin 1 receptor accessory protein	X-linked intellectual disability (XLID)	81470, 81471
IL2RG	IL2RG	Interleukin 2 receptor, gamma	X-linked severe combined immunodeficiency	81405
INF2	INF2	Inverted formin, FH2 and WH2 domain containing	Focal segmental glomerulosclerosis	81406
INS	INS	Insulin	Diabetes mellitus	81404
ISPD	ISPD	Isoprenoid synthase domain containing	Muscle-eye-brain disease, Walker-Warburg syndrome	81405
ITPR1	ITPR1	Inositol 1,4,5-trisphosphate receptor, type 1	Spinocerebellar ataxia	81408
IVD	IVD	Isovaleryl-CoA dehydrogenase	Isovaleric acidemia	81400, 81406
JAG1	JAG1	Jagged 1	Alagille syndrome	81406, 81407
	JAK2	Janus kinase 2	Myeloproliferative disorder	81270
JAK2	JAK2	Janus kinase 2	Myeloproliferative disorder, hematolymphoid neoplasm or disorder, solid organ neoplasm	81403, 81450, 81455
JUP	JUP	Junction plakoglobin	Arrhythmogenic right ventricular dysplasia/cardiomyopathy 11	81406
KCNC3	KCNC3	Potassium voltage-gated channel, Shaw-related subfamily, member 3	Spinocerebellar ataxia	81403
KCNE1	KCNE1	Potassium voltage-gated channel, subfamily E, member 1	Cardiac ion channelopathies	81413
KCNE2	KCNE2	Potassium voltage-gated channel, subfamily E, member 2	Cardiac ion channelopathies	81413
KCNH2	KCNH2	Potassium voltage-gated channel, subfamily H (eag-related), member 2	Short QT syndrome, long QT syndrome, cardiac ion channelopathies	81406, 81413, 81414
KCNJ1	KCNJ1	Potassium inwardly-rectifying channel, subfamily J, member 1	Bartter syndrome	81404
KCNJ2	KCNJ2	Potassium inwardly-rectifying channel, subfamily J, member 2	Andersen-Tawil syndrome, cardiac ion channelopathies	81403, 81413
KCNJ10	KCNJ10	Potassium inwardly-rectifying channel, subfamily J, member 10	SeSAME syndrome, EAST syndrome, sensorineural hearing loss	81404
KCNJ11	KCNJ11	Potassium inwardly-rectifying channel, subfamily J, member 11	Familial hyperinsulinism	81403
KCNQ1	KCNQ1	Potassium voltage-gated channel, KQT-like subfamily, member 1	Short QT syndrome, long QT syndrome, cardiac ion channelopathies	81406, 81413, 81414
KCNQ1OT1	KCNQ1OT1	KCNQ1 overlapping transcript 1 (non-protein coding)	Beckwith-Wiedemann syndrome	81401
KCNQ2	KCNQ2	Potassium voltage-gated channel, KQT-like subfamily, member 2	Epileptic encephalopathy	81406
KDM5C	KDM5C	Lysine (K)-specific demethylase 5C	X-linked mental retardation, X-linked intellectual disability (XLID)	81407, 81470, 81471
KIAA0196	KIAA0196	KIAA0196	Spastic paraplegia	81407
KIR	KIR	Killer cell immunoglobulin-like receptor	Hematopoietic stem cell transplantation	81403
	KIT	v-kit Hardy-Zuckerman 4 feline sarcoma viral oncogene homolog	Gastrointestinal stromal tumor, acute myeloid leukemia, melanoma, solid organ neoplasm, hematolymphoid neoplasm or disorder	81272, 81273, 81445, 81450, 81455
	KRAS	v-Ki-ras2 Kirsten rat sarcoma viral oncogene homolog	Carcinoma, Noonan syndrome	81275, 81276
KRAS	KRAS	Kirsten rat sarcoma viral oncogene homolog	Noonan syndrome, Noonan spectrum disorders, solid organ neoplasm, hematolymphoid neoplasm or disorder	81405, 81442, 81445, 81450, 81455
L1CAM	L1CAM	L1 cell adhesion molecule	MASA syndrome, X-linked hydrocephaly, X-linked intellectual disability (XLID)	81407, 81470, 81471
LAMA2	LAMA2	Laminin, alpha 2	Congenital muscular dystrophy	81408
LAMB2	LAMB2	Laminin, beta 2 (laminin S)	Pierson syndrome	81407

Molecular Pathology Gene Table, *continued*

Claim Designation	Abbreviated Gene Name	Full Gene Name	Commonly Associated Proteins/Diseases (Not a complete list)	CPT Code(s)
LAMP2	LAMP2	Lysosomal-associated membrane protein 2	Danon disease	81405
LCT	LCT	Lactase-phlorizin hydrolase	Lactose intolerance	81400
LDB3	LDB3	LIM domain binding 3	Familial dilated cardiomyopathy, myofibrillar myopathy	81406
LDLR	LDLR	Low density lipoprotein receptor	Familial hypercholesterolemia	81405, 81406
LEPR	LEPR	Leptin receptor	Obesity with hypogonadism	81406
LHCGR	LHCGR	Luteinizing hormone/choriogonadotropin receptor	Precocious male puberty	81406
LINC00518	LINC00518	Long intergenic non-protein coding RNA 518	Melanoma	81401
LITAF	LITAF	Lipopolysaccharide-induced TNF factor	Charcot-Marie-Tooth disease	81404
LMNA	LMNA	Lamin A/C	Emery-Dreifuss muscular dystrophy (EDMD1, 2, and 3) limb-girdle muscular dystrophy (LGMD) type 1B, dilated cardiomyopathy (CMD1A), familial partial lipodystrophy (FPLD2)	81406
LRP5	LRP5	Low density lipoprotein receptor-related protein 5	Osteopetrosis	81406
LRRK2	LRRK2	Leucine-rich repeat kinase 2	Parkinson disease	81401, 81408
MAP2K1	MAP2K1	Mitogen-activated protein kinase 1	Cardiofaciocutaneous syndrome, Noonan spectrum disorders	81406, 81442
MAP2K2	MAP2K2	Mitogen-activated protein kinase 2	Cardiofaciocutaneous syndrome, Noonan spectrum disorders	81406, 81442
MAPT	MAPT	Microtubule-associated protein tau	Frontotemporal dementia	81406
MAX	MAX	MYC-associated factor X	Hereditary neuroendocrine tumor disorders	81437
MC4R	MC4R	Melanocortin 4 receptor	Obesity	81403
MCCC1	MCCC1	Methylcrotonoyl-CoA carboxylase 1 (alpha)	3-methylcrotonyl-CoA carboxylase deficiency	81406
MCCC2	MCCC2	Methylcrotonoyl-CoA carboxylase 2 (beta)	3-methylcrotonyl carboxylase deficiency	81406
	MCOLN1	Mucolipin 1	Mucolipidosis, type IV, Ashkenazi Jewish-associated disorders, severe inherited conditions	81290, 81412, 81443
	MECP2	Methyl CpG binding protein 2	Rett syndrome, X-linked intellectual disability (XLID)	81302, 81303, 81304, 81470, 81471
MED12	MED12	Mediator complex subunit 12	FG syndrome type 1, Lujan syndrome, X-linked intellectual disability (XLID)	81401, 81470, 81471
MEFV	MEFV	Mediterranean fever	Familial Mediterranean fever	81402, 81404
MEG3DLK1	MEG3/DLK1	Maternally expressed 3 (non-protein coding)/delta-like 1 homolog (Drosophila)	Intrauterine growth retardation	81401
MEN1	MEN1	Multiple endocrine neoplasia 1	Multiple endocrine neoplasia type 1, Wermer syndrome	81404, 81405
MET	MET	Met proto-oncogene	Solid organ neoplasm or hematolymphoid neoplasm	81445, 81455
MFN2	MFN2	Mitofusin 2	Charcot-Marie-Tooth disease, hereditary peripheral neuropathies	81406, 81448
	MGMT	O-6-methylguanine-DNA methyltransferase	Glioblastoma multiforme	81287
MICA	MICA	MHC class I polypeptide-related sequence A	Solid organ transplantation	81403
	Microsatellite instability analysis	N/A	Hereditary nonpolyposis colorectal cancer, Lynch syndrome	81301
MID1	MID1	Midline 1	X-linked intellectual disability (XLID)	81470, 81471
	MLH1	mutL homolog 1, colon cancer, nonpolyposis type 2	Hereditary nonpolyposis colorectal cancer, Lynch syndrome, hereditary breast cancer-related disorders, hereditary colon cancer disorders	81288, 81292, 81293, 81294, 81432, 81433, 81435, 81436
MLL	MLL	N/A	Hematolymphoid neoplasm or disorder, solid organ neoplasm	81450, 81455
MLLAFF1	MLL/AFF1	t(4;11)	Acute lymphoblastic leukemia	81401
MLLMLLT3	MLL/MLLT3	t(9;11)	Acute myeloid leukemia	81401
MMAA	MMAA	Methylmalonic aciduria (cobalamine deficiency) type A	MMAA-related methylmalonic acidemia	81405
MMAB	MMAB	Methylmalonic aciduria (cobalamine deficiency) type B	MMAA-related methylmalonic acidemia	81405

Molecular Pathology Gene Table, *continued*

Claim Designation	Abbreviated Gene Name	Full Gene Name	Commonly Associated Proteins/Diseases (Not a complete list)	CPT Code(s)
MMACHC	MMACHC	Methylmalonic aciduria (cobalamin deficiency) cblC type, with homocystinuria	Methylmalonic acidemia and homocystinuria	81404
MPI	MPI	Mannose phosphate isomerase	Congenital disorder of glycosylation 1b	81405
MPL	MPL	Myeloproliferative leukemia virus oncogene, thrombopoietin receptor, TPOR	Myeloproliferative disorder	81402, 81403
MPV17	MPV17	MpV17 mitochondrial inner membrane protein	Mitochondrial DNA depletion syndrome, mitochondrial disorders	81404, 81405, 81440
MPZ	MPZ	Myelin protein zero	Charcot-Marie-Tooth disease, hereditary peripheral neuropathies	81405, 81448
	MSH2	mutS homolog 2, colon cancer, nonpolyposis type 1	Hereditary nonpolyposis colorectal cancer, Lynch syndrome, hereditary breast cancer-related disorders, hereditary colon cancer disorders	81295, 81296, 81297, 81432, 81433, 81435, 81436
	MSH6	mutS homolog 6 (E. coli)	Hereditary nonpolyposis colorectal cancer, Lynch syndrome, hereditary breast cancer-related disorders, hereditary colon cancer disorders	81298, 81299, 81300, 81432, 81435
MTATP6	MT-ATP6	Mitochondrially encoded ATP synthase 6	Neuropathy with ataxia and retinitis pigmentosa (NARP), Leigh syndrome	81401
	MTHFR	5,10-methylenetetrahydrofolate reductase	Hereditary hypercoagulability	81291
MTM1	MTM1	Myotubularin 1	X-linked centronuclear myopathy	81405, 81406
MTND4ND6	MT-ND4, MT-ND6	Mitochondrially encoded NADH dehydrogenase 4, mitochondrially encoded NADH dehydrogenase 6	Leber hereditary optic neuropathy (LHON)	81401
MTND5	MT-ND5	Mitochondrially encoded tRNA leucine 1 (UUA/G), mitochondrially encoded NADH dehydrogenase 5	Mitochondrial encephalopathy with lactic acidosis and stroke-like episodes (MELAS)	81401
MTRNR1	MT-RNR1	Mitochondrially encoded 12S RNA	Nonsyndromic hearing loss	81401, 81403, 81430
MTTK	MT-TK	Mitochondrially encoded tRNA lysine	Myoclonic epilepsy with ragged-red fibers (MERRF)	81401
MTTL1	MT-TL1	Mitochondrially encoded tRNA leucine 1 (UUA/G)	Diabetes and hearing loss	81401
MTTS1	MT-TS1	Mitochondrially encoded tRNA serine 1	Nonsyndromic hearing loss	81403
MTTS1RNR1	MT-TS1, MT-RNR1	Mitochondrially encoded tRNA serine 1 (UCN), mitochondrially encoded 12S RNA	Nonsyndromic sensorineural deafness (including aminoglycoside-induced nonsyndromic deafness)	81401
MUT	MUT	methylmalonyl CoA mutase	methylmalonic acidemia	81406
MUTYH	MUTYH	mutY homolog (E. coli)	MYH-associated polyposis, hereditary colon cancer disorders	81401, 81406, 81435
MYBPC3	MYBPC3	Myosin binding protein C, cardiac	Familial hypertrophic cardiomyopathy, hereditary cardiomyopathy	81407, 81439
MYD88	MYD88	Myeloid differentiation primary response 88	Waldenstrom's macroglobulinemia, lymphoplasmacytic leukemia	81305
MYH6	MYH6	Myosin, heavy chain 6, cardiac muscle, alpha	Familial dilated cardiomyopathy	81407
MYH7	MYH7	Myosin, heavy chain 7, cardiac muscle, beta	Familial hypertrophic cardiomyopathy, Laing distal myopathy, hereditary cardiomyopathy	81407, 81439
MYH11	MYH11	Myosin, heavy chain 11, smooth muscle	Thoracic aortic aneurysms and aortic dissections, aortic dysfunction or dilation	81408, 81410, 81411
MYL2	MYL2	Myosin, light chain 2, regulatory, cardiac, slow	Familial hypertrophic cardiomyopathy	81405
MYL3	MYL3	Myosin, light chain 3, alkali, ventricular, skeletal, slow	Familial hypertrophic cardiomyopathy	81405
MYLK	MYLK	Myosin light chain kinase	Aortic dysfunction or dilation	81410
MYO7A	MYO7A	Myosin VIIA	Usher syndrome, type 1, hearing loss	81407, 81430
MYO15A	MYO15A	Myosin XVA	Hearing loss	81430
MYOT	MYOT	Myotilin	Limb-girdle muscular dystrophy	81405
NDP	NDP	Norrie disease (pseudoglioma)	Norrie disease	81403, 81404
NDUFA1	NDUFA1	NADH dehydrogenase (ubiquinone) 1 alpha subcomplex, 1, 7.5kDa	Leigh syndrome, mitochondrial complex I deficiency	81404
NDUFAF2	NDUFAF2	NADH dehydrogenase (ubiquinone) 1 alpha subcomplex, assembly factor 2	Leigh syndrome, mitochondrial complex I deficiency	81404

Molecular Pathology Gene Table, *continued*

Claim Designation	Abbreviated Gene Name	Full Gene Name	Commonly Associated Proteins/Diseases (Not a complete list)	CPT Code(s)
NDUFS1	NDUFS1	NADH dehydrogenase (ubiquinone) Fe-S protein 1, 75kDa (NADH-coenzyme Q reductase)	Leigh syndrome, mitochondrial complex I deficiency	81406
NDUFS4	NDUFS4	NADH dehydrogenase (ubiquinone) Fe-S protein 4, 18kDa (NADH-coenzyme Q reductase)	Leigh syndrome, mitochondrial complex I deficiency	81404
NDUFS7	NDUFS7	NADH dehydrogenase (ubiquinone) Fe-S protein 7, 20kDa (NADH-coenzyme Q reductase)	Leigh syndrome, mitochondrial complex I deficiency	81405
NDUFS8	NDUFS8	NADH dehydrogenase (ubiquinone) Fe-S protein 8, 23kDa (NADH-coenzyme Q reductase)	Leigh syndrome, mitochondrial complex I deficiency	81405
NDUFV1	NDUFV1	NADH dehydrogenase (ubiquinone) flavoprotein 1, 51kDa	Leigh syndrome, mitochondrial complex I deficiency	81405
NEB	NEB	Nebulin	Nemaline myopathy 2	81400, 81408
NEFL	NEFL	Neurofilament, light polypeptide	Charcot-Marie-Tooth disease	81405
NF1	NF1	Neurofibromin 1	Neurofibromatosis, type 1	81408
NF2	NF2	Neurofibromin 2 (merlin)	Neurofibromatosis, type 2	81405, 81406
NHLRC1	NHLRC1	NHL repeat containing 1	Progressive myoclonus epilepsy	81403
NIPA1	NIPA1	Non-imprinted in Prader-Willi/Angelman syndrome 1	Spastic paraplegia	81404
NLGN3	NLGN3	Neuroligin 3	Autism spectrum disorders	81405
NLGN4X	NLGN4X	Neuroligin 4, X-linked	Autism spectrum disorders	81404, 81405
NOD2	NOD2	Nucleotide-binding oligomerization domain containing 2	Crohn's disease, Blau syndrome	81401
NOS	Known familial variant NOS	N/A	N/A	81403
NOTCH1	NOTCH1	Notch 1	Aortic valve disease, hematolymphoid neoplasm or disorder or solid organ neoplasm	81407, 81450, 81455
NOTCH3	NOTCH3	Notch 3	Cerebral autosomal dominant arteriopathy with subcortical infarcts and leukoencephalopathy (CADASIL)	81406
NPC1	NPC1	Niemann-Pick disease, type C1	Niemann-Pick disease	81406
NPC2	NPC2	Niemann-Pick disease, type C2 (epididymal secretory protein E1)	Niemann-Pick disease type C2	81404
NPHP1	NPHP1	Nephronophthisis 1 (juvenile)	Joubert syndrome	81405, 81406
NPHS1	NPHS1	Nephrosis 1, congenital, Finnish type (nephrin)	Congenital Finnish nephrosis	81407
NPHS2	NPHS2	Nephrosis 2, idiopathic, steroid-resistant (podocin)	Steroid-resistant nephrotic syndrome	81405
	NPM1	Nucleophosmin	Acute myeloid leukemia, hematolymphoid neoplasm or disorder or solid organ neoplasm	81310, 81450, 81455
NPM1ALK	NPM1/ALK	t(2;5)	Anaplastic large cell lymphoma	81401
NR0B1	NR0B1	Nuclear receptor subfamily 0, group B, member 1	Congenital adrenal hypoplasia	81404
	NRAS	Neuroblastoma RAS viral (v-ras) oncogene homolog	Colorectal carcinoma, Noonan spectrum disorders, solid organ neoplasm, hematolymphoid neoplasm or disorder	81311, 81442, 81445, 81450, 81455
NSD1	NSD1	Nuclear receptor binding SET domain protein 1	Sotos syndrome	81405, 81406
	NUDT15	Nudix hydrolase 15	Drug metabolism	81306
OCRL	OCRL	Oculocerebrorenal syndrome of Lowe	X-linked intellectual disability (XLID)	81470, 81471
OPA1	OPA1	Optic atrophy 1	Optic atrophy, mitochondrial disorders	81406, 81407, 81440
OPTN	OPTN	Optineurin	Amyotrophic lateral sclerosis	81406
OTC	OTC	Ornithine carbamoyltransferase	Ornithine transcarbamylase deficiency	81405
OTOF	OTOF	Otoferlin	Hearing loss	81430
PABPN1	PABPN1	Poly(A) binding protein, nuclear 1	Oculopharyngeal muscular dystrophy	81312
PAFAH1B1	PAFAH1B1	Platelet-activating factor acetylhydrolase 1b, regulatory subunit 1 (45kDa)	Lissencephaly, Miller-Dieker syndrome	81405, 81406
PAH	PAH	Phenylalanine hydroxylase	Phenylketonuria, severe inherited conditions	81406, 81443
PALB2	PALB2	Partner and localizer of BRCA2	Breast and pancreatic cancer, hereditary breast cancer-related disorders	81406, 81432

Molecular Pathology Gene Table, *continued*

Claim Designation	Abbreviated Gene Name	Full Gene Name	Commonly Associated Proteins/Diseases (Not a complete list)	CPT Code(s)
PARK2	PARK2	Parkinson protein 2, E3 ubiquitin protein ligase (parkin)	Parkinson disease	81405, 81406
PAX2	PAX2	Paired box 2	Renal coloboma syndrome	81406
PAX8PPARG	PAX8/PPARG	t(2;3) (q13;p25)	Follicular thyroid carcinoma	81401
PC	PC	Pyruvate carboxylase	Pyruvate carboxylase deficiency	81406
	PCA3/KLK3	Prostate cancer antigen 3/kallikrein-related peptidase 3	Prostate cancer	81313
PCCA	PCCA	Propionyl CoA carboxylase, alpha polypeptide	Propionic acidemia, type 1	81405, 81406
PCCB	PCCB	Propionyl CoA carboxylase, beta polypeptide	Propionic acidemia	81406
PCDH15	PCDH15	Protocadherin-related 15	Usher syndrome type 1F, Usher syndrome type 1, hearing loss	81400, 81406, 81407, 81430
PCDH19	PCDH19	Protocadherin 19	Epileptic encephalopathy	81405
PCSK9	PCSK9	Proprotein convertase subtilisin/kexin type 9	Familial hypercholesterolemia	81406
PDE6A	PDE6A	Phosphodiesterase 6A, CGMP-specific, rod, alpha	Hereditary retinal disorders	81434
PDE6B	PDE6B	Phosphodiesterase 6B, CGMP-specific, rod, beta	Hereditary retinal disorders	81434
	PDGFRA	Platelet-derived growth factor receptor, alpha polypeptide	Gastrointestinal stromal tumor, solid organ neoplasm or hematolymphoid neoplasm	81314, 81445, 81455
	PDGFRB	Platelet-derived growth factor receptor, beta polypeptide	Solid organ neoplasm or hematolymphoid neoplasm	81445, 81455
PDHA1	PDHA1	Pyruvate dehydrogenase (lipoamide) alpha 1	Lactic acidosis	81405, 81406
PDHB	PDHB	Pyruvate dehydrogenase (lipoamide) beta	Lactic acidosis	81405
PDHX	PDHX	Pyruvate dehydrogenase complex, component X	Lactic acidosis	81406
PDSS2	PDSS2	Decaprenyl diphosphate synthase subunit 2	Mitochondrial disorders	81440
PDX1	PDX1	Pancreatic and duodenal homeobox 1	Maturity-onset diabetes of the young (MODY)	81404
PGR	PGR	Progesterone receptor	Solid organ or hematolymphoid neoplasm	81445, 81455
PHEX	PHEX	Phosphate regulating endopeptidase homolog, X-linked	Hypophosphatemic rickets	81406
PHOX2B	PHOX2B	Paired-like homeobox 2b	Congenital central hypoventilation syndrome	81403, 81404
PIK3CA	PIK3CA	Phosphatidylinositol-4,5-bisphosphate 3-kinase, catalytic subunit alpha	Colorectal cancer, solid organ neoplasm or hematolymphoid neoplasm	81404, 81445, 81455
PINK1	PINK1	PTEN induced putative kinase 1	Parkinson disease	81405
PKD1	PKD1	Polycystic kidney disease 1 (autosomal dominant)	Polycystic kidney disease	81407
PKD2	PKD2	Polycystic kidney disease 2 (autosomal dominant)	Polycystic kidney disease	81406
PKHD1	PKHD1	Polycystic kidney and hepatic disease 1	Autosomal recessive polycystic kidney disease	81408
PKLR	PKLR	Pyruvate kinase, liver and RBC	Pyruvate kinase deficiency	81405
PKP2	PKP2	Plakophilin 2	Arrhythmogenic right ventricular dysplasia/cardiomyopathy 9, hereditary cardiomyopathy	81406, 81439
PLCE1	PLCE1	Phospholipase C, epsilon 1	Nephrotic syndrome type 3	81407
	PLCG2	Phospholipase C gamma 2	Chronic lymphocytic leukemia	81320
PLN	PLN	Phospholamban	Dilated cardiomyopathy, hypertrophic cardiomyopathy	81403
PLP1	PLP1	Proteolipid protein 1	Pelizaeus-Merzbacher disease, spastic paraplegia	81404, 81405
	PML/RARalpha	t(15;17) promyelocytic leukemia/retinoic acid receptor alpha	Promyelocytic leukemia	81315, 81316
	PMP22	Peripheral myelin protein 22	Charcot-Marie-Tooth disease, hereditary neuropathy with liability to pressure palsies	81324, 81325, 81326
	PMS2	Postmeiotic segregation increased 2 (S. cerevisiae)	Hereditary nonpolyposis colorectal cancer, Lynch syndrome	81317, 81318, 81319
PNKD	PNKD	Paroxysmal nonkinesigenic dyskinesia	Paroxysmal nonkinesigenic dyskinesia	81406
POLG	POLG	Polymerase (DNA directed), gamma	Alpers-Huttenlocher syndrome, autosomal dominant progressive external ophthalmoplegia, mitochondrial disorders	81406, 81440
POLG2	POLG2	Polymerase (DNA directed), gamma 2	Mitochondrial disorders	81440
POMGNT1	POMGNT1	Protein O-linked mannose beta1,2-N acetylglucosaminyltransferase	Muscle-eye-brain disease, Walker-Warburg syndrome	81406

Molecular Pathology Gene Table, *continued*

Claim Designation	Abbreviated Gene Name	Full Gene Name	Commonly Associated Proteins/Diseases (Not a complete list)	CPT Code(s)
POMT1	POMT1	Protein-O-mannosyltransferase 1	Limb-girdle muscular dystrophy (LGMD) type 2K, Walker-Warburg syndrome	81406
POMT2	POMT2	Protein-O-mannosyltransferase 2	Limb-girdle muscular dystrophy (LGMD) type 2N, Walker-Warburg syndrome	81406
POU1F1	POU1F1	POU class 1 homeobox 1	Combined pituitary hormone deficiency	81405
PPOX	PPOX	Protoporphyrinogen oxidase	Variegate porphyria	81406
PPP2R2B	PPP2R2B	Protein phosphatase 2, regulatory subunit B, beta	Spinocerebellar ataxia	81343
PQBP1	PQBP1	Polyglutamine binding protein 1	Renpenning syndrome	81404, 81405
PRAME	PRAME	Preferentially expressed antigen in melanoma	Melanoma	81401
PRKAG2	PRKAG2	Protein kinase, AMP-activated, gamma 2 non-catalytic subunit	Familial hypertrophic cardiomyopathy with Wolff-Parkinson-White syndrome, lethal congenital glycogen storage disease of heart	81406
PRKCG	PRKCG	Protein kinase C, gamma; (sodium channel, voltage-gated, type IV, alpha subunit)	Spinocerebellar ataxia; hyperkalemic periodic paralysis	81406
PRNP	PRNP	Srion protein	Genetic prion disease	81404
PROP1	PROP1	PROP paired-like homeobox 1	Combined pituitary hormone deficiency	81404
PRPF31	PRPF31	Pre-MRNA processing factor 31	Hereditary retinal disorders	81434
PRPH2	PRPH2	Peripherin 2 (retinal degeneration, slow)	Retinitis pigmentosa, hereditary retinal disorders	81404, 81434
PRSS1	PRSS1	Protease, serine, 1 (trypsin 1)	Hereditary pancreatitis	81401, 81404
PRX	PRX	Periaxin	Charcot-Marie-Tooth disease	81405
PSEN1	PSEN1	Presenilin 1	Alzheimer disease	81405
PSEN2	PSEN2	Presenilin 2 (Alzheimer disease 4)	Alzheimer disease	81406
	PTEN	Phosphatase and tensin homolog	Cowden syndrome, PTEN hamartoma tumor syndrome, hereditary breast cancer-related disorders, hereditary colon cancer disorders, solid organ neoplasm or hematolymphoid neoplasm	81321 81322, 81323, 81432, 81435, 81445, 81455
PTPN11	PTPN11	Protein tyrosine phosphatase, non-receptor type 11	Noonan syndrome, LEOPARD syndrome, Noonan spectrum disorders	81406, 81442
PYGM	PYGM	Phosphorylase, glycogen, muscle	Glycogen storage disease type V, McArdle disease	81401, 81406
RAB7A	RAB7A	RAB7A, member RAS oncogene family	Charcot-Marie-Tooth disease	81405
RAF1	RAF1	v-raf-1 murine leukemia viral oncogene homolog 1	LEOPARD syndrome, Noonan spectrum disorder	81404, 81406, 81442
RAI1	RAI1	Retinoic acid induced 1	Smith-Magenis syndrome	81405
RDH12	RDH12	Retinol dehydrogenase 12 (All-Trans/9-Cis/11-Cis)	Hereditary retinal disorders	81434
REEP1	REEP1	Receptor accessory protein 1	Spastic paraplegia, hereditary peripheral neuropathies	81405, 81448
RET	RET	Ret proto-oncogene	Multiple endocrine neoplasia, type 2A and familial medullary thyroid carcinoma, Hirschsprung disease, solid organ neoplasm or hematolymphoid neoplasm	81404, 81405, 81406, 81445, 81455
RHDDA	RHD, deletion analysis	Rh blood group, D antigen	Hemolytic disease of the fetus and newborn, Rh maternal/fetal compatibility	81403
RHDDAMB	RHD, deletion analysis, cell-free fetal DNA in maternal blood	Rh blood group, D antigen	Hemolytic disease of the fetus and newborn, Rh maternal/fetal compatibility	81403
RHO	RHO	Rhodopsin	Retinitis pigmentosa, hereditary retinal disorders	81404, 81434
RIT1	RIT1	Ras-like without CAAX 1	Noonan spectrum disorders	81442
RP1	RP1	Retinitis pigmentosa 1	Retinitis pigmentosa, hereditary retinal disorders	81404, 81434
RP2	RP2	Retinitis pigmentosa 2	Hereditary retinal disorders	81434
RPE65	RPE65	Retinal pigment epithelium-specific protein 65kDa	Retinitis pigmentosa, Leber congenital amaurosis, hereditary retinal disorders	81406, 81434
RPGR	RPGR	Retinitis pigmentosa GTPase regulator	Hereditary retinal disorders	81434
RPS19	RPS19	Ribosomal protein S19	Diamond-Blackfan anemia	81405
RPS6KA3	RPS6KA3	Ribosomal protein S6 kinase, 90kDa, polypeptide 3	X-linked intellectual disability (XLID)	81470, 81471

Molecular Pathology Gene Table, *continued*

Claim Designation	Abbreviated Gene Name	Full Gene Name	Commonly Associated Proteins/Diseases (Not a complete list)	CPT Code(s)
RRM2B	RRM2B	Ribonucleotide reductase M2 B (TP53 inducible)	Mitochondrial DNA depletion, mitochondrial disorders	81405, 81440
RUNX1	RUNX1	Runt related transcription factor 1	Acute myeloid leukemia, familial platelet disorder with associated myeloid malignancy	81334
RUNX1RUNX1T1	RUNX1/RUNX1T1	t(8;21)	Acute myeloid leukemia	81401
RYR1	RYR1	Ryanodine receptor 1, skeletal	Malignant hyperthermia	81406, 81408
RYR2	RYR2	Ryanodine receptor 2 (cardiac)	Catecholaminergic polymorphic ventricular tachycardia, arrhythmogenic right ventricular dysplasia, cardiac ion channelopathies	81408, 81413
SCN1A	SCN1A	Sodium channel, voltage-gated, type 1, alpha subunit	Generalized epilepsy with febrile seizures	81407
SCN1B	SCN1B	Sodium channel, voltage-gated, type I, beta	Brugada syndrome	81404
SCN4A	SCN4A	Sodium channel, voltage-gated, type IV, alpha subunit	Hyperkalemic periodic paralysis	81406
SCN5A	SCN5A	Sodium channel, voltage-gated, type V, alpha subunit	Familial dilated cardiomyopathy, cardiac ion channelopathies	81407, 81413
SCNN1A	SCNN1A	Sodium channel, nonvoltage-gated 1 alpha	Pseudohypoaldosteronism	81406
SCNN1B	SCNN1B	Sodium channel, nonvoltage-gated 1, beta	Liddle syndrome, pseudohypoaldosteronism	81406
SCNN1G	SCNN1G	Sodium channel, nonvoltage-gated 1, gamma	Liddle syndrome, pseudohypoaldosteronism	81406
SCO1	SCO1	SCO cytochrome oxidase deficient homolog 1	Mitochondrial respiratory chain complex IV deficiency, mitochondrial disorders	81405, 81440
SCO2	SCO2	SCO cytochrome oxidase deficient homolog 2 (SCO1L)	Mitochondrial respiratory chain complex IV deficiency, mitochondrial disorders	81404, 81440
SDHA	SDHA	Succinate dehydrogenase complex, subunit A, flavoprotein (Fp)	Leigh syndrome, mitochondrial complex II deficiency	81406
SDHB	SDHB	Succinate dehydrogenase complex, subunit B, iron sulfur	Hereditary paraganglioma, hereditary neuroendocrine tumor disorders	81405, 81437, 81438
SDHC	SDHC	Succinate dehydrogenase complex, subunit C, integral membrane protein, 15kDa	Hereditary paraganglioma-pheochromocytoma syndrome, hereditary neuroendocrine tumor disorders	81404, 81405, 81437, 81438
SDHD	SDHD	Succinate dehydrogenase complex, subunit D, integral membrane protein	Hereditary paraganglioma, hereditary neuroendocrine tumor disorders	81404, 81437, 81438
SEPT9	SEPT9	Septin 9	Colorectal cancer	81327
	SERPINA1	Serpin peptidase inhibitor, clade A, alpha-1 antiproteinase, antitrypsin, member 1	Alpha-1-antitrypsin deficiency	81332
SERPINE1	SERPINE1	Serpine peptidase inhibitor clade E, member 1, plasminogen activator inhibitor -1, PAI-1	Thrombophilia	81400
SETX	SETX	Senataxin	Ataxia	81406
SGCA	SGCA	Sarcoglycan, alpha (50kDa dystrophin-associated glycoprotein)	Limb-girdle muscular dystrophy	81405
SGCB	SGCB	Sarcoglycan, beta (43kDa dystrophin-associated glycoprotein)	Limb-girdle muscular dystrophy	81405
SGCD	SGCD	Sarcoglycan, delta (35kDa dystrophin-associated glycoprotein)	Limb-girdle muscular dystrophy	81405
SGCE	SGCE	Sarcoglycan, epsilon	Myoclonic dystonia	81405, 81406
SGCG	SGCG	Sarcoglycan, gamma (35kDa dystrophin-associated glycoprotein)	Limb-girdle muscular dystrophy	81404, 81405
SH2D1A	SH2D1A	SH2 domain containing 1A	X-linked lymphoproliferative syndrome	81403, 81404
SH3TC2	SH3TC2	SH3 domain and tetratricopeptide repeats 2	Charcot-Marie-Tooth disease	81406
SHOC2	SHOC2	Soc-2 suppressor of clear homolog	Noonan-like syndrome with loose anagen hair, Noonan spectrum disorders	81400, 81405, 81442
	Short Tandem Repeat (STR)	N/A	Pre-transplant recipient, donor germline testing, post-transplant recipient	81265, 81266
SHOX	SHOX	Short stature homeobox	Langer mesomelic dysplasia	81405
SIL1	SIL1	SIL1 homolog, endoplasmic reticulum chaperone (S. cerevisiae)	Ataxia	81405
SLC2A1	SLC2A1	Solute carrier family 2 (facilitated glucose transporter), member 1	Glucose transporter type 1 (GLUT 1) deficiency syndrome	81405

Molecular Pathology Gene Table, *continued*

Claim Designation	Abbreviated Gene Name	Full Gene Name	Commonly Associated Proteins/Diseases (Not a complete list)	CPT Code(s)
SLC2A10	SLC2A10	Solute carrier family 2 (facilitated glucose transporter), member 10	Aortic dysfunction or dilation	81410
SLC9A6	SLC9A6	Solute carrier family 9 (sodium/hydrogen exchanger), member 6	Christianson syndrome	81406
SLC12A1	SLC12A1	Solute carrier family 12 (sodium/potassium/chloride transporters), member 1	Bartter syndrome	81407
SLC12A3	SLC12A3	Solute carrier family 12 (sodium/chloride transporters), member 3	Gitelman syndrome	81407
SLC16A2	SLC16A2	Solute carrier family 16, member 2 (thyroid hormone transporter)	Specific thyroid hormone cell transporter deficiency, Allan-Herndon-Dudley syndrome, X-linked intellectual disability (XLID)	81404, 81405, 81470, 81471
SLC22A5	SLC22A5	Solute carrier family 22 (organic cation/carnitine transporter), member 5	Systemic primary carnitine deficiency	81405
SLC25A4	SLC25A4	Solute carrier family 25 (mitochondrial carrier; adenine nucleotide translocator), member 4	Progressive external ophthalmoplegia, mitochondrial disorders	81404, 81440
SLC25A20	SLC25A20	Solute carrier family 25 (carnitine/acylcarnitine translocase), member 20	Carnitine-acylcarnitine translocase deficiency	81404, 81405
SLC26A4	SLC26A4	Solute carrier family 26, member 4	Pendred syndrome, hearing loss	81406, 81430
SLC37A4	SLC37A4	Solute carrier family 37 (glucose-6-phosphate transporter), member 4	Glycogen storage disease type Ib	81406
SLCO1B1	SLCO1B1	Solute carrier organic anion transporter family, member 1B1	Adverse drug reaction	81328
SMAD3	SMAD3	SMAD family member 3	Aortic dysfunction or dilation	81410
SMAD4	SMAD4	SMAD family member 4	Hemorrhagic telangiectasia syndrome, juvenile polyposis, hereditary colon cancer disorders	81405, 81406, 81435, 81436
SMN1	SMN1	Survival of motor neuron 1, telomeric	Spinal muscular atrophy	81329, 81336, 81337
SMN1SMN2	SMN1/SMN2	Survival of motor neuron 1, telomeric/survival of motor neuron 2, centromeric	Spinal muscular atrophy	81329
	SMPD1	Sphingomyelin phosphodiesterase 1, acid lysosomal	Niemann-Pick disease, type A, Ashkenazi Jewish-associated disorders	81330, 81412
	SNRPN/UBE3A	Small nuclear ribonucleoprotein polypeptide N and ubiquitin protein ligase E3A	Prader-Willi syndrome and/or Angelman syndrome	81331
SOD1	SOD1	Superoxide dismutase 1, soluble	Amyotrophic lateral sclerosis	81404
SOS1	SOS1	Son of sevenless homolog 1	Noonan syndrome, gingival fibromatosis, Noonan spectrum disorders	81406, 81442
SPAST	SPAST	Spastin	Spastic paraplegia, hereditary peripheral neuropathies	81405, 81406, 81448
SPG11	SPG11	Spastic paraplegia 11 (autosomal recessive)	Spastic paraplegia, hereditary peripheral neuropathies	81407, 81448
SPG7	SPG7	Spastic paraplegia 7 (pure and complicated autosomal recessive)	Spastic paraplegia	81405, 81406
SPINK1	SPINK1	Serine peptidase inhibitor, Kazal type 1	Hereditary pancreatitis	81404
SPRED1	SPRED1	Sprouty-related, EVH1 domain containing 1	Legius syndrome	81405
SPTBN2	SPTBN2	Spectrin, beta, non-erythrocytic 2	Spinocerebellar ataxia	81407
SPTLC1	SPTLC1	Serine palmitoyltransferase, long chain base subunit 1	Hereditary peripheral neuropathies	81448
SRY	SRY	Sex determining region Y	46, XX testicular disorder of sex development, gonadal dysgenesis	81400
SS18SSX1	SS18/SSX1	t(X;18)	Synovial sarcoma	81401
SS18SSX2	SS18/SSX2	t(X;18)	Synovial sarcoma	81401
STAT3	STAT3	Signal transducer and activator of transcription 3 (acute-phase response factor)	Autosomal dominant hyper-IgE syndrome	81405
STK11	STK11	Serine/threonine kinase 11	Peutz-Jeghers syndrome, hereditary breast cancer-related disorders, hereditary colon cancer disorders	81404, 81405, 81432, 81433, 81435, 81436
STRC	STRC	Stereocilin	Hearing loss	81431
STXBP1	STXBP1	Syntaxin binding protein 1	Epileptic encephalopathy	81406

Molecular Pathology Gene Table, *continued*

Claim Designation	Abbreviated Gene Name	Full Gene Name	Commonly Associated Proteins/Diseases (Not a complete list)	CPT Code(s)
SUCLA2	SUCLA2	Succinate-CoA ligase ADP-forming beta subunit	Mitochondrial disorders	81440
SUCLG1	SUCLG1	Succinate-CoA ligase alpha subunit	Mitochondrial disorders	81440
SURF1	SURF1	Surfeit 1	Mitochondrial respiratory chain complex IV deficiency	81405
TACO1	TACO1	Translational activator of mitochondrial encoded cytochrome c oxidase I	Mitochondrial respiratory chain complex IV deficiency	81404
TARDBP	TARDBP	TAR DNA binding protein	Amyotrophic lateral sclerosis	81405
TAZ	TAZ	tafazzin	Methylglutaconic aciduria type 2, Barth syndrome, mitochondrial disorders	81406, 81440
TBP	TBP	TATA box binding protein	Spinocerebellar ataxia	81344
TBX5	TBX5	T-box 5	Holt-Oram syndrome	81405
TCF4	TCF4	Transcription factor 4	Pitt-Hopkins syndrome	81405, 81406
	TERT	Telomerase reverse transcriptase	Thyroid carcinoma, glioblastoma multiforme	81345
	TGFBI	Transforming growth factor beta-induced	Corneal dystrophy	81333
TGFBR1	TGFBR1	Transforming growth factor, beta receptor 1	Marfan syndrome, aortic dysfunction or dilation	81405, 81410, 81411
TGFBR2	TGFBR2	Transforming growth factor, beta receptor 2	Marfan syndrome, aortic dysfunction or dilation	81405, 81410, 81411
TH	TH	Tyrosine hydroxylase	Segawa syndrome	81406
THAP1	THAP1	THAP domain containing, apoptosis associated protein 1	Torsion dystonia	81404
THRB	THRB	Thyroid hormone receptor, beta	Thyroid hormone resistance, thyroid hormone beta receptor deficiency	81405
TK2	TK2	Thymidine kinase 2, mitochondrial	Mitochondrial DNA depletion syndrome, mitochondrial disorders	81405, 81440
TMC1	TMC1	Transmembrane channel-like 1	Hearing loss	81430
TMEM43	TMEM43	Transmembrane protein 43	Arrhythmogenic right ventricular cardiomyopathy	81406
TMEM67	TMEM67	Transmembrane protein 67	Joubert syndrome	81407
TMEM127	TMEM127	Transmembrane protein 127	Hereditary neuroendocrine tumor disorders	81437
TMPRSS3	TMPRSS3	Transmembrane protease, serine 3	Hearing loss	81430
TNNC1	TNNC1	Troponin C type 1 (slow)	Hypertrophic cardiomyopathy or dilated cardiomyopathy	81405
TNNI3	TNNI3	Troponin I, type 3 (cardiac)	Familial hypertrophic cardiomyopathy	81405
TNNT2	TNNT2	Troponin T, type 2 (cardiac)	Familial hypertrophic cardiomyopathy	81406
TOR1A	TOR1A	Torsin family 1, member A (torsin A)	Early-onset primary dystonia (DYT1), torsion dystonia	81400, 81404
TP53	TP53	Tumor protein 53	Tumor samples, Li-Fraumeni syndrome, hereditary breast cancer-related disorders	81404, 81405, 81432
TPM1	TPM1	Tropomyosin 1 (alpha)	Familial hypertrophic cardiomyopathy	81405
TPMT	TPMT	Thiopurine S-methyltransferase	Drug metabolism	81335
	TRB@	T cell antigen receptor, beta	Leukemia and lymphoma	81340, 81341
TRD	TRD@	T cell antigen receptor, delta	Leukemia and lymphoma	81402
	TRG@	T cell antigen receptor, gamma	Leukemia and lymphoma	81342
TRPC6	TRPC6	Transient receptor potential cation channel, subfamily C, member 6	Focal segmental glomerulosclerosis	81406
TSC1	TSC1	Tuberous sclerosis 1	Tuberous sclerosis	81405, 81406
TSC2	TSC2	Tuberous sclerosis 2	Tuberous sclerosis	81406, 81407
TTN	TTN	Titin	Hereditary cardiomyopathy	81439
TTPA	TTPA	Tocopherol (alpha) transfer protein	Ataxia	81404
TTR	TTR	Transthyretin	Familial transthyretin amyloidosis	81404
TWIST1	TWIST1	Twist homolog 1 (Drosophila)	Saethre-Chotzen syndrome	81403, 81404
TYMP	TYMP	Thymidine phosphorylase	Mitochondrial DNA depletion syndrome, mitochondrial disorders	81405, 81440

Molecular Pathology Gene Table, *continued*

Claim Designation	Abbreviated Gene Name	Full Gene Name	Commonly Associated Proteins/Diseases (Not a complete list)	CPT Code(s)
TYMS	TYMS	Thymidylate synthetase	5-fluorouracil/5-FU drug metabolism	81346
TYR	TYR	Tyrosinase (oculocutaneous albinism IA)	Oculocutaneous albinism IA	81404
UBA1	UBA1	Ubiquitin-like modifier activating enzyme 1	Spinal muscular atrophy, X-linked	81403
UBE3A	UBE3A	Ubiquitin protein ligase E3A	Angelman syndrome	81406
	UGT1A1	UDP glucuronosyltransferase 1 family, polypeptide A1	Irinotecan metabolism	81350
UMOD	UMOD	Uromodulin	Glomerulocystic kidney disease with hyperuricemia and isosthenuria	81406
UPD	Uniparental disomy	UPD	Russell-Silver syndrome, Prader-Willi/Angelman syndrome	81402
USH1C	USH1C	Usher syndrome 1C (autosomal recessive, severe)	Usher syndrome, type 1, hearing loss	81407, 81430
USH1G	USH1G	Usher syndrome 1G (autosomal recessive)	Usher syndrome, type 1, hearing loss	81404, 81430
USH2A	USH2A	Usher syndrome 2A (autosomal recessive, mild)	Usher syndrome, type 2, hearing loss, hereditary retinal disorders	81408, 81430, 81434
VHL	VHL	Von Hippel-Lindau tumor suppressor	Von Hippel-Lindau familial cancer syndrome, hereditary neuroendocrine tumor disorders	81403, 81404, 81437, 81438
	VKORC1	Vitamin K epoxide reductase complex, subunit 1	Warfarin metabolism	81355
VPS13B	VPS13B	Vacuolar protein sorting 13 homolog B (yeast)	Cohen syndrome	81407, 81408
VWF	VWF	Von Willebrand factor	Von Willebrand disease types 1, 1C, 2A, 2B, 2M, 2N, 3	81401, 81403, 81404, 81405, 81406, 81408
WAS	WAS	Wiskott-Aldrich syndrome (eczema-thrombocytopenia)	Wiskott-Aldrich syndrome	81406
WDR62	WDR62	WD repeat domain 62	Primary autosomal recessive microcephaly	81407
WFS1	WFS1	Wolfram syndrome 1	Hearing loss	81430
WT1	WT1	Wilms tumor 1	Denys-Drash syndrome, familial Wilms tumor	81405
ZEB2	ZEB2	Zinc finger E-box binding homeobox 2	Mowat-Wilson syndrome	81404, 81405
ZNF41	ZNF41	Zinc finger protein 41	X-linked mental retardation 89	81404

Pathology and Laboratory Guidelines

Guidelines to direct general reporting of services are presented in the **Introduction.** Some of the commonalities are repeated here for the convenience of those referring to this section on **Pathology and Laboratory.** Other definitions and items unique to Pathology and Laboratory are also listed.

Services in Pathology and Laboratory

Services in Pathology and Laboratory are provided by a physician or by technologists under responsible supervision of a physician.

Separate or Multiple Procedures

It is appropriate to designate multiple procedures that are rendered on the same date by separate entries.

Unlisted Service or Procedure

A service or procedure may be provided that is not listed in this edition of the CPT codebook. When reporting such a service, the appropriate "Unlisted Procedure" code may be used to indicate the service, identifying it by "Special Report" as discussed below. The "Unlisted Procedures" and accompanying codes for **Pathology and Laboratory** are as follows:

81099 Unlisted urinalysis procedure

81479 Unlisted molecular pathology procedure

81599 Unlisted multianalyte assay with algorithmic analysis

84999 Unlisted chemistry procedure

85999 Unlisted hematology and coagulation procedure

86486 unlisted antigen, each

86849 Unlisted immunology procedure

86999 Unlisted transfusion medicine procedure

87999 Unlisted microbiology procedure

88099 Unlisted necropsy (autopsy) procedure

88199 Unlisted cytopathology procedure

88299 Unlisted cytogenetic study

88399 Unlisted surgical pathology procedure

88749 Unlisted in vivo (eg, transcutaneous) laboratory service

89240 Unlisted miscellaneous pathology test

89398 Unlisted reproductive medicine laboratory procedure

Special Report

A service that is rarely provided, unusual, variable, or new may require a special report. Pertinent information should include an adequate definition or description of the nature, extent, and need for the procedure; and the time, effort, and equipment necessary to provide the service.

Pathology and Laboratory

Organ or Disease-Oriented Panels

These panels were developed for coding purposes only and should not be interpreted as clinical parameters. The tests listed with each panel identify the defined components of that panel.

These panel components are not intended to limit the performance of other tests. If one performs tests in addition to those specifically indicated for a particular panel, those tests should be reported separately in addition to the panel code.

Do not report two or more panel codes that include any of the same constituent tests performed from the same patient collection. If a group of tests overlaps two or more panels, report the panel that incorporates the greater number of tests to fulfill the code definition and report the remaining tests using individual test codes (eg, do not report 80047 in conjunction with 80053).

80047 Basic metabolic panel (Calcium, ionized)

This panel must include the following:

Calcium, ionized (82330)

Carbon dioxide (bicarbonate) (82374)

Chloride (82435)

Creatinine (82565)

Glucose (82947)

Potassium (84132)

Sodium (84295)

Urea Nitrogen (BUN) (84520)

➔ *CPT Changes: An Insider's View* 2008

➔ *CPT Assistant* Apr 08:5, Apr 13:10

80048 Basic metabolic panel (Calcium, total)

This panel must include the following:

Calcium, total (82310)

Carbon dioxide (bicarbonate) (82374)

Chloride (82435)

Creatinine (82565)

Glucose (82947)

Potassium (84132)

Sodium (84295)

Urea nitrogen (BUN) (84520)

➔ *CPT Changes: An Insider's View* 2000, 2008, 2009

➔ *CPT Assistant* Jan 98:6, Sep 99:11, Nov 99:44, Jan 00:7, Aug 05:9

80050 General health panel

This panel must include the following:

Comprehensive metabolic panel (80053)

Blood count, complete (CBC), automated and automated differential WBC count (85025 or 85027 and 85004)

OR

Blood count, complete (CBC), automated (85027) and appropriate manual differential WBC count (85007 or 85009)

Thyroid stimulating hormone (TSH) (84443)

➔ *CPT Changes: An Insider's View* 2001, 2004

➔ *CPT Assistant* Winter 92:14, Summer 93:14, Jun 97:10, Nov 97:28, Jan 98:6, Sep 99:11

80051 Electrolyte panel

This panel must include the following:

Carbon dioxide (bicarbonate) (82374)

Chloride (82435)

Potassium (84132)

Sodium (84295)

➔ *CPT Assistant* Nov 97:28, Jan 98:7, Sep 99:11

80053 Comprehensive metabolic panel

This panel must include the following:

Albumin (82040)

Bilirubin, total (82247)

Calcium, total (82310)

Carbon dioxide (bicarbonate) (82374)

Chloride (82435)

Creatinine (82565)

Glucose (82947)

Phosphatase, alkaline (84075)

Potassium (84132)

Protein, total (84155)

Sodium (84295)

Transferase, alanine amino (ALT) (SGPT) (84460)

Transferase, aspartate amino (AST) (SGOT) (84450)

Urea nitrogen (BUN) (84520)

➔ *CPT Changes: An Insider's View* 2000, 2009

➔ *CPT Assistant* Jan 98:6, Nov 98:23, Sep 99:11, Nov 99:44, May 00:11, Jan 05:46, Apr 08:5, Apr 10:11, Apr 13:10

80055 Obstetric panel

This panel must include the following:

Blood count, complete (CBC), automated and automated differential WBC count (85025 or 85027 and 85004)

OR

Blood count, complete (CBC), automated (85027) and appropriate manual differential WBC count (85007 or 85009)

Hepatitis B surface antigen (HBsAg) (87340)

Antibody, rubella (86762)

Syphilis test, non-treponemal antibody; qualitative (eg, VDRL, RPR, ART) (86592)

Antibody screen, RBC, each serum technique (86850)

Blood typing, ABO (86900) AND

Blood typing, Rh (D) (86901)

➔ *CPT Changes: An Insider's View* 2004

➔ *CPT Assistant* Winter 92:14, Summer 93:14, Jun 97:10, Apr 99:6, Sep 99:11

(When syphilis screening is performed using a treponemal antibody approach [86780], do not use 80055. Use the individual codes for the tests performed in the obstetric panel)

 # 80081 Obstetric panel (includes HIV testing)

This panel must include the following:

Blood count, complete (CBC), and automated differential WBC count (85025 or 85027 and 85004)

OR

Blood count, complete (CBC), automated (85027) and appropriate manual differential WBC count (85007 or 85009)

Hepatitis B surface antigen (HBsAg) (87340)

HIV-1 antigen(s), with HIV-1 and HIV-2 antibodies, single result (87389)

Antibody, rubella (86762)

Syphilis test, non-treponemal antibody; qualitative (eg, VDRL, RPR, ART) (86592)

Antibody screen, RBC, each serum technique (86850)

Blood typing, ABO (86900) AND

Blood typing, Rh (D) (86901)

➔ *CPT Changes: An Insider's View* 2016

(When syphilis screening is performed using a treponemal antibody approach [86780], do not use 80081. Use the individual codes for the tests performed in the Obstetric panel)

80061 Lipid panel

This panel must include the following:

Cholesterol, serum, total (82465)

Lipoprotein, direct measurement, high density cholesterol (HDL cholesterol) (83718)

Triglycerides (84478)

➔ *CPT Assistant* Winter 92:14, Summer 93:14, Jun 97:10, Sep 99:11, Mar 00:11, Feb 05:9, Sep 17:12

80069 Renal function panel

This panel must include the following:

Albumin (82040)

Calcium, total (82310)

Carbon dioxide (bicarbonate) (82374)

Chloride (82435)

Creatinine (82565)

Glucose (82947)

Phosphorus inorganic (phosphate) (84100)

Potassium (84132)

Sodium (84295)

Urea nitrogen (BUN) (84520)

➔ *CPT Changes: An Insider's View* 2000, 2009

➔ *CPT Assistant* Sep 99:11, Nov 99:44

80074 Acute hepatitis panel

This panel must include the following:

Hepatitis A antibody (HAAb), IgM antibody (86709)

Hepatitis B core antibody (HBcAb), IgM antibody (86705)

Hepatitis B surface antigen (HBsAg) (87340)

Hepatitis C antibody (86803)

➔ *CPT Changes: An Insider's View* 2000

➔ *CPT Assistant* Sep 99:11, Nov 99:45

80076 Hepatic function panel

This panel must include the following:

Albumin (82040)

Bilirubin, total (82247)

Bilirubin, direct (82248)

Phosphatase, alkaline (84075)

Protein, total (84155)

Transferase, alanine amino (ALT) (SGPT) (84460)

Transferase, aspartate amino (AST) (SGOT) (84450)

➔ *CPT Changes: An Insider's View* 2000

➔ *CPT Assistant* Winter 92:14, Summer 93:14, Jun 97:10, Jan 98:6, Apr 99:6, Sep 99:11, Nov 99:45, Jan 00:7, Aug 05:9

80081 Code is out of numerical sequence. See 80053-80069

Drug Assay

Drug procedures are divided into three subsections: **Therapeutic Drug Assay**, **Drug Assay**, and **Chemistry**—with code selection dependent on the purpose and type of patient results obtained. Therapeutic Drug Assays are performed to monitor clinical response to a known, prescribed medication. The two major categories for drug testing in the Drug Assay subsection are:

1. **Presumptive Drug Class** procedures are used to identify possible use or non-use of a drug or drug class. A presumptive test may be followed by a definitive test in order to specifically identify drugs or metabolites.
2. **Definitive Drug Class** procedures are qualitative or quantitative test to identify possible use or non-use of a drug. These test identify specific drugs and associated metabolites, if performed. A presumptive test is not required prior to a definitive drug test.

The material for drug class procedures may be any specimen type unless otherwise specified in the code descriptor (eg, urine, blood, oral fluid, meconium, hair). Procedures can be qualitative (eg, positive/negative or present/absent), semi-quantitative, or quantitative (measured) depending on the purpose of the testing. Therapeutic drug assay (TDA) procedures are typically quantitative tests and the specimen type is whole blood, serum, plasma, or cerebrospinal fluid. *(continued on page 542)*

DEFINITIONS AND ACRONYM CONVERSION LISTING

Drug Testing Term/Acronym	Definition
6-MAM	Acronym for the heroin drug metabolite 6-monacetylmorphine
Acid	Descriptor for classifying drug/drug metabolite molecules based upon chemical ionization properties. Laboratory procedures for drug isolation and identification may include acid, base, or neutral groupings.
AM	A category of synthetic marijuana drugs discovered by and named after Alexandros Makriyannis at Northeastern University
Analog	A structural derivative of a parent chemical compound that often differs from it by a single element
Analyte	The substance or chemical constituent that is of interest in an analytical procedure
Base	Descriptor for classifying drug/drug metabolite molecules based upon chemical ionization properties. Laboratory procedures for drug isolation and identification may include acid, base, or neutral groupings.
Card(s)	Multiplexed presumptive drug class(es) immunoassay product that is read by visual observation, including instrumented when performed
Cassette(s)	Multiplexed presumptive drug class immunoassay product(s) that is read by visual observation, including instrumented when performed
CEDIA	Acronym for Cloned-Enzyme-Donor-Immuno-Assay. CEDIA immunoassay is a competitive antibody binding procedure that utilizes enzyme donor fragment-labeled antigens (drugs) to compete for antigens (drugs) contained in the patient sample. Recombination of enzyme donor fragment and enzyme acceptor fragment produces a functional enzyme. CEDIA immunoassay enzyme activity is proportional to concentration of drug(s) detected.
Chromatography	An analytical technique used to separate components of a mixture. See thin layer chromatography, gas chromatography, and high performance chromatography.
Confirmatory	Term used to describe definitive identification/quantitation procedures that are secondary to presumptive screening methods
DART	Acronym for Direct-Analysis-in-Real-Time. DART is an atmospheric pressure ionization method for mass spectrometry analysis
Definitive Drug Procedure	A procedure that provides specific identification of individual drugs and drug metabolites
DESI	Acronym for Desorption-ElectroSpray-Ionization. DESI is a combination of electrospray ionization and desorption ionization methods for mass spectrometry analysis.
Dipstick	A multiplexed presumptive drug class immunoassay product that is read by visual observation, including instrumented when performed
Drug test cup	A multiplexed presumptive drug class immunoassay product that is read by visual observation, including instrumented when performed
EDDP	Acronym for the methadone drug metabolite 2-ethylidene-1,5-dimethyl-3,3-diphenylpyrrolidine

DEFINITIONS AND ACRONYM CONVERSION LISTING

Drug Testing Term/Acronym	Definition
EIA	Acronym for Enzyme-Immuno-Assay. Enzyme immunoassay is a competitive antibody binding procedure that utilizes enzyme-labeled antigens (drugs) to compete for antigens (drugs) contained in the patient sample. Enzyme immunoassay enzyme activity is proportional to concentration of drug(s) detected
ELISA	Acronym for Enzyme-Linked Immunosorbent Assay. ELISA is a competitive binding immunoassay that is designed to measure antigens (drugs) or antibodies. ELISA immunoassay results are proportional to concentration of drug(s) detected.
EMIT	Acronym for Enzyme-Multiplied-Immunoassay-Test. EMIT is a trade name for a type of enzyme immunoassay (EIA).
FPIA	Acronym for Fluorescence-Polarization-Immuno-Assay. FPIA is a competitive binding immunoassay that utilizes fluorescein-labeled antigens (drugs) to compete for antigens (drugs) contained in the patient sample. The measure of polarized light emission is inversely proportional to the concentration of drug(s) detected.
Gas chromatography	Gas chromatography is a chromatography technique in which patient sample preparations are vaporized into a gas (mobile phase) which flows through a tubular column (containing a stationary phase) and into a detector. The retention time of a drug on the column is determined by partitioning characteristics of the drug into the mobile and stationary phases. Chromatography column detectors may be non-specific (eg, flame ionization) or specific (eg, mass spectrometry). The combination of column retention time and specific detector response provides a definitive identification of the drug or drug metabolite.
GC	Acronym for gas chromatography
GC-MS	Acronym for gas chromatography mass spectrometry
GC-MS/MS	Acronym for gas chromatography mass spectrometry/mass spectrometry
High performance liquid chromatography	High performance liquid chromatography is a chromatography technique in which patient sample preparations are injected into a liquid (mobile phase) which flows through a tubular column (containing a stationary phase) and into a detector. The retention time of a drug on the column is determined by partitioning characteristics of the drug into the mobile and stationary phases. Chromatography column detectors may be non-specific (eg, ultra-violet spectrophotometry) or specific (eg, mass spectrometry). The combination of column retention time and specific detector response provides a definitive identification of the drug or drug metabolite. High performance liquid chromatography is also called high pressure liquid chromatography.
HPLC	Acronym for high performance liquid chromatography
HU	A category of synthetic marijuana drugs discovered by and named after Raphael Mechoulam at Hebrew University
IA	Acronym for immunoassay
Immunoassay	Antigen-antibody binding procedures utilized to detect antigens (eg, drugs and/or drug metabolites) in patient samples. Immunoassay designs include competitive or non-competitive with various mechanisms for detection.
Isobaric	In mass spectrometry, ions with the same mass
Isomers	Compounds that have the same molecular formula but differ in structural formula
JWH	A category of synthetic marijuana drugs discovered by and named after John W. Huffman at Clemson University.
KIMS	Acronym for kinetic interaction of microparticles in solution. KIMS immunoassay is a competitive antibody binding procedure that utilizes microparticle-labeled antigens (drugs) to compete for antigens (drugs) contained in the patient sample. Microparticle immunoassay absorbance increase is inversely proportional to concentration of drug(s) detected.
LC-MS	Acronym for liquid chromatography mass spectrometry
LC-MS/MS	Acronym for liquid chromatography mass spectrometry/mass spectrometry
LDTD	Acronym for laser diode thermal desorption. LDTD is a combination of atmospheric pressure chemical ionization and laser diode thermal desorption methods for mass spectrometry analysis.
MALDI	Acronym for matrix assisted laser desorption/Ionization mass spectrometry. MALDI is a soft ionization technique that reduces molecular fragmentation.
MDA	Acronym for the drug 3,4-methylenedioxyamphetamine. MDA is also a drug metabolite of MDMA.
MDEA	Acronym for the drug 3,4-methylenedioxy-N-ethylamphetamine

DEFINITIONS AND ACRONYM CONVERSION LISTING

Drug Testing Term/Acronym	Definition
MDMA	Acronym for the drug 3,4-methylenedioxy-N-methylamphetamine
MDPV	Acronym for the drug methylenedioxypyrovalerone
MS	Acronym for mass spectrometry. MS is an identification technique that measures the charge-to-mass ratio of charged particles. There are several types of mass spectrometry instruments, such as magnetic sectoring, time of flight, quadrapole mass filter, ion traps, and Fourier transformation. Mass spectrometry is used as part of the process to assign definitive identification of drugs and drug metabolites.
MS/MS	Acronym for mass spectrometry/mass spectrometry. MS/MS instruments combine multiple units of mass spectrometry filters into a single instrument. MS/MS is also called tandem mass spectrometry.
MS-TOF	Acronym for mass spectrometry time of flight. Time of flight is a mass spectrometry identification technique that utilizes ion velocity to determine the mass-to-charge ratio.
Multiplexed	Descriptor for a multiple component test device that simultaneously measures multiple analytes (drug classes) in a single analysis.
Neutral	Descriptor for classifying drug/drug metabolite molecules based upon chemical ionization properties. Laboratory procedures for drug isolation and identification may include acid, base, or neutral groupings.
ng/mL	Unit of measure for weight per volume calculated as nanograms per milliliter. The ng/mL unit of measure is equivalent to the ug/L unit of measure.
Optical observation	Optical observation refers to procedure results that are interpreted visually with or without instrumentation assistance.
Opiate	Medicinal category of narcotic alkaloid drugs that are natural products in the opium poppy plant *Papaver somniferum*. This immunoassay class of drugs typically includes detection of codeine, dihydrocodeine, hydrocodone, hydromorphone, and morphine.
Opioids	A category of medicinal synthetic or semi-synthetic narcotic alkaloid opioid receptor stimulating drugs including butorphanol, desomorphine, dextromethorphan, dextrorphan, levorphanol, meperidine, naloxone, naltrexone, normeperidine, and pentazocine.
Presumptive	Drug test results that indicate possible, but not definitive, presence of drugs and/or drug metabolites
QTOF	Acronym for quadrapole-time of flight mass spectrometry. QTOF is a hybrid mass spectrometry identification technique that combines ion velocity with tandem quadrapole mass spectrometry (MS or MS/MS) to determine the mass-to-charge ratio.
RCS	A category of synthetic marijuana drugs that are analogs of JHW compounds. See JWH.
RIA	Acronym for radio-immuno-assay. Radioimmunoassay is a competitive antibody binding procedure that utilizes radioactive-labeled antigens (drugs) to compete for antigens (drugs) contained in the patient sample. The measure of radioactivity is inversely proportional to concentration of drug(s) detected.
Stereoisomers	Isomeric molecules that have the same molecular formula and sequence of bonded atoms (constitution), but that differ only in the three-dimensional orientations of their atoms in space
Substance	A substance is a drug that does not have an established therapeutic use as distinguished from other analytes listed in the Chemistry section (82009-84999).
TDM	Acronym for therapeutic drug monitoring
THC	Acronym for marijuana active drug ingredient tetrahydrocannabinol
Therapeutic Drug Monitoring	Analysis of blood (serum, plasma) drug concentration to monitor clinical response to therapy
Time of flight	Time of flight is a mass spectrometry technique that utilizes ion velocity to determine the mass-to-charge ratio
TLC	Acronym for thin layer chromatography
TOF	Acronym for time of flight
ug/L	Unit of measure for mass per volume calculated as micrograms per liter. The ug/L unit of measure is equivalent to the ng/mL unit of measure.

(continued from page 539)

When the same procedure(s) is performed on more than one specimen type (eg, blood and urine), the appropriate code is reported separately for each specimen type using modifier 59.

Drugs or classes of drugs may be commonly assayed first by a presumptive screening method followed by a definitive drug identification method. Presumptive methods include, but are not limited to, immunoassays (IA, EIA, ELISA, RIA, EMIT, FPIA, etc), enzymatic methods (alcohol dehydrogenase, etc), chromatographic methods without mass spectrometry (TLC, HPLC, GC, etc), or mass spectrometry without adequate drug resolution by chromatography (MS-TOF, DART, DESI, LDTD, MALDI). LC-MS, LCMS/MS, or mass spectrometry without adequate drug resolution by chromatography may also be used for presumptive testing if the chromatographic phase is not adequate to identify individual drugs and distinguish between structural isomers or isobaric compounds. All drug class immunoassays are considered presumptive, whether qualitative, semi-quantitative, or quantitative. Methods that cannot distinguish between structural isomers (such as morphine and hydromorphone or methamphetamine and phentermine) are also considered presumptive.

Definitive drug identification methods are able to identify individual drugs and distinguish between structural isomers but not necessarily stereoisomers. Definitive methods include, but are not limited to, gas chromatography with mass spectrometry (any type, single or tandem) and liquid chromatography mass spectrometry (any type, single or tandem) and excludes immunoassays (eg, IA, EIA, ELISA, RIA, EMIT, FPIA), and enzymatic methods (eg, alcohol dehydrogenase).

For chromatography, each combination of stationary and mobile phase is to be counted as one procedure.

Presumptive Drug Class Screening

Drugs or classes of drugs may be commonly assayed first by a presumptive screening method followed by a definitive drug identification method. The methodology is considered when coding presumptive procedures. Each code (80305, 80306, 80307) represents all drugs and drug classes performed by the respective methodology per date of service. Each code also includes all sample validation procedures performed. Examples of sample validation procedures may include, but are not limited to, pH, specific gravity, and nitrite. The codes (80305, 80306, 80307) represent three different method categories:

1. Code 80305 is used to report procedures in which the results are read by direct optical observation. The results are visually read. Examples of these procedures are dipsticks, cups, cards, and cartridges. Report 80305 once, irrespective of the number of direct observation drug class procedures performed or results on any date of service.
2. Code 80306 is used to report procedures when an instrument is used to assist in determining the result of a direct optical observation methodology. Examples of these procedures are dipsticks, cards, and cartridges inserted into an instrument that determines the final result of an optical observation methodology. Report 80306 once, irrespective of the number of drug class procedures or results on any date of service.
3. Code 80307 is used to report any number of devices or procedures by instrumented chemistry analyzers. There are many different instrumented methodologies available to perform presumptive drug assays. Examples include immunoassay (eg, EIA, ELISA, EMIT, FPIA, IA, KIMS, RIA), chromatography (eg, GC, HPLC), and mass spectrometry, either with or without chromatography (eg, DART, DESI, GC-MS, GC-MS/MS, LC-MS, LC-MS/MS, LDTD, MALDI, TOF). Some of these methodologies may be used for definitive drug testing also, but, for the purpose of presumptive drug testing, the presumptive method is insufficient to provide definitive drug identification. Report 80307 once, irrespective of the number of drug class procedures or results on any date of service.

(80300, 80301, 80302, 80303, 80304 have been deleted. To report, see 80305, 80306, 80307)

 # 80305 Drug test(s), presumptive, any number of drug classes, any number of devices or procedures; capable of being read by direct optical observation only (eg, utilizing immunoassay [eg, dipsticks, cups, cards, or cartridges]), includes sample validation when performed, per date of service

➲ *CPT Changes: An Insider's View* 2017, 2018
➲ *CPT Assistant* Mar 17:6

 # 80306 read by instrument assisted direct optical observation (eg, utilizing immunoassay [eg, dipsticks, cups, cards, or cartridges]), includes sample validation when performed, per date of service

➲ *CPT Changes: An Insider's View* 2017, 2018
➲ *CPT Assistant* Mar 17:6

 # 80307 by instrument chemistry analyzers (eg, utilizing immunoassay [eg, EIA, ELISA, EMIT, FPIA, IA, KIMS, RIA]), chromatography (eg, GC, HPLC), and mass spectrometry either with or without chromatography, (eg, DART, DESI, GC-MS, GC-MS/MS, LC-MS, LC-MS/MS, LDTD, MALDI, TOF) includes sample validation when performed, per date of service

➲ *CPT Changes: An Insider's View* 2017, 2018
➲ *CPT Assistant* Mar 17:6

Definitive Drug Testing

Definitive drug identification methods are able to identify individual drugs and distinguish between structural isomers but not necessarily stereoisomers. Definitive methods include, but are not limited to, gas chromatography with mass spectrometry (any type, single or tandem) and liquid chromatography mass spectrometry (any type, single or tandem) and exclude immunoassays (eg, IA, EIA, ELISA, RIA, EMIT, FPIA) and enzymatic methods (eg, alcohol dehydrogenase).

Use 80320-80377 to report definitive drug class procedures. Definitive testing may be qualitative, quantitative, or a combination of qualitative and quantitative for the same patient on the same date of service.

The **Definitive Drug Classes Listing** provides the drug classes, their associated CPT codes, and the drugs included in each class. Each category of a drug class, including metabolite(s) if performed (except stereoisomers), is reported once per date of service. Metabolites not listed in the table may be reported using the code for the parent drug. Drug class metabolite(s) is not reported separately unless the metabolite(s) is listed as a separate category in **Definitive Drug Classes Listing** (eg, heroin metabolite).

Drug classes may contain one or more codes based on the number of analytes. For example, an analysis in which five or more amphetamines and/or amphetamine metabolites would be reported with 80326. The code is based on the number of reported analytes and not the capacity of the analysis.

Definitive drug procedures that are not specified in 80320-80373 should be reported using the unlisted definitive procedure codes 80375, 80376, 80377, unless the specific analyte is listed in the **Therapeutic Drug Assays** (80150-80203) or **Chemistry** (82009-84830) sections.

See the **Definitive Drug Classes Listing** Table for a listing of the more common analytes within each drug class.

 # 80320 Alcohols
➔ *CPT Changes: An Insider's View* 2015
➔ *CPT Assistant* Apr 15:3

 # 80321 Alcohol biomarkers; 1 or 2
➔ *CPT Changes: An Insider's View* 2015

 # 80322 3 or more
➔ *CPT Changes: An Insider's View* 2015

 # 80323 Alkaloids, not otherwise specified
➔ *CPT Changes: An Insider's View* 2015

 # 80324 Amphetamines; 1 or 2
➔ *CPT Changes: An Insider's View* 2015

 # 80325 3 or 4
➔ *CPT Changes: An Insider's View* 2015

 # 80326 5 or more
➔ *CPT Changes: An Insider's View* 2015

 # 80327 Anabolic steroids; 1 or 2
➔ *CPT Changes: An Insider's View* 2015
➔ *CPT Assistant* Apr 15:5

 # 80328 3 or more
➔ *CPT Changes: An Insider's View* 2015
➔ *CPT Assistant* Apr 15:5

►(For dihydrotestosterone analysis for endogenous hormone levels or therapeutic monitoring, use 82642)◄

 # 80329 Analgesics, non-opioid; 1 or 2
➔ *CPT Changes: An Insider's View* 2015

 # 80330 3-5
➔ *CPT Changes: An Insider's View* 2015

 # 80331 6 or more
➔ *CPT Changes: An Insider's View* 2015

 # 80332 Antidepressants, serotonergic class; 1 or 2
➔ *CPT Changes: An Insider's View* 2015

 # 80333 3-5
➔ *CPT Changes: An Insider's View* 2015

 # 80334 6 or more
➔ *CPT Changes: An Insider's View* 2015

 # 80335 Antidepressants, tricyclic and other cyclicals; 1 or 2
➔ *CPT Changes: An Insider's View* 2015

 # 80336 3-5
➔ *CPT Changes: An Insider's View* 2015

 # 80337 6 or more
➔ *CPT Changes: An Insider's View* 2015

 # 80338 Antidepressants, not otherwise specified
➔ *CPT Changes: An Insider's View* 2015

 # 80339 Antiepileptics, not otherwise specified; 1-3
➔ *CPT Changes: An Insider's View* 2015

 # 80340 4-6
➔ *CPT Changes: An Insider's View* 2015

 # 80341 7 or more
➔ *CPT Changes: An Insider's View* 2015

(To report definitive drug testing for antihistamines, see 80375, 80376, 80377)

 # 80342 Antipsychotics, not otherwise specified; 1-3
➔ *CPT Changes: An Insider's View* 2015

 # 80343 4-6
➔ *CPT Changes: An Insider's View* 2015

 # 80344 7 or more
➔ *CPT Changes: An Insider's View* 2015

 # 80345 Barbiturates
➔ *CPT Changes: An Insider's View* 2015

 # 80346 Benzodiazepines; 1-12
➔ *CPT Changes: An Insider's View* 2015

 # 80347 13 or more
CPT Changes: An Insider's View 2015

 # 80348 Buprenorphine
CPT Changes: An Insider's View 2015

 # 80349 Cannabinoids, natural
CPT Changes: An Insider's View 2015

 # 80350 Cannabinoids, synthetic; 1-3
CPT Changes: An Insider's View 2015

 # 80351 4-6
CPT Changes: An Insider's View 2015

 # 80352 7 or more
CPT Changes: An Insider's View 2015

 # 80353 Cocaine
CPT Changes: An Insider's View 2015

 # 80354 Fentanyl
CPT Changes: An Insider's View 2015

 # 80355 Gabapentin, non-blood
CPT Changes: An Insider's View 2015
CPT Assistant Apr 15:3

(For therapeutic drug assay, use 80171)

 # 80356 Heroin metabolite
CPT Changes: An Insider's View 2015

 # 80357 Ketamine and norketamine
CPT Changes: An Insider's View 2015

 # 80358 Methadone
CPT Changes: An Insider's View 2015

 # 80359 Methylenedioxyamphetamines (MDA, MDEA, MDMA)
CPT Changes: An Insider's View 2015

 # 80360 Methylphenidate
CPT Changes: An Insider's View 2015

 # 80361 Opiates, 1 or more
CPT Changes: An Insider's View 2015

 # 80362 Opioids and opiate analogs; 1 or 2
CPT Changes: An Insider's View 2015

 # 80363 3 or 4
CPT Changes: An Insider's View 2015

 # 80364 5 or more
CPT Changes: An Insider's View 2015

 # 80365 Oxycodone
CPT Changes: An Insider's View 2015

 # 83992 Phencyclidine (PCP)
CPT Assistant Apr 15:3

(Phenobarbital, use 80345)

 # 80366 Pregabalin
CPT Changes: An Insider's View 2015

 # 80367 Propoxyphene
CPT Changes: An Insider's View 2015

 # 80368 Sedative hypnotics (non-benzodiazepines)
CPT Changes: An Insider's View 2015

 # 80369 Skeletal muscle relaxants; 1 or 2
CPT Changes: An Insider's View 2015

 # 80370 3 or more
CPT Changes: An Insider's View 2015

 # 80371 Stimulants, synthetic
CPT Changes: An Insider's View 2015

 # 80372 Tapentadol
CPT Changes: An Insider's View 2015

 # 80373 Tramadol
CPT Changes: An Insider's View 2015

 # 80374 Stereoisomer (enantiomer) analysis, single drug class
CPT Changes: An Insider's View 2015

(Use 80374 in conjunction with an index drug analysis, when performed)

 # 80375 Drug(s) or substance(s), definitive, qualitative or quantitative, not otherwise specified; 1-3
CPT Changes: An Insider's View 2015
CPT Assistant Apr 15:3

 # 80376 4-6
CPT Changes: An Insider's View 2015
CPT Assistant Apr 15:3

 # 80377 7 or more
CPT Changes: An Insider's View 2015
CPT Assistant Apr 15:3

(To report definitive drug testing for antihistamines, see 80375, 80376, 80377)

For Example:

To report amphetamine and methamphetamine using any number of definitive procedures, report 80324 once per facility per date of service.

To report codeine, hydrocodone, hydromorphone, morphine using any number of definitive procedures, report 80361 once per facility per date of service.

To report codeine, hydrocodone, hydromorphone, morphine, oxycodone, oxymorphone, naloxone, naltrexone performed using any number of definitive procedures report 80361 X 1, 80362 X 1, and 80365 X 1 per facility per date of service.

To report benzoylecgonine, cocaine, carboxy-THC, meperidine, normeperidine using any number of definitive procedures, report 80349 X 1, 80353 X 1, and 80362 X 1 per facility per date of service.

Definitive Drug Classes Listing

Drugs and metabolites included in each definitive drug class are listed in the Definitive Drug Classes Listing table. This is not a comprehensive list. FDA classification of drugs not listed should be used where possible within

DEFINITIVE DRUG CLASSES LISTING

Codes	Classes	Drugs
80320	Alcohol(s)	Acetone, ethanol, ethchlorvynol, ethylene glycol, isopropanol, isopropyl alcohol, methanol
80321-80322	Alcohol biomarkers	Ethanol conjugates (ethyl glucuronide [ETG], ethyl sulfate [ETS], fatty acid ethyl esters, phosphatidylethanol)
80323	Alkaloids, not otherwise specified	7-Hydroxymitragynine, atropine, cotinine, lysergic acid diethylamide (LSD), mescaline, mitragynine, nicotine, psilocin, psilocybin, scopolamine
80324-80326	Amphetamines	Amphetamine, ephedrine, lisdexamphetamine, methamphetamine, phentermine, phenylpropanolamine, pseudoephedrine
80327-80328	Anabolic steroids	1-Androstenediol, 1-androstenedione, 1-testosterone, 4-hydroxy-testosterone, 6-oxo, 19-norandrostenedione, androstenedione, androstanolone, bolandiol, bolasterone, boldenone, boldione, calusterone, clostebol, danazol, dehydrochlormethyltestosterone, dihydrotestosterone, drostanolone, epiandrosterone, epitestosterone, fluoxymesterone, furazabol, mestanolone, mesterolone, methandienone, methandriol, methenolone, methydienolone, methyl-1-testosterone, methylnortestosterone, methyltestosterone, mibolerone, nandrolone, norbolethone, norclostebol, norethandrolone, norethindrone, oxabolone, oxandrolone, oxymesterone, oxymetholone, stanozolol, stenbolone, tibolone, trenbolone, zeranol
80329-80331	Analgesics, non-opioid	Acetaminophen, diclofenac ibuprofen, ketoprofen, naproxen, oxaprozin, salicylate
80332-80334	Antidepressants, serotonergic class	Citalopram, duloxetine, escitalopram, fluoxetine, fluvoxamine, paroxetine, sertraline
80335-80337	Antidepressants, tricyclic and other cyclicals	Amitriptyline, amoxapine, clomipramine, demexiptiline, desipramine, doxepin, imipramine, maprotiline, mirtazapine, nortriptyline, protriptyline
80338	Antidepressants, not otherwise specified	Bupropion, desvenlafaxine, isocarboxazid, nefazodone, phenelzine, selegiline, tranylcypromine, trazodone, venlafaxine
80339-80341	Antiepileptics, not otherwise specified	Carbamazepine, clobazam, dimethadione, ethosuximide, ezogabine, lamotrigine, levetiracetam, methsuximide, oxcarbazepine, phenytoin, primidone, rufinamide, tiagabine, topiramate, trimethadione, valproic acid, zonisamide
80342-80344	Antipsychotics, not otherwise specified	Aripiprazole, chlorpromazine, clozapine, fluphenazine, haloperidol, loxapine, mesoridazine, molindone, olanzapine, paliperidone, perphenazine, phenothiazine, pimozide, prochlorperazine, quetiapine, risperidone, trifluoperazine, thiothixene, thioridazine, ziprasidone
80345	Barbiturates	Amobarbital, aprobarbital, butalbital, cyclobarbital, mephobarbital, pentobarbital, phenobarbital, secobarbital, talbutal, thiopental
80346, 80347	Benzodiazepines	Alprazolam, chlordiazepoxide, clonazepam, clorazepate, diazepam, estazolam, flunitrazepam, flurazepam, halazepam, lorazepam, midazolam, nitrazepam, nordazepam, oxazepam, prazepam, quazepam, temazepam
80348	Buprenorphine	Buprenorphine
80349	Cannabinoids, natural	Marijuana, dronabinol carboxy-THC
80350-80352	Cannabinoids, synthetic	CP-47,497, CP497 C8-homolog, JWH-018 and AM678, JWH-073, JWH-019, JWH-200, JWH-210, JWH-250, JWH-081, JWH-122, HWH-398, AM-2201, AM-694, SR-19 and RCS-4, SR-18 and RCS-8, JWH-203, UR-144, XLR-11, MAM-2201, AKB-48
80353	Cocaine	Benzoylecgonine, cocaethylene, cocaine, ecgonine methyl ester, norcocaine
80354	Fentanyls	Acetylfentanyl, alfentanil, fentanyl, remifentanil, sufentanil
80355	Gabapentin, non-blood	Gabapentin
80356	Heroin metabolite	6-acetylmorphine, acetylcodeine, diacetylmorphine

DEFINITIVE DRUG CLASSES LISTING

Codes	Classes	Drugs
80368	Hypnotics, sedative (non-benzodiazepines)	See Sedative Hypnotics
80357	Ketamine and Norketamine	Ketamine, norketamine
80358	Methadone	Methadone and EDDP
80359	Methylenedioxyamphetamines	MDA, MDEA, MDMA
80360	Methylphenidate	Methylphenidate, ritalinic acid
80357	Norketamine	See Ketamine
80368	Non-Benzodiazepines	See Hypnotics, sedative
80361	Opiates	Codeine, dihydrocodeine, hydrocodone, hydromorphone, morphine
80362-80364	Opioids and opiate analogs	Butorphanol, desomorphine, dextromethorphan, dextrorphan, levorphanol, meperidine, naloxone, naltrexone, normeperidine, pentazocine
80365	Oxycodone	Oxycodone, oxymorphone
83992	Phencyclidine	Phencyclidine
80366	Pregabalin	Pregabalin
80367	Propoxyphene	Norpropoxyphene, propoxyphene
80368	Sedative Hypnotics (non-benzodiazepines)	Eszopiclone, zaleplon, zolpidem
80369, 80370	Skeletal muscle relaxants	Baclofen, carisoprodol, cyclobenzaprine, meprobamate, metaxalone, methocarbamol, orphenadrine, tizanidine
80371	Stimulants, synthetic	2C-B, 2C-E, 2C-I, 2C-H, 3TFMPP, 4-methylethcathinone, alpha-PVP, benzylpiperazine, bromodragonfly, cathinone, m-CPP, MDPBP, MDPPP, MDPV, mephedrone, methcathinone, methylone, phenethylamines, salvinorin, tryptamines
80372	Tapentadol	Tapentadol
80373	Tramadol	Tramadol

the defined drug classes. Any metabolites that are not listed should be categorized with the parent drug. Drugs and metabolites not listed may be reported using codes from the Therapeutic Drug Assay (80150-80299) or Chemistry (82009-84999) sections.

Therapeutic Drug Assays

Therapeutic Drug Assays are performed to monitor clinical response to a known, prescribed medication.

The material for examination is whole blood, serum, plasma, or cerebrospinal fluid. Examination is quantitative. Coding is by parent drug; measured metabolites of the drug are included in the code, if performed.

80150 Amikacin
➔ *CPT Changes: An Insider's View* 2015
➔ *CPT Assistant* Aug 05:9, Oct 10:7, Dec 10:7, Mar 11:10, Apr 15:3

(80152 has been deleted. To report definitive drug testing for amitriptyline, see 80335, 80336, 80337)

80155 Caffeine
➔ *CPT Changes: An Insider's View* 2014

80156 Carbamazepine; total
➔ *CPT Changes: An Insider's View* 2001
➔ *CPT Assistant* Oct 10:7, Mar 11:10

80157 free
➔ *CPT Changes: An Insider's View* 2001
➔ *CPT Assistant* Oct 10:7, Mar 11:10

80158 Cyclosporine
➔ *CPT Assistant* Oct 10:7, Mar 11:10

80159 Clozapine
➔ *CPT Changes: An Insider's View* 2014

80162 Digoxin; total
➔ *CPT Changes: An Insider's View* 2015
➔ *CPT Assistant* Oct 10:7, Mar 11:10, Apr 15:3

80163 free
➔ *CPT Changes: An Insider's View* 2015
➔ *CPT Assistant* Apr 15:3

80164 Code is out of numerical sequence. See 80200-80203

80165 Code is out of numerical sequence. See 80200-80203

80168 Ethosuximide
➔ *CPT Assistant* Oct 10:7, Mar 11:10

80169 Everolimus
➔ *CPT Changes: An Insider's View* 2014

 # 80171 Gabapentin, whole blood, serum, or plasma
➔ *CPT Changes: An Insider's View* 2014, 2015
➔ *CPT Assistant* Apr 15:3

80170 Gentamicin
➔ *CPT Assistant* Oct 10:7, Mar 11:10

80171 Code is out of numerical sequence. See 80168-80173

80173 Haloperidol
➔ *CPT Changes: An Insider's View* 2001
➔ *CPT Assistant* Oct 10:7, Mar 11:10

80175 Lamotrigine
➔ *CPT Changes: An Insider's View* 2014

80176 Lidocaine
➔ *CPT Assistant* Oct 10:7, Mar 11:10

80177 Levetiracetam
➔ *CPT Changes: An Insider's View* 2014

80178 Lithium
➔ *CPT Assistant* Oct 10:7, Mar 11:10

80180 Mycophenolate (mycophenolic acid)
➔ *CPT Changes: An Insider's View* 2014

80183 Oxcarbazepine
➔ *CPT Changes: An Insider's View* 2014

80184 Phenobarbital
➔ *CPT Assistant* Oct 10:7, Mar 11:10

80185 Phenytoin; total
➔ *CPT Assistant* Oct 10:7, Mar 11:10

80186 free
➔ *CPT Assistant* Oct 10:7, Mar 11:10

80188 Primidone
➔ *CPT Assistant* Oct 10:7, Mar 11:10

80190 Procainamide;
➔ *CPT Assistant* Oct 10:7, Mar 11:10

80192 with metabolites (eg, n-acetyl procainamide)
➔ *CPT Assistant* Oct 10:7, Mar 11:10

80194 Quinidine
➔ *CPT Assistant* Oct 10:7, Mar 11:10

80195 Sirolimus
➔ *CPT Changes: An Insider's View* 2006
➔ *CPT Assistant* Mar 06:6, Oct 10:7, Mar 11:10

80197 Tacrolimus
➔ *CPT Assistant* Oct 10:7, Mar 11:10

80198 Theophylline
➔ *CPT Assistant* Oct 10:7, Mar 11:10

80199 Tiagabine
➔ *CPT Changes: An Insider's View* 2014

80200 Tobramycin
➔ *CPT Assistant* Oct 10:7, Mar 11:10

80201 Topiramate
➔ *CPT Assistant* Nov 97:28, Oct 10:7, Mar 11:10

 # 80164 Valproic acid (dipropylacetic acid); total
➔ *CPT Changes: An Insider's View* 2015
➔ *CPT Assistant* Oct 10:7, Mar 11:10, Apr 15:3

 # 80165 free
➔ *CPT Changes: An Insider's View* 2015
➔ *CPT Assistant* Apr 15:3

80202 Vancomycin
➔ *CPT Assistant* Oct 10:7, Mar 11:10, Apr 15:3

80203 Zonisamide
➔ *CPT Changes: An Insider's View* 2014

80299 Quantitation of therapeutic drug, not elsewhere specified
➔ *CPT Changes: An Insider's View* 2015
➔ *CPT Assistant* Mar 00:3, Oct 04:14, Aug 05:9, Oct 10:7, Dec 10:3, Mar 11:10, Apr 15:3

80305 Code is out of numerical sequence. See Presumptive Drug Class Screening subsection

80306 Code is out of numerical sequence. See Presumptive Drug Class Screening subsection

80307 Code is out of numerical sequence. See Presumptive Drug Class Screening subsection

80320 Code is out of numerical sequence. See Definitive Drug Testing subsection

80321 Code is out of numerical sequence. See Definitive Drug Testing subsection

80322 Code is out of numerical sequence. See Definitive Drug Testing subsection

80323 Code is out of numerical sequence. See Definitive Drug Testing subsection

80324 Code is out of numerical sequence. See Definitive Drug Testing subsection

80325 Code is out of numerical sequence. See Definitive Drug Testing subsection

80326 Code is out of numerical sequence. See Definitive Drug Testing subsection

80327 Code is out of numerical sequence. See Definitive Drug Testing subsection

80328 Code is out of numerical sequence. See Definitive Drug Testing subsection

80329 Code is out of numerical sequence. See Definitive Drug Testing subsection

80330 Code is out of numerical sequence. See Definitive Drug Testing subsection

80331 Code is out of numerical sequence. See Definitive Drug Testing subsection

80332 Code is out of numerical sequence. See Definitive Drug Testing subsection

80333 Code is out of numerical sequence. See Definitive Drug Testing subsection

80334 Code is out of numerical sequence. See Definitive Drug Testing subsection

80335 Code is out of numerical sequence. See Definitive Drug Testing subsection

80336 Code is out of numerical sequence. See Definitive Drug Testing subsection

80337 Code is out of numerical sequence. See Definitive Drug Testing subsection

80338 Code is out of numerical sequence. See Definitive Drug Testing subsection

80339 Code is out of numerical sequence. See Definitive Drug Testing subsection

80340 Code is out of numerical sequence. See Definitive Drug Testing subsection

80341 Code is out of numerical sequence. See Definitive Drug Testing subsection

80342 Code is out of numerical sequence. See Definitive Drug Testing subsection

80343 Code is out of numerical sequence. See Definitive Drug Testing subsection

80344 Code is out of numerical sequence. See Definitive Drug Testing subsection

80345 Code is out of numerical sequence. See Definitive Drug Testing subsection

80346 Code is out of numerical sequence. See Definitive Drug Testing subsection

80347 Code is out of numerical sequence. See Definitive Drug Testing subsection

80348 Code is out of numerical sequence. See Definitive Drug Testing subsection

80349 Code is out of numerical sequence. See Definitive Drug Testing subsection

80350 Code is out of numerical sequence. See Definitive Drug Testing subsection

80351 Code is out of numerical sequence. See Definitive Drug Testing subsection

80352 Code is out of numerical sequence. See Definitive Drug Testing subsection

80353 Code is out of numerical sequence. See Definitive Drug Testing subsection

80354 Code is out of numerical sequence. See Definitive Drug Testing subsection

80355 Code is out of numerical sequence. See Definitive Drug Testing subsection

80356 Code is out of numerical sequence. See Definitive Drug Testing subsection

80357 Code is out of numerical sequence. See Definitive Drug Testing subsection

80358 Code is out of numerical sequence. See Definitive Drug Testing subsection

80359 Code is out of numerical sequence. See Definitive Drug Testing subsection

80360 Code is out of numerical sequence. See Definitive Drug Testing subsection

80361 Code is out of numerical sequence. See Definitive Drug Testing subsection

80362 Code is out of numerical sequence. See Definitive Drug Testing subsection

80363 Code is out of numerical sequence. See Definitive Drug Testing subsection

80364 Code is out of numerical sequence. See Definitive Drug Testing subsection

80365 Code is out of numerical sequence. See Definitive Drug Testing subsection

80366 Code is out of numerical sequence. See Definitive Drug Testing subsection

80367 Code is out of numerical sequence. See Definitive Drug Testing subsection

80368 Code is out of numerical sequence. See Definitive Drug Testing subsection

80369 Code is out of numerical sequence. See Definitive Drug Testing subsection

80370 Code is out of numerical sequence. See Definitive Drug Testing subsection

80371 Code is out of numerical sequence. See Definitive Drug Testing subsection

80372 Code is out of numerical sequence. See Definitive Drug Testing subsection

80373 Code is out of numerical sequence. See Definitive Drug Testing subsection

80374 Code is out of numerical sequence. See Definitive Drug Testing subsection

80375 Code is out of numerical sequence. See Definitive Drug Testing subsection

80376 Code is out of numerical sequence. See Definitive Drug Testing subsection

80377 Code is out of numerical sequence. See Definitive Drug Testing subsection

Evocative/Suppression Testing

The following test panels involve the administration of evocative or suppressive agents and the baseline and subsequent measurement of their effects on chemical constituents. These codes are to be used for the reporting of the laboratory component of the overall testing protocol. For the administration of the evocative or suppressive agents, see Hydration, Therapeutic, Prophylactic, Diagnostic Injections and Infusions, and Chemotherapy and Other Highly Complex Drug or Highly Complex Biologic Agent Administration (eg, 96365, 96366, 96367, 96368, 96372, 96374, 96375, 96376). In the code descriptors where reference is made to a particular analyte (eg, Cortisol: 82533 x 2) the "x 2" refers to the number of times the test for that particular analyte is performed.

80400 ACTH stimulation panel; for adrenal insufficiency

This panel must include the following:

Cortisol (82533 x 2)

➔ *CPT Assistant* Summer 94:1, Fall 94:10, Aug 05:9

80402 for 21 hydroxylase deficiency

This panel must include the following:

Cortisol (82533 x 2)

17 hydroxyprogesterone (83498 x 2)

➔ *CPT Assistant* Summer 94:1, Fall 94:10

80406 for 3 beta-hydroxydehydrogenase deficiency

This panel must include the following:

Cortisol (82533 x 2)

17 hydroxypregnenolone (84143 x 2)

➔ *CPT Assistant* Summer 94:1, Fall 94:10

80408 Aldosterone suppression evaluation panel (eg, saline infusion)

This panel must include the following:

Aldosterone (82088 x 2)

Renin (84244 x 2)

➔ *CPT Assistant* Summer 94:1, Fall 94:10

80410 Calcitonin stimulation panel (eg, calcium, pentagastrin)

This panel must include the following:

Calcitonin (82308 x 3)

➔ *CPT Assistant* Summer 94:1, Fall 94:11

80412 Corticotropic releasing hormone (CRH) stimulation panel

This panel must include the following:

Cortisol (82533 x 6)

Adrenocorticotropic hormone (ACTH) (82024 x 6)

➔ *CPT Assistant* Summer 94:1, Fall 94:11

80414 Chorionic gonadotropin stimulation panel; testosterone response

This panel must include the following:

Testosterone (84403 x 2 on 3 pooled blood samples)

➔ *CPT Changes: An Insider's View* 2009

➔ *CPT Assistant* Summer 94:1, Fall 94:11

80415 estradiol response

This panel must include the following:

Estradiol (82670 x 2 on 3 pooled blood samples)

➔ *CPT Changes: An Insider's View* 2009

➔ *CPT Assistant* Summer 94:1, Fall 94:11

80416 Renal vein renin stimulation panel (eg, captopril)

This panel must include the following:

Renin (84244 x 6)

➔ *CPT Assistant* Summer 94:1

80417 Peripheral vein renin stimulation panel (eg, captopril)

This panel must include the following:

Renin (84244 x 2)

80418 Combined rapid anterior pituitary evaluation panel

This panel must include the following:

Adrenocorticotropic hormone (ACTH) (82024 x 4)

Luteinizing hormone (LH) (83002 x 4)

Follicle stimulating hormone (FSH) (83001 x 4)

Prolactin (84146 x 4)

Human growth hormone (HGH) (83003 x 4)

Cortisol (82533 x 4)

Thyroid stimulating hormone (TSH) (84443 x 4)

➔ *CPT Assistant* Summer 94:1, Fall 94:13

80420 Dexamethasone suppression panel, 48 hour

This panel must include the following:

Free cortisol, urine (82530 x 2)

Cortisol (82533 x 2)

Volume measurement for timed collection (81050 x 2)

➔ *CPT Assistant* Fall 94:13

(For single dose dexamethasone, use 82533)

80422 Glucagon tolerance panel; for insulinoma

This panel must include the following:

Glucose (82947 x 3)

Insulin (83525 x 3)

➔ *CPT Assistant* Summer 94:1, Fall 94:13

80424 for pheochromocytoma

This panel must include the following:

Catecholamines, fractionated (82384 x 2)

➔ *CPT Assistant* Summer 94:1, Fall 94:14

80426 Gonadotropin releasing hormone stimulation panel

This panel must include the following:

Follicle stimulating hormone (FSH) (83001 x 4)

Luteinizing hormone (LH) (83002 x 4)

➔ *CPT Assistant* Summer 94:1, Fall 94:14

80428 Growth hormone stimulation panel (eg, arginine infusion, l-dopa administration)

This panel must include the following:

Human growth hormone (HGH) (83003 x 4)

➔ *CPT Assistant* Summer 94:1, Fall 94:14

80430 Growth hormone suppression panel (glucose administration)

This panel must include the following:

Glucose (82947 x 3)

Human growth hormone (HGH) (83003 x 4)

➔ *CPT Assistant* Summer 94:1, Fall 94:14

80432 Insulin-induced C-peptide suppression panel

This panel must include the following:

Insulin (83525)

C-peptide (84681 x 5)

Glucose (82947 x 5)

➔ *CPT Assistant* Summer 94:1, Fall 94:15

80434 Insulin tolerance panel; for ACTH insufficiency

This panel must include the following:

Cortisol (82533 x 5)

Glucose (82947 x 5)

➔ *CPT Assistant* Summer 94:1, Fall 94:15

80435 for growth hormone deficiency

This panel must include the following:

Glucose (82947 x 5)

Human growth hormone (HGH) (83003 x 5)

➔ *CPT Assistant* Summer 94:1, Fall 94:15

80436 Metyrapone panel

This panel must include the following:

Cortisol (82533 x 2)

11 deoxycortisol (82634 x 2)

➔ *CPT Assistant* Summer 94:1, Fall 94:16

80438 Thyrotropin releasing hormone (TRH) stimulation panel; 1 hour

This panel must include the following:

Thyroid stimulating hormone (TSH) (84443 x 3)

➔ *CPT Assistant* Summer 94:1, Fall 94:16

80439 2 hour

This panel must include the following:

Thyroid stimulating hormone (TSH) (84443 x 4)

➔ *CPT Assistant* Summer 94:1, Fall 94:16

Consultations (Clinical Pathology)

A clinical pathology consultation is a service, including a written report, rendered by the pathologist in response to a request from a physician or qualified health care professional in relation to a test result(s) requiring additional medical interpretive judgment.

Reporting of a test result(s) without medical interpretive judgment is not considered a clinical pathology consultation.

80500 Clinical pathology consultation; limited, without review of patient's history and medical records

➔ *CPT Assistant* Apr 97:9, Nov 02:9, Aug 05:9

80502 comprehensive, for a complex diagnostic problem, with review of patient's history and medical records

➔ *CPT Assistant* Apr 97:9, Nov 02:9, Aug 05:9

(These codes may also be used for pharmacokinetic consultations)

(For consultations involving the examination and evaluation of the patient, see 99241-99255)

Urinalysis

For specific analyses, see appropriate section.

81000 Urinalysis, by dip stick or tablet reagent for bilirubin, glucose, hemoglobin, ketones, leukocytes, nitrite, pH, protein, specific gravity, urobilinogen, any number of these constituents; non-automated, with microscopy

➔ *CPT Assistant* Winter 91:10, Fall 93:25, Aug 05:9

81001 automated, with microscopy

81002 non-automated, without microscopy

➔ *CPT Assistant* Mar 98:3, Apr 07:1

81003 automated, without microscopy

➔ *CPT Assistant* Apr 07:1

81005 Urinalysis; qualitative or semiquantitative, except immunoassays

➔ *CPT Assistant* Winter 90:, Winter 91:10, Fall 93:25

(For non-immunoassay reagent strip urinalysis, see 81000, 81002)

(For immunoassay, qualitative or semiquantitative, use 83518)

(For microalbumin, see 82043, 82044)

81007 bacteriuria screen, except by culture or dipstick

➔ *CPT Changes: An Insider's View* 2001

(For culture, see 87086-87088)

(For dipstick, use 81000 or 81002)

Pathology and Laboratory 80047-89398, 0001U-0061U

81015 microscopic only
➔ *CPT Assistant* Nov 17:11

(For sperm evaluation for retrograde ejaculation, use 89331)

81020 2 or 3 glass test
➔ *CPT Assistant* Winter 90:, Winter 91:10

81025 Urine pregnancy test, by visual color comparison methods
➔ *CPT Assistant* Mar 98:3

81050 Volume measurement for timed collection, each

81099 Unlisted urinalysis procedure
➔ *CPT Assistant* Aug 05:9

Molecular Pathology

Molecular pathology procedures are medical laboratory procedures involving the analyses of nucleic acid (ie, DNA, RNA) to detect variants in genes that may be indicative of germline (eg, constitutional disorders) or somatic (eg, neoplasia) conditions, or to test for histocompatibility antigens (eg, HLA). Code selection is typically based on the specific gene(s) that is being analyzed. Genes are described using Human Genome Organization (HUGO) approved gene names and are italicized in the code descriptors. Gene names were taken from tables of the HUGO Gene Nomenclature Committee (HGNC) at the time the CPT codes were developed. For the most part, Human Genome Variation Society (HGVS) recommendations were followed for the names of specific molecular variants. The familiar name is used for some variants because defined criteria were not in place when the variant was first described or because HGVS recommendations were changed over time (eg, intronic variants, processed proteins). When the gene name is represented by an abbreviation, the abbreviation is listed first, followed by the full gene name italicized in parentheses (eg, "F5 *[coagulation Factor V]*"), except for the HLA series of codes. Proteins or diseases commonly associated with the genes are listed as examples in the code descriptors. The examples do not represent all conditions in which testing of the gene may be indicated.

Codes that describe tests to assess for the presence of gene variants (see definitions) use common gene variant names. Typically, all of the listed variants would be tested. However, these lists are not exclusive. If other variants are also tested in the analysis, they would be included in the procedure and not reported separately. Full gene sequencing should not be reported using codes that assess for the presence of gene variants unless specifically stated in the code descriptor.

The molecular pathology codes include all analytical services performed in the test (eg, cell lysis, nucleic acid stabilization, extraction, digestion, amplification, and detection). Any procedures required prior to cell lysis (eg, microdissection, codes 88380 and 88381) should be reported separately.

The results of the procedure may require interpretation by a physician or other qualified health care professional. When only the interpretation and report are performed, modifier 26 may be appended to the specific molecular pathology code.

All analyses are qualitative unless otherwise noted.

For microbial identification, see 87149-87153 and 87471-87801, and 87900-87904. For in situ hybridization analyses, see 88271-88275 and 88365-88368.

Molecular pathology procedures that are not specified in 81161, 81200-81383 should be reported using either the appropriate Tier 2 code (81400-81408) or the unlisted molecular pathology procedure code, 81479.

Definitions

For purposes of CPT reporting, the following definitions apply:

Abnormal allele: an alternative form of a gene that contains a disease-related variation from the normal sequence.

Breakpoint: the region at which a chromosome breaks during a translocation (defined elsewhere). These regions are often consistent for a given translocation.

Codon: a discrete unit of three nucleotides of a DNA or mRNA sequence that encodes a specific amino acid within, or signals the termination of, a polypeptide.

Common variants: variants (as defined elsewhere) that are associated with compromised gene function and are interrogated in a single round of laboratory testing (in a single, typically multiplex, assay format or using more than one assay to encompass all variants to be tested). These variants typically fit the definition of a "mutation," and are usually the predominant ones causing disease. Testing for additional uncommon variants may provide additional limited value in assessment of a patient. Often there are professional society recommendations or guidelines for which variants are most appropriate to test (eg, American College of Medical Genetics/American College of Obstetrics and Gynecology guidelines for variants used in population screening for cystic fibrosis).

Constitutional: synonymous with germline, often used in reference to the genetic code that is present at birth.

Copy number variants (CNVs): structural changes in the genome composed of large deletions or duplications. CNVs can be found in the germline, but can also occur in somatic cells. See also Duplication/Deletion (Dup/Del).

Cytogenomic: chromosome analysis using molecular techniques.

▶***DNA methylation:*** the process of adding methyl groups to a DNA sequence, specifically adenine and cytosine nucleotides, thereby affecting transcription of that sequence. DNA hyper-methylation in a gene promoter typically represses gene transcription. DNA methylation serves as a regulatory mechanism in numerous scenarios including development, chromosome inactivation, and carcinogenesis.

DNA methylation analysis: analytical protocols are designed to evaluate the degree of DNA methylation related to specific disease processes. This analysis has various applications, qualitative or quantitative, and could be gene specific or encompass global degrees of methylation. All assays employ specific maneuvers (eg, chemical, enzymatic) that allow for distinguishable evaluation of methylated and non-methylated sequences.◄

Duplication/Deletion (Dup/Del): terms that are usually used together with the "/" to refer to molecular testing, which assesses the dosage of a particular genomic region. The region tested is typically of modest to substantial size — from several dozen to several million or more nucleotides. Normal gene dosage is two copies per cell, except for the sex chromosomes (X and Y). Thus, zero or one copy represents a deletion, and three (or more) copies represent a duplication.

Dynamic mutation: polynucleotide (eg, trinucleotide) repeats that are in or associated with genes that can undergo disease-producing increases or decreases in the numbers of repeats within tissues and across generations.

Exome: DNA sequences within the human genome that code for proteins (coding regions).

Exon: typically, one of multiple nucleic acid sequences used to encode information for a gene product (polypeptide or protein). Exons are separated from each other by non-protein-coding sequences known as introns. Exons at the respective ends of a gene also contain nucleic acid sequence that does not code for the gene's protein product.

Gene: a nucleic acid sequence that typically contains information for coding a protein as well as for the regulated expression of that protein. Human genes usually contain multiple protein coding regions (exons) separated by non-protein coding regions (introns). See also *exon, intron,* and *polypeptide.*

►***Gene expression:*** the sequence of events that results in the production and assembly of a protein product corresponding to the information encoded in a specific gene. The process begins with the transcription of gene sequences to produce an mRNA intermediary, which is subsequently translated to produce a specific protein product.◄

Genome: The total (nuclear) human genetic content.

Heteroplasmy: The copy number of a variant within a cell; it is expressed as a percent. It reflects the varied distribution and dosage of mutant mitochondria in tissues and organs (mitotic segregation).

Intron: a nucleic acid sequence found between exons in human genes. An intron contains essential sequences for its proper removal (by a process known as *splicing*) to join exons together and thus facilitate production of a functional protein from a gene. An intron is sometimes referred to as an intervening sequence (IVS).

Inversion: A defect in a chromosome in which a segment breaks and reinserts in the same place but in the opposite orientation.

Loss of heterozygosity (LOH, allelic imbalance): An event that can occur in dividing cells that are heterozygous for one or more alleles, in which a daughter cell becomes hemizygous or homozygous for the allele(s) through mitotic recombination, deletion, or other chromosomal event.

Microarray: surface(s) on which multiple specific nucleic acid sequences are attached in a known arrangement. Sometimes referred to as a 'gene chip'. Examples of uses of microarrays include evaluation of a patient specimen for gains or losses of DNA sequences (copy number variants, CNVs), identification of the presence of specific nucleotide sequence variants (also known as single nucleotide polymorphisms, SNPs), mRNA expression levels, or DNA sequence analysis.

Mitochondrial DNA (mtDNA): DNA located in the mitochondria, which are cytoplasmic organelles involved with energy production. MtDNA contains 37 genes coding for oxidative phosphorylation enzymes, transfer RNAs (tRNAs) and ribosomal RNAs (rRNAs).

Mutations: typically are variants associated with altered gene function that lead to functional deficits or disease (pathogenic).

Mutation scanning: a technique (eg, single strand conformation polymorphism, temperature gradient gel electrophoresis, etc.) typically employed on multiple PCR amplicons to indicate the presence of DNA sequence variants by differences in physical properties compared to normal. Variants are then further characterized by DNA sequence analysis only in amplicons which demonstrate differences.

Nuclear DNA: DNA located in the nucleus of a cell, generally packaged in chromosomes.

Polymorphisms: typically are variants that do not compromise gene function or produce disease (benign).

Polypeptide: a sequence of amino acids covalently linked in a specified order. Polypeptides alone or in combination with other polypeptide subunits are the building blocks of proteins.

►***Promoter:*** a region of DNA associated with a gene (on the same strand) which regulates gene expression. Promoter regions can affect gene transcription through the binding of specific transcription factors.◄

Short Tandem Repeat (STR): a region of DNA where a pattern of two or more nucleotides are repeated. The number of repeating segments can be used as genetic markers for human identity testing.

Single-nucleotide polymorphism (SNP): a DNA sequence variation existing at a significant frequency in the population, in which a single nucleotide (A, T, C, or G) differs between individuals and/or within an individual's paired chromosomes.

Somatic: synonymous with acquired, referring to genetic code alterations that develop after birth (eg, occurring in neoplastic cells).

Translocation: an abnormality resulting from the breakage of a chromosome and the relocation of a portion of that chromosome's DNA sequence to the same or another chromosome. Most common translocations involve a reciprocal exchange of DNA sequences between two differently numbered (ie, non-homologous) chromosomes, with or without a clinically significant loss of DNA.

Uniparental disomy (UPD): Abnormal inheritance of both members of a chromosome pair from one parent, with absence of the other parent's chromosome for the pair.

Variant: a nucleotide sequence difference from the "normal" (predominant) sequence for a given region. Variants are typically of two types: substitutions of one nucleotide for another, and deletions or insertions of nucleotides. Occasionally, variants reflect several nucleotide sequence changes in reasonably close proximity on the same chromosomal strand of DNA (a haplotype). These nucleotide sequence variants often result in amino acid changes in the protein made by the gene. The term *variant* does not itself carry a functional implication for those protein changes.

Variants in introns are typically described in one of two ways. The altered nucleotide(s) within a defined intervening sequence (eg, IVS3-2A>G) of a gene is listed with a "+" or "-" sign, which indicates the position relative to the first or last nucleotide of the intron. Or, the variant position is indicated relative to the last nucleotide of the preceding exon or first nucleotide of the following exon (eg, c.171+1G>A c.172-1G>T are single nucleotide changes at the first and last nucleotide of a given intron for a specific gene).

The majority of the variants described here are listed by the amino acid change using the single letter amino acid code for the original amino acid followed by the numerical position in the protein product and the amino acid substitution, eg, for *ASPA* E285A, Glutamic acid (E) at position 285 is replaced with an alanine (A). A few of the variants are described by the DNA change using the numerical position followed by the original nucleotide, a greater than sign (>) and the new nucleotide, eg, *MTHFR*. 677C>T.

A known familial variant is a specific mutation that has previously been identified within a patient's family.

Tier 1 Molecular Pathology Procedures

The following codes represent gene-specific and genomic procedures:

81105 Code is out of numerical sequence. See 81255-81270

81106 Code is out of numerical sequence. See 81255-81270

81107 Code is out of numerical sequence. See 81255-81270

81108 Code is out of numerical sequence. See 81255-81270

81109 Code is out of numerical sequence. See 81255-81270

81110 Code is out of numerical sequence. See 81255-81270

81111 Code is out of numerical sequence. See 81255-81270

81112 Code is out of numerical sequence. See 81255-81270

81120 Code is out of numerical sequence. See 81255-81270

81121 Code is out of numerical sequence. See 81255-81270

81161 Code is out of numerical sequence. See 81228-81235

81162 Code is out of numerical sequence. See 81182-81220

81163 Code is out of numerical sequence. See 81182-81220

81164 Code is out of numerical sequence. See 81182-81220

81165 Code is out of numerical sequence. See 81182-81220

81166 Code is out of numerical sequence. See 81182-81220

81167 Code is out of numerical sequence. See 81182-81220

81170 *ABL1 (ABL proto-oncogene 1, non-receptor tyrosine kinase)* (eg, acquired imatinib tyrosine kinase inhibitor resistance), gene analysis, variants in the kinase domain
- *CPT Changes: An Insider's View* 2016
- *CPT Assistant* Aug 16:10

● **81171** *AFF2 (AF4/FMR2 family, member 2 [FMR2])* (eg, fragile X mental retardation 2 [FRAXE]) gene analysis; evaluation to detect abnormal (eg, expanded) alleles
- *CPT Changes: An Insider's View* 2019

● **81172** characterization of alleles (eg, expanded size and methylation status)
- *CPT Changes: An Insider's View* 2019

81173 Code is out of numerical sequence. See 81171-81176

81174 Code is out of numerical sequence. See 81171-81176

\# **81201** *APC (adenomatous polyposis coli)* (eg, familial adenomatosis polyposis [FAP], attenuated FAP) gene analysis; full gene sequence
- *CPT Changes: An Insider's View* 2013
- *CPT Assistant* May 12:4, Sep 13:3, Aug 16:10

\# **81202** known familial variants
- *CPT Changes: An Insider's View* 2013
- *CPT Assistant* May 12:4, Sep 13:3, Aug 16:10

\# **81203** duplication/deletion variants
- *CPT Changes: An Insider's View* 2013
- *CPT Assistant* May 12:4, Sep 13:3, Aug 16:10

#● **81204** *AR (androgen receptor)* (eg, spinal and bulbar muscular atrophy, Kennedy disease, X chromosome inactivation) gene analysis; characterization of alleles (eg, expanded size or methylation status)
➲ *CPT Changes: An Insider's View* 2019

#● **81173** full gene sequence
➲ *CPT Changes: An Insider's View* 2019

#● **81174** known familial variant
➲ *CPT Changes: An Insider's View* 2019

\# **81200** *ASPA (aspartoacylase)* (eg, Canavan disease) gene analysis, common variants (eg, E285A, Y231X)
➲ *CPT Changes: An Insider's View* 2012
➲ *CPT Assistant* May 12:4, Aug 16:10

81175 *ASXL1 (additional sex combs like 1, transcriptional regulator)* (eg, myelodysplastic syndrome, myeloproliferative neoplasms, chronic myelomonocytic leukemia), gene analysis; full gene sequence
➲ *CPT Changes: An Insider's View* 2018

81176 targeted sequence analysis (eg, exon 12)
➲ *CPT Changes: An Insider's View* 2018

● **81177** *ATN1 (atrophin 1)* (eg, dentatorubral-pallidoluysian atrophy) gene analysis, evaluation to detect abnormal (eg, expanded) alleles
➲ *CPT Changes: An Insider's View* 2019

● **81178** *ATXN1 (ataxin 1)* (eg, spinocerebellar ataxia) gene analysis, evaluation to detect abnormal (eg, expanded) alleles
➲ *CPT Changes: An Insider's View* 2019

● **81179** *ATXN2 (ataxin 2)* (eg, spinocerebellar ataxia) gene analysis, evaluation to detect abnormal (eg, expanded) alleles
➲ *CPT Changes: An Insider's View* 2019

● **81180** *ATXN3 (ataxin 3)* (eg, spinocerebellar ataxia, Machado-Joseph disease) gene analysis, evaluation to detect abnormal (eg, expanded) alleles
➲ *CPT Changes: An Insider's View* 2019

● **81181** *ATXN7 (ataxin 7)* (eg, spinocerebellar ataxia) gene analysis, evaluation to detect abnormal (eg, expanded) alleles
➲ *CPT Changes: An Insider's View* 2019

● **81182** *ATXN8OS (ATXN8 opposite strand [non-protein coding])* (eg, spinocerebellar ataxia) gene analysis, evaluation to detect abnormal (eg, expanded) alleles
➲ *CPT Changes: An Insider's View* 2019

● **81183** *ATXN10 (ataxin 10)* (eg, spinocerebellar ataxia) gene analysis, evaluation to detect abnormal (eg, expanded) alleles
➲ *CPT Changes: An Insider's View* 2019

81184 Code is out of numerical sequence. See 81182-81220

81185 Code is out of numerical sequence. See 81182-81220

81186 Code is out of numerical sequence. See 81182-81220

81187 Code is out of numerical sequence. See 81223-81226

81188 Code is out of numerical sequence. See 81223-81226

81189 Code is out of numerical sequence. See 81223-81226

81190 Code is out of numerical sequence. See 81223-81226

81200 Code is out of numerical sequence. See 81171-81176

81201 Code is out of numerical sequence. See 81171-81176

81202 Code is out of numerical sequence. See 81171-81176

81203 Code is out of numerical sequence. See 81171-81176

81204 Code is out of numerical sequence. See 81171-81176

81205 Code is out of numerical sequence. See 81182-81220

81206 Code is out of numerical sequence. See 81182-81220

81207 Code is out of numerical sequence. See 81182-81220

81208 Code is out of numerical sequence. See 81182-81220

81209 Code is out of numerical sequence. See 81182-81220

81210 Code is out of numerical sequence. See 81182-81220

\# **81205** *BCKDHB (branched-chain keto acid dehydrogenase E1, beta polypeptide)* (eg, maple syrup urine disease) gene analysis, common variants (eg, R183P, G278S, E422X)
➲ *CPT Changes: An Insider's View* 2012
➲ *CPT Assistant* May 12:4, Aug 16:10

\# **81206** *BCR/ABL1 (t(9;22))* (eg, chronic myelogenous leukemia) translocation analysis; major breakpoint, qualitative or quantitative
➲ *CPT Changes: An Insider's View* 2012
➲ *CPT Assistant* May 12:4, Aug 16:10

\# **81207** minor breakpoint, qualitative or quantitative
➲ *CPT Changes: An Insider's View* 2012
➲ *CPT Assistant* May 12:4, Aug 16:10

\# **81208** other breakpoint, qualitative or quantitative
➲ *CPT Changes: An Insider's View* 2012
➲ *CPT Assistant* May 12:4, Aug 16:10

\# **81209** *BLM (Bloom syndrome, RecQ helicase-like)* (eg, Bloom syndrome) gene analysis, 2281del6ins7 variant
➲ *CPT Changes: An Insider's View* 2012
➲ *CPT Assistant* May 12:4, Aug 16:10

\# **81210** *BRAF (B-Raf proto-oncogene, serine/threonine kinase)* (eg, colon cancer, melanoma), gene analysis, V600 variant(s)
➲ *CPT Changes: An Insider's View* 2012, 2016
➲ *CPT Assistant* May 12:4, Aug 16:10

#▲ **81162** *BRCA1 (BRCA1, DNA repair associated), BRCA2 (BRCA2, DNA repair associated)* (eg, hereditary breast and ovarian cancer) gene analysis; full sequence analysis and full duplication/deletion analysis (ie, detection of large gene rearrangements)
➲ *CPT Changes: An Insider's View* 2016, 2019
➲ *CPT Assistant* Aug 16:10

►(Do not report 81162 in conjunction with 81163, 81164, 81165, 81166, 81167, 81216, 81217, 81432)◄

#● 81163 full sequence analysis
➲ *CPT Changes: An Insider's View* 2019

#● 81164 full duplication/deletion analysis (ie, detection of large gene rearrangements)
➲ *CPT Changes: An Insider's View* 2019

►(To report *BRCA1, BRCA2* full sequence analysis and full duplication/deletion analysis on the same date of service, use 81162)◄

►(For analysis of common duplication/deletion variant(s) in *BRCA1* [ie, exon 13 del 3.835kb, exon 13 dup 6kb, exon 14-20 del 26kb, exon 22 del 510bp, exon 8-9 del 7.1kb], use 81479)◄

►(Do not report 81163 in conjunction with 81162, 81164, 81165, 81216, 81432)◄

►(Do not report 81164 in conjunction with 81162, 81163, 81166, 81167, 81217)◄

▲ 81212 185delAG, 5385insC, 6174delT variants
➲ *CPT Changes: An Insider's View* 2012, 2019
➲ *CPT Assistant* May 12:4, Aug 16:10

►(81211, 81213 have been deleted. To report see 81162, 81163, 81164)◄

►(81214 has been deleted. To report, see 81165, 81166)◄

#● 81165 *BRCA1 (BRCA1, DNA repair associated)* (eg, hereditary breast and ovarian cancer) gene analysis; full sequence analysis
➲ *CPT Changes: An Insider's View* 2019

#● 81166 full duplication/deletion analysis (ie, detection of large gene rearrangements)
➲ *CPT Changes: An Insider's View* 2019

▲ 81215 known familial variant
➲ *CPT Changes: An Insider's View* 2012, 2019
➲ *CPT Assistant* May 12:4, Aug 16:10

►(For analysis of common duplication/deletion variant(s) in *BRCA1* [ie, exon 13 del 3.835kb, exon 13 dup 6kb, exon 14-20 del 26kb, exon 22 del 510bp, exon 8-9 del 7.1kb], use 81479)◄

►(Do not report 81165 in conjunction with 81162, 81163, 81432)◄

►(Do not report 81166 in conjunction with 81162, 81164)◄

▲ 81216 *BRCA2 (BRCA2, DNA repair associated)* (eg, hereditary breast and ovarian cancer) gene analysis; full sequence analysis
➲ *CPT Changes: An Insider's View* 2012, 2019
➲ *CPT Assistant* May 12:4, Aug 16:10

#● 81167 full duplication/deletion analysis (ie, detection of large gene rearrangements)
➲ *CPT Changes: An Insider's View* 2019

▲ 81217 known familial variant
➲ *CPT Changes: An Insider's View* 2012, 2019
➲ *CPT Assistant* May 12:4, Aug 16:10

►(Do not report 81216 in conjunction with 81162, 81163, 81432)◄

►(Do not report 81167 in conjunction with 81162, 81164, 81217)◄

►(Do not report 81217 in conjunction with 81162, 81164, 81167)◄

#● 81233 *BTK (Bruton's tyrosine kinase)* (eg, chronic lymphocytic leukemia) gene analysis, common variants (eg, C481S, C481R, C481F)
➲ *CPT Changes: An Insider's View* 2019

#● 81184 *CACNA1A (calcium voltage-gated channel subunit alpha1 A)* (eg, spinocerebellar ataxia) gene analysis; evaluation to detect abnormal (eg, expanded) alleles
➲ *CPT Changes: An Insider's View* 2019

#● 81185 full gene sequence
➲ *CPT Changes: An Insider's View* 2019

#● 81186 known familial variant
➲ *CPT Changes: An Insider's View* 2019

81219 *CALR (calreticulin)* (eg, myeloproliferative disorders), gene analysis, common variants in exon 9
➲ *CPT Changes: An Insider's View* 2016
➲ *CPT Assistant* Aug 16:10

81218 *CEBPA (CCAAT/enhancer binding protein [C/EBP], alpha)* (eg, acute myeloid leukemia), gene analysis, full gene sequence
➲ *CPT Changes: An Insider's View* 2016
➲ *CPT Assistant* Aug 16:10

81219 Code is out of numerical sequence. See 81182-81220

81220 *CFTR (cystic fibrosis transmembrane conductance regulator)* (eg, cystic fibrosis) gene analysis; common variants (eg, ACMG/ACOG guidelines)
➲ *CPT Changes: An Insider's View* 2012
➲ *CPT Assistant* May 12:4, Aug 16:10

(When Intron 8 poly-T analysis is performed in conjunction with 81220 in a R117H positive patient, do not report 81224)

81221 known familial variants
➲ *CPT Changes: An Insider's View* 2012
➲ *CPT Assistant* May 12:4, Aug 16:10

81222 duplication/deletion variants
➲ *CPT Changes: An Insider's View* 2012
➲ *CPT Assistant* May 12:4, Aug 16:10

81223 full gene sequence
➲ *CPT Changes: An Insider's View* 2012
➲ *CPT Assistant* May 12:4, Aug 16:10

81224 intron 8 poly-T analysis (eg, male infertility)
➲ *CPT Changes: An Insider's View* 2012
➲ *CPT Assistant* May 12:4, Aug 16:10

 # 81267 Chimerism (engraftment) analysis, post transplantation specimen (eg, hematopoietic stem cell), includes comparison to previously performed baseline analyses; without cell selection
CPT Changes: An Insider's View 2012
CPT Assistant May 12:4, Aug 16:10

 # 81268 with cell selection (eg, CD3, CD33), each cell type
CPT Changes: An Insider's View 2012
CPT Assistant May 12:4, Aug 16:10

(If comparative STR analysis of recipient [using buccal swab or other germline tissue sample] and donor are performed after hematopoietic stem cell transplantation, report 81265, 81266 in conjunction with 81267, 81268 for chimerism testing)

#● 81187 *CNBP (CCHC-type zinc finger nucleic acid binding protein)* (eg, myotonic dystrophy type 2) gene analysis, evaluation to detect abnormal (eg, expanded) alleles
CPT Changes: An Insider's View 2019

 # 81265 Comparative analysis using Short Tandem Repeat (STR) markers; patient and comparative specimen (eg, pre-transplant recipient and donor germline testing, post-transplant non-hematopoietic recipient germline [eg, buccal swab or other germline tissue sample] and donor testing, twin zygosity testing, or maternal cell contamination of fetal cells)
CPT Changes: An Insider's View 2012
CPT Assistant May 12:4, Aug 16:10

#+ 81266 each additional specimen (eg, additional cord blood donor, additional fetal samples from different cultures, or additional zygosity in multiple birth pregnancies) (List separately in addition to code for primary procedure)
CPT Changes: An Insider's View 2012
CPT Assistant May 12:4, Aug 16:10

(Use 81266 in conjunction with 81265)

#● 81188 *CSTB (cystatin B)* (eg, Unverricht-Lundborg disease) gene analysis; evaluation to detect abnormal (eg, expanded) alleles
CPT Changes: An Insider's View 2019

#● 81189 full gene sequence
CPT Changes: An Insider's View 2019

#● 81190 known familial variant(s)
CPT Changes: An Insider's View 2019

 # 81227 *CYP2C9 (cytochrome P450, family 2, subfamily C, polypeptide 9)* (eg, drug metabolism), gene analysis, common variants (eg, *2, *3, *5, *6)
CPT Changes: An Insider's View 2012
CPT Assistant May 12:4, Aug 16:10

81225 *CYP2C19 (cytochrome P450, family 2, subfamily C, polypeptide 19)* (eg, drug metabolism), gene analysis, common variants (eg, *2, *3, *4, *8, *17)
CPT Changes: An Insider's View 2012
CPT Assistant May 12:4, Aug 16:10

81226 *CYP2D6 (cytochrome P450, family 2, subfamily D, polypeptide 6)* (eg, drug metabolism), gene analysis, common variants (eg, *2, *3, *4, *5, *6, *9, *10, *17, *19, *29, *35, *41, *1XN, *2XN, *4XN)
CPT Changes: An Insider's View 2012
CPT Assistant May 12:4, Aug 16:10

81227 Code is out of numerical sequence. See 81223-81226

 # 81230 *CYP3A4 (cytochrome P450 family 3 subfamily A member 4)* (eg, drug metabolism), gene analysis, common variant(s) (eg, *2, *22)
CPT Changes: An Insider's View 2018

 # 81231 *CYP3A5 (cytochrome P450 family 3 subfamily A member 5)* (eg, drug metabolism), gene analysis, common variants (eg, *2, *3, *4, *5, *6, *7)
CPT Changes: An Insider's View 2018

81228 Cytogenomic constitutional (genome-wide) microarray analysis; interrogation of genomic regions for copy number variants (eg, bacterial artificial chromosome [BAC] or oligo-based comparative genomic hybridization [CGH] microarray analysis)
CPT Changes: An Insider's View 2012
CPT Assistant May 12:4, Sep 13:4, 6, Aug 16:10

81229 interrogation of genomic regions for copy number and single nucleotide polymorphism (SNP) variants for chromosomal abnormalities
CPT Changes: An Insider's View 2012
CPT Assistant May 12:4, Sep 13:4, Aug 16:10

(Do not report 81228 in conjunction with 81229)

(When performing cytogenomic constitutional microarray analysis that is not genome-wide [ie, regionally targeted], report the specific code for the targeted analysis if available [eg, 81405] or the unlisted molecular pathology code [81479])

(Do not report analyte-specific molecular pathology procedures separately in conjunction with 81228, 81229 when the specific analytes are included as part of the microarray analysis)

(Do not report 88271 when performing cytogenomic microarray analysis)

(For genomic sequencing procedures or other molecular multianalyte assays for copy number analysis using circulating cell-free fetal DNA in maternal blood, see 81420, 81422, 81479)

81230 Code is out of numerical sequence. See 81225-81229

81231 Code is out of numerical sequence. See 81225-81229

 # 81161 *DMD (dystrophin)* (eg, Duchenne/Becker muscular dystrophy) deletion analysis, and duplication analysis, if performed
CPT Changes: An Insider's View 2013
CPT Assistant Aug 16:10

#● 81234 *DMPK (DM1 protein kinase)* (eg, myotonic dystrophy type 1) gene analysis; evaluation to detect abnormal (expanded) alleles
CPT Changes: An Insider's View 2019

#● 81239 characterization of alleles (eg, expanded size)
CPT Changes: An Insider's View 2019

81232 *DPYD (dihydropyrimidine dehydrogenase)* (eg, 5-fluorouracil/5-FU and capecitabine drug metabolism), gene analysis, common variant(s) (eg, *2A, *4, *5, *6)
CPT Changes: An Insider's View 2018

81233 Code is out of numerical sequence. See 81182-81220

81234 Code is out of numerical sequence. See 81228-81235

81235 *EGFR (epidermal growth factor receptor)* (eg, non-small cell lung cancer) gene analysis, common variants (eg, exon 19 LREA deletion, L858R, T790M, G719A, G719S, L861Q)
CPT Changes: An Insider's View 2013
CPT Assistant Sep 13:3, Aug 16:10

● 81236 *EZH2 (enhancer of zeste 2 polycomb repressive complex 2 subunit)* (eg, myelodysplastic syndrome, myeloproliferative neoplasms) gene analysis, full gene sequence
CPT Changes: An Insider's View 2019

● 81237 *EZH2 (enhancer of zeste 2 polycomb repressive complex 2 subunit)* (eg, diffuse large B-cell lymphoma) gene analysis, common variant(s) (eg, codon 646)
CPT Changes: An Insider's View 2019

81238 Code is out of numerical sequence. See 81240-81248

81239 Code is out of numerical sequence. See 81228-81235

81240 *F2 (prothrombin, coagulation factor II)* (eg, hereditary hypercoagulability) gene analysis, 20210G>A variant
CPT Changes: An Insider's View 2012
CPT Assistant May 12:4, Aug 16:10

81241 *F5 (coagulation factor V)* (eg, hereditary hypercoagulability) gene analysis, Leiden variant
CPT Changes: An Insider's View 2012
CPT Assistant May 12:4, Aug 16:10

 # 81238 *F9 (coagulation factor IX)* (eg, hemophilia B), full gene sequence
CPT Changes: An Insider's View 2018

81242 *FANCC (Fanconi anemia, complementation group C)* (eg, Fanconi anemia, type C) gene analysis, common variant (eg, IVS4+4A>T)
CPT Changes: An Insider's View 2012
CPT Assistant May 12:4, Aug 16:10

 # 81245 *FLT3 (fms-related tyrosine kinase 3)* (eg, acute myeloid leukemia), gene analysis; internal tandem duplication (ITD) variants (ie, exons 14, 15)
CPT Changes: An Insider's View 2012, 2015
CPT Assistant May 12:4, Jan 15:3, Aug 16:10

 # 81246 tyrosine kinase domain (TKD) variants (eg, D835, I836)
CPT Changes: An Insider's View 2015
CPT Assistant Jan 15:3, Aug 16:10

81243 *FMR1 (fragile X mental retardation 1)* (eg, fragile X mental retardation) gene analysis; evaluation to detect abnormal (eg, expanded) alleles
CPT Changes: An Insider's View 2012
CPT Assistant May 12:4, Aug 16:10

(For evaluation to detect and characterize abnormal alleles, see 81243, 81244)

(For evaluation to detect and characterize abnormal alleles using a single assay [eg, PCR], use 81243)

▲ 81244 characterization of alleles (eg, expanded size and promoter methylation status)
CPT Changes: An Insider's View 2012, 2019
CPT Assistant May 12:4, Aug 16:10

81245 Code is out of numerical sequence. See 81240-81248

81246 Code is out of numerical sequence. See 81240-81248

#● 81284 *FXN (frataxin)* (eg, Friedreich ataxia) gene analysis; evaluation to detect abnormal (expanded) alleles
CPT Changes: An Insider's View 2019

#● 81285 characterization of alleles (eg, expanded size)
CPT Changes: An Insider's View 2019

#● 81286 full gene sequence
CPT Changes: An Insider's View 2019

#● 81289 known familial variant(s)
CPT Changes: An Insider's View 2019

 # 81250 *G6PC (glucose-6-phosphatase, catalytic subunit)* (eg, Glycogen storage disease, type 1a, von Gierke disease) gene analysis, common variants (eg, R83C, Q347X)
CPT Changes: An Insider's View 2012
CPT Assistant May 12:4, Aug 16:10

81247 *G6PD (glucose-6-phosphate dehydrogenase)* (eg, hemolytic anemia, jaundice), gene analysis; common variant(s) (eg, A, A-)
CPT Changes: An Insider's View 2018

81248 known familial variant(s)
CPT Changes: An Insider's View 2018

81249 full gene sequence
CPT Changes: An Insider's View 2018

81250 Code is out of numerical sequence. See 81243-81248

81251 *GBA (glucosidase, beta, acid)* (eg, Gaucher disease) gene analysis, common variants (eg, N370S, 84GG, L444P, IVS2+1G>A)
CPT Changes: An Insider's View 2012
CPT Assistant May 12:4, Aug 16:10

81252 *GJB2 (gap junction protein, beta 2, 26kDa, connexin 26)* (eg, nonsyndromic hearing loss) gene analysis; full gene sequence
CPT Changes: An Insider's View 2013
CPT Assistant Sep 13:3, Aug 16:10

81253 known familial variants
CPT Changes: An Insider's View 2013
CPT Assistant Sep 13:3, Aug 16:10

81254 *GJB6 (gap junction protein, beta 6, 30kDa, connexin 30)* (eg, nonsyndromic hearing loss) gene analysis, common variants (eg, 309kb [del(GJB6-D13S1830)] and 232kb [del(GJB6-D13S1854)])
➲ *CPT Changes: An Insider's View* 2013
➲ *CPT Assistant* Sep 13:3, Aug 16:10

 # 81257 *HBA1/HBA2 (alpha globin 1 and alpha globin 2)* (eg, alpha thalassemia, Hb Bart hydrops fetalis syndrome, HbH disease), gene analysis; common deletions or variant (eg, Southeast Asian, Thai, Filipino, Mediterranean, alpha3.7, alpha4.2, alpha20.5, Constant Spring)
➲ *CPT Changes: An Insider's View* 2012, 2018
➲ *CPT Assistant* May 12:4, Aug 16:10

 # 81258 known familial variant
➲ *CPT Changes: An Insider's View* 2018

 # 81259 full gene sequence
➲ *CPT Changes: An Insider's View* 2018

 # 81269 duplication/deletion variants
➲ *CPT Changes: An Insider's View* 2018

 # 81361 *HBB (hemoglobin, subunit beta)* (eg, sickle cell anemia, beta thalassemia, hemoglobinopathy); common variant(s) (eg, HbS, HbC, HbE)
➲ *CPT Changes: An Insider's View* 2018

 # 81362 known familial variant(s)
➲ *CPT Changes: An Insider's View* 2018

 # 81363 duplication/deletion variant(s)
➲ *CPT Changes: An Insider's View* 2018

 # 81364 full gene sequence
➲ *CPT Changes: An Insider's View* 2018

81255 *HEXA (hexosaminidase A [alpha polypeptide])* (eg, Tay-Sachs disease) gene analysis, common variants (eg, 1278insTATC, 1421+1G>C, G269S)
➲ *CPT Changes: An Insider's View* 2012
➲ *CPT Assistant* May 12:4, Aug 16:10

81256 *HFE (hemochromatosis)* (eg, hereditary hemochromatosis) gene analysis, common variants (eg, C282Y, H63D)
➲ *CPT Changes: An Insider's View* 2012
➲ *CPT Assistant* May 12:4, Aug 16:10

81257 Code is out of numerical sequence. See 81253-81256

81258 Code is out of numerical sequence. See 81253-81256

81259 Code is out of numerical sequence. See 81253-81256

#● 81271 *HTT (huntingtin)* (eg, Huntington disease) gene analysis; evaluation to detect abnormal (eg, expanded) alleles
➲ *CPT Changes: An Insider's View* 2019

#● 81274 characterization of alleles (eg, expanded size)
➲ *CPT Changes: An Insider's View* 2019

 # 81105 *Human Platelet Antigen 1 genotyping (HPA-1), ITGB3 (integrin, beta 3 [platelet glycoprotein IIIa], antigen CD61 [GPIIIa])* (eg, neonatal alloimmune thrombocytopenia [NAIT], post-transfusion purpura), gene analysis, common variant, HPA-1a/b (L33P)
➲ *CPT Changes: An Insider's View* 2018

 # 81106 *Human Platelet Antigen 2 genotyping (HPA-2), GP1BA (glycoprotein Ib [platelet], alpha polypeptide [GPIba])* (eg, neonatal alloimmune thrombocytopenia [NAIT], post-transfusion purpura), gene analysis, common variant, HPA-2a/b (T145M)
➲ *CPT Changes: An Insider's View* 2018

 # 81107 *Human Platelet Antigen 3 genotyping (HPA-3), ITGA2B (integrin, alpha 2b [platelet glycoprotein IIb of IIb/IIIa complex], antigen CD41 [GPIIb])* (eg, neonatal alloimmune thrombocytopenia [NAIT], post-transfusion purpura), gene analysis, common variant, HPA-3a/b (I843S)
➲ *CPT Changes: An Insider's View* 2018

 # 81108 *Human Platelet Antigen 4 genotyping (HPA-4), ITGB3 (integrin, beta 3 [platelet glycoprotein IIIa], antigen CD61 [GPIIIa])* (eg, neonatal alloimmune thrombocytopenia [NAIT], post-transfusion purpura), gene analysis, common variant, HPA-4a/b (R143Q)
➲ *CPT Changes: An Insider's View* 2018

 # 81109 *Human Platelet Antigen 5 genotyping (HPA-5), ITGA2 (integrin, alpha 2 [CD49B, alpha 2 subunit of VLA-2 receptor] [GPIa])* (eg, neonatal alloimmune thrombocytopenia [NAIT], post-transfusion purpura), gene analysis, common variant (eg, HPA-5a/b [K505E])
➲ *CPT Changes: An Insider's View* 2018

 # 81110 *Human Platelet Antigen 6 genotyping (HPA-6w), ITGB3 (integrin, beta 3 [platelet glycoprotein IIIa, antigen CD61] [GPIIIa])* (eg, neonatal alloimmune thrombocytopenia [NAIT], post-transfusion purpura), gene analysis, common variant, HPA-6a/b (R489Q)
➲ *CPT Changes: An Insider's View* 2018

 # 81111 *Human Platelet Antigen 9 genotyping (HPA-9w), ITGA2B (integrin, alpha 2b [platelet glycoprotein IIb of IIb/IIIa complex, antigen CD41] [GPIIb])* (eg, neonatal alloimmune thrombocytopenia [NAIT], post-transfusion purpura), gene analysis, common variant, HPA-9a/b (V837M)
➲ *CPT Changes: An Insider's View* 2018

 # 81112 *Human Platelet Antigen 15 genotyping (HPA-15), CD109 (CD109 molecule)* (eg, neonatal alloimmune thrombocytopenia [NAIT], post-transfusion purpura), gene analysis, common variant, HPA-15a/b (S682Y)
➲ *CPT Changes: An Insider's View* 2018

 # 81120 *IDH1 (isocitrate dehydrogenase 1 [NADP+], soluble)* (eg, glioma), common variants (eg, R132H, R132C)
➲ *CPT Changes: An Insider's View* 2018

 # 81121 *IDH2 (isocitrate dehydrogenase 2 [NADP+], mitochondrial)* (eg, glioma), common variants (eg, R140W, R172M)
➲ *CPT Changes: An Insider's View* 2018

 # 81283 *IFNL3 (interferon, lambda 3)* (eg, drug response), gene analysis, rs12979860 variant
➲ *CPT Changes: An Insider's View* 2018

 # 81261 *IGH@ (Immunoglobulin heavy chain locus)* (eg, leukemias and lymphomas, B-cell), gene rearrangement analysis to detect abnormal clonal population(s); amplified methodology (eg, polymerase chain reaction)
➲ *CPT Changes: An Insider's View* 2012
➲ *CPT Assistant* May 12:4, Sep 13:7, Aug 16:10

 # 81262 direct probe methodology (eg, Southern blot)
➲ *CPT Changes: An Insider's View* 2012
➲ *CPT Assistant* May 12:4, Aug 16:10

 # 81263 *IGH@ (Immunoglobulin heavy chain locus)* (eg, leukemia and lymphoma, B-cell), variable region somatic mutation analysis
➲ *CPT Changes: An Insider's View* 2012
➲ *CPT Assistant* May 12:4, Aug 16:10

 # 81264 *IGK@ (Immunoglobulin kappa light chain locus)* (eg, leukemia and lymphoma, B-cell), gene rearrangement analysis, evaluation to detect abnormal clonal population(s)
➲ *CPT Changes: An Insider's View* 2012
➲ *CPT Assistant* May 12:4, Aug 16:10

(For immunoglobulin lambda gene *[IGL@]* rearrangement or immunoglobulin kappa deleting element, *[IGKDEL]* analysis, use 81479)

81260 *IKBKAP (inhibitor of kappa light polypeptide gene enhancer in B-cells, kinase complex-associated protein)* (eg, familial dysautonomia) gene analysis, common variants (eg, 2507+6T>C, R696P)
➲ *CPT Changes: An Insider's View* 2012
➲ *CPT Assistant* May 12:4, Aug 16:10

81261 Code is out of numerical sequence. See 81255-81270

81262 Code is out of numerical sequence. See 81255-81270

81263 Code is out of numerical sequence. See 81255-81270

81264 Code is out of numerical sequence. See 81255-81270

81265 Code is out of numerical sequence. See 81223-81226

81266 Code is out of numerical sequence. See 81223-81226

81267 Code is out of numerical sequence. See 81223-81226

81268 Code is out of numerical sequence. See 81223-81226

81269 Code is out of numerical sequence. See 81253-81256

81270 *JAK2 (Janus kinase 2)* (eg, myeloproliferative disorder) gene analysis, p.Val617Phe (V617F) variant
➲ *CPT Changes: An Insider's View* 2012
➲ *CPT Assistant* May 12:4, Aug 16:10

81271 Code is out of numerical sequence. See 81255-81270

81272 *KIT (v-kit Hardy-Zuckerman 4 feline sarcoma viral oncogene homolog)* (eg, gastrointestinal stromal tumor [GIST], acute myeloid leukemia, melanoma), gene analysis, targeted sequence analysis (eg, exons 8, 11, 13, 17, 18)
➲ *CPT Changes: An Insider's View* 2016
➲ *CPT Assistant* Aug 16:10

81273 *KIT (v-kit Hardy-Zuckerman 4 feline sarcoma viral oncogene homolog)* (eg, mastocytosis), gene analysis, D816 variant(s)
➲ *CPT Changes: An Insider's View* 2016
➲ *CPT Assistant* Aug 16:10

81274 Code is out of numerical sequence. See 81255-81270

81275 *KRAS (Kirsten rat sarcoma viral oncogene homolog)* (eg, carcinoma) gene analysis; variants in exon 2 (eg, codons 12 and 13)
➲ *CPT Changes: An Insider's View* 2012, 2016
➲ *CPT Assistant* May 12:4, Sep 13:6, Aug 16:10

81276 additional variant(s) (eg, codon 61, codon 146)
➲ *CPT Changes: An Insider's View* 2016
➲ *CPT Assistant* Aug 16:10

(81280, 81281, 81282 have been deleted)

81283 Code is out of numerical sequence. See 81255-81270

81284 Code is out of numerical sequence. See 81243-81248

81285 Code is out of numerical sequence. See 81243-81248

81286 Code is out of numerical sequence. See 81243-81248

81287 Code is out of numerical sequence. See 81276-81297

81288 Code is out of numerical sequence. See 81276-81297

81289 Code is out of numerical sequence. See 81243-81248

81290 *MCOLN1 (mucolipin 1)* (eg, Mucolipidosis, type IV) gene analysis, common variants (eg, IVS3-2A>G, del6.4kb)
➲ *CPT Changes: An Insider's View* 2012
➲ *CPT Assistant* May 12:4, Aug 16:10

 # 81302 *MECP2 (methyl CpG binding protein 2)* (eg, Rett syndrome) gene analysis; full sequence analysis
➲ *CPT Changes: An Insider's View* 2012
➲ *CPT Assistant* May 12:4, Aug 16:10

 # 81303 known familial variant
➲ *CPT Changes: An Insider's View* 2012
➲ *CPT Assistant* May 12:4, Aug 16:10

 # 81304 duplication/deletion variants
➲ *CPT Changes: An Insider's View* 2012
➲ *CPT Assistant* May 12:4, Aug 16:10

#▲ 81287 *MGMT (O-6-methylguanine-DNA methyltransferase)* (eg, glioblastoma multiforme) promoter methylation analysis
➲ *CPT Changes: An Insider's View* 2014, 2019
➲ *CPT Assistant* Aug 16:10

 # 81301 Microsatellite instability analysis (eg, hereditary non-polyposis colorectal cancer, Lynch syndrome) of markers for mismatch repair deficiency (eg, BAT25, BAT26), includes comparison of neoplastic and normal tissue, if performed
➲ *CPT Changes: An Insider's View* 2012
➲ *CPT Assistant* May 12:4, Aug 16:10

 # 81292 *MLH1 (mutL homolog 1, colon cancer, nonpolyposis type 2)* (eg, hereditary non-polyposis colorectal cancer, Lynch syndrome) gene analysis; full sequence analysis
➲ *CPT Changes: An Insider's View* 2012
➲ *CPT Assistant* May 12:4, Jan 15:3, Aug 16:10

 # 81288 promoter methylation analysis
➲ *CPT Changes: An Insider's View* 2015
➲ *CPT Assistant* Jan 15:3, Aug 16:10

 # 81293 known familial variants
- CPT Changes: An Insider's View 2012
- CPT Assistant May 12:4, Aug 16:10

 # 81294 duplication/deletion variants
- CPT Changes: An Insider's View 2012
- CPT Assistant May 12:4, Aug 16:10

 # 81295 *MSH2 (mutS homolog 2, colon cancer, nonpolyposis type 1)* (eg, hereditary non-polyposis colorectal cancer, Lynch syndrome) gene analysis; full sequence analysis
- CPT Changes: An Insider's View 2012
- CPT Assistant May 12:4, Aug 16:10

81291 Code is out of numerical sequence. See 81299-81310

81292 Code is out of numerical sequence. See 81276-81297

81293 Code is out of numerical sequence. See 81276-81297

81294 Code is out of numerical sequence. See 81276-81297

81295 Code is out of numerical sequence. See 81276-81297

81296 known familial variants
- CPT Changes: An Insider's View 2012
- CPT Assistant May 12:3, Aug 16:10

81297 duplication/deletion variants
- CPT Changes: An Insider's View 2012
- CPT Assistant May 12:4, Aug 16:10

81298 *MSH6 (mutS homolog 6 [E. coli])* (eg, hereditary non-polyposis colorectal cancer, Lynch syndrome) gene analysis; full sequence analysis
- CPT Changes: An Insider's View 2012
- CPT Assistant May 12:4, Aug 16:10

81299 known familial variants
- CPT Changes: An Insider's View 2012
- CPT Assistant May 12:4, Aug 16:10

81300 duplication/deletion variants
- CPT Changes: An Insider's View 2012
- CPT Assistant May 12:4, Aug 16:10

81301 Code is out of numerical sequence. See 81276-81297

81302 Code is out of numerical sequence. See 81276-81297

81303 Code is out of numerical sequence. See 81276-81297

81304 Code is out of numerical sequence. See 81276-81297

 # 81291 *MTHFR (5,10-methylenetetrahydrofolate reductase)* (eg, hereditary hypercoagulability) gene analysis, common variants (eg, 677T, 1298C)
- CPT Changes: An Insider's View 2012
- CPT Assistant May 12:4, Aug 16:10

● 81305 *MYD88 (myeloid differentiation primary response 88)* (eg, Waldenstrom's macroglobulinemia, lymphoplasmacytic leukemia) gene analysis, p.Leu265Pro (L265P) variant
- CPT Changes: An Insider's View 2019

81306 Code is out of numerical sequence. See 81310-81318

81310 *NPM1 (nucleophosmin)* (eg, acute myeloid leukemia) gene analysis, exon 12 variants
- CPT Changes: An Insider's View 2012
- CPT Assistant May 12:4, Aug 16:10

81311 *NRAS (neuroblastoma RAS viral [v-ras] oncogene homolog)* (eg, colorectal carcinoma), gene analysis, variants in exon 2 (eg, codons 12 and 13) and exon 3 (eg, codon 61)
- CPT Changes: An Insider's View 2016
- CPT Assistant Aug 16:10

81312 Code is out of numerical sequence. See 81310-81318

#● 81306 *NUDT15 (nudix hydrolase 15)* (eg, drug metabolism) gene analysis, common variant(s) (eg, *2, *3, *4, *5, *6)
- CPT Changes: An Insider's View 2019

#● 81312 *PABPN1 (poly[A] binding protein nuclear 1)* (eg, oculopharyngeal muscular dystrophy) gene analysis, evaluation to detect abnormal (eg, expanded) alleles
- CPT Changes: An Insider's View 2019

81313 *PCA3/KLK3 (prostate cancer antigen 3 [non-protein coding]/kallikrein-related peptidase 3 [prostate specific antigen])* ratio (eg, prostate cancer)
- CPT Changes: An Insider's View 2015
- CPT Assistant Jan 15:3, Aug 16:10

81314 *PDGFRA (platelet-derived growth factor receptor, alpha polypeptide)* (eg, gastrointestinal stromal tumor [GIST]), gene analysis, targeted sequence analysis (eg, exons 12, 18)
- CPT Changes: An Insider's View 2016
- CPT Assistant Aug 16:10

#● 81320 *PLCG2 (phospholipase C gamma 2)* (eg, chronic lymphocytic leukemia) gene analysis, common variants (eg, R665W, S707F, L845F)
- CPT Changes: An Insider's View 2019

81315 *PML/RARalpha, (t(15;17)), (promyelocytic leukemia/retinoic acid receptor alpha)* (eg, promyelocytic leukemia) translocation analysis; common breakpoints (eg, intron 3 and intron 6), qualitative or quantitative
- CPT Changes: An Insider's View 2012
- CPT Assistant May 12:4, Aug 16:10

81316 single breakpoint (eg, intron 3, intron 6 or exon 6), qualitative or quantitative
- CPT Changes: An Insider's View 2012
- CPT Assistant May 12:4, Aug 16:10

(For intron 3 and intron 6 [including exon 6 if performed] analysis, use 81315)

(If both intron 6 and exon 6 are analyzed, without intron 3, use one unit of 81316)

 # 81324 *PMP22 (peripheral myelin protein 22)* (eg, Charcot-Marie-Tooth, hereditary neuropathy with liability to pressure palsies) gene analysis; duplication/deletion analysis
- CPT Changes: An Insider's View 2013
- CPT Assistant Sep 13:3, Aug 16:10

 # 81325 full sequence analysis
- CPT Changes: An Insider's View 2013
- CPT Assistant Sep 13:3, Aug 16:10

 # 81326 known familial variant
- CPT Changes: An Insider's View 2013
- CPT Assistant Sep 13:3, Aug 16:10

81317 *PMS2 (postmeiotic segregation increased 2 [S. cerevisiae])* (eg, hereditary non-polyposis colorectal cancer, Lynch syndrome) gene analysis; full sequence analysis
➔ *CPT Changes: An Insider's View* 2012
➔ *CPT Assistant* May 12:4, Aug 16:10

81318 known familial variants
➔ *CPT Changes: An Insider's View* 2012
➔ *CPT Assistant* May 12:4, Aug 16:10

81319 duplication/deletion variants
➔ *CPT Changes: An Insider's View* 2012
➔ *CPT Assistant* May 12:4, Aug 16:10

81320 Code is out of numerical sequence. See 81310-81318

#● **81343** *PPP2R2B (protein phosphatase 2 regulatory subunit Bbeta)* (eg, spinocerebellar ataxia) gene analysis, evaluation to detect abnormal (eg, expanded) alleles
➔ *CPT Changes: An Insider's View* 2019

81321 *PTEN (phosphatase and tensin homolog)* (eg, Cowden syndrome, *PTEN* hamartoma tumor syndrome) gene analysis; full sequence analysis
➔ *CPT Changes: An Insider's View* 2013
➔ *CPT Assistant* Sep 13:3, Aug 16:10

81322 known familial variant
➔ *CPT Changes: An Insider's View* 2013
➔ *CPT Assistant* Sep 13:3, Aug 16:10

81323 duplication/deletion variant
➔ *CPT Changes: An Insider's View* 2013
➔ *CPT Assistant* Sep 13:3, Aug 16:10

81324 Code is out of numerical sequence. See 81310-81318

81325 Code is out of numerical sequence. See 81310-81318

81326 Code is out of numerical sequence. See 81310-81318

\# **81334** *RUNX1 (runt related transcription factor 1)* (eg, acute myeloid leukemia, familial platelet disorder with associated myeloid malignancy) gene analysis, targeted sequence analysis (eg, exons 3-8)
➔ *CPT Changes: An Insider's View* 2018

▲ **81327** *SEPT9 (Septin9)* (eg, colorectal cancer) promoter methylation analysis
➔ *CPT Changes: An Insider's View* 2017, 2019

\# **81332** *SERPINA1 (serpin peptidase inhibitor, clade A, alpha-1 antiproteinase, antitrypsin, member 1)* (eg, alpha-1-antitrypsin deficiency), gene analysis, common variants (eg, *S and *Z)
➔ *CPT Changes: An Insider's View* 2012
➔ *CPT Assistant* May 12:4, Aug 16:10

81328 *SLCO1B1 (solute carrier organic anion transporter family, member 1B1)* (eg, adverse drug reaction), gene analysis, common variant(s) (eg, *5)
➔ *CPT Changes: An Insider's View* 2018

● **81329** *SMN1 (survival of motor neuron 1, telomeric)* (eg, spinal muscular atrophy) gene analysis; dosage/deletion analysis (eg, carrier testing), includes *SMN2 (survival of motor neuron 2, centromeric)* analysis, if performed
➔ *CPT Changes: An Insider's View* 2019

#● **81336** full gene sequence
➔ *CPT Changes: An Insider's View* 2019

#● **81337** known familial sequence variant(s)
➔ *CPT Changes: An Insider's View* 2019

81330 *SMPD1(sphingomyelin phosphodiesterase 1, acid lysosomal)* (eg, Niemann-Pick disease, Type A) gene analysis, common variants (eg, R496L, L302P, fsP330)
➔ *CPT Changes: An Insider's View* 2012
➔ *CPT Assistant* May 12:4, Aug 16:10

81331 *SNRPN/UBE3A (small nuclear ribonucleoprotein polypeptide N and ubiquitin protein ligase E3A)* (eg, Prader-Willi syndrome and/or Angelman syndrome), methylation analysis
➔ *CPT Changes: An Insider's View* 2012
➔ *CPT Assistant* May 12:4, Aug 16:10

81332 Code is out of numerical sequence. See 81318-81335

#● **81344** *TBP (TATA box binding protein)* (eg, spinocerebellar ataxia) gene analysis, evaluation to detect abnormal (eg, expanded) alleles
➔ *CPT Changes: An Insider's View* 2019

#● **81345** *TERT (telomerase reverse transcriptase)* (eg, thyroid carcinoma, glioblastoma multiforme) gene analysis, targeted sequence analysis (eg, promoter region)
➔ *CPT Changes: An Insider's View* 2019

● **81333** *TGFBI (transforming growth factor beta-induced)* (eg, corneal dystrophy) gene analysis, common variants (eg, R124H, R124C, R124L, R555W, R555Q)
➔ *CPT Changes: An Insider's View* 2019

81334 Code is out of numerical sequence. See 81318-81335

81335 *TPMT (thiopurine S-methyltransferase)* (eg, drug metabolism), gene analysis, common variants (eg, *2, *3)
➔ *CPT Changes: An Insider's View* 2018

81336 Code is out of numerical sequence. See 81318-81335

81337 Code is out of numerical sequence. See 81318-81335

81340 *TRB@ (T cell antigen receptor, beta)* (eg, leukemia and lymphoma), gene rearrangement analysis to detect abnormal clonal population(s); using amplification methodology (eg, polymerase chain reaction)
➔ *CPT Changes: An Insider's View* 2012
➔ *CPT Assistant* May 12:4, Aug 16:10

81341 using direct probe methodology (eg, Southern blot)
➔ *CPT Changes: An Insider's View* 2012
➔ *CPT Assistant* May 12:4, Aug 16:10

81342 *TRG@ (T cell antigen receptor, gamma)* (eg, leukemia and lymphoma), gene rearrangement analysis, evaluation to detect abnormal clonal population(s)
➔ *CPT Changes: An Insider's View* 2012
➔ *CPT Assistant* May 12:4, Aug 16:10

(For T cell antigen alpha *[TRA@]* gene rearrangement analysis, use 81479)

(For T cell antigen delta *[TRD@]* gene rearrangement analysis, use 81402)

81343 Code is out of numerical sequence. See 81318-81335

81344 Code is out of numerical sequence. See 81318-81335

81345 Code is out of numerical sequence. See 81318-81335

81346 *TYMS (thymidylate synthetase)* (eg, 5-fluorouracil/5-FU drug metabolism), gene analysis, common variant(s) (eg, tandem repeat variant)
➔ *CPT Changes: An Insider's View* 2018

81350 *UGT1A1 (UDP glucuronosyltransferase 1 family, polypeptide A1)* (eg, irinotecan metabolism), gene analysis, common variants (eg, *28, *36, *37)
➔ *CPT Changes: An Insider's View* 2012
➔ *CPT Assistant* May 12:4, Aug 16:10

81355 *VKORC1 (vitamin K epoxide reductase complex, subunit 1)* (eg, warfarin metabolism), gene analysis, common variant(s) (eg, -1639G>A, c.173+1000C>T)
➔ *CPT Changes: An Insider's View* 2012, 2016
➔ *CPT Assistant* May 12:4, Aug 16:10

81361 Code is out of numerical sequence. See 81253-81256

81362 Code is out of numerical sequence. See 81253-81256

81363 Code is out of numerical sequence. See 81253-81256

81364 Code is out of numerical sequence. See 81253-81256

Human Leukocyte Antigen (HLA) typing is performed to assess compatibility of recipients and potential donors as a part of solid organ and hematopoietic stem cell pretransplant testing. HLA testing is also performed to identify HLA alleles and allele groups (antigen equivalents) associated with specific diseases and individualized responses to drug therapy (eg, HLA-B*27 and ankylosing spondylitis and HLA-B*57:01 and abacavir hypersensitivity), as well as other clinical uses. One or more HLA genes may be tested in specific clinical situations (eg, HLA-DQB1 for narcolepsy and HLA-A, -B, -C, -DRB1, and -DQB1 for kidney transplantation). Each HLA gene typically has multiple variant alleles or allele groups that can be identified by typing. For HLA result reporting, a low resolution HLA type is denoted by a two digit HLA name (eg, A*02) and intermediate resolution typing by a string of alleles or an NMDP (National Marrow Donor Program) code (eg, B*14:01/07N/08/12/14, B*39CKGN). Both low and intermediate resolutions are considered low resolution for code assignment. High resolution typing resolves the common well defined (CWD) alleles and is usually denoted by at least 4 digits (eg, A*02:02, *03:01:01:01, A*26:01:01G, and C*03:04P), however, high resolution typing may include some ambiguities for rare alleles, which may be reported as a string of alleles or an NMDP code.

If additional testing is required to resolve ambiguous allele combinations for high resolution typing, this is included in the base HLA typing codes below. The gene names have been italicized similar to the other molecular pathology codes.

(For HLA antigen typing by non-molecular pathology techniques, see 86812, 86813, 86816, 86817, 86821)

81370 HLA Class I and II typing, low resolution (eg, antigen equivalents); *HLA-A, -B, -C, -DRB1/3/4/5,* and *-DQB1*
➔ *CPT Changes: An Insider's View* 2012
➔ *CPT Assistant* May 12:4, Aug 16:10

81371 *HLA-A, -B, and -DRB1* (eg, verification typing)
➔ *CPT Changes: An Insider's View* 2012, 2014
➔ *CPT Assistant* May 12:4, Aug 16:10

(When HLA typing includes a determination of the presence or absence of the DRB3/4/5 genes, that service is included in the typing and is not separately reported)

81372 HLA Class I typing, low resolution (eg, antigen equivalents); complete *(ie, HLA-A, -B,* and *-C)*
➔ *CPT Changes: An Insider's View* 2012
➔ *CPT Assistant* May 12:4, Aug 16:10

(When performing both Class I and II low resolution *HLA typing for HLA-A,-B,-C, -DRB1/3/4/5,* and *-DQB1*, use 81370)

81373 one locus *(eg, HLA-A, -B, or -C)*, each
➔ *CPT Changes: An Insider's View* 2012
➔ *CPT Assistant* May 12:4, Jun 12:16, Aug 16:10

(When performing a complete Class I *[HLA-A,-B,* and *-C]* low resolution HLA typing, use 81372)

(When the presence or absence of a single antigen equivalent is reported using low resolution testing, use 81374)

81374 one antigen equivalent (eg, *B*27)*, each
➔ *CPT Changes: An Insider's View* 2012
➔ *CPT Assistant* May 12:4, Jun 12:16, Aug 16:10

(When testing for presence or absence of more than 2 antigen equivalents at a locus, use 81373 for each locus tested)

81375 HLA Class II typing, low resolution (eg, antigen equivalents); *HLA-DRB1/3/4/5* and *-DQB1*
➔ *CPT Changes: An Insider's View* 2012
➔ *CPT Assistant* May 12:4, Aug 16:10

(When performing both Class I and II low resolution HLA typing *for HLA-A,-B,-C, -DRB1/3/4/5,* and *–DQB1*, use 81370)

81376 one locus *(eg, HLA-DRB1, -DRB3/4/5, -DQB1, -DQA1, -DPB1, or -DPA1)*, each
➔ *CPT Changes: An Insider's View* 2012, 2014
➔ *CPT Assistant* May 12:4, Jun 12:16, Aug 16:10

(When low resolution typing is performed for *HLA-DRB1/3/4/5* and *-DQB1*, use 81375)

(When HLA typing includes a determination of the presence or absence of the DRB3/4/5 genes, that service is included in the typing and is not separately reported. When low or intermediate resolution typing of any or all of the DRB3/4/5 genes is performed, treat as one locus)

81377 one antigen equivalent, each

➲ *CPT Changes: An Insider's View* 2012

➲ *CPT Assistant* May 12:4, Jun 12:16, Aug 16:10

(When testing for presence or absence of more than 2 antigen equivalents at a locus, use 81376 for each locus)

81378 HLA Class I and II typing, high resolution (ie, alleles or allele groups), *HLA-A, -B, -C,* and *-DRB1*

➲ *CPT Changes: An Insider's View* 2012

➲ *CPT Assistant* May 12:4, Jun 12:16, Aug 16:10

81379 HLA Class I typing, high resolution (ie, alleles or allele groups); complete (ie, *HLA-A, -B,* and *-C)*

➲ *CPT Changes: An Insider's View* 2012

➲ *CPT Assistant* May 12:4, Aug 16:10

81380 one locus (eg, *HLA-A, -B,* or *-C*), each

➲ *CPT Changes: An Insider's View* 2012

➲ *CPT Assistant* May 12:4, Jun 12:16, Aug 16:10

(When a complete Class I high resolution typing for *HLA-A,-B,* and *-C* is performed, use 81379)

(When the presence or absence of a single allele or allele group is reported using high resolution testing, use 81381)

81381 one allele or allele group (eg, *B*57:01P*), each

➲ *CPT Changes: An Insider's View* 2012

➲ *CPT Assistant* May 12:4, Jun 12:16, Aug 16:10

(When testing for the presence or absence of more than 2 alleles or allele groups at a locus, use 81380 for each locus)

81382 HLA Class II typing, high resolution (ie, alleles or allele groups); one locus (eg, *HLA-DRB1, -DRB3/4/5, -DQB1, -DQA1, -DPB1,* or *-DPA1*), each

➲ *CPT Changes: An Insider's View* 2012, 2014

➲ *CPT Assistant* May 12:4, Jun 12:16

(When only the presence or absence of a single allele or allele group is reported using high resolution testing, use 81383)

(When high resolution typing of any or all of the DRB3/4/5 genes is performed, treat as one locus)

81383 one allele or allele group (eg, *HLA-DQB1*06:02P*), each

➲ *CPT Changes: An Insider's View* 2012

➲ *CPT Assistant* May 12:4, Jun 12:16

(When testing for the presence or absence of more than 2 alleles or allele groups at a locus, use 81382 for each locus)

Tier 2 Molecular Pathology Procedures

The following molecular pathology procedure (Tier 2) codes are used to report procedures not listed in the Tier 1 molecular pathology codes (81161, 81200-81383). They represent medically useful procedures that are generally performed in lower volumes than Tier 1 procedures (eg, the incidence of the disease being tested is rare). They are arranged by level of technical resources and interpretive work by the physician or other qualified health care professional. The individual analyses listed under each code (ie, level of procedure) utilize the definitions and coding principles as described in the introduction preceding the Tier 1 molecular pathology codes. The parenthetical examples of methodologies presented near the beginning of each code provide general guidelines used to group procedures for a given level and are not all-inclusive.

Use the appropriate molecular pathology procedure level code that includes the specific analyte listed after the code descriptor. If the analyte tested is not listed under one of the Tier 2 codes or is not represented by a Tier 1 code, use the unlisted molecular pathology procedure code, 81479.

▲ **81400** Molecular pathology procedure, Level 1 (eg, identification of single germline variant [eg, SNP] by techniques such as restriction enzyme digestion or melt curve analysis)

ACADM (acyl-CoA dehydrogenase, C-4 to C-12 straight chain, MCAD) (eg, medium chain acyl dehydrogenase deficiency), K304E variant

ACE (angiotensin converting enzyme) (eg, hereditary blood pressure regulation), insertion/deletion variant

AGTR1 (angiotensin II receptor, type 1) (eg, essential hypertension), 1166A>C variant

BCKDHA (branched chain keto acid dehydrogenase E1, alpha polypeptide) (eg, maple syrup urine disease, type 1A), Y438N variant

CCR5 (chemokine C-C motif receptor 5) (eg, HIV resistance), 32-bp deletion mutation/794 825del32 deletion

CLRN1 (clarin 1) (eg, Usher syndrome, type 3), N48K variant

F2 (coagulation factor 2) (eg, hereditary hypercoagulability), 1199G>A variant

F5 (coagulation factor V) (eg, hereditary hypercoagulability), HR2 variant

F7 (coagulation factor VII [serum prothrombin conversion accelerator]) (eg, hereditary hypercoagulability), R353Q variant

F13B (coagulation factor XIII, B polypeptide) (eg, hereditary hypercoagulability), V34L variant

FGB (fibrinogen beta chain) (eg, hereditary ischemic heart disease), -455G>A variant

FGFR1 (fibroblast growth factor receptor 1) (eg, Pfeiffer syndrome type 1, craniosynostosis), P252R variant

FGFR3 (fibroblast growth factor receptor 3) (eg, Muenke syndrome), P250R variant

FKTN (fukutin) (eg, Fukuyama congenital muscular dystrophy), retrotransposon insertion variant

GNE (glucosamine [UDP-N-acetyl]-2-epimerase/N-acetylmannosamine kinase) (eg, inclusion body myopathy 2 [IBM2], Nonaka myopathy), M712T variant

IVD (isovaleryl-CoA dehydrogenase) (eg, isovaleric acidemia), A282V variant

LCT (lactase-phlorizin hydrolase) (eg, lactose intolerance), 13910 C>T variant

NEB (nebulin) (eg, nemaline myopathy 2), exon 55 deletion variant

PCDH15 (protocadherin-related 15) (eg, Usher syndrome type 1F), R245X variant

SERPINE1 (serpine peptidase inhibitor clade E, member 1, plasminogen activator inhibitor -1, PAI-1) (eg, thrombophilia), 4G variant

SHOC2 (soc-2 suppressor of clear homolog) (eg, Noonan-like syndrome with loose anagen hair), S2G variant

SRY (sex determining region Y) (eg, 46,XX testicular disorder of sex development, gonadal dysgenesis), gene analysis

TOR1A (torsin family 1, member A [torsin A]) (eg, early-onset primary dystonia [DYT1]), 907_909delGAG (904_906delGAG) variant

➲ *CPT Changes: An Insider's View* 2012, 2013, 2014, 2018, 2019

➲ *CPT Assistant* May 12:4, Jul 13:12, Sep 13:4, 5, 8, Jan 15:3, Aug 16:10

▲ **81401** Molecular pathology procedure, Level 2 (eg, 2-10 SNPs, 1 methylated variant, or 1 somatic variant [typically using nonsequencing target variant analysis], or detection of a dynamic mutation disorder/triplet repeat)

ABCC8 (ATP-binding cassette, sub-family C [CFTR/MRP], member 8) (eg, familial hyperinsulinism), common variants (eg, c.3898-9G>A [c.3992-9G>A], F1388del)

ABL1 (ABL proto-oncogene 1, non-receptor tyrosine kinase) (eg, acquired imatinib resistance), T315I variant

ACADM (acyl-CoA dehydrogenase, C-4 to C-12 straight chain, MCAD) (eg, medium chain acyl dehydrogenase deficiency), commons variants (eg, K304E, Y42H)

ADRB2 (adrenergic beta-2 receptor surface) (eg, drug metabolism), common variants (eg, G16R, Q27E)

APOB (apolipoprotein B) (eg, familial hypercholesterolemia type B), common variants (eg, R3500Q, R3500W)

APOE (apolipoprotein E) (eg, hyperlipoproteinemia type III, cardiovascular disease, Alzheimer disease), common variants (eg, *2, *3, *4)

CBFB/MYH11 (inv(16)) (eg, acute myeloid leukemia), qualitative, and quantitative, if performed

CBS (cystathionine-beta-synthase) (eg, homocystinuria, cystathionine beta-synthase deficiency), common variants (eg, I278T, G307S)

CCND1/IGH (BCL1/IgH, t(11;14)) (eg, mantle cell lymphoma) translocation analysis, major breakpoint, qualitative, and quantitative, if performed

CFH/ARMS2 (complement factor H/age-related maculopathy susceptibility 2) (eg, macular degeneration), common variants (eg, Y402H [CFH], A69S [ARMS2])

DEK/NUP214 (t(6;9)) (eg, acute myeloid leukemia), translocation analysis, qualitative, and quantitative, if performed

E2A/PBX1 (t(1;19)) (eg, acute lymphocytic leukemia), translocation analysis, qualitative, and quantitative, if performed

EML4/ALK (inv(2)) (eg, non-small cell lung cancer), translocation or inversion analysis

ETV6/NTRK3 (t(12;15)) (eg, congenital/infantile fibrosarcoma), translocation analysis, qualitative, and quantitative, if performed

ETV6/RUNX1 (t(12;21)) (eg, acute lymphocytic leukemia), translocation analysis, qualitative, and quantitative, if performed

EWSR1/ATF1 (t(12;22)) (eg, clear cell sarcoma), translocation analysis, qualitative, and quantitative, if performed

EWSR1/ERG (t(21;22)) (eg, Ewing sarcoma/peripheral neuroectodermal tumor), translocation analysis, qualitative, and quantitative, if performed

EWSR1/FLI1 (t(11;22)) (eg, Ewing sarcoma/peripheral neuroectodermal tumor), translocation analysis, qualitative, and quantitative, if performed

EWSR1/WT1 (t(11;22)) (eg, desmoplastic small round cell tumor), translocation analysis, qualitative, and quantitative, if performed

F11 (coagulation factor XI) (eg, coagulation disorder), common variants (eg, E117X [Type II], F283L [Type III], IVS14del14, and IVS14+1G>A [Type I])

FGFR3 (fibroblast growth factor receptor 3) (eg, achondroplasia, hypochondroplasia), common variants (eg, 1138G>A, 1138G>C, 1620C>A, 1620C>G)

FIP1L1/PDGFRA (del[4q12]) (eg, imatinib-sensitive chronic eosinophilic leukemia), qualitative, and quantitative, if performed

FLG (filaggrin) (eg, ichthyosis vulgaris), common variants (eg, R501X, 2282del4, R2447X, S3247X, 3702delG)

FOXO1/PAX3 (t(2;13)) (eg, alveolar rhabdomyosarcoma), translocation analysis, qualitative, and quantitative, if performed

FOXO1/PAX7 (t(1;13)) (eg, alveolar rhabdomyosarcoma), translocation analysis, qualitative, and quantitative, if performed

FUS/DDIT3 (t(12;16)) (eg, myxoid liposarcoma), translocation analysis, qualitative, and quantitative, if performed

GALC (galactosylceramidase) (eg, Krabbe disease), common variants (eg, c.857G>A, 30-kb deletion)

GALT (galactose-1-phosphate uridylyltransferase) (eg, galactosemia), common variants (eg, Q188R, S135L, K285N, T138M, L195P, Y209C, IVS2-2A>G, P171S, del5kb, N314D, L218L/N314D)

H19 (imprinted maternally expressed transcript [non-protein coding]) (eg, Beckwith-Wiedemann syndrome), methylation analysis

IGH@/BCL2 (t(14;18)) (eg, follicular lymphoma), translocation analysis; single breakpoint (eg, major breakpoint region [MBR] or minor cluster region [mcr]), qualitative or quantitative

(When both MBR and mcr breakpoints are performed, use 81402)

KCNQ1OT1 (KCNQ1 overlapping transcript 1 [non-protein coding]) (eg, Beckwith-Wiedemann syndrome), methylation analysis

LINC00518 (long intergenic non-protein coding RNA 518) (eg, melanoma), expression analysis

LRRK2 (leucine-rich repeat kinase 2) (eg, Parkinson disease), common variants (eg, R1441G, G2019S, I2020T)

MED12 (mediator complex subunit 12) (eg, FG syndrome type 1, Lujan syndrome), common variants (eg, R961W, N1007S)

MEG3/DLK1 (maternally expressed 3 [non-protein coding]/delta-like 1 homolog [Drosophila]) (eg, intrauterine growth retardation), methylation analysis

MLL/AFF1 (t(4;11)) (eg, acute lymphoblastic leukemia), translocation analysis, qualitative, and quantitative, if performed

MLL/MLLT3 (t(9;11)) (eg, acute myeloid leukemia), translocation analysis, qualitative, and quantitative, if performed

MT-ATP6 (mitochondrially encoded ATP synthase 6) (eg, neuropathy with ataxia and retinitis pigmentosa [NARP], Leigh syndrome), common variants (eg, m.8993T>G, m.8993T>C)

MT-ND4, MT-ND6 (mitochondrially encoded NADH dehydrogenase 4, mitochondrially encoded NADH dehydrogenase 6) (eg, Leber hereditary optic neuropathy [LHON]), common variants (eg, m.11778G>A, m.3460G>A, m.14484T>C)

MT-ND5 (mitochondrially encoded tRNA leucine 1 [UUA/G], mitochondrially encoded NADH dehydrogenase 5) (eg, mitochondrial encephalopathy with lactic acidosis and stroke-like episodes [MELAS]), common variants (eg, m.3243A>G, m.3271T>C, m.3252A>G, m.13513G>A)

MT-RNR1 (mitochondrially encoded 12S RNA) (eg, nonsyndromic hearing loss), common variants (eg, m.1555A>G, m.1494C>T)

MT-TK (mitochondrially encoded tRNA lysine) (eg, myoclonic epilepsy with ragged-red fibers [MERRF]), common variants (eg, m.8344A>G, m.8356T>C)

MT-TL1 (mitochondrially encoded tRNA leucine 1 [UUA/G]) (eg, diabetes and hearing loss), common variants (eg, m.3243A>G, m.14709 T>C) MT-TL1

MT-TS1, MT-RNR1 (mitochondrially encoded tRNA serine 1 [UCN], mitochondrially encoded 12S RNA) (eg, nonsyndromic sensorineural deafness [including aminoglycoside-induced nonsyndromic deafness]), common variants (eg, m.7445A>G, m.1555A>G)

MUTYH (mutY homolog [E. coli]) (eg, MYH-associated polyposis), common variants (eg, Y165C, G382D)

NOD2 (nucleotide-binding oligomerization domain containing 2) (eg, Crohn's disease, Blau syndrome), common variants (eg, SNP 8, SNP 12, SNP 13)

NPM1/ALK (t(2;5)) (eg, anaplastic large cell lymphoma), translocation analysis

PAX8/PPARG (t(2;3) (q13;p25)) (eg, follicular thyroid carcinoma), translocation analysis

PRAME (preferentially expressed antigen in melanoma) (eg, melanoma), expression analysis

PRSS1 (protease, serine, 1 [trypsin 1]) (eg, hereditary pancreatitis), common variants (eg, N29I, A16V, R122H)

PYGM (phosphorylase, glycogen, muscle) (eg, glycogen storage disease type V, McArdle disease), common variants (eg, R50X, G205S)

RUNX1/RUNX1T1 (t(8;21)) (eg, acute myeloid leukemia) translocation analysis, qualitative, and quantitative, if performed

SS18/SSX1 (t(X;18)) (eg, synovial sarcoma), translocation analysis, qualitative, and quantitative, if performed

SS18/SSX2 (t(X;18)) (eg, synovial sarcoma), translocation analysis, qualitative, and quantitative, if performed

VWF (von Willebrand factor) (eg, von Willebrand disease type 2N), common variants (eg, T791M, R816W, R854Q)

➔ *CPT Changes: An Insider's View* 2012, 2013, 2014, 2016, 2017, 2018, 2019

➔ *CPT Assistant* May 12:4, Jul 13:12, Sep 13:5, Jan 15:3, Aug 16:10

81402 Molecular pathology procedure, Level 3 (eg, >10 SNPs, 2-10 methylated variants, or 2-10 somatic variants [typically using non-sequencing target variant analysis], immunoglobulin and T-cell receptor gene rearrangements, duplication/deletion variants of 1 exon, loss of heterozygosity [LOH], uniparental disomy [UPD])

Chromosome 1p-/19q- (eg, glial tumors), deletion analysis

Chromosome 18q- (eg, D18S55, D18S58, D18S61, D18S64, and D18S69) (eg, colon cancer), allelic imbalance assessment (ie, loss of heterozygosity)

COL1A1/PDGFB (t(17;22)) (eg, dermatofibrosarcoma protuberans), translocation analysis, multiple breakpoints, qualitative, and quantitative, if performed

CYP21A2 (cytochrome P450, family 21, subfamily A, polypeptide 2) (eg, congenital adrenal hyperplasia, 21-hydroxylase deficiency), common variants (eg, IVS2-13G, P30L, I172N, exon 6 mutation cluster [I235N, V236E, M238K], V281L, L307FfsX6, Q318X, R356W, P453S, G110VfsX21, 30-kb deletion variant)

ESR1/PGR (receptor 1/progesterone receptor) ratio (eg, breast cancer)

IGH@/BCL2 (t(14;18)) (eg, follicular lymphoma), translocation analysis; major breakpoint region (MBR) and minor cluster region (mcr) breakpoints, qualitative or quantitative

MEFV (Mediterranean fever) (eg, familial Mediterranean fever), common variants (eg, E148Q, P369S, F479L, M680I, I692del, M694V, M694I, K695R, V726A, A744S, R761H)

MPL (myeloproliferative leukemia virus oncogene, thrombopoietin receptor, TPOR) (eg, myeloproliferative disorder), common variants (eg, W515A, W515K, W515L, W515R)

TRD@ (T cell antigen receptor, delta) (eg, leukemia and lymphoma), gene rearrangement analysis, evaluation to detect abnormal clonal population

Uniparental disomy (UPD) (eg, Russell-Silver syndrome, Prader-Willi/Angelman syndrome), short tandem repeat (STR) analysis

➔ *CPT Changes: An Insider's View* 2012, 2013, 2014, 2015, 2016

➔ *CPT Assistant* May 12:4, Jul 13:12, Sep 13:5, 9, Jan 15:3, Aug 16:10

▲ **81403** Molecular pathology procedure, Level 4 (eg, analysis of single exon by DNA sequence analysis, analysis of >10 amplicons using multiplex PCR in 2 or more independent reactions, mutation scanning or duplication/deletion variants of 2-5 exons)

ANG (angiogenin, ribonuclease, RNase A family, 5) (eg, amyotrophic lateral sclerosis), full gene sequence

ARX (aristaless-related homeobox) (eg, X-linked lissencephaly with ambiguous genitalia, X-linked mental retardation), duplication/deletion analysis

CEL (carboxyl ester lipase [bile salt-stimulated lipase]) (eg, maturity-onset diabetes of the young [MODY]), targeted sequence analysis of exon 11 (eg, c.1785delC, c.1686delT)

CTNNB1 (catenin [cadherin-associated protein], beta 1, 88kDa) (eg, desmoid tumors), targeted sequence analysis (eg, exon 3)

DAZ/SRY (deleted in azoospermia and sex determining region Y) (eg, male infertility), common deletions (eg, AZFa, AZFb, AZFc, AZFd)

DNMT3A (DNA [cytosine-5-]-methyltransferase 3 alpha) (eg, acute myeloid leukemia), targeted sequence analysis (eg, exon 23)

EPCAM (epithelial cell adhesion molecule) (eg, Lynch syndrome), duplication/deletion analysis

F8 (coagulation factor VIII) (eg, hemophilia A), inversion analysis, intron 1 and intron 22A

F12 (coagulation factor XII [Hageman factor]) (eg, angioedema, hereditary, type III; factor XII deficiency), targeted sequence analysis of exon 9

FGFR3 (fibroblast growth factor receptor 3) (eg, isolated craniosynostosis), targeted sequence analysis (eg, exon 7)

(For targeted sequence analysis of multiple FGFR3 exons, use 81404)

GJB1 (gap junction protein, beta 1) (eg, Charcot-Marie-Tooth X-linked), full gene sequence

GNAQ (guanine nucleotide-binding protein G[q] subunit alpha) (eg, uveal melanoma), common variants (eg, R183, Q209)

Human erythrocyte antigen gene analyses (eg, SLC14A1 [Kidd blood group], BCAM [Lutheran blood group], ICAM4 [Landsteiner-Wiener blood group], SLC4A1 [Diego blood group], AQP1 [Colton blood group], ERMAP [Scianna blood group], RHCE [Rh blood group, CcEe antigens], KEL [Kell blood group], DARC [Duffy blood group], GYPA, GYPB, GYPE [MNS blood group], ART4 [Dombrock blood group]) (eg, sickle-cell disease, thalassemia, hemolytic transfusion reactions, hemolytic disease of the fetus or newborn), common variants

HRAS (v-Ha-ras Harvey rat sarcoma viral oncogene homolog) (eg, Costello syndrome), exon 2 sequence

JAK2 (Janus kinase 2) (eg, myeloproliferative disorder), exon 12 sequence and exon 13 sequence, if performed

KCNC3 (potassium voltage-gated channel, Shaw-related subfamily, member 3) (eg, spinocerebellar ataxia), targeted sequence analysis (eg, exon 2)

KCNJ2 (potassium inwardly-rectifying channel, subfamily J, member 2) (eg, Andersen-Tawil syndrome), full gene sequence

KCNJ11 (potassium inwardly-rectifying channel, subfamily J, member 11) (eg, familial hyperinsulinism), full gene sequence

Killer cell immunoglobulin-like receptor (KIR) gene family (eg, hematopoietic stem cell transplantation), genotyping of KIR family genes

Known familial variant not otherwise specified, for gene listed in Tier 1 or Tier 2, or identified during a genomic sequencing procedure, DNA sequence analysis, each variant exon

(For a known familial variant that is considered a common variant, use specific common variant Tier 1 or Tier 2 code)

MC4R (melanocortin 4 receptor) (eg, obesity), full gene sequence

MICA (MHC class I polypeptide-related sequence A) (eg, solid organ transplantation), common variants (eg, *001, *002)

MPL (myeloproliferative leukemia virus oncogene, thrombopoietin receptor, TPOR) (eg, myeloproliferative disorder), exon 10 sequence

MT-RNR1 (mitochondrially encoded 12S RNA) (eg, nonsyndromic hearing loss), full gene sequence

MT-TS1 (mitochondrially encoded tRNA serine 1) (eg, nonsyndromic hearing loss), full gene sequence

NDP (Norrie disease [pseudoglioma]) (eg, Norrie disease), duplication/deletion analysis

NHLRC1 (NHL repeat containing 1) (eg, progressive myoclonus epilepsy), full gene sequence

PHOX2B (paired-like homeobox 2b) (eg, congenital central hypoventilation syndrome), duplication/deletion analysis

PLN (phospholamban) (eg, dilated cardiomyopathy, hypertrophic cardiomyopathy), full gene sequence

RHD (Rh blood group, D antigen) (eg, hemolytic disease of the fetus and newborn, Rh maternal/fetal compatibility), deletion analysis (eg, exons 4, 5, and 7, pseudogene)

RHD (Rh blood group, D antigen) (eg, hemolytic disease of the fetus and newborn, Rh maternal/fetal compatibility), deletion analysis (eg, exons 4, 5, and 7, pseudogene), performed on cell-free fetal DNA in maternal blood

(For human erythrocyte gene analysis of RHD, use a separate unit of 81403)

SH2D1A (SH2 domain containing 1A) (eg, X-linked lymphoproliferative syndrome), duplication/deletion analysis

TWIST1 (twist homolog 1 [Drosophila]) (eg, Saethre-Chotzen syndrome), duplication/deletion analysis

UBA1 (ubiquitin-like modifier activating enzyme 1) (eg, spinal muscular atrophy, X-linked), targeted sequence analysis (eg, exon 15)

VHL (von Hippel-Lindau tumor suppressor) (eg, von Hippel-Lindau familial cancer syndrome), deletion/duplication analysis

VWF (von Willebrand factor) (eg, von Willebrand disease types 2A, 2B, 2M), targeted sequence analysis (eg, exon 28)

➔ *CPT Changes: An Insider's View* 2012, 2013, 2014, 2015, 2016, 2017, 2018, 2019

➔ *CPT Assistant* May 12:4, Jul 13:12, Sep 13:3, Jan 15:3, Aug 16:10

▲ **81404** Molecular pathology procedure, Level 5 (eg, analysis of 2-5 exons by DNA sequence analysis, mutation scanning or duplication/deletion variants of 6-10 exons, or characterization of a dynamic mutation disorder/triplet repeat by Southern blot analysis)

ACADS (acyl-CoA dehydrogenase, C-2 to C-3 short chain) (eg, short chain acyl-CoA dehydrogenase deficiency), targeted sequence analysis (eg, exons 5 and 6)

AQP2 (aquaporin 2 [collecting duct]) (eg, nephrogenic diabetes insipidus), full gene sequence

ARX (aristaless related homeobox) (eg, X-linked lissencephaly with ambiguous genitalia, X-linked mental retardation), full gene sequence

AVPR2 (arginine vasopressin receptor 2) (eg, nephrogenic diabetes insipidus), full gene sequence

BBS10 (Bardet-Biedl syndrome 10) (eg, Bardet-Biedl syndrome), full gene sequence

BTD (biotinidase) (eg, biotinidase deficiency), full gene sequence

C10orf2 (chromosome 10 open reading frame 2) (eg, mitochondrial DNA depletion syndrome), full gene sequence

CAV3 (caveolin 3) (eg, CAV3-related distal myopathy, limb-girdle muscular dystrophy type 1C), full gene sequence

CD40LG (CD40 ligand) (eg, X-linked hyper IgM syndrome), full gene sequence

CDKN2A (cyclin-dependent kinase inhibitor 2A) (eg, CDKN2A-related cutaneous malignant melanoma, familial atypical mole-malignant melanoma syndrome), full gene sequence

CLRN1 (clarin 1) (eg, Usher syndrome, type 3), full gene sequence

COX6B1 (cytochrome c oxidase subunit VIb polypeptide 1) (eg, mitochondrial respiratory chain complex IV deficiency), full gene sequence

CPT2 (carnitine palmitoyltransferase 2) (eg, carnitine palmitoyltransferase II deficiency), full gene sequence

CRX (cone-rod homeobox) (eg, cone-rod dystrophy 2, Leber congenital amaurosis), full gene sequence

CYP1B1 (cytochrome P450, family 1, subfamily B, polypeptide 1) (eg, primary congenital glaucoma), full gene sequence

EGR2 (early growth response 2) (eg, Charcot-Marie-Tooth), full gene sequence

EMD (emerin) (eg, Emery-Dreifuss muscular dystrophy), duplication/deletion analysis

EPM2A (epilepsy, progressive myoclonus type 2A, Lafora disease [laforin]) (eg, progressive myoclonus epilepsy), full gene sequence

FGF23 (fibroblast growth factor 23) (eg, hypophosphatemic rickets), full gene sequence

FGFR2 (fibroblast growth factor receptor 2) (eg, craniosynostosis, Apert syndrome, Crouzon syndrome), targeted sequence analysis (eg, exons 8, 10)

FGFR3 (fibroblast growth factor receptor 3) (eg, achondroplasia, hypochondroplasia), targeted sequence analysis (eg, exons 8, 11, 12, 13)

FHL1 (four and a half LIM domains 1) (eg, Emery-Dreifuss muscular dystrophy), full gene sequence

FKRP (fukutin related protein) (eg, congenital muscular dystrophy type 1C [MDC1C], limb-girdle muscular dystrophy [LGMD] type 2I), full gene sequence

FOXG1 (forkhead box G1) (eg, Rett syndrome), full gene sequence

FSHMD1A (facioscapulohumeral muscular dystrophy 1A) (eg, facioscapulohumeral muscular dystrophy), evaluation to detect abnormal (eg, deleted) alleles

FSHMD1A (facioscapulohumeral muscular dystrophy 1A) (eg, facioscapulohumeral muscular dystrophy), characterization of haplotype(s) (ie, chromosome 4A and 4B haplotypes)

GH1 (growth hormone 1) (eg, growth hormone deficiency), full gene sequence

GP1BB (glycoprotein Ib [platelet], beta polypeptide) (eg, Bernard-Soulier syndrome type B), full gene sequence

(For common deletion variants of alpha globin 1 and alpha globin 2 genes, use 81257)

HNF1B (HNF1 homeobox B) (eg, maturity-onset diabetes of the young [MODY]), duplication/deletion analysis

HRAS (v-Ha-ras Harvey rat sarcoma viral oncogene homolog) (eg, Costello syndrome), full gene sequence

HSD3B2 (hydroxy-delta-5-steroid dehydrogenase, 3 beta- and steroid delta-isomerase 2) (eg, 3-beta-hydroxysteroid dehydrogenase type II deficiency), full gene sequence

HSD11B2 (hydroxysteroid [11-beta] dehydrogenase 2) (eg, mineralocorticoid excess syndrome), full gene sequence

HSPB1 (heat shock 27kDa protein 1) (eg, Charcot-Marie-Tooth disease), full gene sequence

INS (insulin) (eg, diabetes mellitus), full gene sequence

KCNJ1 (potassium inwardly-rectifying channel, subfamily J, member 1) (eg, Bartter syndrome), full gene sequence

KCNJ10 (potassium inwardly-rectifying channel, subfamily J, member 10) (eg, SeSAME syndrome, EAST syndrome, sensorineural hearing loss), full gene sequence

LITAF (lipopolysaccharide-induced TNF factor) (eg, Charcot-Marie-Tooth), full gene sequence

MEFV (Mediterranean fever) (eg, familial Mediterranean fever), full gene sequence

MEN1 (multiple endocrine neoplasia I) (eg, multiple endocrine neoplasia type 1, Wermer syndrome), duplication/deletion analysis

MMACHC (methylmalonic aciduria [cobalamin deficiency] cblC type, with homocystinuria) (eg, methylmalonic acidemia and homocystinuria), full gene sequence

MPV17 (MpV17 mitochondrial inner membrane protein) (eg, mitochondrial DNA depletion syndrome), duplication/deletion analysis

NDP (Norrie disease [pseudoglioma]) (eg, Norrie disease), full gene sequence

NDUFA1 (NADH dehydrogenase [ubiquinone] 1 alpha subcomplex, 1, 7.5kDa) (eg, Leigh syndrome, mitochondrial complex I deficiency), full gene sequence

NDUFAF2 (NADH dehydrogenase [ubiquinone] 1 alpha subcomplex, assembly factor 2) (eg, Leigh syndrome, mitochondrial complex I deficiency), full gene sequence

NDUFS4 (NADH dehydrogenase [ubiquinone] Fe-S protein 4, 18kDa [NADH-coenzyme Q reductase]) (eg, Leigh syndrome, mitochondrial complex I deficiency), full gene sequence

NIPA1 (non-imprinted in Prader-Willi/Angelman syndrome 1) (eg, spastic paraplegia), full gene sequence

NLGN4X (neuroligin 4, X-linked) (eg, autism spectrum disorders), duplication/deletion analysis

NPC2 (Niemann-Pick disease, type C2 [epididymal secretory protein E1]) (eg, Niemann-Pick disease type C2), full gene sequence

NR0B1 (nuclear receptor subfamily 0, group B, member 1) (eg, congenital adrenal hypoplasia), full gene sequence

PDX1 (pancreatic and duodenal homeobox 1) (eg, maturity-onset diabetes of the young [MODY]), full gene sequence

PHOX2B (paired-like homeobox 2b) (eg, congenital central hypoventilation syndrome), full gene sequence

PIK3CA (phosphatidylinositol-4,5-bisphosphate 3-kinase, catalytic subunit alpha) (eg, colorectal cancer), targeted sequence analysis (eg, exons 9 and 20)

PLP1 (proteolipid protein 1) (eg, Pelizaeus-Merzbacher disease, spastic paraplegia), duplication/deletion analysis

PQBP1 (polyglutamine binding protein 1) (eg, Renpenning syndrome), duplication/deletion analysis

PRNP (prion protein) (eg, genetic prion disease), full gene sequence

PROP1 (PROP paired-like homeobox 1) (eg, combined pituitary hormone deficiency), full gene sequence

PRPH2 (peripherin 2 [retinal degeneration, slow]) (eg, retinitis pigmentosa), full gene sequence

PRSS1 (protease, serine, 1 [trypsin 1]) (eg, hereditary pancreatitis), full gene sequence

RAF1 (v-raf-1 murine leukemia viral oncogene homolog 1) (eg, LEOPARD syndrome), targeted sequence analysis (eg, exons 7, 12, 14, 17)

RET (ret proto-oncogene) (eg, multiple endocrine neoplasia, type 2B and familial medullary thyroid carcinoma), common variants (eg, M918T, 2647_2648delinsTT, A883F)

RHO (rhodopsin) (eg, retinitis pigmentosa), full gene sequence

RP1 (retinitis pigmentosa 1) (eg, retinitis pigmentosa), full gene sequence

SCN1B (sodium channel, voltage-gated, type I, beta) (eg, Brugada syndrome), full gene sequence

SCO2 (SCO cytochrome oxidase deficient homolog 2 [SCO1L]) (eg, mitochondrial respiratory chain complex IV deficiency), full gene sequence

SDHC (succinate dehydrogenase complex, subunit C, integral membrane protein, 15kDa) (eg, hereditary paraganglioma-pheochromocytoma syndrome), duplication/deletion analysis

SDHD (succinate dehydrogenase complex, subunit D, integral membrane protein) (eg, hereditary paraganglioma), full gene sequence

SGCG (sarcoglycan, gamma [35kDa dystrophin-associated glycoprotein]) (eg, limb-girdle muscular dystrophy), duplication/deletion analysis

SH2D1A (SH2 domain containing 1A) (eg, X-linked lymphoproliferative syndrome), full gene sequence

SLC16A2 (solute carrier family 16, member 2 [thyroid hormone transporter]) (eg, specific thyroid hormone cell transporter deficiency, Allan-Herndon-Dudley syndrome), duplication/deletion analysis

SLC25A20 (solute carrier family 25 [carnitine/acylcarnitine translocase], member 20) (eg, carnitine-acylcarnitine translocase deficiency), duplication/deletion analysis

SLC25A4 (solute carrier family 25 [mitochondrial carrier; adenine nucleotide translocator], member 4) (eg, progressive external ophthalmoplegia), full gene sequence

SOD1 (superoxide dismutase 1, soluble) (eg, amyotrophic lateral sclerosis), full gene sequence

SPINK1 (serine peptidase inhibitor, Kazal type 1) (eg, hereditary pancreatitis), full gene sequence

STK11 (serine/threonine kinase 11) (eg, Peutz-Jeghers syndrome), duplication/deletion analysis

TACO1 (translational activator of mitochondrial encoded cytochrome c oxidase I) (eg, mitochondrial respiratory chain complex IV deficiency), full gene sequence

THAP1 (THAP domain containing, apoptosis associated protein 1) (eg, torsion dystonia), full gene sequence

TOR1A (torsin family 1, member A [torsin A]) (eg, torsion dystonia), full gene sequence

TP53 (tumor protein 53) (eg, tumor samples), targeted sequence analysis of 2-5 exons

TTPA (tocopherol [alpha] transfer protein) (eg, ataxia), full gene sequence

TTR (transthyretin) (eg, familial transthyretin amyloidosis), full gene sequence

TWIST1 (twist homolog 1 [Drosophila]) (eg, Saethre-Chotzen syndrome), full gene sequence

TYR (tyrosinase [oculocutaneous albinism IA]) (eg, oculocutaneous albinism IA), full gene sequence

USH1G (Usher syndrome 1G [autosomal recessive]) (eg, Usher syndrome, type 1), full gene sequence

VHL (von Hippel-Lindau tumor suppressor) (eg, von Hippel-Lindau familial cancer syndrome), full gene sequence

VWF (von Willebrand factor) (eg, von Willebrand disease type 1C), targeted sequence analysis (eg, exons 26, 27, 37)

ZEB2 (zinc finger E-box binding homeobox 2) (eg, Mowat-Wilson syndrome), duplication/deletion analysis

ZNF41 (zinc finger protein 41) (eg, X-linked mental retardation 89), full gene sequence

➔ *CPT Changes: An Insider's View* 2012, 2013, 2014, 2015, 2016, 2018, 2019

➔ *CPT Assistant* May 12:4, Jul 13:12, Sep 13:6, 7, 9, Jan 15:3, Aug 16:10

▲ **81405** Molecular pathology procedure, Level 6 (eg, analysis of 6-10 exons by DNA sequence analysis, mutation scanning or duplication/deletion variants of 11-25 exons, regionally targeted cytogenomic array analysis)

ABCD1 (ATP-binding cassette, sub-family D [ALD], member 1) (eg, adrenoleukodystrophy), full gene sequence

ACADS (acyl-CoA dehydrogenase, C-2 to C-3 short chain) (eg, short chain acyl-CoA dehydrogenase deficiency), full gene sequence

ACTA2 (actin, alpha 2, smooth muscle, aorta) (eg, thoracic aortic aneurysms and aortic dissections), full gene sequence

ACTC1 (actin, alpha, cardiac muscle 1) (eg, familial hypertrophic cardiomyopathy), full gene sequence

ANKRD1 (ankyrin repeat domain 1) (eg, dilated cardiomyopathy), full gene sequence

APTX (aprataxin) (eg, ataxia with oculomotor apraxia 1), full gene sequence

ARSA (arylsulfatase A) (eg, arylsulfatase A deficiency), full gene sequence

BCKDHA (branched chain keto acid dehydrogenase E1, alpha polypeptide) (eg, maple syrup urine disease, type 1A), full gene sequence

BCS1L (BCS1-like [S. cerevisiae]) (eg, Leigh syndrome, mitochondrial complex III deficiency, GRACILE syndrome), full gene sequence

BMPR2 (bone morphogenetic protein receptor, type II [serine/threonine kinase]) (eg, heritable pulmonary arterial hypertension), duplication/deletion analysis

CASQ2 (calsequestrin 2 [cardiac muscle]) (eg, catecholaminergic polymorphic ventricular tachycardia), full gene sequence

CASR (calcium-sensing receptor) (eg, hypocalcemia), full gene sequence

CDKL5 (cyclin-dependent kinase-like 5) (eg, early infantile epileptic encephalopathy), duplication/deletion analysis

CHRNA4 (cholinergic receptor, nicotinic, alpha 4) (eg, nocturnal frontal lobe epilepsy), full gene sequence

CHRNB2 (cholinergic receptor, nicotinic, beta 2 [neuronal]) (eg, nocturnal frontal lobe epilepsy), full gene sequence

COX10 (COX10 homolog, cytochrome c oxidase assembly protein) (eg, mitochondrial respiratory chain complex IV deficiency), full gene sequence

COX15 (COX15 homolog, cytochrome c oxidase assembly protein) (eg, mitochondrial respiratory chain complex IV deficiency), full gene sequence

CPOX (coproporphyrinogen oxidase) (eg, hereditary coproporphyria), full gene sequence

CTRC (chymotrypsin C) (eg, hereditary pancreatitis), full gene sequence

CYP11B1 (cytochrome P450, family 11, subfamily B, polypeptide 1) (eg, congenital adrenal hyperplasia), full gene sequence

CYP17A1 (cytochrome P450, family 17, subfamily A, polypeptide 1) (eg, congenital adrenal hyperplasia), full gene sequence

CYP21A2 (cytochrome P450, family 21, subfamily A, polypeptide2) (eg, steroid 21-hydroxylase isoform, congenital adrenal hyperplasia), full gene sequence

Cytogenomic constitutional targeted microarray analysis of chromosome 22q13 by interrogation of genomic regions for copy number and single nucleotide polymorphism (SNP) variants for chromosomal abnormalities

(When performing genome-wide cytogenomic constitutional microarray analysis, see 81228, 81229)

(Do not report analyte-specific molecular pathology procedures separately when the specific analytes are included as part of the microarray analysis of chromosome 22q13)

(Do not report 88271 when performing cytogenomic microarray analysis)

DBT (dihydrolipoamide branched chain transacylase E2) (eg, maple syrup urine disease, type 2), duplication/deletion analysis

DCX (doublecortin) (eg, X-linked lissencephaly), full gene sequence

DES (desmin) (eg, myofibrillar myopathy), full gene sequence

DFNB59 (deafness, autosomal recessive 59) (eg, autosomal recessive nonsyndromic hearing impairment), full gene sequence

DGUOK (deoxyguanosine kinase) (eg, hepatocerebral mitochondrial DNA depletion syndrome), full gene sequence

DHCR7 (7-dehydrocholesterol reductase) (eg, Smith-Lemli-Opitz syndrome), full gene sequence

EIF2B2 (eukaryotic translation initiation factor 2B, subunit 2 beta, 39kDa) (eg, leukoencephalopathy with vanishing white matter), full gene sequence

EMD (emerin) (eg, Emery-Dreifuss muscular dystrophy), full gene sequence

ENG (endoglin) (eg, hereditary hemorrhagic telangiectasia, type 1), duplication/deletion analysis

EYA1 (eyes absent homolog 1 [Drosophila]) (eg, branchio-oto-renal [BOR] spectrum disorders), duplication/deletion analysis

FGFR1 (fibroblast growth factor receptor 1) (eg, Kallmann syndrome 2), full gene sequence

FH (fumarate hydratase) (eg, fumarate hydratase deficiency, hereditary leiomyomatosis with renal cell cancer), full gene sequence

FKTN (fukutin) (eg, limb-girdle muscular dystrophy [LGMD] type 2M or 2L), full gene sequence

FTSJ1 (FtsJ RNA methyltransferase homolog 1 [E. coli]) (eg, X-linked mental retardation 9), duplication/deletion analysis

GABRG2 (gamma-aminobutyric acid [GABA] A receptor, gamma 2) (eg, generalized epilepsy with febrile seizures), full gene sequence

GCH1 (GTP cyclohydrolase 1) (eg, autosomal dominant dopa-responsive dystonia), full gene sequence

GDAP1 (ganglioside-induced differentiation-associated protein 1) (eg, Charcot-Marie-Tooth disease), full gene sequence

GFAP (glial fibrillary acidic protein) (eg, Alexander disease), full gene sequence

GHR (growth hormone receptor) (eg, Laron syndrome), full gene sequence

GHRHR (growth hormone releasing hormone receptor) (eg, growth hormone deficiency), full gene sequence

GLA (galactosidase, alpha) (eg, Fabry disease), full gene sequence

HNF1A (HNF1 homeobox A) (eg, maturity-onset diabetes of the young [MODY]), full gene sequence

HNF1B (HNF1 homeobox B) (eg, maturity-onset diabetes of the young [MODY]), full gene sequence

HTRA1 (HtrA serine peptidase 1) (eg, macular degeneration), full gene sequence

IDS (iduronate 2-sulfatase) (eg, mucopolysacchridosis, type II), full gene sequence

IL2RG (interleukin 2 receptor, gamma) (eg, X-linked severe combined immunodeficiency), full gene sequence

ISPD (isoprenoid synthase domain containing) (eg, muscle-eye-brain disease, Walker-Warburg syndrome), full gene sequence

KRAS (Kirsten rat sarcoma viral oncogene homolog) (eg, Noonan syndrome), full gene sequence

LAMP2 (lysosomal-associated membrane protein 2) (eg, Danon disease), full gene sequence

LDLR (low density lipoprotein receptor) (eg, familial hypercholesterolemia), duplication/deletion analysis

MEN1 (multiple endocrine neoplasia I) (eg, multiple endocrine neoplasia type 1, Wermer syndrome), full gene sequence

MMAA (methylmalonic aciduria [cobalamine deficiency] type A) (eg, MMAA-related methylmalonic acidemia), full gene sequence

MMAB (methylmalonic aciduria [cobalamine deficiency] type B) (eg, MMAA-related methylmalonic acidemia), full gene sequence

MPI (mannose phosphate isomerase) (eg, congenital disorder of glycosylation 1b), full gene sequence

MPV17 (MpV17 mitochondrial inner membrane protein) (eg, mitochondrial DNA depletion syndrome), full gene sequence

MPZ (myelin protein zero) (eg, Charcot-Marie-Tooth), full gene sequence

MTM1 (myotubularin 1) (eg, X-linked centronuclear myopathy), duplication/deletion analysis

MYL2 (myosin, light chain 2, regulatory, cardiac, slow) (eg, familial hypertrophic cardiomyopathy), full gene sequence

MYL3 (myosin, light chain 3, alkali, ventricular, skeletal, slow) (eg, familial hypertrophic cardiomyopathy), full gene sequence

MYOT (myotilin) (eg, limb-girdle muscular dystrophy), full gene sequence

NDUFS7 (NADH dehydrogenase [ubiquinone] Fe-S protein 7, 20kDa [NADH-coenzyme Q reductase]) (eg, Leigh syndrome, mitochondrial complex I deficiency), full gene sequence

NDUFS8 (NADH dehydrogenase [ubiquinone] Fe-S protein 8, 23kDa [NADH-coenzyme Q reductase]) (eg, Leigh syndrome, mitochondrial complex I deficiency), full gene sequence

NDUFV1 (NADH dehydrogenase [ubiquinone] flavoprotein 1, 51kDa) (eg, Leigh syndrome, mitochondrial complex I deficiency), full gene sequence

NEFL (neurofilament, light polypeptide) (eg, Charcot-Marie-Tooth), full gene sequence

NF2 (neurofibromin 2 [merlin]) (eg, neurofibromatosis, type 2), duplication/deletion analysis

NLGN3 (neuroligin 3) (eg, autism spectrum disorders), full gene sequence

NLGN4X (neuroligin 4, X-linked) (eg, autism spectrum disorders), full gene sequence

NPHP1 (nephronophthisis 1 [juvenile]) (eg, Joubert syndrome), deletion analysis, and duplication analysis, if performed

NPHS2 (nephrosis 2, idiopathic, steroid-resistant [podocin]) (eg, steroid-resistant nephrotic syndrome), full gene sequence

NSD1 (nuclear receptor binding SET domain protein 1) (eg, Sotos syndrome), duplication/deletion analysis

OTC (ornithine carbamoyltransferase) (eg, ornithine transcarbamylase deficiency), full gene sequence

PAFAH1B1 (platelet-activating factor acetylhydrolase 1b, regulatory subunit 1 [45kDa]) (eg, lissencephaly, Miller-Dieker syndrome), duplication/deletion analysis

PARK2 (Parkinson protein 2, E3 ubiquitin protein ligase [parkin]) (eg, Parkinson disease), duplication/deletion analysis

PCCA (propionyl CoA carboxylase, alpha polypeptide) (eg, propionic acidemia, type 1), duplication/deletion analysis

PCDH19 (protocadherin 19) (eg, epileptic encephalopathy), full gene sequence

PDHA1 (pyruvate dehydrogenase [lipoamide] alpha 1) (eg, lactic acidosis), duplication/deletion analysis

PDHB (pyruvate dehydrogenase [lipoamide] beta) (eg, lactic acidosis), full gene sequence

PINK1 (PTEN induced putative kinase 1) (eg, Parkinson disease), full gene sequence

PKLR (pyruvate kinase, liver and RBC) (eg, pyruvate kinase deficiency), full gene sequence

PLP1 (proteolipid protein 1) (eg, Pelizaeus-Merzbacher disease, spastic paraplegia), full gene sequence

POU1F1 (POU class 1 homeobox 1) (eg, combined pituitary hormone deficiency), full gene sequence

PRX (periaxin) (eg, Charcot-Marie-Tooth disease), full gene sequence

PQBP1 (polyglutamine binding protein 1) (eg, Renpenning syndrome), full gene sequence

PSEN1 (presenilin 1) (eg, Alzheimer disease), full gene sequence

RAB7A (RAB7A, member RAS oncogene family) (eg, Charcot-Marie-Tooth disease), full gene sequence

RAI1 (retinoic acid induced 1) (eg, Smith-Magenis syndrome), full gene sequence

REEP1 (receptor accessory protein 1) (eg, spastic paraplegia), full gene sequence

RET (ret proto-oncogene) (eg, multiple endocrine neoplasia, type 2A and familial medullary thyroid carcinoma), targeted sequence analysis (eg, exons 10, 11, 13-16)

RPS19 (ribosomal protein S19) (eg, Diamond-Blackfan anemia), full gene sequence

RRM2B (ribonucleotide reductase M2 B [TP53 inducible]) (eg, mitochondrial DNA depletion), full gene sequence

SCO1 (SCO cytochrome oxidase deficient homolog 1) (eg, mitochondrial respiratory chain complex IV deficiency), full gene sequence

SDHB (succinate dehydrogenase complex, subunit B, iron sulfur) (eg, hereditary paraganglioma), full gene sequence

SDHC (succinate dehydrogenase complex, subunit C, integral membrane protein, 15kDa) (eg, hereditary paraganglioma-pheochromocytoma syndrome), full gene sequence

SGCA (sarcoglycan, alpha [50kDa dystrophin-associated glycoprotein]) (eg, limb-girdle muscular dystrophy), full gene sequence

SGCB (sarcoglycan, beta [43kDa dystrophin-associated glycoprotein]) (eg, limb-girdle muscular dystrophy), full gene sequence

SGCD (sarcoglycan, delta [35kDa dystrophin-associated glycoprotein]) (eg, limb-girdle muscular dystrophy), full gene sequence

SGCE (sarcoglycan, epsilon) (eg, myoclonic dystonia), duplication/deletion analysis

SGCG (sarcoglycan, gamma [35kDa dystrophin-associated glycoprotein]) (eg, limb-girdle muscular dystrophy), full gene sequence

SHOC2 (soc-2 suppressor of clear homolog) (eg, Noonan-like syndrome with loose anagen hair), full gene sequence

SHOX (short stature homeobox) (eg, Langer mesomelic dysplasia), full gene sequence

SIL1 (SIL1 homolog, endoplasmic reticulum chaperone [S. cerevisiae]) (eg, ataxia), full gene sequence

SLC2A1 (solute carrier family 2 [facilitated glucose transporter], member 1) (eg, glucose transporter type 1 [GLUT 1] deficiency syndrome), full gene sequence

SLC16A2 (solute carrier family 16, member 2 [thyroid hormone transporter]) (eg, specific thyroid hormone cell transporter deficiency, Allan-Herndon-Dudley syndrome), full gene sequence

SLC22A5 (solute carrier family 22 [organic cation/carnitine transporter], member 5) (eg, systemic primary carnitine deficiency), full gene sequence

SLC25A20 (solute carrier family 25 [carnitine/acylcarnitine translocase], member 20) (eg, carnitine-acylcarnitine translocase deficiency), full gene sequence

SMAD4 (SMAD family member 4) (eg, hemorrhagic telangiectasia syndrome, juvenile polyposis), duplication/deletion analysis

SPAST (spastin) (eg, spastic paraplegia), duplication/deletion analysis

SPG7 (spastic paraplegia 7 [pure and complicated autosomal recessive]) (eg, spastic paraplegia), duplication/deletion analysis

SPRED1 (sprouty-related, EVH1 domain containing 1) (eg, Legius syndrome), full gene sequence

STAT3 (signal transducer and activator of transcription 3 [acute-phase response factor]) (eg, autosomal dominant hyper-IgE syndrome), targeted sequence analysis (eg, exons 12, 13, 14, 16, 17, 20, 21)

STK11 (serine/threonine kinase 11) (eg, Peutz-Jeghers syndrome), full gene sequence

SURF1 (surfeit 1) (eg, mitochondrial respiratory chain complex IV deficiency), full gene sequence

TARDBP (TAR DNA binding protein) (eg, amyotrophic lateral sclerosis), full gene sequence

TBX5 (T-box 5) (eg, Holt-Oram syndrome), full gene sequence

TCF4 (transcription factor 4) (eg, Pitt-Hopkins syndrome), duplication/deletion analysis

TGFBR1 (transforming growth factor, beta receptor 1) (eg, Marfan syndrome), full gene sequence

TGFBR2 (transforming growth factor, beta receptor 2) (eg, Marfan syndrome), full gene sequence

THRB (thyroid hormone receptor, beta) (eg, thyroid hormone resistance, thyroid hormone beta receptor deficiency), full gene sequence or targeted sequence analysis of >5 exons

TK2 (thymidine kinase 2, mitochondrial) (eg, mitochondrial DNA depletion syndrome), full gene sequence

TNNC1 (troponin C type 1 [slow]) (eg, hypertrophic cardiomyopathy or dilated cardiomyopathy), full gene sequence

TNNI3 (troponin I, type 3 [cardiac]) (eg, familial hypertrophic cardiomyopathy), full gene sequence

TP53 (tumor protein 53) (eg, Li-Fraumeni syndrome, tumor samples), full gene sequence or targeted sequence analysis of >5 exons

TPM1 (tropomyosin 1 [alpha]) (eg, familial hypertrophic cardiomyopathy), full gene sequence

TSC1 (tuberous sclerosis 1) (eg, tuberous sclerosis), duplication/deletion analysis

TYMP (thymidine phosphorylase) (eg, mitochondrial DNA depletion syndrome), full gene sequence

VWF (von Willebrand factor) (eg, von Willebrand disease type 2N), targeted sequence analysis (eg, exons 18-20, 23-25)

WT1 (Wilms tumor 1) (eg, Denys-Drash syndrome, familial Wilms tumor), full gene sequence

ZEB2 (zinc finger E-box binding homeobox 2) (eg, Mowat-Wilson syndrome), full gene sequence

➲ *CPT Changes: An Insider's View* 2012, 2013, 2014, 2015, 2016, 2018, 2019

➲ *CPT Assistant* May 12:4, Jul 13:12, Sep 13:8, 10, Jan 15:3, Aug 16:10

81406 Molecular pathology procedure, Level 7 (eg, analysis of 11-25 exons by DNA sequence analysis, mutation scanning or duplication/deletion variants of 26-50 exons, cytogenomic array analysis for neoplasia)

ACADVL (acyl-CoA dehydrogenase, very long chain) (eg, very long chain acyl-coenzyme A dehydrogenase deficiency), full gene sequence

ACTN4 (actinin, alpha 4) (eg, focal segmental glomerulosclerosis), full gene sequence

AFG3L2 (AFG3 ATPase family gene 3-like 2 [S. cerevisiae]) (eg, spinocerebellar ataxia), full gene sequence

AIRE (autoimmune regulator) (eg, autoimmune polyendocrinopathy syndrome type 1), full gene sequence

ALDH7A1 (aldehyde dehydrogenase 7 family, member A1) (eg, pyridoxine-dependent epilepsy), full gene sequence

ANO5 (anoctamin 5) (eg, limb-girdle muscular dystrophy), full gene sequence

ANOS1 (anosmin-1) (eg, Kallmann syndrome 1), full gene sequence

APP (amyloid beta [A4] precursor protein) (eg, Alzheimer disease), full gene sequence

ASS1 (argininosuccinate synthase 1) (eg, citrullinemia type I), full gene sequence

ATL1 (atlastin GTPase 1) (eg, spastic paraplegia), full gene sequence

ATP1A2 (ATPase, Na+/K+ transporting, alpha 2 polypeptide) (eg, familial hemiplegic migraine), full gene sequence

ATP7B (ATPase, Cu++ transporting, beta polypeptide) (eg, Wilson disease), full gene sequence

BBS1 (Bardet-Biedl syndrome 1) (eg, Bardet-Biedl syndrome), full gene sequence

BBS2 (Bardet-Biedl syndrome 2) (eg, Bardet-Biedl syndrome), full gene sequence

BCKDHB (branched-chain keto acid dehydrogenase E1, beta polypeptide) (eg, maple syrup urine disease, type 1B), full gene sequence

BEST1 (bestrophin 1) (eg, vitelliform macular dystrophy), full gene sequence

BMPR2 (bone morphogenetic protein receptor, type II [serine/threonine kinase]) (eg, heritable pulmonary arterial hypertension), full gene sequence

BRAF (B-Raf proto-oncogene, serine/threonine kinase) (eg, Noonan syndrome), full gene sequence

BSCL2 (Berardinelli-Seip congenital lipodystrophy 2 [seipin]) (eg, Berardinelli-Seip congenital lipodystrophy), full gene sequence

BTK (Bruton agammaglobulinemia tyrosine kinase) (eg, X-linked agammaglobulinemia), full gene sequence

CACNB2 (calcium channel, voltage-dependent, beta 2 subunit) (eg, Brugada syndrome), full gene sequence

CAPN3 (calpain 3) (eg, limb-girdle muscular dystrophy [LGMD] type 2A, calpainopathy), full gene sequence

CBS (cystathionine-beta-synthase) (eg, homocystinuria, cystathionine beta-synthase deficiency), full gene sequence

CDH1 (cadherin 1, type 1, E-cadherin [epithelial]) (eg, hereditary diffuse gastric cancer), full gene sequence

CDKL5 (cyclin-dependent kinase-like 5) (eg, early infantile epileptic encephalopathy), full gene sequence

CLCN1 (chloride channel 1, skeletal muscle) (eg, myotonia congenita), full gene sequence

CLCNKB (chloride channel, voltage-sensitive Kb) (eg, Bartter syndrome 3 and 4b), full gene sequence

CNTNAP2 (contactin-associated protein-like 2) (eg, Pitt-Hopkins-like syndrome 1), full gene sequence

COL6A2 (collagen, type VI, alpha 2) (eg, collagen type VI-related disorders), duplication/deletion analysis

CPT1A (carnitine palmitoyltransferase 1A [liver]) (eg, carnitine palmitoyltransferase 1A [CPT1A] deficiency), full gene sequence

CRB1 (crumbs homolog 1 [Drosophila]) (eg, Leber congenital amaurosis), full gene sequence

CREBBP (CREB binding protein) (eg, Rubinstein-Taybi syndrome), duplication/deletion analysis

Cytogenomic microarray analysis, neoplasia (eg, interrogation of copy number, and loss-of-heterozygosity via single nucleotide polymorphism [SNP]-based comparative genomic hybridization [CGH] microarray analysis)

(Do not report analyte-specific molecular pathology procedures separately when the specific analytes are included as part of the cytogenomic microarray analysis for neoplasia)

(Do not report 88271 when performing cytogenomic microarray analysis)

DBT (dihydrolipoamide branched chain transacylase E2) (eg, maple syrup urine disease, type 2), full gene sequence

DLAT (dihydrolipoamide S-acetyltransferase) (eg, pyruvate dehydrogenase E2 deficiency), full gene sequence

DLD (dihydrolipoamide dehydrogenase) (eg, maple syrup urine disease, type III), full gene sequence

DSC2 (desmocollin) (eg, arrhythmogenic right ventricular dysplasia/cardiomyopathy 11), full gene sequence

DSG2 (desmoglein 2) (eg, arrhythmogenic right ventricular dysplasia/cardiomyopathy 10), full gene sequence

DSP (desmoplakin) (eg, arrhythmogenic right ventricular dysplasia/cardiomyopathy 8), full gene sequence

EFHC1 (EF-hand domain [C-terminal] containing 1) (eg, juvenile myoclonic epilepsy), full gene sequence

EIF2B3 (eukaryotic translation initiation factor 2B, subunit 3 gamma, 58kDa) (eg, leukoencephalopathy with vanishing white matter), full gene sequence

EIF2B4 (eukaryotic translation initiation factor 2B, subunit 4 delta, 67kDa) (eg, leukoencephalopathy with vanishing white matter), full gene sequence

EIF2B5 (eukaryotic translation initiation factor 2B, subunit 5 epsilon, 82kDa) (eg, childhood ataxia with central nervous system hypomyelination/vanishing white matter), full gene sequence

ENG (endoglin) (eg, hereditary hemorrhagic telangiectasia, type 1), full gene sequence

EYA1 (eyes absent homolog 1 [Drosophila]) (eg, branchio-oto-renal [BOR] spectrum disorders), full gene sequence

F8 (coagulation factor VIII) (eg, hemophilia A), duplication/deletion analysis

FAH (fumarylacetoacetate hydrolase [fumarylacetoacetase]) (eg, tyrosinemia, type 1), full gene sequence

FASTKD2 (FAST kinase domains 2) (eg, mitochondrial respiratory chain complex IV deficiency), full gene sequence

FIG4 (FIG4 homolog, SAC1 lipid phosphatase domain containing [S. cerevisiae]) (eg, Charcot-Marie-Tooth disease), full gene sequence

FTSJ1 (FtsJ RNA methyltransferase homolog 1 [E. coli]) (eg, X-linked mental retardation 9), full gene sequence

FUS (fused in sarcoma) (eg, amyotrophic lateral sclerosis), full gene sequence

GAA (glucosidase, alpha; acid) (eg, glycogen storage disease type II [Pompe disease]), full gene sequence

GALC (galactosylceramidase) (eg, Krabbe disease), full gene sequence

GALT (galactose-1-phosphate uridylyltransferase) (eg, galactosemia), full gene sequence

GARS (glycyl-tRNA synthetase) (eg, Charcot-Marie-Tooth disease), full gene sequence

GCDH (glutaryl-CoA dehydrogenase) (eg, glutaricacidemia type 1), full gene sequence

GCK (glucokinase [hexokinase 4]) (eg, maturity-onset diabetes of the young [MODY]), full gene sequence

GLUD1 (glutamate dehydrogenase 1) (eg, familial hyperinsulinism), full gene sequence

GNE (glucosamine [UDP-N-acetyl]-2-epimerase/N-acetylmannosamine kinase) (eg, inclusion body myopathy 2 [IBM2], Nonaka myopathy), full gene sequence

GRN (granulin) (eg, frontotemporal dementia), full gene sequence

HADHA (hydroxyacyl-CoA dehydrogenase/3-ketoacyl-CoA thiolase/enoyl-CoA hydratase [trifunctional protein] alpha subunit) (eg, long chain acyl-coenzyme A dehydrogenase deficiency), full gene sequence

HADHB (hydroxyacyl-CoA dehydrogenase/3-ketoacyl-CoA thiolase/enoyl-CoA hydratase [trifunctional protein], beta subunit) (eg, trifunctional protein deficiency), full gene sequence

HEXA (hexosaminidase A, alpha polypeptide) (eg, Tay-Sachs disease), full gene sequence

HLCS (HLCS holocarboxylase synthetase) (eg, holocarboxylase synthetase deficiency), full gene sequence

HMBS (hydroxymethylbilane synthase) (eg, acute intermittent porphyria), full gene sequence

HNF4A (hepatocyte nuclear factor 4, alpha) (eg, maturity-onset diabetes of the young [MODY]), full gene sequence

IDUA (iduronidase, alpha-L-) (eg, mucopolysaccharidosis type I), full gene sequence

INF2 (inverted formin, FH2 and WH2 domain containing) (eg, focal segmental glomerulosclerosis), full gene sequence

IVD (isovaleryl-CoA dehydrogenase) (eg, isovaleric acidemia), full gene sequence

JAG1 (jagged 1) (eg, Alagille syndrome), duplication/deletion analysis

JUP (junction plakoglobin) (eg, arrhythmogenic right ventricular dysplasia/cardiomyopathy 11), full gene sequence

KCNH2 (potassium voltage-gated channel, subfamily H [eag-related], member 2) (eg, short QT syndrome, long QT syndrome), full gene sequence

KCNQ1 (potassium voltage-gated channel, KQT-like subfamily, member 1) (eg, short QT syndrome, long QT syndrome), full gene sequence

KCNQ2 (potassium voltage-gated channel, KQT-like subfamily, member 2) (eg, epileptic encephalopathy), full gene sequence

LDB3 (LIM domain binding 3) (eg, familial dilated cardiomyopathy, myofibrillar myopathy), full gene sequence

LDLR (low density lipoprotein receptor) (eg, familial hypercholesterolemia), full gene sequence

LEPR (leptin receptor) (eg, obesity with hypogonadism), full gene sequence

LHCGR (luteinizing hormone/choriogonadotropin receptor) (eg, precocious male puberty), full gene sequence

LMNA (lamin A/C) (eg, Emery-Dreifuss muscular dystrophy [EDMD1, 2 and 3] limb-girdle muscular dystrophy [LGMD] type 1B, dilated cardiomyopathy [CMD1A], familial partial lipodystrophy [FPLD2]), full gene sequence

LRP5 (low density lipoprotein receptor-related protein 5) (eg, osteopetrosis), full gene sequence

MAP2K1 (mitogen-activated protein kinase 1) (eg, cardiofaciocutaneous syndrome), full gene sequence

MAP2K2 (mitogen-activated protein kinase 2) (eg, cardiofaciocutaneous syndrome), full gene sequence

MAPT (microtubule-associated protein tau) (eg, frontotemporal dementia), full gene sequence

MCCC1 (methylcrotonoyl-CoA carboxylase 1 [alpha]) (eg, 3-methylcrotonyl-CoA carboxylase deficiency), full gene sequence

MCCC2 (methylcrotonoyl-CoA carboxylase 2 [beta]) (eg, 3-methylcrotonyl carboxylase deficiency), full gene sequence

MFN2 (mitofusin 2) (eg, Charcot-Marie-Tooth disease), full gene sequence

MTM1 (myotubularin 1) (eg, X-linked centronuclear myopathy), full gene sequence

MUT (methylmalonyl CoA mutase) (eg, methylmalonic acidemia), full gene sequence

MUTYH (mutY homolog [E. coli]) (eg, MYH-associated polyposis), full gene sequence

NDUFS1 (NADH dehydrogenase [ubiquinone] Fe-S protein 1, 75kDa [NADH-coenzyme Q reductase]) (eg, Leigh syndrome, mitochondrial complex I deficiency), full gene sequence

NF2 (neurofibromin 2 [merlin]) (eg, neurofibromatosis, type 2), full gene sequence

NOTCH3 (notch 3) (eg, cerebral autosomal dominant arteriopathy with subcortical infarcts and leukoencephalopathy [CADASIL]), targeted sequence analysis (eg, exons 1-23)

NPC1 (Niemann-Pick disease, type C1) (eg, Niemann-Pick disease), full gene sequence

NPHP1 (nephronophthisis 1 [juvenile]) (eg, Joubert syndrome), full gene sequence

NSD1 (nuclear receptor binding SET domain protein 1) (eg, Sotos syndrome), full gene sequence

OPA1 (optic atrophy 1) (eg, optic atrophy), duplication/deletion analysis

OPTN (optineurin) (eg, amyotrophic lateral sclerosis), full gene sequence

PAFAH1B1 (platelet-activating factor acetylhydrolase 1b, regulatory subunit 1 [45kDa]) (eg, lissencephaly, Miller-Dieker syndrome), full gene sequence

PAH (phenylalanine hydroxylase) (eg, phenylketonuria), full gene sequence

PALB2 (partner and localizer of BRCA2) (eg, breast and pancreatic cancer), full gene sequence

PARK2 (Parkinson protein 2, E3 ubiquitin protein ligase [parkin]) (eg, Parkinson disease), full gene sequence

PAX2 (paired box 2) (eg, renal coloboma syndrome), full gene sequence

PC (pyruvate carboxylase) (eg, pyruvate carboxylase deficiency), full gene sequence

PCCA (propionyl CoA carboxylase, alpha polypeptide) (eg, propionic acidemia, type 1), full gene sequence

PCCB (propionyl CoA carboxylase, beta polypeptide) (eg, propionic acidemia), full gene sequence

PCDH15 (protocadherin-related 15) (eg, Usher syndrome type 1F), duplication/deletion analysis

PCSK9 (proprotein convertase subtilisin/kexin type 9) (eg, familial hypercholesterolemia), full gene sequence

PDHA1 (pyruvate dehydrogenase [lipoamide] alpha 1) (eg, lactic acidosis), full gene sequence

PDHX (pyruvate dehydrogenase complex, component X) (eg, lactic acidosis), full gene sequence

PHEX (phosphate-regulating endopeptidase homolog, X-linked) (eg, hypophosphatemic rickets), full gene sequence

PKD2 (polycystic kidney disease 2 [autosomal dominant]) (eg, polycystic kidney disease), full gene sequence

PKP2 (plakophilin 2) (eg, arrhythmogenic right ventricular dysplasia/cardiomyopathy 9), full gene sequence

PNKD (paroxysmal nonkinesigenic dyskinesia) (eg, paroxysmal nonkinesigenic dyskinesia), full gene sequence

POLG (polymerase [DNA directed], gamma) (eg, Alpers-Huttenlocher syndrome, autosomal dominant progressive external ophthalmoplegia), full gene sequence

POMGNT1 (protein O-linked mannose beta1,2-N acetylglucosaminyltransferase) (eg, muscle-eye-brain disease, Walker-Warburg syndrome), full gene sequence

POMT1 (protein-O-mannosyltransferase 1) (eg, limb-girdle muscular dystrophy [LGMD] type 2K, Walker-Warburg syndrome), full gene sequence

POMT2 (protein-O-mannosyltransferase 2) (eg, limb-girdle muscular dystrophy [LGMD] type 2N, Walker-Warburg syndrome), full gene sequence

PPOX (protoporphyrinogen oxidase) (eg, variegate porphyria), full gene sequence

PRKAG2 (protein kinase, AMP-activated, gamma 2 non-catalytic subunit) (eg, familial hypertrophic cardiomyopathy with Wolff-Parkinson-White syndrome, lethal congenital glycogen storage disease of heart), full gene sequence

PRKCG (protein kinase C, gamma) (eg, spinocerebellar ataxia), full gene sequence

PSEN2 (presenilin 2 [Alzheimer disease 4]) (eg, Alzheimer disease), full gene sequence

PTPN11 (protein tyrosine phosphatase, non-receptor type 11) (eg, Noonan syndrome, LEOPARD syndrome), full gene sequence

PYGM (phosphorylase, glycogen, muscle) (eg, glycogen storage disease type V, McArdle disease), full gene sequence

RAF1 (v-raf-1 murine leukemia viral oncogene homolog 1) (eg, LEOPARD syndrome), full gene sequence

RET (ret proto-oncogene) (eg, Hirschsprung disease), full gene sequence

RPE65 (retinal pigment epithelium-specific protein 65kDa) (eg, retinitis pigmentosa, Leber congenital amaurosis), full gene sequence

RYR1 (ryanodine receptor 1, skeletal) (eg, malignant hyperthermia), targeted sequence analysis of exons with functionally-confirmed mutations

SCN4A (sodium channel, voltage-gated, type IV, alpha subunit) (eg, hyperkalemic periodic paralysis), full gene sequence

SCNN1A (sodium channel, nonvoltage-gated 1 alpha) (eg, pseudohypoaldosteronism), full gene sequence

SCNN1B (sodium channel, nonvoltage-gated 1, beta) (eg, Liddle syndrome, pseudohypoaldosteronism), full gene sequence

SCNN1G (sodium channel, nonvoltage-gated 1, gamma) (eg, Liddle syndrome, pseudohypoaldosteronism), full gene sequence

SDHA (succinate dehydrogenase complex, subunit A, flavoprotein [Fp]) (eg, Leigh syndrome, mitochondrial complex II deficiency), full gene sequence

SETX (senataxin) (eg, ataxia), full gene sequence

SGCE (sarcoglycan, epsilon) (eg, myoclonic dystonia), full gene sequence

SH3TC2 (SH3 domain and tetratricopeptide repeats 2) (eg, Charcot-Marie-Tooth disease), full gene sequence

SLC9A6 (solute carrier family 9 [sodium/hydrogen exchanger], member 6) (eg, Christianson syndrome), full gene sequence

SLC26A4 (solute carrier family 26, member 4) (eg, Pendred syndrome), full gene sequence

SLC37A4 (solute carrier family 37 [glucose-6-phosphate transporter], member 4) (eg, glycogen storage disease type Ib), full gene sequence

SMAD4 (SMAD family member 4) (eg, hemorrhagic telangiectasia syndrome, juvenile polyposis), full gene sequence

SOS1 (son of sevenless homolog 1) (eg, Noonan syndrome, gingival fibromatosis), full gene sequence

SPAST (spastin) (eg, spastic paraplegia), full gene sequence

SPG7 (spastic paraplegia 7 [pure and complicated autosomal recessive]) (eg, spastic paraplegia), full gene sequence

STXBP1 (syntaxin-binding protein 1) (eg, epileptic encephalopathy), full gene sequence

TAZ (tafazzin) (eg, methylglutaconic aciduria type 2, Barth syndrome), full gene sequence

TCF4 (transcription factor 4) (eg, Pitt-Hopkins syndrome), full gene sequence

TH (tyrosine hydroxylase) (eg, Segawa syndrome), full gene sequence

TMEM43 (transmembrane protein 43) (eg, arrhythmogenic right ventricular cardiomyopathy), full gene sequence

TNNT2 (troponin T, type 2 [cardiac]) (eg, familial hypertrophic cardiomyopathy), full gene sequence

TRPC6 (transient receptor potential cation channel, subfamily C, member 6) (eg, focal segmental glomerulosclerosis), full gene sequence

TSC1 (tuberous sclerosis 1) (eg, tuberous sclerosis), full gene sequence

TSC2 (tuberous sclerosis 2) (eg, tuberous sclerosis), duplication/deletion analysis

UBE3A (ubiquitin protein ligase E3A) (eg, Angelman syndrome), full gene sequence

UMOD (uromodulin) (eg, glomerulocystic kidney disease with hyperuricemia and isosthenuria), full gene sequence

VWF (von Willebrand factor) (von Willebrand disease type 2A), extended targeted sequence analysis (eg, exons 11-16, 24-26, 51, 52)

WAS (Wiskott-Aldrich syndrome [eczema-thrombocytopenia]) (eg, Wiskott-Aldrich syndrome), full gene sequence

➲ *CPT Changes: An Insider's View* 2012, 2013, 2014, 2016, 2017, 2018

➲ *CPT Assistant* May 12:4, Jul 13:12, Sep 13:5, 6, 8, 11, Jan 15:3, Aug 16:10, Apr 17:10

▲ **81407** Molecular pathology procedure, Level 8 (eg, analysis of 26-50 exons by DNA sequence analysis, mutation scanning or duplication/deletion variants of >50 exons, sequence analysis of multiple genes on one platform)

ABCC8 (ATP-binding cassette, sub-family C [CFTR/MRP], member 8) (eg, familial hyperinsulinism), full gene sequence

AGL (amylo-alpha-1, 6-glucosidase, 4-alpha-glucanotransferase) (eg, glycogen storage disease type III), full gene sequence

AHI1 (Abelson helper integration site 1) (eg, Joubert syndrome), full gene sequence

ASPM (asp [abnormal spindle] homolog, microcephaly associated [Drosophila]) (eg, primary microcephaly), full gene sequence

CHD7 (chromodomain helicase DNA binding protein 7) (eg, CHARGE syndrome), full gene sequence

COL4A4 (collagen, type IV, alpha 4) (eg, Alport syndrome), full gene sequence

COL4A5 (collagen, type IV, alpha 5) (eg, Alport syndrome), duplication/deletion analysis

COL6A1 (collagen, type VI, alpha 1) (eg, collagen type VI-related disorders), full gene sequence

COL6A2 (collagen, type VI, alpha 2) (eg, collagen type VI-related disorders), full gene sequence

COL6A3 (collagen, type VI, alpha 3) (eg, collagen type VI-related disorders), full gene sequence

CREBBP (CREB binding protein) (eg, Rubinstein-Taybi syndrome), full gene sequence

F8 (coagulation factor VIII) (eg, hemophilia A), full gene sequence

JAG1 (jagged 1) (eg, Alagille syndrome), full gene sequence

KDM5C (lysine [K]-specific demethylase 5C) (eg, X-linked mental retardation), full gene sequence

KIAA0196 (KIAA0196) (eg, spastic paraplegia), full gene sequence

L1CAM (L1 cell adhesion molecule) (eg, MASA syndrome, X-linked hydrocephaly), full gene sequence

LAMB2 (laminin, beta 2 [laminin S]) (eg, Pierson syndrome), full gene sequence

MYBPC3 (myosin binding protein C, cardiac) (eg, familial hypertrophic cardiomyopathy), full gene sequence

MYH6 (myosin, heavy chain 6, cardiac muscle, alpha) (eg, familial dilated cardiomyopathy), full gene sequence

MYH7 (myosin, heavy chain 7, cardiac muscle, beta) (eg, familial hypertrophic cardiomyopathy, Liang distal myopathy), full gene sequence

MYO7A (myosin VIIA) (eg, Usher syndrome, type 1), full gene sequence

NOTCH1 (notch 1) (eg, aortic valve disease), full gene sequence

NPHS1 (nephrosis 1, congenital, Finnish type [nephrin]) (eg, congenital Finnish nephrosis), full gene sequence

OPA1 (optic atrophy 1) (eg, optic atrophy), full gene sequence

PCDH15 (protocadherin-related 15) (eg, Usher syndrome, type 1), full gene sequence

PKD1 (polycystic kidney disease 1 [autosomal dominant]) (eg, polycystic kidney disease), full gene sequence

PLCE1 (phospholipase C, epsilon 1) (eg, nephrotic syndrome type 3), full gene sequence

SCN1A (sodium channel, voltage-gated, type 1, alpha subunit) (eg, generalized epilepsy with febrile seizures), full gene sequence

SCN5A (sodium channel, voltage-gated, type V, alpha subunit) (eg, familial dilated cardiomyopathy), full gene sequence

SLC12A1 (solute carrier family 12 [sodium/potassium/chloride transporters], member 1) (eg, Bartter syndrome), full gene sequence

SLC12A3 (solute carrier family 12 [sodium/chloride transporters], member 3) (eg, Gitelman syndrome), full gene sequence

SPG11 (spastic paraplegia 11 [autosomal recessive]) (eg, spastic paraplegia), full gene sequence

SPTBN2 (spectrin, beta, non-erythrocytic 2) (eg, spinocerebellar ataxia), full gene sequence

TMEM67 (transmembrane protein 67) (eg, Joubert syndrome), full gene sequence

TSC2 (tuberous sclerosis 2) (eg, tuberous sclerosis), full gene sequence

USH1C (Usher syndrome 1C [autosomal recessive, severe]) (eg, Usher syndrome, type 1), full gene sequence

VPS13B (vacuolar protein sorting 13 homolog B [yeast]) (eg, Cohen syndrome), duplication/deletion analysis

WDR62 (WD repeat domain 62) (eg, primary autosomal recessive microcephaly), full gene sequence

➔ *CPT Changes: An Insider's View* 2012, 2013, 2014, 2019

➔ *CPT Assistant* May 12:4, Jul 13:12, Sep 13:14, Jan 15:3, Aug 16:10

81408 Molecular pathology procedure, Level 9 (eg, analysis of >50 exons in a single gene by DNA sequence analysis)

ABCA4 (ATP-binding cassette, sub-family A [ABC1], member 4) (eg, Stargardt disease, age-related macular degeneration), full gene sequence

ATM (ataxia telangiectasia mutated) (eg, ataxia telangiectasia), full gene sequence

CDH23 (cadherin-related 23) (eg, Usher syndrome, type 1), full gene sequence

CEP290 (centrosomal protein 290kDa) (eg, Joubert syndrome), full gene sequence

COL1A1 (collagen, type I, alpha 1) (eg, osteogenesis imperfecta, type I), full gene sequence

COL1A2 (collagen, type I, alpha 2) (eg, osteogenesis imperfecta, type I), full gene sequence

COL4A1 (collagen, type IV, alpha 1) (eg, brain small-vessel disease with hemorrhage), full gene sequence

COL4A3 (collagen, type IV, alpha 3 [Goodpasture antigen]) (eg, Alport syndrome), full gene sequence

COL4A5 (collagen, type IV, alpha 5) (eg, Alport syndrome), full gene sequence

DMD (dystrophin) (eg, Duchenne/Becker muscular dystrophy), full gene sequence

DYSF (dysferlin, limb girdle muscular dystrophy 2B [autosomal recessive]) (eg, limb-girdle muscular dystrophy), full gene sequence

FBN1 (fibrillin 1) (eg, Marfan syndrome), full gene sequence

ITPR1 (inositol 1,4,5-trisphosphate receptor, type 1) (eg, spinocerebellar ataxia), full gene sequence

LAMA2 (laminin, alpha 2) (eg, congenital muscular dystrophy), full gene sequence

LRRK2 (leucine-rich repeat kinase 2) (eg, Parkinson disease), full gene sequence

MYH11 (myosin, heavy chain 11, smooth muscle) (eg, thoracic aortic aneurysms and aortic dissections), full gene sequence

NEB (nebulin) (eg, nemaline myopathy 2), full gene sequence

NF1 (neurofibromin 1) (eg, neurofibromatosis, type 1), full gene sequence

PKHD1 (polycystic kidney and hepatic disease 1) (eg, autosomal recessive polycystic kidney disease), full gene sequence

RYR1 (ryanodine receptor 1, skeletal) (eg, malignant hyperthermia), full gene sequence

RYR2 (ryanodine receptor 2 [cardiac]) (eg, catecholaminergic polymorphic ventricular tachycardia, arrhythmogenic right ventricular dysplasia), full gene sequence or targeted sequence analysis of > 50 exons

USH2A (Usher syndrome 2A [autosomal recessive, mild]) (eg, Usher syndrome, type 2), full gene sequence

VPS13B (vacuolar protein sorting 13 homolog B [yeast]) (eg, Cohen syndrome), full gene sequence

VWF (von Willebrand factor) (eg, von Willebrand disease types 1 and 3), full gene sequence

➲ *CPT Changes: An Insider's View* 2012, 2013, 2014

➲ *CPT Assistant* May 12:4, Jul 13:12, Sep 13:4, 5, 14, Jan 15:3, Aug 16:10

 # 81479 Unlisted molecular pathology procedure

➲ *CPT Changes: An Insider's View* 2013

➲ *CPT Assistant* Jul 13:12, Sep 13:4-8, Jan 15:3, Apr 16:4, Aug 16:10, Sep 16:10, Apr 17:10

Genomic Sequencing Procedures and Other Molecular Multianalyte Assays

Genomic sequencing procedures (GSPs) and other molecular multianalyte assays GSPs are DNA or RNA sequence analysis methods that simultaneously assay multiple genes or genetic regions relevant to a clinical situation. They may target specific combinations of genes or genetic material, or assay the exome or genome. The technology used for genomic sequencing is commonly referred to as next generation sequencing (NGS) or massively parallel sequencing (MPS). GSPs are performed on nucleic acids from germline or neoplastic samples. Examples of applications include aneuploidy analysis of cell-free circulating fetal DNA, gene panels for somatic alterations in neoplasms, and sequence analysis of the exome or genome to determine the cause of developmental delay. The exome and genome procedures are designed to evaluate the genetic material in totality or near totality. Although commonly used to identify sequence (base) changes, they can also be used to identify copy number, structural changes, and abnormal zygosity patterns. Another unique feature of GSPs is the ability to "re-query" or re-evaluate the sequence data (eg, complex phenotype such as developmental delay is reassessed when new genetic knowledge is attained, or for a separate unrelated clinical indication). The analyses listed below represent groups of genes that are often performed by GSPs; however, the analyses may also be performed by other molecular techniques (polymerase chain reaction [PCR] methods and microarrays). These codes should be used when the components of the descriptor(s) are fulfilled regardless of the technique used to provide the analysis, unless specifically noted in the code descriptor. When a GSP assay includes gene(s) that is listed in more than one code descriptor, the code for the most specific test for the primary disorder sought should be reported, rather than reporting multiple codes for the same gene(s). When all of the components of the descriptor are not performed, use individual Tier 1 codes, Tier 2 codes, or 81479 (Unlisted molecular pathology procedure).

The assays in this section represent discrete genetic values, properties, or characteristics in which the measurement or analysis of each analyte is potentially of independent medical significance or useful in medical management. In contrast to multianalyte assays with algorithmic analyses (MAAAs), the assays in this section do not represent algorithmically combined results to obtain a risk score or other value, which in itself represents a new and distinct medical property that is of independent medical significance relative to the individual, component test results.

(For cytogenomic microarray analyses, see 81228, 81229, 81405, 81406)

81410 Aortic dysfunction or dilation (eg, Marfan syndrome, Loeys Dietz syndrome, Ehler Danlos syndrome type IV, arterial tortuosity syndrome); genomic sequence analysis panel, must include sequencing of at least 9 genes, including *FBN1, TGFBR1, TGFBR2, COL3A1, MYH11, ACTA2, SLC2A10, SMAD3,* and *MYLK*

➔ *CPT Changes: An Insider's View* 2015
➔ *CPT Assistant* Jan 15:3

81411 duplication/deletion analysis panel, must include analyses for *TGFBR1, TGFBR2, MYH11, and COL3A1*

➔ *CPT Changes: An Insider's View* 2015
➔ *CPT Assistant* Jan 15:3

81412 Ashkenazi Jewish associated disorders (eg, Bloom syndrome, Canavan disease, cystic fibrosis, familial dysautonomia, Fanconi anemia group C, Gaucher disease, Tay-Sachs disease), genomic sequence analysis panel, must include sequencing of at least 9 genes, including *ASPA, BLM, CFTR, FANCC, GBA, HEXA, IKBKAP, MCOLN1,* and *SMPD1*

➔ *CPT Changes: An Insider's View* 2016
➔ *CPT Assistant* Apr 16:4

81413 Cardiac ion channelopathies (eg, Brugada syndrome, long QT syndrome, short QT syndrome, catecholaminergic polymorphic ventricular tachycardia); genomic sequence analysis panel, must include sequencing of at least 10 genes, including *ANK2, CASQ2, CAV3, KCNE1, KCNE2, KCNH2, KCNJ2, KCNQ1, RYR2,* and *SCN5A*

➔ *CPT Changes: An Insider's View* 2017
➔ *CPT Assistant* Apr 17:3

81414 duplication/deletion gene analysis panel, must include analysis of at least 2 genes, including *KCNH2* and *KCNQ1*

➔ *CPT Changes: An Insider's View* 2017
➔ *CPT Assistant* Apr 17:3

(For genomic sequencing panel testing for cardiomyopathies, use 81439)

(Do not report 81413, 81414 in conjunction with 81439 when performed on the same date of service)

81415 Exome (eg, unexplained constitutional or heritable disorder or syndrome); sequence analysis

➔ *CPT Changes: An Insider's View* 2015
➔ *CPT Assistant* Jan 15:3

+ 81416 sequence analysis, each comparator exome (eg, parents, siblings) (List separately in addition to code for primary procedure)

➔ *CPT Changes: An Insider's View* 2015
➔ *CPT Assistant* Jan 15:3

(Use 81416 in conjunction with 81415)

81417 re-evaluation of previously obtained exome sequence (eg, updated knowledge or unrelated condition/syndrome)

➔ *CPT Changes: An Insider's View* 2015
➔ *CPT Assistant* Jan 15:3

(Do not report 81417 for incidental findings)

(For exome-wide copy number assessment by microarray, see 81228, 81229)

81420 Fetal chromosomal aneuploidy (eg, trisomy 21, monosomy X) genomic sequence analysis panel, circulating cell-free fetal DNA in maternal blood, must include analysis of chromosomes 13, 18, and 21

➔ *CPT Changes: An Insider's View* 2015
➔ *CPT Assistant* Jan 15:3, Dec 15:17, Apr 18:11

(Do not report 81228, 81229, 88271 when performing genomic sequencing procedures or other molecular multianalyte assays for copy number analysis)

81422 Fetal chromosomal microdeletion(s) genomic sequence analysis (eg, DiGeorge syndrome, Cri-du-chat syndrome), circulating cell-free fetal DNA in maternal blood

➔ *CPT Changes: An Insider's View* 2017
➔ *CPT Assistant* Apr 17:3

(Do not report 81228, 81229, 88271 when performing genomic sequencing procedures or other molecular multianalyte assays for copy number analysis)

81425 Genome (eg, unexplained constitutional or heritable disorder or syndrome); sequence analysis

➔ *CPT Changes: An Insider's View* 2015
➔ *CPT Assistant* Jan 15:3

+ 81426 sequence analysis, each comparator genome (eg, parents, siblings) (List separately in addition to code for primary procedure)

➔ *CPT Changes: An Insider's View* 2015
➔ *CPT Assistant* Jan 15:3

(Use 81426 in conjunction with 81425)

81427 re-evaluation of previously obtained genome sequence (eg, updated knowledge or unrelated condition/syndrome)

➔ *CPT Changes: An Insider's View* 2015
➔ *CPT Assistant* Jan 15:3

(Do not report 81427 for incidental findings)

(For genome-wide copy number assessment by microarray, see 81228, 81229)

81430 Hearing loss (eg, nonsyndromic hearing loss, Usher syndrome, Pendred syndrome); genomic sequence analysis panel, must include sequencing of at least 60 genes, including *CDH23, CLRN1, GJB2, GPR98, MTRNR1, MYO7A, MYO15A, PCDH15, OTOF, SLC26A4, TMC1, TMPRSS3, USH1C, USH1G, USH2A,* and *WFS1*

➔ *CPT Changes: An Insider's View* 2015
➔ *CPT Assistant* Jan 15:3

81431 duplication/deletion analysis panel, must include copy number analyses for *STRC* and *DFNB1* deletions *in GJB2 and GJB6 genes*
➲ *CPT Changes: An Insider's View* 2015
➲ *CPT Assistant* Jan 15:3

81432 Hereditary breast cancer-related disorders (eg, hereditary breast cancer, hereditary ovarian cancer, hereditary endometrial cancer); genomic sequence analysis panel, must include sequencing of at least 10 genes, always including *BRCA1, BRCA2, CDH1, MLH1, MSH2, MSH6, PALB2, PTEN, STK11*, and *TP53*
➲ *CPT Changes: An Insider's View* 2016, 2018
➲ *CPT Assistant* Apr 16:4

81433 duplication/deletion analysis panel, must include analyses for *BRCA1, BRCA2, MLH1, MSH2*, and *STK11*
➲ *CPT Changes: An Insider's View* 2016
➲ *CPT Assistant* Apr 16:4

81434 Hereditary retinal disorders (eg, retinitis pigmentosa, Leber congenital amaurosis, cone-rod dystrophy), genomic sequence analysis panel, must include sequencing of at least 15 genes, including *ABCA4, CNGA1, CRB1, EYS, PDE6A, PDE6B, PRPF31, PRPH2, RDH12, RHO, RP1, RP2, RPE65, RPGR*, and *USH2A*
➲ *CPT Changes: An Insider's View* 2016
➲ *CPT Assistant* Apr 16:4

81435 Hereditary colon cancer disorders (eg, Lynch syndrome, PTEN hamartoma syndrome, Cowden syndrome, familial adenomatosis polyposis); genomic sequence analysis panel, must include sequencing of at least 10 genes, including *APC, BMPR1A, CDH1, MLH1, MSH2, MSH6, MUTYH, PTEN, SMAD4*, and *STK11*
➲ *CPT Changes: An Insider's View* 2015, 2016
➲ *CPT Assistant* Jan 15:3, Apr 16:4

81436 duplication/deletion analysis panel, must include analysis of at least 5 genes, including *MLH1, MSH2, EPCAM, SMAD4*, and *STK11*
➲ *CPT Changes: An Insider's View* 2015, 2016
➲ *CPT Assistant* Jan 15:3, Apr 16:4

81437 Hereditary neuroendocrine tumor disorders (eg, medullary thyroid carcinoma, parathyroid carcinoma, malignant pheochromocytoma or paraganglioma); genomic sequence analysis panel, must include sequencing of at least 6 genes, including *MAX, SDHB, SDHC, SDHD, TMEM127, and VHL*
➲ *CPT Changes: An Insider's View* 2016
➲ *CPT Assistant* Apr 16:4

81438 duplication/deletion analysis panel, must include analyses for *SDHB, SDHC, SDHD*, and *VHL*
➲ *CPT Changes: An Insider's View* 2016
➲ *CPT Assistant* Apr 16:4

 # 81448 Hereditary peripheral neuropathies (eg, Charcot-Marie-Tooth, spastic paraplegia), genomic sequence analysis panel, must include sequencing of at least 5 peripheral neuropathy-related genes (eg, *BSCL2, GJB1, MFN2, MPZ, REEP1, SPAST, SPG11, SPTLC1*)
➲ *CPT Changes: An Insider's View* 2018

81439 Hereditary cardiomyopathy (eg, hypertrophic cardiomyopathy, dilated cardiomyopathy, arrhythmogenic right ventricular cardiomyopathy), genomic sequence analysis panel, must include sequencing of at least 5 cardiomyopathy-related genes (eg, *DSG2, MYBPC3, MYH7, PKP2, TTN*)
➲ *CPT Changes: An Insider's View* 2017, 2018
➲ *CPT Assistant* Apr 17:3

(Do not report 81439 in conjunction with 81413, 81414 when performed on the same date of service)

(For genomic sequencing panel testing for cardiac ion channelopathies, see 81413, 81414)

81440 Nuclear encoded mitochondrial genes (eg, neurologic or myopathic phenotypes), genomic sequence panel, must include analysis of at least 100 genes, including *BCS1L, C10orf2, COQ2, COX10, DGUOK, MPV17, OPA1, PDSS2, POLG, POLG2, RRM2B, SCO1, SCO2, SLC25A4, SUCLA2, SUCLG1, TAZ, TK2*, and *TYMP*
➲ *CPT Changes: An Insider's View* 2015
➲ *CPT Assistant* Jan 15:3

81442 Noonan spectrum disorders (eg, Noonan syndrome, cardio-facio-cutaneous syndrome, Costello syndrome, LEOPARD syndrome, Noonan-like syndrome), genomic sequence analysis panel, must include sequencing of at least 12 genes, including *BRAF, CBL, HRAS, KRAS, MAP2K1, MAP2K2, NRAS, PTPN11, RAF1, RIT1, SHOC2*, and *SOS1*
➲ *CPT Changes: An Insider's View* 2016
➲ *CPT Assistant* Apr 16:4

● 81443 Genetic testing for severe inherited conditions (eg, cystic fibrosis, Ashkenazi Jewish-associated disorders [eg, Bloom syndrome, Canavan disease, Fanconi anemia type C, mucolipidosis type VI, Gaucher disease, Tay-Sachs disease], beta hemoglobinopathies, phenylketonuria, galactosemia), genomic sequence analysis panel, must include sequencing of at least 15 genes (eg, *ACADM, ARSA, ASPA, ATP7B, BCKDHA, BCKDHB, BLM, CFTR, DHCR7, FANCC, G6PC, GAA, GALT, GBA, GBE1, HBB, HEXA, IKBKAP, MCOLN1, PAH*)
➲ *CPT Changes: An Insider's View* 2019

►(If spinal muscular atrophy testing is performed separately, use 81401)◄

►(If testing is performed only for Ashkenazi Jewish-associated disorders, use 81412)◄

►(If *FMR1* [expanded allele] testing is performed separately, use 81243)◄

►(If hemoglobin A testing is performed separately, use 81257)◄

►(Do not report 81443 in conjunction with 81412)◄

81445 Targeted genomic sequence analysis panel, solid organ neoplasm, DNA analysis, and RNA analysis when performed, 5-50 genes (eg, *ALK, BRAF, CDKN2A, EGFR, ERBB2, KIT, KRAS, NRAS, MET, PDGFRA, PDGFRB, PGR, PIK3CA, PTEN, RET*), interrogation for sequence variants and copy number variants or rearrangements, if performed

CPT Changes: An Insider's View 2015, 2016

CPT Assistant Jan 15:3, Apr 16:4

(For copy number assessment by microarray, use 81406)

81448 Code is out of numerical sequence. See 81437-81440

81450 Targeted genomic sequence analysis panel, hematolymphoid neoplasm or disorder, DNA analysis, and RNA analysis when performed, 5-50 genes (eg, *BRAF, CEBPA, DNMT3A, EZH2, FLT3, IDH1, IDH2, JAK2, KRAS, KIT, MLL, NRAS, NPM1, NOTCH1*), interrogation for sequence variants, and copy number variants or rearrangements, or isoform expression or mRNA expression levels, if performed

CPT Changes: An Insider's View 2015, 2016

CPT Assistant Jan 15:3, Apr 16:4

(For copy number assessment by microarray, use 81406)

81455 Targeted genomic sequence analysis panel, solid organ or hematolymphoid neoplasm, DNA analysis, and RNA analysis when performed, 51 or greater genes (eg, *ALK, BRAF, CDKN2A, CEBPA, DNMT3A, EGFR, ERBB2, EZH2, FLT3, IDH1, IDH2, JAK2, KIT, KRAS, MLL, NPM1, NRAS, MET, NOTCH1, PDGFRA, PDGFRB, PGR, PIK3CA, PTEN, RET*), interrogation for sequence variants and copy number variants or rearrangements, if performed

CPT Changes: An Insider's View 2015, 2016

CPT Assistant Jan 15:3, Apr 16:4

(For copy number assessment by microarray, use 81406)

81460 Whole mitochondrial genome (eg, Leigh syndrome, mitochondrial encephalomyopathy, lactic acidosis, and stroke-like episodes [MELAS], myoclonic epilepsy with ragged-red fibers [MERFF], neuropathy, ataxia, and retinitis pigmentosa [NARP], Leber hereditary optic neuropathy [LHON]), genomic sequence, must include sequence analysis of entire mitochondrial genome with heteroplasmy detection

CPT Changes: An Insider's View 2015

CPT Assistant Jan 15:3

81465 Whole mitochondrial genome large deletion analysis panel (eg, Kearns-Sayre syndrome, chronic progressive external ophthalmoplegia), including heteroplasmy detection, if performed

CPT Changes: An Insider's View 2015

CPT Assistant Jan 15:3

81470 X-linked intellectual disability (XLID) (eg, syndromic and non-syndromic XLID); genomic sequence analysis panel, must include sequencing of at least 60 genes, including *ARX, ATRX, CDKL5, FGD1, FMR1, HUWE1, IL1RAPL, KDM5C, L1CAM, MECP2, MED12, MID1, OCRL, RPS6KA3*, and *SLC16A2*

CPT Changes: An Insider's View 2015

CPT Assistant Jan 15:3

81471 duplication/deletion gene analysis, must include analysis of at least 60 genes, including *ARX, ATRX, CDKL5, FGD1, FMR1, HUWE1, IL1RAPL, KDM5C, L1CAM, MECP2, MED12, MID1, OCRL, RPS6KA3*, and *SLC16A2*

CPT Changes: An Insider's View 2015

CPT Assistant Jan 15:3

81479 Code is out of numerical sequence. See 81407-81411

Multianalyte Assays with Algorithmic Analyses

Multianalyte Assays with Algorithmic Analyses (MAAAs) are procedures that utilize multiple results derived from panels of analyses of various types, including molecular pathology assays, fluorescent in situ hybridization assays, and non-nucleic acid based assays (eg, proteins, polypeptides, lipids, carbohydrates). Algorithmic analysis using the results of these assays as well as other patient information (if used) is then performed and typically reported as a numeric score(s) or as a probability. MAAAs are typically unique to a single clinical laboratory or manufacturer. The results of individual component procedure(s) that are inputs to the MAAAs may be provided on the associated laboratory report; however, these assays are not separately reported using additional codes.

The format for the code descriptors of MAAAs usually include (in order):

- Disease type (eg, oncology, autoimmune, tissue rejection),
- Material(s) analyzed (eg, DNA, RNA, protein, antibody),
- Number of markers (eg, number of genes, number of proteins),
- Methodology(ies) (eg, microarray, real-time [RT]-PCR, in situ hybridization [ISH], enzyme linked immunosorbent assays [ELISA]),
- Number of functional domains (if indicated),
- Specimen type (eg, blood, fresh tissue, formalin-fixed paraffin-embedded),
- Algorithm result type (eg, prognostic, diagnostic),
- Report (eg, probability index, risk score)

In contrast to GSPs and other molecular multianalyte assays, the assays in this section represent algorithmically combined results of analyses of multiple analytes to obtain a risk score or other value which in itself represents a new and distinct medical property that is of independent medical significance relative to the individual component test results in clinical context in which the assay is performed.

MAAAs, including those that do not have a Category I code, may be found in Appendix O. MAAAs that do not have a Category I code are identified in Appendix O by a four-digit number followed by the letter "M." The Category I MAAA codes that are included in this subsection are also included in Appendix O. All MAAA codes are listed in Appendix O along with the procedure's proprietary name. In order to report a MAAA code, the analysis performed must fulfill the code descriptor **and**, if proprietary, must be the test represented by the proprietary name listed in Appendix O.

When a specific MAAA procedure is not listed below or in Appendix O, the procedure must be reported using the Category I MAAA unlisted code (81599).

These codes encompass all analytical services required (eg, cell lysis, nucleic acid stabilization, extraction, digestion, amplification, hybridization, and detection) in addition to the algorithmic analysis itself. Procedures that are required prior to cell lysis (eg, microdissection, codes 88380 and 88381) should be reported separately.

81490 Autoimmune (rheumatoid arthritis), analysis of 12 biomarkers using immunoassays, utilizing serum, prognostic algorithm reported as a disease activity score

➲ *CPT Changes: An Insider's View* 2016

(Do not report 81490 in conjunction with 86140)

81493 Coronary artery disease, mRNA, gene expression profiling by real-time RT-PCR of 23 genes, utilizing whole peripheral blood, algorithm reported as a risk score

➲ *CPT Changes: An Insider's View* 2016

81500 Oncology (ovarian), biochemical assays of two proteins (CA-125 and HE4), utilizing serum, with menopausal status, algorithm reported as a risk score

➲ *CPT Changes: An Insider's View* 2013

(Do not report 81500 in conjunction with 86304, 86305)

81503 Oncology (ovarian), biochemical assays of five proteins (CA-125, apolipoprotein A1, beta-2 microglobulin, transferrin, and pre-albumin), utilizing serum, algorithm reported as a risk score

➲ *CPT Changes: An Insider's View* 2013

(Do not report 81503 in conjunction with 82172, 82232, 84134, 84466, 86304)

81504 Oncology (tissue of origin), microarray gene expression profiling of > 2000 genes, utilizing formalin-fixed paraffin-embedded tissue, algorithm reported as tissue similarity scores

➲ *CPT Changes: An Insider's View* 2014

81506 Endocrinology (type 2 diabetes), biochemical assays of seven analytes (glucose, HbA1c, insulin, hs-CRP, adiponectin, ferritin, interleukin 2-receptor alpha), utilizing serum or plasma, algorithm reporting a risk score

➲ *CPT Changes: An Insider's View* 2013

(Do not report 81506 in conjunction with constituent components [ie, 82728, 82947, 83036, 83525, 86141], 84999 [for adopectin], and 83520 [for interleukin 2-receptor alpha])

81507 Fetal aneuploidy (trisomy 21, 18, and 13) DNA sequence analysis of selected regions using maternal plasma, algorithm reported as a risk score for each trisomy

➲ *CPT Changes: An Insider's View* 2014

➲ *CPT Assistant* Apr 18:11

(Do not report 81228, 81229, 88271 when performing genomic sequencing procedures or other molecular multianalyte assays for copy number analysis)

81508 Fetal congenital abnormalities, biochemical assays of two proteins (PAPP-A, hCG [any form]), utilizing maternal serum, algorithm reported as a risk score

➲ *CPT Changes: An Insider's View* 2013

(Do not report 81508 in conjunction with 84163, 84702)

81509 Fetal congenital abnormalities, biochemical assays of three proteins (PAPP-A, hCG [any form], DIA), utilizing maternal serum, algorithm reported as a risk score

➲ *CPT Changes: An Insider's View* 2013

(Do not report 81509 in conjunction with 84163, 84702, 86336)

81510 Fetal congenital abnormalities, biochemical assays of three analytes (AFP, uE3, hCG [any form]), utilizing maternal serum, algorithm reported as a risk score

➲ *CPT Changes: An Insider's View* 2013

(Do not report 81510 in conjunction with 82105, 82677, 84702)

81511 Fetal congenital abnormalities, biochemical assays of four analytes (AFP, uE3, hCG [any form], DIA) utilizing maternal serum, algorithm reported as a risk score (may include additional results from previous biochemical testing)

➲ *CPT Changes: An Insider's View* 2013

(Do not report 81511 in conjunction with 82105, 82677, 84702, 86336)

81512 Fetal congenital abnormalities, biochemical assays of five analytes (AFP, uE3, total hCG, hyperglycosylated hCG, DIA) utilizing maternal serum, algorithm reported as a risk score

➲ *CPT Changes: An Insider's View* 2013

(Do not report 81512 in conjunction with 82105, 82677, 84702, 86336

● **81518** Oncology (breast), mRNA, gene expression profiling by real-time RT-PCR of 11 genes (7 content and 4 housekeeping), utilizing formalin-fixed paraffin-embedded tissue, algorithms reported as percentage risk for metastatic recurrence and likelihood of benefit from extended endocrine therapy

➲ *CPT Changes: An Insider's View* 2019

81519 Oncology (breast), mRNA, gene expression profiling by real-time RT-PCR of 21 genes, utilizing formalin-fixed paraffin-embedded tissue, algorithm reported as recurrence score

➲ *CPT Changes: An Insider's View* 2015

➲ *CPT Assistant* Jan 15:3

81520 Oncology (breast), mRNA gene expression profiling by hybrid capture of 58 genes (50 content and 8 housekeeping), utilizing formalin-fixed paraffin-embedded tissue, algorithm reported as a recurrence risk score

➔ *CPT Changes: An Insider's View* 2018

81521 Oncology (breast), mRNA, microarray gene expression profiling of 70 content genes and 465 housekeeping genes, utilizing fresh frozen or formalin-fixed paraffin-embedded tissue, algorithm reported as index related to risk of distant metastasis

➔ *CPT Changes: An Insider's View* 2018

81525 Oncology (colon), mRNA, gene expression profiling by real-time RT-PCR of 12 genes (7 content and 5 housekeeping), utilizing formalin-fixed paraffin-embedded tissue, algorithm reported as a recurrence score

81528 Oncology (colorectal) screening, quantitative real-time target and signal amplification of 10 DNA markers (*KRAS* mutations, promoter methylation of *NDRG4* and *BMP3*) and fecal hemoglobin, utilizing stool, algorithm reported as a positive or negative result

➔ *CPT Changes: An Insider's View* 2016

(Do not report 81528 in conjunction with 81275, 82274)

81535 Oncology (gynecologic), live tumor cell culture and chemotherapeutic response by DAPI stain and morphology, predictive algorithm reported as a drug response score; first single drug or drug combination

➔ *CPT Changes: An Insider's View* 2016

+ 81536 each additional single drug or drug combination (List separately in addition to code for primary procedure)

➔ *CPT Changes: An Insider's View* 2016

(Use 81536 in conjunction with 81535)

81538 Oncology (lung), mass spectrometric 8-protein signature, including amyloid A, utilizing serum, prognostic and predictive algorithm reported as good versus poor overall survival

➔ *CPT Changes: An Insider's View* 2016

81539 Oncology (high-grade prostate cancer), biochemical assay of four proteins (Total PSA, Free PSA, Intact PSA, and human kallikrein-2 [hK2]), utilizing plasma or serum, prognostic algorithm reported as a probability score

➔ *CPT Changes: An Insider's View* 2017

➔ *CPT Assistant* Apr 17:4

81540 Oncology (tumor of unknown origin), mRNA, gene expression profiling by real-time RT-PCR of 92 genes (87 content and 5 housekeeping) to classify tumor into main cancer type and subtype, utilizing formalin-fixed paraffin-embedded tissue, algorithm reported as a probability of a predicted main cancer type and subtype

➔ *CPT Changes: An Insider's View* 2016

81541 Oncology (prostate), mRNA gene expression profiling by real-time RT-PCR of 46 genes (31 content and 15 housekeeping), utilizing formalin-fixed paraffin-embedded tissue, algorithm reported as a disease-specific mortality risk score

➔ *CPT Changes: An Insider's View* 2018

81545 Oncology (thyroid), gene expression analysis of 142 genes, utilizing fine needle aspirate, algorithm reported as a categorical result (eg, benign or suspicious)

➔ *CPT Changes: An Insider's View* 2016

81551 Oncology (prostate), promoter methylation profiling by real-time PCR of 3 genes (*GSTP1, APC, RASSF1*), utilizing formalin-fixed paraffin-embedded tissue, algorithm reported as a likelihood of prostate cancer detection on repeat biopsy

➔ *CPT Changes: An Insider's View* 2018

81595 Cardiology (heart transplant), mRNA, gene expression profiling by real-time quantitative PCR of 20 genes (11 content and 9 housekeeping), utilizing subfraction of peripheral blood, algorithm reported as a rejection risk score

➔ *CPT Changes: An Insider's View* 2016

● **81596** Infectious disease, chronic hepatitis C virus (HCV) infection, six biochemical assays (ALT, A2-macroglobulin, apolipoprotein A-1, total bilirubin, GGT, and haptoglobin) utilizing serum, prognostic algorithm reported as scores for fibrosis and necroinflammatory activity in liver

➔ *CPT Changes: An Insider's View* 2019

81599 Unlisted multianalyte assay with algorithmic analysis

➔ *CPT Changes: An Insider's View* 2013

➔ *CPT Assistant* Apr 18:11

(Do not use 81599 for multianalyte assays with algorithmic analyses listed in Appendix O)

Chemistry

The material for examination may be from any source unless otherwise specified in the code descriptor. When an analyte is measured in multiple specimens from different sources, or in specimens that are obtained at different times, the analyte is reported separately for each source and for each specimen. The examination is quantitative unless specified. To report an organ or disease oriented panel, see codes 80048-80076.

Clinical information or mathematically calculated values, which are not specifically requested by the ordering physician and are derived from the results of other ordered or performed laboratory tests, are considered part of the ordered test procedure(s) and therefore are not separately reportable service(s).

When the requested analyte result is derived using a calculation that requires values from nonrequested laboratory analyses, only the requested analyte code should be reported.

When the calculated analyte determination requires values derived from other requested and nonrequested laboratory analyses, the requested analyte codes (including those calculated) should be reported.

An exception to the above is when an analyte (eg, urinary creatinine) is performed to compensate for variations in urine concentration (eg, microalbumin, thromboxane metabolites) in random urine samples; the appropriate CPT code is reported for both the ordered analyte and the additional required analyte. When the calculated result(s) represent an algorithmically derived numeric score or probability, see the appropriate multianalyte assay with algorithmic analyses (MAAA) code or the MAAA unlisted code (81599).

82009 Ketone body(s) (eg, acetone, acetoacetic acid, beta-hydroxybutyrate); qualitative
➔ *CPT Changes: An Insider's View* 2013
➔ *CPT Assistant* Oct 11:11, Jun 15:10

82010 quantitative
➔ *CPT Changes: An Insider's View* 2013
➔ *CPT Assistant* Oct 11:11

82013 Acetylcholinesterase

(For gastric acid analysis, use 82930)

(Acid phosphatase, see 84060-84066)

82016 Acylcarnitines; qualitative, each specimen
➔ *CPT Assistant* Nov 98:23

82017 quantitative, each specimen
➔ *CPT Changes: An Insider's View* 2000
➔ *CPT Assistant* Nov 98:23

(For carnitine, use 82379)

82024 Adrenocorticotropic hormone (ACTH)

82030 Adenosine, 5-monophosphate, cyclic (cyclic AMP)

82040 Albumin; serum, plasma or whole blood
➔ *CPT Changes: An Insider's View* 2009
➔ *CPT Assistant* Dec 99:2

82042 Code is out of numerical sequence. See 82044-82085

82043 urine (eg, microalbumin), quantitative
➔ *CPT Changes: An Insider's View* 2018
➔ *CPT Assistant* Summer 94:2

82044 urine (eg, microalbumin), semiquantitative (eg, reagent strip assay)
➔ *CPT Changes: An Insider's View* 2018
➔ *CPT Assistant* Summer 94:2, Mar 98:3, Sep 02:10

(For prealbumin, use 84134)

82045 ischemia modified
➔ *CPT Changes: An Insider's View* 2005

 # 82042 other source, quantitative, each specimen
➔ *CPT Changes: An Insider's View* 2001, 2018

(For total protein, see 84155, 84156, 84157, 84160)

82075 Alcohol (ethanol), breath
➔ *CPT Changes: An Insider's View* 2015

82085 Aldolase

82088 Aldosterone
➔ *CPT Assistant* Oct 10:7

(Alkaline phosphatase, see 84075, 84080)

(Alphaketoglutarate, see 82009, 82010)

(Alpha tocopherol [Vitamin E], use 84446)

82103 Alpha-1-antitrypsin; total

82104 phenotype

82105 Alpha-fetoprotein (AFP); serum

82106 amniotic fluid

82107 AFP-L3 fraction isoform and total AFP (including ratio)
➔ *CPT Changes: An Insider's View* 2007

82108 Aluminum

82120 Amines, vaginal fluid, qualitative
➔ *CPT Changes: An Insider's View* 2000
➔ *CPT Assistant* Nov 99:45

(For combined pH and amines test for vaginitis, use 82120 and 83986)

82127 Amino acids; single, qualitative, each specimen
➔ *CPT Assistant* Nov 98:24

82128 multiple, qualitative, each specimen
➔ *CPT Assistant* Nov 98:24

82131 single, quantitative, each specimen
➔ *CPT Assistant* May 98:11, Nov 98:24

82135 Aminolevulinic acid, delta (ALA)

82136 Amino acids, 2 to 5 amino acids, quantitative, each specimen
➔ *CPT Assistant* Nov 98:24

82139 Amino acids, 6 or more amino acids, quantitative, each specimen
➔ *CPT Assistant* Nov 98:24

82140 Ammonia

82143 Amniotic fluid scan (spectrophotometric)

(For L/S ratio, use 83661)

(Amobarbital, use 80345)

82150 Amylase

82154 Androstanediol glucuronide
➔ *CPT Assistant* Summer 94:5

82157 Androstenedione

82160 Androsterone

82163 Angiotensin II

82164 Angiotensin I - converting enzyme (ACE)

(Antidiuretic hormone (ADH), use 84588)

(Antimony, use 83015)

(Antitrypsin, alpha-1-, see 82103, 82104)

82172 Apolipoprotein, each

82175 Arsenic

(For heavy metal screening, use 83015)

82180 Ascorbic acid (Vitamin C), blood

(Aspirin, see acetylsalicylic acid, 80329, 80330, 80331)

(Atherogenic index, blood, ultracentrifugation, quantitative, use 83701)

82190 Atomic absorption spectroscopy, each analyte
➲ *CPT Assistant* Oct 10:7

82232 Beta-2 microglobulin

(Bicarbonate, use 82374)

82239 Bile acids; total

82240 cholylglycine

(For bile pigments, urine, see 81000-81005)

82247 Bilirubin; total
➲ *CPT Assistant* Nov 98:24, Apr 99:6, Dec 99:1, Jan 00:7, Dec 08:5, Apr 10:11

82248 direct
➲ *CPT Assistant* Nov 98:24, Apr 99:6, Dec 99:1, Apr 10:11

82252 feces, qualitative

82261 Biotinidase, each specimen
➲ *CPT Assistant* Nov 98:24

82270 Blood, occult, by peroxidase activity (eg, guaiac), qualitative; feces, consecutive collected specimens with single determination, for colorectal neoplasm screening (ie, patient was provided 3 cards or single triple card for consecutive collection)
➲ *CPT Changes: An Insider's View* 2002, 2006
➲ *CPT Assistant* Sep 03:15, Feb 06:7, Apr 08:5

82271 other sources
➲ *CPT Changes: An Insider's View* 2006
➲ *CPT Assistant* Feb 06:7

82272 Blood, occult, by peroxidase activity (eg, guaiac), qualitative, feces, 1-3 simultaneous determinations, performed for other than colorectal neoplasm screening
➲ *CPT Changes: An Insider's View* 2006, 2008
➲ *CPT Assistant* Feb 06:7, Apr 08:5, Jun 09:10

(Blood urea nitrogen [BUN], see 84520, 84525)

82274 Blood, occult, by fecal hemoglobin determination by immunoassay, qualitative, feces, 1-3 simultaneous determinations
➲ *CPT Changes: An Insider's View* 2002

82286 Bradykinin
➲ *CPT Assistant* Oct 10:7

82300 Cadmium
➲ *CPT Assistant* Aug 05:9, Oct 10:7

82306 Vitamin D; 25 hydroxy, includes fraction(s), if performed
➲ *CPT Changes: An Insider's View* 2010

 # 82652 1, 25 dihydroxy, includes fraction(s), if performed
➲ *CPT Changes: An Insider's View* 2010

82308 Calcitonin

82310 Calcium; total
➲ *CPT Assistant* Dec 99:2

82330 ionized
➲ *CPT Assistant* Apr 13:10

82331 after calcium infusion test

82340 urine quantitative, timed specimen

82355 Calculus; qualitative analysis
➲ *CPT Changes: An Insider's View* 2002

82360 quantitative analysis, chemical

82365 infrared spectroscopy

82370 X-ray diffraction
➲ *CPT Changes: An Insider's View* 2001

(Carbamates, see individual listings)

82373 Carbohydrate deficient transferrin
➲ *CPT Changes: An Insider's View* 2001

82374 Carbon dioxide (bicarbonate)
➲ *CPT Assistant* Dec 99:2, Apr 13:10

(See also 82803)

82375 Carboxyhemoglobin; quantitative
➲ *CPT Changes: An Insider's View* 2009

82376 qualitative
➲ *CPT Changes: An Insider's View* 2009

(For transcutaneous measurement of carboxyhemoglobin, use 88740)

82378 Carcinoembryonic antigen (CEA)
➲ *CPT Assistant* Fall 93:25, Aug 96:11

82379 Carnitine (total and free), quantitative, each specimen
➲ *CPT Assistant* Nov 98:24

(For acylcarnitine, see 82016, 82017)

82380 Carotene

82382 Catecholamines; total urine

82383 blood

82384 fractionated

(For urine metabolites, see 83835, 84585)

82387 Cathepsin-D

82390 Ceruloplasmin

82397 Chemiluminescent assay
➲ *CPT Assistant* Fall 93:25, Oct 10:7

82415 Chloramphenicol
➲ *CPT Assistant* Aug 05:9, Oct 10:7

82435 Chloride; blood
➲ *CPT Assistant* Dec 99:2, Apr 13:10

82436 urine

82438 other source
➲ *CPT Assistant* Jul 03:7

(For sweat collection by iontophoresis, use 89230)

82441 Chlorinated hydrocarbons, screen

(Cholecalciferol [Vitamin D], use 82306)

82465 Cholesterol, serum or whole blood, total

➔ *CPT Changes: An Insider's View* 2001

➔ *CPT Assistant* Dec 99:2, Mar 00:11, Feb 05:9

(For high density lipoprotein [HDL], use 83718)

82480 Cholinesterase; serum

82482 RBC

82485 Chondroitin B sulfate, quantitative

(Chorionic gonadotropin, see gonadotropin, 84702, 84703)

(82486 has been deleted. For a qualitative column chromatography procedure, use the appropriate specific analyte code, if available, or 82542)

(82487, 82488 have been deleted. For a paper chromatography procedure, use the appropriate specific analyte code, if available, or 84999)

(82489 has been deleted. For a thin layer chromatography procedure, use the appropriate specific analyte code, if available, or 84999)

(82491 has been deleted. For a quantitative column chromatography procedure, use the appropriate specific analyte code, if available, or 82542)

(82492 has been deleted. For a quantitative column chromatography procedure that detects more than one analyte, use a single specific code that represents all of the analytes, if available, or one unit of 82542 for all of the analytes)

82495 Chromium

➔ *CPT Assistant* Oct 10:7

82507 Citrate

➔ *CPT Assistant* Aug 05:9, Oct 10:7

(Cocaine, qualitative analysis, use 80353)

(Codeine, qualitative analysis, use 80361)

(Complement, see 86160-86162)

82523 Collagen cross links, any method

82525 Copper

(Coproporphyrin, see 84119, 84120)

(Corticosteroids, use 83491)

82528 Corticosterone

82530 Cortisol; free

➔ *CPT Assistant* Summer 94:3

82533 total

➔ *CPT Assistant* Summer 94:3

(C-peptide, use 84681)

82540 Creatine

(82541 has been deleted. For a quantitative chromatography procedure with mass spectrometry that only detects a single specific analyte, use the appropriate specific analyte code, if applicable, or 82542)

82542 Column chromatography, includes mass spectrometry, if performed (eg, HPLC, LC, LC/MS, LC/MS-MS, GC, GC/MS-MS, GC/MS, HPLC/MS), non-drug analyte(s) not elsewhere specified, qualitative or quantitative, each specimen

➔ *CPT Changes: An Insider's View* 2015, 2016

➔ *CPT Assistant* Nov 98:24-25, Apr 15:3

(Do not report more than one unit of 82542 for each specimen)

(82543 has been deleted. For a quantitative chromatography procedure with mass spectrometry that only detects a single specific analyte, use the appropriate specific analyte code, if available, or 82542)

(82544 has been deleted. For a quantitative chromatography procedure with mass spectrometry that detects more than one analyte, use a single specific code that represents all of the analytes, if available, or one unit of 82542 for all of the analytes)

(For column chromatography/mass spectrometry of drugs or substances, see 80305, 80306, 80307, 80320-80377, or specific analyte code[s] in the **Chemistry** section)

82550 Creatine kinase (CK), (CPK); total

➔ *CPT Assistant* Feb 98:1, Dec 99:2

82552 isoenzymes

➔ *CPT Assistant* Feb 98:1

82553 MB fraction only

➔ *CPT Assistant* Feb 98:1

82554 isoforms

➔ *CPT Assistant* Feb 98:1

82565 Creatinine; blood

➔ *CPT Assistant* Dec 99:2, Apr 13:10

82570 other source

82575 clearance

82585 Cryofibrinogen

82595 Cryoglobulin, qualitative or semi-quantitative (eg, cryocrit)

➔ *CPT Changes: An Insider's View* 2001

➔ *CPT Assistant* Oct 10:7

(For quantitative, cryoglobulin, see 82784, 82785)

(Crystals, pyrophosphate vs urate, use 89060)

82600 Cyanide

➔ *CPT Assistant* Aug 05:9, Oct 10:7

82607 Cyanocobalamin (Vitamin B-12);

82608 unsaturated binding capacity

(Cyclic AMP, use 82030)

(Cyclosporine, use 80158)

82610 Cystatin C
➔ *CPT Changes: An Insider's View* 2008
➔ *CPT Assistant* Apr 08:5, Aug 08:13

82615 Cystine and homocystine, urine, qualitative

82626 Dehydroepiandrosterone (DHEA)
➔ *CPT Assistant* Summer 94:4

(Do not report 82626 in conjunction with 80327, 80328 to identify anabolic steroid testing for testosterone)

82627 Dehydroepiandrosterone-sulfate (DHEA-S)
➔ *CPT Assistant* Summer 94:4

(Delta-aminolevulinic acid (ALA), use 82135)

82633 Desoxycorticosterone, 11-

82634 Deoxycortisol, 11-

(Dexamethasone suppression test, use 80420)

(Diastase, urine, use 82150)

82638 Dibucaine number

(Dichloroethane, use 82441)

(Dichloromethane, use 82441)

(Diethylether, use 84600)

● **82642** Dihydrotestosterone (DHT)
➔ *CPT Changes: An Insider's View* 2019

►(For dihydrotestosterone analysis for anabolic drug testing, see 80327, 80328)◄

82652 Code is out of numerical sequence. See 82300-82310

(Dipropylacetic acid, use 80164)

(Dopamine, see 82382-82384)

(Duodenal contents, see individual enzymes; for intubation and collection, see 43756, 43757)

82656 Elastase, pancreatic (EL-1), fecal, qualitative or semi-quantitative
➔ *CPT Changes: An Insider's View* 2005
➔ *CPT Assistant* Sep 05:9

82657 Enzyme activity in blood cells, cultured cells, or tissue, not elsewhere specified; nonradioactive substrate, each specimen
➔ *CPT Assistant* Nov 98:25

82658 radioactive substrate, each specimen
➔ *CPT Assistant* Nov 98:25

82664 Electrophoretic technique, not elsewhere specified

(Endocrine receptor assays, see 84233-84235)

82668 Erythropoietin

82670 Estradiol

82671 Estrogens; fractionated

82672 total

(Estrogen receptor assay, use 84233)

82677 Estriol

82679 Estrone

(Ethanol, use 80320)

82693 Ethylene glycol

82696 Etiocholanolone
➔ *CPT Assistant* Oct 10:7

(For fractionation of ketosteroids, use 83593)

82705 Fat or lipids, feces; qualitative
➔ *CPT Assistant* Aug 05:9, Oct 10:7

82710 quantitative

82715 Fat differential, feces, quantitative

82725 Fatty acids, nonesterified

82726 Very long chain fatty acids
➔ *CPT Assistant* Nov 98:25

(For long-chain [C20-22] omega-3 fatty acids in red blood cell [RBC] membranes, use Category III code 0111T)

82728 Ferritin

(Fetal hemoglobin, see hemoglobin 83030, 83033, and 85460)

(Fetoprotein, alpha-1, see 82105, 82106)

82731 Fetal fibronectin, cervicovaginal secretions, semi-quantitative
➔ *CPT Assistant* Nov 98:25

82735 Fluoride

(Foam stability test, use 83662)

82746 Folic acid; serum

82747 RBC

(Follicle stimulating hormone [FSH], use 83001)

82757 Fructose, semen

(Fructosamine, use 82985)

(Fructose, TLC screen, use 84375)

82759 Galactokinase, RBC

82760 Galactose

82775 Galactose-1-phosphate uridyl transferase; quantitative

82776 screen

82777 Galectin-3
➔ *CPT Changes: An Insider's View* 2013

82784 Gammaglobulin (immunoglobulin); IgA, IgD, IgG, IgM, each
➔ *CPT Changes: An Insider's View* 2010
➔ *CPT Assistant* Spring 94:31, Aug 00:11

82785 IgE
➔ *CPT Changes: An Insider's View* 2010
➔ *CPT Assistant* Spring 94:31

(For allergen specific IgE, see 86003, 86005)

82787 immunoglobulin subclasses (eg, IgG1, 2, 3, or 4), each
➲ *CPT Changes: An Insider's View* 2001, 2010
➲ *CPT Assistant* Oct 10:7

(Gamma-glutamyltransferase [GGT], use 82977)

82800 Gases, blood, pH only
➲ *CPT Assistant* Aug 05:9, Oct 10:7

82803 Gases, blood, any combination of pH, pCO_2, pO_2, CO_2, HCO3 (including calculated O_2 saturation);

(Use 82803 for 2 or more of the above listed analytes)

82805 with O_2 saturation, by direct measurement, except pulse oximetry

82810 Gases, blood, O_2 saturation only, by direct measurement, except pulse oximetry

(For pulse oximetry, use 94760)

82820 Hemoglobin-oxygen affinity (pO_2 for 50% hemoglobin saturation with oxygen)
➲ *CPT Assistant* Oct 10:7

(For gastric acid analysis, use 82930)

82930 Gastric acid analysis, includes pH if performed, each specimen
➲ *CPT Changes: An Insider's View* 2011
➲ *CPT Assistant* Oct 10:7, Dec 10:7, Sep 11:3

82938 Gastrin after secretin stimulation

82941 Gastrin
➲ *CPT Assistant* Aug 05:9

(Gentamicin, use 80170)

(GGT, use 82977)

(For a qualitative column chromatography procedure [eg, gas liquid chromatography], use the appropriate specific analyte code, if available, or 82542)

82943 Glucagon

82945 Glucose, body fluid, other than blood
➲ *CPT Changes: An Insider's View* 2001

82946 Glucagon tolerance test

82947 Glucose; quantitative, blood (except reagent strip)
➲ *CPT Changes: An Insider's View* 2001
➲ *CPT Assistant* Summer 93:14, Summer 94:5, Sep 99:10, Dec 99:2, Jun 02:3, Feb 05:9, Apr 13:10

82948 blood, reagent strip
➲ *CPT Assistant* Summer 94:5, Jan 99:10, Nov 10:10, Oct 11:8

82950 post glucose dose (includes glucose)
➲ *CPT Assistant* Sep 99:10, Jun 02:3, Feb 05:9

82951 tolerance test (GTT), 3 specimens (includes glucose)
➲ *CPT Assistant* Feb 01:10, Feb 05:9, Oct 10:7

+ 82952 tolerance test, each additional beyond 3 specimens (List separately in addition to code for primary procedure)
➲ *CPT Changes: An Insider's View* 2011
➲ *CPT Assistant* Feb 01:10, Oct 10:7, Dec 10:7

(Use 82952 in conjunction with 82951)

(For insulin tolerance test, see 80434, 80435)

(For leucine tolerance test, use 80428)

(For semiquantitative urine glucose, see 81000, 81002, 81005, 81099)

82955 Glucose-6-phosphate dehydrogenase (G6PD); quantitative

82960 screen

(For glucose tolerance test with medication, use 96374 in addition)

82962 Glucose, blood by glucose monitoring device(s) cleared by the FDA specifically for home use
➲ *CPT Assistant* Summer 94:4, Jan 99:10, Nov 10:10, Oct 11:8

82963 Glucosidase, beta

82965 Glutamate dehydrogenase

82977 Glutamyltransferase, gamma (GGT)
➲ *CPT Assistant* Dec 99:1

82978 Glutathione

82979 Glutathione reductase, RBC

(Glycohemoglobin, use 83036)

82985 Glycated protein
➲ *CPT Assistant* Summer 94:2

(Gonadotropin, chorionic, see 84702, 84703)

83001 Gonadotropin; follicle stimulating hormone (FSH)
➲ *CPT Assistant* Aug 05:9, Oct 10:7

83002 luteinizing hormone (LH)

(For luteinizing releasing factor [LRH], use 83727)

83003 Growth hormone, human (HGH) (somatotropin)

(For antibody to human growth hormone, use 86277)

83006 Growth stimulation expressed gene 2 (ST2, Interleukin 1 receptor like-1)
➲ *CPT Changes: An Insider's View* 2015

83009 Helicobacter pylori, blood test analysis for urease activity, non-radioactive isotope (eg, C-13)
➲ *CPT Changes: An Insider's View* 2005

(For H. pylori, breath test analysis for urease activity, see 83013, 83014)

83010 Haptoglobin; quantitative

83012 phenotypes

83013 Helicobacter pylori; breath test analysis for urease activity, non-radioactive isotope (eg, C-13)
➲ *CPT Changes: An Insider's View* 2001, 2002, 2005
➲ *CPT Assistant* Nov 98:25, Feb 99:8, Nov 99:45

83014 drug administration
➲ *CPT Changes: An Insider's View* 2005
➲ *CPT Assistant* Nov 98:25, Feb 99:8, Nov 99:45

(For H. pylori, stool, use 87338. For H. pylori, liquid scintillation counter, see 78267, 78268. For H. pylori, immunoassay, use 87339)

(For H. pylori, blood test analysis for urease activity, use 83009)

83015 Heavy metal (eg, arsenic, barium, beryllium, bismuth, antimony, mercury); qualitative, any number of analytes
CPT Changes: An Insider's View 2017

83018 quantitative, each, not elsewhere specified
CPT Changes: An Insider's View 2017

(Use an analyte-specific heavy metal quantitative code, instead of 83018, when available)

83020 Hemoglobin fractionation and quantitation; electrophoresis (eg, A2, S, C, and/or F)
CPT Assistant Nov 98:25

83021 chromatography (eg, A2, S, C, and/or F)
CPT Assistant Nov 98:25, Dec 99:7

(For glycosylated [A1c] hemoglobin analysis, by electrophoresis or chromatography, in the absence of an identified hemoglobin variant, use 83036)

83026 Hemoglobin; by copper sulfate method, non-automated

83030 F (fetal), chemical

83033 F (fetal), qualitative
CPT Changes: An Insider's View 2001

83036 glycosylated (A1C)
CPT Changes: An Insider's View 2006
CPT Assistant Summer 94:2, Feb 06:7, Oct 06:15

(For glycosylated [A1C] hemoglobin analysis, by electrophoresis or chromatography, in the setting of an identified hemoglobin variant, see 83020, 83021)

(For fecal hemoglobin detection by immunoassay, use 82274)

83037 glycosylated (A1C) by device cleared by FDA for home use
CPT Changes: An Insider's View 2006
CPT Assistant Feb 06:7, Oct 06:15

83045 methemoglobin, qualitative

83050 methemoglobin, quantitative

(For transcutaneous quantitative methemoglobin determination, use 88741)

83051 plasma

83060 sulfhemoglobin, quantitative

83065 thermolabile

83068 unstable, screen

83069 urine

83070 Hemosiderin, qualitative

(HIAA, use 83497)

(For a qualitative column chromatography procedure [eg, high performance liquid chromatography], use the appropriate specific analyte code, if available, or 82542)

83080 b-Hexosaminidase, each assay
CPT Assistant Nov 98:25

83088 Histamine

(Hollander test, see 43754, 43755)

83090 Homocysteine
CPT Changes: An Insider's View 2001
CPT Assistant Jan 01:13, Oct 10:7

83150 Homovanillic acid (HVA)
CPT Assistant Aug 05:9, Oct 10:7

(Hormones, see individual alphabetic listings in **Chemistry** section)

(For hydrogen/methane breath test, use 91065)

83491 Hydroxycorticosteroids, 17- (17-OHCS)
CPT Assistant Aug 05:9, Oct 10:7

(For cortisol, see 82530, 82533. For deoxycortisol, use 82634)

83497 Hydroxyindolacetic acid, 5-(HIAA)

(For urine qualitative test, use 81005)

(5-Hydroxytryptamine, use 84260)

83498 Hydroxyprogesterone, 17-d

(83499 has been deleted)

83500 Hydroxyproline; free
CPT Assistant Aug 05:9, Oct 10:7

83505 total

83516 Immunoassay for analyte other than infectious agent antibody or infectious agent antigen; qualitative or semiquantitative, multiple step method
CPT Changes: An Insider's View 2010
CPT Assistant Nov 98:25

83518 qualitative or semiquantitative, single step method (eg, reagent strip)
CPT Changes: An Insider's View 2010
CPT Assistant Fall 93:26

83519 quantitative, by radioimmunoassay (eg, RIA)
CPT Changes: An Insider's View 2010
CPT Assistant Fall 93:26, Summer 94:2

83520 quantitative, not otherwise specified
CPT Changes: An Insider's View 2010
CPT Assistant Fall 93:26

(For immunoassays for antibodies to infectious agent antigens, see analyte and method specific codes in the **Immunology** section)

(For immunoassay of tumor antigen not elsewhere specified, use 86316)

(Immunoglobulins, see 82784, 82785)

83525 Insulin; total

(For proinsulin, use 84206)

83527 free
➔ *CPT Assistant* Summer 94:5

83528 Intrinsic factor

(For intrinsic factor antibodies, use 86340)

83540 Iron
➔ *CPT Assistant* Fall 93:25

83550 Iron binding capacity

83570 Isocitric dehydrogenase (IDH)

(Isonicotinic acid hydrazide, INH, see code for specific method)

(Isopropyl alcohol, use 80320)

83582 Ketogenic steroids, fractionation

(Ketone bodies, for serum, see 82009, 82010; for urine, see 81000-81003)

83586 Ketosteroids, 17- (17-KS); total

83593 fractionation
➔ *CPT Assistant* Oct 10:7

83605 Lactate (lactic acid)
➔ *CPT Assistant* Aug 05:9, Oct 10:7

83615 Lactate dehydrogenase (LD), (LDH);
➔ *CPT Assistant* Fall 93:25, Feb 98:1, Dec 99:2

83625 isoenzymes, separation and quantitation
➔ *CPT Assistant* Fall 93:25, Feb 98:1

83630 Lactoferrin, fecal; qualitative
➔ *CPT Changes: An Insider's View* 2005, 2006
➔ *CPT Assistant* Feb 06:7

83631 quantitative
➔ *CPT Changes: An Insider's View* 2006
➔ *CPT Assistant* Feb 06:7, Jan 07:29

83632 Lactogen, human placental (HPL) human chorionic somatomammotropin

83633 Lactose, urine, qualitative

(For tolerance, see 82951, 82952)

(For breath hydrogen/methane test for lactase deficiency, use 91065)

83655 Lead

83661 Fetal lung maturity assessment; lecithin sphingomyelin (L/S) ratio
➔ *CPT Changes: An Insider's View* 2001

83662 foam stability test

83663 fluorescence polarization
➔ *CPT Changes: An Insider's View* 2001

83664 lamellar body density
➔ *CPT Changes: An Insider's View* 2001

(For phosphatidylglycerol, use 84081)

83670 Leucine aminopeptidase (LAP)

83690 Lipase

83695 Lipoprotein (a)
➔ *CPT Changes: An Insider's View* 2006
➔ *CPT Assistant* Feb 06:7

83698 Lipoprotein-associated phospholipase A2 (Lp-PLA2)
➔ *CPT Changes: An Insider's View* 2007
➔ *CPT Assistant* Oct 10:7

(For secretory type II phospholipase A2 [sPLA2-IIA], use 0423T)

83700 Lipoprotein, blood; electrophoretic separation and quantitation
➔ *CPT Changes: An Insider's View* 2006
➔ *CPT Assistant* Feb 06:7, Oct 10:7

83701 high resolution fractionation and quantitation of lipoproteins including lipoprotein subclasses when performed (eg, electrophoresis, ultracentrifugation)
➔ *CPT Changes: An Insider's View* 2006
➔ *CPT Assistant* Feb 06:7

83704 quantitation of lipoprotein particle number(s) (eg, by nuclear magnetic resonance spectroscopy), includes lipoprotein particle subclass(es), when performed
➔ *CPT Changes: An Insider's View* 2006, 2017
➔ *CPT Assistant* Feb 06:7

83718 Lipoprotein, direct measurement; high density cholesterol (HDL cholesterol)
➔ *CPT Assistant* Oct 99:11, Mar 00:11, Feb 05:9

83719 VLDL cholesterol
➔ *CPT Assistant* Oct 99:11

83721 LDL cholesterol
➔ *CPT Assistant* Nov 98:25, Oct 99:11

● **83722** small dense LDL cholesterol
➔ *CPT Changes: An Insider's View* 2019

(For fractionation by high resolution electrophoresis or ultracentrifugation, use 83701)

(For lipoprotein particle numbers and subclasses analysis by nuclear magnetic resonance spectroscopy, use 83704)

83727 Luteinizing releasing factor (LRH)

(Luteinizing hormone [LH], use 83002)

(Macroglobulins, alpha-2, use 86329)

83735 Magnesium

83775 Malate dehydrogenase

(Maltose tolerance, see 82951, 82952)

(Mammotropin, use 84146)

83785 Manganese

(83788 has been deleted. For a qualitative mass spectrometry or tandem mass spectrometry procedure, use the specific analyte code, if available, or 83789)

83789 Mass spectrometry and tandem mass spectrometry (eg, MS, MS/MS, MALDI, MS-TOF, QTOF), non-drug analyte(s) not elsewhere specified, qualitative or quantitative, each specimen
CPT Changes: An Insider's View 2016
CPT Assistant Nov 98:26, Oct 10:7

(Do not report more than one unit of 83789 for each specimen)

(For column chromatography/mass spectrometry of drugs or substances, see 80305, 80306, 80307, 80320-80377, or specific analyte code[s] in the **Chemistry** section)

83825 Mercury, quantitative

(Mercury screen, use 83015)

83835 Metanephrines

(For catecholamines, see 82382-82384)

(Methamphetamine, see 80324, 80325, 80326)

(Methane breath test, use 91065)

83857 Methemalbumin

(Methemoglobin, see hemoglobin 83045, 83050)

(Methyl alcohol, use 80320)

(Microalbumin, see 82043 for quantitative, see 82044 for semiquantitative)

83861 Microfluidic analysis utilizing an integrated collection and analysis device, tear osmolarity
CPT Changes: An Insider's View 2011
CPT Assistant Dec 10:7

(Microglobulin, beta-2, use 82232)

(For microfluidic tear osmolarity of both eyes, report 83861 twice)

83864 Mucopolysaccharides, acid, quantitative

83872 Mucin, synovial fluid (Ropes test)

83873 Myelin basic protein, cerebrospinal fluid
CPT Changes: An Insider's View 2002

(For oligoclonal bands, use 83916)

83874 Myoglobin
CPT Assistant Feb 98:1

83876 Myeloperoxidase (MPO)
CPT Changes: An Insider's View 2009

83880 Natriuretic peptide
CPT Changes: An Insider's View 2003
CPT Assistant Jul 03:7

83883 Nephelometry, each analyte not elsewhere specified

83885 Nickel

83915 Nucleotidase 5'-

83916 Oligoclonal immune (oligoclonal bands)
CPT Changes: An Insider's View 2002

83918 Organic acids; total, quantitative, each specimen
CPT Changes: An Insider's View 2001
CPT Assistant Mar 96:11, Nov 98:26

83919 qualitative, each specimen
CPT Assistant Nov 98:26

83921 Organic acid, single, quantitative
CPT Changes: An Insider's View 2001

83930 Osmolality; blood

83935 urine

(For tear osmolarity using microfluidic analysis, use 83861)

83937 Osteocalcin (bone g1a protein)
CPT Assistant Summer 94:5

83945 Oxalate

83950 Oncoprotein; HER-2/neu
CPT Changes: An Insider's View 2002, 2009

(For tissue, see 88342, 88365)

83951 des-gamma-carboxy-prothrombin (DCP)
CPT Changes: An Insider's View 2009

83970 Parathormone (parathyroid hormone)

(Pesticide, quantitative, see code for specific method. For screen for chlorinated hydrocarbons, use 82441)

83986 pH; body fluid, not otherwise specified
CPT Changes: An Insider's View 2010
CPT Assistant Sep 13:13, May 16:14

83987 exhaled breath condensate
CPT Changes: An Insider's View 2010

(For blood pH, see 82800, 82803)

83992 Code is out of numerical sequence. See Definitive Drug Testing subsection

(Phenobarbital, use 80345)

83993 Calprotectin, fecal
CPT Changes: An Insider's View 2008
CPT Assistant Apr 08:5, Oct 10:7

84030 Phenylalanine (PKU), blood

(Phenylalanine-tyrosine ratio, see 84030, 84510)

84035 Phenylketones, qualitative

84060 Phosphatase, acid; total

(84061 has been deleted)

84066 prostatic

84075 Phosphatase, alkaline;
CPT Assistant Dec 99:2

84078 heat stable (total not included)

84080 isoenzymes

84081 Phosphatidylglycerol

(Phosphates inorganic, use 84100)

(Phosphates, organic, see code for specific method. For cholinesterase, see 82480, 82482)

84085 Phosphogluconate, 6-, dehydrogenase, RBC

84087 Phosphohexose isomerase
➲ *CPT Assistant* Oct 10:7

84100 Phosphorus inorganic (phosphate);
➲ *CPT Assistant* Dec 99:2, Aug 05:9, Oct 10:7

84105 urine

(Pituitary gonadotropins, see 83001-83002)

(PKU, see 84030, 84035)

84106 Porphobilinogen, urine; qualitative

84110 quantitative

84112 Evaluation of cervicovaginal fluid for specific amniotic fluid protein(s) (eg, placental alpha microglobulin-1 [PAMG-1], placental protein 12 [PP12], alpha-fetoprotein), qualitative, each specimen
➲ *CPT Changes: An Insider's View* 2011, 2014
➲ *CPT Assistant* Oct 10:8, Dec 10:8

84119 Porphyrins, urine; qualitative

84120 quantitation and fractionation

84126 Porphyrins, feces, quantitative

(Porphyrin precursors, see 82135, 84106, 84110)

(For protoporphyrin, RBC, see 84202, 84203)

84132 Potassium; serum, plasma or whole blood
➲ *CPT Changes: An Insider's View* 2009
➲ *CPT Assistant* Dec 99:2, Jun 02:3, Apr 13:10

84133 urine

84134 Prealbumin

(For microalbumin, see 82043, 82044)

84135 Pregnanediol

84138 Pregnanetriol

84140 Pregnenolone
➲ *CPT Assistant* Summer 94:6

84143 17-hydroxypregnenolone
➲ *CPT Assistant* Summer 94:6

84144 Progesterone

(Progesterone receptor assay, use 84234)

(For proinsulin, use 84206)

84145 Procalcitonin (PCT)
➲ *CPT Changes: An Insider's View* 2010

84146 Prolactin

84150 Prostaglandin, each

84152 Prostate specific antigen (PSA); complexed (direct measurement)
➲ *CPT Changes: An Insider's View* 2001

84153 total
➲ *CPT Assistant* Fall 93:26, May 96:10, Aug 96:10, Jan 97:10, Nov 98:26, Aug 99:5, Dec 99:10

84154 free
➲ *CPT Assistant* Nov 98:26, Aug 99:5, Dec 99:10

84155 Protein, total, except by refractometry; serum, plasma or whole blood
➲ *CPT Changes: An Insider's View* 2004, 2009
➲ *CPT Assistant* Dec 99:2, Jan 00:7

84156 urine
➲ *CPT Changes: An Insider's View* 2004

84157 other source (eg, synovial fluid, cerebrospinal fluid)
➲ *CPT Changes: An Insider's View* 2004

84160 Protein, total, by refractometry, any source
➲ *CPT Changes: An Insider's View* 2004

(For urine total protein by dipstick method, use 81000-81003)

84163 Pregnancy-associated plasma protein-A (PAPP-A)
➲ *CPT Changes: An Insider's View* 2005

84165 Protein; electrophoretic fractionation and quantitation, serum
➲ *CPT Changes: An Insider's View* 2004, 2005

84166 electrophoretic fractionation and quantitation, other fluids with concentration (eg, urine, CSF)
➲ *CPT Changes: An Insider's View* 2005

84181 Western Blot, with interpretation and report, blood or other body fluid

84182 Western Blot, with interpretation and report, blood or other body fluid, immunological probe for band identification, each
➲ *CPT Assistant* Oct 10:7

(For Western Blot tissue analysis, use 88371)

84202 Protoporphyrin, RBC; quantitative
➲ *CPT Assistant* Aug 05:9, Oct 10:7

84203 screen

84206 Proinsulin

(Pseudocholinesterase, use 82480)

84207 Pyridoxal phosphate (Vitamin B-6)

84210 Pyruvate

84220 Pyruvate kinase

84228 Quinine
➲ *CPT Assistant* Apr 15:3

84233 Receptor assay; estrogen

84234 progesterone

84235 endocrine, other than estrogen or progesterone (specify hormone)

84238 non-endocrine (specify receptor)
➲ *CPT Changes: An Insider's View* 2006
➲ *CPT Assistant* Nov 05:14

84244 Renin

84252 Riboflavin (Vitamin B-2)

(Salicylates, see 80329, 80330, 80331)

(Secretin test, see 99070, 43756, 43757 and appropriate analyses)

84255 Selenium

84260 Serotonin

(For urine metabolites (HIAA), use 83497)

84270 Sex hormone binding globulin (SHBG)

➲ *CPT Assistant* Summer 94:4

84275 Sialic acid

(Sickle hemoglobin, use 85660)

84285 Silica

84295 Sodium; serum, plasma or whole blood

➲ *CPT Changes: An Insider's View* 2009

➲ *CPT Assistant* Dec 99:2, Oct 10:7, Apr 13:10

84300 urine

➲ *CPT Assistant* Aug 05:9, Oct 10:7

84302 other source

➲ *CPT Changes: An Insider's View* 2003

➲ *CPT Assistant* Jul 03:7

(Somatomammotropin, use 83632)

(Somatotropin, use 83003)

84305 Somatomedin

➲ *CPT Assistant* Summer 94:4

84307 Somatostatin

➲ *CPT Assistant* Summer 94:4

84311 Spectrophotometry, analyte not elsewhere specified

84315 Specific gravity (except urine)

(For specific gravity, urine, see 81000-81003)

(Stone analysis, see 82355-82370)

(For suppression of growth stimulation expressed gene 2 [ST2] testing, use 83006)

84375 Sugars, chromatographic, TLC or paper chromatography

84376 Sugars (mono-, di-, and oligosaccharides); single qualitative, each specimen

➲ *CPT Assistant* Nov 98:26-27, Dec 99:7

84377 multiple qualitative, each specimen

➲ *CPT Assistant* Nov 98:26-27, Jul 03:7

84378 single quantitative, each specimen

➲ *CPT Assistant* Nov 98:26-27

84379 multiple quantitative, each specimen

➲ *CPT Assistant* Nov 98:26-27, Dec 99:7, Jul 03:7

84392 Sulfate, urine

➲ *CPT Assistant* Oct 10:7

(Sulfhemoglobin, use hemoglobin, 83060)

(T-3, see 84479-84481)

(T-4, see 84436-84439)

84402 Testosterone; free

➲ *CPT Assistant* Aug 05:9, Oct 10:7

84403 total

84410 bioavailable, direct measurement (eg, differential precipitation)

➲ *CPT Changes: An Insider's View* 2017

(Do not report 84402, 84403 in conjunction with 80327, 80328 to identify anabolic steroid testing for testosterone)

84425 Thiamine (Vitamin B-1)

84430 Thiocyanate

84431 Thromboxane metabolite(s), including thromboxane if performed, urine

➲ *CPT Changes: An Insider's View* 2010

(For concurrent urine creatinine determination, use 84431 in conjunction with 82570)

84432 Thyroglobulin

➲ *CPT Assistant* Summer 94:2

(Thyroglobulin, antibody, use 86800)

(Thyrotropin releasing hormone [TRH] test, see 80438, 80439)

84436 Thyroxine; total

➲ *CPT Assistant* Fall 93:25, Summer 94:3

84437 requiring elution (eg, neonatal)

84439 free

84442 Thyroxine binding globulin (TBG)

84443 Thyroid stimulating hormone (TSH)

➲ *CPT Assistant* Summer 94:3

84445 Thyroid stimulating immune globulins (TSI)

➲ *CPT Changes: An Insider's View* 2002

➲ *CPT Assistant* Summer 94:3

(Tobramycin, use 80200)

84446 Tocopherol alpha (Vitamin E)

84449 Transcortin (cortisol binding globulin)

➲ *CPT Assistant* Summer 94:6

84450 Transferase; aspartate amino (AST) (SGOT)

➲ *CPT Assistant* Dec 99:2

84460 alanine amino (ALT) (SGPT)

➲ *CPT Assistant* Dec 99:2

84466 Transferrin

➲ *CPT Assistant* Summer 94:4

(Iron binding capacity, use 83550)

84478 Triglycerides

➲ *CPT Assistant* Dec 99:2, Mar 00:11, Feb 05:9

84479 Thyroid hormone (T3 or T4) uptake or thyroid hormone binding ratio (THBR)
➔ *CPT Assistant* Fall 93:25, Summer 94:3

84480 Triiodothyronine T3; total (TT-3)

84481 free

84482 reverse
➔ *CPT Assistant* Summer 94:2

84484 Troponin, quantitative
➔ *CPT Assistant* Nov 97:29, Jan 98:6, Feb 98:1

(For troponin, qualitative assay, use 84512)

84485 Trypsin; duodenal fluid

84488 feces, qualitative

84490 feces, quantitative, 24-hour collection
➔ *CPT Assistant* Oct 10:7

84510 Tyrosine
➔ *CPT Assistant* Oct 10:7

(Urate crystal identification, use 89060)

84512 Troponin, qualitative
➔ *CPT Assistant* Nov 97:29, Jan 98:6, Feb 98:1

(For troponin, quantitative assay, use 84484)

84520 Urea nitrogen; quantitative
➔ *CPT Assistant* Dec 99:2, Apr 13:10

84525 semiquantitative (eg, reagent strip test)
➔ *CPT Assistant* Mar 98:3

84540 Urea nitrogen, urine

84545 Urea nitrogen, clearance

84550 Uric acid; blood
➔ *CPT Assistant* Dec 99:2

84560 other source

84577 Urobilinogen, feces, quantitative

84578 Urobilinogen, urine; qualitative

84580 quantitative, timed specimen

84583 semiquantitative

(Uroporphyrins, use 84120)

(Valproic acid [dipropylacetic acid], use 80164)

84585 Vanillylmandelic acid (VMA), urine

84586 Vasoactive intestinal peptide (VIP)
➔ *CPT Assistant* Summer 94:6

84588 Vasopressin (antidiuretic hormone, ADH)
➔ *CPT Assistant* Jan 18:7

84590 Vitamin A
➔ *CPT Assistant* Aug 05:9

(Vitamin B-1, use 84425)

(Vitamin B-2, use 84252)

(Vitamin B-6, use 84207)

(Vitamin B-12, use 82607)

(Vitamin C, use 82180)

(Vitamin D, see 82306, 82652)

(Vitamin E, use 84446)

84591 Vitamin, not otherwise specified
➔ *CPT Changes: An Insider's View* 2001

84597 Vitamin K
➔ *CPT Assistant* Oct 10:7

(VMA, use 84585)

84600 Volatiles (eg, acetic anhydride, diethylether)
➔ *CPT Changes: An Insider's View* 2015
➔ *CPT Assistant* Aug 05:9, Oct 10:7

(For carbon tetrachloride, dichloroethane, dichloromethane, use 82441)

(For isopropyl alcohol and methanol, use 80320)

(Volume, blood, RISA or Cr-51, see 78110, 78111)

84620 Xylose absorption test, blood and/or urine

(For administration, use 99070)

84630 Zinc

84681 C-peptide
➔ *CPT Assistant* Oct 10:7

84702 Gonadotropin, chorionic (hCG); quantitative
➔ *CPT Assistant* Oct 10:7

84703 qualitative

(For urine pregnancy test by visual color comparison, use 81025)

84704 free beta chain
➔ *CPT Changes: An Insider's View* 2008
➔ *CPT Assistant* Apr 08:5, Aug 08:13, Oct 10:7

84830 Ovulation tests, by visual color comparison methods for human luteinizing hormone
➔ *CPT Assistant* Oct 10:7, Jun 15:10

84999 Unlisted chemistry procedure
➔ *CPT Assistant* Oct 00:24, Aug 05:9, Oct 10:7, Dec 10:7, Apr 15:3

(For definitive testing of a drug, not otherwise specified, see 80299, 80375, 80376, 80377)

Hematology and Coagulation

(For blood banking procedures, see **Transfusion Medicine**)

(Agglutinins, see **Immunology**)

(Antiplasmin, use 85410)

(Antithrombin III, see 85300, 85301)

85002 Bleeding time
➔ *CPT Assistant* Aug 05:9

85004 Blood count; automated differential WBC count
➲ *CPT Changes: An Insider's View* 2003
➲ *CPT Assistant* Jan 04:26

85007 blood smear, microscopic examination with manual differential WBC count
➲ *CPT Changes: An Insider's View* 2003
➲ *CPT Assistant* Jul 03:7, Jan 04:26

85008 blood smear, microscopic examination without manual differential WBC count
➲ *CPT Changes: An Insider's View* 2003
➲ *CPT Assistant* Jul 03:8, Jan 04:26

(For other fluids [eg, CSF], see 89050, 89051)

85009 manual differential WBC count, buffy coat
➲ *CPT Changes: An Insider's View* 2003
➲ *CPT Assistant* Jul 03:7, Jan 04:26

(Eosinophils, nasal smear, use 89190)

85013 spun microhematocrit

85014 hematocrit (Hct)
➲ *CPT Changes: An Insider's View* 2003
➲ *CPT Assistant* Jul 03:7

85018 hemoglobin (Hgb)
➲ *CPT Changes: An Insider's View* 2003
➲ *CPT Assistant* Jul 03:8

(For other hemoglobin determination, see 83020-83069)

(For immunoassay, hemoglobin, fecal, use 82274)

(For transcutaneous hemoglobin measurement, use 88738)

85025 complete (CBC), automated (Hgb, Hct, RBC, WBC and platelet count) and automated differential WBC count
➲ *CPT Changes: An Insider's View* 2003
➲ *CPT Assistant* Jul 00:11, Jul 03:7, Jan 04:26, Jul 11:16

85027 complete (CBC), automated (Hgb, Hct, RBC, WBC and platelet count)
➲ *CPT Changes: An Insider's View* 2003
➲ *CPT Assistant* Jul 03:8, Jan 04:26

85032 manual cell count (erythrocyte, leukocyte, or platelet) each
➲ *CPT Changes: An Insider's View* 2003
➲ *CPT Assistant* Jul 03:8, Nov 03:15

85041 red blood cell (RBC), automated
➲ *CPT Changes: An Insider's View* 2003
➲ *CPT Assistant* Jul 03:8

(Do not report code 85041 in conjunction with 85025 or 85027)

85044 reticulocyte, manual
➲ *CPT Changes: An Insider's View* 2003
➲ *CPT Assistant* Jul 03:8

85045 reticulocyte, automated
➲ *CPT Changes: An Insider's View* 2003
➲ *CPT Assistant* Jul 03:8

85046 reticulocytes, automated, including 1 or more cellular parameters (eg, reticulocyte hemoglobin content [CHr], immature reticulocyte fraction [IRF], reticulocyte volume [MRV], RNA content), direct measurement
➲ *CPT Changes: An Insider's View* 2005
➲ *CPT Assistant* Nov 98:27

85048 leukocyte (WBC), automated
➲ *CPT Changes: An Insider's View* 2003
➲ *CPT Assistant* Jul 03:8

85049 platelet, automated
➲ *CPT Changes: An Insider's View* 2003

85055 Reticulated platelet assay
➲ *CPT Changes: An Insider's View* 2004

85060 Blood smear, peripheral, interpretation by physician with written report

85097 Bone marrow, smear interpretation
➲ *CPT Changes: An Insider's View* 2002
➲ *CPT Assistant* Winter 92:17, Jul 98:4, Mar 03:22

(For special stains, see 88312, 88313)

(For bone biopsy, see 20220, 20225, 20240, 20245, 20250, 20251)

85130 Chromogenic substrate assay
➲ *CPT Assistant* Aug 05:9

(Circulating anti-coagulant screen [mixing studies], see 85611, 85732)

85170 Clot retraction

85175 Clot lysis time, whole blood dilution

(Clotting factor I [fibrinogen], see 85384, 85385)

85210 Clotting; factor II, prothrombin, specific
➲ *CPT Assistant* Aug 05:9

(See also 85610-85613)

85220 factor V (AcG or proaccelerin), labile factor

85230 factor VII (proconvertin, stable factor)

85240 factor VIII (AHG), 1-stage

85244 factor VIII related antigen

85245 factor VIII, VW factor, ristocetin cofactor

85246 factor VIII, VW factor antigen

85247 factor VIII, von Willebrand factor, multimetric analysis

85250 factor IX (PTC or Christmas)

85260 factor X (Stuart-Prower)

85270 factor XI (PTA)

85280 factor XII (Hageman)

85290 factor XIII (fibrin stabilizing)

85291 factor XIII (fibrin stabilizing), screen solubility

85292 prekallikrein assay (Fletcher factor assay)

85293 high molecular weight kininogen assay (Fitzgerald factor assay)

85300 Clotting inhibitors or anticoagulants; antithrombin III, activity
➔ *CPT Assistant* Aug 05:9

85301 antithrombin III, antigen assay

85302 protein C, antigen

85303 protein C, activity

85305 protein S, total

85306 protein S, free

85307 Activated Protein C (APC) resistance assay
➔ *CPT Changes: An Insider's View* 2001

85335 Factor inhibitor test

85337 Thrombomodulin

(For mixing studies for inhibitors, use 85732)

85345 Coagulation time; Lee and White

85347 activated

85348 other methods

(Differential count, see 85007 et seq)

(Duke bleeding time, use 85002)

(Eosinophils, nasal smear, use 89190)

85360 Euglobulin lysis

(Fetal hemoglobin, see 83030, 83033, 85460)

85362 Fibrin(ogen) degradation (split) products (FDP) (FSP); agglutination slide, semiquantitative

(Immunoelectrophoresis, use 86320)

85366 paracoagulation

85370 quantitative

85378 Fibrin degradation products, D-dimer; qualitative or semiquantitative
➔ *CPT Changes: An Insider's View* 2003
➔ *CPT Assistant* Jul 03:8

85379 quantitative

(For ultrasensitive and standard sensitivity quantitative D-dimer, use 85379)

85380 ultrasensitive (eg, for evaluation for venous thromboembolism), qualitative or semiquantitative
➔ *CPT Changes: An Insider's View* 2003
➔ *CPT Assistant* Jul 03:8

85384 Fibrinogen; activity

85385 antigen

85390 Fibrinolysins or coagulopathy screen, interpretation and report

85396 Coagulation/fibrinolysis assay, whole blood (eg, viscoelastic clot assessment), including use of any pharmacologic additive(s), as indicated, including interpretation and written report, per day
➔ *CPT Changes: An Insider's View* 2004

85397 Coagulation and fibrinolysis, functional activity, not otherwise specified (eg, ADAMTS-13), each analyte
➔ *CPT Changes: An Insider's View* 2009

85400 Fibrinolytic factors and inhibitors; plasmin
➔ *CPT Assistant* Aug 05:9

85410 alpha-2 antiplasmin

85415 plasminogen activator

85420 plasminogen, except antigenic assay

85421 plasminogen, antigenic assay

(Fragility, red blood cell, see 85547, 85555-85557)

85441 Heinz bodies; direct

85445 induced, acetyl phenylhydrazine

(Hematocrit [PCV], see 85014, 85025, 85027)

(Hemoglobin, see 83020-83068, 85018, 85025, 85027)

85460 Hemoglobin or RBCs, fetal, for fetomaternal hemorrhage; differential lysis (Kleihauer-Betke)
➔ *CPT Assistant* Fall 93:25

(See also 83030, 83033)

(Hemolysins, see 86940, 86941)

85461 rosette

85475 Hemolysin, acid

(See also 86940, 86941)

85520 Heparin assay
➔ *CPT Assistant* Aug 05:9

85525 Heparin neutralization
➔ *CPT Assistant* Aug 17:10

85530 Heparin-protamine tolerance test

85536 Iron stain, peripheral blood
➔ *CPT Changes: An Insider's View* 2001

(For iron stains on bone marrow or other tissues with physician evaluation, use 88313)

85540 Leukocyte alkaline phosphatase with count

85547 Mechanical fragility, RBC

85549 Muramidase

(Nitroblue tetrazolium dye test, use 86384)

85555 Osmotic fragility, RBC; unincubated

85557 incubated

(Packed cell volume, use 85013)

(Partial thromboplastin time, see 85730, 85732)

(Parasites, blood [eg, malaria smears], use 87207)

(Plasmin, use 85400)

(Plasminogen, use 85420)

(Plasminogen activator, use 85415)

85576 Platelet, aggregation (in vitro), each agent
➔ *CPT Changes: An Insider's View* 2003
➔ *CPT Assistant* Jul 96:10

(For thromboxane metabolite[s], including thromboxane, if performed, measurement[s] in urine, use 84431)

85597 Phospholipid neutralization; platelet
➔ *CPT Changes: An Insider's View* 2011
➔ *CPT Assistant* Oct 10:8, Dec 10:8, Apr 11:9

85598 hexagonal phospholipid
➔ *CPT Changes: An Insider's View* 2011
➔ *CPT Assistant* Oct 10:8, Dec 10:8, Apr 11:9

85610 Prothrombin time;
➔ *CPT Assistant* Aug 05:9

85611 substitution, plasma fractions, each

85612 Russell viper venom time (includes venom); undiluted

85613 diluted

(Red blood cell count, see 85025, 85027, 85041)

85635 Reptilase test

(Reticulocyte count, see 85044, 85045)

85651 Sedimentation rate, erythrocyte; non-automated

85652 automated

85660 Sickling of RBC, reduction

(Hemoglobin electrophoresis, use 83020)

(Smears [eg, for parasites, malaria], use 87207)

85670 Thrombin time; plasma

85675 titer

85705 Thromboplastin inhibition, tissue
➔ *CPT Assistant* Aug 05:9

(For individual clotting factors, see 85245-85247)

85730 Thromboplastin time, partial (PTT); plasma or whole blood

85732 substitution, plasma fractions, each
➔ *CPT Assistant* Apr 11:9

85810 Viscosity

(von Willebrand factor assay, see 85245-85247)

(WBC count, see 85025, 85027, 85048, 89050)

85999 Unlisted hematology and coagulation procedure
➔ *CPT Assistant* Aug 05:9, Oct 09:12, Aug 17:10

Immunology

(Acetylcholine receptor antibody, see 83519, 86255, 86256)

(Actinomyces, antibodies to, use 86602)

(Adrenal cortex antibodies, see 86255, 86256)

86000 Agglutinins, febrile (eg, Brucella, Francisella, Murine typhus, Q fever, Rocky Mountain spotted fever, scrub typhus), each antigen
➔ *CPT Assistant* Aug 05:9

(For antibodies to infectious agents, see 86602-86804)

86001 Allergen specific IgG quantitative or semiquantitative, each allergen
➔ *CPT Changes: An Insider's View* 2001

(Agglutinins and autohemolysins, see 86940, 86941)

86003 Allergen specific IgE; quantitative or semiquantitative, crude allergen extract, each
➔ *CPT Changes: An Insider's View* 2018
➔ *CPT Assistant* Spring 94:31

(For total quantitative IgE, use 82785)

86005 qualitative, multiallergen screen (eg, disk, sponge, card)
➔ *CPT Changes: An Insider's View* 2018
➔ *CPT Assistant* Spring 94:31

86008 quantitative or semiquantitative, recombinant or purified component, each
➔ *CPT Changes: An Insider's View* 2018

(For total qualitative IgE, use 83518)

(Alpha-1 antitrypsin, see 82103, 82104)

(Alpha-1 feto-protein, see 82105, 82106)

(Anti-AChR [acetylcholine receptor] antibody titer, see 86255, 86256)

(Anticardiolipin antibody, use 86147)

(Anti-DNA, use 86225)

(Anti-deoxyribonuclease titer, use 86215)

86021 Antibody identification; leukocyte antibodies

86022 platelet antibodies

86023 platelet associated immunoglobulin assay

86038 Antinuclear antibodies (ANA);

86039 titer

(Antistreptococcal antibody, ie, anti-DNAse, use 86215)

(Antistreptokinase titer, use 86590)

86060 Antistreptolysin O; titer

(For antibodies to infectious agents, see 86602-86804)

86063 screen

(For antibodies to infectious agents, see 86602-86804)

(Blastomyces, antibodies to, use 86612)

86077 Blood bank physician services; difficult cross match and/or evaluation of irregular antibody(s), interpretation and written report

86078 investigation of transfusion reaction including suspicion of transmissible disease, interpretation and written report

86079 authorization for deviation from standard blood banking procedures (eg, use of outdated blood, transfusion of Rh incompatible units), with written report

(Brucella, antibodies to, use 86622)

(Candida, antibodies to, use 86628. For skin testing, use 86485)

86140 C-reactive protein;
➔ *CPT Changes: An Insider's View* 2002
➔ *CPT Assistant* Aug 05:9

(Candidiasis, use 86628)

86141 high sensitivity (hsCRP)
➔ *CPT Changes: An Insider's View* 2002

86146 Beta 2 Glycoprotein I antibody, each
➔ *CPT Changes: An Insider's View* 2001

86147 Cardiolipin (phospholipid) antibody, each Ig class
➔ *CPT Changes: An Insider's View* 2001

 # 86152 Cell enumeration using immunologic selection and identification in fluid specimen (eg, circulating tumor cells in blood);
➔ *CPT Changes: An Insider's View* 2013

(For physician interpretation and report, use 86153. For cell enumeration with interpretation and report, use 86152 and 86153)

 # 86153 physician interpretation and report, when required
➔ *CPT Changes: An Insider's View* 2013

(For cell enumeration, use 86152. For cell enumeration with interpretation and report, use 86152 and 86153)

(For flow cytometric immunophenotyping, see 88184-88189)

(For flow cytometric quantitation, see 86355, 86356, 86357, 86359, 86360, 86361, 86367)

86148 Anti-phosphatidylserine (phospholipid) antibody
➔ *CPT Assistant* Nov 97:30, Jul 03:8, Nov 03:5

(To report antiprothrombin [phospholipid cofactor] antibody, use 86849)

86152 Code is out of numerical sequence. See 86146-86155

86153 Code is out of numerical sequence. See 86146-86155

86155 Chemotaxis assay, specify method

(Clostridium difficile toxin, use 87230)

(Coccidioides, antibodies to, see 86635. For skin testing, use 86490)

86156 Cold agglutinin; screen

86157 titer

86160 Complement; antigen, each component

86161 functional activity, each component

86162 total hemolytic (CH50)

86171 Complement fixation tests, each antigen

(Coombs test, see 86880-86886)

(86185 has been deleted)

86200 Cyclic citrullinated peptide (CCP), antibody
➔ *CPT Changes: An Insider's View* 2006
➔ *CPT Assistant* Mar 06:6

86215 Deoxyribonuclease, antibody
➔ *CPT Assistant* Aug 05:9

86225 Deoxyribonucleic acid (DNA) antibody; native or double stranded

(Echinococcus, antibodies to, see code for specific method)

(For HIV antibody tests, see 86701-86703)

86226 single stranded

(Anti D.S., DNA, IFA, eg, using C.Lucilae, see 86255 and 86256)

86235 Extractable nuclear antigen, antibody to, any method (eg, nRNP, SS-A, SS-B, Sm, RNP, Sc170, J01), each antibody

(86243 has been deleted)

86255 Fluorescent noninfectious agent antibody; screen, each antibody
➔ *CPT Assistant* Nov 98:27

86256 titer, each antibody

(Fluorescent technique for antigen identification in tissue, use 88346; for indirect fluorescence, see 88346, 88350)

(FTA, use 86780)

(Gel [agar] diffusion tests, use 86331)

86277 Growth hormone, human (HGH), antibody

86280 Hemagglutination inhibition test (HAI)

(For rubella, use 86762)

(For antibodies to infectious agents, see 86602-86804)

86294 Immunoassay for tumor antigen, qualitative or semiquantitative (eg, bladder tumor antigen)
➔ *CPT Changes: An Insider's View* 2001

(For qualitative NMP22 protein, use 86386)

86300 Immunoassay for tumor antigen, quantitative; CA 15-3 (27.29)
➔ *CPT Changes: An Insider's View* 2001
➔ *CPT Assistant* Aug 05:9

86301 CA 19-9
CPT Changes: An Insider's View 2001

86304 CA 125
CPT Changes: An Insider's View 2001

(For measurement of serum HER-2/neu oncoprotein, see 83950)

(For hepatitis delta agent, antibody, use 86692)

86305 Human epididymis protein 4 (HE4)
CPT Changes: An Insider's View 2010

86308 Heterophile antibodies; screening

(For antibodies to infectious agents, see 86602-86804)

86309 titer

(For antibodies to infectious agents, see 86602-86804)

86310 titers after absorption with beef cells and guinea pig kidney

(Histoplasma, antibodies to, use 86698. For skin testing, use 86510)

(For antibodies to infectious agents, see 86602-86804)

(Human growth hormone antibody, use 86277)

86316 Immunoassay for tumor antigen, other antigen, quantitative (eg, CA 50, 72-4, 549), each
CPT Changes: An Insider's View 2001
CPT Assistant May 96:11, Aug 96:11, Apr 98:15, Aug 99:5, Dec 99:10

86317 Immunoassay for infectious agent antibody, quantitative, not otherwise specified
CPT Assistant Nov 97:30-31

(For immunoassay techniques for antigens, see 83516, 83518, 83519, 83520, 87301-87450, 87810-87899)

(For particle agglutination procedures, use 86403)

86318 Immunoassay for infectious agent antibody, qualitative or semiquantitative, single step method (eg, reagent strip)
CPT Assistant Mar 07:10

86320 Immunoelectrophoresis; serum

86325 other fluids (eg, urine, cerebrospinal fluid) with concentration
CPT Changes: An Insider's View 2002

86327 crossed (2-dimensional assay)

86329 Immunodiffusion; not elsewhere specified
CPT Assistant Aug 00:11

86331 gel diffusion, qualitative (Ouchterlony), each antigen or antibody

86332 Immune complex assay

86334 Immunofixation electrophoresis; serum
CPT Changes: An Insider's View 2005

86335 other fluids with concentration (eg, urine, CSF)
CPT Changes: An Insider's View 2005

86336 Inhibin A
CPT Changes: An Insider's View 2002

86337 Insulin antibodies

86340 Intrinsic factor antibodies

(Leptospira, antibodies to, use 86720)

(Leukoagglutinins, use 86021)

86341 Islet cell antibody
CPT Assistant Summer 94:6

86343 Leukocyte histamine release test (LHR)

86344 Leukocyte phagocytosis

86352 Cellular function assay involving stimulation (eg, mitogen or antigen) and detection of biomarker (eg, ATP)
CPT Changes: An Insider's View 2010

86353 Lymphocyte transformation, mitogen (phytomitogen) or antigen induced blastogenesis

(Malaria antibodies, use 86750)

(For cellular function assay involving stimulation and detection of biomarker, use 86352)

86355 B cells, total count
CPT Changes: An Insider's View 2006
CPT Assistant Mar 06:6, Apr 08:5

86356 Mononuclear cell antigen, quantitative (eg, flow cytometry), not otherwise specified, each antigen
CPT Changes: An Insider's View 2008
CPT Assistant Apr 08:5

(Do not report 88187-88189 for interpretation of 86355, 86356, 86357, 86359, 86360, 86361, 86367)

86357 Natural killer (NK) cells, total count
CPT Changes: An Insider's View 2006
CPT Assistant Mar 06:6, Apr 08:5

86359 T cells; total count
CPT Assistant Nov 97:30, Apr 08:5

86360 absolute CD4 and CD8 count, including ratio
CPT Assistant Nov 97:30, Jan 07:29, Apr 08:5

86361 absolute CD4 count
CPT Assistant Nov 97:30, Apr 08:5

86367 Stem cells (ie, CD34), total count
CPT Changes: An Insider's View 2006
CPT Assistant Mar 06:6, Apr 08:5, Oct 13:3

(For flow cytometric immunophenotyping for the assessment of potential hematolymphoid neoplasia, see 88184-88189)

86376 Microsomal antibodies (eg, thyroid or liver-kidney), each

(86378 has been deleted)

86382 Neutralization test, viral

86384 Nitroblue tetrazolium dye test (NTD)

86386 Nuclear Matrix Protein 22 (NMP22), qualitative
CPT Changes: An Insider's View 2012

(Ouchterlony diffusion, use 86331)

(Platelet antibodies, see 86022, 86023)

86403 Particle agglutination; screen, each antibody
CPT Assistant Aug 05:9

86406 titer, each antibody

(Pregnancy test, see 84702, 84703)

(Rapid plasma reagin test (RPR), see 86592, 86593)

86430 Rheumatoid factor; qualitative

86431 quantitative

(Serologic test for syphilis, see 86592, 86593)

86480 Tuberculosis test, cell mediated immunity antigen response measurement; gamma interferon
CPT Changes: An Insider's View 2006, 2011
CPT Assistant Mar 06:6, Oct 10:7, Dec 10:8

86481 enumeration of gamma interferon-producing T-cells in cell suspension
CPT Changes: An Insider's View 2011
CPT Assistant Oct 10:8, Dec 10:8

86485 Skin test; candida

(For antibody, candida, use 86628)

86486 unlisted antigen, each
CPT Changes: An Insider's View 2008

86490 coccidioidomycosis

86510 histoplasmosis
CPT Assistant Aug 05:9

(For histoplasma, antibody, use 86698)

86580 tuberculosis, intradermal

(For tuberculosis test, cell mediated immunity measurement of gamma interferon antigen response, use 86480)

(For skin tests for allergy, see 95012-95199)

(Smooth muscle antibody, see 86255, 86256)

(Sporothrix, antibodies to, see code for specific method)

86590 Streptokinase, antibody

(For antibodies to infectious agents, see 86602-86804)

(Streptolysin O antibody, see antistreptolysin O, 86060, 86063)

86592 Syphilis test, non-treponemal antibody; qualitative (eg, VDRL, RPR, ART)
CPT Changes: An Insider's View 2010

(For antibodies to infectious agents, see 86602-86804)

86593 quantitative
CPT Changes: An Insider's View 2010

(For antibodies to infectious agents, see 86602-86804)

(Tetanus antibody, use 86774)

(Thyroglobulin antibody, use 86800)

(Thyroglobulin, use 84432)

(Thyroid microsomal antibody, use 86376)

(For toxoplasma antibody, see 86777-86778)

The following codes (86602-86804) are qualitative or semiquantitative immunoassays performed by multiple-step methods for the detection of antibodies to infectious agents. For immunoassays by single-step method (eg, reagent strips), use code 86318. Procedures for the identification of antibodies should be coded as precisely as possible. For example, an antibody to a virus could be coded with increasing specificity for virus, family, genus, species, or type. In some cases, further precision may be added to codes by specifying the class of immunoglobulin being detected. When multiple tests are done to detect antibodies to organisms classified more precisely than the specificity allowed by available codes, it is appropriate to code each as a separate service. For example, a test for antibody to an enterovirus is coded as 86658. Coxsackie viruses are enteroviruses, but there are no codes for the individual species of enterovirus. If assays are performed for antibodies to coxsackie A and B species, each assay should be separately coded. Similarly, if multiple assays are performed for antibodies of different immunoglobulin classes, each assay should be coded separately. When a coding option exists for reporting IgM specific antibodies (eg, 86632), the corresponding nonspecific code (eg, 86631) may be reported for performance of either an antibody analysis not specific for a particular immunoglobulin class or for an IgG analysis.

(For the detection of antibodies other than those to infectious agents, see specific antibody [eg, 86021-86023, 86376, 86800, 86850-86870] or specific method [eg, 83516, 86255, 86256]).

(For infectious agent/antigen detection, see 87260-87899)

86602 Antibody; actinomyces
CPT Assistant Aug 05:9

86603 adenovirus

86606 Aspergillus

86609 bacterium, not elsewhere specified

86611 Bartonella
CPT Changes: An Insider's View 2001

86612 Blastomyces

86615 Bordetella

86617 Borrelia burgdorferi (Lyme disease) confirmatory test (eg, Western Blot or immunoblot)

86618 Borrelia burgdorferi (Lyme disease)

86619 Borrelia (relapsing fever)

86622 Brucella

86625 Campylobacter

86628 Candida

(For skin test, candida, use 86485)

86631 Chlamydia

86632 Chlamydia, IgM
➔ *CPT Assistant* Nov 97:31

(For chlamydia antigen, see 87270, 87320. For fluorescent antibody technique, see 86255, 86256)

86635 Coccidioides

86638 Coxiella burnetii (Q fever)

86641 Cryptococcus

86644 cytomegalovirus (CMV)

86645 cytomegalovirus (CMV), IgM
➔ *CPT Assistant* Jul 03:7

86648 Diphtheria

86651 encephalitis, California (La Crosse)

86652 encephalitis, Eastern equine

86653 encephalitis, St. Louis

86654 encephalitis, Western equine

86658 enterovirus (eg, coxsackie, echo, polio)

(Trichinella, antibodies to, use 86784)

(Trypanosoma, antibodies to, see code for specific method)

(Tuberculosis, use 86580 for skin testing)

(Viral antibodies, see code for specific method)

86663 Epstein-Barr (EB) virus, early antigen (EA)

86664 Epstein-Barr (EB) virus, nuclear antigen (EBNA)

86665 Epstein-Barr (EB) virus, viral capsid (VCA)

86666 Ehrlichia
➔ *CPT Changes: An Insider's View* 2001

86668 Francisella tularensis

86671 fungus, not elsewhere specified

86674 Giardia lamblia

86677 Helicobacter pylori
➔ *CPT Assistant* Jan 98:6

86682 helminth, not elsewhere specified

86684 Haemophilus influenza

86687 HTLV-I

86688 HTLV-II

86689 HTLV or HIV antibody, confirmatory test (eg, Western Blot)
➔ *CPT Assistant* Mar 08:3

86692 hepatitis, delta agent
➔ *CPT Assistant* Nov 97:31

(For hepatitis delta agent, antigen, use 87380)

86694 herpes simplex, non-specific type test

86695 herpes simplex, type 1

86696 herpes simplex, type 2
➔ *CPT Changes: An Insider's View* 2001

86698 histoplasma

86701 HIV-1
➔ *CPT Assistant* Aug 05:9, Mar 08:3, Apr 08:5

86702 HIV-2
➔ *CPT Assistant* Mar 08:3, Apr 08:5

86703 HIV-1 and HIV-2, single result
➔ *CPT Changes: An Insider's View* 2012
➔ *CPT Assistant* Nov 97:31, Mar 08:3, Apr 08:5

(For HIV-1 antigen(s) with HIV-1 and HIV-2 antibodies, single result, use 87389)

(When HIV immunoassay [HIV testing 86701-86703 or 87389] is performed using a kit or transportable instrument that wholly or in part consists of a single use, disposable analytical chamber, the service may be identified by adding modifier 92 to the usual code)

(For HIV-1 antigen, use 87390)

(For HIV-2 antigen, use 87391)

(For confirmatory test for HIV antibody (eg, Western Blot), use 86689)

86704 Hepatitis B core antibody (HBcAb); total
➔ *CPT Changes: An Insider's View* 2001
➔ *CPT Assistant* Nov 97:31-32

86705 IgM antibody
➔ *CPT Assistant* Nov 97:31-32

86706 Hepatitis B surface antibody (HBsAb)
➔ *CPT Assistant* Nov 97:31-32

86707 Hepatitis Be antibody (HBeAb)
➔ *CPT Assistant* Nov 97:31-32

86708 Hepatitis A antibody (HAAb)
➔ *CPT Changes: An Insider's View* 2001, 2016
➔ *CPT Assistant* Nov 97:31-32, Jun 00:11

86709 Hepatitis A antibody (HAAb), IgM antibody
➔ *CPT Changes: An Insider's View* 2016
➔ *CPT Assistant* Nov 97:31-32, Jun 00:11

86710 Antibody; influenza virus

86711 JC (John Cunningham) virus
➔ *CPT Changes: An Insider's View* 2013

86713 Legionella

86717 Leishmania

86720 Leptospira

86723 Listeria monocytogenes

86727 lymphocytic choriomeningitis

(86729 has been deleted)

86732 mucormycosis

86735 mumps

86738 mycoplasma

86741 Neisseria meningitidis

86744 Nocardia

86747 parvovirus

86750 Plasmodium (malaria)

86753 protozoa, not elsewhere specified

86756 respiratory syncytial virus

86757 Rickettsia

➔ *CPT Changes: An Insider's View* 2001

86759 rotavirus

86762 rubella

86765 rubeola

86768 Salmonella

86771 Shigella

86774 tetanus

86777 Toxoplasma

86778 Toxoplasma, IgM

86780 Treponema pallidum

➔ *CPT Changes: An Insider's View* 2010

(For syphilis testing by non-treponemal antibody analysis, see 86592-86593)

86784 Trichinella

86787 varicella-zoster

86788 West Nile virus, IgM

➔ *CPT Changes: An Insider's View* 2007

86789 West Nile virus

➔ *CPT Changes: An Insider's View* 2007

86790 virus, not elsewhere specified

86793 Yersinia

86794 Zika virus, IgM

➔ *CPT Changes: An Insider's View* 2018

86800 Thyroglobulin antibody

➔ *CPT Assistant* Aug 05:9

(For thyroglobulin, use 84432)

86803 Hepatitis C antibody;

➔ *CPT Assistant* Nov 97:31-32

86804 confirmatory test (eg, immunoblot)

➔ *CPT Assistant* Nov 97:31-32

Tissue Typing

86805 Lymphocytotoxicity assay, visual crossmatch; with titration

86806 without titration

86807 Serum screening for cytotoxic percent reactive antibody (PRA); standard method

➔ *CPT Assistant* Jun 01:11

86808 quick method

➔ *CPT Assistant* Jun 01:11

86812 HLA typing; A, B, or C (eg, A10, B7, B27), single antigen

➔ *CPT Assistant* Mar 03:23, Jun 06:17

86813 A, B, or C, multiple antigens

➔ *CPT Assistant* Mar 03:23, Jun 06:17

86816 DR/DQ, single antigen

➔ *CPT Assistant* Mar 03:23

86817 DR/DQ, multiple antigens

➔ *CPT Assistant* Mar 03:23

86821 lymphocyte culture, mixed (MLC)

➔ *CPT Assistant* Mar 03:23

(86822 has been deleted)

86825 Human leukocyte antigen (HLA) crossmatch, non-cytotoxic (eg, using flow cytometry); first serum sample or dilution

➔ *CPT Changes: An Insider's View* 2010

+ 86826 each additional serum sample or sample dilution (List separately in addition to primary procedure)

➔ *CPT Changes: An Insider's View* 2010

(Use 86826 in conjunction with 86825)

(Do not report 86825, 86826 in conjunction with 86355, 86359, 88184-88189 for antibody surface markers integral to crossmatch testing)

(For autologous HLA crossmatch, see 86825, 86826)

(For lymphocytotoxicity visual crossmatch, see 86805, 86806)

86828 Antibody to human leukocyte antigens (HLA), solid phase assays (eg, microspheres or beads, ELISA, flow cytometry); qualitative assessment of the presence or absence of antibody(ies) to HLA Class I and Class II HLA antigens

➔ *CPT Changes: An Insider's View* 2013

86829 qualitative assessment of the presence or absence of antibody(ies) to HLA Class I or Class II HLA antigens

➔ *CPT Changes: An Insider's View* 2013

(If solid phase testing is performed to assess presence or absence of antibody to both HLA classes, use 86828)

86830 antibody identification by qualitative panel using complete HLA phenotypes, HLA Class I

➔ *CPT Changes: An Insider's View* 2013

86831 antibody identification by qualitative panel using complete HLA phenotypes, HLA Class II
➔ *CPT Changes: An Insider's View* 2013

86832 high definition qualitative panel for identification of antibody specificities (eg, individual antigen per bead methodology), HLA Class I
➔ *CPT Changes: An Insider's View* 2013

86833 high definition qualitative panel for identification of antibody specificities (eg, individual antigen per bead methodology), HLA Class II
➔ *CPT Changes: An Insider's View* 2013

(If solid phase testing is performed to test for HLA Class I or II antibody after treatment [eg, to remove IgM antibodies or other interfering substances], report 86828-86833 once for each panel with the untreated serum and once for each panel with the treated serum)

86834 semi-quantitative panel (eg, titer), HLA Class I
➔ *CPT Changes: An Insider's View* 2013

86835 semi-quantitative panel (eg, titer), HLA Class II
➔ *CPT Changes: An Insider's View* 2013

86849 Unlisted immunology procedure
➔ *CPT Assistant* Mar 98:10

Transfusion Medicine

(For apheresis, use 36511, 36512)

(For therapeutic phlebotomy, use 99195)

86850 Antibody screen, RBC, each serum technique
➔ *CPT Assistant* Fall 93:25, Aug 05:9, Apr 08:5

86860 Antibody elution (RBC), each elution

86870 Antibody identification, RBC antibodies, each panel for each serum technique
➔ *CPT Assistant* Fall 93:25, Mar 01:10

86880 Antihuman globulin test (Coombs test); direct, each antiserum

86885 indirect, qualitative, each reagent red cell
➔ *CPT Changes: An Insider's View* 2008
➔ *CPT Assistant* Apr 08:5

86886 indirect, each antibody titer
➔ *CPT Changes: An Insider's View* 2008
➔ *CPT Assistant* Apr 08:5

(For indirect antihuman globulin [Coombs] test for RBC antibody screening, use 86850)

(For indirect antihuman globulin [Coombs] test for RBC antibody identification using reagent red cell panels, use 86870)

86890 Autologous blood or component, collection processing and storage; predeposited
➔ *CPT Assistant* Apr 96:2

86891 intra- or postoperative salvage

86900 Blood typing, serologic; ABO
➔ *CPT Changes: An Insider's View* 2015
➔ *CPT Assistant* Aug 05:9

86901 Rh (D)
➔ *CPT Changes: An Insider's View* 2015
➔ *CPT Assistant* Fall 93:25

86902 antigen testing of donor blood using reagent serum, each antigen test
➔ *CPT Changes: An Insider's View* 2011, 2015
➔ *CPT Assistant* Oct 10:8, Dec 10:8

(If multiple blood units are tested for the same antigen, 86902 should be reported once for each antigen for each unit tested)

86904 antigen screening for compatible unit using patient serum, per unit screened
➔ *CPT Changes: An Insider's View* 2015

86905 RBC antigens, other than ABO or Rh (D), each
➔ *CPT Changes: An Insider's View* 2015

86906 Rh phenotyping, complete
➔ *CPT Changes: An Insider's View* 2015

(For human erythrocyte antigen typing by molecular pathology techniques, use 81403)

86910 Blood typing, for paternity testing, per individual; ABO, Rh and MN

86911 each additional antigen system

86920 Compatibility test each unit; immediate spin technique
➔ *CPT Assistant* Mar 06:6

86921 incubation technique
➔ *CPT Assistant* Mar 06:6

86922 antiglobulin technique
➔ *CPT Assistant* Mar 06:6

86923 electronic
➔ *CPT Changes: An Insider's View* 2006
➔ *CPT Assistant* Mar 06:6

(Do not use 86923 in conjunction with 86920-86922 for same unit crossmatch)

86927 Fresh frozen plasma, thawing, each unit

86930 Frozen blood, each unit; freezing (includes preparation)
➔ *CPT Changes: An Insider's View* 2003
➔ *CPT Assistant* Apr 96:2, Jul 03:8

86931 thawing
➔ *CPT Changes: An Insider's View* 2003
➔ *CPT Assistant* Jul 03:8

86932 freezing (includes preparation) and thawing
➔ *CPT Changes: An Insider's View* 2003
➔ *CPT Assistant* Jul 03:8

86940 Hemolysins and agglutinins; auto, screen, each

86941 incubated

86945 Irradiation of blood product, each unit
➲ *CPT Assistant* Dec 07:14

86950 Leukocyte transfusion
➲ *CPT Assistant* Oct 13:3

(For allogeneic lymphocyte infusion, use 38242)

(For leukapheresis, use 36511)

86960 Volume reduction of blood or blood product (eg, red blood cells or platelets), each unit
➲ *CPT Changes: An Insider's View* 2006
➲ *CPT Assistant* Mar 06:6

86965 Pooling of platelets or other blood products
➲ *CPT Assistant* Oct 10:8, Dec 10:8

(For harvesting, preparation, and injection[s] of platelet rich plasma, use 0232T)

For harvesting, preparation, and injection[s] of autologous white blood cell/autologous protein solution, use 0481T

86970 Pretreatment of RBCs for use in RBC antibody detection, identification, and/or compatibility testing; incubation with chemical agents or drugs, each

86971 incubation with enzymes, each

86972 by density gradient separation

86975 Pretreatment of serum for use in RBC antibody identification; incubation with drugs, each

86976 by dilution

86977 incubation with inhibitors, each

86978 by differential red cell absorption using patient RBCs or RBCs of known phenotype, each absorption

86985 Splitting of blood or blood products, each unit
➲ *CPT Assistant* Apr 96:2, May 12:11

86999 Unlisted transfusion medicine procedure
➲ *CPT Assistant* Aug 05:9, Nov 05:14, Mar 09:10, Apr 09:9, May 12:11

Microbiology

Includes bacteriology, mycology, parasitology, and virology.

Presumptive identification of microorganisms is defined as identification by colony morphology, growth on selective media, Gram stains, or up to three tests (eg, catalase, oxidase, indole, urease). Definitive identification of microorganisms is defined as an identification to the genus or species level that requires additional tests (eg, biochemical panels, slide cultures). If additional studies involve molecular probes, nucleic acid sequencing, chromatography, or immunologic techniques, these should be separately coded using 87140-87158, in addition to definitive identification codes. The molecular diagnostic codes (eg, 81161, 81200-81408) are not to be used in combination with or instead of the procedures represented by 87140-87158. For multiple specimens/sites use modifier 59. For repeat laboratory tests performed on the same day, use modifier 91.

87003 Animal inoculation, small animal, with observation and dissection

87015 Concentration (any type), for infectious agents
➲ *CPT Changes: An Insider's View* 2001

(Do not report 87015 in conjunction with 87177)

87040 Culture, bacterial; blood, aerobic, with isolation and presumptive identification of isolates (includes anaerobic culture, if appropriate)
➲ *CPT Changes: An Insider's View* 2001, 2004
➲ *CPT Assistant* Aug 97:18, Jun 02:2, Oct 10:17, Dec 10:17

87045 stool, aerobic, with isolation and preliminary examination (eg, KIA, LIA), Salmonella and Shigella species
➲ *CPT Changes: An Insider's View* 2001, 2002, 2004

87046 stool, aerobic, additional pathogens, isolation and presumptive identification of isolates, each plate
➲ *CPT Changes: An Insider's View* 2001, 2002, 2004, 2005

87070 any other source except urine, blood or stool, aerobic, with isolation and presumptive identification of isolates
➲ *CPT Changes: An Insider's View* 2001, 2004
➲ *CPT Assistant* Aug 97:18, Nov 01:10, Oct 03:10, Nov 11:11

(For urine, use 87088)

87071 quantitative, aerobic with isolation and presumptive identification of isolates, any source except urine, blood or stool
➲ *CPT Changes: An Insider's View* 2001
➲ *CPT Assistant* Jun 02:3, Sep 03:3

(For urine, use 87088)

87073 quantitative, anaerobic with isolation and presumptive identification of isolates, any source except urine, blood or stool
➲ *CPT Changes: An Insider's View* 2001
➲ *CPT Assistant* Jun 02:3

(For definitive identification of isolates, use 87076 or 87077. For typing of isolates see 87140-87158)

87075 any source, except blood, anaerobic with isolation and presumptive identification of isolates
➲ *CPT Changes: An Insider's View* 2001, 2004

87076 anaerobic isolate, additional methods required for definitive identification, each isolate
➲ *CPT Changes: An Insider's View* 2001

87077 aerobic isolate, additional methods required for definitive identification, each isolate
➲ *CPT Changes: An Insider's View* 2001
➲ *CPT Assistant* Nov 01:10, Nov 11:10

87081 Culture, presumptive, pathogenic organisms, screening only;
➲ *CPT Changes: An Insider's View* 2001
➲ *CPT Assistant* Nov 01:10

87084 with colony estimation from density chart

87086 Culture, bacterial; quantitative colony count, urine
- *CPT Changes: An Insider's View* 2001
- *CPT Assistant* Nov 11:10

87088 with isolation and presumptive identification of each isolate, urine
- *CPT Changes: An Insider's View* 2001, 2007
- *CPT Assistant* Nov 11:10

87101 Culture, fungi (mold or yeast) isolation, with presumptive identification of isolates; skin, hair, or nail
- *CPT Changes: An Insider's View* 2001
- *CPT Assistant* Sep 99:10, Aug 05:9

87102 other source (except blood)

87103 blood

87106 Culture, fungi, definitive identification, each organism; yeast
- *CPT Changes: An Insider's View* 2001

87107 mold
- *CPT Changes: An Insider's View* 2001

87109 Culture, mycoplasma, any source

87110 Culture, chlamydia, any source
- *CPT Changes: An Insider's View* 2001

(For immunofluorescence staining of shell vials, use 87140)

87116 Culture, tubercle or other acid-fast bacilli (eg, TB, AFB, mycobacteria) any source, with isolation and presumptive identification of isolates
- *CPT Changes: An Insider's View* 2001

(For concentration, use 87015)

87118 Culture, mycobacterial, definitive identification, each isolate
- *CPT Changes: An Insider's View* 2001

87140 Culture, typing; immunofluorescent method, each antiserum
- *CPT Changes: An Insider's View* 2001
- *CPT Assistant* Nov 01:10, Sep 03:3

87143 gas liquid chromatography (GLC) or high pressure liquid chromatography (HPLC) method
- *CPT Changes: An Insider's View* 2001

87147 immunologic method, other than immunofluorescence (eg, agglutination grouping), per antiserum
- *CPT Changes: An Insider's View* 2001
- *CPT Assistant* Apr 02:18, Oct 03:10

87149 identification by nucleic acid (DNA or RNA) probe, direct probe technique, per culture or isolate, each organism probed
- *CPT Changes: An Insider's View* 2001, 2010
- *CPT Assistant* Nov 01:10, May 12:5, Sep 13:3

(Do not report 87149 in conjunction with 81161, 81200-81408)

87150 identification by nucleic acid (DNA or RNA) probe, amplified probe technique, per culture or isolate, each organism probed
- *CPT Changes: An Insider's View* 2010
- *CPT Assistant* May 12:5, Sep 13:3

(Do not report 87150 in conjunction with 81161, 81200-81408)

87152 identification by pulse field gel typing
- *CPT Changes: An Insider's View* 2001
- *CPT Assistant* May 12:5, Sep 13:3

(Do not report 87152 in conjunction with 81161, 81200-81408)

87153 identification by nucleic acid sequencing method, each isolate (eg, sequencing of the 16S rRNA gene)
- *CPT Changes: An Insider's View* 2010
- *CPT Assistant* May 12:5, Sep 13:3

87158 other methods
- *CPT Assistant* Nov 01:10, Sep 03:3

87164 Dark field examination, any source (eg, penile, vaginal, oral, skin); includes specimen collection

87166 without collection

87168 Macroscopic examination; arthropod
- *CPT Changes: An Insider's View* 2001

87169 parasite
- *CPT Changes: An Insider's View* 2001

87172 Pinworm exam (eg, cellophane tape prep)
- *CPT Changes: An Insider's View* 2001

87176 Homogenization, tissue, for culture
- *CPT Changes: An Insider's View* 2001

87177 Ova and parasites, direct smears, concentration and identification
- *CPT Assistant* Jul 03:8, Nov 03:15, Mar 06:6

(Do not report 87177 in conjunction with 87015)

(For direct smears from a primary source, use 87207)

(For coccidia or microsporidia exam, use 87207)

(For complex special stain (trichrome, iron hematoxylin), use 87209)

(For nucleic acid probes in cytologic material, use 88365)

87181 Susceptibility studies, antimicrobial agent; agar dilution method, per agent (eg, antibiotic gradient strip)
- *CPT Changes: An Insider's View* 2001
- *CPT Assistant* Nov 01:10

87184 disk method, per plate (12 or fewer agents)
- *CPT Changes: An Insider's View* 2001
- *CPT Assistant* Nov 01:10

87185 enzyme detection (eg, beta lactamase), per enzyme
- *CPT Changes: An Insider's View* 2001
- *CPT Assistant* Nov 01:10

87186 microdilution or agar dilution (minimum inhibitory concentration [MIC] or breakpoint), each multi-antimicrobial, per plate
➔ *CPT Changes: An Insider's View* 2001
➔ *CPT Assistant* Nov 01:10

+ 87187 microdilution or agar dilution, minimum lethal concentration (MLC), each plate (List separately in addition to code for primary procedure)
➔ *CPT Changes: An Insider's View* 2001
➔ *CPT Assistant* Nov 01:10

(Use 87187 in conjunction with 87186 or 87188)

87188 macrobroth dilution method, each agent
➔ *CPT Changes: An Insider's View* 2001
➔ *CPT Assistant* Nov 01:10

87190 mycobacteria, proportion method, each agent
➔ *CPT Changes: An Insider's View* 2001

(For other mycobacterial susceptibility studies, see 87181, 87184, 87186, or 87188)

87197 Serum bactericidal titer (Schlichter test)

87205 Smear, primary source with interpretation; Gram or Giemsa stain for bacteria, fungi, or cell types
➔ *CPT Changes: An Insider's View* 2001
➔ *CPT Assistant* Aug 05:9, Oct 09:12

87206 fluorescent and/or acid fast stain for bacteria, fungi, parasites, viruses or cell types
➔ *CPT Changes: An Insider's View* 2001

87207 special stain for inclusion bodies or parasites (eg, malaria, coccidia, microsporidia, trypanosomes, herpes viruses)
➔ *CPT Changes: An Insider's View* 2001, 2003
➔ *CPT Assistant* Jul 03:8, Mar 06:6

(For direct smears with concentration and identification, use 87177)

(For thick smear preparation, use 87015)

(For fat, meat, fibers, nasal eosinophils, and starch, see miscellaneous section)

87209 complex special stain (eg, trichrome, iron hemotoxylin) for ova and parasites
➔ *CPT Changes: An Insider's View* 2006
➔ *CPT Assistant* Mar 06:6

87210 wet mount for infectious agents (eg, saline, India ink, KOH preps)
➔ *CPT Changes: An Insider's View* 2001
➔ *CPT Assistant* May 16:14

(For KOH examination of skin, hair or nails, see 87220)

87220 Tissue examination by KOH slide of samples from skin, hair, or nails for fungi or ectoparasite ova or mites (eg, scabies)
➔ *CPT Changes: An Insider's View* 2001

87230 Toxin or antitoxin assay, tissue culture (eg, Clostridium difficile toxin)

87250 Virus isolation; inoculation of embryonated eggs, or small animal, includes observation and dissection
➔ *CPT Changes: An Insider's View* 2001

87252 tissue culture inoculation, observation, and presumptive identification by cytopathic effect
➔ *CPT Changes: An Insider's View* 2001

87253 tissue culture, additional studies or definitive identification (eg, hemabsorption, neutralization, immunofluorescence stain), each isolate
➔ *CPT Changes: An Insider's View* 2001

(Electron microscopy, use 88348)

(Inclusion bodies in tissue sections, see 88304-88309; in smears, see 87207-87210; in fluids, use 88106)

87254 centrifuge enhanced (shell vial) technique, includes identification with immunofluorescence stain, each virus
➔ *CPT Changes: An Insider's View* 2001, 2003
➔ *CPT Assistant* Jul 03:8

(Report 87254 in addition to 87252 as appropriate)

87255 including identification by non-immunologic method, other than by cytopathic effect (eg, virus specific enzymatic activity)
➔ *CPT Changes: An Insider's View* 2003
➔ *CPT Assistant* Jul 03:9

These codes are intended for primary source only. For similar studies on culture material, refer to codes 87140-87158. Infectious agents by antigen detection, immunofluorescence microscopy, or nucleic acid probe techniques should be reported as precisely as possible. The molecular pathology procedures codes (81161, 81200-81408) are not to be used in combination with or instead of the procedures represented by 87471-87801. The most specific code possible should be reported. If there is no specific agent code, the general methodology code (eg, 87299, 87449, 87450, 87797, 87798, 87799, 87899) should be used. For identification of antibodies to many of the listed infectious agents, see 86602-86804. When separate results are reported for different species or strain of organisms, each result should be coded separately. Use modifier 59 when separate results are reported for different species or strains that are described by the same code.

87260 Infectious agent antigen detection by immunofluorescent technique; adenovirus
➔ *CPT Changes: An Insider's View* 2001
➔ *CPT Assistant* Nov 97:32

87265 Bordetella pertussis/parapertussis
➔ *CPT Assistant* Nov 97:32

87267 Enterovirus, direct fluorescent antibody (DFA)
➔ *CPT Assistant* Jul 03:8

87269 giardia
➔ *CPT Changes: An Insider's View* 2004

Pathology and Laboratory 80047-89398, 0001U-0061U

87270 Chlamydia trachomatis
➲ *CPT Assistant* Nov 97:32

87271 Cytomegalovirus, direct fluorescent antibody (DFA)
➲ *CPT Assistant* Jul 03:7

87272 cryptosporidium
➲ *CPT Changes: An Insider's View* 2004
➲ *CPT Assistant* Nov 97:32

87273 Herpes simplex virus type 2
➲ *CPT Changes: An Insider's View* 2001

87274 Herpes simplex virus type 1
➲ *CPT Changes: An Insider's View* 2001
➲ *CPT Assistant* Nov 97:32

87275 influenza B virus
➲ *CPT Changes: An Insider's View* 2001

87276 influenza A virus
➲ *CPT Assistant* Nov 97:32, May 09:6

(87277 has been deleted)

87278 Legionella pneumophila
➲ *CPT Assistant* Nov 97:32

87279 Parainfluenza virus, each type
➲ *CPT Changes: An Insider's View* 2001

87280 respiratory syncytial virus
➲ *CPT Assistant* Nov 97:32

87281 Pneumocystis carinii
➲ *CPT Changes: An Insider's View* 2001

87283 Rubeola
➲ *CPT Changes: An Insider's View* 2001

87285 Treponema pallidum
➲ *CPT Assistant* Nov 97:32

87290 Varicella zoster virus
➲ *CPT Assistant* Nov 97:32

87299 not otherwise specified, each organism
➲ *CPT Changes: An Insider's View* 2001
➲ *CPT Assistant* Nov 97:32, Nov 01:10

87300 Infectious agent antigen detection by immunofluorescent technique, polyvalent for multiple organisms, each polyvalent antiserum
➲ *CPT Changes: An Insider's View* 2001
➲ *CPT Assistant* Aug 05:9

(For physician evaluation of infectious disease agents by immunofluorescence, use 88346)

87301 Infectious agent antigen detection by immunoassay technique, (eg, enzyme immunoassay [EIA], enzyme-linked immunosorbent assay [ELISA], immunochemiluminometric assay [IMCA]) qualitative or semiquantitative, multiple-step method; adenovirus enteric types 40/41
➲ *CPT Changes: An Insider's View* 2016
➲ *CPT Assistant* Nov 97:32, Nov 99:46

87305 Aspergillus
➲ *CPT Changes: An Insider's View* 2007, 2016

87320 Chlamydia trachomatis
➲ *CPT Changes: An Insider's View* 2016
➲ *CPT Assistant* Nov 97:32

87324 Clostridium difficile toxin(s)
➲ *CPT Changes: An Insider's View* 2001, 2016
➲ *CPT Assistant* Nov 97:32

87327 Cryptococcus neoformans
➲ *CPT Changes: An Insider's View* 2001, 2016

(For Cryptococcus latex agglutination, use 86403)

87328 cryptosporidium
➲ *CPT Changes: An Insider's View* 2004, 2016
➲ *CPT Assistant* Nov 97:32

87329 giardia
➲ *CPT Changes: An Insider's View* 2004, 2016

87332 cytomegalovirus
➲ *CPT Changes: An Insider's View* 2016
➲ *CPT Assistant* Nov 97:32

87335 Escherichia coli 0157
➲ *CPT Changes: An Insider's View* 2016
➲ *CPT Assistant* Nov 97:32

(For giardia antigen, use 87329)

87336 Entamoeba histolytica dispar group
➲ *CPT Changes: An Insider's View* 2001, 2016

87337 Entamoeba histolytica group
➲ *CPT Changes: An Insider's View* 2001, 2016

87338 Helicobacter pylori, stool
➲ *CPT Changes: An Insider's View* 2000, 2016
➲ *CPT Assistant* Nov 99:46

87339 Helicobacter pylori
➲ *CPT Changes: An Insider's View* 2001, 2016

(For H. pylori, stool, use 87338. For H. pylori, breath and blood by mass spectrometry, see 83013, 83014. For H. pylori, liquid scintillation counter, see 78267, 78268)

87340 hepatitis B surface antigen (HBsAg)
➲ *CPT Changes: An Insider's View* 2016
➲ *CPT Assistant* Nov 97:32, Jan 00:11

87341 hepatitis B surface antigen (HBsAg) neutralization
➲ *CPT Changes: An Insider's View* 2001, 2016

87350 hepatitis Be antigen (HBeAg)
➲ *CPT Changes: An Insider's View* 2016
➲ *CPT Assistant* Nov 97:32

87380 hepatitis, delta agent
➲ *CPT Changes: An Insider's View* 2016
➲ *CPT Assistant* Nov 97:32

87385 Histoplasma capsulatum
➲ *CPT Changes: An Insider's View* 2016
➲ *CPT Assistant* Nov 97:32

87389 HIV-1 antigen(s), with HIV-1 and HIV-2 antibodies, single result
➔ *CPT Changes: An Insider's View* 2012, 2016

87390 HIV-1
➔ *CPT Changes: An Insider's View* 2016
➔ *CPT Assistant* Nov 97:32

87391 HIV-2
➔ *CPT Changes: An Insider's View* 2016
➔ *CPT Assistant* Nov 97:32

87400 Influenza, A or B, each
➔ *CPT Changes: An Insider's View* 2001, 2016
➔ *CPT Assistant* Jun 01:11, Dec 01:6, Aug 05:9, May 09:6

87420 respiratory syncytial virus
➔ *CPT Changes: An Insider's View* 2016
➔ *CPT Assistant* Nov 97:32

87425 rotavirus
➔ *CPT Changes: An Insider's View* 2016
➔ *CPT Assistant* Nov 97:32

87427 Shiga-like toxin
➔ *CPT Changes: An Insider's View* 2001, 2016

87430 Streptococcus, group A
➔ *CPT Changes: An Insider's View* 2016
➔ *CPT Assistant* Nov 97:32

87449 Infectious agent antigen detection by immunoassay technique, (eg, enzyme immunoassay [EIA], enzyme-linked immunosorbent assay [ELISA], immunochemiluminometric assay [IMCA]), qualitative or semiquantitative; multiple-step method, not otherwise specified, each organism
➔ *CPT Changes: An Insider's View* 2001, 2016
➔ *CPT Assistant* Nov 97:32, Jan 00:11, Nov 01:10

87450 single step method, not otherwise specified, each organism
➔ *CPT Changes: An Insider's View* 2001, 2016
➔ *CPT Assistant* Nov 97:33

87451 multiple step method, polyvalent for multiple organisms, each polyvalent antiserum
➔ *CPT Changes: An Insider's View* 2001, 2016

(87470 has been deleted)

87471 Infectious agent detection by nucleic acid (DNA or RNA); Bartonella henselae and Bartonella quintana, amplified probe technique
➔ *CPT Assistant* May 12:5, Sep 13:3

87472 Bartonella henselae and Bartonella quintana, quantification
➔ *CPT Assistant* Sep 13:3

87475 Borrelia burgdorferi, direct probe technique
➔ *CPT Assistant* May 12:5, Sep 13:3

87476 Borrelia burgdorferi, amplified probe technique
➔ *CPT Assistant* Sep 13:3

(87477 has been deleted)

87480 Candida species, direct probe technique
➔ *CPT Assistant* May 12:5, Sep 13:3

87481 Candida species, amplified probe technique
➔ *CPT Assistant* Sep 13:3

87482 Candida species, quantification
➔ *CPT Assistant* Sep 13:3

87483 central nervous system pathogen (eg, Neisseria meningitidis, Streptococcus pneumoniae, Listeria, Haemophilus influenzae, E. coli, Streptococcus agalactiae, enterovirus, human parechovirus, herpes simplex virus type 1 and 2, human herpesvirus 6, cytomegalovirus, varicella zoster virus, Cryptococcus), includes multiplex reverse transcription, when performed, and multiplex amplified probe technique, multiple types or subtypes, 12-25 targets
➔ *CPT Changes: An Insider's View* 2017

87485 Chlamydia pneumoniae, direct probe technique
➔ *CPT Assistant* May 12:5, Sep 13:3

87486 Chlamydia pneumoniae, amplified probe technique
➔ *CPT Assistant* Sep 13:3

87487 Chlamydia pneumoniae, quantification
➔ *CPT Assistant* Sep 13:3

87490 Chlamydia trachomatis, direct probe technique
➔ *CPT Assistant* Sep 13:3

87491 Chlamydia trachomatis, amplified probe technique
➔ *CPT Assistant* Jun 13:14, Sep 13:3

87492 Chlamydia trachomatis, quantification
➔ *CPT Assistant* Sep 13:3

87493 Clostridium difficile, toxin gene(s), amplified probe technique
➔ *CPT Changes: An Insider's View* 2010
➔ *CPT Assistant* Sep 10:8, May 12:5, Sep 13:3

87495 cytomegalovirus, direct probe technique
➔ *CPT Assistant* May 12:5, Sep 13:3

87496 cytomegalovirus, amplified probe technique
➔ *CPT Assistant* Sep 13:3

87497 cytomegalovirus, quantification
➔ *CPT Assistant* Sep 13:3

87498 enterovirus, amplified probe technique, includes reverse transcription when performed
➔ *CPT Changes: An Insider's View* 2007, 2013, 2014
➔ *CPT Assistant* May 12:5, Sep 13:3

87500 vancomycin resistance (eg, enterococcus species van A, van B), amplified probe technique
➔ *CPT Changes: An Insider's View* 2008
➔ *CPT Assistant* Apr 08:5, May 12:5, Sep 13:3

87501 influenza virus, includes reverse transcription, when performed, and amplified probe technique, each type or subtype
➔ *CPT Changes: An Insider's View* 2011, 2015
➔ *CPT Assistant* Oct 10:8, Dec 10:8, May 12:5, Sep 13:3

87502 influenza virus, for multiple types or sub-types, includes multiplex reverse transcription, when performed, and multiplex amplified probe technique, first 2 types or sub-types
- *CPT Changes: An Insider's View* 2011, 2012, 2015, 2016
- *CPT Assistant* Oct 10:8, Dec 10:8, Sep 13:3

+ 87503 influenza virus, for multiple types or sub-types, includes multiplex reverse transcription, when performed, and multiplex amplified probe technique, each additional influenza virus type or sub-type beyond 2 (List separately in addition to code for primary procedure)
- *CPT Changes: An Insider's View* 2011, 2015, 2016
- *CPT Assistant* Oct 10:8, Dec 10:8, Sep 13:3

(Use 87503 in conjunction with 87502)

87505 gastrointestinal pathogen (eg, Clostridium difficile, E. coli, Salmonella, Shigella, norovirus, Giardia), includes multiplex reverse transcription, when performed, and multiplex amplified probe technique, multiple types or subtypes, 3-5 targets
- *CPT Changes: An Insider's View* 2015

87506 gastrointestinal pathogen (eg, Clostridium difficile, E. coli, Salmonella, Shigella, norovirus, Giardia), includes multiplex reverse transcription, when performed, and multiplex amplified probe technique, multiple types or subtypes, 6-11 targets
- *CPT Changes: An Insider's View* 2015

87507 gastrointestinal pathogen (eg, Clostridium difficile, E. coli, Salmonella, Shigella, norovirus, Giardia), includes multiplex reverse transcription, when performed, and multiplex amplified probe technique, multiple types or subtypes, 12-25 targets
- *CPT Changes: An Insider's View* 2015, 2018

87510 Gardnerella vaginalis, direct probe technique
- *CPT Assistant* Aug 05:9, May 12:5, Sep 13:3

87511 Gardnerella vaginalis, amplified probe technique
- *CPT Assistant* May 12:5, Sep 13:3

87512 Gardnerella vaginalis, quantification
- *CPT Assistant* Sep 13:3

(87515 has been deleted)

87516 hepatitis B virus, amplified probe technique
- *CPT Assistant* Sep 13:3

87517 hepatitis B virus, quantification
- *CPT Assistant* Sep 13:3

87520 hepatitis C, direct probe technique
- *CPT Assistant* Sep 13:3

87521 hepatitis C, amplified probe technique, includes reverse transcription when performed
- *CPT Changes: An Insider's View* 2013, 2014
- *CPT Assistant* Sep 13:3

87522 hepatitis C, quantification, includes reverse transcription when performed
- *CPT Changes: An Insider's View* 2013, 2014
- *CPT Assistant* Sep 13:3

87525 hepatitis G, direct probe technique
- *CPT Assistant* Sep 13:3

87526 hepatitis G, amplified probe technique
- *CPT Assistant* Sep 13:3

87527 hepatitis G, quantification
- *CPT Assistant* Sep 13:3

87528 Herpes simplex virus, direct probe technique
- *CPT Assistant* May 12:5, Sep 13:3

87529 Herpes simplex virus, amplified probe technique
- *CPT Assistant* Sep 13:3

87530 Herpes simplex virus, quantification
- *CPT Assistant* Sep 13:3

87531 Herpes virus-6, direct probe technique
- *CPT Assistant* Sep 13:3

87532 Herpes virus-6, amplified probe technique
- *CPT Assistant* Sep 13:3

87533 Herpes virus-6, quantification
- *CPT Assistant* Sep 13:3

87534 HIV-1, direct probe technique
- *CPT Assistant* May 12:5, Sep 13:3

87535 HIV-1, amplified probe technique, includes reverse transcription when performed
- *CPT Changes: An Insider's View* 2013, 2014
- *CPT Assistant* Mar 08:3, Sep 13:3

87536 HIV-1, quantification, includes reverse transcription when performed
- *CPT Changes: An Insider's View* 2013, 2014
- *CPT Assistant* Sep 13:3

87537 HIV-2, direct probe technique
- *CPT Assistant* Sep 13:3

87538 HIV-2, amplified probe technique, includes reverse transcription when performed
- *CPT Changes: An Insider's View* 2013, 2014
- *CPT Assistant* Sep 13:3

87539 HIV-2, quantification, includes reverse transcription when performed
- *CPT Changes: An Insider's View* 2013, 2014
- *CPT Assistant* Sep 13:3

 # 87623 Human Papillomavirus (HPV), low-risk types (eg, 6, 11, 42, 43, 44)
- *CPT Changes: An Insider's View* 2015

 # 87624 Human Papillomavirus (HPV), high-risk types (eg, 16, 18, 31, 33, 35, 39, 45, 51, 52, 56, 58, 59, 68)
- *CPT Changes: An Insider's View* 2015
- *CPT Assistant* Oct 15:10

(When both low-risk and high-risk HPV types are performed in a single assay, use only 87624)

 # 87625 Human Papillomavirus (HPV), types 16 and 18 only, includes type 45, if performed
CPT Changes: An Insider's View 2015
CPT Assistant Jun 15:10, Oct 15:10

(For Human Papillomavirus [HPV] detection of five or greater separately reported high-risk HPV types [ie, genotyping], use 0500T)

87540 Legionella pneumophila, direct probe technique
CPT Assistant May 12:5, Sep 13:3

87541 Legionella pneumophila, amplified probe technique
CPT Assistant Sep 13:3

87542 Legionella pneumophila, quantification
CPT Assistant Sep 13:3

87550 Mycobacteria species, direct probe technique
CPT Assistant May 12:5, Sep 13:3

87551 Mycobacteria species, amplified probe technique
CPT Assistant Sep 13:3

87552 Mycobacteria species, quantification
CPT Assistant Sep 13:3

87555 Mycobacteria tuberculosis, direct probe technique
CPT Assistant Sep 13:3

87556 Mycobacteria tuberculosis, amplified probe technique
CPT Assistant Sep 13:3

87557 Mycobacteria tuberculosis, quantification
CPT Assistant Sep 13:3

87560 Mycobacteria avium-intracellulare, direct probe technique
CPT Assistant Sep 13:3

87561 Mycobacteria avium-intracellulare, amplified probe technique
CPT Assistant Sep 13:3

87562 Mycobacteria avium-intracellulare, quantification
CPT Assistant Sep 13:3

87580 Mycoplasma pneumoniae, direct probe technique
CPT Assistant Sep 13:3

87581 Mycoplasma pneumoniae, amplified probe technique
CPT Assistant Sep 13:3

87582 Mycoplasma pneumoniae, quantification
CPT Assistant Sep 13:3

87590 Neisseria gonorrhoeae, direct probe technique
CPT Assistant May 12:5, Sep 13:3

87591 Neisseria gonorrhoeae, amplified probe technique
CPT Assistant Jun 13:14, Sep 13:3

87592 Neisseria gonorrhoeae, quantification
CPT Assistant Sep 13:3

87623 Code is out of numerical sequence. See 87538-87541

87624 Code is out of numerical sequence. See 87538-87541

87625 Code is out of numerical sequence. See 87538-87541

87631 respiratory virus (eg, adenovirus, influenza virus, coronavirus, metapneumovirus, parainfluenza virus, respiratory syncytial virus, rhinovirus), includes multiplex reverse transcription, when performed, and multiplex amplified probe technique, multiple types or subtypes, 3-5 targets
CPT Changes: An Insider's View 2013, 2015
CPT Assistant Sep 13:3

87632 respiratory virus (eg, adenovirus, influenza virus, coronavirus, metapneumovirus, parainfluenza virus, respiratory syncytial virus, rhinovirus), includes multiplex reverse transcription, when performed, and multiplex amplified probe technique, multiple types or subtypes, 6-11 targets
CPT Changes: An Insider's View 2013, 2015
CPT Assistant Sep 13:3

87633 respiratory virus (eg, adenovirus, influenza virus, coronavirus, metapneumovirus, parainfluenza virus, respiratory syncytial virus, rhinovirus), includes multiplex reverse transcription, when performed, and multiplex amplified probe technique, multiple types or subtypes, 12-25 targets
CPT Changes: An Insider's View 2013, 2015
CPT Assistant Sep 13:3

(Use 87631-87633 for nucleic acid assays which detect multiple respiratory viruses in a multiplex reaction [ie, single procedure with multiple results])

(For assays that are used to type or subtype influenza viruses only, see 87501-87503)

(For assays that include influenza viruses with additional respiratory viruses, see 87631-87633)

(For detection of multiple infectious agents not otherwise specified which report a single result, see 87800, 87801)

87634 respiratory syncytial virus, amplified probe technique
CPT Changes: An Insider's View 2018

(For assays that include respiratory syncytial virus with additional respiratory viruses, see 87631, 87632, 87633)

87640 Staphylococcus aureus, amplified probe technique
CPT Changes: An Insider's View 2007
CPT Assistant Aug 07:7, May 12:5, Sep 13:3

87641 Staphylococcus aureus, methicillin resistant, amplified probe technique
CPT Changes: An Insider's View 2007
CPT Assistant Aug 07:7, Sep 13:3

(For assays that detect methicillin resistance and identify Staphylococcus aureus using a single nucleic acid sequence, use 87641)

87650 Streptococcus, group A, direct probe technique
CPT Assistant Sep 13:4

87651 Streptococcus, group A, amplified probe technique
CPT Assistant Sep 13:4

87652 Streptococcus, group A, quantification
CPT Assistant Sep 13:4

87653 Streptococcus, group B, amplified probe technique
➲ *CPT Changes: An Insider's View* 2007
➲ *CPT Assistant* Aug 07:7, Sep 13:3

87660 Trichomonas vaginalis, direct probe technique
➲ *CPT Changes: An Insider's View* 2004
➲ *CPT Assistant* May 12:5, Sep 13:3

87661 Trichomonas vaginalis, amplified probe technique
➲ *CPT Changes: An Insider's View* 2014

87662 Zika virus, amplified probe technique
➲ *CPT Changes: An Insider's View* 2018

87797 Infectious agent detection by nucleic acid (DNA or RNA), not otherwise specified; direct probe technique, each organism
➲ *CPT Changes: An Insider's View* 2001
➲ *CPT Assistant* Nov 97:34, Nov 01:10, Aug 05:9, May 12:5, Sep 13:3, Aug 16:10

87798 amplified probe technique, each organism
➲ *CPT Changes: An Insider's View* 2001
➲ *CPT Assistant* Nov 97:34, Nov 01:10, Aug 07:7, Sep 13:3

87799 quantification, each organism
➲ *CPT Changes: An Insider's View* 2001
➲ *CPT Assistant* Nov 97:34, Sep 13:3

87800 Infectious agent detection by nucleic acid (DNA or RNA), multiple organisms; direct probe(s) technique
➲ *CPT Changes: An Insider's View* 2001
➲ *CPT Assistant* Aug 05:9, May 12:5, Sep 13:3, Aug 16:10

87801 amplified probe(s) technique
➲ *CPT Changes: An Insider's View* 2001
➲ *CPT Assistant* May 12:5, Jun 13:14, Sep 13:3

(For each specific organism nucleic acid detection from a primary source, see 87471-87660. For detection of specific infectious agents not otherwise specified, see 87797, 87798, or 87799 1 time for each agent)

(For detection of multiple infectious agents not otherwise specified which report a single result, see 87800, 87801)

(Do not use 87801 for nucleic acid assays that detect multiple respiratory viruses in a multiplex reaction [ie, single procedure with multiple results], see 87631-87633)

87802 Infectious agent antigen detection by immunoassay with direct optical observation; Streptococcus, group B
➲ *CPT Changes: An Insider's View* 2002
➲ *CPT Assistant* Jun 03:12

87803 Clostridium difficile toxin A
➲ *CPT Changes: An Insider's View* 2002
➲ *CPT Assistant* Jun 03:12

 # 87806 HIV-1 antigen(s), with HIV-1 and HIV-2 antibodies
➲ *CPT Changes: An Insider's View* 2015

87804 Influenza
➲ *CPT Changes: An Insider's View* 2002
➲ *CPT Assistant* Jun 03:11-12, May 09:6

87806 Code is out of numerical sequence. See 87802-87903

87807 respiratory syncytial virus
➲ *CPT Changes: An Insider's View* 2005

87808 Trichomonas vaginalis
➲ *CPT Changes: An Insider's View* 2007

87809 adenovirus
➲ *CPT Changes: An Insider's View* 2008
➲ *CPT Assistant* Apr 08:5

87810 Chlamydia trachomatis
➲ *CPT Changes: An Insider's View* 2009
➲ *CPT Assistant* Nov 97:34, Jan 98:6

87850 Neisseria gonorrhoeae
➲ *CPT Assistant* Nov 97:34, Jan 98:6

87880 Streptococcus, group A
➲ *CPT Assistant* Nov 97:34, Jan 98:6, Dec 98:8

87899 not otherwise specified
➲ *CPT Assistant* Jan 98:6, Jun 01:11

87900 Infectious agent drug susceptibility phenotype prediction using regularly updated genotypic bioinformatics
➲ *CPT Changes: An Insider's View* 2006
➲ *CPT Assistant* Mar 06:6, May 12:5, Sep 13:3, Dec 15:17

 # 87910 Infectious agent genotype analysis by nucleic acid (DNA or RNA); cytomegalovirus
➲ *CPT Changes: An Insider's View* 2013
➲ *CPT Assistant* Sep 13:3

(For infectious agent drug susceptibility phenotype prediction for HIV-1, use 87900)

(For Human Papillomavirus [HPV] for high-risk types [ie, genotyping], of five or greater separately reported HPV types, use 0500T)

87901 HIV-1, reverse transcriptase and protease regions
➲ *CPT Changes: An Insider's View* 2001, 2002, 2011, 2013
➲ *CPT Assistant* Aug 05:9, Mar 06:6, Oct 10:9, Dec 10:9, May 12:5, Sep 13:3

 # 87906 HIV-1, other region (eg, integrase, fusion)
➲ *CPT Changes: An Insider's View* 2011
➲ *CPT Assistant* Oct 10:8, Dec 10:8, Sep 13:3

(For infectious agent drug susceptibility phenotype prediction for HIV-1, use 87900)

 # 87912 Hepatitis B virus
➲ *CPT Changes: An Insider's View* 2013
➲ *CPT Assistant* Sep 13:3

87902 Hepatitis C virus
➲ *CPT Changes: An Insider's View* 2002
➲ *CPT Assistant* May 12:5, Sep 13:3, Nov 15:11, Dec 15:17

87903 Infectious agent phenotype analysis by nucleic acid (DNA or RNA) with drug resistance tissue culture analysis, HIV 1; first through 10 drugs tested
➲ *CPT Changes: An Insider's View* 2001, 2002
➲ *CPT Assistant* Apr 04:15, Mar 06:6, May 12:3, Sep 13:3

+ 87904 each additional drug tested (List separately in addition to code for primary procedure)
➲ *CPT Changes: An Insider's View* 2001, 2002, 2006
➲ *CPT Assistant* Apr 04:15, Mar 06:6, May 12:3, Sep 13:3

(Use 87904 in conjunction with 87903)

87905 Infectious agent enzymatic activity other than virus (eg, sialidase activity in vaginal fluid)
➲ *CPT Changes: An Insider's View* 2009

(For virus isolation including identification by non-immunologic method, other than by cytopathic effect, use 87255)

87906 Code is out of numerical sequence. See 87802-87903

87910 Code is out of numerical sequence. See 87802-87903

87912 Code is out of numerical sequence. See 87802-87903

87999 Unlisted microbiology procedure
➲ *CPT Assistant* Aug 05:9

Anatomic Pathology

Postmortem Examination

Procedures 88000 through 88099 represent physician services only. Use modifier 90 for outside laboratory services.

88000 Necropsy (autopsy), gross examination only; without CNS
➲ *CPT Assistant* Aug 05:9

88005 with brain

88007 with brain and spinal cord

88012 infant with brain

88014 stillborn or newborn with brain

88016 macerated stillborn

88020 Necropsy (autopsy), gross and microscopic; without CNS

88025 with brain

88027 with brain and spinal cord

88028 infant with brain

88029 stillborn or newborn with brain

88036 Necropsy (autopsy), limited, gross and/or microscopic; regional

88037 single organ

88040 Necropsy (autopsy); forensic examination

88045 coroner's call

88099 Unlisted necropsy (autopsy) procedure

Cytopathology

88104 Cytopathology, fluids, washings or brushings, except cervical or vaginal; smears with interpretation
➲ *CPT Assistant* Spring 91:6, Fall 94:3, Aug 05:9

88106 simple filter method with interpretation
➲ *CPT Changes: An Insider's View* 2007
➲ *CPT Assistant* Fall 94:3

(Do not report 88106 in conjunction with 88104)

(For nongynecological selective cellular enhancement including filter transfer techniques, use 88112)

88108 Cytopathology, concentration technique, smears and interpretation (eg, Saccomanno technique)
➲ *CPT Assistant* Fall 94:3, Nov 97:34, Jan 98:6

(For cervical or vaginal smears, see 88150-88155)

(For gastric intubation with lavage, see 43754, 43755)

(For x-ray localization, use 74340)

88112 Cytopathology, selective cellular enhancement technique with interpretation (eg, liquid based slide preparation method), except cervical or vaginal
➲ *CPT Changes: An Insider's View* 2004

(Do not report 88112 with 88108)

88120 Cytopathology, in situ hybridization (eg, FISH), urinary tract specimen with morphometric analysis, 3-5 molecular probes, each specimen; manual
➲ *CPT Changes: An Insider's View* 2011
➲ *CPT Assistant* Oct 10:9, Dec 10:9

88121 using computer-assisted technology
➲ *CPT Changes: An Insider's View* 2011
➲ *CPT Assistant* Oct 10:9, Dec 10:9

(For morphometric in situ hybridization on cytologic specimens other than urinary tract, see 88367, 88368)

(For more than 5 probes, use 88399)

88125 Cytopathology, forensic (eg, sperm)

88130 Sex chromatin identification; Barr bodies

88140 peripheral blood smear, polymorphonuclear drumsticks
➲ *CPT Assistant* Nov 98:27-28, Mar 06:6

(For Guard stain, use 88313)

Codes 88141-88155, 88164-88167, 88174-88175 are used to report cervical or vaginal screening by various methods and to report physician interpretation services. Use codes 88150, 88152, 88153 to report conventional Pap smears that are examined using non-Bethesda reporting. Use codes 88164-88167 to report conventional Pap smears that are examined using the Bethesda System of reporting. Use codes 88142-88143 to report liquid-based specimens processed as thin-layer preparations that are examined using any system of reporting (Bethesda or non-Bethesda). Use codes 88174-88175 to report automated screening of liquid-based specimens that are examined using any system of reporting (Bethesda or non-Bethesda). Within each of these three code families choose the one code that describes the screening method(s) used. Codes 88141 and 88155 should be reported in addition to the screening code chosen when the additional services are provided. Manual rescreening requires a complete visual reassessment of the entire slide initially screened by either an automated or manual process. Manual review represents an assessment of selected cells or regions of a slide identified by initial automated review.

88141 Cytopathology, cervical or vaginal (any reporting system), requiring interpretation by physician

➲ *CPT Assistant* Nov 97:35, Jan 98:6, Jan 99:11, May 99:6, Nov 99:46, Mar 04:6, Mar 05:16, May 11:10, Dec 11:17

(Use 88141 in conjunction with 88142, 88143, 88147, 88148, 88150, 88152, 88153, 88164-88167, 88174-88175)

88142 Cytopathology, cervical or vaginal (any reporting system), collected in preservative fluid, automated thin layer preparation; manual screening under physician supervision

➲ *CPT Assistant* Nov 97:34-35, Jan 98:6, Nov 98:28, May 99:6, Jul 03:7, Mar 04:4

88143 with manual screening and rescreening under physician supervision

➲ *CPT Assistant* Nov 97:34-35, Nov 98:28, May 99:6, Jul 03:7, Mar 04:4, Mar 05:16

(For automated screening of automated thin layer preparation, see 88174, 88175)

88147 Cytopathology smears, cervical or vaginal; screening by automated system under physician supervision

➲ *CPT Assistant* Nov 97:35, Nov 98:28, Jan 99:11, May 99:6, Nov 99:46, Mar 04:6

88148 screening by automated system with manual rescreening under physician supervision

➲ *CPT Changes: An Insider's View* 2000

➲ *CPT Assistant* Jan 99:1, May 99:6, Nov 99:46, Mar 04:6

88150 Cytopathology, slides, cervical or vaginal; manual screening under physician supervision

➲ *CPT Assistant* Winter 91:19, Nov 97:34-35, Nov 98:28, May 99:6, Mar 04:5

88152 with manual screening and computer-assisted rescreening under physician supervision

➲ *CPT Assistant* Nov 97:35, Jan 98:6, May 99:6, Mar 04:5

88153 with manual screening and rescreening under physician supervision

➲ *CPT Assistant* Nov 97:34-35, Nov 98:28, May 99:6, Mar 04:5, Mar 05:16

(88154 has been deleted)

+ 88155 Cytopathology, slides, cervical or vaginal, definitive hormonal evaluation (eg, maturation index, karyopyknotic index, estrogenic index) (List separately in addition to code[s] for other technical and interpretation services)

➲ *CPT Assistant* Nov 97:35, Nov 98:28, May 99:6, Nov 99:46, Mar 04:5, May 11:10

(Use 88155 in conjunction with 88142, 88143, 88147, 88148, 88150, 88152, 88153, 88164-88167, 88174-88175)

88160 Cytopathology, smears, any other source; screening and interpretation

➲ *CPT Assistant* Jan 98:6

88161 preparation, screening and interpretation

➲ *CPT Assistant* Aug 97:18, Jan 98:6

88162 extended study involving over 5 slides and/or multiple stains

(For aerosol collection of sputum, use 89220)

(For special stains, see 88312-88314)

88164 Cytopathology, slides, cervical or vaginal (the Bethesda System); manual screening under physician supervision

➲ *CPT Assistant* Nov 98:28, May 99:6, Mar 04:5

88165 with manual screening and rescreening under physician supervision

➲ *CPT Assistant* Nov 98:28, May 99:6, Mar 04:5, Mar 05:16

88166 with manual screening and computer-assisted rescreening under physician supervision

➲ *CPT Assistant* Nov 98:28, May 99:6, Mar 04:5

88167 with manual screening and computer-assisted rescreening using cell selection and review under physician supervision

➲ *CPT Assistant* Nov 98:28, May 99:6, Jul 03:7, Mar 04:5

►(For collection of specimen via fine needle aspiration biopsy, see 10004, 10005, 10006, 10007, 10008, 10009, 10010, 10011, 10012, 10021)◄

88172 Cytopathology, evaluation of fine needle aspirate; immediate cytohistologic study to determine adequacy for diagnosis, first evaluation episode, each site

➲ *CPT Changes: An Insider's View* 2001, 2011

➲ *CPT Assistant* Fall 93:26, Fall 94:2, Dec 98:8, Aug 07:15, Oct 10:9, Dec 10:9, Jan 16:12

(The evaluation episode represents a complete set of cytologic material submitted for evaluation and is independent of the number of needle passes or slides prepared. A separate evaluation episode occurs if the proceduralist provider obtains additional material from the same site, based on the prior immediate adequacy assessment, or a separate lesion is aspirated)

88173 interpretation and report

➲ *CPT Assistant* Fall 93:26, Fall 94:2, Dec 98:8, Oct 10:9, Dec 10:9

(Report one unit of 88173 for the interpretation and report from each anatomic site, regardless of the number of passes or evaluation episodes performed during the aspiration procedure)

►(For fine needle aspirate biopsy, see 10004, 10005, 10006, 10007, 10008, 10009, 10010, 10011, 10012, 10021)◄

(Do not report 88172, 88173 in conjunction with 88333 and 88334 for the same specimen)

#+ 88177 immediate cytohistologic study to determine adequacy for diagnosis, each separate additional evaluation episode, same site (List separately in addition to code for primary procedure)
➲ *CPT Changes: An Insider's View* 2011
➲ *CPT Assistant* Oct 10:9, Dec 10:9, Jan 16:12

(When repeat immediate evaluation episode(s) is required on subsequent cytologic material from the same site, eg, following determination the prior sampling that was not adequate for diagnosis, use 1 unit of 88177 for each additional evaluation episode)

(Use 88177 in conjunction with 88172)

88174 Cytopathology, cervical or vaginal (any reporting system), collected in preservative fluid, automated thin layer preparation; screening by automated system, under physician supervision
➲ *CPT Changes: An Insider's View* 2003
➲ *CPT Assistant* Jul 03:9, Mar 04:4

88175 with screening by automated system and manual rescreening or review, under physician supervision
➲ *CPT Changes: An Insider's View* 2003, 2006
➲ *CPT Assistant* Jul 03:9, Mar 04:4, Mar 06:6, May 11:10

(For manual screening, see 88142, 88143)

88177 Code is out of numerical sequence. See 88172-88175

88182 Flow cytometry, cell cycle or DNA analysis
➲ *CPT Assistant* Oct 13:3

(For DNA ploidy analysis by morphometric technique, use 88358)

88184 Flow cytometry, cell surface, cytoplasmic, or nuclear marker, technical component only; first marker
➲ *CPT Changes: An Insider's View* 2005
➲ *CPT Assistant* Dec 07:14, Oct 13:3

+ 88185 each additional marker (List separately in addition to code for first marker)
➲ *CPT Changes: An Insider's View* 2005
➲ *CPT Assistant* Dec 07:14, Oct 13:3

(Report 88185 in conjunction with 88184)

88187 Flow cytometry, interpretation; 2 to 8 markers
➲ *CPT Changes: An Insider's View* 2005
➲ *CPT Assistant* Apr 05:14, Oct 13:3

88188 9 to 15 markers
➲ *CPT Changes: An Insider's View* 2005
➲ *CPT Assistant* Apr 05:14, Oct 13:3

88189 16 or more markers
➲ *CPT Changes: An Insider's View* 2005
➲ *CPT Assistant* Apr 05:14, Oct 13:3

(Do not report 88187-88189 for interpretation of 86355, 86356, 86357, 86359, 86360, 86361, 86367)

(For assessment of circulating antibodies by flow cytometric techniques, see analyte and method-specific codes in the Chemistry section [83516-83520] or Immunology section [86000-86849])

(For cell enumeration using immunologic selection and identification in fluid specimen [eg, circulating tumor cells in blood], see 86152, 86153)

88199 Unlisted cytopathology procedure

(For electron microscopy, use 88348)

Cytogenetic Studies

Molecular pathology procedures should be reported using the appropriate code from Tier 1 (81161, 81200-81383), Tier 2 (81400-81408), Genomic Sequencing Procedures and Other Molecular Multianalyte Assays (81410-81471), or Multianalyte Assays with Algorithmic Analyses (81500-81512) sections. If no specific code exists, one of the unlisted codes (81479 or 81599) should be used.

(For acetylcholinesterase, use 82013)

(For alpha-fetoprotein, serum or amniotic fluid, see 82105, 82106)

(For laser microdissection of cells from tissue sample, see 88380)

88230 Tissue culture for non-neoplastic disorders; lymphocyte
➲ *CPT Assistant* Nov 98:29, Oct 99:2, Aug 05:9, May 08:5

88233 skin or other solid tissue biopsy
➲ *CPT Assistant* Nov 98:29, Oct 99:2, May 08:5

88235 amniotic fluid or chorionic villus cells
➲ *CPT Assistant* Nov 98:29, Oct 99:2, May 08:5

88237 Tissue culture for neoplastic disorders; bone marrow, blood cells
➲ *CPT Assistant* Nov 98:29, Oct 99:2, May 08:5

88239 solid tumor
➲ *CPT Assistant* Nov 98:29, Oct 99:2, May 08:5

88240 Cryopreservation, freezing and storage of cells, each cell line
➲ *CPT Assistant* Nov 98:29, Oct 99:2, Jul 03:9, May 08:5, Oct 13:3

(For therapeutic cryopreservation and storage, use 38207)

88241 Thawing and expansion of frozen cells, each aliquot
➲ *CPT Assistant* Nov 98:29, Oct 99:2, Jul 03:9, May 08:5, Oct 13:3

(For therapeutic thawing of previous harvest, use 38208)

88245 Chromosome analysis for breakage syndromes; baseline Sister Chromatid Exchange (SCE), 20-25 cells
➲ *CPT Assistant* Nov 98:29, Oct 99:2, Jul 05:1, May 08:5

88248 baseline breakage, score 50-100 cells, count 20 cells, 2 karyotypes (eg, for ataxia telangiectasia, Fanconi anemia, fragile X)
➲ *CPT Assistant* Nov 98:29, Oct 99:2, Jul 05:1, May 08:5

88249 score 100 cells, clastogen stress (eg, diepoxybutane, mitomycin C, ionizing radiation, UV radiation)
➲ *CPT Assistant* Nov 98:29, Oct 99:2, Jul 05:1, May 08:5

88261 Chromosome analysis; count 5 cells, 1 karyotype, with banding
➔ *CPT Assistant* Nov 98:29, Oct 99:2, Jul 05:1, May 08:5

88262 count 15-20 cells, 2 karyotypes, with banding
➔ *CPT Assistant* Nov 98:29, Oct 99:2, May 08:5, May 11:10

88263 count 45 cells for mosaicism, 2 karyotypes, with banding
➔ *CPT Assistant* Nov 98:29, Oct 99:2, Jul 05:1, May 08:5

88264 analyze 20-25 cells
➔ *CPT Assistant* Nov 98:29, Oct 99:2, Jul 05:1, May 08:5

88267 Chromosome analysis, amniotic fluid or chorionic villus, count 15 cells, 1 karyotype, with banding
➔ *CPT Assistant* Jul 05:1

88269 Chromosome analysis, in situ for amniotic fluid cells, count cells from 6-12 colonies, 1 karyotype, with banding
➔ *CPT Assistant* Jul 05:1

88271 Molecular cytogenetics; DNA probe, each (eg, FISH)
➔ *CPT Assistant* Nov 98:29, Mar 99:10, Oct 99:3, Jun 02:11, Jul 05:1, May 08:5, May 12:5, Sep 13:3

(For cytogenomic microarray analysis, see 81228, 81229, 81405, 81406, 81479)

(For genomic sequencing procedures or other molecular multianalyte assays for copy number analysis using circulating cell-free fetal DNA in maternal blood, see 81420, 81422, 81479)

88272 chromosomal in situ hybridization, analyze 3-5 cells (eg, for derivatives and markers)
➔ *CPT Assistant* Nov 98:29, Mar 99:10, Oct 99:3, Jun 02:11, Jul 05:1, May 08:5, May 12:5, Sep 13:3

88273 chromosomal in situ hybridization, analyze 10-30 cells (eg, for microdeletions)
➔ *CPT Assistant* Nov 98:29, Mar 99:10, Oct 99:3, Jun 02:11, Jul 05:1, May 08:5, May 12:5, Sep 13:3

88274 interphase in situ hybridization, analyze 25-99 cells
➔ *CPT Assistant* Nov 98:29, Mar 99:10, Oct 99:3, Jun 02:11, Jul 05:1, May 08:5, May 12:5, Sep 13:3

88275 interphase in situ hybridization, analyze 100-300 cells
➔ *CPT Assistant* Nov 98:29, Mar 99:10, Oct 99:3, Jun 02:11, Jul 05:1, May 08:5, May 12:5, Sep 13:3

88280 Chromosome analysis; additional karyotypes, each study
➔ *CPT Assistant* Jul 05:1, May 08:5

88283 additional specialized banding technique (eg, NOR, C-banding)
➔ *CPT Assistant* Jul 05:1, May 08:5

88285 additional cells counted, each study
➔ *CPT Assistant* Jul 05:1, Dec 07:14, May 08:5, May 11:10

88289 additional high resolution study
➔ *CPT Assistant* Oct 99:3, Jul 05:1

88291 Cytogenetics and molecular cytogenetics, interpretation and report
➔ *CPT Assistant* Nov 98:29, Oct 99:3, Jul 05:1, May 08:5

88299 Unlisted cytogenetic study
➔ *CPT Assistant* Oct 99:3

Surgical Pathology

Services 88300 through 88309 include accession, examination, and reporting. They do not include the services designated in codes 88311 through 88365 and 88399, which are coded in addition when provided.

The unit of service for codes 88300 through 88309 is the specimen.

A specimen is defined as tissue or tissues that is (are) submitted for individual and separate attention, requiring individual examination and pathologic diagnosis. Two or more such specimens from the same patient (eg, separately identified endoscopic biopsies, skin lesions) are each appropriately assigned an individual code reflective of its proper level of service.

Service code 88300 is used for any specimen that in the opinion of the examining pathologist can be accurately diagnosed without microscopic examination. Service code 88302 is used when gross and microscopic examination is performed on a specimen to confirm identification and the absence of disease. Service codes 88304 through 88309 describe all other specimens requiring gross and microscopic examination, and represent additional ascending levels of physician work. Levels 88302 through 88309 are specifically defined by the assigned specimens.

Any unlisted specimen should be assigned to the code which most closely reflects the physician work involved when compared to other specimens assigned to that code.

(Do not report 88302-88309 on the same specimen as part of Mohs surgery)

88300 **Level I** - Surgical pathology, gross examination only
➔ *CPT Assistant* Winter 91:18, Sep 00:10, Aug 05:9

88302 **Level II** - Surgical pathology, gross and microscopic examination

Appendix, incidental

Fallopian tube, sterilization

Fingers/toes, amputation, traumatic

Foreskin, newborn

Hernia sac, any location

Hydrocele sac

Nerve

Skin, plastic repair

Sympathetic ganglion

Testis, castration

Vaginal mucosa, incidental

Vas deferens, sterilization
➔ *CPT Assistant* Winter 91:18, Sep 00:10, Nov 06:1, Jan 07:29, Dec 11:17, Feb 14:10

Pathology and Laboratory 80047-89398, 0001U-0061U

88304 **Level III** - Surgical pathology, gross and microscopic examination

Abortion, induced

Abscess

Aneurysm - arterial/ventricular

Anus, tag

Appendix, other than incidental

Artery, atheromatous plaque

Bartholin's gland cyst

Bone fragment(s), other than pathologic fracture

Bursa/synovial cyst

Carpal tunnel tissue

Cartilage, shavings

Cholesteatoma

Colon, colostomy stoma

Conjunctiva - biopsy/pterygium

Cornea

Diverticulum - esophagus/small intestine

Dupuytren's contracture tissue

Femoral head, other than fracture

Fissure/fistula

Foreskin, other than newborn

Gallbladder

Ganglion cyst

Hematoma

Hemorrhoids

Hydatid of Morgagni

Intervertebral disc

Joint, loose body

Meniscus

Mucocele, salivary

Neuroma - Morton's/traumatic

Pilonidal cyst/sinus

Polyps, inflammatory - nasal/sinusoidal

Skin - cyst/tag/debridement

Soft tissue, debridement

Soft tissue, lipoma

Spermatocele

Tendon/tendon sheath

Testicular appendage

Thrombus or embolus

Tonsil and/or adenoids

Varicocele

Vas deferens, other than sterilization

Vein, varicosity

➔ *CPT Changes: An Insider's View* 2002

➔ *CPT Assistant* Spring 91:2, Winter 91:18, Aug 97:18, Sep 00:10, Jan 07:29, Dec 11:17

88305 **Level IV** - Surgical pathology, gross and microscopic examination

Abortion - spontaneous/missed

Artery, biopsy

Bone marrow, biopsy

Bone exostosis

Brain/meninges, other than for tumor resection

Breast, biopsy, not requiring microscopic evaluation of surgical margins

Breast, reduction mammoplasty

Bronchus, biopsy

Cell block, any source

Cervix, biopsy

Colon, biopsy

Duodenum, biopsy

Endocervix, curettings/biopsy

Endometrium, curettings/biopsy

Esophagus, biopsy

Extremity, amputation, traumatic

Fallopian tube, biopsy

Fallopian tube, ectopic pregnancy

Femoral head, fracture

Fingers/toes, amputation, non-traumatic

Gingiva/oral mucosa, biopsy

Heart valve

Joint, resection

Kidney, biopsy

Larynx, biopsy

Leiomyoma(s), uterine myomectomy - without uterus

Lip, biopsy/wedge resection

Lung, transbronchial biopsy

Lymph node, biopsy

Muscle, biopsy

Nasal mucosa, biopsy

Nasopharynx/oropharynx, biopsy

Nerve, biopsy

Pathology and Laboratory 80047-89398, 0001U-0061U

Odontogenic/dental cyst

Omentum, biopsy

Ovary with or without tube, non-neoplastic

Ovary, biopsy/wedge resection

Parathyroid gland

Peritoneum, biopsy

Pituitary tumor

Placenta, other than third trimester

Pleura/pericardium - biopsy/tissue

Polyp, cervical/endometrial

Polyp, colorectal

Polyp, stomach/small intestine

Prostate, needle biopsy

Prostate, TUR

Salivary gland, biopsy

Sinus, paranasal biopsy

Skin, other than cyst/tag/debridement/plastic repair

Small intestine, biopsy

Soft tissue, other than tumor/mass/lipoma/debridement

Spleen

Stomach, biopsy

Synovium

Testis, other than tumor/biopsy/castration

Thyroglossal duct/brachial cleft cyst

Tongue, biopsy

Tonsil, biopsy

Trachea, biopsy

Ureter, biopsy

Urethra, biopsy

Urinary bladder, biopsy

Uterus, with or without tubes and ovaries, for prolapse

Vagina, biopsy

Vulva/labia, biopsy

➔ *CPT Changes: An Insider's View* 2002

➔ *CPT Assistant* Winter 90:2, Spring 91:6, Winter 91:18, Winter 92:17, Aug 97:18, Jul 98:4, Nov 98:29-30, Jul 00:4, Sep 00:10, Dec 00:15, Jul 05:13, Nov 06:1, Jan 07:29, Dec 11:17

88307 **Level V** - Surgical pathology, gross and microscopic examination

Adrenal, resection

Bone - biopsy/curettings

Bone fragment(s), pathologic fracture

Brain, biopsy

Brain/meninges, tumor resection

Breast, excision of lesion, requiring microscopic evaluation of surgical margins

Breast, mastectomy - partial/simple

Cervix, conization

Colon, segmental resection, other than for tumor

Extremity, amputation, non-traumatic

Eye, enucleation

Kidney, partial/total nephrectomy

Larynx, partial/total resection

Liver, biopsy - needle/wedge

Liver, partial resection

Lung, wedge biopsy

Lymph nodes, regional resection

Mediastinum, mass

Myocardium, biopsy

Odontogenic tumor

Ovary with or without tube, neoplastic

Pancreas, biopsy

Placenta, third trimester

Prostate, except radical resection

Salivary gland

Sentinel lymph node

Small intestine, resection, other than for tumor

Soft tissue mass (except lipoma) - biopsy/simple excision

Stomach - subtotal/total resection, other than for tumor

Testis, biopsy

Thymus, tumor

Thyroid, total/lobe

Ureter, resection

Urinary bladder, TUR

Uterus, with or without tubes and ovaries, other than neoplastic/prolapse

➔ *CPT Changes: An Insider's View* 2001

➔ *CPT Assistant* Winter 91:18, Winter 92:18, Jul 98:4, Nov 98:29-30, Jul 99:10, Jul 00:4, Sep 00:10, Dec 00:15, Dec 03:11, Nov 06:1, Jan 07:29, Dec 11:17

88309 **Level VI** - Surgical pathology, gross and microscopic examination

Bone resection

Breast, mastectomy - with regional lymph nodes

Colon, segmental resection for tumor

Colon, total resection

Esophagus, partial/total resection

Extremity, disarticulation

Fetus, with dissection

Larynx, partial/total resection - with regional lymph nodes

Lung - total/lobe/segment resection

Pancreas, total/subtotal resection

Prostate, radical resection

Small intestine, resection for tumor

Soft tissue tumor, extensive resection

Stomach - subtotal/total resection for tumor

Testis, tumor

Tongue/tonsil -resection for tumor

Urinary bladder, partial/total resection

Uterus, with or without tubes and ovaries, neoplastic

Vulva, total/subtotal resection

CPT Assistant Spring 91:2, Winter 91:18, Fall 93:2, 26, Jul 00:4, Sep 00:10, Dec 03:11, Nov 06:1, Jan 07:29, Dec 11:18, Feb 14:10

►(For fine needle aspiration biopsy, see 10004, 10005, 10006, 10007, 10008, 10009, 10010, 10011, 10012, 10021)◄

(For evaluation of fine needle aspirate, see 88172-88173)

(Do not report 88302-88309 on the same specimen as part of Mohs surgery)

+ 88311 Decalcification procedure (List separately in addition to code for surgical pathology examination)

CPT Assistant Winter 92:18, Jul 98:4, Jun 02:11, Nov 02:7, Nov 06:1, Dec 11:18

88312 Special stain including interpretation and report; Group I for microorganisms (eg, acid fast, methenamine silver)

CPT Changes: An Insider's View 2004, 2010, 2012

CPT Assistant Winter 91:19, Jun 02:11, Nov 02:7, Nov 06:1, Dec 11:18

(Report one unit of 88312 for each special stain, on each surgical pathology block, cytologic specimen, or hematologic smear)

88313 Group II, all other (eg, iron, trichrome), except stain for microorganisms, stains for enzyme constituents, or immunocytochemistry and immunohistochemistry

CPT Changes: An Insider's View 2010, 2012

CPT Assistant Jun 02:11, Nov 02:7, Mar 03:22, Nov 03:15, Jun 06:17, Nov 06:1, Dec 11:18

(Report one unit of 88313 for each special stain, on each surgical pathology block, cytologic specimen, or hematologic smear)

(For immunocytochemistry and immunohistochemistry, use 88342)

+ 88314 histochemical stain on frozen tissue block (List separately in addition to code for primary procedure)

CPT Changes: An Insider's View 2010, 2012

CPT Assistant Nov 02:7, Nov 06:1, Dec 11:18

(Use 88314 in conjunction with 17311-17315, 88302-88309, 88331, 88332)

(Do not report 88314 with 17311-17315 for routine frozen section stain [eg, hematoxylin and eosin, toluidine blue], performed during Mohs surgery. When a nonroutine histochemical stain on frozen tissue during Mohs surgery is utilized, report 88314 with modifier 59)

(Report one unit of 88314 for each special stain on each frozen surgical pathology block)

(For a special stain performed on frozen tissue section material to identify enzyme constituents, use 88319)

(For determinative histochemistry to identify chemical components, use 88313)

88319 Group III, for enzyme constituents

CPT Changes: An Insider's View 2012

CPT Assistant Dec 11:18

(For each stain on each surgical pathology block, cytologic specimen, or hematologic smear, use one unit of 88319)

(For detection of enzyme constituents by immunohistochemical or immunocytochemical technique, use 88342)

88321 Consultation and report on referred slides prepared elsewhere

CPT Assistant Winter 91:19, Apr 97:9, Oct 00:7, Dec 02:10, Jan 10:11, Dec 11:18, Jun 13:15

88323 Consultation and report on referred material requiring preparation of slides

CPT Assistant Winter 91:19, Apr 97:9, Oct 00:7, Dec 02:10, Dec 11:18, Jun 13:15

88325 Consultation, comprehensive, with review of records and specimens, with report on referred material

CPT Assistant Winter 91:19, Apr 97:9, Dec 02:10, Dec 11:18, Jun 13:15

88329 Pathology consultation during surgery;

CPT Assistant Winter 91:19, Apr 97:12, Aug 97:18, Jan 07:29, Dec 11:18

88331 first tissue block, with frozen section(s), single specimen

CPT Changes: An Insider's View 2001

CPT Assistant Spring 91:2, Winter 91:19, Apr 97:12, Aug 97:18, Jul 00:4, Nov 02:7, Mar 06:6, Nov 06:1, Jan 07:29, Oct 10:9, Dec 10:9, Dec 11:18

+ 88332 each additional tissue block with frozen section(s) (List separately in addition to code for primary procedure)

CPT Changes: An Insider's View 2011

CPT Assistant Winter 91:19, Apr 97:12, Aug 97:18, Jul 00:4, Mar 06:6, Jan 07:29, Oct 10:9, Dec 10:9, Dec 11:18

(Use 88332 in conjunction with 88331)

88333 cytologic examination (eg, touch prep, squash prep), initial site

CPT Changes: An Insider's View 2006

CPT Assistant Mar 06:6, Jan 07:29, Jun 08:15, Dec 10:9, Dec 11:18

+ 88334 cytologic examination (eg, touch prep, squash prep), each additional site (List separately in addition to code for primary procedure)

➲ *CPT Changes: An Insider's View* 2006, 2011

➲ *CPT Assistant* Mar 06:6, Jan 07:29, Oct 10:9, Dec 11:18

(Use 88334 in conjunction with 88331, 88333)

(For intraoperative consultation on a specimen requiring both frozen section and cytologic evaluation, use 88331 and 88334)

(For percutaneous needle biopsy requiring intraprocedural cytologic examination, use 88333)

(Do not report 88333 and 88334 for non-intraoperative cytologic examination, see 88160-88162)

(Do not report 88333 and 88334 for intraprocedural cytologic evaluation of fine needle aspirate, see 88172)

88341 Code is out of numerical sequence. See 88334-88372

88342 Immunohistochemistry or immunocytochemistry, per specimen; initial single antibody stain procedure

➲ *CPT Changes: An Insider's View* 2004, 2014, 2015

➲ *CPT Assistant* Winter 91:17, Jul 00:10, Nov 02:6-7, Nov 06:1, Dec 11:18, Jun 14:15, Jun 15:11

(For quantitative or semiquantitative immunohistochemistry, see 88360, 88361)

#+ 88341 each additional single antibody stain procedure (List separately in addition to code for primary procedure)

➲ *CPT Changes: An Insider's View* 2015

➲ *CPT Assistant* Jun 15:11

(Use 88341 in conjunction with 88342)

(For multiplex antibody stain procedure, use 88344)

88344 each multiplex antibody stain procedure

➲ *CPT Changes: An Insider's View* 2015

➲ *CPT Assistant* Jun 15:11

(Do not use more than one unit of 88341, 88342, or 88344 for the same separately identifiable antibody per specimen)

(Do not report 88341, 88342, 88344 in conjunction with 88360, 88361 unless each procedure is for a different antibody)

(When multiple separately identifiable antibodies are applied to the same specimen [ie, multiplex antibody stain procedure], use one unit of 88344)

(When multiple antibodies are applied to the same slide that are not separately identifiable, [eg, antibody cocktails], use 88342, unless an additional separately identifiable antibody is also used, then use 88344)

88346 Immunofluorescence, per specimen; initial single antibody stain procedure

➲ *CPT Changes: An Insider's View* 2016

➲ *CPT Assistant* Dec 11:18

(88347 has been deleted. To report, see 88346, 88350)

#+ 88350 each additional single antibody stain procedure (List separately in addition to code for primary procedure)

➲ *CPT Changes: An Insider's View* 2016

(Report 88350 in conjunction with 88346)

(Do not report 88346 and 88350 for fluorescent in situ hybridization studies, see 88364, 88365, 88366, 88367, 88368, 88369, 88373, 88374, and 88377)

(Do not report 88346 and 88350 for multiplex immunofluorescence analysis, use 88399)

88348 Electron microscopy, diagnostic

➲ *CPT Assistant* Dec 11:18

88350 Code is out of numerical sequence. See 88334-88372

88355 Morphometric analysis; skeletal muscle

➲ *CPT Assistant* Dec 11:18

88356 nerve

➲ *CPT Assistant* Dec 11:18, Jun 14:15

88358 tumor (eg, DNA ploidy)

➲ *CPT Changes: An Insider's View* 2004

➲ *CPT Assistant* Jul 98:4, Jul 99:11, Jun 02:11, Jun 06:17, Dec 11:18

(Do not report 88358 with 88313 unless each procedure is for a different special stain)

88360 Morphometric analysis, tumor immunohistochemistry (eg, Her-2/neu, estrogen receptor/progesterone receptor), quantitative or semiquantitative, per specimen, each single antibody stain procedure; manual

➲ *CPT Changes: An Insider's View* 2005, 2015

➲ *CPT Assistant* Dec 11:18, Jun 14:15

88361 using computer-assisted technology

➲ *CPT Changes: An Insider's View* 2004, 2005, 2015

➲ *CPT Assistant* Dec 11:18, Jun 14:15

(Do not report 88360, 88361 in conjunction with 88341, 88342, or 88344 unless each procedure is for a different antibody)

(Morphometric analysis of a multiplex antibody stain should be reported with one unit of 88360 or 88361, per specimen)

(For morphometric analysis using in situ hybridization techniques, see 88367, 88368)

(When semi-thin plastic-embedded sections are performed in conjunction with morphometric analysis, only the morphometric analysis should be reported; if performed as an independent procedure, see codes 88300-88309 for surgical pathology.)

88362 Nerve teasing preparations

➲ *CPT Assistant* Dec 11:18

88363 Examination and selection of retrieved archival (ie, previously diagnosed) tissue(s) for molecular analysis (eg, KRAS mutational analysis)

➲ *CPT Changes: An Insider's View* 2011

➲ *CPT Assistant* Oct 10:10, Dec 10:10, Dec 11:18

88364 Code is out of numerical sequence. See 88334-88372

88365 In situ hybridization (eg, FISH), per specimen; initial single probe stain procedure
- ➔ *CPT Changes: An Insider's View* 2005, 2015
- ➔ *CPT Assistant* Jun 02:11, Mar 05:16, Dec 11:18, May 12:3, Sep 13:3

#+ 88364 each additional single probe stain procedure (List separately in addition to code for primary procedure)
- ➔ *CPT Changes: An Insider's View* 2015

(Use 88364 in conjunction with 88365)

88366 each multiplex probe stain procedure
- ➔ *CPT Changes: An Insider's View* 2015

(Do not report 88365, 88366 in conjunction with 88367, 88368, 88374, 88377 for the same probe)

88367 Morphometric analysis, in situ hybridization (quantitative or semi-quantitative), using computer-assisted technology, per specimen; initial single probe stain procedure
- ➔ *CPT Changes: An Insider's View* 2005, 2015
- ➔ *CPT Assistant* Mar 05:16, Oct 10:9, Dec 11:18, May 12:5, Sep 13:3

#+ 88373 each additional single probe stain procedure (List separately in addition to code for primary procedure)
- ➔ *CPT Changes: An Insider's View* 2015

(Use 88373 in conjunction with 88367)

 # 88374 each multiplex probe stain procedure
- ➔ *CPT Changes: An Insider's View* 2015

(Do not report 88367, 88374 in conjunction with 88365, 88366, 88368, 88377 for the same probe)

88368 Morphometric analysis, in situ hybridization (quantitative or semi-quantitative), manual, per specimen; initial single probe stain procedure
- ➔ *CPT Changes: An Insider's View* 2005, 2015
- ➔ *CPT Assistant* Mar 05:16, Oct 10:9, Dec 11:18, May 12:5, Sep 13:3

+ 88369 each additional single probe stain procedure (List separately in addition to code for primary procedure)
- ➔ *CPT Changes: An Insider's View* 2015

(Use 88369 in conjunction with 88368)

 # 88377 each multiplex probe stain procedure
- ➔ *CPT Changes: An Insider's View* 2015

(Do not report 88368 or 88377 in conjunction with 88365, 88366, 88367, 88374 for the same probe)

(For morphometric in situ hybridization evaluation of urinary tract cytologic specimens, see 88120, 88121)

88371 Protein analysis of tissue by Western Blot, with interpretation and report;
- ➔ *CPT Assistant* Dec 11:18, Dec 15:17

88372 immunological probe for band identification, each
- ➔ *CPT Assistant* Dec 11:8

88373 Code is out of numerical sequence. See 88334-88372

88374 Code is out of numerical sequence. See 88334-88372

88375 Optical endomicroscopic image(s), interpretation and report, real-time or referred, each endoscopic session
- ➔ *CPT Changes: An Insider's View* 2013
- ➔ *CPT Assistant* Aug 13:5

(Do not report 88375 in conjunction with 43206, 43252, 0397T)

88377 Code is out of numerical sequence. See 88334-88372

88380 Microdissection (ie, sample preparation of microscopically identified target); laser capture
- ➔ *CPT Changes: An Insider's View* 2002, 2008
- ➔ *CPT Assistant* Apr 02:17, Apr 08:5, Dec 11:18, May 12:8, 10, Sep 13:3

88381 manual
- ➔ *CPT Changes: An Insider's View* 2008
- ➔ *CPT Assistant* Apr 08:5, Dec 11:18, May 12:8, 10, Sep 13:3

(Do not report 88380 in conjunction with 88381)

88387 Macroscopic examination, dissection, and preparation of tissue for non-microscopic analytical studies (eg, nucleic acid-based molecular studies); each tissue preparation (eg, a single lymph node)
- ➔ *CPT Changes: An Insider's View* 2010
- ➔ *CPT Assistant* Dec 11:18

(Do not report 88387 for tissue preparation for microbiologic cultures or flow cytometric studies)

(Do not report 88387 in conjunction with 88388, 88329-88334)

+ 88388 in conjunction with a touch imprint, intraoperative consultation, or frozen section, each tissue preparation (eg, a single lymph node) (List separately in addition to code for primary procedure)
- ➔ *CPT Changes: An Insider's View* 2010
- ➔ *CPT Assistant* Dec 11:18

(Use 88388 in conjunction with 88329-88334)

(Do not report 88387 or 88388 for tissue preparation for microbiologic cultures or flow cytometric studies)

88399 Unlisted surgical pathology procedure
- ➔ *CPT Assistant* Jun 14:15

In Vivo (eg, Transcutaneous) Laboratory Procedures

(For all in vivo measurements not specifically listed, use 88749)

(For wavelength fluorescent spectroscopy of advanced glycation end products [skin], use 88749)

(For transcutaneous oxyhemoglobin measurement in a lower extremity wound by near infrared spectroscopy, use 0493T)

88720 Bilirubin, total, transcutaneous
➔ *CPT Changes: An Insider's View* 2009
➔ *CPT Assistant* Dec 10:10

(For transdermal oxygen saturation, see 94760-94762)

88738 Hemoglobin (Hgb), quantitative, transcutaneous
➔ *CPT Changes: An Insider's View* 2010

(For in vitro hemoglobin measurement, use 85018)

88740 Hemoglobin, quantitative, transcutaneous, per day; carboxyhemoglobin
➔ *CPT Changes: An Insider's View* 2009

(For in vitro carboxyhemoglobin measurement, use 82375)

88741 methemoglobin
➔ *CPT Changes: An Insider's View* 2009

(For in vitro quantitative methemoglobin determination, use 83050)

88749 Unlisted in vivo (eg, transcutaneous) laboratory service
➔ *CPT Changes: An Insider's View* 2011
➔ *CPT Assistant* Oct 10:10, Dec 10:10

Other Procedures

89049 Caffeine halothane contracture test (CHCT) for malignant hyperthermia susceptibility, including interpretation and report
➔ *CPT Changes: An Insider's View* 2006
➔ *CPT Assistant* Mar 06:6, May 06:19, Sep 11:4

89050 Cell count, miscellaneous body fluids (eg, cerebrospinal fluid, joint fluid), except blood;
➔ *CPT Changes: An Insider's View* 2002
➔ *CPT Assistant* Aug 05:9, Sep 11:4

89051 with differential count
➔ *CPT Assistant* Sep 11:4

89055 Leukocyte assessment, fecal, qualitative or semiquantitative
➔ *CPT Changes: An Insider's View* 2003, 2004
➔ *CPT Assistant* Jul 03:9, Sep 11:4

89060 Crystal identification by light microscopy with or without polarizing lens analysis, tissue or any body fluid (except urine)
➔ *CPT Changes: An Insider's View* 2007
➔ *CPT Assistant* Sep 11:4

(Do not report 89060 for crystal identification on paraffin-embedded tissue)

89125 Fat stain, feces, urine, or respiratory secretions
➔ *CPT Changes: An Insider's View* 2001
➔ *CPT Assistant* Sep 11:4

89160 Meat fibers, feces
➔ *CPT Assistant* Sep 11:4

89190 Nasal smear for eosinophils
➔ *CPT Assistant* Sep 11:4

(Occult blood, feces, use 82270)

(Paternity tests, use 86910)

89220 Sputum, obtaining specimen, aerosol induced technique (separate procedure)
➔ *CPT Changes: An Insider's View* 2004
➔ *CPT Assistant* Aug 05:9, Sep 11:4

89230 Sweat collection by iontophoresis
➔ *CPT Changes: An Insider's View* 2004
➔ *CPT Assistant* Sep 11:4

89240 Unlisted miscellaneous pathology test
➔ *CPT Changes: An Insider's View* 2004
➔ *CPT Assistant* Nov 05:14, Jan 07:30, Sep 11:4

Reproductive Medicine Procedures

89250 Culture of oocyte(s)/embryo(s), less than 4 days;
➔ *CPT Changes: An Insider's View* 2004
➔ *CPT Assistant* Nov 97:35-36, Jan 98:6, Oct 98:1, Apr 04:2, May 04:16, Jun 04:9, Sep 11:4

89251 with co-culture of oocyte(s)/embryos
➔ *CPT Changes: An Insider's View* 2004
➔ *CPT Assistant* Nov 97:35-36, Jan 98:6, Oct 98:1, Apr 04:2

(For extended culture of oocyte[s]/embryo[s], see 89272)

89253 Assisted embryo hatching, microtechniques (any method)
➔ *CPT Assistant* Nov 97:35-36, Jan 98:6, Oct 98:1, Apr 04:2, May 04:16, Jun 04:9

89254 Oocyte identification from follicular fluid
➔ *CPT Assistant* Nov 97:35-36, Jan 98:6, Oct 98:1, Apr 04:2, May 04:16, Jun 04:9

89255 Preparation of embryo for transfer (any method)
➔ *CPT Assistant* Nov 97:35-36, Jan 98:6, Oct 98:1, Apr 04:2, May 04:16, Jun 04:9

89257 Sperm identification from aspiration (other than seminal fluid)
➔ *CPT Assistant* Nov 97:35-36, Jan 98:6, Oct 98:1, Nov 98:30, Apr 04:2

(For semen analysis, see 89300-89320)

(For sperm identification from testis tissue, use 89264)

89258 Cryopreservation; embryo(s)
➔ *CPT Changes: An Insider's View* 2004
➔ *CPT Assistant* Nov 97:36, Jan 98:6, Oct 98:1, Apr 04:2, 4

89259 sperm
➔ *CPT Assistant* Nov 97:36, Jan 98:6, Oct 98:1, Apr 04:2, 4

(For cryopreservation of reproductive tissue, testicular, use 89335)

89260 Sperm isolation; simple prep (eg, sperm wash and swim-up) for insemination or diagnosis with semen analysis
➔ *CPT Assistant* Nov 97:36, Jan 98:6, Oct 98:1, Apr 04:3-4

89261 complex prep (eg, Percoll gradient, albumin gradient) for insemination or diagnosis with semen analysis
CPT Assistant Nov 97:36, Jan 98:6, Oct 98:1, Apr 04:3-4

(For semen analysis without sperm wash or swim-up, use 89320)

89264 Sperm identification from testis tissue, fresh or cryopreserved
CPT Assistant Nov 98:30, Apr 04:3-4

(For biopsy of testis, see 54500, 54505)

(For sperm identification from aspiration, use 89257)

(For semen analysis, see 89300-89320)

89268 Insemination of oocytes
CPT Changes: An Insider's View 2004
CPT Assistant Apr 04:3-4

89272 Extended culture of oocyte(s)/embryo(s), 4-7 days
CPT Changes: An Insider's View 2004
CPT Assistant Apr 04:3-4

89280 Assisted oocyte fertilization, microtechnique; less than or equal to 10 oocytes
CPT Changes: An Insider's View 2004
CPT Assistant Apr 04:3-4

89281 greater than 10 oocytes
CPT Changes: An Insider's View 2004
CPT Assistant Apr 04:3-4

89290 Biopsy, oocyte polar body or embryo blastomere, microtechnique (for pre-implantation genetic diagnosis); less than or equal to 5 embryos
CPT Changes: An Insider's View 2004
CPT Assistant Apr 04:5

89291 greater than 5 embryos
CPT Changes: An Insider's View 2004
CPT Assistant Apr 04:3, 5

89300 Semen analysis; presence and/or motility of sperm including Huhner test (post coital)
CPT Assistant Nov 97:36, Jul 98:10, Oct 98:4, Apr 04:3, Aug 05:9

89310 motility and count (not including Huhner test)
CPT Changes: An Insider's View 2003
CPT Assistant Jul 03:9, Apr 04:3

89320 volume, count, motility, and differential
CPT Changes: An Insider's View 2008
CPT Assistant Apr 04:3, Apr 08:5

(Skin tests, see 86485-86580 and 95012-95199)

89321 sperm presence and motility of sperm, if performed
CPT Changes: An Insider's View 2001, 2008

(To report Hyaluronan binding assay [HBA], use 89398)

89322 volume, count, motility, and differential using strict morphologic criteria (eg, Kruger)
CPT Changes: An Insider's View 2008
CPT Assistant Apr 08:5

89325 Sperm antibodies

(For medicolegal identification of sperm, use 88125)

89329 Sperm evaluation; hamster penetration test

89330 cervical mucus penetration test, with or without spinnbarkeit test
CPT Assistant Nov 05:14

89331 Sperm evaluation, for retrograde ejaculation, urine (sperm concentration, motility, and morphology, as indicated)
CPT Changes: An Insider's View 2008
CPT Assistant Apr 08:5

(For semen analysis on concurrent semen specimen, see 89300-89322 in conjunction with 89331)

(For detection of sperm in urine, use 81015)

89335 Cryopreservation, reproductive tissue, testicular
CPT Changes: An Insider's View 2004
CPT Assistant Apr 04:5

(For cryopreservation of embryo[s], use 89258. For cryopreservation of sperm, use 89259)

(For cryopreservation, ovarian tissue, oocytes, use 0058T; for mature oocytes, use 89337; for immature oocytes, use 0357T)

89337 Cryopreservation, mature oocyte(s)
CPT Changes: An Insider's View 2015

(For cryopreservation of immature oocyte[s], use 0357T)

89342 Storage (per year); embryo(s)
CPT Changes: An Insider's View 2004
CPT Assistant Apr 04:5

89343 sperm/semen
CPT Changes: An Insider's View 2004
CPT Assistant Apr 04:5

89344 reproductive tissue, testicular/ovarian
CPT Changes: An Insider's View 2004
CPT Assistant Apr 04:5

89346 oocyte(s)
CPT Changes: An Insider's View 2004, 2005
CPT Assistant Apr 04:5

89352 Thawing of cryopreserved; embryo(s)
CPT Changes: An Insider's View 2004
CPT Assistant Apr 04:5

89353 sperm/semen, each aliquot
CPT Changes: An Insider's View 2004
CPT Assistant Apr 04:5

89354 reproductive tissue, testicular/ovarian
CPT Changes: An Insider's View 2004
CPT Assistant Apr 04:5

89356 oocytes, each aliquot
CPT Changes: An Insider's View 2004
CPT Assistant Apr 04:5, Aug 05:9

89398 Unlisted reproductive medicine laboratory procedure
CPT Changes: An Insider's View 2010

Proprietary Laboratory Analyses

Proprietary laboratory analyses (PLA) codes describe proprietary clinical laboratory analyses and can be either provided by a single ("sole-source") laboratory or licensed or marketed to multiple providing laboratories (eg, cleared or approved by the Food and Drug Administration [FDA]).

This subsection includes advanced diagnostic laboratory tests (ADLTs) and clinical diagnostic laboratory tests (CDLTs), as defined under the Protecting Access to Medicare Act (PAMA) of 2014. These analyses may include a range of medical laboratory tests including, but not limited to, multianalyte assays with algorithmic analyses (MAAA) and genomic sequencing procedures (GSP). The descriptor nomenclature follows, where possible, existing code conventions (eg, MAAA, GSP).

These codes are not required to fulfill the Category I criteria. The standards for inclusion in this section are:

- The test must be commercially available in the United States for use on human specimens and
- The clinical laboratory or manufacturer that offers the test must request the code.

For similar laboratory analyses that fulfill Category I criteria, see codes listed in the numeric 80000 series.

When a PLA code is available to report a given proprietary laboratory service, that PLA code takes precedence. The service should not be reported with any other CPT code(s) and other CPT code(s) should not be used to report services that may be reported with that specific PLA code. These codes encompass all analytical services required for the analysis (eg, cell lysis, nucleic acid stabilization, extraction, digestion, amplification, hybridization and detection). For molecular analyses, additional procedures that are required prior to cell lysis (eg, microdissection [codes 88380 and 88381]) may be reported separately.

Codes in this subsection are released on a quarterly basis to expedite dissemination for reporting. PLA codes will be published electronically on the AMA CPT website (www.ama-assn.org/practice-management/cpt-pla-codes), distributed via CPT data files on a quarterly basis, and, at a minimum, made available in print annually in the CPT codebook. Go to www.ama-assn.org/sites/default/files/media-browser/public/physicians/cpt/cpt-pla-codes-long.pdf for the most current listing.

All codes that are included in this section are also included in Appendix O, with the procedure's proprietary name. In order to report a PLA code, the analysis performed must fulfill the code descriptor and must be the test represented by the proprietary name listed in Appendix O. In some instances, the descriptor language of PLA codes may be identical and the code may only be differentiated by the listed proprietary name in Appendix O. When more than one PLA has an identical descriptor, the codes will be denoted by the symbol "Ӿ."

0001U Red blood cell antigen typing, DNA, human erythrocyte antigen gene analysis of 35 antigens from 11 blood groups, utilizing whole blood, common RBC alleles reported

➔ *CPT Changes: An Insider's View* 2018

0002U Oncology (colorectal), quantitative assessment of three urine metabolites (ascorbic acid, succinic acid and carnitine) by liquid chromatography with tandem mass spectrometry (LC-MS/MS) using multiple reaction monitoring acquisition, algorithm reported as likelihood of adenomatous polyps

➔ *CPT Changes: An Insider's View* 2018

0003U Oncology (ovarian) biochemical assays of five proteins (apolipoprotein A-1, CA 125 II, follicle stimulating hormone, human epididymis protein 4, transferrin), utilizing serum, algorithm reported as a likelihood score

➔ *CPT Changes: An Insider's View* 2018

►(0004U has been deleted)◄

0005U Oncology (prostate) gene expression profile by real-time RT-PCR of 3 genes *(ERG, PCA3, and SPDEF),* urine, algorithm reported as risk score

➔ *CPT Changes: An Insider's View* 2018

▲ **0006U** Detection of interacting medications, substances, supplements and foods, 120 or more analytes, definitive chromatography with mass spectrometry, urine, description and severity of each interaction identified, per date of service

➔ *CPT Changes: An Insider's View* 2018, 2019

Ӿ **0007U** Drug test(s), presumptive, with definitive confirmation of positive results, any number of drug classes, urine, includes specimen verification including DNA authentication in comparison to buccal DNA, per date of service

➔ *CPT Changes: An Insider's View* 2018

►(For additional PLA code with identical clinical descriptor, see 0020U. See Appendix O to determine appropriate code assignment)◄

0008U Helicobacter pylori detection and antibiotic resistance, DNA, 16S and 23S rRNA, gyrA, pbp1, rdxA and rpoB, next generation sequencing, formalin-fixed paraffin-embedded or fresh tissue, predictive, reported as positive or negative for resistance to clarithromycin, fluoroquinolones, metronidazole, amoxicillin, tetracycline and rifabutin

➔ *CPT Changes: An Insider's View* 2018

0009U Oncology (breast cancer), *ERBB2* (HER2) copy number by FISH, tumor cells from formalin-fixed paraffin-embedded tissue isolated using image-based dielectrophoresis (DEP) sorting, reported as *ERBB2* gene amplified or non-amplified

➔ *CPT Changes: An Insider's View* 2018

0010U Infectious disease (bacterial), strain typing by whole genome sequencing, phylogenetic-based report of strain relatedness, per submitted isolate
CPT Changes: An Insider's View 2018

0011U Prescription drug monitoring, evaluation of drugs present by LC-MS/MS, using oral fluid, reported as a comparison to an estimated steady-state range, per date of service including all drug compounds and metabolites
CPT Changes: An Insider's View 2018

0012U Germline disorders, gene rearrangement detection by whole genome next-generation sequencing, DNA, whole blood, report of specific gene rearrangement(s)
CPT Changes: An Insider's View 2018

0013U Oncology (solid organ neoplasia), gene rearrangement detection by whole genome next-generation sequencing, DNA, fresh or frozen tissue or cells, report of specific gene rearrangement(s)
CPT Changes: An Insider's View 2018

0014U Hematology (hematolymphoid neoplasia), gene rearrangement detection by whole genome next-generation sequencing, DNA, whole blood or bone marrow, report of specific gene rearrangement(s)
CPT Changes: An Insider's View 2018

►(0015U has been deleted)◄

0016U Oncology (hematolymphoid neoplasia), RNA, *BCR/ABL1* major and minor breakpoint fusion transcripts, quantitative PCR amplification, blood or bone marrow, report of fusion not detected or detected with quantitation
CPT Changes: An Insider's View 2018

0017U Oncology (hematolymphoid neoplasia), *JAK2* mutation, DNA, PCR amplification of exons 12-14 and sequence analysis, blood or bone marrow, report of *JAK2* mutation not detected or detected
CPT Changes: An Insider's View 2018

● **0018U** Oncology (thyroid), microRNA profiling by RT-PCR of 10 microRNA sequences, utilizing fine needle aspirate, algorithm reported as a positive or negative result for moderate to high risk of malignancy
CPT Changes: An Insider's View 2019

● **0019U** Oncology, RNA, gene expression by whole transcriptome sequencing, formalin-fixed paraffin-embedded tissue or fresh frozen tissue, predictive algorithm reported as potential targets for therapeutic agents
CPT Changes: An Insider's View 2019

⋊● **0020U** Drug test(s), presumptive, with definitive confirmation of positive results, any number of drug classes, urine, with specimen verification including DNA authentication in comparison to buccal DNA, per date of service
CPT Changes: An Insider's View 2019

►(For additional PLA code with identical clinical descriptor, see 0007U. See Appendix O to determine appropriate code assignment)◄

● **0021U** Oncology (prostate), detection of 8 autoantibodies (ARF 6, NKX3-1, 5'-UTR-BMI1, CEP 164, 3'-UTR-Ropporin, Desmocollin, AURKAIP-1, CSNK2A2), multiplexed immunoassay and flow cytometry serum, algorithm reported as risk score
CPT Changes: An Insider's View 2019

● **0022U** Targeted genomic sequence analysis panel, non-small cell lung neoplasia, DNA and RNA analysis, 23 genes, interrogation for sequence variants and rearrangements, reported as presence/absence of variants and associated therapy(ies) to consider
CPT Changes: An Insider's View 2019

● **0023U** Oncology (acute myelogenous leukemia), DNA, genotyping of internal tandem duplication, p.D835, p.I836, using mononuclear cells, reported as detection or non-detection of *FLT3* mutation and indication for or against the use of midostaurin
CPT Changes: An Insider's View 2019

● **0024U** Glycosylated acute phase proteins (GlycA), nuclear magnetic resonance spectroscopy, quantitative
CPT Changes: An Insider's View 2019

● **0025U** Tenofovir, by liquid chromatography with tandem mass spectrometry (LC-MS/MS), urine, quantitative
CPT Changes: An Insider's View 2019

● **0026U** Oncology (thyroid), DNA and mRNA of 112 genes, next-generation sequencing, fine needle aspirate of thyroid nodule, algorithmic analysis reported as a categorical result ("Positive, high probability of malignancy" or "Negative, low probability of malignancy")
CPT Changes: An Insider's View 2019

● **0027U** *JAK2 (Janus kinase 2)* (eg, myeloproliferative disorder) gene analysis, targeted sequence analysis exons 12-15
CPT Changes: An Insider's View 2019

● **0028U** *CYP2D6 (cytochrome P450, family 2, subfamily D, polypeptide 6)* (eg, drug metabolism) gene analysis, copy number variants, common variants with reflex to targeted sequence analysis
CPT Changes: An Insider's View 2019

● **0029U** Drug metabolism (adverse drug reactions and drug response), targeted sequence analysis (ie, *CYP1A2, CYP2C19, CYP2C9, CYP2D6, CYP3A4, CYP3A5, CYP4F2, SLCO1B1, VKORC1* and rs12777823)
CPT Changes: An Insider's View 2019

● **0030U** Drug metabolism (warfarin drug response), targeted sequence analysis (ie, *CYP2C9, CYP4F2, VKORC1*, rs12777823)
CPT Changes: An Insider's View 2019

● **0031U** *CYP1A2 (cytochrome P450 family 1, subfamily A, member 2)* (eg, drug metabolism) gene analysis, common variants (ie, *1F, *1K, *6, *7)
CPT Changes: An Insider's View 2019

● **0032U** *COMT (catechol-O-methyltransferase)* (eg, drug metabolism) gene analysis, c.472G>A (rs4680) variant
CPT Changes: An Insider's View 2019

Pathology and Laboratory 80047-89398, 0001U-0061U

● **0033U** *HTR2A (5-hydroxytryptamine receptor 2A), HTR2C (5-hydroxytryptamine receptor 2C)* (eg, citalopram metabolism) gene analysis, common variants (ie, *HTR2A* rs7997012 [c.614-2211T>C], *HTR2C* rs3813929 [c.-759C>T] and rs1414334 [c.551-3008C>G])

➔ *CPT Changes: An Insider's View* 2019

● **0034U** *TPMT (thiopurine S-methyltransferase), NUDT15 (nudix hydroxylase 15)* (eg, thiopurine metabolism) gene analysis, common variants (ie, *TPMT* *2, *3A, *3B, *3C, *4, *5, *6, *8, *12; *NUDT15* *3, *4, *5)

➔ *CPT Changes: An Insider's View* 2019

● **0035U** Neurology (prion disease), cerebrospinal fluid, detection of prion protein by quaking-induced conformational conversion, qualitative

➔ *CPT Changes: An Insider's View* 2019

● **0036U** Exome (ie, somatic mutations), paired formalin-fixed paraffin-embedded tumor tissue and normal specimen, sequence analyses

➔ *CPT Changes: An Insider's View* 2019

● **0037U** Targeted genomic sequence analysis, solid organ neoplasm, DNA analysis of 324 genes, interrogation for sequence variants, gene copy number amplifications, gene rearrangements, microsatellite instability and tumor mutational burden

➔ *CPT Changes: An Insider's View* 2019

● **0038U** Vitamin D, 25 hydroxy D2 and D3, by LC-MS/MS, serum microsample, quantitative

➔ *CPT Changes: An Insider's View* 2019

● **0039U** Deoxyribonucleic acid (DNA) antibody, double stranded, high avidity

➔ *CPT Changes: An Insider's View* 2019

● **0040U** *BCR/ABL1 (t(9;22))* (eg, chronic myelogenous leukemia) translocation analysis, major breakpoint, quantitative

➔ *CPT Changes: An Insider's View* 2019

● **0041U** Borrelia burgdorferi, antibody detection of 5 recombinant protein groups, by immunoblot, IgM

➔ *CPT Changes: An Insider's View* 2019

● **0042U** Borrelia burgdorferi, antibody detection of 12 recombinant protein groups, by immunoblot, IgG

➔ *CPT Changes: An Insider's View* 2019

● **0043U** Tick-borne relapsing fever Borrelia group, antibody detection to 4 recombinant protein groups, by immunoblot, IgM

➔ *CPT Changes: An Insider's View* 2019

● **0044U** Tick-borne relapsing fever Borrelia group, antibody detection to 4 recombinant protein groups, by immunoblot, IgG

➔ *CPT Changes: An Insider's View* 2019

● **0045U** Oncology (breast ductal carcinoma in situ), mRNA, gene expression profiling by real-time RT-PCR of 12 genes (7 content and 5 housekeeping), utilizing formalin-fixed paraffin-embedded tissue, algorithm reported as recurrence score

➔ *CPT Changes: An Insider's View* 2019

● **0046U** *FLT3 (fms-related tyrosine kinase 3)* (eg, acute myeloid leukemia) internal tandem duplication (ITD) variants, quantitative

➔ *CPT Changes: An Insider's View* 2019

● **0047U** Oncology (prostate), mRNA, gene expression profiling by real-time RT-PCR of 17 genes (12 content and 5 housekeeping), utilizing formalin-fixed paraffin-embedded tissue, algorithm reported as a risk score

➔ *CPT Changes: An Insider's View* 2019

● **0048U** Oncology (solid organ neoplasia), DNA, targeted sequencing of protein-coding exons of 468 cancer-associated genes, including interrogation for somatic mutations and microsatellite instability, matched with normal specimens, utilizing formalin-fixed paraffin-embedded tumor tissue, report of clinically significant mutation(s)

➔ *CPT Changes: An Insider's View* 2019

● **0049U** *NPM1 (nucleophosmin)* (eg, acute myeloid leukemia) gene analysis, quantitative

➔ *CPT Changes: An Insider's View* 2019

● **0050U** Targeted genomic sequence analysis panel, acute myelogenous leukemia, DNA analysis, 194 genes, interrogation for sequence variants, copy number variants or rearrangements

➔ *CPT Changes: An Insider's View* 2019

● **0051U** Prescription drug monitoring, evaluation of drugs present by LC-MS/MS, urine, 31 drug panel, reported as quantitative results, detected or not detected, per date of service

➔ *CPT Changes: An Insider's View* 2019

● **0052U** Lipoprotein, blood, high resolution fractionation and quantitation of lipoproteins, including all five major lipoprotein classes and subclasses of HDL, LDL, and VLDL by vertical auto profile ultracentrifugation

➔ *CPT Changes: An Insider's View* 2019

● **0053U** Oncology (prostate cancer), FISH analysis of 4 genes *(ASAP1, HDAC9, CHD1* and *PTEN)*, needle biopsy specimen, algorithm reported as probability of higher tumor grade

➔ *CPT Changes: An Insider's View* 2019

● **0054U** Prescription drug monitoring, 14 or more classes of drugs and substances, definitive tandem mass spectrometry with chromatography, capillary blood, quantitative report with therapeutic and toxic ranges, including steady-state range for the prescribed dose when detected, per date of service

➔ *CPT Changes: An Insider's View* 2019

● **0055U** Cardiology (heart transplant), cell-free DNA, PCR assay of 96 DNA target sequences (94 single nucleotide polymorphism targets and two control targets), plasma

➔ *CPT Changes: An Insider's View* 2019

● **0056U** Hematology (acute myelogenous leukemia), DNA, whole genome next-generation sequencing to detect gene rearrangement(s), blood or bone marrow, report of specific gene rearrangement(s)

➔ *CPT Changes: An Insider's View* 2019

● **0057U** Oncology (solid organ neoplasia), mRNA, gene expression profiling by massively parallel sequencing for analysis of 51 genes, utilizing formalin-fixed paraffin-embedded tissue, algorithm reported as a normalized percentile rank

➔ *CPT Changes: An Insider's View* 2019

● **0058U** Oncology (Merkel cell carcinoma), detection of antibodies to the Merkel cell polyoma virus oncoprotein (small T antigen), serum, quantitative

➔ *CPT Changes: An Insider's View* 2019

● **0059U** Oncology (Merkel cell carcinoma), detection of antibodies to the Merkel cell polyoma virus capsid protein (VP1), serum, reported as positive or negative

➔ *CPT Changes: An Insider's View* 2019

● **0060U** Twin zygosity, genomic-targeted sequence analysis of chromosome 2, using circulating cell-free fetal DNA in maternal blood

➔ *CPT Changes: An Insider's View* 2019

● **0061U** Transcutaneous measurement of five biomarkers (tissue oxygenation [StO_2], oxyhemoglobin [$ctHbO_2$], deoxyhemoglobin [ctHbR], papillary and reticular dermal hemoglobin concentrations [ctHb1 and ctHb2]), using spatial frequency domain imaging (SFDI) and multi-spectral analysis

➔ *CPT Changes: An Insider's View* 2019

Notes

Medicine Guidelines

Add-on Codes....631
Separate Procedures....631
Unlisted Service or Procedure....631
Special Report....632
Imaging Guidance....632
Supplied Materials....632

Medicine

The following is a listing of headings and subheadings that appear within the Medicine section of the CPT codebook. The subheadings or subsections denoted with asterisks (*) below have special instructions unique to that subsection. Where these are indicated, special notes or guidelines will be presented preceding those procedural terminology listings, referring to that subsection specifically.

Immune Globulins, Serum or Recombinant Products* (90281-90399)....633
Immunization Administration for Vaccines/Toxoids* (90460-90474)....633
Vaccines, Toxoids* (90476-90756)....634
Psychiatry* (90785-90899)....639
Interactive Complexity* (90785)....639
Psychiatric Diagnostic Procedures* (90791-90899)....640
Psychotherapy* (90832-90838)....640
Psychotherapy for Crisis* (90839-90840)....641
Other Psychotherapy (90845-90853)....642
Other Psychiatric Services or Procedures (90863-90899)....642
Biofeedback (90901-90911)....643
Dialysis (90935-90999)....643
Hemodialysis* (90935-90940)....643
Miscellaneous Dialysis Procedures* (90945-90947)....644
End-Stage Renal Disease Services* (90951-90970)....644
Other Dialysis Procedures (90989-90999)....646
Gastroenterology (91010-91299)....646
Gastric Physiology (91132-91133)....647
Other Procedures (91200-91299)....647
Ophthalmology* (92002-92499)....648
General Ophthalmological Services (92002-92014)....648
New Patient (92002-92004)....648
Established Patient (92012-92014)....648
Special Ophthalmological Services (92015-92287)....649
Ophthalmoscopy* (92225-92260)....650
Other Specialized Services* (92265-92287)....651
Contact Lens Services* (92310-92326)....652
Spectacle Services (Including Prosthesis for Aphakia)* (92340-92499)....652
Other Procedures (92499)....652
Special Otorhinolaryngologic Services* (92502-92700)....653
Vestibular Function Tests, Without Electrical Recording (92531-92534)....653
Vestibular Function Tests, With Recording (eg, ENG) (92537-92548)....654
Audiologic Function Tests* (92550-92596)....654
Evaluative and Therapeutic Services* (92597, 92601-92633)....655
Special Diagnostic Procedures (92640)....657

Other Procedures (92700) 657
Cardiovascular (92920-93799) **657**
Therapeutic Services and Procedures (92920-92998) 657
Other Therapeutic Services and Procedures (92950-92998) 658
Coronary Therapeutic Services and Procedures* (92920-92979) 658
Cardiography* (93000-93050) 661
Cardiovascular Monitoring Services* (93224-93278) 662
►Implantable, Insertable, and Wearable Cardiac Device Evaluations*◄ (93264, 93279-93299) 664
Echocardiography* (93303-93355) 669
Cardiac Catheterization* (93451-93592) 671
Injection Procedures* (93561-93572) 678
Repair of Structural Heart Defect (93580-93592) 679
Transcatheter Closure of Paravalvular Leak* (93590-93592) 680
Intracardiac Electrophysiological Procedures/Studies* (93600-93662) 681
Peripheral Arterial Disease Rehabilitation* (93668) 684
Noninvasive Physiologic Studies and Procedures (93701-93790) 684
Home and Outpatient International Normalized Ratio (INR) Monitoring Services* (93792-93793) 685
Other Procedures (93797-93799) 686
Noninvasive Vascular Diagnostic Studies* (93880-93998) **686**
Cerebrovascular Arterial Studies* (93880-93895) 686
Extremity Arterial Studies (Including Digits) (93922-93931) 687
Extremity Venous Studies (Including Digits) (93970-93971) 688
Visceral and Penile Vascular Studies (93975-93981) 688
Extremity Arterial-Venous Studies (93990) 688
Other Noninvasive Vascular Diagnostic Studies (93998) 688
Pulmonary (94002-94799) **689**
Ventilator Management (94002-94005) 689
Pulmonary Diagnostic Testing and Therapies* (94010-94799) 689
Allergy and Clinical Immunology* (95004-95199) **692**
Allergy Testing (95004-95071) 693
Ingestion Challenge Testing* (95076-95079) 693
Allergen Immunotherapy* (95115-95199) 694
Endocrinology* (95249-95251) **695**
Neurology and Neuromuscular Procedures* (95782-96020) **695**
Sleep Medicine Testing* (95782, 95783, 95800-95811) 695
Routine Electroencephalography (EEG)* (95812-95827, 95830) 697
►Electrocorticography*◄ (95829, 95836) 698
Muscle and Range of Motion Testing (95831-95834, 95851-95857) 698
Electromyography* (95860-95872, 95885-95887) 698
Ischemic Muscle Testing and Guidance for Chemodenervation (95873-95875) 700
Nerve Conduction Tests* (95905-95913) 700
Intraoperative Neurophysiology* (95940-95941) 701
Autonomic Function Tests* (95921-95924, 95943) 702
Evoked Potentials and Reflex Tests (95925-95939) 703
Special EEG Tests* (95950-95967) 703
Neurostimulators, Analysis-Programming* (95970-95984) 705
Other Procedures (95990-95999) 708
Motion Analysis* (96000-96004) 708

Functional Brain Mapping* (96020) 709
Medical Genetics and Genetic Counseling Services* (96040) 709
►Adaptive Behavior Services*◄ (97151-97158) 709
►Adaptive Behavior Assessments*◄ (97151-97152) 710
►Adaptive Behavior Treatment*◄ (97153-97158) 711
Central Nervous System Assessments/Tests (eg, Neuro-Cognitive, Mental Status, Speech Testing)* (96105-96146) 712
►Assessment of Aphasia and Cognitive Performance Testing◄ (96105, 96125) 715
►Developmental/Behavioral Screening and Testing◄ (96110-96113, 96127) 715
►Psychological/Neuropsychological Testing◄ (96116, 96121, 96130-96139, 96146) 715
►Neurobehavioral Status Examination◄ (96116, 96121) 715
►Testing Evaluation Services◄ (96130-96133) 715
►Test Administration and Scoring◄ (96136-96139) 716
►Automated Testing and Result◄ (96146) 716
Health and Behavior Assessment/Intervention* (96150-96161) 716
Hydration, Therapeutic, Prophylactic, Diagnostic Injections and Infusions, and Chemotherapy and Other Highly Complex Drug or Highly Complex Biologic Agent Administration* (96360-96549) 717
Hydration* (96360-96361) 718
Therapeutic, Prophylactic, and Diagnostic Injections and Infusions (Excludes Chemotherapy and Other Highly Complex Drug or Highly Complex Biologic Agent Administration)* (96365-96379) 719
Chemotherapy and Other Highly Complex Drug or Highly Complex Biologic Agent Administration* (96401-96549) 720
Injection and Intravenous Infusion Chemotherapy and Other Highly Complex Drug or Highly Complex Biologic Agent Administration* (96401-96417) 721
Intra-Arterial Chemotherapy and Other Highly Complex Drug or Highly Complex Biologic Agent Administration (96420-96425) 722
Other Injection and Infusion Services* (96440-96549) 722
Photodynamic Therapy* (96567-96574) 722
Special Dermatological Procedures* (96900-96999) 723
Physical Medicine and Rehabilitation* (97161-97799) 724
Physical Therapy Evaluations* (97161-97164) 724
Occupational Therapy Evaluations* (97165-97168) 726
Athletic Training Evaluations* (97169-97172) 727
Modalities* (97010-97039) 728
Supervised* (97010-97028) 728
Constant Attendance* (97032-97039) 728
Therapeutic Procedures* (97110-97150, 97530-97546) 729
Active Wound Care Management* (97597-97610) 730
Tests and Measurements* (97750-97755) 731
Orthotic Management and Training and Prosthetic Training (97760-97763) 731
Other Procedures (97799) 731
Medical Nutrition Therapy (97802-97804) 731
Acupuncture* (97810-97814) 731
Osteopathic Manipulative Treatment* (98925-98929) 732
Chiropractic Manipulative Treatment* (98940-98943) 732
Education and Training for Patient Self-Management* (98960-98962) 733

Non-Face-to-Face Nonphysician Services (98966-98969) 734
Telephone Services* (98966-98968) 734
On-line Medical Evaluation* (98969) 734
Special Services, Procedures and Reports* (99000-99082) 734
Miscellaneous Services (99000-99082) 735
Qualifying Circumstances for Anesthesia (99100-99140) 736
Moderate (Conscious) Sedation* (99151-99157) 736
Other Services and Procedures (99170-99199) 738
Home Health Procedures/Services* (99500-99602) 739
Home Infusion Procedures/Services (99601-99602) 740
Medication Therapy Management Services* (99605-99607) 740

Medicine Guidelines

In addition to the definitions and commonly used terms presented in the **Introduction**, several other items unique to this section on **Medicine** are defined or identified here.

Add-on Codes

Some of the listed procedures are commonly carried out in addition to the primary procedure performed. All add-on codes found in the CPT codebook are exempt from the multiple procedure concept. They are exempt from the use of modifier 51, as these procedures are not reported as stand-alone codes. These additional or supplemental procedures are designated as "add-on" codes. Add-on codes in the CPT codebook can be readily identified by specific descriptor nomenclature which includes phrases such as "each additional" or "(List separately in addition to primary procedure)."

Separate Procedures

Some of the procedures or services listed in the CPT codebook that are commonly carried out as an integral component of a total service or procedure have been identified by the inclusion of the term "separate procedure." The codes designated as "separate procedure" should not be reported in addition to the code for the total procedure or service of which it is considered an integral component.

However, when a procedure or service that is designated as a "separate procedure" is carried out independently or considered to be unrelated or distinct from other procedures/services provided at that time, it may be reported by itself, or in addition to other procedures/services by appending modifier 59 to the specific "separate procedure" code to indicate that the procedure is not considered to be a component of another procedure, but is a distinct, independent procedure. This may represent a different session or patient encounter, different procedure or surgery, different site or organ system, separate incision/excision, separate lesion, or separate injury (or area of injury in extensive injuries).

Unlisted Service or Procedure

A service or procedure may be provided that is not listed in this edition of the CPT codebook. When reporting such a service, the appropriate "Unlisted Procedure" code may be used to indicate the service, identifying it by "Special Report" as discussed on the following page. The "Unlisted Procedures" and accompanying codes for **Medicine** are as follows:

90399	Unlisted immune globulin
90749	Unlisted vaccine/toxoid
90899	Unlisted psychiatric service or procedure
90999	Unlisted dialysis procedure, inpatient or outpatient
91299	Unlisted diagnostic gastroenterology procedure
92499	Unlisted ophthalmological service or procedure
92700	Unlisted otorhinolaryngological service or procedure
93799	Unlisted cardiovascular service or procedure
93998	Unlisted noninvasive vascular diagnostic study
94799	Unlisted pulmonary service or procedure
95199	Unlisted allergy/clinical immunologic service or procedure
95999	Unlisted neurological or neuromuscular diagnostic procedure
96379	Unlisted therapeutic, prophylactic, or diagnostic intravenous or intra-arterial injection or infusion
96549	Unlisted chemotherapy procedure
96999	Unlisted special dermatological service or procedure
97039	Unlisted modality (specify type and time if constant attendance)
97139	Unlisted therapeutic procedure (specify)
97799	Unlisted physical medicine/rehabilitation service or procedure
99199	Unlisted special service, procedure or report
99600	Unlisted home visit service or procedure

Special Report

A service that is rarely provided, unusual, variable, or new may require a special report. Pertinent information should include an adequate definition or description of the nature, extent, and need for the procedure; and the time, effort, and equipment necessary to provide the service.

Imaging Guidance

▶When imaging guidance or imaging supervision and interpretation is included in a procedure, guidelines for image documentation and report, included in the guidelines for Radiology (including Nuclear Medicine and Diagnostic Ultrasound) will apply. Imaging guidance should not be reported for use of a non-imaging guided tracking or localizing system (eg, radar signals, electromagnetic signals). Imaging guidance should only be reported when an imaging modality (eg, radiography, fluoroscopy, ultrasonography, magnetic resonance imaging, computed tomography, or nuclear medicine) is used and is appropriately documented.◀

Supplied Materials

Supplies and materials (eg, trays, drug supplies, and materials) over and above those usually included with the procedure(s) rendered are reported separately using code 99070 or a specific supply code.

Medicine

Immune Globulins, Serum or Recombinant Products

Codes 90281-90399 identify the serum globulins, extracted from human blood; or recombinant immune globulin products created in a laboratory through genetic modification of human and/or animal proteins. Both are reported in addition to the administration codes 96365, 96366, 96367, 96368, 96369, 96370, 96371, 96372, 96374, 96375, as appropriate. Modifier 51 should not be reported with this section of products codes when performed with another procedure. The serum or recombinant globulin products listed here include broad-spectrum anti-infective immune globulins, antitoxins, various isoantibodies, and monoclonal antibodies.

90281 Immune globulin (Ig), human, for intramuscular use
➲ *CPT Changes: An Insider's View* 2008
➲ *CPT Assistant* Nov 98:30, Jan 99:3, Sep 99:10

90283 Immune globulin (IgIV), human, for intravenous use
➲ *CPT Changes: An Insider's View* 2008
➲ *CPT Assistant* Nov 98:30, Jan 99:3

90284 Immune globulin (SCIg), human, for use in subcutaneous infusions, 100 mg, each
➲ *CPT Changes: An Insider's View* 2008

90287 Botulinum antitoxin, equine, any route
➲ *CPT Changes: An Insider's View* 2008
➲ *CPT Assistant* Nov 98:30, Jan 99:3

90288 Botulism immune globulin, human, for intravenous use
➲ *CPT Changes: An Insider's View* 2008
➲ *CPT Assistant* Nov 98:30, Jan 99:3

90291 Cytomegalovirus immune globulin (CMV-IgIV), human, for intravenous use
➲ *CPT Changes: An Insider's View* 2008
➲ *CPT Assistant* Nov 98:30, Jan 99:3

90296 Diphtheria antitoxin, equine, any route
➲ *CPT Changes: An Insider's View* 2008
➲ *CPT Assistant* Nov 98:30, Jan 99:3

90371 Hepatitis B immune globulin (HBIg), human, for intramuscular use
➲ *CPT Changes: An Insider's View* 2008
➲ *CPT Assistant* Nov 98:30, Jan 99:3

90375 Rabies immune globulin (RIg), human, for intramuscular and/or subcutaneous use
➲ *CPT Changes: An Insider's View* 2008
➲ *CPT Assistant* Nov 98:30, Jan 99:3

90376 Rabies immune globulin, heat-treated (RIg-HT), human, for intramuscular and/or subcutaneous use
➲ *CPT Changes: An Insider's View* 2008
➲ *CPT Assistant* Nov 98:30, Jan 99:3

90378 Respiratory syncytial virus, monoclonal antibody, recombinant, for intramuscular use, 50 mg, each
➲ *CPT Changes: An Insider's View* 2000, 2001, 2008, 2010
➲ *CPT Assistant* Jan 99:3, Nov 99:47, Jun 00:10

90384 Rho(D) immune globulin (RhIg), human, full-dose, for intramuscular use
➲ *CPT Changes: An Insider's View* 2008
➲ *CPT Assistant* Nov 98:30, Jan 99:3

90385 Rho(D) immune globulin (RhIg), human, mini-dose, for intramuscular use
➲ *CPT Changes: An Insider's View* 2008
➲ *CPT Assistant* Nov 98:30, Jan 99:3

90386 Rho(D) immune globulin (RhIgIV), human, for intravenous use
➲ *CPT Changes: An Insider's View* 2008
➲ *CPT Assistant* Nov 98:30, Jan 99:3

90389 Tetanus immune globulin (TIg), human, for intramuscular use
➲ *CPT Changes: An Insider's View* 2008
➲ *CPT Assistant* Nov 98:30, Jan 99:3

90393 Vaccinia immune globulin, human, for intramuscular use
➲ *CPT Changes: An Insider's View* 2008
➲ *CPT Assistant* Nov 98:30, Jan 99:3

90396 Varicella-zoster immune globulin, human, for intramuscular use
➲ *CPT Changes: An Insider's View* 2008
➲ *CPT Assistant* Nov 98:30, Jan 99:3

90399 Unlisted immune globulin
➲ *CPT Changes: An Insider's View* 2008
➲ *CPT Assistant* Nov 98:30, Jan 99:3, Feb 99:11, Sep 99:10

Immunization Administration for Vaccines/Toxoids

Report vaccine immunization administration codes 90460, 90461, 90471-90474 in addition to the vaccine and toxoid code(s) 90476-90749.

Report codes 90460 and 90461 only when the physician or qualified health care professional provides face-to-face counseling of the patient/family during the administration of a vaccine. For immunization administration of any vaccine that is not accompanied by face-to-face physician or qualified health care professional counseling to the patient/family or for administration of vaccines to patients over 18 years of age, report codes 90471-90474. (See also **Instructions for Use of the CPT Codebook** for definition of reporting qualifications.)

If a significant separately identifiable Evaluation and Management service (eg, new or established patient office or other outpatient services [99201-99215], office or other outpatient consultations [99241-99245], emergency department services [99281-99285], preventive medicine services [99381-99429]) is performed, the appropriate E/M service code should be reported in addition to the vaccine and toxoid administration codes.

A component refers to all antigens in a vaccine that prevent disease(s) caused by one organism (90460 and 90461). Multi-valent antigens or multiple serotypes of antigens against a single organism are considered a single component of vaccines. Combination vaccines are those vaccines that contain multiple vaccine components. Conjugates or adjuvants contained in vaccines are not considered to be component parts of the vaccine as defined above.

(For allergy testing, see 95004 et seq)

(For skin testing of bacterial, viral, fungal extracts, see 86485-86580)

(For therapeutic or diagnostic injections, see 96372-96379)

90460 Immunization administration through 18 years of age via any route of administration, with counseling by physician or other qualified health care professional; first or only component of each vaccine or toxoid administered

➲ *CPT Changes: An Insider's View* 2011, 2012

➲ *CPT Assistant* Mar 11:3, Jun 11:14, Jan 12:43, Jul 12:7, Aug 13:10, Mar 14:10, Apr 15:9, 11, May 15:6, Oct 16:7

+ 90461 each additional vaccine or toxoid component administered (List separately in addition to code for primary procedure)

➲ *CPT Changes: An Insider's View* 2011, 2012

➲ *CPT Assistant* Mar 11:3, Jun 11:14, Jan 12:43, Jul 12:7, Aug 13:10, Mar 14:10, Apr 15:4, May 15:6, Oct 16:7

(Use 90460 for each vaccine administered. For vaccines with multiple components [combination vaccines], report 90460 in conjunction with 90461 for each additional component in a given vaccine)

90471 Immunization administration (includes percutaneous, intradermal, subcutaneous, or intramuscular injections); 1 vaccine (single or combination vaccine/toxoid)

➲ *CPT Changes: An Insider's View* 2002, 2005

➲ *CPT Assistant* Nov 98:31, Jan 99:2, Apr 99:10, Oct 99:9, Nov 99:47-48, Nov 00:10, Feb 01:5, Jul 01:2, Nov 02:11, Mar 04:11, Apr 04:14, Apr 05:1-3, 5, Nov 05:1, Jan 09:8, Jul 09:7, Aug 09:9, Sep 09:7, Oct 09:3, Mar 11:3, Jun 11:14, Jul 12:7, Aug 13:10, Mar 14:10, Apr 15:9, 11, May 15:6, Oct 16:7

(Do not report 90471 in conjunction with 90473)

+ 90472 each additional vaccine (single or combination vaccine/toxoid) (List separately in addition to code for primary procedure)

➲ *CPT Changes: An Insider's View* 2000

➲ *CPT Assistant* Nov 98:31, Jan 99:2, Apr 99:10, Oct 99:9, Nov 99:47-48, Nov 00:10, Feb 01:5, Jul 01:2, Nov 02:11, Mar 04:11, Apr 04:14, Apr 05:1-3, Nov 05:1, Jan 09:3, 8, Jul 09:7, Aug 09:9, Sep 09:7, Oct 09:3, Mar 11:3, Jun 11:14, Jul 12:7, Aug 13:10, Mar 14:10, Apr 15:9, 11, May 15:6, Oct 16:7

(Use 90472 in conjunction with 90460, 90471, 90473)

(For immune globulins, see 90281-90399. For administration of immune globulins, see 96365, 96366, 96367, 96368, 96369, 96370, 96371, 96374)

(For intravesical administration of BCG vaccine, see 51720, 90586)

90473 Immunization administration by intranasal or oral route; 1 vaccine (single or combination vaccine/toxoid)

➲ *CPT Changes: An Insider's View* 2002

➲ *CPT Assistant* Feb 01:5, Nov 02:11, Apr 04:14, Apr 05:1-3, Jan 09:3, 8, Jul 09:7, Aug 09:9, Oct 09:3, Mar 11:3, Jun 11:14, Jul 12:7, Aug 13:10, Mar 14:10, Apr 15:9, May 15:6

(Do not report 90473 in conjunction with 90471)

+ 90474 each additional vaccine (single or combination vaccine/toxoid) (List separately in addition to code for primary procedure)

➲ *CPT Changes: An Insider's View* 2002

➲ *CPT Assistant* Feb 01:5, Nov 02:11, Apr 04:14, Apr 05:1-3, Jan 09:3, 8, Jul 09:7, Aug 09:9, Oct 09:3, Mar 11:3, Jun 11:14, Jul 12:7, Aug 13:10, Mar 14:10, Apr 15:9, May 15:6

(Use 90474 in conjunction with 90460, 90471, 90473)

Vaccines, Toxoids

To assist users to report the most recent new or revised vaccine product codes, the American Medical Association (AMA) currently uses the CPT website, which features updates of CPT Editorial Panel actions regarding these products. Once approved by the CPT Editorial Panel, these codes will be made available for release on a semi-annual (twice a year: July 1 and January 1) basis. As part of the electronic distribution, there is a six-month implementation period from the initial release date (ie, codes released on January 1 are eligible for use on July 1 and codes released on July 1 are eligible for use January 1).

The CPT Editorial Panel, in recognition of the public health interest in vaccine products, has chosen to publish new vaccine product codes prior to approval by the US Food and Drug Administration (FDA). These codes are indicated with the ⚡ symbol and will be tracked by the AMA to monitor FDA approval status. Once the FDA status changes to approval, the ⚡ symbol will be removed. CPT users should refer to the AMA CPT website (www.ama-assn.org/go/cpt-vaccine) for the most up-to-date information on codes with the ⚡ symbol.

Codes 90476-90749 identify the vaccine product **only**. To report the administration of a vaccine/toxoid, the vaccine/toxoid product codes 90476-90749 must be used in addition to an immunization administration code(s) 90460, 90461, 90471, 90472, 90473, 90474. Modifier 51 should not be reported with vaccine/toxoid codes 90476-90749, when reported in conjunction with administration codes 90460, 90461, 90471, 90472, 90473, 90474.

If a significantly separately identifiable Evaluation and Management (E/M) service (eg, office or other outpatient services, preventive medicine services) is performed, the appropriate E/M service code should be reported in addition to the vaccine and toxoid administration codes.

To meet the reporting requirements of immunization registries, vaccine distribution programs, and reporting systems (eg, Vaccine Adverse Event Reporting System) the exact vaccine product administered needs to be reported. Multiple codes for a particular vaccine are provided in the CPT codebook when the schedule (number of doses or timing) differs for two or more products of the same vaccine type (eg, hepatitis A, Hib) or the vaccine product is available in more than one chemical formulation, dosage, or route of administration.

The "when administered to" age descriptions included in CPT vaccine codes are not intended to identify a product's licensed age indication. The term "preservative free" includes use for vaccines that contain no preservative and vaccines that contain trace amounts of preservative agents that are not present in a sufficient concentration for the purpose of preserving the final vaccine formulation. The absence of a designation regarding a preservative does not necessarily indicate the presence or absence of preservative in the vaccine. Refer to the product's prescribing information (PI) for the licensed age indication before administering vaccine to a patient.

Separate codes are available for combination vaccines (eg, Hib-HepB, DTap-IPV/Hib). It is inappropriate to code each component of a combination vaccine separately. If a specific vaccine code is not available, the unlisted procedure code should be reported, until a new code becomes available.

The vaccine/toxoid abbreviations listed in codes 90476-90748 reflect the most recent US vaccine abbreviations references used in the Advisory Committee on Immunization Practices (ACIP) recommendations at the time of CPT code set publication. Interim updates to vaccine code descriptors will be made following abbreviation approval by the ACIP on a timely basis via the AMA CPT website (www.ama-assn.org/go/cpt-vaccine). The accuracy of the ACIP vaccine abbreviation designations in the CPT code set does not affect the validity of the vaccine code and its reporting function.

(For immune globulins, see 90281-90399. For administration of immune globulins, see 96365-96375)

90476 Adenovirus vaccine, type 4, live, for oral use
- *CPT Changes: An Insider's View* 2008
- *CPT Assistant* Nov 98:31-33, Jan 99:2, Sep 99:10, Oct 99:9, Nov 99:48, Mar 11:4, Aug 13:10, May 15:6, Oct 16:6

90477 Adenovirus vaccine, type 7, live, for oral use
- *CPT Changes: An Insider's View* 2008
- *CPT Assistant* Nov 98:31-33, Jan 99:2, Oct 99:9, Mar 11:4, Aug 13:10

90581 Anthrax vaccine, for subcutaneous or intramuscular use
- *CPT Changes: An Insider's View* 2008, 2012
- *CPT Assistant* Nov 98:31-33, Jan 99:2, Oct 99:9, Mar 11:4, Aug 13:10

90585 Bacillus Calmette-Guerin vaccine (BCG) for tuberculosis, live, for percutaneous use
- *CPT Changes: An Insider's View* 2008
- *CPT Assistant* Nov 98:31-33, Jan 99:2, Oct 99:9, Mar 11:4, Aug 13:10

90586 Bacillus Calmette-Guerin vaccine (BCG) for bladder cancer, live, for intravesical use
- *CPT Changes: An Insider's View* 2008
- *CPT Assistant* Nov 98:31-33, Jan 99:2, Oct 99:9, Nov 02:11, Mar 11:4, Aug 13:10

⚡ **90587** Dengue vaccine, quadrivalent, live, 3 dose schedule, for subcutaneous use
- *CPT Changes: An Insider's View* 2018

90620 Code is out of numerical sequence. See 90717-90739

90621 Code is out of numerical sequence. See 90717-90739

90625 Code is out of numerical sequence. See 90717-90739

90630 Code is out of numerical sequence. See 90653-90656

90632 Hepatitis A vaccine (HepA), adult dosage, for intramuscular use
- *CPT Changes: An Insider's View* 2008, 2016
- *CPT Assistant* Nov 98:31-33, Jan 99:2, Oct 99:9, Mar 11:4, Aug 13:10

90633 Hepatitis A vaccine (HepA), pediatric/adolescent dosage-2 dose schedule, for intramuscular use
- *CPT Changes: An Insider's View* 2008, 2016
- *CPT Assistant* Nov 98:31-33, Jan 99:2, Oct 99:9, Mar 11:4, Aug 13:10

90634 Hepatitis A vaccine (HepA), pediatric/adolescent dosage-3 dose schedule, for intramuscular use
- *CPT Changes: An Insider's View* 2008, 2016
- *CPT Assistant* Nov 98:31-33, Jan 99:2, Oct 99:9, Mar 11:4, Aug 13:10

90636 Hepatitis A and hepatitis B vaccine (HepA-HepB), adult dosage, for intramuscular use
- *CPT Changes: An Insider's View* 2008
- *CPT Assistant* Nov 98:31-33, Jan 99:2, Oct 99:9, Mar 11:4, Aug 13:10

90644 Code is out of numerical sequence. See 90717-90739

(90645 has been deleted)

(90646 has been deleted)

90647 Haemophilus influenzae type b vaccine (Hib), PRP-OMP conjugate, 3 dose schedule, for intramuscular use
- *CPT Changes: An Insider's View* 2008, 2016
- *CPT Assistant* Nov 98:31-33, Jan 99:2, Oct 99:9, Mar 11:4, Aug 13:10

90648 Haemophilus influenzae type b vaccine (Hib), PRP-T conjugate, 4 dose schedule, for intramuscular use
- *CPT Changes: An Insider's View* 2008, 2016
- *CPT Assistant* Nov 98:31-33, Jan 99:2, Oct 99:9, Sep 09:7, Mar 11:4, Aug 13:10

90649 Human Papillomavirus vaccine, types 6, 11, 16, 18, quadrivalent (4vHPV), 3 dose schedule, for intramuscular use
- *CPT Changes: An Insider's View* 2006, 2008, 2016
- *CPT Assistant* Dec 05:9, Jun 06:8, Sep 06:14, Jul 07:13, Mar 11:4, Aug 13:10

90650 Human Papillomavirus vaccine, types 16, 18, bivalent (2vHPV), 3 dose schedule, for intramuscular use
- *CPT Changes: An Insider's View* 2009, 2011, 2016
- *CPT Assistant* Mar 11:4, Aug 13:10

90651 Human Papillomavirus vaccine types 6, 11, 16, 18, 31, 33, 45, 52, 58, nonavalent (9vHPV), 2 or 3 dose schedule, for intramuscular use
- *CPT Changes: An Insider's View* 2015, 2016, 2018
- *CPT Assistant* May 15:6

90653 Influenza vaccine, inactivated (IIV), subunit, adjuvanted, for intramuscular use
- *CPT Changes: An Insider's View* 2013, 2016
- *CPT Assistant* Aug 13:10, Oct 16:6

90654 Influenza virus vaccine, trivalent (IIV3), split virus, preservative-free, for intradermal use
- *CPT Changes: An Insider's View* 2012, 2015
- *CPT Assistant* Aug 13:10, Apr 15:9, May 15:6, Oct 16:6

 # 90630 Influenza virus vaccine, quadrivalent (IIV4), split virus, preservative free, for intradermal use
- *CPT Changes: An Insider's View* 2015
- *CPT Assistant* May 15:6

90655 Influenza virus vaccine, trivalent (IIV3), split virus, preservative free, 0.25 mL dosage, for intramuscular use
- *CPT Changes: An Insider's View* 2004, 2007, 2008, 2013, 2016, 2017
- *CPT Assistant* Oct 99:9, Feb 04:2, Apr 07:12, Apr 08:8, Oct 09:3, Mar 11:4, Aug 13:10, May 16:9, Oct 16:6

90656 Influenza virus vaccine, trivalent (IIV3), split virus, preservative free, 0.5 mL dosage, for intramuscular use
- *CPT Changes: An Insider's View* 2005, 2007, 2008, 2013, 2016, 2017
- *CPT Assistant* Apr 08:8, Oct 09:3, Mar 11:4, Aug 13:10, May 16:9, Oct 16:6

90657 Influenza virus vaccine, trivalent (IIV3), split virus, 0.25 mL dosage, for intramuscular use
- *CPT Changes: An Insider's View* 2004, 2007, 2008, 2013, 2016, 2017
- *CPT Assistant* Nov 98:31-33, Jan 99:2, Oct 99:9, Feb 02:10, Feb 04:2, Apr 05:5, Apr 08:8, Oct 09:3, Mar 11:4, Aug 13:10, May 16:9, Oct 16:6

90658 Influenza virus vaccine, trivalent (IIV3), split virus, 0.5 mL dosage, for intramuscular use
- *CPT Changes: An Insider's View* 2004, 2007, 2008, 2013, 2016, 2017
- *CPT Assistant* Nov 98:31-33, Jan 99:2, Oct 99:9, Feb 04:2, Apr 07:12, Apr 08:8, Oct 09:3, Mar 11:4, Aug 13:10, May 16:9, Oct 16:6

90660 Influenza virus vaccine, trivalent, live (LAIV3), for intranasal use
- *CPT Changes: An Insider's View* 2008, 2013, 2016
- *CPT Assistant* Nov 98:31-33, Jan 99:2, Oct 99:9, Mar 04:11, Apr 04:14, Oct 09:3, Mar 11:4, Aug 13:10

 # 90672 Influenza virus vaccine, quadrivalent, live (LAIV4), for intranasal use
- *CPT Changes: An Insider's View* 2013, 2016
- *CPT Assistant* Aug 13:10

90661 Influenza virus vaccine, trivalent (ccIIV3), derived from cell cultures, subunit, preservative and antibiotic free, 0.5 mL dosage, for intramuscular use
- *CPT Changes: An Insider's View* 2008, 2016, 2017
- *CPT Assistant* Apr 08:8, Oct 09:3, Mar 11:4, Aug 13:10, Oct 16:6

 # 90674 Influenza virus vaccine, quadrivalent (ccIIV4), derived from cell cultures, subunit, preservative and antibiotic free, 0.5 mL dosage, for intramuscular use
- *CPT Changes: An Insider's View* 2017
- *CPT Assistant* Oct 16:6

 # 90756 Influenza virus vaccine, quadrivalent (ccIIV4), derived from cell cultures, subunit, antibiotic free, 0.5 mL dosage, for intramuscular use
- *CPT Changes: An Insider's View* 2018

 # 90673 Influenza virus vaccine, trivalent (RIV3), derived from recombinant DNA, hemagglutinin (HA) protein only, preservative and antibiotic free, for intramuscular use
- *CPT Changes: An Insider's View* 2014, 2016
- *CPT Assistant* Mar 14:10

90662 Influenza virus vaccine (IIV), split virus, preservative free, enhanced immunogenicity via increased antigen content, for intramuscular use
- *CPT Changes: An Insider's View* 2008, 2011, 2016
- *CPT Assistant* Apr 08:8, Oct 09:3, 6, Mar 11:4, Aug 13:10

90664 Influenza virus vaccine, live (LAIV), pandemic formulation, for intranasal use
- *CPT Changes: An Insider's View* 2011, 2016
- *CPT Assistant* Mar 11:4, Aug 13:10

⚡ 90666 Influenza virus vaccine (IIV), pandemic formulation, split virus, preservative free, for intramuscular use
- *CPT Changes: An Insider's View* 2011, 2016
- *CPT Assistant* May 11:4, Aug 13:10

⚡ 90667 Influenza virus vaccine (IIV), pandemic formulation, split virus, adjuvanted, for intramuscular use
- *CPT Changes: An Insider's View* 2011, 2016
- *CPT Assistant* Mar 11:4, Aug 13:10

ꟿ **90668** Influenza virus vaccine (IIV), pandemic formulation, split virus, for intramuscular use
- *CPT Changes: An Insider's View* 2011, 2016
- *CPT Assistant* Mar 11:4, Aug 13:10

(90669 has been deleted)

90670 Pneumococcal conjugate vaccine, 13 valent (PCV13), for intramuscular use
- *CPT Changes: An Insider's View* 2010, 2011, 2016
- *CPT Assistant* Mar 11:4, Aug 13:10

90672 Code is out of numerical sequence. See 90658-90664

90673 Code is out of numerical sequence. See 90658-90664

90674 Code is out of numerical sequence. See 90658-90664

90675 Rabies vaccine, for intramuscular use
- *CPT Changes: An Insider's View* 2008
- *CPT Assistant* Nov 98:31-33, Jan 99:2, Oct 99:9, Mar 11:4, Aug 13:10

90676 Rabies vaccine, for intradermal use
- *CPT Changes: An Insider's View* 2008
- *CPT Assistant* Nov 98:31-33, Jan 99:2, Oct 99:9, Mar 11:4, Jul 12:7, Aug 13:10

90680 Rotavirus vaccine, pentavalent (RV5), 3 dose schedule, live, for oral use
- *CPT Changes: An Insider's View* 2006, 2008, 2016
- *CPT Assistant* Nov 98:31-33, Jan 99:2, Oct 99:9, Jun 05:6, Dec 05:9, Jun 06:8, Mar 11:4, Aug 13:10

90681 Rotavirus vaccine, human, attenuated (RV1), 2 dose schedule, live, for oral use
- *CPT Changes: An Insider's View* 2009, 2016
- *CPT Assistant* Mar 11:4, Jul 12:7, Aug 13:10

90682 Influenza virus vaccine, quadrivalent (RIV4), derived from recombinant DNA, hemagglutinin (HA) protein only, preservative and antibiotic free, for intramuscular use
- *CPT Changes: An Insider's View* 2018

90685 Influenza virus vaccine, quadrivalent (IIV4), split virus, preservative free, 0.25 mL dosage, for intramuscular use
- *CPT Changes: An Insider's View* 2014, 2016, 2017
- *CPT Assistant* Mar 14:10, May 16:9, Oct 16:6

90686 Influenza virus vaccine, quadrivalent (IIV4), split virus, preservative free, 0.5 mL dosage, for intramuscular use
- *CPT Changes: An Insider's View* 2014, 2016, 2017
- *CPT Assistant* Mar 14:10, May 16:9, Oct 16:6

90687 Influenza virus vaccine, quadrivalent (IIV4), split virus, 0.25 mL dosage, for intramuscular use
- *CPT Changes: An Insider's View* 2014, 2016, 2017
- *CPT Assistant* Mar 14:10, May 16:9, Oct 16:6

90688 Influenza virus vaccine, quadrivalent (IIV4), split virus, 0.5 mL dosage, for intramuscular use
- *CPT Changes: An Insider's View* 2014, 2016, 2017
- *CPT Assistant* Mar 14:10, May 16:9, Oct 16:6

ꟿ● **90689** Influenza virus vaccine, quadrivalent (IIV4), inactivated, adjuvanted, preservative free, 0.25 mL dosage, for intramuscular use
- *CPT Changes: An Insider's View* 2019

90690 Typhoid vaccine, live, oral
- *CPT Changes: An Insider's View* 2008
- *CPT Assistant* Nov 98:31-33, Jan 99:2, Oct 99:9, Mar 11:4, Aug 13:10

90691 Typhoid vaccine, Vi capsular polysaccharide (ViCPs), for intramuscular use
- *CPT Changes: An Insider's View* 2008
- *CPT Assistant* Nov 98:31-33, Jan 99:2, Oct 99:9, Mar 11:4, Aug 13:10

(90692 has been deleted)

(90693 has been deleted)

90696 Diphtheria, tetanus toxoids, acellular pertussis vaccine and inactivated poliovirus vaccine (DTaP-IPV), when administered to children 4 through 6 years of age, for intramuscular use
- *CPT Changes: An Insider's View* 2009, 2016
- *CPT Assistant* Mar 11:4, Aug 13:10

ꟿ **90697** Diphtheria, tetanus toxoids, acellular pertussis vaccine, inactivated poliovirus vaccine, Haemophilus influenzae type b PRP-OMP conjugate vaccine, and hepatitis B vaccine (DTaP-IPV-Hib--HepB), for intramuscular use
- *CPT Changes: An Insider's View* 2016

90698 Diphtheria, tetanus toxoids, acellular pertussis vaccine, Haemophilus influenzae type b, and inactivated poliovirus vaccine, (DTaP-IPV/Hib), for intramuscular use
- *CPT Changes: An Insider's View* 2008, 2009, 2016
- *CPT Assistant* Oct 99:9, Dec 05:9, Jun 06:8, Mar 11:4, Aug 13:10

90700 Diphtheria, tetanus toxoids, and acellular pertussis vaccine (DTaP), when administered to individuals younger than 7 years, for intramuscular use
- *CPT Changes: An Insider's View* 2005, 2007, 2008
- *CPT Assistant* Jan 96:5, Apr 97:10, Nov 98:31-33, Jan 99:2, Oct 99:9, Nov 03:13, Mar 11:4, Jul 12:7, Aug 13:10

90702 Diphtheria and tetanus toxoids adsorbed (DT) when administered to individuals younger than 7 years, for intramuscular use
- *CPT Changes: An Insider's View* 2001, 2007, 2008, 2016
- *CPT Assistant* Jan 96:6, Aug 96:10, Apr 97:10, Nov 98:31-33, Jan 99:2, Sep 99:10, Oct 99:9, Jun 00:10, Feb 07:11, Mar 11:4, Aug 13:10

(90703 has been deleted)

(90704 has been deleted)

(90705 has been deleted)

(90706 has been deleted)

90707 Measles, mumps and rubella virus vaccine (MMR), live, for subcutaneous use
- *CPT Changes: An Insider's View* 2004, 2008
- *CPT Assistant* Jan 96:6, May 96:10, Apr 97:10, Nov 98:31-33, Jan 99:2, Oct 99:9, Apr 05:1, 5, Mar 11:4, Jul 12:7, Aug 13:10

(90708 has been deleted)

90710 Measles, mumps, rubella, and varicella vaccine (MMRV), live, for subcutaneous use
- *CPT Changes: An Insider's View* 2008
- *CPT Assistant* May 96:10, Apr 97:10, Nov 98:31-33, Jan 99:2, Oct 99:9, Dec 05:9, Jun 06:8, Mar 11:4, Aug 13:10

(90712 has been deleted)

90713 Poliovirus vaccine, inactivated (IPV), for subcutaneous or intramuscular use

CPT Changes: An Insider's View 2006, 2008

CPT Assistant Apr 97:10, Nov 98:31-33, Jan 99:2, Oct 99:9, Jun 05:6, Mar 11:4, Aug 13:10

90714 Tetanus and diphtheria toxoids adsorbed (Td), preservative free, when administered to individuals 7 years or older, for intramuscular use

CPT Changes: An Insider's View 2006, 2007, 2008, 2016

CPT Assistant Jun 05:6, Mar 11:4, Aug 13:10

90715 Tetanus, diphtheria toxoids and acellular pertussis vaccine (Tdap), when administered to individuals 7 years or older, for intramuscular use

CPT Changes: An Insider's View 2006, 2007, 2008

CPT Assistant Oct 99:9, Jun 05:6, Dec 05:9, Jun 06:8, Mar 11:4, Aug 13:10

90716 Varicella virus vaccine (VAR), live, for subcutaneous use

CPT Changes: An Insider's View 2008, 2016

CPT Assistant Jan 96:6, May 96:10, Apr 97:10, Nov 98:31-33, Jan 99:2, Oct 99:9, Mar 11:4, Aug 13:10

90717 Yellow fever vaccine, live, for subcutaneous use

CPT Changes: An Insider's View 2008

CPT Assistant Apr 97:10, Nov 98:31-33, Jan 99:2, Oct 99:9, Mar 11:4, Aug 13:10

(90719 has been deleted)

(90720 has been deleted)

(90721 has been deleted)

90723 Diphtheria, tetanus toxoids, acellular pertussis vaccine, hepatitis B, and inactivated poliovirus vaccine (DTaP-HepB-IPV), for intramuscular use

CPT Changes: An Insider's View 2001, 2008, 2015

CPT Assistant Apr 97:10, Oct 99:9, Mar 11:4, Aug 13:10, May 15:6

(90725 has been deleted)

 # 90625 Cholera vaccine, live, adult dosage, 1 dose schedule, for oral use

CPT Changes: An Insider's View 2016

CPT Assistant Oct 16:6

(90727 has been deleted)

90732 Pneumococcal polysaccharide vaccine, 23-valent (PPSV23), adult or immunosuppressed patient dosage, when administered to individuals 2 years or older, for subcutaneous or intramuscular use

CPT Changes: An Insider's View 2002, 2007, 2008, 2016

CPT Assistant Apr 97:10, Nov 98:31-33, Jan 99:2, Oct 99:9, Mar 11:4, Aug 13:10

 # 90644 Meningococcal conjugate vaccine, serogroups C & Y and Haemophilus influenzae type b vaccine (Hib-MenCY), 4 dose schedule, when administered to children 6 weeks-18 months of age, for intramuscular use

CPT Changes: An Insider's View 2011, 2012, 2016, 2017

CPT Assistant Mar 11:4, Aug 13:10

90733 Meningococcal polysaccharide vaccine, serogroups A, C, Y, W-135, quadrivalent (MPSV4), for subcutaneous use

CPT Changes: An Insider's View 2001, 2004, 2008, 2016

CPT Assistant Apr 97:10, Nov 98:31-33, Jan 99:2, Oct 99:9, Dec 99:7, Mar 11:4, Aug 13:10

90734 Meningococcal conjugate vaccine, serogroups A, C, Y and W-135, quadrivalent (MCV4 or MenACWY), for intramuscular use

CPT Changes: An Insider's View 2008, 2015, 2016, 2017

CPT Assistant Oct 99:9, Mar 11:4, Aug 13:10, May 15:6, Oct 16:6

 # 90620 Meningococcal recombinant protein and outer membrane vesicle vaccine, serogroup B (MenB-4C), 2 dose schedule, for intramuscular use

CPT Changes: An Insider's View 2016, 2018

 # 90621 Meningococcal recombinant lipoprotein vaccine, serogroup B (MenB-FHbp), 2 or 3 dose schedule, for intramuscular use

CPT Changes: An Insider's View 2016, 2018

(90735 has been deleted)

90736 Zoster (shingles) vaccine (HZV), live, for subcutaneous injection

CPT Changes: An Insider's View 2006, 2008, 2016

CPT Assistant Dec 05:9, Jun 06:8, Jul 07:13, Mar 11:4, Aug 13:10

 # 90750 Zoster (shingles) vaccine (HZV), recombinant, subunit, adjuvanted, for intramuscular use

CPT Changes: An Insider's View 2018

90738 Japanese encephalitis virus vaccine, inactivated, for intramuscular use

CPT Changes: An Insider's View 2009, 2010

CPT Assistant Mar 11:4, Aug 13:10

90739 Hepatitis B vaccine (HepB), adult dosage, 2 dose schedule, for intramuscular use

CPT Changes: An Insider's View 2013, 2016

CPT Assistant Aug 13:10

90740 Hepatitis B vaccine (HepB), dialysis or immunosuppressed patient dosage, 3 dose schedule, for intramuscular use

CPT Changes: An Insider's View 2001, 2008, 2016

CPT Assistant Apr 97:10, Oct 99:9, Apr 01:10, Mar 11:4, Aug 13:10

90743 Hepatitis B vaccine (HepB), adolescent, 2 dose schedule, for intramuscular use

CPT Changes: An Insider's View 2001, 2008, 2016

CPT Assistant Apr 97:10, Oct 99:9, Mar 11:4, Aug 13:10

90744 Hepatitis B vaccine (HepB), pediatric/adolescent dosage, 3 dose schedule, for intramuscular use

CPT Changes: An Insider's View 2000, 2001, 2008, 2016

CPT Assistant Jan 96:5, Apr 97:10, Jun 97:10, Nov 98:31-33, Jan 99:2, Oct 99:9, Nov 99:48-49, Jun 00:10, Mar 11:4, Aug 13:10

90746 Hepatitis B vaccine (HepB), adult dosage, 3 dose schedule, for intramuscular use

CPT Changes: An Insider's View 2008, 2013, 2016

CPT Assistant Jan 96:5, Apr 97:10, Nov 98:31-33, Jan 99:2, Oct 99:9, Mar 11:4, Aug 13:10

90747 Hepatitis B vaccine (HepB), dialysis or immunosuppressed patient dosage, 4 dose schedule, for intramuscular use

CPT Changes: An Insider's View 2001, 2008, 2016

CPT Assistant Jan 96:5, Apr 97:10, Jun 97:10, Nov 98:31-33, Jan 99:2, Oct 99:9, Jun 00:10, Apr 01:10, Mar 11:4, Aug 13:10

90748 Hepatitis B and Haemophilus influenzae type b vaccine (Hib-HepB), for intramuscular use

CPT Changes: An Insider's View 2008, 2016

CPT Assistant Apr 97:10, Nov 97:37, Nov 98:31-33, Jan 99:2, Sep 99:10, Oct 99:9, Mar 11:4, Jul 12:7, Aug 13:10, Oct 16:6

90749 Unlisted vaccine/toxoid

CPT Changes: An Insider's View 2008

CPT Assistant Jan 96:6, Apr 97:10, Jun 97:10, Nov 98:31-33, Jan 99:2, Oct 99:9, Nov 02:11, Mar 11:4, May 15:6

90750 Code is out of numerical sequence. See 90717-90739

90756 Code is out of numerical sequence. See 90658-90664

Psychiatry

Psychiatry services include diagnostic services, psychotherapy, and other services to an individual, family, or group. Patient condition, characteristics, or situational factors may require services described as being with interactive complexity. Services may be provided to a patient in crisis. Services are provided in all settings of care and psychiatry services codes are reported without regard to setting. Services may be provided by a physician or other qualified health care professional. Some psychiatry services may be reported with **Evaluation and Management Services** (99201-99255, 99281-99285, 99304-99337, 99341-99350) or other services when performed. **Evaluation and Management Services** (99201-99285, 99304-99337, 99341-99350) may be reported for treatment of psychiatric conditions, rather than using **Psychiatry Services** codes, when appropriate.

Hospital care in treating a psychiatric inpatient or partial hospitalization may be initial or subsequent in nature (see 99221-99233).

Some patients receive hospital evaluation and management services only and others receive hospital evaluation and management services and other procedures. If other procedures such as electroconvulsive therapy or psychotherapy are rendered in addition to hospital evaluation and management services, these may be listed separately (eg, hospital care services [99221-99223, 99231-99233] plus electroconvulsive therapy [90870]), or when psychotherapy is done, with appropriate code(s) defining psychotherapy services.

Consultation for psychiatric evaluation of a patient includes examination of a patient and exchange of information with the primary physician and other informants such as nurses or family members, and preparation of a report. These services may be reported using consultation codes (see **Consultations**).

►(Do not report 90785-90899 in conjunction with 90839, 90840, 97151, 97152, 97153, 97154, 97155, 97156, 97157, 97158, 0362T, 0373T)◄

Interactive Complexity

Code 90785 is an add-on code for interactive complexity to be reported in conjunction with codes for diagnostic psychiatric evaluation (90791, 90792), psychotherapy (90832, 90834, 90837), psychotherapy when performed with an evaluation and management service (90833, 90836, 90838, 99201-99255, 99304-99337, 99341-99350), and group psychotherapy (90853).

Interactive complexity refers to specific communication factors that complicate the delivery of a psychiatric procedure. Common factors include more difficult communication with discordant or emotional family members and engagement of young and verbally undeveloped or impaired patients. Typical patients are those who have third parties, such as parents, guardians, other family members, interpreters, language translators, agencies, court officers, or schools involved in their psychiatric care.

These factors are typically present with patients who:

- Have other individuals legally responsible for their care, such as minors or adults with guardians, or
- Request others to be involved in their care during the visit, such as adults accompanied by one or more participating family members or interpreter or language translator, or
- Require the involvement of other third parties, such as child welfare agencies, parole or probation officers, or schools.

Psychiatric procedures may be reported "with interactive complexity" when at least one of the following is present:

1. The need to manage maladaptive communication (related to, eg, high anxiety, high reactivity, repeated questions, or disagreement) among participants that complicates delivery of care.
2. Caregiver emotions or behavior that interferes with the caregiver's understanding and ability to assist in the implementation of the treatment plan.
3. Evidence or disclosure of a sentinel event and mandated report to third party (eg, abuse or neglect with report to state agency) with initiation of discussion of the sentinel event and/or report with patient and other visit participants.
4. Use of play equipment, other physical devices, interpreter, or translator to communicate with the patient to overcome barriers to therapeutic or diagnostic interaction between the physician or other qualified health care professional and a patient who:
   - Is not fluent in the same language as the physician or other qualified health care professional, or

- Has not developed, or has lost, either the expressive language communication skills to explain his/her symptoms and response to treatment, or the receptive communication skills to understand the physician or other qualified health care professional if he/she were to use typical language for communication.

When provided in conjunction with the psychotherapy services (90832-90838), the amount of time spent by a physician or other qualified health care professional providing interactive complexity services should be reflected in the timed service code for psychotherapy (90832, 90834, 90837) or the psychotherapy add-on code performed with an evaluation and management service (90833, 90836, 90838) and must relate to the psychotherapy service only. Interactive complexity is not a factor for evaluation and management services selection (99201-99255, 99281-99285, 99304-99337, 99341-99350), except as it directly affects key components as defined in the Evaluation and Management Services Guidelines (ie, history, examination, and medical decision making).

+ 90785 Interactive complexity (List separately in addition to the code for primary procedure)

➔ *CPT Changes: An Insider's View* 2013

➔ *CPT Assistant* May 13:12, Jun 13:3, Apr 14:6

(Use 90785 in conjunction with codes for diagnostic psychiatric evaluation [90791, 90792], psychotherapy [90832, 90834, 90837], psychotherapy when performed with an evaluation and management service [90833, 90836, 90838, 99201-99255, 99304-99337, 99341-99350], and group psychotherapy [90853])

(Do not report 90785 in conjunction with 90839, 90840, or in conjunction with E/M services when no psychotherapy service is also reported)

►(Do not report 90785 in conjunction with 90839, 90840, 97151, 97152, 97153, 97154, 97155, 97156, 97157, 97158, 0362T, 0373T)◄

Psychiatric Diagnostic Procedures

Psychiatric diagnostic evaluation is an integrated biopsychosocial assessment, including history, mental status, and recommendations. The evaluation may include communication with family or other sources and review and ordering of diagnostic studies.

Psychiatric diagnostic evaluation with medical services is an integrated biopsychosocial and medical assessment, including history, mental status, other physical examination elements as indicated, and recommendations. The evaluation may include communication with family or other sources, prescription of medications, and review and ordering of laboratory or other diagnostic studies.

In certain circumstances one or more other informants (family members, guardians, or significant others) may be seen in lieu of the patient. Codes 90791, 90792 may be reported more than once for the patient when separate diagnostic evaluations are conducted with the patient and other informants. Report services as being provided to the patient and not the informant or other party in such circumstances. Codes 90791, 90792 may be reported once per day and not on the same day as an evaluation and management service performed by the same individual for the same patient.

The psychiatric diagnostic evaluation may include interactive complexity services when factors exist that complicate the delivery of the psychiatric procedure. These services should be reported with add-on code 90785 used in conjunction with the diagnostic psychiatric evaluation codes 90791, 90792.

Codes 90791, 90792 are used for the diagnostic assessment(s) or reassessment(s), if required, and do not include psychotherapeutic services. Psychotherapy services, including for crisis, may not be reported on the same day.

►(Do not report 90791-90899 in conjunction with 90839, 90840, 97151, 97152, 97153, 97154, 97155, 97156, 97157, 97158, 0362T, 0373T)◄

★ 90791 Psychiatric diagnostic evaluation

➔ *CPT Changes: An Insider's View* 2013, 2017

➔ *CPT Assistant* May 13:12, Jun 13:3, Dec 13:18, Jun 14:3, Nov 17:3

★ 90792 Psychiatric diagnostic evaluation with medical services

➔ *CPT Changes: An Insider's View* 2013, 2017

➔ *CPT Assistant* Jun 13:3, Dec 13:18, Jun 14:3, Nov 17:3

►(Do not report 90791 or 90792 in conjunction with 99201-99337, 99341-99350, 99366-99368, 99401-99444, 97151, 97152, 97153, 97154, 97155, 97156, 97157, 97158, 0362T, 0373T)◄

(Use 90785 in conjunction with 90791, 90792 when the diagnostic evaluation includes interactive complexity services)

Psychotherapy

Psychotherapy is the treatment of mental illness and behavioral disturbances in which the physician or other qualified health care professional, through definitive therapeutic communication, attempts to alleviate the emotional disturbances, reverse or change maladaptive patterns of behavior, and encourage personality growth and development.

The psychotherapy service codes 90832-90838 include ongoing assessment and adjustment of psychotherapeutic interventions, and may include involvement of informants in the treatment process.

Codes 90832, 90833, 90834, 90836, 90837, 90838 describe psychotherapy for the individual patient, although times are for face-to-face services with patient and may include informant(s). The patient must be present for all or a majority of the service.

See codes 90846, 90847 when utilizing family psychotherapy techniques, such as focusing on family dynamics. Do not report 90846, 90847 for family psychotherapy services less than 26 minutes. Codes 90832, 90833, 90834, 90836, 90837, 90838 may be reported on the same day as codes 90846, 90847, when the services are separate and distinct.

In reporting, choose the code closest to the actual time (ie, 16-37 minutes for 90832 and 90833, 38-52 minutes for 90834 and 90836, and 53 or more minutes for 90837 and 90838). Do not report psychotherapy of less than 16 minutes duration. (See instructions for the usage of time in the Introduction of the CPT code set.)

Psychotherapy provided to a patient in a crisis state is reported with codes 90839 and 90840 and cannot be reported in addition to the psychotherapy codes 90832-90838. For psychotherapy for crisis, see "Other Psychotherapy."

Code 90785 is an add-on code to report interactive complexity services when provided in conjunction with the psychotherapy codes 90832-90838. For family psychotherapy, see 90846, 90847. The amount of time spent by a physician or other qualified health care professional providing interactive complexity services should be reflected in the timed service code for psychotherapy (90832, 90834, 90837) or the psychotherapy add-on code performed with an evaluation and management service (90833, 90836, 90838).

Some psychiatric patients receive a medical evaluation and management (E/M) service on the same day as a psychotherapy service by the same physician or other qualified health care professional. To report both E/M and psychotherapy, the two services must be significant and separately identifiable. These services are reported by using codes specific for psychotherapy when performed with evaluation and management services (90833, 90836, 90838) as add-on codes to the evaluation and management service.

Medical symptoms and disorders inform treatment choices of psychotherapeutic interventions, and data from therapeutic communication are used to evaluate the presence, type, and severity of medical symptoms and disorders. For the purposes of reporting, the medical and psychotherapeutic components of the service may be separately identified as follows:

1. The type and level of E/M service is selected first based upon the key components of history, examination, and medical decision-making.
2. Time associated with activities used to meet criteria for the E/M service is not included in the time used for reporting the psychotherapy service (ie, time spent on history, examination and medical decision making **when used for the E/M service** is not psychotherapy time). Time may not be used as the basis of E/M code selection and Prolonged Services may not be reported when psychotherapy with E/M (90833, 90836, 90838) are reported.
3. A separate diagnosis is not required for the reporting of E/M and psychotherapy on the same date of service.

★ **90832** Psychotherapy, 30 minutes with patient

➔ *CPT Changes: An Insider's View* 2013, 2017

➔ *CPT Assistant* Jan 13:3, May 13:12, Jun 13:3, Aug 13:14, Feb 14:3, Aug 14:5, Oct 15:9, Dec 16:11, Sep 17:12

★+ **90833** Psychotherapy, 30 minutes with patient when performed with an evaluation and management service (List separately in addition to the code for primary procedure)

➔ *CPT Changes: An Insider's View* 2013, 2017

➔ *CPT Assistant* Jan 13:3, May 13:12, Jun 13:3, Aug 13:14, Aug 14:5, Oct 15:9, Dec 16:11

(Use 90833 in conjunction with 99201-99255, 99304-99337, 99341-99350)

★ **90834** Psychotherapy, 45 minutes with patient

➔ *CPT Changes: An Insider's View* 2013, 2017

➔ *CPT Assistant* Jan 13:3, May 13:12, Jun 13:3, Aug 13:14, Jun 14:3, Oct 15:9, Dec 16:11

★+ **90836** Psychotherapy, 45 minutes with patient when performed with an evaluation and management service (List separately in addition to the code for primary procedure)

➔ *CPT Changes: An Insider's View* 2013, 2017

➔ *CPT Assistant* Jan 13:3, May 13:12, Jun 13:3, Aug 13:14, Oct 15:9, Dec 16:11

(Use 90836 in conjunction with 99201-99255, 99304-99337, 99341-99350)

★ **90837** Psychotherapy, 60 minutes with patient

➔ *CPT Changes: An Insider's View* 2013, 2017

➔ *CPT Assistant* Jan 13:3, May 13:12, Jun 13:3, Aug 13:14, Apr 14:6, Oct 15:3, 9, Dec 16:11

(Use the appropriate prolonged services code [99354, 99355, 99356, 99357] for psychotherapy services not performed with an E/M service of 90 minutes or longer face-to-face with the patient)

★+ **90838** Psychotherapy, 60 minutes with patient when performed with an evaluation and management service (List separately in addition to the code for primary procedure)

➔ *CPT Changes: An Insider's View* 2013, 2017

➔ *CPT Assistant* Jan 13:3, May 13:12, Jun 13:3, Aug 13:14, Feb 14:3, Apr 14:6, Oct 15:9, Dec 16:11

(Use 90838 in conjunction with 99201-99255, 99304-99337, 99341-99350)

(Use 90785 in conjunction with 90832, 90833, 90834, 90836, 90837, 90838 when psychotherapy includes interactive complexity services)

Psychotherapy for Crisis

Psychotherapy for crisis is an urgent assessment and history of a crisis state, a mental status exam, and a disposition. The treatment includes psychotherapy, mobilization of resources to defuse the crisis and restore safety, and implementation of psychotherapeutic interventions to minimize the potential for psychological trauma. The presenting problem is typically life threatening or complex and requires immediate attention to a patient in high distress.

Codes 90839, 90840 are used to report the total duration of time face-to-face with the patient and/or family spent by the physician or other qualified health care professional providing psychotherapy for crisis, even if the time spent on that date is not continuous. For any given period of time spent providing psychotherapy for crisis state, the physician or other qualified health care professional must devote his or her full attention to the patient and, therefore, cannot provide services to any other patient during the same time period. The patient must be present for all or some of the service. Do not report with 90791 or 90792.

Code 90839 is used to report the first 30-74 minutes of psychotherapy for crisis on a given date. It should be used only once per date even if the time spent by the physician or other health care professional is not continuous on that date. Psychotherapy for crisis of less than 30 minutes total duration on a given date should be reported with 90832 or 90833 (when provided with evaluation and management services).

Code 90840 is used to report additional block(s) of time, of up to 30 minutes each beyond the first 74 minutes.

90839 Psychotherapy for crisis; first 60 minutes

➲ *CPT Changes: An Insider's View* 2013

➲ *CPT Assistant* Jun 13:3, Aug 14:5, Oct 15:9

+ 90840 each additional 30 minutes (List separately in addition to code for primary service)

➲ *CPT Changes: An Insider's View* 2013

➲ *CPT Assistant* Jun 13:3, Aug 14:5, Oct 15:9

(Use 90840 in conjunction with 90839)

(Do not report 90839, 90840 in conjunction with 90791, 90792, psychotherapy codes 90832-90838 or other psychiatric services, or 90785-90899)

Other Psychotherapy

★ 90845 Psychoanalysis

➲ *CPT Changes: An Insider's View* 2017

➲ *CPT Assistant* Summer 92:15, Nov 97:40-41, Mar 01:8, Mar 02:4, May 05:1, Feb 06:15, Mar 10:6, Oct 15:9

★ 90846 Family psychotherapy (without the patient present), 50 minutes

➲ *CPT Changes: An Insider's View* 2017

➲ *CPT Assistant* Summer 92:15, Nov 97:40-41, Mar 01:8, Mar 02:4, May 05:1, Sep 09:11, Mar 10:6, Jun 13:3, Dec 13:18, Oct 15:9, Dec 16:11, Mar 17:11

★ 90847 Family psychotherapy (conjoint psychotherapy) (with patient present), 50 minutes

➲ *CPT Changes: An Insider's View* 2017

➲ *CPT Assistant* Summer 92:15, Nov 97:40-41, Mar 01:5, Mar 02:4, May 05:1, Mar 10:6, Jun 13:3, Dec 13:18, Oct 15:9, Dec 16:11

(Do not report 90846, 90847 for family psychotherapy services less than 26 minutes)

►(Do not report 90846, 90847 in conjunction with 97151, 97152, 97153, 97154, 97155, 97156, 97157, 97158, 0362T, 0373T)◄

90849 Multiple-family group psychotherapy

➲ *CPT Assistant* Summer 92:15, Nov 97:40-41, Mar 01:5, Mar 02:4, May 05:1, Mar 10:6, Aug 14:15, Oct 15:9

90853 Group psychotherapy (other than of a multiple-family group)

➲ *CPT Assistant* Summer 92:15, Nov 97:40-41, Mar 01:8, Mar 02:4, May 05:1, Mar 10:6, Jun 13:3, Jun 14:3, Aug 14:15, Oct 15:9, Mar 17:11

(Use 90853 in conjunction with 90785 for the specified patient when group psychotherapy includes interactive complexity)

►(Do not report 90853 in conjunction with 97151, 97152, 97153, 97154, 97155, 97156, 97157, 97158, 0362T, 0373T)◄

Other Psychiatric Services or Procedures

►(For electronic analysis with programming, when performed, of vagal nerve neurostimulators, see 95970, 95976, 95977)◄

★+ 90863 Pharmacologic management, including prescription and review of medication, when performed with psychotherapy services (List separately in addition to the code for primary procedure)

➲ *CPT Changes: An Insider's View* 2013, 2017

➲ *CPT Assistant* Jun 13:3

(Use 90863 in conjunction with 90832, 90834, 90837)

(For pharmacologic management with psychotherapy services performed by a physician or other qualified health care professional who may report evaluation and management codes, use the appropriate evaluation and management codes 99201-99255, 99281-99285, 99304-99337, 99341-99350 and the appropriate psychotherapy with evaluation and management service 90833, 90836, 90838)

(Do not count time spent on providing pharmacologic management services in the time used for selection of the psychotherapy service)

90865 Narcosynthesis for psychiatric diagnostic and therapeutic purposes (eg, sodium amobarbital (Amytal) interview)

➲ *CPT Assistant* Nov 97:41, Mar 01:5, Mar 02:4, May 05:1

90867 Therapeutic repetitive transcranial magnetic stimulation (TMS) treatment; initial, including cortical mapping, motor threshold determination, delivery and management

➲ *CPT Changes: An Insider's View* 2011, 2012

(Report only once per course of treatment)

(Do not report 90867 in conjunction with 90868, 90869, 95860, 95870, 95928, 95929, 95939)

90868 subsequent delivery and management, per session

➔ *CPT Changes: An Insider's View* 2011, 2012

90869 subsequent motor threshold re-determination with delivery and management

➔ *CPT Changes: An Insider's View* 2012

(Do not report 90869 in conjunction with 90867, 90868, 95860-95870, 95928, 95929, 95939)

(If a significant, separately identifiable evaluation and management, medication management, or psychotherapy service is performed, the appropriate E/M or psychotherapy code may be reported in addition to 90867-90869. Evaluation and management activities directly related to cortical mapping, motor threshold determination, delivery and management of TMS are not separately reported)

90870 Electroconvulsive therapy (includes necessary monitoring)

➔ *CPT Changes: An Insider's View* 2006

➔ *CPT Assistant* Summer 92:16, Mar 01:5, Mar 02:4, May 05:1, Mar 10:6, Feb 13:3

90875 Individual psychophysiological therapy incorporating biofeedback training by any modality (face-to-face with the patient), with psychotherapy (eg, insight oriented, behavior modifying or supportive psychotherapy); 30 minutes

➔ *CPT Changes: An Insider's View* 2013

➔ *CPT Assistant* Nov 96:15, Sep 97:11, Nov 97:41, Apr 98:14, Jun 99:5, Mar 01:5, Mar 02:4, Mar 05:16, May 05:1

90876 45 minutes

➔ *CPT Changes: An Insider's View* 2013

➔ *CPT Assistant* Nov 96:15, Sep 97:11, Nov 97:41, Jun 99:5, Mar 01:5, Mar 05:16, May 05:1

90880 Hypnotherapy

➔ *CPT Assistant* Summer 92:16, Nov 97:41, Mar 01:5, Mar 02:4, May 05:1

90882 Environmental intervention for medical management purposes on a psychiatric patient's behalf with agencies, employers, or institutions

➔ *CPT Assistant* Summer 92:16, Mar 01:5, Mar 02:4, May 05:1

90885 Psychiatric evaluation of hospital records, other psychiatric reports, psychometric and/or projective tests, and other accumulated data for medical diagnostic purposes

➔ *CPT Assistant* Nov 97:41, Mar 01:5, Mar 02:4, Oct 04:10, May 05:1

90887 Interpretation or explanation of results of psychiatric, other medical examinations and procedures, or other accumulated data to family or other responsible persons, or advising them how to assist patient

➔ *CPT Assistant* Summer 92:17, Mar 01:5, Mar 02:4, Oct 02:11, May 05:1

►(Do not report 90887 in conjunction with 97151, 97152, 97153, 97154, 97155, 97156, 97157, 97158, 0362T, 0373T)◄

90889 Preparation of report of patient's psychiatric status, history, treatment, or progress (other than for legal or consultative purposes) for other individuals, agencies, or insurance carriers

➔ *CPT Changes: An Insider's View* 2013

➔ *CPT Assistant* Summer 92:17, Mar 01:5, Mar 02:4, May 05:1

90899 Unlisted psychiatric service or procedure

➔ *CPT Assistant* Mar 01:5, Mar 02:4, May 05:1, Jan 10:11, Apr 14:6

Biofeedback

(For psychophysiological therapy incorporating biofeedback training, see 90875, 90876)

90901 Biofeedback training by any modality

➔ *CPT Assistant* Sep 97:11, Apr 98:14, Jun 98:10, Jun 99:5, May 02:18, Sep 04:13, Mar 05:16

90911 Biofeedback training, perineal muscles, anorectal or urethral sphincter, including EMG and/or manometry

➔ *CPT Assistant* Sep 97:11, Nov 97:41, Jun 98:10, Jun 99:5, Sep 14:14

(For testing of rectal sensation, tone and compliance, use 91120)

(For incontinence treatment by pulsed magnetic neuromodulation, use 53899)

Dialysis

(For therapeutic apheresis for white blood cells, red blood cells, platelets and plasma pheresis, see 36511, 36512, 36513, 36514)

(For therapeutic apheresis extracorporeal adsorption procedures, use 36516)

(90918, 90922 have been deleted. To report ESRD-related services for patients younger than 2 years of age, see 90951-90953, 90963, 90967)

(90919, 90923 have been deleted. To report ESRD-related services for patients between 2 and 11 years of age, see 90954-90956, 90964, 90968)

(90920, 90924 have been deleted. To report ESRD-related services for patients between 12 and 19 years of age, see 90957-90959, 90965, 90969)

(90921, 90925 have been deleted. To report ESRD-related services for patients 20 years of age and older, see 90960-90962, 90966, 90970)

Hemodialysis

Codes 90935, 90937 are reported to describe the hemodialysis procedure with all evaluation and management services related to the patient's renal disease on the day of the hemodialysis procedure. These codes are used for inpatient ESRD and non-ESRD procedures or for outpatient non-ESRD dialysis services. Code 90935 is reported if only one evaluation of the patient is required related to that hemodialysis procedure. Code 90937 is reported when patient re-evaluation(s) is required during a hemodialysis procedure. Use modifier 25 with evaluation and management codes including new or established patient office or other outpatient services (99201-99215), office or other outpatient consultations (99241-99245), observation care (99217-99220, 99224-99226), observation or inpatient care including admission and discharge (99234-99236), initial hospital care (99221-99226, 99231-99239), new or established patient emergency department services (99281-99285), critical care services (99291, 99292), inpatient neonatal intensive care services and pediatric and neonatal critical care services (99466-99480), nursing facility services (99304-99318), domiciliary, rest home services, or custodial care (99324-99337), and home services (99341-99350), for separately identifiable services unrelated to the dialysis procedure or renal failure which cannot be rendered during the dialysis session.

(For home visit hemodialysis services performed by a non-physician health care professional, use 99512)

(For cannula declotting, see 36831, 36833, 36860, 36861)

(For declotting of implanted vascular access device or catheter by thrombolytic agent, use 36593)

(For collection of blood specimen from a partially or completely implantable venous access device, use 36591)

(For prolonged attendance by a physician or other qualified health care professional, see 99354-99360)

90935 Hemodialysis procedure with single evaluation by a physician or other qualified health care professional

➲ *CPT Changes: An Insider's View* 2013

➲ *CPT Assistant* Fall 93:2, May 02:17, Jan 03:22

90937 Hemodialysis procedure requiring repeated evaluation(s) with or without substantial revision of dialysis prescription

➲ *CPT Assistant* Fall 93:2, May 02:17, Jan 03:22

90940 Hemodialysis access flow study to determine blood flow in grafts and arteriovenous fistulae by an indicator method

➲ *CPT Changes: An Insider's View* 2001, 2006

➲ *CPT Assistant* Jan 03:22, May 06:18

➲ *Clinical Examples in Radiology* Summer 06:7, 12

(For duplex scan of hemodialysis access, use 93990)

Miscellaneous Dialysis Procedures

Codes 90945, 90947 describe dialysis procedures other than hemodialysis (eg, peritoneal dialysis, hemofiltration or continuous renal replacement therapies), and all evaluation and management services related to the patient's renal disease on the day of the procedure. Code 90945 is reported if only one evaluation of the patient is required related to that procedure. Code 90947 is reported when patient re-evaluation(s) is required during a procedure. Use modifier 25 with Evaluation and Management codes including office or other outpatient services (99201-99215), office or other outpatient consultations (99241-99245), observation care (99217-99220, 99224-99226), observation or inpatient care including admission and discharge (99234-99239), hospital care (99221-99226, 99231-99239), new or established patient emergency department services (99281-99285), critical care services (99291, 99292), inpatient neonatal intensive care services and pediatric and neonatal critical care services (99466-99480), nursing facility services (99304-99318), domiciliary, rest home, or custodial care services (99324-99337), and home services (99341-99350) for separately identifiable services unrelated to the procedure or the renal failure which cannot be rendered during the dialysis session.

(For percutaneous insertion of intraperitoneal tunneled catheter, use 49418. For open insertion of tunneled intraperitoneal catheter, use 49421)

(For prolonged attendance by a physician or other qualified health care professional, see 99354-99360)

90945 Dialysis procedure other than hemodialysis (eg, peritoneal dialysis, hemofiltration, or other continuous renal replacement therapies), with single evaluation by a physician or other qualified health care professional

➲ *CPT Changes: An Insider's View* 2001, 2013

➲ *CPT Assistant* Fall 93:2, Nov 97:41, Jul 98:10, Oct 01:11, Jan 03:22

(For home infusion of peritoneal dialysis, use 99601, 99602)

90947 Dialysis procedure other than hemodialysis (eg, peritoneal dialysis, hemofiltration, or other continuous renal replacement therapies) requiring repeated evaluations by a physician or other qualified health care professional, with or without substantial revision of dialysis prescription

➲ *CPT Changes: An Insider's View* 2001, 2013

➲ *CPT Assistant* Fall 93:2, Nov 97:41, Jul 98:10, Oct 01:11, Jan 03:22

End-Stage Renal Disease Services

Codes 90951-90962 are reported **once** per month to distinguish age-specific services related to the patient's end-stage renal disease (ESRD) performed in an outpatient setting with three levels of service based on the number of face-to-face visits. ESRD-related services by a physician or other qualified health care professional include establishment of a dialyzing cycle, outpatient evaluation and management of the dialysis visits, telephone calls, and patient management during the dialysis provided during a full month. In the circumstances in which the patient has had a complete assessment visit during the month and services are provided over a period of less than a month, 90951-90962 may be used according to the number of visits performed.

Codes 90963-90966 are reported once per month for a full month of service to distinguish age-specific services for end-stage renal disease (ESRD) services for home dialysis patients.

For ESRD and non-ESRD dialysis services performed in an inpatient setting, and for non-ESRD dialysis services performed in an outpatient setting, see 90935-90937 and 90945-90947.

Evaluation and management services unrelated to ESRD services that cannot be performed during the dialysis session may be reported separately.

Codes 90967-90970 are reported to distinguish age-specific services for end-stage renal disease (ESRD) services for less than a full month of service, per day, for services provided under the following circumstances: transient patients, partial month where there was one or more face-to-face visits without the complete assessment, the patient was hospitalized before a complete assessment was furnished, dialysis was stopped due to recovery or death, or the patient received a kidney transplant. For reporting purposes, each month is considered 30 days.

Examples:

ESRD-related services:

ESRD-related services are initiated on July 1 for a 57-year-old male. On July 11, he is admitted to the hospital as an inpatient and is discharged on July 27. He has had a complete assessment and the physician or other qualified health care professional has performed two face-to-face visits prior to admission. Another face-to-face visit occurs after discharge during the month.

In this example, 90961 is reported for the three face-to-face outpatient visits. Report inpatient E/M services as appropriate. Dialysis procedures rendered during the hospitalization (July 11-27) should be reported as appropriate (90935-90937, 90945-90947).

If the patient did not have a complete assessment during the month or was a transient or dialysis was stopped due to recovery or death, 90970 would be used to report each day outside the inpatient hospitalization as described in the home dialysis example below.

ESRD-related services for the home dialysis patient:

Home ESRD-related services are initiated on July 1 for a 57-year-old male. On July 11, he is admitted to the hospital as an inpatient and is discharged on July 27.

Report inpatient E/M services as appropriate. Dialysis procedures rendered during the hospitalization (July 11-27) should be reported as appropriate (90935-90937, 90945-90947).

(Do not report 90951-90970 during the same month in conjunction with 99487-99489)

(Do not report 90951-90970 during the service time of 99495, 99496)

★ **90951** End-stage renal disease (ESRD) related services monthly, for patients younger than 2 years of age to include monitoring for the adequacy of nutrition, assessment of growth and development, and counseling of parents; with 4 or more face-to-face visits by a physician or other qualified health care professional per month

➲ *CPT Changes: An Insider's View* 2009, 2013, 2017

➲ *CPT Assistant* Apr 13:3, Nov 13:3, Oct 14:3, Feb 18:12

★ **90952** with 2-3 face-to-face visits by a physician or other qualified health care professional per month

➲ *CPT Changes: An Insider's View* 2009, 2013, 2017

➲ *CPT Assistant* Apr 13:3, Feb 18:12

90953 with 1 face-to-face visit by a physician or other qualified health care professional per month

➲ *CPT Changes: An Insider's View* 2009, 2013

➲ *CPT Assistant* Apr 13:3, Feb 18:12

★ **90954** End-stage renal disease (ESRD) related services monthly, for patients 2-11 years of age to include monitoring for the adequacy of nutrition, assessment of growth and development, and counseling of parents; with 4 or more face-to-face visits by a physician or other qualified health care professional per month

➲ *CPT Changes: An Insider's View* 2009, 2013, 2017

➲ *CPT Assistant* Apr 13:3, Feb 18:12

★ **90955** with 2-3 face-to-face visits by a physician or other qualified health care professional per month

➲ *CPT Changes: An Insider's View* 2009, 2013, 2017

➲ *CPT Assistant* Apr 13:3, Feb 18:12

90956 with 1 face-to-face visit by a physician or other qualified health care professional per month

➲ *CPT Changes: An Insider's View* 2009, 2013

➲ *CPT Assistant* Apr 13:3, Feb 18:12

★ **90957** End-stage renal disease (ESRD) related services monthly, for patients 12-19 years of age to include monitoring for the adequacy of nutrition, assessment of growth and development, and counseling of parents; with 4 or more face-to-face visits by a physician or other qualified health care professional per month

➲ *CPT Changes: An Insider's View* 2009, 2013, 2017

➲ *CPT Assistant* Apr 13:3, Feb 18:12

★ **90958** with 2-3 face-to-face visits by a physician or other qualified health care professional per month

➲ *CPT Changes: An Insider's View* 2009, 2013, 2017

➲ *CPT Assistant* Apr 13:3, Feb 18:12

90959 with 1 face-to-face visit by a physician or other qualified health care professional per month

➲ *CPT Changes: An Insider's View* 2009, 2013

➲ *CPT Assistant* Apr 13:3, Feb 18:12

★ **90960** End-stage renal disease (ESRD) related services monthly, for patients 20 years of age and older; with 4 or more face-to-face visits by a physician or other qualified health care professional per month

➲ *CPT Changes: An Insider's View* 2009, 2013, 2017

➲ *CPT Assistant* Apr 13:3, Feb 18:12

★ 90961 with 2-3 face-to-face visits by a physician or other qualified health care professional per month
CPT Changes: An Insider's View 2009, 2013, 2017
CPT Assistant Apr 13:3, Feb 18:12

90962 with 1 face-to-face visit by a physician or other qualified health care professional per month
CPT Changes: An Insider's View 2009, 2013
CPT Assistant Apr 13:3, Feb 18:12

90963 End-stage renal disease (ESRD) related services for home dialysis per full month, for patients younger than 2 years of age to include monitoring for the adequacy of nutrition, assessment of growth and development, and counseling of parents
CPT Changes: An Insider's View 2009
CPT Assistant Apr 13:3, Feb 18:12

90964 End-stage renal disease (ESRD) related services for home dialysis per full month, for patients 2-11 years of age to include monitoring for the adequacy of nutrition, assessment of growth and development, and counseling of parents
CPT Changes: An Insider's View 2009
CPT Assistant Apr 13:3, Feb 18:12

90965 End-stage renal disease (ESRD) related services for home dialysis per full month, for patients 12-19 years of age to include monitoring for the adequacy of nutrition, assessment of growth and development, and counseling of parents
CPT Changes: An Insider's View 2009
CPT Assistant Apr 13:3, Feb 18:12

90966 End-stage renal disease (ESRD) related services for home dialysis per full month, for patients 20 years of age and older
CPT Changes: An Insider's View 2009
CPT Assistant Apr 13:3, Feb 18:12

90967 End-stage renal disease (ESRD) related services for dialysis less than a full month of service, per day; for patients younger than 2 years of age
CPT Changes: An Insider's View 2009
CPT Assistant Apr 13:3, Feb 18:12

90968 for patients 2-11 years of age
CPT Changes: An Insider's View 2009
CPT Assistant Apr 13:3, Feb 18:12

90969 for patients 12-19 years of age
CPT Changes: An Insider's View 2009
CPT Assistant Apr 13:3, Feb 18:12

90970 for patients 20 years of age and older
CPT Changes: An Insider's View 2009
CPT Assistant Apr 13:3, Nov 13:3, Oct 14:3, Feb 18:12

Other Dialysis Procedures

90989 Dialysis training, patient, including helper where applicable, any mode, completed course
CPT Assistant Fall 93:5, Jun 01:10

90993 Dialysis training, patient, including helper where applicable, any mode, course not completed, per training session
CPT Assistant Winter 90:11, Fall 93:5, Jun 01:10

90997 Hemoperfusion (eg, with activated charcoal or resin)

90999 Unlisted dialysis procedure, inpatient or outpatient

Gastroenterology

91010 Esophageal motility (manometric study of the esophagus and/or gastroesophageal junction) study with interpretation and report;
CPT Changes: An Insider's View 2011, 2012
CPT Assistant Nov 97:42

+ 91013 with stimulation or perfusion (eg, stimulant, acid or alkali perfusion) (List separately in addition to code for primary procedure)
CPT Changes: An Insider's View 2011, 2012

(Use 91013 in conjunction with 91010)

(Do not report 91013 more than once per session)

(To report esophageal motility studies with high resolution esophageal pressure topography, use 91299)

91020 Gastric motility (manometric) studies
CPT Assistant Nov 97:42, Sep 13:13

91022 Duodenal motility (manometric) study
CPT Changes: An Insider's View 2006
CPT Assistant Sep 13:13

(If gastrointestinal endoscopy is performed, use 43235)

(If fluoroscopy is performed, use 76000)

(If gastric motility study is performed, use 91020)

(Do not report 91020, 91022 in conjunction with 91112)

91030 Esophagus, acid perfusion (Bernstein) test for esophagitis

91034 Esophagus, gastroesophageal reflux test; with nasal catheter pH electrode(s) placement, recording, analysis and interpretation
CPT Changes: An Insider's View 2005
CPT Assistant May 05:3, Feb 14:11

91035 with mucosal attached telemetry pH electrode placement, recording, analysis and interpretation
CPT Changes: An Insider's View 2005
CPT Assistant May 05:3, Feb 14:11

91037 Esophageal function test, gastroesophageal reflux test with nasal catheter intraluminal impedance electrode(s) placement, recording, analysis and interpretation;
CPT Changes: An Insider's View 2005
CPT Assistant May 05:3

91038 prolonged (greater than 1 hour, up to 24 hours)
CPT Changes: An Insider's View 2005
CPT Assistant May 05:3, Feb 14:11

Esophageal Acid Reflux Test

91034

A catheter with a pH electrode is placed into the esophagus, either through the nares or swallowed, to measure intraesophageal pH (an indicator of gastric reflux).

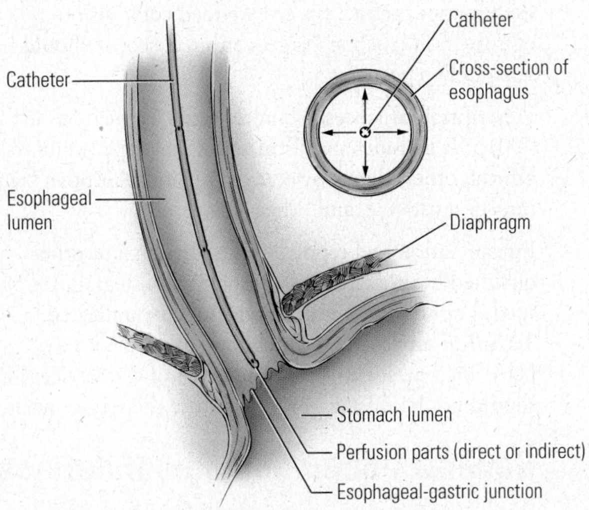

91040 Esophageal balloon distension study, diagnostic, with provocation when performed

➔ *CPT Changes: An Insider's View* 2005, 2016

➔ *CPT Assistant* May 05:3, Jan 17:7

(Do not report 91040 more than once per session)

91065 Breath hydrogen or methane test (eg, for detection of lactase deficiency, fructose intolerance, bacterial overgrowth, or oro-cecal gastrointestinal transit)

➔ *CPT Changes: An Insider's View* 2005, 2014

➔ *CPT Assistant* May 05:3

(Report 91065 once for each administered challenge)

(For H. pylori breath test analysis, use 83013 for non-radioactive (C-13) isotope or 78268 for radioactive (C-14) isotope)

(To report placement of an esophageal tamponade tube for management of variceal bleeding, use 43460. To report placement of a long intestinal Miller-Abbott tube, use 44500)

(For abdominal paracentesis, see 49082, 49083, 49084; with instillation of medication, see 96440, 96446)

(For peritoneoscopy, use 49320; with biopsy, use 49321)

(For splenoportography, see 38200, 75810)

91110 Gastrointestinal tract imaging, intraluminal (eg, capsule endoscopy), esophagus through ileum, with interpretation and report

➔ *CPT Changes: An Insider's View* 2004, 2013

➔ *CPT Assistant* Oct 04:15, Aug 05:14, May 09:8, Sep 13:13

(Do not report 91110 in conjunction with 91111, 0355T)

(Visualization of the colon is not reported separately)

(Append modifier 52 if the ileum is not visualized)

91111 Gastrointestinal tract imaging, intraluminal (eg, capsule endoscopy), esophagus with interpretation and report

➔ *CPT Changes: An Insider's View* 2007, 2013

➔ *CPT Assistant* Sep 13:13

(Do not report 91111 in conjunction with 91110, 0355T)

(For measurement of gastrointestinal tract transit times or pressure using wireless capsule, use 91112)

91112 Gastrointestinal transit and pressure measurement, stomach through colon, wireless capsule, with interpretation and report

➔ *CPT Changes: An Insider's View* 2013

➔ *CPT Assistant* Sep 13:13

(Do not report 91112 in conjunction with 83986, 91020, 91022, 91117)

91117 Colon motility (manometric) study, minimum 6 hours continuous recording (including provocation tests, eg, meal, intracolonic balloon distension, pharmacologic agents, if performed), with interpretation and report

➔ *CPT Changes: An Insider's View* 2011

➔ *CPT Assistant* Sep 13:13

(For wireless capsule pressure measurements, use 91112)

(Do not report 91117 in conjunction with 91120, 91122)

91120 Rectal sensation, tone, and compliance test (ie, response to graded balloon distention)

➔ *CPT Changes: An Insider's View* 2005

➔ *CPT Assistant* May 05:3

(For biofeedback training, use 90911)

(For anorectal manometry, use 91122)

91122 Anorectal manometry

(Do not report 91120, 91122 in conjunction with 91117)

Gastric Physiology

91132 Electrogastrography, diagnostic, transcutaneous;

➔ *CPT Changes: An Insider's View* 2001

91133 with provocative testing

➔ *CPT Changes: An Insider's View* 2001

Other Procedures

91200 Liver elastography, mechanically induced shear wave (eg, vibration), without imaging, with interpretation and report

➔ *CPT Changes: An Insider's View* 2015

➔ *CPT Assistant* Oct 17:9

➔ *Clinical Examples in Radiology* Spring 15:4

►(Do not report 91200 in conjunction with 76981, 76982, 76983)◄

91299 Unlisted diagnostic gastroenterology procedure

➔ *CPT Assistant* Aug 05:14

Ophthalmology

(For surgical procedures, see **Surgery,** Eye and Ocular Adnexa, 65091 et seq)

Definitions

Intermediate ophthalmological services describes an evaluation of a new or existing condition complicated with a new diagnostic or management problem not necessarily relating to the primary diagnosis, including history, general medical observation, external ocular and adnexal examination and other diagnostic procedures as indicated; may include the use of mydriasis for ophthalmoscopy.

For example:

a. Review of history, external examination, ophthalmoscopy, biomicroscopy for an acute complicated condition (eg, iritis) not requiring comprehensive ophthalmological services.

b. Review of interval history, external examination, ophthalmoscopy, biomicroscopy and tonometry in established patient with known cataract not requiring comprehensive ophthalmological services.

Comprehensive ophthalmological services describes a general evaluation of the complete visual system. The comprehensive services constitute a single service entity but need not be performed at one session. The service includes history, general medical observation, external and ophthalmoscopic examinations, gross visual fields and basic sensorimotor examination. It often includes, as indicated: biomicroscopy, examination with cycloplegia or mydriasis and tonometry. It always includes initiation of diagnostic and treatment programs.

Intermediate and comprehensive ophthalmological services constitute integrated services in which medical decision making cannot be separated from the examining techniques used. Itemization of service components, such as slit lamp examination, keratometry, routine ophthalmoscopy, retinoscopy, tonometry, or motor evaluation is not applicable.

For example:

The comprehensive services required for diagnosis and treatment of a patient with symptoms indicating possible disease of the visual system, such as glaucoma, cataract or retinal disease, or to rule out disease of the visual system, new or established patient.

Initiation of diagnostic and treatment program includes the prescription of medication, and arranging for special ophthalmological diagnostic or treatment services, consultations, laboratory procedures and radiological services.

Special ophthalmological services describes services in which a special evaluation of part of the visual system is made, which goes beyond the services included under general ophthalmological services, or in which special treatment is given. Special ophthalmological services may be reported in addition to the general ophthalmological services or evaluation and management services.

For example:

Fluorescein angioscopy, quantitative visual field examination, refraction or extended color vision examination (such as Nagel's anomaloscope) should be separately reported.

Prescription of lenses, when required, is included in 92015. It includes specification of lens type (monofocal, bifocal, other), lens power, axis, prism, absorptive factor, impact resistance, and other factors.

Interpretation and report by the physician or other qualified health care professional is an integral part of special ophthalmological services where indicated. Technical procedures (which may or may not be performed personally) are often part of the service, but should not be mistaken to constitute the service itself.

General Ophthalmological Services

New Patient

(For distinguishing between new and established patients, see **Evaluation and Management** guidelines)

92002 Ophthalmological services: medical examination and evaluation with initiation of diagnostic and treatment program; intermediate, new patient

➲ *CPT Assistant* Feb 97:6, Aug 98:3, Jun 05:11, Dec 05:10, Jan 07:30, Jan 08:1, Sep 08:7, Feb 11:10, Aug 12:9, Oct 12:9, Sep 17:15, Feb 18:3

(Do not report 92002 in conjunction with 99173, 99174, 99177, 0469T)

92004 comprehensive, new patient, 1 or more visits

➲ *CPT Assistant* Feb 97:6, Aug 98:3, Jun 05:11, Dec 05:10, Jan 07:30, Jan 08:1, Sep 08:7, Nov 10:8, Jan 11:9, Feb 11:10, Aug 12:9, Nov 16:9, Sep 17:15, Feb 18:3

(Do not report 92004 in conjunction with 99173, 99174, 99177, 0469T)

Established Patient

(For distinguishing between new and established patients, see **Evaluation and Management** guidelines)

92012 Ophthalmological services: medical examination and evaluation, with initiation or continuation of diagnostic and treatment program; intermediate, established patient

➲ *CPT Assistant* Feb 97:6, Aug 98:3, Jun 05:11, Dec 05:10, Jan 07:30, Jan 08:1, Sep 08:7, Feb 11:10, Aug 12:9, Sep 17:15, Feb 18:3

(Do not report 92012 in conjunction with 99173, 99174, 99177, 0469T)

92014 comprehensive, established patient, 1 or more visits

➔ *CPT Assistant* Feb 97:6, Aug 98:3, Dec 99:10, Jun 05:11, Dec 05:10, Jan 07:30, Jan 08:1, Sep 08:7, Nov 10:8, Jan 11:9, Feb 11:10, Aug 12:9, Oct 12:9, Nov 16:9, Sep 17:15, Feb 18:3

(Do not report 92014 in conjunction with 99173, 99174, 99177, 0469T)

(For surgical procedures, see **Surgery**, Eye and Ocular Adnexa, 65091 et seq)

Special Ophthalmological Services

92015 Determination of refractive state

➔ *CPT Assistant* Mar 96:11, Feb 97:6, Aug 98:3, Aug 06:11, Mar 13:6, Mar 16:11

(Do not report 92015 in conjunction with 99173, 99174, 99177)

(For instrument-based ocular screening, use 99174, 99177)

92018 Ophthalmological examination and evaluation, under general anesthesia, with or without manipulation of globe for passive range of motion or other manipulation to facilitate diagnostic examination; complete

➔ *CPT Assistant* Feb 97:6, Aug 98:3

92019 limited

➔ *CPT Assistant* Feb 97:6, Aug 98:3

92020 Gonioscopy (separate procedure)

➔ *CPT Assistant* Feb 97:6, Aug 98:3

(For gonioscopy under general anesthesia, use 92018)

92025 Computerized corneal topography, unilateral or bilateral, with interpretation and report

➔ *CPT Changes: An Insider's View* 2007

➔ *CPT Assistant* Oct 10:10, Oct 12:9

(Do not report 92025 in conjunction with 65710-65771)

(92025 is not used for manual keratoscopy, which is part of a single system Evaluation and Management or ophthalmological service)

92060 Sensorimotor examination with multiple measurements of ocular deviation (eg, restrictive or paretic muscle with diplopia) with interpretation and report (separate procedure)

➔ *CPT Assistant* Feb 97:6, Aug 98:3

92065 Orthoptic and/or pleoptic training, with continuing medical direction and evaluation

➔ *CPT Assistant* Feb 97:6, Jun 98:10, Aug 98:3

92071 Fitting of contact lens for treatment of ocular surface disease

➔ *CPT Changes: An Insider's View* 2012

➔ *CPT Assistant* Aug 12:9

(Do not report 92071 in conjunction with 92072)

(Report supply of lens separately with 99070 or appropriate supply code)

92072 Fitting of contact lens for management of keratoconus, initial fitting

➔ *CPT Changes: An Insider's View* 2012

➔ *CPT Assistant* Aug 12:9, Sep 17:15

(For subsequent fittings, report using evaluation and management services or general ophthalmological services)

(Do not report 92072 in conjunction with 92071)

(Report supply of lens separately with 99070 or appropriate supply code)

92081 Visual field examination, unilateral or bilateral, with interpretation and report; limited examination (eg, tangent screen, Autoplot, arc perimeter, or single stimulus level automated test, such as Octopus 3 or 7 equivalent)

➔ *CPT Assistant* Feb 97:6, Aug 98:3, Sep 10:10, Oct 12:9

92082 intermediate examination (eg, at least 2 isopters on Goldmann perimeter, or semiquantitative, automated suprathreshold screening program, Humphrey suprathreshold automatic diagnostic test, Octopus program 33)

➔ *CPT Assistant* Feb 97:6, Aug 98:3, Oct 12:9

92083 extended examination (eg, Goldmann visual fields with at least 3 isopters plotted and static determination within the central 30°, or quantitative, automated threshold perimetry, Octopus program G-1, 32 or 42, Humphrey visual field analyzer full threshold programs 30-2, 24-2, or 30/60-2)

➔ *CPT Assistant* Feb 97:6, Aug 98:3, Oct 12:9

(Gross visual field testing (eg, confrontation testing) is a part of general ophthalmological services and is not reported separately)

(For visual field assessment by patient activated data transmission to a remote surveillance center, see 0378T, 0379T)

92100 Serial tonometry (separate procedure) with multiple measurements of intraocular pressure over an extended time period with interpretation and report, same day (eg, diurnal curve or medical treatment of acute elevation of intraocular pressure)

➔ *CPT Assistant* Feb 97:6, Jun 98:10, Aug 98:3, Aug 12:9, 15, Oct 12:9, May 14:5

(For monitoring of intraocular pressure for 24 hours or longer, use 0329T)

(Ocular blood flow measurements are reported with 0198T. Single-episode tonometry is a component of general ophthalmological service or E/M service)

92132 Scanning computerized ophthalmic diagnostic imaging, anterior segment, with interpretation and report, unilateral or bilateral

➔ *CPT Changes: An Insider's View* 2011

➔ *CPT Assistant* Feb 11:6, Oct 12:9, Mar 13:6, Apr 13:7, May 14:5

(For specular microscopy and endothelial cell analysis, use 92286)

(For tear film imaging, use 0330T)

92133 Scanning computerized ophthalmic diagnostic imaging, posterior segment, with interpretation and report, unilateral or bilateral; optic nerve
- ➲ *CPT Changes: An Insider's View* 2011
- ➲ *CPT Assistant* Feb 11:6, Oct 12:9, Nov 14:10

92134 retina
- ➲ *CPT Changes: An Insider's View* 2011
- ➲ *CPT Assistant* Feb 11:6, Oct 12:9, Nov 14:10

(Do not report 92133 and 92134 at the same patient encounter)

(For scanning computerized ophthalmic diagnostic imaging of the optic nerve and retina, see 92133, 92134)

92136 Ophthalmic biometry by partial coherence interferometry with intraocular lens power calculation
- ➲ *CPT Changes: An Insider's View* 2002
- ➲ *CPT Assistant* Aug 98:3, Apr 02:18, Sep 09:5, May 14:5

(For tear film imaging, use 0330T)

(92140 has been deleted)

92145 Corneal hysteresis determination, by air impulse stimulation, unilateral or bilateral, with interpretation and report
- ➲ *CPT Changes: An Insider's View* 2015

Ophthalmoscopy

Routine ophthalmoscopy is part of general and special ophthalmologic services whenever indicated. It is a non-itemized service and is not reported separately.

92225 Ophthalmoscopy, extended, with retinal drawing (eg, for retinal detachment, melanoma), with interpretation and report; initial
- ➲ *CPT Assistant* Feb 97:6, Aug 98:2, Dec 99:10, Feb 11:6, Oct 12:9

92226 subsequent
- ➲ *CPT Assistant* Feb 97:6, Aug 98:2, Feb 11:6

★ **92227** Remote imaging for detection of retinal disease (eg, retinopathy in a patient with diabetes) with analysis and report under physician supervision, unilateral or bilateral
- ➲ *CPT Changes: An Insider's View* 2011, 2017
- ➲ *CPT Assistant* Feb 11:7, May 11:9, Oct 12:9, Jul 16:9

(Do not report 92227 in conjunction with 92002-92014, 92133, 92134, 92250, 92228 or with the evaluation and management of the single organ system, the eye, 99201-99350)

★ **92228** Remote imaging for monitoring and management of active retinal disease (eg, diabetic retinopathy) with physician review, interpretation and report, unilateral or bilateral
- ➲ *CPT Changes: An Insider's View* 2011, 2017
- ➲ *CPT Assistant* Feb 11:7, May 11:9, Oct 12:9

(Do not report 92228 in conjunction with 92002-92014, 92133, 92134, 92250, 92227 or with the evaluation and management of the single organ system, the eye, 99201-99350)

Extended Ophthalmoscopy
92225, 92226

Illustration of retinal structures to document for comparison with future examinations

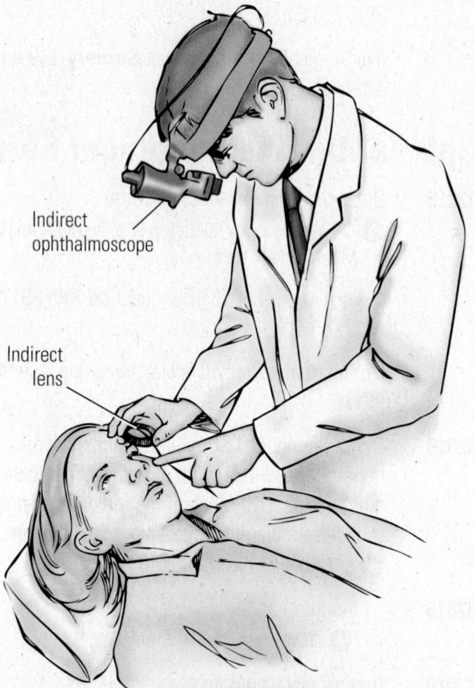

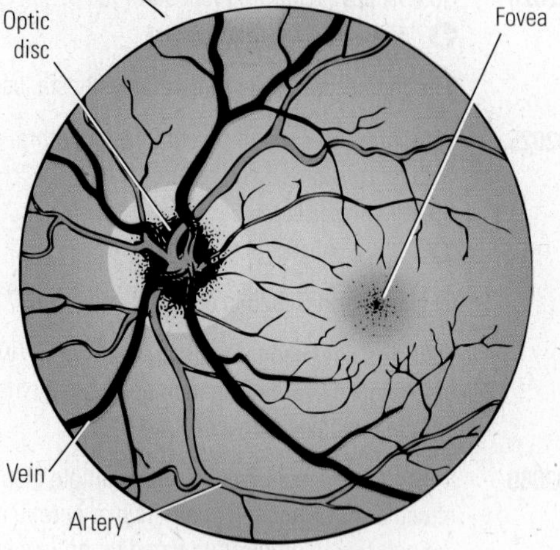

Ophthalmoscopic appearance of retina

92230 Fluorescein angioscopy with interpretation and report
- ➲ *CPT Assistant* Feb 97:6, Feb 11:6

92235 Fluorescein angiography (includes multiframe imaging) with interpretation and report, unilateral or bilateral
- ➲ *CPT Changes: An Insider's View* 2017
- ➲ *CPT Assistant* Feb 97:6, Feb 11:6, Jun 17:8

(When fluorescein and indocyanine-green angiography are performed at the same patient encounter, use 92242)

Fluorescein Angiography
92235

Fluorescein dye is injected in a peripheral vein to enhance imaging. Serial multiframe angiography is performed to evaluate choroidal and retinal circulation. In this illustration, arteries display an even fluorescence, while veins appear striped from the laminar dye flow.

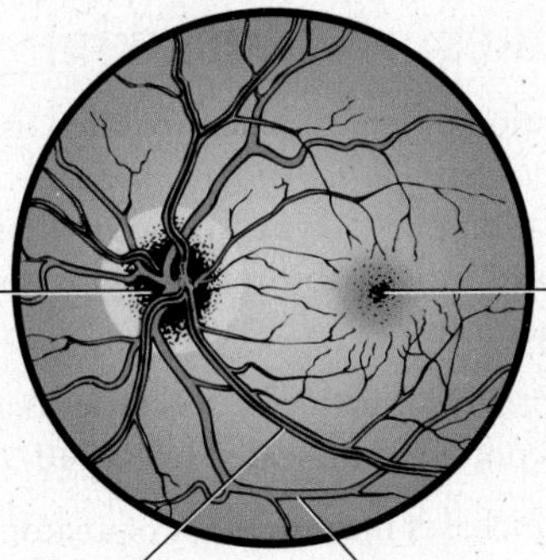

92240 Indocyanine-green angiography (includes multiframe imaging) with interpretation and report, unilateral or bilateral
➔ *CPT Changes: An Insider's View* 2017
➔ *CPT Assistant* Feb 11:6, Oct 12:9, Jun 17:8

(When indocyanine-green and fluorescein angiography are performed at the same patient encounter, use 92242)

92242 Fluorescein angiography and indocyanine-green angiography (includes multiframe imaging) performed at the same patient encounter with interpretation and report, unilateral or bilateral
➔ *CPT Changes: An Insider's View* 2017
➔ *CPT Assistant* Jun 17:8

(To report fluorescein angiography and indocyanine-green angiography not performed at the same patient encounter, see 92235, 92240)

92250 Fundus photography with interpretation and report
➔ *CPT Assistant* Feb 97:6, Apr 99:10, Feb 11:6, Oct 12:9, Nov 14:10, Dec 14:17, May 15:9, Jul 16:9

92260 Ophthalmodynamometry
➔ *CPT Assistant* Feb 97:6, Feb 11:6

(For ophthalmoscopy under general anesthesia, use 92018)

Other Specialized Services

For prescription, fitting, and/or medical supervision of ocular prosthetic (artificial eye) adaptation by a physician, see evaluation and management services including office or other outpatient services (99201-99215), office or other outpatient consultations (99241-99245) or general ophthalmological service codes 92002-92014.

►Electroretinography (ERG) is used to evaluate function of the retina and optic nerve of the eye, including photoreceptors and ganglion cells. A number of techniques are used which target different areas of the eye, including full field (flash and flicker) (92273) for a global response of photoreceptors of the retina, multifocal (92274) for photoreceptors in multiple separate locations in the retina including the macula, and pattern (0509T) for retinal ganglion cells. Multiple additional terms and techniques are used to describe various types of ERG. If the technique used is not specifically named in the code descriptors for 92273, 92274, or 0509T, use the unlisted procedure code 92499.◄

92265 Needle oculoelectromyography, 1 or more extraocular muscles, 1 or both eyes, with interpretation and report
➔ *CPT Assistant* Feb 97:6, Oct 12:9

92270 Electro-oculography with interpretation and report
➔ *CPT Assistant* Feb 97:6, Aug 08:12, May 09:9, Oct 12:9, Sep 15:7

(For vestibular function tests with recording, see 92537, 92538, 92540, 92541, 92542, 92544, 92545, 92546, 92547, 92548)

(Do not report 92270 in conjunction with 92537, 92538, 92540, 92541, 92542, 92544, 92545, 92546, 92547, 92548)

(To report saccadic eye movement testing with recording, use 92700)

● **92273** Electroretinography (ERG), with interpretation and report; full field (ie, ffERG, flash ERG, Ganzfeld ERG)
➔ *CPT Changes: An Insider's View* 2019

● **92274** multifocal (mfERG)
➔ *CPT Changes: An Insider's View* 2019

►(For pattern ERG, use 0509T)◄

►(92275 has been deleted. To report electroretinography, see 92273, 92274, 0509T)◄

(For electronystagmography for vestibular function studies, see 92541 et seq)

(For ophthalmic echography (diagnostic ultrasound), see 76511-76529)

92283 Color vision examination, extended, eg, anomaloscope or equivalent
➔ *CPT Assistant* Feb 97:6, Oct 12:9

(Color vision testing with pseudoisochromatic plates [such as HRR or Ishihara] is not reported separately. It is included in the appropriate general or ophthalmological service, or 99172)

92284 Dark adaptation examination with interpretation and report
➔ *CPT Assistant* Feb 97:6, Oct 12:9

92285 External ocular photography with interpretation and report for documentation of medical progress (eg, close-up photography, slit lamp photography, goniophotography, stereo-photography)
➔ *CPT Assistant* Feb 97:6, Sep 97:10, Oct 12:9, May 14:5

(For tear film imaging, use 0330T)

►(For meibomian gland imaging, use 0507T)◄

92286 Anterior segment imaging with interpretation and report; with specular microscopy and endothelial cell analysis
➲ *CPT Changes: An Insider's View* 2013
➲ *CPT Assistant* Feb 97:6, Oct 12:9, Mar 13:6

92287 with fluorescein angiography
➲ *CPT Changes: An Insider's View* 2013
➲ *CPT Assistant* Feb 97:6, Mar 13:6

Contact Lens Services

The prescription of contact lens includes specification of optical and physical characteristics (such as power, size, curvature, flexibility, gas-permeability). It is **not** a part of the general ophthalmological services.

The fitting of contact lens includes instruction and training of the wearer and incidental revision of the lens during the training period.

Follow-up of successfully fitted extended wear lenses is reported as part of a general ophthalmological service (92012 et seq).

The supply of contact lenses may be reported as part of the service of fitting. It may also be reported separately by using the appropriate supply codes.

(For therapeutic or surgical use of contact lens, see 68340, 92071, 92072)

92310 Prescription of optical and physical characteristics of and fitting of contact lens, with medical supervision of adaptation; corneal lens, both eyes, except for aphakia
➲ *CPT Assistant* Feb 97:6, Oct 12:9

(For prescription and fitting of 1 eye, add modifier 52)

92311 corneal lens for aphakia, 1 eye
➲ *CPT Assistant* Feb 97:6, Oct 12:9

92312 corneal lens for aphakia, both eyes
➲ *CPT Assistant* Feb 97:6, Oct 12:9

92313 corneoscleral lens
➲ *CPT Assistant* Feb 97:7, Mar 03:1

92314 Prescription of optical and physical characteristics of contact lens, with medical supervision of adaptation and direction of fitting by independent technician; corneal lens, both eyes except for aphakia
➲ *CPT Assistant* Feb 97:7, Oct 12:9

(For prescription and fitting of 1 eye, add modifier 52)

92315 corneal lens for aphakia, 1 eye
➲ *CPT Assistant* Feb 97:7, Oct 12:9

92316 corneal lens for aphakia, both eyes
➲ *CPT Assistant* Feb 97:7, Oct 12:9

92317 corneoscleral lens
➲ *CPT Assistant* Feb 97:7

92325 Modification of contact lens (separate procedure), with medical supervision of adaptation
➲ *CPT Assistant* Feb 97:7, Oct 12:9

92326 Replacement of contact lens
➲ *CPT Assistant* Feb 97:7

Spectacle Services (Including Prosthesis for Aphakia)

Prescription of lenses, when required, is included in 92015, *Determination of refractive state*. It includes specification of lens type (monofocal, bifocal, other), lens power, axis, prism, absorptive factor, impact resistance, and other factors.

When provided, fitting of spectacles is a separate service and is reported as indicated by 92340-92371.

Fitting includes measurement of anatomical facial characteristics, the writing of laboratory specifications, and the final adjustment of the spectacles to the visual axes and anatomical topography. Presence of the physician or other qualified health care professional is not required.

Supply of materials is a separate service component; it is not part of the service of fitting spectacles.

92340 Fitting of spectacles, except for aphakia; monofocal
➲ *CPT Assistant* Feb 97:7, Aug 98:4, Mar 13:6

92341 bifocal
➲ *CPT Assistant* Feb 97:7, Aug 98:4, Mar 13:6

92342 multifocal, other than bifocal
➲ *CPT Assistant* Feb 97:7, Aug 98:4, Mar 13:6

92352 Fitting of spectacle prosthesis for aphakia; monofocal
➲ *CPT Assistant* Feb 97:7, Aug 98:4, Mar 13:6

92353 multifocal
➲ *CPT Assistant* Feb 97:7, Aug 98:4, Mar 13:6

92354 Fitting of spectacle mounted low vision aid; single element system
➲ *CPT Assistant* Feb 97:7, Aug 98:4, Mar 13:6

92355 telescopic or other compound lens system
➲ *CPT Assistant* Feb 97:7, Aug 98:4, Mar 13:6

92358 Prosthesis service for aphakia, temporary (disposable or loan, including materials)
➲ *CPT Assistant* Feb 97:7, Aug 98:4, Mar 13:6

92370 Repair and refitting spectacles; except for aphakia
➲ *CPT Assistant* Feb 97:7, Mar 13:6

92371 spectacle prosthesis for aphakia
➲ *CPT Assistant* Feb 97:7, Aug 98:4, Mar 13:6

Other Procedures

92499 Unlisted ophthalmological service or procedure
➲ *CPT Assistant* Feb 97:7

Special Otorhinolaryngologic Services

Diagnostic or treatment procedures that are reported as evaluation and management services (eg, otoscopy, anterior rhinoscopy, tuning fork test, removal of non-impacted cerumen) are not reported separately.

Special otorhinolaryngologic services are those diagnostic and treatment services not included in an evaluation and management service, including office or other outpatient services (99201-99215), or office or other outpatient consultations (99241-99245).

Codes 92507, 92508, 92520, 92521, 92522, 92523, 92524, and 92526 are used to report evaluation and treatment of speech sound production, receptive language, and expressive language abilities, voice and resonance production, speech fluency, and swallowing. Evaluations may include examination of speech sound production, articulatory movements of oral musculature, oral-pharyngeal swallowing function, qualitative analysis of voice and resonance, and measures of frequency, type, and duration of stuttering. Evaluations may also include the patient's ability to understand the meaning and intent of written and verbal expressions, as well as the appropriate formulation and utterance of expressive thought. In contrast, 92626 and 92627 are reported for an evaluation of auditory rehabilitation status determining the patient's ability to use residual hearing in order to identify the acoustic characteristics of sounds associated with speech communication.

(For laryngoscopy with stroboscopy, use 31579)

92502 Otolaryngologic examination under general anesthesia
➔ *CPT Assistant* Sep 16:6

92504 Binocular microscopy (separate diagnostic procedure)
➔ *CPT Assistant* Jul 05:14, Oct 11:10, Oct 13:14, Sep 16:6

92507 Treatment of speech, language, voice, communication, and/or auditory processing disorder; individual
➔ *CPT Changes: An Insider's View* 2006
➔ *CPT Assistant* Dec 04:14, Jan 06:7, Oct 13:7, Sep 16:6

►(Do not report 92507 in conjunction with 97153, 97155)◄

92508 group, 2 or more individuals
➔ *CPT Assistant* Dec 04:14, Oct 13:7, Sep 16:6

►(Do not report 92508 in conjunction with 97154, 97158)◄

(For auditory rehabilitation, prelingual hearing loss, use 92630)

(For auditory rehabilitation, postlingual hearing loss, use 92633)

(For cochlear implant programming, see 92601-92604)

92511 Nasopharyngoscopy with endoscope (separate procedure)
➔ *CPT Assistant* Sep 16:6

(Do not report 92511 in conjunction with 31575, 43197, 43198)

92512 Nasal function studies (eg, rhinomanometry)
➔ *CPT Assistant* Sep 16:6

92516 Facial nerve function studies (eg, electroneuronography)
➔ *CPT Assistant* Sep 16:6

92520 Laryngeal function studies (ie, aerodynamic testing and acoustic testing)
➔ *CPT Changes: An Insider's View* 2006
➔ *CPT Assistant* Dec 04:17, Jan 06:7, Sep 16:6

(For performance of a single test, use modifier 52)

(To report flexible fiberoptic laryngeal evaluation of swallowing and laryngeal sensory testing, see 92611-92617)

(To report other testing of laryngeal function (eg, electroglottography), use 92700)

92521 Evaluation of speech fluency (eg, stuttering, cluttering)
➔ *CPT Changes: An Insider's View* 2014
➔ *CPT Assistant* Jun 14:3, Sep 16:6

92522 Evaluation of speech sound production (eg, articulation, phonological process, apraxia, dysarthria)
➔ *CPT Changes: An Insider's View* 2014
➔ *CPT Assistant* Jun 14:3

92523 with evaluation of language comprehension and expression (eg, receptive and expressive language)
➔ *CPT Changes: An Insider's View* 2014
➔ *CPT Assistant* Jun 14:3, Sep 16:6

92524 Behavioral and qualitative analysis of voice and resonance
➔ *CPT Changes: An Insider's View* 2014
➔ *CPT Assistant* Jun 14:3, Sep 16:6

92526 Treatment of swallowing dysfunction and/or oral function for feeding
➔ *CPT Assistant* Sep 16:6

Vestibular Function Tests, Without Electrical Recording

92531 Spontaneous nystagmus, including gaze

92532 Positional nystagmus test
➔ *CPT Changes: An Insider's View* 2002

(Do not report 92531, 92532 with evaluation and management services including office or other outpatient services [99201-99215], observation care [99218-99220, 99224-99226], observation or inpatient care including admission and discharge [99234-99236], hospital care [99221-99223, 99231-99233], office or other outpatient consultations [99241-99245], nursing facility services [99304-99318], and domiciliary, rest home, or custodial care services [99324-99337])

92533 Caloric vestibular test, each irrigation (binaural, bithermal stimulation constitutes 4 tests)
➔ *CPT Assistant* May 96:5

92534 Optokinetic nystagmus test
➲ *CPT Changes: An Insider's View* 2002

Vestibular Function Tests, With Recording (eg, ENG)

92537 Caloric vestibular test with recording, bilateral; bithermal (ie, one warm and one cool irrigation in each ear for a total of four irrigations)
➲ *CPT Changes: An Insider's View* 2016

(Do not report 92537 in conjunction with 92270, 92538)

(For three irrigations, use modifier 52)

(For monothermal caloric vestibular testing, use 92538)

92538 monothermal (ie, one irrigation in each ear for a total of two irrigations)
➲ *CPT Changes: An Insider's View* 2016

(Do not report 92538 in conjunction with 92270, 92537)

(For one irrigation, use modifier 52)

(For bilateral, bithermal caloric vestibular testing, use 92537)

92540 Basic vestibular evaluation, includes spontaneous nystagmus test with eccentric gaze fixation nystagmus, with recording, positional nystagmus test, minimum of 4 positions, with recording, optokinetic nystagmus test, bidirectional foveal and peripheral stimulation, with recording, and oscillating tracking test, with recording
➲ *CPT Changes: An Insider's View* 2010
➲ *CPT Assistant* Sep 15:7

(Do not report 92540 in conjunction with 92270, 92541, 92542, 92544, 92545)

92541 Spontaneous nystagmus test, including gaze and fixation nystagmus, with recording
➲ *CPT Assistant* Feb 05:13, Aug 08:12, May 11:10, Sep 15:7

(Do not report 92541 in conjunction with 92270, 92540 or the set of 92542, 92544, and 92545)

92542 Positional nystagmus test, minimum of 4 positions, with recording
➲ *CPT Assistant* Feb 05:13, Aug 08:12, Sep 10:9, Sep 15:7

(Do not report 92542 in conjunction with 92270, 92540 or the set of 92541, 92544, and 92545)

(92543 has been deleted. To report caloric vestibular testing, see 92537, 92538)

92544 Optokinetic nystagmus test, bidirectional, foveal or peripheral stimulation, with recording
➲ *CPT Assistant* Feb 05:13, Aug 08:12, Sep 15:7

(Do not report 92544 in conjunction with 92270, 92540 or the set of 92541, 92542, and 92545)

92545 Oscillating tracking test, with recording
➲ *CPT Assistant* Feb 05:13, Aug 08:12, May 11:10, Sep 15:7

(Do not report 92545 in conjunction with 92270, 92540 or the set of 92541, 92542, and 92544)

92546 Sinusoidal vertical axis rotational testing
➲ *CPT Assistant* Sep 04:13, Feb 05:13, Aug 08:12, May 11:10, Jun 13:14, Sep 15:7

(Do not report 92546 in conjunction with 92270)

+ 92547 Use of vertical electrodes (List separately in addition to code for primary procedure)
➲ *CPT Assistant* May 04:14, Feb 05:13, Aug 08:12, Sep 15:7

(Use 92547 in conjunction with 92540-92546)

(For unlisted vestibular tests, use 92700)

(Do not report 92547 in conjunction with 92270)

92548 Computerized dynamic posturography
➲ *CPT Assistant* May 11:10, Sep 15:7

(Do not report 92548 in conjunction with 92270)

Audiologic Function Tests

The audiometric tests listed below require the use of calibrated electronic equipment, recording of results and a report with interpretation. Hearing tests (such as whispered voice, tuning fork) that are otorhinolaryngologic Evaluation and Management services are not reported separately. All services include testing of both ears. Use modifier 52 if a test is applied to one ear instead of two ears. All codes (except 92559) apply to testing of individuals. For testing of groups, use 92559 and specify test(s) used.

(For evaluation of speech, language, and/or hearing problems through observation and assessment of performance, see 92521, 92522, 92523, 92524)

92550 Tympanometry and reflex threshold measurements
➲ *CPT Changes: An Insider's View* 2010
➲ *CPT Assistant* Aug 14:3

(Do not report 92550 in conjunction with 92567, 92568)

92551 Screening test, pure tone, air only
➲ *CPT Assistant* Aug 14:3

92552 Pure tone audiometry (threshold); air only
➲ *CPT Assistant* Aug 14:3

92553 air and bone
➲ *CPT Assistant* Mar 11:8, Aug 14:3

92555 Speech audiometry threshold;
➲ *CPT Assistant* Aug 14:3

92556 with speech recognition
➲ *CPT Assistant* Mar 11:8, Aug 14:3

92557 Comprehensive audiometry threshold evaluation and speech recognition (92553 and 92556 combined)
➲ *CPT Assistant* Sep 07:11, Mar 11:8, Aug 14:3

(For hearing aid evaluation and selection, see 92590-92595)

(For automated audiometry, see 0208T-0212T)

Coding Tip

Instructions for Reporting Group Testing

For testing of groups, use 92559 and specify test(s) used.

CPT Coding Guidelines, Special Otorhinolaryngologic Service, Audiologic Function Tests

92558 Code is out of numerical sequence. See 92585-92588

92559 Audiometric testing of groups
CPT Assistant Aug 14:3

92560 Bekesy audiometry; screening
CPT Assistant Aug 14:3

92561 diagnostic
CPT Assistant Aug 14:3

92562 Loudness balance test, alternate binaural or monaural
CPT Assistant Mar 05:7, 9, Aug 14:3

92563 Tone decay test
CPT Assistant Aug 14:3

92564 Short increment sensitivity index (SISI)
CPT Assistant Oct 96:9, Aug 14:3

92565 Stenger test, pure tone
CPT Assistant Aug 14:3

92567 Tympanometry (impedance testing)
CPT Assistant Winter 90:11, Aug 14:3

92568 Acoustic reflex testing, threshold
CPT Changes: An Insider's View 2006, 2010
CPT Assistant Jan 06:7, Sep 07:11, Jun 09:10, Aug 14:3

92570 Acoustic immittance testing, includes tympanometry (impedance testing), acoustic reflex threshold testing, and acoustic reflex decay testing
CPT Changes: An Insider's View 2010
CPT Assistant Aug 14:3

(Do not report 92570 in conjunction with 92567, 92568)

92571 Filtered speech test
CPT Assistant Mar 05:7, Aug 14:3

92572 Staggered spondaic word test
CPT Assistant Mar 05:7, Aug 14:3

92575 Sensorineural acuity level test
CPT Assistant Aug 14:3

92576 Synthetic sentence identification test
CPT Assistant Mar 05:7, Aug 14:3

92577 Stenger test, speech
CPT Assistant Aug 14:3

92579 Visual reinforcement audiometry (VRA)
CPT Assistant Aug 14:3

92582 Conditioning play audiometry
CPT Assistant Aug 14:3

92583 Select picture audiometry

92584 Electrocochleography
CPT Assistant Jul 11:17, Aug 14:3

92585 Auditory evoked potentials for evoked response audiometry and/or testing of the central nervous system; comprehensive
CPT Changes: An Insider's View 2001
CPT Assistant Winter 90:11, May 13:8, Aug 14:3

92586 limited
CPT Changes: An Insider's View 2001
CPT Assistant Aug 14:3

 # 92558 Evoked otoacoustic emissions, screening (qualitative measurement of distortion product or transient evoked otoacoustic emissions), automated analysis
CPT Changes: An Insider's View 2012
CPT Assistant Aug 14:3

92587 Distortion product evoked otoacoustic emissions; limited evaluation (to confirm the presence or absence of hearing disorder, 3-6 frequencies) or transient evoked otoacoustic emissions, with interpretation and report
CPT Changes: An Insider's View 2012
CPT Assistant Sep 07:11

92588 comprehensive diagnostic evaluation (quantitative analysis of outer hair cell function by cochlear mapping, minimum of 12 frequencies), with interpretation and report
CPT Changes: An Insider's View 2012
CPT Assistant Aug 14:3

(For central auditory function evaluation, see 92620, 92621)

92590 Hearing aid examination and selection; monaural
CPT Assistant Jul 14:4, Aug 14:3

92591 binaural

92592 Hearing aid check; monaural

92593 binaural

92594 Electroacoustic evaluation for hearing aid; monaural

92595 binaural
CPT Assistant Aug 14:3

92596 Ear protector attenuation measurements
CPT Assistant Aug 14:3

92597 Code is out of numerical sequence. See 92603-92607

Evaluative and Therapeutic Services

Codes 92601 and 92603 describe post-operative analysis and fitting of previously placed external devices, connection to the cochlear implant, and programming of the stimulator. Codes 92602 and 92604 describe subsequent sessions for measurements and adjustment of the external transmitter and re-programming of the internal stimulator.

(For placement of cochlear implant, use 69930)

92601 Diagnostic analysis of cochlear implant, patient younger than 7 years of age; with programming
➲ *CPT Changes: An Insider's View* 2003
➲ *CPT Assistant* Mar 03:1, Jan 06:7, Jul 11:17, Oct 13:7, Jul 14:4

92602 subsequent reprogramming
➲ *CPT Changes: An Insider's View* 2003
➲ *CPT Assistant* Mar 03:1, 21, Jan 06:7, Oct 13:7

(Do not report 92602 in addition to 92601)

(For aural rehabilitation services following cochlear implant, including evaluation of rehabilitation status, see 92626-92627, 92630-92633)

92603 Diagnostic analysis of cochlear implant, age 7 years or older; with programming
➲ *CPT Changes: An Insider's View* 2003
➲ *CPT Assistant* Mar 03:2, 4, Jan 06:7, Jul 11:17, Oct 13:7

92604 subsequent reprogramming
➲ *CPT Changes: An Insider's View* 2003
➲ *CPT Assistant* Mar 03:2, 21, Jan 06:7, Jul 11:17, Oct 13:7, Jul 14:4

(Do not report 92604 in addition to 92603)

A View of the Outer Cochlear Implant

92601-92604

An example of the elements that are addressed in the diagnostic analysis and reprogramming of the cochlear implant

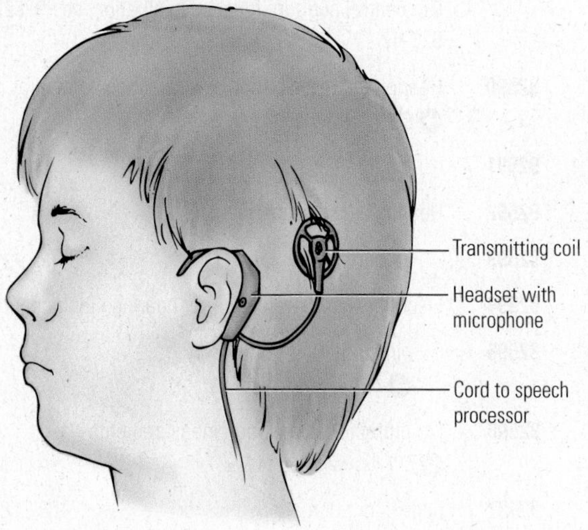

 # 92597 Evaluation for use and/or fitting of voice prosthetic device to supplement oral speech

(To report augmentative and alternative communication device services, see 92605, 92607, 92608, 92618)

92605 Evaluation for prescription of non-speech-generating augmentative and alternative communication device, face-to-face with the patient; first hour
➲ *CPT Changes: An Insider's View* 2003, 2012
➲ *CPT Assistant* Mar 03:2, 4, Oct 13:7

(To report evaluation for use and/or fitting of voice prosthetic device, use 92597)

#+ 92618 each additional 30 minutes (List separately in addition to code for primary procedure)
➲ *CPT Changes: An Insider's View* 2012

(Use 92618 in conjunction with 92605)

92606 Therapeutic service(s) for the use of non-speech-generating device, including programming and modification
➲ *CPT Changes: An Insider's View* 2003
➲ *CPT Assistant* Mar 03:2, 4

92607 Evaluation for prescription for speech-generating augmentative and alternative communication device, face-to-face with the patient; first hour
➲ *CPT Changes: An Insider's View* 2003
➲ *CPT Assistant* Mar 03:2, 4, Dec 04:16, Oct 13:7

(To report evaluation for use and/or fitting of voice prosthetic device, use 92597)

(For evaluation for prescription of a non-speech-generating device, use 92605)

+ 92608 each additional 30 minutes (List separately in addition to code for primary procedure)
➲ *CPT Changes: An Insider's View* 2003
➲ *CPT Assistant* Mar 03:2, 5, Dec 04:16, Oct 13:7

(Use 92608 in conjunction with 92607)

92609 Therapeutic services for the use of speech-generating device, including programming and modification
➲ *CPT Changes: An Insider's View* 2003
➲ *CPT Assistant* Mar 03:2, 4, Dec 04:16

(For therapeutic service(s) for the use of a non-speech-generating device, use 92606)

92610 Evaluation of oral and pharyngeal swallowing function
➲ *CPT Changes: An Insider's View* 2003
➲ *CPT Assistant* Mar 03:2, 5, Dec 04:17
➲ *Clinical Examples in Radiology* Spring 18:15

(For motion fluoroscopic evaluation of swallowing function, use 92611)

(For flexible endoscopic examination, use 92612-92617)

92611 Motion fluoroscopic evaluation of swallowing function by cine or video recording
➲ *CPT Changes: An Insider's View* 2003
➲ *CPT Assistant* Mar 03:2, 5, Dec 04:17, Jan 06:7, Jul 14:5, Apr 17:8
➲ *Clinical Examples in Radiology* Summer 06:4-5, Spring 18:14

(For radiological supervision and interpretation, use 74230)

(For evaluation of oral and pharyngeal swallowing function, use 92610)

(For flexible diagnostic laryngoscopy, use 31575)

92612 Flexible endoscopic evaluation of swallowing by cine or video recording
➲ *CPT Changes: An Insider's View* 2003, 2017
➲ *CPT Assistant* Mar 03:6, Jan 06:7, Apr 17:8

(If flexible endoscopic evaluation of swallowing is performed without cine or video recording, use 92700)

(Do not report 92612 in conjunction with 31575)

92613 interpretation and report only
➲ *CPT Changes: An Insider's View* 2003, 2013, 2017
➲ *CPT Assistant* Jan 06:7, Apr 17:8

(To report an evaluation of oral and pharyngeal swallowing function, use 92610)

(To report motion fluoroscopic evaluation of swallowing function, use 92611)

92614 Flexible endoscopic evaluation, laryngeal sensory testing by cine or video recording
➲ *CPT Changes: An Insider's View* 2003, 2017
➲ *CPT Assistant* Mar 03:6, Jan 06:7, Apr 17:8

(If flexible endoscopic evaluation of swallowing is performed without cine or video recording, use 92700)

(Do not report 92614 in conjunction with 31575)

92615 interpretation and report only
➲ *CPT Changes: An Insider's View* 2003, 2013, 2017
➲ *CPT Assistant* Mar 03:6, Jan 06:7, Apr 17:8

92616 Flexible endoscopic evaluation of swallowing and laryngeal sensory testing by cine or video recording
➲ *CPT Changes: An Insider's View* 2003, 2017
➲ *CPT Assistant* Mar 03:6, Jan 06:7, Apr 17:8

(If flexible endoscopic evaluation of swallowing is performed without cine or video recording, use 92700)

(Do not report 92616 in conjunction with 31575)

92617 interpretation and report only
➲ *CPT Changes: An Insider's View* 2003, 2013, 2017
➲ *CPT Assistant* Mar 03:6, Jan 06:7, Apr 17:8

92618 Code is out of numerical sequence. See 92603-92607

92620 Evaluation of central auditory function, with report; initial 60 minutes
➲ *CPT Changes: An Insider's View* 2005
➲ *CPT Assistant* Mar 05:7-8, Aug 14:3

+ 92621 each additional 15 minutes (List separately in addition to code for primary procedure)
➲ *CPT Changes: An Insider's View* 2005, 2012
➲ *CPT Assistant* Mar 05:7, Aug 14:3

(Use 92621 in conjunction with 92620)

(Do not report 92620, 92621 in conjunction with 92521, 92522, 92523, 92524)

92625 Assessment of tinnitus (includes pitch, loudness matching, and masking)
➲ *CPT Changes: An Insider's View* 2005
➲ *CPT Assistant* Mar 05:7-10, Aug 14:3

(Do not report 92625 in conjunction with 92562)

(For unilateral assessment, use modifier 52)

92626 Evaluation of auditory rehabilitation status; first hour
➲ *CPT Changes: An Insider's View* 2006
➲ *CPT Assistant* Jan 06:7, May 14:10, Jul 14:4, Sep 16:7

+ 92627 each additional 15 minutes (List separately in addition to code for primary procedure)
➲ *CPT Changes: An Insider's View* 2006
➲ *CPT Assistant* Jan 06:7, Jul 14:4, Sep 16:7

(Use 92627 in conjunction with 92626)

(When reporting 92626, 92627, use the face-to-face time with the patient or family)

92630 Auditory rehabilitation; prelingual hearing loss
➲ *CPT Changes: An Insider's View* 2006
➲ *CPT Assistant* Jan 06:7, Oct 13:7

92633 postlingual hearing loss
➲ *CPT Changes: An Insider's View* 2006
➲ *CPT Assistant* Jan 06:7, Oct 13:7

Special Diagnostic Procedures

92640 Diagnostic analysis with programming of auditory brainstem implant, per hour
➲ *CPT Changes: An Insider's View* 2007

(Report nonprogramming services separately [eg, cardiac monitoring])

Other Procedures

92700 Unlisted otorhinolaryngological service or procedure
➲ *CPT Changes: An Insider's View* 2003
➲ *CPT Assistant* Sep 04:14, Oct 04:10, Jan 06:7, Sep 06:13, Sep 07:11, Mar 11:10, Jul 11:17, May 14:10, Sep 15:15, Apr 17:8

Cardiovascular

Therapeutic Services and Procedures

92920 Code is out of numerical sequence. See 92997-93005

92921 Code is out of numerical sequence. See 92997-93005

92924 Code is out of numerical sequence. See 92997-93005

92925 Code is out of numerical sequence. See 92997-93005

92928 Code is out of numerical sequence. See 92997-93005

92929 Code is out of numerical sequence. See 92997-93005

92933 Code is out of numerical sequence. See 92997-93005

92934 Code is out of numerical sequence. See 92997-93005

92937 Code is out of numerical sequence. See 92997-93005

92938 Code is out of numerical sequence. See 92997-93005

92941 Code is out of numerical sequence. See 92997-93005

92943 Code is out of numerical sequence. See 92997-93005

92944 Code is out of numerical sequence. See 92997-93005

Other Therapeutic Services and Procedures

92950 Cardiopulmonary resuscitation (eg, in cardiac arrest)
➔ *CPT Assistant* Jan 96:7, Oct 04:14, Nov 07:5, Jul 12:13, Sep 12:17

(See also critical care services, 99291, 99292)

92953 Temporary transcutaneous pacing
➔ *CPT Changes: An Insider's View* 2017
➔ *CPT Assistant* Nov 99:49, Feb 07:10, Jul 07:1, May 14:4

(For direction of ambulance or rescue personnel outside the hospital by a physician or other qualified health care professional, use 99288)

92960 Cardioversion, elective, electrical conversion of arrhythmia; external
➔ *CPT Changes: An Insider's View* 2000, 2017
➔ *CPT Assistant* Summer 93:13, Nov 99:49, Jun 00:5, Nov 00:9, Jul 01:11, Jan 12:13

92961 internal (separate procedure)
➔ *CPT Changes: An Insider's View* 2000, 2017
➔ *CPT Assistant* Summer 93:13, Nov 99:49, Jun 00:5, Jul 00:5, Nov 00:9, Feb 15:3

(Do not report 92961 in conjunction with 93282-93284, 93287, 93289, 93295, 93296, 93618-93624, 93631, 93640-93642, 93650, 93653-93657, 93662)

92970 Cardioassist-method of circulatory assist; internal

92971 external

(For balloon atrial-septostomy, use 92992)

(For placement of catheters for use in circulatory assist devices such as intra-aortic balloon pump, use 33970)

92973 Code is out of numerical sequence. See 92997-93005

92974 Code is out of numerical sequence. See 92997-93005

92975 Code is out of numerical sequence. See 92997-93005

92977 Code is out of numerical sequence. See 92997-93005

92978 Code is out of numerical sequence. See 92997-93005

92979 Code is out of numerical sequence. See 92997-93005

92986 Percutaneous balloon valvuloplasty; aortic valve
➔ *CPT Changes: An Insider's View* 2017
➔ *CPT Assistant* Jan 13:6, Feb 15:3

92987 mitral valve
➔ *CPT Changes: An Insider's View* 2017
➔ *CPT Assistant* Feb 15:3

92990 pulmonary valve
➔ *CPT Assistant* Winter 91:3, Feb 15:3, Jul 15:11

92992 Atrial septectomy or septostomy; transvenous method, balloon (eg, Rashkind type) (includes cardiac catheterization)
➔ *CPT Assistant* Nov 97:44, Apr 98:3, 10, Nov 07:9, Jul 16:4

92993 blade method (Park septostomy) (includes cardiac catheterization)
➔ *CPT Assistant* Apr 98:10, Jul 16:4

92997 Percutaneous transluminal pulmonary artery balloon angioplasty; single vessel
➔ *CPT Assistant* Nov 97:44, Feb 15:3, Mar 16:5

+ 92998 each additional vessel (List separately in addition to code for primary procedure)
➔ *CPT Assistant* Nov 97:44, Feb 15:3, Mar 16:5

(Use 92998 in conjunction with 92997)

Coronary Therapeutic Services and Procedures

Codes 92920-92944 describe percutaneous revascularization services performed for occlusive disease of the coronary vessels (major coronary arteries, coronary artery branches, or coronary artery bypass grafts). These percutaneous coronary intervention (PCI) codes are built on progressive hierarchies with more intensive services inclusive of lesser intensive services. These PCI codes all include the work of accessing and selectively catheterizing the vessel, traversing the lesion, radiological supervision and interpretation directly related to the intervention(s) performed, closure of the arteriotomy when performed through the access sheath, and imaging performed to document completion of the intervention in addition to the intervention(s) performed. These codes include angioplasty (eg, balloon, cutting balloon, wired balloons, cryoplasty), atherectomy (eg, directional, rotational, laser), and stenting (eg, balloon expandable, self-expanding, bare metal, drug eluting, covered). Each code in this family includes balloon angioplasty, when performed. Diagnostic coronary angiography may be reported separately under specific circumstances.

Diagnostic coronary angiography codes (93454-93461) and injection procedure codes (93563-93564) should not be used with percutaneous coronary revascularization services (92920-92944) to report:

1. Contrast injections, angiography, roadmapping, and/or fluoroscopic guidance for the coronary intervention,
2. Vessel measurement for the coronary intervention, **or**
3. Post-coronary angioplasty/stent/atherectomy angiography, as this work is captured in the percutaneous coronary revascularization services codes (92920-92944).

Diagnostic angiography performed at the time of a coronary interventional procedure may be separately reportable if:

1. No prior catheter-based coronary angiography study is available, and a full diagnostic study is performed, and a decision to intervene is based on the diagnostic angiography, **or**
2. A prior study is available, but as documented in the medical record:
   a. The patient's condition with respect to the clinical indication has changed since the prior study, **or**
   b. There is inadequate visualization of the anatomy and/or pathology, **or**
   c. There is a clinical change during the procedure that requires new evaluation outside the target area of intervention.

Diagnostic coronary angiography performed at a separate session from an interventional procedure is separately reportable.

Major coronary arteries: The major coronary arteries are the left main, left anterior descending, left circumflex, right, and ramus intermedius arteries. All PCI procedures performed in all segments (proximal, mid, distal) of a single major coronary artery through the native coronary circulation are reported with one code. When one segment of a major coronary artery is treated through the native circulation and treatment of another segment of the same artery requires access through a coronary artery bypass graft, the intervention through the bypass graft is reported separately.

Coronary artery branches: Up to two coronary artery branches of the left anterior descending (diagonals), left circumflex (marginals), and right (posterior descending, posterolaterals) coronary arteries are recognized. The left main and ramus intermedius coronary arteries do not have recognized branches for reporting purposes. All PCI(s) performed in any segment (proximal, mid, distal) of a coronary artery branch is reported with one code. PCI is reported for up to two branches of a major coronary artery. Additional PCI in a third branch of the same major coronary artery is not separately reportable.

Coronary artery bypass grafts: Each coronary artery bypass graft represents a coronary vessel. A sequential bypass graft with more than one distal anastomosis represents only one graft. A branching bypass graft (eg, Y graft) represents a coronary vessel for the main graft, and each branch off the main graft constitutes an additional coronary vessel. PCI performed on major coronary arteries or coronary artery branches by access through a bypass graft is reported using the bypass graft PCI codes. All bypass graft PCI codes include the use of coronary artery embolic protection devices when performed.

Only one base code from this family may be reported for revascularization of a major coronary artery and its recognized branches. Only one base code should be reported for revascularization of a coronary artery bypass graft, its subtended coronary artery, and recognized branches of the subtended coronary artery. If one segment of a major coronary artery and its recognized branches is treated through the native circulation, and treatment of another segment of the same vessel requires access through a coronary artery bypass graft, an additional base code is reported to describe the intervention performed through the bypass graft. The PCI base codes are 92920, 92924, 92928, 92933, 92937, 92941, and 92943. The PCI base code that includes the most intensive service provided for the target vessel should be reported. The hierarchy of these services is built on an intensity of service ranked from highest to lowest as 92943 = 92941 = 92933 > 92924 > 92937 = 92928 > 92920.

PCI performed during the same session in additional recognized branches of the target vessel should be reported using the applicable add-on code(s). The add-on codes are 92921, 92925, 92928, 92934, 92938, and 92944 and follow the same principle in regard to reporting the most intensive service provided. The intensity of service is ranked from highest to lowest as 92944 = 92938 > 92934 > 92925 > 92929 > 92921.

PCI performed during the same session in additional major coronary or in additional coronary artery bypass grafts should be reported using the applicable additional base code(s). PCI performed during the same session in additional coronary artery branches should be reported using the applicable additional add-on code(s).

If a single lesion extends from one target vessel (major coronary artery, coronary artery bypass graft, or coronary artery branch) into another target vessel, but can be revascularized with a single intervention bridging the two vessels, this PCI should be reported with a single code despite treating more than one vessel. For example, if a left main coronary lesion extends into the proximal left circumflex coronary artery and a single stent is placed to treat the entire lesion, this PCI should be reported as a single vessel stent (92928). In this example, a code for additional vessel treatment (92929) would not be additionally reported.

When bifurcation lesions are treated, PCI is reported for both vessels treated. For example, when a bifurcation lesion involving the left anterior descending artery and the first diagonal artery is treated by stenting both vessels, 92928 and 92929 are both reported.

Target vessel PCI for acute myocardial infarction is inclusive of all balloon angioplasty, atherectomy, stenting, manual aspiration thrombectomy, distal protection, and intracoronary rheolytic agent administration performed. Mechanical thrombectomy is reported separately.

Chronic total occlusion of a coronary vessel is present when there is no antegrade flow through the true lumen, accompanied by suggestive angiographic and clinical criteria (eg, antegrade "bridging" collaterals present, calcification at the occlusion site, no current presentation with ST elevation or Q wave acute myocardial infarction attributable to the occluded target lesion). Current presentation with ST elevation or Q wave acute myocardial infarction attributable to the occluded target lesion, subtotal occlusion, and occlusion with dye staining at the site consistent with fresh thrombus are not considered chronic total occlusion.

Codes 92973 (percutaneous transluminal coronary thrombectomy, mechanical), 92974 (coronary brachytherapy), 92978 and 92979 (intravascular ultrasound/optical coherence tomography), and 93571 and 93572 (intravascular Doppler velocity and/or pressure [fractional flow reserve (FFR) or coronary flow reserve (CFR)]) are add-on codes for reporting procedures performed in addition to coronary and bypass graft diagnostic and interventional services, unless included in the base code. Non-mechanical, aspiration thrombectomy is not reported with 92973, and is included in the PCI code for acute myocardial infarction (92941), when performed.

(To report transcatheter placement of radiation delivery device for coronary intravascular brachytherapy, use 92974)

(For intravascular radioelement application, see 77770, 77771, 77772)

(For nonsurgical septal reduction therapy [eg, alcohol ablation], use 93799)

 # 92920 Percutaneous transluminal coronary angioplasty; single major coronary artery or branch
- *CPT Changes: An Insider's View* 2013, 2017
- *CPT Assistant* Jan 13:3, Dec 14:6

#+ 92921 each additional branch of a major coronary artery (List separately in addition to code for primary procedure)
- *CPT Changes: An Insider's View* 2013, 2017
- *CPT Assistant* Jan 13:3, Sep 14:14, Dec 14:6

(Use 92921 in conjunction with 92920, 92924, 92928, 92933, 92937, 92941, 92943)

 # 92924 Percutaneous transluminal coronary atherectomy, with coronary angioplasty when performed; single major coronary artery or branch
- *CPT Changes: An Insider's View* 2013, 2017
- *CPT Assistant* Jan 13:3, Dec 14:6

#+ 92925 each additional branch of a major coronary artery (List separately in addition to code for primary procedure)
- *CPT Changes: An Insider's View* 2013, 2017
- *CPT Assistant* Jan 13:3, Sep 14:14, Dec 14:6

(Use 92925 in conjunction with 92924, 92928, 92933, 92937, 92941, 92943)

 # 92928 Percutaneous transcatheter placement of intracoronary stent(s), with coronary angioplasty when performed; single major coronary artery or branch
- *CPT Changes: An Insider's View* 2013, 2017
- *CPT Assistant* Jan 13:3, Jan 14:3, Mar 14:14, Sep 14:14, Dec 14:6, Jan 17:7, Feb 17:15

#+ 92929 each additional branch of a major coronary artery (List separately in addition to code for primary procedure)
- *CPT Changes: An Insider's View* 2013, 2017
- *CPT Assistant* Jan 13:3, Sep 14:14, Dec 14:6, Jan 17:7

(Use 92929 in conjunction with 92928, 92933, 92937, 92941, 92943)

 # 92933 Percutaneous transluminal coronary atherectomy, with intracoronary stent, with coronary angioplasty when performed; single major coronary artery or branch
- *CPT Changes: An Insider's View* 2013, 2017
- *CPT Assistant* Jan 13:3, Dec 14:6

#+ 92934 each additional branch of a major coronary artery (List separately in addition to code for primary procedure)
- *CPT Changes: An Insider's View* 2013, 2017
- *CPT Assistant* Jan 13:3, Sep 14:14, Dec 14:6

(Use 92934 in conjunction with 92933, 92937, 92941, 92943)

 # 92937 Percutaneous transluminal revascularization of or through coronary artery bypass graft (internal mammary, free arterial, venous), any combination of intracoronary stent, atherectomy and angioplasty, including distal protection when performed; single vessel
- *CPT Changes: An Insider's View* 2013, 2017
- *CPT Assistant* Jan 13:3, Mar 14:14, Dec 14:6, Feb 17:15

#+ 92938 each additional branch subtended by the bypass graft (List separately in addition to code for primary procedure)
- *CPT Changes: An Insider's View* 2013, 2017
- *CPT Assistant* Jan 13:3, Mar 14:14, Sep 14:14, Dec 14:6

(Use 92938 in conjunction with 92937)

 # 92941 Percutaneous transluminal revascularization of acute total/subtotal occlusion during acute myocardial infarction, coronary artery or coronary artery bypass graft, any combination of intracoronary stent, atherectomy and angioplasty, including aspiration thrombectomy when performed, single vessel
- *CPT Changes: An Insider's View* 2013, 2017
- *CPT Assistant* Jan 13:3, Jan 14:3, Mar 14:14, Dec 14:6, Feb 17:14

(For additional vessels treated, see 92920-92938, 92943, 92944)

 # 92943 Percutaneous transluminal revascularization of chronic total occlusion, coronary artery, coronary artery branch, or coronary artery bypass graft, any combination of intracoronary stent, atherectomy and angioplasty; single vessel
- *CPT Changes: An Insider's View* 2013, 2017
- *CPT Assistant* Jan 13:3, Dec 14:6

#+ 92944 each additional coronary artery, coronary artery branch, or bypass graft (List separately in addition to code for primary procedure)
- *CPT Changes: An Insider's View* 2013, 2017
- *CPT Assistant* Jan 13:3, Sep 14:14, Dec 14:6

(Use 92944 in conjunction with 92924, 92928, 92933, 92937, 92941, 92943)

(To report transcatheter placement of radiation delivery device for coronary intravascular brachytherapy, use 92974)

(For intravascular radioelement application, see 77770, 77771, 77772)

#+ 92973 Percutaneous transluminal coronary thrombectomy mechanical (List separately in addition to code for primary procedure)

➔ *CPT Changes: An Insider's View* 2002, 2013, 2017

➔ *CPT Assistant* Mar 02:2, 10, Mar 04:10, Dec 14:6, Feb 17:14

(Use 92973 in conjunction with 92920, 92924, 92928, 92933, 92937, 92941, 92943, 92975, 93454-93461, 93563, 93564)

(Do not report 92973 for aspiration thrombectomy)

#+ 92974 Transcatheter placement of radiation delivery device for subsequent coronary intravascular brachytherapy (List separately in addition to code for primary procedure)

➔ *CPT Changes: An Insider's View* 2002, 2017

➔ *CPT Assistant* Mar 02:2, Dec 14:6, Feb 17:15

(Use 92974 in conjunction with 92920, 92924, 92928, 92933, 92937, 92941, 92943, 93454-93461)

(For intravascular radioelement application, see 77770, 77771, 77772)

 # 92975 Thrombolysis, coronary; by intracoronary infusion, including selective coronary angiography

➔ *CPT Changes: An Insider's View* 2017

 # 92977 by intravenous infusion

(For thrombolysis of vessels other than coronary, see 37211-37214)

(For cerebral thrombolysis, use 37195)

#+ 92978 Endoluminal imaging of coronary vessel or graft using intravascular ultrasound (IVUS) or optical coherence tomography (OCT) during diagnostic evaluation and/or therapeutic intervention including imaging supervision, interpretation and report; initial vessel (List separately in addition to code for primary procedure)

➔ *CPT Changes: An Insider's View* 2000, 2017

➔ *CPT Assistant* Nov 97:43-44, Nov 99:49, Dec 13:18, Dec 14:6

(Report 92978 once per session)

(Use 92978 in conjunction with 92975, 92920, 92924, 92928, 92933, 92937, 92941, 92943, 93454-93461, 93563, 93564)

Intravascular Ultrasound (Coronary Vessel or Graft)
92978

A catheter with a transducer at its tip is inserted and threaded through a selected coronary artery(s) or coronary bypass graft(s).

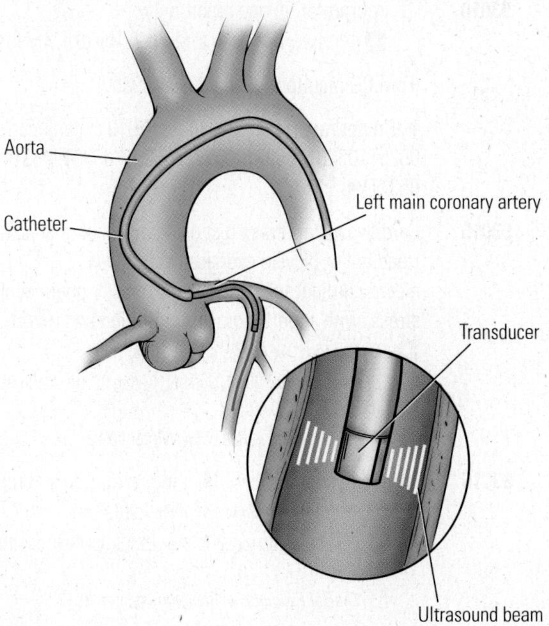

#+ 92979 each additional vessel (List separately in addition to code for primary procedure)

➔ *CPT Changes: An Insider's View* 2000, 2017

➔ *CPT Assistant* Nov 97:43-44, Nov 99:49, Dec 13:18, Dec 14:6

(Report 92979 once per additional vessel)

(Use 92979 in conjunction with 92978)

(Intravascular ultrasound and optical coherence tomography services include all transducer manipulations and repositioning within the specific vessel being examined, both before and after therapeutic intervention [eg, stent placement])

(For intravascular spectroscopy, use 0205T)

Cardiography

Codes 93040-93042 are appropriate when an order for the test is triggered by an event, the rhythm strip is used to help diagnose the presence or absence of an arrhythmia, and a report is generated. There must be a specific order for an electrocardiogram or rhythm strip followed by a separate, signed, written, and retrievable report. It is not appropriate to use these codes for reviewing the telemetry monitor strips taken from a monitoring system. The need for an electrocardiogram or rhythm strip should be supported by documentation in the patient medical record.

(For echocardiography, see 93303-93350)

(For acoustic cardiography services, use 93799)

93000 Electrocardiogram, routine ECG with at least 12 leads; with interpretation and report
CPT Assistant Aug 97:9, Feb 05:9, Mar 05:1, 11, Jul 08:3

93005 tracing only, without interpretation and report
CPT Assistant Aug 97:9, Mar 05:1, Apr 16:8

93010 interpretation and report only
CPT Assistant Aug 97:9, Mar 05:1, Apr 07:1, Apr 16:8

(For ECG monitoring, see 99354-99360)

►(Do not report 93000, 93005, 93010 in conjunction with 0525T, 0526T, 0527T, 0528T, 0529T, 0530T, 0531T, 0532T)◄

93015 Cardiovascular stress test using maximal or submaximal treadmill or bicycle exercise, continuous electrocardiographic monitoring, and/or pharmacological stress; with supervision, interpretation and report
CPT Changes: An Insider's View 2013
CPT Assistant Apr 96:11, Jun 96:10, Aug 02:10, Jul 08:3, Jan 10:8, May 10:6
Clinical Examples in Radiology Winter 10:12

93016 supervision only, without interpretation and report
CPT Changes: An Insider's View 2013
CPT Assistant Apr 96:11, Aug 02:10, Jul 08:3, Jan 10:8, May 10:6
Clinical Examples in Radiology Winter 10:12

93017 tracing only, without interpretation and report
CPT Assistant Aug 02:10, Jul 08:3, Jan 10:8, May 10:6
Clinical Examples in Radiology Winter 10:12

93018 interpretation and report only
CPT Assistant Apr 96:11, Jun 96:10, Jul 08:3, Jan 10:8, May 10:6
Clinical Examples in Radiology Winter 10:12

93024 Ergonovine provocation test

93025 Microvolt T-wave alternans for assessment of ventricular arrhythmias
CPT Changes: An Insider's View 2002
CPT Assistant Mar 02:3

Coding Tip

Instructions for Reporting Electrocardiographic Recording

Codes 93040-93042 are appropriate when an order for the test is triggered by an event, the rhythm strip is used to help diagnose the presence or absence of an arrhythmia, and a report is generated. There must be a specific order for an electrocardiogram or rhythm strip followed by a separate, signed, written, and retrievable report. It is not appropriate to use these codes for reviewing the telemetry monitor strips taken from a monitoring system. The need for an electrocardiogram or rhythm strip should be supported by documentation in the patient medical record.

CPT Coding Guidelines, Cardiovascular, Cardiography

93040 Rhythm ECG, 1-3 leads; with interpretation and report
CPT Assistant Apr 04:8, Oct 10:10, Nov 12:6

93041 tracing only without interpretation and report
CPT Assistant Apr 04:8, Oct 10:10

93042 interpretation and report only
CPT Assistant Apr 04:8, Oct 10:10, Oct 11:7

Coding Tip

Instructions for Reporting Electrocardiographic Recording

Do not report 93268-93272 when performing 93279-93289, 93291-93296, or 93298-93299. Do not report 93040-93042 *when performing 93279-93289, 93291-93296, or 93298-93299.*

CPT Coding Guidelines, Cardiovascular, Cardiography Implantable and Wearable Cardiac Device Evaluations

93050 Arterial pressure waveform analysis for assessment of central arterial pressures, includes obtaining waveform(s), digitization and application of nonlinear mathematical transformations to determine central arterial pressures and augmentation index, with interpretation and report, upper extremity artery, non-invasive
CPT Changes: An Insider's View 2016

(Do not report 93050 in conjunction with diagnostic or interventional intra-arterial procedures)

Cardiovascular Monitoring Services

Cardiovascular monitoring services are diagnostic medical procedures using in-person and remote technology to assess cardiovascular rhythm (ECG) data. Holter monitors (93224-93227) include up to 48 hours of continuous recording. Mobile cardiac telemetry monitors (93228, 93229) have the capability of transmitting a tracing at any time, always have internal ECG analysis algorithms designed to detect major arrhythmias, and transmit to an attended surveillance center. Event monitors (93268-93272) record segments of ECGs with recording initiation triggered either by patient activation or by an internal automatic, pre-programmed detection algorithm (or both) and transmit the recorded electrocardiographic data when requested (but cannot transmit immediately based upon the patient or algorithmic activation rhythm) and require attended surveillance.

Attended surveillance: is the immediate availability of a remote technician to respond to rhythm or device alert transmissions from a patient, either from an implanted or wearable monitoring or therapy device, as they are generated and transmitted to the remote surveillance location or center.

Electrocardiographic rhythm derived elements: elements derived from recordings of the electrical activation of the heart including, but not limited to heart rhythm, rate, ST analysis, heart rate variability, T-wave alternans.

Mobile cardiovascular telemetry (MCT): continuously records the electrocardiographic rhythm from external electrodes placed on the patient's body. Segments of the ECG data are automatically (without patient intervention) transmitted to a remote surveillance location by cellular or landline telephone signal. The segments of the rhythm, selected for transmission, are triggered automatically (MCT device algorithm) by rapid and slow heart rates or by the patient during a symptomatic episode. There is continuous real time data analysis by preprogrammed algorithms in the device and attended surveillance of the transmitted rhythm segments by a surveillance center technician to evaluate any arrhythmias and to determine signal quality. The surveillance center technician reviews the data and notifies the physician or other qualified health care professional depending on the prescribed criteria.

►ECG rhythm derived elements are distinct from physiologic data, even when the same device is capable of producing both. Implantable cardiovascular physiologic monitor device services are always separately reported from implantable cardioverter-defibrillator (ICD) service.◄

93224 External electrocardiographic recording up to 48 hours by continuous rhythm recording and storage; includes recording, scanning analysis with report, review and interpretation by a physician or other qualified health care professional

➲ *CPT Changes: An Insider's View* 2009, 2011, 2013

➲ *CPT Assistant* Oct 05:14, Apr 07:3, Mar 08:4, Mar 09:5, Oct 11:5, Nov 11:11

93225 recording (includes connection, recording, and disconnection)

➲ *CPT Changes: An Insider's View* 2009, 2011

➲ *CPT Assistant* Oct 05:14, Apr 07:3, Mar 09:5, Oct 11:5

93226 scanning analysis with report

➲ *CPT Changes: An Insider's View* 2009, 2011

➲ *CPT Assistant* Oct 05:14, Apr 07:3, Mar 09:5, Oct 11:5

93227 review and interpretation by a physician or other qualified health care professional

➲ *CPT Changes: An Insider's View* 2009, 2011, 2013

➲ *CPT Assistant* Apr 07:3, Mar 09:5, Apr 09:7, Oct 11:5, Mar 18:5

(For less than 12 hours of continuous recording, use modifier 52)

(For greater than 48 hours of monitoring, see Category III codes 0295T-0298T)

★ **93228** External mobile cardiovascular telemetry with electrocardiographic recording, concurrent computerized real time data analysis and greater than 24 hours of accessible ECG data storage (retrievable with query) with ECG triggered and patient selected events transmitted to a remote attended surveillance center for up to 30 days; review and interpretation with report by a physician or other qualified health care professional

➲ *CPT Changes: An Insider's View* 2009, 2011, 2013, 2017

➲ *CPT Assistant* Oct 11:5

(Report 93228 only once per 30 days)

(Do not report 93228 in conjunction with 93224, 93227)

★ **93229** technical support for connection and patient instructions for use, attended surveillance, analysis and transmission of daily and emergent data reports as prescribed by a physician or other qualified health care professional

➲ *CPT Changes: An Insider's View* 2009, 2011, 2013, 2017

➲ *CPT Assistant* Oct 11:5

(Report 93229 only once per 30 days)

(Do not report 93229 in conjunction with 93224, 93226)

(For external cardiovascular monitors that do not perform automatic ECG triggered transmissions to an attended surveillance center, see 93224-93227, 93268-93272)

93260 Code is out of numerical sequence. See 93283-93291

93261 Code is out of numerical sequence. See 93283-93291

93264 Code is out of numerical sequence. See 93272-93280

★ **93268** External patient and, when performed, auto activated electrocardiographic rhythm-derived event recording with symptom-related memory loop with remote download capability up to 30 days, 24-hour attended monitoring; includes transmission, review and interpretation by a physician or other qualified health care professional

➲ *CPT Changes: An Insider's View* 2003, 2009, 2011, 2013, 2017

➲ *CPT Assistant* Jun 96:2, Nov 99:49-50, Oct 05:14, Apr 07:3, Mar 08:4, Mar 09:5, Oct 11:5

★ **93270** recording (includes connection, recording, and disconnection)

➲ *CPT Changes: An Insider's View* 2009, 2011, 2017

➲ *CPT Assistant* Jun 96:2, Oct 05:14, Apr 07:3, Mar 09:5, Aug 10:13, Oct 11:5

★ **93271** transmission and analysis

➲ *CPT Changes: An Insider's View* 2009, 2011, 2017

➲ *CPT Assistant* Jun 96:2, Oct 05:14, Apr 07:3, Mar 09:5, Oct 11:5

★ **93272** review and interpretation by a physician or other qualified health care professional

➲ *CPT Changes: An Insider's View* 2009, 2011, 2013, 2017

➲ *CPT Assistant* Jun 96:2, Apr 98:14, Nov 99:49-50, Oct 05:14, Apr 07:3, Mar 09:5, Apr 09:7, Oct 11:5, Mar 18:5

►(For subcutaneous cardiac rhythm monitoring, see 33285, 93285, 93291, 93298, 93299)◄

93278 Signal-averaged electrocardiography (SAECG), with or without ECG

➔ *CPT Assistant* Oct 11:5

(For interpretation and report only, use 93278 with modifier 26)

(For unlisted cardiographic procedure, use 93799)

▸Implantable, Insertable, and Wearable Cardiac Device Evaluations◂

▶Cardiac device evaluation services are diagnostic medical procedures using in-person and remote technology to assess device therapy and cardiovascular physiologic data. Codes 93260, 93261, 93279-93299 describe this technology and technical/professional and service center practice. Codes 93260, 93261, 93279-93292 are reported per procedure. Codes 93293, 93294, 93295, 93296 are reported no more than **once** every 90 days. Do not report 93293, 93294, 93295, 93296, if the monitoring period is less than 30 days. Codes 93297, 93298 are reported no more than **once** up to every 30 days, per patient. Do not report 93297-93299, if the monitoring period is less than 10 days. Do not report 93264 if the monitoring period is less than 30 days. Code 93264 is reported no more than once up to every 30 days, per patient.

A service center may report 93296 or 93299 during a period in which a physician or other qualified health care professional performs an in-person interrogation device evaluation. The same individual may not report an in-person and remote interrogation of the same device during the same period. Report only remote services when an in-person interrogation device evaluation is performed during a period of remote interrogation device evaluation. A period is established by the initiation of the remote monitoring or the 91st day of a pacemaker or implantable defibrillator monitoring or the 31st day of monitoring a subcutaneous cardiac rhythm monitor or implantable cardiovascular physiologic monitor, and extends for the subsequent 90 or 30 days respectively, for which remote monitoring is occurring. Programming device evaluations and in-person interrogation device evaluations may not be reported on the same date by the same individual. Programming device evaluations and remote interrogation device evaluations may both be reported during the remote interrogation device evaluation period.◀

For monitoring by wearable devices, see 93224-93272.

▶ECG rhythm derived elements are distinct from physiologic data, even when the same device is capable of producing both. Implantable cardiovascular physiologic monitor services are always separately reported from implantable defibrillator services. When cardiac rhythm data are derived from an implantable defibrillator or pacemaker, do not report subcutaneous cardiac rhythm monitor services with pacemaker or implantable defibrillator services.◀

Do not report 93268-93272 when performing 93260, 93261, 93279-93289, 93291-93296, or 93298-93299. Do not report 93040, 93041, 93042 when performing 93260, 93261, 93279-93289, 93291-93296, or 93298-93299.

The pacemaker and implantable defibrillator interrogation device evaluations, peri-procedural device evaluations and programming, and programming device evaluations may not be reported in conjunction with pacemaker or implantable defibrillator device and/or lead insertion or revision services by the same individual.

The following definitions and instructions apply to codes 93260, 93261, 93279-93299.

▶***Attended surveillance:*** the immediate availability of a remote technician to respond to rhythm or device alert transmissions from a patient, either from an implanted, inserted, or wearable monitoring or therapy device, as they are generated and transmitted to the remote surveillance location or center.

Device, leadless: a leadless cardiac pacemaker system that includes a pulse generator with built-in battery and electrode for implantation into the cardiac chamber via a transcatheter approach.◀

Device, single lead: a pacemaker or implantable defibrillator with pacing and sensing function in only one chamber of the heart or a subcutaneous electrode.

Device, dual lead: a pacemaker or implantable defibrillator with pacing and sensing function in only two chambers of the heart.

Device, multiple lead: a pacemaker or implantable defibrillator with pacing and sensing function in three or more chambers of the heart.

Electrocardiographic rhythm derived elements: elements derived from recordings of the electrical activation of the heart including, but not limited to heart rhythm, rate, ST analysis, heart rate variability, T-wave alternans.

▶***Implantable cardiovascular physiologic monitor:*** an implantable cardiovascular device used to assist the physician or other qualified health care professional in the management of non-rhythm related cardiac conditions such as heart failure. The device collects longitudinal physiologic cardiovascular data elements from one or more internal sensors (such as right ventricular pressure, pulmonary artery pressure, left atrial pressure, or an index of lung water) and/or external sensors (such as blood pressure or body weight) for patient assessment and management. The data are stored and transmitted by either local telemetry or remotely to an Internet-based file server or surveillance technician. The function of the implantable cardiovascular physiologic monitor may be an additional function of an implantable cardiac device (eg, implantable defibrillator) or a function of a stand-alone device. When implantable cardiovascular physiologic monitor functionality is included in an implantable defibrillator device or pacemaker, the implantable cardiovascular physiologic monitor data and the implantable defibrillator or pacemaker, heart rhythm data such as sensing, pacing, and tachycardia detection therapy are distinct and, therefore, the monitoring processes are distinct.

Implantable defibrillator: two general categories of implantable defibrillators exist: transvenous implantable pacing cardioverter-defibrillator (ICD) and subcutaneous implantable defibrillator (SICD). An implantable pacing cardioverter-defibrillator device provides high-energy and low-energy stimulation to one or more chambers of the heart to terminate rapid heart rhythms called tachycardia or fibrillation. Implantable pacing cardioverter-defibrillators also have pacemaker functions to treat slow heart rhythms called bradycardia. In addition to the tachycardia and bradycardia functions, the implantable pacing cardioverter-defibrillator may or may not include the functionality of an implantable cardiovascular physiologic monitor or a subcutaneous cardiac rhythm monitor. The subcutaneous implantable defibrillator uses a single subcutaneous electrode to treat ventricular tachyarrhythmias. Subcutaneous implantable defibrillators differ from transvenous implantable pacing cardioverter-defibrillators in that subcutaneous implantable defibrillators do not provide antitachycardia pacing or chronic pacing. For subcutaneous implantable defibrillator device evaluation, see 93260, 93261.

Interrogation device evaluation: an evaluation of an implantable device such as a cardiac pacemaker, implantable defibrillator, implantable cardiovascular physiologic monitor, or subcutaneous cardiac rhythm monitor. Using an office, hospital, or emergency room instrument or via a remote interrogation system, stored and measured information about the lead(s) when present, sensor(s) when present, battery and the implanted device function, as well as data collected about the patient's heart rhythm and heart rate is retrieved. The retrieved information is evaluated to determine the current programming of the device and to evaluate certain aspects of the device function such as battery voltage, lead impedance, tachycardia detection settings, and rhythm treatment settings.

The components that must be evaluated for the various types of implantable or insertable cardiac devices are listed below. (The required components for both remote and in-person interrogations are the same.)

Pacemaker: programmed parameters, with or without lead(s), battery, capture and sensing function and heart rhythm.◄

Implantable defibrillator: programmed parameters, lead(s), battery, capture and sensing function, presence or absence of therapy for ventricular tachyarrhythmias and underlying heart rhythm.

►***Implantable cardiovascular physiologic monitor:*** programmed parameters and analysis of at least one recorded physiologic cardiovascular data element from either internal or external sensors.

Subcutaneous cardiac rhythm monitor: programmed parameters and the heart rate and rhythm during recorded episodes from both patient initiated and device algorithm detected events, when present.

Interrogation device evaluation (remote): a procedure performed for patients with pacemakers, implantable defibrillators, or subcutaneous cardiac rhythm monitors using data obtained remotely. All device functions, including the programmed parameters, lead(s), battery, capture and sensing function, presence or absence of therapy for ventricular tachyarrhythmias (for implantable defibrillators) and underlying heart rhythm are evaluated.

The components that must be evaluated for the various types of implantable or insertable cardiac devices are listed below. (The required components for both remote and in person interrogations are the same.)

Pacemaker: programmed parameters, with or without lead(s), battery, capture and sensing function, and heart rhythm.◄

Implantable defibrillator: programmed parameters, lead(s), battery, capture and sensing function, presence or absence of therapy for ventricular tachyarrhythmias, and underlying heart rhythm.

►***Implantable cardiovascular physiologic monitor:*** programmed parameters and analysis of at least one recorded physiologic cardiovascular data element from either internal or external sensors.

Subcutaneous cardiac rhythm monitor: programmed parameters and the heart rate and rhythm during recorded episodes from both patient-initiated and device algorithm detected events, when present.

Pacemaker: an implantable device that provides low energy localized stimulation to one or more chambers of the heart to initiate contraction in that chamber. Two general categories of pacemakers exist: (1) pacemakers with a subcutaneous generator plus transvenous/epicardial lead(s); and (2) leadless pacemakers. A leadless pacemaker does not require a subcutaneous pocket for the generator. It combines a miniaturized generator with an integrated electrode for implantation in a heart chamber via a transcatheter approach.

Peri-procedural device evaluation and programming: an evaluation of an implantable device system (either a pacemaker or implantable defibrillator) to adjust the device to settings appropriate for the patient prior to a surgery, procedure, or test. The device system data are interrogated to evaluate the lead(s) when present, sensor(s), and battery in addition to review of stored information, including patient and system measurements. The device is programmed to settings appropriate for the surgery, procedure, or test, as required. A second evaluation and programming are performed after the surgery, procedure, or test to provide settings appropriate to the post procedural situation, as required. If one performs both the pre- and post-evaluation and programming service, the appropriate code, either 93286 or 93287, would be reported two times. If one performs the pre-surgical service and a separate individual performs the post-surgical service, each reports either 93286 or 93287 only one time.◀

Physiologic cardiovascular data elements: data elements from one or more internal sensors (such as right ventricular pressure, left atrial pressure or an index of lung water) and/or external sensors (such as blood pressure or body weight) for patient assessment and management. It does not include ECG rhythm derived data elements.

▶***Programming device evaluation (in person):*** a procedure performed for patients with a pacemaker, implantable defibrillator, or subcutaneous cardiac rhythm monitor. All device functions, including the battery, programmable settings and lead(s), when present, are evaluated. To assess capture thresholds, iterative adjustments (eg, progressive changes in pacing output of a pacing lead) of the programmable parameters are conducted. The iterative adjustments provide information that permits the operator to assess and select the most appropriate final program parameters to provide for consistent delivery of the appropriate therapy and to verify the function of the device. The final program parameters may or may not change after evaluation.◀

The programming device evaluation includes all of the components of the interrogation device evaluation (remote) or the interrogation device evaluation (in person), and it includes the selection of patient specific programmed parameters depending on the type of device.

The components that must be evaluated for the various types of programming device evaluations are listed below. (See also required interrogation device evaluation [remote and in person] components above.)

▶***Pacemaker:*** programmed parameters, lead(s) when present, battery, capture and sensing function, and heart rhythm. Often, but not always, the sensor rate response, lower and upper heart rates, AV intervals, pacing voltage and pulse duration, sensing value, and diagnostics will be adjusted during a programming evaluation.◀

Implantable defibrillator: programmed parameters, lead(s), battery, capture and sensing function, presence or absence of therapy for ventricular tachyarrhythmias and underlying heart rhythm. Often, but not always, the sensor rate response, lower and upper heart rates, AV intervals, pacing voltage and pulse duration, sensing value, and diagnostics will be adjusted during a programming evaluation. In addition, ventricular tachycardia detection and therapies are sometimes altered depending on the interrogated data, patient's rhythm, symptoms, and condition.

▶***Subcutaneous cardiac rhythm monitor:*** programmed parameters and the heart rhythm during recorded episodes from both patient initiated and device algorithm detected events. Often, but not always, the tachycardia and bradycardia detection criteria will be adjusted during a programming evaluation.

Subcutaneous cardiac rhythm monitor: an implantable or insertable device that continuously records the electrocardiographic rhythm triggered automatically by rapid, irregular, and/or slow heart rates or by the patient during a symptomatic episode. The cardiac rhythm monitor function may be the only function of the device or it may be part of a pacemaker or implantable defibrillator device. The data are stored and transmitted by either local telemetry or remotely to an Internet-based file server or surveillance technician. Extraction of data and compilation or report for physician or qualified health care professional interpretation is usually performed in the office setting.

Transtelephonic rhythm strip pacemaker evaluation: service of transmission of an electrocardiographic rhythm strip over the telephone by the patient using a transmitter and recorded by a receiving location using a receiver/recorder (also commonly known as transtelephonic pacemaker monitoring). The electrocardiographic rhythm strip is recorded both with and without a magnet applied over the pacemaker. The rhythm strip is evaluated for heart rate and rhythm, atrial and ventricular capture (if observed) and atrial and ventricular sensing (if observed). In addition, the battery status of the pacemaker is determined by measurement of the paced rate on the electrocardiographic rhythm strip recorded with the magnet applied. For remote monitoring of an implantable wireless pulmonary artery pressure sensor, use 93264.

Implantable wireless pulmonary artery sensor: an implantable cardiovascular device used to assist the physician or other qualified health care professional in monitoring heart failure. The device collects longitudinal physiologic cardiovascular data elements from an internal sensor located in the pulmonary artery. The data are transmitted and stored remotely to an Internet-based file server.

#● 93264 Remote monitoring of a wireless pulmonary artery pressure sensor for up to 30 days, including at least weekly downloads of pulmonary artery pressure recordings, interpretation(s), trend analysis, and report(s) by a physician or other qualified health care professional

CPT Changes: An Insider's View 2019

▶(Report 93264 only once per 30 days)◀

▶(Do not report 93264 if download[s], interpretation[s], trend analysis, and report[s] do not occur at least weekly during the 30-day time period)◀

▶(Do not report 93264 if review does not occur at least weekly during the 30-day time period)◀

▶(Do not report 93264 if monitoring period is less than 30 days)◀

▲ **93279** Programming device evaluation (in person) with iterative adjustment of the implantable device to test the function of the device and select optimal permanent programmed values with analysis, review and report by a physician or other qualified health care professional; single lead pacemaker system or leadless pacemaker system in one cardiac chamber

➲ *CPT Changes: An Insider's View* 2009, 2010, 2013, 2019

➲ *CPT Assistant* Jun 12:4, Jun 13:6, Jul 13:7, Apr 14:3, Jul 14:3, Nov 14:5, Aug 16:5

(Do not report 93279 in conjunction with 93286, 93288)

93280 dual lead pacemaker system

➲ *CPT Changes: An Insider's View* 2009, 2010, 2013

➲ *CPT Assistant* Jun 12:4, Jun 13:6, Jul 13:7, Apr 14:3, Aug 16:5

(Do not report 93280 in conjunction with 93286, 93288)

93281 multiple lead pacemaker system

➲ *CPT Changes: An Insider's View* 2009, 2010, 2013

➲ *CPT Assistant* Jun 12:4, Jun 13:6, Jul 13:7, Apr 14:3, Aug 16:5

(Do not report 93281 in conjunction with 93286, 93288)

93282 single lead transvenous implantable defibrillator system

➲ *CPT Changes: An Insider's View* 2009, 2010, 2013, 2015

➲ *CPT Assistant* Jun 13:6, Jul 13:7, Apr 14:3, Aug 16:5

(Do not report 93282 in conjunction with 93260, 93287, 93289, 93745)

93283 dual lead transvenous implantable defibrillator system

➲ *CPT Changes: An Insider's View* 2009, 2010, 2013, 2015

➲ *CPT Assistant* Jun 13:6, Jul 13:7, Apr 14:3, Aug 16:5

(Do not report 93283 in conjunction with 93287, 93289)

93284 multiple lead transvenous implantable defibrillator system

➲ *CPT Changes: An Insider's View* 2009, 2010, 2013, 2015

➲ *CPT Assistant* Jun 13:6, Jul 13:7, Apr 14:3, Aug 16:5

(Do not report 93284 in conjunction with 93287, 93289)

 # 93260 implantable subcutaneous lead defibrillator system

➲ *CPT Changes: An Insider's View* 2015

➲ *CPT Assistant* Nov 14:5, Aug 16:5

(Do not report 93260 in conjunction with 93261, 93282, 93287)

(Do not report 93260 in conjunction with pulse generator and lead insertion or repositioning codes 33240, 33241, 33262, 33270, 33271, 33272, 33273)

▲ **93285** subcutaneous cardiac rhythm monitor system

➲ *CPT Changes: An Insider's View* 2009, 2010, 2013, 2019

➲ *CPT Assistant* Aug 16:5

▶(Do not report 93285 in conjunction with 33285, 93279-93284, 93291)◀

▲ **93286** Peri-procedural device evaluation (in person) and programming of device system parameters before or after a surgery, procedure, or test with analysis, review and report by a physician or other qualified health care professional; single, dual, or multiple lead pacemaker system, or leadless pacemaker system

➲ *CPT Changes: An Insider's View* 2009, 2010, 2013, 2019

➲ *CPT Assistant* Jun 13:6, Jul 13:7, Apr 14:3, Aug 16:5

(Report 93286 once before and once after surgery, procedure, or test, when device evaluation and programming is performed before and after surgery, procedure, or test)

(Do not report 93286 in conjunction with 93279-93281, 93288, 0408T, 0409T, 0410T, 0411T, 0414T, 0415T)

93287 single, dual, or multiple lead implantable defibrillator system

➲ *CPT Changes: An Insider's View* 2009, 2010, 2013, 2015

➲ *CPT Assistant* Jun 13:6, Jul 13:7, Apr 14:3, Jul 14:3, Aug 16:5

(Report 93287 once before and once after surgery, procedure, or test, when device evaluation and programming is performed before and after surgery, procedure, or test)

(Do not report 93287 in conjunction with 93260, 93261, 93282, 93283, 93284, 93289, 0408T, 0409T, 0410T, 0411T, 0414T, 0415T)

▲ **93288** Interrogation device evaluation (in person) with analysis, review and report by a physician or other qualified health care professional, includes connection, recording and disconnection per patient encounter; single, dual, or multiple lead pacemaker system, or leadless pacemaker system

➲ *CPT Changes: An Insider's View* 2009, 2013, 2019

➲ *CPT Assistant* Jun 12:4, Jun 13:6, Jul 13:7, Apr 14:3, Aug 16:5

(Do not report 93288 in conjunction with 93279-93281, 93286, 93294, 93296)

93289 single, dual, or multiple lead transvenous implantable defibrillator system, including analysis of heart rhythm derived data elements

➲ *CPT Changes: An Insider's View* 2009, 2013, 2015

➲ *CPT Assistant* Jun 13:6, Jul 13:7, Apr 14:3, Aug 16:5

(For monitoring physiologic cardiovascular data elements derived from an implantable defibrillator, use 93290)

(Do not report 93289 in conjunction with 93261, 93282, 93283, 93284, 93287, 93295, 93296)

 # 93261 implantable subcutaneous lead defibrillator system

➲ *CPT Changes: An Insider's View* 2015

➲ *CPT Assistant* Nov 14:5, Aug 16:5

(Do not report 93261 in conjunction with 93260, 93287, 93289)

(Do not report 93261 in conjunction with pulse generator and lead insertion or repositioning codes 33240, 33241, 33262, 33270, 33271, 33272, 33273)

▲ **93290** implantable cardiovascular physiologic monitor system, including analysis of 1 or more recorded physiologic cardiovascular data elements from all internal and external sensors

➲ *CPT Changes: An Insider's View* 2009, 2013, 2019

➲ *CPT Assistant* Feb 10:13, Apr 13:11, Aug 16:5

(For heart rhythm derived data elements, use 93289)

(Do not report 93290 in conjunction with 93297, 93299)

▲ **93291** subcutaneous cardiac rhythm monitor system, including heart rhythm derived data analysis

➲ *CPT Changes: An Insider's View* 2009, 2013, 2019

➲ *CPT Assistant* Aug 16:5

►(Do not report 93291 in conjunction with 33285, 93288-93290, 93298, 93299)◄

93292 wearable defibrillator system

➲ *CPT Changes: An Insider's View* 2009, 2013

➲ *CPT Assistant* Aug 16:5

(Do not report 93292 in conjunction with 93745)

Coding Tip

Instructions for Reporting Pacemaker and Interrogation Device Evaluations

Codes 93293-93296 are reported no more than once every 90 days. Do not report 93293-93296 if the monitoring period is less than 30 days.

CPT Coding Guidelines, Cardiovascular, Cardiography Implantable and Wearable Cardiac Device Evaluations

93293 Transtelephonic rhythm strip pacemaker evaluation(s) single, dual, or multiple lead pacemaker system, includes recording with and without magnet application with analysis, review and report(s) by a physician or other qualified health care professional, up to 90 days

➲ *CPT Changes: An Insider's View* 2009, 2013

➲ *CPT Assistant* Aug 16:5

(Do not report 93293 in conjunction with 93294)

(For in person evaluation, see 93040, 93041, 93042)

(Report 93293 only once per 90 days)

▲ **93294** Interrogation device evaluation(s) (remote), up to 90 days; single, dual, or multiple lead pacemaker system, or leadless pacemaker system with interim analysis, review(s) and report(s) by a physician or other qualified health care professional

➲ *CPT Changes: An Insider's View* 2009, 2013, 2019

➲ *CPT Assistant* Jun 12:4, Aug 16:5

(Do not report 93294 in conjunction with 93288, 93293)

(Report 93294 only once per 90 days)

93295 single, dual, or multiple lead implantable defibrillator system with interim analysis, review(s) and report(s) by a physician or other qualified health care professional

➲ *CPT Changes: An Insider's View* 2009, 2013, 2015

➲ *CPT Assistant* Aug 16:5

(For remote monitoring of physiologic cardiovascular data elements derived from an ICD, use 93297)

(Do not report 93295 in conjunction with 93289)

(Report 93295 only once per 90 days)

▲ **93296** single, dual, or multiple lead pacemaker system, leadless pacemaker system, or implantable defibrillator system, remote data acquisition(s), receipt of transmissions and technician review, technical support and distribution of results

➲ *CPT Changes: An Insider's View* 2009, 2015, 2019

➲ *CPT Assistant* Aug 16:5

(Do not report 93296 in conjunction with 93288, 93289, 93299)

(Report 93296 only once per 90 days)

▲ **93297** Interrogation device evaluation(s), (remote) up to 30 days; implantable cardiovascular physiologic monitor system, including analysis of 1 or more recorded physiologic cardiovascular data elements from all internal and external sensors, analysis, review(s) and report(s) by a physician or other qualified health care professional

➲ *CPT Changes: An Insider's View* 2009, 2013, 2019

➲ *CPT Assistant* Feb 09:9-12, Apr 13:11, Aug 16:5

(For heart rhythm derived data elements, use 93295)

►(Do not report 93297 in conjunction with 93264, 93290, 93298)◄

(Report 93297 only once per 30 days)

★▲ **93298** subcutaneous cardiac rhythm monitor system, including analysis of recorded heart rhythm data, analysis, review(s) and report(s) by a physician or other qualified health care professional

➲ *CPT Changes: An Insider's View* 2009, 2013, 2017, 2019

➲ *CPT Assistant* Feb 09:9-12, Aug 16:5

►(Do not report 93298 in conjunction with 33285, 93291, 93297)◄

(Report 93298 only once per 30 days)

★▲ **93299** implantable cardiovascular physiologic monitor system or subcutaneous cardiac rhythm monitor system, remote data acquisition(s), receipt of transmissions and technician review, technical support and distribution of results

➲ *CPT Changes: An Insider's View* 2009, 2017, 2019

➲ *CPT Assistant* Feb 09:9-12, Apr 13:11, Jul 14:3, Nov 14:5, Aug 16:5

►(For remote monitoring of an implantable wireless pulmonary artery pressure sensor, use 93264)◄

►(Do not report 93299 in conjunction with 93264, 93290, 93291, 93296)◄

(Report 93299 only once per 30 days)

Echocardiography

Echocardiography includes obtaining ultrasonic signals from the heart and great vessels, with real time image and/or Doppler ultrasonic signal documentation, with interpretation and report. When interpretation is performed separately, use modifier 26.

A complete transthoracic echocardiogram without spectral or color flow Doppler (93307) is a comprehensive procedure that includes 2-dimensional and, when performed, selected M-mode examination of the left and right atria, left and right ventricles, the aortic, mitral, and tricuspid valves, the pericardium, and adjacent portions of the aorta. Multiple views are required to obtain a complete functional and anatomic evaluation, and appropriate measurements are obtained and recorded. Despite significant effort, identification and measurement of some structures may not always be possible. In such instances, the reason that an element could not be visualized must be documented. Additional structures that may be visualized (eg, pulmonary veins, pulmonary artery, pulmonic valve, inferior vena cava) would be included as part of the service.

A complete transthoracic echocardiogram with spectral and color flow Doppler (93306) is a comprehensive procedure that includes spectral Doppler and color flow Doppler in addition to the 2-dimensional and selected M-mode examinations, when performed. Spectral Doppler (93320, 93321) and color flow Doppler (93325) provide information regarding intracardiac blood flow and hemodynamics.

A follow-up or limited echocardiographic study (93308) is an examination that does not evaluate or document the attempt to evaluate all the structures that comprise the complete echocardiographic exam. This is typically limited to, or performed in follow-up of a focused clinical concern.

In stress echocardiography, echocardiographic images are recorded from multiple cardiac windows before, after, and in some protocols, during stress. The stress is achieved by (1) walking on a treadmill; (2) using a bicycle (supine or upright); or (3) the administration of pharmacological agents that either simulate exercise (by increasing heart rate, blood pressure, or myocardial contractility) or alter coronary flow (vasodilation). The patient's ECG, heart rate, and blood pressure are monitored at baseline, throughout the procedure and during recovery. Reports are prepared to evaluate (1) the duration of stress, the reason for stopping, and the hemodynamic response to stress; (2) the electrocardiographic response to stress; and (3) the echocardiographic response to stress.

When a stress echocardiogram is performed with a complete cardiovascular stress test (continuous electrocardiographic monitoring, supervision, interpretation and report by a physician or other qualified health care professional), use 93351. When only the professional components of a complete stress test and a stress echocardiogram are provided (eg, in a facility setting) by the same physician, use 93351 with modifier 26. When all professional services of a stress test are not performed by the same physician performing the stress echocardiogram, use 93350 in conjunction with the appropriate codes (93016-93018) for the components of the cardiovascular stress test that are provided.

When left ventricular endocardial borders cannot be adequately identified by standard echocardiographic imaging, echocardiographic contrast may be infused intravenously both at rest and with stress to achieve that purpose. Code 93352 is used to report the administration of echocardiographic contrast agent in conjunction with the stress echocardiography codes (93350 or 93351). Supply of contrast agent and/or drugs used for pharmacological stress is reported separately in addition to the procedure code.

Code 93355 is used to report transesophageal echocardiography (TEE) services during transcatheter intracardiac therapies. Code 93355 is reported once per intervention and only by an individual who is not performing the interventional procedure. Code 93355 includes the work of passing the endoscopic ultrasound transducer through the mouth into the esophagus, when performed by the individual performing the TEE, diagnostic transesophageal echocardiography and ongoing manipulation of the transducer to guide sizing and/or placement of implants, determination of adequacy of the intervention, and assessment for potential complications. Real-time image acquisition, measurements, and interpretation of image(s), documentation of completion of the intervention, and final written report are included in this code.

A range of intracardiac therapies may be performed with TEE guidance. Code 93355 describes TEE during advanced transcatheter structural heart procedures (eg, transcatheter aortic valve replacement [TAVR], left atrial appendage closure [LAA], or percutaneous mitral valve repair).

See 93313 for separate reporting of the probe insertion by a physician other than the physician performing the TEE.

Report of an echocardiographic study, whether complete or limited, includes an interpretation of all obtained information, documentation of all clinically relevant findings including quantitative measurements obtained, plus a description of any recognized abnormalities. Pertinent images, videotape, and/or digital data are archived for permanent storage and are available for subsequent review. Use of echocardiography not meeting these criteria is not separately reportable.

Use of ultrasound, without thorough evaluation of organ(s) or anatomic region, image documentation and final, written report, is not separately reportable.

(For fetal echocardiography, see 76825-76828)

93303 Transthoracic echocardiography for congenital cardiac anomalies; complete

➲ *CPT Assistant* Nov 97:44, Dec 97:5, Sep 05:10-11, Mar 08:4, Oct 10:17, Dec 10:17, Aug 13:3, Dec 13:15, May 15:10

➲ *Clinical Examples in Radiology* Fall 06:9-10

93304 follow-up or limited study

➲ *CPT Assistant* Nov 97:44, Dec 97:5, Jan 10:8, Oct 10:17, Dec 10:17, Aug 13:3, Dec 13:15, May 15:10

➲ *Clinical Examples in Radiology* Fall 06:9-10

93306 Echocardiography, transthoracic, real-time with image documentation (2D), includes M-mode recording, when performed, complete, with spectral Doppler echocardiography, and with color flow Doppler echocardiography

➲ *CPT Changes: An Insider's View* 2009

➲ *CPT Assistant* Oct 10:17, Dec 10:17, Aug 13:3, May 15:10, Apr 16:9

(For transthoracic echocardiography without spectral and color Doppler, use 93307)

93307 Echocardiography, transthoracic, real-time with image documentation (2D), includes M-mode recording, when performed, complete, without spectral or color Doppler echocardiography

➲ *CPT Changes: An Insider's View* 2009

➲ *CPT Assistant* Dec 97:5, Sep 05:11, Oct 10:17, Dec 10:17, Aug 13:3, May 15:10, Apr 16:9

➲ *Clinical Examples in Radiology* Fall 06:9-10

(Do not report 93307 in conjunction with 93320, 93321, 93325)

93308 Echocardiography, transthoracic, real-time with image documentation (2D), includes M-mode recording, when performed, follow-up or limited study

➲ *CPT Changes: An Insider's View* 2009

➲ *CPT Assistant* Dec 97:5, Sep 05:11, Jan 10:8, Oct 10:17, Dec 10:17, Mar 12:10, Aug 13:3, May 15:10, Apr 16:9

➲ *Clinical Examples in Radiology* Fall 06:9-10

93312 Echocardiography, transesophageal, real-time with image documentation (2D) (with or without M-mode recording); including probe placement, image acquisition, interpretation and report

➲ *CPT Changes: An Insider's View* 2017

➲ *CPT Assistant* Dec 97:5, Jan 00:10, Jan 10:8, Oct 12:15, Aug 13:3, Jul 14:9

(Do not report 93312 in conjunction with 93355)

93313 placement of transesophageal probe only

➲ *CPT Changes: An Insider's View* 2017

➲ *CPT Assistant* Dec 97:5, Mar 08:4, Jan 10:8, Aug 13:3

(The same individual may not report 93313 in conjunction with 93355)

93314 image acquisition, interpretation and report only

➲ *CPT Changes: An Insider's View* 2017

➲ *CPT Assistant* Dec 97:5, Jan 00:10, Jan 10:8, Aug 13:3

(Do not report 93314 in conjunction with 93355)

Transesophageal Echocardiography (TEE)
93312-93318

An endoscopic ultrasound transducer is passed through the mouth into the esophagus and 2-dimensional images are obtained from the posterior aspect of the heart.

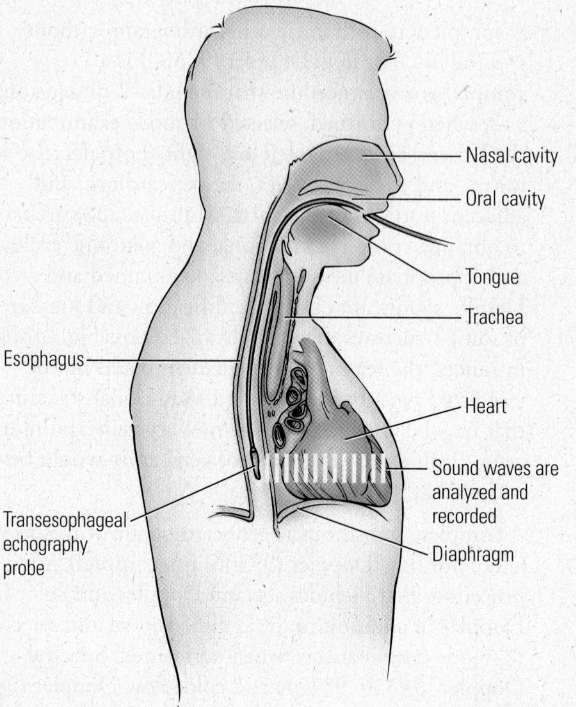

93315 Transesophageal echocardiography for congenital cardiac anomalies; including probe placement, image acquisition, interpretation and report

➲ *CPT Changes: An Insider's View* 2017

➲ *CPT Assistant* Nov 97:44, Dec 97:5, Jan 10:8, Aug 13:3, Dec 13:15, Jul 14:9

(Do not report 93315 in conjunction with 93355)

93316 placement of transesophageal probe only

➲ *CPT Changes: An Insider's View* 2017

➲ *CPT Assistant* Nov 97:44, Dec 97:5, Jan 10:8, Aug 13:3

(Do not report 93316 in conjunction with 93355)

93317 image acquisition, interpretation and report only

➲ *CPT Changes: An Insider's View* 2017

➲ *CPT Assistant* Nov 97:44, Dec 97:5, Jan 10:8, Aug 13:3, Dec 13:15

(Do not report 93317 in conjunction with 93355)

93318 Echocardiography, transesophageal (TEE) for monitoring purposes, including probe placement, real time 2-dimensional image acquisition and interpretation leading to ongoing (continuous) assessment of (dynamically changing) cardiac pumping function and to therapeutic measures on an immediate time basis

➲ *CPT Changes: An Insider's View* 2001, 2017

➲ *CPT Assistant* Jan 10:8, Apr 10:6, Aug 13:3

(Do not report 93318 in conjunction with 93355)

+ 93320 Doppler echocardiography, pulsed wave and/or continuous wave with spectral display (List separately in addition to codes for echocardiographic imaging); complete

➲ *CPT Assistant* Nov 97:44, Dec 97:5, Aug 13:3

➲ *Clinical Examples in Radiology* Fall 06:9-10

(Use 93320 in conjunction with 93303, 93304, 93312, 93314, 93315, 93317, 93350, 93351)

(Do not report 93320 in conjunction with 93355)

+ 93321 follow-up or limited study (List separately in addition to codes for echocardiographic imaging)

➲ *CPT Assistant* Nov 97:44, Dec 97:5, Jan 10:8, Aug 13:3

➲ *Clinical Examples in Radiology* Fall 06:9-10

(Use 93321 in conjunction with 93303, 93304, 93308, 93312, 93314, 93315, 93317, 93350, 93351)

(Do not report 93321 in conjunction with 93355)

+ 93325 Doppler echocardiography color flow velocity mapping (List separately in addition to codes for echocardiography)

➲ *CPT Assistant* Nov 97:44, Dec 97:5, Aug 13:3, Jul 16:9

➲ *Clinical Examples in Radiology* Fall 06:9-10

(Use 93325 in conjunction with 76825, 76826, 76827, 76828, 93303, 93304, 93308, 93312, 93314, 93315, 93317, 93350, 93351)

(Do not report 93325 in conjunction with 93355)

93350 Echocardiography, transthoracic, real-time with image documentation (2D), includes M-mode recording, when performed, during rest and cardiovascular stress test using treadmill, bicycle exercise and/or pharmacologically induced stress, with interpretation and report;

➲ *CPT Changes: An Insider's View* 2009

➲ *CPT Assistant* Aug 02:11, Jan 10:8, Oct 10:17, Dec 10:17, Aug 13:3, Jul 14:9, Apr 16:9

(Stress testing codes 93016-93018 should be reported, when appropriate, in conjunction with 93350 to capture the cardiovascular stress portion of the study)

(Do not report 93350 in conjunction with 93015)

93351 including performance of continuous electrocardiographic monitoring, with supervision by a physician or other qualified health care professional

➲ *CPT Changes: An Insider's View* 2009, 2013

➲ *CPT Assistant* Jan 10:8, Oct 10:17, Dec 10:17, Aug 13:3, Jul 14:9, Apr 16:9

(Do not report 93351 in conjunction with 93015-93018, 93350. Do not report 93351-26 in conjunction with 93016, 93018, 93350-26)

+ 93352 Use of echocardiographic contrast agent during stress echocardiography (List separately in addition to code for primary procedure)

➲ *CPT Changes: An Insider's View* 2009

➲ *CPT Assistant* Jan 10:8, Oct 10:17, Dec 10:17, Aug 13:3

(Do not report 93352 more than once per stress echocardiogram)

(Use 93352 in conjunction with 93350, 93351)

93355 Echocardiography, transesophageal (TEE) for guidance of a transcatheter intracardiac or great vessel(s) structural intervention(s) (eg, TAVR, transcatheter pulmonary valve replacement, mitral valve repair, paravalvular regurgitation repair, left atrial appendage occlusion/closure, ventricular septal defect closure) (peri-and intra-procedural), real-time image acquisition and documentation, guidance with quantitative measurements, probe manipulation, interpretation, and report, including diagnostic transesophageal echocardiography and, when performed, administration of ultrasound contrast, Doppler, color flow, and 3D

➲ *CPT Changes: An Insider's View* 2015

(To report placement of transesophageal probe by separate physician, use 93313)

(Do not report 93355 in conjunction with 76376, 76377, 93312, 93313, 93314, 93315, 93316, 93317, 93318, 93320, 93321, 93325)

Cardiac Catheterization

Cardiac catheterization is a diagnostic medical procedure which includes introduction, positioning and repositioning, when necessary, of catheter(s), within the vascular system, recording of intracardiac and/or intravascular pressure(s), and final evaluation and report of procedure. There are two code families for cardiac catheterization: one for congenital heart disease and one for all other conditions. Anomalous coronary arteries, patent foramen ovale, mitral valve prolapse, and bicuspid aortic valve are to be reported with 93451-93464, 93566-93568.

Right heart catheterization includes catheter placement in one or more right-sided cardiac chamber(s) or structures (ie, the right atrium, right ventricle, pulmonary artery, pulmonary wedge), obtaining blood samples for measurement of blood gases, and cardiac output measurements (Fick or other method), when performed. Left heart catheterization involves catheter placement in a left-sided (systemic) cardiac chamber(s) (left ventricle or left atrium) and includes left ventricular injection(s) when performed. Do not report 93503 in conjunction with other diagnostic cardiac catheterization codes. When right heart catheterization is performed in conjunction with other cardiac catheterization services, report 93453, 93456, 93457, 93460, or 93461. For placement of a flow directed catheter (eg, Swan-Ganz) performed for hemodynamic monitoring purposes not in conjunction with other catheterization services, use 93503. Right heart catheterization does not include right ventricular or right atrial angiography (93566). When left heart catheterization is performed using either transapical puncture of the left ventricle or transseptal puncture of an intact septum, report 93462 in conjunction with 93452,

93453, 93458-93461, 93653, 93654. Catheter placement(s) in coronary artery(ies) involves selective engagement of the origins of the native coronary artery(ies) for the purpose of coronary angiography. Catheter placement(s) in bypass graft(s) (venous, internal mammary, free arterial graft[s]) involve selective engagement of the origins of the graft(s) for the purpose of bypass angiography. It is typically performed only in conjunction with coronary angiography of native vessels.

The cardiac catheterization codes (93452-93461), other than those for congenital heart disease, include contrast injection(s), imaging supervision, interpretation, and report for imaging typically performed. Codes for left heart catheterization (93452, 93453, 93458-93461), other than those for congenital heart disease, include intraprocedural injection(s) for left ventricular/left atrial angiography, imaging supervision, and interpretation, when performed. Codes for coronary catheter placement(s) (93454-93461), other than those for congenital heart disease, include intraprocedural injection(s) for coronary angiography, imaging supervision, and interpretation. Codes for catheter placement(s) in bypass graft(s) (93455, 93457, 93459, 93461), other than those for congenital heart disease, include intraprocedural injection(s) for bypass graft angiography, imaging supervision, and interpretation. Do not report 93563-93565 in conjunction with 93452-93461.

For cardiac catheterization for congenital cardiac anomalies, see 93530-93533. When contrast injection(s) are performed in conjunction with cardiac catheterization for congenital anomalies, see 93563-93568.

Cardiac catheterization (93451-93461) includes all roadmapping angiography in order to place the catheters, including any injections and imaging supervision, interpretation, and report. It does not include contrast injection(s) and imaging supervision, interpretation, and report for imaging that is separately identified by specific procedure code(s). For right ventricular or right atrial angiography performed in conjunction with cardiac catheterization for congenital or noncongenital heart disease (93451-93461, 93530-93533), use 93566. For aortography, use 93567. For pulmonary angiography, use 93568. For angiography of noncoronary arteries and veins, performed as a distinct service, use appropriate codes from the Radiology section and the Vascular Injection Procedures section.

When cardiac catheterization is combined with pharmacologic agent administration with the specific purpose of repeating hemodynamic measurements to evaluate hemodynamic response, use 93463 in conjunction with 93451-93453 and 93456-93461. Do not report 93463 for intracoronary administration of pharmacologic agents during percutaneous coronary interventional procedures, during intracoronary assessment of coronary pressure, flow or resistance, or during intracoronary imaging procedures. Do not report 93463 in conjunction with 92920-92944, 92975, 92977.

When cardiac catheterization is combined with exercise (eg, walking or arm or leg ergometry protocol) with the specific purpose of repeating hemodynamic measurements to evaluate hemodynamic response, report 93464 in conjunction with 93451-93453, 93456-93461, and 93530-93533.

Contrast injection to image the access site(s) for the specific purpose of placing a closure device is inherent to the catheterization procedure and not separately reportable. Closure device placement at the vascular access site is inherent to the catheterization procedure and not separately reportable.

Modifier 51 should not be appended to 93451, 93456, 93503.

Please see the cardiac catheterization table located on page 675.

⊘ **93451** Right heart catheterization including measurement(s) of oxygen saturation and cardiac output, when performed

➲ *CPT Changes: An Insider's View* 2011, 2017

➲ *CPT Assistant* Aug 11:5, Mar 12:10, May 13:12, Jul 14:3, Sep 15:3, Mar 16:5, Dec 17:16

►(Do not report 93451 in conjunction with 33289, 93453, 93456, 93457, 93460, 93461)◄

(Do not report 93451 in conjunction with 0345T for diagnostic left and right heart catheterization procedures intrinsic to the valve repair procedure)

Right Heart Catheterization

93451

The physician introduces a cardiac catheter into the venous system. The catheter is directed into the right atrium, right ventricle, and pulmonary artery.

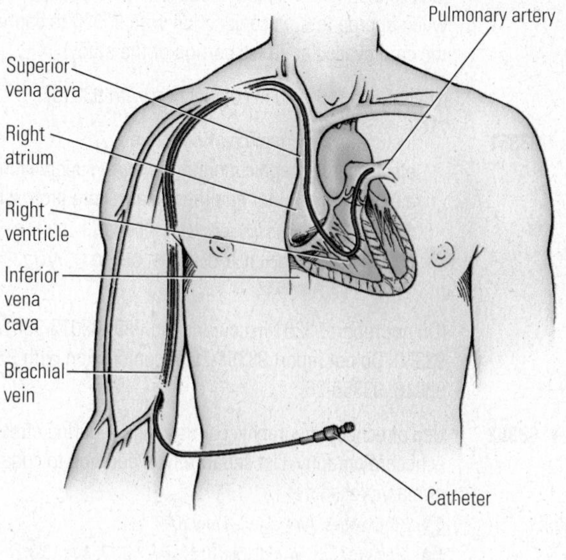

Right Heart Catheterization—Infant

Catheter is advanced retrograde through the arterial system to the ascending aorta; pressures are measured in the aortic root; the catheter is manipulated using fluoroscopic guidance into the ostium of a coronary artery, arterial bypass conduit, or venous coronary bypass graft.

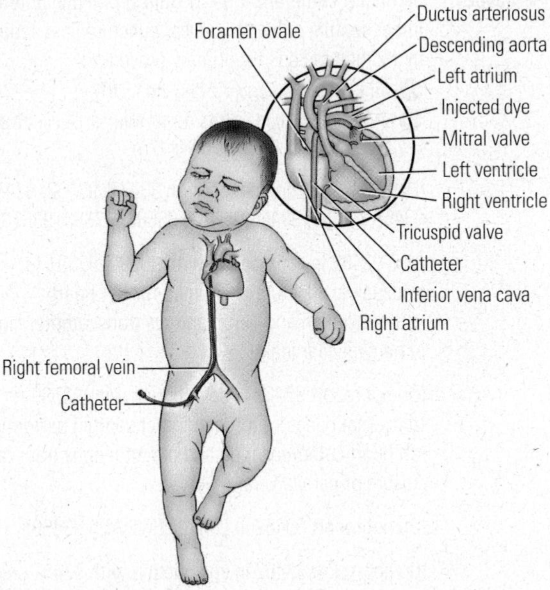

93452 Left heart catheterization including intraprocedural injection(s) for left ventriculography, imaging supervision and interpretation, when performed

➲ *CPT Changes: An Insider's View* 2011, 2017

➲ *CPT Assistant* Aug 11:3, Mar 12:10, Jan 13:6, May 13:12, Sep 15:3

(Do not report 93452 in conjunction with 93453, 93458-93461, 0408T, 0409T, 0410T, 0411T, 0414T, 0415T)

Left Heart Catheterization
93452

A catheter is inserted into the arterial system and then into the left ventricle.

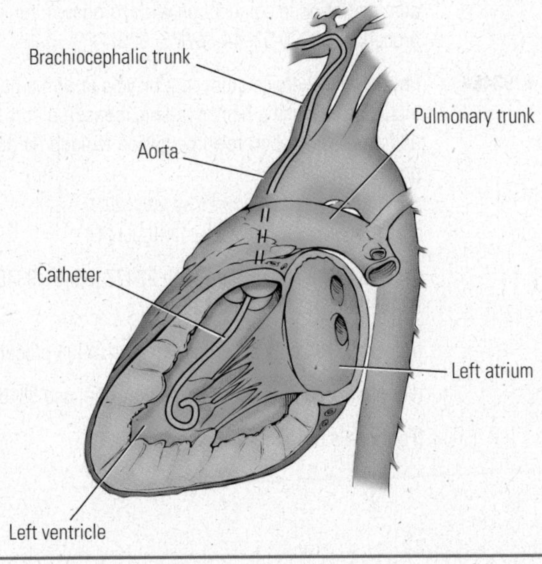

93453 Combined right and left heart catheterization including intraprocedural injection(s) for left ventriculography, imaging supervision and interpretation, when performed

➲ *CPT Changes: An Insider's View* 2011, 2017

➲ *CPT Assistant* Aug 11:3, Mar 12:10, Jan 13:6, May 13:12, Sep 15:3, Mar 16:5

(Do not report 93453 in conjunction with 93451, 93452, 93456-93461, 0408T, 0409T, 0410T, 0411T, 0414T, 0415T)

(Do not report 93453 in conjunction with 0345T for diagnostic left and right heart catheterization procedures intrinsic to the valve repair procedure)

93454 Catheter placement in coronary artery(s) for coronary angiography, including intraprocedural injection(s) for coronary angiography, imaging supervision and interpretation;

➲ *CPT Changes: An Insider's View* 2011, 2017

➲ *CPT Assistant* Aug 11:3, Mar 12:10, May 13:12, Dec 14:6, Mar 16:5, Feb 17:15

(Do not report 93453, 93454 in conjunction with 0345T for coronary angiography intrinsic to the valve repair procedure)

Coronary Angiography Without Concomitant Left Heart Catheterization
93454

Cardiac catheterization procedure performed wherein the catheter does not cross the aortic valve into the left ventricle (left heart catheterization).

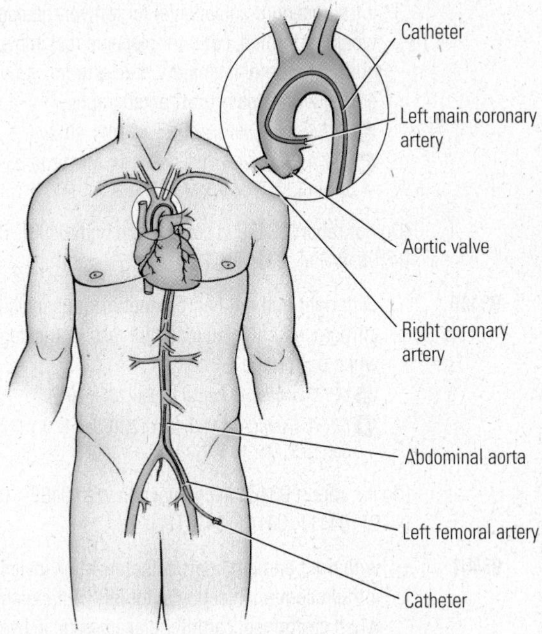

Medicine / Cardiovascular 92920-93799

93455 with catheter placement(s) in bypass graft(s) (internal mammary, free arterial, venous grafts) including intraprocedural injection(s) for bypass graft angiography

➲ *CPT Changes: An Insider's View* 2011, 2017

➲ *CPT Assistant* Aug 11:3, Dec 11:9, Mar 12:10, May 13:12, Mar 16:5

⊘ **93456** with right heart catheterization

➲ *CPT Changes: An Insider's View* 2011, 2017

➲ *CPT Assistant* Aug 11:3, Mar 12:10, May 13:12, Sep 15:3, Mar 16:5

(Do not report 93456 in conjunction with 0345T for diagnostic left and right heart catheterization procedures intrinsic to the valve repair procedure)

93457 with catheter placement(s) in bypass graft(s) (internal mammary, free arterial, venous grafts) including intraprocedural injection(s) for bypass graft angiography and right heart catheterization

➲ *CPT Changes: An Insider's View* 2011, 2017

➲ *CPT Assistant* Aug 11:3, Dec 11:9, Mar 12:10, May 13:12, Sep 15:3, Mar 16:5

93458 with left heart catheterization including intraprocedural injection(s) for left ventriculography, when performed

➲ *CPT Changes: An Insider's View* 2011, 2017

➲ *CPT Assistant* Aug 11:3, Mar 12:10, Jan 13:6, May 13:12, Sep 15:3, Mar 16:5

(Do not report 93458 in conjunction with 0408T, 0409T, 0410T, 0411T, 0414T, 0415T)

93459 with left heart catheterization including intraprocedural injection(s) for left ventriculography, when performed, catheter placement(s) in bypass graft(s) (internal mammary, free arterial, venous grafts) with bypass graft angiography

➲ *CPT Changes: An Insider's View* 2011, 2017

➲ *CPT Assistant* Aug 11:3, Dec 11:11, Mar 12:10, Jan 13:6, May 13:12, Sep 15:3, Mar 16:5

(Do not report 93459 in conjunction with 0408T, 0409T, 0410T, 0411T, 0414T, 0415T)

93460 with right and left heart catheterization including intraprocedural injection(s) for left ventriculography, when performed

➲ *CPT Changes: An Insider's View* 2011, 2017

➲ *CPT Assistant* Aug 11:3, Mar 12:10, Jan 13:6, May 13:12, Sep 15:3, Mar 16:5

(Do not report 93460 in conjunction with 0408T, 0409T, 0410T, 0411T, 0414T, 0415T)

93461 with right and left heart catheterization including intraprocedural injection(s) for left ventriculography, when performed, catheter placement(s) in bypass graft(s) (internal mammary, free arterial, venous grafts) with bypass graft angiography

➲ *CPT Changes: An Insider's View* 2011, 2017

➲ *CPT Assistant* Aug 11:3, Dec 11:9, Mar 12:10, Jan 13:6, May 13:12, Jul 14:3, Dec 14:6, Sep 15:3, Mar 16:5

(Do not report 93461 in conjunction with 0345T for diagnostic left and right heart catheterization procedures intrinsic to the valve repair procedure)

(Do not report 93461 in conjunction with 0408T, 0409T, 0410T, 0411T, 0414T, 0415T)

+ 93462 Left heart catheterization by transseptal puncture through intact septum or by transapical puncture (List separately in addition to code for primary procedure)

➲ *CPT Changes: An Insider's View* 2011, 2017

➲ *CPT Assistant* Aug 11:3, Mar 12:10, May 13:12, Jun 13:6, Jul 14:3, Sep 15:3, Jul 17:3, Sep 17:3

(Use 93462 in conjunction with 33477, 93452, 93453, 93458, 93459, 93460, 93461, 93582, 93653, 93654)

(Use 93462 in conjunction with 93590, 93591 for transapical puncture performed for left heart catheterization and percutaneous transcatheter closure of paravalvular leak)

(Do not report 93462 in conjunction with 93590 for transeptal puncture through intact septum performed for left heart catheterization and percutaneous transcatheter closure of paravalvular leak)

(Do not report 93462 in conjunction with 93656)

(Do not report 93462 in conjunction with 0345T unless transapical puncture is performed)

+ 93463 Pharmacologic agent administration (eg, inhaled nitric oxide, intravenous infusion of nitroprusside, dobutamine, milrinone, or other agent) including assessing hemodynamic measurements before, during, after and repeat pharmacologic agent administration, when performed (List separately in addition to code for primary procedure)

➲ *CPT Changes: An Insider's View* 2011, 2017

➲ *CPT Assistant* Aug 11:3, Mar 12:10, Dec 14:6

(Use 93463 in conjunction with 33477, 93451-93453, 93456-93461, 93530, 93531, 93532, 93533, 93580, 93581)

(Report 93463 only once per catheterization procedure)

(Do not report 93463 for pharmacologic agent administration in conjunction with coronary interventional procedure 92920-92944, 92975, 92977)

+ 93464 Physiologic exercise study (eg, bicycle or arm ergometry) including assessing hemodynamic measurements before and after (List separately in addition to code for primary procedure)

➲ *CPT Changes: An Insider's View* 2011, 2017

➲ *CPT Assistant* Aug 11:3, Mar 12:10, Jul 14:3

(Use 93464 in conjunction with 33477, 93451-93453, 93456-93461, 93530-93533)

(Report 93464 only once per catheterization procedure)

(For pharmacologic agent administration, use 93463)

(For bundle of His recording, use 93600)

Cardiac Catheterization Codes

		Catheter Placement Type				Add-on Procedures (Can Be Reported Separately)					
CPT Code	Code Descriptor	RHC	LHC	Coronary Artery Placement	Bypass Graft(s)	With Transseptal or Transapical Puncture	With Pharmacological Study	With Exercise Study	Injection Procedure for Selective Right Ventricular or Right Atrial Angiography	Injection Procedure for Supravalvular Aortography	Injection Procedure for Pulmonary Angiography
						93462	93463	93464	93566	93567	93568
93451	Right heart catheterization including measurement(s) of oxygen saturation and cardiac output, when performed	X					X	X	X		X
93452	Left heart catheterization including intraprocedural injection(s) for left ventriculography, imaging supervision and interpretation, when performed		X			X	X	X		X	
93453	Combined right and left heart catheterization including intraprocedural injection(s) for left ventriculography, imaging supervision and interpretation, when performed	X	X			X	X	X	X	X	X
93454	Catheter placement in coronary artery(s) for coronary angiography, including intraprocedural injection(s) for coronary angiography, imaging supervision and interpretation;			X						X	
93455	Catheter placement in coronary artery(s) for coronary angiography, including intraprocedural injection(s) for coronary angiography, imaging supervision and interpretation; with catheter placement(s) in bypass graft(s), (internal mammary, free arterial, venous grafts) including intraprocedural injection(s) for bypass graft angiography			X	X					X	

Cardiac Catheterization Codes, *continued*

		Catheter Placement Type				Add-on Procedures (Can Be Reported Separately)					
CPT Code	Code Descriptor	RHC	LHC	Coronary Artery Placement	Bypass Graft(s)	With Transseptal or Transapical Puncture	With Pharmacological Study	With Exercise Study	Injection Procedure for Selective Right Ventricular or Right Atrial Angiography	Injection Procedure for Supravalvular Aortography	Injection Procedure for Pulmonary Angiography
						93462	93463	93464	93566	93567	93568
93456	Catheter placement in coronary artery(s) for coronary angiography, including intraprocedural injection(s) for coronary angiography, imaging supervision and interpretation; **with right heart catheterization**	X		X			X	X	X	X	X
93457	Catheter placement in coronary artery(s) for coronary angiography, including intraprocedural injection(s) for coronary angiography, imaging supervision and interpretation; **with catheter placement(s) in bypass graft(s) (internal mammary, free arterial, venous grafts) including intraprocedural injection(s) for bypass graft angiography and right heart catheterization**	X		X	X		X	X	X	X	X
93458	Catheter placement in coronary artery(s) for coronary angiography, including intraprocedural injection(s) for coronary angiography, imaging supervision and interpretation; **with left heart catheterization including intraprocedural injection(s) for left ventriculography, when performed**		X	X		X	X	X		X	

Cardiac Catheterization Codes, *continued*

		Catheter Placement Type				Add-on Procedures (Can Be Reported Separately)					
CPT Code	Code Descriptor	RHC	LHC	Coronary Artery Placement	Bypass Graft(s)	With Transseptal or Transapical Puncture	With Pharmacological Study	With Exercise Study	Injection Procedure for Selective Right Ventricular or Right Atrial Angiography	Injection Procedure for Supravalvular Aortography	Injection Procedure for Pulmonary Angiography
						93462	93463	93464	93566	93567	93568
93459	Catheter placement in coronary artery(s) for coronary angiography, including intraprocedural injection(s) for coronary angiography, imaging supervision and interpretation; **with left heart catheterization including intraprocedural injection(s) for left ventriculography, when performed, catheter placement(s) in bypass graft(s) (internal mammary, free arterial, venous grafts) with bypass graft angiography**		X	X	X	X	X	X		X	
93460	Catheter placement in coronary artery(s) for coronary angiography, including intraprocedural injection(s) for coronary angiography, imaging supervision and interpretation; **with right and left heart catheterization including intraprocedural injection(s) for left ventriculography, when performed**	X	X	X		X	X	X	X	X	X
93461	Catheter placement in coronary artery(s) for coronary angiography, including intraprocedural injection(s) for coronary angiography, imaging supervision and interpretation; with right and left heart catheterization including intraprocedural injection(s) for left ventriculography, when performed, catheter placement(s) in bypass graft(s) (internal mammary, free arterial, venous grafts) with bypass graft angiography	X	X	X	X	X	X	X	X	X	X

⊘ **93503** Insertion and placement of flow directed catheter (eg, Swan-Ganz) for monitoring purposes

➲ *CPT Assistant* Winter 91:3, Fall 95:8, Feb 97:5, Apr 98:2, Mar 08:4, Aug 11:3, Dec 11:18

(For subsequent monitoring, see 99356-99357)

93505 Endomyocardial biopsy

➲ *CPT Changes: An Insider's View* 2008, 2017

➲ *CPT Assistant* Apr 98:2, Apr 00:10, Aug 11:3, Dec 17:16

93530 Right heart catheterization, for congenital cardiac anomalies

➲ *CPT Changes: An Insider's View* 2008, 2017

➲ *CPT Assistant* Nov 97:45, Jan 98:11, Mar 98:11, Apr 98:3, 6-7, Aug 11:3, Dec 11:11, Mar 12:10, May 13:12, Jul 14:3, Sep 15:3, Mar 16:5

93531 Combined right heart catheterization and retrograde left heart catheterization, for congenital cardiac anomalies

➲ *CPT Changes: An Insider's View* 2008

➲ *CPT Assistant* Nov 97:45, Jan 98:11, Mar 98:11, Apr 98:8, 10-11, Aug 11:3, Dec 11:11, Mar 12:10, Sep 15:3, Mar 16:5

93532 Combined right heart catheterization and transseptal left heart catheterization through intact septum with or without retrograde left heart catheterization, for congenital cardiac anomalies

➲ *CPT Changes: An Insider's View* 2008

➲ *CPT Assistant* Nov 97:45, Jan 98:11, Mar 98:11, Apr 98:10-11, Aug 11:3, Dec 11:11, Mar 12:10, Sep 15:3, Mar 16:5

93533 Combined right heart catheterization and transseptal left heart catheterization through existing septal opening, with or without retrograde left heart catheterization, for congenital cardiac anomalies

➲ *CPT Changes: An Insider's View* 2008

➲ *CPT Assistant* Nov 97:45, Jan 98:11, Mar 98:11, Apr 98:12-13, Aug 11:3, Dec 11:11, Mar 12:10, Jul 14:3, Sep 15:3, Mar 16:5

Injection Procedures

All injection codes include radiological supervision, interpretation, and report. Cardiac catheterization codes (93452-93461), other than those for congenital heart disease, include contrast injection(s) for imaging typically performed during these procedures (see Cardiac Catheterization above). Do not report 93563-93565 in conjunction with 93452-93461. When injection procedures for right ventricular, right atrial, aortic, or pulmonary angiography are performed in conjunction with cardiac catheterization, these services are reported separately (93566-93568). When right ventricular or right atrial angiography is performed at the time of heart catheterization, use 93566 with the appropriate catheterization code (93451, 93453, 93456, 93457, 93460, or 93461). Use 93567 when supravalvular ascending aortography is performed at the time of heart catheterization. Use 93568 with the appropriate right heart catheterization code when pulmonary angiography is performed. Separately reported injection procedures do not include introduction of catheters but do include repositioning of catheters when necessary and use of automatic power injectors, when performed.

When contrast injection(s) are performed in conjunction with cardiac catheterization for congenital cardiac anomalies (93530-93533), see 93563-93568. Injection procedure codes 93563-93568 include imaging supervision, interpretation, and report.

Injection procedures 93563-93568 represent separate identifiable services and may be coded in conjunction with one another when appropriate. The technical details of angiography, supervision of imaging and processing, interpretation, and report are included.

93561 Indicator dilution studies such as dye or thermodilution, including arterial and/or venous catheterization; with cardiac output measurement (separate procedure)

➲ *CPT Changes: An Insider's View* 2012, 2017

➲ *CPT Assistant* Winter 91:25, Summer 95:2, Aug 00:2, Feb 07:10, Jul 07:1, Aug 11:3, Jul 14:3

93562 subsequent measurement of cardiac output

➲ *CPT Changes: An Insider's View* 2012, 2017

➲ *CPT Assistant* Winter 91:25, Summer 95:2, Aug 00:2, Feb 07:10, Jul 07:1, Aug 11:3, May 14:4, Jul 14:3

(Do not report 93561, 93562 in conjunction with 93451-93462, 93582)

(For radioisotope method of cardiac output, see 78472, 78473, or 78481)

+ 93563 Injection procedure during cardiac catheterization including imaging supervision, interpretation, and report; for selective coronary angiography during congenital heart catheterization (List separately in addition to code for primary procedure)

➲ *CPT Changes: An Insider's View* 2011, 2017

➲ *CPT Assistant* Aug 11:3, Dec 11:11, Jan 13:6, Dec 14:6, Mar 16:5

+ 93564 for selective opacification of aortocoronary venous or arterial bypass graft(s) (eg, aortocoronary saphenous vein, free radial artery, or free mammary artery graft) to one or more coronary arteries and in situ arterial conduits (eg, internal mammary), whether native or used for bypass to one or more coronary arteries during congenital heart catheterization, when performed (List separately in addition to code for primary procedure)

➲ *CPT Changes: An Insider's View* 2011, 2017

➲ *CPT Assistant* Aug 11:3, Dec 11:11, Jan 13:6, Dec 14:6, Mar 16:5

(Do not report 93563, 93564 in conjunction with 0345T for coronary angiography intrinsic to the valve repair procedure)

+ 93565 for selective left ventricular or left atrial angiography (List separately in addition to code for primary procedure)

➲ *CPT Changes: An Insider's View* 2011, 2017

➲ *CPT Assistant* Aug 11:3, Dec 11:9, Jan 13:6

(Do not report 93563-93565 in conjunction with 93452-93461)

(Use 93563-93565 in conjunction with 93530-93533)

+ 93566 for selective right ventricular or right atrial angiography (List separately in addition to code for primary procedure)

CPT Changes: An Insider's View 2011, 2017

CPT Assistant Aug 11:3, Dec 11:9, Jan 13:6, May 15:3, Mar 16:5, May 16:5

(Use 93566 in conjunction with 93451, 93453, 93456, 93457, 93460, 93461, 93530-93533)

►(Do not report 93566 in conjunction with 33274 for right ventriculography performed during leadless pacemaker insertion)◄

+ 93567 for supravalvular aortography (List separately in addition to code for primary procedure)

CPT Changes: An Insider's View 2011, 2017

CPT Assistant Aug 11:3, Dec 11:9, Jan 13:6, Mar 16:5

(Use 93567 in conjunction with 93451-93461, 93530-93533)

(For non-supravalvular thoracic aortography or abdominal aortography performed at the time of cardiac catheterization, use the appropriate radiological supervision and interpretation codes [36221, 75600-75630])

+ 93568 for pulmonary angiography (List separately in addition to code for primary procedure)

CPT Changes: An Insider's View 2011, 2017

CPT Assistant Aug 11:3, Dec 11:9, Jan 13:6, Mar 16:5

(Use 93568 in conjunction with 93451, 93453, 93456, 93457, 93460, 93461, 93530-93533, 93582, 93583)

+ 93571 Intravascular Doppler velocity and/or pressure derived coronary flow reserve measurement (coronary vessel or graft) during coronary angiography including pharmacologically induced stress; initial vessel (List separately in addition to code for primary procedure)

CPT Changes: An Insider's View 2017

CPT Assistant Nov 98:33, Apr 00:2, Mar 08:4, Aug 11:3, Dec 14:6, May 15:10, Dec 15:17

(Use 93571 in conjunction with 92920, 92924, 92928, 92933, 92937, 92941, 92943, 92975, 93454-93461, 93563, 93564)

►(Do not report 93571 in conjunction with 0523T)◄

+ 93572 each additional vessel (List separately in addition to code for primary procedure)

CPT Changes: An Insider's View 2017

CPT Assistant Nov 98:34, Apr 00:2, Aug 11:5, Dec 14:6, May 15:10, Dec 15:17

(Use 93572 in conjunction with 93571)

(Intravascular distal coronary blood flow velocity measurements include all Doppler transducer manipulations and repositioning within the specific vessel being examined, during coronary angiography or therapeutic intervention [eg, angioplasty])

(For unlisted cardiac catheterization procedure, use 93799)

►(Do not report 93572 in conjunction with 0523T)◄

Intravascular Distal Blood Flow Velocity
93571

A Doppler guidewire is positioned in a proximal coronary artery with the transducer beam parallel to blood flow to measure blood flow velocity.

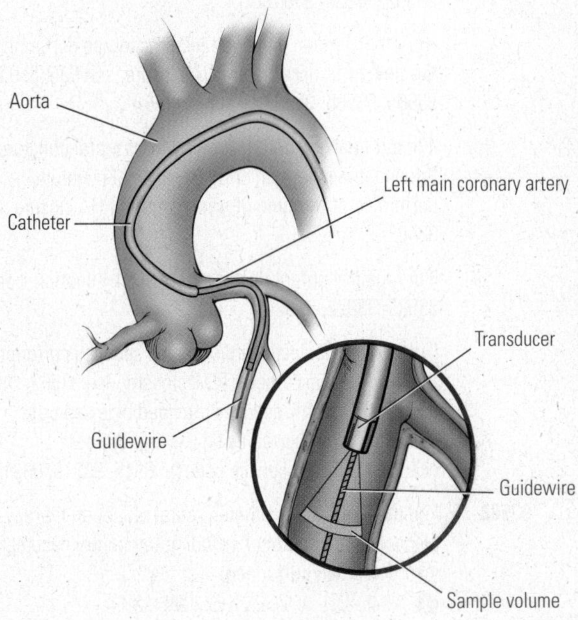

Repair of Structural Heart Defect

93580 Percutaneous transcatheter closure of congenital interatrial communication (ie, Fontan fenestration, atrial septal defect) with implant

CPT Changes: An Insider's View 2003

CPT Assistant Mar 03:23

(Percutaneous transcatheter closure of atrial septal defect includes a right heart catheterization procedure. Code 93580 includes injection of contrast for atrial and ventricular angiograms. Codes 93451-93453, 93455-93461, 93530-93533, 93564-93566 should not be reported separately in addition to code 93580)

93581 Percutaneous transcatheter closure of a congenital ventricular septal defect with implant

CPT Changes: An Insider's View 2003

CPT Assistant Mar 03:23, Mar 08:4

(Percutaneous transcatheter closure of ventricular septal defect includes a right heart catheterization procedure. Code 93581 includes injection of contrast for atrial and ventricular angiograms. Codes 93451-93453, 93455-93461, 93530-93533, 93564-93566 should not be reported separately in addition to code 93581)

(For echocardiographic services performed in addition to 93580, 93581, see 93303-93317, 93662 as appropriate)

93582 Percutaneous transcatheter closure of patent ductus arteriosus

CPT Changes: An Insider's View 2014, 2017

CPT Assistant Jul 14:3

(93582 includes congenital right and left heart catheterization, catheter placement in the aorta, and aortic arch angiography, when performed)

(Do not report 93582 in conjunction with 36013, 36014, 36200, 75600, 75605, 93451-93461, 93530, 93531, 93532, 93533, 93567)

(For other cardiac angiographic procedures performed at the time of transcatheter PDA closure, see 93563, 93564, 93565, 93566, 93568 as appropriate)

(For left heart catheterization by transseptal puncture through intact septum or by transapical puncture performed at the time of transcatheter PDA closure, use 93462)

(For repair of patent ductus arteriosus by ligation, see 33820, 33822, 33824)

(For intracardiac echocardiographic services performed at the time of transcatheter PDA closure, use 93662. Other echocardiographic services provided by a separate individual are reported using the appropriate echocardiography service codes, 93315, 93316, 93317)

93583 Percutaneous transcatheter septal reduction therapy (eg, alcohol septal ablation) including temporary pacemaker insertion when performed

➲ *CPT Changes: An Insider's View* 2014, 2017

(93583 includes insertion of temporary pacemaker, when performed, and left heart catheterization)

(Do not report 93583 in conjunction with 33210, 93452, 93453, 93458, 93459, 93460, 93461, 93531, 93532, 93533, 93565)

(93583 includes left anterior descending coronary angiography for the purpose of roadmapping to guide the intervention. Do not report 93454, 93455, 93456, 93457, 93458, 93459, 93460, 93461, 93563 for coronary angiography performed during alcohol septal ablation for the purpose of roadmapping, guidance of the intervention, vessel measurement, and completion angiography)

(Diagnostic cardiac catheterization procedures may be separately reportable when no prior catheter-based diagnostic study of the treatment zone is available, the prior diagnostic study is inadequate, or the patient's condition with respect to the clinical indication has changed since the prior study or during the intervention. Use the appropriate codes from 93451, 93454, 93455, 93456, 93457, 93530, 93563, 93564, 93566, 93567, 93568)

(Do not report 93583 in conjunction with 33210, 33211)

(Do not report 93463 for the injection of alcohol for this procedure)

(For intracardiac echocardiographic services performed at the time of alcohol septal ablation, use 93662)

(Other echocardiographic services provided by a separate physician are reported using the appropriate echocardiography services codes, 93312, 93313, 93314, 93315, 93316, 93317)

(For surgical ventriculomyotomy [-myectomy] for idiopathic hypertrophic subaortic stenosis, use 33416)

Transcatheter Closure of Paravalvular Leak

Codes 93590, 93591, 93592 are used to report transcatheter closure of paravalvular leak (PVL). Codes 93590 and 93591 include, when performed, percutaneous access, placing the access sheath(s), advancing the delivery system to the paravalvular leak, positioning the closure device, repositioning the closure device as needed, and deploying the device.

Codes 93590 and 93591 include, when performed, fluoroscopy (76000), angiography, radiological supervision and interpretation services performed to guide the PVL closure (eg, guiding the device placement and documenting completion of the intervention).

Code 93590 includes transseptal puncture, and left heart catheterization/left ventriculography (93452, 93453, 93458, 93459, 93460, 93461, 93531, 93532, 93533, 93565), when performed. Transapical left heart catheterization (93462) may be reported separately, when performed.

Code 93591 includes, when performed, supravalvular aortography (93567), left heart catheterization/left ventriculography (93452, 93453, 93458, 93459, 93460, 93461, 93531, 93532, 93533, 93565). Transapical left heart catheterization (93462) may be reported separately, when performed.

Diagnostic right heart catheterization codes (93451, 93456, 93457, 93530) and diagnostic coronary angiography codes (93454, 93455, 93456, 93457, 93563, 93564) may be reported with 93590, 93591, representing separate and distinct services from PVL closure, if:

1. No prior study is available and a full diagnostic study is performed, or
2. A prior study is available, but as documented in the medical record:
   a. there is inadequate visualization of the anatomy and/or pathology, or
   b. the patient's condition with respect to the clinical indication has changed since the prior study, or
   c. there is a clinical change during the procedure that requires new evaluation.

Other cardiac catheterization services may be reported separately, when performed for diagnostic purposes not intrinsic to PVL closure.

For same session/same day diagnostic cardiac catheterization services, report the appropriate diagnostic cardiac catheterization code(s) appended with modifier 59 indicating separate and distinct procedural service from PVL closure.

93590 Percutaneous transcatheter closure of paravalvular leak; initial occlusion device, mitral valve

➔ *CPT Changes: An Insider's View* 2017

➔ *CPT Assistant* Sep 17:3

(Do not report 93590 in conjunction with 93462 for transseptal puncture)

(For transapical puncture performed in conjunction with 93590, use 93462)

93591 initial occlusion device, aortic valve

➔ *CPT Changes: An Insider's View* 2017

➔ *CPT Assistant* Sep 17:3

(For transseptal or transapical puncture performed in conjunction with 93591, use 93462)

+ 93592 each additional occlusion device (List separately in addition to code for primary procedure)

➔ *CPT Changes: An Insider's View* 2017

➔ *CPT Assistant* Sep 17:3

(Use 93592 in conjunction with 93590, 93591)

Intracardiac Electrophysiological Procedures/Studies

Intracardiac electrophysiologic studies (EPS) are invasive diagnostic medical procedures which include the insertion and repositioning of electrode catheters, recording of electrograms before and during pacing, programmed stimulation of multiple locations in the heart, analysis of recorded information, and report of the procedure. In many circumstances, patients with arrhythmias are evaluated and treated at the same encounter. In this situation, a diagnostic *electrophysiologic study* is performed, induced tachycardia(s) are *mapped*, and on the basis of the diagnostic and mapping information, the tissue is *ablated*.

Definitions

Arrhythmia Induction: In most electrophysiologic studies, an attempt is made to induce arrhythmia(s) from single or multiple sites within the heart. Arrhythmia induction may be achieved by multiple techniques, eg, by performing pacing at different rates or programmed stimulation (introduction of critically timed electrical impulses). Because arrhythmia induction occurs via the same catheter(s) inserted for the electrophysiologic study(ies), catheter insertion and temporary pacemaker codes are not additionally reported. Codes 93600-93603, 93610, 93612, and 93618 are used to describe unusual situations where there may be recording, pacing, or an attempt at arrhythmia induction from only one site in the heart. Code 93619 describes only evaluation of the sinus node, atrioventricular node, and His-Purkinje conduction system, without arrhythmia induction. Codes 93620-93624, 93640-93642, 93653, 93654, and 93656 all include recording, pacing, and attempted arrhythmia induction from one or more site(s) in the heart.

Mapping: When a tachycardia is induced, the site of tachycardia origination or its electrical path through the heart is often defined by mapping. Mapping creates a multidimensional depiction of a tachycardia by recording multiple electrograms obtained sequentially or simultaneously from multiple catheter sites in the heart. Depending upon the technique, certain types of mapping catheters may be repositioned from point-to-point within the heart, allowing sequential recording from the various sites to construct maps. Other types of mapping catheters allow mapping without a point-to-point technique by allowing simultaneous recording from many electrodes on the same catheter and computer-assisted three-dimensional reconstruction of the tachycardia activation sequence.

Mapping is a distinct procedure performed in addition to a diagnostic electrophysiologic study or ablation procedure and may be separately reported using 93609 or 93613. Do not report standard mapping (93609) in addition to 3-dimensional mapping (93613).

Ablation: Once the part of the heart involved in the tachycardia is localized, the tachycardia may be treated by ablation (the delivery of a radiofrequency or cryo-energy to the area to selectively destroy cardiac tissue). Ablation procedures (93653-93657) are performed at the same session as electrophysiology studies and therefore represent a combined code description. When reporting ablation therapy codes (93653-93657), the single site electrophysiology studies (93600-93603, 93610, 93612, 93618) and the comprehensive electrophysiology studies (93619, 93620) may not be reported separately. Code 93622 may be reported separately with 93653 and 93656. Code 93623 may be reported separately with 93653, 93654, and 93656. However, 93621 for left atrial pacing and recording from coronary sinus or left atrium should not be reported in conjunction with 93656, as this procedure is a component of 93656. Codes 93653 and 93654 include right ventricular pacing and recording and His bundle recording when clinically indicated. When performance of one or more components is not possible or indicated, document the reason for not performing. Code 93656 includes each of left atrial pacing/recording, right ventricular pacing/recording, and His bundle recording when clinically indicated. When performance of one or more components is not possible or indicated, document the reason for not performing.

The differences in the techniques involved for ablation of supraventricular arrhythmias, ventricular arrhythmias, and atrial fibrillation are reflected within the descriptions for 93653-93657. Code 93653 is a primary code for catheter ablation for treatment of supraventricular tachycardia caused by dual atrioventricular nodal pathways, accessory atrioventricular connections, or other atrial foci. Code 93654 describes catheter ablation for treatment of ventricular tachycardia or focus of ventricular ectopy. Code 93656 is a primary code for reporting treatment of atrial fibrillation by ablation to achieve complete pulmonary vein electrical isolation. Codes 93653, 93654, and 93656 are distinct primary procedure codes and may not be reported together.

Codes 93655 and 93657 are add-on codes listed in addition to the primary ablation code to report ablation of sites distinct from the primary ablation site. After ablation of the primary target site, post-ablation electrophysiologic evaluation is performed as part of those ablation services (93653, 93654, 93656) and additional mechanisms of tachycardia may be identified. For example, if the primary tachycardia ablated was atrioventricular nodal reentrant tachycardia and during post-ablation testing an atrial tachycardia, atrial flutter, or accessory pathway with orthodromic reentry tachycardia was identified, this would be considered a separate mechanism of tachycardia. Pacing maneuvers are performed to define the mechanism(s) of the new tachycardia(s). Catheter ablation of this distinct mechanism of tachycardia is then performed at the newly discovered atrial or ventricular origin. Appropriate post-ablation attempts at re-induction and observation are again performed. Code 93655 is listed in conjunction with 93653 when repeat ablation is for treatment of an additional supraventricular tachycardia mechanism and with 93654 when the repeat ablation is for treatment of an additional ventricular tachycardia mechanism. Code 93655 may be reported with 93656 when an additional non-atrial fibrillation tachycardia is separately diagnosed after pulmonary vein isolation. Code 93657 is reported in conjunction with 93656 when successful pulmonary vein isolation is achieved, attempts at re-induction of atrial fibrillation identify an additional left or right atrial focus for atrial fibrillation, and further ablation of this new focus is performed.

In certain circumstances, depending on the chamber of origin, a catheter or catheters may be maneuvered into the left ventricle to facilitate arrhythmia diagnosis. This may be accomplished via a retrograde aortic approach by means of the arterial access or through a transseptal puncture. For ablation treatment of supraventricular tachycardia (93653) and ventricular tachycardia (93654), the left heart catheterization by transseptal puncture through intact septum (93462) may be reported separately as an add-on code. However, for ablation treatment of atrial fibrillation (93656), the transseptal puncture (93462) is a standard component of the procedure and may not be reported separately. Do not report 93462 in conjunction with 93656.

Modifier 51 should not be appended to 93600-93603, 93610, 93612, 93615-93618, 93631.

⊘ **93600** Bundle of His recording

➲ *CPT Assistant* Summer 94:12, Aug 97:9, Apr 04:9, Jul 04:13, Aug 05:13, Dec 07:16, Mar 08:4, Jun 13:6, Jul 13:7, Apr 14:3

(Do not report 93600 in conjunction with 93619, 93620, 93653, 93654, 93656)

⊘ **93602** Intra-atrial recording

➲ *CPT Assistant* Summer 94:12, Aug 97:9, Apr 04:9, Jul 04:13, Aug 05:13, Jun 13:6, Jul 13:7, Apr 14:3

(Do not report 93602 in conjunction with 93619, 93620, 93653, 93654, 93656)

⊘ **93603** Right ventricular recording

➲ *CPT Assistant* Summer 94:12, Aug 97:9, Apr 04:9, Jul 04:13, Aug 05:13, Jun 13:6, Jul 13:7, Apr 14:3

(Do not report 93603 in conjunction with 93619, 93620, 93653, 93654, 93656)

+ 93609 Intraventricular and/or intra-atrial mapping of tachycardia site(s) with catheter manipulation to record from multiple sites to identify origin of tachycardia (List separately in addition to code for primary procedure)

➲ *CPT Changes: An Insider's View* 2002, 2017

➲ *CPT Assistant* Summer 94:12, Aug 97:9, Apr 04:9, Aug 05:13, Jun 13:6, Jul 13:7, Apr 14:3

(Use 93609 in conjunction with 93620, 93653, 93656)

(Do not report 93609 in conjunction with 93613, 93654)

⊘ **93610** Intra-atrial pacing

➲ *CPT Assistant* Summer 94:12, Aug 97:9, Apr 04:9, Jul 04:13, Jun 13:6, Jul 13:7, Apr 14:3

(Do not report 93610 in conjunction with 93619, 93620, 93653, 93654, 93656)

⊘ **93612** Intraventricular pacing

➲ *CPT Assistant* Summer 94:12, Aug 97:9, Apr 04:9, Jul 04:13, Jun 13:6, Jul 13:7, Apr 14:3

(Do not report 93612 in conjunction with 93619, 93620, 93621, 93622, 93653, 93654, 93656)

+ 93613 Intracardiac electrophysiologic 3-dimensional mapping (List separately in addition to code for primary procedure)

➲ *CPT Changes: An Insider's View* 2002, 2017

➲ *CPT Assistant* Apr 04:8, Aug 05:13, Jun 13:6, Jul 13:7, Apr 14:3

(Use 93613 in conjunction with 93620, 93653, 93656)

(Do not report 93613 in conjunction with 93609, 93654)

⊘ **93615** Esophageal recording of atrial electrogram with or without ventricular electrogram(s);

➲ *CPT Changes: An Insider's View* 2017

➲ *CPT Assistant* Summer 94:12, Aug 97:9, Apr 04:9, Aug 05:13, Apr 14:3

⊘ **93616** with pacing

➲ *CPT Changes: An Insider's View* 2017

➲ *CPT Assistant* Summer 94:12, Aug 97:9, Apr 04:9, Aug 05:13, Apr 14:3

⊘ **93618** Induction of arrhythmia by electrical pacing

➲ *CPT Changes: An Insider's View* 2017

➲ *CPT Assistant* Summer 94:12, Aug 97:9, Oct 97:10, Apr 99:10, Jun 00:5, Nov 00:9, Apr 04:9, Jul 04:13, Aug 05:13, Dec 07:16, Jun 13:6, Jul 13:7, Apr 14:3

(Do not report 93618 in conjunction with 93619, 93620, 93621, 93622, 93653, 93654, 93656)

(For intracardiac phonocardiogram, use 93799)

93619 Comprehensive electrophysiologic evaluation with right atrial pacing and recording, right ventricular pacing and recording, His bundle recording, including insertion and repositioning of multiple electrode catheters, without induction or attempted induction of arrhythmia

➔ *CPT Changes: An Insider's View* 2002, 2008, 2017

➔ *CPT Assistant* Aug 97:9, Oct 97:10, Nov 00:9, Apr 04:9, Jul 04:13, Aug 05:13, Dec 07:16, Nov 12:6, Jun 13:6, Jul 13:7, Apr 14:3

(Do not report 93619 in conjunction with 93600, 93602, 93603, 93610, 93612, 93618, 93620, 93621, 93622, 93653, 93654, 93655, 93656, 93657)

93620 Comprehensive electrophysiologic evaluation including insertion and repositioning of multiple electrode catheters with induction or attempted induction of arrhythmia; with right atrial pacing and recording, right ventricular pacing and recording, His bundle recording

➔ *CPT Changes: An Insider's View* 2002, 2003, 2008, 2017

➔ *CPT Assistant* Summer 94:12, Aug 97:9, Oct 97:10, Jul 98:10, Aug 98:7, Nov 00:9, Apr 04:9, Jul 04:13, Aug 05:13, Dec 07:16, Oct 08:10, Nov 12:6, Jun 13:6, Jul 13:7, Apr 14:3

(Do not report 93620 in conjunction with 93600, 93602, 93603, 93610, 93612, 93618, 93619, 93653, 93654, 93655, 93656, 93657)

+ 93621 with left atrial pacing and recording from coronary sinus or left atrium (List separately in addition to code for primary procedure)

➔ *CPT Changes: An Insider's View* 2002, 2017

➔ *CPT Assistant* Summer 94:12, Aug 97:9, Oct 97:10, Jul 98:10, Aug 98:7, Nov 98:34, Nov 00:9, Apr 04:9, Jul 04:13, Aug 05:13, Dec 07:16, Oct 08:10, Nov 12:6, Jun 13:6, Jul 13:7, Apr 14:3

(Use 93621 in conjunction with 93620, 93653, 93654)

(Do not report 93621 in conjunction with 93656)

+ 93622 with left ventricular pacing and recording (List separately in addition to code for primary procedure)

➔ *CPT Changes: An Insider's View* 2002, 2017

➔ *CPT Assistant* Summer 94:14, Aug 97:9, Oct 97:10, Jul 98:10, Aug 98:7, Nov 98:34, Nov 00:9, Apr 04:9, Jul 04:13, Aug 05:13, Dec 07:16, Mar 08:4, Nov 12:6, Jun 13:6, Jul 13:7, Apr 14:3

(Use 93622 in conjunction with 93620, 93653, 93656)

(Do not report 93622 in conjunction with 93654)

+ 93623 Programmed stimulation and pacing after intravenous drug infusion (List separately in addition to code for primary procedure)

➔ *CPT Assistant* Summer 94:14, Aug 97:9, Nov 00:9, Aug 05:13, Dec 07:16, Oct 08:10, Apr 14:3

(Use 93623 in conjunction with 93610, 93612, 93619, 93620, 93653, 93654, 93656)

93624 Electrophysiologic follow-up study with pacing and recording to test effectiveness of therapy, including induction or attempted induction of arrhythmia

➔ *CPT Changes: An Insider's View* 2008, 2017

➔ *CPT Assistant* Summer 94:14, Aug 97:9, Nov 00:9, Aug 05:13, Dec 07:16

⊘ **93631** Intra-operative epicardial and endocardial pacing and mapping to localize the site of tachycardia or zone of slow conduction for surgical correction

➔ *CPT Assistant* Summer 94:14, Aug 97:9, Nov 00:9, Aug 05:13, Dec 07:16

(For operative ablation of an arrhythmogenic focus or pathway by a separate individual, see 33250-33261)

93640 Electrophysiologic evaluation of single or dual chamber pacing cardioverter-defibrillator leads including defibrillation threshold evaluation (induction of arrhythmia, evaluation of sensing and pacing for arrhythmia termination) at time of initial implantation or replacement;

➔ *CPT Changes: An Insider's View* 2000, 2008, 2017

➔ *CPT Assistant* Summer 94:14, Aug 97:9, Apr 99:10, Nov 99:50, Nov 00:9, Aug 05:13, Jun 12:3

93641 with testing of single or dual chamber pacing cardioverter-defibrillator pulse generator

➔ *CPT Changes: An Insider's View* 2000, 2008, 2017

➔ *CPT Assistant* Summer 94:14, Aug 97:9, Apr 99:10, Nov 99:50, Jun 00:5, Jul 00:5, Nov 00:9, Aug 05:13, Jun 12:3, Apr 14:3

(For subsequent or periodic electronic analysis and/or reprogramming of single or dual chamber pacing cardioverter-defibrillators, see 93282, 93283, 93289, 93292, 93295, 93642)

93642 Electrophysiologic evaluation of single or dual chamber transvenous pacing cardioverter-defibrillator (includes defibrillation threshold evaluation, induction of arrhythmia, evaluation of sensing and pacing for arrhythmia termination, and programming or reprogramming of sensing or therapeutic parameters)

➔ *CPT Changes: An Insider's View* 2000, 2008, 2015, 2017

➔ *CPT Assistant* Summer 94:14, Aug 97:9, Nov 99:50, Jun 00:5, Nov 00:9, Aug 05:13, Jun 13:6, Jul 13:7, Apr 14:3

93644 Electrophysiologic evaluation of subcutaneous implantable defibrillator (includes defibrillation threshold evaluation, induction of arrhythmia, evaluation of sensing for arrhythmia termination, and programming or reprogramming of sensing or therapeutic parameters)

➔ *CPT Changes: An Insider's View* 2015, 2017

(Do not report 93644 in conjunction with 33270 at the time of subcutaneous implantable defibrillator device insertion)

(For subsequent or periodic electrophysiologic evaluation of a subcutaneous implantable defibrillator device, see 93260, 93261)

93650 Intracardiac catheter ablation of atrioventricular node function, atrioventricular conduction for creation of complete heart block, with or without temporary pacemaker placement

➔ *CPT Changes: An Insider's View* 2008, 2017

➔ *CPT Assistant* Summer 94:15, Aug 97:9, Nov 00:9, Aug 05:13, Apr 12:18, May 12:15

93653 Comprehensive electrophysiologic evaluation including insertion and repositioning of multiple electrode catheters with induction or attempted induction of an arrhythmia with right atrial pacing and recording, right ventricular pacing and recording (when necessary), and His bundle recording (when necessary) with intracardiac catheter ablation of arrhythmogenic focus; with treatment of supraventricular tachycardia by ablation of fast or slow atrioventricular pathway, accessory atrioventricular connection, cavo-tricuspid isthmus or other single atrial focus or source of atrial re-entry

➔ *CPT Changes: An Insider's View* 2013, 2014, 2017

➔ *CPT Assistant* Jun 13:6, Jul 13:7, Apr 14:3

(Do not report 93653 in conjunction with 93600-93603, 93610, 93612, 93618-93620, 93642, 93654, 93656)

93654 with treatment of ventricular tachycardia or focus of ventricular ectopy including intracardiac electrophysiologic 3D mapping, when performed, and left ventricular pacing and recording, when performed

➔ *CPT Changes: An Insider's View* 2013, 2014, 2017

➔ *CPT Assistant* Jun 13:6, Jul 13:7, Apr 14:3

(Do not report 93654 in conjunction with 93279-93284, 93286-93289, 93600-93603, 93609, 93610, 93612, 93613, 93618-93620, 93622, 93642, 93653, 93656)

+ 93655 Intracardiac catheter ablation of a discrete mechanism of arrhythmia which is distinct from the primary ablated mechanism, including repeat diagnostic maneuvers, to treat a spontaneous or induced arrhythmia (List separately in addition to code for primary procedure)

➔ *CPT Changes: An Insider's View* 2013, 2017

➔ *CPT Assistant* Jun 13:6, Jul 13:7

(Use 93655 in conjunction with 93653, 93654, 93656)

93656 Comprehensive electrophysiologic evaluation including transseptal catheterizations, insertion and repositioning of multiple electrode catheters with induction or attempted induction of an arrhythmia including left or right atrial pacing/recording when necessary, right ventricular pacing/recording when necessary, and His bundle recording when necessary with intracardiac catheter ablation of atrial fibrillation by pulmonary vein isolation

➔ *CPT Changes: An Insider's View* 2013, 2014, 2017

➔ *CPT Assistant* Jun 13:6, Jul 13:7, Apr 14:3

(Do not report 93656 in conjunction with 93279-93284, 93286-93289, 93462, 93600, 93602, 93603, 93610, 93612, 93618, 93619, 93620, 93621, 93653, 93654)

+ 93657 Additional linear or focal intracardiac catheter ablation of the left or right atrium for treatment of atrial fibrillation remaining after completion of pulmonary vein isolation (List separately in addition to code for primary procedure)

➔ *CPT Changes: An Insider's View* 2013, 2017

➔ *CPT Assistant* Jun 13:6, Jul 13:7, Apr 14:3

(Use 93657 in conjunction with 93656)

93660 Evaluation of cardiovascular function with tilt table evaluation, with continuous ECG monitoring and intermittent blood pressure monitoring, with or without pharmacological intervention

➔ *CPT Changes: An Insider's View* 2008

➔ *CPT Assistant* Nov 12:6

(For testing of autonomic nervous system function, see 95921, 95924, 95943)

+ 93662 Intracardiac echocardiography during therapeutic/diagnostic intervention, including imaging supervision and interpretation (List separately in addition to code for primary procedure)

➔ *CPT Changes: An Insider's View* 2001

➔ *CPT Assistant* Mar 03:23

(Use 93662 in conjunction with 92987, 93453, 93460-93462, 93532, 93580, 93581, 93620, 93621, 93622, 93653, 93654, 93656 as appropriate)

(Do not report 92961 in addition to 93662)

Peripheral Arterial Disease Rehabilitation

Peripheral arterial disease (PAD) rehabilitative physical exercise consists of a series of sessions, lasting 45-60 minutes per session, involving use of either a motorized treadmill or a track to permit each patient to achieve symptom-limited claudication. Each session is supervised by an exercise physiologist or nurse. The supervising provider monitors the individual patient's claudication threshold and other cardiovascular limitations for adjustment of workload. During this supervised rehabilitation program, the development of new arrhythmias, symptoms that might suggest angina or the continued inability of the patient to progress to an adequate level of exercise may require review and examination of the patient by a physician or other qualified health care professional. These services would be separately reported with an appropriate level E/M service code including office or other outpatient services (99201-99215), initial hospital care (99221-99223), subsequent hospital care (99231-99233), critical care services (99291-99292).

93668 Peripheral arterial disease (PAD) rehabilitation, per session

➔ *CPT Changes: An Insider's View* 2001

Noninvasive Physiologic Studies and Procedures

(For arterial cannulization and recording of direct arterial pressure, use 36620)

(For radiographic injection procedures, see 36000-36299)

(For vascular cannulization for hemodialysis, see 36800-36821)

(For chemotherapy for malignant disease, see 96409-96549)

(For penile plethysmography, use 54240)

93701 Bioimpedance-derived physiologic cardiovascular analysis

➔ *CPT Changes: An Insider's View* 2002, 2010

➔ *CPT Assistant* Mar 02:3, Mar 08:4

(For bioelectrical impedance analysis whole body composition, use 0358T. For left ventricular filling pressure indirect measurement by computerized calibration of the arterial waveform response to Valsalva, use 93799)

93702 Bioimpedance spectroscopy (BIS), extracellular fluid analysis for lymphedema assessment(s)

➔ *CPT Changes: An Insider's View* 2015

(For bioelectrical impedance analysis whole body composition, use 0358T)

(For bioimpedance-derived physiological cardiovascular analysis, use 93701)

93724 Electronic analysis of antitachycardia pacemaker system (includes electrocardiographic recording, programming of device, induction and termination of tachycardia via implanted pacemaker, and interpretation of recordings)

➔ *CPT Assistant* Summer 94:23

93740 Temperature gradient studies

93745 Initial set-up and programming by a physician or other qualified health care professional of wearable cardioverter-defibrillator includes initial programming of system, establishing baseline electronic ECG, transmission of data to data repository, patient instruction in wearing system and patient reporting of problems or events

➔ *CPT Changes: An Insider's View* 2005, 2013

(Do not report 93745 in conjunction with 93282, 93292)

93750 Interrogation of ventricular assist device (VAD), in person, with physician or other qualified health care professional analysis of device parameters (eg, drivelines, alarms, power surges), review of device function (eg, flow and volume status, septum status, recovery), with programming, if performed, and report

➔ *CPT Changes: An Insider's View* 2010, 2013

➔ *CPT Assistant* Apr 10:6

(Do not report 93750 in conjunction with 33975, 33976, 33979, 33981-33983)

(93760, 93762 have been deleted)

93770 Determination of venous pressure

(For central venous cannulization see 36555-36556, 36500)

93784 Ambulatory blood pressure monitoring, utilizing a system such as magnetic tape and/or computer disk, for 24 hours or longer; including recording, scanning analysis, interpretation and report

93786 recording only

93788 scanning analysis with report

93790 review with interpretation and report

➔ *CPT Changes: An Insider's View* 2013

Home and Outpatient International Normalized Ratio (INR) Monitoring Services

Home and outpatient international normalized ratio (INR) monitoring services describe the management of warfarin therapy, including ordering, review, and interpretation of new INR test result(s), patient instructions, and dosage adjustments as needed.

If a significantly, separately identifiable evaluation and management (E/M) service is performed on the same day as 93792, the appropriate E/M service may be reported using modifier 25.

Do not report 93793 on the same day as an E/M service.

Do not report 93792, 93793 in conjunction with 98966, 98967, 98968, 98969, 99441, 99442, 99443, 99444, when telephone or online services address home and outpatient INR monitoring.

Do not report 93792, 93793 when performed during the service time of 99487, 99489, 99490, 99495, 99496.

93792 Patient/caregiver training for initiation of home international normalized ratio (INR) monitoring under the direction of a physician or other qualified health care professional, face-to-face, including use and care of the INR monitor, obtaining blood sample, instructions for reporting home INR test results, and documentation of patient's/caregiver's ability to perform testing and report results

➔ *CPT Changes: An Insider's View* 2018

➔ *CPT Assistant* Mar 18:7

(For provision of test materials and equipment for home INR monitoring, see 99070 or the appropriate supply code)

93793 Anticoagulant management for a patient taking warfarin, must include review and interpretation of a new home, office, or lab international normalized ratio (INR) test result, patient instructions, dosage adjustment (as needed), and scheduling of additional test(s), when performed

➔ *CPT Changes: An Insider's View* 2018

➔ *CPT Assistant* Nov 17:11, Mar 18:7

(Do not report 93793 in conjunction with 99201, 99202, 99203, 99204, 99205, 99211, 99212, 99213, 99214, 99215, 99241, 99242, 99243, 99244, 99245)

(Report 93793 no more than once per day, regardless of the number of tests reviewed)

Other Procedures

93797 Physician or other qualified health care professional services for outpatient cardiac rehabilitation; without continuous ECG monitoring (per session)

➲ *CPT Changes: An Insider's View* 2013

93798 with continuous ECG monitoring (per session)

➲ *CPT Changes: An Insider's View* 2013

93799 Unlisted cardiovascular service or procedure

➲ *CPT Assistant* Mar 98:11, Mar 02:10, Nov 05:15, Apr 09:9, Jul 10:10, Oct 11:7, Nov 11:11, Dec 13:18

Noninvasive Vascular Diagnostic Studies

Vascular studies include patient care required to perform the studies, supervision of the studies and interpretation of study results with copies for patient records of hard copy output with analysis of all data, including bidirectional vascular flow or imaging when provided.

The use of a simple hand-held or other Doppler device that does not produce hard copy output, or that produces a record that does not permit analysis of bidirectional vascular flow, is considered to be part of the physical examination of the vascular system and is not separately reported. The Ankle-Brachial Index (or ABI) is reportable with 93922 or 93923 as long as simultaneous Doppler recording and analysis of bidirectional blood flow, volume plethysmography, or transcutaneous oxygen tension measurements are also performed.

Duplex scan (eg, 93880, 93882) describes an ultrasonic scanning procedure for characterizing the pattern and direction of blood flow in arteries or veins with the production of real-time images integrating B-mode two-dimensional vascular structure, Doppler spectral analysis, and color flow Doppler imaging.

Physiologic studies Noninvasive physiologic studies are performed using equipment separate and distinct from the duplex ultrasound imager. Codes 93922, 93923, 93924 describe the evaluation of non-imaging physiologic recordings of pressures with Doppler analysis of bi-directional blood flow, plethysmography, and/or oxygen tension measurements appropriate for the anatomic area studied.

Limited studies for lower extremity require either:

(1) ankle/brachial indices at distal posterior tibial and anterior tibial/dorsalis pedis arteries plus bidirectional Doppler waveform recording and analysis at 1-2 levels; or (2) ankle/brachial indices at distal posterior tibial and anterior tibial/dorsalis pedis arteries plus volume plethysmography at 1-2 levels; or (3) ankle/brachial indices at distal posterior tibial and anterior tibial/dorsalis pedis arteries with transcutaneous oxygen tension measurements at 1-2 levels. Potential levels include high thigh, low thigh, calf, ankle, metatarsal and toes.

Limited studies for upper extremity require either:

(1) Doppler-determined systolic pressures and bidirectional Doppler waveform recording and analysis at 1-2 levels; or (2) Doppler-determined systolic pressures and volume plethysmography at 1-2 levels; or (3) Doppler-determined systolic pressures and transcutaneous oxygen tension measurements at 1-2 levels. Potential levels include arm, forearm, wrist, and digits.

Complete studies for lower extremity require either:

(1) ankle/brachial indices at distal posterior tibial and anterior tibial/dorsalis pedis arteries plus bidirectional Doppler waveform recording and analysis at 3 or more levels; or (2) ankle/brachial indices at distal posterior tibial and anterior tibial/dorsalis pedis arteries plus volume plethysmography at 3 or more levels; or (3) ankle/brachial indices at distal posterior tibial and anterior tibial/dorsalis pedis arteries with transcutaneous oxygen tension measurements at 3 or more levels. Alternatively, a complete study may be reported with measurements at a single level if provocative functional maneuvers (eg, measurements with postural provocative tests, or measurements with reactive hyperemia) are performed.

Complete studies for upper extremity require either:

(1) Doppler-determined systolic pressures and bidirectional Doppler waveform recording and analysis at 3 or more levels; or (2) Doppler-determined systolic pressures and volume plethysmography at 3 or more levels; or (3) Doppler-determined systolic pressures and transcutaneous oxygen tension measurements at 3 or more levels. Potential levels include arm, forearm, wrist, and digits. Alternatively, a complete study may be reported with measurements at a single level if provocative functional maneuvers (eg, measurements with postural provocative tests, or measurements with cold stress) are performed.

Cerebrovascular Arterial Studies

A complete transcranial Doppler (TCD) study (93886) includes ultrasound evaluation of the right and left anterior circulation territories and the posterior circulation territory (to include vertebral arteries and basilar artery). In a limited TCD study (93888) there is ultrasound evaluation of two or fewer of these territories. For TCD, ultrasound evaluation is a reasonable and concerted attempt to identify arterial signals through an acoustic window.

Code 93895 includes the acquisition and storage of images of the common carotid arteries, carotid bulbs, and internal carotid arteries bilaterally with quantification of intima media thickness (common carotid artery mean and maximal values) and determination of presence of atherosclerotic plaque. When any of these elements are not obtained, use 0126T.

93880 Duplex scan of extracranial arteries; complete bilateral study

➔ *CPT Assistant* Jun 96:9, Dec 05:3

➔ *Clinical Examples in Radiology* Fall 07:6, Winter 09:2, Winter 13:8, Winter 18:15

(Do not report 93880 in conjunction with 93895, 0126T)

93882 unilateral or limited study

➔ *CPT Assistant* Jun 96:9, Dec 05:3

➔ *Clinical Examples in Radiology* Fall 07:6, Winter 09:2, Winter 13:8, Winter 18:15

(Do not report 93882 in conjunction with 93895, 0126T)

(To report common carotid intima-media thickness (IMT) study for evaluation of atherosclerotic burden or coronary heart disease risk factor assessment, use Category III code 0126T)

93886 Transcranial Doppler study of the intracranial arteries; complete study

➔ *CPT Assistant* Jun 96:9, Dec 05:3

➔ *Clinical Examples in Radiology* Winter 18:15

93888 limited study

➔ *CPT Assistant* Jun 96:9, Dec 05:3

➔ *Clinical Examples in Radiology* Winter 18:15

93890 vasoreactivity study

➔ *CPT Changes: An Insider's View* 2005

➔ *CPT Assistant* Dec 05:3

➔ *Clinical Examples in Radiology* Winter 18:15

93892 emboli detection without intravenous microbubble injection

➔ *CPT Changes: An Insider's View* 2005

➔ *CPT Assistant* Dec 05:3

➔ *Clinical Examples in Radiology* Winter 18:15

93893 emboli detection with intravenous microbubble injection

➔ *CPT Changes: An Insider's View* 2005

➔ *CPT Assistant* Dec 05:3

➔ *Clinical Examples in Radiology* Winter 18:15

93895 Quantitative carotid intima media thickness and carotid atheroma evaluation, bilateral

➔ *CPT Changes: An Insider's View* 2015

➔ *Clinical Examples in Radiology* Winter 18:15

(Do not report 93895 in conjunction with 93880, 93882, 0126T)

(Do not report 93890-93893 in conjunction with 93888)

Extremity Arterial Studies (Including Digits)

93922 Limited bilateral noninvasive physiologic studies of upper or lower extremity arteries, (eg, for lower extremity: ankle/brachial indices at distal posterior tibial and anterior tibial/dorsalis pedis arteries plus bidirectional, Doppler waveform recording and analysis at 1-2 levels, or ankle/brachial indices at distal posterior tibial and anterior tibial/dorsalis pedis arteries plus volume plethysmography at 1-2 levels, or ankle/brachial indices at distal posterior tibial and anterior tibial/dorsalis pedis arteries with, transcutaneous oxygen tension measurement at 1-2 levels)

➔ *CPT Changes: An Insider's View* 2011

➔ *CPT Assistant* Jun 96:9, Dec 05:3, Aug 09:3, Jun 12:16, Jun 13:14, Jan 14:10

➔ *Clinical Examples in Radiology* Spring 11:5, 6, Summer 11:11, Winter 18:15

(When only 1 arm or leg is available for study, report 93922 with modifier 52 for a unilateral study when recording 1-2 levels. Report 93922 when recording 3 or more levels or performing provocative functional maneuvers)

(Report 93922 only once in the upper extremity(s) and/or once in the lower extremity(s). When both the upper and lower extremities are evaluated in the same setting, 93922 may be reported twice by adding modifier 59 to the second procedure)

(For transcutaneous oxyhemoglobin measurement in a lower extremity wound by near infrared spectroscopy, use 0493T)

93923 Complete bilateral noninvasive physiologic studies of upper or lower extremity arteries, 3 or more levels (eg, for lower extremity: ankle/brachial indices at distal posterior tibial and anterior tibial/dorsalis pedis arteries plus segmental blood pressure measurements with bidirectional Doppler waveform recording and analysis, at 3 or more levels, or ankle/brachial indices at distal posterior tibial and anterior tibial/dorsalis pedis arteries plus segmental volume plethysmography at 3 or more levels, or ankle/brachial indices at distal posterior tibial and anterior tibial/dorsalis pedis arteries plus segmental transcutaneous oxygen tension measurements at 3 or more levels), or single level study with provocative functional maneuvers (eg, measurements with postural provocative tests, or measurements with reactive hyperemia)

➔ *CPT Changes: An Insider's View* 2011

➔ *CPT Assistant* Jun 96:9, Jun 01:10, Dec 05:3, Aug 09:3, Jun 12:16, Jan 14:10

➔ *Clinical Examples in Radiology* Spring 11:5, 6, Summer 11:11, Winter 18:15

(When only 1 arm or leg is available for study, report 93922 for a unilateral study when recording 3 or more levels or when performing provocative functional maneuvers)

(Report 93923 only once in the upper extremity(s) and/or once in the lower extremity(s). When both the upper and lower extremities are evaluated in the same setting, 93923 may be reported twice by adding modifier 59 to the second procedure)

93924 Noninvasive physiologic studies of lower extremity arteries, at rest and following treadmill stress testing, (ie, bidirectional Doppler waveform or volume plethysmography recording and analysis at rest with ankle/brachial indices immediately after and at timed intervals following performance of a standardized protocol on a motorized treadmill plus recording of time of onset of claudication or other symptoms, maximal walking time, and time to recovery) complete bilateral study

CPT Changes: An Insider's View 2011

CPT Assistant Jun 96:9, Dec 05:3, Aug 09:3, Jun 12:16, Jan 14:10

Clinical Examples in Radiology Spring 11:5, 6, Winter 18:15

(Do not report 93924 in conjunction with 93922, 93923)

93925 Duplex scan of lower extremity arteries or arterial bypass grafts; complete bilateral study

CPT Assistant Jun 96:9, Dec 05:3, Sep 16:9

Clinical Examples in Radiology Winter 18:15

93926 unilateral or limited study

CPT Assistant Jun 96:9, Oct 01:2, Dec 05:3, Sep 16:9

Clinical Examples in Radiology Fall 09:4, 5, Winter 18:15

93930 Duplex scan of upper extremity arteries or arterial bypass grafts; complete bilateral study

CPT Assistant Jun 96:9, Dec 05:3, Sep 16:9

Clinical Examples in Radiology Winter 18:15

93931 unilateral or limited study

CPT Assistant Jun 96:9, Oct 01:2, Dec 05:3, Sep 16:9

Clinical Examples in Radiology Winter 18:15

Extremity Venous Studies (Including Digits)

(93965 has been deleted)

93970 Duplex scan of extremity veins including responses to compression and other maneuvers; complete bilateral study

CPT Assistant Jun 96:9, Dec 05:3, Jan 12:13, Feb 12:11, Oct 14:6, Sep 16:9

Clinical Examples in Radiology Spring 12:8, Spring 17:11, Winter 18:15

93971 unilateral or limited study

CPT Assistant Jun 96:9, Oct 01:2, Mar 03:21, Dec 05:3, Jul 10:6, Apr 11:13, Jan 12:13, Feb 12:11, Oct 14:6, Aug 15:8, Sep 16:9

Clinical Examples in Radiology Winter 08:11, Fall 09:4, 5, Spring 17:11, Winter 18:15

(Do not report 93970, 93971 in conjunction with 36475, 36476, 36478, 36479)

Visceral and Penile Vascular Studies

93975 Duplex scan of arterial inflow and venous outflow of abdominal, pelvic, scrotal contents and/or retroperitoneal organs; complete study

CPT Assistant Apr 96:11, Jun 96:9, Dec 05:3, Jun 14:15, Mar 15:10, Aug 16:10

Clinical Examples in Radiology Spring 08:9, Winter 08:10, Summer 09:12, Summer 12:7, Summer 15:10, Winter 15:11, Winter 18:15

93976 limited study

CPT Assistant Apr 96:11, Jun 96:9, Dec 05:3, Mar 15:10, Aug 16:10

Clinical Examples in Radiology Spring 08:10, Summer 09:12, Summer 12:7, Summer 15:10, Winter 18:15

93978 Duplex scan of aorta, inferior vena cava, iliac vasculature, or bypass grafts; complete study

CPT Assistant Jun 96:9, Dec 05:3

Clinical Examples in Radiology Spring 07:5-6, Spring 17:5, Winter 18:15

93979 unilateral or limited study

CPT Assistant Jun 96:9, Dec 05:3, Jun 14:15

Clinical Examples in Radiology Winter 15:11, Spring 17:5, Winter 18:15

(For ultrasound screening study for abdominal aortic aneurysm [AAA], real time with image documentation, use 76706)

93980 Duplex scan of arterial inflow and venous outflow of penile vessels; complete study

CPT Assistant Jun 96:9, Dec 05:3

Clinical Examples in Radiology Winter 18:15

93981 follow-up or limited study

CPT Assistant Jun 96:9, Dec 05:3

Clinical Examples in Radiology Winter 18:15

(93982 has been deleted)

Extremity Arterial-Venous Studies

93990 Duplex scan of hemodialysis access (including arterial inflow, body of access and venous outflow)

CPT Assistant Jun 96:9, Dec 05:3

Clinical Examples in Radiology Spring 07:5-6, Winter 18:15

(For measurement of hemodialysis access flow using indicator dilution methods, use 90940)

Other Noninvasive Vascular Diagnostic Studies

93998 Unlisted noninvasive vascular diagnostic study

CPT Changes: An Insider's View 2012

CPT Assistant Sep 12:9, Jan 14:10

Pulmonary

Ventilator Management

94002 Ventilation assist and management, initiation of pressure or volume preset ventilators for assisted or controlled breathing; hospital inpatient/observation, initial day

➔ *CPT Changes: An Insider's View* 2007

➔ *CPT Assistant* Feb 07:10, Mar 07:10, Apr 07:3, Jul 07:1, Nov 08:5, May 14:4, Oct 14:9

94003 hospital inpatient/observation, each subsequent day

➔ *CPT Changes: An Insider's View* 2007

➔ *CPT Assistant* Feb 07:10, Apr 07:3, Jul 07:1, Nov 08:5, May 14:4

94004 nursing facility, per day

➔ *CPT Changes: An Insider's View* 2007

➔ *CPT Assistant* Feb 07:10, Apr 07:3, Jul 07:1, Nov 08:5

(Do not report 94002-94004 in conjunction with Evaluation and Management services 99201-99499)

94005 Home ventilator management care plan oversight of a patient (patient not present) in home, domiciliary or rest home (eg, assisted living) requiring review of status, review of laboratories and other studies and revision of orders and respiratory care plan (as appropriate), within a calendar month, 30 minutes or more

➔ *CPT Changes: An Insider's View* 2007

➔ *CPT Assistant* Mar 07:11, Apr 07:3, Nov 08:5, Oct 14:9

(Do not report 94005 in conjunction with 99339, 99340, 99374-99378)

(Ventilator management care plan oversight is reported separately from home or domiciliary, rest home [eg, assisted living] services. A physician or other qualified health care professional may report 94005, when performed, including when a different individual reports 99339, 99340, 99374-99378 for the same 30 days)

Pulmonary Diagnostic Testing and Therapies

Codes 94010-94799 include laboratory procedure(s) and interpretation of test results. If a separate identifiable evaluation and management service is performed, the appropriate E/M service code including new or established patient office or other outpatient services (99201-99215), office or other outpatient consultations (99241-99245), emergency department services (99281-99285), nursing facility services (99304-99318), domiciliary, rest home, or custodial care services (99324-99337), and home services (99341-99350) may be reported in addition to 94010-94799.

Spirometry (94010) measures expiratory airflow and volumes and forms the basis of most pulmonary function testing. When spirometry is performed before and after administration of a bronchodilator, report 94060. Measurement of vital capacity (94150) is a component of spirometry and is only reported when performed alone. The flow-volume loop (94375) is used to identify patterns of inspiratory and/or expiratory obstruction in central or peripheral airways. Spirometry (94010, 94060) includes maximal breathing capacity (94200) and flow-volume loop (94375), when performed.

Measurement of lung volumes may be performed using plethysmography, helium dilution or nitrogen washout. Plethysmography (94726) is utilized to determine total lung capacity, residual volume, functional residual capacity, and airway resistance. Nitrogen washout or helium dilution (94727) may be used to measure lung volumes, distribution of ventilation and closing volume. Impulse oscillometry (94728) assesses airway resistance and may be reported in addition to gas dilution techniques. Spirometry (94010, 94060) and bronchial provocation (94070) are not included in 94726 and 94727 and may be reported separately.

Diffusing capacity (94729) is most commonly performed in conjunction with lung volumes or spirometry and is an add-on code to 94726-94728, 94010, 94060, 94070, and 94375.

Pulmonary function tests (94011-94013) are reported for measurements in infants and young children through 2 years of age.

Pulmonary function testing measurements are reported as actual values and as a percent of predicted values by age, gender, height, and race.

Chest wall manipulation for the mobilization of secretions and improvement in lung function can be performed using manual (94667, 94668) or mechanical (94669) methods. Manual techniques include cupping, percussing, and use of a hand-held vibration device. A mechanical technique is the application of an external vest or wrap that delivers mechanical oscillation.

94010 Spirometry, including graphic record, total and timed vital capacity, expiratory flow rate measurement(s), with or without maximal voluntary ventilation

➔ *CPT Assistant* Summer 91:16, Summer 95:4, Feb 96:9, Mar 96:10, Nov 97:45, Nov 98:35, Jan 99:8, Feb 99:9, Aug 03:15, Jul 05:11, Nov 08:5, Oct 10:15, Dec 10:15, Aug 12:6, 7, Nov 12:14, Dec 13:12, Mar 14:11, Sep 15:9

(Do not report 94010 in conjunction with 94150, 94200, 94375, 94728)

94011 Measurement of spirometric forced expiratory flows in an infant or child through 2 years of age

➔ *CPT Changes: An Insider's View* 2010, 2017

➔ *CPT Assistant* May 10:7, Aug 12:6, Dec 13:12

94012 Measurement of spirometric forced expiratory flows, before and after bronchodilator, in an infant or child through 2 years of age

➔ *CPT Changes: An Insider's View* 2010, 2017

➔ *CPT Assistant* May 10:7, Aug 12:6

94013 Measurement of lung volumes (ie, functional residual capacity [FRC], forced vital capacity [FVC], and expiratory reserve volume [ERV]) in an infant or child through 2 years of age

➔ *CPT Changes: An Insider's View* 2010, 2017

➔ *CPT Assistant* May 10:7, Aug 12:6, Dec 13:12

94014 Patient-initiated spirometric recording per 30-day period of time; includes reinforced education, transmission of spirometric tracing, data capture, analysis of transmitted data, periodic recalibration and review and interpretation by a physician or other qualified health care professional

➔ *CPT Changes: An Insider's View* 2000, 2013

➔ *CPT Assistant* Summer 95:4, Nov 98:34, Jan 99:8, Jul 05:11, Nov 08:5

94015 recording (includes hook-up, reinforced education, data transmission, data capture, trend analysis, and periodic recalibration)

➔ *CPT Assistant* Summer 95:4, Nov 98:34, Jan 99:8, Jul 05:11, Nov 08:5

94016 review and interpretation only by a physician or other qualified health care professional

➔ *CPT Changes: An Insider's View* 2013

➔ *CPT Assistant* Summer 95:4, Nov 98:34, Jan 99:8, Jul 05:11, Nov 08:5

94060 Bronchodilation responsiveness, spirometry as in 94010, pre- and post-bronchodilator administration

➔ *CPT Changes: An Insider's View* 2005

➔ *CPT Assistant* Summer 95:4, Feb 96:9, Feb 97:10, Nov 98:34, Jan 99:8, Feb 99:9, Jul 05:11, Nov 08:5, Dec 10:15, Aug 12:6, 7, Mar 14:11, Sep 15:9

(Do not report 94060 in conjunction with 94150, 94200, 94375, 94640, 94728)

(Report bronchodilator supply separately with 99070 or appropriate supply code)

(For exercise test for bronchospasm with pre- and post-spirometry, use 94617)

94070 Bronchospasm provocation evaluation, multiple spirometric determinations as in 94010, with administered agents (eg, antigen[s], cold air, methacholine)

➔ *CPT Changes: An Insider's View* 2005

➔ *CPT Assistant* Summer 91:16, Summer 95:4, Feb 96:9, Nov 97:45, Jan 99:8, Jul 05:11, Nov 08:5, Aug 12:6, Nov 12:11, Sep 15:9

(Do not report 94070 in conjunction with 94640)

(Report antigen[s] administration separately with 99070 or appropriate supply code)

94150 Vital capacity, total (separate procedure)

➔ *CPT Assistant* Summer 95:4, Feb 96:9, Jul 05:11, Nov 08:5, Dec 10:15, Aug 12:6, Mar 14:11

(Do not report 94150 in conjunction with 94010, 94060, 94728. To report thoracic gas volumes, see 94726, 94727)

94200 Maximum breathing capacity, maximal voluntary ventilation

➔ *CPT Assistant* Summer 95:4, Feb 96:9, Aug 03:15, Jul 05:11, Nov 08:5, Dec 10:15, Aug 12:6, 7, Mar 14:11

(Do not report 94200 in conjunction with 94010, 94060)

94250 Expired gas collection, quantitative, single procedure (separate procedure)

➔ *CPT Assistant* Summer 95:4, Feb 96:9, Jul 05:11, Nov 08:5, Dec 15:17

(Do not report 94250 in conjunction with 94621)

94375 Respiratory flow volume loop

➔ *CPT Assistant* Summer 95:4, Feb 96:9, Oct 03:2, Jul 05:11, Jul 06:4, Jul 07:1, Nov 08:5, Aug 12:6, 7, Mar 14:11

(Do not report 94375 in conjunction with 94010, 94060, 94728)

94400 Breathing response to CO2 (CO2 response curve)

➔ *CPT Assistant* Summer 95:4, Feb 96:9, Jul 05:11, Nov 08:5, Dec 10:15, Mar 14:11, Sep 15:9

(Do not report 94400 in conjunction with 94640)

94450 Breathing response to hypoxia (hypoxia response curve)

➔ *CPT Assistant* Summer 95:4, Feb 96:9, Jul 05:11, Nov 08:5

(For high altitude simulation test [HAST], see 94452, 94453)

94452 High altitude simulation test (HAST), with interpretation and report by a physician or other qualified health care professional;

➔ *CPT Changes: An Insider's View* 2005, 2013

➔ *CPT Assistant* Jul 05:11, Nov 08:5

(For obtaining arterial blood gases, use 36600)

(Do not report 94452 in conjunction with 94453, 94760, 94761)

94453 with supplemental oxygen titration

➔ *CPT Changes: An Insider's View* 2005, 2013

➔ *CPT Assistant* Jul 05:11, Nov 08:5

(For obtaining arterial blood gases, use 36600)

(Do not report 94453 in conjunction with 94452, 94760, 94761)

⊘ **94610** Intrapulmonary surfactant administration by a physician or other qualified health care professional through endotracheal tube

➔ *CPT Changes: An Insider's View* 2007, 2013

➔ *CPT Assistant* Apr 07:3, Jul 08:7, Nov 08:5, Dec 10:15

(Do not report 94610 in conjunction with 99468-99472)

(For endotracheal intubation, use 31500)

(Report 94610 once per dosing episode)

94617 Exercise test for bronchospasm, including pre- and post-spirometry, electrocardiographic recording(s), and pulse oximetry

➔ *CPT Changes: An Insider's View* 2018

➔ *CPT Assistant* Oct 17:3

94618 Pulmonary stress testing (eg, 6-minute walk test), including measurement of heart rate, oximetry, and oxygen titration, when performed

➔ *CPT Changes: An Insider's View* 2018

➔ *CPT Assistant* Oct 17:3

(94620 has been deleted. To report pulmonary stress testing, use 94618)

94621 Cardiopulmonary exercise testing, including measurements of minute ventilation, CO2 production, O2 uptake, and electrocardiographic recordings

➲ *CPT Changes: An Insider's View* 2018

➲ *CPT Assistant* Summer 95:4, Nov 98:35, Jan 99:8, Aug 02:10, Jul 05:11, Nov 08:5, Nov 12:14, Oct 17:3

(Do not report 94617, 94621 in conjunction with 93000, 93005, 93010, 93040, 93041, 93042 for ECG monitoring performed during the same session)

(Do not report 94617, 94621 in conjunction with 93015, 93016, 93017, 93018)

(Do not report 94621 in conjunction with 94250, 94680, 94681, 94690)

(Do not report 94617, 94618, 94621 in conjunction with 94760, 94761)

94640 Pressurized or nonpressurized inhalation treatment for acute airway obstruction for therapeutic purposes and/or for diagnostic purposes such as sputum induction with an aerosol generator, nebulizer, metered dose inhaler or intermittent positive pressure breathing (IPPB) device

➲ *CPT Changes: An Insider's View* 2003, 2016

➲ *CPT Assistant* Summer 95:4, Feb 96:9, May 98:10, Apr 00:11, Jul 05:11, Apr 07:3, Nov 08:5, Sep 10:3, Dec 13:12, Mar 14:11, Sep 15:9

(Do not report 94640 in conjunction with 94060, 94070, or 94400)

(For more than 1 inhalation treatment performed on the same date, append modifier 76)

(For continuous inhalation treatment of 1 hour or more, see 94644, 94645)

94642 Aerosol inhalation of pentamidine for pneumocystis carinii pneumonia treatment or prophylaxis

➲ *CPT Assistant* Summer 95:4, Feb 96:9, Jul 05:11, Nov 08:5

94644 Continuous inhalation treatment with aerosol medication for acute airway obstruction; first hour

➲ *CPT Changes: An Insider's View* 2007

➲ *CPT Assistant* Apr 07:3, Nov 08:5, Mar 14:11, Sep 15:9

(For services of less than 1 hour, use 94640)

+ 94645 each additional hour (List separately in addition to code for primary procedure)

➲ *CPT Changes: An Insider's View* 2007

➲ *CPT Assistant* Apr 07:3, Nov 08:5, Mar 14:11, Sep 15:9

(Use 94645 in conjunction with 94644)

94660 Continuous positive airway pressure ventilation (CPAP), initiation and management

➲ *CPT Assistant* Fall 92:30, Spring 95:4, Summer 95:4, Feb 96:9, Jan 99:10, Aug 00:2, Oct 03:2, Jul 05:11, Jul 06:4, Feb 07:10, Jul 07:1, Nov 08:5, May 14:4, Oct 14:9

94662 Continuous negative pressure ventilation (CNP), initiation and management

➲ *CPT Assistant* Fall 92:30, Spring 94:4, Summer 95:4, Feb 96:9, Aug 00:2, Jul 05:11, Feb 07:10, Jul 07:1, Nov 08:5, May 14:4

94664 Demonstration and/or evaluation of patient utilization of an aerosol generator, nebulizer, metered dose inhaler or IPPB device

➲ *CPT Changes: An Insider's View* 2003

➲ *CPT Assistant* Summer 95:4, Feb 96:9, May 98:10, Apr 00:11, Jul 05:11, Nov 08:5, Sep 10:3, Dec 13:12

(94664 can be reported 1 time only per day of service)

94667 Manipulation chest wall, such as cupping, percussing, and vibration to facilitate lung function; initial demonstration and/or evaluation

➲ *CPT Assistant* Summer 95:4, Feb 96:9, Jul 05:11, Nov 08:5, Sep 10:3, Dec 13:12, Mar 14:11, Sep 15:9

94668 subsequent

➲ *CPT Assistant* Summer 95:4, Feb 96:9, Jul 05:11, Sep 10:3, Dec 13:12, Mar 14:11, Sep 15:9

94669 Mechanical chest wall oscillation to facilitate lung function, per session

➲ *CPT Changes: An Insider's View* 2014

94680 Oxygen uptake, expired gas analysis; rest and exercise, direct, simple

➲ *CPT Assistant* Summer 95:4, Feb 96:9, Jul 05:11

94681 including CO2 output, percentage oxygen extracted

➲ *CPT Assistant* Summer 95:4, Feb 96:9, Jul 05:11

94690 rest, indirect (separate procedure)

➲ *CPT Assistant* Summer 95:4, Feb 96:9, Jul 05:11

(For single arterial puncture, use 36600)

(Do not report 94680, 94681, 94690 in conjunction with 94621)

94726 Plethysmography for determination of lung volumes and, when performed, airway resistance

➲ *CPT Changes: An Insider's View* 2012

➲ *CPT Assistant* Jan 12:3, Aug 12:6, May 13:11

(Do not report 94726 in conjunction with 94727, 94728)

94727 Gas dilution or washout for determination of lung volumes and, when performed, distribution of ventilation and closing volumes

➲ *CPT Changes: An Insider's View* 2012

➲ *CPT Assistant* Jan 12:3, Aug 12:6, May 13:11

(Do not report 94727 in conjunction with 94726)

94728 Airway resistance by impulse oscillometry

➲ *CPT Changes: An Insider's View* 2012

➲ *CPT Assistant* Jan 12:3, Aug 12:6, May 13:11, Mar 14:11

(Do not report 94728 in conjunction with 94010, 94060, 94070, 94375, 94726)

+ 94729 Diffusing capacity (eg, carbon monoxide, membrane) (List separately in addition to code for primary procedure)

➲ *CPT Changes: An Insider's View* 2012

➲ *CPT Assistant* Jan 12:3, Aug 12:6, Dec 13:12

(Report 94729 in conjunction with 94010, 94060, 94070, 94375, 94726-94728)

94750 Pulmonary compliance study (eg, plethysmography, volume and pressure measurements)
➲ *CPT Changes: An Insider's View* 2002
➲ *CPT Assistant* Summer 95:4, Feb 96:9, Jul 05:11

94760 Noninvasive ear or pulse oximetry for oxygen saturation; single determination
➲ *CPT Assistant* Summer 95:4, Feb 96:9, Feb 97:10, Jul 98:2, Oct 03:2, Jul 05:11, Feb 06:9, Jul 06:4, Feb 07:10, Apr 07:1, Jul 07:1, Dec 10:15, May 14:4

(For blood gases, see 82803-82810)

94761 multiple determinations (eg, during exercise)
➲ *CPT Assistant* Summer 95:4, Feb 96:9, Jul 98:2, Jun 99:10, Jul 05:11, Feb 06:9, Jul 06:4, Feb 07:10, Apr 07:1, Jun 07:11, Jul 07:1, Dec 08:5, May 14:4

(Do not report 94760, 94761 in conjunction with 94617, 94618, 94621)

94762 by continuous overnight monitoring (separate procedure)
➲ *CPT Assistant* Summer 95:4, Feb 96:9, Jul 98:2, Oct 03:2, Jul 05:11, Feb 06:9, Jul 06:4, Feb 07:10, Apr 07:1, Jul 07:1, Dec 08:5, May 14:4

(For other in vivo laboratory procedures, see 88720-88741)

94770 Carbon dioxide, expired gas determination by infrared analyzer
➲ *CPT Assistant* Summer 95:4, Feb 96:9, Jul 05:11, Mar 14:11

(For bronchoscopy, see 31622-31654)

(For placement of flow directed catheter, use 93503)

(For venipuncture, use 36410)

(For central venous catheter placement, see 36555-36556)

(For arterial puncture, use 36600)

(For arterial catheterization, use 36620)

(For thoracentesis, use 32554, 32555)

(For phlebotomy, therapeutic, use 99195)

(For lung biopsy, needle, use 32405)

(For intubation, orotracheal or nasotracheal, use 31500)

94772 Circadian respiratory pattern recording (pediatric pneumogram), 12-24 hour continuous recording, infant
➲ *CPT Assistant* Summer 95:4, Feb 96:9, Jul 05:11

(Separate procedure codes for electromyograms, EEG, ECG, and recordings of respiration are excluded when 94772 is reported)

94774 Pediatric home apnea monitoring event recording including respiratory rate, pattern and heart rate per 30-day period of time; includes monitor attachment, download of data, review, interpretation, and preparation of a report by a physician or other qualified health care professional
➲ *CPT Changes: An Insider's View* 2007, 2013
➲ *CPT Assistant* Apr 07:3, Mar 08:4

(Do not report 94774 in conjunction with 94775-94777 during the same reporting period)

94775 monitor attachment only (includes hook-up, initiation of recording and disconnection)
➲ *CPT Changes: An Insider's View* 2007
➲ *CPT Assistant* Apr 07:3, Mar 08:4

94776 monitoring, download of information, receipt of transmission(s) and analyses by computer only
➲ *CPT Changes: An Insider's View* 2007
➲ *CPT Assistant* Apr 07:3, Mar 08:4

94777 review, interpretation and preparation of report only by a physician or other qualified health care professional
➲ *CPT Changes: An Insider's View* 2007, 2013
➲ *CPT Assistant* Apr 07:3, Mar 08:4

(When oxygen saturation monitoring is used in addition to heart rate and respiratory monitoring, it is not reported separately)

(Do not report 94774-94777 in conjunction with 93224-93272)

(Do not report apnea recording device separately)

(For sleep study, see 95805-95811)

▲ **94780** Car seat/bed testing for airway integrity, for infants through 12 months of age, with continual clinical staff observation and continuous recording of pulse oximetry, heart rate and respiratory rate, with interpretation and report; 60 minutes
➲ *CPT Changes: An Insider's View* 2012, 2019
➲ *CPT Assistant* Aug 12:6, May 15:11

(Do not report 94780 for less than 60 minutes)

(Do not report 94780 in conjunction with 93040-93042, 94760, 94761, 99468-99472, 99477-99480)

+▲ **94781** each additional full 30 minutes (List separately in addition to code for primary procedure)
➲ *CPT Changes: An Insider's View* 2012, 2019
➲ *CPT Assistant* Aug 12:6, May 15:11

(Use 94781 in conjunction with 94780)

94799 Unlisted pulmonary service or procedure
➲ *CPT Assistant* Summer 95:4, Feb 96:9, Mar 96:10, Jul 05:11, Dec 10:15, Nov 12:14, Dec 13:12, May 15:11, Dec 15:17

Allergy and Clinical Immunology

Definitions

Immunotherapy (desensitization, hyposensitization): is the parenteral administration of allergenic extracts as antigens at periodic intervals, usually on an increasing dosage scale to a dosage which is maintained as maintenance therapy. Indications for immunotherapy are determined by appropriate diagnostic procedures coordinated with clinical judgment and knowledge of the natural history of allergic diseases.

Other therapy: for medical conferences on the use of mechanical and electronic devices (precipitators, air conditioners, air filters, humidifiers, dehumidifiers), climatotherapy, physical therapy, occupational and recreational therapy, see Evaluation and Management services.

Do not report Evaluation and Management (E/M) services for test interpretation and report. If a significant separately identifiable E/M service is performed, the appropriate E/M service code, which may include new or established patient office or other outpatient services (99201-99215), hospital observation services (99217-99220, 99224-99226), hospital care (99221-99223, 99231-99233), consultations (99241-99255), emergency department services (99281-99285), nursing facility services (99304-99318), domiciliary, rest home, or custodial care services (99324-99337), home services (99341-99350), or preventive medicine services (99381-99429), should be reported using modifier 25.

Allergy Testing

(For allergy laboratory tests, see 86000-86999)

(For administration of medications [eg, epinephrine, steroidal agents, antihistamines] for therapy for severe or intractable allergic reaction, use 96372)

95004 Percutaneous tests (scratch, puncture, prick) with allergenic extracts, immediate type reaction, including test interpretation and report, specify number of tests
- *CPT Changes: An Insider's View* 2007, 2008, 2013
- *CPT Assistant* Summer 91:15, May 10:3, Jan 13:9

95012 Nitric oxide expired gas determination
- *CPT Changes: An Insider's View* 2007
- *CPT Assistant* Mar 07:11, Apr 07:6, Jan 13:9, Mar 14:11

95017 Allergy testing, any combination of percutaneous (scratch, puncture, prick) and intracutaneous (intradermal), sequential and incremental, with venoms, immediate type reaction, including test interpretation and report, specify number of tests
- *CPT Changes: An Insider's View* 2013
- *CPT Assistant* Jan 13:9, Jul 15:9

95018 Allergy testing, any combination of percutaneous (scratch, puncture, prick) and intracutaneous (intradermal), sequential and incremental, with drugs or biologicals, immediate type reaction, including test interpretation and report, specify number of tests
- *CPT Changes: An Insider's View* 2013
- *CPT Assistant* Jan 13:9, Jul 15:9

95024 Intracutaneous (intradermal) tests with allergenic extracts, immediate type reaction, including test interpretation and report, specify number of tests
- *CPT Changes: An Insider's View* 2003, 2008, 2013
- *CPT Assistant* Summer 91:15, May 10:3, Jan 13:9

95027 Intracutaneous (intradermal) tests, sequential and incremental, with allergenic extracts for airborne allergens, immediate type reaction, including test interpretation and report, specify number of tests
- *CPT Changes: An Insider's View* 2003, 2008, 2013
- *CPT Assistant* Summer 91:15, Jun 97:10, Dec 07:9, May 10:3, Jan 13:9

95028 Intracutaneous (intradermal) tests with allergenic extracts, delayed type reaction, including reading, specify number of tests
- *CPT Changes: An Insider's View* 2003
- *CPT Assistant* Summer 91:14, May 10:3, Jan 13:9

95044 Patch or application test(s) (specify number of tests)
- *CPT Assistant* Summer 91:15, Spring 94:31, Jan 13:9

95052 Photo patch test(s) (specify number of tests)
- *CPT Assistant* Spring 94:31, Jan 13:9

95056 Photo tests
- *CPT Assistant* Summer 91:16, Jan 13:9

95060 Ophthalmic mucous membrane tests
- *CPT Assistant* Summer 91:16, Jan 13:9

95065 Direct nasal mucous membrane test
- *CPT Assistant* Summer 91:15, Jan 13:9

95070 Inhalation bronchial challenge testing (not including necessary pulmonary function tests); with histamine, methacholine, or similar compounds
- *CPT Assistant* Summer 91:16, Nov 12:11, Jan 13:9

95071 with antigens or gases, specify
- *CPT Assistant* Summer 91:16, Nov 12:11, Jan 13:9

(For pulmonary function tests, see 94060, 94070)

Ingestion Challenge Testing

Codes 95076 and 95079 are used to report ingestion challenge testing. Report 95076 for initial 120 minutes of testing time (ie, not physician face-to-face time). Report 95079 for each additional 60 minutes of testing time (ie, not physician face-to-face time). For total testing time less than 61 minutes (eg, positive challenge resulting in cessation of testing), report an evaluation and management service, if appropriate. Patient assessment/monitoring activities for allergic reaction (eg, blood pressure testing, peak flow meter testing) are not separately reported. Intervention therapy (eg, injection of steroid or epinephrine) may be reported separately as appropriate.

For purposes of reporting testing times, if an evaluation and management service is required, then testing time ends.

95076 Ingestion challenge test (sequential and incremental ingestion of test items, eg, food, drug or other substance); initial 120 minutes of testing
- *CPT Changes: An Insider's View* 2013
- *CPT Assistant* Jan 13:9

+ 95079 each additional 60 minutes of testing (List separately in addition to code for primary procedure)
➔ *CPT Changes: An Insider's View* 2013
➔ *CPT Assistant* Jan 13:9

(Use 95079 in conjunction with 95076)

Allergen Immunotherapy

Codes 95115-95199 include the professional services necessary for allergen immunotherapy. Office visit codes may be used in addition to allergen immunotherapy if other identifiable services are provided at that time.

95115 Professional services for allergen immunotherapy not including provision of allergenic extracts; single injection
➔ *CPT Assistant* Fall 91:19, Spring 94:30, Summer 95:4, May 96:1, Nov 98:35, Apr 00:4, Feb 05:10-12, Nov 05:1, Nov 06:23, Dec 07:9, Jan 13:9

95117 2 or more injections
➔ *CPT Assistant* Fall 91:19, Spring 94:30, Summer 95:4, May 96:1, Aug 96:10, Nov 98:35, Apr 00:4, Feb 05:10-12, Nov 05:1, Nov 06:23, Dec 07:9, Jan 13:9

95120 Professional services for allergen immunotherapy in the office or institution of the prescribing physician or other qualified health care professional, including provision of allergenic extract; single injection
➔ *CPT Changes: An Insider's View* 2013
➔ *CPT Assistant* Fall 91:19, Spring 94:30, Summer 95:4, May 96:2, Nov 98:35, Feb 05:10-12, Jan 13:9

95125 2 or more injections
➔ *CPT Changes: An Insider's View* 2013
➔ *CPT Assistant* Fall 91:19, Spring 94:30, Summer 95:4, May 96:2, Aug 96:10, Nov 98:35, Feb 05:10, 12, Jan 13:9

95130 single stinging insect venom
➔ *CPT Changes: An Insider's View* 2013
➔ *CPT Assistant* Fall 91:19, Summer 95:4, May 96:2, Jun 96:10, Nov 98:35, Sep 99:10, Feb 05:10, 12, Jan 13:9

95131 2 stinging insect venoms
➔ *CPT Changes: An Insider's View* 2013
➔ *CPT Assistant* Fall 91:19, Summer 95:4, May 96:2, Jun 96:10, Nov 98:35, Sep 99:10, Feb 05:10, 12, Jan 13:9

95132 3 stinging insect venoms
➔ *CPT Changes: An Insider's View* 2013
➔ *CPT Assistant* Fall 91:19, Summer 95:4, May 96:2, Nov 98:35, Sep 99:11, Feb 05:10, 12, Jan 13:9

95133 4 stinging insect venoms
➔ *CPT Changes: An Insider's View* 2013
➔ *CPT Assistant* Fall 91:19, Summer 95:4, May 96:2, Nov 98:35, Sep 99:11, Feb 05:10, 12, Jan 13:9

95134 5 stinging insect venoms
➔ *CPT Changes: An Insider's View* 2013
➔ *CPT Assistant* Fall 91:19, Summer 95:4, May 96:2, Nov 98:35, Sep 99:11, Feb 05:10, 12, Jan 13:9

95144 Professional services for the supervision of preparation and provision of antigens for allergen immunotherapy, single dose vial(s) (specify number of vials)
➔ *CPT Changes: An Insider's View* 2002
➔ *CPT Assistant* Fall 91:19, Spring 94:30, Summer 95:4, May 96:11, Nov 98:35, Feb 05:10-11, Jan 13:9

(A single dose vial contains a single dose of antigen administered in 1 injection)

95145 Professional services for the supervision of preparation and provision of antigens for allergen immunotherapy (specify number of doses); single stinging insect venom
➔ *CPT Changes: An Insider's View* 2002
➔ *CPT Assistant* Fall 91:19, Summer 95:4, May 96:11, Nov 98:35, Feb 05:10-12, Jan 13:9

95146 2 single stinging insect venoms
➔ *CPT Assistant* Fall 91:19, Summer 95:4, May 96:11, Nov 98:35, Feb 05:10-12, Jan 13:9

95147 3 single stinging insect venoms
➔ *CPT Assistant* Fall 91:19, Summer 95:4, May 96:11, Nov 98:35, Feb 05:10-12, Jan 13:9

95148 4 single stinging insect venoms
➔ *CPT Assistant* Fall 91:19, Summer 95:4, May 96:11, Nov 98:35, Feb 05:10-12, Jan 13:9

95149 5 single stinging insect venoms
➔ *CPT Assistant* Fall 91:19, Summer 95:4, May 96:11, Nov 98:35, Feb 05:10-12, Jan 13:9

95165 Professional services for the supervision of preparation and provision of antigens for allergen immunotherapy; single or multiple antigens (specify number of doses)
➔ *CPT Changes: An Insider's View* 2002
➔ *CPT Assistant* Fall 91:19, Spring 94:30, Summer 95:4, May 96:11, Nov 98:35, Apr 00:4, Apr 01:11, Feb 05:10-12, Jun 05:9, Jan 13:9

95170 whole body extract of biting insect or other arthropod (specify number of doses)
➔ *CPT Assistant* Fall 91:19, Spring 94:30, Summer 95:4, May 96:12, Apr 01:11, Feb 05:10-12, Jun 05:9, Jan 13:9

(For allergy immunotherapy reporting, a dose is the amount of antigen[s] administered in a single injection from a multiple dose vial)

95180 Rapid desensitization procedure, each hour (eg, insulin, penicillin, equine serum)
➔ *CPT Changes: An Insider's View* 2002
➔ *CPT Assistant* Summer 95:4, Jan 13:9

95199 Unlisted allergy/clinical immunologic service or procedure
➔ *CPT Assistant* Summer 95:4, Nov 98:35, Jan 13:9

(For skin testing of bacterial, viral, fungal extracts, see 86485-86580, 95028)

(For special reports on allergy patients, use 99080)

(For testing procedures such as radioallergosorbent testing [RAST], rat mast cell technique [RMCT], mast cell degranulation test [MCDT], lymphocytic transformation test [LTT], leukocyte histamine release [LHR], migration inhibitory factor test [MIF], transfer factor test [TFT], nitroblue tetrazolium dye test [NTD], see Immunology section in **Pathology** or use 95199)

Endocrinology

Codes 95249 and 95250 are used to report the service for subcutaneous interstitial sensor placement, hook-up of the sensor to the transmitter, calibration of continuous glucose monitoring (CGM) device, patient training on CGM device functions and management, removal of the interstitial sensor, and the print-out of captured data recordings. For the CGM device owned by the physician's or other qualified health care professional's office, use 95250 for the data capture occurring over a **minimum** period of 72 hours.

Code 95249 may be reported only once during the time that a patient owns a given data receiver, including the initial episode of data collection.

Code 95249 may not be reported for subsequent episodes of data collection, unless the patient obtains a new and/or different model of data receiver. Obtaining a new sensor and/or transmitter without a change in receiver may not be reported with 95249.

Code 95249 may not be reported unless the patient brings the data receiver to the physician's or other qualified health care professional's office with the entire initial data collection procedure conducted in the physician's or other qualified health care professional's office.

95249 Code is out of numerical sequence. See 95199-95803

95250 Ambulatory continuous glucose monitoring of interstitial tissue fluid via a subcutaneous sensor for a minimum of 72 hours; physician or other qualified health care professional (office) provided equipment, sensor placement, hook-up, calibration of monitor, patient training, removal of sensor, and printout of recording

➲ *CPT Changes: An Insider's View* 2002, 2006, 2009, 2016, 2018

➲ *CPT Assistant* Mar 18:5

(Do not report 95250 more than once per month)

(Do not report 95250 in conjunction with 99091, 0446T)

 # 95249 patient-provided equipment, sensor placement, hook-up, calibration of monitor, patient training, and printout of recording

➲ *CPT Changes: An Insider's View* 2018

(Do not report 95249 more than once for the duration that the patient owns the data receiver)

(Do not report 95249 in conjunction with 99091, 0446T)

95251 analysis, interpretation and report

➲ *CPT Changes: An Insider's View* 2006, 2009, 2016, 2018

➲ *CPT Assistant* Mar 18:5

(Do not report 95251 more than once per month)

(Do not report 95251 in conjunction with 99091)

Neurology and Neuromuscular Procedures

Neurologic services are typically consultative, and any of the levels of consultation (99241-99255) may be appropriate.

In addition, services and skills outlined under **Evaluation and Management** levels of service appropriate to neurologic illnesses should be reported similarly.

The EEG, autonomic function, evoked potential, reflex tests, EMG, NCV, and MEG services (95812-95829 and 95860-95967) include recording, interpretation, and report by a physician or other qualified health care professional. For interpretation only, use modifier 26. For EMG guidance, see 95873, 95874.

Codes 95812-95822, 95950-95953 and 95956 use recording time as a basis for code use. Recording time is when the recording is underway and data is being collected. Recording time excludes set up and take down time. Codes 95961-95962 use physician or other qualified health care professional attendance time as a basis for code use.

(Do not report codes 95860-95875 in addition to 96000-96004)

Sleep Medicine Testing

Sleep medicine services include procedures that evaluate adult and pediatric patients for a variety of sleep disorders. Sleep medicine testing services are diagnostic procedures using in-laboratory and portable technology to assess physiologic data and therapy.

All sleep services (95800-95811) include recording, interpretation, and report. (Report with modifier 52 if less than 6 hours of recording for 95800, 95801 and 95806, 95807, 95810, 95811; if less than 7 hours of recording for 95782, 95783, or if less than four nap opportunities are recorded for 95805).

Definitions

For purposes of CPT reporting of sleep medicine testing services, the following definitions apply:

Actigraphy: the use of a portable, non-invasive, device that continuously records gross motor movement over an extended period of time. The periods of activity and rest are indirect parameters for estimates of the periods of wakefulness and sleep of an individual.

Attended: a technologist or qualified health care professional is physically present (ie, sufficient proximity such that the qualified health care professional can physically respond to emergencies, to other appropriate patient needs or to technical problems at the bedside) throughout the recording session.

Electrooculogram (EOG): a recording of electrical activity indicative of eye movement.

Maintenance of wakefulness test (MWT): a standardized objective test used to determine a person's ability to stay awake. MWT requires sleep staging of the trials that are performed at defined intervals and is attended by a qualified health care professional.

Multiple sleep latency test (MSLT): a standardized objective test of the tendency to fall asleep. MSLT requires sleep staging of the nap opportunities that are performed at defined intervals and is attended by a technologist or qualified health care professional.

Peripheral arterial tonometry (PAT): a plethysmography technique that continuously measures pulsatile volume changes in a digit. This reflects the relative change of blood volume as an indirect measure of sympathetic nervous system activity which is used in respiratory analysis.

Physiological measurements of sleep as used in 95805: the parameters measured are a frontal, central and occipital lead of EEG (3 leads), submental EMG lead and a left and right EOG. These parameters are used together for staging sleep.

Polysomnography: a sleep test involving the continuous, simultaneous, recording of physiological parameters for a period of at least 6 hours that is performed in a sleep laboratory and attended by a technologist or qualified health care professional. The parameters measured are a frontal, central and occipital lead of EEG (3 leads), submental EMG lead and a left and right EOG, (from which sleep is staged), plus four or more additional parameters. The additional parameters typically required in polysomnography are listed below:

a. Electrocardiogram (ECG)

b. Nasal and/or oral airflow

c. Respiratory effort

d. Oxyhemoglobin saturation, SpO2

e. Bilateral anterior tibialis EMG

Positive airway pressure (PAP): a device used to treat sleep-related breathing disorders with the use of non-invasive delivery of positive pressure to the airway. Examples include but are not limited to: CPAP (continuous positive airway pressure), bilevel PAP, AutoPAP (autotitrating or adjusting PAP), ASV (adaptive-servo ventilation).

Remote: the site of service is distant from the monitoring center. Neither a technologist nor a qualified health care professional is physically present at the testing site.

Respiratory airflow (ventilation): the movement of air during inhaled and exhaled breaths. This is typically assessed using thermistor and nasal pressure sensors.

Respiratory analysis: generation of derived parameters that describe components of respiration obtained by using direct or indirect parameters, eg, by airflow or peripheral arterial tone.

Respiratory effort: contraction of the diaphragmatic and/or intercostal muscles to cause (or attempt to cause) respiratory airflow. This is typically measured using transducers that estimate motion of the thorax and abdomen such as respiratory inductive plethysmography, transducers that estimate pressures generated by breathing muscles such as esophageal manometry, or by contraction of breathing muscles, such as diaphragmatic/intercostal EMG.

Respiratory (thoracoabdominal) movement: movement of the chest and abdomen during respiratory effort.

Sleep latency: the length of time it takes to transition from wakefulness to sleep. In the sleep laboratory it is the time from "lights out" to the first epoch scored as any stage of sleep.

Sleep staging: the delineation of the distinct sleep levels through the simultaneous evaluation of physiologic measures including a frontal, central and occipital lead of EEG (3 leads), submental EMG lead and a left and right EOG.

Sleep testing (or sleep study): the continuous, simultaneous monitoring of physiological parameters during sleep (eg, polysomnography, EEG).

Total sleep time: a derived parameter obtained by sleep staging or may be estimated indirectly using actigraphy or other methods.

Unattended: a technologist or qualified health care professional is not physically present with the patient during the recording session.

(Report with modifier 52 if less than 6 hours of recording or in other cases of reduced services as appropriate)

(For unattended sleep study, use 95806)

95782 Code is out of numerical sequence. See 95805-95813

95783 Code is out of numerical sequence. See 95805-95813

95800 Code is out of numerical sequence. See 95805-95813

95801 Code is out of numerical sequence. See 95805-95813

95803 Actigraphy testing, recording, analysis, interpretation, and report (minimum of 72 hours to 14 consecutive days of recording)

➲ *CPT Changes: An Insider's View* 2009

➲ *CPT Assistant* Nov 11:3

(Do not report 95803 more than once in any 14 day period)

(Do not report 95803 in conjunction with 95806-95811)

95805 Multiple sleep latency or maintenance of wakefulness testing, recording, analysis and interpretation of physiological measurements of sleep during multiple trials to assess sleepiness

➲ *CPT Assistant* Nov 97:45-46, Nov 98:35, Dec 01:3, Sep 02:2-3, Mar 08:4, Nov 11:3

95806 Sleep study, unattended, simultaneous recording of, heart rate, oxygen saturation, respiratory airflow, and respiratory effort (eg, thoracoabdominal movement)

➲ *CPT Changes: An Insider's View* 2010

➲ *CPT Assistant* Nov 97:45-46, Aug 98:10, Nov 98:35, Jan 11:7, Nov 11:3, Feb 13:14, Jul 13:11

(Do not report 95806 in conjunction with 93041-93227, 93228, 93229, 93268-93272, 95800, 95801)

(For unattended sleep study that measures heart rate, oxygen saturation, respiratory analysis, and sleep time, use 95800)

(For unattended sleep study that measures a minimum heart rate, oxygen saturation, and respiratory analysis, use 95801)

 # 95800 Sleep study, unattended, simultaneous recording; heart rate, oxygen saturation, respiratory analysis (eg, by airflow or peripheral arterial tone), and sleep time

➲ *CPT Changes: An Insider's View* 2011

➲ *CPT Assistant* Jan 11:6, Nov 11:3, Feb 13:14

(Do not report 95800 in conjunction with 93041-93227, 93228, 93229, 93268-93272, 95801, 95803, 95806)

(For unattended sleep study that measures a minimum of heart rate, oxygen saturation, and respiratory analysis, use 95801)

 # 95801 minimum of heart rate, oxygen saturation, and respiratory analysis (eg, by airflow or peripheral arterial tone)

➲ *CPT Changes: An Insider's View* 2011

➲ *CPT Assistant* Jan 11:7, Nov 11:3, Feb 13:14

(Do not report 95801 in conjunction with 93041-93227, 93228, 93229, 93268-93272, 95800, 95806)

(For unattended sleep study that measures heart rate, oxygen saturation, respiratory analysis and sleep time, use 95800)

95807 Sleep study, simultaneous recording of ventilation, respiratory effort, ECG or heart rate, and oxygen saturation, attended by a technologist

➲ *CPT Assistant* Nov 97:46, Nov 98:35, Mar 08:4, Nov 11:3, Feb 13:14

95808 Polysomnography; any age, sleep staging with 1-3 additional parameters of sleep, attended by a technologist

➲ *CPT Changes: An Insider's View* 2013

➲ *CPT Assistant* Sep 96:11, Nov 97:46, Feb 98:6, Nov 98:35, Sep 02:2-3, Mar 08:4, Nov 11:3, Feb 13:14

95810 age 6 years or older, sleep staging with 4 or more additional parameters of sleep, attended by a technologist

➲ *CPT Changes: An Insider's View* 2013

➲ *CPT Assistant* Feb 98:6, Nov 98:35, Sep 02:2-3, Nov 11:3, Feb 13:14

95811 age 6 years or older, sleep staging with 4 or more additional parameters of sleep, with initiation of continuous positive airway pressure therapy or bilevel ventilation, attended by a technologist

➲ *CPT Changes: An Insider's View* 2013

➲ *CPT Assistant* Nov 97:46, Feb 98:6, Nov 98:35, Sep 02:2-3, Mar 08:4, Nov 11:3, Feb 13:14, Oct 14:9

 # 95782 younger than 6 years, sleep staging with 4 or more additional parameters of sleep, attended by a technologist

➲ *CPT Changes: An Insider's View* 2013

➲ *CPT Assistant* Feb 13:14

 # 95783 younger than 6 years, sleep staging with 4 or more additional parameters of sleep, with initiation of continuous positive airway pressure therapy or bi-level ventilation, attended by a technologist

➲ *CPT Changes: An Insider's View* 2013

➲ *CPT Assistant* Feb 13:14, Oct 14:9

Routine Electroencephalography (EEG)

EEG codes 95812-95822 include hyperventilation and/or photic stimulation when appropriate. Routine EEG codes 95816-95822 include 20 to 40 minutes of recording. Extended EEG codes 95812-95813 include reporting times longer than 40 minutes.

95812 Electroencephalogram (EEG) extended monitoring; 41-60 minutes

➲ *CPT Changes: An Insider's View* 2003

➲ *CPT Assistant* Winter 94:18, Nov 98:35, May 11:3, 10

95813 greater than 1 hour

➲ *CPT Assistant* Winter 94:18, Nov 98:35, May 11:3, 10

95816 Electroencephalogram (EEG); including recording awake and drowsy

➲ *CPT Changes: An Insider's View* 2000, 2003

➲ *CPT Assistant* Sep 96:11, Nov 98:35, Nov 99:51, Jul 00:1, May 11:3, Dec 15:17

95819 including recording awake and asleep

➲ *CPT Changes: An Insider's View* 2000, 2003

➲ *CPT Assistant* Nov 98:35, Nov 99:51, Jul 00:1, May 11:3, Dec 15:17

95822 recording in coma or sleep only

➲ *CPT Changes: An Insider's View* 2003

➲ *CPT Assistant* Nov 98:35, May 11:3, May 13:8, Dec 14:19

95824 cerebral death evaluation only

➲ *CPT Assistant* Nov 98:35

95827 all night recording

➲ *CPT Changes: An Insider's View* 2003

➲ *CPT Assistant* Nov 98:35

(For 24-hour EEG monitoring, see 95950-95953 or 95956)

(For EEG during nonintracranial surgery, use 95955)

(For Wada test, use 95958)

(For digital analysis of EEG, use 95957)

95829 Code is out of numerical sequence. See 95827-95832

95830 Insertion by physician or other qualified health care professional of sphenoidal electrodes for electroencephalographic (EEG) recording

➔ *CPT Changes: An Insider's View* 2013

►Electrocorticography◄

►Electrocorticography (ECoG) is the recording of EEG from electrodes directly on or in the brain.

Code 95829 describes intraoperative recordings of ECoG from electrode arrays implanted in or placed directly on the brain exposed during surgery. Code 95829 includes review and interpretation during surgery.

Code 95836 describes recording of ECoG from electrodes chronically implanted on or in the brain. Chronically implanted electrodes allow for intracranial recordings to continue after the patient has been discharged from the hospital. Code 95836 includes unattended ECoG recording with storage for later review and interpretation during a single 30-day period. Code 95836 may be reported only once for each 30-day period. The dates encompassed by the 30-day period must be documented in the report.

For report of programming for a brain neurostimulator pulse generator/transmitter during the ECoG (95836) 30-day period, see 95983, 95984.◄

 # 95829 Electrocorticogram at surgery (separate procedure)

➔ *CPT Assistant* Nov 98:35

#● 95836 Electrocorticogram from an implanted brain neurostimulator pulse generator/transmitter, including recording, with interpretation and written report, up to 30 days

➔ *CPT Changes: An Insider's View* 2019

►(Report 95836 only once per 30 days)◄

►(Do not report 95836 in conjunction with 95957)◄

►(For programming a brain neurostimulator pulse generator/transmitter when performed in conjunction with ECoG [95836], see 95983, 95984)◄

Muscle and Range of Motion Testing

95831 Muscle testing, manual (separate procedure) with report; extremity (excluding hand) or trunk

➔ *CPT Changes: An Insider's View* 2000

➔ *CPT Assistant* Nov 99:51, Dec 99:10, Mar 00:11, Jul 00:2, Nov 01:5, Apr 03:28, Dec 03:7, Feb 04:5, May 08:9, Aug 13:7, Dec 16:16

95832 hand, with or without comparison with normal side

➔ *CPT Assistant* Nov 99:51, Dec 99:10, Mar 00:11, Jul 00:2, Nov 01:5, Apr 03:28, Dec 03:7, Feb 04:5, May 08:9, Aug 13:7, Dec 16:16

95833 total evaluation of body, excluding hands

➔ *CPT Assistant* Nov 99:51, Dec 99:10, Jul 00:2, Nov 01:5, Jul 02:2, Apr 03:28, Dec 03:7, Feb 04:5, May 08:9, Sep 12:16, Aug 13:7, Dec 16:16

95834 total evaluation of body, including hands

➔ *CPT Assistant* Nov 99:51, Dec 99:10, Jul 00:2, Nov 01:5, Apr 03:28, Dec 03:7, Feb 04:5, May 08:9, Aug 13:7

95836 Code is out of numerical sequence. See 95827-95832

95851 Range of motion measurements and report (separate procedure); each extremity (excluding hand) or each trunk section (spine)

➔ *CPT Assistant* Sep 99:10, Nov 01:5, Apr 03:28, Dec 03:7, Feb 04:5, Dec 07:16, May 08:9, Aug 13:7, Dec 16:16

95852 hand, with or without comparison with normal side

➔ *CPT Assistant* Nov 01:5, Apr 03:28, Dec 03:7, May 08:9, Aug 13:7

95857 Cholinesterase inhibitor challenge test for myasthenia gravis

➔ *CPT Changes: An Insider's View* 2011

➔ *CPT Assistant* Feb 11:3

Electromyography

Needle electromyographic (EMG) procedures include the interpretation of electrical waveforms measured by equipment that produces both visible and audible components of electrical signals recorded from the muscle(s) studied by the needle electrode.

Use 95870 or 95885 when four or fewer muscles are tested in an extremity. Use 95860-95864 or 95886 when five or more muscles are tested in an extremity.

Use EMG codes (95860-95864 and 95867-95870) when no nerve conduction studies (95907-95913) are performed on that day. Use 95885, 95886, and 95887 for EMG services when nerve conduction studies (95907-95913) are performed in conjunction with EMG on the same day.

Report either 95885 or 95886 once per extremity. Codes 95885 and 95886 can be reported together up to a combined total of four units of service per patient when all four extremities are tested.

Report 95887 once per anatomic site (ie, cervical paraspinal muscle[s], thoracic paraspinal muscle[s], lumbar paraspinal muscle[s], chest wall muscle[s], and abdominal wall muscle[s]). Use 95887 for a unilateral study of the cranial nerve innervated muscles (excluding extra-ocular and larynx); when performed bilaterally, 95887 may be reported twice.

Use 95887 when a study of the cervical paraspinal muscle(s), or the lumbar paraspinal muscle(s) is performed with no corresponding limb study (95885 or 95886) on the same day.

(For needle electromyography of anal or urethral sphincter, use 51785)

(For non-needle electromyography of anal or urethral sphincter, use 51784)

(For needle electromyography of larynx, use 95865)

(For needle electromyography of hemidiaphragm, use 95866)

(For needle electromyography of extra-ocular muscles, use 92265)

95860 Needle electromyography; 1 extremity with or without related paraspinal areas

➔ *CPT Changes: An Insider's View* 2003

➔ *CPT Assistant* Nov 97:46, Jul 00:2, Apr 02:2, May 03:20, Jun 03:3, Feb 04:4, Jul 04:6, Oct 04:15, Jun 06:8, Sep 06:5, Aug 08:12, Jan 09:8, Oct 10:15, Dec 10:15, Feb 12:8, Mar 13:3, May 13:8, Mar 15:6

95861 2 extremities with or without related paraspinal areas

➔ *CPT Changes: An Insider's View* 2003

➔ *CPT Assistant* Nov 97:46, Jul 00:2, Apr 02:2, May 03:20, Jun 03:3, Feb 04:4, Jul 04:6, Oct 04:15, Jun 05:9, Jun 06:8, Sep 06:5, Aug 08:12, Jan 09:8, Oct 10:15, Dec 10:15, Feb 12:8, Mar 13:3, May 13:8

(For dynamic electromyography performed during motion analysis studies, see 96002-96003)

95863 3 extremities with or without related paraspinal areas

➔ *CPT Changes: An Insider's View* 2003

➔ *CPT Assistant* Nov 97:46, Jul 00:2, Apr 02:2, May 03:20, Jun 03:3, Feb 04:4, Jul 04:6, Oct 04:15, Jun 06:8, Sep 06:5, Oct 10:15, Dec 10:15, Feb 12:8, Mar 13:3, May 13:8

95864 4 extremities with or without related paraspinal areas

➔ *CPT Changes: An Insider's View* 2003

➔ *CPT Assistant* Nov 97:46, Jul 00:2, Jan 02:11, Apr 02:2, May 03:20, Jun 03:3, Feb 04:4, Jul 04:6, Oct 04:15, Jun 06:8, Sep 06:5, Aug 08:12, Jan 09:8, Oct 10:15, Dec 10:15, Feb 12:8, Mar 13:3, May 13:8

95865 larynx

➔ *CPT Changes: An Insider's View* 2006

➔ *CPT Assistant* Sep 06:5, Dec 07:16, Jan 09:8, May 13:8, Jan 14:6

(Do not report modifier 50 in conjunction with 95865)

(For unilateral procedure, report modifier 52 in conjunction with 95865)

95866 hemidiaphragm

➔ *CPT Changes: An Insider's View* 2006

➔ *CPT Assistant* May 13:8

95867 cranial nerve supplied muscle(s), unilateral

➔ *CPT Changes: An Insider's View* 2003

➔ *CPT Assistant* Apr 02:2, May 03:20, Jun 03:3, Jun 06:8, Sep 06:5, Dec 07:16, Aug 08:12, Jan 09:8, Feb 12:8, Mar 13:3, May 13:8

95868 cranial nerve supplied muscles, bilateral

➔ *CPT Changes: An Insider's View* 2003

➔ *CPT Assistant* Apr 02:2, May 03:20, Jun 03:3, Jun 06:8, Sep 06:5, Dec 07:16, Jan 09:8, Feb 12:8, Mar 13:3, May 13:8

95869 thoracic paraspinal muscles (excluding T1 or T12)

➔ *CPT Changes: An Insider's View* 2003

➔ *CPT Assistant* Nov 97:46, Apr 02:2, May 03:20, Jun 03:3, Feb 04:4, Jun 06:8, Sep 06:5, Jan 09:8, May 10:9, Feb 12:8, Mar 13:3, May 13:8

95870 limited study of muscles in 1 extremity or non-limb (axial) muscles (unilateral or bilateral), other than thoracic paraspinal, cranial nerve supplied muscles, or sphincters

➔ *CPT Changes: An Insider's View* 2000

➔ *CPT Assistant* Nov 97:46, Nov 99:51, Jul 00:2, Apr 02:2, May 03:20, Jun 03:3, Feb 04:4, Jul 04:6, Jun 05:9, Jun 06:8, Sep 06:5, Jan 09:8, Feb 12:8, Mar 13:3, May 13:8

(To report a complete study of the extremities, see 95860-95864)

(For anal or urethral sphincter, detrusor, urethra, perineum musculature, see 51785-51792)

(For eye muscles, use 92265)

95872 Needle electromyography using single fiber electrode, with quantitative measurement of jitter, blocking and/or fiber density, any/all sites of each muscle studied

➔ *CPT Assistant* Apr 02:2, May 03:20, Jun 03:3, Sep 06:5, Jan 09:8

#+ 95885 Needle electromyography, each extremity, with related paraspinal areas, when performed, done with nerve conduction, amplitude and latency/velocity study; limited (List separately in addition to code for primary procedure)

➔ *CPT Changes: An Insider's View* 2012

➔ *CPT Assistant* Feb 12:8, Mar 13:3, May 13:8, Sep 13:18, Mar 15:6, Jul 17:10

#+ 95886 complete, five or more muscles studied, innervated by three or more nerves or four or more spinal levels (List separately in addition to code for primary procedure)

➔ *CPT Changes: An Insider's View* 2012

➔ *CPT Assistant* Feb 12:8, Mar 13:3, May 13:8, Sep 13:18, Mar 15:6, Jul 17:10

(Use 95885, 95886 in conjunction with 95907-95913)

(Do not report 95885, 95886 in conjunction with 95860-95864, 95870, 95905)

#+ 95887 Needle electromyography, non-extremity (cranial nerve supplied or axial) muscle(s) done with nerve conduction, amplitude and latency/velocity study (List separately in addition to code for primary procedure)

➔ *CPT Changes: An Insider's View* 2012

➔ *CPT Assistant* Feb 12:8, Jul 12:12, Mar 13:3, Jan 14:8, Mar 15:6, Jul 17:11

(Use 95887 in conjunction with 95907-95913)

(Do not report 95887 in conjunction with 95867-95870, 95905)

Ischemic Muscle Testing and Guidance for Chemodenervation

+ 95873 Electrical stimulation for guidance in conjunction with chemodenervation (List separately in addition to code for primary procedure)

➲ *CPT Changes: An Insider's View* 2006

➲ *CPT Assistant* Apr 13:5, Jan 14:6

(Do not report 95873 in conjunction with 64617, 95860-95870, 95874)

+ 95874 Needle electromyography for guidance in conjunction with chemodenervation (List separately in addition to code for primary procedure)

➲ *CPT Changes: An Insider's View* 2006

➲ *CPT Assistant* Apr 13:5, Jan 14:6, Oct 14:15

(Use 95873, 95874 in conjunction with 64612, 64615, 64616, 64642, 64643, 64644, 64645, 64646, 64647)

(Do not report more than one guidance code for each corresponding chemodenervation code)

(Do not report 95874 in conjunction with 64617, 95860-95870, 95873)

95875 Ischemic limb exercise test with serial specimen(s) acquisition for muscle(s) metabolite(s)

➲ *CPT Changes: An Insider's View* 2002, 2003

➲ *CPT Assistant* Jun 03:3

(For listing of nerves considered for separate study, see **Appendix J**)

95885 Code is out of numerical sequence. See 95870-95874

95886 Code is out of numerical sequence. See 95870-95874

95887 Code is out of numerical sequence. See 95870-95874

Nerve Conduction Tests

The following applies to nerve conduction tests (95907-95913): Codes 95907-95913 describe nerve conduction tests when performed with individually placed stimulating, recording, and ground electrodes. The stimulating, recording, and ground electrode placement and the test design must be individualized to the patient's unique anatomy. Nerves tested must be limited to the specific nerves and conduction studies needed for the particular clinical question being investigated. The stimulating electrode must be placed directly over the nerve to be tested, and stimulation parameters properly adjusted to avoid stimulating other nerves or nerve branches. In most motor nerve conduction studies, and in some sensory and mixed nerve conduction studies, both proximal and distal stimulation will be used. Motor nerve conduction study recordings must be made from electrodes placed directly over the motor point of the specific muscle to be tested. Sensory nerve conduction study recordings must be made from electrodes placed directly over the specific nerve to be tested. Waveforms must be reviewed on site in real time, and the technique (stimulus site, recording site, ground site, filter settings) must be adjusted, as appropriate, as the test proceeds in order to minimize artifact, and to minimize the chances of unintended stimulation of adjacent nerves and the unintended recording from adjacent muscles or nerves. Reports must be prepared on site by the examiner, and consist of the work product of the interpretation of numerous test results, using well-established techniques to assess the amplitude, latency, and configuration of waveforms elicited by stimulation at each site of each nerve tested. This includes the calculation of nerve conduction velocities, sometimes including specialized F-wave indices, along with comparison to normal values, summarization of clinical and electrodiagnostic data, and physician or other qualified health care professional interpretation. Codes 95907-95913 describe one or more nerve conduction studies. For the purposes of coding, a single conduction study is defined as a sensory conduction test, a motor conduction test with or without an F wave test, or an H-reflex test. Each type of study (sensory, motor with or without F wave, H-reflex) for each nerve includes all orthodromic and antidromic impulses associated with that nerve and constitutes a distinct study when determining the number of studies in each grouping (eg, 1-2 or 3-4 nerve conduction studies). Each type of nerve conduction study is counted only once when multiple sites on the same nerve are stimulated or recorded. The numbers of these separate tests should be added to determine which code to use. For a list of nerves, see Appendix J. Use 95885-95887 in conjunction with 95907-95913 when performing electromyography with nerve conduction studies.

Code 95905 describes nerve conduction tests when performed with preconfigured electrodes customized to a specific anatomic site.

⊘ 95905 Motor and/or sensory nerve conduction, using preconfigured electrode array(s), amplitude and latency/velocity study, each limb, includes F-wave study when performed, with interpretation and report;

➲ *CPT Changes: An Insider's View* 2010

➲ *CPT Assistant* Mar 13:3

(Report 95905 only once per limb studied)

(Do not report 95905 in conjunction with 95885, 95886, 95907-95913)

95907 Nerve conduction studies; 1-2 studies

➲ *CPT Changes: An Insider's View* 2013

➲ *CPT Assistant* Mar 13:3, May 13:8, Sep 13:18, Dec 17:15

95908 3-4 studies

➲ *CPT Changes: An Insider's View* 2013

➲ *CPT Assistant* Mar 13:3, May 13:8, Sep 13:18, Mar 15:6

95909 5-6 studies
➲ *CPT Changes: An Insider's View* 2013
➲ *CPT Assistant* Mar 13:3, May 13:8, Sep 13:18

95910 7-8 studies
➲ *CPT Changes: An Insider's View* 2013
➲ *CPT Assistant* Mar 13:3, May 13:8, Sep 13:18

95911 9-10 studies
➲ *CPT Changes: An Insider's View* 2013
➲ *CPT Assistant* Mar 13:3, May 13:8, Sep 13:18

95912 11-12 studies
➲ *CPT Changes: An Insider's View* 2013
➲ *CPT Assistant* Mar 13:3, May 13:8, Sep 13:18

95913 13 or more studies
➲ *CPT Changes: An Insider's View* 2013
➲ *CPT Assistant* Mar 13:3, May 13:8, Sep 13:18

Intraoperative Neurophysiology

Codes 95940, 95941 describe ongoing neurophysiologic monitoring, testing, and data interpretation distinct from performance of specific type(s) of baseline neurophysiologic study(s) performed during surgical procedures. When the service is performed by the surgeon or anesthesiologist, the professional services are included in the surgeon's or anesthesiologist's primary service code(s) for the procedure and are not reported separately. Do not report these codes for automated monitoring devices that do not require continuous attendance by a professional qualified to interpret the testing and monitoring.

Recording and testing are performed either personally or by a technologist who is physically present with the patient during the service. Supervision is performed either in the operating room or by real time connection outside the operating room. The monitoring professional must be solely dedicated to performing the intraoperative neurophysiologic monitoring and must be available to intervene at all times during the service as necessary, for the reported time period(s). For any given period of time spent providing these services, the service takes full attention and, therefore, other clinical activities beyond providing and interpreting of monitoring cannot be provided during the same period of time.

Throughout the monitoring, there must be provisions for continuous and immediate communication directly with the operating room team in the surgical suite. One or more simultaneous cases may be reported (95941). When monitoring more than one procedure, there must be the immediate ability to transfer patient monitoring to another monitoring professional during the surgical procedure should that individual's exclusive attention be required for another procedure. Report 95941 for all remote or non-one-on-one monitoring time connected to each case regardless of overlap with other cases.

Codes 95940, 95941 include only the ongoing neurophysiologic monitoring time distinct from performance of specific type(s) of baseline neurophysiologic study(s), or other services such as intraoperative functional cortical or subcortical mapping. Codes 95940 and 95941 are reported based upon the time spent monitoring only, and not the number of baseline tests performed or parameters monitored. The time spent performing or interpreting the baseline neurophysiologic study(ies) should not be counted as intraoperative monitoring, but represents separately reportable procedures. When reporting 95940 and 95941, the same neurophysiologic study(ies) performed at baseline should be reported not more than once per operative session. Baseline study reporting is based upon the total unique studies performed. For example, if during the course of baseline testing and one-on-one monitoring, two separate nerves have motor testing performed in conjunction with limited single extremity EMG, then 95885 and 95907 would be reported in addition to 95940. Time spent monitoring (95940, 95941) excludes time to set up, record, and interpret the baseline studies, and to remove electrodes at the end of the procedure. To report time spent waiting on standby for a case to start, use 99360. For procedures that last beyond midnight, report services using the day on which the monitoring began and using the total time monitored.

Code 95940 is reported per 15 minutes of service. Code 95940 requires reporting only the portion of time the monitoring professional was physically present in the operating room providing one-on-one patient monitoring, and no other cases may be monitored at the same time. Time spent in the operating room is cumulative. To determine units of service of 95940, use the total minutes monitoring in the operating room one-on-one. Monitoring may begin prior to incision (eg, when positioning on the table is a time of risk). Report continuous intraoperative neurophysiologic monitoring in the operating room (95940) in addition to the services related to monitoring from outside the operating room (95941).

Code 95941 should be used once per hour even if multiple methods of neurophysiologic monitoring are used during the time. Code 95941 requires the monitoring of neurophysiological data that is collected from the operating room continuously on-line in real time via a secure data link. When reporting 95941, real-time ability must be available through sufficient data bandwidth transfer rates to view and interrogate the neurophysiologic data contemporaneously.

Report 95941 for all cases in which there was no physical presence by the monitoring professional in the operating room during the monitoring time or when monitoring more than one case in an operating room. It is also used to report the time of monitoring physically performed outside of the operating room in those cases where monitoring occurred both within and outside the operating room. Do not report 95941 if the monitoring lasts 30 minutes or less.

Intraoperative neurophysiology monitoring codes 95940 and 95941 are each used to report the total duration of respective time spent providing each service, even if that time is not in a single continuous block.

#+ 95940 Continuous intraoperative neurophysiology monitoring in the operating room, one on one monitoring requiring personal attendance, each 15 minutes (List separately in addition to code for primary procedure)

➲ *CPT Changes: An Insider's View* 2013

➲ *CPT Assistant* May 13:8, 9, 10, Apr 14:5, 11, Aug 17:8

(Use 95940 in conjunction with the study performed, 92585, 95822, 95860-95870, 95907-95913, 95925, 95926, 95927, 95928, 95929, 95930-95937, 95938, 95939)

#+ 95941 Continuous intraoperative neurophysiology monitoring, from outside the operating room (remote or nearby) or for monitoring of more than one case while in the operating room, per hour (List separately in addition to code for primary procedure)

➲ *CPT Changes: An Insider's View* 2013

➲ *CPT Assistant* Feb 13:16, May 13:8, Apr 14:5, 11, Dec 14:19, Aug 17:8

(Use 95941 in conjunction with the study performed, 92585, 95822, 95860-95870, 95907-95913, 95925, 95926, 95927, 95928, 95929, 95930-95937, 95938, 95939)

(For time spent waiting on standby before monitoring, use 99360)

(For electrocorticography, use 95829)

(For intraoperative EEG during nonintracranial surgery, use 95955)

(For intraoperative functional cortical or subcortical mapping, see 95961-95962)

►(For intraoperative neurostimulator programming, see 95971, 95972, 95976, 95977, 95983, 95984)◄

Autonomic Function Tests

The purpose of autonomic nervous system function testing is to determine the presence of autonomic dysfunction, the site of autonomic dysfunction, and the various autonomic subsystems that may be disordered.

Code 95921 should be reported only when electrocardiographic monitoring of heart rate derived from the time elapsing between two consecutive R waves in the electrocardiogram, or the R-R interval, is displayed on a monitor and stored for subsequent analysis of waveforms. Testing is typically performed in the prone position. A tilt table may be used, but is not required equipment for testing of the parasympathetic function. At least two of the following components need to be included in testing:

1. Heart rate response to deep breathing derived from a visual quantitative analysis of recordings with subject breathing at a rate of 5-6 breaths per minute.
2. Valsalva ratio determined by dividing the maximum heart rate by the lowest heart rate. The initial heart rate responses to sustained oral pressure (blowing into a tube with an open glottis) consist of tachycardia followed by a bradycardia at 15-45 seconds after the Valsalva pressure has been released. A minimum of two Valsalva maneuvers are to be performed. The initial cardioacceleration is an exercise reflex while the subsequent tachycardia and bradycardia are baroreflex-mediated.
3. A 30:15 ratio (R-R interval at beat 30)/(R-R interval at beat 15) used as an index of cardiovascular function.

Code 95922 should be reported only when all of the following components are included in testing:

1. Continuous recording of beat-to-beat BP and heart rate. The heart rate needs to be derived from an electrocardiogram (ECG) unit such that an accurate quantitative graphical measurement of the R-R interval is obtained.
2. A period of supine rest of at least 20 minutes prior to testing.
3. The performance and recording of beat-to-beat blood pressure and heart rate during a minimum of two (2) Valsalva maneuvers.
4. The performance of passive head-up tilt with continuous recording of beat-to-beat blood pressure and heart rate for a minimum of five minutes, followed by passive tilt-back to the supine position. This must be performed using a tilt table.

Code 95924 should be reported only when both the parasympathetic function and the adrenergic function are tested together with the use of a tilt table.

(To report autonomic function testing that does not include beat-to-beat recording or for testing without use of a tilt table, use 95943)

95921 Testing of autonomic nervous system function; cardiovagal innervation (parasympathetic function), including 2 or more of the following: heart rate response to deep breathing with recorded R-R interval, Valsalva ratio, and 30:15 ratio

➲ *CPT Assistant* Nov 98:35-36, Apr 02:2, Oct 03:11, Feb 06:15, Nov 12:6

95922 vasomotor adrenergic innervation (sympathetic adrenergic function), including beat-to-beat blood pressure and R-R interval changes during Valsalva maneuver and at least 5 minutes of passive tilt

➲ *CPT Assistant* Nov 98:35-36, Apr 02:2, Jun 03:11, Feb 06:15, Nov 06:23, Dec 08:4, Nov 12:6

(Do not report 95922 in conjunction with 95921)

95923 sudomotor, including 1 or more of the following: quantitative sudomotor axon reflex test (QSART), silastic sweat imprint, thermoregulatory sweat test, and changes in sympathetic skin potential
➲ *CPT Assistant* Nov 98:35-36, Apr 02:2, Feb 06:15, Nov 12:6

95924 combined parasympathetic and sympathetic adrenergic function testing with at least 5 minutes of passive tilt
➲ *CPT Changes: An Insider's View* 2013
➲ *CPT Assistant* Nov 12:6

(Do not report 95924 in conjunction with 95921 or 95922)

 # 95943 Simultaneous, independent, quantitative measures of both parasympathetic function and sympathetic function, based on time-frequency analysis of heart rate variability concurrent with time-frequency analysis of continuous respiratory activity, with mean heart rate and blood pressure measures, during rest, paced (deep) breathing, Valsalva maneuvers, and head-up postural change
➲ *CPT Changes: An Insider's View* 2013
➲ *CPT Assistant* Nov 12:6

(Do not report 95943 in conjunction with 93040, 95921, 95922, 95924)

Evoked Potentials and Reflex Tests

95925 Short-latency somatosensory evoked potential study, stimulation of any/all peripheral nerves or skin sites, recording from the central nervous system; in upper limbs
➲ *CPT Assistant* Nov 98:35-36, Apr 02:2, Apr 12:17, May 13:8

(Do not report 95925 in conjunction with 95926)

95926 in lower limbs
➲ *CPT Assistant* May 01:11, Apr 02:2, Apr 12:17, May 13:8

(Do not report 95926 in conjunction with 95925)

 # 95938 in upper and lower limbs
➲ *CPT Changes: An Insider's View* 2012
➲ *CPT Assistant* Apr 12:17, 18, Feb 13:17, May 13:8

(Do not report 95938 in conjunction with 95925, 95926)

95927 in the trunk or head
➲ *CPT Assistant* Apr 02:2, May 13:8

(To report a unilateral study, use modifier 52)

(For auditory evoked potentials, use 92585)

95928 Central motor evoked potential study (transcranial motor stimulation); upper limbs
➲ *CPT Changes: An Insider's View* 2005
➲ *CPT Assistant* May 13:8

(Do not report 95928 in conjunction with 95929)

95929 lower limbs
➲ *CPT Changes: An Insider's View* 2005
➲ *CPT Assistant* May 13:8

(Do not report 95929 in conjunction with 95928)

 # 95939 in upper and lower limbs
➲ *CPT Changes: An Insider's View* 2012
➲ *CPT Assistant* Apr 12:17, 18, May 13:8

(Do not report 95939 in conjunction with 95928, 95929)

95930 Visual evoked potential (VEP) checkerboard or flash testing, central nervous system except glaucoma, with interpretation and report
➲ *CPT Changes: An Insider's View* 2018
➲ *CPT Assistant* May 13:8, Aug 14:8, Feb 18:3

(For visual evoked potential testing for glaucoma, use 0464T)

(For screening of visual acuity using automated visual evoked potential devices, use 0333T)

95933 Orbicularis oculi (blink) reflex, by electrodiagnostic testing
➲ *CPT Assistant* Nov 98:35-36, May 13:8, Jul 17:10

95937 Neuromuscular junction testing (repetitive stimulation, paired stimuli), each nerve, any 1 method
➲ *CPT Assistant* Nov 98:35-36, Apr 02:2, Jun 06:8, Mar 13:3, May 13:8, Feb 16:14

95938 Code is out of numerical sequence. See 95912-95933

95939 Code is out of numerical sequence. See 95912-95933

95940 Code is out of numerical sequence. See 95912-95933

95941 Code is out of numerical sequence. See 95912-95933

95943 Code is out of numerical sequence. See 95912-95933

Special EEG Tests

Codes 95950-95953 and 95956 are used per 24 hours of recording. For recording more than 12 hours, do not use modifier 52. For recording 12 hours or less, use modifier 52. Codes 95951 and 95956 are used for recordings in which interpretations can be made throughout the recording time, with interventions to alter or end the recording or to alter the patient care during the recordings as needed.

Codes 95961 and 95962 use physician or other qualified health care professional time as a basis for unit of service. Report 95961 for the first hour of attendance. Use modifier 52 with 95961 for 30 minutes or less. Report 95962 for each additional hour of attendance.

95950 Monitoring for identification and lateralization of cerebral seizure focus, electroencephalographic (eg, 8 channel EEG) recording and interpretation, each 24 hours
➲ *CPT Assistant* Nov 98:35, Feb 11:3

95951 Monitoring for localization of cerebral seizure focus by cable or radio, 16 or more channel telemetry, combined electroencephalographic (EEG) and video recording and interpretation (eg, for presurgical localization), each 24 hours

➲ *CPT Assistant* Nov 98:35, Mar 03:21, Dec 04:18, Dec 09:3, Nov 10:6, Feb 11:3, Aug 13:14, Dec 14:17

Electroencephalographic (EEG) Monitoring and Video Recording

95951

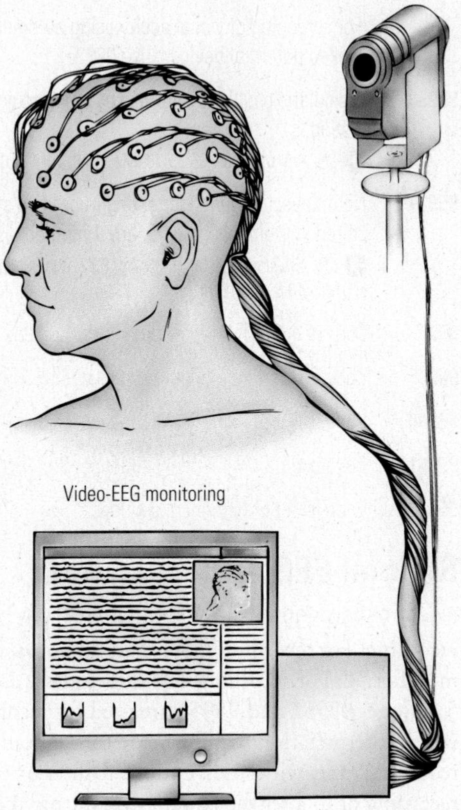

Video-EEG monitoring

95953 Monitoring for localization of cerebral seizure focus by computerized portable 16 or more channel EEG, electroencephalographic (EEG) recording and interpretation, each 24 hours, unattended

➲ *CPT Changes: An Insider's View* 2011

➲ *CPT Assistant* Nov 98:35, Dec 09:3, Feb 11:3, Dec 14:17

95954 Pharmacological or physical activation requiring physician or other qualified health care professional attendance during EEG recording of activation phase (eg, thiopental activation test)

➲ *CPT Changes: An Insider's View* 2013

➲ *CPT Assistant* Winter 94:18, Nov 98:35

95955 Electroencephalogram (EEG) during nonintracranial surgery (eg, carotid surgery)

➲ *CPT Assistant* Nov 98:35, Dec 14:19

95956 Monitoring for localization of cerebral seizure focus by cable or radio, 16 or more channel telemetry, electroencephalographic (EEG) recording and interpretation, each 24 hours, attended by a technologist or nurse

➲ *CPT Changes: An Insider's View* 2011

➲ *CPT Assistant* Nov 98:35, Dec 09:3, Feb 11:3

95957 Digital analysis of electroencephalogram (EEG) (eg, for epileptic spike analysis)

➲ *CPT Assistant* Winter 94:18, Nov 98:35, Nov 10:6

95958 Wada activation test for hemispheric function, including electroencephalographic (EEG) monitoring

➲ *CPT Assistant* Nov 98:35

95961 Functional cortical and subcortical mapping by stimulation and/or recording of electrodes on brain surface, or of depth electrodes, to provoke seizures or identify vital brain structures; initial hour of attendance by a physician or other qualified health care professional

➲ *CPT Changes: An Insider's View* 2000, 2013

➲ *CPT Assistant* Winter 94:18, Nov 98:35, Nov 99:52-53, Apr 10:10, Aug 10:13, Feb 11:3

+ 95962 each additional hour of attendance by a physician or other qualified health care professional (List separately in addition to code for primary procedure)

➲ *CPT Changes: An Insider's View* 2013

➲ *CPT Assistant* Winter 94:18, Nov 98:35, Nov 99:52-53, Apr 10:10, Aug 10:13, Feb 11:3

(Use 95962 in conjunction with 95961)

95965 Magnetoencephalography (MEG), recording and analysis; for spontaneous brain magnetic activity (eg, epileptic cerebral cortex localization)

➲ *CPT Changes: An Insider's View* 2002

95966 for evoked magnetic fields, single modality (eg, sensory, motor, language, or visual cortex localization)

➲ *CPT Changes: An Insider's View* 2002

+ 95967 for evoked magnetic fields, each additional modality (eg, sensory, motor, language, or visual cortex localization) (List separately in addition to code for primary procedure)

➲ *CPT Changes: An Insider's View* 2002

(Use 95967 in conjunction with 95966)

(For electroencephalography performed in addition to magnetoencephalography, see 95812-95827)

(For somatosensory evoked potentials, auditory evoked potentials, and visual evoked potentials performed in addition to magnetic evoked field responses, see 92585, 95925, 95926, and/or 95930)

(For computerized tomography performed in addition to magnetoencephalography, see 70450-70470, 70496)

(For magnetic resonance imaging performed in addition to magnetoencephalography, see 70551-70553)

►Physician or Other Qualified Health Care Professional Face-to-Face Time for Brain Neurostimulator Analysis With Programming	Code(s)
Less than 8 minutes	Not reported
8-22 minutes	95983 X 1
23-37 minutes	95983 X 1 + 95984 X 1
38-52 minutes	95983 X 1 + 95984 X 2
53-67 minutes	95983 X 1 + 95984 X 3
68 minutes or longer	add units of 95984◄

Neurostimulators, Analysis-Programming

►Electronic analysis of an implanted neurostimulator pulse generator/transmitter involves documenting settings and electrode impedances of the system parameters prior to programming. Programming involves adjusting the system parameter(s) to address clinical signs and patient symptoms. Parameters available for programming can vary between systems and may need to be adjusted multiple times during a single programming session. The iterative adjustments to parameters provide information that is required for the physician or other qualified health care professional to assess and select the most appropriate final program parameters to provide for consistent delivery of appropriate therapy. The values of the final program parameters may differ from the starting values after the programming session.

Examples of parameters include: contact group(s), interleaving, amplitude, pulse width, frequency (Hz), on/off cycling, burst, magnet mode, dose lockout, patient-selectable parameters, responsive neurostimulation, detection algorithms, closed-loop parameters, and passive parameters. Not all parameters are available for programming in every neurostimulator pulse generator/transmitter.

For coding purposes, a neurostimulator system is considered implanted when the electrode array(s) is inserted into the target area for either permanent or trial placement.

There are several types of implantable neurostimulator pulse generator/transmitters and they are differentiated by the nervous system region that is stimulated. A brain neurostimulator may stimulate either brain surface regions (cortical stimulation) or deep brain structures (deep brain stimulation). A brain neurostimulation system consists of array(s) that targets one or more of these regions.

A cranial nerve neurostimulator targets the fibers of the cranial nerves or their branches and divisions. There are 12 pairs of cranial nerves (see nerve anatomy figure on page 706). Each cranial nerve has its origin in the brain and passes through one or more foramina in the skull to innervate extracranial structures. A cranial nerve neurostimulator stimulates the nerve fibers of either the extracranial or intracranial portion(s) of one or more cranial nerve(s) (eg, vagus nerve, trigeminal nerve).

A spinal cord or peripheral nerve neurostimulator targets nerve(s) that originate in the spinal cord and exit the spine through neural foramina and gives rise to peripheral nerves. The peripheral nervous system consists of the nerves and ganglia outside of the brain and spinal cord. Peripheral nerves may give rise to independent branches or branches that combine with other peripheral nerves in neural plexuses (ie, brachial plexus, lumbosacral plexus). Under the lumbosacral plexus, the sacral nerves (specifically S2, S3, S4) are located in the lower back just above the tailbone. Neurostimulation of the sacral nerves affect pelvic floor muscles and urinary organs (eg, bladder, urinary sphincter).

Cranial nerve, spinal cord, peripheral nerve, and sacral nerve neurostimulator analysis with programming (95971, 95972, 95976, 95977) are reported based on the number of parameters adjusted during a programming session. Brain neurostimulator analysis with programming (95983, 95984) is reported based on physician or other qualified health care professional face-to-face time.

Code 95970 describes electronic analysis of the implanted brain, cranial nerve, spinal cord, peripheral nerve, or sacral nerve neurostimulator pulse generator/transmitter without programming. Electronic analysis is inherent to implantation codes 43647, 43648, 43881, 43882, 61850, 61860, 61863, 61864, 61867, 61868, 61870, 61880, 61885, 61886, 61888, 63650, 63655, 63661, 63662, 63663, 63664, 63685, 63688, 64553, 64555, 64561, 64566, 64568, 64569, 64570, 64575, 64580, 64581, 64585, 64590, 64595, and is not separately reportable at the same operative session.

The Cranial Nerves

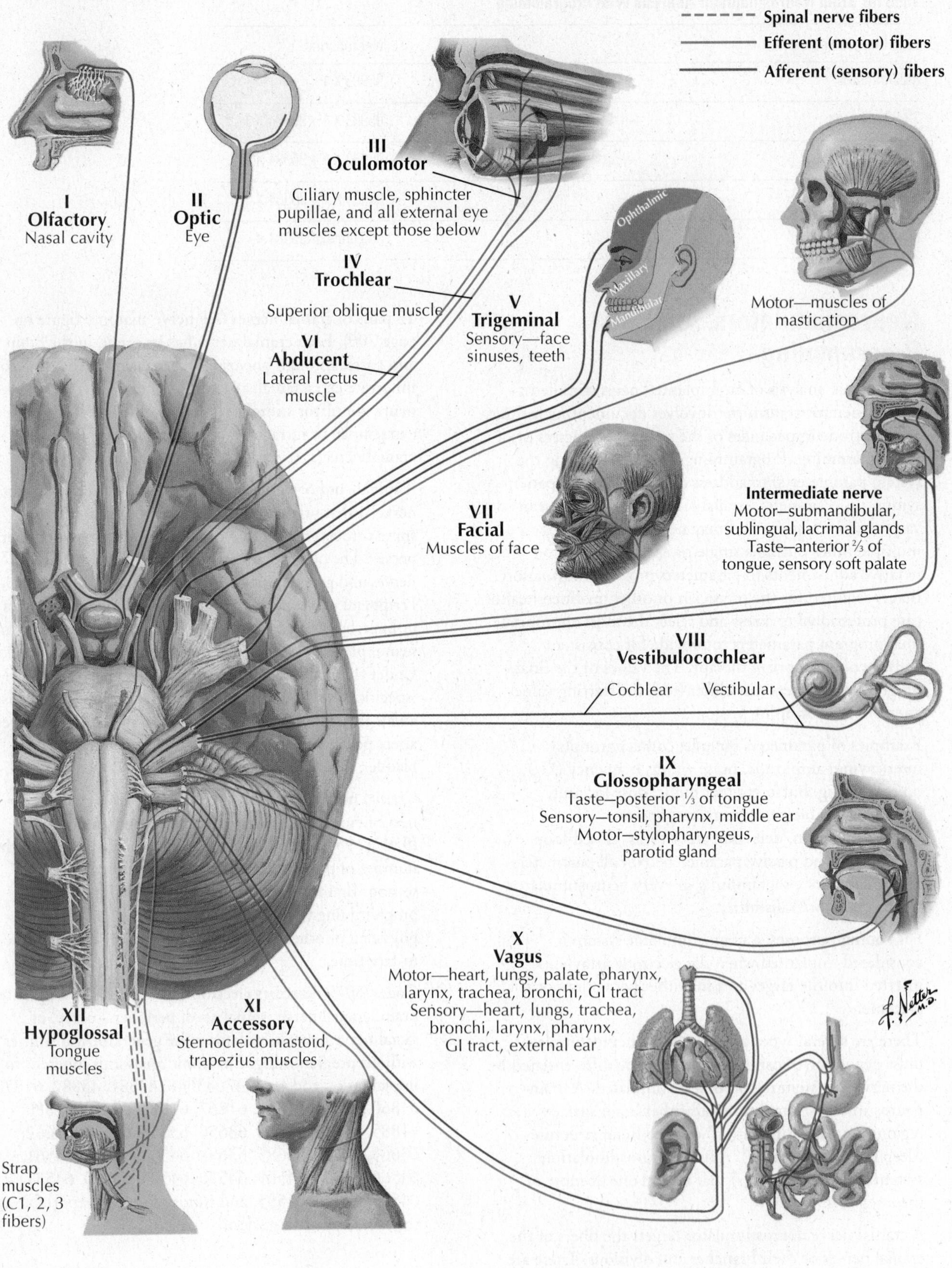

Codes 95971, 95972, 95976, 95977 describe electronic analysis with simple or complex programming of the implanted neurostimulator pulse generator/transmitter. *Simple* programming of a neurostimulator pulse generator/transmitter includes adjustment of one to three parameter(s). *Complex* programming includes adjustment of more than three parameters. For purposes of counting the number of parameters being programmed, a single parameter that is adjusted two or more times during a programming session counts as one parameter.

Code 95971 describes electronic analysis with simple programming of an implanted spinal cord or peripheral nerve (eg, sacral nerve) neurostimulator pulse generator/transmitter.

Code 95972 describes electronic analysis with complex programming of an implanted spinal cord or peripheral nerve (eg, sacral nerve) neurostimulator pulse generator/transmitter.

Code 95976 describes electronic analysis with simple programming of an implanted cranial nerve neurostimulator pulse generator/transmitter.

Code 95977 describes electronic analysis with complex programming of an implanted cranial nerve neurostimulator pulse generator/transmitter.

Codes 95983, 95984 describe electronic analysis with programming of an implanted brain neurostimulator pulse generator/transmitter. Code 95983 is reported for the first 15 minutes of physician or other qualified health care professional face-to-face time for analysis and programming. Code 95984 is reported for each additional 15 minutes. A unit of service is attained when the mid-point is passed. Physician or other qualified health care professional face-to-face time of less than eight minutes is not separately reportable.◄

Code 95980 describes intraoperative electronic analysis of an implanted gastric neurostimulator pulse generator system, with programming; code 95981 describes subsequent analysis of the device; code 95982 describes subsequent analysis and reprogramming. For electronic analysis and reprogramming of gastric neurostimulator, lesser curvature, see 95980-95982.

►Codes 95971, 95972, 95976, 95977, 95983, 95984 are reported when programming a neurostimulator is performed by a physician or other qualified health care professional. Programming may be performed in the operating room, postoperative care unit, inpatient, and/or outpatient setting. Programming a neurostimulator in the operating room is not inherent in the service represented by the implantation code and may be reported by either the implanting surgeon or other qualified health care professional, when performed.

Test stimulations are typically performed during an implantation procedure (43647, 43648, 43881, 43882, 61850, 61860, 61863, 61864, 61867, 61868, 61870, 61880, 61885, 61886, 61888, 63650, 63655, 63661, 63662, 63663, 63664, 63685, 63688, 64553, 64555, 64561, 64566, 64568, 64569, 64570, 64575, 64580, 64581, 64585, 64590, 64595) to confirm correct target site placement of the electrode array(s) and/or to confirm the functional status of the system. Test stimulation is not considered electronic analysis or programming of the neurostimulator system (test stimulation is included in the service described by the implantation code) and should not be reported with 95970, 95971, 95972, 95980, 95981, 95982, 95983, 95984. Electronic analysis of a device (95970) is not reported separately at the time of implantation.◄

►(For insertion of neurostimulator pulse generator, see 61885, 61886, 63685, 64568, 64590)◄

►(For revision or removal of neurostimulator pulse generator or receiver, see 61888, 63688, 64569, 64570, 64595)◄

►(For implantation of neurostimulator electrodes, see 43647, 43881, 61850-61870, 63650, 63655, 64553-64581. For revision or removal of neurostimulator electrodes, see 43648, 43882, 61880, 63661, 63662, 63663, 63664, 64569, 64570, 64585)◄

▲ **95970** Electronic analysis of implanted neurostimulator pulse generator/transmitter (eg, contact group[s], interleaving, amplitude, pulse width, frequency [Hz], on/off cycling, burst, magnet mode, dose lockout, patient selectable parameters, responsive neurostimulation, detection algorithms, closed loop parameters, and passive parameters) by physician or other qualified health care professional; with brain, cranial nerve, spinal cord, peripheral nerve, or sacral nerve, neurostimulator pulse generator/transmitter, without programming

CPT Changes: An Insider's View 2000, 2012, 2019

CPT Assistant Nov 98:36-37, Sep 99:1, Nov 99:53-54, Aug 05:7, Sep 05:10, Oct 12:15, Jul 16:7

►(Do not report 95970 in conjunction with 43647, 43648, 43881, 43882, 61850, 61860, 61863, 61864, 61867, 61868, 61870, 61880, 61885, 61886, 61888, 63650, 63655, 63661, 63662, 63663, 63664, 63685, 63688, 64553, 64555, 64561, 64566, 64568, 64569, 64570, 64575, 64580, 64581, 64585, 64590, 64595, during the same operative session)◄

►(Do not report 95970 in conjunction with 95971, 95972, 95976, 95977, 95983, 95984)◄

▲ **95971** with simple spinal cord or peripheral nerve (eg, sacral nerve) neurostimulator pulse generator/transmitter programming by physician or other qualified health care professional

CPT Changes: An Insider's View 2000, 2005, 2012, 2019

CPT Assistant Nov 98:36-37, Sep 99:1, Nov 99:53-54, Aug 05:7, Oct 10:14, Dec 10:14, Apr 11:11, Oct 12:15, Jul 16:7

►(Do not report 95971 in conjunction with 95972)◄

▲ **95972** with complex spinal cord or peripheral nerve (eg, sacral nerve) neurostimulator pulse generator/transmitter programming by physician or other qualified health care professional

➔ *CPT Changes: An Insider's View* 2000, 2005, 2012, 2015, 2016, 2019

➔ *CPT Assistant* Nov 98:36-37, Sep 99:1, Nov 99:53-54, Aug 05:7, Apr 11:10, Oct 12:15, Aug 14:5, Jul 16:7

►(95974, 95975 have been deleted. To report, see 95976, 95977)◄

● **95976** with simple cranial nerve neurostimulator pulse generator/transmitter programming by physician or other qualified health care professional

➔ *CPT Changes: An Insider's View* 2019

►(Do not report 95976 in conjunction with 95977)◄

● **95977** with complex cranial nerve neurostimulator pulse generator/transmitter programming by physician or other qualified health care professional

➔ *CPT Changes: An Insider's View* 2019

#● **95983** with brain neurostimulator pulse generator/transmitter programming, first 15 minutes face-to-face time with physician or other qualified health care professional

➔ *CPT Changes: An Insider's View* 2019

#+● **95984** with brain neurostimulator pulse generator/transmitter programming, each additional 15 minutes face-to-face time with physician or other qualified health care professional (List separately in addition to code for primary procedure)

➔ *CPT Changes: An Insider's View* 2019

►(Use 95984 in conjunction with 95983)◄

►(95978, 95979 have been deleted. To report, see 95983, 95984)◄

95980 Electronic analysis of implanted neurostimulator pulse generator system (eg, rate, pulse amplitude and duration, configuration of wave form, battery status, electrode selectability, output modulation, cycling, impedance and patient measurements) gastric neurostimulator pulse generator/transmitter; intraoperative, with programming

➔ *CPT Changes: An Insider's View* 2008

➔ *CPT Assistant* Jan 08:8, Nov 10:8, Jul 16:7

95981 subsequent, without reprogramming

➔ *CPT Changes: An Insider's View* 2008

➔ *CPT Assistant* Jan 08:8, Jul 16:7

95982 subsequent, with reprogramming

➔ *CPT Changes: An Insider's View* 2008

➔ *CPT Assistant* Jan 08:8, Jul 16:7

(For intraoperative or subsequent analysis, with programming, when performed, of vagus nerve trunk stimulator used for blocking therapy [morbid obesity], see 0312T, 0317T)

95983 Code is out of numerical sequence. See 95976-95981

95984 Code is out of numerical sequence. See 95976-95981

Other Procedures

95990 Refilling and maintenance of implantable pump or reservoir for drug delivery, spinal (intrathecal, epidural) or brain (intraventricular), includes electronic analysis of pump, when performed;

➔ *CPT Changes: An Insider's View* 2003, 2012

➔ *CPT Assistant* Nov 02:4, Nov 05:1, Jul 06:1, Jul 12:6, Aug 12:10, 11, 12, 15

95991 requiring skill of a physician or other qualified health care professional

➔ *CPT Changes: An Insider's View* 2004, 2012, 2013

➔ *CPT Assistant* Nov 05:1, Jul 06:1, Jul 12:6, Aug 12:10, 11, 12, 15

(Do not report 95990, 95991 in conjunction with 62367-62370. For analysis and/or reprogramming of implantable infusion pump, see 62367-62370)

(For refill and maintenance of implanted infusion pump or reservoir for systemic drug therapy [eg, chemotherapy], use 96522)

Coding Tip

Instructions for Use of the CPT Codebook

When advanced practice nurses and physician assistants are working with physicians, they are considered as working in the exact same specialty and exact same subspecialties as the physician. A "physician or other qualified health care professional" is an individual who is qualified by education, training, licensure/regulation (when applicable), and facility privileging (when applicable) who performs a professional service within his or her scope of practice and independently reports that professional service. These professionals are distinct from "clinical staff." A clinical staff member is a person who works under the supervision of a physician or other qualified health care professional, and who is allowed by law, regulation, and facility policy to perform or assist in the performance of a specific professional service, but does not individually report that professional service. Other policies may also affect who may report specific services.

CPT Coding Guidelines, Introduction, Instructions for Use of the CPT Codebook

⊘ **95992** Canalith repositioning procedure(s) (eg, Epley maneuver, Semont maneuver), per day

➔ *CPT Changes: An Insider's View* 2009

(Do not report 95992 in conjunction with 92531, 92532)

95999 Unlisted neurological or neuromuscular diagnostic procedure

➔ *CPT Assistant* Feb 99:11, Jan 02:11, Mar 07:4, Apr 07:7, Dec 08:10, Aug 15:8

Motion Analysis

Codes 96000-96004 describe services performed as part of a major therapeutic or diagnostic decision making process. Motion analysis is performed in a dedicated motion analysis laboratory (ie, a facility capable of performing videotaping from the front, back and both sides, computerized 3D kinematics, 3D kinetics, and dynamic electromyography). Code 96000 may include 3D kinetics and stride characteristics. Codes 96002-96003 describe dynamic electromyography.

Code 96004 should only be reported once regardless of the number of study(ies) reviewed/interpreted.

(For performance of needle electromyography procedures, see 95860-95870, 95872, 95885-95887)

(For gait training, use 97116)

96000 Comprehensive computer-based motion analysis by video-taping and 3D kinematics;

➔ *CPT Changes: An Insider's View* 2002

➔ *CPT Assistant* Aug 02:5, Jun 03:2

96001 with dynamic plantar pressure measurements during walking

➔ *CPT Changes: An Insider's View* 2002

➔ *CPT Assistant* Aug 02:5, Jun 03:2

96002 Dynamic surface electromyography, during walking or other functional activities, 1-12 muscles

➔ *CPT Changes: An Insider's View* 2002

➔ *CPT Assistant* Aug 02:5, Jun 03:3, Aug 15:8

96003 Dynamic fine wire electromyography, during walking or other functional activities, 1 muscle

➔ *CPT Changes: An Insider's View* 2002

➔ *CPT Assistant* Aug 02:5, Jun 03:3

(Do not report 96002, 96003 in conjunction with 95860-95866, 95869-95872, 95885-95887)

96004 Review and interpretation by physician or other qualified health care professional of comprehensive computer-based motion analysis, dynamic plantar pressure measurements, dynamic surface electromyography during walking or other functional activities, and dynamic fine wire electromyography, with written report

➔ *CPT Changes: An Insider's View* 2002, 2013

➔ *CPT Assistant* Aug 02:5, Jun 03:3, Aug 15:8

Functional Brain Mapping

Code 96020 includes selection and administration of testing of language, memory, cognition, movement, sensation, and other neurological functions when conducted in association with functional neuroimaging, monitoring of performance of this testing, and determination of validity of neurofunctional testing relative to separately interpreted functional magnetic resonance images.

96020 Neurofunctional testing selection and administration during noninvasive imaging functional brain mapping, with test administered entirely by a physician or other qualified health care professional (ie, psychologist), with review of test results and report

➔ *CPT Changes: An Insider's View* 2007, 2013

➔ *CPT Assistant* Feb 07:6

(For functional magnetic resonance imaging [fMRI], brain, use 70555)

►(Do not report 96020 in conjunction with 96112, 96113, 96116, 96121, 96130, 96131, 96132, 96133)◄

(Do not report 96020 in conjunction with 70554)

(Evaluation and Management services codes should not be reported on the same day as 96020)

Medical Genetics and Genetic Counseling Services

These services are provided by trained genetic counselors and may include obtaining a structured family genetic history, pedigree construction, analysis for genetic risk assessment, and counseling of the patient and family. These activities may be provided during one or more sessions and may include review of medical data and family information, face-to-face interviews, and counseling services.

Code 96040 is reported for each 30-minute increment of face-to-face time. Do not report 96040 for 15 minutes or less of face-to-face time. Report 96040 once for 16 to 30 minutes of face-to-face time.

★ **96040** Medical genetics and genetic counseling services, each 30 minutes face-to-face with patient/family

➔ *CPT Changes: An Insider's View* 2007, 2017

➔ *CPT Assistant* Aug 07:9

(For genetic counseling and education provided to an individual by a physician or other qualified health care professional who may report evaluation and management services, see the appropriate Evaluation and Management codes)

(For genetic counseling and education to a group by a physician or other qualified health care professional, use 99078)

(For education regarding genetic risks by a nonphysician to a group, see 98961, 98962)

(For genetic counseling and/or risk factor reduction intervention provided to patient(s) without symptoms or established disease, by a physician or other qualified health care professional who may report evaluation and management services, see 99401-99412)

►Adaptive Behavior Services◄

►Adaptive behavior services address deficient adaptive behaviors (eg, impaired social, communication, or self-care skills), maladaptive behaviors (eg, repetitive and stereotypic behaviors, behaviors that risk physical harm to the patient, others, and/or property), or other impaired functioning secondary to deficient adaptive or maladaptive behaviors, including, but not limited to, instruction-following, verbal and nonverbal communication, imitation, play and leisure, social interactions, self-care, daily living, and personal safety.

Definitions

Functional behavior assessment: comprises descriptive assessment procedures designed to identify environmental events that occur just before and just after occurrences of potential target behaviors and that may influence those behaviors. That information may be gathered by interviewing the patient's caregivers; having caregivers complete checklists, rating scales, or questionnaires; and/or observing and recording occurrences of target behaviors and environmental events in everyday situations.

Functional analysis: an assessment procedure for evaluating the separate effects of each of several environmental events on a potential target behavior by systematically presenting and withdrawing each event to a patient multiple times and observing and measuring occurrences of the behavior in response to those events. Graphed data are analyzed visually to determine which events produced relatively high and low occurrences of the behavior.

Standardized instruments and procedures: include, but not limited to, behavior checklists, rating scales, and adaptive skill assessment instruments that comprise a fixed set of items and are administered and scored in a uniform way with all patients (eg, Pervasive Developmental Disabilities Behavior Inventory, Brigance Inventory of Early Development, Vineland Adaptive Behavior Scales).

Nonstandardized instruments and procedures: include, but not limited to, curriculum-referenced assessments, stimulus preference–assessment procedures, and other procedures for assessing behaviors and associated environmental events that are specific to the individual patient and behaviors.◄

►Adaptive Behavior Assessments◄

►**Behavior identification assessment** (97151) is conducted by the physician or other qualified health care professional and may include analysis of pertinent past data (including medical diagnosis), a detailed behavioral history, patient observation, administration of standardized and/or nonstandardized instruments and procedures, functional behavior assessment, functional analysis, and/or guardian/caregiver interview to identify and describe deficient adaptive behaviors, maladaptive behaviors, and other impaired functioning secondary to deficient adaptive or maladaptive behaviors. Code 97151 includes the physician's or other qualified health care professional's scoring of assessments, interpretation of results, discussion of findings and recommendations with the primary guardian(s)/caregiver(s), preparation of report, and development of plan of care, which may include behavior identification supporting assessment (97152) or behavior identification–supporting assessment with four required components (0362T).

Behavior identification supporting assessment (97152) is administered by a technician under the direction of a physician or other qualified health care professional. The physician or other qualified health care professional may or may not be on site during the face-to-face assessment process. Code 97152 includes the physician's or other qualified health care professional's interpretation of results and may include functional behavior assessment, functional analysis, and other structured observations and/or standardized and/or nonstandardized instruments and procedures to determine levels of adaptive and maladaptive behavior.

Codes 97152, 0362T may be reported separately with 97151 based on the time that the patient is face-to-face with one or more technician(s). Only count the time of one technician when two or more are present.

For behavior identification–supporting assessment with four required components, use 0362T.◄

Coding Tip

If the physician or other qualified health care professional personally performs the technician activities, his or her time engaged in these activities should be included as part of the required technician time to meet the components of the code.

#● **97151** **Behavior identification assessment,** administered by a physician or other qualified health care professional, each 15 minutes of the physician's or other qualified health care professional's time face-to-face with patient and/or guardian(s)/caregiver(s) administering assessments and discussing findings and recommendations, and non-face-to-face analyzing past data, scoring/interpreting the assessment, and preparing the report/treatment plan

➲ *CPT Changes: An Insider's View* 2019

#● **97152** **Behavior identification–supporting assessment,** administered by one technician under the direction of a physician or other qualified health care professional, face-to-face with the patient, each 15 minutes

➲ *CPT Changes: An Insider's View* 2019

►(97151, 97152, 0362T may be repeated on the same or different days until the behavior identification assessment [97151] and, if necessary, supporting assessment[s] [97152, 0362T], is complete)◄

►(For psychiatric diagnostic evaluation, see 90791, 90792)◄

►(For speech evaluations, see 92521, 92522, 92523, 92524)◄

►Guide to Selection of Codes 97152 and 0362T

	97152	0362T
Physician or other qualified health care professional required to be on site		✓
Physician or other qualified health care professional not required to be on site	✓	
Number of technicians	1	2 or more
Deficient adaptive behavior(s), maladaptive behavior(s), or other impaired functioning secondary to deficient adaptive or maladaptive behaviors	✓	
Destructive behavior(s)		✓
May include functional behavior assessment	✓	✓
May include functional analysis	✓	✓
Environment customized to patient and behavior		✓◄

►(For occupational therapy evaluation, see 97165, 97166, 97167, 97168)◄

►(For medical team conference, see 99366, 99367, 99368)◄

►(For health and behavior assessment/intervention, see 96150, 96151, 96152, 96153, 96154, 96155)◄

►(For neurobehavioral status examination, see 96116, 96121)◄

►(For neuropsychological testing, see 96132, 96133, 96136, 96137, 96138, 96139, 96146)◄

►Adaptive Behavior Treatment◄

►**Adaptive behavior treatment** codes 97153, 97154, 97155, 97156, 97157, 97158, 0373T describe services that address specific treatment targets and goals based on results of previous assessments (see 97151, 97152, 0362T), and include ongoing assessment and adjustment of treatment protocols, targets, and goals.

Adaptive behavior treatment by protocol (97153) and **group adaptive behavior treatment by protocol** (97154) are administered by a technician under the direction of a physician or other qualified health care professional, utilizing a treatment protocol designed in advance by the physician or other qualified health care professional, who may or may not provide direction during the treatment. Code 97153 describes face-to-face services with one patient and code 97154 describes face-to-face services with two or more patients. Do not report 97154 if the group has more than eight patients.

Adaptive behavior treatment with protocol modification (97155) is administered by a physician or other qualified health care professional face-to-face with a single patient. The physician or other qualified health care professional resolves one or more problems with the protocol and may simultaneously direct a technician in administering the modified protocol while the patient is present. Physician or other qualified health care professional direction to the technician without the patient present is not reported separately.

Family adaptive behavior treatment guidance and **multiple-family group adaptive behavior treatment guidance** (97156, 97157) are administered by a physician or other qualified health care professional face-to-face with guardian(s)/caregiver(s) and involve identifying potential treatment targets and training guardian(s)/caregiver(s) of one patient (97156) or multiple patients (97157) to implement treatment protocols designed to address deficient adaptive or maladaptive behaviors. Services described by 97156 may be performed with or without the patient present. Services described by 97157 are performed without the patient present. Do not report 97157 if the group has more than eight patients' guardian(s)/caregiver(s).

Group adaptive behavior treatment with protocol modification (97158) is administered by a physician or other qualified health care professional face-to-face with multiple patients. The physician or other qualified health care professional monitors the needs of individual patients and adjusts the treatment techniques during the group sessions, as needed. In contrast to group adaptive behavior treatment by protocol (97154), protocol adjustments are made in real time rather than for a subsequent service. Do not report 97158 if the group has more than eight patients.

For adaptive behavior treatment with protocol modification with four required components, use 0373T.◄

Coding Tip

If the physician or other qualified health care professional personally performs the technician activities, his or her time engaged in these activities should be reported as technician time.

#● 97153 **Adaptive behavior treatment by protocol,** administered by technician under the direction of a physician or other qualified health care professional, face-to-face with one patient, each 15 minutes

➲ *CPT Changes: An Insider's View* 2019

►(Do not report 97153 in conjunction with 90785-90899, 92507, 96105-96155)◄

►Guide to Selection of Codes 97153, 97155, and 0373T

	97153	97155	0373T
By protocol	✓		
With protocol modification		✓	✓
Physician or other qualified health care professional face-to-face with patient		✓	
Physician or other qualified health care professional required to be on site			✓
Physician or other qualified health care professional not required to be on site	✓		
Number of technicians	1	0-1	2 or more
Deficient adaptive behavior(s), maladaptive behavior(s), or other impaired functioning secondary to deficient adaptive or maladaptive behaviors	✓	✓	
Destructive behavior(s)		✓	✓
Environment customized to patient and behavior			✓◄

#● **97154** **Group adaptive behavior treatment by protocol,** administered by technician under the direction of a physician or other qualified health care professional, face-to-face with two or more patients, each 15 minutes

➲ *CPT Changes: An Insider's View* 2019

►(Do not report 97154 if the group has more than 8 patients)◄

►(Do not report 97154 in conjunction with 90785-90899, 92508, 96105-96155, 97150)◄

#● **97155** **Adaptive behavior treatment with protocol modification,** administered by physician or other qualified health care professional, which may include simultaneous direction of technician, face-to-face with one patient, each 15 minutes

➲ *CPT Changes: An Insider's View* 2019

►(Do not report 97155 in conjunction with 90785-90899, 96105-96155, 92507)◄

#● **97156** **Family adaptive behavior treatment guidance,** administered by physician or other qualified health care professional (with or without the patient present), face-to-face with guardian(s)/caregiver(s), each 15 minutes

➲ *CPT Changes: An Insider's View* 2019

►(Do not report 97156 in conjunction with 90785-90899, 96105-96155)◄

#● **97157** **Multiple-family group adaptive behavior treatment guidance,** administered by physician or other qualified health care professional (without the patient present), face-to-face with multiple sets of guardians/caregivers, each 15 minutes

➲ *CPT Changes: An Insider's View* 2019

►(Do not report 97157 if the group has more than 8 families)◄

►(Do not report 97156, 97157 in conjunction with 90785-90899, 96105-96155)◄

#● **97158** **Group adaptive behavior treatment with protocol modification,** administered by physician or other qualified health care professional, face-to-face with multiple patients, each 15 minutes

➲ *CPT Changes: An Insider's View* 2019

►(Do not report 97158 if the group has more than 8 patients)◄

►(Do not report 97158 in conjunction with 90785-90899, 96105-96155, 92508, 97150)◄

Central Nervous System Assessments/Tests (eg, Neuro-Cognitive, Mental Status, Speech Testing)

►The following codes are used to report the services provided during testing of the central nervous system functions. The central nervous system assessments include, but are not limited to, memory, language, visual motor responses, and abstract reasoning/problem-solving abilities. It is accomplished by the combination of several types of testing procedures. Testing procedures include assessment of aphasia and cognitive performance testing, developmental screening and behavioral assessments and testing, and psychological/neuropsychological testing. The administration of these tests will generate material that will be formulated into a report or an automated result.◄

(For development of cognitive skills, see 97127, 97533)

(For dementia screens, [eg, Folstein Mini-Mental State Examination, by a physician or other qualified health care professional], see **Evaluation and Management** services codes)

►(Do not report assessment of aphasia and cognitive performance testing services [96105, 96125], developmental/behavioral screening and testing services [96110, 96112, 96113, 96127], and psychological/neuropsychological testing services [96116, 96121, 96130, 96131, 96132, 96133, 96136, 96137, 96138, 96139, 96146] in conjunction with 97151, 97152, 97153, 97154, 97155, 97156, 97157, 97158, 0362T, 0373T)◄

►Definitions

Codes in this family (96105-96146) describe a number of services that are defined below:

Cognitive performance testing: assesses the patient's ability to complete specific functional tasks applicable to the patient's environment in order to identify or quantify specific cognitive deficits. The results are used to determine impairments and develop therapeutic goals and objectives.

Interactive feedback: used to convey the implications of psychological or neuropsychological test findings and diagnostic formulation. Based on patient-specific cognitive and emotional strengths and weaknesses, interactive feedback may include promoting adherence to medical and/or psychological treatment plans; educating and engaging the patient about his or her condition to maximize patient collaboration in their care; addressing safety issues; facilitating psychological coping; coordinating care; and engaging the patient in planning given the expected course of illness or condition, when performed.

Interpretation and report: performed by a physician or other qualified health care professional. In some circumstances, a result is generated through the use of a computer, tablet computer, or other device(s).

Neurobehavioral status examination: a clinical assessment of cognitive functions and behavior, and may include an interview with the patient, other informant(s), and/or staff, as well as integration of prior history and other sources of clinical data with clinical decision making, further assessment and/or treatment planning and report. Evaluation domains may include acquired knowledge, attention, language, memory, planning and problem solving, and visual spatial abilities.

Neuropsychological testing evaluation services: typically include integration of patient data with other sources of clinical data, interpretation, clinical decision making, and treatment planning and report. It may include interactive feedback to the patient, family member(s) or caregiver(s), when performed. Evaluation domains for neuropsychological evaluation may include intellectual function, attention, executive function, language and communication, memory, visual-spatial function, sensorimotor function, emotional and personality features, and adaptive behavior.

Psychological testing evaluation services: typically include integration of patient data with other sources of clinical data, interpretation, clinical decision making, and treatment planning and report. It may include interactive feedback to the patient, family member(s) or caregiver(s), when performed. Evaluation domains for psychological evaluation may include emotional and interpersonal functioning, intellectual function, thought processes, personality, and psychopathology.

Standardized instruments: used in the performance of these services. Standardized instruments are validated tests that are administered and scored in a consistent or "standard" manner consistent with their validation.

Testing: administered by a physician, other qualified health care professional, and technician, or completed by the patient. The mode of completion can be manual (eg, paper and pencil) or via automated means.

Assessment of aphasia and cognitive performance testing, which includes interpretation and report, are described by 96105, 96125.

Developmental screening services are described by 96110. Developmental/behavioral testing services, which include interpretation and report, are described by 96112, 96113.

Neurobehavioral status examination, which includes interpretation and report, is described by 96116, 96121.

Psychological and neuropsychological test evaluation services, which include integration of patient data, interpretation of test results and clinical data, treatment planning and report, and interactive feedback, are described by 96130, 96131, 96132, 96133.

Testing and administration services (96136, 96137) are performed by a physician or other qualified health care professional. For 96136, 96137, do not include time for evaluation services (eg, integration of patient data or interpretation of test results). This time is included with psychological and neuropsychological test evaluation services (96130, 96131, 96132, 96133). Testing and administration services (96138, 96139) are performed by a technician. The tests selected, test administration and method of testing and scoring are the same, regardless whether the testing is performed by a physician, other qualified health care professional, or a technician, for 96136, 96137, 96138, 96139. Automated testing and result code 96146 describes testing performed by a single automated instrument with an automated result.

Some of these services are typically performed together. For example, psychological/neuropsychological testing evaluation services (96130, 96131, 96132, 96133) may be reported with psychological/neuropsychological test administration and scoring services (96136, 96137, 96138, 96139).

Central Nervous System Assessments/Tests (eg, Neuro-Cognitive, Mental Status, Speech Testing) Tables

Assessment of Aphasia and Cognitive Performance Testing

		Cognitive Services		Test Administration/Scoring		Interpretation and Report or Automated Result	
Code	**Unit**	**Evaluation**	**Interactive Feedback**	**Physician or Qualified Health Care Professional**	**Technician**	**Physician or Qualified Health Care Professional**	**Automated Result**
96105	Per hour	X		X		X	
96125	Per hour	X		X		X	

Developmental/Behavioral Screening and Testing

		Cognitive Services		Test Administration/Scoring		Interpretation and Report or Automated Result	
Code	**Unit**	**Evaluation**	**Interactive Feedback**	**Physician or Qualified Health Care Professional**	**Clinical Staff**	**Physician or Qualified Health Care Professional**	**Automated Result**
96110	Per instrument				X		
96112	Per hour	X		X		X	
+96113	Per hour (add-on)	X		X		X	
96127	Per instrument				X		

Psychological/Neuropsychological Testing

		Cognitive Services		Test Administration/ Scoring		Interpretation and Report or Automated Result	
Code	**Unit**	**Evaluation**	**Interactive Feedback**	**Physician or Qualified Health Care Professional**	**Technician**	**Physician or Qualified Health Care Professional**	**Automated Result**
Neurobehavioral Status Examination							
96116	Per hour	X		X		X	
+96121	Per hour (add-on)	X		X		X	
Testing Evaluation Services							
96130	Per hour	X	X	Not included in Code	Not Included in Code	X	
+96131	Per hour (add-on)	X	X	Not included in Code	Not Included in Code	X	
96132	Per hour	X	X	Not included in Code	Not Included in Code	X	
+96133	Per hour (add-on)	X	X	Not included in Code	Not Included in Code	X	
Test Administration & Scoring							
96136	Per 30 min	Not included in Code	Not Included in Code	X		Not included in Code	Not Included in Code
+96137	Per 30 min (add-on)	Not included in Code	Not included in Code	X		Not included in Code	Not Included in Code
96138	Per 30 min	Not included in Code	Not included in Code		X	Not included in Code	Not Included in Code
+96139	Per 30 min (add-on)	Not included in Code	Not included in Code		X	Not included in Code	Not Included in Code
Automated Testing and Result							
96146	Automated report(s)	Not included in Code	Not Included in Code				X

A requirement of testing services (96105, 96125, 96112, 96113, 96130, 96131, 96132, 96133, 96146) is that there is an interpretation and report when performed by a qualified health care professional, or a result when generated by automation. These services follow standard CPT time definitions (ie, a minimum of 16 minutes for 30 minutes codes and 31 minutes for 1-hour codes must be provided to report any per hour code). The time reported in 96116, 96121, 96130, 96131, 96132, 96133, 96125 is the face-to-face time with the patient and the time spent integrating and interpreting data.

Report the total time at the completion of the entire episode of evaluation.◄

►(96101, 96102, 96103 have been deleted.)◄

►(To report psychological testing evaluation and administration and scoring services, see 96130, 96131, 96136, 96137, 96138, 96139, 96146)◄

►(To report psychological test administration using a single automated instrument, use 96146)◄

►Assessment of Aphasia and Cognitive Performance Testing◄

96105 Assessment of aphasia (includes assessment of expressive and receptive speech and language function, language comprehension, speech production ability, reading, spelling, writing, eg, by Boston Diagnostic Aphasia Examination) with interpretation and report, per hour

➲ *CPT Assistant* Jul 96:8, May 05:1, Nov 09:10

 # 96125 Standardized cognitive performance testing (eg, Ross Information Processing Assessment) per hour of a qualified health care professional's time, both face-to-face time administering tests to the patient and time interpreting these test results and preparing the report

➲ *CPT Changes: An Insider's View* 2008

➲ *CPT Assistant* Oct 11:4

►(To report neuropsychological testing evaluation and administration and scoring services, see 96132, 96133, 96136, 96137, 96138, 96139, 96146)◄

►Developmental/Behavioral Screening and Testing◄

96110 Developmental screening (eg, developmental milestone survey, speech and language delay screen), with scoring and documentation, per standardized instrument

➲ *CPT Changes: An Insider's View* 2012, 2015

➲ *CPT Assistant* Jul 96:9, May 05:1, Nov 09:10, Jun 14:3, Aug 15:5, Feb 17:15

(For an emotional/behavioral assessment, use 96127)

►(96111 has been deleted)◄

►(To report developmental testing, see 96112, 96113)◄

● 96112 Developmental test administration (including assessment of fine and/or gross motor, language, cognitive level, social, memory and/or executive functions by standardized developmental instruments when performed), by physician or other qualified health care professional, with interpretation and report; first hour

➲ *CPT Changes: An Insider's View* 2019

+● 96113 each additional 30 minutes (List separately in addition to code for primary procedure)

➲ *CPT Changes: An Insider's View* 2019

 # 96127 Brief emotional/behavioral assessment (eg, depression inventory, attention-deficit/hyperactivity disorder [ADHD] scale), with scoring and documentation, per standardized instrument

➲ *CPT Changes: An Insider's View* 2015

➲ *CPT Assistant* Aug 15:5, Feb 17:15

(For developmental screening, use 96110)

►Psychological/Neuropsychological Testing◄

►Neurobehavioral Status Examination◄

★▲ 96116 Neurobehavioral status examination (clinical assessment of thinking, reasoning and judgment, [eg, acquired knowledge, attention, language, memory, planning and problem solving, and visual spatial abilities]), by physician or other qualified health care professional, both face-to-face time with the patient and time interpreting test results and preparing the report; first hour

➲ *CPT Changes: An Insider's View* 2006, 2017, 2019

➲ *CPT Assistant* Oct 11:4, Jun 14:3

►(96118, 96119, 96120 have been deleted)◄

►(To report neuropsychological testing evaluation and administration and scoring services, see 96132, 96133, 96136, 96137, 96138, 96139, 96146)◄

►(To report neuropsychological test administration using a single automated instrument, use 96146)◄

+● 96121 each additional hour (List separately in addition to code for primary procedure)

➲ *CPT Changes: An Insider's View* 2019

►(Use 96121 in conjunction with 96116)◄

96125 Code is out of numerical sequence. See 96020-96121

96127 Code is out of numerical sequence. See 96020-96121

►Testing Evaluation Services◄

● 96130 Psychological testing evaluation services by physician or other qualified health care professional, including integration of patient data, interpretation of standardized test results and clinical data, clinical decision making, treatment planning and report, and interactive feedback to the patient, family member(s) or caregiver(s), when performed; first hour

➲ *CPT Changes: An Insider's View* 2019

+● 96131 each additional hour (List separately in addition to code for primary procedure)

CPT Changes: An Insider's View 2019

● 96132 Neuropsychological testing evaluation services by physician or other qualified health care professional, including integration of patient data, interpretation of standardized test results and clinical data, clinical decision making, treatment planning and report, and interactive feedback to the patient, family member(s) or caregiver(s), when performed; first hour

CPT Changes: An Insider's View 2019

+● 96133 each additional hour (List separately in addition to code for primary procedure)

CPT Changes: An Insider's View 2019

▸Test Administration and Scoring◂

● 96136 Psychological or neuropsychological test administration and scoring by physician or other qualified health care professional, two or more tests, any method; first 30 minutes

CPT Changes: An Insider's View 2019

+● 96137 each additional 30 minutes (List separately in addition to code for primary procedure)

CPT Changes: An Insider's View 2019

▶(96136, 96137 may be reported in conjunction with 96130, 96131, 96132, 96133 on the same or different days)◀

● 96138 Psychological or neuropsychological test administration and scoring by technician, two or more tests, any method; first 30 minutes

CPT Changes: An Insider's View 2019

+● 96139 each additional 30 minutes (List separately in addition to code for primary procedure)

CPT Changes: An Insider's View 2019

▶(96138, 96139 may be reported in conjunction with 96130, 96131, 96132, 96133 on the same or different days)◀

▶(For 96136, 96137, 96138, 96139, do not include time for evaluation services [eg, integration of patient data or interpretation of test results]. This time is included in 96130, 96131, 96132, 96133)◀

▸Automated Testing and Result◂

● 96146 Psychological or neuropsychological test administration, with single automated, standardized instrument via electronic platform, with automated result only

CPT Changes: An Insider's View 2019

▶(If test is administered by physician, other qualified health care professional, or technician, do not report 96146. To report, see 96127, 96136, 96137, 96138, 96139)◀

Health and Behavior Assessment/Intervention

Health and behavior assessment procedures are used to identify the psychological, behavioral, emotional, cognitive, and social factors important to the prevention, treatment, or management of physical health problems.

The focus of the assessment is not on mental health but on the biopsychosocial factors important to physical health problems and treatments. The focus of the intervention is to improve the patient's health and well-being utilizing cognitive, behavioral, social, and/or psychophysiological procedures designed to ameliorate specific disease-related problems.

Codes 96150-96155 describe services offered to patients who present with primary physical illnesses, diagnoses, or symptoms and may benefit from assessments and interventions that focus on the biopsychosocial factors related to the patient's health status. These services do not represent preventive medicine counseling and risk factor reduction interventions.

For patients that require psychiatric services (90785-90899) as well as health and behavior assessment/intervention (96150-96155), report the predominant service performed. Do not report 96150-96155 in conjunction with 90785-90899 on the same date.

▶Evaluation and management services codes (including counseling risk factor reduction and behavior change intervention [99401-99412]), should not be reported on the same day as health and behavior assessment/intervention codes 96150, 96151, 96152, 96153, 96154, 96155.◀

▶(For health and behavior assessment and/or intervention services [96150, 96151, 96152, 96153, 96154, 96155] performed by a physician or other qualified health care professional who may report evaluation and management services, see **Evaluation and Management** or **Preventive Medicine Services** codes)◀

▶(Do not report 96150, 96151, 96152, 96153, 96154, 96155 in conjunction with 97151, 97152, 97153, 97154, 97155, 97156, 97157, 97158, 0362T, 0373T)◀

★ 96150 Health and behavior assessment (eg, health-focused clinical interview, behavioral observations, psychophysiological monitoring, health-oriented questionnaires), each 15 minutes face-to-face with the patient; initial assessment

CPT Changes: An Insider's View 2002, 2017

CPT Assistant Mar 02:4, Feb 04:11, Mar 04:10, May 05:1, Jun 05:10, Aug 09:9, May 13:12, Jun 14:3, Sep 14:15

★ 96151 re-assessment

CPT Changes: An Insider's View 2002, 2017

CPT Assistant Mar 02:4, Feb 04:11, Mar 04:10, May 05:1, Jun 05:10, Aug 09:9, May 13:12, Jun 14:3, Sep 14:15

★ **96152** Health and behavior intervention, each 15 minutes, face-to-face; individual

➲ *CPT Changes: An Insider's View* 2002, 2017

➲ *CPT Assistant* Mar 02:4, Feb 04:11, Mar 04:10, May 05:1, Jun 05:10, Aug 09:9, May 13:12, Jun 14:3, Sep 14:15, Oct 17:5

★ **96153** group (2 or more patients)

➲ *CPT Changes: An Insider's View* 2002, 2017

➲ *CPT Assistant* Mar 02:4, Feb 04:11, Mar 04:10, May 05:1, Jun 05:10, Aug 09:9, May 13:12, Jun 14:3, Sep 14:15

★ **96154** family (with the patient present)

➲ *CPT Changes: An Insider's View* 2002, 2017

➲ *CPT Assistant* Mar 02:4, Feb 04:11, Mar 04:10, May 05:1, Jun 05:10, Aug 09:9, May 13:12, Jun 14:3, Sep 14:15

96155 family (without the patient present)

➲ *CPT Changes: An Insider's View* 2002

➲ *CPT Assistant* Mar 02:4, 12, Feb 04:11, Mar 04:10, May 05:1, Jun 05:10, Aug 09:9, May 13:12, Jun 14:3, Sep 14:15

96160 Administration of patient-focused health risk assessment instrument (eg, health hazard appraisal) with scoring and documentation, per standardized instrument

➲ *CPT Changes: An Insider's View* 2017

➲ *CPT Assistant* Feb 17:15

96161 Administration of caregiver-focused health risk assessment instrument (eg, depression inventory) for the benefit of the patient, with scoring and documentation, per standardized instrument

➲ *CPT Changes: An Insider's View* 2017

➲ *CPT Assistant* Feb 17:15

Hydration, Therapeutic, Prophylactic, Diagnostic Injections and Infusions, and Chemotherapy and Other Highly Complex Drug or Highly Complex Biologic Agent Administration

Physician or other qualified health care professional work related to hydration, injection, and infusion services predominantly involves affirmation of treatment plan and direct supervision of staff.

Codes 96360-96379, 96401, 96402, 96409-96425, 96521-96523 are not intended to be reported by the physician in the facility setting. If a significant, separately identifiable office or other outpatient Evaluation and Management service is performed, the appropriate E/M service (99201-99215, 99241-99245, 99354-99355) should be reported using modifier 25 in addition to 96360-96549. For same day E/M service, a different diagnosis is not required.

If performed to facilitate the infusion or injection, the following services are included and are not reported separately:

a. Use of local anesthesia

b. IV start

c. Access to indwelling IV, subcutaneous catheter or port

d. Flush at conclusion of infusion

e. Standard tubing, syringes, and supplies

(For declotting a catheter or port, use 36593)

When multiple drugs are administered, report the service(s) and the specific materials or drugs for each.

When administering multiple infusions, injections or combinations, only one "initial" service code should be reported for a given date, unless protocol requires that two separate IV sites must be used. Do not report a second initial service on the same date due to an intravenous line requiring a re-start, an IV rate not being able to be reached without two lines, or for accessing a port of a multi-lumen catheter. If an injection or infusion is of a subsequent or concurrent nature, even if it is the first such service within that group of services, then a subsequent or concurrent code from the appropriate section should be reported (eg, the first IV push given subsequent to an initial one-hour infusion is reported using a subsequent IV push code).

Initial infusion: For physician or other qualified health care professional reporting, an initial infusion is the *key or primary reason for the encounter* reported irrespective of the temporal order in which the infusion(s) or injection(s) are administered. For facility reporting, an initial infusion is based using the hierarchy. For both physician or other qualified health care professional and facility reporting, only one *initial* service code (eg, 96365) should be reported unless the protocol or patient condition requires that two separate IV sites must be utilized. The difference in time and effort in providing this second IV site access is also reported using the *initial* service code with modifier 59 appended (eg, 96365, 96365-59).

Sequential infusion: A sequential infusion is an infusion or IV push of a new substance or drug following a primary or initial service. All sequential services require that there be a new substance or drug, except that facilities may report a sequential intravenous push of the same drug using 96376.

Concurrent infusion: A concurrent infusion is an infusion of a new substance or drug infused at the same time as another substance or drug. A concurrent infusion service is not time based and is only reported once per day regardless of whether an additional new drug or substance is administered concurrently. Hydration may not be reported concurrently with any other service. A separate subsequent concurrent administration of another new drug or substance (the third substance or drug) is not reported.

In order to determine which service should be reported as the initial service when there is more than one type of service, hierarchies have been created. These vary by whether the physician or other qualified health care professional or a facility is reporting. The order of selection for reporting is based upon the physician's or other qualified health care professional's knowledge of the clinical condition(s) and treatment(s). The hierarchy that facilities are to use is based upon a structural algorithm. When these codes are reported by the physician or other qualified health care professional, the "initial" code that best describes the key or primary reason for the encounter should always be reported irrespective of the order in which the infusions or injections occur.

When these codes are reported *by the facility*, the following instructions apply. The initial code should be selected using a hierarchy whereby chemotherapy services are primary to therapeutic, prophylactic, and diagnostic services which are primary to hydration services. Infusions are primary to pushes, which are primary to injections. This hierarchy is to be followed by facilities and supersedes parenthetical instructions for add-on codes that suggest an add-on of a higher hierarchical position may be reported in conjunction with a base code of a lower position. (For example, the hierarchy would not permit reporting 96376 with 96360, as 96376 is a higher order code. IV push is primary to hydration.)

When reporting multiple infusions of the same drug/substance on the same date of service, the initial code should be selected. The second and subsequent infusion(s) should be reported based on the individual time(s) of each additional infusion(s) of the same drug/substance using the appropriate add-on code.

Example: In the outpatient observation setting, a patient receives one-hour intravenous infusions of the same antibiotic every 8 hours on the same date of service through the same IV access. The hierarchy for facility reporting permits the reporting of code 96365 for the first one-hour dose administered. Add-on 96366 would be reported twice (once for the second and third one-hour infusions of the same drug).

When reporting codes for which infusion time is a factor, use the actual time over which the infusion is administered. Intravenous or intra-arterial push is defined as: (a) an injection in which the individual who administers the drug/substance is continuously present to administer the injection and observe the patient, or (b) an infusion of 15 minutes or less. If intravenous hydration (96360, 96361) is given from 11 PM to 2 AM, 96360 would be reported once and 96361 twice. For continuous services that last beyond midnight, use the date in which the service began and report the total units of time provided continuously. However, if instead of a continuous infusion, a medication was given by intravenous push at 10 PM and 2 AM, as the service was not continuous, the two administrations would be reported as an initial service (96374) and sequential (96376) as: (1) no other infusion services were performed; and (2) the push of the same drug was performed more than 30 minutes beyond the initial administration. A "keep open" infusion of any type is not separately reported.

Hydration

Codes 96360-96361 are intended to report a hydration IV infusion to consist of a pre-packaged fluid and electrolytes (eg, normal saline, D5-1/2 normal saline+30mEq KCl/liter), but are not used to report infusion of drugs or other substances. Hydration IV infusions typically require direct supervision for purposes of consent, safety oversight, or intraservice supervision of staff. Typically such infusions require little special handling to prepare or dispose of, and staff that administer these do not typically require advanced practice training. After initial set-up, infusion typically entails little patient risk and thus little monitoring. These codes are not intended to be reported by the physician or other qualified health care professional in the facility setting.

Some chemotherapeutic agents and other therapeutic agents require pre- and/or post-hydration to be given in order to avoid specific toxicities. A minimum time duration of 31 minutes of hydration infusion is required to report the service. However, the hydration codes 96360 or 96361 are not used when the purpose of the intravenous fluid is to "keep open" an IV line prior or subsequent to a therapeutic infusion, or as a free-flowing IV during chemotherapy or other therapeutic infusion.

96360 Intravenous infusion, hydration; initial, 31 minutes to 1 hour

➔ *CPT Changes: An Insider's View* 2009

➔ *CPT Assistant* May 10:8, May 11:7, Oct 11:3, Dec 11:3, Oct 13:3, May 14:11

(Do not report 96360 if performed as a concurrent infusion service)

(Do not report intravenous infusion for hydration of 30 minutes or less)

+ 96361 each additional hour (List separately in addition to code for primary procedure)

➔ *CPT Changes: An Insider's View* 2009

➔ *CPT Assistant* May 10:8, May 11:7, Oct 11:3, Dec 11:3, Oct 13:3,.May 14:11

(Use 96361 in conjunction with 96360)

(Report 96361 for hydration infusion intervals of greater than 30 minutes beyond 1 hour increments)

(Report 96361 to identify hydration if provided as a secondary or subsequent service after a different initial service [96360, 96365, 96374, 96409, 96413] is administered through the same IV access)

Therapeutic, Prophylactic, and Diagnostic Injections and Infusions (Excludes Chemotherapy and Other Highly Complex Drug or Highly Complex Biologic Agent Administration)

A therapeutic, prophylactic, or diagnostic IV infusion or injection (other than hydration) is for the administration of substances/drugs. When fluids are used to administer the drug(s), the administration of the fluid is considered incidental hydration and is not separately reportable. These services typically require direct supervision for any or all purposes of patient assessment, provision of consent, safety oversight, and intra-service supervision of staff. Typically, such infusions require special consideration to prepare, dose or dispose of, require practice training and competency for staff who administer the infusions, and require periodic patient assessment with vital sign monitoring during the infusion. These codes are not intended to be reported by the physician or other qualified health care professional in the facility setting.

See codes 96401-96549 for the administration of chemotherapy or other highly complex drug or highly complex biologic agent services. These highly complex services require advanced practice training and competency for staff who provide these services; special considerations for preparation, dosage or disposal; and commonly, these services entail significant patient risk and frequent monitoring. Examples are frequent changes in the infusion rate, prolonged presence of nurse administering the solution for patient monitoring and infusion adjustments, and frequent conferring with the physician or other qualified health care professional about these issues.

(Do not report 96365-96379 with codes for which IV push or infusion is an inherent part of the procedure [eg, administration of contrast material for a diagnostic imaging study])

Coding Tip

Instructions for Reporting Medication Administration With Chemotherapy and Other Highly Complex Drug or Highly Complex Biologic Agent Administration

The administration of medications (eg, antibiotics, steroidal agents, antiemetics, narcotics, analgesics) administered independently or sequentially as supportive management of chemotherapy administration, should be separately reported using 96360, 96361, 96365, 96379 as appropriate.

CPT Coding Guidelines, Chemotherapy and Other Highly Complex Drug or Highly Complex Biologic Agent Administration

96365 Intravenous infusion, for therapy, prophylaxis, or diagnosis (specify substance or drug); initial, up to 1 hour

➲ *CPT Changes: An Insider's View* 2009

➲ *CPT Assistant* May 10:8, May 11:7, Oct 11:4, Dec 11:3

➲ *Clinical Examples in Radiology* Spring 10:10

+ 96366 each additional hour (List separately in addition to code for primary procedure)

➲ *CPT Changes: An Insider's View* 2009

➲ *CPT Assistant* May 11:7, Dec 11:3

(Report 96366 in conjunction with 96365, 96367)

(Report 96366 for additional hour[s] of sequential infusion)

(Report 96366 for infusion intervals of greater than 30 minutes beyond 1 hour increments)

(Report 96366 in conjunction with 96365 to identify each second and subsequent infusions of the same drug/substance)

+ 96367 additional sequential infusion of a new drug/substance, up to 1 hour (List separately in addition to code for primary procedure)

➲ *CPT Changes: An Insider's View* 2009, 2012

➲ *CPT Assistant* May 11:7, Dec 11:3

(Report 96367 in conjunction with 96365, 96374, 96409, 96413 to identify the infusion of a new drug/substance provided as a secondary or subsequent service after a different initial service is administered through the same IV access. Report 96367 only once per sequential infusion of same infusate mix)

+ 96368 concurrent infusion (List separately in addition to code for primary procedure)

➲ *CPT Changes: An Insider's View* 2009

➲ *CPT Assistant* May 10:8, May 11:7, Dec 11:3

(Report 96368 only once per date of service)

(Report 96368 in conjunction with 96365, 96366, 96413, 96415, 96416)

96369 Subcutaneous infusion for therapy or prophylaxis (specify substance or drug); initial, up to 1 hour, including pump set-up and establishment of subcutaneous infusion site(s)

➲ *CPT Changes: An Insider's View* 2009

➲ *CPT Assistant* May 11:7

(For infusions of 15 minutes or less, use 96372)

+ 96370 each additional hour (List separately in addition to code for primary procedure)

➲ *CPT Changes: An Insider's View* 2009

➲ *CPT Assistant* May 11:7

(Use 96370 in conjunction with 96369)

(Use 96370 for infusion intervals of greater than 30 minutes beyond 1 hour increments)

+ 96371 additional pump set-up with establishment of new subcutaneous infusion site(s) (List separately in addition to code for primary procedure)

➲ *CPT Changes: An Insider's View* 2009

➲ *CPT Assistant* May 11:7

(Use 96371 in conjunction with 96369)

(Use 96369, 96371 only once per encounter)

96372 Therapeutic, prophylactic, or diagnostic injection (specify substance or drug); subcutaneous or intramuscular

CPT Changes: An Insider's View 2009

CPT Assistant May 10:9, May 11:7, Jan 13:9, Jan 14:10, Oct 16:9

(For administration of vaccines/toxoids, see 90460, 90461, 90471, 90472)

(Report 96372 for non-antineoplastic hormonal therapy injections)

(Report 96401 for anti-neoplastic nonhormonal injection therapy)

(Report 96402 for anti-neoplastic hormonal injection therapy)

(Do not report 96372 for injections given without direct physician or other qualified health care professional supervision. To report, use 99211. Hospitals may report 96372 when the physician or other qualified health care professional is not present)

(96372 does not include injections for allergen immunotherapy. For allergen immunotherapy injections, see 95115-95117)

96373 intra-arterial

CPT Changes: An Insider's View 2009

CPT Assistant May 11:7

96374 intravenous push, single or initial substance/drug

CPT Changes: An Insider's View 2009

CPT Assistant May 10:8, May 11:7, Oct 11:3, Dec 11:4, Feb 13:3, Jun 13:9

Clinical Examples in Radiology Spring 10:10, Summer 16:10

+ 96375 each additional sequential intravenous push of a new substance/drug (List separately in addition to code for primary procedure)

CPT Changes: An Insider's View 2009

CPT Assistant May 10:8, May 11:7, Feb 13:3

Clinical Examples in Radiology Summer 16:10

(Use 96375 in conjunction with 96365, 96374, 96409, 96413)

(Report 96375 to identify intravenous push of a new substance/drug if provided as a secondary or subsequent service after a different initial service is administered through the same IV access)

+ 96376 each additional sequential intravenous push of the same substance/drug provided in a facility (List separately in addition to code for primary procedure)

CPT Changes: An Insider's View 2009

CPT Assistant May 10:6, May 11:7, Dec 11:3, Nov 14:15

Clinical Examples in Radiology Summer 16:10

(Do not report 96376 for a push performed within 30 minutes of a reported push of the same substance or drug)

(96376 may be reported by facilities only)

(Report 96376 in conjunction with 96365, 96374, 96409, 96413)

96377 Application of on-body injector (includes cannula insertion) for timed subcutaneous injection

CPT Changes: An Insider's View 2017

CPT Assistant Oct 16:9

96379 Unlisted therapeutic, prophylactic, or diagnostic intravenous or intra-arterial injection or infusion

CPT Changes: An Insider's View 2009

CPT Assistant May 11:7, Dec 11:19

(For allergy immunology, see 95004 et seq)

Chemotherapy and Other Highly Complex Drug or Highly Complex Biologic Agent Administration

Chemotherapy administration codes 96401-96549 apply to parenteral administration of non-radionuclide anti-neoplastic drugs; and also to anti-neoplastic agents provided for treatment of noncancer diagnoses (eg, cyclophosphamide for auto-immune conditions) or to substances such as certain monoclonal antibody agents, and other biologic response modifiers. The highly complex infusion of chemotherapy or other drug or biologic agents requires physician or other qualified health care professional work and/or clinical staff monitoring well beyond that of therapeutic drug agents (96360-96379) because the incidence of severe adverse patient reactions are typically greater. These services can be provided by any physician or other qualified health care professional. Chemotherapy services are typically highly complex and require direct supervision for any or all purposes of patient assessment, provision of consent, safety oversight, and intraservice supervision of staff. Typically, such chemotherapy services require advanced practice training and competency for staff who provide these services; special considerations for preparation, dosage, or disposal; and commonly, these services entail significant patient risk and frequent monitoring. Examples are frequent changes in the infusion rate, prolonged presence of the nurse administering the solution for patient monitoring and infusion adjustments, and frequent conferring with the physician or other qualified health care professional about these issues. When performed to facilitate the infusion of injection, preparation of chemotherapy agent(s), highly complex agent(s), or other highly complex drugs is included and is not reported separately. To report infusions that do not require this level of complexity, see 96360-96379. Codes 96401-96402, 96409-96425, 96521-96523 are not intended to be reported by the individual physician or other qualified health care professional in the facility setting.

The term "chemotherapy" in 96401-96549 includes other highly complex drugs or highly complex biologic agents.

Report separate codes for each parenteral method of administration employed when chemotherapy is administered by different techniques. The administration of medications (eg, antibiotics, steroidal agents, antiemetics, narcotics, analgesics) administered independently or sequentially as supportive management of chemotherapy administration, should be separately reported using 96360, 96361, 96365, 96379 as appropriate.

Report both the specific service as well as code(s) for the specific substance(s) or drug(s) provided. The fluid used to administer the drug(s) is considered incidental hydration and is not separately reportable.

Regional (isolation) chemotherapy perfusion should be reported using the codes for arterial infusion (96420-96425). Placement of the intra-arterial catheter should be reported using the appropriate code from the **Cardiovascular Surgery** section. Placement of arterial and venous cannula(s) for extracorporeal circulation via a membrane oxygenator perfusion pump should be reported using 36823. Code 36823 includes dose calculation and administration of the chemotherapy agent by injection into the perfusate. Do not report 96409-96425 in conjunction with 36823.

(For home infusion services, see 99601-99602)

Injection and Intravenous Infusion Chemotherapy and Other Highly Complex Drug or Highly Complex Biologic Agent Administration

Intravenous or intra-arterial push is defined as: (a) an injection in which the healthcare professional who administers the substance/drug is continuously present to administer the injection and observe the patient, or (b) an infusion of 15 minutes or less.

96401 Chemotherapy administration, subcutaneous or intramuscular; non-hormonal anti-neoplastic
- *CPT Changes: An Insider's View* 2006
- *CPT Assistant* Nov 05:1, Jan 06:47, Jan 07:30, May 07:3, Jun 07:4, Feb 09:17, Aug 11:9, Dec 11:3
- *Clinical Examples in Radiology* Winter 18:12

96402 hormonal anti-neoplastic
- *CPT Changes: An Insider's View* 2006
- *CPT Assistant* Nov 05:1, Jan 07:30, May 07:3, Feb 09:17, Dec 11:3
- *Clinical Examples in Radiology* Winter 18:12

96405 Chemotherapy administration; intralesional, up to and including 7 lesions
- *CPT Changes: An Insider's View* 2006
- *CPT Assistant* Sep 96:5, Aug 97:19, Feb 01:10, Jul 01:2, Nov 05:1, Jan 07:30, May 07:3, Feb 09:17

96406 intralesional, more than 7 lesions
- *CPT Changes: An Insider's View* 2006
- *CPT Assistant* Sep 96:5, Aug 97:19, Feb 01:10, Jul 01:2, Nov 05:1, Jan 07:30, May 07:3, Feb 09:17

96409 intravenous, push technique, single or initial substance/drug
- *CPT Changes: An Insider's View* 2006
- *CPT Assistant* Nov 05:1, Jan 07:30, May 07:3, Feb 09:17, May 10:8, May 11:17, Dec 11:3
- *Clinical Examples in Radiology* Winter 18:12

+ 96411 intravenous, push technique, each additional substance/drug (List separately in addition to code for primary procedure)
- *CPT Changes: An Insider's View* 2006
- *CPT Assistant* Nov 05:1, Jan 07:30, May 07:3, Feb 09:17, Dec 11:3
- *Clinical Examples in Radiology* Winter 18:12

(Use 96411 in conjunction with 96409, 96413)

96413 Chemotherapy administration, intravenous infusion technique; up to 1 hour, single or initial substance/drug
- *CPT Changes: An Insider's View* 2006
- *CPT Assistant* Nov 05:1, Jan 07:30, May 07:3, Sep 07:3, Dec 07:15, Feb 09:17, May 10:8, May 11:7, Dec 11:4
- *Clinical Examples in Radiology* Winter 18:12

(Report 96361 to identify hydration if administered as a secondary or subsequent service in association with 96413 through the same IV access)

(Report 96366, 96367, 96375 to identify therapeutic, prophylactic, or diagnostic drug infusion or injection, if administered as a secondary or subsequent service in association with 96413 through the same IV access)

+ 96415 each additional hour (List separately in addition to code for primary procedure)
- *CPT Changes: An Insider's View* 2006, 2007
- *CPT Assistant* Nov 05:1, Jan 07:30, May 07:3, Sep 07:3, Dec 07:15, Feb 09:17, Dec 11:3
- *Clinical Examples in Radiology* Winter 18:12

(Use 96415 in conjunction with 96413)

(Report 96415 for infusion intervals of greater than 30 minutes beyond 1-hour increments)

96416 initiation of prolonged chemotherapy infusion (more than 8 hours), requiring use of a portable or implantable pump
- *CPT Changes: An Insider's View* 2006
- *CPT Assistant* Nov 05:1, Jan 07:30, May 07:3, Sep 07:3, Dec 07:15, Feb 09:17, Dec 11:3
- *Clinical Examples in Radiology* Winter 18:12

(For refilling and maintenance of a portable pump or an implantable infusion pump or reservoir for drug delivery, see 96521-96523)

+ 96417 each additional sequential infusion (different substance/drug), up to 1 hour (List separately in addition to code for primary procedure)
- *CPT Changes: An Insider's View* 2006
- *CPT Assistant* Nov 05:1, Jan 07:30, May 07:3, Jun 07:4, Feb 09:17, Aug 11:9, Dec 11:3
- *Clinical Examples in Radiology* Winter 18:12

(Use 96417 in conjunction with 96413)

(Report only once per sequential infusion. Report 96415 for additional hour(s) of sequential infusion)

Intra-Arterial Chemotherapy and Other Highly Complex Drug or Highly Complex Biologic Agent Administration

96420 Chemotherapy administration, intra-arterial; push technique

➔ *CPT Assistant* Aug 97:19, Nov 98:37, Nov 99:54, Feb 01:10, Jul 01:2, Nov 05:1, Jan 07:30, May 07:3, Jun 07:4, Feb 09:17, Aug 11:9, Dec 11:3, Nov 13:6

➔ *Clinical Examples in Radiology* Summer 08:1, 2, 4, Winter 18:11

96422 infusion technique, up to 1 hour

➔ *CPT Assistant* Dec 96:10, Aug 97:19, Nov 98:37, Feb 01:10, Jul 01:2, Nov 05:1, Jan 07:30, May 07:3, Dec 07:15, Feb 09:17, Aug 11:9, Dec 11:3

➔ *Clinical Examples in Radiology* Winter 18:12

+ 96423 infusion technique, each additional hour (List separately in addition to code for primary procedure)

➔ *CPT Changes: An Insider's View* 2006, 2007

➔ *CPT Assistant* Dec 96:10, Nov 98:37, Feb 01:10, Jul 01:2, Nov 05:1, Jan 07:30, May 07:3, Dec 07:15, Feb 09:17, Dec 11:3

➔ *Clinical Examples in Radiology* Winter 18:12

(Use 96423 in conjunction with 96422)

(Report 96423 for infusion intervals of greater than 30 minutes beyond 1-hour increments)

(For regional chemotherapy perfusion via membrane oxygenator perfusion pump to an extremity, use 36823)

96425 infusion technique, initiation of prolonged infusion (more than 8 hours), requiring the use of a portable or implantable pump

➔ *CPT Assistant* Nov 99:54, Feb 01:10, Jul 01:2, Nov 05:1, Jan 07:30, May 07:3, Jun 07:4, Feb 09:17, Aug 11:9, Dec 11:3

➔ *Clinical Examples in Radiology* Winter 18:12

(For refilling and maintenance of a portable pump or an implantable infusion pump or reservoir for drug delivery, see 96521-96523)

Other Injection and Infusion Services

Code 96523 does not require direct supervision. Codes 96521-96523 may be reported when these devices are used for therapeutic drugs other than chemotherapy.

(For collection of blood specimen from a completely implantable venous access device, use 36591)

96440 Chemotherapy administration into pleural cavity, requiring and including thoracentesis

➔ *CPT Assistant* Feb 01:10, Jul 01:2, Nov 05:1, Jan 07:30, May 07:3, Jun 07:4, Feb 09:17

96446 Chemotherapy administration into the peritoneal cavity via indwelling port or catheter

➔ *CPT Changes: An Insider's View* 2011

➔ *CPT Assistant* Oct 10:16, Dec 10:16

96450 Chemotherapy administration, into CNS (eg, intrathecal), requiring and including spinal puncture

➔ *CPT Changes: An Insider's View* 2002

➔ *CPT Assistant* Feb 01:10, Jul 01:2, Nov 05:1, Jan 07:30, May 07:3, Feb 09:17

➔ *Clinical Examples in Radiology* Spring 11:10, Winter 14:10

(For intravesical (bladder) chemotherapy administration, use 51720)

(For insertion of subarachnoid catheter and reservoir for infusion of drug, see 62350, 62351, 62360-62362; for insertion of intraventricular catheter and reservoir, see 61210, 61215)

(If fluoroscopic guidance is performed, use 77003)

96521 Refilling and maintenance of portable pump

➔ *CPT Changes: An Insider's View* 2006

➔ *CPT Assistant* Nov 05:1, Jan 07:30, May 07:3, Feb 09:17, Dec 11:3

➔ *Clinical Examples in Radiology* Winter 18:12

96522 Refilling and maintenance of implantable pump or reservoir for drug delivery, systemic (eg, intravenous, intra-arterial)

➔ *CPT Changes: An Insider's View* 2006

➔ *CPT Assistant* Jul 06:1, Jan 07:30, May 07:3, Feb 09:17, Dec 11:3

➔ *Clinical Examples in Radiology* Winter 18:12

(For refilling and maintenance of an implantable infusion pump for spinal or brain drug infusion, use 95990-95991)

96523 Irrigation of implanted venous access device for drug delivery systems

➔ *CPT Changes: An Insider's View* 2006

➔ *CPT Assistant* Jan 07:30, May 07:3, Feb 09:17, Jul 11:16, Dec 11:3

➔ *Clinical Examples in Radiology* Winter 18:12

(Do not report 96523 in conjunction with other services. To report collection of blood specimen, use 36591)

96542 Chemotherapy injection, subarachnoid or intraventricular via subcutaneous reservoir, single or multiple agents

➔ *CPT Assistant* Aug 97:19, Jul 01:2, Nov 05:1, Jan 07:30, May 07:3, Feb 09:17

(For radioactive isotope therapy, use 79005)

96549 Unlisted chemotherapy procedure

➔ *CPT Assistant* Aug 97:19, Jul 01:2, Nov 05:1, Jan 07:30, May 07:3, Jun 07:4, Oct 10:16, Dec 10:16

Photodynamic Therapy

Codes 96573, 96574 should be used to report nonsurgical treatment of cutaneous lesions using photodynamic therapy by external application of light to destroy premalignant lesion(s) of the skin and adjacent mucosa (eg, face, scalp) by activation of photosensitizing drug(s).

A treatment session is defined as an application of photosensitizer to all lesions within an anatomic area (eg, face, scalp), with or without debridement of all premalignant hyperkeratotic lesions in that area, followed by illumination/activation with an appropriate light source to the same area.

►Do not report codes for debridement (11000, 11001, 11004, 11005), lesion shaving (11300-11313), biopsy (11102, 11103, 11104, 11105, 11106, 11107), or lesion excision (11400-11471) within the treatment area(s) on the same day as photodynamic therapy (96573, 96574).◄

(To report ocular photodynamic therapy, use 67221)

96567 Photodynamic therapy by external application of light to destroy premalignant lesions of the skin and adjacent mucosa with application and illumination/activation of photosensitive drug(s), per day

➲ *CPT Changes: An Insider's View* 2002, 2018

➲ *CPT Assistant* Feb 18:10

(Use 96567 for reporting photodynamic therapy when physician or other qualified health care professional is not directly involved in the delivery of the photodynamic therapy service)

+ 96570 Photodynamic therapy by endoscopic application of light to ablate abnormal tissue via activation of photosensitive drug(s); first 30 minutes (List separately in addition to code for endoscopy or bronchoscopy procedures of lung and gastrointestinal tract)

➲ *CPT Changes: An Insider's View* 2000, 2010

➲ *CPT Assistant* Nov 99:54, Sep 00:5, Oct 11:11, Apr 13:8

(Report 96570 with modifier 52 for service of less than 23 minutes with report)

+ 96571 each additional 15 minutes (List separately in addition to code for endoscopy or bronchoscopy procedures of lung and gastrointestinal tract)

➲ *CPT Changes: An Insider's View* 2000, 2010

➲ *CPT Assistant* Nov 99:54, Sep 00:5, Oct 11:11, Apr 13:8

(For 23-37 minutes of service, use 96570. For 38-52 minutes of service, use 96570 in conjunction with 96571)

(96570, 96571 are to be used in addition to bronchoscopy, endoscopy codes)

(Use 96570, 96571 in conjunction with 31641, 43229 as appropriate)

96573 Photodynamic therapy by external application of light to destroy premalignant lesions of the skin and adjacent mucosa with application and illumination/activation of photosensitizing drug(s) provided by a physician or other qualified health care professional, per day

➲ *CPT Changes: An Insider's View* 2018

➲ *CPT Assistant* Feb 18:10

(Do not report 96573 in conjunction with 96567, 96574 for the same anatomic area)

96574 Debridement of premalignant hyperkeratotic lesion(s) (ie, targeted curettage, abrasion) followed with photodynamic therapy by external application of light to destroy premalignant lesions of the skin and adjacent mucosa with application and illumination/activation of photosensitizing drug(s) provided by a physician or other qualified health care professional, per day

➲ *CPT Changes: An Insider's View* 2018

➲ *CPT Assistant* Feb 18:10

(Do not report 96574 in conjunction with 96567, 96573 for the same anatomic area)

Special Dermatological Procedures

See the **Evaluation and Management coding guidelines** for further instructions on reporting that is appropriate for management of dermatologic illnesses.

(For intralesional injections, see 11900, 11901)

(For Tzanck smear, see 88160-88161)

96900 Actinotherapy (ultraviolet light)

➲ *CPT Assistant* Jul 12:9, Sep 16:3, Nov 16:9

(For rhinophototherapy, intranasal application of ultraviolet and visible light, use 30999)

96902 Microscopic examination of hairs plucked or clipped by the examiner (excluding hair collected by the patient) to determine telogen and anagen counts, or structural hair shaft abnormality

➲ *CPT Assistant* Nov 97:46-47

96904 Whole body integumentary photography, for monitoring of high risk patients with dysplastic nevus syndrome or a history of dysplastic nevi, or patients with a personal or familial history of melanoma

➲ *CPT Changes: An Insider's View* 2007

96910 Photochemotherapy; tar and ultraviolet B (Goeckerman treatment) or petrolatum and ultraviolet B

➲ *CPT Assistant* Jul 12:9, Sep 16:3

96912 psoralens and ultraviolet A (PUVA)

➲ *CPT Assistant* Jul 12:9, Sep 16:3

96913 Photochemotherapy (Goeckerman and/or PUVA) for severe photoresponsive dermatoses requiring at least 4-8 hours of care under direct supervision of the physician (includes application of medication and dressings)

➲ *CPT Assistant* Sep 16:3

96920 Laser treatment for inflammatory skin disease (psoriasis); total area less than 250 sq cm

➲ *CPT Changes: An Insider's View* 2003

➲ *CPT Assistant* Oct 10:9, Jul 12:9, May 13:12, Sep 16:3

96921 250 sq cm to 500 sq cm

➲ *CPT Changes: An Insider's View* 2003

➲ *CPT Assistant* Oct 10:9, Jul 12:9, May 13:12, Sep 16:3

96922 over 500 sq cm
CPT Changes: An Insider's View 2003
CPT Assistant Oct 10:9, Jul 12:9, May 13:12, Sep 16:3

(For laser destruction of premalignant lesions, see 17000-17004)

(For laser destruction of cutaneous vascular proliferative lesions, see 17106-17108)

(For laser destruction of benign lesions, see 17110-17111)

(For laser destruction of malignant lesions, see 17260-17286)

Codes 96931, 96932, 96933, 96934, 96935, 96936 describe the acquisition and/or diagnostic interpretation of the device generated stitched image mosaics related to a single lesion. Do not report 96931, 96932, 96933, 96934, 96935, 96936 for a reflectance confocal microscopy examination that does not produce mosaic images. For services rendered using reflectance confocal microscopy not generating mosaic images, use 96999.

(For optical coherence tomography [OCT] for microstructural and morphological imaging of skin, see 0470T, 0471T)

96931 Reflectance confocal microscopy (RCM) for cellular and sub-cellular imaging of skin; image acquisition and interpretation and report, first lesion
CPT Changes: An Insider's View 2016
CPT Assistant Sep 17:9

96932 image acquisition only, first lesion
CPT Changes: An Insider's View 2016
CPT Assistant Sep 17:9

96933 interpretation and report only, first lesion
CPT Changes: An Insider's View 2016
CPT Assistant Sep 17:9

+ 96934 image acquisition and interpretation and report, each additional lesion (List separately in addition to code for primary procedure)
CPT Changes: An Insider's View 2016
CPT Assistant Sep 17:9

(Use 96934 in conjunction with 96931)

+ 96935 image acquisition only, each additional lesion (List separately in addition to code for primary procedure)
CPT Changes: An Insider's View 2016
CPT Assistant Sep 17:9

(Use 96935 in conjunction with 96932)

+ 96936 interpretation and report only, each additional lesion (List separately in addition to code for primary procedure)
CPT Changes: An Insider's View 2016
CPT Assistant Sep 17:9

(Use 96936 in conjunction with 96933)

96999 Unlisted special dermatological service or procedure
CPT Assistant Jul 12:9, May 13:12, Sep 17:9

Physical Medicine and Rehabilitation

Codes 97010-97763 should be used to report each distinct procedure performed. Do not append modifier 51 to 97010-97763.

The work of the physician or other qualified health care professional consists of face-to-face time with the patient (and caregiver, if applicable) delivering skilled services. For the purpose of determining the total time of a service, incremental intervals of treatment at the same visit may be accumulated.

The meanings of terms in the Physical Medicine and Rehabilitation section are not the same as those in the Evaluation and Management Services section (99201-99350). Do not use the Definitions of Commonly Used Terms in the Evaluation and Management (E/M) Guidelines for Physical Medicine and Rehabilitation services.

(For muscle testing, range of joint motion, electromyography, see 95831 et seq)

(For biofeedback training by EMG, use 90901)

►(For transcutaneous nerve stimulation [TENS], use 97014 for electrical stimulation requiring supervision only, or use 97032 for electrical stimulation requiring constant attendance)◄

Physical Therapy Evaluations

Physical therapy evaluations include a patient history and an examination with development of a plan of care, conducted by the physician or other qualified health care professional, which is based on the composite of the patient's presentation.

Coordination, consultation, and collaboration of care with physicians, other qualified health care professionals, or agencies is provided consistent with the nature of the problem(s) and the needs of the patient, family, and/or other caregivers.

At a minimum, each of the following components noted in the code descriptors must be documented, in order to report the selected level of physical therapy evaluation.

Physical therapy evaluations include the following components:

- History
- Examination
- Clinical decision making
- Development of plan of care

Report 97164 for performance of patient re-evaluation that is based on an established and ongoing plan of care.

Definitions

The level of the physical therapy evaluation performed is dependent on clinical decision making and on the nature of the patient's condition (severity). For the purpose of reporting physical therapy evaluations, the body regions and body systems are defined as follows:

Body regions: head, neck, back, lower extremities, upper extremities, and trunk.

Body systems: musculoskeletal, neuromuscular, cardiovascular pulmonary, and integumentary.

A review of body systems include the following:

- For the musculoskeletal system: the assessment of gross symmetry, gross range of motion, gross strength, height, and weight
- For the neuromuscular system: a general assessment of gross coordinated movement (eg, balance, gait, locomotion, transfers, and transitions) and motor function (motor control and motor learning)
- For the cardiovascular pulmonary system: the assessment of heart rate, respiratory rate, blood pressure, and edema
- For the integumentary system: the assessment of pliability (texture), presence of scar formation, skin color, and skin integrity

A review of any of the body systems also includes the assessment of the ability to make needs known, consciousness, orientation (person, place, and time), expected emotional/behavioral responses, and learning preferences (eg, learning barriers, education needs)

Body structures: The structural or anatomical parts of the body, such as organs, limbs, and their components, classified according to body systems.

Personal factors: Factors that include sex, age, coping styles, social background, education, profession, past and current experience, overall behavior pattern, character, and other factors that influence how disability is experienced by the individual. Personal factors that exist but do not impact the physical therapy plan of care are not to be considered, when selecting a level of service.

 # 97161 Physical therapy evaluation: low complexity, requiring these components:

- A history with no personal factors and/or comorbidities that impact the plan of care;
- An examination of body system(s) using standardized tests and measures addressing 1-2 elements from any of the following: body structures and functions, activity limitations, and/or participation restrictions;
- A clinical presentation with stable and/or uncomplicated characteristics; and
- Clinical decision making of low complexity using standardized patient assessment instrument and/or measurable assessment of functional outcome.

Typically, 20 minutes are spent face-to-face with the patient and/or family.

➲ *CPT Changes: An Insider's View* 2017

➲ *CPT Assistant* Aug 17:3

 # 97162 Physical therapy evaluation: moderate complexity, requiring these components:

- A history of present problem with 1-2 personal factors and/or comorbidities that impact the plan of care;
- An examination of body systems using standardized tests and measures in addressing a total of 3 or more elements from any of the following: body structures and functions, activity limitations, and/or participation restrictions;
- An evolving clinical presentation with changing characteristics; and
- Clinical decision making of moderate complexity using standardized patient assessment instrument and/or measurable assessment of functional outcome.

Typically, 30 minutes are spent face-to-face with the patient and/or family.

➲ *CPT Changes: An Insider's View* 2017

➲ *CPT Assistant* Aug 17:3

 # 97163 Physical therapy evaluation: high complexity, requiring these components:

- A history of present problem with 3 or more personal factors and/or comorbidities that impact the plan of care;
- An examination of body systems using standardized tests and measures addressing a total of 4 or more elements from any of the following: body structures and functions, activity limitations, and/or participation restrictions;
- A clinical presentation with unstable and unpredictable characteristics; and
- Clinical decision making of high complexity using standardized patient assessment instrument and/or measurable assessment of functional outcome.

Typically, 45 minutes are spent face-to-face with the patient and/or family.

➲ *CPT Changes: An Insider's View* 2017

➲ *CPT Assistant* Aug 17:3

 # 97164 Re-evaluation of physical therapy established plan of care, requiring these components:

- An examination including a review of history and use of standardized tests and measures is required; and
- Revised plan of care using a standardized patient assessment instrument and/or measurable assessment of functional outcome

Typically, 20 minutes are spent face-to-face with the patient and/or family.

➲ *CPT Changes: An Insider's View* 2017

➲ *CPT Assistant* Aug 17:3

Occupational Therapy Evaluations

Occupational therapy evaluations include an occupational profile, medical and therapy history, relevant assessments, and development of a plan of care, which reflects the therapist's clinical reasoning and interpretation of the data.

Coordination, consultation, and collaboration of care with physicians, other qualified health care professionals, or agencies is provided consistent with the nature of the problem(s) and the needs of the patient, family and/or other caregivers.

At a minimum, each of the following components noted in the code descriptors must be documented, in order to report the selected level of occupational therapy evaluation.

Occupational therapy evaluations include the following components:

- Occupational profile and client history (medical and therapy)
- Assessments of occupational performance
- Clinical decision making
- Development of plan of care

Report 97168 for performance of a re-evaluation that is based on an established and ongoing plan of care.

Definitions

The level of the occupational therapy evaluation performed is determined by patient condition, complexity of clinical decision making, and the scope and nature of the patient's performance deficits relating to physical, cognitive, or psychosocial skills to be assessed. The patient's plan of treatment should reflect assessment of each of the identified performance deficits.

Performance deficits: performance deficits refer to the inability to complete activities due to the lack of skills in one or more of the categories below (ie, relating to physical, cognitive, or psychosocial skills):

- ***Physical skills:*** Physical skills refer to impairments of body structure or body function (eg, balance, mobility, strength, endurance, fine or gross motor coordination, sensation, dexterity).
- ***Cognitive skills:*** Cognitive skills refer to the ability to attend, perceive, think, understand, problem solve, mentally sequence, learn, and remember resulting in the ability to organize occupational performance in a timely and safe manner. These skills are observed when: (1) a person attends to and selects, interacts with, and uses task tools and materials; (2) carries out individual actions and steps; and (3) modifies performance when problems are encountered.
- ***Psychosocial skills:*** Psychosocial skills refer to interpersonal interactions, habits, routines and behaviors, active use of coping strategies, and/or environmental adaptations to develop skills necessary to successfully and appropriately participate in everyday tasks and social situations.

 # 97165 Occupational therapy evaluation, low complexity, requiring these components:

- An occupational profile and medical and therapy history, which includes a brief history including review of medical and/or therapy records relating to the presenting problem;
- An assessment(s) that identifies 1-3 performance deficits (ie, relating to physical, cognitive, or psychosocial skills) that result in activity limitations and/or participation restrictions; and
- Clinical decision making of low complexity, which includes an analysis of the occupational profile, analysis of data from problem-focused assessment(s), and consideration of a limited number of treatment options. Patient presents with no comorbidities that affect occupational performance. Modification of tasks or assistance (eg, physical or verbal) with assessment(s) is not necessary to enable completion of evaluation component.

Typically, 30 minutes are spent face-to-face with the patient and/or family.

➲ *CPT Changes: An Insider's View* 2017
➲ *CPT Assistant* Feb 17:3

 # 97166 Occupational therapy evaluation, moderate complexity, requiring these components:

- An occupational profile and medical and therapy history, which includes an expanded review of medical and/or therapy records and additional review of physical, cognitive, or psychosocial history related to current functional performance;
- An assessment(s) that identifies 3-5 performance deficits (ie, relating to physical, cognitive, or psychosocial skills) that result in activity limitations and/or participation restrictions; and
- Clinical decision making of moderate analytic complexity, which includes an analysis of the occupational profile, analysis of data from detailed assessment(s), and consideration of several treatment options. Patient may present with comorbidities that affect occupational performance. Minimal to moderate modification of tasks or assistance (eg, physical or verbal) with assessment(s) is necessary to enable patient to complete evaluation component.

Typically, 45 minutes are spent face-to-face with the patient and/or family.

➲ *CPT Changes: An Insider's View* 2017
➲ *CPT Assistant* Feb 17:3

 # 97167 Occupational therapy evaluation, high complexity, requiring these components:

- An occupational profile and medical and therapy history, which includes review of medical and/or therapy records and extensive additional review of physical, cognitive, or psychosocial history related to current functional performance;
- An assessment(s) that identifies 5 or more performance deficits (ie, relating to physical, cognitive, or psychosocial skills) that result in activity limitations and/or participation restrictions; and
- Clinical decision making of high analytic complexity, which includes an analysis of the patient profile, analysis of data from comprehensive assessment(s), and consideration of multiple treatment options. Patient presents with comorbidities that affect occupational performance. Significant modification of tasks or assistance (eg, physical or verbal) with assessment(s) is necessary to enable patient to complete evaluation component.

Typically, 60 minutes are spent face-to-face with the patient and/or family.

➔ *CPT Changes: An Insider's View* 2017

➔ *CPT Assistant* Feb 17:3

 # 97168 Re-evaluation of occupational therapy established plan of care, requiring these components:

- An assessment of changes in patient functional or medical status with revised plan of care;
- An update to the initial occupational profile to reflect changes in condition or environment that affect future interventions and/or goals; and
- A revised plan of care. A formal reevaluation is performed when there is a documented change in functional status or a significant change to the plan of care is required.

Typically, 30 minutes are spent face-to-face with the patient and/or family.

➔ *CPT Changes: An Insider's View* 2017

➔ *CPT Assistant* Feb 17:3

Athletic Training Evaluations

Athletic training evaluations include a patient history and an examination with development of a plan of care, conducted by the physician or other qualified health care professional.

Coordination, consultation, and collaboration of care with physicians, other qualified health care professionals, or agencies is provided consistent with the nature of the problem(s) and the needs of the patient, family, and/or other caregivers.

At a minimum, each of the following components noted in the code descriptors must be documented, in order to report the selected level of athletic training evaluation.

Athletic training evaluations include the following components:

- History and physical activity profile
- Examination
- Clinical decision making
- Development of plan of care

Report 97172 for performance of patient re-evaluation that is based on an established and ongoing plan of care.

Definitions

For the purpose of reporting athletic training evaluations, the body areas and body systems are defined as follows:

Body areas: head, neck, back, lower extremities, upper extremities, and trunk.

Body systems: musculoskeletal, neuromuscular, cardiovascular pulmonary, and integumentary.

The body systems review includes the following:

- For the musculoskeletal system: the assessment of gross symmetry, gross range of motion, gross strength, height, and weight
- For the neuromuscular system: a general assessment of gross coordinated movement (eg, balance, gait, locomotion, transfers, and transitions) and motor function (motor control and motor learning)
- For the cardiovascular pulmonary system: the assessment of heart rate, respiratory rate, blood pressure, and edema
- For the integumentary system: the assessment of pliability (texture), presence of scar formation, skin color, and skin integrity

 # 97169 Athletic training evaluation, low complexity, requiring these components:

- A history and physical activity profile with no comorbidities that affect physical activity;
- An examination of affected body area and other symptomatic or related systems addressing 1-2 elements from any of the following: body structures, physical activity, and/or participation deficiencies; and
- Clinical decision making of low complexity using standardized patient assessment instrument and/or measurable assessment of functional outcome.

Typically, 15 minutes are spent face-to-face with the patient and/or family.

➔ *CPT Changes: An Insider's View* 2017

➔ *CPT Assistant* Jun 17:6

 # 97170 Athletic training evaluation, moderate complexity, requiring these components:

- A medical history and physical activity profile with 1-2 comorbidities that affect physical activity;
- An examination of affected body area and other symptomatic or related systems addressing a total of 3 or more elements from any of the following: body structures, physical activity, and/or participation deficiencies; and

- Clinical decision making of moderate complexity using standardized patient assessment instrument and/or measurable assessment of functional outcome.

Typically, 30 minutes are spent face-to-face with the patient and/or family.

➲ *CPT Changes: An Insider's View* 2017

➲ *CPT Assistant* Jun 17:6

 # 97171 Athletic training evaluation, high complexity, requiring these components:

- A medical history and physical activity profile, with 3 or more comorbidities that affect physical activity;
- A comprehensive examination of body systems using standardized tests and measures addressing a total of 4 or more elements from any of the following: body structures, physical activity, and/or participation deficiencies;
- Clinical presentation with unstable and unpredictable characteristics; and
- Clinical decision making of high complexity using standardized patient assessment instrument and/or measurable assessment of functional outcome.

Typically, 45 minutes are spent face-to-face with the patient and/or family.

➲ *CPT Changes: An Insider's View* 2017

➲ *CPT Assistant* Jun 17:6

 # 97172 Re-evaluation of athletic training established plan of care requiring these components:

- An assessment of patient's current functional status when there is a documented change; and
- A revised plan of care using a standardized patient assessment instrument and/or measurable assessment of functional outcome with an update in management options, goals, and interventions.

Typically, 20 minutes are spent face-to-face with the patient and/or family.

➲ *CPT Changes: An Insider's View* 2017

➲ *CPT Assistant* Jun 17:6

(97001, 97002, 97003, 97004, 97005, 97006 have been deleted. To report, see 97161-97172)

Modalities

Any physical agent applied to produce therapeutic changes to biologic tissue; includes but not limited to thermal, acoustic, light, mechanical, or electric energy.

Supervised

The application of a modality that does not require direct (one-on-one) patient contact.

97010 Application of a modality to 1 or more areas; hot or cold packs

➲ *CPT Assistant* Summer 95:5, Apr 96:11, Nov 97:47, Dec 98:1, Nov 01:5, Aug 02:11, Aug 06:11, Nov 09:10, Jun 10:8, Aug 10:13, Nov 10:8, Jun 16:9

97012 traction, mechanical

➲ *CPT Assistant* Summer 95:5, Apr 96:11, Nov 97:47, Dec 98:1, May 99:11, Nov 01:5, Aug 02:11, Dec 03:4, Oct 04:9, Jun 10:8, Aug 10:13, Nov 10:8, Jun 16:9

97014 electrical stimulation (unattended)

➲ *CPT Assistant* Summer 95:5, Apr 96:11, Nov 97:47, May 98:10, Nov 01:5, Jan 02:11, Apr 02:18, Aug 02:11, Dec 03:4, Nov 09:10, Jun 10:8, Aug 10:13, Nov 10:8, Aug 11:6

(For acupuncture with electrical stimulation, see 97813, 97814)

97016 vasopneumatic devices

➲ *CPT Assistant* Summer 95:6, Apr 96:11, Dec 98:1, Nov 01:5, Aug 02:11, May 05:14, Jun 10:8, Aug 10:13, Nov 10:8

97018 paraffin bath

➲ *CPT Assistant* Summer 95:6, Apr 96:11, Dec 98:1, Nov 01:5, Aug 02:11, Nov 09:10, Jun 10:8, Aug 10:13, Nov 10:8

97022 whirlpool

➲ *CPT Assistant* Summer 95:6, Apr 96:11, May 98:10, Dec 98:1, Nov 01:5, Aug 02:11, Nov 09:10, Jun 10:8, Aug 10:13, Nov 10:8

97024 diathermy (eg, microwave)

➲ *CPT Changes: An Insider's View* 2006

➲ *CPT Assistant* Summer 95:6, Apr 96:11, Dec 98:1, Nov 01:5, Aug 02:11, Nov 09:10, Jun 10:8, Aug 10:13, Nov 10:8

97026 infrared

➲ *CPT Assistant* Summer 95:6, Apr 96:11, Dec 98:1, Nov 01:5, Aug 02:11, Nov 09:10, Feb 10:12, Jun 10:8, Aug 10:13, Nov 10:8

97028 ultraviolet

➲ *CPT Assistant* Summer 95:6, Apr 96:11, Dec 98:1, Nov 01:5, Aug 02:11, Nov 09:10, Jun 10:8, Aug 10:13, Nov 10:8

Constant Attendance

The application of a modality that requires direct (one-on-one) patient contact.

97032 Application of a modality to 1 or more areas; electrical stimulation (manual), each 15 minutes

➲ *CPT Assistant* Summer 95:6, Dec 98:1, Nov 01:5, Apr 02:18, Jul 04:14, Nov 09:10, Jun 10:8, Aug 10:13, Nov 10:8

(For transcutaneous electrical modulation pain reprocessing [TEMPR/scrambler therapy], use 0278T)

97033 iontophoresis, each 15 minutes

➲ *CPT Assistant* Summer 95:7, Dec 98:1, Nov 01:5, Nov 09:10, Jun 10:8, Aug 10:13, Nov 10:8

97034 contrast baths, each 15 minutes

➲ *CPT Assistant* Summer 95:7, Dec 98:1, Nov 01:5, Jun 10:8, Aug 10:13, Nov 10:8

97035 ultrasound, each 15 minutes

➲ *CPT Assistant* Summer 95:7, Sep 96:10, Dec 98:1, Nov 01:5, Nov 09:10, Jun 10:8, Aug 10:13, Nov 10:8

97036 Hubbard tank, each 15 minutes

➲ *CPT Assistant* Summer 95:7, Dec 98:1, Nov 01:5, Nov 09:10, Jun 10:8, Aug 10:13, Nov 10:8

97039 Unlisted modality (specify type and time if constant attendance)

➔ *CPT Assistant* Summer 95:7, May 98:10, Dec 98:1, Jan 00:10, Nov 01:5, May 05:14, Nov 09:10, Feb 10:12, Jun 10:8, Aug 10:13, Nov 10:8, Jun 16:9, Nov 16:10

Therapeutic Procedures

A manner of effecting change through the application of clinical skills and/or services that attempt to improve function.

Physician or other qualified health care professional (ie, therapist) required to have direct (one-on-one) patient contact.

97110 Therapeutic procedure, 1 or more areas, each 15 minutes; therapeutic exercises to develop strength and endurance, range of motion and flexibility

➔ *CPT Assistant* Summer 95:7, Feb 97:10, Nov 98:37, Dec 99:11, Mar 05:11, Apr 05:14, Aug 05:11, Dec 05:8, Mar 06:15, Aug 06:11, May 08:13, Dec 09:15, May 10:9, Mar 12:9, Mar 14:15, Aug 14:6, Jun 16:9, Dec 17:15

97112 neuromuscular reeducation of movement, balance, coordination, kinesthetic sense, posture, and/or proprioception for sitting and/or standing activities

➔ *CPT Changes: An Insider's View* 2002

➔ *CPT Assistant* Summer 95:7, Feb 97:10, Apr 05:14, Aug 05:11, Mar 06:15, Aug 06:11, May 08:13, Oct 09:10, May 10:9, Mar 12:9, Mar 14:15

97113 aquatic therapy with therapeutic exercises

➔ *CPT Assistant* Summer 95:7, Feb 97:10, Apr 05:14, Mar 06:15, Aug 06:11, Oct 09:10, May 10:9, Mar 14:15

97116 gait training (includes stair climbing)

➔ *CPT Assistant* Summer 95:8, Sep 96:7, Feb 97:10, Jun 03:3, Apr 05:14, Mar 06:15, Aug 06:11, Oct 09:10, May 10:9, Mar 14:15

(Use 96000-96003 to report comprehensive gait and motion analysis procedures)

97124 massage, including effleurage, petrissage and/or tapotement (stroking, compression, percussion)

➔ *CPT Assistant* Summer 95:8, May 96:10, Feb 97:10, Dec 99:7, Apr 05:14, May 05:14, Mar 06:15, Aug 06:11, Oct 09:10, May 10:9, Mar 14:15, Jun 16:9

(For myofascial release, use 97140)

97127 Therapeutic interventions that focus on cognitive function (eg, attention, memory, reasoning, executive function, problem solving, and/or pragmatic functioning) and compensatory strategies to manage the performance of an activity (eg, managing time or schedules, initiating, organizing and sequencing tasks), direct (one-on-one) patient contact

➔ *CPT Changes: An Insider's View* 2018

(Report 97127 only once per day)

►(Do not report 97127 in conjunction with 97153, 97155)◄

97139 Unlisted therapeutic procedure (specify)

➔ *CPT Assistant* Summer 95:8, Feb 97:10, Apr 05:14, Aug 06:11, Mar 14:15

97140 Manual therapy techniques (eg, mobilization/manipulation, manual lymphatic drainage, manual traction), 1 or more regions, each 15 minutes

➔ *CPT Assistant* Nov 98:37, Feb 99:10, Mar 99:1, Jul 99:11, Aug 01:10, Dec 03:5, May 09:9, Oct 09:10, Mar 14:15, Mar 15:10, Aug 16:11, Sep 16:11, Nov 16:9

97150 Therapeutic procedure(s), group (2 or more individuals)

➔ *CPT Assistant* Summer 95:8, Dec 96:10, Feb 97:10, Oct 99:10, Nov 99:54-55, Dec 99:11, Apr 05:14, Aug 06:11, Mar 14:15, Nov 16:9

(Report 97150 for each member of group)

(Group therapy procedures involve constant attendance of the physician or other qualified health care professional [ie, therapist], but by definition do not require one-on-one patient contact by the same physician or other qualified health care professional)

(For manipulation under general anesthesia, see appropriate anatomic section in **Musculoskeletal System**)

(For osteopathic manipulative treatment [OMT], see 98925-98929)

►(Do not report 97150 in conjunction with 97154, 97158)◄

97151 Code is out of numerical sequence. See 96020-96112

97152 Code is out of numerical sequence. See 96020-96112

97153 Code is out of numerical sequence. See 96020-96112

97154 Code is out of numerical sequence. See 96020-96112

97155 Code is out of numerical sequence. See 96020-96112

97156 Code is out of numerical sequence. See 96020-96112

97157 Code is out of numerical sequence. See 96020-96112

97158 Code is out of numerical sequence. See 96020-96112

97161 Code is out of numerical sequence. See Physical Therapy Evaluations subsection

97162 Code is out of numerical sequence. See Physical Therapy Evaluations subsection

97163 Code is out of numerical sequence. See Physical Therapy Evaluations subsection

97164 Code is out of numerical sequence. See Physical Therapy Evaluations subsection

97165 Code is out of numerical sequence. See Occupational Therapy Evaluations subsection

97166 Code is out of numerical sequence. See Occupational Therapy Evaluations subsection

97167 Code is out of numerical sequence. See Occupational Therapy Evaluations subsection

97168 Code is out of numerical sequence. See Occupational Therapy Evaluations subsection

97169 Code is out of numerical sequence. See Athletic Training Evaluations subsection

97170 Code is out of numerical sequence. See Athletic Training Evaluations subsection

97171 Code is out of numerical sequence. See Athletic Training Evaluations subsection

97172 Code is out of numerical sequence. See Athletic Training Evaluations subsection

97530 Therapeutic activities, direct (one-on-one) patient contact (use of dynamic activities to improve functional performance), each 15 minutes

➲ *CPT Changes: An Insider's View* 2013

➲ *CPT Assistant* Summer 95:9, Dec 01:6, Apr 03:26, Jul 03:15, Aug 05:11, May 08:13, Mar 14:15

(97532 has been deleted. To report, use 97127)

97533 Sensory integrative techniques to enhance sensory processing and promote adaptive responses to environmental demands, direct (one-on-one) patient contact, each 15 minutes

➲ *CPT Changes: An Insider's View* 2001, 2013

➲ *CPT Assistant* Dec 01:1, Mar 14:15

97535 Self-care/home management training (eg, activities of daily living (ADL) and compensatory training, meal preparation, safety procedures, and instructions in use of assistive technology devices/adaptive equipment) direct one-on-one contact, each 15 minutes

➲ *CPT Changes: An Insider's View* 2002, 2013

➲ *CPT Assistant* Sep 96:7, Apr 00:11, Dec 03:6, Mar 14:15, Mar 15:10, Jun 15:11, Aug 16:3

97537 Community/work reintegration training (eg, shopping, transportation, money management, avocational activities and/or work environment/modification analysis, work task analysis, use of assistive technology device/adaptive equipment), direct one-on-one contact, each 15 minutes

➲ *CPT Changes: An Insider's View* 2004, 2013

➲ *CPT Assistant* Sep 96:7, Dec 03:6, Mar 14:15

(For wheelchair management/propulsion training, use 97542)

97542 Wheelchair management (eg, assessment, fitting, training), each 15 minutes

➲ *CPT Changes: An Insider's View* 2006

➲ *CPT Assistant* Sep 96:8, Mar 14:15, Jun 15:11

97545 Work hardening/conditioning; initial 2 hours

➲ *CPT Assistant* Apr 03:26, Jul 03:15, May 08:13, Mar 14:15

+ 97546 each additional hour (List separately in addition to code for primary procedure)

➲ *CPT Assistant* Mar 14:15

(Use 97546 in conjunction with 97545)

Active Wound Care Management

Active wound care procedures are performed to remove devitalized and/or necrotic tissue and promote healing. Chemical cauterization (17250) to achieve wound hemostasis is included in active wound care procedures (97597, 97598, 97602) and should not be separately reported for the same lesion. Services require direct (one-on-one) contact with the patient.

(Do not report 97597-97602 in conjunction with 11042-11047 for the same wound)

(For debridement of burn wounds, see 16020-16030)

97597 Debridement (eg, high pressure waterjet with/without suction, sharp selective debridement with scissors, scalpel and forceps), open wound, (eg, fibrin, devitalized epidermis and/or dermis, exudate, debris, biofilm), including topical application(s), wound assessment, use of a whirlpool, when performed and instruction(s) for ongoing care, per session, total wound(s) surface area; first 20 sq cm or less

➲ *CPT Changes: An Insider's View* 2005, 2011

➲ *CPT Assistant* Jun 05:1, 10, Nov 09:10, Jun 10:8, Nov 10:9, May 11:3, Sep 11:11, Jan 12:8, Mar 12:11, Oct 12:3, Jun 14:11, Aug 16:9, Oct 16:3

+ 97598 each additional 20 sq cm, or part thereof (List separately in addition to code for primary procedure)

➲ *CPT Changes: An Insider's View* 2005, 2011

➲ *CPT Assistant* Jun 05:1, 10, May 11:3, Sep 11:11, Jan 12:8, Mar 12:11, Jun 14:11, Aug 16:9, Oct 16:3

(Use 97598 in conjunction with 97597)

97602 Removal of devitalized tissue from wound(s), non-selective debridement, without anesthesia (eg, wet-to-moist dressings, enzymatic, abrasion, larval therapy), including topical application(s), wound assessment, and instruction(s) for ongoing care, per session

➲ *CPT Changes: An Insider's View* 2001, 2017

➲ *CPT Assistant* May 02:5, Jun 05:1, 10, Sep 08:11, May 11:4, Aug 11:7, Jan 12:9, Mar 12:11, Dec 12:15, Jun 14:11, Oct 16:3

97605 Negative pressure wound therapy (eg, vacuum assisted drainage collection), utilizing durable medical equipment (DME), including topical application(s), wound assessment, and instruction(s) for ongoing care, per session; total wound(s) surface area less than or equal to 50 square centimeters

➲ *CPT Changes: An Insider's View* 2005, 2015

➲ *CPT Assistant* Apr 05:13, Jun 05:1, 10, May 11:4, Nov 14:8, Feb 16:14

97606 total wound(s) surface area greater than 50 square centimeters

➲ *CPT Changes: An Insider's View* 2005, 2015

➲ *CPT Assistant* Apr 05:13, Jun 05:1, 10, May 11:4, Nov 14:8, Feb 16:14

97607 Negative pressure wound therapy, (eg, vacuum assisted drainage collection), utilizing disposable, non-durable medical equipment including provision of exudate management collection system, topical application(s), wound assessment, and instructions for ongoing care, per session; total wound(s) surface area less than or equal to 50 square centimeters

➲ *CPT Changes: An Insider's View* 2015

➲ *CPT Assistant* Nov 14:8

97608 total wound(s) surface area greater than 50 square centimeters
➲ *CPT Changes: An Insider's View* 2015
➲ *CPT Assistant* Nov 14:8

(Do not report 97607, 97608 in conjunction with 97605, 97606)

97610 Low frequency, non-contact, non-thermal ultrasound, including topical application(s), when performed, wound assessment, and instruction(s) for ongoing care, per day
➲ *CPT Changes: An Insider's View* 2014
➲ *CPT Assistant* Jun 14:11

Tests and Measurements

Requires direct one-on-one patient contact.

(For muscle testing, manual or electrical, joint range of motion, electromyography, or nerve velocity determination, see 95831-95857, 95860-95872, 95885-95887, 95907-95913)

97750 Physical performance test or measurement (eg, musculoskeletal, functional capacity), with written report, each 15 minutes
➲ *CPT Assistant* Summer 95:5, Feb 97:10, Aug 98:11, Mar 00:11, Nov 01:5, May 02:18, Apr 03:28, Dec 03:7, Feb 04:5, Feb 07:12, May 08:9, Aug 13:7

97755 Assistive technology assessment (eg, to restore, augment or compensate for existing function, optimize functional tasks and/or maximize environmental accessibility), direct one-on-one contact, with written report, each 15 minutes
➲ *CPT Changes: An Insider's View* 2004, 2013

(To report augmentative and alternative communication devices, see 92605, 92607)

Orthotic Management and Training and Prosthetic Training

97760 Orthotic(s) management and training (including assessment and fitting when not otherwise reported), upper extremity(ies), lower extremity(ies) and/or trunk, initial orthotic(s) encounter, each 15 minutes
➲ *CPT Changes: An Insider's View* 2006, 2018
➲ *CPT Assistant* Dec 05:8, 11, Feb 07:8

(Code 97760 should not be reported with 97116 for the same extremity[ies])

97761 Prosthetic(s) training, upper and/or lower extremity(ies), initial prosthetic(s) encounter, each 15 minutes
➲ *CPT Changes: An Insider's View* 2006, 2018
➲ *CPT Assistant* Dec 05:8, 11, Feb 07:8

(97762 has been deleted. To report, use 97763)

97763 Orthotic(s)/prosthetic(s) management and/or training, upper extremity(ies), lower extremity(ies), and/or trunk, subsequent orthotic(s)/prosthetic(s) encounter, each 15 minutes
➲ *CPT Changes: An Insider's View* 2018

(Do not report 97763 in conjunction with 97760, 97761)

Other Procedures

(For extracorporeal shock wave musculoskeletal therapy, see 0101T, 0102T)

97799 Unlisted physical medicine/rehabilitation service or procedure
➲ *CPT Assistant* Summer 95:5, Oct 99:10, Nov 16:10

Medical Nutrition Therapy

★ **97802** Medical nutrition therapy; initial assessment and intervention, individual, face-to-face with the patient, each 15 minutes
➲ *CPT Changes: An Insider's View* 2001, 2017
➲ *CPT Assistant* Apr 03:10, Nov 03:1, Feb 09:13

★ **97803** re-assessment and intervention, individual, face-to-face with the patient, each 15 minutes
➲ *CPT Changes: An Insider's View* 2001, 2017
➲ *CPT Assistant* Apr 03:10, Nov 03:1, Feb 09:13

★ **97804** group (2 or more individual(s)), each 30 minutes
➲ *CPT Changes: An Insider's View* 2001, 2017
➲ *CPT Assistant* Apr 03:10, Nov 03:1, Feb 09:13

(Physicians and other qualified health care professionals who may report evaluation and management services should use the appropriate evaluation and management codes)

Acupuncture

Acupuncture is reported based on 15-minute increments of personal (face-to-face) contact with the patient, not the duration of acupuncture needle(s) placement.

If no electrical stimulation is used during a 15-minute increment, use 97810, 97811. If electrical stimulation of any needle is used during a 15-minute increment, use 97813, 97814.

Only one code may be reported for each 15-minute increment. Use either 97810 or 97813 for the initial 15-minute increment. Only one initial code is reported per day.

Evaluation and management services may be reported in addition to acupuncture procedures when performed by physicians or other health care professionals, who may report evaluation and management services, including new or established patient office or other outpatient services (99201-99215), hospital observation care (99217-99220, 99224-99226), hospital care (99221-99223, 99231-99233), office or other outpatient consultations (99241-99245), inpatient consultations (99251-99255), critical care services (99291, 99292), inpatient neonatal intensive care services and pediatric and neonatal critical care services (99466-99480), emergency department services (99281-99285), nursing facility services (99304-99318), domiciliary, rest home, or custodial care services (99324-99337), and home services (99341-99350) may be reported separately using modifier 25 if the patient's condition requires a significant, separately identifiable E/M service above and beyond the usual preservice and postservice work associated with the acupuncture services. The time of the E/M service is not included in the time of the acupuncture service.

97810 Acupuncture, 1 or more needles; without electrical stimulation, initial 15 minutes of personal one-on-one contact with the patient

➲ *CPT Changes: An Insider's View* 2005

➲ *CPT Assistant* Jan 05:16-17, Jun 05:5, Jun 06:20, Aug 06:4

(Do not report 97810 in conjunction with 97813)

+ 97811 without electrical stimulation, each additional 15 minutes of personal one-on-one contact with the patient, with re-insertion of needle(s) (List separately in addition to code for primary procedure)

➲ *CPT Changes: An Insider's View* 2005, 2006

➲ *CPT Assistant* Jan 05:16, Jun 05:5, Aug 06:4

(Use 97811 in conjunction with 97810, 97813)

Acupuncture, Needle
97810-97811

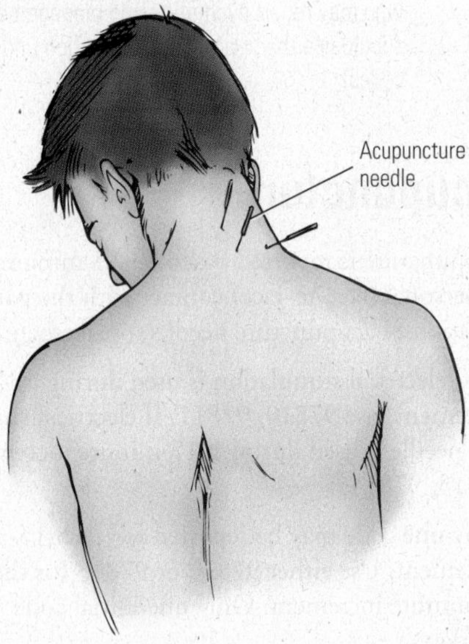

97813 with electrical stimulation, initial 15 minutes of personal one-on-one contact with the patient

➲ *CPT Changes: An Insider's View* 2005, 2006

➲ *CPT Assistant* Jan 05:16-18, Jun 05:5, Jun 06:20, Aug 06:4

(Do not report 97813 in conjunction with 97810)

+ 97814 with electrical stimulation, each additional 15 minutes of personal one-on-one contact with the patient, with re-insertion of needle(s) (List separately in addition to code for primary procedure)

➲ *CPT Changes: An Insider's View* 2005, 2006

➲ *CPT Assistant* Jan 05:16, Jun 05:5, Aug 06:4

(Use 97814 in conjunction with 97810, 97813)

Osteopathic Manipulative Treatment

Osteopathic manipulative treatment (OMT) is a form of manual treatment applied by a physician or other qualified health care professional to eliminate or alleviate somatic dysfunction and related disorders. This treatment may be accomplished by a variety of techniques.

Evaluation and Management services including new or established patient office or other outpatient services (99201-99215), hospital observation care (99217-99220, 99224-99226), hospital care (99221-99223, 99231-99233), critical care services (99291, 99292), observation or inpatient care services (99234-99236), office or other outpatient consultations (99241-99245), emergency department services (99281-99285), nursing facility services (99304-99318), domiciliary, rest home, or custodial care services (99324-99337), and home services (99341-99350) may be reported separately using modifier 25 if the patient's condition requires a significant, separately identifiable E/M service above and beyond the usual preservice and postservice work associated with the procedure. The E/M service may be caused or prompted by the same symptoms or condition for which the OMT service was provided. As such, different diagnoses are not required for the reporting of the OMT and E/M service on the same date.

Body regions referred to are: head region; cervical region; thoracic region; lumbar region; sacral region; pelvic region; lower extremities; upper extremities; rib cage region; abdomen and viscera region.

98925 Osteopathic manipulative treatment (OMT); 1-2 body regions involved

➲ *CPT Assistant* May 96:10, Jan 97:8, 10, Jul 98:10, Aug 00:11, Dec 00:15, Oct 09:10, Dec 17:15

98926 3-4 body regions involved

➲ *CPT Assistant* May 96:10, Jan 97:8, Aug 00:11, Dec 00:15, Oct 09:10

98927 5-6 body regions involved

➲ *CPT Assistant* May 96:10, Jan 97:8, Aug 00:11, Dec 00:15, Oct 09:10

98928 7-8 body regions involved

➲ *CPT Assistant* May 96:10, Jan 97:8, Aug 00:11, Dec 00:15, Oct 09:10, Mar 12:14, May 12:14

98929 9-10 body regions involved

➲ *CPT Assistant* May 96:10, Jan 97:8, 10, Aug 00:11, Oct 09:10

Chiropractic Manipulative Treatment

Chiropractic manipulative treatment (CMT) is a form of manual treatment to influence joint and neurophysiological function. This treatment may be accomplished using a variety of techniques.

The chiropractic manipulative treatment codes include a pre-manipulation patient assessment. Additional evaluation and management services including office or other outpatient services (99201-99215), subsequent observation care (99224-99226), subsequent hospital care (99231-99233), office or other outpatient consultations (99241-99245), subsequent nursing facility services (99307-99310), domiciliary, rest home, or custodial care services (99324-99337), and home services (99341-99350) may be reported separately using modifier 25 if the patient's condition requires a significant, separately identifiable E/M service above and beyond the usual preservice and postservice work associated with the procedure. The E/M service may be caused or prompted by the same symptoms or condition for which the CMT service was provided. As such, different diagnoses are not required for the reporting of the CMT and E/M service on the same date.

For purposes of CMT, the five spinal regions referred to are: cervical region (includes atlanto-occipital joint); thoracic region (includes costovertebral and costotransverse joints); lumbar region; sacral region; and pelvic (sacro-iliac joint) region. The five extraspinal regions referred to are: head (including temporomandibular joint, excluding atlanto-occipital) region; lower extremities; upper extremities; rib cage (excluding costotransverse and costovertebral joints) and abdomen.

98940 Chiropractic manipulative treatment (CMT); spinal, 1-2 regions

➲ *CPT Assistant* Jan 97:7, 11, Feb 99:10, Dec 00:15, Mar 06:15, Dec 07:16, 17, Oct 09:10, May 10:9, Dec 13:15

98941 spinal, 3-4 regions

➲ *CPT Assistant* Jan 97:7, 11, Mar 97:10, Feb 99:10, Dec 00:15, Mar 06:15, Dec 07:16, 17, Oct 09:10, May 10:9

98942 spinal, 5 regions

➲ *CPT Assistant* Jan 97:7, 11, Feb 99:10, Dec 00:15, Mar 06:15, Dec 07:16, 17, Oct 09:10, May 10:9

98943 extraspinal, 1 or more regions

➲ *CPT Assistant* Jan 97:7, 11, Mar 97:10, Feb 99:10, Dec 00:15, Mar 06:15, Dec 07:16, 17, Oct 09:10, May 10:9, Dec 13:15

Education and Training for Patient Self-Management

The following codes are used to report educational and training services prescribed by a physician or other qualified health care professional and provided by a qualified, nonphysician health care professional using a standardized curriculum to an individual or a group of patients for the treatment of established illness(s)/disease(s) or to delay comorbidity(s). Education and training for patient self-management may be reported with these codes only when using a standardized curriculum as described below. This curriculum may be modified as necessary for the clinical needs, cultural norms and health literacy of the individual patient(s).

The purpose of the educational and training services is to teach the patient (may include caregiver[s]) how to effectively self-manage the patient's illness(s)/disease(s) or delay disease comorbidity(s) in conjunction with the patient's professional healthcare team. Education and training related to subsequent reinforcement or due to changes in the patient's condition or treatment plan are reported in the same manner as the original education and training. The type of education and training provided for the patient's clinical condition will be identified by the appropriate diagnosis code(s) reported.

The qualifications of the nonphysician healthcare professionals and the content of the educational and training program must be consistent with guidelines or standards established or recognized by a physician society, nonphysician healthcare professional society/association, or other appropriate source.

(For counseling and education provided by a physician to an individual, see the appropriate evaluation and management codes including office or other outpatient services [99201-99215], hospital observation care [99217-99220, 99224-99226], hospital care [99221-99223, 99231-99233], new or established patient office or other outpatient consultations [99241-99245], inpatient consultations [99251-99255], emergency department services [99281-99285], nursing facility services [99304-99318], domiciliary, rest home, or custodial care services [99324-99337], home services [99341-99350], and counseling risk factor reduction and behavior change intervention [99401-99429]. See also **Instructions for Use of the CPT Codebook** for definition of reporting qualifications)

(For counseling and education provided by a physician to a group, use 99078)

(For counseling and/or risk factor reduction intervention provided by a physician to patient[s] without symptoms or established disease, see 99401-99412)

(For medical nutrition therapy, see 97802-97804)

(For health and behavior assessment/intervention that is not part of a standardized curriculum, see 96150-96155)

(For education provided as genetic counseling services, use 96040. For education to a group regarding genetic risks, see 98961, 98962)

★ **98960** Education and training for patient self-management by a qualified, nonphysician health care professional using a standardized curriculum, face-to-face with the patient (could include caregiver/family) each 30 minutes; individual patient

➲ *CPT Changes: An Insider's View* 2006, 2017

➲ *CPT Assistant* Apr 13:3, Nov 13:3, Oct 14:3

★ **98961** 2-4 patients

➲ *CPT Changes: An Insider's View* 2006, 2017

➲ *CPT Assistant* Aug 07:9, Aug 08:3, Feb 09:13, Apr 13:3

★ **98962** 5-8 patients

➲ *CPT Changes: An Insider's View* 2006, 2017

➲ *CPT Assistant* Aug 07:9, Aug 08:3, Feb 09:13, Apr 13:3, Nov 13:3, Oct 14:3

Non-Face-to-Face Nonphysician Services

Telephone Services

Telephone services are non-face-to-face assessment and management services provided by a qualified health care professional to a patient using the telephone. These codes are used to report episodes of care by the qualified health care professional initiated by an established patient or guardian of an established patient. If the telephone service ends with a decision to see the patient within 24 hours or the next available urgent visit appointment, the code is not reported; rather the encounter is considered part of the preservice work of the subsequent assessment and management service, procedure, and visit. Likewise, if the telephone call refers to a service performed and reported by the qualified health care professional within the previous seven days (either qualified health care professional requested or unsolicited patient follow-up) or within the postoperative period of the previously completed procedure, then the service(s) are considered part of that previous service or procedure. (Do not report 98966-98969 if reporting 98966-98969 performed in the previous seven days.)

(For telephone services provided by a physician, see 99441-99443)

98966 Telephone assessment and management service provided by a qualified nonphysician health care professional to an established patient, parent, or guardian not originating from a related assessment and management service provided within the previous 7 days nor leading to an assessment and management service or procedure within the next 24 hours or soonest available appointment; 5-10 minutes of medical discussion

➲ *CPT Changes: An Insider's View* 2008

➲ *CPT Assistant* Apr 13:3, Oct 13:11, Nov 13:3, Oct 14:3, Mar 18:7

98967 11-20 minutes of medical discussion

➲ *CPT Changes: An Insider's View* 2008

➲ *CPT Assistant* Apr 13:3, Oct 13:11, Mar 18:7

98968 21-30 minutes of medical discussion

➲ *CPT Changes: An Insider's View* 2008

➲ *CPT Assistant* Apr 13:3, Oct 13:11, Nov 13:3, Oct 14:3, Mar 18:7

(Do not report 98966-98968 during the same month with 99487-99489)

(Do not report 98966-98968 when performed during the service time of codes 99495, 99496)

(Do not report 98966, 98967, 98968 in conjunction with 93792, 93793)

On-line Medical Evaluation

An on-line electronic medical evaluation is a non-face-to-face assessment and management service by a qualified health care professional to a patient using Internet resources in response to a patient's on-line inquiry. Reportable services involve the qualified health care professional's personal timely response to the patient's inquiry and must involve permanent storage (electronic or hard copy) of the encounter. This service is reported only once for the same episode of care during a seven-day period, although multiple qualified health care professionals could report their exchange with the same patient. If the on-line medical evaluation refers to an assessment and management service previously performed and reported by the qualified health care professional within the previous seven days (either qualified health care professional requested or unsolicited patient follow-up) or within the postoperative period of the previously completed procedure, then the service(s) are considered covered by the previous assessment and management office service or procedure. A reportable service encompasses the sum of communication (eg, related telephone calls, prescription provision, laboratory orders) pertaining to the on-line patient encounter.

(For an on-line medical evaluation provided by a physician, use 99444)

98969 Online assessment and management service provided by a qualified nonphysician health care professional to an established patient or guardian, not originating from a related assessment and management service provided within the previous 7 days, using the Internet or similar electronic communications network

➲ *CPT Changes: An Insider's View* 2008, 2013

➲ *CPT Assistant* Apr 13:3, Oct 13:11, Nov 13:3, Oct 14:3, Mar 18:7

(Do not report 98969 when using 99339-99340, 99374-99380 for the same communication[s])

(Do not report 98969 for home and outpatient INR monitoring when reporting 93792, 93793)

(Do not report 98969 during the same month with 99487-99489)

(Do not report 98969 when performed during the service time of codes 99495, 99496)

Special Services, Procedures and Reports

►The procedures with code numbers 99000 through 99082 provide the reporting physician or other qualified health care professional with the means to identify the completion of special reports and services that are an adjunct to the basic services rendered. The specific number assigned indicates the special circumstances under which a basic procedure is performed.◄

Codes 99050-99060 are reported in addition to an associated basic service. Do not append modifier 51 to 99050-99060. Typically only a single adjunct code from among 99050-99060 would be reported per patient encounter. However, there may be circumstances in which reporting multiple adjunct codes per patient encounter may be appropriate.

Miscellaneous Services

99000 Handling and/or conveyance of specimen for transfer from the office to a laboratory
- *CPT Changes: An Insider's View* 2013
- *CPT Assistant* Winter 94:26, Feb 99:10, Oct 99:11, May 02:19, Aug 06:6, Sep 06:15, Jan 07:30

99001 Handling and/or conveyance of specimen for transfer from the patient in other than an office to a laboratory (distance may be indicated)
- *CPT Changes: An Insider's View* 2013
- *CPT Assistant* Winter 94:26, May 02:19, Aug 06:6, Sep 06:15, Jan 07:30

99002 Handling, conveyance, and/or any other service in connection with the implementation of an order involving devices (eg, designing, fitting, packaging, handling, delivery or mailing) when devices such as orthotics, protectives, prosthetics are fabricated by an outside laboratory or shop but which items have been designed, and are to be fitted and adjusted by the attending physician or other qualified health care professional
- *CPT Changes: An Insider's View* 2013
- *CPT Assistant* Winter 94:26, May 02:19, Aug 06:6, Sep 06:15, Jan 07:30

(For routine collection of venous blood, use 36415)

99024 Postoperative follow-up visit, normally included in the surgical package, to indicate that an evaluation and management service was performed during a postoperative period for a reason(s) related to the original procedure
- *CPT Changes: An Insider's View* 2004
- *CPT Assistant* Winter 94:26, Sep 97:10, Aug 98:5, May 02:19, Nov 03:13, Aug 06:6, Sep 06:15, Jan 07:30, Mar 15:3, Jan 17:3, Jul 17:9

(As a component of a surgical "package," see **Surgery Guidelines**)

99026 Hospital mandated on call service; in-hospital, each hour
- *CPT Changes: An Insider's View* 2003
- *CPT Assistant* Jun 03:10, Aug 06:6, Sep 06:15, Jan 07:30

99027 out-of-hospital, each hour
- *CPT Changes: An Insider's View* 2003
- *CPT Assistant* Jun 03:10, Aug 06:6, Sep 06:15, Jan 07:30

(For standby services requiring prolonged attendance, use 99360, as appropriate. Time spent performing separately reportable procedure(s) or service(s) should not be included in the time reported as mandated on-call service)

99050 Services provided in the office at times other than regularly scheduled office hours, or days when the office is normally closed (eg, holidays, Saturday or Sunday), in addition to basic service
- *CPT Changes: An Insider's View* 2004, 2006
- *CPT Assistant* Winter 94:27, May 02:19, Jun 03:10, May 06:18, Aug 06:6, Sep 06:15, Jan 07:30, Aug 10:9

99051 Service(s) provided in the office during regularly scheduled evening, weekend, or holiday office hours, in addition to basic service
- *CPT Changes: An Insider's View* 2006
- *CPT Assistant* May 06:18, Aug 06:6, Sep 06:15, Jan 07:30, Aug 10:9

99053 Service(s) provided between 10:00 PM and 8:00 AM at 24-hour facility, in addition to basic service
- *CPT Changes: An Insider's View* 2006
- *CPT Assistant* May 06:18, Aug 06:6, Sep 06:15, Jan 07:30

99056 Service(s) typically provided in the office, provided out of the office at request of patient, in addition to basic service
- *CPT Changes: An Insider's View* 2006
- *CPT Assistant* Winter 94:27, May 02:19, May 06:18, Aug 06:6, Sep 06:15, Jan 07:30

99058 Service(s) provided on an emergency basis in the office, which disrupts other scheduled office services, in addition to basic service
- *CPT Changes: An Insider's View* 2006
- *CPT Assistant* Winter 94:27, May 02:19, May 06:18, Aug 06:6, Sep 06:15, Jan 07:30, Aug 10:9

99060 Service(s) provided on an emergency basis, out of the office, which disrupts other scheduled office services, in addition to basic service
- *CPT Changes: An Insider's View* 2006
- *CPT Assistant* May 06:18, Aug 06:6, Sep 06:15, Jan 07:30

99070 Supplies and materials (except spectacles), provided by the physician or other qualified health care professional over and above those usually included with the office visit or other services rendered (list drugs, trays, supplies, or materials provided)
- *CPT Changes: An Insider's View* 2013
- *CPT Assistant* Winter 94:28, May 98:10, Jun 99:10, Jun 00:11, Jul 01:2, May 02:19, Aug 02:11, Jun 05:1, Jul 06:1, Aug 06:6, Sep 06:15, Jan 07:30, 31, Feb 07:8, Sep 08:11, May 09:8, Sep 09:5, May 10:10, Jun 10:8, Sep 10:11, Apr 12:10, Nov 12:11, Mar 13:6, Dec 13:12, Mar 14:11, Jan 17:6, Sep 17:15, Jan 18:3, Mar 18:7

(For supply of spectacles, use the appropriate supply codes)

99071 Educational supplies, such as books, tapes, and pamphlets, for the patient's education at cost to physician or other qualified health care professional
- *CPT Changes: An Insider's View* 2013
- *CPT Assistant* Winter 94:28, May 02:19, Aug 06:6, Sep 06:15, Jan 07:30, Apr 13:3, Nov 13:3, Oct 14:3

Medicine / Special Services, Procedures and Reports 99000-99082

99075 Medical testimony

➲ *CPT Assistant* Winter 94:28, May 02:19, Aug 06:6, Sep 06:15, Jan 07:30

99078 Physician or other qualified health care professional qualified by education, training, licensure/regulation (when applicable) educational services rendered to patients in a group setting (eg, prenatal, obesity, or diabetic instructions)

➲ *CPT Changes: An Insider's View* 2013

➲ *CPT Assistant* Winter 94:28, Jan 98:12, May 02:19, Aug 06:6, Sep 06:15, Jan 07:30, Aug 07:9, Apr 13:3, Nov 13:3, Oct 14:3

99080 Special reports such as insurance forms, more than the information conveyed in the usual medical communications or standard reporting form

➲ *CPT Assistant* Winter 94:28, May 02:19, Aug 06:6, Sep 06:15, Jan 07:30, Apr 13:3, Nov 13:3, Oct 14:3

(Do not report 99080 in conjunction with 99455, 99456 for the completion of Workmen's Compensation forms)

99082 Unusual travel (eg, transportation and escort of patient)

➲ *CPT Assistant* May 02:19, Jan 03:24, Nov 03:14, Aug 06:6, Sep 06:15, Jan 07:30

►(99090 has been deleted)◄

99091 Code is out of numerical sequence. See 99448-99455

Qualifying Circumstances for Anesthesia

(For explanation of these services, see **Anesthesia Guidelines**)

+ 99100 Anesthesia for patient of extreme age, younger than 1 year and older than 70 (List separately in addition to code for primary anesthesia procedure)

➲ *CPT Assistant* Apr 08:3, Dec 17:8

(For procedure performed on infants younger than 1 year of age at time of surgery, see 00326, 00561, 00834, 00836)

+ 99116 Anesthesia complicated by utilization of total body hypothermia (List separately in addition to code for primary anesthesia procedure)

➲ *CPT Assistant* Apr 08:3, Dec 17:8

+ 99135 Anesthesia complicated by utilization of controlled hypotension (List separately in addition to code for primary anesthesia procedure)

➲ *CPT Assistant* Apr 08:3, Dec 17:8

+ 99140 Anesthesia complicated by emergency conditions (specify) (List separately in addition to code for primary anesthesia procedure)

➲ *CPT Assistant* Mar 01:10, Apr 08:3, Dec 17:8

(An emergency is defined as existing when delay in treatment of the patient would lead to a significant increase in the threat to life or body part)

Moderate (Conscious) Sedation

Moderate (also known as conscious) sedation is a drug-induced depression of consciousness during which patients respond purposefully to verbal commands, either alone or accompanied by light tactile stimulation. No interventions are required to maintain cardiovascular function or a patent airway, and spontaneous ventilation is adequate.

Moderate sedation codes 99151, 99152, 99153, 99155, 99156, 99157 are not used to report administration of medications for pain control, minimal sedation (anxiolysis), deep sedation, or monitored anesthesia care (00100-01999).

For purposes of reporting, intraservice time of moderate sedation is used to select the appropriate code(s). The following definitions are used to determine intraservice time (compared to pre- and postservice time).

An independent trained observer is an individual who is qualified to monitor the patient during the procedure, who has no other duties (eg, assisting at surgery) during the procedure.

Preservice Work

The preservice activities required for moderate sedation are included in the work described by each of these codes (99151, 99152, 99153, 99155, 99156, 99157) and are not reported separately. The following preservice work components are not included when determining intra-service time for reporting:

- Assessment of the patient's past medical and surgical history with particular emphasis on cardiovascular, pulmonary, airway, or neurological conditions;
- Review of the patient's previous experiences with anesthesia and/or sedation;
- Family history of sedation complications;
- Summary of the patient's present medication list;
- Drug allergy and intolerance history;
- Focused physical examination of the patient with emphasis on:
  - Mouth, jaw, oropharynx, neck and airway for Mallampati score assessment;
  - Chest and lungs;
  - Heart and circulation;
- Vital signs, including heart rate, respiratory rate, blood pressure, and oxygenation with end tidal CO2 when indicated;
- Review of any pre-sedation diagnostic tests;
- Completion of a pre-sedation assessment form (with an American Society of Anesthesiologists [ASA] Physical Status classification);

		Moderate sedation (MS) provided by physician or other qualified health care professional (same physician or qualified health care professional also performing the procedure MS is supporting)	MS provided by different physician or other qualified health care professional (not the physician or qualified health care professional who is performing the procedure MS is supporting)
Total Intra-service Time for Moderate Sedation	**Patient Age**	**Code(s)**	**Code(s)**
Less than 10 minutes	Any age	Not reported separately	Not reported separately
10-22 minutes	< 5 years	99151	99155
10-22 minutes	5 years or older	99152	99156
23-37 minutes	< 5 years	99151 + 99153 X 1	99155 + 99157 X 1
23-37 minutes	5 years or older	99152 + 99153 X 1	99156 + 99157 X 1
38-52 minutes	< 5 years	99151 + 99153 X 2	99155 + 99157 X 2
38-52 minutes	5 years or older	99152 + 99153 X 2	99156 + 99157 X 2
53-67 minutes (53 min. - 1 hr. 7 min.)	< 5 years	99151 + 99153 X 3	99155 + 99157 X 3
53-67 minutes (53 min. - 1 hr. 7 min.)	5 years or older	99152 + 99153 X 3	99156 + 99157 X 3
68-82 minutes (1 hr. 8 min. - 1 hr. 22 min.)	< 5 years	99151 + 99153 X 4	99155 + 99157 X 4
68-82 minutes (1 hr. 8 min. - 1 hr. 22 min.)	5 years or older	99152 + 99153 X 4	99156 + 99157 X 4
83 minutes or longer (1 hr. 23 min. - etc.)	< 5 years	99153	Add 99157
83 minutes or longer (1 hr. 23 min. - etc.)	5 years or older	Add 99153	Add 99157

- Patient informed consent;
- Immediate pre-sedation assessment prior to first sedating doses; and
- Initiation of IV access and fluids to maintain patency.

Intraservice Work

Intraservice time is used to determine the appropriate CPT code to report moderate sedation services:

- Begins with the administration of the sedating agent(s);
- Ends when the procedure is completed, the patient is stable for recovery status, and the physician or other qualified health care professional providing the sedation ends personal continuous face-to-face time with the patient;
- Includes ordering and/or administering the initial and subsequent doses of sedating agents;
- Requires continuous face-to-face attendance of the physician or other qualified health care professional;
- Requires monitoring patient response to the sedating agents, including:
  - Periodic assessment of the patient;
  - Further administration of agent(s) as needed to maintain sedation; and
  - Monitoring of oxygen saturation, heart rate, and blood pressure.

If the physician or other qualified health care professional who provides the sedation services also performs the procedure supported by sedation (99151, 99152, 99153), the physician or other qualified health care professional will supervise and direct an independent trained observer who will assist in monitoring the patient's level of consciousness and physiological status throughout the procedure.

Postservice Work

The postservice activities required for moderate sedation are included in the work described by each of these codes (99151, 99152, 99153, 99155, 99156, 99157) and are not reported separately. Once continuous face-to-face time with the patient has ended, additional face-to-face time with the patient is not added to the intraservice time, however, it is considered as part of the postservice work. The following postservice work components are not included, when determining intraservice time for reporting:

- Assessment of the patient's vital signs, level of consciousness, neurological, cardiovascular, and pulmonary stability in the post-sedation recovery period;

- Assessment of the patient's readiness for discharge following the procedure;
- Preparation of documentation regarding sedation service; and
- Communication with family/caregiver regarding sedation service.

Postservice work/times are not used to select the appropriate code.

Do not report 99151, 99152, 99153, 99155, 99156, 99157 in conjunction with 94760, 94761, 94762.

Codes 99151, 99152, 99155, 99156 are reported for the first 15 minutes of intraservice time providing moderate sedation. Codes 99153, 99157 are reported for each additional 15 minutes, in addition to the code for the primary service.

(99143, 99144, 99145 have been deleted. To report moderate sedation services provided by the same physician or other qualified health care professional performing the diagnostic or therapeutic service that the sedation supports, see 99151, 99152, 99153)

(99148, 99149, 99150 have been deleted. To report moderate sedation services provided by a physician or other qualified health care professional other than the physician or other qualified health care professional performing the diagnostic or therapeutic service that the sedation supports, see 99155, 99156, 99157)

⊘ **99151** Moderate sedation services provided by the same physician or other qualified health care professional performing the diagnostic or therapeutic service that the sedation supports, requiring the presence of an independent trained observer to assist in the monitoring of the patient's level of consciousness and physiological status; initial 15 minutes of intraservice time, patient younger than 5 years of age
- *CPT Changes: An Insider's View* 2017
- *CPT Assistant* Jan 17:3, May 17:3, Jun 17:3, Sep 17:11
- *Clinical Examples in Radiology* Winter 17:5, Spring 18:8, Winter 18:11

⊘ **99152** initial 15 minutes of intraservice time, patient age 5 years or older
- *CPT Changes: An Insider's View* 2017
- *CPT Assistant* Jan 17:3, May 17:3, Jun 17:3, Sep 17:11
- *Clinical Examples in Radiology* Spring 17:2, Fall 17:2, Winter 17:5, Spring 18:4, Winter 18:3

+ **99153** each additional 15 minutes intraservice time (List separately in addition to code for primary service)
- *CPT Changes: An Insider's View* 2017
- *CPT Assistant* Jan 17:3, May 17:3, Jun 17:3, Sep 17:11
- *Clinical Examples in Radiology* Spring 17:2, Fall 17:2, Winter 17:5, Spring 18:4, Winter 18:3

(Use 99153 in conjunction with 99151, 99152)

(Do not report 99153 in conjunction with 99155, 99156)

99155 Moderate sedation services provided by a physician or other qualified health care professional other than the physician or other qualified health care professional performing the diagnostic or therapeutic service that the sedation supports; initial 15 minutes of intraservice time, patient younger than 5 years of age
- *CPT Changes: An Insider's View* 2017
- *CPT Assistant* Jan 17:3, May 17:3, Jun 17:3, Sep 17:11
- *Clinical Examples in Radiology* Winter 17:5, Spring 18:10

99156 initial 15 minutes of intraservice time, patient age 5 years or older
- *CPT Changes: An Insider's View* 2017
- *CPT Assistant* Jan 17:3, May 17:3, Jun 17:3, Sep 17:11
- *Clinical Examples in Radiology* Winter 17:5, Spring 18:10

+ **99157** each additional 15 minutes intraservice time (List separately in addition to code for primary service)
- *CPT Changes: An Insider's View* 2017
- *CPT Assistant* Jan 17:3, May 17:3, Jun 17:3, Sep 17:11
- *Clinical Examples in Radiology* Winter 17:5, Spring 18:10

(Use 99157 in conjunction with 99155, 99156)

(Do not report 99157 in conjunction with 99151, 99152)

Other Services and Procedures

99170 Anogenital examination, magnified, in childhood for suspected trauma, including image recording when performed
- *CPT Changes: An Insider's View* 2014
- *CPT Assistant* Nov 99:55, Apr 06:1, Sep 14:7

(For moderate sedation, see 99151, 99152, 99153, 99155, 99156, 99157)

99172 Visual function screening, automated or semi-automated bilateral quantitative determination of visual acuity, ocular alignment, color vision by pseudoisochromatic plates, and field of vision (may include all or some screening of the determination[s] for contrast sensitivity, vision under glare)
- *CPT Changes: An Insider's View* 2001
- *CPT Assistant* Feb 01:7, Mar 05:1, 3

(This service must employ graduated visual acuity stimuli that allow a quantitative determination of visual acuity [eg, Snellen chart]. This service may not be used in addition to a general ophthalmological service or an E/M service)

(Do not report 99172 in conjunction with 99173, 99174, 99177, 0469T)

99173 Screening test of visual acuity, quantitative, bilateral
- *CPT Changes: An Insider's View* 2000
- *CPT Assistant* Nov 99:55, May 02:2, Mar 05:1, 3

(The screening test used must employ graduated visual acuity stimuli that allow a quantitative estimate of visual acuity [eg, Snellen chart]. Other identifiable services unrelated to this screening test provided at the same time may be reported separately [eg, preventive medicine services]. When acuity is measured as part of a general ophthalmological service or of an E/M service of the eye, it is a diagnostic examination and not a screening test.)

(Do not report 99173 in conjunction with 99172, 99174, 99177)

99174 Instrument-based ocular screening (eg, photoscreening, automated-refraction), bilateral; with remote analysis and report

➔ *CPT Changes: An Insider's View* 2008, 2013, 2016

➔ *CPT Assistant* Mar 13:6, Mar 16:11, Feb 18:3

(Do not report 99174 in conjunction with 92002-92014, 99172, 99173, 99177)

 # 99177 with on-site analysis

➔ *CPT Changes: An Insider's View* 2016

➔ *CPT Assistant* Mar 16:11, Feb 18:3

(Do not report 99177 in conjunction with 92002-92014, 99172, 99173, 99174)

(For retinal polarization scan, use 0469T)

99175 Ipecac or similar administration for individual emesis and continued observation until stomach adequately emptied of poison

(For diagnostic intubation, see 43754, 43755)

(For gastric lavage for diagnostic purposes, see 43754, 43755)

99177 Code is out of numerical sequence. See 99173-99183

99183 Physician or other qualified health care professional attendance and supervision of hyperbaric oxygen therapy, per session

➔ *CPT Changes: An Insider's View* 2013

➔ *CPT Assistant* Jan 03:23

(Evaluation and Management services and/or procedures [eg, wound debridement] provided in a hyperbaric oxygen treatment facility in conjunction with a hyperbaric oxygen therapy session should be reported separately)

99184 Initiation of selective head or total body hypothermia in the critically ill neonate, includes appropriate patient selection by review of clinical, imaging and laboratory data, confirmation of esophageal temperature probe location, evaluation of amplitude EEG, supervision of controlled hypothermia, and assessment of patient tolerance of cooling

➔ *CPT Changes: An Insider's View* 2015

➔ *CPT Assistant* Oct 15:8

(Do not report 99184 more than once per hospital stay)

(99185, 99186 have been deleted)

99188 Application of topical fluoride varnish by a physician or other qualified health care professional

➔ *CPT Changes: An Insider's View* 2015

99190 Assembly and operation of pump with oxygenator or heat exchanger (with or without ECG and/or pressure monitoring); each hour

99191 45 minutes

99192 30 minutes

99195 Phlebotomy, therapeutic (separate procedure)

➔ *CPT Assistant* Apr 96:3, Jun 96:10

99199 Unlisted special service, procedure or report

➔ *CPT Changes: An Insider's View* 2000

➔ *CPT Assistant* Nov 99:55, Jun 12:16, Sep 12:9

Home Health Procedures/ Services

These codes are used by non-physician health care professionals. Physicians should utilize the home visit codes 99341-99350 and utilize CPT codes other than 99500-99600 for any additional procedure/service provided to a patient living in a residence.

The following codes are used to report services provided in a patient's residence (including assisted living apartments, group homes, nontraditional private homes, custodial care facilities, or schools).

Health care professionals who are authorized to use Evaluation and Management (E/M) Home Visit codes (99341-99350) may report 99500-99600 in addition to 99341-99350 if both services are performed. E/M services may be reported separately, using modifier 25, if the patient's condition requires a significant separately identifiable E/M service, above and beyond the home health service(s)/procedure(s) codes 99500-99600.

99500 Home visit for prenatal monitoring and assessment to include fetal heart rate, non-stress test, uterine monitoring, and gestational diabetes monitoring

➔ *CPT Changes: An Insider's View* 2002

➔ *CPT Assistant* Oct 03:7, Jan 07:30

99501 Home visit for postnatal assessment and follow-up care

➔ *CPT Changes: An Insider's View* 2002

➔ *CPT Assistant* Oct 03:7, Jan 07:30

99502 Home visit for newborn care and assessment

➔ *CPT Changes: An Insider's View* 2002

➔ *CPT Assistant* Oct 03:7, Jan 07:30

99503 Home visit for respiratory therapy care (eg, bronchodilator, oxygen therapy, respiratory assessment, apnea evaluation)

➔ *CPT Changes: An Insider's View* 2002

➔ *CPT Assistant* Oct 03:7, Jan 07:30

99504 Home visit for mechanical ventilation care
➲ *CPT Changes: An Insider's View* 2002, 2003
➲ *CPT Assistant* Oct 03:7, Jan 07:30

99505 Home visit for stoma care and maintenance including colostomy and cystostomy
➲ *CPT Changes: An Insider's View* 2002
➲ *CPT Assistant* Oct 03:7, Jan 07:30

99506 Home visit for intramuscular injections
➲ *CPT Changes: An Insider's View* 2002
➲ *CPT Assistant* Oct 03:7, Jan 07:30

99507 Home visit for care and maintenance of catheter(s) (eg, urinary, drainage, and enteral)
➲ *CPT Changes: An Insider's View* 2002
➲ *CPT Assistant* Oct 03:7, Jan 07:30

99509 Home visit for assistance with activities of daily living and personal care
➲ *CPT Changes: An Insider's View* 2002
➲ *CPT Assistant* Oct 03:7, Jan 07:30

(To report self-care/home management training, see 97535)

(To report home medical nutrition assessment and intervention services, see 97802-97804)

(To report home speech therapy services, see 92507-92508)

99510 Home visit for individual, family, or marriage counseling
➲ *CPT Changes: An Insider's View* 2002
➲ *CPT Assistant* Oct 03:7, Jan 07:30

99511 Home visit for fecal impaction management and enema administration
➲ *CPT Changes: An Insider's View* 2002
➲ *CPT Assistant* Oct 03:7, Jan 07:30

99512 Home visit for hemodialysis
➲ *CPT Changes: An Insider's View* 2002, 2004
➲ *CPT Assistant* Oct 03:7, Jan 07:30

(For home infusion of peritoneal dialysis, use 99601, 99602)

99600 Unlisted home visit service or procedure
➲ *CPT Changes: An Insider's View* 2003
➲ *CPT Assistant* Oct 03:7, Jan 07:30

Home Infusion Procedures/Services

99601 Home infusion/specialty drug administration, per visit (up to 2 hours);
➲ *CPT Changes: An Insider's View* 2004
➲ *CPT Assistant* Nov 05:1

+ 99602 each additional hour (List separately in addition to code for primary procedure)
➲ *CPT Changes: An Insider's View* 2004
➲ *CPT Assistant* Nov 05:1

(Use 99602 in conjunction with 99601)

Medication Therapy Management Services

Medication therapy management service(s) (MTMS) describe face-to-face patient assessment and intervention as appropriate, by a pharmacist, upon request. MTMS is provided to optimize the response to medications or to manage treatment-related medication interactions or complications.

MTMS includes the following documented elements: review of the pertinent patient history, medication profile (prescription and nonprescription), and recommendations for improving health outcomes and treatment compliance. These codes are not to be used to describe the provision of product-specific information at the point of dispensing or any other routine dispensing-related activities.

99605 Medication therapy management service(s) provided by a pharmacist, individual, face-to-face with patient, with assessment and intervention if provided; initial 15 minutes, new patient
➲ *CPT Changes: An Insider's View* 2008
➲ *CPT Assistant* Apr 13:3, Nov 13:3, Oct 14:3

99606 initial 15 minutes, established patient
➲ *CPT Changes: An Insider's View* 2008
➲ *CPT Assistant* Apr 13:3

+ 99607 each additional 15 minutes (List separately in addition to code for primary service)
➲ *CPT Changes: An Insider's View* 2008
➲ *CPT Assistant* Apr 13:3, Nov 13:3, Oct 14:3

(Use 99607 in conjunction with 99605, 99606)

Notes

Notes

Category II Codes

The following section of *Current Procedural Terminology* (CPT) contains a set of supplemental tracking codes that can be used for performance measurement. It is anticipated that the use of Category II codes for performance measurement will decrease the need for record abstraction and chart review, and thereby minimize administrative burden on physicians, other health care professionals, hospitals, and entities seeking to measure the quality of patient care. These codes are intended to facilitate data collection about the quality of care rendered by coding certain services and test results that support nationally established performance measures and that have an evidence base as contributing to quality patient care.

The use of these codes is optional. The codes are not required for correct coding and may not be used as a substitute for Category I codes.

These codes describe clinical components that may be typically included in evaluation and management services or clinical services and, therefore, do not have a relative value associated with them. Category II codes may also describe results from clinical laboratory or radiology tests and other procedures, identified processes intended to address patient safety practices, or services reflecting compliance with state or federal law.

Category II codes described in this section make use of alphabetical characters as the 5th character in the string (ie, 4 digits followed by the letter **F**). These digits are not intended to reflect the placement of the code in the regular (Category I) part of the CPT code set. To promote understanding of these codes and their associated measures, users are referred to the Alphabetical Clinical Topics Listing, which contains information about performance measurement exclusion modifiers, measures, and the measure's source.

Cross-references to the measures associated with each Category II code and their source are included for reference in the Alphabetical Clinical Topics Listing. In addition, acronyms for the related diseases or clinical condition(s) have been added at the end of each code descriptor to identify the topic or clinical category in which that code is included. A complete listing of the diseases/clinical conditions, and their acronyms are provided in alphabetical order in the Alphabetical Clinical Topics Listing. The Alphabetical Clinical Topics Listing can be accessed on the website at www.ama-assn.org, under the Category II link. Users should review the complete measure(s) associated with each code prior to implementation.

Requests for Category II CPT codes will be reviewed by the CPT/HCPAC Advisory Committee just as requests for Category I CPT codes are reviewed. In developing new and revised performance measurement codes, requests for codes are considered from:

- measurements that were developed and tested by a national organization;
- evidenced-based measurements with established ties to health outcomes;
- measurements that address clinical conditions of high prevalence, high risk, or high cost; and
- well-established measurements that are currently being used by large segments of the health care industry across the country.

In addition, all of the following are required:

- Definition or purpose of the measure is consistent with its intended use (quality improvement and accountability, or solely quality improvement)
- Aspect of care measured is substantially influenced by the physician (or other qualified health care professional or entity for which the code may be relevant)
- Reduces data collection burden on physicians (or other qualified health care professional or entities)
- Significant
  - Affects a large segment of health care community
  - Tied to health outcomes
  - Addresses clinical conditions of high prevalence, high costs, high risks
- Evidence-based
  - Agreed upon
  - Definable
  - Measurable
- Risk-adjustment specifications and instructions for all outcome measures submitted or compelling evidence as to why risk adjustment is not relevant
- Sufficiently detailed to make it useful for multiple purposes
- Facilitates reporting of performance measure(s)
- Inclusion of select patient history, testing (eg, glycohemoglobin), other process measures, cognitive or procedure services within CPT, or physiologic measures (eg, blood pressure) to support performance measurements
- Performance measure-development process that includes
  - Nationally recognized expert panel
  - Multidisciplinary
  - Vetting process

The most current listing of Category II codes, including guidelines, code change application forms, and release and implementation dates for Category II codes may be accessed at www.ama-assn.org/go/cpt.

The superscripted numbers included at the end of each code descriptor direct users to the measure developers that are associated with these footnotes, whose names and Web addresses are listed below.

1 Physician Consortium for Performance Improvement®(PCPI), www.physicianconsortium.org.

2 National Committee on Quality Assurance (NCQA), Health Employer Data Information Set (HEDIS®), www.ncqa.org.

3 The Joint Commission (TJC), ORYX Initiative Performance Measures, www.jointcommission.org/performancemeasurement/aspx.

4 National Diabetes Quality Improvement Alliance (NDQIA), www.nationaldiabetesalliance.org.

5 Joint measure from The Physician Consortium for Performance Improvement, www.physicianconsortium.org, and National Committee on Quality Assurance (NCQA), www.ncqa.org.

6 The Society of Thoracic Surgeons at www.sts.org and National Quality Forum, www.qualityforum.org.

7 Optum, www.optum.com.

8 American Academy of Neurology, www.aan.com/go/practice/quality/measurements or quality@aan.com.

9 College of American Pathologists (CAP), www.cap.org/apps/docs/advocacy/pathology performance measurement.pdf.

10 American Gastroenterological Association (AGA), www.gastro.org/quality.

11 American Society of Anesthesiologists (ASA), www.asahq.org.

12 American College of Gastroenterology (ACG), www.gi.org; American Gastroenterological Association (AGA), www.gastro.org; and American Society for Gastrointestinal Endoscopy (ASGE), www.asge.org.

Modifiers

The following performance measurement modifiers may be used for Category II codes to indicate that a service specified in the associated measure(s) was considered but, due to either medical, patient, or system circumstance(s) documented in the medical record, the service was not provided. These modifiers serve as denominator exclusions from the performance measure. The user should note that not all listed measures provide for exclusions (see Alphabetical Clinical Topics Listing for more discussion regarding exclusion criteria).

Category II modifiers should only be reported with Category II codes—they should not be reported with Category I or Category III codes. In addition, the modifiers in the Category II section should only be used where specified in the guidelines, reporting instructions, parenthetic notes, or code descriptor language listed in the Category II section (code listing and the Alphabetical Clinical Topics Listing).

1P Performance Measure Exclusion Modifier due to Medical Reasons

Reasons include:

- Not indicated (absence of organ/limb, already received/performed, other)
- Contraindicated (patient allergic history, potential adverse drug interaction, other)
- Other medical reasons

2P Performance Measure Exclusion Modifier due to Patient Reasons

Reasons include:

- Patient declined
- Economic, social, or religious reasons
- Other patient reasons

3P Performance Measure Exclusion Modifier due to System Reasons

Reasons include:

- Resources to perform the services not available
- Insurance coverage/payor-related limitations
- Other reasons attributable to health care delivery system

Modifier 8P is intended to be used as a "reporting modifier" to allow the reporting of circumstances when an action described in a measure's numerator is not performed and the reason is not otherwise specified.

8P Performance measure reporting modifier–action not performed, reason not otherwise specified

Composite Codes

Composite codes combine several measures grouped within a single code descriptor to facilitate reporting for a clinical condition when all components are met. If only some of the components are met or if services are provided in addition to those included in the composite code, they may be reported individually using the corresponding CPT Category II codes for those services.

0001F Heart failure assessed (includes assessment of all the following components) (CAD)[1]:

Blood pressure measured (2000F)[1]

Level of activity assessed (1003F)[1]

Clinical symptoms of volume overload (excess) assessed (1004F)[1]

Weight, recorded (2001F)[1]

Clinical signs of volume overload (excess) assessed (2002F)[1]

➲ *CPT Changes: An Insider's View* 2006, 2007

➲ *CPT Assistant* Oct 05:1

(To report blood pressure measured, use 2000F)

0005F Osteoarthritis assessed (OA)[1]

Includes assessment of all the following components:

Osteoarthritis symptoms and functional status assessed (1006F)[1]

Use of anti-inflammatory or over-the-counter (OTC) analgesic medications assessed (1007F)[1]

Initial examination of the involved joint(s) (includes visual inspection, palpation, range of motion) (2004F)[1]

➲ *CPT Changes: An Insider's View* 2006, 2007, 2009

➲ *CPT Assistant* Oct 05:1, 6

(To report tobacco use cessation intervention, use 4001F)

0012F Community-acquired bacterial pneumonia assessment (includes all of the following components) (CAP)[1]:

Co-morbid conditions assessed (1026F)[1]

Vital signs recorded (2010F)[1]

Mental status assessed (2014F)[1]

Hydration status assessed (2018F)[1]

➲ *CPT Changes: An Insider's View* 2007

0014F Comprehensive preoperative assessment performed for cataract surgery with intraocular lens (IOL) placement (includes assessment of all of the following components) (EC)[5]:

Dilated fundus evaluation performed within 12 months prior to cataract surgery (2020F)[5]

Pre-surgical (cataract) axial length, corneal power measurement and method of intraocular lens power calculation documented (must be performed within 12 months prior to surgery) (3073F)[5]

Preoperative assessment of functional or medical indication(s) for surgery prior to the cataract surgery with intraocular lens placement (must be performed within 12 months prior to cataract surgery) (3325F)[5]

➲ *CPT Changes: An Insider's View* 2009

0015F Melanoma follow up completed (includes assessment of all of the following components) (ML)[5]:

History obtained regarding new or changing moles (1050F)[5]

Complete physical skin exam performed (2029F)[5]

Patient counseled to perform a monthly self skin examination (5005F)[5]

➲ *CPT Changes: An Insider's View* 2009

Patient Management

Patient management codes describe utilization measures or measures of patient care provided for specific clinical purposes (eg, prenatal care, pre- and post-surgical care).

0500F Initial prenatal care visit (report at first prenatal encounter with health care professional providing obstetrical care. Report also date of visit and, in a separate field, the date of the last menstrual period [LMP]) (Prenatal)[2]

➲ *CPT Changes: An Insider's View* 2005

➲ *CPT Assistant* Oct 05:1, 6, Aug 07:1

0501F Prenatal flow sheet documented in medical record by first prenatal visit (documentation includes at minimum blood pressure, weight, urine protein, uterine size, fetal heart tones, and estimated date of delivery). Report also: date of visit and, in a separate field, the date of the last menstrual period [LMP] (Note: If reporting 0501F Prenatal flow sheet, it is not necessary to report 0500F Initial prenatal care visit) (Prenatal)[1]

➲ *CPT Changes: An Insider's View* 2005

➲ *CPT Assistant* Oct 05:6

0502F Subsequent prenatal care visit (Prenatal)[2]

[Excludes: patients who are seen for a condition unrelated to pregnancy or prenatal care (eg, an upper respiratory infection; patients seen for consultation only, not for continuing care)]

➲ *CPT Changes: An Insider's View* 2005, 2007

➲ *CPT Assistant* Oct 05:6

0503F Postpartum care visit (Prenatal)[2]

➲ *CPT Changes: An Insider's View* 2005

➲ *CPT Assistant* Oct 05:6

0505F Hemodialysis plan of care documented (ESRD, P-ESRD)[1]

➲ *CPT Changes: An Insider's View* 2008

0507F Peritoneal dialysis plan of care documented (ESRD)[1]

➲ *CPT Changes: An Insider's View* 2008

0509F Urinary incontinence plan of care documented (GER)[5]

➲ *CPT Changes: An Insider's View* 2008

0513F Elevated blood pressure plan of care documented (CKD)[1]

➲ *CPT Changes: An Insider's View* 2009

0514F Plan of care for elevated hemoglobin level documented for patient receiving Erythropoiesis-Stimulating Agent therapy (ESA) (CKD)[1]

➲ *CPT Changes: An Insider's View* 2009

0516F Anemia plan of care documented (ESRD)[1]

➲ *CPT Changes: An Insider's View* 2009

0517F Glaucoma plan of care documented (EC)[5]

➲ *CPT Changes: An Insider's View* 2009

0518F Falls plan of care documented (GER)[5]

➲ *CPT Changes: An Insider's View* 2009

0519F Planned chemotherapy regimen, including at a minimum: drug(s) prescribed, dose, and duration, documented prior to initiation of a new treatment regimen (ONC)[1]
➲ *CPT Changes: An Insider's View* 2009, 2010

0520F Radiation dose limits to normal tissues established prior to the initiation of a course of 3D conformal radiation for a minimum of 2 tissue/organ (ONC)[1]
➲ *CPT Changes: An Insider's View* 2009, 2010

0521F Plan of care to address pain documented (COA)[2] (ONC)[1]
➲ *CPT Changes: An Insider's View* 2009, 2010

0525F Initial visit for episode (BkP)[2]
➲ *CPT Changes: An Insider's View* 2009

0526F Subsequent visit for episode (BkP)[2]
➲ *CPT Changes: An Insider's View* 2009

0528F Recommended follow-up interval for repeat colonoscopy of at least 10 years documented in colonoscopy report (End/Polyp)[5]
➲ *CPT Changes: An Insider's View* 2010

0529F Interval of 3 or more years since patient's last colonoscopy, documented (End/Polyp)[5]
➲ *CPT Changes: An Insider's View* 2010

0535F Dyspnea management plan of care, documented (Pall Cr)[5]
➲ *CPT Changes: An Insider's View* 2010

0540F Glucorticoid Management Plan Documented (RA)[5]
➲ *CPT Changes: An Insider's View* 2010

0545F Plan for follow-up care for major depressive disorder, documented (MDD ADOL)[1]
➲ *CPT Changes: An Insider's View* 2011

0550F Cytopathology report on routine nongynecologic specimen finalized within two working days of accession date (PATH)[9]
➲ *CPT Changes: An Insider's View* 2012

0551F Cytopathology report on nongynecologic specimen with documentation that the specimen was non-routine (PATH)[9]
➲ *CPT Changes: An Insider's View* 2012

0555F Symptom management plan of care documented (HF)[1]
➲ *CPT Changes: An Insider's View* 2012

0556F Plan of care to achieve lipid control documented (CAD)[1]
➲ *CPT Changes: An Insider's View* 2012

0557F Plan of care to manage anginal symptoms documented (CAD)[1]
➲ *CPT Changes: An Insider's View* 2012

0575F HIV RNA control plan of care, documented (HIV)[5]
➲ *CPT Changes: An Insider's View* 2010

0580F Multidisciplinary care plan developed or updated (ALS)[8]
➲ *CPT Changes: An Insider's View* 2014

0581F Patient transferred directly from anesthetizing location to critical care unit (Peri2)[11]
➲ *CPT Changes: An Insider's View* 2014

0582F Patient not transferred directly from anesthetizing location to critical care unit (Peri2)[11]
➲ *CPT Changes: An Insider's View* 2014

0583F Transfer of care checklist used (Peri2)[11]
➲ *CPT Changes: An Insider's View* 2014

0584F Transfer of care checklist not used (Peri2)[11]
➲ *CPT Changes: An Insider's View* 2014

Patient History

Patient history codes describe measures for select aspects of patient history or review of systems.

1000F Tobacco use assessed (CAD, CAP, COPD, PV)[1] (DM)[4]
➲ *CPT Changes: An Insider's View* 2005, 2007
➲ *CPT Assistant* Oct 05:1, 6

1002F Anginal symptoms and level of activity assessed (NMA-No Measure Associated)
➲ *CPT Changes: An Insider's View* 2005
➲ *CPT Assistant* Oct 05:6

1003F Level of activity assessed (NMA-No Measure Associated)
➲ *CPT Changes: An Insider's View* 2006
➲ *CPT Assistant* Oct 05:6

1004F Clinical symptoms of volume overload (excess) assessed (NMA-No Measure Associated)
➲ *CPT Changes: An Insider's View* 2006
➲ *CPT Assistant* Oct 05:6

1005F Asthma symptoms evaluated (includes documentation of numeric frequency of symptoms or patient completion of an asthma assessment tool/survey/questionnaire) (NMA-No Measure Associated)
➲ *CPT Changes: An Insider's View* 2006, 2013
➲ *CPT Assistant* Oct 05:6

1006F Osteoarthritis symptoms and functional status assessed (may include the use of a standardized scale or the completion of an assessment questionnaire, such as the SF-36, AAOS Hip & Knee Questionnaire) (OA)[1]
[Instructions: Report when osteoarthritis is addressed during the patient encounter]
➲ *CPT Changes: An Insider's View* 2006
➲ *CPT Assistant* Oct 05:6

1007F Use of anti-inflammatory or analgesic over-the-counter (OTC) medications for symptom relief assessed (OA)[1]
➲ *CPT Changes: An Insider's View* 2006
➲ *CPT Assistant* Oct 05:6

1008F Gastrointestinal and renal risk factors assessed for patients on prescribed or OTC non-steroidal anti-inflammatory drug (NSAID) (OA)[1]
➲ *CPT Changes: An Insider's View* 2006
➲ *CPT Assistant* Oct 05:6

1010F Severity of angina assessed by level of activity (CAD)[1]
➲ *CPT Changes: An Insider's View* 2012

1011F Angina present (CAD)[1]
➲ *CPT Changes: An Insider's View* 2012

1012F Angina absent (CAD)[1]
CPT Changes: An Insider's View 2012

1015F Chronic obstructive pulmonary disease (COPD) symptoms assessed (Includes assessment of at least 1 of the following: dyspnea, cough/sputum, wheezing), or respiratory symptom assessment tool completed (COPD)[1]
CPT Changes: An Insider's View 2007

1018F Dyspnea assessed, not present (COPD)[1]
CPT Changes: An Insider's View 2007

1019F Dyspnea assessed, present (COPD)[1]
CPT Changes: An Insider's View 2007

1022F Pneumococcus immunization status assessed (CAP, COPD)[1]
CPT Changes: An Insider's View 2007

1026F Co-morbid conditions assessed (eg, includes assessment for presence or absence of: malignancy, liver disease, congestive heart failure, cerebrovascular disease, renal disease, chronic obstructive pulmonary disease, asthma, diabetes, other co-morbid conditions) (CAP)[1]
CPT Changes: An Insider's View 2007

1030F Influenza immunization status assessed (CAP)[1]
CPT Changes: An Insider's View 2007

1031F Smoking status and exposure to second hand smoke in the home assessed (Asthma)[1]
CPT Changes: An Insider's View 2012

1032F Current tobacco smoker **or** currently exposed to secondhand smoke (Asthma)[1]
CPT Changes: An Insider's View 2012

1033F Current tobacco non-smoker **and** not currently exposed to secondhand smoke (Asthma)[1]
CPT Changes: An Insider's View 2012

1034F Current tobacco smoker (CAD, CAP, COPD, PV)[1] (DM)[4]
CPT Changes: An Insider's View 2007

1035F Current smokeless tobacco user (eg, chew, snuff) (PV)[1]
CPT Changes: An Insider's View 2007

1036F Current tobacco non-user (CAD, CAP, COPD, PV)[1] (DM)[4] (IBD)[10]
CPT Changes: An Insider's View 2007

1038F Persistent asthma (mild, moderate or severe) (Asthma)[1]
CPT Changes: An Insider's View 2007
CPT Assistant Jul 10:3

1039F Intermittent asthma (Asthma)[1]
CPT Changes: An Insider's View 2007
CPT Assistant Jul 10:3

1040F DSM-5 criteria for major depressive disorder documented at the initial evaluation (MDD, MDD ADOL)[1]
CPT Changes: An Insider's View 2008, 2009, 2014, 2015

1050F History obtained regarding new or changing moles (ML)[5]
CPT Changes: An Insider's View 2008

1052F Type, anatomic location, and activity all assessed (IBD)[10]
CPT Changes: An Insider's View 2013

1055F Visual functional status assessed (EC)[5]
CPT Changes: An Insider's View 2008

1060F Documentation of permanent **or** persistent **or** paroxysmal atrial fibrillation (STR)[5]
CPT Changes: An Insider's View 2008

1061F Documentation of absence of permanent **and** persistent **and** paroxysmal atrial fibrillation (STR)[5]
CPT Changes: An Insider's View 2008

1065F Ischemic stroke symptom onset of less than 3 hours prior to arrival (STR)[5]
CPT Changes: An Insider's View 2008

1066F Ischemic stroke symptom onset greater than or equal to 3 hours prior to arrival (STR)[5]
CPT Changes: An Insider's View 2008

1070F Alarm symptoms (involuntary weight loss, dysphagia, or gastrointestinal bleeding) assessed; none present (GERD)[5]
CPT Changes: An Insider's View 2008

1071F 1 or more present (GERD)[5]
CPT Changes: An Insider's View 2008

1090F Presence or absence of urinary incontinence assessed (GER)[5]
CPT Changes: An Insider's View 2008

1091F Urinary incontinence characterized (eg, frequency, volume, timing, type of symptoms, how bothersome) (GER)[5]
CPT Changes: An Insider's View 2008

1100F Patient screened for future fall risk; documentation of 2 or more falls in the past year or any fall with injury in the past year (GER)[5]
CPT Changes: An Insider's View 2008

1101F documentation of no falls in the past year or only 1 fall without injury in the past year (GER)[5]
CPT Changes: An Insider's View 2008

1110F Patient discharged from an inpatient facility (eg, hospital, skilled nursing facility, or rehabilitation facility) within the last 60 days (GER)[5]
CPT Changes: An Insider's View 2008

1111F Discharge medications reconciled with the current medication list in outpatient medical record (COA)[2] (GER)[5]
CPT Changes: An Insider's View 2008

1116F Auricular or periauricular pain assessed (AOE)[1]
CPT Changes: An Insider's View 2009

1118F GERD symptoms assessed after 12 months of therapy (GERD)[5]
CPT Changes: An Insider's View 2009

1119F Initial evaluation for condition (HEP C)[1](EPI, DSP)[8]
CPT Changes: An Insider's View 2009

1121F Subsequent evaluation for condition (HEP C)[1](EPI)[8]
CPT Changes: An Insider's View 2009

1123F Advance Care Planning discussed and documented advance care plan or surrogate decision maker documented in the medical record (DEM)[1] (GER, Pall Cr)[5]
➲ *CPT Changes: An Insider's View* 2009

1124F Advance Care Planning discussed and documented in the medical record, patient did not wish or was not able to name a surrogate decision maker or provide an advance care plan (DEM)[1] (GER, Pall Cr)[5]
➲ *CPT Changes: An Insider's View* 2009

1125F Pain severity quantified; pain present (COA)[2] (ONC)[1]
➲ *CPT Changes: An Insider's View* 2009

1126F no pain present (COA)[2] (ONC)[1]
➲ *CPT Changes: An Insider's View* 2009, 2010

1127F New episode for condition (NMA-No Measure Associated)
➲ *CPT Changes: An Insider's View* 2009, 2012

1128F Subsequent episode for condition (NMA-No Measure Associated)
➲ *CPT Changes: An Insider's View* 2009, 2012

1130F Back pain and function assessed, including all of the following: Pain assessment **and** functional status **and** patient history, including notation of presence or absence of "red flags" (warning signs) **and** assessment of prior treatment and response, **and** employment status (BkP)[2]
➲ *CPT Changes: An Insider's View* 2009

1134F Episode of back pain lasting 6 weeks or less (BkP)[2]
➲ *CPT Changes: An Insider's View* 2009

1135F Episode of back pain lasting longer than 6 weeks (BkP)[2]
➲ *CPT Changes: An Insider's View* 2009

1136F Episode of back pain lasting 12 weeks or less (BkP)[2]
➲ *CPT Changes: An Insider's View* 2009

1137F Episode of back pain lasting longer than 12 weeks (BkP)[2]
➲ *CPT Changes: An Insider's View* 2009

1150F Documentation that a patient has a substantial risk of death within 1 year (Pall Cr)[5]
➲ *CPT Changes: An Insider's View* 2010

1151F Documentation that a patient does not have a substantial risk of death within one year (Pall Cr)[5]
➲ *CPT Changes: An Insider's View* 2010

1152F Documentation of advanced disease diagnosis, goals of care prioritize comfort (Pall Cr)[5]
➲ *CPT Changes: An Insider's View* 2010

1153F Documentation of advanced disease diagnosis, goals of care do not prioritize comfort (Pall Cr)[5]
➲ *CPT Changes: An Insider's View* 2010

1157F Advance care plan or similar legal document present in the medical record (COA)[2]
➲ *CPT Changes: An Insider's View* 2010

1158F Advance care planning discussion documented in the medical record (COA)[2]
➲ *CPT Changes: An Insider's View* 2010

1159F Medication list documented in medical record (COA)[2]
➲ *CPT Changes: An Insider's View* 2010

1160F Review of all medications by a prescribing practitioner or clinical pharmacist (such as, prescriptions, OTCs, herbal therapies and supplements) documented in the medical record (COA)[2]
➲ *CPT Changes: An Insider's View* 2010

1170F Functional status assessed (COA)[2] (RA)[5]
➲ *CPT Changes: An Insider's View* 2010

1175F Functional status for dementia assessed and results reviewed (DEM)[1]
➲ *CPT Changes: An Insider's View* 2012

1180F All specified thromboembolic risk factors assessed (AFIB)[1]
➲ *CPT Changes: An Insider's View* 2010

1181F Neuropsychiatric symptoms assessed and results reviewed (DEM)[1]
➲ *CPT Changes: An Insider's View* 2012

1182F Neuropsychiatric symptoms, one or more present (DEM)[1]
➲ *CPT Changes: An Insider's View* 2012

1183F Neuropsychiatric symptoms, absent (DEM)[1]
➲ *CPT Changes: An Insider's View* 2012

1200F Seizure type(s) and current seizure frequency(ies) documented (EPI)[8]
➲ *CPT Changes: An Insider's View* 2011

1205F Etiology of epilepsy or epilepsy syndrome(s) reviewed and documented (EPI)[8]
➲ *CPT Changes: An Insider's View* 2011

1220F Patient screened for depression (SUD)[5]
➲ *CPT Changes: An Insider's View* 2010

1400F Parkinson's disease diagnosis reviewed (Prkns)[8]
➲ *CPT Changes: An Insider's View* 2011

1450F Symptoms improved or remained consistent with treatment goals since last assessment (HF)[1]
➲ *CPT Changes: An Insider's View* 2012

1451F Symptoms demonstrated clinically important deterioration since last assessment (HF)[1]
➲ *CPT Changes: An Insider's View* 2012

1460F Qualifying cardiac event/diagnosis in previous 12 months (CAD)[1]
➲ *CPT Changes: An Insider's View* 2012

1461F No qualifying cardiac event/diagnosis in previous 12 months (CAD)[1]
➲ *CPT Changes: An Insider's View* 2012

1490F Dementia severity classified, mild (DEM)[1]
➲ *CPT Changes: An Insider's View* 2012

1491F Dementia severity classified, moderate (DEM)[1]
➲ *CPT Changes: An Insider's View* 2012

1493F Dementia severity classified, severe (DEM)[1]
➲ *CPT Changes: An Insider's View* 2012

1494F Cognition assessed and reviewed (DEM)[1]
➲ *CPT Changes: An Insider's View* 2012

1500F Symptoms and signs of distal symmetric polyneuropathy reviewed and documented (DSP)[8]
➲ *CPT Changes: An Insider's View* 2014

1501F Not initial evaluation for condition (DSP)[8]
➲ *CPT Changes: An Insider's View* 2014

1502F Patient queried about pain and pain interference with function using a valid and reliable instrument (DSP)[8]
➲ *CPT Changes: An Insider's View* 2014

1503F Patient queried about symptoms of respiratory insufficiency (ALS)[8]
➲ *CPT Changes: An Insider's View* 2014

1504F Patient has respiratory insufficiency (ALS)[8]
➲ *CPT Changes: An Insider's View* 2014

1505F Patient does not have respiratory insufficiency (ALS)[8]
➲ *CPT Changes: An Insider's View* 2014

Physical Examination

Physical examination codes describe aspects of physical examination or clinical assessment.

2000F Blood pressure measured (CKD)[1](DM)[2,4]
➲ *CPT Changes: An Insider's View* 2005, 2009
➲ *CPT Assistant* Oct 05:1, 6, Aug 07:1

2001F Weight recorded (PAG)[1]
➲ *CPT Changes: An Insider's View* 2006
➲ *CPT Assistant* Oct 05:6

2002F Clinical signs of volume overload (excess) assessed (NMA–No Measure Associated)
➲ *CPT Changes: An Insider's View* 2006
➲ *CPT Assistant* Oct 05:6

2004F Initial examination of the involved joint(s) (includes visual inspection, palpation, range of motion) (OA)[1]

[Instructions: Report only for initial osteoarthritis visit or for visits for new joint involvement]
➲ *CPT Changes: An Insider's View* 2006
➲ *CPT Assistant* Oct 05:6

2010F Vital signs (temperature, pulse, respiratory rate, and blood pressure) documented and reviewed (CAP)[1] (EM)[5]
➲ *CPT Changes: An Insider's View* 2007, 2008

2014F Mental status assessed (CAP)[1] (EM)[5]
➲ *CPT Changes: An Insider's View* 2007, 2008

2015F Asthma impairment assessed (Asthma)[1]
➲ *CPT Changes: An Insider's View* 2012

2016F Asthma risk assessed (Asthma)[1]
➲ *CPT Changes: An Insider's View* 2012

2018F Hydration status assessed (normal/mildly dehydrated/severely dehydrated) (CAP)[1]
➲ *CPT Changes: An Insider's View* 2007

2019F Dilated macular exam performed, including documentation of the presence or absence of macular thickening or hemorrhage **and** the level of macular degeneration severity (EC)[5]
➲ *CPT Changes: An Insider's View* 2008

2020F Dilated fundus evaluation performed within 12 months prior to cataract surgery (EC)[5]
➲ *CPT Changes: An Insider's View* 2008, 2009

2021F Dilated macular or fundus exam performed, including documentation of the presence or absence of macular edema **and** level of severity of retinopathy (EC)[5]
➲ *CPT Changes: An Insider's View* 2008

2022F Dilated retinal eye exam with interpretation by an ophthalmologist or optometrist documented and reviewed (DM)[2,4]
➲ *CPT Changes: An Insider's View* 2007, 2009

2024F 7 standard field stereoscopic photos with interpretation by an ophthalmologist or optometrist documented and reviewed (DM)[2,4]
➲ *CPT Changes: An Insider's View* 2007, 2009

2026F Eye imaging validated to match diagnosis from 7 standard field stereoscopic photos results documented and reviewed (DM)[2,4]
➲ *CPT Changes: An Insider's View* 2007, 2009

2027F Optic nerve head evaluation performed (EC)[5]
➲ *CPT Changes: An Insider's View* 2008

2028F Foot examination performed (includes examination through visual inspection, sensory exam with monofilament, and pulse exam – report when any of the 3 components are completed) (DM)[4]
➲ *CPT Changes: An Insider's View* 2007

2029F Complete physical skin exam performed (ML)[5]
➲ *CPT Changes: An Insider's View* 2008

2030F Hydration status documented, normally hydrated (PAG)[1]
➲ *CPT Changes: An Insider's View* 2008

2031F Hydration status documented, dehydrated (PAG)[1]
➲ *CPT Changes: An Insider's View* 2008

2035F Tympanic membrane mobility assessed with pneumatic otoscopy or tympanometry (OME)[1]
➲ *CPT Changes: An Insider's View* 2009

2040F Physical examination on the date of the initial visit for low back pain performed, in accordance with specifications (BkP)[2]
➲ *CPT Changes: An Insider's View* 2009

2044F Documentation of mental health assessment prior to intervention (back surgery or epidural steroid injection) or for back pain episode lasting longer than 6 weeks (BkP)[2]
➲ *CPT Changes: An Insider's View* 2009

2050F Wound characteristics including size **and** nature of wound base tissue **and** amount of drainage prior to debridement documented (CWC)[5]
➲ *CPT Changes: An Insider's View* 2010

2060F Patient interviewed directly on or before date of diagnosis of major depressive disorder (MDD ADOL)[1]
➔ *CPT Changes: An Insider's View* 2011, 2013

Diagnostic/Screening Processes or Results

Diagnostic/screening processes or results codes describe results of tests ordered (clinical laboratory tests, radiological or other procedural examinations, and conclusions of medical decision-making).

3006F Chest X-ray results documented and reviewed (CAP)[1]
➔ *CPT Changes: An Insider's View* 2007
➔ *CPT Assistant* Aug 07:1

3008F Body Mass Index (BMI), documented (PV)[1]
➔ *CPT Changes: An Insider's View* 2011

3011F Lipid panel results documented and reviewed (must include total cholesterol, HDL-C, triglycerides and calculated LDL-C) (CAD)[1]
➔ *CPT Changes: An Insider's View* 2007

3014F Screening mammography results documented and reviewed (PV)[1,2]
➔ *CPT Changes: An Insider's View* 2007, 2009

3015F Cervical cancer screening results documented and reviewed (PV)[1]
➔ *CPT Changes: An Insider's View* 2011

3016F Patient screened for unhealthy alcohol use using a systematic screening method (PV)[1] (DSP)[8]
➔ *CPT Changes: An Insider's View* 2010

3017F Colorectal cancer screening results documented and reviewed (PV)[12]
➔ *CPT Changes: An Insider's View* 2009

3018F Pre-procedure risk assessment **and** depth of insertion **and** quality of the bowel prep **and** complete description of polyp(s) found, including location of each polyp, size, number and gross morphology **and** recommendations for follow-up in final colonoscopy report documented (End/Polyp)[5]
➔ *CPT Changes: An Insider's View* 2010

3019F Left ventricular ejection fraction (LVEF) assessment planned post discharge (HF)[1]
➔ *CPT Changes: An Insider's View* 2012

3020F Left ventricular function (LVF) assessment (eg, echocardiography, nuclear test, or ventriculography) documented in the medical record (Includes quantitative or qualitative assessment results) (NMA–No Measure Associated)
➔ *CPT Changes: An Insider's View* 2007

3021F Left ventricular ejection fraction (LVEF) less than 40% or documentation of moderately or severely depressed left ventricular systolic function (CAD, HF)[1]
➔ *CPT Changes: An Insider's View* 2007

3022F Left ventricular ejection fraction (LVEF) greater than or equal to 40% or documentation as normal or mildly depressed left ventricular systolic function (CAD, HF)[1]
➔ *CPT Changes: An Insider's View* 2007

3023F Spirometry results documented and reviewed (COPD)[1]
➔ *CPT Changes: An Insider's View* 2007

3025F Spirometry test results demonstrate FEV_1/FVC less than 70% with COPD symptoms (eg, dyspnea, cough/sputum, wheezing) (CAP, COPD)[1]
➔ *CPT Changes: An Insider's View* 2007

3027F Spirometry test results demonstrate FEV_1/FVC greater than or equal to 70% or patient does not have COPD symptoms (COPD)[1]
➔ *CPT Changes: An Insider's View* 2007

3028F Oxygen saturation results documented and reviewed (includes assessment through pulse oximetry or arterial blood gas measurement) (CAP, COPD)[1] (EM)[5]
➔ *CPT Changes: An Insider's View* 2007

3035F Oxygen saturation less than or equal to 88% or a PaO_2 less than or equal to 55 mm Hg (COPD)[1]
➔ *CPT Changes: An Insider's View* 2007

3037F Oxygen saturation greater than 88% or PaO_2 greater than 55 mm Hg (COPD)[1]
➔ *CPT Changes: An Insider's View* 2007

3038F Pulmonary function test performed within 12 months prior to surgery (Lung/Esop Cx)[6]
➔ *CPT Changes: An Insider's View* 2011

3040F Functional expiratory volume (FEV_1) less than 40% of predicted value (COPD)[1]
➔ *CPT Changes: An Insider's View* 2007

3042F Functional expiratory volume (FEV_1) greater than or equal to 40% of predicted value (COPD)[1]
➔ *CPT Changes: An Insider's View* 2007

3044F Most recent hemoglobin A1c (HbA1c) level less than 7.0% (DM)[2,4]
➔ *CPT Changes: An Insider's View* 2008

3045F Most recent hemoglobin A1c (HbA1c) level 7.0–9.0% (DM)[2,4]
➔ *CPT Changes: An Insider's View* 2008

3046F Most recent hemoglobin A1c level greater than 9.0% (DM)[4]
➔ *CPT Changes: An Insider's View* 2007

(To report most recent hemoglobin A1c level less than or equal to 9.0%, see codes 3044F-3045F)

3048F Most recent LDL-C less than 100 mg/dL (CAD)[1] (DM)[4]
➔ *CPT Changes: An Insider's View* 2007

3049F Most recent LDL-C 100-129 mg/dL (CAD)[1] (DM)[4]
➔ *CPT Changes: An Insider's View* 2007

3050F Most recent LDL-C greater than or equal to 130 mg/dL (CAD)[1] (DM)[4]
➔ *CPT Changes: An Insider's View* 2007

3055F Left ventricular ejection fraction (LVEF) less than or equal to 35% (HF)[1]
CPT Changes: An Insider's View 2012

3056F Left ventricular ejection fraction (LVEF) greater than 35% or no LVEF result available (HF)[1]
CPT Changes: An Insider's View 2012

3060F Positive microalbuminuria test result documented and reviewed (DM)[2,4]
CPT Changes: An Insider's View 2007

3061F Negative microalbuminuria test result documented and reviewed (DM)[2,4]
CPT Changes: An Insider's View 2007

3062F Positive macroalbuminuria test result documented and reviewed (DM)[2,4]
CPT Changes: An Insider's View 2007

3066F Documentation of treatment for nephropathy (eg, patient receiving dialysis, patient being treated for ESRD, CRF, ARF, or renal insufficiency, any visit to a nephrologist) (DM)[2,4]
CPT Changes: An Insider's View 2007

3072F Low risk for retinopathy (no evidence of retinopathy in the prior year) (DM)[2,4]
CPT Changes: An Insider's View 2007

3073F Pre-surgical (cataract) axial length, corneal power measurement and method of intraocular lens power calculation documented within 12 months prior to surgery (EC)[5]
CPT Changes: An Insider's View 2008, 2009

3074F Most recent systolic blood pressure less than 130 mm Hg (DM)[2,4] (HTN, CKD, CAD)[1]
CPT Changes: An Insider's View 2008

3075F Most recent systolic blood pressure 130-139 mm Hg (DM)[2,4](HTN, CKD, CAD)[1]
CPT Changes: An Insider's View 2008

(To report most recent systolic blood pressure less than 140 mm Hg, see codes 3074F-3075F)

3077F Most recent systolic blood pressure greater than or equal to 140 mm Hg (HTN, CKD, CAD)[1] (DM)[2,4]
CPT Changes: An Insider's View 2007

3078F Most recent diastolic blood pressure less than 80 mm Hg (HTN, CKD, CAD)[1] (DM)[2,4]
CPT Changes: An Insider's View 2007

3079F Most recent diastolic blood pressure 80-89 mm Hg (HTN, CKD, CAD)[1] (DM)[2,4]
CPT Changes: An Insider's View 2007

3080F Most recent diastolic blood pressure greater than or equal to 90 mm Hg (HTN, CKD, CAD)[1] (DM)[2,4]
CPT Changes: An Insider's View 2007, 2012

3082F Kt/V less than 1.2 (Clearance of urea [Kt]/volume [V]) (ESRD, P-ESRD)[1]
CPT Changes: An Insider's View 2008

3083F Kt/V equal to or greater than 1.2 and less than 1.7 (Clearance of urea [Kt]/volume [V]) (ESRD, P-ESRD)[1]
CPT Changes: An Insider's View 2008

3084F Kt/V greater than or equal to 1.7 (Clearance of urea [Kt]/volume [V]) (ESRD, P-ESRD)[1]
CPT Changes: An Insider's View 2008

3085F Suicide risk assessed (MDD, MDD ADOL)[1]
CPT Changes: An Insider's View 2008

3088F Major depressive disorder, mild (MDD)[1]
CPT Changes: An Insider's View 2008

3089F Major depressive disorder, moderate (MDD)[1]
CPT Changes: An Insider's View 2008

3090F Major depressive disorder, severe without psychotic features (MDD)[1]
CPT Changes: An Insider's View 2008

3091F Major depressive disorder, severe with psychotic features (MDD)[1]
CPT Changes: An Insider's View 2008

3092F Major depressive disorder, in remission (MDD)[1]
CPT Changes: An Insider's View 2008

3093F Documentation of new diagnosis of initial or recurrent episode of major depressive disorder (MDD)[1]
CPT Changes: An Insider's View 2008

3095F Central dual-energy X-ray absorptiometry (DXA) results documented (OP)[5](IBD)[10]
CPT Changes: An Insider's View 2008

3096F Central dual-energy X-ray absorptiometry (DXA) ordered (OP)[5](IBD)[10]
CPT Changes: An Insider's View 2008

3100F Carotid imaging study report (includes direct or indirect reference to measurements of distal internal carotid diameter as the denominator for stenosis measurement) (STR, RAD)[5]
CPT Changes: An Insider's View 2008

3110F Documentation in final CT or MRI report of presence or absence of hemorrhage and mass lesion and acute infarction (STR)[5]
CPT Changes: An Insider's View 2008, 2011
Clinical Examples in Radiology Winter 08:6

3111F CT or MRI of the brain performed in the hospital within 24 hours of arrival **or** performed in an outpatient imaging center, to confirm initial diagnosis of stroke, TIA or intracranial hemorrhage (STR)[5]
CPT Changes: An Insider's View 2008, 2011, 2012

3112F CT or MRI of the brain performed greater than 24 hours after arrival to the hospital **or** performed in an outpatient imaging center for purpose other than confirmation of initial diagnosis of stroke, TIA, or intracranial hemorrhage (STR)[5]
CPT Changes: An Insider's View 2008, 2011, 2012
Clinical Examples in Radiology Winter 08:6

3115F Quantitative results of an evaluation of current level of activity and clinical symptoms (HF)[1]

CPT Changes: An Insider's View 2012

3117F Heart failure disease specific structured assessment tool completed (HF)[1]

CPT Changes: An Insider's View 2012

3118F New York Heart Association (NYHA) Class documented (HF)[1]

CPT Changes: An Insider's View 2012

3119F No evaluation of level of activity or clinical symptoms (HF)[1]

CPT Changes: An Insider's View 2012

3120F 12-Lead ECG Performed (EM)[5]

CPT Changes: An Insider's View 2008

3126F Esophageal biopsy report with a statement about dysplasia (present, absent, or indefinite, and if present, contains appropriate grading) (PATH)[9]

CPT Changes: An Insider's View 2015

3130F Upper gastrointestinal endoscopy performed (GERD)[5]

CPT Changes: An Insider's View 2008

3132F Documentation of referral for upper gastrointestinal endoscopy (GERD)[5]

CPT Changes: An Insider's View 2008

3140F Upper gastrointestinal endoscopy report indicates suspicion of Barrett's esophagus (GERD)[5]

CPT Changes: An Insider's View 2008

3141F Upper gastrointestinal endoscopy report indicates no suspicion of Barrett's esophagus (GERD)[5]

CPT Changes: An Insider's View 2008

3142F Barium swallow test ordered (GERD)[1]

CPT Changes: An Insider's View 2008

(To report documentation of barium swallow study, use 3142F)

3150F Forceps esophageal biopsy performed (GERD)[5]

CPT Changes: An Insider's View 2008

3155F Cytogenetic testing performed on bone marrow at time of diagnosis or prior to initiating treatment (HEM)[1]

CPT Changes: An Insider's View 2008

3160F Documentation of iron stores prior to initiating erythropoietin therapy (HEM)[1]

CPT Changes: An Insider's View 2008

3170F Flow cytometry studies performed at time of diagnosis or prior to initiating treatment (HEM)[1]

CPT Changes: An Insider's View 2008

3200F Barium swallow test not ordered (GERD)[5]

CPT Changes: An Insider's View 2008

3210F Group A Strep Test Performed (PHAR)[2]

CPT Changes: An Insider's View 2008

3215F Patient has documented immunity to Hepatitis A (HEP-C)[1]

CPT Changes: An Insider's View 2009

3216F Patient has documented immunity to Hepatitis B (HEP-C)[1](IBD)[10]

CPT Changes: An Insider's View 2009

3218F RNA testing for Hepatitis C documented as performed within 6 months prior to initiation of antiviral treatment for Hepatitis C (HEP-C)[1]

CPT Changes: An Insider's View 2009

3220F Hepatitis C quantitative RNA testing documented as performed at 12 weeks from initiation of antiviral treatment (HEP-C)[1]

CPT Changes: An Insider's View 2009

3230F Documentation that hearing test was performed within 6 months prior to tympanostomy tube insertion (OME)[1]

CPT Changes: An Insider's View 2009

3250F Specimen site other than anatomic location of primary tumor (PATH)[1]

CPT Changes: An Insider's View 2010

3260F pT category (primary tumor), pN category (regional lymph nodes), and histologic grade documented in pathology report (PATH)[1]

CPT Changes: An Insider's View 2009

3265F Ribonucleic acid (RNA) testing for Hepatitis C viremia ordered or results documented (HEP C)[1]

CPT Changes: An Insider's View 2009

3266F Hepatitis C genotype testing documented as performed prior to initiation of antiviral treatment for Hepatitis C (HEP C)[1]

CPT Changes: An Insider's View 2009

3267F Pathology report includes pT category, pN category, Gleason score, and statement about margin status (PATH)[9]

CPT Changes: An Insider's View 2012

3268F Prostate-specific antigen (PSA), **and** primary tumor (T) stage, **and** Gleason score documented prior to initiation of treatment (PRCA)[1]

CPT Changes: An Insider's View 2009

3269F Bone scan performed prior to initiation of treatment or at any time since diagnosis of prostate cancer (PRCA)[1]

CPT Changes: An Insider's View 2009

3270F Bone scan not performed prior to initiation of treatment nor at any time since diagnosis of prostate cancer (PRCA)[1]

CPT Changes: An Insider's View 2009

3271F Low risk of recurrence, prostate cancer (PRCA)[1]

CPT Changes: An Insider's View 2009

3272F Intermediate risk of recurrence, prostate cancer (PRCA)[1]

CPT Changes: An Insider's View 2009

3273F High risk of recurrence, prostate cancer (PRCA)[1]

CPT Changes: An Insider's View 2009

3274F Prostate cancer risk of recurrence not determined or neither low, intermediate nor high (PRCA)[1]

CPT Changes: An Insider's View 2009

3278F Serum levels of calcium, phosphorus, intact Parathyroid Hormone (PTH) and lipid profile ordered (CKD)[1]

➔ *CPT Changes: An Insider's View* 2009

3279F Hemoglobin level greater than or equal to 13 g/dL (CKD, ESRD)[1]

➔ *CPT Changes: An Insider's View* 2009

3280F Hemoglobin level 11 g/dL to 12.9 g/dL (CKD, ESRD)[1]

➔ *CPT Changes: An Insider's View* 2009

3281F Hemoglobin level less than 11 g/dL (CKD, ESRD)[1]

➔ *CPT Changes: An Insider's View* 2009

3284F Intraocular pressure (IOP) reduced by a value of greater than or equal to 15% from the pre-intervention level (EC)[5]

➔ *CPT Changes: An Insider's View* 2009

3285F Intraocular pressure (IOP) reduced by a value less than 15% from the pre-intervention level (EC)[5]

➔ *CPT Changes: An Insider's View* 2009

3288F Falls risk assessment documented (GER)[5]

➔ *CPT Changes: An Insider's View* 2009

3290F Patient is D (Rh) negative and unsensitized (Pre-Cr)[1]

➔ *CPT Changes: An Insider's View* 2009

3291F Patient is D (Rh) positive or sensitized (Pre-Cr)[1]

➔ *CPT Changes: An Insider's View* 2009

3292F HIV testing ordered or documented and reviewed during the first or second prenatal visit (Pre-Cr)[1]

➔ *CPT Changes: An Insider's View* 2009

3293F ABO and Rh blood typing documented as performed (Pre-Cr)[7]

➔ *CPT Changes: An Insider's View* 2011

3294F Group B Streptococcus (GBS) screening documented as performed during week 35-37 gestation (Pre-Cr)[7]

➔ *CPT Changes: An Insider's View* 2011

3300F American Joint Committee on Cancer (AJCC) stage documented and reviewed (ONC)[1]

➔ *CPT Changes: An Insider's View* 2009

3301F Cancer stage documented in medical record as metastatic and reviewed (ONC)[1]

➔ *CPT Changes: An Insider's View* 2009

(To report measures for cancer staging, see 3321F-3390F)

3315F Estrogen receptor (ER) or progesterone receptor (PR) positive breast cancer (ONC)[1]

➔ *CPT Changes: An Insider's View* 2009

3316F Estrogen receptor (ER) and progesterone receptor (PR) negative breast cancer (ONC)[1]

➔ *CPT Changes: An Insider's View* 2009

3317F Pathology report confirming malignancy documented in the medical record and reviewed prior to the initiation of chemotherapy (ONC)[1]

➔ *CPT Changes: An Insider's View* 2009

3318F Pathology report confirming malignancy documented in the medical record and reviewed prior to the initiation of radiation therapy (ONC)[1]

➔ *CPT Changes: An Insider's View* 2009

3319F 1 of the following diagnostic imaging studies ordered: chest x-ray, CT, Ultrasound, MRI, PET, or nuclear medicine scans (ML)[5]

➔ *CPT Changes: An Insider's View* 2009, 2010

3320F None of the following diagnostic imaging studies ordered: chest X-ray, CT, Ultrasound, MRI, PET, or nuclear medicine scans (ML)[5]

➔ *CPT Changes: An Insider's View* 2009

3321F AJCC Cancer Stage 0 or IA Melanoma, documented (ML)[5]

➔ *CPT Changes: An Insider's View* 2010

3322F Melanoma greater than AJCC Stage 0 or IA (ML)[5]

➔ *CPT Changes: An Insider's View* 2010

3323F Clinical tumor, node and metastases (TNM) staging documented and reviewed prior to surgery (Lung/Esop Cx)[6]

➔ *CPT Changes: An Insider's View* 2011

3324F MRI or CT scan ordered, reviewed or requested (EPI)[8]

➔ *CPT Changes: An Insider's View* 2011

3325F Preoperative assessment of functional or medical indication(s) for surgery prior to the cataract surgery with intraocular lens placement (must be performed within 12 months prior to cataract surgery) (EC)[5]

➔ *CPT Changes: An Insider's View* 2009

3328F Performance status documented and reviewed within 2 weeks prior to surgery (Lung/Esop Cx)[6]

➔ *CPT Changes: An Insider's View* 2011

3330F Imaging study ordered (BkP)[2]

➔ *CPT Changes: An Insider's View* 2009

3331F Imaging study not ordered (BkP)[2]

➔ *CPT Changes: An Insider's View* 2009

3340F Mammogram assessment category of "incomplete: need additional imaging evaluation" documented (RAD)[5]

➔ *CPT Changes: An Insider's View* 2009

3341F Mammogram assessment category of "negative," documented (RAD)[5]

➔ *CPT Changes: An Insider's View* 2009

3342F Mammogram assessment category of "benign," documented (RAD)[5]

➔ *CPT Changes: An Insider's View* 2009

3343F Mammogram assessment category of "probably benign," documented (RAD)[5]

➔ *CPT Changes: An Insider's View* 2009

3344F Mammogram assessment category of "suspicious," documented (RAD)[5]

➔ *CPT Changes: An Insider's View* 2009

3345F Mammogram assessment category of "highly suggestive of malignancy," documented (RAD)[5]

➔ *CPT Changes: An Insider's View* 2009

3350F Mammogram assessment category of "known biopsy proven malignancy," documented (RAD)[5]

➔ *CPT Changes: An Insider's View* 2009

3351F Negative screen for depressive symptoms as categorized by using a standardized depression screening/assessment tool (MDD)[2]
➔ *CPT Changes: An Insider's View* 2009

3352F No significant depressive symptoms as categorized by using a standardized depression assessment tool (MDD)[2]
➔ *CPT Changes: An Insider's View* 2009

3353F Mild to moderate depressive symptoms as categorized by using a standardized depression screening/assessment tool (MDD)[2]
➔ *CPT Changes: An Insider's View* 2009

3354F Clinically significant depressive symptoms as categorized by using a standardized depression screening/assessment tool (MDD)[2]
➔ *CPT Changes: An Insider's View* 2009

3370F AJCC Breast Cancer Stage 0 documented (ONC)[1]
➔ *CPT Changes: An Insider's View* 2010

3372F AJCC Breast Cancer Stage I: T1mic, T1a or T1b (tumor size ≤ 1 cm) documented (ONC)[1]
➔ *CPT Changes: An Insider's View* 2010

3374F AJCC Breast Cancer Stage I: T1c (tumor size > 1 cm to 2 cm) documented (ONC)[1]
➔ *CPT Changes: An Insider's View* 2010

3376F AJCC Breast Cancer Stage II documented (ONC)[1]
➔ *CPT Changes: An Insider's View* 2010

3378F AJCC Breast Cancer Stage III documented (ONC)[1]
➔ *CPT Changes: An Insider's View* 2010

3380F AJCC Breast Cancer Stage IV documented (ONC)[1]
➔ *CPT Changes: An Insider's View* 2010

3382F AJCC colon cancer, Stage 0 documented (ONC)[1]
➔ *CPT Changes: An Insider's View* 2010

3384F AJCC colon cancer, Stage I documented (ONC)[1]
➔ *CPT Changes: An Insider's View* 2010

3386F AJCC colon cancer, Stage II documented (ONC)[1]
➔ *CPT Changes: An Insider's View* 2010

3388F AJCC colon cancer, Stage III documented (ONC)[1]
➔ *CPT Changes: An Insider's View* 2010

3390F AJCC colon cancer, Stage IV documented (ONC)[1]
➔ *CPT Changes: An Insider's View* 2010

3394F Quantitative HER2 immunohistochemistry (IHC) evaluation of breast cancer consistent with the scoring system defined in the ASCO/CAP guidelines (PATH)[9]
➔ *CPT Changes: An Insider's View* 2012

3395F Quantitative non-HER2 immunohistochemistry (IHC) evaluation of breast cancer (eg, testing for estrogen or progesterone receptors [ER/PR]) performed (PATH)[9]
➔ *CPT Changes: An Insider's View* 2012

3450F Dyspnea screened, no dyspnea or mild dyspnea (Pall Cr)[5]
➔ *CPT Changes: An Insider's View* 2010

3451F Dyspnea screened, moderate or severe dyspnea (Pall Cr)[5]
➔ *CPT Changes: An Insider's View* 2010

3452F Dyspnea not screened (Pall Cr)[5]
➔ *CPT Changes: An Insider's View* 2010

3455F TB screening performed and results interpreted within six months prior to initiation of first-time biologic disease modifying anti-rheumatic drug therapy for RA (RA)[5]
➔ *CPT Changes: An Insider's View* 2010

3470F Rheumatoid arthritis (RA) disease activity, low (RA)[5]
➔ *CPT Changes: An Insider's View* 2010

3471F Rheumatoid arthritis (RA) disease activity, moderate (RA)[5]
➔ *CPT Changes: An Insider's View* 2010

3472F Rheumatoid arthritis (RA) disease activity, high (RA)[5]
➔ *CPT Changes: An Insider's View* 2010

3475F Disease prognosis for rheumatoid arthritis assessed, poor prognosis documented (RA)[5]
➔ *CPT Changes: An Insider's View* 2010

3476F Disease prognosis for rheumatoid arthritis assessed, good prognosis documented (RA)[5]
➔ *CPT Changes: An Insider's View* 2010

3490F History of AIDS-defining condition (HIV)[5]
➔ *CPT Changes: An Insider's View* 2010

3491F HIV indeterminate (infants of undetermined HIV status born of HIV-infected mothers) (HIV)[5]
➔ *CPT Changes: An Insider's View* 2010

3492F History of nadir CD4+ cell count <350 cells/mm^3 (HIV)[5]
➔ *CPT Changes: An Insider's View* 2010

3493F No history of nadir CD4+ cell count <350 cells/mm^3 **and** no history of AIDS-defining condition (HIV)[5]
➔ *CPT Changes: An Insider's View* 2010

3494F CD4+ cell count <200 cells/mm^3 (HIV)[5]
➔ *CPT Changes: An Insider's View* 2010

3495F CD4+ cell count 200 – 499 cells/mm^3 (HIV)[5]
➔ *CPT Changes: An Insider's View* 2010

3496F CD4+ cell count ≥500 cells/mm^3 (HIV)[5]
➔ *CPT Changes: An Insider's View* 2010

3497F CD4+ cell percentage <15% (HIV)[5]
➔ *CPT Changes: An Insider's View* 2010

3498F CD4+ cell percentage ≥15% (HIV)[5]
➔ *CPT Changes: An Insider's View* 2010

3500F CD4+ cell count or CD4+ cell percentage documented as performed (HIV)[5]
➔ *CPT Changes: An Insider's View* 2010

3502F HIV RNA viral load below limits of quantification (HIV)[5]
➔ *CPT Changes: An Insider's View* 2010

3503F HIV RNA viral load not below limits of quantification (HIV)[5]
➔ *CPT Changes: An Insider's View* 2010

3510F Documentation that tuberculosis (TB) screening test performed and results interpreted (HIV)[5] (IBD)[10]
➔ *CPT Changes: An Insider's View* 2010

3511F Chlamydia and gonorrhea screenings documented as performed (HIV)[5]
CPT Changes: An Insider's View 2010

3512F Syphilis screening documented as performed (HIV)[5]
CPT Changes: An Insider's View 2010

3513F Hepatitis B screening documented as performed (HIV)[5]
CPT Changes: An Insider's View 2010

3514F Hepatitis C screening documented as performed (HIV)[5]
CPT Changes: An Insider's View 2010

3515F Patient has documented immunity to Hepatitis C (HIV)[5]
CPT Changes: An Insider's View 2010

3517F Hepatitis B Virus (HBV) status assessed and results interpreted within one year prior to receiving a first course of anti-TNF (tumor necrosis factor) therapy (IBD)[10]
CPT Changes: An Insider's View 2013

3520F Clostridium difficile testing performed (IBD)[10]
CPT Changes: An Insider's View 2013

3550F Low risk for thromboembolism (AFIB)[1]
CPT Changes: An Insider's View 2010

3551F Intermediate risk for thromboembolism (AFIB)[1]
CPT Changes: An Insider's View 2010

3552F High risk for thromboembolism (AFIB)[1]
CPT Changes: An Insider's View 2010

3555F Patient had International Normalized Ratio (INR) measurement performed (AFIB)[1]
CPT Changes: An Insider's View 2010

3570F Final report for bone scintigraphy study includes correlation with existing relevant imaging studies (eg, X ray, MRI, CT) corresponding to the same anatomical region in question (NUC_MED)[1]
CPT Changes: An Insider's View 2010

3572F Patient considered to be potentially at risk for fracture in a weight-bearing site (NUC_MED)[1]
CPT Changes: An Insider's View 2010

3573F Patient not considered to be potentially at risk for fracture in a weight-bearing site (NUC_MED)[1]
CPT Changes: An Insider's View 2010

3650F Electroencephalogram (EEG) ordered, reviewed or requested (EPI)[8]
CPT Changes: An Insider's View 2011

3700F Psychiatric disorders or disturbances assessed (Prkns)[8]
CPT Changes: An Insider's View 2011

3720F Cognitive impairment or dysfunction assessed (Prkns)[8]
CPT Changes: An Insider's View 2011

3725F Screening for depression performed (DEM)[1]
CPT Changes: An Insider's View 2012

3750F Patient not receiving dose of corticosteroids greater than or equal to 10 mg/day for 60 or greater consecutive days (IBD)[10]
CPT Changes: An Insider's View 2013

3751F Electrodiagnostic studies for distal symmetric polyneuropathy conducted (or requested), documented, and reviewed within 6 months of initial evaluation for condition (DSP)[8]
CPT Changes: An Insider's View 2014

3752F Electrodiagnostic studies for distal symmetric polyneuropathy **not** conducted (or requested), documented, or reviewed within 6 months of initial evaluation for condition (DSP)[8]
CPT Changes: An Insider's View 2014

3753F Patient has clear clinical symptoms and signs that are highly suggestive of neuropathy AND cannot be attributed to another condition, AND has an obvious cause for the neuropathy (DSP)[8]
CPT Changes: An Insider's View 2014

3754F Screening tests for diabetes mellitus reviewed, requested, or ordered (DSP)[8]
CPT Changes: An Insider's View 2014

3755F Cognitive and behavioral impairment screening performed (ALS)[8]
CPT Changes: An Insider's View 2014

3756F Patient has pseudobulbar affect, sialorrhea, or ALS-related symptoms (ALS)[8]
CPT Changes: An Insider's View 2014

3757F Patient does not have pseudobulbar affect, sialorrhea, or ALS-related symptoms (ALS)[8]
CPT Changes: An Insider's View 2014

3758F Patient referred for pulmonary function testing or peak cough expiratory flow (ALS)[8]
CPT Changes: An Insider's View 2014

3759F Patient screened for dysphagia, weight loss, and impaired nutrition, and results documented (ALS)[8]
CPT Changes: An Insider's View 2014

3760F Patient exhibits dysphagia, weight loss, or impaired nutrition (ALS)[8]
CPT Changes: An Insider's View 2014

3761F Patient does not exhibit dysphagia, weight loss, or impaired nutrition (ALS)[8]
CPT Changes: An Insider's View 2014

3762F Patient is dysarthric (ALS)[8]
CPT Changes: An Insider's View 2014

3763F Patient is not dysarthric (ALS)[8]
CPT Changes: An Insider's View 2014

3775F Adenoma(s) or other neoplasm detected during screening colonoscopy (SCADR)
CPT Changes: An Insider's View 2015

3776F Adenoma(s) or other neoplasm not detected during screening colonoscopy (SCADR)
CPT Changes: An Insider's View 2015

Therapeutic, Preventive, or Other Interventions

Therapeutic, preventive, or other interventions codes describe pharmacologic, procedural, or behavioral therapies, including preventive services such as patient education and counseling.

4000F Tobacco use cessation intervention, counseling (COPD, CAP, CAD, Asthma)[1] (DM)[4] (PV)[2]
- *CPT Changes: An Insider's View* 2005
- *CPT Assistant* Oct 05:1

4001F Tobacco use cessation intervention, pharmacologic therapy (COPD, CAD, CAP, PV, Asthma)[1] (DM)[4] (PV)[2]
- *CPT Changes: An Insider's View* 2005
- *CPT Assistant* Oct 05:6

4003F Patient education, written/oral, appropriate for patients with heart failure, performed (NMA–No Measure Associated)[1]
- *CPT Changes: An Insider's View* 2006
- *CPT Assistant* Oct 05:6

4004F Patient screened for tobacco use **and** received tobacco cessation intervention (counseling, pharmacotherapy, or both), if identified as a tobacco user (PV, CAD)[1]
- *CPT Changes: An Insider's View* 2011, 2012

4005F Pharmacologic therapy (other than minerals/vitamins) for osteoporosis prescribed (OP)[5] (IBD)[10]
- *CPT Changes: An Insider's View* 2008

4008F Beta-blocker therapy prescribed or currently being taken (CAD,HF)[1]
- *CPT Changes: An Insider's View* 2012

4010F Angiotensin Converting Enzyme (ACE) Inhibitor or Angiotensin Receptor Blocker (ARB) therapy prescribed or currently being taken (CAD, CKD, HF)[1] (DM)[2]
- *CPT Changes: An Insider's View* 2012

4011F Oral antiplatelet therapy prescribed (CAD)[1]
- *CPT Changes: An Insider's View* 2005, 2010
- *CPT Assistant* Oct 05:6

4012F Warfarin therapy prescribed (NMA-No Measure Associated)
- *CPT Changes: An Insider's View* 2006
- *CPT Assistant* Oct 05:6

4013F Statin therapy prescribed or currently being taken (CAD)[1]
- *CPT Changes: An Insider's View* 2012

4014F Written discharge instructions provided to heart failure patients discharged home (Instructions include all of the following components: activity level, diet, discharge medications, follow-up appointment, weight monitoring, what to do if symptoms worsen) (NMA-No Measure Associated)
- *CPT Changes: An Insider's View* 2006, 2007, 2009

4015F Persistent asthma, preferred long term control medication or an acceptable alternative treatment, prescribed (NMA–No Measure Associated)
- *CPT Changes: An Insider's View* 2006, 2007, 2009

(Note: There are no medical exclusion criteria)

(Do not report modifier 1P with 4015F)

(To report patient reasons for not prescribing, use modifier 2P)

4016F Anti-inflammatory/analgesic agent prescribed (OA)[1]

(Use for prescribed or continued medication[s], including over-the-counter medication[s])
- *CPT Changes: An Insider's View* 2006
- *CPT Assistant* Oct 05:6

4017F Gastrointestinal prophylaxis for NSAID use prescribed (OA)[1]
- *CPT Changes: An Insider's View* 2006
- *CPT Assistant* Oct 05:6

4018F Therapeutic exercise for the involved joint(s) instructed or physical or occupational therapy prescribed (OA)[1]
- *CPT Changes: An Insider's View* 2006
- *CPT Assistant* Oct 05:6

4019F Documentation of receipt of counseling on exercise **and** either both calcium and vitamin D use or counseling regarding both calcium and vitamin D use (OP)[5]
- *CPT Changes: An Insider's View* 2008

4025F Inhaled bronchodilator prescribed (COPD)[1]
- *CPT Changes: An Insider's View* 2007

4030F Long-term oxygen therapy prescribed (more than 15 hours per day) (COPD)[1]
- *CPT Changes: An Insider's View* 2007

4033F Pulmonary rehabilitation exercise training recommended (COPD)[1]
- *CPT Changes: An Insider's View* 2007

(Report 4033F with 1019F)

4035F Influenza immunization recommended (COPD)[1] (IBD)[10]
- *CPT Changes: An Insider's View* 2007

4037F Influenza immunization ordered or administered (COPD, PV, CKD, ESRD)[1](IBD)[10]
- *CPT Changes: An Insider's View* 2007

4040F Pneumococcal vaccine administered or previously received (COPD)[1] (PV)[1,2] (IBD)[10]
- *CPT Changes: An Insider's View* 2007, 2009

4041F Documentation of order for cefazolin OR cefuroxime for antimicrobial prophylaxis (PERI 2)[5]
- *CPT Changes: An Insider's View* 2008

4042F Documentation that prophylactic antibiotics were neither given within 4 hours prior to surgical incision nor given intraoperatively (PERI 2)[5]
- *CPT Changes: An Insider's View* 2008

4043F Documentation that an order was given to discontinue prophylactic antibiotics within 48 hours of surgical end time, cardiac procedures (PERI 2)[5]

➔ *CPT Changes: An Insider's View* 2008

4044F Documentation that an order was given for venous thromboembolism (VTE) prophylaxis to be given within 24 hours prior to incision time or 24 hours after surgery end time (PERI 2)[5]

➔ *CPT Changes: An Insider's View* 2008

4045F Appropriate empiric antibiotic prescribed (CAP)[1], (EM)[5]

➔ *CPT Changes: An Insider's View* 2007, 2008

4046F Documentation that prophylactic antibiotics were given within 4 hours prior to surgical incision or given intraoperatively (PERI 2)[5]

➔ *CPT Changes: An Insider's View* 2008

4047F Documentation of order for prophylactic parenteral antibiotics to be given within 1 hour (if fluoroquinolone or vancomycin, 2 hours) prior to surgical incision (or start of procedure when no incision is required) (PERI 2)[5]

➔ *CPT Changes: An Insider's View* 2008, 2011

4048F Documentation that administration of prophylactic parenteral antibiotic was initiated within 1 hour (if fluoroquinolone or vancomycin, 2 hours) prior to surgical incision (or start of procedure when no incision is required) as ordered (PERI 2)[5]

➔ *CPT Changes: An Insider's View* 2008, 2011

4049F Documentation that order was given to discontinue prophylactic antibiotics within 24 hours of surgical end time, non-cardiac procedure (PERI 2)[5]

➔ *CPT Changes: An Insider's View* 2008

4050F Hypertension plan of care documented as appropriate (NMA-No Measure Associated)[1]

➔ *CPT Changes: An Insider's View* 2007

4051F Referred for an arteriovenous (AV) fistula (ESRD, CKD)[1]

➔ *CPT Changes: An Insider's View* 2008

4052F Hemodialysis via functioning arteriovenous (AV) fistula (ESRD)[1]

➔ *CPT Changes: An Insider's View* 2008

4053F Hemodialysis via functioning arteriovenous (AV) graft (ESRD)[1]

➔ *CPT Changes: An Insider's View* 2008

4054F Hemodialysis via catheter (ESRD)[1]

➔ *CPT Changes: An Insider's View* 2008

4055F Patient receiving peritoneal dialysis (ESRD)[1]

➔ *CPT Changes: An Insider's View* 2008

4056F Appropriate oral rehydration solution recommended (PAG)[1]

➔ *CPT Changes: An Insider's View* 2008

4058F Pediatric gastroenteritis education provided to caregiver (PAG)[1]

➔ *CPT Changes: An Insider's View* 2008

4060F Psychotherapy services provided (MDD, MDD ADOL)[1]

➔ *CPT Changes: An Insider's View* 2008, 2011

4062F Patient referral for psychotherapy documented (MDD, MDD ADOL)[1]

➔ *CPT Changes: An Insider's View* 2008

4063F Antidepressant pharmacotherapy considered and not prescribed (MDD ADOL)[1]

➔ *CPT Changes: An Insider's View* 2011

4064F Antidepressant pharmacotherapy prescribed (MDD, MDD ADOL)[1]

➔ *CPT Changes: An Insider's View* 2008

4065F Antipsychotic pharmacotherapy prescribed (MDD)[1]

➔ *CPT Changes: An Insider's View* 2008

4066F Electroconvulsive therapy (ECT) provided (MDD)[1]

➔ *CPT Changes: An Insider's View* 2008

4067F Patient referral for electroconvulsive therapy (ECT) documented (MDD)[1]

➔ *CPT Changes: An Insider's View* 2008

4069F Venous thromboembolism (VTE) prophylaxis received (IBD)[10]

➔ *CPT Changes: An Insider's View* 2013

4070F Deep vein thrombosis (DVT) prophylaxis received by end of hospital day 2 (STR)[5]

➔ *CPT Changes: An Insider's View* 2008

4073F Oral antiplatelet therapy prescribed at discharge (STR)[5]

➔ *CPT Changes: An Insider's View* 2008

4075F Anticoagulant therapy prescribed at discharge (STR)[5]

➔ *CPT Changes: An Insider's View* 2008

4077F Documentation that tissue plasminogen activator (t-PA) administration was considered (STR)[5]

➔ *CPT Changes: An Insider's View* 2008

4079F Documentation that rehabilitation services were considered (STR)[5]

➔ *CPT Changes: An Insider's View* 2008

4084F Aspirin received within 24 hours before emergency department arrival or during emergency department stay (EM)[5]

➔ *CPT Changes: An Insider's View* 2008

4086F Aspirin or clopidogrel prescribed or currently being taken (CAD)[1]

➔ *CPT Changes: An Insider's View* 2012

4090F Patient receiving erythropoietin therapy (HEM)[1]

➔ *CPT Changes: An Insider's View* 2008

4095F Patient not receiving erythropoietin therapy (HEM)[1]

➔ *CPT Changes: An Insider's View* 2008

4100F Bisphosphonate therapy, intravenous, ordered or received (HEM)[1]

➔ *CPT Changes: An Insider's View* 2008

4110F Internal mammary artery graft performed for primary, isolated coronary artery bypass graft procedure (CABG)[6]
➲ *CPT Changes: An Insider's View* 2008

4115F Beta blocker administered within 24 hours prior to surgical incision (CABG)[6]
➲ *CPT Changes: An Insider's View* 2008

4120F Antibiotic prescribed or dispensed (URI, PHAR)[2], (A-BRONCH)[2]
➲ *CPT Changes: An Insider's View* 2008

4124F Antibiotic neither prescribed nor dispensed (URI, PHAR)[2], (A-BRONCH)[2]
➲ *CPT Changes: An Insider's View* 2008

4130F Topical preparations (including OTC) prescribed for acute otitis externa (AOE)[1]
➲ *CPT Changes: An Insider's View* 2009

4131F Systemic antimicrobial therapy prescribed (AOE)[1]
➲ *CPT Changes: An Insider's View* 2009

4132F Systemic antimicrobial therapy not prescribed (AOE)[1]
➲ *CPT Changes: An Insider's View* 2009

4133F Antihistamines or decongestants prescribed or recommended (OME)[1]
➲ *CPT Changes: An Insider's View* 2009

4134F Antihistamines or decongestants neither prescribed nor recommended (OME)[1]
➲ *CPT Changes: An Insider's View* 2009

4135F Systemic corticosteroids prescribed (OME)[1]
➲ *CPT Changes: An Insider's View* 2009

4136F Systemic corticosteroids not prescribed (OME)[1]
➲ *CPT Changes: An Insider's View* 2009

4140F Inhaled corticosteroids prescribed (Asthma)[1]
➲ *CPT Changes: An Insider's View* 2012

4142F Corticosteroid sparing therapy prescribed (IBD)[10]
➲ *CPT Changes: An Insider's View* 2013

4144F Alternative long-term control medication prescribed (Asthma)[1]
➲ *CPT Changes: An Insider's View* 2012

4145F Two or more anti-hypertensive agents prescribed or currently being taken (CAD, HTN)[1]
➲ *CPT Changes: An Insider's View* 2012

4148F Hepatitis A vaccine injection administered or previously received (HEP-C)[1]
➲ *CPT Changes: An Insider's View* 2010

4149F Hepatitis B vaccine injection administered or previously received (HEP-C, HIV)[1] (IBD)[10]
➲ *CPT Changes: An Insider's View* 2010, 2012

4150F Patient receiving antiviral treatment for Hepatitis C (HEP-C)[1]
➲ *CPT Changes: An Insider's View* 2009

4151F Patient did not start or is not receiving antiviral treatment for Hepatitis C during the measurement period (HEP-C)[1]
➲ *CPT Changes: An Insider's View* 2009, 2017

4153F Combination peginterferon and ribavirin therapy prescribed (HEP-C)[1]
➲ *CPT Changes: An Insider's View* 2009

4155F Hepatitis A vaccine series previously received (HEP-C)[1]
➲ *CPT Changes: An Insider's View* 2009

4157F Hepatitis B vaccine series previously received (HEP-C)[1]
➲ *CPT Changes: An Insider's View* 2009

4158F Patient counseled about risks of alcohol use (HEP-C)[1]
➲ *CPT Changes: An Insider's View* 2009, 2010

4159F Counseling regarding contraception received prior to initiation of antiviral treatment (HEP-C)[1]
➲ *CPT Changes: An Insider's View* 2009

4163F Patient counseling at a minimum on all of the following treatment options for clinically localized prostate cancer: active surveillance, **and** interstitial prostate brachytherapy, **and** external beam radiotherapy, **and** radical prostatectomy, provided prior to initiation of treatment (PRCA)[1]
➲ *CPT Changes: An Insider's View* 2009

4164F Adjuvant (ie, in combination with external beam radiotherapy to the prostate for prostate cancer) hormonal therapy (gonadotropin-releasing hormone [GnRH] agonist or antagonist) prescribed/administered (PRCA)[1]
➲ *CPT Changes: An Insider's View* 2009

4165F 3-dimensional conformal radiotherapy (3D-CRT) or intensity modulated radiation therapy (IMRT) received (PRCA)[1]
➲ *CPT Changes: An Insider's View* 2009

4167F Head of bed elevation (30-45 degrees) on first ventilator day ordered (CRIT)[1]
➲ *CPT Changes: An Insider's View* 2009

4168F Patient receiving care in the intensive care unit (ICU) and receiving mechanical ventilation, 24 hours or less (CRIT)[1]
➲ *CPT Changes: An Insider's View* 2009

4169F Patient either not receiving care in the intensive care unit (ICU) OR not receiving mechanical ventilation OR receiving mechanical ventilation greater than 24 hours (CRIT)[1]
➲ *CPT Changes: An Insider's View* 2009

4171F Patient receiving erythropoiesis-stimulating agents (ESA) therapy (CKD)[1]
➲ *CPT Changes: An Insider's View* 2009

4172F Patient not receiving erythropoiesis-stimulating agents (ESA) therapy (CKD)[1]
➲ *CPT Changes: An Insider's View* 2009

4174F Counseling about the potential impact of glaucoma on visual functioning and quality of life, and importance of treatment adherence provided to patient and/or caregiver(s) (EC)[5]
➲ *CPT Changes: An Insider's View* 2009

4175F Best-corrected visual acuity of 20/40 or better (distance or near) achieved within the 90 days following cataract surgery (EC)[5]

➔ *CPT Changes: An Insider's View* 2009

4176F Counseling about value of protection from UV light and lack of proven efficacy of nutritional supplements in prevention or progression of cataract development provided to patient and/or caregiver(s) (NMA-No Measure Associated)

➔ *CPT Changes: An Insider's View* 2009

4177F Counseling about the benefits and/or risks of the Age-Related Eye Disease Study (AREDS) formulation for preventing progression of age-related macular degeneration (AMD) provided to patient and/or caregiver(s) (EC)[5]

➔ *CPT Changes: An Insider's View* 2009

4178F Anti-D immune globulin received between 26 and 30 weeks gestation (Pre-Cr)[1]

➔ *CPT Changes: An Insider's View* 2009

4179F Tamoxifen or aromatase inhibitor (AI) prescribed (ONC)[1]

➔ *CPT Changes: An Insider's View* 2009

4180F Adjuvant chemotherapy referred, prescribed, or previously received for Stage III colon cancer (ONC)[1]

➔ *CPT Changes: An Insider's View* 2009, 2010

4181F Conformal radiation therapy received (NMA-No Measure Associated)

➔ *CPT Changes: An Insider's View* 2009

4182F Conformal radiation therapy not received (NMA-No Measure Associated)

➔ *CPT Changes: An Insider's View* 2009

4185F Continuous (12-months) therapy with proton pump inhibitor (PPI) or histamine H2 receptor antagonist (H2RA) received (GERD)[5]

➔ *CPT Changes: An Insider's View* 2009

4186F No continuous (12-months) therapy with either proton pump inhibitor (PPI) or histamine H2 receptor antagonist (H2RA) received (GERD)[5]

➔ *CPT Changes: An Insider's View* 2009

4187F Disease modifying anti-rheumatic drug therapy prescribed or dispensed (RA)[2]

➔ *CPT Changes: An Insider's View* 2009

4188F Appropriate angiotensin converting enzyme (ACE)/ angiotensin receptor blockers (ARB) therapeutic monitoring test ordered or performed (AM)[2]

➔ *CPT Changes: An Insider's View* 2009

4189F Appropriate digoxin therapeutic monitoring test ordered or performed (AM)[2]

➔ *CPT Changes: An Insider's View* 2009

4190F Appropriate diuretic therapeutic monitoring test ordered or performed (AM)[2]

➔ *CPT Changes: An Insider's View* 2009

4191F Appropriate anticonvulsant therapeutic monitoring test ordered or performed (AM)[2]

➔ *CPT Changes: An Insider's View* 2009

4192F Patient not receiving glucocorticoid therapy (RA)[5]

➔ *CPT Changes: An Insider's View* 2010

4193F Patient receiving <10 mg daily prednisone (or equivalent), or RA activity is worsening, or glucocorticoid use is for less than 6 months (RA)[5]

➔ *CPT Changes: An Insider's View* 2010

4194F Patient receiving ≥10 mg daily prednisone (or equivalent) for longer than 6 months, and improvement or no change in disease activity (RA)[5]

➔ *CPT Changes: An Insider's View* 2010

4195F Patient receiving first-time biologic disease modifying anti-rheumatic drug therapy for rheumatoid arthritis (RA)[5]

➔ *CPT Changes: An Insider's View* 2010

4196F Patient not receiving first-time biologic disease modifying anti-rheumatic drug therapy for rheumatoid arthritis (RA)[5]

➔ *CPT Changes: An Insider's View* 2010

4200F External beam radiotherapy as primary therapy to prostate with or without nodal irradiation (PRCA)[1]

➔ *CPT Changes: An Insider's View* 2009, 2010

4201F External beam radiotherapy with or without nodal irradiation as adjuvant or salvage therapy for prostate cancer patient (PRCA)[1]

➔ *CPT Changes: An Insider's View* 2009, 2010

4210F Angiotensin converting enzyme (ACE) or angiotensin receptor blockers (ARB) medication therapy for 6 months or more (MM)[2]

➔ *CPT Changes: An Insider's View* 2009

4220F Digoxin medication therapy for 6 months or more (MM)[2]

➔ *CPT Changes: An Insider's View* 2009

4221F Diuretic medication therapy for 6 months or more (MM)[2]

➔ *CPT Changes: An Insider's View* 2009

4230F Anticonvulsant medication therapy for 6 months or more (MM)[2]

➔ *CPT Changes: An Insider's View* 2009

4240F Instruction in therapeutic exercise with follow-up provided to patients during episode of back pain lasting longer than 12 weeks (BkP)[2]

➔ *CPT Changes: An Insider's View* 2009, 2013

4242F Counseling for supervised exercise program provided to patients during episode of back pain lasting longer than 12 weeks (BkP)[2]

➔ *CPT Changes: An Insider's View* 2009

4245F Patient counseled during the initial visit to maintain or resume normal activities (BkP)[2]

➔ *CPT Changes: An Insider's View* 2009

4248F Patient counseled during the initial visit for an episode of back pain against bed rest lasting 4 days or longer (BkP)[2]

➔ *CPT Changes: An Insider's View* 2009

4250F Active warming used intraoperatively for the purpose of maintaining normothermia, **or** at least 1 body temperature equal to or greater than 36 degrees Centigrade (or 96.8 degrees Fahrenheit) recorded within the 30 minutes immediately before or the 15 minutes immediately after anesthesia end time (CRIT)[1]

➲ *CPT Changes: An Insider's View* 2009, 2010

4255F Duration of general or neuraxial anesthesia 60 minutes or longer, as documented in the anesthesia record (CRIT)[5] (Peri2)[11]

➲ *CPT Changes: An Insider's View* 2011

4256F Duration of general or neuraxial anesthesia less than 60 minutes, as documented in the anesthesia record (CRIT)[5] (Peri2)[11]

➲ *CPT Changes: An Insider's View* 2011

4260F Wound surface culture technique used (CWC)[5]

➲ *CPT Changes: An Insider's View* 2010

4261F Technique other than surface culture of the wound exudate used (eg, Levine/deep swab technique, semi-quantitative or quantitative swab technique) **or** wound surface culture technique not used (CWC)[5]

➲ *CPT Changes: An Insider's View* 2010

4265F Use of wet to dry dressings prescribed or recommended (CWC)[5]

➲ *CPT Changes: An Insider's View* 2010

4266F Use of wet to dry dressings neither prescribed nor recommended (CWC)[5]

➲ *CPT Changes: An Insider's View* 2010

4267F Compression therapy prescribed (CWC)[5]

➲ *CPT Changes: An Insider's View* 2010

4268F Patient education regarding the need for long term compression therapy including interval replacement of compression stockings received (CWC)[5]

➲ *CPT Changes: An Insider's View* 2010

4269F Appropriate method of offloading (pressure relief) prescribed (CWC)[5]

➲ *CPT Changes: An Insider's View* 2010

4270F Patient receiving potent antiretroviral therapy for 6 months or longer (HIV)[5]

➲ *CPT Changes: An Insider's View* 2010

4271F Patient receiving potent antiretroviral therapy for less than 6 months or not receiving potent antiretroviral therapy (HIV)[5]

➲ *CPT Changes: An Insider's View* 2010

4274F Influenza immunization administered or previously received (HIV)[5] (P-ESRD)[1]

➲ *CPT Changes: An Insider's View* 2010

4276F Potent antiretroviral therapy prescribed (HIV)[5]

➲ *CPT Changes: An Insider's View* 2010

4279F Pneumocystis jiroveci pneumonia prophylaxis prescribed (HIV)[5]

➲ *CPT Changes: An Insider's View* 2010

4280F Pneumocystis jiroveci pneumonia prophylaxis prescribed within 3 months of low CD4+ cell count or percentage (HIV)[5]

➲ *CPT Changes: An Insider's View* 2010

4290F Patient screened for injection drug use (HIV)[5]

➲ *CPT Changes: An Insider's View* 2010

4293F Patient screened for high-risk sexual behavior (HIV)[5]

➲ *CPT Changes: An Insider's View* 2010

4300F Patient receiving warfarin therapy for nonvalvular atrial fibrillation or atrial flutter (AFIB)[1]

➲ *CPT Changes: An Insider's View* 2010

4301F Patient not receiving warfarin therapy for nonvalvular atrial fibrillation or atrial flutter (AFIB)[1]

➲ *CPT Changes: An Insider's View* 2010

4305F Patient education regarding appropriate foot care **and** daily inspection of the feet received (CWC)[5]

➲ *CPT Changes: An Insider's View* 2010

4306F Patient counseled regarding psychosocial **and** pharmacologic treatment options for opioid addiction (SUD)[1]

➲ *CPT Changes: An Insider's View* 2010

4320F Patient counseled regarding psychosocial **and** pharmacologic treatment options for alcohol dependence (SUD)[5]

➲ *CPT Changes: An Insider's View* 2010

4322F Caregiver provided with education and referred to additional resources for support (DEM)[1]

➲ *CPT Changes: An Insider's View* 2012

4324F Patient (or caregiver) queried about Parkinson's disease medication related motor complications (Prkns)[8]

➲ *CPT Changes: An Insider's View* 2011

4325F Medical and surgical treatment options reviewed with patient (or caregiver) (Prkns)[8]

➲ *CPT Changes: An Insider's View* 2011

4326F Patient (or caregiver) queried about symptoms of autonomic dysfunction (Prkns)[8]

➲ *CPT Changes: An Insider's View* 2011

4328F Patient (or caregiver) queried about sleep disturbances (Prkns)[8]

➲ *CPT Changes: An Insider's View* 2011

4330F Counseling about epilepsy specific safety issues provided to patient (or caregiver(s)) (EPI)[8]

➲ *CPT Changes: An Insider's View* 2011

4340F Counseling for women of childbearing potential with epilepsy (EPI)[8]

➲ *CPT Changes: An Insider's View* 2011

4350F Counseling provided on symptom management, end of life decisions, and palliation (DEM)[1]

➲ *CPT Changes: An Insider's View* 2012

4400F Rehabilitative therapy options discussed with patient (or caregiver) (Prkns)[8]

➲ *CPT Changes: An Insider's View* 2011

4450F Self-care education provided to patient (HF)[1]
➲ *CPT Changes: An Insider's View* 2012

4470F Implantable cardioverter-defibrillator (ICD) counseling provided (HF)[1]
➲ *CPT Changes: An Insider's View* 2012

4480F Patient receiving ACE inhibitor/ARB therapy and beta-blocker therapy for 3 months or longer (HF)[1]
➲ *CPT Changes: An Insider's View* 2012

4481F Patient receiving ACE inhibitor/ARB therapy and beta-blocker therapy for less than 3 months or patient not receiving ACE inhibitor/ARB therapy and beta-blocker therapy (HF)[1]
➲ *CPT Changes: An Insider's View* 2012

4500F Referred to an outpatient cardiac rehabilitation program (CAD)[1]
➲ *CPT Changes: An Insider's View* 2012

4510F Previous cardiac rehabilitation for qualifying cardiac event completed (CAD)[1]
➲ *CPT Changes: An Insider's View* 2012

4525F Neuropsychiatric intervention ordered (DEM)[1]
➲ *CPT Changes: An Insider's View* 2012

4526F Neuropsychiatric intervention received (DEM)[1]
➲ *CPT Changes: An Insider's View* 2012

4540F Disease modifying pharmacotherapy discussed (ALS)[8]
➲ *CPT Changes: An Insider's View* 2014

4541F Patient offered treatment for pseudobulbar affect, sialorrhea, or ALS-related symptoms (ALS)[8]
➲ *CPT Changes: An Insider's View* 2014

4550F Options for noninvasive respiratory support discussed with patient (ALS)[8]
➲ *CPT Changes: An Insider's View* 2014

4551F Nutritional support offered (ALS)[8]
➲ *CPT Changes: An Insider's View* 2014

4552F Patient offered referral to a speech language pathologist (ALS)[8]
➲ *CPT Changes: An Insider's View* 2014

4553F Patient offered assistance in planning for end of life issues (ALS)[8]
➲ *CPT Changes: An Insider's View* 2014

4554F Patient received inhalational anesthetic agent (Peri2)[11]
➲ *CPT Changes: An Insider's View* 2014

4555F Patient did not receive inhalational anesthetic agent (Peri2)[11]
➲ *CPT Changes: An Insider's View* 2014

4556F Patient exhibits 3 or more risk factors for post-operative nausea and vomiting (Peri2)[11]
➲ *CPT Changes: An Insider's View* 2014

4557F Patient does not exhibit 3 or more risk factors for post-operative nausea and vomiting (Peri2)[11]
➲ *CPT Changes: An Insider's View* 2014

4558F Patient received at least 2 prophylactic pharmacologic anti-emetic agents of different classes preoperatively and intraoperatively (Peri2)[11]
➲ *CPT Changes: An Insider's View* 2014

4559F At least 1 body temperature measurement equal to or greater than 35.5 degrees Celsius (or 95.9 degrees Fahrenheit) recorded within the 30 minutes immediately before or the 15 minutes immediately after anesthesia end time (Peri2)[11]
➲ *CPT Changes: An Insider's View* 2014

4560F Anesthesia technique did not involve general or neuraxial anesthesia (Peri2)[11]
➲ *CPT Changes: An Insider's View* 2014

4561F Patient has a coronary artery stent (Peri2)[11]
➲ *CPT Changes: An Insider's View* 2014

4562F Patient does not have a coronary artery stent (Peri2)[11]
➲ *CPT Changes: An Insider's View* 2014

4563F Patient received aspirin within 24 hours prior to anesthesia start time (Peri2)[11]
➲ *CPT Changes: An Insider's View* 2014

Follow-up or Other Outcomes

Follow-up or other outcomes codes describe review and communication of test results to patients, patient satisfaction or experience with care, patient functional status, and patient morbidity and mortality.

5005F Patient counseled on self-examination for new or changing moles (ML)[5]
➲ *CPT Changes: An Insider's View* 2008

5010F Findings of dilated macular or fundus exam communicated to the physician or other qualified health care professional managing the diabetes care (EC)[5]
➲ *CPT Changes: An Insider's View* 2008, 2013

5015F Documentation of communication that a fracture occurred and that the patient was or should be tested or treated for osteoporosis (OP)[5]
➲ *CPT Changes: An Insider's View* 2008

5020F Treatment summary report communicated to physician(s) or other qualified health care professional(s) managing continuing care and to the patient within 1 month of completing treatment (ONC)[1]
➲ *CPT Changes: An Insider's View* 2009, 2010, 2013

5050F Treatment plan communicated to provider(s) managing continuing care within 1 month of diagnosis (ML)[5]
➲ *CPT Changes: An Insider's View* 2009

5060F Findings from diagnostic mammogram communicated to practice managing patient's on-going care within 3 business days of exam interpretation (RAD)[5]
➲ *CPT Changes: An Insider's View* 2009

5062F Findings from diagnostic mammogram communicated to the patient within 5 days of exam interpretation (RAD)[5]
➲ *CPT Changes: An Insider's View* 2009

5100F Potential risk for fracture communicated to the referring physician or other qualified health care professional within 24 hours of completion of the imaging study (NUC_MED)[1]

CPT Changes: An Insider's View 2010, 2013

5200F Consideration of referral for a neurological evaluation of appropriateness for surgical therapy for intractable epilepsy within the past 3 years (EPI)[8]

CPT Changes: An Insider's View 2011

5250F Asthma discharge plan provided to patient (Asthma)[1]

CPT Changes: An Insider's View 2012

Patient Safety

Patient safety codes that describe patient safety practices.

6005F Rationale (eg, severity of illness and safety) for level of care (eg, home, hospital) documented (CAP)[1]

CPT Changes: An Insider's View 2007

CPT Assistant Aug 07:1

6010F Dysphagia screening conducted prior to order for or receipt of any foods, fluids, or medication by mouth (STR)[5]

CPT Changes: An Insider's View 2008

6015F Patient receiving or eligible to receive foods, fluids, or medication by mouth (STR)[5]

CPT Changes: An Insider's View 2008

6020F NPO (nothing by mouth) ordered (STR)[5]

CPT Changes: An Insider's View 2008

6030F All elements of maximal sterile barrier technique, hand hygiene, skin preparation and, if ultrasound is used, sterile ultrasound techniques followed (CRIT)[1]

CPT Changes: An Insider's View 2009, 2010, 2016

6040F Use of appropriate radiation dose reduction devices OR manual techniques for appropriate moderation of exposure, documented (RAD)[5]

CPT Changes: An Insider's View 2009

6045F Radiation exposure or exposure time in final report for procedure using fluoroscopy, documented (RAD)[5]

CPT Changes: An Insider's View 2009

Clinical Examples in Radiology Summer 10:1, Spring 11:2, 9-10, Summer 11:2, Fall 11:2-3, Winter 11:2, Spring 13:2, 3, 6, Summer 13:2, 3, 5, 6, Spring 14:7, Fall 14:6

6070F Patient queried and counseled about anti-epileptic drug (AED) side effects (EPI)[8]

CPT Changes: An Insider's View 2011

6080F Patient (or caregiver) queried about falls (Prkns, DSP)[8]

CPT Changes: An Insider's View 2011

6090F Patient (or caregiver) counseled about safety issues appropriate to patient's stage of disease (Prkns)[8]

CPT Changes: An Insider's View 2011

6100F Timeout to verify correct patient, correct site, and correct procedure, documented (PATH)[9]

CPT Changes: An Insider's View 2012

6101F Safety counseling for dementia provided (DEM)[1]

CPT Changes: An Insider's View 2012

6102F Safety counseling for dementia ordered (DEM)[1]

CPT Changes: An Insider's View 2012

6110F Counseling provided regarding risks of driving and the alternatives to driving (DEM)[1]

CPT Changes: An Insider's View 2012

6150F Patient not receiving a first course of anti-TNF (tumor necrosis factor) therapy (IBD)[10]

CPT Changes: An Insider's View 2013

Structural Measures

Structural measures codes are used to identify measures that address the setting or system of the delivered care. These codes also address aspects of the capabilities of the organization or health care professional providing the care.

7010F Patient information entered into a recall system that includes: target date for the next exam specified **and** a process to follow up with patients regarding missed or unscheduled appointments (ML)[5]

CPT Changes: An Insider's View 2009, 2011

7020F Mammogram assessment category (eg, Mammography Quality Standards Act [MQSA], Breast Imaging Reporting and Data System [BI-RADS®], or FDA approved equivalent categories) entered into an internal database to allow for analysis of abnormal interpretation (recall) rate (RAD)[5]

CPT Changes: An Insider's View 2009

7025F Patient information entered into a reminder system with a target due date for the next mammogram (RAD)[5]

CPT Changes: An Insider's View 2009

Nonmeasure Code Listing

The following codes are included for reporting of certain aspects of care. These factors are not represented by measures developed by existing measures organizations or recognized measures-development processes at the time they are placed in the CPT code set, but may ultimately be associated with measures approved by an appropriate quality improvement organization.

9001F Aortic aneurysm less than 5.0 cm maximum diameter on centerline formatted CT or minor diameter on axial formatted CT (NMA–No Measure Associated)

CPT Changes: An Insider's View 2014

9002F Aortic aneurysm 5.0 - 5.4 cm maximum diameter on centerline formatted CT or minor diameter on axial formatted CT (NMA–No Measure Associated)

CPT Changes: An Insider's View 2014

9003F Aortic aneurysm 5.5 - 5.9 cm maximum diameter on centerline formatted CT or minor diameter on axial formatted CT (NMA–No Measure Associated)

CPT Changes: An Insider's View 2014

9004F Aortic aneurysm 6.0 cm or greater maximum diameter on centerline formatted CT or minor diameter on axial formatted CT (NMA–No Measure Associated)

CPT Changes: An Insider's View 2014

9005F Asymptomatic carotid stenosis: No history of any transient ischemic attack or stroke in any carotid or vertebrobasilar territory (NMA–No Measure Associated)

CPT Changes: An Insider's View 2014

9006F Symptomatic carotid stenosis: Ipsilateral carotid territory TIA or stroke less than 120 days prior to procedure (NMA–No Measure Associated)

CPT Changes: An Insider's View 2014

9007F Other carotid stenosis: Ipsilateral TIA or stroke 120 days or greater prior to procedure or any prior contralateral carotid territory or vertebrobasilar TIA or stroke (NMA–No Measure Associated)

CPT Changes: An Insider's View 2014

Notes

Category III Codes

The following section contains a set of temporary codes for emerging technology, services, procedures, and service paradigms. Category III codes allow data collection for these services/procedures. Use of unlisted codes does not offer the opportunity for the collection of specific data. If a Category III code is available, this code must be reported instead of a Category I unlisted code. This is an activity that is critically important in the evaluation of health care delivery and the formation of public and private policy. The use of the codes in this section allows physicians and other qualified health care professionals, insurers, health services researchers, and health policy experts to identify emerging technology, services, procedures, and service paradigms for clinical efficacy, utilization and outcomes.

The inclusion of a service or procedure in this section does not constitute a finding of support, or lack thereof, with regard to clinical efficacy, safety, applicability to clinical practice, or payer coverage. The codes in this section may not conform to the usual requirements for CPT Category I codes established by the Editorial Panel. For Category I codes, the Panel requires that the service/procedure be performed by many health care professionals in clinical practice in multiple locations and that FDA approval, as appropriate, has already been received. The nature of emerging technology, services, procedures, and service paradigms is such that these requirements may not be met. For these reasons, temporary codes for emerging technology, services, procedures, and service paradigms have been placed in a separate section of the CPT code set and the codes are differentiated from Category I CPT codes by the use of alphanumeric characters.

▶Services and procedures described in this section make use of alphanumeric characters. These codes have an alpha character as the 5th character in the string (ie, four digits followed by the letter T). The digits are not intended to reflect the placement of the code in the Category I section of CPT nomenclature. Codes in this section may or may not eventually receive a Category I CPT code. In either case, in general, a given Category III code will be archived five years from the date of initial publication or extension unless a modification of the archival date is specifically noted at the time of a revision or change to a code (eg, addition of parenthetical instructions, reinstatement). Services and procedures described by Category III codes which have been archived after five years, without conversion, must be reported using the Category I unlisted code unless another specific cross-reference is established at the time of archiving. New codes or revised codes in this section are released semi-annually via the AMA CPT website to expedite dissemination for reporting. Codes approved for deletion are published annually with the full set of temporary codes for emerging technology, services, procedures, and service paradigms in the CPT code set. Go to www.ama-assn.org/go/cpt for the most current listing.◀

(For destruction of localized lesion of choroid by transpupillary thermotherapy, use 67299)

(For destruction of macular drusen, photocoagulation, use 67299)

(0019T has been deleted)

(For extracorporeal shock wave involving musculoskeletal system, not otherwise specified, low energy, use 20999)

(For application of high energy extracorporeal shock wave involving musculoskeletal system not otherwise specified, use 0101T)

(For application of high energy extracorporeal shock wave involving lateral humeral epicondyle, use 0102T)

(For non-surgical septal reduction therapy, use 93799)

(For lipoprotein, direct measurement, intermediate density lipoproteins [IDL] [remnant lipoprotein], use 84999)

(For endoscopic lysis of epidural adhesions with direct visualization using mechanical means or solution injection [eg, normal saline], use 64999)

(For dual energy x-ray absorptiometry [DXA] body composition study, use 76499)

(For pulsed magnetic neuromodulation incontinence treatment, use 53899)

(To report antiprothrombin [phospholipid cofactor] antibody, use 86849)

(0031T, 0032T have been deleted)

(For speculoscopy, including sampling, use 58999)

(For urinalysis infectious agent detection, semi-quantitative analysis of volatile compounds, use 81099)

0042T Cerebral perfusion analysis using computed tomography with contrast administration, including post-processing of parametric maps with determination of cerebral blood flow, cerebral blood volume, and mean transit time

Sunset January 2024

➲ *CPT Changes: An Insider's View* 2003

(For carbon monoxide, expired gas analysis [eg, ETCOc/hemolysis breath test], use 84999)

(0046T, 0047T have been deleted)

(For mammary duct[s] catheter lavage, use 19499)

(0051T, 0052T, 0053T have been deleted. To report, see 33927, 33928, 33929)

+ 0054T Computer-assisted musculoskeletal surgical navigational orthopedic procedure, with image-guidance based on fluoroscopic images (List separately in addition to code for primary procedure)
Sunset January 2024
➔ *CPT Changes: An Insider's View* 2004
➔ *CPT Assistant* May 04:14, Jun 04:8

+ 0055T Computer-assisted musculoskeletal surgical navigational orthopedic procedure, with image-guidance based on CT/MRI images (List separately in addition to code for primary procedure)
Sunset January 2024
➔ *CPT Changes: An Insider's View* 2004, 2005
➔ *CPT Assistant* May 04:14, Jun 04:8

(When CT and MRI are both performed, report 0055T only once)

0058T Cryopreservation; reproductive tissue, ovarian
Sunset January 2021
➔ *CPT Changes: An Insider's View* 2004, 2011

(For cryopreservation of mature oocyte(s), use 89337. For cryopreservation of immature oocyte(s), use 0357T)

 # 0357T immature oocyte(s)
Sunset January 2020
➔ *CPT Changes: An Insider's View* 2015

(For cryopreservation of mature oocyte(s), use 89337)

(For cryopreservation of embryo(s), sperm and testicular reproductive tissue, see 89258, 89259, 89335)

(For electrical impedance breast scan, use 76499)

(For destruction/reduction of malignant breast tumor, microwave phased array thermotherapy, use 19499)

(0062T, 0063T have been deleted)

(For percutaneous intradiscal annuloplasty, any method other than electrothermal, use 22899)

(For intradiscal electrothermal annuloplasty, see 22526, 22527)

(To report CT colon, screening, use 74263)

(To report CT colon, diagnostic, see 74261-74262)

(0068T-0070T have been deleted)

(For acoustic heart sound recording and computer analysis, use 93799)

0071T Focused ultrasound ablation of uterine leiomyomata, including MR guidance; total leiomyomata volume less than 200 cc of tissue
Sunset January 2020
➔ *CPT Changes: An Insider's View* 2005
➔ *CPT Assistant* Mar 05:1, 5, Dec 05:3

0072T total leiomyomata volume greater or equal to 200 cc of tissue
Sunset January 2020
➔ *CPT Changes: An Insider's View* 2005
➔ *CPT Assistant* Mar 05:1, 5, Dec 05:3

(Do not report 0071T, 0072T in conjunction with 51702 or 77022)

0075T Transcatheter placement of extracranial vertebral artery stent(s), including radiologic supervision and interpretation, open or percutaneous; initial vessel
Sunset January 2020
➔ *CPT Changes: An Insider's View* 2005, 2015
➔ *CPT Assistant* May 05:7, Mar 14:8

+ 0076T each additional vessel (List separately in addition to code for primary procedure)
Sunset January 2020
➔ *CPT Changes: An Insider's View* 2005, 2015
➔ *CPT Assistant* May 05:7, Mar 14:8

(Use 0076T in conjunction with 0075T)

(When the ipsilateral extracranial vertebral arteriogram (including imaging and selective catheterization) confirms the need for stenting, then 0075T and 0076T include all ipsilateral extracranial vertebral catheterization, all diagnostic imaging for ipsilateral extracranial vertebral artery stenting, and all related radiologic supervision and interpretation. If stenting is not indicated, then the appropriate codes for selective catheterization and imaging should be reported in lieu of 0075T or 0076T)

0085T Breath test for heart transplant rejection
Sunset January 2021
➔ *CPT Changes: An Insider's View* 2005
➔ *CPT Assistant* May 05:7

(To report total disc lumbar arthroplasty, use 22857)

(For cervical arthroplasty procedure on three or more levels, use 0375T)

+ 0095T Removal of total disc arthroplasty (artificial disc), anterior approach, each additional interspace, cervical (List separately in addition to code for primary procedure)
Sunset January 2024
➔ *CPT Changes: An Insider's View* 2006, 2009
➔ *CPT Assistant* Jun 05:6, Feb 06:1

(Use 0095T in conjunction with 22864)

(To report revision of total disc lumbar arthroplasty, use 22862)

+ 0098T Revision including replacement of total disc arthroplasty (artificial disc), anterior approach, each additional interspace, cervical (List separately in addition to code for primary procedure)
Sunset January 2024
➔ *CPT Changes: An Insider's View* 2006, 2009
➔ *CPT Assistant* Jun 05:6, Feb 06:1

(Use 0098T in conjunction with 22861)

(Do not report 0098T in conjunction with 0095T)

(Do not report 0098T in conjunction with 22853, 22854, 22859 when performed at the same level)

(For decompression, see 63001-63048)

(0099T has been deleted. To report, use 65785)

0100T Placement of a subconjunctival retinal prosthesis receiver and pulse generator, and implantation of intraocular retinal electrode array, with vitrectomy
Sunset January 2021
➲ *CPT Changes: An Insider's View* 2006
➲ *CPT Assistant* Jun 05:6, Feb 06:1, Jun 11:13, Feb 18:3

(For initial programming of implantable intraocular retinal electrode array device, use 0472T)

0101T Extracorporeal shock wave involving musculoskeletal system, not otherwise specified, high energy
Sunset January 2021
➲ *CPT Changes: An Insider's View* 2006
➲ *CPT Assistant* Jun 05:6, Mar 06:1, Jun 11:13

►(For extracorporeal shock wave therapy involving integumentary system not otherwise specified, see 0512T, 0513T)◄

►(Do not report 0101T in conjunction 0512T, 0513T, when treating same area)◄

0102T Extracorporeal shock wave, high energy, performed by a physician, requiring anesthesia other than local, involving lateral humeral epicondyle
Sunset January 2021
➲ *CPT Changes: An Insider's View* 2006
➲ *CPT Assistant* Jun 05:6, Mar 06:1, Jun 11:13

#● 0512T Extracorporeal shock wave for integumentary wound healing, high energy, including topical application and dressing care; initial wound
Sunset January 2024
➲ *CPT Changes: An Insider's View* 2019

#+● 0513T each additional wound (List separately in addition to code for primary procedure)
Sunset January 2024
➲ *CPT Changes: An Insider's View* 2019

►(Use 0513T in conjunction with 0512T)◄

(0103T has been deleted)

(For holotranscobalamin, quantitative, use 84999)

(For inert gas rebreathing for cardiac output measurement during rest, use 93799)

(For inert gas rebreathing for cardiac output measurement during exercise, use 93799)

0106T Quantitative sensory testing (QST), testing and interpretation per extremity; using touch pressure stimuli to assess large diameter sensation
Sunset January 2021
➲ *CPT Changes: An Insider's View* 2006
➲ *CPT Assistant* Jun 05:6, Mar 06:1, May 11:10, Jun 11:13

0107T using vibration stimuli to assess large diameter fiber sensation
Sunset January 2021
➲ *CPT Changes: An Insider's View* 2006
➲ *CPT Assistant* Jun 05:6, Mar 06:1, May 11:10, Jun 11:13

0108T using cooling stimuli to assess small nerve fiber sensation and hyperalgesia
Sunset January 2021
➲ *CPT Changes: An Insider's View* 2006
➲ *CPT Assistant* Jun 05:6, Mar 06:1, May 11:10, Jun 11:13

0109T using heat-pain stimuli to assess small nerve fiber sensation and hyperalgesia
Sunset January 2021
➲ *CPT Changes: An Insider's View* 2006
➲ *CPT Assistant* Jun 05:6, Mar 06:1, May 11:10, Jun 11:13

0110T using other stimuli to assess sensation
Sunset January 2021
➲ *CPT Changes: An Insider's View* 2006
➲ *CPT Assistant* Jun 05:6, Mar 06:1, May 11:10, Jun 11:13

0111T Long-chain (C20-22) omega-3 fatty acids in red blood cell (RBC) membranes
Sunset January 2021
➲ *CPT Changes: An Insider's View* 2006
➲ *CPT Assistant* Jun 05:6, Mar 06:1, Jun 11:13

(For very long chain fatty acids, use 82726)

(0123T has been deleted)

(For fistulization of sclera for glaucoma, through ciliary body, use 66999)

(For conjunctival incision with posterior extrascleral placement of pharmacological agent, use 68399)

0126T Common carotid intima-media thickness (IMT) study for evaluation of atherosclerotic burden or coronary heart disease risk factor assessment
Sunset January 2021
➲ *CPT Changes: An Insider's View* 2006
➲ *CPT Assistant* Jun 11:13

(Do not report 0126T in conjunction with 93880, 93882, 93895)

(For bilateral quantitative carotid intima media thickness and carotid atheroma evaluation that includes all required elements, use 93895)

(For validated, statistically reliable, randomized, controlled, single-patient clinical investigation of FDA approved chronic care drugs, provided by a pharmacist, interpretation and report to the prescribing health care professional, use 99199)

(To report pancreatic islet cell transplantation, use 48999)

(0144T-0151T have been deleted. To report, see 75571-75574)

(For laparoscopic implantation, replacement, revision, or removal of gastric stimulation electrodes, lesser curvature, use 43659)

(For open implantation, replacement, revision, or removal of gastric stimulation electrodes, lesser curvature, use 43999)

►(0159T has been deleted. To report, see 77048, 77049)◄

+ 0163T Total disc arthroplasty (artificial disc), anterior approach, including discectomy to prepare interspace (other than for decompression), each additional interspace, lumbar (List separately in addition to code for primary procedure)

Sunset January 2024

➔ *CPT Changes: An Insider's View* 2007, 2009

➔ *CPT Assistant* Jun 07:1

(Use 0163T in conjunction with 22857)

+ 0164T Removal of total disc arthroplasty, (artificial disc), anterior approach, each additional interspace, lumbar (List separately in addition to code for primary procedure)

Sunset January 2024

➔ *CPT Changes: An Insider's View* 2007, 2009

➔ *CPT Assistant* Jun 07:1

(Use 0164T in conjunction with 22865)

+ 0165T Revision including replacement of total disc arthroplasty (artificial disc), anterior approach, each additional interspace, lumbar (List separately in addition to code for primary procedure)

Sunset January 2024

➔ *CPT Changes: An Insider's View* 2007, 2009

➔ *CPT Assistant* Jun 07:1

(Use 0165T in conjunction with 22862)

(Do not report 0163T, 0164T, 0165T in conjunction with 22853, 22854, 22859, 49010, when performed at the same level)

(For decompression, see 63001-63048)

(For transmyocardial transcatheter closure of ventricular septal defect, with implant, including cardiopulmonary bypass if performed, use 33999)

(For rhinophototherapy, intranasal application of ultraviolet and visible light, use 30999)

(0169T has been deleted)

(For stereotactic placement of infusion catheter[s] in the brain for delivery of therapeutic agent[s], use 64999)

(0171T has been deleted)

(To report insertion of interlaminar/interspinous process stabilization/distraction device, without fusion, including image guidance when performed, with open decompression, lumbar, single level, use 22867. To report insertion of interlaminar/interspinous process stabilization/distraction device, without open decompression or fusion, including image guidance when performed, lumbar, single level, use 22869)

(0172T has been deleted)

(To report insertion of interlaminar/interspinous process stabilization/distraction device, without fusion, including image guidance when performed, with open decompression, lumbar, second level, use 22868. To report insertion of interlaminar/interspinous process stabilization/distraction device, without open decompression or fusion, including image guidance when performed, lumbar, second level use, 22870)

+ 0174T Computer-aided detection (CAD) (computer algorithm analysis of digital image data for lesion detection) with further physician review for interpretation and report, with or without digitization of film radiographic images, chest radiograph(s), performed concurrent with primary interpretation (List separately in addition to code for primary procedure)

Sunset January 2022

➔ *CPT Changes: An Insider's View* 2008

➔ *CPT Assistant* Apr 18:7

(Use 0174T in conjunction with 71045, 71046, 71047, 71048)

0175T Computer-aided detection (CAD) (computer algorithm analysis of digital image data for lesion detection) with further physician review for interpretation and report, with or without digitization of film radiographic images, chest radiograph(s), performed remote from primary interpretation

Sunset January 2022

➔ *CPT Changes: An Insider's View* 2008

➔ *CPT Assistant* Apr 18:7

(Do not report 0175T in conjunction with 71045, 71046, 71047, 71048)

(0178T, 0179T, 0180T have been deleted)

(For electrocardiogram, 64 leads or greater, with graphic presentation and analysis, use 93799)

(For electrocardiogram routine, with at least 12 leads separately performed, see 93000-93010)

(0182T has been deleted. To report, see 0394T, 0395T)

0184T Excision of rectal tumor, transanal endoscopic microsurgical approach (ie, TEMS), including muscularis propria (ie, full thickness)

Sunset January 2024

➔ *CPT Changes: An Insider's View* 2009, 2011

➔ *CPT Assistant* Jun 10:3, Feb 18:11

(For non-endoscopic excision of rectal tumor, see 45160, 45171, 45172)

(Do not report 0184T in conjunction with 45300, 45308, 45309, 45315, 45317, 45320, 69990)

(For multivariate analysis of patient-specific findings with quantifiable computer probability assessment, including report, use 99199)

(For suprachoroidal delivery of pharmacologic agent, use 67299)

Remote Real-Time Interactive Video-conferenced Critical Care Services

►(0188T, 0189T have been deleted)◄

►(For remote real-time interactive video-conferenced critical care, evaluation and management of the critically ill or critically injured patient, use 99499)◄

►(0190T has been deleted)◄

►(For placement of intraocular radiation source applicator, use 67299)◄

(For application of the source by radiation oncologist, see Clinical Brachytherapy section)

0191T Insertion of anterior segment aqueous drainage device, without extraocular reservoir, internal approach, into the trabecular meshwork; initial insertion
Sunset January 2024
➲ *CPT Changes: An Insider's View* 2009, 2011, 2015
➲ *CPT Assistant* Dec 12:14, Feb 18:3

#+ 0376T each additional device insertion (List separately in addition to code for primary procedure)
Sunset January 2024
➲ *CPT Changes: An Insider's View* 2015
➲ *CPT Assistant* Feb 18:3

(Use 0376T in conjunction with 0191T)

 # 0253T Insertion of anterior segment aqueous drainage device, without extraocular reservoir, internal approach, into the suprachoroidal space
Sunset January 2024
➲ *CPT Changes: An Insider's View* 2011, 2015

(To report insertion of drainage device by external approach, use 66183)

►(0195T, 0196T have been deleted)◄

►(For arthrodesis, pre-sacral interbody technique, disc space preparation, discectomy, without instrumentation, with image guidance, includes bone graft when performed, L4-L5 interspace, L5-S1 interspace, use 22899)◄

0198T Measurement of ocular blood flow by repetitive intraocular pressure sampling, with interpretation and report
Sunset January 2020
➲ *CPT Changes: An Insider's View* 2010
➲ *CPT Assistant* Mar 11:10, Aug 12:9

(For tremor measurement with accelerometer(s) and/or gyroscope(s), use 95999)

0200T Percutaneous sacral augmentation (sacroplasty), unilateral injection(s), including the use of a balloon or mechanical device, when used, 1 or more needles, includes imaging guidance and bone biopsy, when performed
Sunset January 2020
➲ *CPT Changes: An Insider's View* 2010, 2015, 2017
➲ *CPT Assistant* Apr 15:8, Dec 15:17
➲ *Clinical Examples in Radiology* Fall 14:3

0201T Percutaneous sacral augmentation (sacroplasty), bilateral injections, including the use of a balloon or mechanical device, when used, 2 or more needles, includes imaging guidance and bone biopsy, when performed
Sunset January 2020
➲ *CPT Changes: An Insider's View* 2010, 2015, 2017
➲ *CPT Assistant* Apr 15:8, Dec 15:19

(Do not report 0200T, 0201T in conjunction with 20225 when performed at the same level)

0202T Posterior vertebral joint(s) arthroplasty (eg, facet joint[s] replacement), including facetectomy, laminectomy, foraminotomy, and vertebral column fixation, injection of bone cement, when performed, including fluoroscopy, single level, lumbar spine
Sunset January 2020
➲ *CPT Changes: An Insider's View* 2015

(Do not report 0202T in conjunction with 22511, 22514, 22840, 22853, 22854, 22857, 22859, 63005, 63012, 63017, 63030, 63042, 63047, 63056 at the same level)

+ 0205T Intravascular catheter-based coronary vessel or graft spectroscopy (eg, infrared) during diagnostic evaluation and/or therapeutic intervention including imaging supervision, interpretation, and report, each vessel (List separately in addition to code for primary procedure)
Sunset January 2020
➲ *CPT Changes: An Insider's View* 2010

(Use 0205T in conjunction with 92920, 92924, 92928, 92933, 92937, 92941, 92943, 92975, 93454-93461, 93563, 93564)

0206T Computerized database analysis of multiple cycles of digitized cardiac electrical data from two or more ECG leads, including transmission to a remote center, application of multiple nonlinear mathematical transformations, with coronary artery obstruction severity assessment
Sunset January 2020
➲ *CPT Changes: An Insider's View* 2010, 2013

(When a 12-lead ECG is performed, 93000-93010 may be reported, as appropriate)

0207T Evacuation of meibomian glands, automated, using heat and intermittent pressure, unilateral
Sunset January 2020
➲ *CPT Changes: An Insider's View* 2010
➲ *CPT Assistant* May 14:5

0208T Pure tone audiometry (threshold), automated; air only
Sunset January 2021
➲ *CPT Changes: An Insider's View* 2011
➲ *CPT Assistant* Aug 14:3

0209T air and bone
Sunset January 2021
➲ *CPT Changes: An Insider's View* 2011
➲ *CPT Assistant* Mar 11:8, Aug 14:3

0210T Speech audiometry threshold, automated;
Sunset January 2021
➔ *CPT Changes: An Insider's View* 2011

0211T with speech recognition
Sunset January 2021
➔ *CPT Changes: An Insider's View* 2011
➔ *CPT Assistant* Mar 11:8

0212T Comprehensive audiometry threshold evaluation and speech recognition (0209T, 0211T combined), automated
Sunset January 2021
➔ *CPT Changes: An Insider's View* 2011
➔ *CPT Assistant* Mar 11:8, Aug 14:3

(For audiometric testing using audiometers performed manually by a qualified health care professional, see 92551-92557)

0213T Injection(s), diagnostic or therapeutic agent, paravertebral facet (zygapophyseal) joint (or nerves innervating that joint) with ultrasound guidance, cervical or thoracic; single level
Sunset January 2021
➔ *CPT Changes: An Insider's View* 2011
➔ *CPT Assistant* Feb 11:5, Jul 11:14
➔ *Clinical Examples in Radiology* Winter 10:15

(To report bilateral procedure, use 0213T with modifier 50)

+ 0214T second level (List separately in addition to code for primary procedure)
Sunset January 2021
➔ *CPT Changes: An Insider's View* 2011
➔ *CPT Assistant* Jul 11:14
➔ *Clinical Examples in Radiology* Winter 10:15

(Use 0214T in conjunction with 0213T)

(To report bilateral procedure, use 0214T with modifier 50)

+ 0215T third and any additional level(s) (List separately in addition to code for primary procedure)
Sunset January 2021
➔ *CPT Changes: An Insider's View* 2011
➔ *CPT Assistant* Jul 11:14
➔ *Clinical Examples in Radiology* Winter 10:14

(Do not report 0215T more than once per day)

(Use 0215T in conjunction with 0213T, 0214T)

(To report bilateral procedure, use 0215T with modifier 50)

0216T Injection(s), diagnostic or therapeutic agent, paravertebral facet (zygapophyseal) joint (or nerves innervating that joint) with ultrasound guidance, lumbar or sacral; single level
Sunset January 2021
➔ *CPT Changes: An Insider's View* 2011
➔ *CPT Assistant* Jul 11:14
➔ *Clinical Examples in Radiology* Winter 10:14

(To report bilateral procedure, use 0216T with modifier 50)

+ 0217T second level (List separately in addition to code for primary procedure)
Sunset January 2021
➔ *CPT Changes: An Insider's View* 2011
➔ *CPT Assistant* Jul 11:14
➔ *Clinical Examples in Radiology* Winter 10:14

(Use 0217T in conjunction with 0216T)

(To report bilateral procedure, use 0217T with modifier 50)

+ 0218T third and any additional level(s) (List separately in addition to code for primary procedure)
Sunset January 2021
➔ *CPT Changes: An Insider's View* 2011
➔ *CPT Assistant* Feb 11:5, Jul 11:14
➔ *Clinical Examples in Radiology* Winter 10:14

(Do not report 0218T more than once per day)

(Use 0218T in conjunction with 0216T, 0217T)

(If injection(s) are performed using fluoroscopy or CT, see 64490-64495)

(To report bilateral procedure, use 0218T with modifier 50)

0219T Placement of a posterior intrafacet implant(s), unilateral or bilateral, including imaging and placement of bone graft(s) or synthetic device(s), single level; cervical
Sunset January 2021
➔ *CPT Changes: An Insider's View* 2011
➔ *CPT Assistant* Nov 10:8, Jul 11:18

0220T thoracic
Sunset January 2021
➔ *CPT Changes: An Insider's View* 2011
➔ *CPT Assistant* Nov 10:8, Jul 11:18

0221T lumbar
Sunset January 2021
➔ *CPT Changes: An Insider's View* 2011
➔ *CPT Assistant* Nov 10:8, Jul 11:18

(Do not report 0219T-0221T in conjunction with any radiological service)

(Do not report 0219T, 0220T, 0221T in conjunction with 20930, 20931, 22600-22614, 22840, 22853, 22854, 22859 at the same level)

+ 0222T each additional vertebral segment (List separately in addition to code for primary procedure)
Sunset January 2021
➔ *CPT Changes: An Insider's View* 2011
➔ *CPT Assistant* Nov 10:6, Jul 11:18

(Use 0222T in conjunction with 0219T-0221T)

(For posterior or posterolateral arthrodesis technique, see 22600-22614)

Category III 0042T-0542T

0228T Injection(s), anesthetic agent and/or steroid, transforaminal epidural, with ultrasound guidance, cervical or thoracic; single level
Sunset January 2021
➲ *CPT Changes: An Insider's View* 2011
➲ *CPT Assistant* Feb 11:4, Jul 11:16
➲ *Clinical Examples in Radiology* Winter 18:8

+ 0229T each additional level (List separately in addition to code for primary procedure)
Sunset January 2021
➲ *CPT Changes: An Insider's View* 2011
➲ *CPT Assistant* Feb 11:4, Jul 11:16
➲ *Clinical Examples in Radiology* Winter 18:8

(Use 0229T in conjunction with 0228T)

0230T Injection(s), anesthetic agent and/or steroid, transforaminal epidural, with ultrasound guidance, lumbar or sacral; single level
Sunset January 2021
➲ *CPT Changes: An Insider's View* 2011
➲ *CPT Assistant* Feb 11:4, Jul 11:16, Nov 11:11
➲ *Clinical Examples in Radiology* Winter 18:8

+ 0231T each additional level (List separately in addition to code for primary procedure)
Sunset January 2021
➲ *CPT Changes: An Insider's View* 2011
➲ *CPT Assistant* Feb 11:4, Jul 11:16
➲ *Clinical Examples in Radiology* Winter 18:8

(Use 0231T in conjunction with 0230T)

(For transforaminal epidural injections performed under fluoroscopy or CT, see 64479–64484)

(Do not report 0228T-0231T in conjunction with 76942, 76998, 76999)

0232T Injection(s), platelet rich plasma, any site, including image guidance, harvesting and preparation when performed
Sunset January 2022
➲ *CPT Changes: An Insider's View* 2011
➲ *CPT Assistant* Oct 10:8, Dec 10:8, May 12:11, Oct 12:14
➲ *Clinical Examples in Radiology* Spring 18:6

(Do not report 0232T in conjunction with 20550, 20551, 20600, 20604, 20605, 20606, 20610, 20611, 20926, 36415, 36592, 76942, 77002, 77012, 77021, 86965, 0481T)

(Do not report 38220-38230 for bone marrow aspiration for platelet rich stem cell injection. For bone marrow aspiration for platelet rich stem cell injection, use 0232T)

(0233T has been deleted. To report skin advanced glycation endproducts measurement by multi-wavelength fluorescent spectroscopy, use 88749)

Atherectomy (Open or Percutaneous) for Supra-Inguinal Arteries

Codes 0234T-0238T describe atherectomy performed by any method (eg, directional, rotational, laser) in arteries above the inguinal ligaments. These codes are structured differently than the codes describing atherectomy performed below the inguinal ligaments (37225, 37227, 37229, 37231, 37233, 37235).

These supra-inguinal atherectomy codes all include the surgical work of performing the atherectomy plus the radiological supervision and interpretation of the atherectomy. Unlike the atherectomy codes for infra-inguinal arteries, this set of Category III codes does not include accessing and selectively catheterizing the vessel, traversing the lesion, embolic protection if used, other intervention used to treat the same or other vessels, or closure of the arteriotomy by any method. These codes describe endovascular procedures performed percutaneously and/or through an open surgical exposure.

0234T Transluminal peripheral atherectomy, open or percutaneous, including radiological supervision and interpretation; renal artery
Sunset January 2021
➲ *CPT Changes: An Insider's View* 2011
➲ *CPT Assistant* Jul 11:3
➲ *Clinical Examples in Radiology* Spring 11:3

0235T visceral artery (except renal), each vessel
Sunset January 2021
➲ *CPT Changes: An Insider's View* 2011
➲ *CPT Assistant* Jul 11:3
➲ *Clinical Examples in Radiology* Spring 11:3

0236T abdominal aorta
Sunset January 2021
➲ *CPT Changes: An Insider's View* 2011
➲ *CPT Assistant* Jul 11:3
➲ *Clinical Examples in Radiology* Spring 11:3

0237T brachiocephalic trunk and branches, each vessel
Sunset January 2021
➲ *CPT Changes: An Insider's View* 2011
➲ *CPT Assistant* Jul 11:3
➲ *Clinical Examples in Radiology* Spring 11:3

0238T iliac artery, each vessel
Sunset January 2021
➲ *CPT Changes: An Insider's View* 2011
➲ *CPT Assistant* Jul 11:3
➲ *Clinical Examples in Radiology* Spring 11:3

(To report esophageal motility studies without high resolution esophageal pressure topography, use 91010 and with stimulant or perfusion, use 91013)

0249T Ligation, hemorrhoidal vascular bundle(s), including ultrasound guidance
Sunset January 2021
➲ *CPT Changes: An Insider's View* 2011

(Do not report 0249T in conjunction with 46020, 46221, 46250-46262, 46600, 46945, 46946, 76872, 76942, 76998)

0253T Code is out of numerical sequence. See 0184T-0200T

0254T Endovascular repair of iliac artery bifurcation (eg, aneurysm, pseudoaneurysm, arteriovenous malformation, trauma, dissection) using bifurcated endograft from the common iliac artery into both the external and internal iliac artery, including all selective and/or nonselective catheterization(s) required for device placement and all associated radiological supervision and interpretation, unilateral

Sunset January 2021

➔ *CPT Changes: An Insider's View* 2011, 2018

➔ *CPT Assistant* Dec 13:8

(0255T has been deleted. To report, use 0254T)

(0262T has been deleted. To report transcatheter pulmonary valve implantation, use 33477)

0263T Intramuscular autologous bone marrow cell therapy, with preparation of harvested cells, multiple injections, one leg, including ultrasound guidance, if performed; complete procedure including unilateral or bilateral bone marrow harvest

Sunset January 2022

➔ *CPT Changes: An Insider's View* 2012

(Do not report 0263T in conjunction with 38204-38242, 76942, 93925, 93926)

0264T complete procedure excluding bone marrow harvest

Sunset January 2022

➔ *CPT Changes: An Insider's View* 2012

(Do not report 0264T in conjunction with 38204-38242, 76942, 93925, 93926, 0265T)

0265T unilateral or bilateral bone marrow harvest only for intramuscular autologous bone marrow cell therapy

Sunset January 2022

➔ *CPT Changes: An Insider's View* 2012

(Do not report 0265T in conjunction with 38204-38242, 0264T. For complete procedure, use 0263T)

0266T Implantation or replacement of carotid sinus baroreflex activation device; total system (includes generator placement, unilateral or bilateral lead placement, intra-operative interrogation, programming, and repositioning, when performed)

Sunset January 2022

➔ *CPT Changes: An Insider's View* 2012

0267T lead only, unilateral (includes intra-operative interrogation, programming, and repositioning, when performed)

Sunset January 2022

➔ *CPT Changes: An Insider's View* 2012

(For bilateral lead implantation or replacement, use 0267T with modifier 50)

0268T pulse generator only (includes intra-operative interrogation, programming, and repositioning, when performed)

Sunset January 2022

➔ *CPT Changes: An Insider's View* 2012

(Do not report 0267T, 0268T in conjunction with 0266T, 0269T-0273T)

0269T Revision or removal of carotid sinus baroreflex activation device; total system (includes generator placement, unilateral or bilateral lead placement, intra-operative interrogation, programming, and repositioning, when performed)

Sunset January 2022

➔ *CPT Changes: An Insider's View* 2012

(Do not report 0269T in conjunction with 0266T-0268T, 0270T-0273T)

0270T lead only, unilateral (includes intra-operative interrogation, programming, and repositioning, when performed)

Sunset January 2022

➔ *CPT Changes: An Insider's View* 2012

(Do not report 0270T in conjunction with 0266T-0269T, 0271T-0273T)

(For bilateral lead removal, use 0270T with modifier 50)

(For removal of total carotid sinus baroreflex activation device, use 0269T)

0271T pulse generator only (includes intra-operative interrogation, programming, and repositioning, when performed)

Sunset January 2022

➔ *CPT Changes: An Insider's View* 2012

(Do not report 0271T in conjunction with 0266T-0270T, 0272T, 0273T)

(For removal and replacement, see 0266T, 0267T, 0268T)

0272T Interrogation device evaluation (in person), carotid sinus baroreflex activation system, including telemetric iterative communication with the implantable device to monitor device diagnostics and programmed therapy values, with interpretation and report (eg, battery status, lead impedance, pulse amplitude, pulse width, therapy frequency, pathway mode, burst mode, therapy start/stop times each day);

Sunset January 2022

➔ *CPT Changes: An Insider's View* 2012

(Do not report 0272T in conjunction with 0266T-0271T, 0273T)

0273T with programming

Sunset January 2022

➔ *CPT Changes: An Insider's View* 2012

(Do not report 0273T in conjunction with 0266T-0272T)

0274T Percutaneous laminotomy/laminectomy (interlaminar approach) for decompression of neural elements, (with or without ligamentous resection, discectomy, facetectomy and/or foraminotomy), any method, under indirect image guidance (eg, fluoroscopic, CT), single or multiple levels, unilateral or bilateral; cervical or thoracic
Sunset January 2022
➔ *CPT Changes: An Insider's View* 2012, 2017
➔ *CPT Assistant* Jan 12:14, Jul 12:3, 4, Feb 17:12

0275T lumbar
Sunset January 2022
➔ *CPT Changes: An Insider's View* 2012, 2017
➔ *CPT Assistant* Jan 12:14, Jul 12:3, 4, Feb 17:12

(For percutaneous decompression of the nucleus pulposus of intervertebral disc utilizing needle based technique, use 62287)

0278T Transcutaneous electrical modulation pain reprocessing (eg, scrambler therapy), each treatment session (includes placement of electrodes)
Sunset January 2022
➔ *CPT Changes: An Insider's View* 2012

(0281T has been deleted. To report, use 33340)

(0282T, 0283T, 0284T, 0285T have been deleted)

(For implantation of trial or permanent electrode arrays or pulse generators for peripheral subcutaneous field stimulation, use 64999)

(0286T has been deleted)

(0287T has been deleted)

(0288T has been deleted)

(For delivery of thermal energy to the muscle of the anal canal, use 46999)

(0289T has been deleted)

+ 0290T Corneal incisions in the recipient cornea created using a laser, in preparation for penetrating or lamellar keratoplasty (List separately in addition to code for primary procedure)
Sunset January 2022
➔ *CPT Changes: An Insider's View* 2012
➔ *CPT Assistant* Aug 12:15

(Use 0290T in conjunction with 65710, 65730, 65750, 65755)

(0291T, 0292T have been deleted. To report, see 92978, 92979)

(0293T, 0294T have been deleted)

0295T External electrocardiographic recording for more than 48 hours up to 21 days by continuous rhythm recording and storage; includes recording, scanning analysis with report, review and interpretation
Sunset January 2023
➔ *CPT Changes: An Insider's View* 2013
➔ *CPT Assistant* Feb 13:17

0296T recording (includes connection and initial recording)
Sunset January 2023
➔ *CPT Changes: An Insider's View* 2013
➔ *CPT Assistant* Feb 13:17

0297T scanning analysis with report
Sunset January 2023
➔ *CPT Changes: An Insider's View* 2013
➔ *CPT Assistant* Feb 13:17

0298T review and interpretation
Sunset January 2023
➔ *CPT Changes: An Insider's View* 2013
➔ *CPT Assistant* Feb 13:17

(Do not report 0295T-0298T in conjunction with 93224-93272 for same monitoring period)

(0299T, 0300T have been deleted)

(For extracorporeal shock wave for integumentary wound healing, high energy, use 28899)

(0301T has been deleted)

(For focused microwave thermotherapy of the breast, use 19499)

(0302T, 0303T, 0304T, 0305T, 0306T, 0307T have been deleted)

0308T Insertion of ocular telescope prosthesis including removal of crystalline lens or intraocular lens prosthesis
Sunset January 2021
➔ *CPT Changes: An Insider's View* 2013, 2016, 2017
➔ *CPT Assistant* Mar 13:6

(Do not report 0308T in conjunction with 65800-65815, 66020, 66030, 66600-66635, 66761, 66825, 66982-66986, 69990)

(0309T has been deleted)

(For arthrodesis, pre-sacral interbody technique, including disc space preparation, discectomy, with posterior instrumentation, with image guidance, including bone graft, when performed, lumbar, L4-L5 interspace, use 22899)

(0310T has been deleted)

(For motor function mapping using non-invasive navigated transcranial magnetic stimulation [nTMS] for therapeutic treatment planning, upper and lower extremity, use 64999)

(0311T has been deleted. To report, use 93050)

0312T Vagus nerve blocking therapy (morbid obesity); laparoscopic implantation of neurostimulator electrode array, anterior and posterior vagal trunks adjacent to esophagogastric junction (EGJ), with implantation of pulse generator, includes programming
Sunset January 2023
➔ *CPT Changes: An Insider's View* 2013
➔ *CPT Assistant* Jan 13:11

0313T laparoscopic revision or replacement of vagal trunk neurostimulator electrode array, including connection to existing pulse generator
Sunset January 2023
➔ *CPT Changes: An Insider's View* 2013
➔ *CPT Assistant* Jan 13:11

0314T laparoscopic removal of vagal trunk neurostimulator electrode array and pulse generator
Sunset January 2023
➔ *CPT Changes: An Insider's View* 2013
➔ *CPT Assistant* Jan 13:11

0315T removal of pulse generator
Sunset January 2023
➔ *CPT Changes: An Insider's View* 2013
➔ *CPT Assistant* Jan 13:11

0316T replacement of pulse generator
Sunset January 2023
➔ *CPT Changes: An Insider's View* 2013
➔ *CPT Assistant* Jan 13:11

(Do not report 0315T in conjunction with 0316T)

0317T neurostimulator pulse generator electronic analysis, includes reprogramming when performed
Sunset January 2023
➔ *CPT Changes: An Insider's View* 2013
➔ *CPT Assistant* Jan 13:11

(For implantation, revision, replacement, and/or removal of vagus [cranial] nerve neurostimulator electrode array and/or pulse generator for vagus nerve stimulation performed other than at the EGJ [eg, epilepsy], see 64568-64570)

►(For electronic analysis with programming, when performed, of vagal nerve neurostimulators, see 95970, 95976, 95977. Test stimulation to confirm correct target site placement of the electrode array[s] and/or to confirm the functional status of the system is inherent to placement, and is not separately reported as electronic analysis or programming of the neurostimulator system. Electronic analysis [95970] at the time of implantation is not separately reported.)◄

0329T Monitoring of intraocular pressure for 24 hours or longer, unilateral or bilateral, with interpretation and report
Sunset January 2024
➔ *CPT Changes: An Insider's View* 2014
➔ *CPT Assistant* May 14:5

0330T Tear film imaging, unilateral or bilateral, with interpretation and report
Sunset January 2024
➔ *CPT Changes: An Insider's View* 2014
➔ *CPT Assistant* May 14:5

0331T Myocardial sympathetic innervation imaging, planar qualitative and quantitative assessment
Sunset January 2024
➔ *CPT Changes: An Insider's View* 2014
➔ *CPT Assistant* Jun 14:15
➔ *Clinical Examples in Radiology* Summer 13:11

0332T with tomographic SPECT
Sunset January 2024
➔ *CPT Changes: An Insider's View* 2014
➔ *CPT Assistant* Jun 14:15
➔ *Clinical Examples in Radiology* Summer 13:11

(For myocardial infarct avid imaging, see 78466, 78468, 78469)

0333T Visual evoked potential, screening of visual acuity, automated, with report
Sunset January 2024
➔ *CPT Changes: An Insider's View* 2014, 2018
➔ *CPT Assistant* Aug 14:8, Feb 18:3

(For visual evoked potential testing for glaucoma, use 0464T)

 # 0464T Visual evoked potential, testing for glaucoma, with interpretation and report
Sunset January 2023
➔ *CPT Changes: An Insider's View* 2018
➔ *CPT Assistant* Feb 18:3

(To report percutaneous/minimally invasive [indirect visualization] arthrodesis of the sacroiliac joint with image guidance, use 27279)

(For visual evoked potential screening of visual acuity, use 0333T)

▲ 0335T Insertion of sinus tarsi implant
Sunset January 2024
➔ *CPT Changes: An Insider's View* 2019

►(Do not report 0335T in conjunction with 28585, 28725, 29907)◄

#● 0510T Removal of sinus tarsi implant
Sunset January 2024
➔ *CPT Changes: An Insider's View* 2019

#● 0511T Removal and reinsertion of sinus tarsi implant
Sunset January 2024
➔ *CPT Changes: An Insider's View* 2019

(0336T has been deleted. To report laparoscopy, surgical, ablation of uterine fibroid[s], use 58674)

►(0337T has been deleted)◄

►(For unilateral or bilateral endothelial function assessments, using peripheral vascular response to reactive hyperemia, noninvasive [eg, brachial artery ultrasound, peripheral artery tonometry], use 93998)◄

0338T Transcatheter renal sympathetic denervation, percutaneous approach including arterial puncture, selective catheter placement(s) renal artery(ies), fluoroscopy, contrast injection(s), intraprocedural roadmapping and radiological supervision and interpretation, including pressure gradient measurements, flush aortogram and diagnostic renal angiography when performed; unilateral
Sunset January 2024
➲ *CPT Changes: An Insider's View* 2014

0339T bilateral
Sunset January 2024
➲ *CPT Changes: An Insider's View* 2014

(Do not report 0338T, 0339T in conjunction with 36251, 36252, 36253, 36254)

(0340T has been deleted. To report, use 32994)

0341T Quantitative pupillometry with interpretation and report, unilateral or bilateral
Sunset January 2020
➲ *CPT Changes: An Insider's View* 2015

0342T Therapeutic apheresis with selective HDL delipidation and plasma reinfusion
Sunset January 2024
➲ *CPT Changes: An Insider's View* 2015

►Fluoroscopy (76000) and radiologic supervision and interpretation are inherent to the transcatheter mitral valve repair (TMVR) procedure and are not separately reportable. Diagnostic cardiac catheterization (93451, 93452, 93453, 93454, 93455, 93456, 93457, 93458, 93459, 93460, 93461, 93530, 93531, 93532, 93533) should **not** be reported with transcatheter mitral valve repair (0345T) for:◄

- Contrast injections, angiography, roadmapping, and/or fluoroscopic guidance for the transcatheter mitral valve repair (TMVR),
- Left ventricular angiography to assess mitral regurgitation, for guidance of TMVR, or
- Right and left heart catheterization for hemodynamic measurements before, during, and after TMVR for guidance of TMVR.

Diagnostic right and left heart catheterization (93451, 93452, 93453, 93456, 93457, 93458, 93459, 93460, 93461, 93530, 93531, 93532, 93533), and diagnostic coronary angiography (93454, 93455, 93456, 93457, 93458, 93459, 93460, 93461, 93563, 93564) not inherent to the TMVR, may be reported with 0345T, appended with modifier 59 if:

1. No prior study is available and a full diagnostic study is performed, or
2. A prior study is available, but as documented in the medical record:
   a. There is inadequate visualization of the anatomy and/or pathology, or
   b. The patient's condition with respect to the clinical indication has changed since the prior study, or
   c. There is a clinical change during the procedure that requires new evaluation.

Percutaneous coronary interventional procedures may be reported separately, when performed.

Other cardiac catheterization services may be reported separately, when performed for diagnostic purposes not intrinsic to the TMVR.

When transcatheter ventricular support is required, the appropriate code may be reported with the appropriate ventricular assist device (VAD) procedure (33990, 33991, 33992, 33993) or balloon pump insertion (33967, 33970, 33973).

0345T Transcatheter mitral valve repair percutaneous approach via the coronary sinus
Sunset January 2020
➲ *CPT Changes: An Insider's View* 2015
➲ *CPT Assistant* Sep 15:3

(For transcatheter mitral valve repair percutaneous approach including transseptal puncture when performed, see 33418, 33419)

(Do not report 0345T in conjunction with 93451, 93452, 93453, 93456, 93457, 93458, 93459, 93460, 93461 for diagnostic left and right heart catheterization procedures intrinsic to the valve repair procedure)

(Do not report 0345T in conjunction with 93453, 93454, 93563, 93564 for coronary angiography intrinsic to the valve repair procedure)

(For transcatheter mitral valve implantation/replacement [TMVI], see 0483T, 0484T)

►(0346T has been deleted. To report, see 76981, 76982, 76983)◄

0347T Placement of interstitial device(s) in bone for radiostereometric analysis (RSA)
Sunset January 2020
➲ *CPT Changes: An Insider's View* 2015
➲ *CPT Assistant* Jun 15:8

0348T Radiologic examination, radiostereometric analysis (RSA); spine, (includes cervical, thoracic and lumbosacral, when performed)
Sunset January 2020
➲ *CPT Changes: An Insider's View* 2015
➲ *CPT Assistant* Jun 15:8

0349T upper extremity(ies), (includes shoulder, elbow, and wrist, when performed)
Sunset January 2020
➲ *CPT Changes: An Insider's View* 2015
➲ *CPT Assistant* Jun 15:8

0350T lower extremity(ies), (includes hip, proximal femur, knee, and ankle, when performed)
Sunset January 2020
➲ *CPT Changes: An Insider's View* 2015
➲ *CPT Assistant* Jun 15:8

0351T Optical coherence tomography of breast or axillary lymph node, excised tissue, each specimen; real-time intraoperative
Sunset January 2020
➔ *CPT Changes: An Insider's View* 2015
➔ *CPT Assistant* Apr 15:6

0352T interpretation and report, real-time or referred
Sunset January 2020
➔ *CPT Changes: An Insider's View* 2015
➔ *CPT Assistant* Apr 15:6

(Do not report 0352T in conjunction with 0351T, when performed by the same physician)

0353T Optical coherence tomography of breast, surgical cavity; real-time intraoperative
Sunset January 2020
➔ *CPT Changes: An Insider's View* 2015
➔ *CPT Assistant* Apr 15:6

(Report 0353T once per session)

0354T interpretation and report, real-time or referred
Sunset January 2020
➔ *CPT Changes: An Insider's View* 2015
➔ *CPT Assistant* Apr 15:6

(Do not report 0354T in conjunction with 0353T, when performed by the same physician)

0355T Gastrointestinal tract imaging, intraluminal (eg, capsule endoscopy), colon, with interpretation and report
Sunset January 2020
➔ *CPT Changes: An Insider's View* 2015

(Use 0355T for imaging of distal ileum, when performed)

(Do not report 0355T in conjunction with 91110, 91111)

0356T Insertion of drug-eluting implant (including punctal dilation and implant removal when performed) into lacrimal canaliculus, each
Sunset January 2020
➔ *CPT Changes: An Insider's View* 2015
➔ *CPT Assistant* Aug 17:7

(For placement of drug-eluting insert under the eyelid[s], see 0444T, 0445T)

0357T Code is out of numerical sequence. See 0055T-0072T

0358T Bioelectrical impedance analysis whole body composition assessment, with interpretation and report
Sunset January 2020
➔ *CPT Changes: An Insider's View* 2015, 2016

(For bioimpedance-derived physiological cardiovascular analysis, use 93701)

(For bioimpedance spectroscopy (BIS), use 93702)

▸Adaptive Behavior Assessments and Treatment◂

▸**Behavior identification supporting assessment** (0362T) and **adaptive behavior treatment with protocol modification** (0373T) include the following required components:

- administration by the physician or other qualified health care professional who is on-site but not necessarily face-to-face with the patient;
- with the assistance of two or more technicians;
- for a patient with destructive behavior that requires the presence of a team;
- completion in an environment that is customized to the patient's behavior.

"On-site" is defined as immediately available and interruptible to provide assistance and direction throughout the performance of the procedure, however, the physician or other qualified health care professional does not need to be present in the room when the procedure is performed.

Typical patients for 0362T and 0373T present with one or more specific destructive behavior(s) (ie, maladaptive behaviors associated with high risk of medical consequences or property damage [eg, elopement, pica, or self-injury requiring medical attention, aggression with injury to other{s}, or breaking furniture, walls, or windows]). Code 0362T may include functional behavior assessment, functional analysis, other structured observations, and standardized and/or nonstandardized instruments and procedures to determine levels of adaptive and maladaptive behavior as well as other impairments in functioning.

Only count the time of one technician when two or more are present. For assistance with code selection of 97152, 0362T, see the Guide to Selection of Codes 97152 and 0362T on page 711. For assistance with code selection of 97153, 97155, 0373T, see Guide to Selection of Codes 97153, 97155, 0373T on page 712.◂

▸(0359T, 0360T, 0361T have been deleted. To report, see 97151, 97152)◂

▲ **0362T** **Behavior identification supporting assessment,** each 15 minutes of technicians' time face-to-face with a patient, requiring the following components:

- administration by the physician or other qualified health care professional who is on site;
- with the assistance of two or more technicians;
- for a patient who exhibits destructive behavior;
- completion in an environment that is customized to the patient's behavior.

Sunset January 2024
➔ *CPT Changes: An Insider's View* 2015, 2019
➔ *CPT Assistant* Jun 14:4

►(0362T is reported based on a single technician's face-to-face time with the patient and not the combined time of multiple technicians [eg, one hour with three technicians equals one hour of service])◄

►(0362T may be repeated on different days until the behavior identification assessment [97151] and, if necessary, supporting assessment[s] [97152, 0362T], is complete)◄

►(For psychiatric diagnostic evaluation, see 90791, 90792)◄

►(For speech evaluations, see 92521, 92522, 92523, 92524)◄

►(For occupational therapy evaluation, see 97165, 97166, 97167, 97168)◄

►(For medical team conference, see 99366, 99367, 99368)◄

►(For health and behavior assessment/intervention, see 96150, 96151, 96152, 96153, 96154, 96155)◄

►(For neurobehavioral status examination, see 96116, 96121)◄

►(For neuropsychological testing, see 96132, 96133, 96136, 96137, 96138, 96139, 96146)◄

►(0363T, 0364T, 0365T, 0366T, 0367T, 0368T, 0369T, 0370T, 0371T, 0372T have been deleted. To report, see 97153, 97154, 97155, 97156, 97157, 97158, 0373T)◄

▲ **0373T** **Adaptive behavior treatment with protocol modification,** each 15 minutes of technicians' time face-to-face with a patient, requiring the following components:

- administration by the physician or other qualified health care professional who is on site;
- with the assistance of two or more technicians;
- for a patient who exhibits destructive behavior;
- completion in an environment that is customized to the patient's behavior.

Sunset January 2024

➲ *CPT Changes: An Insider's View* 2015, 2019

➲ *CPT Assistant* Jun 14:4, 6, 9

►(0373T is reported based on a single technician's face-to-face time with the patient and not the combined time of multiple technicians)◄

►(Do not report 0373T in conjunction with 90785-90899, 96105, 96110, 96116, 96121, 96150, 96151, 96152, 96153, 96154, 96155)◄

►(0374T has been deleted. To report, use 0373T)◄

0375T Total disc arthroplasty (artificial disc), anterior approach, including discectomy with end plate preparation (includes osteophytectomy for nerve root or spinal cord decompression and microdissection), cervical, three or more levels

Sunset January 2020

➲ *CPT Changes: An Insider's View* 2015

➲ *CPT Assistant* Apr 15:7

(Do not report 0375T in conjunction with 22853, 22854, 22856, 22858, 22859 when performed at the same level)

0376T Code is out of numerical sequence. See 0184T-0200T

0377T Anoscopy with directed submucosal injection of bulking agent for fecal incontinence

Sunset January 2020

➲ *CPT Changes: An Insider's View* 2015

(Do not report 0377T in conjunction with 46600)

0378T Visual field assessment, with concurrent real time data analysis and accessible data storage with patient initiated data transmitted to a remote surveillance center for up to 30 days; review and interpretation with report by a physician or other qualified health care professional

Sunset January 2020

➲ *CPT Changes: An Insider's View* 2015

0379T technical support and patient instructions, surveillance, analysis, and transmission of daily and emergent data reports as prescribed by a physician or other qualified health care professional

Sunset January 2020

➲ *CPT Changes: An Insider's View* 2015

0380T Computer-aided animation and analysis of time series retinal images for the monitoring of disease progression, unilateral or bilateral, with interpretation and report

Sunset January 2020

➲ *CPT Changes: An Insider's View* 2015

0381T External heart rate and 3-axis accelerometer data recording up to 14 days to assess changes in heart rate and to monitor motion analysis for the purposes of diagnosing nocturnal epilepsy seizure events; includes report, scanning analysis with report, review and interpretation by a physician or other qualified health care professional

Sunset January 2021

➲ *CPT Changes: An Insider's View* 2016

0382T review and interpretation only

Sunset January 2021

➲ *CPT Changes: An Insider's View* 2016

(Do not report 0381T, 0382T in conjunction with 0383T, 0384T, 0385T, 0386T)

0383T External heart rate and 3-axis accelerometer data recording from 15 to 30 days to assess changes in heart rate and to monitor motion analysis for the purposes of diagnosing nocturnal epilepsy seizure events; includes report, scanning analysis with report, review and interpretation by a physician or other qualified health care professional

Sunset January 2021

➲ *CPT Changes: An Insider's View* 2016

0384T review and interpretation only

Sunset January 2021

➲ *CPT Changes: An Insider's View* 2016

(Do not report 0383T, 0384T in conjunction with 0381T, 0382T, 0385T, 0386T)

0385T External heart rate and 3-axis accelerometer data recording more than 30 days to assess changes in heart rate and to monitor motion analysis for the purposes of diagnosing nocturnal epilepsy seizure events; includes report, scanning analysis with report, review and interpretation by a physician or other qualified health care professional

Sunset January 2021

➲ *CPT Changes: An Insider's View* 2016

0386T review and interpretation only

Sunset January 2021

➲ *CPT Changes: An Insider's View* 2016

(Do not report 0385T, 0386T in conjunction with 0381T, 0382T, 0383T, 0384T)

Pacemaker-Leadless and Pocketless System

►(0387T, 0388T have been deleted. To report, see 33274, 33275)◄

►(0389T, 0390T, 0391T have been deleted. To report, see 33274, 33275, 93279, 93286, 93288, 93294, 93296)◄

(0392T has been deleted. To report, use 43284)

(0393T has been deleted. To report, use 43285)

(Electronic brachytherapy is a form of radiation therapy in which an electrically generated X-ray source of ionizing radiation is placed inside or in close proximity to the tumor or target tissue to deliver therapeutic radiation dosage)

0394T High dose rate electronic brachytherapy, skin surface application, per fraction, includes basic dosimetry, when performed

Sunset January 2021

➲ *CPT Changes: An Insider's View* 2016

(Do not report 0394T in conjunction with 77261, 77262, 77263, 77300, 77306, 77307, 77316, 77317, 77318, 77332, 77333, 77334, 77336, 77427, 77431, 77432, 77435, 77469, 77470, 77499, 77761, 77762, 77763, 77767, 77768, 77770, 77771, 77772, 77778, 77789)

(For high dose rate radionuclide surface brachytherapy, see 77767, 77768)

(For non-brachytherapy superficial [eg, ≤200 kV] radiation treatment delivery, use 77401)

0395T High dose rate electronic brachytherapy, interstitial or intracavitary treatment, per fraction, includes basic dosimetry, when performed

Sunset January 2021

➲ *CPT Changes: An Insider's View* 2016

(Do not report 0395T in conjunction with 77261, 77262, 77263, 77300, 77306, 77307, 77316, 77317, 77318, 77332, 77333, 77334, 77336, 77427, 77431, 77432, 77435, 77469, 77470, 77499, 77761, 77762, 77763, 77767, 77768, 77770, 77771, 77772, 77778, 77789)

(For skin surface application of high dose rate electronic brachytherapy, use 0394T)

+ 0396T Intra-operative use of kinetic balance sensor for implant stability during knee replacement arthroplasty (List separately in addition to code for primary procedure)

Sunset January 2021

➲ *CPT Changes: An Insider's View* 2016

(Use 0396T in conjunction with 27445, 27446, 27447, 27486, 27487, 27488)

+ 0397T Endoscopic retrograde cholangiopancreatography (ERCP), with optical endomicroscopy (List separately in addition to code for primary procedure)

Sunset January 2021

➲ *CPT Changes: An Insider's View* 2016, 2017

(Use 0397T in conjunction with 43260, 43261, 43262, 43263, 43264, 43265, 43274, 43275, 43276, 43277, 43278)

(Do not report 0397T in conjunction with 88375)

(Do not report optical endomicroscopy more than once per session)

0398T Magnetic resonance image guided high intensity focused ultrasound (MRgFUS), stereotactic ablation lesion, intracranial for movement disorder including stereotactic navigation and frame placement when performed

Sunset January 2021

➲ *CPT Changes: An Insider's View* 2016

(Do not report 0398T in conjunction with 61781, 61800)

+ 0399T Myocardial strain imaging (quantitative assessment of myocardial mechanics using image-based analysis of local myocardial dynamics) (List separately in addition to code for primary procedure)

Sunset January 2021

➲ *CPT Changes: An Insider's View* 2016

(Use 0399T in conjunction with 93303, 93304, 93306, 93307, 93308, 93312, 93314, 93315, 93317, 93350, 93351, 93355)

(Report 0399T once per session)

0400T Multi-spectral digital skin lesion analysis of clinically atypical cutaneous pigmented lesions for detection of melanomas and high risk melanocytic atypia; one to five lesions
Sunset January 2021
➲ *CPT Changes: An Insider's View* 2016

0401T six or more lesions
Sunset January 2021
➲ *CPT Changes: An Insider's View* 2016

(Do not report 0401T in conjunction with 0400T)

0402T Collagen cross-linking of cornea (including removal of the corneal epithelium and intraoperative pachymetry when performed)
Sunset January 2021
➲ *CPT Changes: An Insider's View* 2016
➲ *CPT Assistant* Feb 16:12

(Do not report 0402T in conjunction with 65435, 69990, 76514)

A diabetes prevention program consists of intensive behavioral counseling that is provided in person, online, or via electronic technology, or a combination of both modalities.

Intensive behavioral counseling consists of care management, lifestyle coaching, facilitation of a peer-support group, and provision of clinically validated educational lessons based on a standardized curriculum that is focused on nutrition, exercise, stress, and weight management. Lifestyle coaches must complete a nationally recognized training program. The lifestyle coach is available to interact with the participants.

Codes 0403T and 0488T describe diabetes prevention programs that use a standardized diabetes prevention curriculum. For educational services that use a standardized curriculum provided to patients with an established illness/disease, see 98960, 98961, 98962. Use 0403T for diabetes prevention programs that are provided only in-person. Use 0488T for programs that are provided online or via electronic technology. Code 0488T includes in person components, if provided.

0403T Preventive behavior change, intensive program of prevention of diabetes using a standardized diabetes prevention program curriculum, provided to individuals in a group setting, minimum 60 minutes, per day
Sunset January 2021
➲ *CPT Changes: An Insider's View* 2016

(Do not report 0403T in conjunction with 98960, 98961, 98962, 0488T)

 # 0488T Preventive behavior change, online/electronic structured intensive program for prevention of diabetes using a standardized diabetes prevention program curriculum, provided to an individual, per 30 days
Sunset January 2023
➲ *CPT Changes: An Insider's View* 2018

(Do not report 0488T in conjunction with 98960, 98961, 98962, 0403T)

0404T Transcervical uterine fibroid(s) ablation with ultrasound guidance, radiofrequency
Sunset January 2021
➲ *CPT Changes: An Insider's View* 2016

0405T Oversight of the care of an extracorporeal liver assist system patient requiring review of status, review of laboratories and other studies, and revision of orders and liver assist care plan (as appropriate), within a calendar month, 30 minutes or more of non-face-to-face time
Sunset January 2021
➲ *CPT Changes: An Insider's View* 2016

►(0406T, 0407T have been deleted)◄

►(To report endoscopic placement of a drug-eluting implant in the ethmoid sinus without any other nasal/sinus endoscopic surgical service, use 31299. To report endoscopic placement of a drug-eluting implant in the ethmoid sinus in conjunction with biopsy, polypectomy, or debridement, use 31237)◄

Codes 0408T-0418T describe procedures related to cardiac contractility modulation systems (CCM). These systems consist of a pulse generator plus one atrial and two ventricular pacemaker electrodes (leads). In contrast to a pacemaker or a defibrillator, which modulate the heart's rhythm, the CCM system's impulses are designed to modulate the strength of contraction of the heart muscle. Unlike pacemakers, these systems stimulate for specific time intervals in order to improve myocardial function.

All catheterization and imaging guidance required to complete a CCM procedure are included in the work of each code. Left heart catheterization with a high fidelity transducer is intrinsic to the CCM procedure. Left heart catheterization codes (93452, 93453, 93458, 93459, 93460, 93461) at the time of CCM placement, replacement, or revision may not be reported separately. Removal of only the CCM pulse generator is reported with 0412T. If only the pulse generator is removed and replaced at the same session without any right atrial and/or right ventricular lead(s) inserted or replaced, report 0414T. For removal and replacement of the pulse generator and leads, individual codes for removal of the generator (0412T) and removal of the leads (0413T for each lead removed) are used in conjunction with the insertion/replacement system code (0408T). When individual transvenous electrodes are inserted or replaced, report using 0410T and 0411T, as appropriate. When the entire system is inserted or replaced, report with 0408T.

Revision of the CCM generator skin pocket is included in 0408T, 0412T, 0414T. Relocation of a skin pocket for a CCM may be necessary for various clinical situations such as infection or erosion. Relocation is reported with 0416T, and follows conventions for pacemaker skin pocket relocation.

Repositioning of a CCM electrode is reported using 0415T.

CCM device evaluation codes 0417T, 0418T may not be reported in conjunction with pulse generator and lead insertion or revision codes.

0408T Insertion or replacement of permanent cardiac contractility modulation system, including contractility evaluation when performed, and programming of sensing and therapeutic parameters; pulse generator with transvenous electrodes
Sunset January 2022
CPT Changes: An Insider's View 2017

0409T pulse generator only
Sunset January 2022
CPT Changes: An Insider's View 2017

0410T atrial electrode only
Sunset January 2022
CPT Changes: An Insider's View 2017

0411T ventricular electrode only
Sunset January 2022
CPT Changes: An Insider's View 2017

(Report 0410T, 0411T once for each transvenous electrode inserted or replaced)

(If the entire system is inserted or replaced, report 0408T)

0412T Removal of permanent cardiac contractility modulation system; pulse generator only
Sunset January 2022
CPT Changes: An Insider's View 2017

0413T transvenous electrode (atrial or ventricular)
Sunset January 2022
CPT Changes: An Insider's View 2017

(Report 0413T once for each transvenous electrode removed)

(For removal of the pulse generator and all 3 leads, use 0412T plus 0413T once for each electrode removed)

(If transvenous electrodes are removed and replaced, report 0413T once for each electrode removed in conjunction with 0410T, 0411T, as appropriate)

0414T Removal and replacement of permanent cardiac contractility modulation system pulse generator only
Sunset January 2022
CPT Changes: An Insider's View 2017

(For removal and replacement of the pulse generator plus all three electrodes, report 0408T in conjunction with 0412T, 0413T once for each transvenous electrode removed)

0415T Repositioning of previously implanted cardiac contractility modulation transvenous electrode (atrial or ventricular lead)
Sunset January 2022
CPT Changes: An Insider's View 2017

(Do not report 0408T, 0409T, 0410T, 0411T, 0414T, 0415T in conjunction with 93286, 93287, 93452, 93453, 93458, 93459, 93460, 93461)

(Do not report 0415T in conjunction with 0408T, 0410T, 0411T)

0416T Relocation of skin pocket for implanted cardiac contractility modulation pulse generator
Sunset January 2022
CPT Changes: An Insider's View 2017

0417T Programming device evaluation (in person) with iterative adjustment of the implantable device to test the function of the device and select optimal permanent programmed values with analysis, including review and report, implantable cardiac contractility modulation system
Sunset January 2022
CPT Changes: An Insider's View 2017

(Do not report 0417T in conjunction with 0408T, 0409T, 0410T, 0411T, 0412T, 0413T, 0414T, 0415T, 0418T)

0418T Interrogation device evaluation (in person) with analysis, review and report, includes connection, recording and disconnection per patient encounter, implantable cardiac contractility modulation system
Sunset January 2022
CPT Changes: An Insider's View 2017

(Do not report 0418T in conjunction with 0408T, 0409T, 0410T, 0411T, 0412T, 0413T, 0414T, 0415T, 0417T)

0419T Destruction of neurofibroma, extensive (cutaneous, dermal extending into subcutaneous); face, head and neck, greater than 50 neurofibromas
Sunset January 2022
CPT Changes: An Insider's View 2017
CPT Assistant Apr 16:3

(For excision of neurofibroma, use 64792)

(Report 0419T once per session regardless of the number of lesions treated)

0420T trunk and extremities, extensive, greater than 100 neurofibromas
Sunset January 2022
CPT Changes: An Insider's View 2017
CPT Assistant Apr 16:3

(For excision of neurofibroma, use 64792)

(Report 0420T once per session regardless of the number of lesions treated)

0421T Transurethral waterjet ablation of prostate, including control of post-operative bleeding, including ultrasound guidance, complete (vasectomy, meatotomy, cystourethroscopy, urethral calibration and/or dilation, and internal urethrotomy are included when performed)
Sunset January 2022
CPT Changes: An Insider's View 2017

(Do not report 0421T in conjunction with 52500, 52630, 76872)

0422T Tactile breast imaging by computer-aided tactile sensors, unilateral or bilateral
Sunset January 2022
CPT Changes: An Insider's View 2017

0423T Secretory type II phospholipase A2 (sPLA2-IIA)
Sunset January 2022
CPT Changes: An Insider's View 2017

(For lipoprotein-associated phospholipase A2 [Lp-PLA2], use 83698)

Phrenic Nerve Stimulation System

A phrenic nerve stimulation system includes a pulse generator (containing electronics and a battery), one stimulation lead (electrode), and one sensing lead (electrode). Pulse generators are placed in a submuscular or subcutaneous "pocket" in the pectoral region. The stimulation lead is placed transvenously into the right brachiocephalic vein or left pericardiophrenic vein. The sensing lead is placed transvenously into the azygos vein.

If replacing less than a complete system, report 0425T, 0426T, and/or 0427T (for sensing lead, stimulation lead or pulse generator respectively). If all three components are replaced, report only 0424T in conjunction with codes for removal of each of the components (0428T, 0429T, 0430T).

Codes 0424T-0433T include vessel catheterization, all image guidance required for the procedure, and interrogation and programming, when performed. Interrogation device evaluation and programming device evaluation include parameters of rate, pulse amplitude, pulse duration, configuration of waveform, battery status, electrode selectability, output modulation, cycling, impedance, and patient compliance measurements. For patients that require programming during an overnight sleep study, report 0436T once, regardless of how many programming changes are made during the sleep study.

0424T Insertion or replacement of neurostimulator system for treatment of central sleep apnea; complete system (transvenous placement of right or left stimulation lead, sensing lead, implantable pulse generator)
Sunset January 2022
CPT Changes: An Insider's View 2017

0425T sensing lead only
Sunset January 2022
CPT Changes: An Insider's View 2017

0426T stimulation lead only
Sunset January 2022
CPT Changes: An Insider's View 2017

0427T pulse generator only
Sunset January 2022
CPT Changes: An Insider's View 2017

(Do not report 0425T, 0426T, 0427T in conjunction with 0424T)

0428T Removal of neurostimulator system for treatment of central sleep apnea; pulse generator only
Sunset January 2022
CPT Changes: An Insider's View 2017

0429T sensing lead only
Sunset January 2022
CPT Changes: An Insider's View 2017

0430T stimulation lead only
Sunset January 2022
CPT Changes: An Insider's View 2017

(Report 0429T, 0430T once for each transvenous sensing or stimulation lead removed)

(For removal of the entire system, report 0428T for pulse generator removal plus 0429T or 0430T for each transvenous lead removal)

0431T Removal and replacement of neurostimulator system for treatment of central sleep apnea, pulse generator only
Sunset January 2022
CPT Changes: An Insider's View 2017

(For removal and replacement of the pulse generator plus all three leads, report 0424T in conjunction with 0428T, 0429T, 0430T)

0432T Repositioning of neurostimulator system for treatment of central sleep apnea; stimulation lead only
Sunset January 2022
CPT Changes: An Insider's View 2017

0433T sensing lead only
Sunset January 2022
CPT Changes: An Insider's View 2017

(Do not report 0432T, 0433T in conjunction with 0424T, 0425T, 0426T, 0427T)

0434T Interrogation device evaluation implanted neurostimulator pulse generator system for central sleep apnea
Sunset January 2022
CPT Changes: An Insider's View 2017

0435T Programming device evaluation of implanted neurostimulator pulse generator system for central sleep apnea; single session
Sunset January 2022
CPT Changes: An Insider's View 2017

0436T during sleep study
Sunset January 2022
CPT Changes: An Insider's View 2017

(Do not report 0434T, 0435T, 0436T in conjunction with 0424T, 0425T, 0426T, 0427T, 0428T, 0429T, 0430T, 0431T, 0432T, 0433T)

(Do not report 0436T in conjunction with 0435T)

(Report 0436T once per sleep study)

+ 0437T Implantation of non-biologic or synthetic implant (eg, polypropylene) for fascial reinforcement of the abdominal wall (List separately in addition to code for primary procedure)
Sunset January 2022
CPT Changes: An Insider's View 2017

(For implantation of mesh or other prosthesis for open incisional or ventral hernia repair, use 49568 in conjunction with 49560, 49561, 49565, 49566)

(For insertion of mesh or other prosthesis for closure of a necrotizing soft tissue infection wound, use 49568 in conjunction with 11004, 11005, 11006)

(0438T has been deleted. To report, use 55874)

+ 0439T Myocardial contrast perfusion echocardiography, at rest or with stress, for assessment of myocardial ischemia or viability (List separately in addition to code for primary procedure)
Sunset January 2022
➔ *CPT Changes: An Insider's View* 2017
➔ *CPT Assistant* Apr 16:9

(Use 0439T in conjunction with 93306, 93307, 93308, 93350, 93351)

0440T Ablation, percutaneous, cryoablation, includes imaging guidance; upper extremity distal/peripheral nerve
Sunset January 2022
➔ *CPT Changes: An Insider's View* 2017
➔ *CPT Assistant* May 17:3
➔ *Clinical Examples in Radiology* Spring 17:13, Winter 17:3

0441T lower extremity distal/peripheral nerve
Sunset January 2022
➔ *CPT Changes: An Insider's View* 2017
➔ *CPT Assistant* May 17:3
➔ *Clinical Examples in Radiology* Spring 17:13, Winter 17:2

0442T nerve plexus or other truncal nerve (eg, brachial plexus, pudendal nerve)
Sunset January 2022
➔ *CPT Changes: An Insider's View* 2017
➔ *CPT Assistant* May 17:3
➔ *Clinical Examples in Radiology* Spring 17:13, Winter 17:3

+ 0443T Real-time spectral analysis of prostate tissue by fluorescence spectroscopy, including imaging guidance (List separately in addition to code for primary procedure)
Sunset January 2022
➔ *CPT Changes: An Insider's View* 2017

(Use 0443T in conjunction with 55700)

(Report 0443T only once per session)

0444T Initial placement of a drug-eluting ocular insert under one or more eyelids, including fitting, training, and insertion, unilateral or bilateral
Sunset January 2022
➔ *CPT Changes: An Insider's View* 2017
➔ *CPT Assistant* Aug 17:7

0445T Subsequent placement of a drug-eluting ocular insert under one or more eyelids, including re-training, and removal of existing insert, unilateral or bilateral
Sunset January 2022
➔ *CPT Changes: An Insider's View* 2017
➔ *CPT Assistant* Aug 17:7

(For insertion and removal of drug-eluting implant into lacrimal canaliculus, use 0356T)

0446T Creation of subcutaneous pocket with insertion of implantable interstitial glucose sensor, including system activation and patient training
Sunset January 2022
➔ *CPT Changes: An Insider's View* 2017

(Do not report 0446T in conjunction with 95251, 0447T, 0448T)

0447T Removal of implantable interstitial glucose sensor from subcutaneous pocket via incision
Sunset January 2022
➔ *CPT Changes: An Insider's View* 2017

0448T Removal of implantable interstitial glucose sensor with creation of subcutaneous pocket at different anatomic site and insertion of new implantable sensor, including system activation
Sunset January 2022
➔ *CPT Changes: An Insider's View* 2017

(Do not report 0448T in conjunction with 0446T, 0447T)

(For placement of non-implantable interstitial glucose sensor without pocket, use 95250)

0449T Insertion of aqueous drainage device, without extraocular reservoir, internal approach, into the subconjunctival space; initial device
Sunset January 2022
➔ *CPT Changes: An Insider's View* 2017

+ 0450T each additional device (List separately in addition to code for primary procedure)
Sunset January 2022
➔ *CPT Changes: An Insider's View* 2017

(Use 0450T in conjunction with 0449T)

(For removal of aqueous drainage device without extraocular reservoir, placed into the subconjunctival space via internal approach, use 92499)

Codes 0451T-0463T describe a family of services related to the placement and maintenance of permanent aortic counterpulsation ventricular assistance devices. These devices are used to treat congestive heart failure, and they employ a counterpulsation device that is implanted in the aorta, which inflates during diastole to reduce end diastolic ventricular pressure on a long-term basis without rerouting blood flow. The counterpulsation assistance device implantation is achieved by surgically placing a subclavian arterial graft and creating of a subcutaneous pocket to implant a mechano-electrical interface, without requiring access to the heart. The counterpulsation device's mechano-electrical skin interface receives ECG signals from the subcutaneous electrodes and digitizes and transmits a signal through an external driveline to an external "driver," which is carried by the patient. The "driver" receives the ECG signal and determines the location of the dichrotic notch. The "driver" then activates a bellows, which sends compressed air through the external driveline to the mechano-electrical skin interface in which the compressed air enters the internal driveline and inflates the balloon. After diastole, the bellows creates suction that deflates the balloon through the same pathway.

These services differ from those performed for the implantation, revision, and removal of existing aortic balloon pumps in several ways in that they: (1) use a permanently implanted balloon that is intended for long-term use; (2) require surgical placement of a vascular graft; (3) use a vascular hemostatic seal; (4) implant a mechano-electrical skin interface that contains a programmable processor; and (5) implant subcutaneous electrodes. In addition, they also differ from procedures to insert, revise, and remove extracorporeal and intracorporeal ventricular assist devices because these procedures require access to the heart and include inflow or outflow grafts into the heart, which divert blood flow from either the left and/or right cardiac chambers into a pump that then pumps blood directly into the corresponding artery (either aorta and/or pulmonary artery).

Codes 0451T-0463T are inclusive of all vessel catheterization, diagnostic angiography, radiological supervision and interpretation, and imaging guidance. Removal of a counterpulsation assistance device at the same session as insertion is not separately reportable.

0451T Insertion or replacement of a permanently implantable aortic counterpulsation ventricular assist system, endovascular approach, and programming of sensing and therapeutic parameters; complete system (counterpulsation device, vascular graft, implantable vascular hemostatic seal, mechano-electrical skin interface and subcutaneous electrodes)

Sunset January 2022

➲ *CPT Changes: An Insider's View* 2017

(Do not report 0451T in conjunction with 33973, 33979, 33990, 33991, 0452T, 0453T, 0454T, 0455T, 0456T, 0457T, 0458T)

(For insertion of intra-aortic balloon assist device, see 33967, 33970, 33973)

(For insertion or replacement of extracorporeal ventricular assist device, see 33975, 33976, 33981)

(For insertion or replacement of intracorporeal ventricular assist device, see 33979, 33982, 33983)

(For percutaneous insertion of ventricular assist device, see 33990, 33991)

0452T aortic counterpulsation device and vascular hemostatic seal

Sunset January 2022

➲ *CPT Changes: An Insider's View* 2017

(Do not report 0452T in conjunction with 33973, 33979, 33990, 33991, 0451T, 0455T, 0456T)

(For insertion or replacement of intracorporeal ventricular assist device, see 33979, 33982, 33983)

0453T mechano-electrical skin interface

Sunset January 2022

➲ *CPT Changes: An Insider's View* 2017

(Do not report 0453T in conjunction with 33973, 33979, 33990, 33991, 0451T, 0455T, 0457T)

(For insertion or replacement of intracorporeal ventricular assist device, see 33979, 33982, 33983)

0454T subcutaneous electrode

Sunset January 2022

➲ *CPT Changes: An Insider's View* 2017

(Report 0454T once for each subcutaneous electrode inserted or replaced)

(If the entire system is inserted or replaced, use 0451T)

(Do not report 0454T in conjunction with 33973, 33979, 33990, 33991, 0451T, 0455T, 0458T)

(For insertion or replacement of intracorporeal ventricular assist device, see 33979, 33982, 33983)

0455T Removal of permanently implantable aortic counterpulsation ventricular assist system; complete system (aortic counterpulsation device, vascular hemostatic seal, mechano-electrical skin interface and electrodes)

Sunset January 2022

➲ *CPT Changes: An Insider's View* 2017

(Do not report 0455T in conjunction with 33974, 33980, 33992, 0451T, 0452T, 0453T, 0454T, 0456T, 0457T, 0458T)

(For removal of intra-aortic balloon assist device, see 33968, 33971, 33974)

(For removal of extracorporeal ventricular assist device, see 33977, 33978)

(For removal of intracorporeal ventricular assist device, use 33980)

(For removal of percutaneous ventricular assist device, use 33992)

0456T aortic counterpulsation device and vascular hemostatic seal

Sunset January 2022

➲ *CPT Changes: An Insider's View* 2017

(Do not report 0456T in conjunction with 33974, 33980, 33992, 0451T, 0452T, 0455T)

0457T mechano-electrical skin interface

Sunset January 2022

➲ *CPT Changes: An Insider's View* 2017

(Do not report 0457T in conjunction with 33974, 33980, 33992, 0451T, 0453T, 0455T)

0458T subcutaneous electrode

Sunset January 2022

➲ *CPT Changes: An Insider's View* 2017

(Report 0458T once for each subcutaneous electrode removed)

(Do not report 0458T in conjunction with 33974, 33980, 33992, 0451T, 0454T, 0455T)

0459T Relocation of skin pocket with replacement of implanted aortic counterpulsation ventricular assist device, mechano-electrical skin interface and electrodes

Sunset January 2022

➔ *CPT Changes: An Insider's View* 2017

(Do not report 0459T in conjunction with 33993)

(For repositioning of percutaneous ventricular assist device, use 33993)

0460T Repositioning of previously implanted aortic counterpulsation ventricular assist device; subcutaneous electrode

Sunset January 2022

➔ *CPT Changes: An Insider's View* 2017

(Report 0460T once for each subcutaneous electrode repositioned)

(Do not report 0460T in conjunction with 33993, 0451T, 0454T)

(For repositioning of percutaneous ventricular assist device, use 33993)

0461T aortic counterpulsation device

Sunset January 2022

➔ *CPT Changes: An Insider's View* 2017

(Do not report 0461T in conjunction with 33993)

(For repositioning of percutaneous ventricular assist device, use 33993)

0462T Programming device evaluation (in person) with iterative adjustment of the implantable mechano-electrical skin interface and/or external driver to test the function of the device and select optimal permanent programmed values with analysis, including review and report, implantable aortic counterpulsation ventricular assist system, per day

Sunset January 2022

➔ *CPT Changes: An Insider's View* 2017

(Do not report 0462T in conjunction with 0451T-0461T, 0463T)

0463T Interrogation device evaluation (in person) with analysis, review and report, includes connection, recording and disconnection per patient encounter, implantable aortic counterpulsation ventricular assist system, per day

Sunset January 2022

➔ *CPT Changes: An Insider's View* 2017

(Do not report 0463T in conjunction with 0451T-0462T)

►(Do not report 0451T-0463T in conjunction with 36000, 36002, 36005, 36010, 36200-36228, 75600-75774, 76000, 76936, 76937, 77001, 77002, 77011, 77012, 77021, 93451-93533, 93561-93572)◄

0464T Code is out of numerical sequence. See 0332T-0339T

0465T Suprachoroidal injection of a pharmacologic agent (does not include supply of medication)

Sunset January 2023

➔ *CPT Changes: An Insider's View* 2018

➔ *CPT Assistant* Feb 18:3

(To report intravitreal injection/implantation, see 67025, 67027, 67028)

+ 0466T Insertion of chest wall respiratory sensor electrode or electrode array, including connection to pulse generator (List separately in addition to code for primary procedure)

Sunset January 2023

➔ *CPT Changes: An Insider's View* 2018

➔ *CPT Assistant* Nov 16:6, Mar 18:9

(Use 0466T in conjunction with 64568)

0467T Revision or replacement of chest wall respiratory sensor electrode or electrode array, including connection to existing pulse generator

Sunset January 2023

➔ *CPT Changes: An Insider's View* 2018

➔ *CPT Assistant* Nov 16:6, Mar 18:9

(Do not report 0467T in conjunction with 0466T, 0468T)

(For revision or replacement of cranial nerve [eg, vagus nerve] neurostimulator electrode array, including connection to existing pulse generator, use 64569)

0468T Removal of chest wall respiratory sensor electrode or electrode array

Sunset January 2023

➔ *CPT Changes: An Insider's View* 2018

➔ *CPT Assistant* Nov 16:6, Mar 18:9

(Do not report 0468T in conjunction with 0466T, 0467T)

(For removal of cranial nerve [eg, vagus nerve] neurostimulator electrode array and pulse generator, use 64570)

0469T Retinal polarization scan, ocular screening with on-site automated results, bilateral

Sunset January 2023

➔ *CPT Changes: An Insider's View* 2018

➔ *CPT Assistant* Feb 18:3

(Do not report 0469T in conjunction with 92002, 92004, 92012, 92014)

(For ocular photoscreening, see 99174, 99177)

0470T Optical coherence tomography (OCT) for microstructural and morphological imaging of skin, image acquisition, interpretation, and report; first lesion

Sunset January 2023

➔ *CPT Changes: An Insider's View* 2018

+ 0471T each additional lesion (List separately in addition to code for primary procedure)

Sunset January 2023

➔ *CPT Changes: An Insider's View* 2018

(Use 0471T in conjunction with 0470T)

(For optical coherence tomography for coronary vessel or graft, see 92978, 92979)

(For reflectance confocal microscopy [RCM] of the skin, see 96931, 96932, 96933, 96934, 96935, 96936)

0472T Device evaluation, interrogation, and initial programming of intraocular retinal electrode array (eg, retinal prosthesis), in person, with iterative adjustment of the implantable device to test functionality, select optimal permanent programmed values with analysis, including visual training, with review and report by a qualified health care professional

Sunset January 2023

➲ *CPT Changes: An Insider's View* 2018

➲ *CPT Assistant* Feb 18:3

0473T Device evaluation and interrogation of intraocular retinal electrode array (eg, retinal prosthesis), in person, including reprogramming and visual training, when performed, with review and report by a qualified health care professional

Sunset January 2023

➲ *CPT Changes: An Insider's View* 2018

➲ *CPT Assistant* Feb 18:3

(For implantation of intraocular electrode array, use 0100T)

(For reprogramming of implantable intraocular retinal electrode array device, use 0473T)

0474T Insertion of anterior segment aqueous drainage device, with creation of intraocular reservoir, internal approach, into the supraciliary space

Sunset January 2023

➲ *CPT Changes: An Insider's View* 2018

➲ *CPT Assistant* Feb 18:3

0475T Recording of fetal magnetic cardiac signal using at least 3 channels; patient recording and storage, data scanning with signal extraction, technical analysis and result, as well as supervision, review, and interpretation of report by a physician or other qualified health care professional

Sunset January 2023

➲ *CPT Changes: An Insider's View* 2018

0476T patient recording, data scanning, with raw electronic signal transfer of data and storage

Sunset January 2023

➲ *CPT Changes: An Insider's View* 2018

0477T signal extraction, technical analysis, and result

Sunset January 2023

➲ *CPT Changes: An Insider's View* 2018

0478T review, interpretation, report by physician or other qualified health care professional

Sunset January 2023

➲ *CPT Changes: An Insider's View* 2018

0479T Fractional ablative laser fenestration of burn and traumatic scars for functional improvement; first 100 cm^2 or part thereof, or 1% of body surface area of infants and children

Sunset January 2023

➲ *CPT Changes: An Insider's View* 2018

➲ *CPT Assistant* Dec 17:13

+ 0480T each additional 100 cm^2, or each additional 1% of body surface area of infants and children, or part thereof (List separately in addition to code for primary procedure)

Sunset January 2023

➲ *CPT Changes: An Insider's View* 2018

➲ *CPT Assistant* Dec 17:13

(Use 0480T in conjunction with 0479T)

(Report 0479T, 0480T only once per day)

(Do not report 0479T, 0480T in conjunction with 0492T)

(For excision of cicatricial lesion[s] [eg, full thickness excision, through the dermis], see 11400-11446)

0481T Injection(s), autologous white blood cell concentrate (autologous protein solution), any site, including image guidance, harvesting and preparation, when performed

Sunset January 2023

➲ *CPT Changes: An Insider's View* 2018

(Do not report 0481T in conjunction with 20550, 20551, 20600, 20604, 20605, 20606, 20610, 20611, 20926, 36415, 36592, 76942, 77002, 77012, 77021, 86965, 0232T)

(Do not report 38220, 38221, 38222, 38230 for bone marrow aspiration for autologous white blood cell concentrate [autologous protein solution] injection. For bone marrow aspiration for autologous white blood cell concentrate [autologous protein solution] injection, use 0481T)

+ 0482T Absolute quantitation of myocardial blood flow, positron emission tomography (PET), rest and stress (List separately in addition to code for primary procedure)

Sunset January 2023

➲ *CPT Changes: An Insider's View* 2018

(Use 0482T in conjunction with 78491, 78492)

(For myocardial imaging metabolic evaluation, use 78459)

(For positron emission tomography [PET] myocardial perfusion study, see 78491, 78492)

Codes 0483T, 0484T include vascular access, catheterization, balloon valvuloplasty, deploying the valve, repositioning the valve as needed, temporary pacemaker insertion for rapid pacing, and access site closure, when performed.

Angiography, radiological supervision and interpretation, intraprocedural roadmapping (eg, contrast injections, fluoroscopy) to guide the TMVI, left ventriculography (eg, to assess mitral regurgitation for guidance of TMVI), and completion angiography are included in codes 0483T,0484T.

Diagnostic right and left heart catheterization codes (93451, 93452, 93453, 93456, 93457, 93458, 93459, 93460, 93461, 93530, 93531, 93532, 93533) should **not** be used with 0483T, 0484T to report:

1. contrast injections, angiography, roadmapping, and/or fluoroscopic guidance for the transcatheter mitral valve implantation (TMVI),
2. left ventricular angiography to assess or confirm valve positioning and function,
3. right and left heart catheterization for hemodynamic measurements before, during, and after TMVI for guidance of TMVI.

Diagnostic right and left heart catheterization codes (93451, 93452, 93453, 93456, 93457, 93458, 93459, 93460, 93461, 93530, 93531, 93532, 93533) and diagnostic coronary angiography codes (93454, 93455, 93456, 93457, 93458, 93459, 93460, 93461, 93563, 93564) performed at the time of TMVI may be separately reportable, if:

1. no prior study is available and a full diagnostic study is performed, or
2. a prior study is available, but as documented in the medical record:
   a. there is inadequate visualization of the anatomy and/or pathology, or
   b. the patient's condition with respect to the clinical indication has changed since the prior study, or
   c. there is a clinical change during the procedure that requires new evaluation.

For same session/same day diagnostic cardiac catheterization services, report the appropriate diagnostic cardiac catheterization code(s) appended with modifier 59, indicating separate and distinct procedural service from TMVI.

When cardiopulmonary bypass is performed in conjunction with TMVI, 0483T, 0484T may be reported with the appropriate add-on code for percutaneous peripheral bypass (33367), open peripheral bypass (33368), or central bypass (33369).

0483T Transcatheter mitral valve implantation/replacement (TMVI) with prosthetic valve; percutaneous approach, including transseptal puncture, when performed
Sunset January 2023
➔ *CPT Changes: An Insider's View* 2018

0484T transthoracic exposure (eg, thoracotomy, transapical)
Sunset January 2023
➔ *CPT Changes: An Insider's View* 2018

0485T Optical coherence tomography (OCT) of middle ear, with interpretation and report; unilateral
Sunset January 2023
➔ *CPT Changes: An Insider's View* 2018

0486T bilateral
Sunset January 2023
➔ *CPT Changes: An Insider's View* 2018

0487T Biomechanical mapping, transvaginal, with report
Sunset January 2023
➔ *CPT Changes: An Insider's View* 2018

0488T Code is out of numerical sequence. See 0402T-0405T

0489T Autologous adipose-derived regenerative cell therapy for scleroderma in the hands; adipose tissue harvesting, isolation and preparation of harvested cells including incubation with cell dissociation enzymes, removal of non-viable cells and debris, determination of concentration and dilution of regenerative cells
Sunset January 2023
➔ *CPT Changes: An Insider's View* 2018

(Do not report 0489T in conjunction with 15876, 15877, 15878, 15879, 20600, 20604, 20926)

0490T multiple injections in one or both hands
Sunset January 2023
➔ *CPT Changes: An Insider's View* 2018

(Do not report 0490T in conjunction with 15876, 15877, 15878, 15879, 20600, 20604, 20926)

(Do not report 0490T for a single injection)

(For complete procedure, use 0490T in conjunction with 0489T)

0491T Ablative laser treatment, non-contact, full field and fractional ablation, open wound, per day, total treatment surface area; first 20 sq cm or less
Sunset January 2023
➔ *CPT Changes: An Insider's View* 2018

+ 0492T each additional 20 sq cm, or part thereof (List separately in addition to code for primary procedure)
Sunset January 2023
➔ *CPT Changes: An Insider's View* 2018

(Use 0492T in conjunction with 0491T)

(Do not report 0492T in conjunction with 0479T, 0480T)

0493T Near-infrared spectroscopy studies of lower extremity wounds (eg, for oxyhemoglobin measurement)
Sunset January 2023
➔ *CPT Changes: An Insider's View* 2018

0494T Surgical preparation and cannulation of marginal (extended) cadaver donor lung(s) to ex vivo organ perfusion system, including decannulation, separation from the perfusion system, and cold preservation of the allograft prior to implantation, when performed
Sunset January 2023
➔ *CPT Changes: An Insider's View* 2018

0495T Initiation and monitoring marginal (extended) cadaver donor lung(s) organ perfusion system by physician or qualified health care professional, including physiological and laboratory assessment (eg, pulmonary artery flow, pulmonary artery pressure, left atrial pressure, pulmonary vascular resistance, mean/peak and plateau airway pressure, dynamic compliance and perfusate gas analysis), including bronchoscopy and X ray when performed; first two hours in sterile field

Sunset January 2023

➔ *CPT Changes: An Insider's View* 2018

+ 0496T each additional hour (List separately in addition to code for primary procedure)

Sunset January 2023

➔ *CPT Changes: An Insider's View* 2018

(Report 0496T in conjunction with 0495T)

0497T External patient-activated, physician- or other qualified health care professional-prescribed, electrocardiographic rhythm derived event recorder without 24-hour attended monitoring; in-office connection

Sunset January 2023

➔ *CPT Changes: An Insider's View* 2018

0498T review and interpretation by a physician or other qualified health care professional per 30 days with at least one patient-generated triggered event

Sunset January 2023

➔ *CPT Changes: An Insider's View* 2018

(Do not report 0497T, 0498T in conjunction with 93040, 93041, 93042, 93228, 93229, 93268, 93271, 93272, 0295T, 0296T, 0297T, 0298T)

0499T Cystourethroscopy, with mechanical dilation and urethral therapeutic drug delivery for urethral stricture or stenosis, including fluoroscopy, when performed

Sunset January 2023

➔ *CPT Changes: An Insider's View* 2018

(Do not report 0499T in conjunction with 52281, 52283)

0500T Infectious agent detection by nucleic acid (DNA or RNA), Human Papillomavirus (HPV) for five or more separately reported high-risk HPV types (eg, 16, 18, 31, 33, 35, 39, 45, 51, 52, 56, 58, 59, 68) (ie, genotyping)

Sunset January 2023

➔ *CPT Changes: An Insider's View* 2018

(For reporting four or fewer separately reported high-risk HPV types, see 87624, 87625)

(For reporting of separately reported high-risk Human Papillomavirus [HPV] types 16, 18 and 45, if performed, use 87625)

(Do not report 0500T in conjunction with 87624 or 87625 for the same procedure)

0501T Noninvasive estimated coronary fractional flow reserve (FFR) derived from coronary computed tomography angiography data using computation fluid dynamics physiologic simulation software analysis of functional data to assess the severity of coronary artery disease; data preparation and transmission, analysis of fluid dynamics and simulated maximal coronary hyperemia, generation of estimated FFR model, with anatomical data review in comparison with estimated FFR model to reconcile discordant data, interpretation and report

Sunset January 2023

➔ *CPT Changes: An Insider's View* 2018

0502T data preparation and transmission

Sunset January 2023

➔ *CPT Changes: An Insider's View* 2018

0503T analysis of fluid dynamics and simulated maximal coronary hyperemia, and generation of estimated FFR model

Sunset January 2023

➔ *CPT Changes: An Insider's View* 2018

0504T anatomical data review in comparison with estimated FFR model to reconcile discordant data, interpretation and report

Sunset January 2023

➔ *CPT Changes: An Insider's View* 2018

(Report 0501T, 0502T, 0503T, 0504T one time per coronary CT angiogram)

►(Do not report 0501T in conjunction with 0502T, 0503T, 0504T, 0523T)◄

#+● 0523T Intraprocedural coronary fractional flow reserve (FFR) with 3D functional mapping of color-coded FFR values for the coronary tree, derived from coronary angiogram data, for real-time review and interpretation of possible atherosclerotic stenosis(es) intervention (List separately in addition to code for primary procedure)

Sunset January 2024

➔ *CPT Changes: An Insider's View* 2019

►(Use 0523T in conjunction with 93454, 93455, 93456, 93457, 93458, 93459, 93460, 93461)◄

►(Do not report 0523T more than once per session)◄

►(Do not report 0523T in conjunction with 76376, 76377, 93571, 93572, 0501T, 0502T, 0503T, 0504T)◄

● 0505T Endovenous femoral-popliteal arterial revascularization, with transcatheter placement of intravascular stent graft(s) and closure by any method, including percutaneous or open vascular access, ultrasound guidance for vascular access when performed, all catheterization(s) and intraprocedural roadmapping and imaging guidance necessary to complete the intervention, all associated radiological supervision and interpretation, when performed, with crossing of the occlusive lesion in an extraluminal fashion

Sunset January 2024

➔ *CPT Changes: An Insider's View* 2019

►(0505T includes all ipsilateral selective arterial and venous catheterization, all diagnostic imaging for ipsilateral, lower extremity arteriography, and all related radiological supervision and interpretation)◄

►(Do not report 0505T in conjunction with 37224, 37225, 37226, 37227, 37238, 37239, 37248, 37249, within the femoral-popliteal segment)◄

►(Do not report 0505T in conjunction with 76937, for ultrasound guidance for vascular access)◄

● **0506T** Macular pigment optical density measurement by heterochromatic flicker photometry, unilateral or bilateral, with interpretation and report

Sunset January 2024

➲ *CPT Changes: An Insider's View* 2019

● **0507T** Near infrared dual imaging (ie, simultaneous reflective and transilluminated light) of meibomian glands, unilateral or bilateral, with interpretation and report

Sunset January 2024

➲ *CPT Changes: An Insider's View* 2019

►(For external ocular photography, use 92285)◄

►(For tear film imaging, use 0330T)◄

● **0508T** Pulse-echo ultrasound bone density measurement resulting in indicator of axial bone mineral density, tibia

Sunset January 2024

➲ *CPT Changes: An Insider's View* 2019

►Electroretinography (ERG) is used to evaluate function of the retina and optic nerve of the eye, including photoreceptors and ganglion cells. A number of techniques that target different areas of the eye, including full field (flash and flicker) (92273) for a global response of photoreceptors of the retina, multifocal (92274) for photoreceptors in multiple separate locations in the retina, including the macula, and pattern (0509T) for retinal ganglion cells are used. Multiple additional terms and techniques are used to describe various types of ERG. If the technique used is not specifically named in the code descriptors for 92273, 92274, 0509T, use the unlisted procedure code 92499.◄

● **0509T** Electroretinography (ERG) with interpretation and report, pattern (PERG)

Sunset January 2024

➲ *CPT Changes: An Insider's View* 2019

►(For full-field ERG, use 92273)◄

►(For multifocal ERG, use 92274)◄

0510T Code is out of numerical sequence. See 0332T-0339T

0511T Code is out of numerical sequence. See 0332T-0339T

0512T Code is out of numerical sequence. See 0101T-0107T

0513T Code is out of numerical sequence. See 0101T-0107T

+● **0514T** Intraoperative visual axis identification using patient fixation (List separately in addition to code for primary procedure)

Sunset January 2024

➲ *CPT Changes: An Insider's View* 2019

►(Use 0514T in conjunction with 66982, 66984)◄

►Wireless Cardiac Stimulation System for Left Ventricular Pacing◄

►A wireless cardiac stimulator system provides biventricular pacing by sensing right ventricular pacing output from a previously implanted conventional device (pacemaker or defibrillator, with univentricular or biventricular leads), and then transmitting an ultrasound pulse to a wireless electrode implanted on the endocardium of the left ventricle, which then emits a left ventricular pacing pulse.

The complete system consists of two components: a wireless endocardial left ventricle electrode and a pulse generator. The pulse generator has two components: a transmitter and a battery. The electrode is implanted transarterially into the left ventricular wall and powered wirelessly using ultrasound delivered by a subcutaneously implanted transmitter. Two subcutaneous pockets are created on the chest wall, one for the battery and one for the transmitter, and these two components are connected by a subcutaneously tunneled cable.

Patients with a wireless cardiac stimulator require programming/interrogation of their existing conventional device, as well as the wireless device. The wireless cardiac stimulator is programmed and interrogated with its own separate programmer and settings.

Code 0515T describes insertion of a complete wireless cardiac stimulator system (electrode and pulse generator, which includes transmitter and battery), including interrogation, programming, pocket creation, revision and repositioning, and all echocardiography and other imaging to guide the procedure, when performed. Use 0516T only when insertion of the electrode is a stand-alone procedure. For insertion of only a new generator or generator component (battery and/or transmitter), use 0517T.

For removal of only the generator or a generator component (battery and/or transmitter) without replacement, use 0518T. For removal and replacement of a generator or a generator component (battery and/or transmitter), use 0519T. For battery and/or generator removal and reinsertion performed together with a new electrode insertion, use 0520T.

All catheterization and imaging guidance (including transthoracic or transesophageal echocardiography) required to complete a wireless cardiac stimulator procedure is included in 0515T, 0516T, 0517T, 0518T, 0519T, 0520T. Do not report 76000, 76998, 93303-93355 in conjunction with 0515T, 0516T, 0517T, 0518T, 0519T, 0520T.

Do not report left heart catheterization codes (93452, 93453, 93458, 93459, 93460, 93461, 93531, 93532, 93533) for delivery of a wireless cardiac stimulator electrode into the left ventricle.◄

● **0515T** Insertion of wireless cardiac stimulator for left ventricular pacing, including device interrogation and programming, and imaging supervision and interpretation, when performed; complete system (includes electrode and generator [transmitter and battery])

Sunset January 2024

➲ *CPT Changes: An Insider's View* 2019

● **0516T** electrode only

Sunset January 2024

➲ *CPT Changes: An Insider's View* 2019

● **0517T** pulse generator component(s) (battery and/or transmitter) only

Sunset January 2024

➲ *CPT Changes: An Insider's View* 2019

►(Do not report 0515T, 0516T, 0517T in conjunction with 0518T, 0519T, 0520T, 0521T, 0522T)◄

● **0518T** Removal of only pulse generator component(s) (battery and/or transmitter) of wireless cardiac stimulator for left ventricular pacing

Sunset January 2024

➲ *CPT Changes: An Insider's View* 2019

►(Do not report 0518T in conjunction with 0515T, 0516T, 0517T, 0519T, 0520T, 0521T, 0522T)◄

● **0519T** Removal and replacement of wireless cardiac stimulator for left ventricular pacing; pulse generator component(s) (battery and/or transmitter)

Sunset January 2024

➲ *CPT Changes: An Insider's View* 2019

● **0520T** pulse generator component(s) (battery and/or transmitter), including placement of a new electrode

Sunset January 2024

➲ *CPT Changes: An Insider's View* 2019

►(Do not report 0519T, 0520T in conjunction with 0515T, 0516T, 0517T, 0518T, 0521T, 0522T)◄

● **0521T** Interrogation device evaluation (in person) with analysis, review and report, includes connection, recording, and disconnection per patient encounter, wireless cardiac stimulator for left ventricular pacing

Sunset January 2024

➲ *CPT Changes: An Insider's View* 2019

►(Do not report 0521T in conjunction with 0515T, 0516T, 0517T, 0518T, 0519T, 0520T, 0522T)◄

● **0522T** Programming device evaluation (in person) with iterative adjustment of the implantable device to test the function of the device and select optimal permanent programmed values with analysis, including review and report, wireless cardiac stimulator for left ventricular pacing

Sunset January 2024

➲ *CPT Changes: An Insider's View* 2019

►(Do not report 0522T in conjunction with 0515T, 0516T, 0517T, 0518T, 0519T, 0520T, 0521T)◄

0523T ►Code is out of numerical sequence. See 0503T-0506T◄

● **0524T** Endovenous catheter directed chemical ablation with balloon isolation of incompetent extremity vein, open or percutaneous, including all vascular access, catheter manipulation, diagnostic imaging, imaging guidance and monitoring

Sunset January 2024

➲ *CPT Changes: An Insider's View* 2019

● **0525T** Insertion or replacement of intracardiac ischemia monitoring system, including testing of the lead and monitor, initial system programming, and imaging supervision and interpretation; complete system (electrode and implantable monitor)

Sunset January 2024

➲ *CPT Changes: An Insider's View* 2019

● **0526T** electrode only

Sunset January 2024

➲ *CPT Changes: An Insider's View* 2019

● **0527T** implantable monitor only

Sunset January 2024

➲ *CPT Changes: An Insider's View* 2019

►(Do not report 0525T, 0526T, 0527T in conjunction with 93000, 93005, 93010, 0528T, 0529T)◄

►(For removal and replacement of intracardiac ischemia monitoring system or its components, see 0525T, 0526T, 0527T in conjunction with 0530T, 0531T, 0532T, as appropriate)◄

● **0528T** Programming device evaluation (in person) of intracardiac ischemia monitoring system with iterative adjustment of programmed values, with analysis, review, and report

Sunset January 2024

➲ *CPT Changes: An Insider's View* 2019

►(Do not report 0528T in conjunction with 93000, 93005, 93010, 0525T, 0526T, 0527T, 0529T, 0530T, 0531T, 0532T)◄

● **0529T** Interrogation device evaluation (in person) of intracardiac ischemia monitoring system with analysis, review, and report

Sunset January 2024

➲ *CPT Changes: An Insider's View* 2019

►(Do not report 0529T in conjunction with 93000, 93005, 93010, 0525T, 0526T, 0527T, 0528T, 0530T, 0531T, 0532T)◄

● **0530T** Removal of intracardiac ischemia monitoring system, including all imaging supervision and interpretation; complete system (electrode and implantable monitor)

Sunset January 2024

➲ *CPT Changes: An Insider's View* 2019

● **0531T** electrode only

Sunset January 2024

➲ *CPT Changes: An Insider's View* 2019

● **0532T** implantable monitor only

Sunset January 2024

CPT Changes: An Insider's View 2019

►(Do not report 0530T, 0531T, 0532T in conjunction with 0528T, 0529T)◄

● **0533T** Continuous recording of movement disorder symptoms, including bradykinesia, dyskinesia, and tremor for 6 days up to 10 days; includes set-up, patient training, configuration of monitor, data upload, analysis and initial report configuration, download review, interpretation and report

Sunset January 2024

CPT Changes: An Insider's View 2019

● **0534T** set-up, patient training, configuration of monitor

Sunset January 2024

CPT Changes: An Insider's View 2019

● **0535T** data upload, analysis and initial report configuration

Sunset January 2024

CPT Changes: An Insider's View 2019

● **0536T** download review, interpretation and report

Sunset January 2024

CPT Changes: An Insider's View 2019

►Cellular and Gene Therapy◄

►Cellular and gene therapies involve the collection, processing and handling of cells or other tissues, genetic modification of those cells or tissues, and administration of the genetically modified cells or tissues with the intent to treat, modify, reverse or cure a serious or life-threatening disease or condition.

Codes 0537T, 0538T, 0539T, 0540T describe the various steps required to collect, prepare, transport, receive, and administer genetically modified T cells. The collection and handling code (0537T) may be reported only once per day, regardless of the number of collections or quantity of cells collected. Similarly, the administration code (0540T) may only be reported once per day, regardless of the number of units administered. The development of genetically modified cells is not reported with this family of codes.

Chimeric antigen receptor therapy (CAR-T) with genetically modified T cells begins with the collection of cells from the patient by peripheral blood leukocyte cell harvesting. The cells are then cryopreserved and/or otherwise prepared for processing or shipping to a manufacturing or cell processing facility, if applicable, where gene modification and expansion of the cells is performed. When gene modification and expansion of the cells by the manufacturer is complete, the genetically modified cells are returned to the physician or other qualified health care professional in which additional preparation occurs, including thawing of the cryopreserved CAR-T cells, if necessary, before the cells are administered to the patient.

The procedure to administer CAR-T cells includes physician monitoring of multiple physiologic parameters, physician verification of cell processing, evaluation of the patient during, as well as immediately before and after the administration of the CAR-T cells, physician presence during the administration and direct supervision of clinical staff, and management of any adverse events during the administration. Care on the same date of service that is not directly related to the service of administration of the CAR-T cells (eg, care provided after the administration is complete, care for the patient's underlying condition or for other medical problems) may be separately reported using the appropriate evaluation and management code with modifier 25. Management of uncomplicated adverse events (eg, nausea, urticaria) during the infusion is not reported separately.

The fluid used to administer the cells and other infusions for incidental hydration (eg, 96360, 96361) are not reported separately. Similarly, infusion(s) of any supportive medication(s) (eg, steroids) concurrently with the CAR-T cell administration are not reported separately. However, hydration or administration of medications (eg, antibiotics, opioids) unrelated to the CAR-T administration may be reported separately with modifier 59.◄

● **0537T** Chimeric antigen receptor T-cell (CAR-T) therapy; harvesting of blood-derived T lymphocytes for development of genetically modified autologous CAR-T cells, per day

Sunset January 2024

CPT Changes: An Insider's View 2019

● **0538T** preparation of blood-derived T lymphocytes for transportation (eg, cryopreservation, storage)

Sunset January 2024

CPT Changes: An Insider's View 2019

● **0539T** receipt and preparation of CAR-T cells for administration

Sunset January 2024

CPT Changes: An Insider's View 2019

● **0540T** CAR-T cell administration, autologous

Sunset January 2024

CPT Changes: An Insider's View 2019

● **0541T** Myocardial imaging by magnetocardiography (MCG) for detection of cardiac ischemia, by signal acquisition using minimum 36 channel grid, generation of magnetic-field time-series images, quantitative analysis of magnetic dipoles, machine learning–derived clinical scoring, and automated report generation, single study;

Sunset January 2024

CPT Changes: An Insider's View 2019

● **0542T** interpretation and report

Sunset January 2024

CPT Changes: An Insider's View 2019

Notes

Appendix A

Modifiers

This list includes all of the modifiers applicable to CPT 2019 codes.

A modifier provides the means to report or indicate that a service or procedure that has been performed has been altered by some specific circumstance but not changed in its definition or code. Modifiers also enable health care professionals to effectively respond to payment policy requirements established by other entities.

22 **Increased Procedural Services:** When the work required to provide a service is substantially greater than typically required, it may be identified by adding modifier 22 to the usual procedure code. Documentation must support the substantial additional work and the reason for the additional work (ie, increased intensity, time, technical difficulty of procedure, severity of patient's condition, physical and mental effort required). **Note:** This modifier should not be appended to an E/M service.

➲ *CPT Changes: An Insider's View* 2008

➲ *CPT Assistant* Jan 09:8, Apr 09:8, Jun 09:8,10, Aug 13:4

23 **Unusual Anesthesia:** Occasionally, a procedure, which usually requires either no anesthesia or local anesthesia, because of unusual circumstances must be done under general anesthesia. This circumstance may be reported by adding modifier 23 to the procedure code of the basic service.

24 **Unrelated Evaluation and Management Service by the Same Physician or Other Qualified Health Care Professional During a Postoperative Period:** The physician or other qualified health care professional may need to indicate that an evaluation and management service was performed during a postoperative period for a reason(s) unrelated to the original procedure. This circumstance may be reported by adding modifier 24 to the appropriate level of E/M service.

➲ *CPT Changes: An Insider's View* 2013

25 **Significant, Separately Identifiable Evaluation and Management Service by the Same Physician or Other Qualified Health Care Professional on the Same Day of the Procedure or Other Service:** It may be necessary to indicate that on the day a procedure or service identified by a CPT code was performed, the patient's condition required a significant, separately identifiable E/M service above and beyond the other service provided or beyond the usual preoperative and postoperative care associated with the procedure that was performed. A significant, separately identifiable E/M service is defined or substantiated by documentation that satisfies the relevant criteria for the respective E/M service to be reported (see **Evaluation and Management Services Guidelines** for instructions on determining level of E/M service). The E/M service may be prompted by the symptom or condition for which the procedure and/or service was provided. As such, different diagnoses are not required for reporting of the E/M services on the same date. This circumstance may be reported by adding modifier 25 to the appropriate level of E/M service. **Note:** This modifier is not used to report an E/M service that resulted in a decision to perform surgery. See modifier 57. For significant, separately identifiable non-E/M services, see modifier 59.

➲ *CPT Changes: An Insider's View* 2008, 2013

➲ *CPT Assistant* Feb 09:22, Mar 09:3, Apr 09:4; Jun 09:11

26 **Professional Component:** Certain procedures are a combination of a physician or other qualified health care professional component and a technical component. When the physician or other qualified health care professional component is reported separately, the service may be identified by adding modifier 26 to the usual procedure number.

➲ *CPT Changes: An Insider's View* 2013

➲ *CPT Assistant* Jan 09:7, Apr 09:4, May 09:7

32 **Mandated Services:** Services related to *mandated* consultation and/or related services (eg, third party payer, governmental, legislative or regulatory requirement) may be identified by adding modifier 32 to the basic procedure.

➲ *CPT Assistant* Aug 13:12

33 **Preventive Services:** When the primary purpose of the service is the delivery of an evidence based service in accordance with a US Preventive Services Task Force A or B rating in effect and other preventive services identified in preventive services mandates (legislative or regulatory), the service may be identified by adding 33 to the procedure. For separately reported services specifically identified as preventive, the modifier should not be used.

➲ *CPT Changes: An Insider's View* 2012

47 **Anesthesia by Surgeon:** Regional or general anesthesia provided by the surgeon may be reported by adding modifier 47 to the basic service. (This does not include local anesthesia.) **Note:** Modifier 47 would not be used as a modifier for the anesthesia procedures.

50 **Bilateral Procedure:** Unless otherwise identified in the listings, bilateral procedures that are performed at the same session, should be identified by adding modifier 50 to the appropriate 5 digit code.

➲ *CPT Changes: An Insider's View* 2011

➲ *CPT Assistant* Apr 09:9, Jun 13:15

51 **Multiple Procedures:** When multiple procedures, other than E/M services, Physical Medicine and Rehabilitation services or provision of supplies (eg, vaccines), are performed at the same session by the same individual, the primary procedure or service may be reported as listed. The additional procedure(s) or service(s) may be identified by appending modifier 51 to the additional procedure or

service code(s). **Note:** This modifier should not be appended to designated "add-on" codes (see Appendix D).

➲ *CPT Changes: An Insider's View* 2008, 2013

➲ *CPT Assistant* Feb 09:6, Mar 09:10, Apr 09:8

52 Reduced Services: Under certain circumstances a service or procedure is partially reduced or eliminated at the discretion of the physician or other qualified health care professional. Under these circumstances the service provided can be identified by its usual procedure number and the addition of modifier 52, signifying that the service is reduced. This provides a means of reporting reduced services without disturbing the identification of the basic service. **Note:** For hospital outpatient reporting of a previously scheduled procedure/service that is partially reduced or cancelled as a result of extenuating circumstances or those that threaten the well-being of the patient prior to or after administration of anesthesia, see modifiers 73 and 74 (see modifiers approved for ASC hospital outpatient use).

➲ *CPT Changes: An Insider's View* 2013

➲ *CPT Assistant* Mar 09:11, Apr 09:5, May 09:8, Jun 09:10, Jun 13:7

53 Discontinued Procedure: Under certain circumstances, the physician or other qualified health care professional may elect to terminate a surgical or diagnostic procedure. Due to extenuating circumstances or those that threaten the well being of the patient, it may be necessary to indicate that a surgical or diagnostic procedure was started but discontinued. This circumstance may be reported by adding modifier 53 to the code reported by the individual for the discontinued procedure. **Note:** This modifier is not used to report the elective cancellation of a procedure prior to the patient's anesthesia induction and/or surgical preparation in the operating suite. For outpatient hospital/ambulatory surgery center (ASC) reporting of a previously scheduled procedure/service that is partially reduced or cancelled as a result of extenuating circumstances or those that threaten the well being of the patient prior to or after administration of anesthesia, see modifiers 73 and 74 (see modifiers approved for ASC hospital outpatient use).

➲ *CPT Changes: An Insider's View* 2013

➲ *CPT Assistant* Feb 14:11

54 Surgical Care Only: When 1 physician or other qualified health care professional performs a surgical procedure and another provides preoperative and/or postoperative management, surgical services may be identified by adding modifier 54 to the usual procedure number.

➲ *CPT Changes: An Insider's View* 2013

55 Postoperative Management Only: When 1 physician or other qualified health care professional performed the postoperative management and another performed the surgical procedure, the postoperative component may be identified by adding modifier 55 to the usual procedure number.

➲ *CPT Changes: An Insider's View* 2013

56 Preoperative Management Only: When 1 physician or other qualified health care professional performed the preoperative care and evaluation and another performed the surgical procedure, the preoperative component may be identified by adding modifier 56 to the usual procedure number.

➲ *CPT Changes: An Insider's View* 2013

57 Decision for Surgery: An evaluation and management service that resulted in the initial decision to perform the surgery may be identified by adding modifier 57 to the appropriate level of E/M service.

➲ *CPT Assistant* May 09:9

58 Staged or Related Procedure or Service by the Same Physician or Other Qualified Health Care Professional During the Postoperative Period: It may be necessary to indicate that the performance of a procedure or service during the postoperative period was: (a) planned or anticipated (staged); (b) more extensive than the original procedure; or (c) for therapy following a surgical procedure. This circumstance may be reported by adding modifier 58 to the staged or related procedure. **Note:** For treatment of a problem that requires a return to the operating/procedure room (eg, unanticipated clinical condition), see modifier 78.

➲ *CPT Changes: An Insider's View* 2008, 2013

59 Distinct Procedural Service: Under certain circumstances, it may be necessary to indicate that a procedure or service was distinct or independent from other non-E/M services performed on the same day. Modifier 59 is used to identify procedures/services, other than E/M services, that are not normally reported together, but are appropriate under the circumstances. Documentation must support a different session, different procedure or surgery, different site or organ system, separate incision/excision, separate lesion, or separate injury (or area of injury in extensive injuries) not ordinarily encountered or performed on the same day by the same individual. However, when another already established modifier is appropriate it should be used rather than modifier 59. Only if no more descriptive modifier is available, and the use of modifier 59 best explains the circumstances, should modifier 59 be used. **Note:** Modifier 59 should not be appended to an E/M service. To report a separate and distinct E/M service with a non-E/M service performed on the same date, see modifier 25.

➲ *CPT Changes: An Insider's View* 2008

➲ *CPT Assistant* Feb 09:17, Apr 09:4,8, May 09:6, Jun 09:8

62 Two Surgeons: When 2 surgeons work together as primary surgeons performing distinct part(s) of a procedure, each surgeon should report his/her distinct operative work by adding modifier 62 to the procedure code and any associated add-on code(s) for that procedure as long as both surgeons continue to work together as primary surgeons. Each surgeon should report the co-surgery once using the same procedure code. If additional procedure(s) (including add-on procedure[s]) are performed during the same surgical session, separate code(s) may also be reported with modifier 62 added. **Note:** If a co-surgeon acts as an assistant in the performance of additional procedure(s), other than those reported with the modifier 62, during the same surgical session, those services may be reported using separate procedure code(s) with modifier 80 or modifier 82 added, as appropriate.

➲ *CPT Changes: An Insider's View* 2013

63 ►Procedure Performed on Infants less than 4 kg: Procedures performed on neonates and infants up to a present body weight of 4 kg may involve significantly increased complexity and physician or other qualified health care professional work commonly associated with these patients. This circumstance may be reported by adding modifier 63 to the procedure number. **Note:** Unless otherwise designated, this modifier may only be appended to procedures/services listed in the 20100-69990 code series. Modifier 63 should not be appended to any CPT codes listed in the **Evaluation and Management Services, Anesthesia, Radiology, Pathology/Laboratory,** or **Medicine** sections.◄

➲ *CPT Changes: An Insider's View* 2013, 2019

66 Surgical Team: Under some circumstances, highly complex procedures (requiring the concomitant services of several physicians or other qualified health care professionals, often of different specialties, plus other highly skilled, specially trained personnel, various types of complex equipment) are carried out under the "surgical team" concept. Such circumstances may be identified by each participating individual with the addition of modifier 66 to the basic procedure number used for reporting services.

➲ *CPT Changes: An Insider's View* 2013

76 Repeat Procedure or Service by Same Physician or Other Qualified Health Care Professional: It may be necessary to indicate that a procedure or service was repeated by the same physician or other qualified health care professional subsequent to the original procedure or service. This circumstance may be reported by adding modifier 76 to the repeated procedure or service. **Note:** This modifier should not be appended to an E/M service.

➲ *CPT Changes: An Insider's View* 2008, 2011, 2013

➲ *CPT Assistant* Feb 09:6

77 Repeat Procedure by Another Physician or Other Qualified Health Care Professional: It may be necessary to indicate that a basic procedure or service was repeated by another physician or other qualified health care professional subsequent to the original procedure or service. This circumstance may be reported by adding modifier 77 to the repeated procedure or service. **Note:** This modifier should not be appended to an E/M service.

➲ *CPT Changes: An Insider's View* 2008, 2011, 2013

78 Unplanned Return to the Operating/Procedure Room by the Same Physician or Other Qualified Health Care Professional Following Initial Procedure for a Related Procedure During the Postoperative Period: It may be necessary to indicate that another procedure was performed during the postoperative period of the initial procedure (unplanned procedure following initial procedure). When this procedure is related to the first, and requires the use of an operating/procedure room, it may be reported by adding modifier 78 to the related procedure. (For repeat procedures, see modifier 76.)

➲ *CPT Changes: An Insider's View* 2008, 2011, 2013

79 Unrelated Procedure or Service by the Same Physician or Other Qualified Health Care Professional During the Postoperative Period: The individual may need to indicate that the performance of a procedure or service during the postoperative period was unrelated to the original procedure. This circumstance may be reported by using modifier 79. (For repeat procedures on the same day, see modifier 76.)

➲ *CPT Changes: An Insider's View* 2013

80 Assistant Surgeon: Surgical assistant services may be identified by adding modifier 80 to the usual procedure number(s).

81 Minimum Assistant Surgeon: Minimum surgical assistant services are identified by adding modifier 81 to the usual procedure number.

82 Assistant Surgeon (when qualified resident surgeon not available): The unavailability of a qualified resident surgeon is a prerequisite for use of modifier 82 appended to the usual procedure code number(s).

90 Reference (Outside) Laboratory: When laboratory procedures are performed by a party other than the treating or reporting physician or other qualified health care professional, the procedure may be identified by adding modifier 90 to the usual procedure number.

➲ *CPT Changes: An Insider's View* 2013

91 Repeat Clinical Diagnostic Laboratory Test: In the course of treatment of the patient, it may be necessary to repeat the same laboratory test on the same day to obtain subsequent (multiple) test results. Under these circumstances, the laboratory test performed can be identified by its usual procedure number and the addition of modifier 91. **Note:** This modifier may not be used when tests are rerun to confirm initial results; due to testing problems with specimens or equipment; or for any other reason when a normal, one-time, reportable result is all that is required. This modifier may not be used when other code(s) describe a series of test results (eg, glucose tolerance tests, evocative/suppression testing). This modifier may only be used for laboratory test(s) performed more than once on the same day on the same patient.

➲ *CPT Assistant* May 09:6, Sept 13:7

92 Alternative Laboratory Platform Testing: When laboratory testing is being performed using a kit or transportable instrument that wholly or in part consists of a single use, disposable analytical chamber, the service may be identified by adding modifier 92 to the usual laboratory procedure code (HIV testing 86701-86703, and 87389). The test does not require permanent dedicated space, hence by its design may be hand carried or transported to the vicinity of the patient for immediate testing at that site, although location of the testing is not in itself determinative of the use of this modifier.

➲ *CPT Changes: An Insider's View* 2008, 2012

Appendix A

95 Synchronous Telemedicine Service Rendered Via a Real-Time Interactive Audio and Video Telecommunications System: Synchronous telemedicine service is defined as a **real-time** interaction between a physician or other qualified health care professional and a patient who is located at a distant site from the physician or other qualified health care professional. The totality of the communication of information exchanged between the physician or other qualified health care professional and the patient during the course of the synchronous telemedicine service must be of an amount and nature that would be sufficient to meet the key components and/or requirements of the same service when rendered via a face-to-face interaction. Modifier 95 may only be appended to the services listed in Appendix P. Appendix P is the list of CPT codes for services that are typically performed face-to-face, but may be rendered via a real-time (synchronous) interactive audio and video telecommunications system.

CPT Changes: An Insider's View 2017

96 Habilitative Services: When a service or procedure that may be either habilitative or rehabilitative in nature is provided for habilitative purposes, the physician or other qualified health care professional may add modifier 96 to the service or procedure code to indicate that the service or procedure provided was a habilitative service. Habilitative services help an individual learn skills and functioning for daily living that the individual has not yet developed, and then keep and/or improve those learned skills. Habilitative services also help an individual keep, learn, or improve skills and functioning for daily living.

CPT Changes: An Insider's View 2018

97 Rehabilitative Services: When a service or procedure that may be either habilitative or rehabilitative in nature is provided for rehabilitative purposes, the physician or other qualified health care professional may add modifier 97 to the service or procedure code to indicate that the service or procedure provided was a rehabilitative service. Rehabilitative services help an individual keep, get back, or improve skills and functioning for daily living that have been lost or impaired because the individual was sick, hurt, or disabled.

CPT Changes: An Insider's View 2018

99 Multiple Modifiers: Under certain circumstances 2 or more modifiers may be necessary to completely delineate a service. In such situations modifier 99 should be added to the basic procedure, and other applicable modifiers may be listed as part of the description of the service.

Anesthesia Physical Status Modifiers

The Physical Status modifiers are consistent with the American Society of Anesthesiologists ranking of patient physical status, and distinguishing various levels of complexity of the anesthesia service provided. All anesthesia services are reported by use of the anesthesia five-digit procedure code (00100-01999) with the appropriate physical status modifier appended.

Example: 00100-P1

Under certain circumstances, when another established modifier(s) is appropriate, it should be used in addition to the physical status modifier.

Example: 00100-P4-53

Physical Status Modifier P1: A normal healthy patient

Physical Status Modifier P2: A patient with mild systemic disease

Physical Status Modifier P3: A patient with severe systemic disease

Physical Status Modifier P4: A patient with severe systemic disease that is a constant threat to life

Physical Status Modifier P5: A moribund patient who is not expected to survive without the operation

Physical Status Modifier P6: A declared brain-dead patient whose organs are being removed for donor purposes

Modifiers Approved for Ambulatory Surgery Center (ASC) Hospital Outpatient Use

CPT Level I Modifiers

25 Significant, Separately Identifiable Evaluation and Management Service by the Same Physician or Other Qualified Health Care Professional on the Same Day of the Procedure or Other Service: It may be necessary to indicate that on the day a procedure or service identified by a CPT code was performed, the patient's condition required a significant, separately identifiable E/M service above and beyond the other service provided or beyond the usual preoperative and postoperative care associated with the procedure that was performed. A significant, separately identifiable E/M service is defined or substantiated by documentation that satisfies the relevant criteria for the respective E/M service to be reported (see **Evaluation and Management Services Guidelines** for instructions on determining level of E/M service). The E/M service may be prompted by the symptom or condition for which the procedure and/or service was provided. As such, different diagnoses are not required for reporting of the E/M services on the same date. This circumstance may be reported by adding modifier 25 to the appropriate level of E/M service. **Note:** This modifier is not used to report an E/M service that resulted in a decision to perform surgery. See modifier 57. For significant, separately identifiable non-E/M services, see modifier 59.

CPT Changes: An Insider's View 2013

27 Multiple Outpatient Hospital E/M Encounters on the Same Date: For hospital outpatient reporting purposes, utilization of hospital resources related to separate and distinct E/M encounters performed in multiple outpatient hospital settings on the same date may be reported by adding modifier 27 to each appropriate level outpatient and/or emergency department E/M code(s). This modifier provides a means of reporting circumstances involving evaluation and management services provided by physician(s) in more than one (multiple) outpatient hospital setting(s) (eg, hospital emergency department, clinic). **Note:** This modifier is not to be used for physician reporting of multiple E/M services performed by the same physician on the same date. For physician reporting of all outpatient evaluation and management services provided by the same physician on the same date and performed in multiple outpatient setting(s) (eg, hospital emergency department, clinic), see **Evaluation and Management, Emergency Department,** or **Preventive Medicine Services** codes.

33 Preventive Services: When the primary purpose of the service is the delivery of an evidence based service in accordance with a US Preventive Services Task Force A or B rating in effect and other preventive services identified in preventive services mandates (legislative or regulatory), the service may be identified by adding 33 to the procedure. For separately reported services specifically identified as preventive, the modifier should not be used.

➲ *CPT Changes: An Insider's View* 2012

50 Bilateral Procedure: Unless otherwise identified in the listings, bilateral procedures that are performed at the same session, should be identified by adding modifier 50 to the appropriate 5 digit code.

➲ *CPT Assistant* Jun 13:15

52 Reduced Services: Under certain circumstances a service or procedure is partially reduced or eliminated at the discretion of the physician or other qualified health care professional. Under these circumstances the service provided can be identified by its usual procedure number and the addition of modifier 52, signifying that the service is reduced. This provides a means of reporting reduced services without disturbing the identification of the basic service. **Note:** For hospital outpatient reporting of a previously scheduled procedure/service that is partially reduced or cancelled as a result of extenuating circumstances or those that threaten the well-being of the patient prior to or after administration of anesthesia, see modifiers 73 and 74 (see modifiers approved for ASC hospital outpatient use).

➲ *CPT Changes: An Insider's View* 2013

➲ *CPT Assistant* Jun 13:7

58 Staged or Related Procedure or Service by the Same Physician or Other Qualified Health Care Professional During the Postoperative Period: It may be necessary to indicate that the performance of a procedure or service during the postoperative period was: (a) planned or anticipated (staged); (b) more extensive than the original procedure; or (c) for therapy following a surgical procedure. This circumstance may be reported by adding modifier 58 to the staged or related procedure. **Note:** For treatment of a problem that requires a return to the operating/procedure room (eg, unanticipated clinical condition), see modifier 78.

➲ *CPT Changes: An Insider's View* 2013

59 Distinct Procedural Service: Under certain circumstances, it may be necessary to indicate that a procedure or service was distinct or independent from other non-E/M services performed on the same day. Modifier 59 is used to identify procedures/services, other than E/M services, that are not normally reported together, but are appropriate under the circumstances. Documentation must support a different session, different procedure or surgery, different site or organ system, separate incision/excision, separate lesion, or separate injury (or area of injury in extensive injuries) not ordinarily encountered or performed on the same day by the same individual. However, when another already established modifier is appropriate it should be used rather than modifier 59. Only if no more descriptive modifier is available, and the use of modifier 59 best explains the circumstances, should modifier 59 be used. **Note:** Modifier 59 should not be appended to an E/M service. To report a separate and distinct E/M service with a non-E/M service performed on the same date, see modifier 25.

73 Discontinued Out-Patient Hospital/Ambulatory Surgery Center (ASC) Procedure Prior to the Administration of Anesthesia: Due to extenuating circumstances or those that threaten the well being of the patient, the physician may cancel a surgical or diagnostic procedure subsequent to the patient's surgical preparation (including sedation when provided, and being taken to the room where the procedure is to be performed), but prior to the administration of anesthesia (local, regional block(s) or general). Under these circumstances, the intended service that is prepared for but cancelled can be reported by its usual procedure number and the addition of modifier 73. **Note:** The elective cancellation of a service prior to the administration of anesthesia and/or surgical preparation of the patient should not be reported. For physician reporting of a discontinued procedure, see modifier 53.

74 Discontinued Out-Patient Hospital/Ambulatory Surgery Center (ASC) Procedure After Administration of Anesthesia: Due to extenuating circumstances or those that threaten the well being of the patient, the physician may terminate a surgical or diagnostic procedure after the administration of anesthesia (local, regional block(s), general) or after the procedure was started (incision made, intubation started, scope inserted, etc). Under these circumstances, the procedure started but terminated can be reported by its usual procedure number and the addition of modifier 74. **Note:** The elective cancellation of a service prior to the administration of anesthesia and/or surgical preparation of the patient should not be reported. For physician reporting of a discontinued procedure, see modifier 53.

➲ *CPT Assistant* Jun 13:7

76 Repeat Procedure or Service by Same Physician or Other Qualified Health Care Professional: It may be necessary to indicate that a procedure or service was repeated by the same physician or other qualified health care professional subsequent to the original procedure or service. This circumstance may be reported by adding modifier 76 to the repeated procedure or service. **Note:** This modifier should not be appended to an E/M service.

CPT Changes: An Insider's View 2013

77 Repeat Procedure by Another Physician or Other Qualified Health Care Professional: It may be necessary to indicate that a basic procedure or service was repeated by another physician or other qualified health care professional subsequent to the original procedure or service. This circumstance may be reported by adding modifier 77 to the repeated procedure or service. **Note:** This modifier should not be appended to an E/M service.

CPT Changes: An Insider's View 2013

78 Unplanned Return to the Operating/Procedure Room by the Same Physician or Other Qualified Health Care Professional Following Initial Procedure for a Related Procedure During the Postoperative Period: It may be necessary to indicate that another procedure was performed during the postoperative period of the initial procedure (unplanned procedure following initial procedure). When this procedure is related to the first, and requires the use of an operating/procedure room, it may be reported by adding modifier 78 to the related procedure. (For repeat procedures, see modifier 76.)

CPT Changes: An Insider's View 2013

79 Unrelated Procedure or Service by the Same Physician or Other Qualified Health Care Professional During the Postoperative Period: The individual may need to indicate that the performance of a procedure or service during the postoperative period was unrelated to the original procedure. This circumstance may be reported by using modifier 79. (For repeat procedures on the same day, see modifier 76.)

CPT Changes: An Insider's View 2008, 2011

91 Repeat Clinical Diagnostic Laboratory Test: In the course of treatment of the patient, it may be necessary to repeat the same laboratory test on the same day to obtain subsequent (multiple) test results. Under these circumstances, the laboratory test performed can be identified by its usual procedure number and the addition of modifier 91. **Note:** This modifier may not be used when tests are rerun to confirm initial results; due to testing problems with specimens or equipment; or for any other reason when a normal, one-time, reportable result is all that is required. This modifier may not be used when other code(s) describe a series of test results (eg, glucose tolerance tests, evocative/suppression testing). This modifier may only be used for laboratory test(s) performed more than once on the same day on the same patient.

Category II Modifiers

The following performance measurement modifiers may be used for Category II codes to indicate that a service specified in the associated measure(s) was considered but, due to either medical, patient, or system circumstance(s) documented in the medical record, the service was not provided. These modifiers serve as denominator exclusions from the performance measure. The user should note that not all listed measures provide for exclusions (see Alphabetical Clinical Topics Listing for more discussion regarding exclusion criteria).

Category II modifiers should only be reported with Category II codes—they should not be reported with Category I or Category III codes. In addition, the modifiers in the Category II section should only be used where specified in the guidelines, reporting instructions, parenthetic notes, or code descriptor language listed in the Category II section (code listing and the Alphabetical Clinical Topics Listing).

1P Performance Measure Exclusion Modifier due to Medical Reasons:

Reasons include:

- Not indicated (absence of organ/limb, already received/performed, other)
- Contraindicated (patient allergic history, potential adverse drug interaction, other)
- Other medical reasons

2P Performance Measure Exclusion Modifier due to Patient Reasons:

Reasons include:

- Patient declined
- Economic, social, or religious reasons
- Other patient reasons

3P Performance Measure Exclusion Modifier due to System Reasons:

Reasons include:

- Resources to perform the services not available
- Insurance coverage/payor-related limitations
- Other reasons attributable to health care delivery system

Modifier 8P is intended to be used as a "reporting modifier" to allow the reporting of circumstances when an action described in a measure's numerator is not performed and the reason is not otherwise specified.

8P Performance measure reporting modifier–action not performed, reason not otherwise specified

Level II (HCPCS/National) Modifiers

E1 Upper left, eyelid

E2 Lower left, eyelid

E3 Upper right, eyelid

E4 Lower right, eyelid

F1 Left hand, second digit

F2 Left hand, third digit

F3 Left hand, fourth digit

F4 Left hand, fifth digit

F5 Right hand, thumb

F6 Right hand, second digit

F7 Right hand, third digit

F8 Right hand, fourth digit

F9 Right hand, fifth digit

FA Left hand, thumb

GG Performance and payment of a screening mammogram and diagnostic mammogram on the same patient, same day

GH Diagnostic mammogram converted from screening mammogram on same day

LC Left circumflex coronary artery

LD Left anterior descending coronary artery

LM Left main coronary artery

LT Left side (used to identify procedures performed on the left side of the body)

QM Ambulance service provided under arrangement by a provider of services

QN Ambulance service furnished directly by a provider of services

RC Right coronary artery

RI Ramus intermedius coronary artery

RT Right side (used to identify procedures performed on the right side of the body)

T1 Left foot, second digit

T2 Left foot, third digit

T3 Left foot, fourth digit

T4 Left foot, fifth digit

T5 Right foot, great toe

T6 Right foot, second digit

T7 Right foot, third digit

T8 Right foot, fourth digit

T9 Right foot, fifth digit

TA Left foot, great toe

XE Separate Encounter *

XS Separate Structure *

XP Separate Practitioner *

XU Unusual Non-Overlapping Service *

(*HCPCS modifiers for selective identification of subsets of Distinct Procedural Services [59 modifier])

Appendix B

Summary of Additions, Deletions, and Revisions

▶Appendix B shows the actual changes that were made to the code descriptors. New codes appear with a bullet (●) and are indicated as "Code added." Revised codes are preceded with a triangle (▲). Within revised codes, the deleted language appears with a ~~strikethrough~~, while new text appears underlined. The symbol ⚡ is used to identify codes for vaccines that are pending FDA approval (see **Appendix K**).The symbol # is used to identify codes that have been resequenced (see **Appendix N**). The symbol ♓ is used to identify codes that are duplicate PLA tests. CPT add-on codes are annotated by the symbol ✚ (see **Appendix D**). The symbol ⊘ is used to identify codes that are exempt from the use of modifier 51 (see **Appendix E**). The symbol ★ is used to identify codes that may be used for reporting telemedicine services (see **Appendix P**).◀

Evaluation and Management

▲ 99446	Interprofessional telephone/Internet/electronic health record assessment and management service provided by a consultative physician, including a verbal and written report to the patient's treating/requesting physician or other qualified health care professional; 5-10 minutes of medical consultative discussion and review
▲ 99447	11-20 minutes of medical consultative discussion and review
▲ 99448	21-30 minutes of medical consultative discussion and review
▲ 99449	31 minutes or more of medical consultative discussion and review
#● 99451	Code added
#● 99452	Code added
#● 99453	Code added
#● 99454	Code added
#▲ 99091	Collection and interpretation of physiologic data (eg, ECG, blood pressure, glucose monitoring) digitally stored and/or transmitted by the patient and/or caregiver to the physician or other qualified health care professional, qualified by education, training, licensure/regulation (when applicable) requiring a minimum of 30 minutes of time, each 30 days
#● 99457	Code added
#● 99491	Code added

Surgery

▲ 10021	Fine needle aspiration biopsy, without imaging guidance; ~~without imaging guidance~~first lesion
~~10022~~	~~with imaging guidance~~
#✚● 10004	Code added
#● 10005	Code added
#✚● 10006	Code added
#● 10007	Code added
#✚● 10008	Code added
#● 10009	Code added
#✚● 10010	Code added
#● 10011	Code added
#✚● 10012	Code added
~~11100~~	~~Biopsy of skin, subcutaneous tissue and/or mucous membrane (including simple closure), unless otherwise listed; single lesion~~
~~11101~~	~~each separate/additional lesion (List separately in addition to code for primary procedure)~~
● 11102	Code added
✚● 11103	Code added
● 11104	Code added
✚● 11105	Code added
● 11106	Code added
✚● 11107	Code added

20005 ~~Incision and drainage of soft tissue abscess, subfascial (ie, involves the soft tissue below the deep fascia)~~

+● **20932** Code added

+● **20933** Code added

+● **20934** Code added

● **27369** Code added

27370 ~~Injection of contrast for knee arthrography~~

31595 ~~Section recurrent laryngeal nerve, therapeutic (separate procedure), unilateral~~

#● **33274** Code added

#● **33275** Code added

33282 ~~Implantation of patient-activated cardiac event recorder~~

33284 ~~Removal of an implantable, patient-activated cardiac event recorder~~

● **33285** Code added

● **33286** Code added

● **33289** Code added

#● **33440** Code added

+● **33866** Code added

▲ **36568** Insertion of peripherally inserted central venous catheter (PICC), without subcutaneous port or pump, without imaging guidance; younger than 5 years of age

▲ **36569** age 5 years or older

#● **36572** Code added

#● **36573** Code added

▲ **36584** Replacement, complete, of a peripherally inserted central venous catheter (PICC), without subcutaneous port or pump, through same venous access, including all imaging guidance, image documentation, and all associated radiological supervision and interpretation required to perform the replacement

● **38531** Code added

41500 ~~Fixation of tongue, mechanical, other than suture (eg, K-wire)~~

43760 ~~Change of gastrostomy tube, percutaneous, without imaging or endoscopic guidance~~

● **43762** Code added

● **43763** Code added

46762 ~~implantation artificial sphincter~~

50395 ~~Introduction of guide into renal pelvis and/or ureter with dilation to establish nephrostomy tract, percutaneous~~

#● **50436** Code added

#● **50437** Code added

● **53854** Code added

61332 ~~Exploration of orbit (transcranial approach); with biopsy~~

61480 ~~for mesencephalic tractotomy or pedunculotomy~~

61610 ~~Transection or ligation, carotid artery in cavernous sinus, with repair by anastomosis or graft (List separately in addition to code for primary procedure)~~

61612 ~~with repair by anastomosis or graft (List separately in addition to code for primary procedure)~~

+▲ **61641** each additional vessel in same vascular ~~family~~territory (List separately in addition to code for primary procedure)

+▲ **61642** each additional vessel in different vascular ~~family~~territory (List separately in addition to code for primary procedure)

63615 ~~Stereotactic biopsy, aspiration, or excision of lesion, spinal cord~~

64508 ~~carotid sinus (separate procedure)~~

64550 ~~Application of surface (transcutaneous) neurostimulator (eg, TENS unit)~~

66220 ~~Repair of scleral staphyloma; without graft~~

Radiology

▲ **74485** Dilation of ~~nephrostomy, ureters,~~ureter(s) or urethra, radiological supervision and interpretation

76001 ~~Fluoroscopy, physician or other qualified health care professional time more than 1 hour, assisting a nonradiologic physician or other qualified health care professional (eg, nephrostolithotomy, ERCP, bronchoscopy, transbronchial biopsy)~~

● **76391** Code added

● **76978** Code added

+● **76979** Code added

● **76981** Code added

● **76982** Code added

+● **76983** Code added

▲ **77021** Magnetic resonance imaging guidance for needle placement (eg, for biopsy, needle aspiration, injection, or placement of localization device) radiological supervision and interpretation

▲ **77022** Magnetic resonance imaging guidance for, and monitoring of, parenchymal tissue ablation

● **77046** Code added

● **77047** Code added

● **77048** Code added

● **77049** Code added

77058 ~~Magnetic resonance imaging, breast,without and/or with contrast material(s); unilateral~~

77059 ~~bilateral~~

#▲ **77387** Guidance for localization of target volume for delivery of radiation treatment ~~delivery~~, includes intrafraction tracking, when performed

78270 ~~Vitamin B-12 absorption study (eg, Schilling test); without intrinsic factor~~

78271 ~~with intrinsic factor~~

78272 ~~Vitamin B-12 absorption studies combined, with and without intrinsic factor~~

Pathology and Laboratory

● **81171** Code added

● **81172** Code added

#● **81204** Code added

#● **81173** Code added

#● **81174** Code added

● **81177** Code added

● **81178** Code added

● **81179** Code added

● **81180** Code added

● **81181** Code added

● **81182** Code added

● **81183** Code added

~~**81211**~~ ~~*BRCA1, BRCA2* (breast cancer 1 and 2) (eg, hereditary breast and ovarian cancer) gene analysis; full sequence analysis and common duplication/deletion variants in BRCA1 (ie, exon 13 del 3.835kb, exon 13 dup 6kb, exon 14-20 del 26kb, exon 22 del 510bp, exon 8-9 del 7.1kb)~~

#▲ **81162** *BRCA1* (*BRCA1, DNA repair associated*), *BRCA2* (*BRCA2, DNA repair associated*)~~(breast cancer 1 and 2)~~ (eg, hereditary breast and ovarian cancer) gene analysis; full sequence analysis and full duplication/deletion analysis (ie, detection of large gene rearrangements)

#● **81163** Code added

#● **81164** Code added

▲ **81212** 185delAG, 5385insC, 6174delT variants

~~**81213**~~ ~~uncommon duplication/deletion variants~~

~~**81214**~~ ~~*BRCA1 (breast cancer 1)* (eg, hereditary breast and ovarian cancer) gene analysis; full sequence analysis and common duplication/deletion variants (ie, exon 13 del 3.835kb, exon 13 dup 6kb, exon 14-20 del 26kb, exon 22 del 510bp, exon 8-9 del 7.1kb)~~

#● **81165** Code added

#● **81166** Code added

▲ **81215** known familial variant

▲ **81216** *BRCA2* (~~*breast cancer 2*~~*BRCA2, DNA repair associated*) (eg, hereditary breast and ovarian cancer) gene analysis; full sequence analysis

#● **81167** Code added

▲ **81217** known familial variant

#● **81233** Code added

#● **81184** Code added

#● **81185** Code added

#● **81186** Code added

#● **81187** Code added

#● **81188** Code added

#● **81189** Code added

#● **81190** Code added

#● **81234** Code added

#● **81239** Code added

● **81236** Code added

● **81237** Code added

▲ **81244** characterization of alleles (eg, expanded size and promoter methylation status)

#● **81284** Code added

#● **81285** Code added

#● **81286** Code added

#● **81289** Code added

#● **81271** Code added

#● **81274** Code added

#▲ **81287** *MGMT (O-6-methylguanine-DNA methyltransferase)* (eg, glioblastoma multiforme)~~,~~; promoter methylation analysis

● **81305** Code added

#● **81306** Code added

#● **81312** Code added

#● **81320** Code added

#● **81343** Code added

▲ **81327** *SEPT9 (Septin9)* (eg, colorectal cancer) promoter methylation analysis

● **81329** Code added

#● **81336** Code added

#● **81337** Code added

#● **81344** Code added

#● **81345** Code added

● **81333** Code added

▲ **81400** Molecular pathology procedure, Level 1 (eg, identification of single germline variant [eg, SNP] by techniques such as restriction enzyme digestion or melt curve analysis)

~~*SMN1 (survival of motor neuron 1, telomeric)* (eg, spinal muscular atrophy), exon 7 deletion~~

▲ **81401** Molecular pathology procedure, Level 2 (eg, 2-10 SNPs, 1 methylated variant, or 1 somatic variant [typically using nonsequencing target variant analysis], or detection of a dynamic mutation disorder/triplet repeat)

~~*AFF2 (AF4/FMR2 family, member 2 [FMR2])* (eg, fragile X mental retardation 2 [FRAXE]), evaluation to detect abnormal (eg, expanded) alleles~~

~~*AR (androgen receptor)* (eg, spinal and bulbar muscular atrophy, Kennedy disease, X chromosome inactivation), characterization of alleles (eg, expanded size or methylation status)~~

~~*ATN1 (atrophin 1)* (eg, dentatorubral-pallidoluysian atrophy), evaluation to detect abnormal (eg, expanded) alleles~~

~~*ATXN1 (ataxin 1)* (eg, spinocerebellar ataxia), evaluation to detect abnormal (eg, expanded) alleles~~

~~*ATXN2 (ataxin 2)* (eg, spinocerebellar ataxia), evaluation to detect abnormal (eg, expanded) alleles~~

~~*ATXN3 (ataxin 3)* (eg, spinocerebellar ataxia, Machado-Joseph disease), evaluation to detect abnormal (eg, expanded) alleles~~

~~*ATXN7 (ataxin 7)* (eg, spinocerebellar ataxia), evaluation to detect abnormal (eg, expanded) alleles~~

~~*ATXN8OS (ATXN8 opposite strand [non-protein coding])* (eg, spinocerebellar ataxia), evaluation to detect abnormal (eg, expanded) alleles~~

~~*ATXN10 (ataxin 10)* (eg, spinocerebellar ataxia), evaluation to detect abnormal (eg, expanded) alleles~~

~~*CACNA1A (calcium channel, voltage-dependent, P/Q type, alpha 1A subunit)* (eg, spinocerebellar ataxia), evaluation to detect abnormal (eg, expanded) alleles~~

~~*CNBP (CCHC-type zinc finger, nucleic acid binding protein)* (eg, myotonic dystrophy type 2), evaluation to detect abnormal (eg, expanded) alleles~~

~~*CSTB (cystatin B [stefin B])* (eg, Unverricht-Lundborg disease), evaluation to detect abnormal (eg, expanded) alleles~~

~~*DMPK (dystrophia myotonica-protein kinase)* (eg, myotonic dystrophy, type 1), evaluation to detect abnormal (eg, expanded) alleles~~

Appendix B

~~*FXN (frataxin) (eg, Friedreich ataxia)*, evaluation to detect abnormal (expanded) alleles~~

~~*HTT (huntingtin) (eg, Huntington disease)*, evaluation to detect abnormal (eg, expanded) alleles~~

~~*PABPN1 (poly[A] binding protein, nuclear 1)* (eg, oculopharyngeal muscular dystrophy), evaluation to detect abnormal (eg, expanded) alleles~~

~~*PPP2R2B (protein phosphatase 2, regulatory subunit B, beta)* (eg, spinocerebellar ataxia), evaluation to detect abnormal (eg, expanded) alleles~~

~~*SMN1/SMN2 (survival of motor neuron 1, telomeric/survival of motor neuron 2, centromeric)* (eg, spinal muscular atrophy), dosage analysis (eg, carrier testing)~~

~~*TBP (TATA box binding protein)* (eg, spinocerebellar ataxia), evaluation to detect abnormal (eg, expanded) alleles~~

▲ **81403** Molecular pathology procedure, Level 4 (eg, analysis of single exon by DNA sequence analysis, analysis of >10 amplicons using multiplex PCR in 2 or more independent reactions, mutation scanning or duplication/deletion variants of 2-5 exons)

~~*SMN1 (survival of motor neuron 1, telomeric)* (eg, spinal muscular atrophy), known familial sequence variant(s)~~

▲ **81404** Molecular pathology procedure, Level 5 (eg, analysis of 2-5 exons by DNA sequence analysis, mutation scanning or duplication/deletion variants of 6-10 exons, or characterization of a dynamic mutation disorder/triplet repeat by Southern blot analysis)

~~*AFF2 (AF4/FMR2 family, member 2 [FMR2])* (eg, fragile X mental retardation 2 [FRAXE]), characterization of alleles (eg, expanded size and methylation status)~~

~~*CSTB (cystatin B [stefin B])* (eg, Unverricht-Lundborg disease), full gene sequence~~

~~*DMPK (dystrophia myotonica-protein kinase)* (eg, myotonic dystrophy type 1), characterization of abnormal (eg, expanded) alleles~~

~~*FXN (frataxin) (eg, Friedreich ataxia)*, full gene sequence~~

▲ **81405** Molecular pathology procedure, Level 6 (eg, analysis of 6-10 exons by DNA sequence analysis, mutation scanning or duplication/deletion variants of 11-25 exons, regionally targeted cytogenomic array analysis)

~~*AR (androgen receptor)* (eg, androgen insensitivity syndrome), full gene sequence~~

~~*SMN1 (survival of motor neuron 1, telomeric)* (eg, spinal muscular atrophy), full gene sequence~~

▲ **81407** Molecular pathology procedure, Level 8 (eg, analysis of 26-50 exons by DNA sequence analysis, mutation scanning or duplication/deletion variants of >50 exons, sequence analysis of multiple genes on one platform)

~~*CACNA1A (calcium channel, voltage-dependent, P/Q type, alpha 1A subunit)* (eg, familial hemiplegic migraine), full gene sequence~~

● **81443** Code added

● **81518** Code added

● **81596** Code added

● **82642** Code added

● **83722** Code added

~~**0004U**~~ ~~Infectious disease (bacterial), DNA, 27 resistance genes, PCR amplification and probe hybridization in microarray format (molecular detection and identification of AmpC, carbapenemase and ESBL coding genes), bacterial culture colonies, report of genes detected or not detected, per isolate~~

▲ **0006U** ~~Prescrip~~Detection ~~drug monitoring~~ of interacting medications, substances, supplements and foods, 120 or more ~~drugs and substances,~~ analytes, definitive ~~tandem mass spectrometry with~~ chromatography~~, urine, qualitative report of presence (including quantitative levels, when detected) or absence of each drug or substance~~ with mass spectrometry, urine, description and severity of ~~potential~~ each interactions~~, with~~ identified ~~substances~~, per date of service

~~**0015U**~~ ~~Drug metabolism (adverse drug reactions), DNA, 22 drug metabolism and transporter genes, real-time PCR, blood or buccal swab, genotype and metabolizer status for therapeutic decision support~~

● **0018U** Code added

● **0019U** Code added

⚹● **0020U** Code added

● **0021U** Code added

● **0022U** Code added

● **0023U** Code added

● **0024U** Code added

● **0025U** Code added

● **0026U** Code added

● **0027U** Code added

● **0028U** Code added

● **0029U** Code added

● **0030U** Code added

● **0031U** Code added

● **0032U** Code added

● **0033U** Code added

● **0034U** Code added

● **0035U** Code added

● **0036U** Code added

● **0037U** Code added

● **0038U** Code added

● **0039U** Code added

● **0040U** Code added

● **0041U** Code added

● **0042U** Code added

● **0043U** Code added

● **0044U** Code added

● **0045U** Code added

● **0046U** Code added

● **0047U** Code added

● **0048U** Code added

● **0049U** Code added

● **0050U** Code added

● **0051U** Code added

● **0052U** Code added

● **0053U** Code added

● **0054U** Code added

● **0055U** Code added

Appendix B

● **0056U** Code added

● **0057U** Code added

● **0058U** Code added

● **0059U** Code added

● **0060U** Code added

● **0061U** Code added

Medicine

⚡● **90689** Code added

● **92273** Code added

● **92274** Code added

~~**92275**~~ ~~Electroretinography with interpretation and report~~

#● **93264** Code added

▲ **93279** Programming device evaluation (in person) with iterative adjustment of the implantable device to test the function of the device and select optimal permanent programmed values with analysis, review and report by a physician or other qualified health care professional; single lead pacemaker system or leadless pacemaker system in one cardiac chamber

▲ **93285** ~~implantable loop recorder system~~subcutaneous cardiac rhythm monitor system

▲ **93286** Peri-procedural device evaluation (in person) and programming of device system parameters before or after a surgery, procedure, or test with analysis, review and report by a physician or other qualified health care professional; single, dual, or multiple lead pacemaker system, or leadless pacemaker system

▲ **93288** Interrogation device evaluation (in person) with analysis, review and report by a physician or other qualified health care professional, includes connection, recording and disconnection per patient encounter; single, dual, or multiple lead pacemaker system, or leadless pacemaker system

▲ **93290** implantable cardiovascular physiologic monitor system, including analysis of 1 or more recorded physiologic cardiovascular data elements from all internal and external sensors

▲ **93291** ~~implantable loop recorder system~~subcutaneous cardiac rhythm monitor system, including heart rhythm derived data analysis

▲ **93294** Interrogation device evaluation(s) (remote), up to 90 days; single, dual, or multiple lead pacemaker system, or leadless pacemaker system with interim analysis, review(s) and report(s) by a physician or other qualified health care professional

▲ **93296** single, dual, or multiple lead pacemaker system, leadless pacemaker system, or implantable defibrillator system, remote data acquisition(s), receipt of transmissions and technician review, technical support and distribution of results

▲ **93297** Interrogation device evaluation(s), (remote) up to 30 days; implantable cardiovascular physiologic monitor system, including analysis of 1 or more recorded physiologic cardiovascular data elements from all internal and external sensors, analysis, review(s) and report(s) by a physician or other qualified health care professional

★▲ **93298** ~~implantable loop recorder system~~subcutaneous cardiac rhythm monitor system, including analysis of recorded heart rhythm data, analysis, review(s) and report(s) by a physician or other qualified health care professional

★▲ **93299** implantable cardiovascular physiologic monitor system or ~~implantable loop recorder system~~subcutaneous cardiac rhythm monitor system, remote data acquisition(s), receipt of transmissions and technician review, technical support and distribution of results

▲ **94780** Car seat/bed testing for airway integrity, ~~neonate~~for infants through 12 months of age, with continual ~~nursing~~clinical staff observation and continuous recording of pulse oximetry, heart rate and respiratory rate, with interpretation and report; 60 minutes

+▲ **94781** each additional full 30 minutes (List separately in addition to code for primary procedure)

#● **95836** Code added

▲ **95970** Electronic analysis of implanted neurostimulator pulse generator-~~system~~/transmitter (eg, ~~rate~~contact group[s], ~~pulse~~interleaving, amplitude, pulse ~~duration~~width, frequency [Hz], ~~configuration of wave form~~on/off cycling, burst, magnet mode, ~~battery status~~dose lockout, ~~electrode selectability~~patient selectable parameters, ~~output modulation~~responsive neurostimulation, ~~cycling~~detection algorithms, ~~impedance~~closed loop parameters, and ~~patient compliance measurements)~~passive parameters) by physician or other qualified health care professional; ~~simple or complex brain~~with brain, cranial nerve, spinal cord, ~~or~~ peripheral ~~(ie, cranial~~ nerve, ~~peripheral nerve,~~or sacral nerve, ~~neuromuscular)~~ neurostimulator pulse generator/transmitter, without ~~reprogramming~~programming

▲ **95971** with simple spinal cord~~,~~ or ~~peripheral (ie,~~ peripheral nerve (eg, sacral nerve~~, neuromuscular~~) neurostimulator pulse generator/transmitter~~, with intraoperative~~ programming by physician or ~~subsequent programming~~other qualified health care professional

▲ **95972** with complex spinal cord~~,~~ or ~~peripheral (ie,~~ peripheral ~~nerve, sacral~~ nerve, ~~neuromuscular) (except cranial~~eg, sacral nerve) neurostimulator pulse generator/transmitter~~, with intraoperative~~ programming by physician or ~~subsequent programming~~other qualified health care professional

~~**95974**~~ ~~complex cranial nerve neurostimulator pulse generator/transmitter, with intraoperative or subsequent programming, with or without nerve interface testing, first hour~~

~~**95975**~~ ~~complex cranial nerve neurostimulator pulse generator/transmitter, with intraoperative or subsequent programming, each additional 30 minutes after first hour (List separately in addition to code for primary procedure)~~

● **95976** Code added

● **95977** Code added

#● **95983** Code added

#+● **95984** Code added

~~**95978**~~ ~~Electronic analysis of implanted neurostimulator pulse generator system (eg, rate, pulse amplitude and duration, battery status, electrode selectability and polarity, impedance and patient compliance measurements), complex deep brain neurostimulator pulse generator/transmitter, with initial or subsequent programming; first hour~~

~~**95979**~~ ~~each additional 30 minutes after first hour (List separately in addition to code for primary procedure)~~

#● **97151** Code added

#● **97152** Code added

#● **97153** Code added

#● **97154** Code added

#● **97155** Code added

#● **97156** Code added

#● **97157** Code added

#● **97158** Code added

~~**96101** Psychological testing (includes psychodiagnostic assessment of emotionality, intellectual abilities, personality and psychopathology, eg, MMPI, Rorschach, WAIS), per hour of the psychologist's or physician's time, both face-to-face time administering tests to the patient and time interpreting these test results and preparing the report~~

~~**96102** Psychological testing (includes psychodiagnostic assessment of emotionality, intellectual abilities, personality and psychopathology, eg, MMPI and WAIS), with qualified health care professional interpretation and report, administered by technician, per hour of technician time, face-to-face~~

~~**96103** Psychological testing (includes psychodiagnostic assessment of emotionality, intellectual abilities, personality and psychopathology, eg, MMPI), administered by a computer, with qualified health care professional interpretation and report~~

~~**96111** Developmental testing, (includes assessment of motor, language, social, adaptive, and/or cognitive functioning by standardized developmental instruments) with interpretation and report~~

● **96112** Code added

+● **96113** Code added

★▲ **96116** Neurobehavioral status exam (clinical assessment of thinking, reasoning and judgment, [eg, acquired knowledge, attention, language, memory, planning and problem solving, and visual spatial abilities]), ~~per hour of the psychologist's or physician's time~~by physician or other qualified health care professional, both face-to-face time with the patient and time interpreting test results and preparing the report; first hour

~~**96118** Neuropsychological testing (eg, Halstead-Reitan Neuropsychological Battery, Wechsler Memory Scales and Wisconsin Card Sorting Test), per hour of the psychologist's or physician's time, both face-to-face time administering tests to the patient and time interpreting these test results and preparing the report~~

~~**96119** Neuropsychological testing (eg, Halstead-Reitan Neuropsychological Battery, Wechsler Memory Scales and Wisconsin Card Sorting Test), with qualified health care professional interpretation and report, administered by technician, per hour of technician time, face-to-face~~

~~**96120** Neuropsychological testing (eg, Wisconsin Card Sorting Test), administered by a computer, with qualified health care professional interpretation and report~~

+● **96121** Code added

● **96130** Code added

+● **96131** Code added

● **96132** Code added

+● **96133** Code added

● **96136** Code added

+● **96137** Code added

● **96138** Code added

+● **96139** Code added

● **96146** Code added

~~**99090** Analysis of clinical data stored in computers (eg, ECGs, blood pressures, hematologic data)~~

Category III Codes

#● **0512T** Code added

#+● **0513T** Code added

~~**0159T** Computer-aided detection, including computer algorithm analysis of MRI image data for lesion detection/characterization, pharmacokinetic analysis, with further physician review for interpretation, breast MRI (List separately in addition to code for primary procedure)~~

~~**0188T** Remote real-time interactive video-conferenced critical care, evaluation and management of the critically ill or critically injured patient; first 30-74 minutes~~

~~**0189T** each additional 30 minutes (List separately in addition to code for primary service)~~

~~**0190T** Placement of intraocular radiation source applicator (List separately in addition to primary procedure)~~

~~**0195T** Arthrodesis, pre-sacral interbody technique, disc space preparation, discectomy, without instrumentation, with image guidance, includes bone graft when performed; L5-S1 interspace~~

~~**0196T** L4-L5 interspace (List separately in addition to code for primary procedure)~~

▲ **0335T** Insertion of sinus tarsi implant~~Extra-osseous subtalar joint implant for talotarsal stabilization~~

#● **0510T** Code added

#● **0511T** Code added

~~**0337T** Endothelial function assessment, using peripheral vascular response to reactive hyperemia, non-invasive (eg, brachial artery ultrasound, peripheral artery tonometry), unilateral or bilateral~~

~~**0346T** Ultrasound, elastography (List separately in addition to code for primary procedure)~~

~~**0359T** **Behavior identification assessment,** by the physician or other qualified health care professional, face-to-face with patient and caregiver(s), includes administration of standardized and non-standardized tests, detailed behavioral history, patient observation and caregiver interview, interpretation of test results, discussion of findings and recommendations with the primary guardian(s)/caregiver(s), and preparation of report~~

~~**0360T** **Observational behavioral follow-up assessment,** includes physician or other qualified health care professional direction with interpretation and report, administered by one technician; first 30 minutes of technician time, face-to-face with the patient~~

~~**0361T** each additional 30 minutes of technician time, face-to-face with the patient (List separately in addition to code for primary service)~~

▲ **0362T** **~~Exposure behavioral follow-up~~Behavior identification supporting assessment,** ~~includes physician or other qualified health care professional direction with interpretation and report, administered by physician or other qualified health care professional with the assistance of one or more technicians~~each 15 minutes of technicians' time face-to-face with a patient, requiring the following components:

- administration by the physician or other qualified health care professional who is on site;
- with the assistance of two or more technicians;
- for a patient who exhibits destructive behavior;
- completion in an environment that is customized to the patient's behavior.

~~first 30 minutes of technician(s) time, face-to-face with the patient~~

~~0363T~~ ~~each additional 30 minutes of technician(s) time, face-to-face with the patient (List separately in addition to code for primary procedure)~~

~~0364T~~ ~~Adaptive behavior treatment by protocol, administered by technician, face-to-face with one patient; first 30 minutes of technician time~~

~~0365T~~ ~~each additional 30 minutes of technician time (List separately in addition to code for primary procedure)~~

~~0366T~~ ~~Group adaptive behavior treatment by protocol, administered by technician, face-to-face with two or more patients; first 30 minutes of technician time~~

~~0367T~~ ~~each additional 30 minutes of technician time (List separately in addition to code for primary procedure~~

~~0368T~~ ~~Adaptive behavior treatment with protocol modification administered by physician or other qualified health care professional with one patient; first 30 minutes of patient face-to-face time~~

~~0369T~~ ~~each additional 30 minutes of patient face-to-face time (List separately in addition to code for primary procedure)~~

~~0370T~~ ~~Family adaptive behavior treatment guidance, administered by physician or other qualified health care professional (without the patient present)~~

~~0371T~~ ~~Multiple-family group adaptive behavior treatment guidance, administered by physician or other qualified health care professional (without the patient present)~~

~~0372T~~ ~~Adaptive behavior treatment social skills group, administered by physician or other qualified health care professional face-to-face with multiple patients~~

▲ **0373T** ~~Exposure adaptive behavior treatment with protocol modification~~**Adaptive behavior treatment with protocol modification,** each 15 minutes of technicians' time face-to-face with a patient, requiring ~~two or more technicians for severe maladaptive behavior(s)~~the following components:

- administration by the physician or other qualified health care professional who is on site;
- with the assistance of two or more technicians;
- for a patient who exhibits destructive behavior;
- completion in an environment that is customized to the patient's behavior.

~~first 60 minutes of technicians' time, face-to-face with patient~~

~~0374T~~ ~~each additional 30 minutes of technicians' time face-to-face with patient (List separately in addition to code for primary procedure)~~

~~0387T~~ ~~Transcatheter insertion or replacement of permanent leadless pacemaker, ventricular~~

~~0388T~~ ~~Transcatheter removal of permanent leadless pacemaker, ventricular~~

~~0389T~~ ~~Programming device evaluation (in person) with iterative adjustment of the implantable device to test the function of the device and select optimal permanent programmed values with analysis, review and report, leadless pacemaker system~~

~~0390T~~ ~~Peri-procedural device evaluation (in person) and programming of device system parameters before or after a surgery, procedure or test with analysis, review and report, leadless pacemaker system~~

~~0391T~~ ~~Interrogation device evaluation (in person) with analysis, review and report, includes connection, recording and disconnection per patient encounter, leadless pacemaker system~~

~~0406T~~ ~~Nasal endoscopy, surgical, ethmoid sinus, placement of drug eluting implant~~

~~0407T~~ ~~with biopsy, polypectomy or debridement~~

#+● **0523T** Code added

● **0505T** Code added

● **0506T** Code added

● **0507T** Code added

● **0508T** Code added

● **0509T** Code added

+● **0514T** Code added

● **0515T** Code added

● **0516T** Code added

● **0517T** Code added

● **0518T** Code added

● **0519T** Code added

● **0520T** Code added

● **0521T** Code added

● **0522T** Code added

● **0524T** Code added

● **0525T** Code added

● **0526T** Code added

● **0527T** Code added

● **0528T** Code added

● **0529T** Code added

● **0530T** Code added

● **0531T** Code added

● **0532T** Code added

● **0533T** Code added

● **0534T** Code added

● **0535T** Code added

● **0536T** Code added

● **0537T** Code added

● **0538T** Code added

● **0539T** Code added

● **0540T** Code added

● **0541T** Code added

● **0542T** Code added

Appendix B

Appendix C

Clinical Examples

As described in the CPT 2019 code set, clinical examples of the CPT codes for Evaluation and Management (E/M) services are intended to be an important element of the coding system. The clinical examples, when used with the E/M descriptors contained in the full text of the CPT code set, provide a useful tool and guidance for individuals to report the services provided to their patients. Clinical examples of the codes for E/M services are provided to assist physicians in understanding the meaning of the descriptors and selecting the correct code. Each example was developed by physicians in the specialties shown.

The same problem, when seen by physicians in different specialties, may involve different amounts of work. Therefore, the appropriate level of encounter should be reported using the descriptors rather than the examples.

The American Medical Association is pleased to provide you with these clinical examples for the CPT 2019 code set. The clinical examples that are provided in this supplement are limited to Office or Other Outpatient Services, Hospital Inpatient Services, Consultations, Critical Care, Prolonged Services, and Care Plan Oversight.

These clinical examples are used to describe presenting problems that are frequently encountered in a given specialty. Typical patients with such problems may commonly require the listed Evaluation and Management (E/M) service. Therefore, these examples are **not** appropriately used for any review of correct coding or estimating physician or qualified health care professional work. These clinical examples do not encompass the entire scope of medical practice. Inclusion or exclusion of any particular specialty group does not infer any judgment of importance or lack thereof; nor does it limit the applicability of the example to any particular specialty. We present these examples to provide additional educational context when used in conjunction with the E/M descriptors and guidelines.

Of utmost importance is that these clinical examples are just that: examples. A particular patient encounter, depending on the specific circumstances, must be judged by the services provided by the physician or other qualified health care professional for that particular patient. Simply because the patient's complaints, symptoms, or diagnoses match those of a particular clinical example does not automatically assign that patient encounter to that particular level of service. Moreover, simply because the patient's complaints, symptoms, or diagnoses **do not** match those of a particular clinical example does not automatically **exclude** that patient encounter from a particular level of service. The three components (history, examination, and medical decision making) must be met, consistent with the Nature of Presenting Problem, and documented in the medical record to report a particular level of service.

Office or Other Outpatient Service

New Patient

99201 Initial office visit for a 50-year-old male from out-of-town who needs a prescription refill for a nonsteroidal anti-inflammatory drug. (Anesthesiology)

Initial office visit for a 40-year-old female, new patient, requesting information about local pain clinics. (Anesthesiology/Pain Medicine)

Initial office visit for a 10-year-old female for determination of visual acuity as part of a summer camp physical (does not include determination of refractive error). (Ophthalmology)

Initial office visit for an out-of-town patient requiring topical refill. (Dermatology/Podiatry Surgery)

Initial office visit for a 65-year-old male for reassurance about an isolated seborrheic keratosis on upper back. (Dermatology)

Initial office visit for an out-of-state visitor who needs refill of topical steroid to treat lichen planus. (Dermatology)

Initial office visit for an 86-year-old male, out-of-town visitor, who needs prescription refilled for an anal skin preparation that he forgot. (Colon & Rectal Surgery)

Initial office visit for a patient following surgery in another OMS practice. Timing and symptoms suggest diagnosis of alveolar osteitis for which packing will be indicated. (Oral & Maxillofacial Surgery)

Initial office visit for a patient with a pedunculated lesion of the neck which is unsightly. (Dermatology)

Initial office visit for a 10-year-old male, for limited subungual hematoma not requiring drainage. (Podiatry Surgery)

Initial office visit with a 9-month-old female with diaper rash. (Pediatrics)

Initial office visit with a 5-year-old female to remove sutures from simple wound placed by another physician. (Dermatology)

Initial office visit for a patient with a small area of sunburn requiring first aid. (Dermatology)

Appendix C

Initial office visit for the evaluation and management of a contusion of a finger. (Orthopaedic Surgery)

Initial office visit for a 22-year-old male with a small area of sunburn requiring first aid. (Family Medicine/Internal Medicine)

Initial office visit for a 25-year-old female, presents with complaints of skin tags on her neck. (Plastic Surgery)

Initial office visit for an 86-year-old male with a 2 cm lipoma on back that he is concerned is infected. (General Surgery)

Initial office visit with a 5-year-old female who had absorbable sutures, in for a wound check with no complications. (Plastic Surgery)

Initial office visit for an 85-year-old patient with a history of cigarette smoking now with an asymmetrical neck mass, referred by primary care physician for fine-needle aspiration. (Pathology)

Initial office visit for a 25-year-old patient with brief history of cigarette smoking now with a symmetrical neck enlargement, referred by primary care physician for fine-needle aspiration. (Pathology)

Initial office visit for a 55-year-old male, out-of-town visitor, with treated sleep apnea who requests a prescription for a replacement CPAP interface. (Sleep Medicine)

99202 Initial office visit for a 13-year-old patient with comedopapular acne of the face unresponsive to over-the-counter medications. (Family Medicine)

Initial office visit for a patient with a clinically benign lesion or nodule of the lower leg that has been present for many years. (Dermatology)

Initial office visit for a patient with a circumscribed patch of dermatitis of the leg. (Dermatology)

Initial office visit for a patient with papulosquamous eruption of elbows. (Dermatology)

Initial office visit for a 9-year-old patient with erythematous grouped, vesicular eruption of the lip of three days' duration. (Pediatrics)

Initial office visit for an 18-year-old male referred by an orthodontist for advice regarding removal of four wisdom teeth. (Oral & Maxillofacial Surgery)

Initial office visit for a 14-year-old male, who was referred by his orthodontist, for advice on the exposure of impacted maxillary cuspids. (Oral & Maxillofacial Surgery)

Initial office visit for a patient presenting with itching patches on the wrists and ankles. (Dermatology)

Initial office visit for a 30-year-old male with a two-week-old burn of the hand, now healed but patient concerned with redness and swelling. (Plastic Surgery)

Initial evaluation and management of recurrent urinary infection in female. (Internal Medicine)

Initial office visit with a 10-year-old female with history of chronic otitis media and a draining ear. (Pediatrics)

Initial office visit for a 10-year-old female with acute maxillary sinusitis. (Family Medicine)

Initial office visit for a patient with papulopustular and comedonal acne. (Dermatology)

Initial office visit for a patient with recurring episodes of herpes simplex who has developed a clustering of vesicles on the upper lip. (Internal Medicine)

Initial office visit with a 10-year-old male with severe rash and itching for the past 24 hours, positive history for contact with poison oak 48 hours prior to the visit. (Family Medicine)

Initial office visit for a 65-year-old female with low hemoglobin level, no evidence of clinical bleeding, who was referred by her internist for possible bone marrow aspiration. (Pathology)

Initial office visit for a 55-year-old patient with a history of cigarette smoking now with an asymmetrical neck mass, referred by primary care physician for fine-needle aspiration. (Pathology)

Initial office visit for a 45-year-old male with known sleep apnea and an inability to tolerate CPAP due to dry mouth. (Sleep Medicine)

Initial office visit for an 18-year-old male with cellulitis around a superficial puncture wound of the skin. (General Surgery)

Initial office visit for a 61-year-old male with a macerated, itching rash between the toes that has been present for three weeks. (Podiatry Surgery)

Initial office visit for a healthy 16-year-old male with an ingrown nail with paronychia. (Podiatry Surgery)

99203 Initial office visit of a 76-year-old male with a stasis ulcer of three months' duration. (Dermatology)

Initial office visit for a 30-year-old female with pain in the lateral aspect of the forearm. (Physical Medicine & Rehabilitation)

Initial office visit for a patient with cystic acne of the face, chest, and back. Discussion of use of systemic medication. (Dermatology)

Initial office visit for a patient with a patchy, scaly erythematous eruption of the extremities. (Dermatology)

Initial office visit for a 57-year-old female who complains of painful parotid swelling of one week's duration. (Oral & Maxillofacial Surgery)

Initial office visit for a diffusely photodamaged patient with multiple crusted lesions. (Dermatology)

Initial office visit for a patient with dermatitis of the antecubital and popliteal fossae. (Dermatology)

Initial office visit for a 22-year-old female with irregular menses. (Family Medicine)

Initial office visit for a 50-year-old female with dyspepsia and nausea. (Family Medicine)

Initial office visit for a 53-year-old laborer with degenerative joint disease of the knee with no prior treatment. (Orthopaedic Surgery)

Initial office visit for a 60-year-old male with Dupuytren's contracture of one hand with multiple digit involvement. (Orthopaedic Surgery)

Initial office visit for a 33-year-old male with painless gross hematuria without cystoscopy. (Internal Medicine)

Initial office visit for a 55-year-old female with chronic blepharitis. There is a history of use of many medications. (Ophthalmology)

Initial office visit for an 18-year-old female with a two-day history of acute conjunctivitis. Extensive history of possible exposures, prior normal ocular history, and medication use is obtained. (Ophthalmology)

Initial office visit for a 14-year-old male with unilateral anterior knee pain. (Physical Medicine & Rehabilitation)

Initial office visit of an adult who presents with symptoms of an upper-respiratory infection that has progressed to unilateral purulent nasal discharge and discomfort in the right maxillary teeth. (Otolaryngology/Head & Neck Surgery)

Initial office visit of a 65-year-old with long-standing nasal stuffiness on multiple medications and continuous positive airway pressure (CPAP) for obstructive sleep apnea syndrome (OSAS). (Otolaryngology/Head & Neck Surgery)

Initial office visit for a 35-year-old female with postprandial right upper quadrant abdominal pain. (General Surgery)

Initial office visit with couple for counseling concerning voluntary vasectomy for sterility. Spent 30 minutes discussing procedure, risks and benefits, and answering questions. (Urology)

Initial office visit for evaluation, diagnosis, and management of painless gross hematuria in a new patient, without cystoscopy. (Internal Medicine)

Initial office visit for evaluation of a 13-year-old female with progressive scoliosis. (Physical Medicine & Rehabilitation)

Initial office visit for a 21-year-old female desiring counseling and evaluation of initiation of contraception. (Family Practice/Internal Medicine/Obstetrics & Gynecology)

Initial office visit for a 49-year-old male presenting with painless blood per rectum associated with bowel movement. (Colon & Rectal Surgery)

Initial office visit for a 19-year-old football player with three-day-old acute knee injury; now with swelling and pain. (Orthopaedic Surgery)

Initial office visit of a 49-year-old male with nasal obstruction. Detailed exam with topical anesthesia. (Plastic Surgery)

Initial office evaluation for gradual symmetric hearing loss, without other otologic symptoms or history, 58-year-old male, history and physical examination, with interpretation of complete audiogram, air bone, etc. (Otolaryngology)

25-year-old male with back pain of six weeks' duration. (Neurology)

Initial office visit for a 61-year-old female whose husband reports loud disruptive snoring that interferes with his sleep. (Sleep Medicine)

Initial office evaluation of a 58-year-old male, gradual symmetric hearing loss, without other otologic symptoms or history. (Otolaryngology)

Initial office visit for a 45-year-old hypertensive female with a two-month history of plantar heel pain. (Podiatry Surgery)

Initial office visit for a 12-year-old male athlete with retrocalcaneal pain and swelling with no prior treatment. (Podiatry Surgery)

99204 Initial office visit for a 13-year-old female with progressive scoliosis. (Orthopaedic Surgery)

Initial office visit for a 34-year-old female with primary infertility for evaluation and counseling. (Obstetrics & Gynecology)

Initial office visit for a patient with a personal history of multiple non-melanoma skin cancers who presents with a rapidly enlarging 2 cm nodule located on the left temple along with associated tingling in the area and fullness of the subcutaneous tissue in the left preauricular region. (Dermatology)

Initial office visit for an adolescent who was referred by school counselor because of repeated skipping school and declining grades. (Psychiatry)

Initial office visit for a 50-year-old machinist with a generalized eruption. (Dermatology)

Initial office visit for a 45-year-old female who has been abstinent from alcohol and benzodiazepines for three months but complains of headaches, insomnia, and anxiety. (Psychiatry)

Initial office visit for a 60-year-old male with recent change in bowel habits, weight loss, and abdominal pain. (Abdominal Surgery/Colon & Rectal Surgery)

Initial office visit for a 50-year-old male with an aortic aneurysm who is considering surgery. (General Surgery)

Initial office visit for a 17-year-old female with depression. (Internal Medicine)

Initial office visit of a 40-year-old with chronic draining ear, progressive hearing loss and imbalance, with findings consistent with chronic otitis media and cholesteatoma. (Otolaryngology/Head & Neck Surgery)

Initial office visit for initial evaluation of a 63-year-old male with chest pain on exertion. (Cardiology/Internal Medicine)

Initial office visit for evaluation of a 70-year-old patient with recent onset of episodic confusion. (Internal Medicine)

Initial office visit for a 7-year-old female with juvenile diabetes mellitus, new to area, past history of hospitalization times three. (Pediatrics)

Initial office visit of a 50-year-old female with progressive solid food dysphagia. (Gastroenterology)

Initial office visit for a 34-year-old patient with primary infertility, including counseling. (Obstetrics & Gynecology)

Initial office visit for evaluation of a 70-year-old female with polyarthralgia. (Rheumatology)

Initial office visit for a patient with papulosquamous eruption involving 60 percent of the cutaneous surface with joint pain. Combinations of topical and systemic treatments discussed. (Dermatology)

Initial office visit of a 40-year-old female with symptoms of atopic allergies including eye and sinus congestion, often associated with infections. She would like to be tested for allergies. (Otolaryngology/Head & Neck Surgery)

An 8-year-old healthy male with attention problems in school. (Neurology)

Initial office visit for a 67-year-old male with nocturnal choking, witnessed apneas, and excessive daytime sleepiness. (Sleep Medicine)

Initial office visit for a 42-year-old female with Charcot-Marie-Tooth disease, pes cavus, and worsening painful hammer toes. (Podiatry Surgery)

Initial office visit for a 55-year-old-male with progressive rheumatoid arthritis and deformity of the ankle secondary to previous injury. (Podiatry Surgery)

99205 Initial office visit for a patient with disseminated lupus erythematosus with kidney disease, edema, purpura, and scarring lesions on the extremities plus cardiac symptoms. (Dermatology/Internal Medicine)

Initial office visit for a 25-year-old female with systemic lupus erythematosus, fever, seizures, and profound thrombocytopenia. (Rheumatology)

Initial office visit for an adult with multiple cutaneous blisters, denuded secondarily infected ulcerations, oral lesions, weight loss, and increasing weakness refractory to high dose corticosteroid. Initiation of new immunosuppressive therapy. (Dermatology)

Initial office visit for a 28-year-old male with systemic vasculitis and compromised circulation to the limbs. (Rheumatology)

Initial office visit for a 41-year-old female new to the area requesting rheumatologic care, on disability due to scleroderma and recent hospitalization for malignant hypertension. (Rheumatology)

Initial office visit for a 52-year-old female with acute four extremity weakness and shortness of breath one week post-flu vaccination. (Physical Medicine & Rehabilitation)

Initial office visit for a 60-year-old male with previous back surgery; now presents with back and pelvic pain, two-month history of bilateral progressive calf and thigh tightness and weakness when walking, causing several falls. (Orthopaedic Surgery)

Initial office visit for an adolescent referred from emergency department after taking a near-lethal overdose that required hospitalization. (Psychiatry)

Initial office visit for a 49-year-old female with a history of headaches and dependence on opioids. She reports weight loss, progressive headache, and depression. (Psychiatry)

Initial office visit for a 34-year-old uremic Type I diabetic patient referred for ESRD modality assessment and planning. (Nephrology)

Initial office visit for a 75-year-old female with neck and bilateral shoulder pain, brisk deep tendon reflexes, and stress incontinence. (Physical Medicine & Rehabilitation)

Initial office visit for an 8-year-old male with cerebral palsy and spastic quadriparesis. (Physical Medicine & Rehabilitation)

Initial office visit for a 73-year-old male with known prostate malignancy, who presents with severe back pain and a recent onset of lower extremity weakness. (Physical Medicine & Rehabilitation)

Initial office visit for a 38-year-old male with paranoid delusions and a history of alcohol abuse. (Psychiatry)

Initial office visit for a 12-week-old with bilateral hip dislocations and bilateral club feet. (Orthopaedic Surgery)

Initial office visit for a 29-year-old female with acute orbital congestion, eyelid retraction, and bilateral visual loss from optic neuropathy. (Ophthalmology)

Initial office visit for a 70-year-old diabetic patient with progressive visual field loss, advanced optic disc cupping, and neovascularization of retina. (Ophthalmology)

Initial office visit for a newly diagnosed Type I diabetic patient. (Endocrinology)

Initial office evaluation of a 65-year-old female with exertional chest pain, intermittent claudication, syncope, and a murmur of aortic stenosis. (Cardiology)

Initial office visit for a 73-year-old male with an unexplained 20 lb weight loss. (Hematology/Oncology)

Initial office evaluation and management of patient with systemic vasculitis and compromised circulation to the limbs. (Rheumatology)

Initial office visit for a 24-year-old with risk factors for HIV infection who has a fever, cough, and shortness of breath. (Infectious Disease)

Initial outpatient evaluation of a 69-year-old male with severe chronic obstructive pulmonary disease, congestive heart failure, and hypertension. (Family Medicine)

Initial office visit for a 17-year-old female who is having school problems and has told a friend that she is considering suicide. She has recently cut herself. The patient and her family are consulted in regard to treatment options. (Psychiatry)

Initial office visit for a female with severe hirsutism, amenorrhea, weight loss, and a desire to have children. (Obstetrics & Gynecology)

Initial office visit for a 42-year-old male on hypertensive medication, newly arrived to the area, with diastolic blood pressure of 110, history of recurrent calculi, episodic headaches, intermittent chest pain, and orthopnea. (Internal Medicine)

Initial office visit for 70-year-old female with hypertension, diabetes, morbid obesity and recurrent incisional hernia that has become increasingly painful. (General Surgery)

57-year-old man with new-onset dementia. (Neurology)

Initial office visit for a 25-year-old female with a history of depression who presents with complaints of difficulty maintaining sleep, excessive daytime somnolence, and fatigue. She also complains of episodes of muscle weakness. (Sleep Medicine)

Initial office visit for a 75-year-old febrile female with an infected posterior heel ulceration penetrating to bone with comorbidities of diabetes and peripheral vascular disease. (Podiatry Surgery)

Initial office visit for a 36-year-old hypertensive laborer with inability to bear weight due to multiple metatarsal fractures and forefoot compartment syndrome stemming from a crush injury suffered two days prior. (Podiatry Surgery)

Initial office visit for a child with a long history of bipolar disorder, ADHD, anxiety, and school problems, relatively stable and recently moved from another state. (Psychiatry)

Initial office visit for 61-year-old male with depression and a history of diabetes mellitus, arthritis, hypertension, and coronary artery disease. (Psychiatry)

Initial office visit of a 40-year-old with chronic draining ear, progressive hearing loss, and imbalance, with findings consistent with chronic otitis media and cholesteatoma. (Head & Neck Surgery/Otolaryngology)

Established Patient

99211 Office visit for an 82-year-old female, established patient, for a monthly B12 injection with documented Vitamin B12 deficiency. (Geriatrics/Internal Medicine/Family Medicine)

Office visit for a 50-year-old male, established patient, for removal of uncomplicated facial sutures. (Plastic Surgery)

Office visit for an established patient who lost prescription for lichen planus. Returned for new copy. (Dermatology)

Office visit for an established patient undergoing orthodontics who complains of a wire and is irritating his/her cheek and asks you to check it. (Oral & Maxillofacial Surgery)

Office visit for a 50-year-old female, established patient, seen for her gold injection by the nurse. (Rheumatology)

Office visit for a 73-year-old female, established patient, with pernicious anemia for weekly B12 injection. (Gastroenterology)

Office visit for an established patient for dressing change on a skin biopsy. (Dermatology/Podiatry Surgery)

Office visit for a 19-year-old, established patient, three days postirrigation and drainage of an infected sebaceous cyst, for removal of packing. (Plastic Surgery)

Office visit of a 20-year-old female, established patient, who receives an allergy vaccine injection and is observed for a reaction by the nurse. (Otolaryngology/Head & Neck Surgery)

Office visit for a 45-year-old male, established patient, with chronic renal failure for the administration of erythropoietin. (Nephrology)

Office visit for an established patient, a Peace Corps enlistee, who requests documentation that third molars have been removed. (Oral & Maxillofacial Surgery)

Office visit for a 45-year-old female, established patient, three weeks post simple repair of scalp laceration, noted a retained suture in healed wound, removed by nurse. (Plastic Surgery)

Office visit for a 9-year-old, established patient, successfully treated for impetigo, requiring release to return to school. (Dermatology/Pediatrics)

Office visit for an established patient requesting a return-to-work certificate for resolving contact dermatitis. (Dermatology)

Office visit for an established patient who is performing glucose monitoring and wants to check accuracy of machine with lab blood glucose by technician who checks accuracy and function of patient machine. (Endocrinology)

Follow-up office visit for a 65-year-old female with a chronic indwelling percutaneous nephrostomy catheter seen for routine pericatheter skin care and dressing change. (Interventional Radiology)

Outpatient visit with 19-year-old male, established patient, for supervised drug screen. (Addiction Medicine)

Appendix C

Office visit with 12-year-old male, established patient, for cursory check of hematoma one day after venipuncture. (Internal Medicine)

Office visit with 31-year-old female, established patient, for return to work certificate. (Anesthesiology)

Office visit for 14-year-old, established patient, to re-dress an abrasion. (Orthopaedic Surgery)

Office visit for a 45-year-old female, established patient, for a blood pressure check. (Obstetrics & Gynecology)

Office visit for prescription refill for a 35-year-old female, established patient, with schizophrenia who is stable but has run out of neuroleptic and is scheduled to be seen in a week. (Psychiatry)

Office visit with a nurse for a 6-year-old asthmatic patient who brings his nebulizer to learn how to use it with the new medicine he was prescribed. (Allergy & Immunology)

Office visit for a 38-year-old male, established patient, for evaluation of resolving nasal erythema from use of CPAP interface. (Sleep Medicine)

Office visit for a 58-year-old male presenting for nursing examination of wound. Patient had incision and drainage of abscess in ER. (General Surgery)

Office visit for a patient treated four months ago. He presents as scheduled for examination of final healing of an intraoral incision at a bone graft site. (Oral & Maxillofacial Surgery)

99212 Office visit for an 11-year-old, established patient, seen in follow-up for mild comedonal acne of the cheeks on topical desquamating agents. (Dermatology/Family Medicine/Pediatrics)

Office visit for a 10-year-old female, established patient, who has been swimming in a lake, now presents with a one-day history of left ear pain with purulent drainage. (Family Medicine)

Office visit for an established patient seen in follow-up of clearing patch of localized contact dermatitis. (Family Medicine/Dermatology)

Office visit for an established patient returning for evaluation of response to treatment of lichen planus on wrists and ankles. (Dermatology)

Office visit for an established patient with tinea pedis being treated with topical therapy. (Dermatology)

Office visit for an established patient with localized erythematous plaque of psoriasis with topical hydration. (Dermatology)

Office visit for a 23-year-old healthy female fully recovered from Bell's palsy, seen one week after onset and initial visit. (Neurology)

Office visit for an established patient with recurring episodes of herpes simplex who has developed a clustering of vesicles on the upper lip. (Oral & Maxillofacial Surgery)

Evaluation of a 50-year-old male, established patient, who has experienced a recurrence of knee pain after he discontinued NSAID. (Anesthesiology/Pain Medicine)

Office visit for an established patient with an irritated skin tag for reassurance. (Dermatology)

Office visit for a 33-year-old, established patient, for contusion and abrasion of lower extremity. (Orthopaedic Surgery)

Office visit for a 22-year-old male, established patient, one month after incision and drainage of sebaceous cyst. (Plastic Surgery)

Office visit for a 21-year-old, established patient, who is seen in follow-up after antibiotic therapy for acute bacterial tonsillitis with resolution of symptoms. (Otolaryngology/Head & Neck Surgery)

Office visit, established patient, 6-year-old with sore throat and headache. (Family Medicine/Pediatrics)

Office evaluation for possible purulent bacterial conjunctivitis with one- to two-day history of redness and discharge, 16-year-old female, established patient. (Pediatrics/Internal Medicine/Family Medicine)

Office visit for a 65-year-old female, established patient, returns for three-week follow-up for resolving severe ankle sprain. (Orthopaedic Surgery)

Office visit, sore throat, fever, and fatigue in a 19-year-old college student, established patient. (Internal Medicine)

Office visit for 66-year-old male, with sebaceous cyst on shoulder. (General Surgery)

Office visit with a 36-year-old male, established patient, for follow-up on effectiveness of medicine management of oral candidiasis. (Oral & Maxillofacial Surgery)

Office visit for a 27-year-old female, established patient, with complaints of vaginal itching. (Obstetrics & Gynecology)

Office visit with a 36-year-old male, established patient, for follow-up on effectiveness of medicine management of oral candidiasis, with improvement in symptoms. (Oral & Maxillofacial Surgery)

Office visit for a 32-year-old patient who has allergic rhinitis that is controlled with intranasal steroids but now is having eye symptoms. (Allergy & Immunology)

Office visit for a 45-year-old asthmatic patient who is seen for renewal of inhaler prescription. She is noted to have wheezing on exam and the dose of medication is increased. (Allergy & Immunology)

Office visit for a 65-year-old, established patient, for CPAP compliance data review. (Sleep Medicine)

Office visit for 66-year-old male with sebaceous cyst on shoulder. (General Surgery)

Office visit for an established patient returning for evaluation of response to medication prescribed for plantar warts. (Podiatry Surgery)

Office visit for an established patient with tinea pedis being treated with topical therapy. (Dermatology/Podiatry Surgery)

Office visit for a 65-year-old female, established patient, returns for three-week follow-up for resolving severe ankle sprain. (Orthopaedic Surgery/Podiatry Surgery)

99213 Office visit for a child, established patient, with chronic secretory otitis media history and physical exam, with interpretation of audiogram. (Otolaryngology/Head & Neck Surgery)

Office visit, established patient, for evaluation and treatment of an acutely draining ear in a 5-year-old with tympanotomy tubes. (Otolaryngology/Head & Neck Surgery)

Office visit for an established patient with new lesions of lichen planus in spite of topical therapies. (Dermatology)

Office visit for a 13-year-old, established patient, with comedopapular acne of the face that has shown poor response to topical medication. Discussion of use of systemic medication. (Dermatology)

Office visit for a 62-year-old female, established patient, for follow-up for stable cirrhosis of the liver. (Internal Medicine/Family Medicine)

Office visit for an 80-year-old female, established patient, to evaluate medical management of osteoarthritis of the temporomandibular joint. (Rheumatology)

Office visit for a healthy 45-year-old female, established patient. Presents with suspicious lesion on the back. (Plastic Surgery)

Office visit for a 68-year-old female, established patient, with polymyalgia rheumatic, maintained on chronic low-dose corticosteroid, with no new complaints. (Rheumatology)

Office visit for a 3-year-old female, established patient, for earache and dyshidrosis of feet. (Pediatrics/Family Medicine)

Office visit for an established patient for 18-months post-operative follow-up of TMJ repair. (Oral & Maxillofacial Surgery)

Office visit for a 45-year-old male, established patient, being re-evaluated for recurrent acute prostatitis. (Urology)

Office visit for a 43-year-old male, established patient, with known reflex sympathetic dystrophy. (Anesthesiology)

Office visit for an established patient with an evenly pigmented superficial nodule of leg that is symptomatic. (Dermatology)

Office visit for an established patient with psoriasis involvement of the elbows, pitting of the nails, and itchy scalp. (Dermatology)

Office visit for a 27-year-old male, established patient, with deep follicular and perifollicular inflammation unable to tolerate systemic antibiotics due to GI upset, requires change of systemic medication. (Dermatology)

Office visit for a 60-year-old, established patient, with chronic essential hypertension on multiple drug regimen, for blood pressure check. (Family Medicine)

Office visit for a 20-year-old male, established patient, for removal of sutures in hand. (Family Medicine)

Office visit for a 58-year-old female, established patient, with unilateral painful bunion. (Orthopaedic Surgery)

Office visit for a 45-year-old female, established patient, with known osteoarthritis and painful swollen knees. (Rheumatology)

Office visit for a 25-year-old female, established patient, complaining of bleeding and heavy menses. (Obstetrics & Gynecology)

Office visit for a 55-year-old male, established patient, with hypertension managed by a beta blocker/thiazide regime; now experiencing mild fatigue. (Nephrology)

Office visit for a 65-year-old female, established patient, with primary glaucoma for interval determination of intraocular pressure and possible adjustment of medication. (Ophthalmology)

Office visit for a 56-year-old male, established patient, with stable exertional angina who complains of new onset of calf pain while walking. (Cardiology)

Office visit for a 63-year-old female, established patient, with rheumatoid arthritis on auranofin and ibuprofen, seen for routine follow-up visit. (Rheumatology)

Office visit for an established patient with Graves' disease, three months post I-131 therapy, who presents with lassitude and malaise. (Endocrinology)

Office visit for the quarterly follow-up of a 63-year-old male, established patient, with chronic myofascial pain syndrome, effectively managed by doxepin, who presents with new onset urinary hesitancy. (Pain Medicine)

Office visit for the biannual follow-up of an established patient with migraine variant having infrequent, intermittent, moderate to severe headaches with nausea and vomiting, which are sometimes effectively managed by ergotamine tartrate and an antiemetic, but occasionally requiring visits to an emergency department. (Pain Medicine)

Office visit for an established patient after discharge from a pain rehabilitation program to review and adjust medication dosage. (Pain Medicine)

Office visit with 55-year-old male, established patient, for management of hypertension, mild fatigue, on beta blocker/thiazide regimen. (Family Medicine/Internal Medicine)

Appendix C

Outpatient visit for a 35-year-old female who had plastic surgery in Mexico two weeks before, presents for wound evaluation and suture removal. (General Surgery)

Office visit for a 70-year-old diabetic hypertensive established patient with recent change in insulin requirement. (Internal Medicine/Nephrology)

Office visit with 80-year-old female, established patient, for follow-up osteoporosis, status-post compression fractures. (Rheumatology)

Office visit for an established patient with stable cirrhosis of the liver. (Gastroenterology)

Routine, follow-up office evaluation at a three-month interval for a 77-year-old female, established patient, with nodular small cleaved-cell lymphoma. (Hematology/Oncology)

Quarterly follow-up office visit for a 45-year-old male, established patient, with stable chronic asthma, on steroid and bronchodilator therapy. (Pulmonary Medicine)

Office visit for a 50-year-old female, established patient, with insulin-dependent diabetes mellitus and stable coronary artery disease, for monitoring. (Family Medicine/Internal Medicine)

Office visit for a patient followed for a diagnosis of allergic rhinitis who recently acquired a cat. Oral nasal medicines are no longer controlling symptoms. Head congestion and yellow drainage are constant. (Allergy & Immunology)

Office visit for a 60-year-old asthmatic who recently developed high blood pressure and is now on BP medicine is seen for worsening asthma and found to have reduced pulmonary function tests compared to last year. (Allergy & Immunology)

Office visit for a 40-year-old female with well-controlled migraine who desires to remain on the same medication. (Neurology)

Office visit for a 25-year-old male, established patient, for periodic follow-up of narcolepsy, stable on stimulant medication. (Sleep Medicine)

Office visit for an established patient with photodamage and a new onset of a bleeding papulonodule on the leg. (Dermatology)

Quarterly follow-up office visit for a 45-year-old male, established patient, with stable chronic asthma, on steroid and bronchodilator therapy. (Pulmonary Medicine)

Office visit for an established diabetic patient, reevaluation of a worsening plantar fasciitis requiring a change in therapy. (Podiatry Surgery)

Office visit for a 58-year-old female, established patient, with unilateral painful bunion. (Orthopaedic Surgery/Podiatry Surgery)

Office visit for a 9-year-old male, established patient, with ADHD. Mild symptoms and minimal medication side effects. (Psychiatry)

Office visit for a 27-year-old female, established patient, with stable depression and anxiety. Intermittent moderate stress. (Psychiatry)

Office visit for a 16-year-old female, established patient, with intermittent moderate depression. (Psychiatry)

99214 Office visit, established patient, presenting with a new onset of a generalized pruritic to painful eruption and mouth sores. (Dermatology)

Office visit for a 32-year-old female, established patient, with new onset right lower quadrant pain. (Family Medicine)

Office visit for reassessment and reassurance/counseling of a 40-year-old female, established patient, who is experiencing increased symptoms while on a pain management treatment program. (Pain Medicine)

Office visit for a 30-year-old, established patient, under management for intractable low back pain, who now presents with new onset right posterior thigh pain. (Pain Medicine)

Office visit for an established patient with frequent intermittent, moderate to severe headaches requiring beta blocker or tricyclic antidepressant prophylaxis, as well as four symptomatic treatments, but who is still experiencing headaches at a frequency of several times a month that are unresponsive to treatment. (Pain Medicine)

Office visit for an established patient with psoriasis with extensive involvement of scalp, trunk, palms, and soles with joint pain. Combinations of topical and systemic treatments discussed and instituted. (Dermatology)

Office visit for a 55-year-old male, established patient, with increasing night pain, limp, and progressive varus of both knees. (Orthopaedic Surgery)

Follow-up visit for a 15-year-old withdrawn patient with four-year history of papulocystic acne of the face, chest, and back with early scarring and poor response to past treatment. Discussion of use of systemic medication. (Dermatology)

Office visit for a 28-year-old male, established patient, with regional enteritis, diarrhea, and low-grade fever. (Internal Medicine)

Office visit for a 25-year-old female, established patient, following recent arthrogram and MR imaging for TMJ pain. (Oral & Maxillofacial Surgery)

Office visit for a 32-year-old female, established patient, with large obstructing stone in left mid-ureter, to discuss management options including urethroscopy with extraction or ESWL. (Urology)

Evaluation for a 28-year-old male, established patient, with new onset of low back pain. (Anesthesiology/Pain Medicine)

Office visit for a 28-year-old female, established patient, with right lower quadrant abdominal pain, fever, and anorexia. (Internal Medicine/Family Medicine)

Appendix C

Office visit for a 45-year-old male, established patient, four months follow-up of L4-5 diskectomy, with persistent incapacitating low back and leg pain. (Orthopaedic Surgery)

Outpatient visit for a 77-year-old male, established patient, with hypertension, presenting with a three-month history of episodic substernal chest pain on exertion. (Cardiology)

Office visit for a 25-year-old female, established patient, for evaluation of progressive saddle nose deformity of unknown etiology. (Plastic Surgery)

Office visit for a 65-year-old male, established patient, with BPH and severe bladder outlet obstruction, to discuss management options such as TURP. (Urology)

Office visit for an established patient with lichen planus and 60% of the cutaneous surface involved, not responsive to systemic steroids, as well as developing symptoms of progressive heartburn and paranoid ideation. (Dermatology)

Office visit for a 52-year-old male, established patient, with a 12-year history of bipolar disorder responding to lithium carbonate and brief psychotherapy. Psychotherapy and prescription provided. (Psychiatry)

Office visit for a 63-year-old female, established patient, with a history of familial polyposis, status post-colectomy with sphincter sparing procedure, who now presents with rectal bleeding and increase in stooling frequency. (General Surgery)

Office visit for a 68-year-old male, established patient, with the sudden onset of multiple flashes and floaters in the right eye due to a posterior vitreous detachment. (Ophthalmology)

Office visit for a 55-year-old female, established patient, on cyclosporin for treatment of resistant, small vessel vasculitis. (Rheumatology)

Follow-up office visit for a 55-year-old male, two months after iliac angioplasty with new onset of contralateral extremity claudication. (Interventional Radiology)

Office visit for a 68-year-old male, established patient, with stable angina, two months post myocardial infarction, who is not tolerating one of his medications. (Cardiology)

Weekly office visit for 5FU therapy for an ambulatory established patient with metastatic colon cancer and increasing shortness of breath. (Hematology/Oncology)

Office visit for a 65-year-old male with Parkinson disease, on medication with sleep disturbance after medication increase. (Neurology)

Office visit for a 32-year-old female with obesity and diabetes. presents with new onset right lower quadrant pain. (Urology/General Surgery/Internal Medicine/Family Medicine)

Office evaluation of 28-year-old, established patient, with regional enteritis, diarrhea, and low-grade fever. (Family Medicine/Internal Medicine)

Office visit with 50-year-old female, established patient, diabetic, blood sugar controlled by diet. She now complains of frequency of urination and weight loss, blood sugar of 320 and negative ketones on dipstick. (Internal Medicine)

Follow-up office visit for a 45-year-old, established patient, with rheumatoid arthritis on gold, methotrexate, or immunosuppressive therapy. (Rheumatology)

Office visit for a 60-year-old male, established patient, two years post-removal of intracranial meningioma, now with new headaches and visual disturbance. (Neurosurgery)

Office visit for a 68-year-old female, established patient, for routine review and follow-up of non-insulin dependent diabetes, obesity, hypertension, and congestive heart failure. Complains of vision difficulties and admits dietary noncompliance. Patient is counseled concerning diet and current medications adjusted. (Family Medicine)

Office visit for an established patient who presents with severe dysphagia, odynophagia, and trismus and is found on physical exam to have a peritonsillar abscess. (Otolaryngology/Head & Neck Surgery)

Office visit for a 65-year-old male with hypertension, BPH, and allergic rhinitis seen because he cannot sleep due to nasal congestion. He was told by his PCP not to use decongestant pills so he uses a nasal decongestant spray regularly to breathe. He has been using the spray daily for the past six months. (Allergy & Immunology)

Office visit for an asthmatic patient who has missed three days of work due to asthma exacerbation and is found to have acute maxillary sinusitis and nocturnal asthma requiring treatment of both the sinusitis and altering the medication regimen. (Allergy & Immunology)

Office visit for an established diabetic patient with peripheral vascular disease with a new noninfected deep plantar ulceration. (Podiatry Surgery)

Office visit for a 48-year-old male, established patient, with bipolar disorder, marital problems, chronic insomnia, and several medical conditions. Mild psychiatric symptoms and minimal medication side effects. (Psychiatry)

Office visit for 7-year-old female, established patient, with ADHD. The patient has been disruptive in school, resulting in daily phone calls to parents over the last two weeks. Low appetite from the medication has been improving. (Psychiatry)

Office visit for a 13-year-old male, established patient, with depression, anxiety, and anger outbursts. (Psychiatry)

Office visit for a 22-year-old female, established patient, with bipolar disorder and obesity. The patient wants to stop the medication because of resulting weight gain. (Psychiatry)

Office visit for a 70-year-old male, established patient, with stable depression and recent mild forgetfulness. (Psychiatry)

Quarterly follow-up office visit for a 45-year-old male, established patient, with chronic asthma, on steroid and bronchodilator therapy. (Pulmonary Medicine)

Office visit for a 70-year-old female, established patient with sleep apnea and diabetes, who continues to have difficulty staying awake during the day despite treatment. (Sleep Medicine)

99215 Office visit for an adult diabetic established patient with a past history of recurrent sinusitis who presents with a one-week history of double vision and CT scan consistent with periorbital abscess. (Otolaryngology/Head & Neck Surgery)

Office visit for an established patient with disseminated lupus erythematosus, extensive edema of extremities, kidney disease, and weakness requiring monitored course on azathioprine and corticosteroid and complicated by acute depression. (Internal Medicine/ Rheumatology)

Office visit for a patient with history of metastatic melanoma presenting with clinical lymphadenopathy distant to the primary tumor and subcutaneous nodules requiring a detailed discussion of treatment alternatives. (Dermatology)

Office visit for an established male patient with dermatomyositis, accelerated weakness, recent onset of fever, diffuse skin rash, nasal speech, and dysphagia with burning retrosternal pain. (Dermatology)

Office visit for an established adolescent patient with history of bipolar disorder treated with lithium; seen on urgent basis at family's request because of severe depressive symptoms. (Psychiatry)

Office visit for an established patient having acute migraine with new onset neurological symptoms and whose headaches are unresponsive to previous attempts at management with a combination of preventive and abortive medication. (Pain Medicine)

Office visit for an established patient with exfoliative lichen planus with daily fever spikes, disorientation, and shortness of breath. (Dermatology)

Office visit for a 25-year-old, established patient, two years post-burn with bilateral ectropion, hypertrophic facial burn scars, near absence of left breast, and burn syndactyly of both hands. Discussion of treatment options following examination. (Plastic Surgery)

Office visit for a 36-year-old, established patient, three-month status post-transplant, with new onset of peripheral edema, increased blood pressure, and progressive fatigue. (Nephrology)

Office visit for a 27-year-old female, established patient, with bipolar disorder who was stable on lithium carbonate and monthly supportive psychotherapy but now has developed symptoms of hypomania. (Psychiatry)

Office visit for a 25-year-old male, established patient with a history of schizophrenia who has been seen bi-monthly but is complaining of auditory hallucinations. (Psychiatry)

Office visit for a 62-year-old male, established patient, three years postoperative abdominal perineal resection, now with a rising carcinoembryonic antigen, weight loss, and pelvic pain. (Abdominal Surgery)

Office visit for a 42-year-old male, established patient, nine months postoperative emergency vena cava shunt for variceal bleeding, now presents with complaints of one episode of "dark" bowel movement, weight gain, tightness in abdomen, whites of eyes seem yellow, and occasional drowsiness after eating hamburgers. (Abdominal Surgery)

Office visit for a 68-year-old male with biopsy-proven rectal carcinoma, for evaluation and discussion of treatment options. (General Surgery)

Office visit for a 60-year-old, established patient, with diabetic nephropathy with increasing edema and dyspnea. (Endocrinology)

Office visit with 30-year-old male, established patient for three-month history of fatigue, weight loss, intermittent fever, and presenting with diffuse adenopathy and splenomegaly. (Family Medicine)

Office visit for restaging of an established patient with new lymphadenopathy one year post-therapy for lymphoma. (Hematology/Oncology)

Office visit for evaluation of recent onset syncopal attacks in a 70-year-old female, established patient. (Internal Medicine)

Follow-up visit, 40-year-old female mother of three, established patient, with acute rheumatoid arthritis, anatomical Stage 3, ARA function Class 3 rheumatoid arthritis, and deteriorating function. (Rheumatology)

Follow-up office visit for a 65-year-old male with a fever of recent onset while on outpatient antibiotic therapy for endocarditis. (Infectious Disease)

Office visit for a healthy 16-year-old male who suffered a concussion a week ago, now fully recovered, needing an evaluation to return to playing football. (Neurology)

Office visit for a 70-year-old female, established patient, with diabetes mellitus and hypertension, presenting with a two-month history of increasing confusion, agitation, and short-term memory loss. (Family Medicine/Internal Medicine)

Office visit for a 28-year-old female, established patient, who is abstinent from previous cocaine dependence but reports progressive panic attacks and chest pains. (Psychiatry)

Office visit for a 10-year-old asthmatic who has been to the emergency room for severe persistent asthma and is on combination therapy and oral steroids but has not stopped wheezing or coughing at night. (Allergy & Immunology)

Office visit, established patient, female with systemic lupus erythematosus and renal disease requiring combination systemic immunosuppressive therapy presents with a new onset of peripheral edema, diffuse skin rash, weakness, and acute depression. (Dermatology)

Office visit for a 53-year-old female, established patient, with sleep apnea and new-onset heart failure, who presents with a recent weight gain as well as recurrence of symptoms of daytime sleepiness and frequent nocturnal awakenings. (Sleep Medicine)

Office visit for an established diabetic patient with a cellulitic deep plantar abscess and history of previous forefoot amputation on the contralateral side. (Podiatry Surgery)

Hospital Inpatient Services

Initial Hospital Care

New or Established Patient

99221 Initial hospital visit following admission for a 42-year-old male for observation following institution of IV antibiotics for a cellulitis of the forearm. (Plastic Surgery/Oral & Maxillofacial Surgery)

Initial hospital visit for a 40-year-old patient with a thrombosed synthetic arteriovenous conduit. (Nephrology)

Initial hospital visit for a healthy 24-year-old male with an acute onset of low back pain following a lifting injury. (Internal Medicine/Anesthesiology/Pain Medicine)

Initial hospital visit for a 69-year-old female with controlled hypertension, scheduled for surgery. (Internal Medicine/Cardiology)

Initial hospital visit for a 24-year-old healthy female with benign tumor of palate. (Oral & Maxillofacial Surgery)

Initial hospital visit for a 14-year-old female with infectious mononucleosis and dehydration. (Internal Medicine)

Initial hospital visit for a 62-year-old female with stable rheumatoid arthritis, admitted for total joint replacement. (Rheumatology)

Initial hospital visit for a 6-month-old infant admitted for observation for apnea after craniofacial CT scan with sedation. (Plastic Surgery)

Initial hospital visit for a 69-year-old female with controlled hypertension, scheduled for surgery. (Cardiology)

Hospital admission, examination, and initiation of treatment program for a 67-year-old male with uncomplicated pneumonia who requires IV antibiotic therapy. (Internal Medicine)

Hospital admission for a 12-year-old with a laceration of the upper eyelid involving the lid margin admitted prior to surgery for IV antibiotic therapy. (Ophthalmology)

Hospital admission for a 32-year-old female with severe flank pain, hematuria, and presumed diagnosis of ureteral calculus as determined by Emergency Department physician. (Urology)

Initial hospital visit for a patient with several large venous stasis ulcers not responding to outpatient therapy. (Dermatology)

Initial hospital visit for 21-year-old pregnant patient (nine-weeks gestation) with hyperemesis gravidarum. (Obstetrics & Gynecology)

Initial hospital visit for a 73-year-old female with acute pyelonephritis who is otherwise generally healthy. (Geriatrics)

Initial hospital visit for 62-year-old patient with cellulitis of the foot requiring bedrest and intravenous antibiotics. (Orthopaedic Surgery)

Initial hospital visit for a 55-year-old female admitted to the hospital with nausea and vomiting, has a benign exam and a nonspecific bowel gas pattern on X ray. (General Surgery)

99222 Hospital admission for an 18-month-old with 10% dehydration. (Pediatrics)

Initial hospital visit for a 65-year-old female with right upper quadrant pain, mild jaundice, and gallstones. (General Surgery/Abdominal Surgery/Colon & Rectal Surgery)

Initial hospital visit for airway management, due to a benign laryngeal mass. (Otolaryngology/Head & Neck Surgery)

Initial hospital visit for a 66-year-old female with an L-2 vertebral compression fracture with acute onset of paralytic ileus; seen in the office two days previously. (Orthopaedic Surgery)

Initial hospital visit and evaluation of a 15-year-old male admitted with peritonsillar abscess or cellulitis requiring intravenous antibiotic therapy. (Otolaryngology/Head & Neck Surgery)

Initial hospital visit for a 42-year-old male with vertebral compression fracture following a motor vehicle accident. (Orthopaedic Surgery)

Initial hospital evaluation of a patient with a diffuse erythematous maculopapular eruption of new onset. Patient has multiple medical problems requiring various medications. (Dermatology)

Initial hospital visit for a 3-year-old patient with high temperature, limp, and painful hip motion of 18 hours' duration. (Pediatrics/Orthopaedic Surgery)

Initial hospital visit for an 18-year-old male who has suppurative sialadenitis and dehydration. (Oral & Maxillofacial Surgery)

Initial hospital visit for a 65-year-old female for acute onset of thrombotic cerebrovascular accident with contralateral paralysis and aphasia. (Neurology)

Initial hospital visit for a 50-year-old male chronic paraplegic patient with pain and spasm below the lesion. (Anesthesiology)

Partial hospital admission for an adolescent patient from chaotic blended family, transferred from inpatient setting, for continued treatment to maintain symptomatic control of hostility and depression. (Psychiatry)

Initial hospital visit for a 61-year-old male with history of previous myocardial infarction, who now complains of chest pain. (Internal Medicine)

Initial hospital visit of a 15-year-old on medications for a sore throat over the last two weeks. The sore throat has worsened and patient now has dysphagia. The exam shows large necrotic tonsils with an adequate airway and small palpable nodes. The initial mono test was negative. (Otolaryngology/Head & Neck Surgery)

Initial hospital evaluation of a 23-year-old allergy patient admitted with eyelid edema and pain on fifth day of oral antibiotic therapy. (Otolaryngology/Head & Neck Surgery)

Hospital admission for a 30-year-old female with epilepsy, not compliant with medication, admitted after three seizures. (Neurology)

Hospital admission, examination, and initiation of treatment program for a 66-year-old chronic hemodialysis patient with fever. (Nephrology)

Hospital admission for a 40-year-old male with submaxillary cellulitis and trismus from infected lower molar. (Oral & Maxillofacial Surgery)

Initial hospital visit following admission for a 42-year-old male for observation following an uncomplicated mandible fracture. (Oral & Maxillofacial Surgery)

Initial hospital visit for a 24-year-old healthy female with benign tumor of palate. (Oral & Maxillofacial Surgery)

Initial hospital visit for a 15-year-old male with acute status asthmaticus, unresponsive to outpatient therapy. (Internal Medicine)

99223 Hospital admission of a 62-year-old smoker, established patient, with bronchitis in acute respiratory distress. (Internal Medicine/Pulmonary Medicine)

Initial hospital visit for a 45-year-old female, who has a history of rheumatic fever as a child and now has anemia, fever, and congestive heart failure. (Cardiology)

Initial hospital visit for a 50-year-old male with acute chest pain and diagnostic electrocardiographic changes of an acute anterior myocardial infarction. (Cardiology/Family Medicine/Internal Medicine)

Initial hospital visit of a 75-year-old with progressive stridor and dysphagia with history of cancer of the larynx treated by radiation therapy in the past. Exam shows a large recurrent tumor of the glottis with a mass in the neck. (Otolaryngology/Head & Neck Surgery)

Initial hospital visit for a 70-year-old male admitted with chest pain, complete heart block, and congestive heart failure. (Cardiology)

Initial hospital visit for an 82-year-old male who presents with syncope, chest pain, and ventricular arrhythmias. (Cardiology)

Initial hospital visit for a 75-year-old male with history of arteriosclerotic coronary vascular disease, who is severely dehydrated, disoriented, and confused. (Psychiatry)

Initial hospital visit for a 70-year-old male with alcohol and sedative-hypnotic dependence, admitted by family for severe withdrawal, hypertension, and diabetes mellitus. (Psychiatry)

Initial hospital visit for a persistently suicidal latency-aged child whose parents have requested admission to provide safety but are anxious about separation from her. (Psychiatry)

Initial psychiatric visit for an adolescent patient without previous psychiatric history, who was transferred from the medical ICU after an overdose. (Psychiatry)

Initial hospital visit for a 35-year-old female with severe systemic lupus erythematosus on corticosteroid and cyclophosphamide, with new onset of fever, chills, rash, and chest pain. (Rheumatology)

Initial hospital visit for a 52-year-old male with known rheumatic heart disease who presents with anasarca, hypertension, and history of alcohol abuse. (Cardiology)

Initial hospital visit for a 55-year-old female with a history of congenital heart disease; now presents with cyanosis. (Cardiology)

Initial hospital visit for a psychotic, hostile, violently combative adolescent, involuntarily committed for his and other's safety. (Psychiatry)

Initial hospital visit for a now subdued and sullen teenage male with six-month history of declining school performance, increasing self-endangerment, and resistance of parental expectations, including running away past weekend after physical fight with father. (Psychiatry)

Initial partial hospital admission for a 17-year-old female with history of borderline mental retardation who has developed auditory hallucinations. Parents are known to abuse alcohol, and Child Protective Services is investigating allegations of sexual abuse of a younger sibling. (Psychiatry)

Initial hospital visit of a 67-year-old male admitted with a large neck mass, dysphagia, and history of myocardial infarction three months before. (Otolaryngology/Head & Neck Surgery)

Initial hospital visit for a patient with suspected cerebrospinal fluid rhinorrhea that developed two weeks after head injury. (Otolaryngology/Head & Neck Surgery)

Initial hospital visit for a 25-year-old female with history of poly-substance abuse and psychiatric disorder. The patient appears to be psychotic with markedly elevated vital signs. (Psychiatry)

Initial hospital visit for a 70-year-old male with cutaneous T-cell lymphoma who has developed fever and lymphadenopathy. (Internal Medicine)

Initial hospital visit for a 62-year-old female with known coronary artery disease, for evaluation of increasing edema, dyspnea on exertion, confusion, and sudden onset of fever with productive cough. (Internal Medicine)

Initial hospital visit for a 3-year-old female with 36-hour history of sore throat and high fever; now with sudden onset of lethargy, irritability, photophobia, and nuchal rigidity. (Pediatrics)

Initial hospital visit for a 26-year-old female for evaluation of severe facial fractures (LeFort's II/III). (Plastic Surgery)

Initial hospital visit for a 55-year-old female for bilateral mandibular fractures resulting in flail mandible and airway obstruction. (Plastic Surgery)

Initial hospital visit for a 71-year-old patient with a red painful eye four days following uncomplicated cataract surgery due to endophthalmitis. (Ophthalmology)

Initial hospital visit for a 45-year-old patient involved in a motor vehicle accident who suffered a perforating corneoscleral laceration with loss of vision. (Ophthalmology)

Initial hospital visit for a 58-year-old male who has Ludwig's angina and progressive airway compromise. (Oral & Maxillofacial Surgery)

Initial hospital visit for an adult with multiple cutaneous blisters, denuded secondarily infected ulcerations, oral lesions, weight loss, and increasing weakness refractory to high-dose corticosteroid. Initiation of new immunosuppressive therapy. (Dermatology)

Initial hospital visit for an 82-year-old male who presents with syncope, chest pain, and ventricular arrhythmias. (Cardiology)

Initial hospital visit for a 62-year-old male with history of previous myocardial infarction, comes in with recurrent, sustained ventricular tachycardia. (Cardiology)

Initial hospital visit for a chronic dialysis patient with infected PTFE fistula, septicemia, and shock. (Nephrology)

Initial hospital visit for a 1-year-old male, victim of child abuse, with central nervous system depression, skull fracture, and retinal hemorrhage. (Neurology)

Initial hospital visit for a 25-year-old female with recent C4-C5 quadriplegia, admitted for rehabilitation. (Physical Medicine & Rehabilitation)

Initial hospital visit for an 18-year-old male, post-traumatic brain injury with multiple impairment. (Physical Medicine & Rehabilitation)

Initial partial hospital admission for 16-year-old male, sullen and subdued, with six-month history of declining school performance, increasing self-endangerment, and resistance to parental expectations. (Psychiatry)

Initial hospital visit for a 16-year-old primigravida at 32 weeks gestation with severe hypertension (200/110), thrombocytopenia, and headache. (Obstetrics & Gynecology)

Initial hospital visit for a 49-year-old male with cirrhosis of liver with hematemesis, hepatic encephalopathy, and fever. (Gastroenterology)

Initial hospital visit for a 55-year-old female in chronic pain who has attempted suicide. (Psychiatry)

Initial hospital visit for a 70-year-old male, with multiple organ system disease, admitted with history of being anuric and septic for 24 hours prior to admission. (Urology)

Initial hospital visit for a 3-year-old female with 36-hour history of sore throat and high fever, now with sudden onset of lethargy, irritability, photophobia, and nuchal rigidity. (Pediatrics/Critical Care)

Initial hospital visit for a 78-year-old male, transfers from nursing home with dysuria and pyuria, increasing confusion, and high fever. (Internal Medicine)

Initial hospital visit for a 1-day-old male with cyanosis, respiratory distress, and tachypnea. (Cardiology)

Initial hospital visit for a 3-year-old female with recurrent tachycardia and syncope. (Cardiology)

Initial hospital visit for a thyrotoxic patient who presents with fever, atrial fibrillation, and delirium. (Endocrinology)

Initial hospital visit for a 50-year-old Type I diabetic who presents with diabetic ketoacidosis with fever and obtundation. (Endocrinology)

Initial hospital visit for a 40-year-old female with anatomical stage 3, ARA functional class 3 rheumatoid arthritis on methotrexate, corticosteroid, and nonsteroidal anti-inflammatory drugs. Patient presents with severe arthritis flare, new oral ulcers, abdominal pain, and leukopenia. (Rheumatology)

Initial hospital exam of a pediatric patient with high fever and proptosis. (Otolaryngology/Head & Neck Surgery)

Initial hospital visit for a 25-year-old patient admitted for the first time to the rehab unit, with recent C4-C5 quadriplegia. (Physical Medicine & Rehabilitation)

Hospital admission, examination, and initiation of treatment program for a previously unknown 58-year-old male who presents with acute chest pain. (Cardiology)

Hospital admission, examination, and initiation of induction chemotherapy for a 42-year-old patient with newly diagnosed acute myelogenous leukemia. (Hematology/Oncology)

Hospital admission following a motor vehicle accident of a 24-year-old male with fracture dislocation of C5-C6; neurologically intact. (Neurosurgery)

Hospital admission for a 78-year-old female with left lower lobe pneumonia and a history of coronary artery disease, congestive heart failure, osteoarthritis, and gout. (Family Medicine)

Hospital admission, examination, and initiation of treatment program for a 65-year-old immunosuppressed male with confusion, fever, and a headache. (Infectious Disease)

Hospital admission for a 9-year-old with vomiting, dehydration, fever, tachypnea, and an admitting diagnosis of diabetic ketoacidosis. (Pediatrics)

Initial hospital visit for a 65-year-old male who presents with acute myocardial infarction, oliguria, hypotension, and altered state of consciousness. (Cardiology)

Initial hospital visit for a 15-year-old male with acute status asthmaticus, unresponsive to outpatient therapy. (Internal Medicine/Pediatrics/Pulmonary Medicine)

Initial hospital visit for a hostile/resistant adolescent patient who is severely depressed and involved in poly-substance abuse. Patient is experiencing significant conflict in his chaotic family situation and was suspended from school following an attack on a teacher with a baseball bat. (Psychiatry)

Initial hospital visit for 89-year-old female with fulminant hepatic failure and encephalopathy. (Gastroenterology)

Initial hospital visit for a patient with congestive heart failure, type 1 diabetes mellitus, and renal failure who has developed an acute onset of fever and a generalized bullous erythematous and purpuric eruption. (Dermatology)

Hospital admission for a 50-year-old male with new-onset left hemiparesis (Neurology)

Hospital admission for an 18-year-old male admitted to the trauma service following a motor vehicle accident for treatment of a closed head injury, liver laceration, and long bone fractures. (General Surgery)

First hour of critical care of a 15-year-old with acute respiratory failure from asthma. (Pulmonary Medicine)

Hospital admission of a 62-year-old smoker, established patient, with bronchitis in acute respiratory distress. (Pulmonary Medicine/Critical Care)

Initial hospital visit for a 15-year-old male with acute status asthmaticus, unresponsive to outpatient therapy. (Cardiology/Family Practice/General Surgery/Pulmonary Medicine/Critical Care)

Initial hospital visit for a 42-year-old female with rapidly progressing scleroderma, malignant hypertension, digital infarcts, and oliguria. (Cardiology/Family Practice/General Surgery/Pulmonary Medicine/Rheumatology/Critical Care)

Subsequent Hospital Care

99231 Subsequent hospital visit for a 65-year-old female, post-open reduction and internal fixation of a fracture. (Physical Medicine & Rehabilitation)

Subsequent hospital visit for a 33-year-old patient with pelvic pain who is responding to pain medication and observation. (Obstetrics & Gynecology)

Subsequent hospital visit for a 21-year-old female with hyperemesis who has responded well to intravenous fluids. (Obstetrics & Gynecology)

Subsequent hospital visit to re-evaluate postoperative pain and titrate patient-controlled analgesia for a 27-year-old female. (Anesthesiology)

Follow-up hospital visit for a 35-year-old female, status post-epidural analgesia. (Anesthesiology/Pain Medicine)

Subsequent hospital visit for a 56-year-old male, post-gastrectomy, for maintenance of analgesia using an intravenous dilaudid infusion. (Anesthesiology)

Subsequent hospital visit for a male with improving venous stasis ulcers. (Dermatology)

Subsequent hospital visit for a 24-year-old female with otitis externa, seen two days before in consultation, now to have otic wick removal. (Otolaryngology/Head & Neck Surgery)

Subsequent hospital visit for a 62-year-old patient with resolving cellulitis of the foot. (Orthopaedic Surgery)

Subsequent hospital visit for a 25-year-old male admitted for supra-ventricular tachycardia and converted on medical therapy. (Cardiology)

Subsequent hospital visit for a 27-year-old male with nasal fracture who was intoxicated and uncooperative on admission exam. Patient confirms no difficulty breathing and no change in nasal appearance, exam normal other than mild tenderness. (Plastic Surgery)

Subsequent hospital visit for a 76-year-old male with venous stasis ulcers. (Geriatrics)

Subsequent hospital visit for a 67-year-old female admitted three days ago with bleeding gastric ulcer; now stable. (Gastroenterology)

Subsequent hospital visit for stable 33-year-old male following a motor vehicle accident who is stable with bruised ribs and improving dyspnea. (General Surgery/Gastroenterology)

Subsequent hospital visit for a 29-year-old male with effort thrombosis of left upper extremity. (General Surgery)

Subsequent hospital visit for a 14-year-old female in middle phase of residential or day treatment who is now behaviorally stable and making satisfactory progress in treatment. (Psychiatry)

Subsequent hospital visit for a 55-year-old male with rheumatoid arthritis, two days following an uncomplicated total joint replacement. (Rheumatology)

Subsequent hospital visit for a 60-year-old dialysis patient with an access infection, now afebrile on antibiotic. (Nephrology)

Subsequent hospital visit for a 23-year-old female admitted for cellulitis following dog bite to hand, redness, pain, and swelling resolving. (Plastic Surgery)

Subsequent hospital visit for a 66-year-old female with L-2 vertebral compression fracture with resolving ileus. (Orthopaedic Surgery)

Subsequent hospital visit for an 18-year-old female responding to intravenous antibiotic therapy for ear or sinus infection. (Otolaryngology/Head & Neck Surgery)

Subsequent hospital visit for a 70-year-old male admitted with congestive heart failure who has responded to therapy. (Cardiology)

Follow-up hospital visit for a 32-year-old female with left ureteral calculus; being followed in anticipation of spontaneous passage. (Urology)

Subsequent hospital visit for a 42-year-old female, admitted for acute gastroenteritis and dehydration, requiring IV hydration; now stable but refusing oral intake. (Family Medicine/Pediatrics)

Subsequent hospital visit for a 50-year-old Type II diabetic who is clinically stable and without complications requiring regulation of a single dose of insulin daily. (Endocrinology)

Subsequent hospital visit to reassesses the status of a 65-year-old patient post-open reduction and internal fixation of hip fracture, on the rehab unit. (Physical Medicine & Rehabilitation)

Subsequent hospital visit for a 78-year-old male with cholangiocarcinoma managed by biliary drainage. (Interventional Radiology)

Subsequent hospital visit for a 50-year-old male with uncomplicated myocardial infarction who is clinically stable and without chest pain. (Family Medicine/Cardiology/Internal Medicine)

Subsequent hospital visit for a stable 72-year-old lung cancer patient undergoing a five-day course of infusion chemotherapy. (Hematology/Oncology)

Subsequent hospital visit, two days post admission for a 65-year-old male with a CVA (cerebral vascular accident) and left hemiparesis, who is clinically stable. (Neurology/Physical Medicine & Rehabilitation)

Subsequent hospital visit for now stable, 33-year-old male, status post lower gastrointestinal bleeding. (General Surgery)

Subsequent hospital visit for a 3-year-old patient in traction for a congenital dislocation of the hip. (Orthopaedic Surgery)

Subsequent hospital visit for a 4-year-old female, admitted for acute gastroenteritis and dehydration, requiring IV hydration; now stable. (Family Medicine/Internal Medicine)

Subsequent hospital visit for 50-year-old female with resolving uncomplicated acute pancreatitis. (Gastroenterology)

Subsequent hospital visit for a 30-day-old male admitted for sepsis evaluation and IV antibiotics due to fever; afebrile now with cultures pending. (Family Medicine/Pediatrics)

Subsequent hospital visit for a 10-year-old male admitted for lobar pneumonia with vomiting and dehydration; is becoming afebrile and tolerating oral fluids. (Pulmonary Medicine)

Subsequent visit on third day of hospitalization for a 60-year-old female recovering from an uncomplicated lower extremity cellulitis. (Infectious Disease/Internal Medicine/Pulmonary Medicine)

Subsequent visit for a 75-year-old female, now three days after onset of left hemiparesis, awaiting placement in a rehabilitation unit. (Neurology)

99232 Subsequent visit on third day of hospitalization for a 60-year-old female recovering from an uncomplicated pneumonia. (Infectious Disease/Internal Medicine/Pulmonary Medicine)

Subsequent hospital visit for a patient with peritonsillar cellulitis, with slow response to antibiotic therapy, with consideration for additional testing and changes in treatment plan. (Otolaryngology/Head & Neck Surgery)

Subsequent hospital visit for a 27-year-old with acute vertigo, with review of laboratory and imaging studies. (Otolaryngology/Head & Neck Surgery)

Subsequent hospital visit for a patient with venous stasis ulcers who developed fever and red streaks adjacent to the ulcer. (Dermatology/Internal Medicine/Family Medicine)

Subsequent hospital visit for a 45-year-old male admitted for IV antibiotics for cellulitis post dog bite to hand. Increased redness and fluctuance found. (Plastic Surgery)

Subsequent hospital visit for a 54-year-old female admitted for myocardial infarction, but who is now having frequent premature ventricular contractions. (Internal Medicine)

Subsequent hospital visit for an 80-year-old patient with a pelvic rim fracture, inability to walk, and severe pain; now 36 hours post-injury, experiencing urinary retention. (Orthopaedic Surgery)

Subsequent hospital visit for a 17-year-old female with fever, pharyngitis, and airway obstruction, who after 48 hours develops a maculopapular rash. (Pediatrics/Family Medicine)

Follow-up visit for a 67-year-old male with congestive heart failure who has responded to antibiotics and diuretics and has now developed a monoarthropathy. (Internal Medicine)

Follow-up hospital visit for a 58-year-old male receiving continuous opioids who is experiencing severe nausea and vomiting. (Pain Medicine)

Subsequent hospital visit for a patient after an auto accident who is slow to respond to ambulation training. (Physical Medicine & Rehabilitation)

Subsequent hospital visit for a 50-year-old diabetic, hypertensive male with back pain not responding to conservative inpatient management with continued radiation of pain to the lower left extremity. (Orthopaedic Surgery)

Subsequent hospital visit for a 37-year-old female on day five of antibiotics for bacterial endocarditis, who still has low-grade fever. (Cardiology)

Subsequent hospital visit for a 54-year-old patient, post MI (myocardial infarction), who is out of the CCU (coronary care unit) but is now having frequent premature ventricular contractions on telemetry. (Cardiology/Internal Medicine)

Subsequent hospital visit for a patient with neutropenia, a fever responding to antibiotics, and continued slow gastrointestinal bleeding on platelet support. (Hematology/Oncology)

Subsequent hospital visit for a 50-year-old male admitted two days ago for sub-acute renal allograft rejection. (Nephrology)

Subsequent hospital visit for a 35-year-old drug addict, not responding to initial antibiotic therapy for pyelonephritis. (Urology)

Subsequent hospital visit for a 79-year-old male with worsening jaundice and a pancreatic mass. (General Surgery)

Subsequent hospital care for a 62-year-old female with congestive heart failure, who remains dyspneic and febrile. (Internal Medicine)

Subsequent hospital visit for a 73-year-old female with recently diagnosed lung cancer, who complains of unsteady gait. (Pulmonary Medicine)

Subsequent hospital visit for a 20-month-old male with bacterial meningitis treated one week with antibiotic therapy; has now developed a temperature of 101 degrees. (Pediatrics)

Subsequent hospital visit for 13-year-old male admitted with left lower quadrant abdominal pain and fever, not responding to therapy. (General Surgery)

Subsequent hospital visit for a 65-year-old male with hemiplegia and painful paretic shoulder. (Physical Medicine & Rehabilitation)

Subsequent hospital visit for a patient admitted for treatment of congestive heart failure, on multiple medications, whose previous pale, diffuse rash has now generalized, brightened, and is intensely pruritic. (Dermatology)

Subsequent hospital visit for a 41-year-old female whose altered mental status improved. (General Surgery)

Subsequent hospital visit for adolescent female who continues to struggle with suicidal thoughts and has multiple questions about her antidepressant medication. (Psychiatry)

Subsequent partial hospital visit for a child with depression and severe anxiety. (Psychiatry)

Subsequent hospital visit for 59-year-old male with depression, anxiety, and medication side effects. (Psychiatry)

Subsequent partial hospital visit for a 25-year-old female with body image ruminations and high anxiety about following the prescribed meal plan. (Psychiatry)

99233 Subsequent hospital visit for a 38-year-old male, quadriplegic with acute autonomic hyperreflexia, who is not responsive to initial care. (Physical Medicine & Rehabilitation)

Follow-up hospital visit for a teenage female who continues to experience severely disruptive, violent, and life-threatening symptoms in a complicated multi-system illness. Family/social circumstances also a contributing factor. (Psychiatry)

Subsequent hospital visit for a 42-year-old female with progressive systemic sclerosis (scleroderma), renal failure on dialysis, congestive heart failure, cardiac arrhythmias, and digital ulcers. (Allergy & Immunology)

Subsequent hospital visit for a 50-year-old diabetic, hypertensive male with nonresponding back pain and radiating pain to the lower left extremity, who develops chest pain, cough, and bloody sputum. (Orthopaedic Surgery)

Subsequent hospital visit for a 64-year-old female, status post-abdominal aortic aneurysm resection, with non-responsive coagulopathy, who has now developed lower GI bleeding. (Abdominal Surgery/Colon & Rectal Surgery/General Surgery)

Follow-up hospital care of a patient with pansinusitis infection complicated by a brain abscess and asthma; no response to current treatment. (Otolaryngology/Head & Neck Surgery)

Subsequent hospital visit for a patient with a laryngeal neoplasm who develops airway compromise, suspected metastasis. (Otolaryngology/Head & Neck Surgery)

Subsequent hospital visit for a 49-year-old male with significant rectal bleeding, etiology undetermined, not responding to treatment. (Abdominal Surgery/General Surgery/Colon & Rectal Surgery)

Subsequent hospital visit for a 50-year-old male, post-aortocoronary bypass surgery; now develops hypotension and oliguria. (Cardiology)

Subsequent hospital visit for an adolescent patient who is violent, unsafe, and noncompliant, with multiple expectations for participation in treatment plan and behavior on the treatment unit. (Psychiatry)

Subsequent hospital visit for an 18-year-old male being treated for presumed PCP-induced psychosis. Patient still has moderate auditory hallucinations and is insisting on signing out against medical advice. (Psychiatry)

Subsequent hospital visit for an 8-year-old female with caustic ingestion, who now has fever, dyspnea, and dropping hemoglobin. (Gastroenterology)

Subsequent hospital visit for a 44-year-old patient with electrical burns to the left arm with ascending infection. (Orthopaedic Surgery)

Subsequent hospital visit for a type 1 diabetes mellitus patient with a new onset of fever, change in mental status, and a diffuse petechial, purpuric eruption. (Internal Medicine)

Subsequent hospital visit for a 65-year-old female, status postoperative resection of abdominal aortic aneurysm, with suspected ischemic bowel. (General Surgery)

Subsequent hospital visit for a 50-year-old male, post-aortocoronary bypass surgery, now develops hypotension and oliguria. (Cardiology)

Subsequent hospital visit for a 65-year-old male, following an acute myocardial infarction, who complains of shortness of breath and new chest pain. (Cardiology)

Subsequent hospital visit for a 65-year-old female with rheumatoid arthritis (stage 3, class 3) admitted for urosepsis. On the third hospital day, chest pain, dyspnea, and fever develop. (Rheumatology)

Follow-up hospital care of a pediatric case with stridor, laryngomalacia, established tracheostomy, complicated by multiple medical problems in PICU. (Otolaryngology/Head & Neck Surgery)

Subsequent hospital visit for a 60-year-old female, four days post uncomplicated inferior myocardial infarction who has developed severe chest pain, dyspnea, diaphoresis, and nausea. (Family Medicine)

Subsequent hospital visit for a patient with AML (acute myelogenous leukemia), fever, elevated white count and uric acid undergoing induction chemotherapy. (Hematology/Oncology)

Subsequent hospital visit for a 38-year-old quadriplegic male with acute autonomic hyperreflexia, who is not responsive to initial care. (Physical Medicine & Rehabilitation)

Subsequent hospital visit for a 65-year-old female postoperative resection of abdominal aortic aneurysm, with suspected ischemic bowel. (General Surgery)

Subsequent hospital visit for a 60-year-old female with persistent leukocytosis, fever, abdominal pain, and hypotension seven days after a sigmoid colon resection for carcinoma. (Infectious Disease)

Subsequent hospital visit for a chronic renal failure patient on dialysis, who develops chest pain, shortness of breath. (Nephrology)

Subsequent hospital visit for a 65-year-old male with acute myocardial infarction who now demonstrates complete heart block and congestive heart failure. (Cardiology)

Subsequent hospital visit for a 55-year-old male with severe chronic obstructive pulmonary disease and bronchospasm; initially admitted for acute respiratory distress requiring ventilatory support in the ICU. The patient was stabilized, extubated, and transferred to the floor but has now developed acute fever, dyspnea, left lower lobe rhonchi, and laboratory evidence of carbon dioxide retention and hypoxemia. (Family Medicine/Internal Medicine)

Subsequent hospital visit for 46-year-old female, known liver cirrhosis patient, with recent upper gastrointestinal hemorrhage from varices; now with worsening ascites and encephalopathy. (Gastroenterology)

Subsequent hospital visit for 62-year-old female admitted with acute subarachnoid hemorrhage, negative cerebral arteriogram, increased lethargy, and hemiparesis with fever. (Neurosurgery)

Subsequent partial hospital visit for an adolescent female who cut herself over the weekend following an intense family argument. (Psychiatry)

Subsequent hospital visit for an adolescent patient who is actively suicidal and experiencing significant medication side effects. (Psychiatry)

Subsequent hospital visit for a 70-year-old male with depression who had a syncopal episode on the unit. (Psychiatry)

Subsequent hospital visit for a 43-year-old male with new onset foot drop after removing a cast from his leg. (Neurology)

Consultations

Office or Other Outpatient Consultations

New or Established Patient

99241 Initial office consultation for a 40-year-old female in pain from blister on lip following a cold. (Oral & Maxillofacial Surgery)

Initial office consultation for a 62-year-old construction worker with olecranon bursitis. (Orthopaedic Surgery)

Office consultation with 25-year-old postpartum female with suspected hemorrhoids. (General Surgery)

Office consultation with 58-year-old male, referred for follow-up of creatinine level and evaluation of obstructive uropathy, relieved two months ago. (Nephrology)

Office consultation for 30-year-old female tennis player with sprain or contusion of the forearm. (Orthopaedic Surgery)

Office consultation for a 45-year-old male, requested by his internist, with asymptomatic torus palatinus requiring no further treatment. (Oral & Maxillofacial Surgery)

99242 Initial office consultation for a 29-year-old soccer player with painful proximal thigh/groin injury. (Orthopaedic Surgery)

Initial office consultation for an 8-year-old female with a five-day-old second-degree scald burn of the foot. (Plastic Surgery)

Initial office consultation for a patient with a history of discoid lupus erythematosus who has developed a new erythematous nodule on a cheek. (Dermatology)

Office consultation for management of systolic hypertension in a 70-year-old male scheduled for elective prostate resection. (Geriatrics)

Office consultation with 27-year-old female, with old amputation, for evaluation of existing above-knee prosthesis. (Physical Medicine & Rehabilitation)

Office consultation with 66-year-old female with wrist and hand pain, and finger numbness, secondary to suspected carpal tunnel syndrome. (Orthopaedic Surgery)

Office consultation for 61-year-old female, recently on antibiotic therapy, now with diarrhea and leukocytosis. (Abdominal Surgery)

Office consultation for a patient with papulosquamous eruption of elbow with pitting of nails and itchy scalp. (Dermatology)

Office consultation for a 25-year-old female seen in consultation for complaints of breast pain, with no nipple discharge, mass, or family history of breast cancer. (General Surgery)

Initial office consultation for a 60-year-old female with ptosis, muscle weakness, and thymic tumor who was referred by her neurologist for possible therapeutic plasmapheresis. (Pathology)

99243 Initial office consultation for a 60-year-old male with avascular necrosis of the left femoral head with increasing pain. (Orthopaedic Surgery)

Office consultation for a 31-year-old female complaining of palpitations and chest pains. Her internist had described a mild systolic click. (Cardiology)

Office consultation for a 65-year-old female with recurrent upper extremity cellulitis following axillary lymph node dissection for breast carcinoma. (Infectious Disease)

Office consultation for a 65-year-old male with chronic low-back pain radiating to the leg. (Neurosurgery)

Office consultation for 23-year-old female with Crohn's disease not responding to therapy. (Abdominal Surgery/ Colon & Rectal Surgery)

Office consultation for 25-year-old patient with symptomatic knee pain and swelling, with torn anterior cruciate ligament and/or torn meniscus. (Orthopaedic Surgery)

Office consultation for a 67-year-old patient with osteoporosis and mandibular atrophy with regard to reconstructive alternatives. (Oral & Maxillofacial Surgery)

Office consultation for 39-year-old patient referred at a perimenopausal age for irregular menses and menopausal symptoms. (Obstetrics & Gynecology)

Office consultation for a patient with a papulosquamous eruption of the elbows, pitting of the nails, an itchy, scaly scalp, and localized joint pains. (Dermatology)

Initial office consultation for a 40-year-old female in pain from blister on lip following a cold. (Oral & Maxillofacial Surgery)

Office consultation for a 45-year-old male, requested by his internist, with asymptomatic torus palatinus requiring no further treatment. (Oral & Maxillofacial Surgery)

Office consultation for a 16-year-old male who suffered a concussion a week ago, now fully recovered, needing an evaluation to return to playing football. (Neurology)

99244 Initial office consultation for a 28-year-old male, HIV+, with a recent change in visual acuity. (Ophthalmology)

Initial office consultation for a 15-year-old male with failing grades, suspected drug abuse. (Pediatrics)

Initial office consultation for a 36-year-old factory worker, status four months post-occupational low back injury and requires management of intractable low back pain. (Pain Medicine)

Initial office consultation for a 45-year-old female with a history of chronic arthralgia of TMJ and associated myalgia and sudden progressive symptomatology over last two to three months. (Oral & Maxillofacial Surgery)

Initial office consultation for a 23-year-old female with developmental facial skeletal anomaly and subsequent abnormal relationship of jaw(s) to cranial base. (Oral & Maxillofacial Surgery)

Initial office consultation for a 45-year-old myopic patient with a one-week history of floaters and a partial retinal detachment. (Ophthalmology)

Initial office consultation for a 65-year-old female with moderate dementia, mild unsteadiness, back pain fatigue on ambulation, intermittent urinary incontinence. (Neurosurgery)

Initial office consultation for a 33-year-old female referred by endocrinologist with amenorrhea and galactorrhea, for evaluation of pituitary tumor. (Neurosurgery)

Initial office consultation for a 34-year-old male with new onset nephrotic syndrome. (Nephrology)

Initial office consultation for a patient with multiple giant tumors of jaws. (Oral & Maxillofacial Surgery)

Initial office consultation for a patient with a failed total hip replacement with loosening and pain upon walking. (Orthopaedic Surgery)

Initial office consultation for a 60-year-old female with three-year history of intermittent tic-like unilateral facial pain; now constant pain for six weeks without relief by adequate carbamazepine dosage. (Neurosurgery)

Initial office consultation for a 45-year-old male heavy construction worker with prior lumbar disk surgery two years earlier; now gradually recurring low back and unilateral leg pain for three months, unable to work for two weeks. (Neurosurgery)

Office consultation with 38-year-old female with inflammatory bowel disease, complaints of pain in the right lower quadrant, and suspected intra-abdominal abscess. (General Surgery/Colon & Rectal Surgery)

Office consultation with 72-year-old male with esophageal carcinoma, symptoms of dysphagia and reflux. (Thoracic Surgery)

Office consultation for discussion of treatment options for a 40-year-old female with a 2 cm adenocarcinoma of the breast. (Radiation Oncology)

Office consultation for 66-year-old female, history of colon resection for adenocarcinoma six years earlier, now with severe mid-back pain; X-rays showing osteoporosis and multiple vertebral compression fractures. (Neurosurgery)

Office consultation for a patient with chronic pelvic inflammatory disease who now has left lower quadrant pain with a palpable pelvic mass. (Obstetrics & Gynecology)

Office consultation for a patient with long-standing psoriasis with acute onset of erythroderma, pustular lesions, chills, and fever. Combinations of topical and systemic treatments discussed and instituted. (Dermatology)

Office consultation for a 39-year-old female with persistent migraines failing medications prescribed by her primary care provider. (Neurology)

99245 Office consultation for young patient referred by pediatrician because of patient's short attention span, easy distractibility, and hyperactivity after a failed stimulant trial. (Psychiatry)

Initial office consultation for evaluation of a 70-year-old male with multiple medical problems and recent unexplained appetite loss and diminished energy. (Psychiatry)

Initial office consultation for an elementary school-aged patient, referred by pediatrician, with multiple somatic complaints and recent onset of behavioral discontrol. (Psychiatry)

Initial office consultation of a patient who presents with a 30-year history of smoking, hypertension, chronic obstructive pulmonary disease, and a hard, fixed right neck mass. Patient on other meds for conditions. Patient presents with CT ordered by PCP. (Otolaryngology/Head & Neck Surgery)

Initial office consultation for a 35-year-old multiple-trauma male patient with complex pelvic fractures, for evaluation and formulation of management plan. (Orthopaedic Surgery)

Initial emergency room consultation for 10-year-old male in status epilepticus, recent closed head injury, information about medication not available. (Neurosurgery)

Initial emergency room consultation for a 23-year-old patient with severe abdominal pain, guarding, febrile, and unstable vital signs. (Obstetrics & Gynecology)

Office consultation for a 67-year-old female longstanding uncontrolled diabetic who presents with retinopathy, nephropathy, and a foot ulcer. (Endocrinology)

Office consultation for a 37-year-old male for initial evaluation and management of Cushing's disease. (Endocrinology)

Office consultation for a 60-year-old male who presents with thyrotoxicosis, exophthalmos, frequent premature ventricular contractions, and congestive heart failure. (Endocrinology)

Initial office consultation for a 36-year-old patient, one year status post occupational herniated cervical disk treated by laminectomy, requiring management of multiple sites of intractable pain, depression, and narcotic dependence. (Pain Medicine)

Office consultation for a 58-year-old male with a history of MI and CHF who complains of the recent onset of rest angina and shortness of breath. The patient has a systolic blood pressure of 90 mmHG and is in Class IV heart failure. (Cardiology)

Emergency room consultation for a 1-year-old with a three-day history of fever with increasing respiratory distress who is thought to have cardiac tamponade by the ER physician. (Cardiology)

Office consultation in the emergency room for a 25-year-old male with severe, acute, closed head injury. (Neurosurgery)

Office consultation for a 53-year-old female with advanced head and neck cancer. (Radiation Oncology)

Office consultation for a 27-year-old juvenile diabetic patient with severe diabetic retinopathy, gastric atony, nephrotic syndrome, and progressive renal failure, now with a serum creatinine of 2.7, and a blood pressure of 170/114. (Nephrology)

Office consultation for independent medical evaluation of a patient with a history of complicated low back and neck problems with previous multiple failed back surgeries. (Orthopaedic Surgery)

Office consultation for an adolescent referred by pediatrician PCP for recent onset of violent and self-injurious behavior. (Psychiatry)

Office consultation for a 6-year-old male for evaluation of severe muscle and joint pain and a diffuse rash. Patient well until 4-6 weeks earlier, when he developed arthralgia, myalgias, and a fever of 102 degrees for one week. (Rheumatology)

Office consultation for a 70-year-old male with COPD, congestive heart failure, and diabetes, who presents with rectal bleeding and pain, and worsening constipation. The patient has a fixed, partially obstructing rectal mass. (General Surgery)

Office consultation for a 57-year-old male with recent onset of three events of left arm weakness lasting 30 minutes each. (Neurology)

Initial office consultation of a patient who presents with a 30 year history of smoking and hard, fixed right neck mass, HTN, COPD for which he is on other meds and/or a suspicious epiglottic lesion on indirect laryngoscopy. He brings a CT ordered by his PCP. (Otolaryngology)

Inpatient Consultations

New or Established Patient

99251 Initial hospital consultation for a 27-year-old female with fractured incisor post-intubation. (Oral & Maxillofacial Surgery)

Initial hospital consultation for an orthopaedic patient on IV antibiotics who has developed an apparent candida infection of the oral cavity. (Oral & Maxillofacial Surgery)

Initial inpatient consultation for a 30-year-old female complaining of vaginal itching, post orthopaedic surgery. (Obstetrics & Gynecology)

Initial inpatient consultation for a 36-year-old male on orthopaedic service with complaint of localized dental pain. (Oral & Maxillofacial Surgery)

Initial hospital consultation for a 20-year-old male following a motor vehicle accident who developed cellulitis around a laceration that was sutured in the emergency room. (General Surgery)

Initial inpatient consultation for a 64-year-old bedridden male with skin irritation and pain in posterior heel. (Podiatry Surgery)

99252 Initial hospital consultation for a 45-year-old male, previously abstinent alcoholic, who relapsed and was admitted for management of gastritis. The patient readily accepts the need for further treatment. (Addiction Medicine)

Inpatient consultation for a 28-year-old female with thrombocytopenia and neurologic symptoms who was referred by her hematologist for possible therapeutic plasmapheresis for thrombotic thrombocytopenic purpura. (Pathology)

Initial hospital consultation for a 35-year-old dialysis patient with episodic oral ulcerations. (Oral & Maxillofacial Surgery)

Initial inpatient preoperative consultation for a 43-year-old female with cholecystitis and well-controlled hypertension. (Cardiology)

Initial inpatient consultation for recommendation of antibiotic prophylaxis for a patient with a synthetic heart valve who will undergo urologic surgery. (Internal Medicine)

Initial inpatient consultation for possible drug induced skin eruption in 50-year-old male. (Dermatology)

Preoperative inpatient consultation for evaluation of hypertension in a 60-year-old male who will undergo a cholecystectomy. Patient had a normal annual check-up in your office four months ago. (Internal Medicine)

Initial inpatient consultation for 66-year-old patient with wrist and hand pain and finger numbness, secondary to carpal tunnel syndrome. (Orthopaedic Surgery/Plastic Surgery)

Initial inpatient consultation for a 66-year-old male smoker referred for pain management immediately status post-biliary tract surgery done via sub-costal incision. (Anesthesiology/Pain Medicine)

Initial inpatient consultation for an asymptomatic patient with an established diagnosis of allergic rhinitis, who has gone six weeks since last allergy injection and needs a dose adjustment before the next dose is given. (Allergy & Immunology)

Initial office visit for an 86-year old male with a 2 cm lipoma on back that he is concerned is infected. (General Surgery)

Initial inpatient consultation for a 70-year-old female who has had no bowel sounds for two days following an orthopedic operation. (General Surgery)

Initial hospital consultation for a 56-year-old stroke patient with ankle venous stasis ulcerations. (Podiatry Surgery)

Initial consultation for 66-year-old patient with a grade 1 sacral decubitus following a six-hour abdominal surgical procedure. (Orthopaedic Surgery/Plastic Surgery)

99253 Initial hospital consultation for a 50-year-old female with incapacitating knee pain due to generalized rheumatoid arthritis. (Orthopaedic Surgery)

Initial hospital consultation for a 60-year-old male with avascular necrosis of the left femoral heel with increasing pain. (Orthopaedic Surgery)

Initial hospital consultation for a 45-year-old female with compound mandibular fracture and concurrent head, abdominal, and/or orthopaedic injuries. (Oral & Maxillofacial Surgery)

Initial hospital consultation for a 22-year-old female, paraplegic, to evaluate wrist and hand pain. (Orthopaedic Surgery)

Initial hospital consultation for a 40-year-old male with 10-day history of incapacitating unilateral sciatica, unable to walk now, not improved by bed rest. (Neurosurgery)

Initial hospital consultation, requested by pediatrician, for treatment recommendations for a patient admitted with persistent inability to walk following soft tissue injury to ankle. (Physiatry)

Initial hospital consultation for a 27-year-old previously healthy male who vomited during IV sedation and may have aspirated gastric contents. (Anesthesiology)

Initial hospital consultation for a 33-year-old female, post-abdominal surgery, who now has a fever. (Internal Medicine)

Initial inpatient consultation for a 57-year-old male admitted for severe abdominal pain and fever two days post lower endoscopy. (General Surgery)

Initial inpatient consultation for rehabilitation of a 73-year-old female one week after surgical management of a hip fracture. (Physical Medicine & Rehabilitation)

Initial inpatient consultation for diagnosis/management of fever following abdominal surgery. (Internal Medicine)

Initial inpatient consultation for a 42-year-old non-diabetic patient, postoperative cholecystectomy, now with an acute urinary tract infection. (Nephrology)

Initial inpatient consultation for 53-year-old female with moderate uncomplicated pancreatitis. (Gastroenterology)

Initial inpatient consultation for 45-year-old patient with chronic neck pain with radicular pain of the left arm. (Orthopaedic Surgery)

Initial inpatient consultation for a 43-year-old male with new onset foot drop after removing a cast from his leg. (Neurology)

Initial hospital consultation for an orthopaedic patient on IV antibiotics who has developed an apparent candida infection of the oral cavity. (Oral & Maxillofacial Surgery)

Initial inpatient consultation for a 36-year-old male on orthopaedic service with complaint of localized dental pain. (Oral & Maxillofacial Surgery)

Initial hospital consultation for a 35-year-old dialysis patient with episodic oral ulcerations. (Oral & Maxillofacial Surgery)

Initial hospital consultation for a 55-year-old diabetic patient on dialysis with infected ingrown toenail. (Podiatry Surgery)

99254 Initial inpatient consultation for a 35-year-old female with a fever and pulmonary infiltrate following cesarean section. (Pulmonary Medicine)

Initial hospital consultation for a 15-year-old patient with painless swelling of proximal humerus with lytic lesion by X-ray. (Orthopaedic Surgery)

Initial hospital consultation for evaluation of a 29-year-old female with a diffusely positive medical review of systems and history of multiple surgeries. (Psychiatry)

Initial hospital consultation for a 70-year-old diabetic female with gangrene of the foot. (Orthopaedic Surgery)

Initial inpatient consultation for a 47-year-old female with progressive pulmonary infiltrate, hypoxemia, and diminished urine output. (Anesthesiology)

Initial hospital consultation for a patient with failed total hip replacement with loosening and pain upon walking. (Orthopaedic Surgery)

Initial hospital consultation for a 62-year-old female with metastatic breast cancer to the femoral neck and thoracic vertebra. (Orthopaedic Surgery)

Initial hospital consultation for a 39-year-old female with nephrolithiasis requiring extensive opioid analgesics, whose vital signs are now elevated. She initially denied any drug use but today gives history of multiple substance abuse, including opioids and prior treatment for a personality disorder. (Psychiatry)

Initial inpatient consultation for evaluation of a 63-year-old in the ICU with diabetes and chronic renal failure who develops acute respiratory distress syndrome 36 hours after a mitral valve replacement. (Anesthesiology)

Initial inpatient consultation for a 66-year-old female with enlarged supraclavicular lymph nodes, found on biopsy to be malignant. (Hematology/Oncology)

Initial inpatient consultation for a 43-year-old female for evaluation of sudden painful visual loss, optic neuritis, and episodic paresthesia. (Ophthalmology)

Initial inpatient consultation for evaluation of a 71-year-old male with hyponatremia (serum sodium 114) who was admitted to the hospital with pneumonia. (Nephrology)

Initial inpatient consultation for a 72-year-old male with emergency admission for possible bowel obstruction. (Internal Medicine/General Surgery)

Initial inpatient consultation for a 35-year-old female with fever, swollen joints, and rash of one-week duration. (Rheumatology)

Initial hospital consultation for a 45-year-old female with compound mandibular fracture and concurrent head, abdominal, and/or orthopaedic injuries. (Oral & Maxillofacial Surgery)

Initial hospital consultation for a 70-year-old diabetic female with gangrene of the foot. (Podiatry Surgery)

Initial hospital consultation for a 39-year-old female with myasthenia admitted for a thymectomy surgery tomorrow. (Neurology)

99255 Initial hospital consultation for a 70-year-old female without previous psychiatric history who is now experiencing nocturnal confusion and visual hallucinations following hip replacement surgery. (Psychiatry)

Initial inpatient consultation for a 76-year-old female with massive, life-threatening gastrointestinal hemorrhage and chest pain. (Gastroenterology)

Initial inpatient consultation for a 75-year-old female, admitted to intensive care with acute respiratory distress syndrome, who is hypersensitive, and has a moderate metabolic acidosis, and a rising serum creatinine. (Nephrology)

Initial hospital consultation for patient with a history of complicated low back pain and neck problems with previous multiple failed back surgeries. (Orthopaedic Surgery/Neurosurgery)

Initial hospital consultation for a 66-year-old female, two days post-abdominal aneurysm repair, with oliguria and hypertension of one-day duration. (Nephrology/Internal Medicine)

Initial hospital consultation for a patient with shotgun wound to face with massive facial trauma and airway obstruction. (Oral & Maxillofacial Surgery)

Initial hospital consultation for patient with severe pancreatitis complicated by respiratory insufficiency, acute renal failure, and abscess formation. (General Surgery/Colon & Rectal Surgery)

Initial hospital consultation for a 35-year-old multiple-trauma male patient with complex pelvic fractures to evaluate and formulate management plan. (Orthopaedic Surgery)

Initial inpatient consultation for adolescent patient with fractured femur and pelvis who pulled out IVs and disconnected traction in attempt to elope from hospital. (Psychiatry)

Initial hospital consultation for a 16-year-old primigravida at 32-weeks gestation requested by a family practitioner for evaluation of severe hypertension, thrombocytopenia, and headache. (Obstetrics & Gynecology)

Initial hospital consultation for a 58-year-old insulin-dependent diabetic with multiple antibiotic allergies, now with multiple fascial plane abscesses and airway obstruction. (Oral & Maxillofacial Surgery)

Initial inpatient consultation for a 55-year-old male with known cirrhosis and ascites, now with jaundice, encephalopathy, and massive hematemesis. (Gastroenterology)

Initial hospital consultation for a 25-year-old male, seen in emergency room with severe, closed head injury. (Neurosurgery)

Initial hospital consultation for a 2-day-old male with single ventricle physiology and subaortic obstruction. Family counseling following evaluation for multiple, staged surgical procedures. (Thoracic Surgery)

Initial hospital consultation for a 45-year-old male admitted with subarachnoid hemorrhage and intracranial aneurysm on angiogram. (Neurosurgery)

Initial inpatient consultation for myxedematous patient who is hypoventilating and obtunded. (Endocrinology)

Initial hospital consultation for a 45-year-old patient with widely metastatic lung carcinoma, intractable back pain, and a history that includes substance dependence, NSAID allergy, and two prior laminectomies with fusion for low back pain. (Pain Medicine)

Initial hospital consultation for evaluation of treatment options in a 50-year-old patient with cirrhosis, known peptic ulcer disease, hypotension, encephalopathy, and massive acute upper gastrointestinal bleeding that cannot be localized by endoscopy. (Interventional Radiology)

Initial inpatient consultation in the ICU for a 70-year-old male who experienced a cardiac arrest during surgery and was resuscitated. (Cardiology)

Initial inpatient consultation for a patient with severe pancreatitis complicated by respiratory insufficiency, acute renal failure, and abscess formation. (Gastroenterology)

Initial inpatient consultation for a 70-year-old cirrhotic male admitted with ascites, jaundice, encephalopathy, and massive hematemesis. (Gastroenterology)

Initial inpatient consultation in the ICU for a 51-year-old patient who has a fever, respiratory failure requiring mechanical ventilation, and bilateral pulmonary infiltrates on chest radiograph two weeks after a renal transplantation. (Infectious Disease)

Initial inpatient consultation for evaluation and formulation of plan for management of multiple-trauma patient with complex pelvic fracture, 35-year-old male. (General Surgery/Orthopaedic Surgery)

Initial inpatient consultation for a 50-year-old male with a history of previous myocardial infarction, now with acute pulmonary edema and hypotension. (Cardiology)

Initial inpatient consultation for 45-year-old male with recent, acute subarachnoid hemorrhage, hesitant speech, mildly confused, drowsy. High risk group for HIV+ status. (Neurosurgery)

Initial inpatient consultation for 36-year-old female referred by her internist to evaluate a patient being followed for abdominal pain and fever. The patient has developed diffuse abdominal pain, guarding, rigidity, and increased fever. (Obstetrics & Gynecology)

Initial inpatient consultation for adolescent patient with fractured femur and pelvis who expressed feeling hopeless and suicidal. (Psychiatry)

Initial inpatient consultation for a 35-year-old male with closed head injury, pulmonary contusion, liver laceration, and complex pelvic fracture. (General Surgery)

Initial hospital consultation for a 35-year-old male patient with acute partial traumatic amputation of the forefoot for evaluation and formulation of a management plan. (Podiatry Surgery)

Initial hospital consultation for a 57-year-old male with new-onset right hemiparesis and aphasia. (Neurology)

Emergency Department Services

New or Established Patient

99281 Emergency department visit for a patient for removal of sutures from a well-healed, uncomplicated laceration. (Emergency Medicine)

Emergency department visit for a patient for tetanus toxoid immunization. (Emergency Medicine)

Emergency department visit for a patient with several uncomplicated insect bites. (Pediatrics)

99282 Emergency department visit for a 20-year-old student who presents with a painful sunburn with blister formation on the back. (Emergency Medicine)

Emergency department visit for a child presenting with impetigo localized to the face. (Emergency Medicine)

Emergency department visit for a patient with a minor traumatic injury of an extremity with localized pain, swelling, and bruising. (Emergency Medicine)

Emergency department visit for an otherwise healthy patient whose chief complaint is a red, swollen cystic lesion on his/her back. (Emergency Medicine)

Emergency department visit for a patient presenting with a rash on both legs after exposure to poison ivy. (Emergency Medicine)

Emergency department visit for a child presenting with impetigo localized to the face with use of topical OTC treatment. (Pediatrics)

Emergency department visit for a patient with a minor traumatic injury of an extremity with localized pain, swelling, and bruising (no imaging done). (Pediatrics)

99283 Emergency department visit for a sexually active female complaining of vaginal discharge who is afebrile and denies experiencing abdominal or back pain. (Emergency Medicine)

Emergency department visit for a well-appearing 8-year-old who has a fever, diarrhea, and abdominal cramps; is tolerating oral fluids and is not vomiting. (Pediatrics)

Emergency department visit for a patient with an inversion ankle injury, who is unable to bear weight on the injured foot and ankle. (Emergency Medicine)

Emergency department visit for a patient who has a complaint of acute pain associated with a suspected foreign body in the painful eye. (Emergency Medicine)

Emergency department visit for a healthy, young adult patient who sustained a blunt head injury with local swelling and bruising without subsequent confusion, loss of consciousness, or memory deficit. (Emergency Medicine)

99284 Emergency department visit for a 4-year-old who fell off a bike sustaining a head injury with brief loss of consciousness. (Emergency Medicine)

Emergency department visit for a patient with flank pain and hematuria. (Emergency Medicine)

Emergency department visit for a female presenting with lower abdominal pain and a vaginal discharge. (Emergency Medicine)

99285 Emergency department visit for a patient with a complicated overdose requiring aggressive management to prevent side effects from the ingested materials. (Emergency Medicine)

Emergency department visit for a patient exhibiting active, upper gastrointestinal bleeding. (Emergency Medicine)

Emergency department visit for a previously healthy young adult patient who is injured in an automobile accident and is brought to the emergency department immobilized and has symptoms compatible with intra-abdominal injuries or multiple extremity injuries. (Emergency Medicine)

Emergency department visit for a patient with an acute onset of chest pain compatible with symptoms of cardiac ischemia and/or pulmonary embolus. (Emergency Medicine)

Emergency department visit for a patient who presents with a sudden onset of "the worst headache of her life," and complains of a stiff neck, nausea, and inability to concentrate. (Emergency Medicine)

Emergency department visit for a patient with a new onset of a cerebral vascular accident. (Emergency Medicine)

Emergency department visit for acute febrile illness in an adult, associated with shortness of breath and an altered level of alertness. (Emergency Medicine)

Initial hospital visit for a 15-year-old male with acute status asthmaticus, unresponsive to outpatient therapy. (Pulmonary Medicine)

Initial hospital visit for a 62-year-old male with history of previous myocardial infarction, comes in with recurrent, sustained ventricular tachycardia. (Cardiology)

Critical Care Services

99291 First hour of critical care of a 65-year-old male with septic shock following relief of ureteral obstruction caused by a stone. (Cardiology/Emergency Medicine/Family Practice/General Surgery/Internal Medicine/Pulmonary Medicine)

First hour of critical care of a 15-year-old with acute respiratory failure from asthma. (Cardiology/Emergency Medicine/Family Practice/General Surgery/Internal Medicine/Pulmonary Medicine)

First hour of critical care of a 45-year-old who sustained a liver laceration, cerebral hematoma, flailed chest, and pulmonary contusion after being struck by an automobile. (Cardiology/Emergency Medicine/Family Practice/General Surgery/Internal Medicine/Pulmonary Medicine)

First hour of critical care of a 65-year-old female who, following a hysterectomy, suffered a cardiac arrest associated with a pulmonary embolus. (Cardiology/Emergency Medicine/Family Practice/General Surgery/Internal Medicine/Pulmonary Medicine)

First hour of critical care of a 6-month-old with hypovolemic shock secondary to diarrhea and dehydration. (Cardiology/Emergency Medicine/Family Practice/General Surgery/Internal Medicine/Pulmonary Medicine/Critical Care)

First hour of critical care of a 3-year-old with respiratory failure secondary to pneumocystis carinii pneumonia. (Cardiology/Emergency Medicine/Family Practice/General Surgery/Internal Medicine/Pulmonary Medicine/Critical Care)

First hour of critical care of a 13-year-old with hypovolemic shock secondary to diarrhea and dehydration. (Cardiology/Emergency Medicine/Family Practice/General Surgery/Internal Medicine/Pediatrics/Pulmonary Medicine/Critical Care)

First hour of critical care of a 13-year-old with respiratory failure secondary to pneumocystis carinii pneumonia (Pediatrics)

Subsequent hospital visit for a 55-year-old male with severe chronic obstructive pulmonary disease and bronchospasm; initially admitted for acute respiratory distress requiring ventilatory support in the ICU. The patient was stabilized, extubated, and transferred to the floor but has now developed acute fever, dyspnea, left lower lobe rhonchi, and laboratory evidence of carbon dioxide retention and hypoxemia. (Family Medicine)

Prolonged Services

Prolonged Service With Direct Patient Contact

Office or Other Outpatient

99354 A 20-year-old female with history of asthma presents with acute bronchospasm and moderate respiratory distress. Initial evaluation shows respiratory rate 30, labored breathing and wheezing heard in all lung fields. Office treatment is initiated which includes intermittent bronchial dilation and subcutaneous epinephrine. Requires intermittent time with patient over a period of 2-3 hours. (Family Medicine/Internal Medicine)

99355 A 20-year-old female with history of asthma presents with acute bronchospasm and moderate respiratory distress. Initial evaluation shows respiratory rate 30, labored breathing, and wheezing heard in all lung fields. Office treatment is initiated that includes intermittent bronchial dilation and subcutaneous epinephrine. Requires intermittent time with patient over a period of 2-3 hours. (Family Medicine/Internal Medicine/Pulmonary Medicine)

Inpatient

99356 A 34-year-old primigravida female presents to hospital in early labor. Admission history and physical reveals severe preeclampsia. Physician supervises management of preeclampsia, IV magnesium initiation and maintenance, labor augmentation with pitocin, and close maternal-fetal monitoring. Involvement includes 40 minutes of continuous bedside care until the patient is stable, then is intermittent over several hours until the delivery. (Family Medicine/Internal Medicine/Obstetrics & Gynecology)

Prolonged Service Without Direct Patient Contact

99358 An 85-year-old new patient with multiple complicated medical problems has moved to the area to live closer to her daughter. She is brought to the primary care office by her daughter and has been seen and examined by the physician. The physician indicated that past medical records would be obtained from the patient's prior physicians' and that he will communicate further with the daughter upon review of them. (Family Medicine/Internal Medicine)

99359 An 85-year-old new patient with multiple complicated medical problems has moved to the area to live closer to her daughter. She is brought to the primary care office by her daughter and has been seen and examined by the physician. The physician indicated that past medical records would be obtained from the patient's prior physicians' and that he will communicate further with the daughter upon review of them. (Family Medicine/Internal Medicine)

Physician Standby Services

99360 A 24-year-old patient is admitted to OB unit attempting VBAC. Fetal monitoring shows increasing fetal distress. Patient's blood pressure is rising and labor progressing slowly. A primary care physician is requested by the OB/GYN to standby in the unit for possible cesarean delivery and neonatal resuscitation. (Family Medicine/Internal Medicine)

Care Plan Oversight Services

99375 First month of care plan oversight for terminal care of a 58-year-old female with advanced intraabdominal ovarian cancer. Care plan includes home oxygen, diuretics IV for edema and ascites control and pain control management involving IV morphine infusion when progressive ileus occurred. Physician phone contacts with nurse, family, and MSW. Discussion with MSW concerning plans to withdraw supportive measures per patient wishes. Documentation includes review and modification of care plan and certifications from nursing, MSW, pharmacy, and DME. (Family Medicine/Internal Medicine)

Prolonged Clinical Staff Services with Physician or Other Qualified Health Care Professional Supervision

99415 A 52-year-old female presents with gastroenteritis and persistent vomiting. She is unable to tolerate food or liquid by mouth. She presents with signs and symptoms of clinical dehydration. Evaluation and management is performed by the physician. The decision is made to begin IV hydration in the office. A hydration IV is initiated, consisting of normal saline. Prolonged monitoring and observation for 2 hours ensues with intermittent evaluation of the patient by the physician.

Inpatient Neonatal Intensive Care Service and Pediatric and Neonatal Critical Care Services

99477 Initial hospital visit for a 1-day-old male with cyanosis, respiratory distress, and tachypnea. (Cardiology)

Appendix D

Summary of CPT Add-on Codes

This listing is a summary of CPT add-on codes for CPT 2019. The codes listed below are identified in CPT 2019 with a ✚ symbol.

01953	15156	20937	26861
01968	15157	20938	26863
01969	15201	20939	27358
10004	15221	20985	27692
10006	15241	22103	29826
10008	15261	22116	31627
10010	15272	22208	31632
10012	15274	22216	31633
10036	15276	22226	31637
11001	15278	22328	31649
11008	15777	22512	31651
11045	15787	22515	31654
11046	15847	22527	32501
11047	16036	22534	32506
11103	17003	22552	32507
11105	17312	22585	32667
11107	17314	22614	32668
11201	17315	22632	32674
11732	19001	22634	33141
11922	19082	22840	33225
13102	19084	22841	33257
13122	19086	22842	33258
13133	19126	22843	33259
13153	19282	22844	33367
14302	19284	22845	33368
15003	19286	22846	33369
15005	19288	22847	33419
15101	19294	22848	33508
15111	19297	22853	33517
15116	20930	22854	33518
15121	20931	22858	33519
15131	20932	22859	33521
15136	20933	22868	33522
15151	20934	22870	33523
15152	20936	26125	33530

33572	37186	51797	64492
33768	37222	52442	64494
33866	37223	56606	64495
33884	37232	57267	64634
33924	37233	58110	64636
33929	37234	58611	64643
33987	37235	59525	64645
34709	37237	60512	64727
34711	37239	61316	64778
34713	37247	61517	64783
34714	37249	61611	64787
34715	37252	61641	64832
34716	37253	61642	64837
34808	38102	61651	64859
34812	38746	61781	64872
34813	38747	61782	64874
34820	38900	61783	64876
34833	43273	61797	64901
34834	43283	61799	64902
35306	43338	61800	64913
35390	43635	61864	65757
35400	44015	61868	66990
35500	44121	62148	67225
35572	44128	62160	67320
35600	44139	63035	67331
35681	44203	63043	67332
35682	44213	63044	67334
35683	44701	63048	67335
35685	44955	63057	67340
35686	47001	63066	69990
35697	47542	63076	74301
35700	47543	63078	74713
36218	47544	63082	75565
36227	47550	63086	75774
36228	48400	63088	76125
36248	49326	63091	76802
36474	49327	63103	76810
36476	49412	63295	76812
36479	49435	63308	76814
36483	49568	63621	76937
36907	49905	64462	76979
36908	50606	64480	76983
36909	50705	64484	77001
37185	50706	64491	77002

77003	92925	95941	99416
77063	92929	95962	99467
77293	92934	95967	99486
78020	92938	95984	99489
78496	92944	96113	99494
78730	92973	96121	99498
81266	92974	96131	99602
81416	92978	96133	99607
81426	92979	96137	0054T
81536	92998	96139	0055T
82952	93320	96361	0076T
86826	93321	96366	0095T
87187	93325	96367	0098T
87503	93352	96368	0163T
87904	93462	96370	0164T
88155	93463	96371	0165T
88177	93464	96375	0174T
88185	93563	96376	0205T
88311	93564	96411	0214T
88314	93565	96415	0215T
88332	93566	96417	0217T
88334	93567	96423	0218T
88341	93568	96570	0222T
88350	93571	96571	0229T
88364	93572	96934	0231T
88369	93592	96935	0290T
88373	93609	96936	0376T
88388	93613	97546	0396T
90461	93621	97598	0397T
90472	93622	97811	0399T
90474	93623	97814	0437T
90785	93655	99100	0439T
90833	93657	99116	0443T
90836	93662	99135	0450T
90838	94645	99140	0466T
90840	94729	99153	0471T
90863	94781	99157	0480T
91013	95079	99292	0482T
92547	95873	99354	0492T
92608	95874	99355	0496T
92618	95885	99356	0513T
92621	95886	99357	0514T
92627	95887	99359	0523T
92921	95940	99415	

Appendix E

Summary of CPT Codes Exempt from Modifier 51

This listing is a summary of CPT codes that are exempt from the use of modifier 51. Procedures on this list are typically performed with another procedure but may be a stand-alone procedure and not always performed with other specified procedures. For add-on codes, see Appendix D. This is not an exhaustive list of procedures that are typically exempt from multiple procedure reductions. The codes listed below are identified in CPT 2019 with a ⊘ symbol.

17004	93456	93618
20697	93503	93631
20974	93600	94610
20975	93602	95905
31500	93603	95992
36620	93610	99151
44500	93612	99152
61107	93615	
93451	93616	

Appendix E

Appendix F

Summary of CPT Codes Exempt from Modifier 63

The listing is a summary of CPT codes that are exempt from the use of modifier 63. The codes listed below are additionally identified in CPT 2019 with the parenthetical instruction "(Do not report modifier 63 in conjunction with…)."

30540	**36420**	**49496**
30545	**36450**	**49600**
31520	**36456**	**49605**
33470	**36460**	**49606**
33502	**36510**	**49610**
33503	**36660**	**49611**
33505	**39503**	**53025**
33506	**43313**	**54000**
33610	**43314**	**54150**
33611	**43520**	**54160**
33619	**43831**	**63700**
33647	**44055**	**63702**
33670	**44126**	**63704**
33690	**44127**	**63706**
33694	**44128**	**65820**
33730	**46070**	
33732	**46705**	
33735	**46715**	
33736	**46716**	
33750	**46730**	
33755	**46735**	
33762	**46740**	
33778	**46742**	
33786	**46744**	
33922	**47700**	
33946	**47701**	
33947	**49215**	
33948	**49491**	
33949	**49492**	
36415	**49495**	

Appendix G

Summary of CPT Codes That Include Moderate (Conscious) Sedation

The summary of CPT codes that include moderate (conscious) sedation (formerly Appendix G) has been removed from the CPT code set.

The codes that were previously included in the former **Appendix G** have been revised with the removal of the moderate (conscious) sedation symbol. For information/guidance on reporting moderate (conscious) sedation services with codes formerly listed in **Appendix G**, please refer to the guidelines for codes 99151, 99152, 99153, 99155, 99156, 99157.

Appendix H

Alphabetical Clinical Topics Listing (AKA – Alphabetical Listing)

The **Alphabetical Clinical Topics Listing** (formerly Appendix H) has been removed from the CPT codebook. Since this document is a dynamic and rapidly expanding source of information to link CPT Category II codes, clinical conditions, and measure abstracts, the Alphabetical Listing is now solely accessed on the AMA CPT website at https://www.ama-assn.org/sites/default/files/media-browser/public/cpt/cpt-cat2-codes-alpha-listing-clinical-topics_0.pdf.

In addition, new codes for the publication cycle (ie, the **Update to the List of Category II Codes**) will continue to be located on the AMA CPT website prior to publication in the next edition of the CPT codebook (subsequent to its listing on the Web).

Appendix I

Genetic Testing Code Modifiers

The **Genetic Testing Code Modifiers** (formerly Appendix I) has been removed from the CPT code set.

The addition of more than 100 molecular pathology codes to the 2012 code set and still more codes to the 2013 CPT code set resulted in the deletion of the stacking codes (83890–83914). The genetic testing code modifiers formerly described in Appendix I applied to those stacking codes, and therefore, the Appendix and modifiers have been removed from the code set.

For the most up-to-date information on future updates for molecular pathology coding in the CPT code set, see the AMA CPT website (https://www.ama-assn.org/practice-management/newly-released-codes).

Appendix J

Electrodiagnostic Medicine Listing of Sensory, Motor, and Mixed Nerves

This summary assigns each sensory, motor, and mixed nerve with its appropriate nerve conduction study code in order to enhance accurate reporting of codes 95907-95913. Each nerve constitutes one unit of service.

Motor Nerves Assigned to Codes 95907-95913

I. Upper extremity, cervical plexus, and brachial plexus motor nerves
  A. Axillary motor nerve to the deltoid
  B. Long thoracic motor nerve to the serratus anterior
  C. Median nerve
    1. Median motor nerve to the abductor pollicis brevis
    2. Median motor nerve, anterior interosseous branch, to the flexor pollicis longus
    3. Median motor nerve, anterior interosseous branch, to the pronator quadratus
    4. Median motor nerve to the first lumbrical
    5. Median motor nerve to the second lumbrical
  D. Musculocutaneous motor nerve to the biceps brachii
  E. Radial nerve
    1. Radial motor nerve to the extensor carpi ulnaris
    2. Radial motor nerve to the extensor digitorum communis
    3. Radial motor nerve to the extensor indicis proprius
    4. Radial motor nerve to the brachioradialis
  F. Suprascapular nerve
    1. Suprascapular motor nerve to the supraspinatus
    2. Suprascapular motor nerve to the infraspinatus
  G. Thoracodorsal motor nerve to the latissimus dorsi
  H. Ulnar nerve
    1. Ulnar motor nerve to the abductor digiti minimi
    2. Ulnar motor nerve to the palmar interosseous
    3. Ulnar motor nerve to the first dorsal interosseous
    4. Ulnar motor nerve to the flexor carpi ulnaris
  I. Other
II. Lower extremity motor nerves
  A. Femoral motor nerve to the quadriceps
    1. Femoral motor nerve to vastus medialis
    2. Femoral motor nerve to vastus lateralis
    3. Femoral motor nerve to vastus intermedialis
    4. Femoral motor nerve to rectus femoris
  B. Ilioinguinal motor nerve
  C. Peroneal (fibular) nerve
    1. Peroneal motor nerve to the extensor digitorum brevis
    2. Peroneal motor nerve to the peroneus brevis
    3. Peroneal motor nerve to the peroneus longus
    4. Peroneal motor nerve to the tibialis anterior
  D. Plantar motor nerve
  E. Sciatic nerve
  F. Tibial nerve
    1. Tibial motor nerve, inferior calcaneal branch, to the abductor digiti minimi
    2. Tibial motor nerve, medial plantar branch, to the abductor hallucis
    3. Tibial motor nerve, lateral plantar branch, to the flexor digiti minimi brevis
  G. Other
III. Cranial nerves and trunk
  A. Cranial nerve VII (facial motor nerve)
    1. Facial nerve to the frontalis
    2. Facial nerve to the nasalis
    3. Facial nerve to the orbicularis oculi
    4. Facial nerve to the orbicularis oris
  B. Cranial nerve XI (spinal accessory motor nerve)
  C. Cranial nerve XII (hypoglossal motor nerve)
  D. Intercostal motor nerve
  E. Phrenic motor nerve to the diaphragm
  F. Recurrent laryngeal nerve
  G. Other
IV. Nerve Roots
  A. Cervical nerve root stimulation
    1. Cervical level 5 (CT)
    2. Cervical level 6 (C6)
    3. Cervical level 7 (C7)
    4. Cervical level 8 (C8)

B. Thoracic nerve root stimulation
  1. Thoracic level 1 (T1)
  2. Thoracic level 2 (T2)
  3. Thoracic level 3 (T3)
  4. Thoracic level 4 (T4)
  5. Thoracic level 5 (T5)
  6. Thoracic level 6 (T6)
  7. Thoracic level 7 (T7)
  8. Thoracic level 8 (T8)
  9. Thoracic level 9 (T9)
  10. Thoracic level 10 (T10)
  11. Thoracic level 11 (T11)
  12. Thoracic level 12 (T12)

C. Lumbar nerve root stimulation
  1. Lumbar level 1 (L1)
  2. Lumbar level 2 (L2)
  3. Lumbar level 3 (L3)
  4. Lumbar level 4 (L4)
  5. Lumbar level 5 (L5)

D. Sacral nerve root stimulation
  1. Sacral level 1 (S1)
  2. Sacral level 2 (S2)
  3. Sacral level 3 (S3)
  4. Sacral level 4 (S4)

Sensory and Mixed Nerves Assigned to Codes 95907-95913

I. Upper extremity sensory and mixed nerves

A. Lateral antebrachial cutaneous sensory nerve

B. Medial antebrachial cutaneous sensory nerve

C. Medial brachial cutaneous sensory nerve

D. Median nerve
  1. Median sensory nerve to the first digit
  2. Median sensory nerve to the second digit
  3. Median sensory nerve to the third digit
  4. Median sensory nerve to the fourth digit
  5. Median palmar cutaneous sensory nerve
  6. Median palmar mixed nerve

E. Posterior antebrachial cutaneous sensory nerve

F. Radial sensory nerve
  1. Radial sensory nerve to the base of the thumb
  2. Radial sensory nerve to digit 1

G. Ulnar nerve
  1. Ulnar dorsal cutaneous sensory nerve
  2. Ulnar sensory nerve to the fourth digit
  3. Ulnar sensory nerve to the fifth digit
  4. Ulnar palmar mixed nerve

H. Intercostal sensory nerve

I. Other

II. Lower extremity sensory and mixed nerves

A. Lateral femoral cutaneous sensory nerve

B. Medial calcaneal sensory nerve

C. Medial femoral cutaneous sensory nerve

D. Peroneal nerve
  1. Deep peroneal sensory nerve
  2. Superficial peroneal sensory nerve, medial dorsal cutaneous branch
  3. Superficial peroneal sensory nerve, intermediate dorsal cutaneous branch

E. Posterior femoral cutaneous sensory nerve

F. Saphenous nerve
  1. Saphenous sensory nerve (distal technique)
  2. Saphenous sensory nerve (proximal technique)

G. Sural nerve
  1. Sural sensory nerve, lateral dorsal cutaneous branch
  2. Sural sensory nerve

H. Tibial sensory nerve (digital nerve to toe 1)

I. Tibial sensory nerve (medial plantar nerve)

J. Tibial sensory nerve (lateral plantar nerve)

K. Other

III. Head and trunk sensory nerves

A. Dorsal nerve of the penis

B. Greater auricular nerve

C. Ophthalmic branch of the trigeminal nerve

D. Pudendal sensory nerve

E. Suprascapular sensory nerves

F. Other

The following table provides a reasonable maximum number of studies performed per diagnostic category necessary for a physician to arrive at a diagnosis in 90% of patients with that final diagnosis. The numbers in each column represent the number of studies recommended. The appropriate number of studies to be performed is based upon the physician's discretion.

	Type of Study/Maximum Number of Studies		
Indication	**Limbs Studied by Needle EMG (95860-95864, 95867-95870, 95885-95887)**	**Nerve Conduction Studies (Total Nerves Studied, 95907-95913)**	**Neuromuscular Junction Testing (Repetitive Stimulation, 95937)**
Carpal Tunnel (Unilateral)	1	7	—
Carpal Tunnel (Bilateral)	2	10	—
Radiculopathy	2	7	—
Mononeuropathy	1	8	—
Polyneuropathy/Mononeuropathy Multiplex	3	10	—
Myopathy	2	4	2
Motor Neuronopathy (eg, ALS)	4	6	2
Plexopathy	2	12	—
Neuromuscular Junction	2	4	3
Tarsal Tunnel Syndrome (Unilateral)	1	8	—
Tarsal Tunnel Syndrome (Bilateral)	2	11	—
Weakness, Fatigue, Cramps, or Twitching (Focal)	2	7	2
Weakness, Fatigue, Cramps, or Twitching (General)	4	8	2
Pain, Numbness, or Tingling (Unilateral)	1	9	—
Pain, Numbness, or Tingling (Bilateral)	2	12	—

Appendix K

Product Pending FDA Approval

Some vaccine products have been assigned a CPT Category I code in anticipation of future approval from the Food and Drug Administration (FDA). Following is a list of the vaccine product codes pending FDA approval status that are identified in the CPT code set with the (✗) symbol. Upon revision of the approval status by the FDA, notation of this revision will be provided via the AMA CPT "Category I Vaccine Codes" website listing (www.ama-assn.org/go/cpt-vaccine) and in subsequent publications of the CPT code set.

90587
90666
90667
90668
90689
90697

Appendix L

Vascular Families

►Appendix L is a vascular branching model that assumes the aorta, vena cava, pulmonary artery, or portal vein is the starting point of catheterization. Accordingly, branches have been categorized into first, second, third order, and beyond. (Note that this categorization does not apply, for instance, if a femoral or carotid artery were catheterized directly in an antegrade direction.) Common branching patterns of typical anatomy are shown in the charts and illustrations.

No specific coding instructions should be inferred from Appendix L. End-users must determine how best to code any specific procedure based on variant anatomy and different vascular access point relative to vessel(s) selectively catheterized (eg, antegrade femoral artery, radial artery, retrograde femoral to ipsilateral internal iliac artery catheterization, transsplenic splenic vein access to portal venous system, etc).◄

Arterial Vascular Family

Abbreviations:	
R = Right	Asc = Ascending
L = Left	Desc = Descending
Ant = Anterior	Lat = Lateral
Post = Posterior	Int = Internal
Sup = Superior	Ext = External
Inf = Inferior	Transv = Transverse
	Tr = Trunk

First Order / Second Order / Third Order / Beyond Third Order

- **Thoracic aorta**
  - R. & L. coronary
  - Innominate (brachiocephalic)
    - R. common carotid
      - R. int. carotid
        - R. vidian
        - R. caroticotympanic
        - R. meningohypophyseal tr.
        - R. inferolateral tr.
        - R. inf. hypophyseal
        - R. ophthalmic
        - R. sup. hypophyseal
        - R. ant. choroidal
        - R. post. communicating
        - R. middle cerebral
        - R. ant. cerebral
      - R. ext. carotid
        - R. sup. thyroid
        - R. asc. pharyngeal
        - R. lingual
        - R. facial
        - R. occipital
        - R. post. auricular
        - R. superficial temporal
        - R. internal maxillary
          - R. middle meningeal
    - R. subclavian
      - R. vertebral
        - Basilar and branches
        - Post. cerebral
      - R. int. thoracic (int. mammary)
        - R. sup. epigastric
      - R. thyrocervical tr.
        - R. inf. thyroid
        - R. asc. cervical
        - R. transv. cervical
        - R. suprascapular
      - R. costocervical tr.
        - R. deep cervical
        - R. supreme intercostal
    - (Considered 1 vessel for coding purposes)
    - R. axillary
      - R. sup. thoracic
      - R. thoracoacromial
      - R. lat. thoracic
      - R. ant. & post. circumflex humeral
      - R. subscapular
        - R. circumflex scapular
        - R. thoracodorsal
      - R. brachial
        - R. profunda brachii
        - R. ulnar
          - R. common interosseous
        - R. radial
          - R. deep palmar arch
          - R. superficial palmar arch
          - R. metacarpal(s)
          - R. digital(s)
  - L. common carotid
    - L. int. carotid
      - L. vidian
      - L. caroticotympanic
      - L. meningohypophyseal tr.
      - L. inferolateral tr.
      - L. inf. hypophyseal
      - L. ophthalmic
      - L. sup. hypophyseal
      - L. ant. choroidal
      - L. post. communicating
      - L. middle cerebral
      - L. ant. cerebral
    - L. ext carotid
      - L. sup. thyroid
      - L. asc. pharyngeal
      - L. lingual
      - L. facial
      - L. occipital
      - L. post. auricular
      - L. superficial temporal
      - L. internal maxillary
        - L. middle meningeal

First Order | Second Order | Third Order | Beyond Third Order

- **Thoracic aorta** *(continued)*
  - L. subclavian
    - L. vertebral
      - Basilar and branches
      - Post. cerebral
    - L. int. thoracic (int. mammary)
      - L. sup. epigastric
    - L. thyrocervical tr.
      - L. inferior thyroid
      - L. asc. cervical
      - L. transv. cervical
      - L. suprascapular
    - L. costocervical tr.
      - L. deep cervical
      - L. supreme intercostal
  - (Considered 1 vessel for coding purposes)
  - L. axillary
    - L. sup. thoracic
    - L. thoracoacromial
    - L. lat. thoracic
    - L. ant. & post. circumflex humeral
    - L. subscapular
      - L. circumflex subscapular
      - L. thoracodorsal
    - L. brachial
      - L. profunda brachii
      - L. ulnar
      - L. radial
        - L. common interosseous
        - L. deep palmar arch
        - L. superficial palmar arch
        - L. metacarpal(s)
        - L. digital(s)
  - L. sup. bronchial
  - L. inf. bronchial
  - R. 3rd intercostal
    - R. bronchial
  - Intercostal(s)
  - Esophageal

Diaphragm

- **Abdominal aorta**
  - Inf. phrenic
    - Sup. suprarenal (adrenal)
  - Celiac
    - L. gastric
      - Esophageal
    - Splenic
      - Dorsal pancreatic
        - Transv. pancreatic (inf. pancreatic)
      - Greater pancreatic (pancreatica magna)
      - Caudal pancreatic
      - L. gastroepiploic
      - Short gastric(s)
    - Common hepatic
      - Gastroduodenal
        - Post. & ant. superior pancreaticoduodenal
        - R. gastroepiploic
      - Proper hepatic
        - Supraduodenal
        - R. gastric
        - L. hepatic
          - Middle hepatic
            - Falciform
        - R. hepatic
          - Cystic
  - Middle suprarenal (adrenal)
  - Sup. mesenteric
    - Inf. pancreaticoduodenal
      - Ant. inf. pancreaticoduodenal
      - Post. inf. pancreaticoduodenal
    - Middle colic
      - Colic marginal(s)
    - R. colic
      - Colic marginal(s)
    - Ileocolic
      - Sup. ileocolic
        - Colic marginal(s)
      - Inf. ileocolic
        - Ant. & post. cecal
        - Appendicular
        - Ileal
    - Jejunal
  - Renal
    - Inf. suprarenal (adrenal)
    - Renal polar
      - Renal cortical
  - Testicular/ovarian
  - Lumbar
  - Inf. mesenteric
    - L. colic
      - Asc. L. colic
        - Colic marginal(s)
      - Desc. L. colic
        - Colic marginal(s)
    - Sigmoid
    - Sup. rectal
  - Middle (median) sacral

First Order | Second Order | Third Order | Beyond Third Order

- Common iliac
  - Int. iliac
    - Post. division
      - Iliolumbar
      - Lat. sacral
      - Sup. gluteal
    - Ant. division
      - Obturator
      - Umbilical
        - Sup. vesical
      - Uterine
      - Vaginal
      - Inf. vesical
      - Middle rectal
        - Prostate
      - Int. pudendal
        - Inf. rectal
      - Inf. gluteal
  - Ext. iliac
    - Deep circumflex iliac
    - Inf. epigastric
      - Cremasteric
  - (Considered 1 vessel for coding purposes)
  - Common femoral
    - Profunda femoris
      - Med. femoral circumflex
      - Lat. femoral circumflex
    - Deep ext. pudendal
    - Superficial ext. pudendal
    - Superficial femoral
    - (Considered 1 vessel for coding purposes)
    - Popliteal
      - Geniculate
      - Ant. tibial
      - Post. tibial
      - Peroneal
      - Pedal arch
      - Digital(s)

Venous Vascular Family

First Order | Second Order | Beyond Second Order

- Sup. vena cava
  - Innominate (R. brachiocephalic)
    - R. int. jugular
      - R. inf. petrosal sinus
      - R. sigmoid sinus
      - Retromandibular
      - Facial
      - Lingual
      - Sup. thyroid
      - Middle thyroid
      - Pharyngeal
    - R. subclavian
      - R. ext. jugular
    - (Considered one vessel for coding purposes)
    - R. axillary
      - Shoulder & arm veins (eg, brachial, basilic, ulnar, radial)
  - L. brachiocephalic
    - L. int. jugular
      - L. inf. petrosal sinus
      - L. sigmoid sinus
      - Retromandibular
      - Facial
      - Lingual
      - Sup. thyroid
      - Middle thyroid
      - Pharyngeal
    - L. subclavian
      - L. ext. jugular
    - (Considered one vessel for coding purposes)
    - L. axillary
      - Shoulder & arm veins (eg, brachial, basilic, ulnar, radial)
  - Azygos
    - Intercostal(s)
    - Hemiazygos
      - L. asc. lumbar
    - R. asc. lumbar

First Order → Second Order → Beyond Second Order

- **Inf. vena cava**
  - Hepatic (right, middle, left)
  - Segment I (liver)
  - R. inf. phrenic
  - R. suprarenal (R. adrenal)
  - R. renal
  - L. renal
    - L. inf. phrenic
    - L. suprarenal (adrenal)
    - L. gonadal (ovarian/testicular)
  - R. gonadal (ovarian/testicular)
  - Lumbar
  - Common iliac
    - Median (middle) sacral
    - Int. iliac (hypogastric)
      - **Post. division**
        - Iliolumbar
        - Sup. gluteal
        - Lat. sacral
      - **Ant. division**
        - Inf. gluteal
        - Obturator
        - Uterine
        - Sup. and inf. vesical
        - Vaginal/prostate
        - Middle rectal
        - Int. pudendal
        - Rectal plexus
    - Ext. iliac
      - Inf. epigastric
      - Deep circumflex iliac
      - (Considered 1 vessel for coding purposes)
      - Common femoral
        - **Deep system**
          - Deep femoral
          - Femoral (superficial)
            - Popliteal
            - Ant. tibial
            - Post. tibial
            - Peroneal
        - **Superficial system**
          - Great saphenous
          - Small saphenous

- **Portal vein**

  Intrahepatic
  - R. portal
    - Ant. segmental
      - Segment V
      - Segment VIII
    - Post. segmental
      - Segment VI
      - Segment VII
  - L. portal
    - Segment II
    - Segment III
    - Segment IV

  Extrahepatic
  - L. gastric
    - Esophageal
  - R. gastric
  - Cystic
  - Sup. mesenteric
    - R. gastroepiploic
    - Pancreaticoduodenal
    - Jejunal
    - Ileal
    - Middle colic
    - R. colic
    - Ileocolic
      - Appendicular
  - Splenic
    - Short gastric(s)
    - L. gastroepiploic
    - Pancreatic
    - Inf. mesenteric
      - L. colic
      - Sup. rectal

- **Pulmonary artery system**
  - Main pulmonary artery
    - R. pulmonary artery
      - Pulmonary artery segmental branches
    - L. pulmonary artery
      - Pulmonary artery segmental branches

Reference: Standstring, S. *Gray's Anatomy: The Anatomical Basis of Clinical Practice*. 41st ed. New York: Elsevier Limited; 2016.

Arterial Vascular Family: Thorax and Abdomen

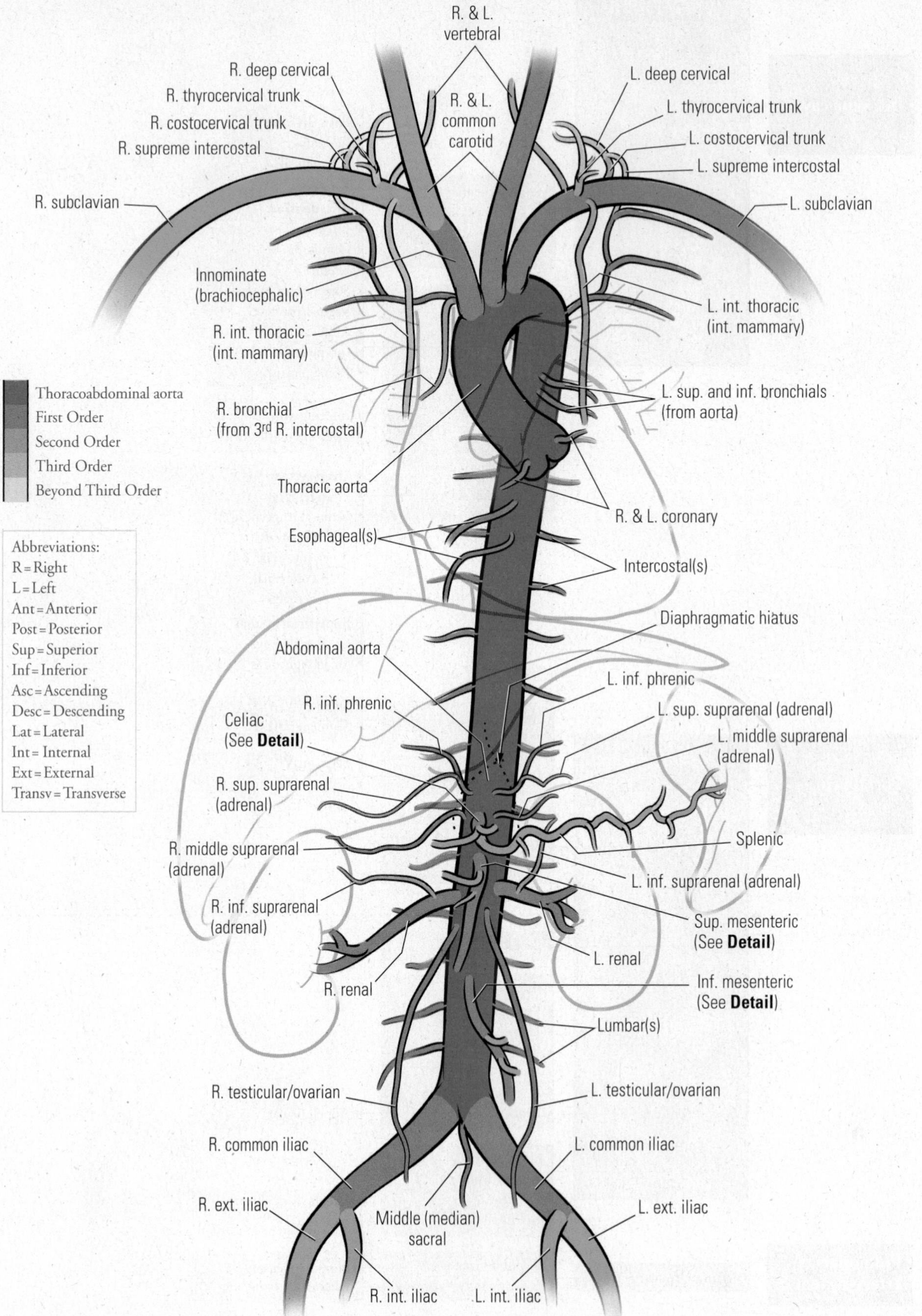

Venous Vascular Family: Thorax and Abdomen

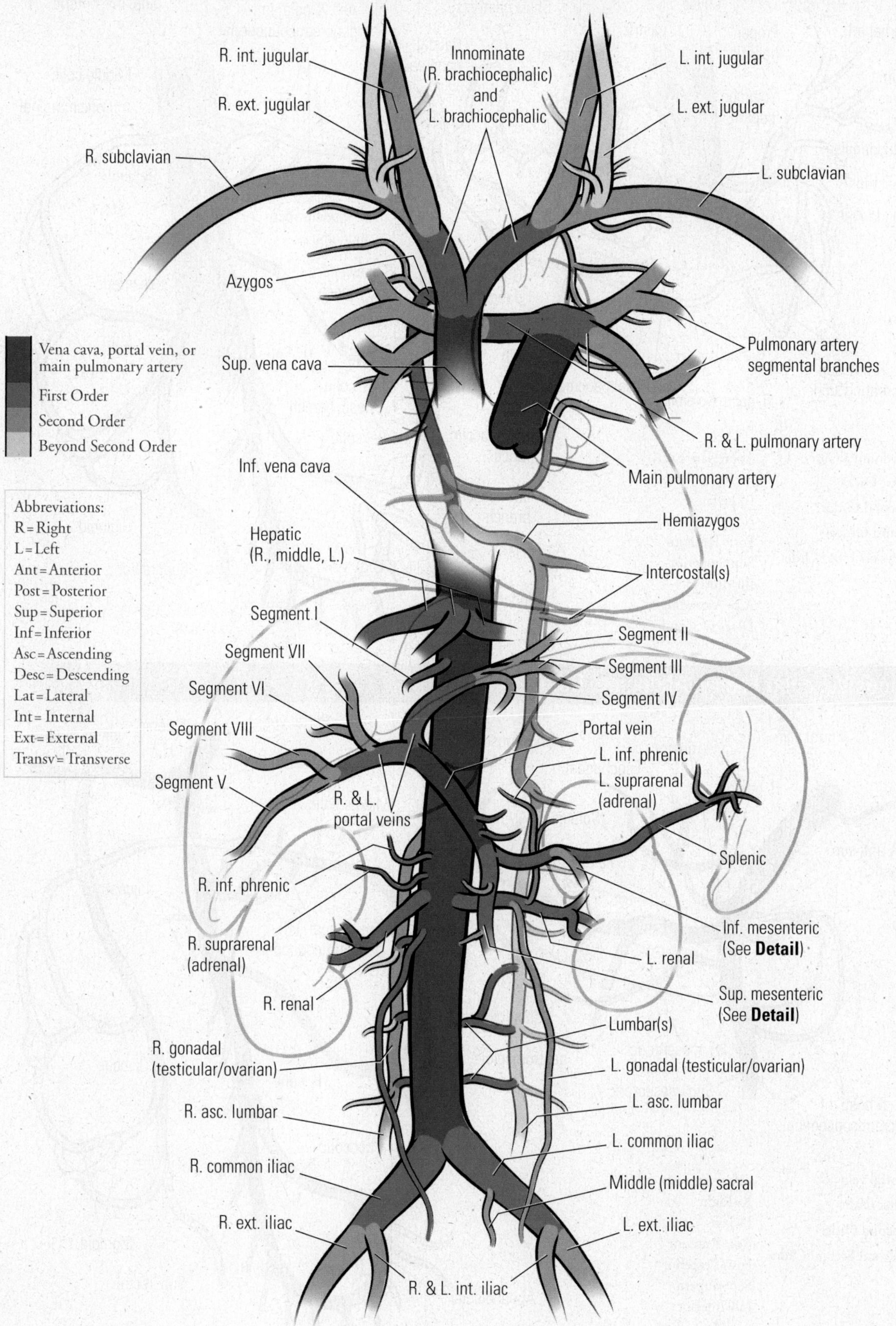

Arterial Vascular Family: Abdomen, Detail

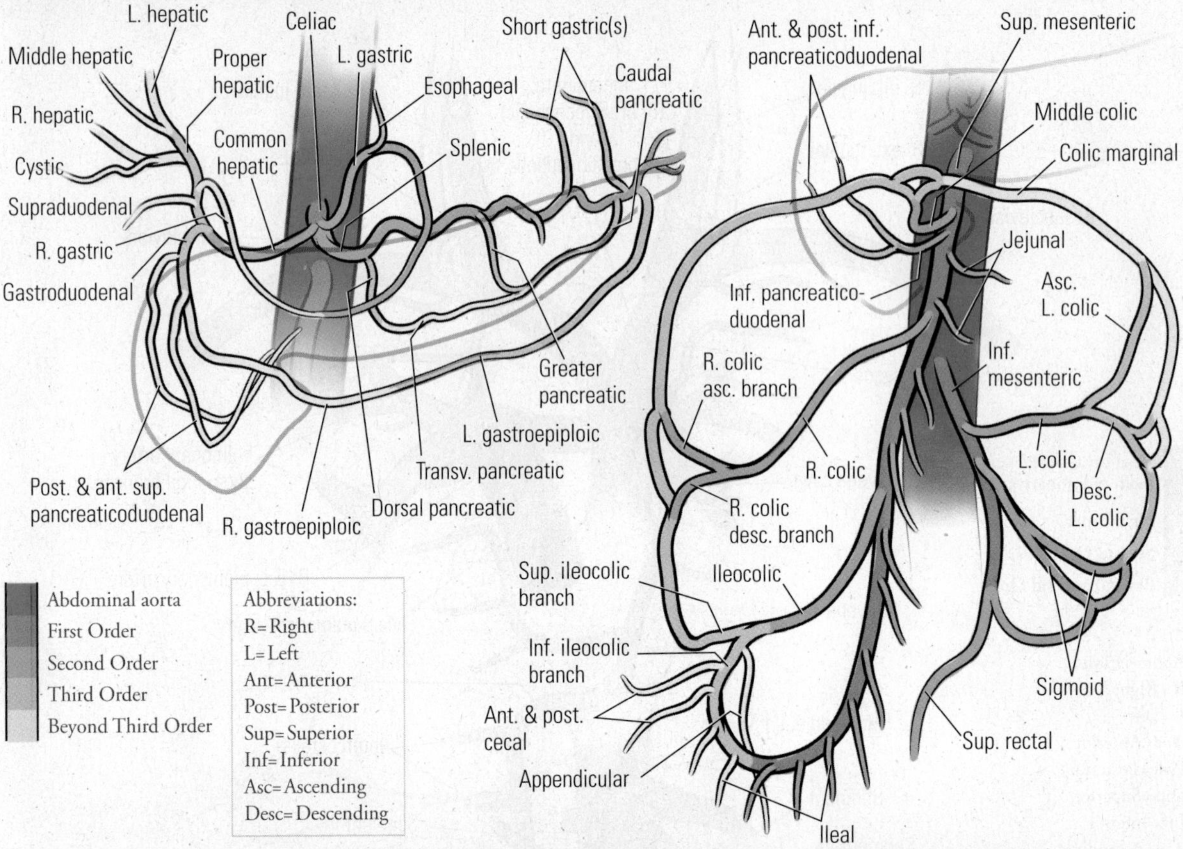

- Abdominal aorta
- First Order
- Second Order
- Third Order
- Beyond Third Order

Abbreviations:
R=Right
L=Left
Ant=Anterior
Post=Posterior
Sup=Superior
Inf=Inferior
Asc=Ascending
Desc=Descending

Venous Vascular Family: Abdomen, Detail

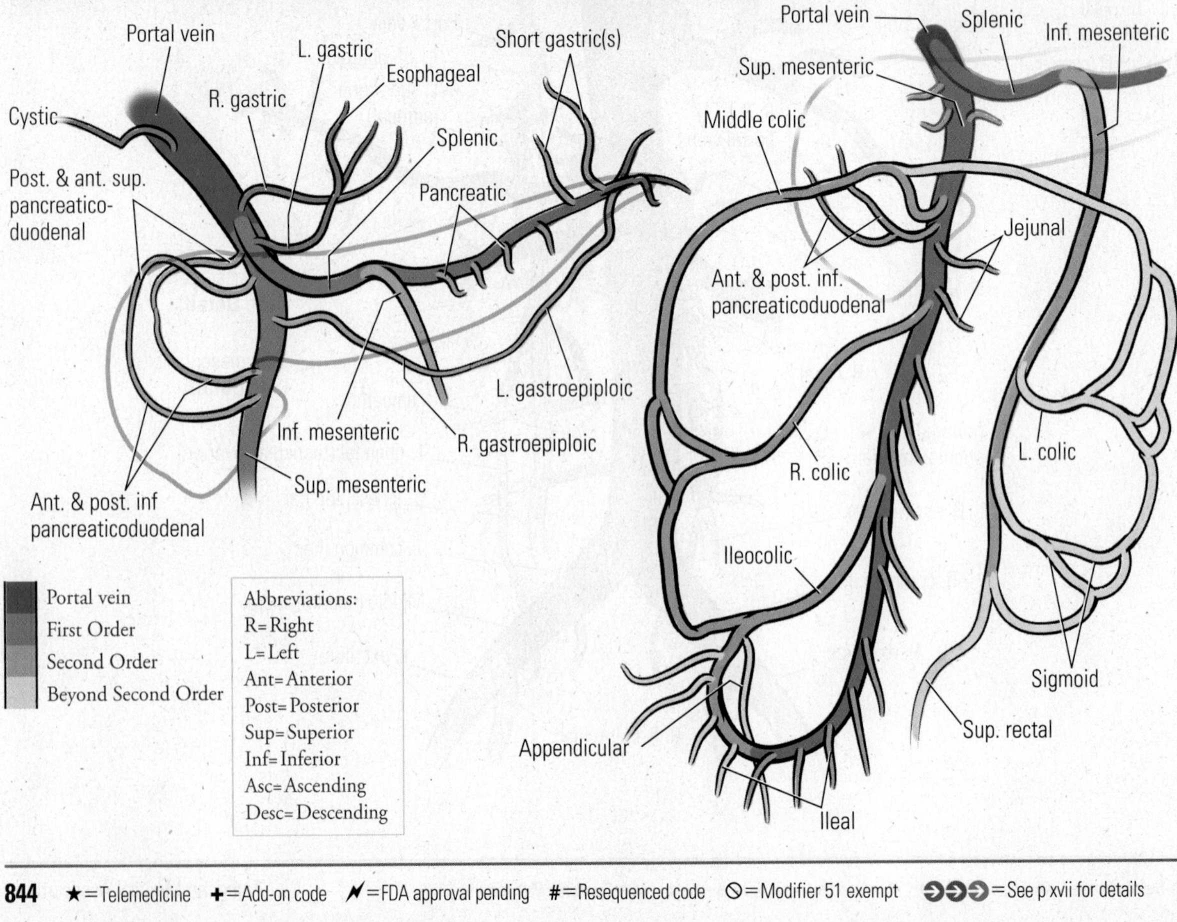

- Portal vein
- First Order
- Second Order
- Beyond Second Order

Abbreviations:
R=Right
L=Left
Ant=Anterior
Post=Posterior
Sup=Superior
Inf=Inferior
Asc=Ascending
Desc=Descending

Arterial Vascular Family: Upper Limb

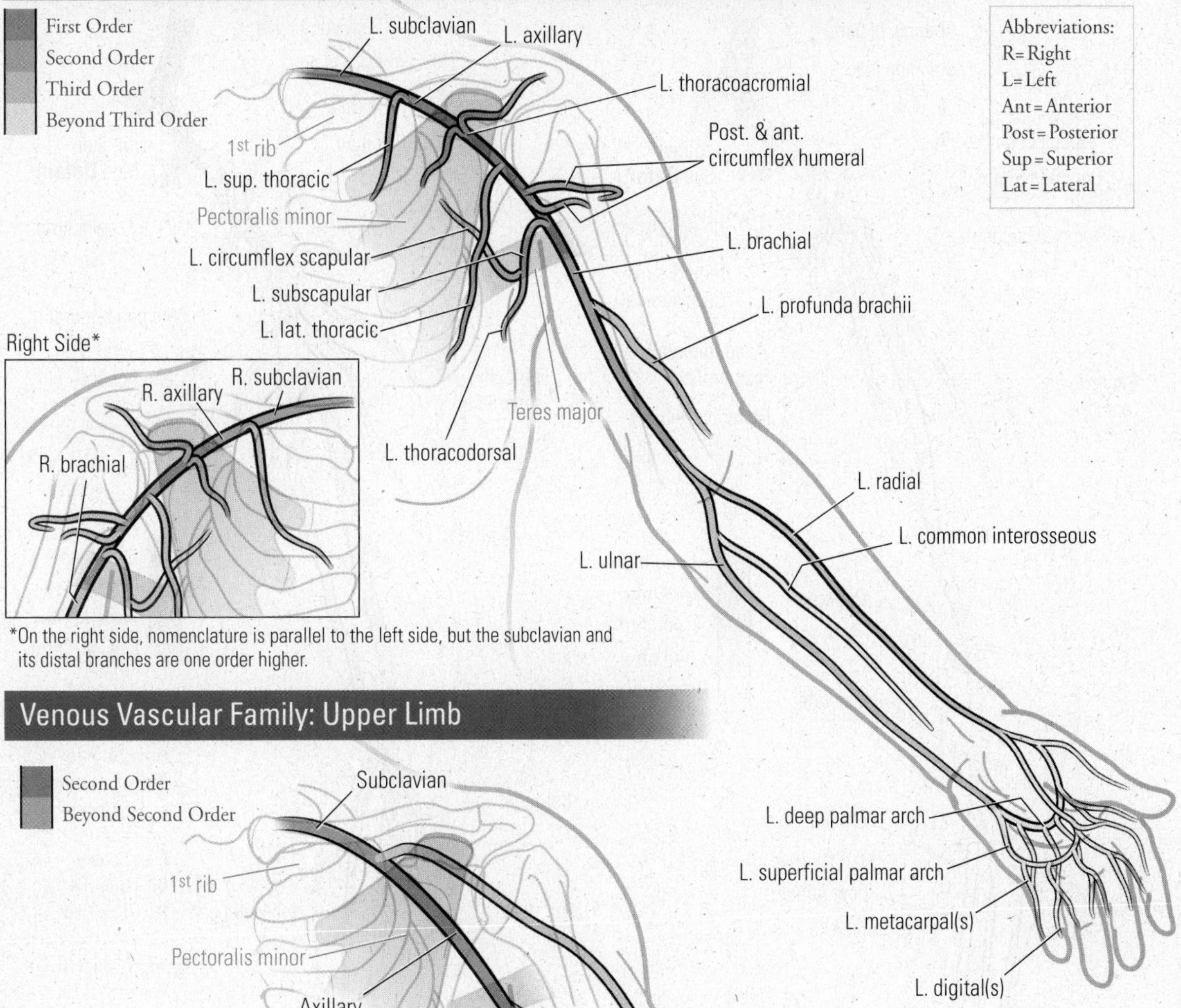

*On the right side, nomenclature is parallel to the left side, but the subclavian and its distal branches are one order higher.

Venous Vascular Family: Upper Limb

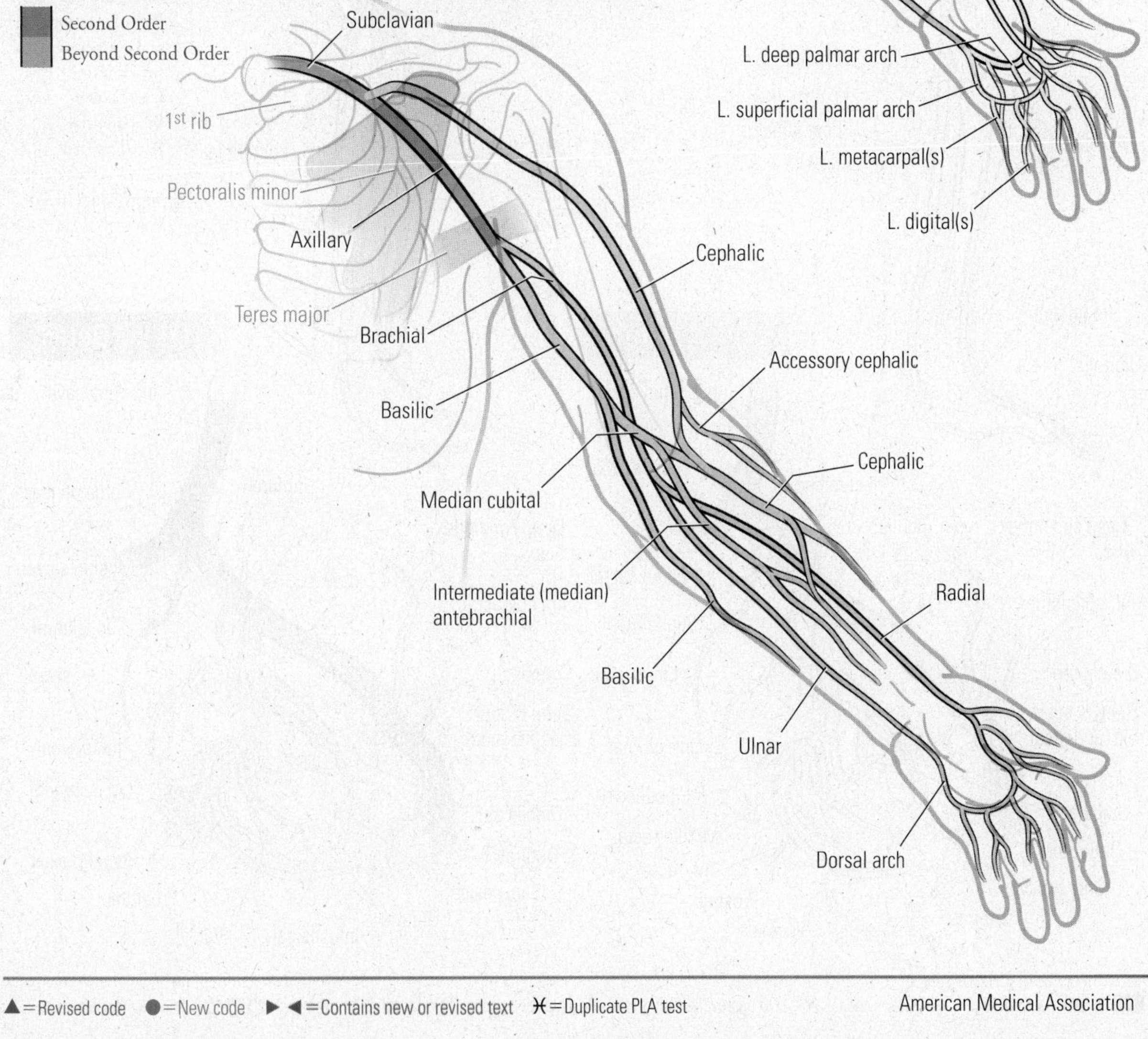

Arterial Vascular Family: Lower Limb

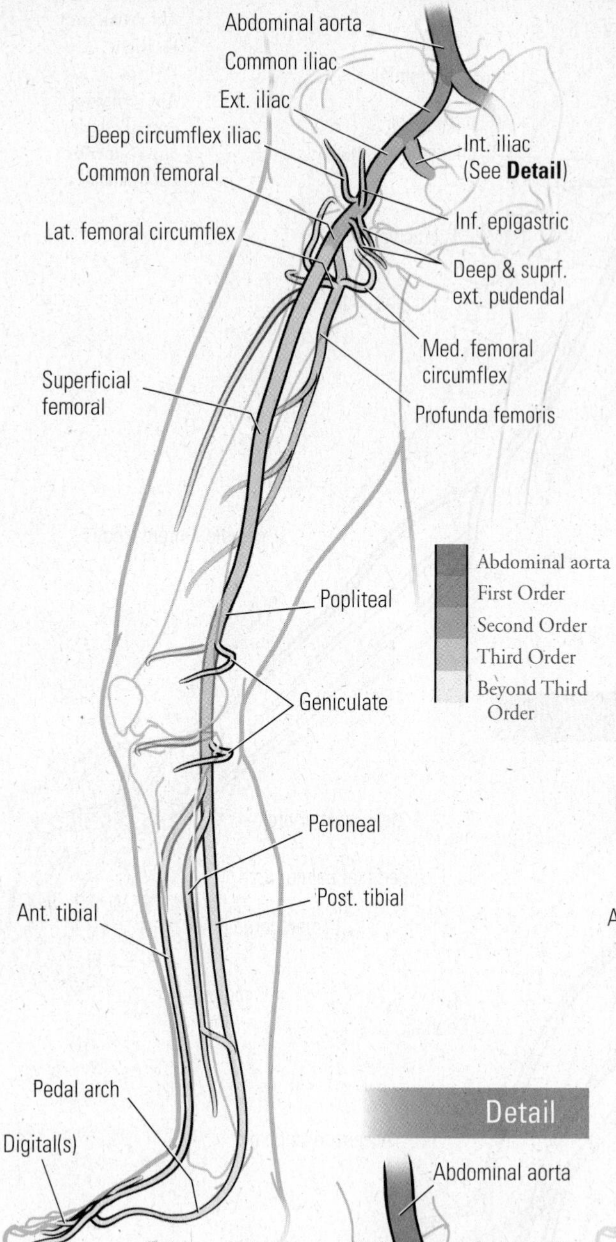

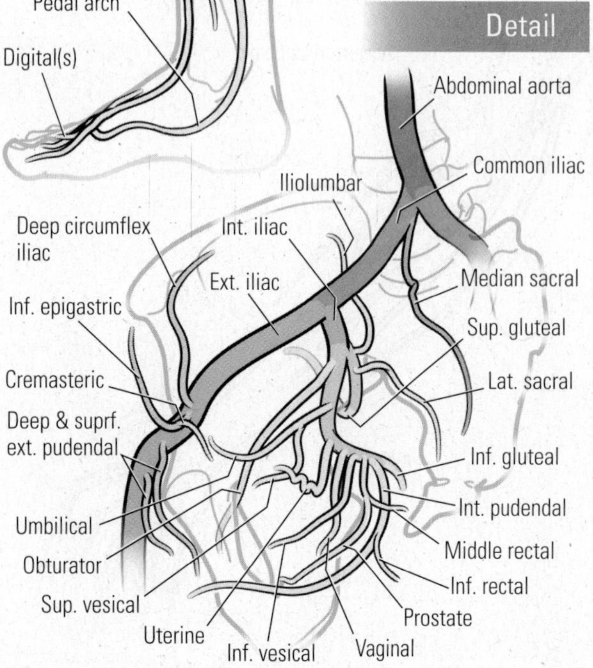

Venous Vascular Family: Lower Limb

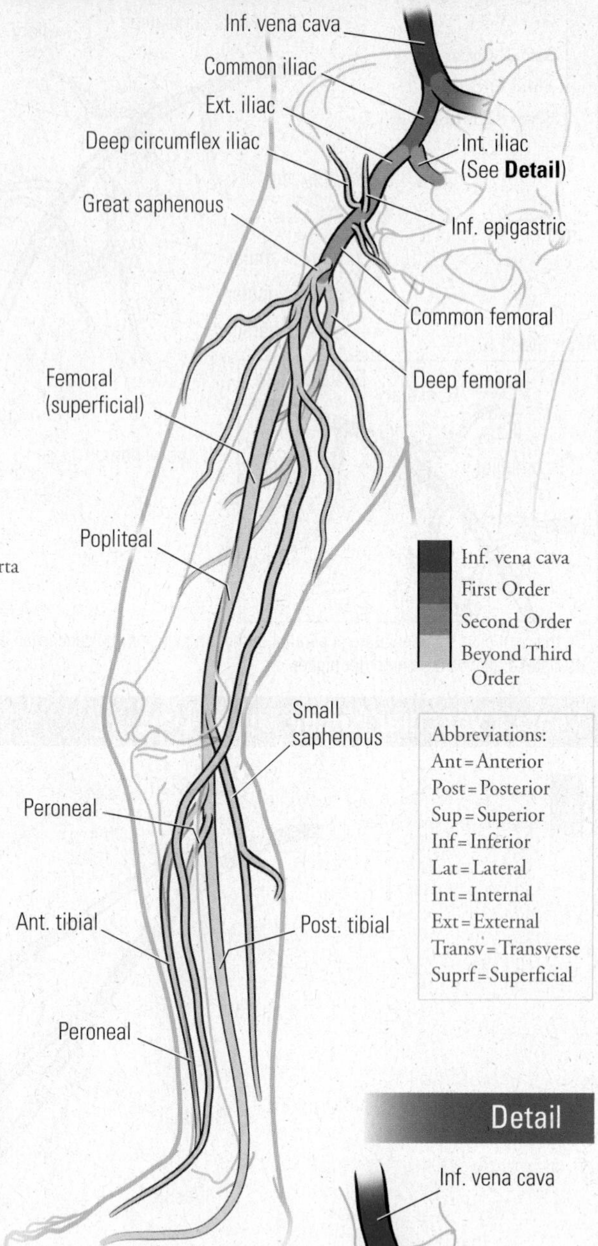

Abbreviations:
Ant = Anterior
Post = Posterior
Sup = Superior
Inf = Inferior
Lat = Lateral
Int = Internal
Ext = External
Transv = Transverse
Suprf = Superficial

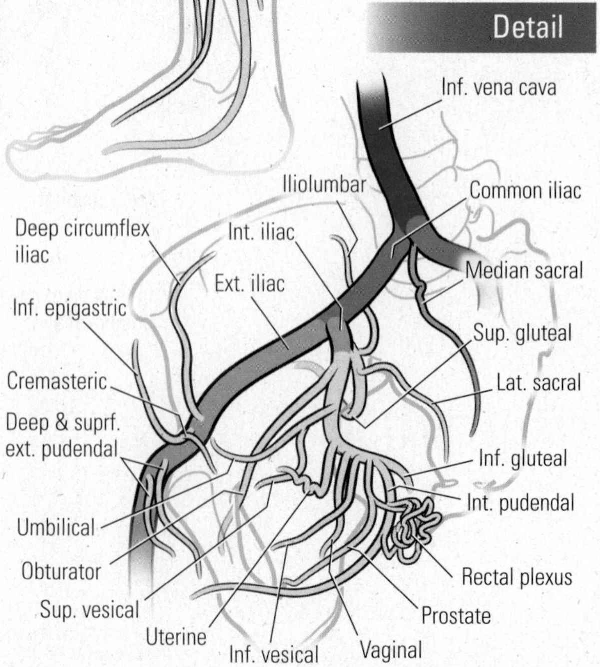

Arterial Vascular Family: Head and Neck

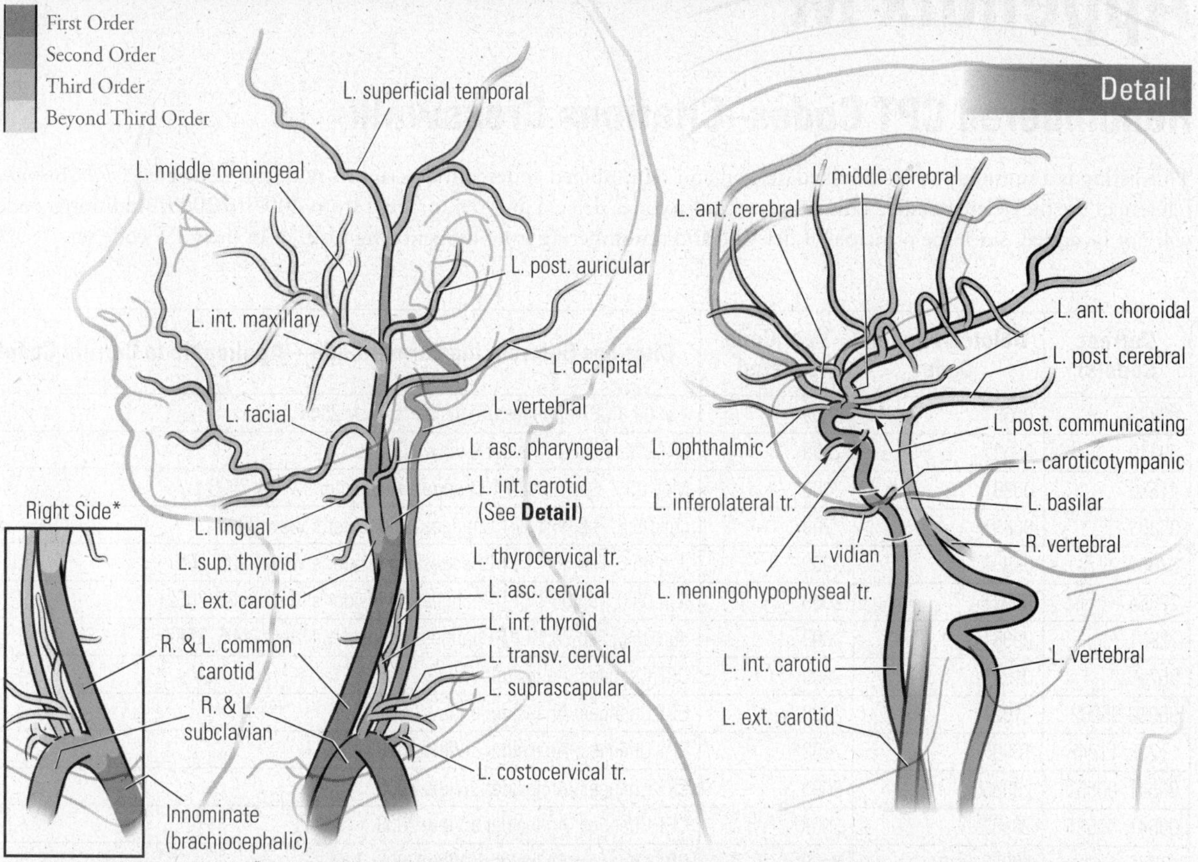

*On the right side, nomenclature is parallel to the left side, but the subclavian and common carotid and their distal branches are one order higher.

Venous Vascular Family: Head and Neck

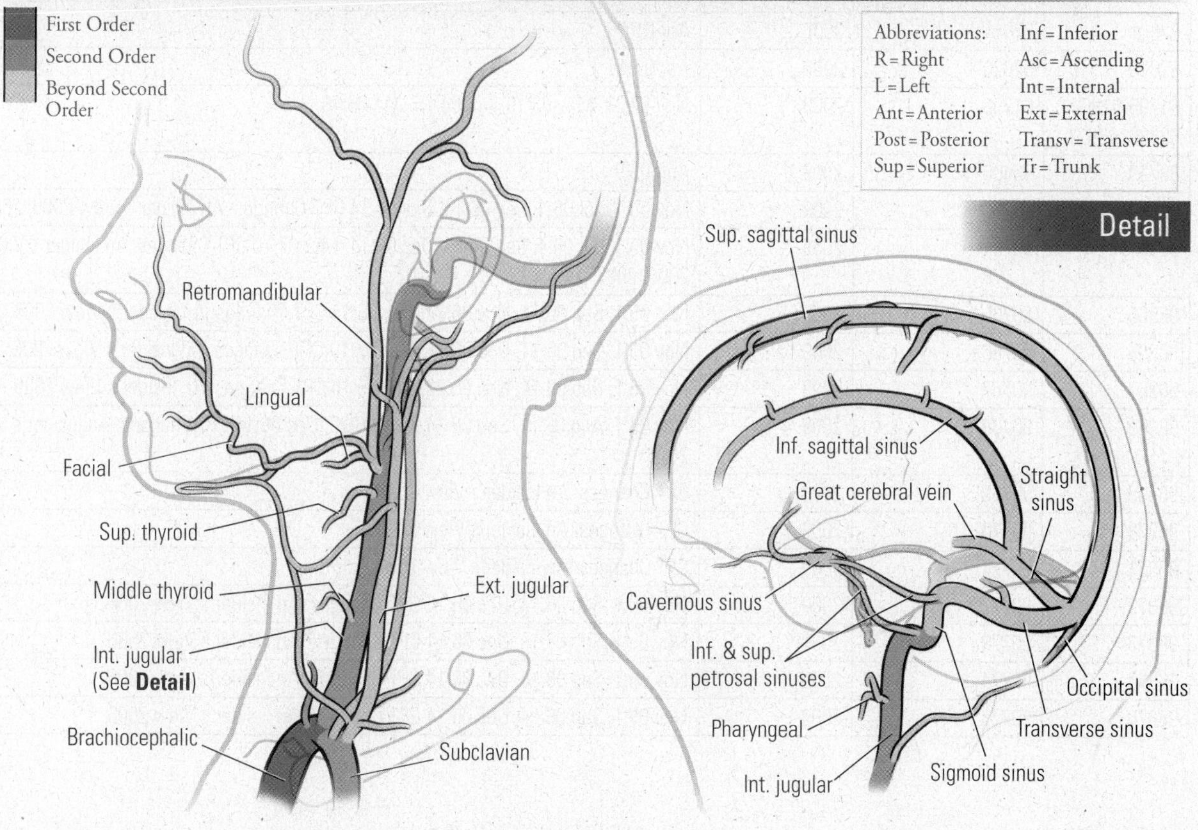

Abbreviations:	
R = Right	Inf = Inferior
L = Left	Asc = Ascending
Ant = Anterior	Int = Internal
Post = Posterior	Ext = External
Sup = Superior	Transv = Transverse
	Tr = Trunk

Appendix M

Renumbered CPT Codes–Citations Crosswalk

This listing is a summary of crosswalked deleted and renumbered codes and descriptors with the associated *CPT Assistant* references for the deleted codes. This listing includes codes deleted and renumbered from 2007 to 2009. Additional codes will not be added, since the principle of deleting and renumbering is no longer being utilized in the CPT code set.

Current Code(s)	Deleted/Former Code	Year Code Deleted	Citations Referencing Former Code—Applicable to Current Code(s)
89240	0058T	2009	Jun 04:8 CPT Changes: An Insider's View 2004
89240	0059T	2009	CPT Changes: An Insider's View 2004
41530	0088T	2009	May 05:7, Sep 05:9 CPT Changes: An Insider's View 2005
95803	0089T	2009	Jun 05:6, Feb 06:1 CPT Changes: An Insider's View 2006
22856	0090T	2009	Jun 05:6, Feb 06:1 CPT Changes: An Insider's View 2006, 2007
22864	0093T	2009	Jun 05:6, Feb 06:1 CPT Changes: An Insider's View 2006, 2007
22861	0096T	2009	Jun 05:6, Feb 06:1 CPT Changes: An Insider's View 2006, 2007
55706	0137T	2009	CPT Changes: An Insider's View 2006
95980-95982	0162T	2009	CPT Changes: An Insider's View 2007
1123F, 1124F	1080F	2009	CPT Changes: An Insider's View 2008
0054T, 0055T	20986	2009	CPT Changes: An Insider's View 2008
0054T, 0055T	20987	2009	CPT Changes: An Insider's View 2008
4177F	4007F	2009	CPT Changes: An Insider's View 2008
52214	52606	2009	Apr 01:4
52601	52612	2009	Apr 01:4
52601	52614	2009	Apr 01:4
52630	52620	2009	Apr 01:4
61796-61800, 63620, 63621	61793	2009	Nov 97:23, May 03:19, Apr 04:15, Jan 06:46
88720	88400	2009	Aug 05:9
96360	90760	2009	Nov 05:1, Jul 06:4, Sep 06:14, Dec 06:14 CPT Changes: An Insider's View 2006, 2008
96361	90761	2009	Nov 05:1, Jul 06:4, Sep 06:14, Dec 06:14, Mar 07:10 CPT Changes: An Insider's View 2006, 2007
96365	90765	2009	Nov 05:1, Sep 06:14, Nov 06:22, Dec 06:14 CPT Changes: An Insider's View 2006
96366	90766	2009	Nov 05:1, Sep 06:14, Dec 06:14, Mar 07:10 CPT Changes: An Insider's View 2006, 2007
96367	90767	2009	Nov 05:1, Sep 06:14, Nov 06:22, Dec 06:14 CPT Changes: An Insider's View 2006
96368	90768	2009	Nov 05:1, Aug 06:11, Sep 06:14, Nov 06:22, Dec 06:14 CPT Changes: An Insider's View 2006
96369	90769	2009	CPT Changes: An Insider's View 2008
96370	90770	2009	CPT Changes: An Insider's View 2008
96371	90771	2009	CPT Changes: An Insider's View 2008
96372	90772	2009	Nov 05:1, Sep 06:14, Dec 06:14 CPT Changes: An Insider's View 2006
96373	90773	2009	Nov 05:1, Sep 06:14, Dec 06:14 CPT Changes: An Insider's View 2006
96374	90774	2009	Nov 05:1, Sep 06:14, Dec 06:14 CPT Changes: An Insider's View 2006
96375	90775	2009	Nov 05:1, Sep 06:14, Dec 06:14 CPT Changes: An Insider's View 2006

Current Code(s)	Deleted/Former Code	Year Code Deleted	Citations Referencing Former Code—Applicable to Current Code(s)
96376	90776	2009	CPT Changes: An Insider's View 2008
96379	90779	2009	Nov 05:1, Sep 06:14, Dec 06:14 CPT Changes: An Insider's View 2006
90951-90953, 90963, 90967	90918	2009	Fall 93:5, May 96:4, May 02:17, Jan 03:22
90954-90956, 90964, 90968	90919	2009	Fall 93:5, May 96:5, May 02:17, Jan 03:22
90957-90959, 90965, 90969	90920	2009	Fall 93:5, May 96:5, May 02:17, Jan 03:22
90960-90962, 90966, 90970	90921	2009	Fall 93:5, May 96:5, May 02:17, Jan 03:22
90951-90953, 90963, 90967	90922	2009	Fall 93:5, May 96:5, May 02:17, Jan 03:22
90954-90956, 90964, 90968	90923	2009	May 96:5, May 02:17, Jan 03:22
90957-90959, 90965, 90969	90924	2009	May 96:5, May 02:17, Jan 03:22
90960-90962, 90966, 90970	90925	2009	May 96:5, May 02:17, Jan 03:22
93285, 93291, 93298	93727	2009	Nov 99:50, Jul 00:5, CPT Changes: An Insider's View 2000
93280, 93288, 93294	93731	2009	Summer 94:23, Feb 98:11
93280, 93288, 93294	93732	2009	Summer 94:23, Feb 98:11, Mar 00:10
93293	93733	2009	Summer 94:23
93279, 93288, 93294	93734	2009	Summer 94:23, Feb 98:11
93279, 93288, 93294	93735	2009	Summer 94:23, Feb 98:11
93293	93736	2009	Summer 94:23
93282, 93289, 93292, 93295	93741	2009	Nov 99:50-51, Jul 00:5, Nov 00:9, Sep 05:8 CPT Changes: An Insider's View 2000, 2005
93282, 93289, 93292, 93295	93742	2009	Nov 99:50-51, Jul 00:5, Nov 00:9 CPT Changes: An Insider's View 2000, 2005
93283, 93289, 93295	93743	2009	Nov 99:50-51, Jul 00:5, Nov 00:9, Sep 05:8 CPT Changes: An Insider's View 2000
93283, 93289, 93295	93744	2009	Nov 99:50-51, Jul 00:5, Nov 00:9 CPT Changes: An Insider's View 2000
99466	99289	2009	May 05:1, Jul 06:4 CPT Changes: An Insider's View 2002, 2003
99467	99290	2009	CPT Changes: An Insider's View 2002
99468	99295	2009	Summer 93:1, Nov 97:4-5, Mar 98:11, Nov 99:5-6, Dec 00:14, Feb 03:15, Oct 03:1, May 05:1, Nov 05:10, CPT Changes: An Insider's View 2000, 2003, 2004, 2005
99469	99296	2009	Summer 93:1, Nov 97:4-5, Mar 98:11, Nov 99:5-6, Dec 00:14, Feb 03:15, Oct 03:1, Nov 05:10, CPT Changes: An Insider's View 2000, 2003, 2004, 2005, 2008
99471	99293	2009	Feb 03:15, Oct 03:2, Aug 04:7, 10, May 05:1, Nov 05:10, Jul 06:4, Apr 07:3 CPT Changes: An Insider's View 2003, 2004, 2005
99472	99294	2009	Feb 03:15, Oct 03:2, Aug 04:7, Nov 05:10, Jul 06:4, Apr 07:3 CPT Changes: An Insider's View 2003, 2004, 2005

Current Code(s)	Deleted/Former Code	Year Code Deleted	Citations Referencing Former Code—Applicable to Current Code(s)
99478	99298	2009	Nov 98:2-3, Nov 99: 5-6, Aug 00:4, Dec 00:15, Oct 03:2, May 05:1, Nov 05:10; CPT Changes: An Insider's View 2000, 2003
99479	99299	2009	Oct 03:2, Nov 05:10; CPT Changes: An Insider's View 2003
99480	99300	2009	CPT Changes: An Insider's View 2006
99460	99431	2009	Apr 97:10, Nov 97:9, Sep 98:5, Apr 04:14, May 05:1
99461	99432	2009	Sep 98:5, May 99:11, Apr 04:14
99462	99433	2009	Sep 98:5, Apr 03:27
99463	99435	2009	Sep 98:5, Apr 04:14
99464	99436	2009	Nov 97:9-10, Sep 98:5, Nov 99:5-6, Aug 00:3, Aug 04:9, Nov 05:15
99465	99440	2009	Summer 93:3, Mar 96:10, Nov 97:9, Sep 98:5, Nov 99:5-6, Aug 00:3, Oct 03:3, Aug 04:9, Apr 07:3
20985	0054T	2008	May 04:14, Jun 04:8 CPT Changes: An Insider's View 2004
20985	0055T	2008	May 04:14, Jun 04:8 CPT Changes: An Insider's View 2004, 2005
20985	0056T	2008	May 04:14, Jun 04:8 CPT Changes: An Insider's View 2004
99174	0065T	2008	Mar 05:1, 3-4 CPT Changes: An Insider's View 2005
99444	0074T	2008	May 05:7, Sep 05:6 CPT Changes: An Insider's View 2005
99605-99607	0115T	2008	CPT Changes: An Insider's View 2006
99605-99607	0116T	2008	CPT Changes: An Insider's View 2006
99605-99607	0117T	2008	CPT Changes: An Insider's View 2006
50593	0135T	2008	CPT Changes: An Insider's View 2006, Clinical Examples in Radiology Winter 06:18
01935, 01936	01905	2008	Mar 06:15 CPT Changes: An Insider's View 2002
24357-24359	24350	2008	
24357-24359	24351	2008	
24357-24359	24352	2008	
24357-24359	24354	2008	
24357-24359	24356	2008	
3044F-3045F	3047F	2008	CPT Changes: An Insider's View 2007
3074F-3075F	3076F	2008	CPT Changes: An Insider's View 2007
32560	32005	2008	
32550	32019	2008	CPT Changes: An Insider's View 2005
32551	32020	2008	Fall 92:13, Nov 03:14
36591	36540	2008	Jan 02:11, Nov 02:3, Apr 03:26, Nov 05:1 CPT Changes: An Insider's View 2001, 2003
36593	36550	2008	Nov 99:20, Nov 05:1 CPT Changes: An Insider's View 2000
49203-49205, 58957, 58958	49200	2008	CPT Changes: An Insider's View 2003
49203-49205, 58957, 58958	49201	2008	
51100	51000	2008	Nov 99:32-33, Aug 00:3, Oct 03:2
51101	51005	2008	
51102	51010	2008	
60300	60001	2008	
67041, 67042, 67043	67038	2008	Aug 03:15, Sep 05:12
75557, 75559, 75561,75563	75552	2008	Fall 95:2

Current Code(s)	Deleted/Former Code	Year Code Deleted	Citations Referencing Former Code—Applicable to Current Code(s)
75557, 75559, 75561,75563	75553	2008	Fall 95:2
75557, 75559, 75561,75563	75554	2008	Fall 95:2
75557, 75559, 75561,75563	75555	2008	Fall 95:2
75557, 75559, 75561,75563	75556	2008	Fall 95:2
78610	78615	2008	CPT Changes: An Insider's View 2002
86356, 86486	86586	2008	Jul 98:11
99366-99368	99361	2008	May 05:1
99366-99368	99362	2008	
99441-99443	99371	2008	Spring 94:34, May 00:11, May 05:1, Nov 05:10
99441-99443	99372	2008	Spring 94:34, May 00:11, Nov 05:10
99441-99443	99373	2008	Spring 94:34, May 00:11, Nov 05:10
96904	0044T	2007	CPT Changes: An Insider's View 2003, 2004
96904	0045T	2007	Jul 04:7 CPT Changes: An Insider's View 2004
77371-77373	0082T	2007	CPT Changes: An Insider's View 2005
77371-77373	0083T	2007	CPT Changes: An Insider's View 2005
22857	0091T	2007	CPT Changes: An Insider's View 2006
22865	0094T	2007	CPT Changes: An Insider's View 2006
22862	0097T	2007	CPT Changes: An Insider's View 2006
19105	0120T	2007	CPT Changes: An Insider's View 2006
15002, 15004	15000	2007	Fall 93:7, Apr 97:4, Aug 97:6, Sep 97:2, Nov 98:5, Jan 99:4, Apr 99:10, May 99:10, Nov 02:7, Aug 03:14 CPT Changes: An Insider's View 2001, 2006
15003, 15005	15001	2007	Nov 98:5-6, Jan 99:4, May 99:10, Aug 03:14
15830, 15847, 17999	15831	2007	May 01:11 CPT Changes: An Insider's View 2007
17311	17304	2007	Winter 94:19, Mar 99:11, Jun 99:10, Nov 02:7, Nov 03:15, Feb 04:11, Jul 04:2 CPT Changes: An Insider's View 2003
17312, 17314	17305	2007	Winter 94:19, Mar 99:11, Jun 99:10, Nov 02:7, Feb 04:11, Jul 04:3
17312, 17314	17306	2007	Winter 94:19, Mar 99:11, Jun 99:10, Nov 02:7, Feb 04:11, Jul 04:4
17312, 17314	17307	2007	Winter 94:19, Mar 99:11, Jun 99:10, Nov 02:7, Nov 03:15, Feb 04:11, Jul 04:4
17315	17310	2007	Winter 94:19, Mar 99:11, Jun 99:10, Nov 02:7, Feb 04:11, May 04:14, Jul 04:4 CPT Changes: An Insider's View 2003
19300	19140	2007	Feb 96:9, Apr 05:13
19301	19160	2007	Apr 05:7 CPT Changes: An Insider's View 2005
19302	19162	2007	Jun 00:11, Apr 05:7
19303	19180	2007	Apr 05:7
19304	19182	2007	Apr 05:7
19305	19200	2007	Apr 05:7
19306	19220	2007	Apr 05:7
19307	19240	2007	Apr 05:7
25606	25611	2007	Fall 93:23, Oct 99:5
25607-25609	25620	2007	
26390	26504	2007	

Appendix M

Current Code(s)	Deleted/Former Code	Year Code Deleted	Citations Referencing Former Code—Applicable to Current Code(s)
27325	27315	2007	
27326	27320	2007	
28055	28030	2007	
33254-33256	33253	2007	
35302-35306	35381	2007	
35506	35507	2007	
35537, 35538	35541	2007	
35539, 35540	35546	2007	
35637, 35638	35641	2007	Dec 01:7
44799	44152	2007	
44799	44153	2007	
48105	48005	2007	
48548	48180	2007	
49402	49085	2007	
54150	54152	2007	Sep 96:11, Dec 96:10, May 98:11, Apr 03:27 CPT Changes: An Insider's View 2007
54865	54820	2007	Oct 01:8
55875	55859	2007	Apr 04:6
56442	56720	2007	
57558	57820	2007	
67346	67350	2007	
77001	75998	2007	Dec 04:12-13 CPT Changes: An Insider's View 2004 Clinical Examples in Radiology Inaugural 04:1-2, Winter 05:9
77002	76003	2007	Fall 93:14, Jul 01:7 CPT Changes: An Insider's View 2001 Clinical Examples in Radiology Spring 05:5-6
77003	76005	2007	Nov 99:32, 34, 41, Jan 00:2, Feb 00:6, Aug 00:8, Sep 02:11, Sep 04:5 CPT Changes: An Insider's View 2000
77071	76006	2007	Nov 98:21 CPT Changes: An Insider's View 2003
77072	76020	2007	
77073	76040	2007	
77074	76061	2007	
77075	76062	2007	
77076	76065	2007	
77077	76066	2007	CPT Changes: An Insider's View 2002
77078	76070	2007	Nov 97:24 CPT Changes: An Insider's View 2002, 2003
77080	76075	2007	Nov 97:24, Jun 03:11 CPT Changes: An Insider's View 2005
77081	76076	2007	Nov 97:24
77053	76086	2007	
77054	76088	2007	
77011	76355	2007	CPT Changes: An Insider's View 2002, 2003
77012	76360	2007	Fall 93:12, Fall 94:2, Jan 01:9-10, Mar 05:2 CPT Changes: An Insider's View 2001, 2002, 2003
77013	76362	2007	Oct 02:4 CPT Changes: An Insider's View 2002, 2004
77014	76370	2007	Fall 91:12 CPT Changes: An Insider's View 2002, 2003

Current Code(s)	Deleted/Former Code	Year Code Deleted	Citations Referencing Former Code—Applicable to Current Code(s)
77021	76393	2007	Jan 01:10, Mar 05:2 CPT Changes: An Insider's View 2001, 2002
77022	76394	2007	Oct 02:4, Mar 05:5 CPT Changes: An Insider's View 2002, 2004
77084	76400	2007	
76775, 76776	76778	2007	CPT Changes: An Insider's View 2002
76998	76986	2007	CPT Changes: An Insider's View 2001
78707-78709	78704	2007	
78701, 78707, 78708, 78709	78715	2007	
78761	78760	2007	
92700	92573	2007	
94002, 94004	94656	2007	Fall 92:30, Spring 95:4, Summer 95:4, Feb 96:9, Aug 00:2, Oct 03:2
94003, 94004	94657	2007	Fall 92:30, Spring 95:4, Summer 95:4, Feb 96:9, Aug 00:2, Oct 03:2

Appendix N

Appendix N

Summary of Resequenced CPT Codes

This is a table of CPT codes that do not appear in numeric sequence in the listing of CPT codes and the code ranges with their corresponding locations. Rather than deleting and renumbering, resequencing allows existing codes to be relocated to an appropriate location for the code concept, regardless of the numeric sequence. The codes listed below are identified in the CPT 2019 code set with a # symbol for the location of the resequenced number within the family of related concepts. Numerically placed references (eg, **Code is out of numerical sequence. See...**) are used as navigational alerts to direct the user to the location of an out-of-sequence code.

Resequenced Code	Corresponding Locations of Resequenced Code
10004	10021-10035
10005	10021-10035
10006	10021-10035
10007	10021-10035
10008	10021-10035
10009	10021-10035
10010	10021-10035
10011	10021-10035
10012	10021-10035
11045	11012-11047
11046	11012-11047
21552	21550-21558
21554	21550-21558
22858	22853-22861
22859	22853-22861
23071	23066-23078
23073	23066-23078
24071	24066-24079
24073	24066-24079
25071	25066-25078
25073	25066-25078
26111	26110-26118
26113	26110-26118
27043	27041-27052
27045	27041-27052
27059	27041-27052
27329	27358-27365
27337	27326-27331
27339	27326-27331
27632	27616-27625

Resequenced Code	Corresponding Locations of Resequenced Code
27634	27616-27625
28039	28035-28047
28041	28035-28047
28295	28292-28298
29914	29862-29867
29915	29862-29867
29916	29862-29867
31253	31254-31267
31257	31254-31267
31259	31254-31267
31551	31579-31587
31552	31579-31587
31553	31579-31587
31554	31579-31587
31572	31577-31580
31573	31577-31580
31574	31577-31580
31651	31646-31649
32994	32997-32999
33221	33212-33215
33227	33226-33244
33228	33226-33244
33229	33226-33244
33230	33226-33244
33231	33226-33244
33262	33226-33244
33263	33226-33244
33264	33226-33244
33270	33244-33251
33271	33244-33251

Resequenced Code	Corresponding Locations of Resequenced Code
33272	33244-33251
33273	33244-33251
33274	33244-33251
33275	33244-33251
33440	33406-33412
33962	33958-33968
33963	33958-33968
33964	33958-33968
33965	33958-33968
33966	33958-33968
33969	33958-33968
33984	33958-33968
33985	33958-33968
33986	33958-33968
33987	33958-33968
33988	33958-33968
33989	33958-33968
34812	34712-34716
34820	34712-34716
34833	34712-34716
34834	34712-34716
36465	36470-36474
36466	36470-36474
36482	36478-36500
36483	36478-36500
36572	36568-36571
36573	36568-36571
37246	37234-37237
37247	37234-37237
37248	37234-37237

Resequenced Code	Corresponding Locations of Resequenced Code
37249	37234-37237
38243	38240-38300
43210	43254-43261
43211	43216-43227
43212	43216-43227
43213	43216-43227
43214	43216-43227
43233	43248-43251
43266	43254-43261
43270	43254-43261
43274	43264-43279
43275	43264-43279
43276	43264-43279
43277	43264-43279
43278	43264-43279
44381	44380-44385
44401	44391-44402
45346	45337-45341
45388	45381-45385
45390	45391-45397
45398	45391-45397
45399	45910-45999
46220	46200-46255
46320	46200-46255
46945	46200-46255
46946	46200-46255
46947	46760-46910
50430	50390-50405
50431	50390-50405
50432	50390-50405

Resequenced Code	Corresponding Locations of Resequenced Code
50433	50390-50405
50434	50390-50405
50435	50390-50405
50436	50390-50405
50437	50390-50405
51797	51728-51741
52356	52352-52355
58674	58520-58542
64461	64483-64487
64462	64483-64487
64463	64483-64487
64633	64617-64632
64634	64617-64632
64635	64617-64632
64636	64617-64632
67810	67710-67801
77085	77080-77261
77086	77080-77261
77295	77293-77301
77385	77412-77427
77386	77412-77427
77387	77412-77427
77424	77412-77427
77425	77412-77427
80081	80053-80069
80164	80200-80203
80165	80200-80203
80171	80168-80173
80305	See Presumptive Drug Class Screening subsection
80306	See Presumptive Drug Class Screening subsection
80307	See Presumptive Drug Class Screening subsection
80320	See Definitive Drug Testing subsection
80321	See Definitive Drug Testing subsection
80322	See Definitive Drug Testing subsection
80323	See Definitive Drug Testing subsection
80324	See Definitive Drug Testing subsection
80325	See Definitive Drug Testing subsection
80326	See Definitive Drug Testing subsection
80327	See Definitive Drug Testing subsection
80328	See Definitive Drug Testing subsection
80329	See Definitive Drug Testing subsection
80330	See Definitive Drug Testing subsection
80331	See Definitive Drug Testing subsection
80332	See Definitive Drug Testing subsection
80333	See Definitive Drug Testing subsection
80334	See Definitive Drug Testing subsection
80335	See Definitive Drug Testing subsection
80336	See Definitive Drug Testing subsection
80337	See Definitive Drug Testing subsection
80338	See Definitive Drug Testing subsection
80339	See Definitive Drug Testing subsection
80340	See Definitive Drug Testing subsection
80341	See Definitive Drug Testing subsection
80342	See Definitive Drug Testing subsection
80343	See Definitive Drug Testing subsection
80344	See Definitive Drug Testing subsection
80345	See Definitive Drug Testing subsection
80346	See Definitive Drug Testing subsection
80347	See Definitive Drug Testing subsection
80348	See Definitive Drug Testing subsection
80349	See Definitive Drug Testing subsection
80350	See Definitive Drug Testing subsection
80351	See Definitive Drug Testing subsection
80352	See Definitive Drug Testing subsection
80353	See Definitive Drug Testing subsection
80354	See Definitive Drug Testing subsection
80355	See Definitive Drug Testing subsection
80356	See Definitive Drug Testing subsection
80357	See Definitive Drug Testing subsection
80358	See Definitive Drug Testing subsection
80359	See Definitive Drug Testing subsection
80360	See Definitive Drug Testing subsection
80361	See Definitive Drug Testing subsection
80362	See Definitive Drug Testing subsection
80363	See Definitive Drug Testing subsection
80364	See Definitive Drug Testing subsection
80365	See Definitive Drug Testing subsection
80366	See Definitive Drug Testing subsection
80367	See Definitive Drug Testing subsection
80368	See Definitive Drug Testing subsection
80369	See Definitive Drug Testing subsection
80370	See Definitive Drug Testing subsection
80371	See Definitive Drug Testing subsection
80372	See Definitive Drug Testing subsection
80373	See Definitive Drug Testing subsection
80374	See Definitive Drug Testing subsection
80375	See Definitive Drug Testing subsection

Resequenced Code	Corresponding Locations of Resequenced Code
80376	See Definitive Drug Testing subsection
80377	See Definitive Drug Testing subsection
81105	81255-81270
81106	81255-81270
81107	81255-81270
81108	81255-81270
81109	81255-81270
81110	81255-81270
81111	81255-81270
81112	81255-81270
81120	81255-81270
81121	81255-81270
81161	81228-81235
81162	81182-81220
81163	81182-81220
81164	81182-81220
81165	81182-81220
81166	81182-81220
81167	81182-81220
81173	81171-81176
81174	81171-81176
81184	81182-81220
81185	81182-81220
81186	81182-81220
81187	81223-81226
81188	81223-81226
81189	81223-81226
81190	81223-81226
81200	81171-81176
81201	81171-81176
81202	81171-81176
81203	81171-81176
81204	81171-81176
81205	81182-81220
81206	81182-81220
81207	81182-81220
81208	81182-81220
81209	81182-81220
81210	81182-81220
81219	81182-81220
81227	81223-81226

Resequenced Code	Corresponding Locations of Resequenced Code
81230	81225-81229
81231	81225-81229
81233	81182-81220
81234	81228-81235
81238	81240-81248
81239	81228-81235
81245	81240-81248
81246	81240-81248
81250	81243-81248
81257	81253-81256
81258	81253-81256
81259	81253-81256
81261	81255-81270
81262	81255-81270
81263	81255-81270
81264	81255-81270
81265	81223-81226
81266	81223-81226
81267	81223-81226
81268	81223-81226
81269	81253-81256
81271	81255-81270
81274	81255-81270
81283	81255-81270
81284	81243-81248
81285	81243-81248
81286	81243-81248
81287	81276-81297
81288	81276-81297
81289	81243-81248
81291	81299-81310
81292	81276-81297
81293	81276-81297
81294	81276-81297
81295	81276-81297
81301	81276-81297
81302	81276-81297
81303	81276-81297
81304	81276-81297
81306	81310-81318
81312	81310-81318
81320	81310-81318
81324	81310-81318
81325	81310-81318

Resequenced Code	Corresponding Locations of Resequenced Code
81326	81310-81318
81332	81318-81335
81334	81318-81335
81336	81318-81335
81337	81318-81335
81343	81318-81335
81344	81318-81335
81345	81318-81335
81361	81253-81256
81362	81253-81256
81363	81253-81256
81364	81253-81256
81448	81437-81440
81479	81407-81411
82042	82044-82085
82652	82300-82310
83992	See Definitive Drug Testing subsection
86152	86146-86155
86153	86146-86155
87623	87538-87541
87624	87538-87541
87625	87538-87541
87806	87802-87903
87906	87802-87903
87910	87802-87903
87912	87802-87903
88177	88172-88175
88341	88334-88372
88350	88334-88372
88364	88334-88372
88373	88334-88372
88374	88334-88372
88377	88334-88372
90620	90717-90739
90621	90717-90739
90625	90717-90739
90630	90653-90656
90644	90717-90739
90672	90658-90664
90673	90658-90664
90674	90658-90664
90750	90717-90739
90756	90658-90664

Resequenced Code	Corresponding Locations of Resequenced Code
92558	92585-92588
92597	92603-92607
92618	92603-92607
92920	92997-93005
92921	92997-93005
92924	92997-93005
92925	92997-93005
92928	92997-93005
92929	92997-93005
92933	92997-93005
92934	92997-93005
92937	92997-93005
92938	92997-93005
92941	92997-93005
92943	92997-93005
92944	92997-93005
92973	92997-93005
92974	92997-93005
92975	92997-93005
92977	92997-93005
92978	92997-93005
92979	92997-93005
93260	93283-93291
93261	93283-93291
93264	93272-93280
95249	95199-95803
95782	95805-95813
95783	95805-95813
95800	95805-95813
95801	95805-95813
95836	95827-95832
95885	95870-95874
95886	95870-95874
95887	95870-95874
95938	95912-95933
95939	95912-95933
95940	95912-95933
95941	95912-95933
95943	95912-95933
95983	95976-95981
95984	95976-95981
96125	96020-96121
96127	96020-96121
97151	96020-96112
97152	96020-96112

Resequenced Code	Corresponding Locations of Resequenced Code
97153	96020-96112
97154	96020-96112
97155	96020-96112
97156	96020-96112
97157	96020-96112
97158	96020-96112
97161	See Physical Therapy Evaluations subsection
97162	See Physical Therapy Evaluations subsection
97163	See Physical Therapy Evaluations subsection
97164	See Physical Therapy Evaluations subsection
97165	See Occupational Therapy Evaluations subsection
97166	See Occupational Therapy Evaluations subsection
97167	See Occupational Therapy Evaluations subsection
97168	See Occupational Therapy Evaluations subsection
97169	See Athletic Training Evaluations subsection

Resequenced Code	Corresponding Locations of Resequenced Code
97170	See Athletic Training Evaluations subsection
97171	See Athletic Training Evaluations subsection
97172	See Athletic Training Evaluations subsection
99091	99448-99455
99177	99173-99183
99224	99219-99222
99225	99219-99222
99226	99219-99222
99415	99358-99366
99416	99358-99366
99451	99448-99455
99452	99448-99455
99453	99448-99455
99454	99448-99455
99457	99448-99455
99484	99497-99499
99485	99466-99469
99486	99466-99469
99490	99480-99489
99491	99480-99489
0253T	0184T-0200T
0357T	0055T-0072T
0376T	0184T-0200T
0464T	0332T-0339T
0488T	0402T-0405T
0510T	0332T-0339T
0511T	0332T-0339T
0512T	0101T-0107T
0513T	0101T-0107T
0523T	0503T-0506T

Appendix O

Multianalyte Assays with Algorithmic Analyses

The following list includes three types of CPT codes:

1. Multianalyte assays with algorithmic analyses (MAAA) administrative codes
2. Category I MAAA codes
3. Proprietary laboratory analyses (PLA) codes

1. Multianalyte assays with algorithmic analyses (MAAAs) are procedures that utilize multiple results derived from assays of various types, including molecular pathology assays, fluorescent in situ hybridization assays and non-nucleic acid based assays (eg, proteins, polypeptides, lipids, carbohydrates). Algorithmic analysis using the results of these assays as well as other patient information (if used) is then performed and reported typically as a numeric score(s) or as a probability. MAAAs are typically unique to a single clinical laboratory or manufacturer. The results of individual component procedure(s) that are inputs to the MAAAs may be provided on the associated laboratory report, however these assays are not reported separately using additional codes. MAAAs, by nature, are typically unique to a single clinical laboratory or manufacturer.

   The list includes a proprietary name and clinical laboratory or manufacturer in the first column, an alpha-numeric code in the second column and code descriptor in the third column. The format for the code descriptor usually includes (in order):The list includes a proprietary name and clinical laboratory or manufacturer in the first column, an alpha-numeric code in the second column and code descriptor in the third column. The format for the code descriptor usually includes (in order):

   - Disease type (eg, oncology, autoimmune, tissue rejection),
   - Chemical(s) analyzed (eg, DNA, RNA, protein, antibody),
   - Number of markers (eg, number of genes, number of proteins),
   - Methodology(s) (eg, microarray, real-time [RT]-PCR, in situ hybridization [ISH], enzyme linked immunosorbent assays [ELISA]),
   - Number of functional domains (if indicated),
   - Specimen type (eg, blood, fresh tissue, formalin-fixed paraffin-embedded),
   - Algorithm result type (eg, prognostic, diagnostic),
   - Report (eg, probability index, risk score).

   MAAA procedures that have been assigned a Category I code are noted in the list below and additionally listed in the Category I MAAA section (81500-81599). The Category I MAAA section introductory language and associated parenthetical instruction(s) should be used to govern the appropriate use for Category I MAAA codes. If a specific MAAA procedure has not been assigned a Category I code, it is indicated as a four-digit number followed by the letter M.

   When a specific MAAA procedure is not included in either the list below or in the Category I MAAA section, report the analysis using the Category I MAAA unlisted code (81599). The codes below are specific to the assays identified in Appendix O by proprietary name. In order to report an MAAA code, the analysis performed must fulfill the code descriptor **and**, if proprietary, must be the test represented by the proprietary name listed in Appendix O. When an analysis is performed that may potentially fall within a specific descriptor, however the proprietary name is not included in the list below, the MAAA unlisted code (81599) should be used.

   Additions in this section may be released tri-annually (or quarterly for PLA codes) via the AMA CPT website to expedite dissemination for reporting. The list will be published annually in the CPT codebook. Go to www.ama-assn.org/go/cpt for the most current listing.

   These administrative codes encompass all analytical services required for the algorithmic analysis (eg, cell lysis, nucleic acid stabilization, extraction, digestion, amplification, hybridization and detection) in addition to the algorithmic analysis itself, when applicable. Procedures that are required prior to cell lysis (eg, micro-dissection, codes 88380 and 88381) should be reported separately.

   The codes in this list are provided as an administrative coding set to facilitate accurate reporting of MAAA services. The minimum standard for inclusion in this list is that an analysis is generally available for patient care. The AMA has not reviewed procedures in the administrative coding set for clinical utility. The list is not a complete list of all MAAA procedures.

2. Category I MAAA codes are included below along with their proprietary names. These codes are also listed in the Pathology and Laboratory section of the CPT code set (81490-81599).

3. PLA codes created in response to the Protecting Access to Medicare Act (PAMA) of 2014 are listed along with their proprietary names. These codes are also located at the end of the Pathology and Laboratory section of the CPT code set. In some instances, the descriptor language of PLA codes may be identical, which are differentiated only by the listed propriety names.

Proprietary Name and Clinical Laboratory or Manufacturer	Alpha-Numeric Code	Code Descriptor
Administrative Codes for Multianalyte Assays with Algorithmic Analyses (MAAA)		
—	►(0001M has been deleted. To report, use 81596◄	—
ASH FibroSURE™, LabCorp	0002M	Liver disease, ten biochemical assays (ALT, A2-macroglobulin, apolipoprotein A-1, total bilirubin, GGT, haptoglobin, AST, glucose, total cholesterol and triglycerides) utilizing serum, prognostic algorithm reported as quantitative scores for fibrosis, steatosis and alcoholic steatohepatitis (ASH)
NASH FibroSURE™, LabCorp	0003M	Liver disease, ten biochemical assays (ALT, A2-macroglobulin, apolipoprotein A-1, total bilirubin, GGT, haptoglobin, AST, glucose, total cholesterol and triglycerides) utilizing serum, prognostic algorithm reported as quantitative scores for fibrosis, steatosis and nonalcoholic steatohepatitis (NASH)
ScoliScore™ Transgenomic	0004M	Scoliosis, DNA analysis of 53 single nucleotide polymorphisms (SNPs), using saliva, prognostic algorithm reported as a risk score
HeproDX™, GoPath Laboratories, LLC	0006M	Oncology (hepatic), mRNA expression levels of 161 genes, utilizing fresh hepatocellular carcinoma tumor tissue, with alpha-fetoprotein level, algorithm reported as a risk classifier
NETest, Wren Laboratories, LLC	0007M	Oncology (gastrointestinal neuroendocrine tumors), real-time PCR expression analysis of 51 genes, utilizing whole peripheral blood, algorithm reported as a nomogram of tumor disease index
—	(0008M has been deleted, use 81520)	—
VisibiliT test, Sequenom Center for Molecular Medicine, LLC	0009M	Fetal aneuploidy (trisomy 21, and 18) DNA sequence analysis of selected regions using maternal plasma, algorithm reported as a risk score for each trisomy
—	(0010M has been deleted, use 81539)	—
►NeoLAB™ Prostate Liquid Biopsy, NeoGenomics Laboratories◄	●0011M	►Oncology, prostate cancer, mRNA expression assay of 12 genes (10 content and 2 housekeeping), RT-PCR test utilizing blood plasma and/or urine, algorithms to predict high-grade prostate cancer risk◄
►Cxbladder™ Detect, Pacific Edge Diagnostics USA, Ltd◄	●0012M	►Oncology (urothelial), mRNA, gene expression profiling by real-time quantitative PCR of five genes *(MDK, HOXA13, CDC2 [CDK1], IGFBP5,* and *CXCR2),* utilizing urine, algorithm reported as a risk score for having urothelial carcinoma◄

(*Continued on page 860*)

Proprietary Name and Clinical Laboratory or Manufacturer	Alpha-Numeric Code	Code Descriptor
▶Cxbladder™ Monitor, Pacific Edge Diagnostics USA, Ltd◀	●0013M	▶Oncology (urothelial), mRNA, gene expression profiling by real-time quantitative PCR of five genes (*MDK, HOXA13, CDC2 [CDK1], IGFBP5,* and *CXCR2),* utilizing urine, algorithm reported as a risk score for having recurrent urothelial carcinoma◀
Category I Codes for Multianalyte Assays with Algorithmic Analyses (MAAA)		
Vectra® DA, Crescendo Bioscience, Inc	81490	Autoimmune (rheumatoid arthritis), analysis of 12 biomarkers using immunoassays, utilizing serum, prognostic algorithm reported as a disease activity score (Do not report 81490 in conjunction with 86140)
Corus® CAD, CardioDx, Inc	81493	Coronary artery disease, mRNA, gene expression profiling by real-time RT-PCR of 23 genes, utilizing whole peripheral blood, algorithm reported as a risk score
AlloMap®, CareDx, Inc	81595	Cardiology (heart transplant), mRNA, gene expression profiling by real-time quantitative PCR of 20 genes (11 content and 9 housekeeping), utilizing subfraction of peripheral blood, algorithm reported as a rejection risk score
Risk of Ovarian Malignancy Algorithm (ROMA)™, Fujirebio Diagnostics	81500	Oncology (ovarian), biochemical assays of two proteins (CA-125 and HE4), utilizing serum, with menopausal status, algorithm reported as a risk score
OVA1™, Vermillion, Inc	81503	Oncology (ovarian), biochemical assays of five proteins (CA-125, apolipoprotein A1, beta-2 microglobulin, transferrin, and pre-albumin), utilizing serum, algorithm reported as a risk score
Tissue of Origin Test Kit-FFPE, Cancer Genetics, Inc	81504	Oncology (tissue of origin), microarray gene expression profiling of >2000 genes, utilizing formalin-fixed paraffin-embedded tissue, algorithm reported as tissue similarity scores
PreDx Diabetes Risk Score™, Tethys Clinical Laboratory	81506	Endocrinology (type 2 diabetes), biochemical assays of seven analytes (glucose, HbA1c, insulin, hs-CRP, adiponectin, ferritin, interleukin 2-receptor alpha), utilizing serum or plasma, algorithm reporting a risk score
Harmony™ Prenatal Test, Ariosa Diagnostics	81507	Fetal aneuploidy (trisomy 21, 18, and 13) DNA sequence analysis of selected regions using maternal plasma, algorithm reported as a risk score for each trisomy

Proprietary Name and Clinical Laboratory or Manufacturer	Alpha-Numeric Code	Code Descriptor
No proprietary name and clinical laboratory or manufacturer. Maternal serum screening procedures are well-established procedures and are performed by many laboratories throughout the country. The concept of prenatal screens has existed and evolved for over 10 years and is not exclusive to any one facility.	81508	Fetal congenital abnormalities, biochemical assays of two proteins (PAPP-A, hCG [any form]), utilizing maternal serum, algorithm reported as a risk score
	81509	Fetal congenital abnormalities, biochemical assays of three proteins (PAPP-A, hCG [any form], DIA), utilizing maternal serum, algorithm reported as a risk score
	81510	Fetal congenital abnormalities, biochemical assays of three analytes (AFP, uE3, hCG [any form]), utilizing maternal serum, algorithm reported as a risk score
	81511	Fetal congenital abnormalities, biochemical assays of four analytes (AFP, uE3, hCG [any form], DIA) utilizing maternal serum, algorithm reported as a risk score (may include additional results from previous biochemical testing)
	81512	Fetal congenital abnormalities, biochemical assays of five analytes (AFP, uE3, total hCG, hyperglycosylated hCG, DIA) utilizing maternal serum, algorithm reported as a risk score
▶Breast Cancer Index, Biotheranostics, Inc◀	●81518	▶Oncology (breast), mRNA, gene expression profiling by real-time RT-PCR of 11 genes (7 content and 4 housekeeping), utilizing formalin-fixed paraffin-embedded tissue, algorithms reported as percentage risk for metastatic recurrence and likelihood of benefit from extended endocrine therapy◀
Oncotype DX®, Genomic Health	81519	Oncology (breast), mRNA, gene expression profiling by real-time RT-PCR of 21 genes, utilizing formalin-fixed paraffin-embedded tissue, algorithm reported as recurrence score
Prosigna® Breast Cancer Assay, NanoString Technologies, Inc	81520	Oncology (breast), mRNA gene expression profiling by hybrid capture of 58 genes (50 content and 8 housekeeping), utilizing formalin-fixed paraffin-embedded tissue, algorithm reported as a recurrence risk score
MammaPrint®, Agendia, Inc	81521	Oncology (breast), mRNA, microarray gene expression profiling of 70 content genes and 465 housekeeping genes, utilizing fresh frozen or formalin-fixed paraffin-embedded tissue, algorithm reported as index related to risk of distant metastasis
Oncotype DX® Colon Cancer Assay, Genomic Health	81525	Oncology (colon), mRNA, gene expression profiling by real-time RT-PCR of 12 genes (7 content and 5 housekeeping), utilizing formalin-fixed paraffin-embedded tissue, algorithm reported as a recurrence score

(Continued on page 862)

Proprietary Name and Clinical Laboratory or Manufacturer	Alpha-Numeric Code	Code Descriptor
Cologuard™, Exact Sciences, Inc	81528	Oncology (colorectal) screening, quantitative real-time target and signal amplification of 10 DNA markers (KRAS mutations, promoter methylation of NDRG4 and BMP3) and fecal hemoglobin, utilizing stool, algorithm reported as a positive or negative result (Do not report 81528 in conjunction with 81275, 82274)
ChemoFX®, Helomics, Corp	81535	Oncology (gynecologic), live tumor cell culture and chemotherapeutic response by DAPI stain and morphology, predictive algorithm reported as a drug response score; first single drug or drug combination
	+81536	each additional single drug or drug combination (List separately in addition to code for primary procedure) (Use 81536 in conjunction with 81535)
VeriStrat, Biodesix, Inc	81538	Oncology (lung), mass spectrometric 8-protein signature, including amyloid A, utilizing serum, prognostic and predictive algorithm reported as good versus poor overall survival
4Kscore test, OPKO Health, Inc	81539	Oncology (high-grade prostate cancer), biochemical assay of four proteins (Total PSA, Free PSA, Intact PSA and human kallikrein-2 [hK2]), utilizing plasma or serum, prognostic algorithm reported as a probability score
CancerTYPE ID, bioTheranostics, Inc	81540	Oncology (tumor of unknown origin), mRNA, gene expression profiling by real-time RT-PCR of 92 genes (87 content and 5 housekeeping) to classify tumor into main cancer type and subtype, utilizing formalin-fixed paraffin-embedded tissue, algorithm reported as a probability of a predicted main cancer type and subtype
Prolaris®, Myriad Genetic Laboratories, Inc	81541	Oncology (prostate), mRNA gene expression profiling by real-time RT-PCR of 46 genes (31 content and 15 housekeeping), utilizing formalin-fixed paraffin-embedded tissue, algorithm reported as a disease-specific mortality risk score
Afirma® Gene Expression Classifier, Veracyte, Inc	81545	Oncology (thyroid), gene expression analysis of 142 genes, utilizing fine needle aspirate, algorithm reported as a categorical result (eg, benign or suspicious)
ConfirmMDx® for Prostate Cancer, MDxHealth, Inc	81551	Oncology (prostate), promoter methylation profiling by real-time PCR of 3 genes *(GSTP1, APC, RASSF1)*, utilizing formalin-fixed paraffin-embedded tissue, algorithm reported as a likelihood of prostate cancer detection on repeat biopsy
►HCV FibroSURE™, FibroTest™, BioPredictive S.A.S.◄	●81596	►Infectious disease, chronic hepatitis C virus (HCV) infection, six biochemical assays (ALT, A2-macroglobulin, apolipoprotein A-1, total bilirubin, GGT, and haptoglobin) utilizing serum, prognostic algorithm reported as scores for fibrosis and necroinflammatory activity in liver◄

Proprietary Name and Clinical Laboratory or Manufacturer	Alpha-Numeric Code	Code Descriptor
	81599	Unlisted multianalyte assay with algorithmic analysis
Proprietary Laboratory Analyses (PLA)		
PreciseType® HEA Test, Immucor, Inc	0001U	Red blood cell antigen typing, DNA, human erythrocyte antigen gene analysis of 35 antigens from 11 blood groups, utilizing whole blood, common RBC alleles reported
PolypDX™, Atlantic Diagnostic Laboratories, LLC, Metabolomic Technologies, Inc	0002U	Oncology (colorectal), quantitative assessment of three urine metabolites (ascorbic acid, succinic acid and carnitine) by liquid chromatography with tandem mass spectrometry (LC-MS/MS) using multiple reaction monitoring acquisition, algorithm reported as likelihood of adenomatous polyps
Overa (OVA1 Next Generation), Asprira Labs, Inc, Vermillion, Inc	0003U	Oncology (ovarian) biochemical assays of five proteins (apolipoprotein A-1, CA 125 II, follicle stimulating hormone, human epididymis protein 4, transferrin), utilizing serum, algorithm reported as a likelihood score
	►(0004U has been deleted)◄	
ExosomeDx® Prostate (IntelliScore), Exosome Diagnostics, Inc	0005U	Oncology (prostate) gene expression profile by real-time RT-PCR of 3 genes *(ERG, PCA3,* and *SPDEF),* urine, algorithm reported as risk score
►Drug-drug, Drug-substance Identification and Interaction, Aegis Sciences Corporation◄	▲0006U	►Detection of interacting medications, substances, supplements and foods, 120 or more analytes, definitive chromatography with mass spectrometry, urine, description and severity of each interaction identified, per date of service◄
ToxProtect, Genotox Laboratories Ltd	Ӿ0007U	Drug test(s), presumptive, with definitive confirmation of positive results, any number of drug classes, urine, includes specimen verification including DNA authentication in comparison to buccal DNA, per date of service ►(For additional PLA code with identical clinical descriptor, see 0020U. See Appendix O to determine appropriate code assignment)◄
AmHPR Helicobacter pylori Antibiotic Resistance Next Generation Sequencing Panel, American Molecular Laboratories, Inc	0008U	Helicobacter pylori detection and antibiotic resistance, DNA, 16S and 23S rRNA, gyrA, pbp1,rdxA and rpoB, next generation sequencing, formalin-fixed paraffin-embedded or fresh tissue, predictive, reported as positive or negative for resistance to clarithromycin, fluoroquinolones, metronidazole, amoxicillin, tetracycline and rifabutin
DEPArray™ HER2, PacificDx	0009U	Oncology (breast cancer), *ERBB2* (HER2) copy number by FISH, tumor cells from formalin-fixed paraffin-embedded tissue isolated using image-based dielectrophoresis (DEP) sorting, reported as *ERBB2* gene amplified or non-amplified
Bacterial Typing by Whole Genome Sequencing, Mayo Clinic	0010U	Infectious disease (bacterial), strain typing by whole genome sequencing, phylogenetic-based report of strain relatedness, per submitted isolate

(Continued on page 864)

▲=Revised code ●=New code ►◄=Contains new or revised text Ӿ=Duplicate PLA test

Proprietary Name and Clinical Laboratory or Manufacturer	Alpha-Numeric Code	Code Descriptor
Cordant CORE™, Cordant Health Solutions	0011U	Prescription drug monitoring, evaluation of drugs present by LC-MS/MS, using oral fluid, reported as a comparison to an estimated steady-state range, per date of service including all drug compounds and metabolites
MatePair Targeted Rearrangements, Congenital, Mayo Clinic	0012U	Germline disorders, gene rearrangement detection by whole genome next-generation sequencing, DNA, whole blood, report of specific gene rearrangement(s)
MatePair Targeted Rearrangements, Oncology, Mayo Clinic	0013U	Oncology (solid organ neoplasia), gene rearrangement detection by whole genome next-generation sequencing, DNA, fresh or frozen tissue or cells, report of specific gene rearrangement(s)
MatePair Targeted Rearrangements, Hematologic, Mayo Clinic	0014U	Hematology (hematolymphoid neoplasia), gene rearrangement detection by whole genome next-generation sequencing, DNA, whole blood or bone marrow, report of specific gene rearrangement(s)
	▶(0015U has been deleted)◀	
BCR-ABL1 major and minor breakpoint fusion transcripts, University of Iowa, Department of Pathology, Asuragen	0016U	Oncology (hematolymphoid neoplasia), RNA, *BCR/ABL1* major and minor breakpoint fusion transcripts, quantitative PCR amplification, blood or bone marrow, report of fusion not detected or detected with quantitation
JAK2 Mutation, University of Iowa, Department of Pathology	0017U	Oncology (hematolymphoid neoplasia), *JAK2* mutation, DNA, PCR amplification of exons 12-14 and sequence analysis, blood or bone marrow, report of *JAK2* mutation not detected or detected
▶ThyraMIR™, Interpace Diagnostics, Interpace Diagnostics◀	●0018U	▶Oncology (thyroid), microRNA profiling by RT-PCR of 10 microRNA sequences, utilizing fine needle aspirate, algorithm reported as a positive or negative result for moderate to high risk of malignancy◀
▶OncoTarget/OncoTreat, Columbia University Department of Pathology and Cell Biology, Darwin Health◀	●0019U	▶Oncology, RNA, gene expression by whole transcriptome sequencing, formalin-fixed paraffin-embedded tissue or fresh frozen tissue, predictive algorithm reported as potential targets for therapeutic agents◀
▶ToxLok, InSource Diagnostics, InSource Diagnostics◀	✱●0020U	▶Drug test(s), presumptive, with definitive confirmation of positive results, any number of drug classes, urine, with specimen verification including DNA authentication in comparison to buccal DNA, per date of service (For additional PLA code with identical clinical descriptor, see 0007U. See Appendix O to determine appropriate code assignment)◀
▶Apifiny®, Armune BioScience, Inc◀	●0021U	▶Oncology (prostate), detection of 8 autoantibodies (ARF 6, NKX3-1, 5'-UTR-BMI1, CEP 164, 3'-UTR-Ropporin, Desmocollin, AURKAIP-1, CSNK2A2), multiplexed immunoassay and flow cytometry serum, algorithm reported as risk score◀

Proprietary Name and Clinical Laboratory or Manufacturer	Alpha-Numeric Code	Code Descriptor
▶Oncomine™ Dx Target Test, Thermo Fisher Scientific◀	●0022U	▶Targeted genomic sequence analysis panel, non-small cell lung neoplasia, DNA and RNA analysis, 23 genes, interrogation for sequence variants and rearrangements, reported as presence/absence of variants and associated therapy(ies) to consider◀
▶LeukoStrat® CDx *FLT3* Mutation Assay, LabPMM LLC, an Invivoscribe Technologies, Inc Company, Invivoscribe Technologies, Inc◀	●0023U	▶Oncology (acute myelogenous leukemia), DNA, genotyping of internal tandem duplication, p. D835, p.I836, using mononuclear cells, reported as detection or non-detection of *FLT3* mutation and indication for or against the use of midostaurin◀
▶GlycA, Laboratory Corporation of America, Laboratory Corporation of America◀	●0024U	▶Glycosylated acute phase proteins (GlycA), nuclear magnetic resonance spectroscopy, quantitative◀
▶UrSure Tenofovir Quantification Test, Synergy Medical Laboratories, UrSure Inc◀	●0025U	▶Tenofovir, by liquid chromatography with tandem mass spectrometry (LC-MS/MS), urine, quantitative◀
▶Thyroseq Genomic Classifier, CBLPath, Inc, University of Pittsburgh Medical Center◀	●0026U	▶Oncology (thyroid), DNA and mRNA of 112 genes, next-generation sequencing, fine needle aspirate of thyroid nodule, algorithmic analysis reported as a categorical result ("Positive, high probability of malignancy" or "Negative, low probability of malignancy")◀
▶*JAK2* Exons 12 to 15 Sequencing, Mayo Clinic, Mayo Clinic◀	●0027U	▶*JAK2 (Janus kinase 2)* (eg, myeloproliferative disorder) gene analysis, targeted sequence analysis exons 12-15◀
▶CYP2D6 Genotype Cascade, Mayo Clinic, Mayo Clinic◀	●0028U	▶*CYP2D6 (cytochrome P450, family 2, subfamily D, polypeptide 6)* (eg, drug metabolism) gene analysis, copy number variants, common variants with reflex to targeted sequence analysis◀
▶Focused Pharmacogenomics Panel, Mayo Clinic, Mayo Clinic◀	●0029U	▶Drug metabolism (adverse drug reactions and drug response), targeted sequence analysis (ie, *CYP1A2, CYP2C19, CYP2C9, CYP2D6, CYP3A4, CYP3A5, CYP4F2, SLCO1B1, VKORC1* and rs12777823)◀
▶Warfarin Response Genotype, Mayo Clinic, Mayo Clinic◀	●0030U	▶Drug metabolism (warfarin drug response), targeted sequence analysis (ie, *CYP2C9, CYP4F2, VKORC1,* rs12777823)◀
▶Cytochrome P450 1A2 Genotype, Mayo Clinic, Mayo Clinic◀	●0031U	▶*CYP1A2 (cytochrome P450 family 1, subfamily A, member 2)* (eg, drug metabolism) gene analysis, common variants (ie, *1F, *1K, *6, *7)◀
▶Catechol-O-Methyltransferase *(COMT)* Genotype, Mayo Clinic, Mayo Clinic◀	●0032U	▶*COMT (catechol-O-methyltransferase)* (eg, drug metabolism) gene analysis, c.472G>A (rs4680) variant◀
▶Serotonin Receptor Genotype *(HTR2A* and *HTR2C)*, Mayo Clinic, Mayo Clinic◀	●0033U	▶*HTR2A (5-hydroxytryptamine receptor 2A), HTR2C (5-hydroxytryptamine receptor 2C)* (eg, citalopram metabolism) gene analysis, common variants (ie, *HTR2A* rs7997012 [c.614-2211T>C], *HTR2C* rs3813929 [c.-759C>T] and rs1414334 [c.551-3008C>G])◀

(Continued on page 866)

Proprietary Name and Clinical Laboratory or Manufacturer	Alpha-Numeric Code	Code Descriptor
▶Thiopurine Methyltransferase *(TPMT)* and Nudix Hydrolase *(NUDT15)* Genotyping, Mayo Clinic, Mayo Clinic◀	●0034U	▶*TPMT (thiopurine S-methyltransferase), NUDT15 (nudix hydroxylase 15)* (eg, thiopurine metabolism) gene analysis, common variants (ie, *TPMT* *2, *3A, *3B, *3C, *4, *5, *6, *8, *12; *NUDT15* *3, *4, *5)◀
▶Real-time quaking-induced conversion for prion detection (RT-QuIC), National Prion Disease Pathology Surveillance Center◀	●0035U	▶Neurology (prion disease), cerebrospinal fluid, detection of prion protein by quaking-induced conformational conversion, qualitative◀
▶EXaCT-1 Whole Exome Testing, Lab of Oncology-Molecular Detection, Weill Cornell Medicine-Clinical Genomics Laboratory◀	●0036U	▶Exome (ie, somatic mutations), paired formalin-fixed paraffin-embedded tumor tissue and normal specimen, sequence analyses◀
▶FoundationOne CDx™ (F1CDx), Foundation Medicine, Inc, Foundation Medicine, Inc◀	●0037U	▶Targeted genomic sequence analysis, solid organ neoplasm, DNA analysis of 324 genes, interrogation for sequence variants, gene copy number amplifications, gene rearrangements, microsatellite instability and tumor mutational burden◀
▶Sensieva™ Droplet 25OH Vitamin D2/D3 Microvolume LC/MS Assay, InSource Diagnostics, InSource Diagnostics◀	●0038U	▶Vitamin D, 25 hydroxy D2 and D3, by LC-MS/MS, serum microsample, quantitative◀
▶Anti-dsDNA, High Salt/Avidity, University of Washington, Department of Laboratory Medicine, Bio-Rad◀	●0039U	▶Deoxyribonucleic acid (DNA) antibody, double stranded, high avidity◀
▶MRDx BCR-ABL Test, MolecularMD, MolecularMD◀	●0040U	▶*BCR/ABL1 (t(9;22))* (eg, chronic myelogenous leukemia) translocation analysis, major breakpoint, quantitative◀
▶Lyme ImmunoBlot IgM, IGeneX Inc ID-FISH Technology Inc (ASR) (Lyme ImmunoBlot IgM Strips Only)◀	●0041U	▶Borrelia burgdorferi, antibody detection of 5 recombinant protein groups, by immunoblot, IgM◀
▶Lyme ImmunoBlot IgG, IGeneX Inc ID-FISH Technology Inc (ASR) (Lyme ImmunoBlot IgG Strips Only)◀	●0042U	▶Borrelia burgdorferi, antibody detection of 12 recombinant protein groups, by immunoblot, IgG◀
▶Tick-Borne Relapsing Fever (TBRF) Borrelia ImmunoBlots IgM Test, IGeneX Inc ID-FISH Technology◀	●0043U	▶Tick-borne relapsing fever Borrelia group, antibody detection to 4 recombinant protein groups, by immunoblot, IgM◀
▶Tick-Borne Relapsing Fever (TBRF) Borrelia ImmunoBlots IgG Test, IGeneX Inc ID-FISH Technology Inc (Provides TBRF ImmunoBlot IgG Strips)◀	●0044U	▶Tick-borne relapsing fever Borrelia group, antibody detection to 4 recombinant protein groups, by immunoblot, IgG◀

Proprietary Name and Clinical Laboratory or Manufacturer	Alpha-Numeric Code	Code Descriptor
►The Oncotype DX® Breast DCIS Score™ Test, Genomic Health, Inc, Genomic Health, Inc◄	●0045U	►Oncology (breast ductal carcinoma in situ), mRNA, gene expression profiling by real-time RT-PCR of 12 genes (7 content and 5 housekeeping), utilizing formalin-fixed paraffin-embedded tissue, algorithm reported as recurrence score◄
►*FLT3* ITD MRD by NGS, LabPMM LLC, an Invivoscribe Technologies, Inc Company◄	●0046U	►*FLT3 (fms-related tyrosine kinase 3)* (eg, acute myeloid leukemia) internal tandem duplication (ITD) variants, quantitative◄
►Oncotype DX Genomic Prostate Score, Genomic Health, Inc, Genomic Health, Inc◄	●0047U	►Oncology (prostate), mRNA, gene expression profiling by real-time RT-PCR of 17 genes (12 content and 5 housekeeping), utilizing formalin-fixed paraffin-embedded tissue, algorithm reported as a risk score◄
►MSK-IMPACT (Integrated Mutation Profiling of Actionable Cancer Targets), Memorial Sloan Kettering Cancer Center◄	●0048U	►Oncology (solid organ neoplasia), DNA, targeted sequencing of protein-coding exons of 468 cancer-associated genes, including interrogation for somatic mutations and microsatellite instability, matched with normal specimens, utilizing formalin-fixed paraffin-embedded tumor tissue, report of clinically significant mutation(s)◄
►NPM1 MRD by NGS, LabPMM LLC, an Invivoscribe Technologies, Inc Company◄	●0049U	►*NPM1 (nucleophosmin)* (eg, acute myeloid leukemia) gene analysis, quantitative◄
►MyAML NGS Panel, LabPMM LLC, an Invivoscribe Technologies, Inc Company◄	●0050U	►Targeted genomic sequence analysis panel, acute myelogenous leukemia, DNA analysis, 194 genes, interrogation for sequence variants, copy number variants or rearrangements◄
►UCompliDx, Elite Medical Laboratory Solutions, LLC, Elite Medical Laboratory Solutions, LLC (LDT)◄	●0051U	►Prescription drug monitoring, evaluation of drugs present by LC-MS/MS, urine, 31 drug panel, reported as quantitative results, detected or not detected, per date of service◄
►VAP Cholesterol Test, VAP Diagnostics Laboratory, Inc, VAP Diagnostics Laboratory, Inc◄	●0052U	►Lipoprotein, blood, high resolution fractionation and quantitation of lipoproteins including all five major lipoprotein classes and the subclasses of HDL, LDL, and VLDL by vertical auto profile ultracentrifugation◄
►Prostate Cancer Risk Panel, Mayo Clinic, Laboratory Developed Test◄	●0053U	►Oncology (prostate cancer), FISH analysis of 4 genes *(ASAP1, HDAC9, CHD1* and *PTEN)*, needle biopsy specimen, algorithm reported as probability of higher tumor grade◄
►AssuranceRx Micro Serum, Firstox Laboratories, LLC, Firstox Laboratories, LLC◄	●0054U	►Prescription drug monitoring, 14 or more classes of drugs and substances, definitive tandem mass spectrometry with chromatography, capillary blood, quantitative report with therapeutic and toxic ranges, including steady-state range for the prescribed dose when detected, per date of service◄
►myTAIHEART, TAI Diagnostics, Inc, TAI Diagnostics, Inc◄	●0055U	►Cardiology (heart transplant), cell-free DNA, PCR assay of 96 DNA target sequences (94 single nucleotide polymorphism targets and two control targets), plasma◄

(Continued on page 868)

Proprietary Name and Clinical Laboratory or Manufacturer	Alpha-Numeric Code	Code Descriptor
▶MatePair Acute Myeloid Leukemia Panel, Mayo Clinic, Laboratory Developed Test◀	●0056U	▶Hematology (acute myelogenous leukemia), DNA, whole genome next-generation sequencing to detect gene rearrangement(s), blood or bone marrow, report of specific gene rearrangement(s)◀
▶RNA-Sequencing by NGS, OmniSeq, Inc, Life Technologies Corporation◀	●0057U	▶Oncology (solid organ neoplasia), mRNA, gene expression profiling by massively parallel sequencing for analysis of 51 genes, utilizing formalin-fixed paraffin-embedded tissue, algorithm reported as a normalized percentile rank◀
▶Merkel SmT Oncoprotein Antibody Titer, University of Washington, Department of Laboratory Medicine◀	●0058U	▶Oncology (Merkel cell carcinoma), detection of antibodies to the Merkel cell polyoma virus oncoprotein (small T antigen), serum, quantitative◀
▶Merkel Virus VP1 Capsid Antibody, University of Washington, Department of Laboratory Medicine◀	●0059U	▶Oncology (Merkel cell carcinoma), detection of antibodies to the Merkel cell polyoma virus capsid protein (VP1), serum, reported as positive or negative◀
▶Twins Zygosity PLA, Natera, Inc, Natera, Inc◀	●0060U	▶Twin zygosity, genomic-targeted sequence analysis of chromosome 2, using circulating cell-free fetal DNA in maternal blood◀
▶Transcutaneous multispectral measurement of tissue oxygenation and hemoglobin using spatial frequency domain imaging (SFDI), Modulated Imaging, Inc, Modulated Imaging, Inc◀	●0061U	▶Transcutaneous measurement of five biomarkers (tissue oxygenation [StO_2], oxyhemoglobin [$ctHbO_2$], deoxyhemoglobin [ctHbR], papillary and reticular dermal hemoglobin concentrations [ctHb1 and ctHb2]), using spatial frequency domain imaging (SFDI) and multi-spectral analysis◀

Appendix P

CPT Codes That May Be Used For Synchronous Telemedicine Services

This listing is a summary of CPT codes that may be used for reporting synchronous (real-time) telemedicine services when appended by modifier 95. Procedures on this list involve electronic communication using interactive telecommunications equipment that includes, at a minimum, audio and video. The codes listed below are identified in CPT 2019 with the ★ symbol.

90791	93298	99242
90792	93299	99243
90832	96040	99244
90833	96116	99245
90834	96150	99251
90836	96151	99252
90837	96152	99253
90838	96153	99254
90845	96154	99255
90846	97802	99307
90847	97803	99308
90863	97804	99309
90951	98960	99310
90952	98961	99354
90954	98962	99355
90955	99201	99406
90957	99202	99407
90958	99203	99408
90960	99204	99409
90961	99205	99495
92227	99212	99496
92228	99213	
93228	99214	
93229	99215	
93268	99231	
93270	99232	
93271	99233	
93272	99241	

Notes

Index

Instructions for the Use of the CPT Index

The alphabetic index is **not** a substitute for the main text of the CPT codebook. Even if only one code is present, the user must refer to the main text to ensure that the code selected accurately identifies the service(s) performed.

Main Terms

The index is organized by main terms. Each main term can stand alone or can be followed by up to three modifying terms. There are four primary classes of main entries:

1. Procedure or service.
   For example: Endoscopy; Anastomosis; Splint
2. Organ or other anatomical site.
   For example: Tibia; Colon; Salivary Gland
3. Condition.
   For example: Abscess; Entropion; Tetralogy of Fallot
4. Synonyms, Eponyms, and Abbreviations.
   For example: EEG; Brock Operation; Clagett Procedure

The Anesthesia-section codes are indexed under the Anesthesia main entry and are not double-entered under the anatomical sites. Only codes within the Surgery, Medicine, Category II, and Category III sections that specifically reference the service of anesthesia are indexed under the anatomical sites.

Modifying Terms

A main term may be followed by up to three indented terms that modify the terms they follow. For example, the main term *Endoscopy* is subdivided by the anatomical sites in which the procedure is used, and within these anatomical sites, the specific purpose of the procedure is identified. In the following example, the code for an endoscopic removal of a foreign body from the bile duct could be located:

Bile Duct
  Removal
    Foreign Body 43275

Note that in this entry, the inclusion of a subentry under "Removal" implies the reading "Removal [of]" the term that follows it. If no subheads followed "Removal," the procedure would relate to the subhead that preceded it, as in this entry for the endoscopic removal of the spleen:

Spleen
  Removal 38120

When modifying terms appear, one should review the list, as these subterms further qualify the selection of the appropriate code for the procedure.

Code Ranges

Whenever more than one code applies to a given index entry, a code range is listed. If several nonsequential codes apply, they will be separated by a comma. In the following example, three nonsequential codes apply:

Esophagus
  Reconstruction 43300, 43310, 43313

If three or more sequential codes apply, they will be separated by a hyphen. If more than one code range applies, the code ranges will be separated by a comma as in the following example:

Anesthesia
  Forearm 01810-01820, 01830-01860

Conventions

As a space-saving convention, certain terms carry meaning inferred from the context. This convention is primarily used when a procedure or service is listed as a subterm. For example:

Knee
  Exploration [of] 27310, 27331

In this example, the bracketed qualifier "[of]" does not appear in the index; "of" is understood in the context of the term "Exploration." As another example:

Pelvis
  Halo [Application of]. 20662

In this example, as there is no such entity as "pelvis halo," the bracketed words are inferred.

Pathology and Laboratory

The Pathology and Laboratory listing in the index presents the headings, subheadings, procedures, and analytes in the Pathology and Laboratory section of the CPT codebook. Analytes are either listed alphabetically (for example, the Chemistry analytes) or cross-referenced to the index main heads where they are alphabetically listed (for example, to reference infectious agent analytes, the entry will indicate "*See* Infectious Agents").

Index

A

A Vitamin
See Vitamin, A

A-II
See Angiotensin II

Abbe-Estlander Procedure
Lip Reconstruction 40527, 40761
See Reconstruction; Repair, Cleft Lip

Abdomen
Abdominal Aorta
  Angiography 75635
Abdominal Wall
  Debridement
    Infected 11005, 11006
  Fascial Reinforcement
    with Implant 0437T
  Implantation
    Non-biologic or Synthetic Implant 0437T
  Removal
    Mesh 11008
    Prosthesis 11008
  Repair
    Hernia 49491-49496, 49501, 49507, 49521, 49590
  Tumor
    Excision 22900-22903
    Radical Resection 22904, 22905
Abscess
  Incision and Drainage
    Open 49020, 49040
Anesthesia
  See Anesthesia, Abdomen
Angiography 74174, 74175, 74185, 75635
Aorta
  See Abdomen, Abdominal Aorta; Aorta, Abdominal
Aortic Aneurysm
  See Aorta, Abdominal, Aneurysm
Artery
  Ligation 37617
Biopsy 49000
Bypass Graft
  Excision 35907
Catheter
  Removal 49422
Celiotomy
  See Laparotomy
  for Staging 49220
CT Scan 74150, 74160, 74170, 74174-74178, 75635
Cyst
  Destruction/Excision 49203-49205
Deliveries
  See Cesarean Delivery
Drainage
  Fluid 49082, 49083
Ectopic Pregnancy 59130
Endometrioma
  Destruction/Excision 49203-49205
Exploration 49000, 49010
  Blood Vessel 35840
  Staging 58960
Hysterectomy
  See Hysterectomy, Abdominal
Incision 49000-49084
  Staging 58960
Incision and Drainage
  Pancreatitis 48000
Infraumbilical Panniculectomy 15830
Injection
  Air 49400
  Contrast Material 49400
Insertion
  Catheter 49324, 49418, 49419, 49421
  Venous Shunt 49425
Intraperitoneal
  Catheter Exit Site 49436
  Catheter Insertion 49418-49421, 49435
  Catheter Removal 49422
  Catheter Revision 49325
  Shunt
    Insertion 49425
    Ligation 49428
    Removal 49429
    Revision 49426
Laparoscopy 49320-49327, 49329
Laparotomy
  Reopening 49002
  Staging 49220, 58960
Lymphangiogram
  See Lymphangiography, Abdomen
Magnetic Resonance Imaging (MRI) . . 74181-74183
Needle Biopsy (Mass) 49180
Paracentesis 49082, 49083
Radical Resection 51597
Radiation Therapy
  Placement of Guidance Devices . . 49411, 49412
Radiographies
  See Abdomen, X ray
Removal
  Node(s) 49220
Repair
  Blood Vessel 35221
    with Other Graft 35281
    with Vein Graft 35251
  Hernia 49491-49525, 49560-49587, 49590
  Suture 49900
Revision
  Venous Shunt 49426
Suture 49900
Tumor
  Destruction/Excision 49203-49205
Ultrasound 76700-76705
Unlisted Services and Procedures 49999
Wall
  See Abdomen, Abdominal Wall
Wound Exploration
  Penetrating 20102
X ray 74018, 74019, 74021, 74022

Abdominal
See Abdomen
Aorta
  See Abdomen, Abdominal Aorta; Aorta, Abdominal
Aortic Aneurysm
  See Aorta, Abdominal, Aneurysm
Deliveries
  See Cesarean Delivery
Hysterectomy
  See Hysterectomy, Abdominal
Lymphangiogram
  See Lymphangiography, Abdomen
Paracentesis
  See Abdomen, Drainage
Radiographies
  See Abdomen, X ray
Wall
  See Abdomen, Abdominal Wall

Abdominohysterectomy
See Hysterectomy, Abdominal

Abdominopelvic Amputation
See Amputation, Interpelviabdominal

Abdominoplasty
See Panniculectomy
Excision, Skin and Tissue 15830, 15847
Unlisted Procedure 17999

Ablation
Anus
  Polyp 46615
  Tumor 46615
Bone
  Tumor
    with Adjacent Soft Tissue 20982, 20983
Colon
  Lesion 44401, 45346, 45388
  Polyp 44401, 45346, 45388
  Tumor 44401, 45346, 45388
Cryosurgical
  Fibroadenoma 19105
  Liver Tumor 47381, 47383
  Renal Mass 50250
  Renal Tumor
    Percutaneous 50593
CT Scan Guidance 77013
Endometrial 58353, 58356, 58563
  with Ultrasound Guidance 58356
Heart
  Arrhythmogenic Focus 33250, 33251, 33261, 93653, 93654, 93655
  Atrioventricular 93650, 93653, 93654
Larynx
  Lesion 31572
Laser
  Wound 0491T, 0492T
Liver (Tumor)
  Cryosurgical 47381, 47383
  Laparoscopic 47370, 47371
  Radiofrequency 47380-47382
Lung
  Tumor
    Radiofrequency 32998
Nerve
  Percutaneous 0440T-0442T
Parenchymal Tissue
  CT Scan Guidance 77013
  Magnetic Resonance Imaging Guidance 77022
  Ultrasound Guidance 76940
Prostate
  Cryosurgical 55873
  Waterjet 0421T
Pulmonary Tumor 32994, 32998
Radiofrequency
  Liver Tumor 47382
  Lung Tumor 32998
  Renal Tumor 50592
  Tongue Base 41530
  Uterine Fibroid 0404T
Rectum
  Lesion 45346
  Polyp 45346
  Tumor 45346
Renal Cyst 50541
Renal Mass 50542
Renal Tumor
  Cryotherapy
    Percutaneous 50593
  Radiofrequency 50592
Stereotactic
  Intracranial Lesion
    Magnetic Resonance Image Guided High Intensity Focused Ultrasound (MRgFUS) 0398T

Tongue Base
Radiofrequency . . . 41530
Turbinate Mucosa . . . 30801, 30802
Uterine Fibroids
Laparoscopic . . . 58674
Radiofrequency . . . 0404T
Uterine Tumor
Ultrasound, Focused . . . 0071T, 0072T
Vein
Endovenous
Chemical Adhesive . . . 36482, 36483
Laser . . . 36478, 36479
Mechanochemical . . . 36473, 36474
Radiofrequency . . . 36475, 36476

Abortion
See Obstetrical Care
Incomplete . . . 59812
Induced
by Dilation and Curettage . . . 59840
by Dilation and Evacuation . . . 59841
by Saline . . . 59850, 59851
by Vaginal Suppositories . . . 59855, 59856
with Hysterotomy . . . 59100, 59852, 59857
Missed
First Trimester . . . 59820
Second Trimester . . . 59821
Septic . . . 59830
Spontaneous
Complete
See Hospital Services
Incomplete . . . 59812
Therapeutic
by Saline . . . 59850
with Dilation and Curettage . . . 59851
with Hysterotomy . . . 59852

Abrasion (Skin)
Chemical Peel . . . 15788, 15789, 15792, 15793
Dermabrasion . . . 15780-15783
Lesion . . . 15786, 15787

Abscess
Bone
Ankle
Incision . . . 27607
Clavicle
Sequestrectomy . . . 23170
Elbow
Incision . . . 23930, 23935
Facial
Excision . . . 21026
Femur
Incision . . . 27303
Finger
Incision . . . 26034
Foot
Incision . . . 28005
Forearm
Incision . . . 25035
Sequestrectomy . . . 25145
Humeral Head
Incision . . . 23174
Humerus
Excision . . . 24134
Incision and Drainage . . . 23935
Knee
Incision . . . 27303
Leg, Lower
Incision . . . 27607
Olecranon Process . . . 24138
Sequestrectomy . . . 24136
Pelvis
Incision . . . 26992
Radius
Incision, Deep . . . 25035
Sequestrectomy . . . 24136
Scapula
Sequestrectomy . . . 23172
Shoulder
Incision . . . 23035
Thorax
Incision . . . 21510
Wrist
Incision . . . 25035
Sequestrectomy . . . 25145
Drainage
with X ray . . . 75989
Localization
Nuclear Medicine . . . 78806, 78807
Tissue
Abdomen . . . 49040
Incision and Drainage . . . 49040
Anus
Incision and Drainage . . . 46045-46060
Ankle
Incision and Drainage . . . 27603
Appendix
Incision and Drainage . . . 44900
Arm, Lower
Incision and Drainage . . . 25028
Auditory Canal, External
Incision and Drainage . . . 69020
Bartholin's Gland
Incision and Drainage . . . 56420
Bladder
Incision and Drainage . . . 51080
Brain
Drainage via Burr Hole . . . 61150, 61151
Drainage via Craniotomy . . . 61320, 61321
Excision . . . 61514, 61522
Breast
Incision and Drainage . . . 19020
Ear, External
Incision and Drainage . . . 69000, 69005
Elbow
Incision and Drainage . . . 23930, 23931
Epididymis
Incision and Drainage . . . 54700
Eyelid
Incision and Drainage . . . 67700
Finger
Incision and Drainage . . . 26010, 26011
Forearm
Incision and Drainage . . . 25028
Gums
Incision and Drainage . . . 41800
Hand
Incision and Drainage . . . 26034
Hip
Incision and Drainage . . . 26990-26992
Kidney
Incision and Drainage . . . 50020
Knee
Incision and Drainage . . . 27301
Leg, Lower
Incision and Drainage . . . 27603
Liver
Drainage
Open . . . 47010
Injection . . . 47015
Marsupialization . . . 47300
Lung
Percutaneous Drainage . . . 32200
Lymph Node
Incision and Drainage . . . 38300, 38305
Mandible
Excision . . . 21025
Mouth . . . 41015-41018
Incision and Drainage
Dentoalveolar . . . 41800
Lingual . . . 41000
Masticator Space . . . 41009, 41018
Sublingual . . . 41005, 41006, 41015
Submandibular . . . 41008, 41017
Submental . . . 41007, 41016
Vestibular . . . 40800, 40801
Nasal
Incision and Drainage . . . 30000, 30020
Neck
Incision and Drainage . . . 21501, 21502
Olecranon Process
Excision . . . 24138
Ovary
Abdominal Approach . . . 58822
Incision and Drainage . . . 58820, 58822
Vaginal Approach . . . 58820
Palate
Incision and Drainage . . . 42000
Paraurethral Gland
Incision and Drainage . . . 53060
Parotid Gland
Drainage . . . 42300, 42305
Pelvis
Incision and Drainage . . . 26990, 26991, 45000
Perineum
Incision and Drainage . . . 56405
Perirenal or Renal
Incision and Drainage . . . 50020
Peritoneum
Incision and Drainage . . . 49020
Pharynx
Incision and Drainage . . . 42720, 42725
Prostate
Incision and Drainage . . . 55720, 55725
Transurethral Drainage . . . 52700
Rectum
Incision and Drainage . . . 45005, 45020, 46040, 46060
Renal
Incision and Drainage . . . 50020
Retroperitoneal
Incision and Drainage . . . 49060
Salivary Gland
Drainage . . . 42300-42320
Scrotum
Incision and Drainage . . . 54700, 55100
Shoulder
Incision and Drainage . . . 23030
Skene's Gland
Incision and Drainage . . . 53060
Skin/Superficial
Incision and Drainage . . . 10060, 10061
Puncture Aspiration . . . 10160
Spine
Incision and Drainage . . . 22010, 22015
Subdiaphragmatic
Drainage . . . 49040
Sublingual Gland
Drainage . . . 42310-42320
Submaxillary Gland
Drainage . . . 42310, 42320
Subphrenic
Drainage . . . 49040
Testis
Incision and Drainage . . . 54700
Thigh
Incision and Drainage . . . 27301

Thorax
  Incision and Drainage........21501, 21502
Throat
  Incision and Drainage........42700-42725
Tongue
  Incision and Drainage........41000-41006
Tonsil
  Incision and Drainage........42700
Urethra
  Incision and Drainage........53040
Uvula
  Incision and Drainage........42000
Vagina
  Incision and Drainage........57010
Vulva
  Incision and Drainage........56405
Wrist
  Incision and Drainage........25028, 25035
X ray........76080

Abscess, Nasal
See Nose, Abscess

Abscess, Parotid Gland
See Parotid Gland, Abscess

Absorptiometry, X-ray (DXA)
Bone Density Study
  Dual-Energy
    Appendicular........77081
    Axial Skeleton........77080
    Vertebral........77085, 77086
  Dual Photon........78351
  Single Photon........78350
Diagnostic Screening........3095F, 3096F

Absorption Spectrophotometry, Atomic
See Atomic Absorption Spectroscopy

Accessory Nerve, Spinal
Anastomosis, Facial-Spinal........64866
Avulsion........64772
Chemodenervation, Muscles........64615
Laminectomy........63191
Transection........64772

Accessory, Toe
See Polydactyly, Toe

ACE
See Angiotensin Converting Enzyme (ACE)

Acetabuloplasty........27120-27122, 29915

Acetabulum
Fracture
  Closed Treatment........27220-27222
    with Manipulation........27222
    without Manipulation........27220
  Open Treatment........27226-27228
Reconstruction........27120
  with Resection, Femoral Head........27122
Tumor
  Excision........27076

Acetic Anhydride
Analyte........84600

Acetylcholinesterase
Blood or Urine........82013

AcG (Accelerator Globulin)
See Clotting Factor

Achilles Tendon
Incision........27605, 27606
Lengthening........27612
Repair........27650-27654

Achillotomy
See Tenotomy, Achilles Tendon

Acid
Gastric........82930

Acid Diethylamide, Lysergic
See Lysergic Acid Diethylamide

Acid-Fast Bacilli (AFB)
Culture........87116

Acid-Fast Bacillus Culture
See Culture, Acid-Fast Bacilli

Acid-Fast Stain
Analysis........88312

Acid Perfusion Study
Esophagus........91013, 91030

Acid Phosphatase........84060, 84066

Acid Probes, Nucleic
See Nucleic Acid Probe

Acid Reflux Test
Esophagus........91034, 91035, 91037, 91038
Gastroesophageal....91034, 91035, 91037, 91038

Acid, Adenylic
See Adenosine Monophosphate (AMP), 5-Monophosphate, Cyclic

Acid, Aminolevulinic
See Aminolevulinic Acid (ALA)

Acid, Ascorbic
See Ascorbic Acid

Acid, Deoxyribonucleic (DNA)
See Deoxyribonucleic Acid (DNA)

Acid, Folic
See Folic Acid

Acid, Glycocholic
See Cholylglycine

Acid, Lactic
See Lactic Acid

Acid, N-Acetylneuraminic
See Sialic Acid

Acid, Phenylethylbarbituric
See Phenobarbital

Acid, Uric
See Uric Acid

Acidity/Alkalinity
See Blood Gases, pH

Acids, Amino
See Amino Acids

Acids, Bile
See Bile Acids

Acids, Fatty
See Fatty Acid

Acne Surgery
Incision and Drainage
  Abscess........10060, 10061
  Comedones........10040
  Cyst........10040
  Milia, Multiple........10040
  Pustules........10040

Acne Treatment
Abrasion........15786, 15787
Chemical Peel........15788-15793
Cryotherapy........17340
Dermabrasion........15780-15783
Exfoliation
  Chemical........17360

Acoustic Cardiography........93799

Acoustic Evoked Brain Stem Potential
See Evoked Potentials, Auditory Brainstem

Acoustic Neuroma
See Brain, Tumor, Excision; Brainstem; Mesencephalon; Skull Base Surgery

Acoustic Recording
Heart Sounds
  with Computer Analysis........93799

Acoustic Respiratory Measurements
for Wheeze Rate........94799

Acromioclavicular Joint
Arthrocentesis........20605, 20606
Arthrotomy........23044
  with Biopsy........23101
Dislocation........23540-23552
  Open Treatment........23550-23552
X ray........73050

Acromion
Excision........23130

Acromionectomy
Partial........23130

Acromioplasty........23415-23420
Partial........23130

ACTH
See Adrenocorticotropic Hormone (ACTH)

ACTH Releasing Factor
See Corticotropic Releasing Hormone (CRH)

Actigraphy
Sleep Study........95803

Actinomyces
Antibody Detection........86602

Actinomycosis
Antibody Detection........86602

Actinomycotic Infection
See Actinomycosis

Actinotherapy........96900
See Dermatology

Activated Factor X
See Stuart-Prower Factor

Activated Partial Thromboplastin Time (aPTT)
See Thromboplastin, Partial Thromboplastin Time (PTT)

Activation, Lymphocyte
See Blastogenesis

Activities of Daily Living
See Physical Medicine/Therapy/Occupational Therapy

Activity, Glomerular Procoagulant
See Thromboplastin

Acupuncture
with Electrical Stimulation........97813, 97814
without Electrical Stimulation........97810, 97811

Acute Poliomyelitis
See Polio

Acylcarnitines........82016, 82017

Index

Adamantinoma, Pituitary
See Craniopharyngioma

Adaptive Behavior Services
Assessment
  Administered by Physician/QHP 0362T, 97151
  Supporting, Administered by Technician . . . 0362T, 97152
Treatment
  Group . . . 97154, 97158
  Individual . . . 0373T, 97153, 97155
Treatment Guidance . . . 97156, 97157

Addam Operation
See Dupuytren's Contracture

Adductor Tenotomy of Hip
See Tenotomy, Hip, Adductor

Adenoidectomy
See Adenoids, Excision

Adenoids
Excision . . . 42830-42836
  with Tonsils . . . 42820, 42821
Unlisted Services and Procedures . . . 42999

Adenoma
Pancreas
  Excision . . . 48120
Parathyroid
  Localization
    Injection Procedure . . . 78808
Thyroid Gland Excision . . . 60200

Adenosine 3'5' Monophosphate
See Cyclic AMP

Adenosine Diphosphate
Blood . . . 82030

Adenosine Monophosphate (AMP)
5-Monophosphate, Cyclic
  Blood . . . 82030

Adenovirus
Antibody Detection . . . 86603
Antigen Detection
  Immunoassay . . . 87301
  Immunofluorescence . . . 87260

Adenovirus Vaccine
See Vaccines and Toxoids

Adenylic Acid
See Adenosine Monophosphate (AMP)

ADH
See Antidiuretic Hormone

Adhesions
Construction . . . 67880
  Transposition of Tarsal Plate . . . 67882
Epidural . . . 62263, 62264
Eye
  Corneovitreal . . . 65880
  Incision
    Anterior Segment . . . 65860, 65870
    Posterior Segment . . . 65875
Intestinal
  Enterolysis . . . 44005
    Laparoscopic . . . 44180
Intracranial
  Dissection . . . 62161
Intrauterine
  Lysis . . . 58559
Labial
  Lysis . . . 56441
Liver
  Lysis . . . 58660
Lungs
  Pneumonolysis . . . 32124, 32940
Nose
  Lysis . . . 30560
Pelvic
  Lysis . . . 58660, 58740
Penile
  Lysis
    Post-circumcision . . . 54162
Preputial
  Lysis . . . 54450
Urethral
  Lysis . . . 53500

Adipectomy
See Lipectomy

ADL
See Activities of Daily Living

Administration
Immunization
  Each Additional Vaccine/Toxoid 90472, 90474
    with Counseling . . . 90461
  One Vaccine/Toxoid . . . 90471, 90473
    with Counseling . . . 90460
Occlusive Substance . . . 31634
Pharmacologic Agent . . . 93463

ADP
See Adenosine Diphosphate

ADP Phosphocreatine Phosphotransferase
See CPK

Adrenal Cortex Hormone
See Corticosteroids

Adrenal Gland
Biopsy . . . 60540-60545
Excision . . . 60540
  Laparoscopy . . . 60650
  Retroperitoneal Tumor . . . 60545
Exploration . . . 60540, 60545
Nuclear Medicine
  Imaging . . . 78075

Adrenal Medulla
See Medulla

Adrenalectomy
Anesthesia . . . 00866
Complete . . . 60540, 60545, 60650
Laparoscopic . . . 50545
Partial . . . 60540, 60545, 60650

Adrenalin
See Catecholamines
Blood . . . 82383
Urine . . . 82382, 82384

Adrenaline-Noradrenaline
Testing . . . 82382-82384

Adrenocorticotropic Hormone (ACTH) . . . 80400-80406, 80412, 80418, 82024
Blood or Urine . . . 82024
Stimulation Panel . . . 80400-80406

Adrenogenital Syndrome . . . 56805, 57335

Adult T Cell Leukemia Lymphoma Virus I
See HTLV-I

Advanced Life Support
Physician/Health Care Professional Direction 99288

Advancement
Genioglossus . . . 21199
Tendon
  Tibia . . . 28238

Advancement Flap
See Skin, Adjacent Tissue Transfer

Aerosol Inhalation
See Pulmonology, Therapeutic
Pentamidine . . . 94642

AFB
See Acid-Fast Bacilli (AFB)

Afferent Nerve
See Sensory Nerve

AFP
See Alpha-Fetoprotein (AFP)

After Hours Medical Services . . . 99050

Agents, Anticoagulant
See Clotting Inhibitors

Agglutinin
Cold . . . 86156, 86157
Febrile . . . 86000

Aggregation
Platelet . . . 85576

AHG
See Clotting Factor

AICD (Automated Implantable Cardioverter-Defibrillator)
See Cardiac Assist Devices, Subcutaneous Implantable Defibrillator (SICD) and Transvenous Implantable Pacing Defibrillator (ICD)

Aid, Hearing
See Hearing Aid

AIDS Antibodies
See Antibody, Detection, Human Immunodeficiency Virus (HIV)

AIDS Virus
See HIV-1

Airway
Leak
  See Bronchoscopy
Obstruction
  Inhalation Treatment . . . 94640

Akin Operation
See Bunion Repair

ALA
See Aminolevulinic Acid (ALA)

Alanine 2 Oxoglutarate Aminotransferase
See Transaminase, Glutamic-Pyruvic

Alanine Amino Transferase (ALT) . . 84460

Alanine Transaminase
See Transaminase, Glutamic-Pyruvic

Albumin
Ischemia modified . . . 82045
Other Source . . . 82042
Serum, Plasma or Whole Blood . . . 82040
Urine . . . 82043, 82044

Alcohol
Breath . . . 82075
  Ethylene Glycol . . . 82693

Index

Alcohol Dehydrogenase
See Antidiuretic Hormone

Alcohol, Isopropyl
See Isopropyl Alcohol

Alcohol, Methyl
See Methanol

Aldolase
Blood ... 82085

Aldosterone
Blood ... 82088
Suppression Evaluation ... 80408
Urine ... 82088

Alimentary Canal
See Gastrointestinal Tract

Alkaline Phosphatase .. 84075, 84078, 84080
Leukocyte ... 85540
WBC ... 85540

Allergen Bronchial Provocation Tests
See Allergy Tests; Bronchial Challenge Test

Allergen Challenge, Endobronchial
See Bronchial Challenge Test

Allergen Immunotherapy
Allergen
  IgE ... 86003, 86005, 86008
  IgG ... 86001
  Multiallergen Screen ... 86005
Allergenic Extracts
  Injection ... 95115, 95117
  Injection and Provision ... 95120-95134
    Insect Venom ... 95130-95134
Antigens
  Preparation and Provision ... 95144-95165
    Insect Venom ... 95145-94149
Insect, Whole Body Extract ... 95170
Rapid Desensitization ... 95180

Allergy Services/Procedures
See Allergen Immunotherapy; Office and/or Other Outpatient Services
Education and Counseling ... 99201-99215
Unlisted Services and Procedures ... 95199

Allergy Tests
Challenge Test
  Bronchial ... 95070, 95071
  Ingestion ... 95076, 95079
Eye Allergy ... 95060
Food Allergy ... 95076, 95079
Intradermal
  Allergen Extract ... 95024-95028
  Biologicals ... 95018
  Drugs ... 95018
  Incremental ... 95027
  Venoms ... 95017
Nasal Mucous Membrane Test ... 95065
Nose Allergy ... 95065
Patch
  Application Tests ... 95044
  Photo Patch ... 95052
Photosensitivity ... 95056
Skin Tests
  Allergen Extract ... 95004, 95024, 95027
  Biologicals ... 95018
  Drugs ... 95018
  Venoms ... 95017

Allogeneic Donor
Lymphocyte Infusion ... 38242

Allogeneic Transplantation
Hematopoietic Progenitor Cells (HPCs) ... 38240
See Homograft

Allograft
Aortic Valve ... 33406, 33413
Bone
  Elbow Joint ... 24370, 24371
  Hemicortical/Hemicylindrical ... 20933
  Intercalary ... 20933, 20934
  Osteoarticular ... 20932
  Shoulder Joint ... 23473, 23474
  Spine Surgery
    Morselized ... 20930
    Structural ... 20931
Cartilage
  Knee ... 27415
Cornea
  Amniotic Membrane ... 65780
    Endothelial ... 65756
    Lamellar ... 65710
    Penetrating ... 65730, 65750, 65755
  for Aphakia ... 65750
Lung Transplant ... 32850
Nerve ... 64910, 64912, 64913
Skin Substitute
  Arms ... 15271-15274
  Digits ... 15275-15278
  Eyelids ... 15275-15278
  Face ... 15275-15278
  Feet ... 15275-15278
  Genitalia ... 15275-15278
  Hands ... 15275-15278
  Legs ... 15271-15274
  Mouth ... 15275-15278
  Orbits ... 15275-15278
  Scalp ... 15275-15278
  Trunk ... 15271-15274

Allograft Preparation
Cornea ... 65757
Heart ... 33933, 33944
Intestines ... 44715-44721
Kidney ... 50323-50329
Liver ... 47143-47147
Lung ... 32855, 32856, 33933
Pancreas ... 48551, 48552
Renal ... 50323-50329

Allotransplantation
Intestines ... 44135, 44136
  Removal ... 44137
Renal ... 50360-50365
  Removal ... 50370

Almen Test
See Blood, Feces

Alpha-1 Antitrypsin ... 82103, 82104

Alpha-2 Antiplasmin ... 85410

Alpha-Fetoprotein (AFP)
Amniotic Fluid ... 82106
Serum ... 82105, 82107

Alpha-tocopherol ... 84446

ALT
See Transaminase, Glutamic-Pyruvic

Altemeier Procedure
See Procidentia, Rectum; Rectum, Prolapse, Excision

Aluminum
Blood ... 82108

Alveola
Fracture
  Closed Treatment ... 21421
  Open Treatment ... 21422, 21423

Alveolar Cleft
Ungrafted Bilateral ... 21147
Ungrafted Unilateral ... 21146

Alveolar Nerve
Avulsion ... 64738
Incision ... 64738
Transection ... 64738

Alveolar Ridge
Fracture
  Closed Treatment ... 21440
  Open Treatment ... 21445

Alveolectomy ... 41830

Alveoloplasty ... 41874

Alveolus
Excision ... 41830

Amide, Procaine
See Procainamide

Amikacin
Assay ... 80150

Amine
Vaginal Fluid ... 82120

Amino Acids ... 82127-82139

Aminolevulinic Acid (ALA)
Blood or Urine ... 82135

Aminotransferase
See Transaminase

Aminotransferase, Alanine
See Transaminase, Glutamic-Pyruvic

Aminotransferase, Aspartate
See Transaminase, Glutamic-Oxaloacetic

Ammonia
Blood ... 82140

Amniocenteses
See Amniocentesis

Amniocentesis
See Chromosome Analysis
Diagnostic ... 59000
Induced Abortion ... 59850
  with Dilation and Curettage ... 59851
  with Dilation and Evacuation ... 59851
  with Hysterotomy ... 59852
Therapeutic
  Amniotic Fluid Reduction ... 59001

Amnioinfusion
Transabdominal ... 59070

Amnion
Amniocentesis ... 59000
  with Amniotic Fluid Reduction ... 59001
Amnioinfusion
  Transabdominal ... 59070
Membrane Placement
  Eye ... 65778, 65779

Amniotic Fluid
Alpha-Fetoprotein ... 82106
Scan ... 82143
Testing ... 83661, 83663, 83664

Amniotic Membrane
See Amnion

AMP
See Adenosine Monophosphate (AMP)

AMP, Cyclic
See Cyclic AMP

Amputation
See Radical Resection; Replantation
Ankle . . . 27888
Arm, Lower . . . 25900-25905, 25915
Revision . . . 25907, 25909
Arm, Upper . . . 24900-24920
and Shoulder . . . 23900-23921
Cineplasty . . . 24940
Revision . . . 24925-24930
with Implant . . . 24931-24935
Cervix
Total . . . 57530
Ear
Partial . . . 69110
Total . . . 69120
Finger . . . 26910-26952
Foot . . . 28800-28805
Hand at Metacarpal . . . 25927
at Wrist . . . 25920
Revision . . . 25922
Revision . . . 25924, 25929, 25931
Interpelviabdominal . . . 27290
Interthoracoscapular . . . 23900
Leg, Lower . . . 27598, 27880-27882
Revision . . . 27884, 27886
Leg, Upper . . . 27590-27592
at Hip . . . 27290, 27295
Revision . . . 27594, 27596
Metacarpal . . . 26910
Metatarsal . . . 28810
Penis
Partial . . . 54120
Radical . . . 54130, 54135
Total . . . 54125
Thumb . . . 26910, 26951, 26952
Toe . . . 28810, 28820, 28825
Upper Extremity . . . 24900-24940
Cineplasty . . . 24940
Revision . . . 24925, 24930, 24935
with Implant . . . 24931-24935

Amputation through Hand
See Hand, Amputation

Amputation, Nose
See Resection, Nose

Amylase
Blood . . . 82150
Urine . . . 82150

ANA
See Antinuclear Antibodies (ANA)

Anabolic Steroid
See Androstenedione

Anal Abscess
See Abscess, Tissue, Anus

Anal Bleeding
See Anus, Hemorrhage

Anal Fistula
Closure . . . 46288
Repair . . . 46706
Surgical Treatment . . . 46270, 46275, 46280, 46285

Anal Fistulectomy
See Excision, Fistula, Anal

Anal Fistulotomy
See Fistulotomy, Anal

Anal Sphincter
Dilation . . . 45905
Incision . . . 46080

Anal Ulceration
See Anus, Fissure

Analgesia
See Anesthesia; Sedation

Analgesic Cutaneous Electrostimulation
See Application, Neurostimulation

Analysis
Cardiac Devices
See Electronic Analysis, Cardiac Devices
Electrocardiograph
Data Analysis . . . 0206T
Electroencephalogram
Digital . . . 95957
Electronic
Drug Infusion Pump . . . 62367-62370
Neurostimulator Pulse Generator System
Brain . . . 95970, 95983, 95984
Cranial Nerve . . . 95970, 95976, 95977
Gastric . . . 95980-95982
Peripheral Nerve . . . 95970-95972
Spinal Cord . . . 95970-95972
with Programming . . . 95971, 95972, 95976, 95977, 95980, 95982-95984
without Reprogramming . . . 95970, 95981
with Vagus Nerve Blocking Therapy . . 0317T
Pacing Cardioverter-Defibrillator
See Electronic Analysis, Cardiac Devices
Multianalyte Assays with Algorithmic Analysis (MAAA)
Risk Score
Endocrinology Analytes . . . 81506
Fetal Aneuploidy DNA Sequence . . . 81507
Fetal Congenital Abnormalities 81508-81512
Ovarian Oncology Proteins . . . 81500, 81503
Tissue Similarity Score
Gene Expression for Oncology . . . 81504
Unlisted Assay . . . 81599
Physiologic Data, Remote . . . 99091
Proprietary Laboratory . . . 0001U-0003U, 0005U-0014U, 0016U-0061U
Protein
Tissue
Western Blot . . . 88372
Semen . . . 89320-89322
Sperm Isolation . . . 89260, 89261
Waveform
Central Arterial Pressure . . . 93050

Analysis, Spectrum
See Spectrophotometry

Anaspadias
See Epispadias

Anastomosis
Aortic . . . 33866
Atria to Pulmonary Artery . . . 33615
Arteriovenous Fistula
Direct . . . 36821
with Bypass Graft . . . 35686
with Graft . . . 36825, 36830, 36832
Artery
to Aorta . . . 33606
to Artery
Cranial . . . 61711
Bile Duct
to Bile Duct . . . 47800
to Intestines . . . 47760, 47780
Bile Duct to Gastrointestinal Tract . . . 47780, 47785
Broncho-Bronchial . . . 32486
Caval to Mesenteric . . . 37160
Cavopulmonary . . . 33622, 33768
Colorectal . . . 44626
Epididymis
to Vas Deferens
Bilateral . . . 54901
Unilateral . . . 54900
Excision
Trachea . . . 31780, 31781
Fallopian Tube . . . 58750
Gallbladder to Intestines . . . 47720-47740
Hepatic Duct to Intestines . . . 47765, 47802
Ileum to Anus . . . 45113
Intestine to Intestine . . . 44130
Intestines
Colon to Anus . . . 45119
Cystectomy . . . 51590
Enterocystoplasty . . . 51960
Ileoanal . . . 44157, 44158
Resection
Laparoscopic . . . 44202-44205
Intrahepatic Portosystemic . . . 37182, 37183
Jejunum . . . 43820-43825
Microvascular
Free Transfer
Jejunum . . . 43496
Nerve
Facial to Hypoglossal . . . 64868
Oviduct . . . 58750
Pancreas to Intestines . . . 48520, 48540, 48548
Portocaval . . . 37140
Pulmonary . . . 33606
Renoportal . . . 37145
Splenorenal . . . 35636, 37180, 37181
Stomach
to Duodenum . . . 43810, 43855
Revision . . . 43850
to Jejunum . . . 43820-43825, 43860-43865
Tubotubal . . . 58750
Ureter
to Bladder . . . 50780-50785
to Colon . . . 50810-50815
Removal . . . 50830
to Intestine . . . 50800, 50820, 50825
Removal . . . 50830
to Kidney . . . 50727-50750
to Ureter . . . 50725-50727, 50760, 50770
Vein
Saphenopopliteal . . . 34530
Vein to Vein . . . 37140-37160, 37182, 37183
Vena Cava to Pulmonary Artery . . . 33615

Anastomosis of Lacrimal Sac to Conjunctival Sac
See Conjunctivorhinostomy

Anastomosis of Pancreas
See Pancreas, Anastomosis

Anastomosis, Aorta-Pulmonary Artery
See Aorta, Anastomosis, to Pulmonary Artery

Anastomosis, Bladder, to Intestine
See Enterocystoplasty

Anastomosis, Hepatic Duct
See Hepatic Duct, Anastomosis

Anderson Tibial Lengthening . . . 27715
See Ankle; Tibia, Osteoplasty, Lengthening

Androstanediol Glucuronide . . . 82154

Androstenedione
Blood or Urine . . . 82157

Index

Androstenolone
- *See* Dehydroepiandrosterone

Androsterone
- Blood or Urine ... 82160

Anesthesia
- *See* Analgesia
- Abbe-Estlander Procedure ... 00102
- Abdomen
  - Abdominal Wall ... 00700, 00730, 00800-00802, 00820, 00836
    - Halsted Repair ... 00750-00756
  - Blood Vessels ... 00770, 00880-00882
  - Endoscopy ... 00731, 00732, 00811-00813
  - Extraperitoneal ... 00860-00870
  - Hernia Repair ... 00830-00836
    - Halsted Repair ... 00750-00756
  - Intraperitoneal ... 00790-00797, 00840-00851
- Abdominoperineal Resection ... 00844
- Abortion
  - Incomplete ... 01965
  - Induced ... 01966
- Achilles Tendon Repair ... 01472
- Acromioclavicular Joint ... 01620
- Adrenalectomy ... 00866
- Amniocentesis ... 00842
- Aneurysm
  - Axillary-Brachial ... 01652
  - Knee ... 01444
  - Popliteal Artery ... 01444
- Angiography ... 01920
- Ankle ... 00400, 01462-01522
- Anorectal Procedure ... 00902
- Anus ... 00902
- Arm
  - Lower ... 00400, 01810-01820, 01830-01860
  - Upper ... 00400, 01710-01782
- Arrhythmias ... 00410
- Arteriography ... 01916
- Arteriovenous Fistula ... 01432
- Arthrography
- Arthroplasty
  - Hip ... 01214, 01215
  - Knee ... 01402
- Arthroscopic Procedures
  - Ankle ... 01464
  - Elbow ... 01732-01740
  - Foot ... 01464
  - Hip ... 01202
  - Knee ... 01382, 01400
  - Shoulder ... 01622-01638
  - Wrist ... 01829, 01830
- Axilla ... 00400, 01610, 01650, 01652, 01654, 01656, 01670
- Back Skin ... 00300
- Batch-Spittler-McFaddin Operation ... 01404
- Biopsy
  - Ear ... 00120
  - Liver ... 00702
  - Salivary Glands ... 00100
- Bladder ... 00870, 00912
- Brain ... 00210-00218, 00220-00222
- Breast ... 00402-00406
- Bronchi ... 00542
  - Intrathoracic Repair of Trauma ... 00548
  - Reconstruction ... 00539
- Bronchoscopy ... 00520
- Burns
  - Debridement and/or Excision ... 01951-01953
- Burr Hole ... 00214
- Bypass Graft
  - Leg, Lower ... 01500
  - Leg, Upper ... 01270
  - Shoulder, Axillary ... 01654, 01656
- Cardiac Catheterization ... 01920
- Cast
  - Knee ... 01420
- Cast Application
  - Forearm, Wrist, and Hand ... 01860
  - Leg ... 01490
  - Pelvis ... 01130
  - Shoulder ... 01680
- Central Venous Circulation ... 00532
- Cervical Cerclage ... 00948
- Cervix ... 00948
- Cesarean Delivery ... 01961, 01963
- Chest ... 00410, 00470-00474, 00522, 00530-00539, 00542-00548, 00550
- Chest Skin ... 00400
- Childbirth
  - Cesarean Delivery ... 01961, 01963, 01968, 01969
  - External Cephalic Version ... 01958
  - Vaginal Delivery ... 01960, 01967
- Clavicle ... 00450, 00454
- Cleft Lip Repair ... 00102
- Cleft Palate Repair ... 00172
- Colonoscopy, Screening ... 00812
- Colpectomy ... 00942
- Colporrhaphy ... 00942
- Colpotomy ... 00942
- Corneal Transplant ... 00144
- Craniectomy ... 00211
- Cranioplasty ... 00215
- Craniotomy ... 00211
- Culdoscopy ... 00950
- Cystectomy ... 00864
- Cystolithotomy ... 00870
- Decortication ... 00542
- Defibrillator ... 00534, 00560
- Diaphragm ... 00540, 00541
- Disarticulation
  - Hip ... 01212
  - Knee ... 01404
  - Shoulder ... 01634
- Drug Administration
  - Epidural or Subarachnoid ... 01996
- Ear ... 00120-00126
- Elbow ... 00400, 01710-01782
- Electrocoagulation
  - Intracranial Nerve ... 00222
- Electroconvulsive Therapy ... 00104
- Embolectomy
  - Arm, Upper ... 01772
  - Femoral ... 01274
  - Femoral Artery ... 01274
  - Forearm, Wrist, and Hand ... 01842
  - Leg, Lower ... 01502
- Endoscopy
  - Arm, Lower ... 01830
  - Gastrointestinal ... 00731, 00732, 00813
  - Intestines ... 00811-00812
  - Uterus ... 00952
  - Vagina ... 00950
- Esophagus ... 00320, 00500
- External Cephalic Version ... 01958
- Eye ... 00140-00148
  - Cornea ... 00144
  - Iridectomy ... 00147
  - Iris ... 00147
  - Lens ... 00142
- Eyelid ... 00103
- Facial Bones ... 00190, 00192
- Fallopian Tube
  - Ligation ... 00851
- Femoral Artery
  - Embolectomy ... 01274
  - Ligation ... 01272
- Femur ... 01220-01234, 01340, 01360
- Fibula ... 01390-01392
- Foot ... 01462-01522
- Forearm ... 01810-01820, 01830-01860
- Fowler-Stephens Orchiopexy ... 00930
- Gastrocnemius Recession ... 01474
- Gastrointestinal Endoscopy ... 00731, 00732, 00813
- Genitalia
  - Female ... 00940-00952
  - Male ... 00920-00938
- Great Vessels of Chest ... 00560-00563
- Hand ... 00400, 01810-01820, 01830-01860
- Harrington Rod Technique ... 00670
- Head ... 00210-00222, 00300
  - Muscles ... 00300
  - Nerves ... 00300
- Heart ... 00560-00567, 00580
  - Coronary Artery Bypass Grafting ... 00566, 00567
  - Electrophysiology/Ablation ... 00537
  - Transplant ... 00580
- Hepatectomy
  - Partial ... 00792
- Hernia Repair
  - Abdomen
    - Lower ... 00830-00836
    - Upper ... 00750-00752, 00756
- Hip ... 01200-01215
- Humerus ... 01620, 01730, 01742-01744, 01758
- Hysterectomy ... 01962
  - Cesarean ... 01963, 01969
  - Radical ... 00846
  - Vaginal ... 00944
- Hysterosalpingography ... 00952
- Hysteroscopy ... 00952
- Induced Abortion ... 01966
- Inferior Vena Cava Ligation ... 00882
  - Nerve ... 01991, 01992
- Integumentary System
  - Anterior Trunk ... 00400
  - Arm, Upper ... 00400
  - Axilla ... 00400
  - Elbow ... 00400
  - Extremity ... 00400
  - Forearm ... 00400
  - Hand ... 00400
  - Head ... 00300
  - Knee ... 00400
  - Leg, Lower ... 00400
  - Leg, Upper ... 00400
  - Neck ... 00300
  - Perineum ... 00400
  - Popliteal Area ... 00400
  - Posterior Pelvis ... 00300
  - Posterior Trunk ... 00300
  - Shoulder ... 00400
  - Wrist ... 00400
- Intestines
  - Endoscopy ... 00811-00813
- Intracranial Procedures ... 00210-00218, 00220-00222
- Intraoral Procedures ... 00170-00176
- Intrathoracic Procedures
  - Bronchi ... 00539, 00548
  - Trachea ... 00539, 00548
- Intrathoracic System ... 00500, 00520-00529, 00530-00539, 00540-00548, 00550, 00560-00567, 00580
- Iridectomy ... 00147
- Keen Operation ... 00604
- Kidney ... 00862, 00868, 00872, 00873

Knee 00400, 01320, 01340, 01360, 01380-01404, 01420, 01430-01432, 01440-01444
Knee Skin 00400
Laminectomy............ 00604
Laparoscopy 00790-00792, 00840
Larynx 00320, 00326
Leg
Lower 01462-01522
Upper 01200-01274
Life Support for Organ Donor 01990
Ligation
Fallopian Tube 00851
Lithotripsy 00872, 00873
Liver............ 00702, 00796
Transplant 00796
Liver Hemorrhage 00792
Lumbar Puncture............ 00635
Lungs............ 00522, 00539, 00540-00548
Transplant 00580
Lymphadenectomy 00934, 00936
Lymphatic System............ 00320
Mammoplasty............ 00402
Manipulation of Temporomandibular Joint(s) (TMJ)
Therapeutic 21073
Mediastinoscopy............ 00528, 00529
Mediastinum........ 00528, 00529, 00540, 00541
Mouth 00170, 00172
Neck 00300, 00320-00322, 00350-00352
Nephrectomy............ 00862
Neuraxial
Cesarean Delivery 01968, 01969
Labor 01967-01969
Vaginal Delivery............ 01967
Nose 00160-00164
Removal
Foreign Body............ 30310
Omphalocele............ 00754
Ophthalmoscopy............ 00148
Orchiectomy 00926, 00928
Orchiopexy 00930
Torek Procedure............ 00930
Organ Harvesting
Brain-Dead Patient............ 01990
Osteoplasty
Tibia/Fibula 01484
Osteotomy
Humerus............ 01742
Tibia/Fibula 01484
Other Procedures 01990, 01996-01999
Otoscopy............ 00124
Pacemaker Insertion 00530
Pacing Cardioverter-Defibrillator
Insertion/Replacement............ 00534
Pancreas 00794
Pancreatectomy 00794
Panniculectomy............ 00802
Patella............ 01390-01392
Pectus Excavatum............ 00474
Pelvic Exenteration............ 00848
Pelvis............ 00400, 00865, 01112
Amputation 01140
Bone............ 01120
Bone Marrow............ 01112
Examination 57400
Extraperitoneal............ 00864
Intraperitoneal 00844-00848
Repair............ 01173
Skin 00300, 00400
Penis 00932-00938
Pericardial Sac 00560-00563
Perineum............ 00904-00908
Pharynx 00174, 00176
Phleborrhaphy
Arm, Upper............ 01782
Forearm, Wrist, and Hand 01852
Pleura 00540, 00541
Needle Biopsy 00522
Pneumocentesis 00524
Popliteal Area 00400, 01320, 01430-01444
Prognathism 00192
Prostate............ 00865, 00908, 00914
Prostatectomy
Perineal 00908
Radical 00865
Walsh Modified Radical 00865
Radiological Procedures 01916-01936
Arterial
Therapeutic............ 01924-01926
Spine and Spinal Cord
Percutaneous Image Guided .. 01935, 01936
Venous/Lymphatic
Therapeutic............ 01930-01933
Renal Procedures 00862
Repair of Skull............ 00215
Replacement
Ankle 01486
Elbow 01760
Hip 01212, 01214, 01215
Knee............ 01402
Shoulder............ 01638
Wrist 01832
Restriction
Gastric
for Obesity 00797
Retropharyngeal Tumor Excision 00174
Rib Resection 00470, 00472, 00474
Sacroiliac Joint............ 01160, 01170
Salivary Glands............ 00100
Scapula 00450
Scheie Procedure 00147
Sedation
Moderate........ 99151-99153, 99155-99157
with Independent Observation 99151-99153
Seminal Vesicles............ 00922
Shoulder
Arteries 01650, 01652, 01654, 01656
Arthroscopic Procedures 01622, 01630, 01634, 01636, 01638
Bursae 01610
Fascia............ 01610
Integumentary System............ 00400
Joint............ 01620
Muscles 01610
Nerves 01610
Tendons 01610
Veins 01670
Shunt
Spinal Fluid............ 00220
Sinuses
Accessory............ 00160-00164
Skull 00190
Skull Fracture
Elevation 00215
Special Circumstances
Emergency 99140
Extreme Age............ 99100
Hypotension............ 99135
Hypothermia............ 99116
Spinal Instrumentation 00670
Spinal Manipulation 00640
Spine and Spinal Cord 00600-00604, 00620, 00670
Cervical 00600-00604, 00640, 00670
Injection............ 62320-62327
Lumbar 00630-00635, 00640, 00670
Percutaneous Image Guided 01935, 01936
Thoracic 00620-00626, 00640, 00670
Vascular............ 00670
Sternoclavicular Joint............ 01620
Sternum............ 00550
Stomach
Restriction
for Obesity 00797
Strayer Procedure............ 01474
Subdural Taps............ 00212
Sympathectomy
Lumbar............ 00632
Symphysis Pubis............ 01160, 01170
Tenodesis 01716
Tenoplasty............ 01714
Tenotomy 01712
Testis............ 00924-00928, 00930
Thoracoplasty 00472
Thoracoscopy 00528, 00529, 00540, 00541
Thoracotomy............ 00540, 00541
Thorax .. 00400-00410, 00450, 00454, 00470-00474
Thromboendarterectomy............ 01442
Thyroid 00320-00322
Tibia 01390-01392, 01484
Trachea............ 00320, 00326, 00542
Reconstruction............ 00539
Transplantation
Cornea 00144
Heart 00580
Kidney 00868
Liver............ 00796, 01990
Lungs 00580
Organ Harvesting............ 01990
Transurethral Procedures 00910-00918
Tubal Ligation 00851
Tuffier Vaginal Hysterectomy............ 00944
TURP 00914
Tympanostomy 00120
Tympanotomy 00126
Unlisted Services and Procedures 01999
Urethra 00910, 00918-00920, 00942
Urethrocystoscopy 00910
Urinary Bladder............ 00864, 00870, 00912
Urinary Tract............ 00860
Uterus............ 00952
Vagina............ 00940-00942, 00950
Vaginal Delivery 01960
Vas Deferens
Excision 00921
Vascular Access 00532
Vascular Shunt 01844
Vascular Surgery
Abdomen, Lower 00880-00882
Abdomen, Upper 00770
Arm, Lower............ 01840-01852
Arm, Upper............ 01770-01782
Brain............ 00216
Elbow 01770-01782
Hand............ 01840-01852
Knee............ 01430-01444
Leg, Lower 01500-01522
Leg, Upper 01260, 01270-01274
Neck............ 00350-00352
Shoulder............ 01650-01670
Wrist 01840-01852
Vasectomy............ 00921
Venography............ 01916
Ventriculography............ 00214, 01920
Vertebroplasty............ 01936
Vitrectomy............ 00145
Vitreoretinal Surgery............ 00145
Vitreous Body 00145
Vulva............ 00906
Vulvectomy 00906

Wertheim Operation 00846
Wrist 00400, 01810-01860

Anesthesia, Local
See Injection, Anesthetic Agent

Aneurysm Repair
See Aorta; Artery
Abdominal Aorta 34830-34832, 34845-34848, 35081-35103
Axillary Artery 35011, 35013
Basilar Artery 61698, 61702
Brachial Artery 35011, 35013
Carotid Artery 35001, 35002, 61613, 61697, 61700, 61703
Celiac Artery 35121, 35122
Femoral Artery 35141, 35142
Hepatic Artery 35121, 35122
Iliac Artery 34703-34708, 35131, 35132
Infrarenal Aorta 34701-34706, 34709-34711
Innominate Artery 35021, 35022
Intracranial Artery 61705-61708
Mesenteric Artery 35121, 35122
Popliteal Artery 35151, 35152
Radial Artery 35045
Renal Artery 35121, 35122
Splenic Artery 35111, 35112
Subclavian Artery 35001, 35002, 35021, 35022
Thoracoabdominal Aorta 33877
Ulnar Artery 35045
Vertebral Artery 61698, 61702

Angel Dust
See Phencyclidine

Angina Assessment
Performance Measures 1002F
  Coronary Artery Disease . . 0557F, 1010F-1012F

Angiocardiographies
See Angiography, specific structure or vessel

Angiography
See Aortography
Abdomen 74174, 74175, 74185, 75635, 75726
Adrenal 75731, 75733
Arm Artery 73206, 75710, 75716
Brain 70496
Bypass Graft 93455, 93457, 93459, 93461
Carotid Artery 36221, 36222, 36223, 36224, 36225, 36226, 37227, 36228
Cervicocerebral Arch 36221, 36222, 36223, 36224, 36225, 36226
Chest 71275, 71555
Common Carotid
  Selective Catheterization 36222, 36223
Endovascular Repair 75956, 75957
Extracranial Carotid
  Non-selective 36221
  Selective 36222, 36223, 36224
Extremity, Lower 73725
Extremity, Upper 73225
Fluorescein 92235, 92242
Head 70496, 70544-70546
Heart
  Abdominal Aorta 75635
  Aorta
    Injection 93567
  Atrial 93565, 93566
  Congenital Heart 93563, 93564
  Coronary Artery 93454-93461, 93563
    Flow Velocity Measurement . . 93571, 93572
  Left Heart
    Injection 93565
      See Cardiac Catheterization, Injection
  Right Heart
    Injection 93566
Injection 93454-93461, 93563, 93565, 93566
Indocyanine-green 92240, 92242
Innominate Artery 36222, 36223, 36225
Intracranial 36221, 36223, 36224
  with Endovascular Infusion 61640, 61650, 61651
  with Thrombectomy 61645
Leg Artery 73706, 75635, 75710-75716
Lung
  Injection 93568
    See Cardiac Catheterization, Injection
Magnetic Resonance (MRA)
  See Magnetic Resonance Angiography (MRA)
Mammary Artery 75756
  See Aortography
Neck 70498, 70547-70549
Non-Cardiac Vascular Flow 78445
Other Artery 75774
Pelvis 72191, 72198, 74174, 75736
Pulmonary 75741-75746, 93568
Renal Artery 36251-36254
Selective Catheterization
  See Selective Catheterization, specific vessel
Spinal Artery 75705
Spinal Canal 72159
Subclavian Artery 36225
Thorax 71275
Transcatheter Therapy
  Embolization 75894, 75898
  Infusion 75898
Ventricular 93565, 93566
Vertebral Artery 36221, 36225, 36226, 36228

Angioma
See Lesion, Skin

Angioplasties, Coronary Balloon
See Percutaneous Transluminal Angioplasty

Angioplasty
Aorta
  Intraoperative 37246, 37247
  Percutaneous 37246, 37247
Axillary Artery
  Intraoperative 37246, 37247
Brachiocephalic Artery
  Intraoperative 37246, 37247
  Percutaneous 37246, 37247
Coronary Artery
  Percutaneous Transluminal 92920, 92921
  with Atherectomy 92937, 92938, 92941, 92943, 92944
  with Stent Placement . . 92928, 92929, 92937, 92938, 92941, 92943, 92944
Femoral Artery
  Intraoperative 37224
for Revascularization
  Intracoronary 92937, 92938, 92941, 92943, 92944
Iliac Artery
  Intraoperative 37220, 37222
Intracranial
  Percutaneous 61630
Patch
  Blood Vessel 35201-35286
  Vein 35879
Percutaneous Transluminal
  See Percutaneous Transluminal Angioplasty
Perineal Artery 37228
Popliteal Artery
  Intraoperative 37224
Pulmonary Artery
  Percutaneous Transluminal 92997, 92998
Renal Artery
  Open 37246-37249
  Percutaneous 37246-37249
Subclavian Artery
  Intraoperative 37246, 37247
Tibial/Peroneal Artery
  Intraoperative 37228
  Balloon
    Open 37246-37249
    Percutaneous 37246-37249
  Dialysis Circuit 36902, 36907
  Venous 37248, 37249
Venous
  Open 37248, 37249
  Percutaneous 37248, 37249
Visceral Artery
  Open 37246, 37247
  Percutaneous 37246, 37247
with Endovascular Repair 34841-34848
with Intravascular Stent Placement . . 37215-37218, 37236-37239

Angioscopy
Noncoronary Vessels 35400

Angiotensin Converting Enzyme (ACE)
Angiotensin I
  Quantitative 82164
Angiotensin II
  Quantitative 82163
Receptor, Gene Analysis 81400
Therapy
  Performance Measures 4188F, 4210F
    Angiotensin Converting Enzyme
    Inhibitor 4010F, 4480F, 4481F
    Angiotensin Receptor Blocker
    (ARB) . . . 4010F, 4188F, 4210F, 4480F, 4481F

Angiotensin Forming Enzyme
See Renin

Angiotensin I 84244
Riboflavin 84252

Angiotensin II
Blood or Urine 82163

Angle Deformity
Toe
  Reconstruction 28313

Anhydride, Carbonic
See Carbon Dioxide

Anhydrides, Acetic
See Acetic Anhydride

Animal Inoculation 87003, 87250

Ankle
See Fibula; Leg, Lower; Tibia; Tibiofibular Joint
Abscess
  Incision and Drainage 27603
Amputation 27888
Arthrocentesis 20605, 20606
Arthrodesis 27870
Arthrography 73615
Arthroplasty 27700, 27702, 27703
Arthroscopy
  Surgical 29891, 29894-29899
Arthrotomy 27610-27612, 27620-27626
Biopsy 27613, 27614, 27620
Bursa
  Incision and Drainage 27604
Disarticulation 27889
Dislocation
  Closed Treatment 27840, 27842
  Open Treatment 27846, 27848

Exploration 27610, 27620
Fracture
Bimalleolar 27808-27814
Lateral 27786-27814
Medial 27760-27766, 27808-27814
Posterior 27767-27769, 27808-27814
Trimalleolar 27816-27823
Fusion 27870
Hematoma
Incision and Drainage 27603
Incision 27607
Injection
Radiological 27648
Lesion
Excision 27630
Magnetic Resonance Imaging (MRI) . . 73721-73723
Manipulation 27860
Removal
Foreign Body 27610, 27620
Implant 27704
Loose Body 27620
Repair
Achilles Tendon 27650-27654
Ligament 27695-27698
Tendon 27612, 27680-27687
Strapping 29540
Synovium
Excision 27625, 27626
Tenotomy 27605, 27606
Tumor
Soft Tissue
Excision . . 27618, 27619, 27630, 27632, 27634
Radical Resection 27615, 27616
Unlisted Services and Procedures 27899
X ray 73600-73610
with Contrast 73615

Ankylosis (Surgical)
See Arthrodesis

Annuloplasty
Intradiscal
Percutaneous 22526, 22527

Anogenital Region
See Perineum

Anoplasty
Stricture 46700, 46705

Anorectal Biofeedback 90911

Anorectal Exam (Surgical) 45990

Anorectal Fistula
Repair 46706, 46707

Anorectal Myectomy
See Myomectomy, Anorectal

Anorectovaginoplasty 46744-46746

Anoscopy
Ablation
Polyp 46615
Tumor 46615
Biopsy 46606
Collection of Specimen 46600, 46601
Dilation 46604
Exploration 46600
Hemorrhage 46614
High Resolution Anoscopy (HRA)
Diagnostic 46601
with Biopsy(ies) 46607
Injection
Bulking Agent 0377T
Removal
Foreign Body 46608
Polyp 46610-46612
Tumor 46610-46612

Antebrachium
See Forearm

Antecedent, Plasma Thromboplastin
See Plasma Thromboplastin, Antecedent

Antepartum Care
Cesarean Delivery 59510
Previous 59610, 59618
Vaginal Delivery 59400, 59425, 59426

Anterior Chamber Fluid, Eye
See Paracentesis, Eye

Anterior Ramus of Thoracic Nerve
See Intercostal Nerve

Anthrax Vaccine
See Vaccines and Toxoids

Anthrogon
See Follicle Stimulating Hormone (FSH)

Anti-Australia Antigens
See Hepatitis Antigen, Detection, Immunoassay, B Surface (HBsAg)

Anti-D Immunoglobulin
See Immune Globulins, Rho(D)

Antihuman Globulin Consumption Test
See Coombs Test

Antiphospholipid Antibody
See Antibody, Detection, Anti-phosphatidylserine (Phospholipid)

Antiactivator, Plasmin
See Alpha-2 Antiplasmin

Antibiotic Administration
Injection 96372-96379
Prescribed or Dispensed 4120F, 4124F

Antibiotic Sensitivity
Susceptibility Studies 87181-87184, 87188
Enzyme Detection 87185
Minimum Inhibitory Concentration (MIC) 87186
Minimum Lethal Concentration (MLC) . . . 87187

Antibodies, Thyroid-Stimulating
See Immunoglobulin, Thyroid Stimulating

Antibodies, Viral
See Viral Antibodies

Antibody
See Antibody Identification; Microsomal Antibody Detection
Actinomyces 86602
Adenovirus 86603
Antinuclear 86038, 86039
Anti-phosphatidylserine (Phospholipid) . . 86148
Antistreptolysin O 86060, 86063
Aspergillus 86606
Bacterium 86609
Bartonella 86611
Beta-2 Glycoprotein I 86146
Blastomyces 86612
Blood Crossmatch 86920-86923
Bordetella 86615
Borrelia 86617-86619
Brucella 86622
Campylobacter 86625
Candida 86628
Cardiolipin 86147
Chlamydia 86631, 86632
Coccidioides 86635
Coxiella Burnetii 86638
C-Reactive Protein (CRP) 86140, 86141
Cryptococcus 86641
Cyclic Citrullinated Peptide (CCP) 86200
Cytomegalovirus (CMV) 86644, 86645
Cytotoxic Screen 86807, 86808
Deoxyribonuclease 86215
Deoxyribonucleic Acid (DNA) 86225, 86226
Diphtheria 86648
Ehrlichia 86666
Encephalitis 86651-86654
Enterovirus 86658
Epstein-Barr Virus 86663-86665
Fluorescent 86255, 86256
Francisella Tularensis 86668
Fungus, Other 86671
Giardia Lamblia 86674
Growth Hormone 86277
Helicobacter Pylori 86677
Helminth 86682
Haemophilus Influenzae 86684
Hepatitis
Delta Agent 86692
Hepatitis A (HAAb) 86708, 86709
Hepatitis B
Core (HBcAb) 86704
IgM 86705
Surface (HBsAb) 86706
Hepatitis Be (HBeAb) 86707
Hepatitis C Virus (HCV) 86803, 86804
Herpes Simplex 86694-86696
Heterophile 86308-86310
Histoplasma 86698
Human Immunodeficiency Virus (HIV)
HIV 86689, 86701-86703
HIV-1 . . . . . 86701, 86703, 87389
HIV-2 . . . . . 86702, 86703, 87389
HTLV-I 86687, 86689
HTLV-II 86688
HTLV-III
Human Leukocyte Antigens (HLA) 86828-86835
Infectious Agent, Other 86317
Influenza Virus 86710
Insulin 86337
Intrinsic Factor 86340
Islet Cell 86341
JC (John Cunningham) Virus 86711
Legionella 86713
Leishmania 86717
Leptospira 86720
Listeria Monocytogenes 86723
Lyme Disease 86617
Lymphocytic Choriomeningitis 86727
Malaria 86750
Microsomal 86376
Mucormycosis 86732
Mumps 86735
Mycoplasma 86738
Neisseria Meningitidis 86741
Nocardia 86744
Nuclear Antigen 86235
Parvovirus 86747
Phospholipid 85597, 86147
Neutralization 85597, 85598
Plasmodium 86750
Platelet 85597, 86022, 86023
Protozoa 86753
Red Blood Cell 86850, 86860, 86870
Respiratory Syncytial Virus 86756
Rickettsia 86757
Rotavirus 86759
Rubella 86762
Rubeola 86765

Index

Salmonella . . . 86768
Shigella . . . 86771
Sperm . . . 89325
Streptokinase . . . 86590
Tetanus . . . 86774
Thyroglobulin . . . 86800
Toxoplasma . . . 86777, 86778
Treponema Pallidum . . . 86780
Trichinella . . . 86784
Tuberculosis . . . 86580
Varicella-Zoster . . . 86787
Virus, Other . . . 86790
West Nile Virus . . . 86788, 86789
White Blood Cell . . . 86021
Yersinia . . . 86793
Zika Virus, IgM . . . 86794

Antibody Identification
Fluorescent . . . 86255, 86256
Immunoassay . . . 83516, 83518-83520
Immunocytochemistry . . . 88341, 88342, 88344
Immunoelectrophoresis . . . 86320, 86325, 86327, 86334, 86335
Leukocyte Antibodies . . . 86021, 86828-86835
Platelet . . . 86022, 86023
Red Blood Cell . . . 86850, 86860, 86870
Pretreatment . . . 86970-86972, 86975-86978
Solid Phase Assay . . . 86828-86835

Antibody Neutralization Test
See Neutralization Test

Antibody Receptor
See Fc Receptor

Antibody Screening
Fluorescent Noninfectious . . . 86255
Cytotoxic Percent Reactive Antibody (PRA) . . . 86807, 86808

Anticoagulant
See Clotting Inhibitors

Anticoagulant Management
Home and Outpatient . . . 93793

Antidiabetic Hormone
See Glucagon

Antidiuretic Hormone
Measurement
Vasopressin . . . 84588

AntiDNA Autoantibody
See Antinuclear Antibodies (ANA)

Antigen
See Antigen Detection
Allergen Immunotherapy . . . 95144-95149, 95165, 95170
Carcinoembryonic . . . 82378
Prostate Specific . . . 84152, 84153

Antigen Bronchial Provocation Tests
See Bronchial Challenge Test

Antigen Detection
Direct Fluorescence
Cytomegalovirus . . . 87271
Enterovirus . . . 87267
Immunoassay
Adenovirus . . . 87301
Aspergillus . . . 87305
Chlamydia Trachomatis . . . 87320
Clostridium Difficile . . . 87324
Cryptococcus Neoformans . . . 87327
Cryptosporidium . . . 87328
Cytomegalovirus . . . 87332
Entamoeba Histolytica Dispar Group . . . 87336
Entamoeba Histolytica Group . . . 87337
Escherichia coli 0157 . . . 87335
Giardia . . . 87329
Helicobacter Pylori . . . 87338, 87339
Hepatitis B Surface Antigen (HBsAg) . . . 87340
Neutralization . . . 87341
Hepatitis Be Antigen (HBeAg) . . . 87350
Hepatitis Delta Agent . . . 87380
Histoplasma capsulatum . . . 87385
HIV-1 . . . 87389, 87390
HIV-2 . . . 87391
Infectious Agent, Otherwise . . . 87449, 87450
Influenza A . . . 87400
Influenza B . . . 87400
Polyvalent . . . 87451
Respiratory Syncytial Virus . . . 87420
Rotavirus . . . 87425
Shiga-like Toxin . . . 87427
Streptococcus, Group A . . . 87430
Immunoassay with Direct Optical Observation
Clostridium Difficile Toxin A . . . 87803
Influenza . . . 87804
Respiratory Syncytial Virus . . . 87807
Streptococcus, Group B . . . 87802
Trichomonas Vaginalis . . . 87808
Immunofluorescence
Adenovirus . . . 87260
Bordetella Pertussis . . . 87265
Chlamydia Trachomatis . . . 87270
Cryptosporidium . . . 87272
Giardia . . . 87269
Herpes Simplex . . . 87273, 87274
Influenza A . . . 87276
Influenza B . . . 87275
Legionella Pneumophila . . . 87278
Organism, Other . . . 87299
Parainfluenza Virus . . . 87279
Pneumocystis Carinii . . . 87281
Polyvalent . . . 87300
Respiratory Syncytial Virus . . . 87280
Rubeola . . . 87283
Treponema Pallidum . . . 87285
Varicella Zoster . . . 87290

Antigen, Australia
See Hepatitis Antigen, Detection, Immunoassay, B Surface (HBsAg)

Antigen, CD4
See CD4

Antigen, CD8
See CD8

Antigens, CD142
See Thromboplastin

Antigens, CD143
See Angiotensin Converting Enzyme (ACE)

Antigens, E
See Hepatitis Antigen, Detection, Immunoassay, Be (HBeAg)

Antigens, Hepatitis
See Hepatitis Antigen

Antigens, Hepatitis B
See Hepatitis Antigen, Detection, Nucleic Acid, B

Antihemophilic Factor B
See Christmas Factor

Antihemophilic Factor C
See Plasma Thromboplastin, Antecedent

Antihemophilic Globulin (AHG) . . . 85240

Antihuman Globulin . . . 86880-86886

Antinuclear Antibodies (ANA) . . . 86038, 86039

Antiplasmin, Alpha-2 . . . 85410

Antiplatelet Therapy
Performance Measures
Coronary Artery Disease . . . 4011F
Stroke and Stroke Rehabilitation . . . 4073F

Antiprotease, Alpha-1
See Alpha-1 Antitrypsin

Antistreptococcal Antibody . . . 86215

Antistreptokinase Titer . . . 86590

Antistreptolysin O . . . 86060-86063

Antithrombin III . . . 85300, 85301

Antithrombin VI
See Fibrin Degradation Products

Antitoxin Assay . . . 87230

Antiviral Antibody
See Viral Antibodies

Antrostomy
Sinus
Maxillary . . . 31256, 31267

Antrotomy
Sinus
Maxillary . . . 31020, 31030, 31032
Transmastoid . . . 69501

Antrum of Highmore
See Sinus/Sinuses, Maxillary

Antrum Puncture
Sinus
Maxillary . . . 31000
Sphenoid . . . 31002

Anus
See Hemorrhoids; Rectum
Ablation . . . 46615
Abscess
Incision and Drainage . . . 46045, 46050
Anoscopy
See Anoscopy
Biofeedback . . . 90911
Biopsy
Endoscopy . . . 46606
Crypt
Excision . . . 46999
Dilation
Endoscopy . . . 46604
Endoscopy
Biopsy . . . 46606
Dilation . . . 46604
Exploration . . . 46600
Hemorrhage . . . 46614
High Resolution Anoscopy (HRA) 46601, 46607
Injection
Bulking Agent . . . 0377T
Removal
Foreign Body . . . 46608
Polyp . . . 46610, 46612
Tumor . . . 46610, 46612
Excision
Tag . . . 46220, 46230
Exploration
Endoscopy . . . 46600
Surgical . . . 45990
Fissure
Destruction . . . 46940, 46942
Excision . . . 46200

Fistula
 Closure . . . 46288
 Excision . . . 46270-46285
 Repair . . . 46706
Hemorrhage
 Endoscopic Control . . . 46614
Hemorrhoids
 Clot Excision . . . 46320
 Destruction . . . 46930
 Excision . . . 46250-46262
 Injection . . . 46500
 Ligation . . . 0249T, 46221, 46945, 46946
 Stapling . . . 46947
 Suture . . . 46945, 46946
Imperforated
 Repair . . . 46715-46742
Incision
 Septum . . . 46070
 Sphincterotomy . . . 46200
Lesion
 Destruction . . . 46900-46917, 46924
 Excision . . . 45108, 46922
Manometry . . . 91122
Placement
 Seton . . . 46020
Reconstruction
 Congenital Absence . . . 46730-46740
 Sphincter . . . 46750, 46751, 46760-46761
 with Graft . . . 46753
Removal
 Foreign Body . . . 46608
 Seton . . . 46030
 Suture . . . 46754
 Wire . . . 46754
Repair
 Anoperineal Fistula . . . 46715, 46716
 Cloacal Anomaly . . . 46744, 46746, 46748
 Fistula . . . 46706
 Stricture . . . 46700, 46705
Sphincter
 Chemodenervation . . . 46505
 Electromyography . . . 51784, 51785
 Needle . . . 51785
 Sphincterotomy . . . 46200
Unlisted Services and Procedures . . . 46999

Aorta
Abdominal
 Aneurysm
  Endovascular Repair . . . 34845-34848
  Screening . . . 76706
 Angiography . . . 75635
 Thromboendarterectomy . . . 35331
Anastomosis
 to Pulmonary Artery . . . 33606
 with Excision of Coarctation . . . 33840
Angiogram
 Radiological Injection . . . 93567
  See Cardiac Catheterization, Injection
Angioplasty . . . 37246, 37247
Aortography . . . 75600, 75605, 75625, 75630
Ascending
 Graft . . . 33864
Balloon Assist Device
 Insertion . . . 33967, 33970, 33973
 Removal . . . 33968, 33971, 33974
Catheterization
 Catheter . . . 36200
 Intracatheter/Needle . . . 36160
Circulation Assist Device
 Insertion . . . 33967, 33970, 33973
 Removal . . . 33968, 33971, 33974
Conduit to Heart . . . 33404
Endograft
 Fenestrated . . . 34839, 34841-34848
Excision
 Coarctation . . . 33840, 33845, 33851
Graft
 Descending Thoracic . . . 33875
 Hemiarch . . . 33866
 Transverse Arch . . . 33870
Implantable Counterpulsation Ventricular Assist System
 Insertion . . . 0451T-0454T
 Interrogation Device Evaluation . . . 0463T
 Programming Device Evaluation . . . 0462T
 Relocation . . . 0459T
 Removal . . . 0455T-0458T
 Replacement . . . 0451T-0454T
 Repositioning . . . 0460T, 0461T
Infrarenal Abdominal
 Repair
  Endovascular . . . 34701-34706, 34709-34711, 34845-34848
Insertion
 Balloon Device . . . 33967, 33970, 33973
 Catheter . . . 36200
 Graft . . . 33330, 33335, 33864, 33866
 Intracatheter/Needle . . . 36160
Removal
 Balloon Assist Device . . . 33968, 33971, 33974
Repair . . . 33320-33322, 33802, 33803
 Coarctation . . . 33840, 33845, 33851
 Aneurysm
  Ascending . . . 33860, 33863, 33864
  Sinus of Valsalva . . . 33720
  Thoracic . . . 33875, 33877
  Transverse Arch . . . 33870
 Hypoplastic or Interrupted Aortic Arch . . . 33852, 33853
 Sinus of Valsalva . . . 33702, 33710, 33720
Suspension . . . 33800
Suture . . . 33320-33322
Thoracic
 Catheterization . . . 36221
 Repair . . . 33875, 33877, 75956-75959
  Endovascular . . . 33880, 33881, 33883, 33884, 33886, 33889, 33891
Translocation
 Aortic Root . . . 33782, 33783
Valve
 Implantation . . . 33361-33369
 Incision . . . 33415
 Repair . . . 33390, 33391
  Left Ventricle . . . 33414
  Supravalvular Stenosis . . . 33417
 Replacement
  See Aortic Valve Replacement
Visceral
 Repair
  Endovascular . . . 34839, 34841-34848
X ray with Contrast . . . 75600, 75605, 75625, 75630

Aortopulmonary Transposition
See Transposition, Great Arteries

Aortic Sinus
See Sinus/Sinuses, Sinus of Valsalva

Aortic Stenosis
Repair . . . 33415
 Nikaidoh Procedure . . . 33782, 33783
 Supravalvular . . . 33417

Aortic Valve
Closure
 Paravalvular Leak . . . 93591, 93592
Construction
 Apical-Aortic Conduit . . . 33404
Implantation
 Transcatheter . . . 33361-33369
Occlusion
 Paravalvular Leak . . . 93591, 93592
Repair
 Gusset Aortoplasty . . . 33417
 Outflow Tract Obstruction
  Left Ventricle . . . 33414
 Stenosis
  Idiopathic Hypertrophic . . . 33416
  Subvalvular . . . 33415
  Supravalvular . . . 33417
 Valvuloplasty
  Open, with Cardiopulmonary Bypass . . . 33390, 33391
Replacement
 See Aortic Valve Replacement

Aortic Valve Replacement
Open
 with Allograft Valve . . . 33406
 with Cardiopulmonary Bypass . . . 33405, 33406, 33410
 with Prosthesis . . . 33405
 with Stentless Tissue Valve . . . 33410
Ross-Konno Procedure . . . 33440
Ross Procedure . . . 33413
Transcatheter
 See Transcatheter Aortic Valve Replacement (TAVR/TAVI)
with Allograft Valve . . . 33406
with Aortic Annulus Enlargement . . . 33411, 33412
with Cardiopulmonary Bypass . . . 33367-33369, 33405, 33406, 33410
with Prosthesis . . . 33405, 33361-33369
with Stentless Tissue Valve . . . 33410
with Translocation, Pulmonary Valve . . . 33413

Aortocoronary Bypass
See Coronary Artery Bypass Graft (CABG)

Aortocoronary Bypass for Heart Revascularization
See Artery, Coronary, Bypass

Aortography
Aorta Imaging . . . 75600-75630, 93567
See Angiography
Serial . . . 75625
with Iliofemoral Artery . . . 75630, 75635

Aortoiliac
Embolectomy . . . 34151, 34201
Thrombectomy . . . 34151, 34201

Aortopexy
Tracheal Decompression . . . 33800

Aortoplasty
Supravalvular Stenosis . . . 33417

AP (Abdominal Pressure)
See Voiding Pressure Studies

Apert-Gallais Syndrome
See Adrenogenital Syndrome

Aphasia Testing
Speech and Language Function . . . 96105
See Neurology, Diagnostic

Apheresis
Therapeutic . . . 0342T, 36511-36516

Apical-Aortic Conduit . . . 33404

Apicectomy
with Mastoidectomy 69605
Petrous 69530

Apoaminotransferase, Aspartate
See Transaminase, Glutamic-Oxaloacetic

Apolipoprotein
Blood or Urine 82172

Appendectomy
Appendix Excision 44950, 44955, 44960
Laparoscopic 44970

Appendiceal Abscess
See Appendix, Abscess

Appendico-Vesicostomy
Cutaneous 50845

Appendix
Abscess
Incision and Drainage
Open 44900
Excision 44950, 44955, 44960, 44970

Application
Allergy (Percutaneous) Tests 95044
Bone Fixation Device
Multiplane 20692
Stereotactic Computer
Assisted 20696, 20697
Uniplane 20690
Caliper 20660
Cranial Tongs 20660
Fixation Device
See Fixation (Device)
Halo
Cranial 20661
Thin Skull Osteology 20664
Femoral 20663
Maxillofacial Fixation
See Fixation (Device), Maxillofacial
Pelvic 20662
Injector Device
for Timed Subcutaneous Injection 96377
Interdental Fixation Device 21110
Neurostimulation 64566
Radioelement
Infusion or Instillation 77750
Interstitial 77770-77772, 77778
Intracavitary 77761-77763, 77770-77772, 77790, 77799
Surface 77767, 77768, 77789
with Ultrasound 76965
Stereotactic Frame 20660
Headframe 61800
Strapping
Multi-layer Compression System
Arm 29584
Leg 29581

Application of External Fixation Device
See Fixation (Device)

APPT (Activated Partial Thromboplastin Time)
See Thromboplastin, Partial Thromboplastin Time (PTT)

Aquatic Therapy
See Physical Medicine/Therapy/Occupational Therapy

Aqueous Shunt
to Extraocular Equatorial Plate
Reservoir 66179, 66180
Revision 66184, 66185
without Extraocular Reservoir 0376T, 66183

Arch Ligament
See Coracoacromial Ligament

Arch, Zygomatic
See Zygomatic Arch

Arm
See Radius; Ulna; Wrist
Lower
Abscess 25028
Amputation 25900, 25905, 25909, 25915
Cineplasty 24940
Revision 25907, 25909
Angiography 73206
Artery
Ligation 37618
Biopsy 25065, 25066
Bursa
Incision and Drainage 25031
Bypass Graft 35903
Cast 29075
CT Scan 73200-73202, 73206
Decompression 25020, 25023-25025
Exploration
Blood Vessel 35860
Fasciotomy 24495, 25020, 25023-25025
Hematoma 25028
Implant 24931
Lesion, Tendon Sheath
Excision 25110
Magnetic Resonance Imaging (MRI) 73218-73220, 73221-73223, 73225
Reconstruction
Ulna 25337
Removal
Foreign Body 25248
Repair
Blood Vessel with Other Graft 35266
Blood Vessel with Vein Graft 35236
Decompression 24495
Muscle 25260-25263, 25270
Secondary 25265
Secondary
Muscle 25272-25274
Tendon 25272-25274
Tendon 25260-25263, 25270, 25280-25295, 25310-25316
Secondary 25265
Tendon Sheath 25275
Replantation 20805
Splint 29125, 29126
Tendon
Excision 25109
Lengthening 25280
Shortening 25280
Transplantation 25310-25312
Tenotomy 25290
Tumor
Excision 25071-25076
Radical Resection 25077, 25078
Ultrasound
Complete 76881
Limited 76882
Unlisted Services and Procedures 25999
X ray 73090
with Upper Arm 73092
Removal
Foreign Body
Forearm or Wrist 25248
Repair
Muscle 24341
Tendon 24341
Strapping
Multi-layer Compression System 29584
Upper
Abscess
Incision and Drainage 23930
See Elbow; Humerus
Amputation 23900-23920, 24900, 24920, 24930, 24931
Cineplasty 24940
Revision 23921, 24925, 24935
with Implant 24931
Angiography 73206
Artery
Ligation 37618
Biopsy 24065, 24066
Bypass Graft 35903
Cast 29065
CT Scan 73200-73206
Exploration
Blood Vessel 35860
Hematoma
Incision and Drainage 23930
Magnetic Resonance Imaging (MRI) 73218-73223
Muscle Revision 24330, 24331
Removal
Cast 29705
Foreign Body 24200, 24201
Repair
Blood Vessel with Other Graft 35266
Blood Vessel with Vein Graft 35236
Muscle Transfer 24301, 24320
Tendon 24332
Tendon Lengthening 24305
Tendon Revision 24320
Tendon Transfer 24301
Tenotomy 24310
Replantation 20802
Splint 29105
Tumor
Soft Tissue
Excision 24071-24076
Radical Resection 24077-24079
Ultrasound
Complete 76881
Limited 76882
Unlisted Services and Procedures 24999
Wound Exploration
Penetrating 20103
X ray
Infant 73092

Arnold-Chiari Malformation Repair
See Decompression, Skull

Arrest, Epiphyseal
See Epiphyseal Arrest

Arrhythmogenic Focus
Heart
Ablation 33250, 33251, 33261, 93653, 93654, 93656
Catheter 93655

Arsenic
Blood or Urine 82175
Qualitative 83015
Quantitative 82175, 83018

ART (Automated Reagin Test)
See Syphilis Test

Arterial Catheterization
See Cannulation, Arterial

Arterial Dilatation, Transluminal
See Angioplasty, Transluminal

Arterial Grafting for Coronary Artery Bypass
See Bypass Graft, Arterial, Coronary

Arterial Infusion, Thrombolysis
See Transcatheter, Therapy, Infusion (Arterial or Venous)

Arterial Pressure
See Blood Pressure
Noninvasive WaveformAnalysis........... 93050

Arterial Puncture
for Diagnosis........................... 36600

Arteriography, Aorta
See Aortography

Arteriosus, Ductus
Closure
  Transcatheter Percutaneous.......... 93582
Repair......................... 33820-33824

Arteriosus, Truncus
Repair............................... 33786

Arteriotomy
See Incision, Artery; Transection, Artery

Arteriovenous Anastomosis
for Increased Blood Flow.......... 36818-36821

Arteriovenous Fistula
Cannulization
  Vein............................. 36815
Creation........................ 36825-36830
Hemodialysis via Fistula................. 4052F
Referral............................ 4051F
Repair
  Abdomen.................. 35182, 35189
  Head...................... 35180, 35188
  Lower Extremity............. 35184, 35190
  Neck...................... 35180, 35188
  Thorax.................... 35182, 35189
  Upper Extremity............. 35184, 35190
Revision
  with Thrombectomy................. 36833
  without Thrombectomy.............. 36832
Thrombectomy
  Dialysis Graft
    without Revision.................. 36831

Arteriovenous Malformation
Carotid
  Obliteration....................... 61613
  Occlusion......................... 61705
Cranial
  Repair
    Carotid Artery Occlusion........... 61705
    Dural..................... 61690, 61692
    Electrothrombosis................. 61708
    Infratentorial.............. 61684, 61686
    Supratentorial.............. 61680, 61682
Iliac Artery
  Repair................ 0254T, 34707, 34708
Spinal
  Excision.................... 63250-63252
  Occlusion............. 63250-63252, 62294

Arteriovenous Shunt
Aorta to Pulmonary Artery......... 33755, 33762
Blalock-Taussig Shunt................. 33750
Intrahepatic Portosystemic
  Insertion.......................... 37182
  Revision.......................... 37183
Patency............................. 78291
Peritoneal-Venous
  Evaluation........................ 49427
  Insertion......................... 49425
  Ligation.......................... 49428
  Removal.......................... 49429
  Revision.......................... 49426
Potts-Smith Shunt..................... 33762
Subclavian to Pulmonary Artery........... 33750
Thomas Shunt......................... 36835
Waterston Shunt...................... 33755

Artery
Abdomen
  Angiography....................... 75726
  Catheterization.............. 36245-36248
  Ligation.......................... 37617
Adrenal
  Angiography................. 75731-75733
Anastomosis
  Cranial........................... 61711
Angioplasty
  See Angioplasty
Aorta
  Angioplasty................. 37246, 37247
Aortobi-iliac
  Bypass Graft................ 35538, 35638
Aortobifemoral
  Bypass Graft...................... 35540
Aortocarotid
  Bypass Graft................ 35526, 35626
Aortofemoral
  Bypass Graft...................... 35539
Aortoiliac
  Bypass Graft................ 35537, 35637
  Embolectomy................ 34151-34201
  Thrombectomy............... 34151-34201
Aortoiliofemoral
  Thromboendarterectomy............. 35363
Aortoinnominate
  Bypass Graft................ 35526, 35626
Aortosubclavian
  Bypass Graft................ 35526, 35626
Arm
  Angiography................. 75710-75716
  Harvest........................... 35600
Atherectomy
  Brachiocephalic................... 0237T
  Coronary....... 92924, 92925, 92933, 92934, 92937, 92938, 92941, 92943, 92944
  Femoral.................... 37225, 37227
  Iliac............................. 0238T
  Peroneal................... 37229, 37231
  Popliteal................... 37225, 37227
  Renal............................ 0234T
  Tibial..................... 37229, 37231
  Visceral.......................... 0235T
  Transluminal......... 0234T-0238T, 92924, 92925, 92933, 92934, 92937, 92938, 92941, 92943, 92944
Axillary
  Aneurysm................... 35011-35013
  Angioplasty................ 37246, 37247
  Bypass Graft............... 35616, 35621, 35623, 35650, 35654
  Embolectomy...................... 34101
  Thrombectomy..................... 34101
  Thromboendarterectomy............. 35321
Basilar
  Aneurysm................... 61698, 61702
Biopsy............................. 75970
Brachial
  Aneurysm................... 35011-35013
  Bypass Graft..... 35510, 35512, 35522-35525
  Embolectomy...................... 34101
  Exploration....................... 24495
  Exposure......................... 34834
  Thrombectomy..................... 34101
  Thromboendarterectomy............. 35321
Brachiocephalic
  Angioplasty................ 37246, 37247
  Atherectomy...................... 0237T
  Catheterization.............. 36215-36218
Bypass Graft
  with Composite Graft.......... 35681-35683
Cannulization
  for Extracorporeal Circulation......... 36823
  to Vein..................... 36810-36815
Carotid
  Aneurysm...... 35001, 35002, 61697, 61700, 61703, 61705, 61708, 61710
  Baroreflex Activation Device
    Implantation/Replacement.... 0266T-0268T
    Interrogation Evaluation...... 0272T, 0273T
    Revision/Removal........... 0269T-0271T
  Bypass Graft.......... 33891, 35501-35510, 35601-35606, 35642
  Carotid Cavernous Fistula 61705, 61708, 61710
  Catheterization................... 36100, 36221-36224, 36227, 36228
  Decompression........ 61590, 61591, 61596
  Embolectomy...................... 34001
  Evaluation
    Atheroma....................... 93895
    Intima Media Thickness........... 93895
  Excision......................... 60605
  Exploration....................... 35701
  Ligation............. 37600-37606, 61611
  Reimplantation......... 35691, 35694-36595
  Stenosis
    Imaging Study Measurement........ 3100F
  Stent Placement
    Transcatheter............. 37217, 37218
  Thrombectomy..................... 34001
  Thromboendarterectomy....... 35301, 35390
  Transection....................... 61611
  Transposition.... 33889, 35691, 35694, 35695
  Vascular Malformation.. 61705, 61708, 61710
Carotid, Common
  Intima-Media Thickness (IMT) Study.... 0126T
Celiac
  Aneurysm.................. 35121, 35122
  Bypass Graft................ 35531, 35631
  Embolectomy...................... 34151
  Endoprosthesis............... 34841-34848
  Thrombectomy..................... 34151
  Thromboendarterectomy............. 35341
Chest
  Ligation.......................... 37616
Coronary
  Angiography................ 93454-93461, 92924-92295, 92933, 92934
  Atherectomy..... 92924, 92925, 92933, 92934
  Bypass..................... 33510-33536
    Internal Mammary Artery Graft...... 4110F
  Fractional Flow Reserve.. 0501T-0504T, 0523T
  Graft..................... 33503, 33504
  Ligation......................... 33502
  Obstruction Severity Assessment...... 0206T
  Repair..................... 33500-33507
  Thrombectomy..................... 92973
  Thrombolysis............... 92975, 92977
  Translocation............... 33506, 33507
  Unroofing........................ 33507
Digital
  Sympathectomy.................... 64820
Endothelial Function Assessment
  Noninvasive...................... 93998
Ethmoidal
  Ligation.......................... 30915

Extracorporeal Circulation
for Regional Chemotherapy of
Extremity 36823
Extracranial
Anastomosis 61711
Extremities
Bypass Graft Revision 35879-35884
Catheterization. . . . 36140, 36245-36248
Ligation 37618
Vascular Studies 93922-93931
Bypass Grafts 93925-93931
Femoral
Aneurysm 35141, 35142
Angiography 73706
Angioplasty 37224
Approach
Transcatheter Aortic Valve
Replacement 33361-33366
Atherectomy 37225, 37227
Bypass Graft 35621, 35646, 35647, 35654, 35656, 35661, 35665, 35666
Revision 35883, 35884
Bypass In-Situ 35583-35585
Embolectomy 34201
Exploration 35721
Exposure 34812
Thrombectomy 34201
Thromboendarterectomy 35371, 35372
Great Vessel
Repair 33770-33781
Hepatic
Aneurysm 35121, 35122
Bypass Graft 35535
Iliac
Aneurysm
Direct Repair 35001, 35131, 35132
Endovascular Repair 34703-34711
Angioplasty 37220, 37222
Atherectomy 0238T
Bypass Graft 35563, 35632-35634, 35637, 35663
Embolectomy 34151-34201
Endograft 0254T
Exposure 34820, 34833
Occlusion Device 34808
Revascularization 37220-37222
Thrombectomy 34151-34201
Thromboendarterectomy 35351, 35361-35363
Ilio-celiac
Bypass Graft 35632
Iliofemoral
Bypass Graft 35565
Thromboendarterectomy 35355, 35363
X ray with Contrast 75630
Ilio-mesenteric
Bypass Graft 35633
Iliorenal
Bypass Graft 35634
Innominate
Aneurysm 35021, 35022
Catheterization 36222, 36223, 36225
Embolectomy 34001-34101
Stent Placement
Transcatheter 37217
Thrombectomy 34001-34101
Thromboendarterectomy 35311
Intracranial
Anastomosis 33606
Aneurysm 61705, 61708
Angiography
with Thrombectomy 61645
Angioplasty 61630
Infusion
for Other Than Thrombolysis . . 61650, 61651
for Thrombolysis 61645
Thrombectomy 61645
Leg
Angiography 73706, 75710-75716
Catheterization 36245-36248
Mammary
Angiography 75756
Maxillary
Ligation 30920
Mesenteric
Aneurysm 35121, 35122
Bypass Graft 35531, 35631
Embolectomy 34151
Endoprosthesis 34841-34848
Thrombectomy 34151
Thromboendarterectomy 35341
Middle Cerebral Artery, Fetal
Ligation 37615
Vascular Studies 76821
Nose
Incision 30915-30920
Other Angiography 75774
Other Artery
Angiography 75774
Exploration 35761
Pelvic
Angiography 72198, 75736
Catheterization 36245-36248
Peripheral Arterial Rehabilitation 93668
Peroneal
Angioplasty 37228-37235
Atherectomy 37229, 37231
Bypass Graft 35566-35571, 35666-35671
Bypass In-Situ 35585-35587
Embolectomy 34203
Thrombectomy 34203
Thromboendarterectomy 35305, 35306
Popliteal
Aneurysm 35151, 35152
Angioplasty 37224
Atherectomy 37225, 37227
Bypass Graft 35623, 35656, 35671
Bypass In-Situ 35583, 35587
Embolectomy 34201-34203
Exploration 35741
Thrombectomy 34201-34203
Thromboendarterectomy 35303
Pressure
Waveform Analysis 93050
Pulmonary
Anastomosis 33606
Angiography 75741-75746
Angioplasty 92997, 92998
Banding 33620, 33622, 33690
Embolectomy 33910, 33915, 33916
Endarterectomy 33916
Ligation 33924
Repair
Arborization Anomalies 33925, 33926
Atresia 33920
Stenosis 33917
Radial
Aneurysm 35045
Bypass Graft 35523
Embolectomy 34111
Sympathectomy 64821
Thrombectomy 34111
Rehabilitation 93668
Reimplantation
Carotid 35691, 35694, 35695
Subclavian 35693-35695
Vertebral 35691-35693
Visceral 35697
Renal
Aneurysm 35121, 35122
Angiography 36251-36254
Angioplasty 37246, 37247
Atherectomy 0234T
Bypass Graft 35631, 35634, 35636
Catheterization 36251-36254
Embolectomy 34151
Endoprosthesis 34841-34848
Fluoroscopy (included) 36251-36254
Thrombectomy 34151
Thromboendarterectomy 35341
Repair
Aneurysm 61697-61708
Angioplasty
Radiological Supervision 37246, 37247
Revision
Hemodialysis Graft or Fistula . . . 36831-36833
Spine
Angiography 75705
Splenic
Aneurysm 35111, 35112
Bypass Graft 35536, 35636
Stent Placement
Carotid 37215-37218, 37236, 37237
Coronary 37236, 37237, 92928, 92929
Dialysis Circuit 36903, 36906, 36908
Extracranial Vertebral 0075T, 0076T, 37236, 37237
Femoral-Popliteal 0505T, 37226, 37227
Iliac 37221, 37223
Innominate 37217, 37218
Intracranial 61635
Tibial-Peroneal . . . 37230, 37231, 37234, 37235
Subclavian
Aneurysm 35001, 35002, 35021, 35022
Angioplasty 37246, 37247
Bypass Graft 35506, 35511-35516, 35606-35616, 35645
Catheterization 36225
Embolectomy 34001-34101
Reimplantation 35693-35695
Thrombectomy 34001-34101
Thromboendarterectomy 35301, 35311
Transposition 33889, 35693-35695
Unlisted Services and Procedures 37799
Superficial Femoral
Thromboendarterectomy 35302
Superficial Palmar Arch
Sympathectomy 64823
Temporal
Biopsy 37609
Ligation 37609
Thoracic
Catheterization 33621, 36215-36218
Thrombectomy
Coronary 92973
Dialysis Circuit 36904-36906
Intracranial 61645
Noncoronary 37184-37186
Hemodialysis Graft or Fistula 36831
Other than Hemodialysis Graft or
Fistula 35875, 36830-36833
Thrombolysis
Intracranial 61645
Noncoronary 37211, 37213, 37214
Tibial
Angiography 73706
Angioplasty 37228
Atherectomy 37229, 37231

Bypass Graft . . . 35566-35571, 35623, 35666-35671
Bypass In-Situ . . . 35585-35587
Embolectomy . . . 34203
Thrombectomy . . . 34203
Thromboendarterectomy . . . 35305, 35306
Tibial/Peroneal Trunk-Tibial Bypass Graft . . . 35570
Tibial-Tibial Bypass Graft . . . 35570
Tibioperoneal
Angioplasty . . . 37228-37235
Atherectomy . . . 37233-37235
Tibioperoneal Trunk
Thromboendarterectomy . . . 35304
Transcatheter Therapy
with Angiography . . . 75894-75898
Transposition
Carotid . . . 33889, 35691, 35694, 35695
Subclavian . . . 33889, 35693-35695
Vertebral . . . 35691-35693
Ulnar
Aneurysm . . . 35045
Bypass Graft . . . 35523
Embolectomy . . . 34111
Sympathectomy . . . 64822
Thrombectomy . . . 34111
Umbilical
Vascular Study . . . 76820
Unlisted Services and Procedures . . . 37799
Vertebral
Aneurysm . . . 35005, 61698, 61702
Bypass Graft . . . 35508, 35515, 35642-35645
Catheterization . . . 36100, 36221, 36225, 36226, 36228
Decompression . . . 61597
Reimplantation . . . 35691-35693
Thromboendarterectomy . . . 35301
Transposition . . . 35691-35693
Visceral
Angioplasty . . . 37246, 37247
Atherectomy . . . 0235T
Reimplantation . . . 35697

Artery Catheterization, Pulmonary
See Catheterization, Pulmonary Artery

Arthrectomy
Elbow . . . 24155

Arthrocentesis
Bursa . . . 20600
with Recording and Reporting . . . 20604, 20606, 20611
with Ultrasound Guidance . . . 20604, 20606, 20611
Intermediate Joint . . . 20605, 20606
Large Joint . . . 20610, 20611
Small Joint . . . 20600, 20604

Arthrodeses
See Arthrodesis

Arthrodesis
Ankle . . . 27870
Carpometacarpal Joint
Hand . . . 26843, 26844
Thumb . . . 26841, 26842
Cervical
Atlas-Axis . . . 22548, 22585, 22595
below C2 22551-22554, 22585, 22595, 22600
Clivus-C1-C2 . . . 22548, 22585, 22595
Occiput-C2 . . . 22590
Elbow . . . 24800-24802
Finger Joint . . . 26850-26852
Interphalangeal . . . 26860-26863
Metacarpophalangeal . . . 26850
Foot Joint . . . 28730-28735, 28740
Pantalar . . . 28705
Subtalar . . . 28725
Triple . . . 28715
with Advancement . . . 28737
with Lengthening . . . 28737
Hand Joint . . . 26843, 26844
Hip Joint . . . 27284-27286
Intercarpal Joint . . . 25800-25820
with Autograft . . . 25825
Interphalangeal Joint . . . 26860-26863
Great Toe . . . 28755
with Tendon Transfer . . . 28760
Knee . . . 27580
Metacarpophalangeal Joint . . . 26850-26852
Metatarsophalangeal Joint
Great Toe . . . 28750
Pubic Symphysis . . . 27282
Radioulnar Joint . . . 25830
Sacroiliac Joint
Minimally Invasive . . . 27279
Open . . . 27280
Percutaneous . . . 27279
Shoulder
See Shoulder, Arthrodesis
Shoulder Joint . . . 23800-23802
Subtalar Joint . . . 29907
Talus
Pantalar . . . 28705
Subtalar . . . 28725
Triple . . . 28715
Tarsal Joint . . . 28730-28737, 28740
Tarsometatarsal Joint . . . 28730-28735, 28740
Thumb Joint . . . 26841, 26842
Tibiofibular Joint . . . 27871
Vertebra
Additional Interspace
Anterior/Anterolateral Approach . . . 22585
Lateral Extracavitary . . . 22534
Posterior . . . 22614, 22634
Cervical
Anterior/Anterolateral Approach . . . 22548
Posterior/Posterolateral/Lateral Transverse . . . 22590-22600
Lumbar
Anterior/Anterolateral Approach . . . 22558
Lateral Extracavitary . . . 22533, 22534
Presacral Interbody . . . 22586, 22899
Posterior/Interbody . . . 22630
Posterior/Posterolateral and/or Lateral Transverse Technique . . . 22612, 22633, 22634
Sacroiliac
Presacral Interbody . . . 22899
Spinal Deformity
Anterior Approach . . . 22808-22812
Posterior Approach . . . 22800-22804
Spinal Fusion
Exploration . . . 22830
Thoracic
Anterior/Anterolateral Approach . . . 22556
Lateral Extracavitary . . . 22532, 22534
Posterior/Posterolateral/Lateral Transverse . . . 22610
with Insertion of Biomechanical Device . . . 22853, 22854
with Bunionectomy . . . 28295, 28296, 28298, 28299
Wrist . . . 25800-25825

Arthrography
Ankle . . . 73615
Injection . . . 27648
Elbow . . . 73085
Injection . . . 24220
Hip . . . 73525
Injection . . . 27093-27095
Knee . . . 73580
Injection . . . 27369
Sacroiliac Joint
Injection . . . 27096
Shoulder . . . 73040
Injection . . . 23350
Temporomandibular Joint (TMJ) . . . 70332
Injection . . . 21116
Wrist . . . 73115
Injection . . . 25246

Arthroplasties, Knee Replacement
See Prosthesis, Knee

Arthroplasty
Ankle . . . 27700-27703
Elbow . . . 24360-24363
Revision . . . 24370, 24371
Hip . . . 27132
Partial Replacement . . . 27125
Revision . . . 27134-27138
Total Replacement . . . 27130
Implant
Radiostereometric Analysis (RSA) . . . 0348T-0350T
Interphalangeal Joint . . . 26535, 26536
Intervertebral Disc
Cervical . . . 0375T, 22856, 22858
Removal . . . 0095T, 22864
Revision . . . 0098T, 22861
Lumbar . . . 0163T, 22857
Removal . . . 0164T, 22865
Revision . . . 0165T, 22862
Knee . . . 27437-27447
Revision . . . 27486, 27487
Metacarpophalangeal Joint . . . 26530, 26531
Radius . . . 24365, 24366
Shoulder Joint . . . 23470, 23472-23474
Subtalar Joint
Sinus Tarsi Implant
Insertion . . . 0335T
Removal . . . 0510T
Removal and Reinsertion . . . 0511T
Temporomandibular Joint . . . 21240-21243
Vertebral Joint
Lumbar Spine . . . 0202T
Wrist . . . 25332
Carpal . . . 25443
Carpometacarpal Joint . . . 25447
Lunate . . . 25444
Navicular . . . 25443
Radius . . . 25441
Revision . . . 25449
Total Replacement . . . 25446
Trapezium . . . 25445
Ulna . . . 25442
with Implant . . . 25441-25445

Arthroplasty, Hip, Total
See Hip, Total Replacement

Arthroplasty, Shoulder
See Repair, Shoulder

Arthropods
Examination . . . 87168

Arthroscopy
Diagnostic
Elbow . . . 29830
Hip . . . 29860
Knee . . . 29870
Metacarpophalangeal Joint . . . 29900
Shoulder . . . 29805

Temporomandibular Joint 29800
Wrist 29840
Surgical
Ankle 29891-29899
Elbow 29834-29838
Hip 29861-29916
Knee 29866-29868, 29871-29889
Metacarpophalangeal Joint 29901, 29902
Shoulder 29806-29828
Subtalar Joint 29904-29907
with Acetabuloplasty 29915
Temporomandibular Joint 29804
Wrist 29843-29847
Unlisted Services and Procedures 29999

Arthroscopy of Ankle
See Ankle, Arthroscopy

Arthrotomy
Acromioclavicular Joint 23044
Ankle 27610-27612, 27620
Ankle Joint 27625, 27626
Carpometacarpal Joint 26070, 26100
Elbow 24000
Capsular Release 24006
with Joint Exploration 24101
with Synovectomy 24102
with Synovial Biopsy 24100
Finger Joint 26075
Interphalangeal 26110
Metacarpophalangeal 26105
Glenohumeral Joint . . 23040, 23100, 23105, 23800
Hip 27030, 27033, 27054
Interphalangeal Joint 26080, 26110
Toe 28024, 28054
Intertarsal Joint 28020, 28050
Knee 27310, 27330-27335, 27403, 29868
Metacarpophalangeal Joint 26075, 26105
Metatarsophalangeal Joint 28022, 28052
Shoulder 23044, 23105-23107
Shoulder Joint 23100, 23101
Sternoclavicular Joint 23044, 23101, 23106
Tarsometatarsal Joint 28020, 28050
Temporomandibular Joint 21010
with Biopsy
Acromioclavicular Joint 23101
Glenohumeral Joint 23100
Hip Joint 27052-27054
Knee Joint 27330
Sacroiliac Joint 27050
Sternoclavicular Joint 23101
with Synovectomy
Glenohumeral Joint 23105
Sternoclavicular Joint 23106
Wrist 25040, 25100-25107

Arthrotomy for Removal of Prosthesis of Ankle
See Ankle, Removal, Implant

Arthrotomy for Removal of Prosthesis of Hip
See Hip, Removal, Prosthesis

Arthrotomy for Removal of Prosthesis of Wrist
See Wrist, Removal, Prosthesis

Articular Ligament
See Ligament

Artificial Abortion
See Abortion

Artificial Cardiac Pacemaker
See Heart, Pacemaker

Artificial Eye
See Prosthesis

Artificial Genitourinary Sphincter
See Prosthesis, Urethral Sphincter

Artificial Insemination
Intracervical 58321
Intrauterine 58322
Sperm Washing 58323

Artificial Knee Joints
See Prosthesis, Knee

Artificial Penis
See Penile Prosthesis

Artificial Pneumothorax
See Pneumothorax, Therapeutic

Arytenoid
Excision 31400, 31560
Fixation 31400

Arytenoidectomy
Arytenoid Excision 31400
Endoscopic 31560

Arytenoidopexy
Arytenoid Fixation 31400

Ascorbic Acid
Blood 82180

Aspartate Aminotransferase
See Transaminase, Glutamic-Oxaloacetic

Aspergillus
Detection
Antibody 86606
Antigen 87305

Aspiration
Abdomen 49322
Amniotic Fluid
Diagnostic 59000
Therapeutic 59001
Aspirate Evaluation 88172, 88173, 88177
Bladder 51100-51102
Bone Marrow 38220, 38222
Spine Surgery 20939
Brain Lesion 61750, 61751
Breast 19000, 19001
Bronchi 31629, 31633, 31645, 31646, 31725
Bursa . . 20600, 20604, 20605, 20606, 20610, 20611
with Recording and Reporting 20604, 20606, 20611
with Ultrasound Guidance 20604, 20606, 20611
Catheter
Nasotracheal 31720
Tracheobronchial 31725
Cyst
Bone 20615
Breast 19000, 19001
Ganglion 20612
Kidney 50390
Pelvis 50390
Spinal Cord 62268
Thyroid 60300
Duodenal 43756, 43757
Fetal Fluid 59074
Fine Needle 67415
Aspirate Evaluation 88172, 88173, 88177
Fine Needle, Biopsy
See Fine Needle Aspiration (FNA) Biopsy
Gastric 43753, 43754
Hydrocele
Tunica Vaginalis 55000
Joint 20600, 20604-20606, 20610, 20611
with Recording and Reporting 20604, 20606, 20611
with Ultrasound Guidance 20604, 20606, 20611
Laryngoscopy 31515
Lens Material 66840
Liver 47015
Orbital Contents 67415
Pericardium 33010, 33011
Pleural Cavity 32554, 32555
with Imaging Guidance 32555
Puncture
See Puncture Aspiration
Spinal Cord
Syrinx 62268
Stomach
Diagnostic 43754, 43755
Therapeutic 43753
Syrinx
Spinal Cord 62268
Thyroid 60300
Trachea 31612, 31629
Nasotracheal 31720
Tracheobronchial 31645, 31646, 31725
Tunica Vaginalis
Hydrocele 55000
Vertebral
Disc 62267
Nucleus Pulposus 62267
Tissue 62267
Vitreous 67015

Aspiration Lipectomies
See Liposuction

Aspiration of Bone Marrow from Donor for Transplant
See Bone Marrow, Harvesting

Aspiration, Chest
Thoracentesis 32554, 32555
with Imaging Guidance 32555

Aspiration, Nail
See Evacuation, Hematoma, Subungual

Aspiration, Spinal Puncture
See Spinal Tap

Assay, Tobramycin
See Tobramycin

Assay, Very Long Chain Fatty Acids
See Fatty Acid, Very Long Chain

Assisted Circulation
See Circulation Assist

AST
See Transaminase, Glutamic-Oxaloacetic

Astragalectomy
Talectomy 28130

Astragalus
See Talus

Asymmetry, Face
See Hemifacial Microsomia

Ataxia Telangiectasia
Chromosome Analysis 88248

Ataxy, Telangiectasia
See Ataxia Telangiectasia

Atherectomies, Coronary
See Artery, Coronary, Atherectomy

Atherectomy
See Revascularization, Artery
Abdominal Aorta 0236T
Brachiocephalic 0237T
Coronary 92924, 92925, 92937, 92938, 92941, 92943, 92944
Femoral 37225, 37227
Iliac 0238T
Peroneal 37229, 37231, 37233, 37235
Popliteal 37225, 37227
Renal 0234T
Tibial 37229, 37231, 37233, 37235
Visceral 0235T

Athletic Training
Evaluation 97169-97171
Re-evaluation 97172

ATLV (Adult T Cell Leukemia Virus)
See HTLV-I

ATLV Antibodies
See HTLV-I, Antibody

Atomic Absorption Spectroscopy
Each Analyte 82190

ATP Creatine Phosphotransferase
See CPK

Atresia
Choanal 30540-30545
Congenital
  Auditory Canal, External 69320
  Bile Duct 47700
  Small Intestine 44126, 44127
Pulmonary Artery 33920
Tetralogy of Fallot 33697
Tricuspid 33615

Atria
Anastomosis
  Pulmonary Artery 33615
Ablation
  Operative Tissue .. 33254-33256, 33265, 33266
Baffle Procedure 33774
Blalock-Hanlon Operation 33735
Cor Triatriatum
  Repair 33732
Cuff Preparation 32855, 32856
Electrogram 93615, 93616
Fibrillation
  See Fibrillation, Atrial
Endoscopy 33265, 33266
Left Atrial Appendage
  Closure 33340
Membrane Resection 33732
Pacemaker
  Electrode
    Removal 33229, 33236
    Repositioning 33215
  Insertion 33206, 33208
Rashkind Procedure 92992
Reconstruction 33254-33256, 33265, 33266
Septal Defect
  See Septal Defect, Atrial
Septectomy 33735, 92992, 92993
Septostomy 33735, 92992, 92993
Shunt 62190, 62220
Thrombus 33310

Atrial Electrogram
See Cardiology, Diagnostic
Esophageal Recording 93615, 93616

Atrial Fibrillation
See Fibrillation, Atrial

Atrioseptopexy
See Septal Defect, Atrial, Repair

Atrioseptoplasty
See Septal Defect, Atrial, Repair

Attachment
See Fixation

Atticotomy
Tympanic Incision 69631, 69635

Audiologic Function Tests
Acoustic Immittance 92570
Acoustic Reflex 92568, 92570
Audiometry
  Automated 0208T-0212T
  Bekesy 92560, 92561
  Comprehensive 0212T, 92557
  Conditioning Play 92582
  Groups 92559
  Pure Tone 0208T, 0209T, 92552, 92553
  Select Picture 92583
  Speech 0210T, 0211T, 92555, 92556
  Visual Reinforcement (VRA) 92579
Auditory Brainstem Implant 92640
Auditory Processing
  Treatment 92507, 92508
Central Auditory Function 92620, 92621
Ear Protector Attenuation 92596
Electrocochleography 92584
Evoked Otoacoustic Emission 92558, 92587, 92588
Filtered Speech 92571
Hearing Aid Evaluation 92590-92595
Loudness Balance 92562
Screening 92551
Sensorineural Acuity 92575
Short Increment Sensitivity Index (SISI) 92564
Staggered Spondaic Word Test 92572
Stenger Test 92565, 92577
Synthetic Sentence Test 92576
Tinnitus Assessment 92625
Tone Decay 92563
Tympanometry 92550, 92567, 92570

Audiometry
Bekesy 92560, 92561
Brainstem Evoked Response 92585, 92586
Comprehensive 0212T, 92557
Conditioning Play 92582
Groups 92559
Pure Tone 92552, 92553
  Automated 0208T, 0209T
Select Picture 92583
Speech 0210T, 0211T, 92555, 92556
Tympanometry 92550, 92567, 92570
Voice Prosthesis Fitting 92597

Auditory Brainstem Evoked Response
See Evoked Potentials, Auditory Brainstem

Auditory Canal
Decompression 61591
External
  Abscess
    Incision and Drainage ... 69000, 69005, 69020
  Biopsy 69105
  Excision 69110, 69120
    Lesion 69140, 69145, 69150, 69155
  Hematoma 69000, 69005
  Reconstruction
    for Congenital Atresia 69320
    for Stenosis 69310
  Removal
    Cerumen 69209, 69210
    Ear Wax 69209, 69210
    Foreign Body 69200-69205
Internal
  Decompression 69960
  Exploration 69440

Auditory Canal Atresia, External
See Atresia, Congenital, Auditory Canal, External

Auditory Evoked Otoacoustic Emission
Screening 92558, 92587, 92588

Auditory Evoked Potentials
See Audiometry

Auditory Labyrinth
See Ear, Inner Ear

Auditory Meatus
X ray 70134

Auditory Tube
See Eustachian Tube

Augmentation
Breast
  See Breast, Augmentation
Chin 21120, 21123
Cruciate Ligament 29888, 29889
Facial Bones 21208
Knee Ligament 27427, 27556-27558
Larynx 31574
Malar 21210, 21270
Mandibular Body 21127-21125
Palate 21082
Pulmonary Valve Outflow 33478
Spine
  Lumbar 22514, 22515
  Thoracic 22513, 22515

Augmentation Mammoplasty
See Breast, Augmentation

Aural Rehabilitation
Status Evaluation 92626, 92627, 92630, 92633

Auricle (Heart)
See Atria

Auricular Fibrillation
See Fibrillation, Atrial

Auricular Prosthesis
Custom Preparation 21086

Australia Antigen
See Hepatitis Antigen, Detection, Immunoassay, B Surface (HBsAg)

Autograft
Bone 20936-20938
Bone Marrow 20939
Chondrocytes
  Knee 27412
Osteochondral
  Knee 27416
  Talus 28446
Skin
  Dermal 15130-15136
  Epidermal 15110-15116
  Tissue Cultured 15150-15157
    Harvesting 15040
Spine 20936-20939

Autologous Blood Transfusion
See Autotransfusion

Autologous Transplantation
See Autograft
Hematopoietic Progenitor Cells
  See Hematopoietic Progenitor Cell (HPC), Transplantation

Autonomic Nervous System Function
See Neurology, Diagnostic; Neurophysiologic Testing

Autoprothrombin C
See Thrombokinase

Autoprothrombin I
See Proconvertin

Autoprothrombin II
See Christmas Factor

Autoprothrombin III
See Stuart-Prower Factor

Autopsy
Coroner's Exam 88045
Forensic Exam 88040
Gross and Micro Exam 88020-88037
Gross Exam 88000-88016
Organ 88037
Regional 88036
Unlisted Services and Procedures 88099

Autotransfusion
Blood 86890, 86891

Autotransplant
See Autograft

Autotransplantation
Renal 50380

AV Fistula
See Arteriovenous Fistula

AV Shunt
See Arteriovenous Shunt

Avulsion
Nails 11730-11732
Nerve 64732-64772

Axilla
Artery
See Artery, Axillary
Nerve
Injection
Anesthetic 64417
Skin Graft
Dermal 15130, 15131
Full-thickness 15200, 15201
Tissue Cultured 15150-15152
Tissue Transfer
Adjacent 14040, 14041
Flap 15574, 15620
Wound Repair 13131-13133

Axillary Nerve
Injection
Anesthetic 64417

Axis, Dens
See Odontoid Process

B

B Antibodies, Hepatitis
See Hepatitis Antibody, B

B Antigens, Hepatitis
See Hepatitis Antigen, Detection, Nucleic Acid, B

B Cells
Count 86355

B-DNA
See Deoxyribonucleic Acid (DNA)

b-Hexosaminidase 83080

B-1 Vitamin
See Thiamine

B-6 Vitamin
See Vitamin, B-6

B-12 Vitamin
See Cyanocobalamin

Bacillus Calmette Guerin Vaccine
See BCG Vaccine

Back/Flank
Biopsy 21920-21925
Penetrating Wound
Exploration 20102
Repair
Hernia 49540
Tumor
Excision 21930-21933
Radical Resection 21935, 21936

Backbone
See Spine

Bacteria Culture
Aerobic 87040-87071, 87077
Anaerobic 87073-87076
Mycobacterial 87118
Screening 87081
Specimen
Blood 87040
Other Source 87070, 87071, 87073, 87075
Stool 87045, 87046
Urine 87086-87088
Typing 87140, 87143, 87147, 87149, 87150, 87152, 87153, 87158

Bacterial Endotoxins 87176, 87205

Bacterial Overgrowth Breath Test 91065

Bactericidal Titer, Serum 87197

Bacterium
Antibody 86609

BAER
See Evoked Potentials, Auditory Brainstem

Baker Tube
Intestine Decompression 44021

Baker's Cyst 27345

Balanoplasty
See Penis, Repair

Balkan Grippe
See Q Fever

Balloon Angioplasties, Coronary
See Percutaneous Transluminal Angioplasty

Balloon Angioplasty
See Angioplasty

Balloon Assisted Device
Aorta 33967-33974
Bronchoscopy 31647, 31648, 31649, 31651

Band, Pulmonary Artery
See Banding, Artery, Pulmonary

Banding
Artery
Fistula 37607
Pulmonary 33610, 33622, 33690

Bank, Blood
See Blood Banking

Bankart Procedure
See Capsulorrhaphy, Anterior

Barany Caloric Test
See Caloric Vestibular Test

Bardenheurer Operation
See Ligation, Artery, Chest

Bariatric Surgery
Gastric Bypass 43644, 43645, 43846, 43847
Gastric Restriction 43644, 43645, 43842, 43843, 43845, 43846, 43847, 43848
Device
Placement 43770
Removal 43772-43774
Replacement 43773
Revision 43771
Port Component 43886-43888
Sleeve Gastrectomy 43775
Surgically Altered Stomach
Ultrasound Examination 43242

Barium Enema 74270-74280

Barker Operation
See Talus, Excision

Baroreflex Activation Device
Implantation/Replacement 0266T-0268T
Interrogation Evaluation 0272T, 0273T
Revision/Removal 0269T-0271T

Barr Bodies 88130

Barr Procedure
See Tendon, Transfer

Bartholin's Gland
Abscess
Incision and Drainage 56420
Cyst
Marsupialization 56440
Excision 56740

Bartonella Detection
Antibody 86611
Nucleic Acid Probe 87471, 87472

Basic Proteins, Myelin
See Myelin Basic Protein

Basilar Arteries
See Artery, Basilar

Batch-Spittler-McFaddin Operation
See Disarticulation, Knee

BCG Vaccine 90585, 90586
See Vaccines and Toxoids

Be Antigens, Hepatitis
See Hepatitis Antigen, Detection, Immunoassay, Be (HBeAg)

Bed Sores
See Pressure, Ulcer (Decubitus)

Bed Testing
See Pulmonology, Diagnostic

Bekesy Audiometry
See Audiometry, Bekesy

Belsey IV Procedure
See Fundoplasty

Benedict Test for Urea
See Urinalysis, Qualitative

Benign Cystic Mucinous Tumor
See Ganglion

Benign Neoplasm of Cranial Nerves
See Nerves, Neurofibroma

Bennett Fracture
Treatment 26645, 26650, 26665

Bennett Procedure
Quadricepsplasty 27430

Benzidine Test
See Blood, Feces

Benzoyl Cholinesterase
See Cholinesterase

Bernstein Test
See Acid Perfusion Study, Esophagus

Beta 2 Glycoprotein I Antibody 86146

Beta-Blocker Therapy
Performance Measures
Coronary Artery Disease 4008F
Heart Failure 4008F, 4480F, 4481F

Beta Glucosidase 82963

Beta Hypophamine
See Antidiuretic Hormone

Beta Lipoproteins
See Lipoprotein, LDL

Beta Test
See Psychiatric Diagnosis

Beta-2-Microglobulin
Blood 82232
Urine 82232

Beta-hydroxydehydrogenase 80406

Bethesda System 88164-88167

Bicarbonate 82374

Biceps Tendon
Reinsertion 24342
Resection 23440
Tenodesis 23430, 29828
Transplantation 23440

Bichloride, Methylene
See Dichloromethane

Bicuspid Valve
See Mitral Valve

Bifrontal Craniotomy
for Craniosynostosis 61557

Bilaminate Skin Substitute/Neodermis
See Tissue, Substitute

Bile Acids 82239
Blood 82240

Bile Duct
See Gallbladder
Anastomosis
with Intestines 47760, 47780-47785
Biopsy
Endoluminal 47543
Endoscopy 47553
Cholangiography
Injection 47531, 47532
with Catheterization 47533-47537
with Placement of Access to Small Bowel 47541
with Stent Placement 47538-47540
Cyst
Excision 47715
Destruction
Calculus (Stone) 43265, 47544
Dilation
Endoscopy 43277, 47555, 47556
Percutaneous 47542
X ray 74360
Drainage
Catheter
Change 75984
Conversion of External to Internal-External 47535
Exchange 47536
Placement 47533, 47534
Removal 47537
Endoscopic Retrograde Cholangiopancreatography (ERCP)
with Optical Endomicroscopy 0397T
Endoscopy
Biopsy 47553
Cannulation 43273
Destruction
Calculus (Stone) 43265
Dilation 43277, 47555, 47556
Exploration 47552
Intraoperative 47550
Placement
Stent 43274
Removal
Calculus (Stone) 43264, 47554
Foreign Body 43275
Specimen Collection 43260
Sphincter Pressure 43263
Sphincterotomy 43262, 43274
Exploration
Atresia 47700
Endoscopy 47552
Incision
Sphincter 43262, 47460
Incision and Drainage 47420-47425
Nuclear Medicine
Imaging 78226, 78227
Pharmacologic Intervention 78227
Placement
Access to Small Bowel 47541
Catheter
Drainage 47533, 47534
Stent 43274, 47801
Reconstruction
Anastomosis 47800
Removal
Calculus (Stone) . . 43264, 47420, 47425, 47544
Foreign Body 43275
Stent 43275
Repair 47701
Gastrointestinal Tract 47785
with Intestines 47760, 47780
Stent Placement 47538-47540, 47801
Tumor
Ablation 43278
Excision 47711, 47712
Unlisted Services and Procedures 47999
X ray
Guide Dilation 74360
with Contrast 47532, 74300, 74301
Calculus Removal 47544
Guide Catheter 74328, 74330

Bile Duct, Common, Cystic Dilatation
See Cyst, Choledochal

Bilirubin
Blood 82247, 82248
Feces 82252
Total
Direct 82247, 82248
Transcutaneous 88720

Billroth I or II
See Gastrectomy, Partial

Bilobectomy 32482
Thoracoscopic 32670

Bimone
See Testosterone

Binding Globulin, Testosterone-Estradiol
See Globulin, Sex Hormone Binding

Binocular Microscopy 92504

Biofeedback
See Biofeedback Training

Biofeedback Training
Anorectal 90911
Psychophysiological 90875, 90876

Bioimpedance
Body Composition Analysis 0358T
Cardiovascular Analysis 93701

Biological Skin Grafts
See Skin Substitute Graft

Biometry
Eye 76516-76519, 92136
Pupillometry 0341T

Biomechanical Mapping
Transvaginal 0487T

Biopsies, Needle
See Needle Biopsy

Biopsy
See Brush Biopsy; Needle Biopsy
Abdomen 49000, 49321
Mass 49180
Adrenal Gland 60540-60545, 60650
Anal
Endoscopy 46606
High-Resolution Magnification (HRA) . . 46607
Ankle 27613, 27614, 27620
Arm, Lower 25065, 25066
Arm, Upper 24065, 24066
Artery
Temporal 37609
Auditory Canal, External 69105
Back/Flank 21920-21925
Bile Duct
Endoluminal 47543
Endoscopy 47553
with Transhepatic Guided Cholangiography
Laparoscopic 47579
Bladder 52354
Cystourethroscopy 52204, 52224, 52250
Blood Vessel
Transcatheter 75970
Bone . . . 0200T, 0201T, 20220-20245, 22510-22512
Bone Marrow 38221, 38222, 88305
Brain 61140
Stereotactic 61750, 61751
Brainstem 61575, 61576
Breast 19100, 19101
Imaging of Specimen with Localization Device
Placement 19081-19086
with Magnetic Resonance Guidance 19085, 19086
with Stereotactic Guidance . . . 19081, 19082
with Ultrasound Guidance 19083, 19084
Bronchi
Catheterization 31717
Endoscopic 31625-31629, 31632, 31633

Index

- Brush
  - Bronchi ... 31717
  - Renal Pelvis ... 52007
  - Ureter ... 52007
  - with Cystourethroscopy ... 52204
- Carpometacarpal Joint
  - Synovium ... 26100
- Cervix ... 57421, 57454, 57455, 57460, 57500
- Chorionic Villus ... 59015
- Colon ... 44025, 44100
  - Endoscopy ... 44389, 45380, 45392
  - Multiple
    - with Colostomy, Cecostomy ... 44322
- Colon-Sigmoid
  - Endoscopy ... 45305, 45331
- Conjunctiva ... 68100
- Cornea ... 65410
- Duodenum ... 44010
- Ear, External ... 69100
- Elbow ... 24065, 24066, 24101, 29830
  - Synovium ... 24100
- Embryo Blastomere ... 89290, 89291
- Endometrium ... 58100-58110, 58558
- Epididymis ... 54800, 54865
- Esophagus
  - Endoscopy ... 43193, 43198, 43202, 43238, 43239, 43242
  - Forceps ... 3150F
- Eye Muscle ... 67346
- Eyelid ... 67810
  - Margin ... 67810
- Fallopian Tube ... 49321
- Femur ... 27323, 27324
- Foot
  - Interphalangeal Joint ... 28054
  - Intertarsal Joint ... 28050
  - Metatarsophalangeal Joint ... 28052
  - Tarsometatarsal Joint ... 28050
- Forearm ... 25065, 25066
- Gallbladder
  - Endoscopy ... 43261
- Gastrointestinal, Upper
  - Endoscopy ... 43239
- Glenohumeral Joint ... 23105
- Hand
  - Interphalangeal Joint ... 26110
  - Metacarpophalangeal Joint ... 26105, 29900
  - Synovium ... 26100
- Heart ... 93505
- Hip ... 27040, 27041
  - Joint ... 27052
  - Synovium ... 29860
- Ileum
  - Endoscopy ... 44382
- Interphalangeal Joint
  - Finger ... 26110
  - Toe ... 28054
- Intertarsal Joint ... 28050
- Intervertebral Disc ... 62267
- Intestines ... 44010, 44020, 44100
  - Endoscopy ... 44361, 44377, 44382, 44386
- Intracranial Lesion ... 61140, 61750
- Kidney ... 50200-50205
  - Endoscopic ... 50555-50557, 50574, 50576, 52354
- Knee ... 27323, 27324, 29870
  - Synovium ... 27330
- Knee Joint
  - Synovium ... 27331
- Lacrimal Gland ... 68510
- Lacrimal Sac ... 68525
- Larynx
  - Endoscopy ... 31510, 31535, 31536, 31576
- Leg
  - Lower ... 27613, 27614
  - Upper ... 27323, 27324
- Lip ... 40490
- Liver ... 47000, 47001, 47100, 47700
- Lung
  - Needle ... 32405
  - Thoracoscopy ... 32607, 32608
  - Thoracotomy ... 32096, 32097
- Lymph Nodes
  - Endobronchial Ultrasound (EBUS) Guided ... 31652, 31653
  - Injection Procedure
    - Radioactive Tracer ... 38792
  - Laparoscopic ... 38570-38573
  - Needle ... 38505
  - Open ... 38500, 38510, 38520, 38525, 38530, 38531
    - Superficial ... 38500
  - Para-aortic ... 57109, 57112, 57531, 58210, 58548
  - Prostate ... 55812, 55842, 55862
  - Transbronchial ... 31652, 31653
  - Transtracheal ... 31652, 31653
- Mediastinum
  - Mediastinoscopy ... 39401, 39402
  - Mediastinotomy ... 39000, 39010
  - Needle ... 32405
- Metacarpophalangeal Joint ... 26105, 29900
- Metatarsophalangeal Joint ... 28052
- Mouth ... 40808, 41108
- Muscle ... 20200-20206
- Nail ... 11755
- Nasopharynx ... 42804-42806
- Neck ... 21550
- Nerve ... 64795
- Nose
  - Endoscopic ... 31237
  - Intranasal ... 30100
- Nucleus Pulposus ... 62267
- Omentum ... 49321
- Oocyte Polar Body ... 89290, 89291
- Orbit
  - Exploration ... 67400, 67450
- Oropharynx ... 42800
- Ovary ... 49321, 58900
- Palate ... 42100
- Pancreas ... 48100-48102
- Paravertebral Tissue ... 62267
- Pelvis ... 27040, 27041
- Penis ... 54100
  - Deep Structures ... 54105
- Pericardial Sac
  - Thorascopic ... 32604
- Pericardium ... 39010
- Perineum ... 56605, 56606
- Peritoneum
  - Endoscopic ... 49321
- Pharynx ... 42800-42806
- Pleura
  - Needle ... 32400
  - Thoracoscopic ... 32609
  - Thoracotomy ... 32098
- Prostate
  - Incisional ... 55705
  - Lymph Nodes ... 55812, 55842, 55862
  - Needle or Punch ... 55700, 55706
  - Stereotactic ... 55706
- Rectum ... 45100, 45305, 45331
- Renal Pelvis
  - Endoluminal, Non-endoscopic ... 50606
- Retroperitoneal Area ... 49010, 49180
- Sacroiliac Joint ... 27050
- Salivary Gland ... 42400, 42405
- Shoulder ... 23065, 23066
- Shoulder Joint ... 23100, 23101, 23106, 29805
- Sinus ... 31237
  - Sphenoid ... 31050
- Skin Lesion
  - Fine Needle Aspiration (FNA) ... 10004-10012, 10021
  - Incisional ... 11106, 11107
  - Punch ... 11104, 11105
  - Tangential ... 11102, 11103
- Skull Base ... 61575, 61576
- Spinal Cord
  - Needle ... 62269
  - Neoplasm ... 63275-63290
  - Transoral ... 61575, 61576
  - Percutaneous ... 62269
- Stomach ... 43605
- Tarsometatarsal Joint
  - Synovium ... 28050
- Temporomandibular Joint ... 29800
- Testis ... 54500-54505
- Thigh ... 27323, 27324
- Thorax ... 21550
- Throat ... 42800-42806
- Thyroid ... 60100
- Tongue ... 41100-41105
- Transcatheter ... 37200
- Ureter ... 52354
  - Endoluminal, Non-endoscopic ... 50606
  - Endoscopic ... 50955-50957, 50974-50976
- Urethra ... 52204, 52250, 52354, 53200
- Uterus
  - Endometrial ... 58100-58110
  - Endoscopic ... 58558
- Uvula ... 42100
- Vagina ... 57100-57105, 57109, 57421
- Vein ... 37200, 75970
- Vertebral Body
  - Open ... 20250, 20251
  - Percutaneous ... 22510-22515
- Vulva ... 56605, 56606, 56821
- with Arthrotomy
  - Acromioclavicular Joint ... 23101
  - Glenohumeral Joint ... 23100, 23105
  - Sternoclavicular Joint ... 23101
- with Cystourethroscopy ... 52354
- Wrist ... 25065, 25066, 25100, 25101, 29840

Biopsy, Skin
See Skin, Biopsy

Biopsy, Vein
See Vein, Biopsy

Biostatistics
See Biometry

Biosterol
See Vitamin, A

Biotinidase ... 82261

Birthing Room
- Newborn Care ... 99460, 99463
  - Attendance at Delivery ... 99464
  - Resuscitation ... 99465

Bischof Procedure
See Laminectomy, with Myelotomy

Bizzozero's Corpuscle/Cell
See Blood, Platelet

Bladder
- Abscess
  - Incision and Drainage ... 51080
- Anastomosis ... 50780-50782, 51960

Aspiration 51100-51102
Biopsy 52204
Calculus
  Litholapaxy 52317, 52318
  Lithotripsy 51065, 52353
  Manipulation 52352
  Removal . . 51050, 51065, 52310-52315, 52352
Catheterization 51045, 51102, 51701-51703
Chemodenervation 52287
Cuff 50234, 50650
Cyst
  Urachal
    Excision 51500
Cystostomy Tube 51705-51710
Cystourethroscopy
  See Endoscopy
Destruction
  Lesion 51030
Dilation 52260-52265
  Ureter
    See Ureter, Dilation
Diverticulum
  Excision 51525
  Incision 52305
  Resection 52305
Endoscopy 52000
  Biopsy 52204, 52224, 52250, 52354
  Dilation 52260-52265
  Diverticulum 52305
  Evacuation
    Clot 52001
  Excision
    Tumor 52234, 52235, 52240, 52355
  Exploration 52351
  Instillation 52005, 52010
  Fulguration 52214-52224, 52400
    Tumor 52234, 52235, 52240
  Injection, Steroid 52283
  Irrigation
    Clot 52001
  Lithotripsy 52353
  Radiotracer 52250
  Removal
    Calculus 52310-52315, 52352
    Foreign Body 52310-52315
  Tumor
    Excision 52234-52240, 52355
    Fulguration 52234, 52235, 52240
Excision
  Partial 51550-51565
  Total 45126, 51570, 51580, 51590-51597
    with Nodes 51575, 51585, 51595
  Transurethral 52640
  Ureterocele 51535
Flap 50785
Fulguration 52214-52224, 52354
Incision and Drainage 51040
Injection
  Radiological 51600-51610
Insertion
  Stent 51045, 52334
Instillation 51700
  Anticarcinogenic Agent 51720
Interstitial Cystitis
  Dilation 52260-52265
Irrigation 51700
Laparoscopy 51999
Lesion
  Destruction 51030
  Fulguration 52224
Neck
  Excision 51520
  Injection of Implant Material 51715
  Remodel for Urinary Incontinence 53860
Nuclear Medicine
  Residual Study 78730
Pressure
  Cystometrogram (CMG) 51725-51729
  Uroflowmetry 51736-51741
  Voiding Study 51728, 51729, 51797
Radiotracer 51020, 52250
Reconstruction
  and Urethra 51800-51820
    Radiofrequency Micro-Remodeling . . . 53860
  with Intestines 51960
Removal
  Calculus . . 51050, 51065, 52310-52315, 52352
  Foreign Body 52310-52315
  Urethral Stent 52310-52315
Repair 51800-51980
  Diverticulum 52305
  Exstrophy 51940
  Fistula 44660, 44661, 45800-45805, 51880-51925
  Neck 51845
  Wound 51860-51865
Resection 52500
Tumor
  Excision 51530
  Fulguration 52234-52240
  Resection 52234-52240
Unlisted Services and Procedures 53899
Ureterocele 51535
Urethrocystography 74450-74455
Urethrotomy 52270-52276
Urinary Incontinence Procedures
  Neck Micro-remodel 53860
  Plan of Care 0509F
  Sling Operation 51992
  Urethral Suspension 51990
X ray 74430, 74450-74455

Bladder Voiding Pressure Studies 51728, 51729

Blalock-Hanlon Procedure . . 33735-33737
See Septostomy, Atrial

Blalock-Taussig Procedure
Shunt, Great Vessel 33750

Blast Cells
See Stem Cell

Blast Transformation
See Blastogenesis

Blastocyst Implantation
See Implantation, Embryo

Blastocyst Transfer
See Embryo Transfer

Blastogenesis 86353

Blastomyces
Antibody 86612

Blastomycosis, European
See Cryptococcus

Bleeding
See Hemorrhage
Disorder
  See Coagulopathy
Time 85002
Uterine
  Postpartum 59160
Vaginal 57180

Blepharoplasty 15820-15823
See Canthoplasty
Anesthesia 00103
Eyelid Reconstruction 15820-15823

Blepharoptosis
Repair 67901-67909
  Frontalis Muscle Technique 67901
    with Fascial Sling 67902
  Superior Rectus Technique with Fascial Sling 67906
  Tarso Levator Resection/Advancement
    External Approach 67904
    Internal Approach 67903

Blepharorrhaphy
See Tarsorrhaphy

Blepharospasm
Chemodenervation 64612

Blepharotomy
Drainage of Abscess 67700

Blister
See Bulla

Blom-Singer Prosthesis 31611

Blood
Apheresis
  See Apheresis
Banking
  See Blood Banking
Bleeding Time 85002
Blood-derived Peripheral Stem Cells
  See Hematopoietic Progenitor Cell (HPC)
Blood Cell Count
  See Blood Cell Count, Complete (CBC)
Blood Clotting
  Assay 85396
    Activity 85397
    ADAMTS-13 85397
  Coagulation Time 85345-85348
  Factor
    See Clotting Factor
  Inhibitors 85300-85303, 85306, 85307, 85335, 85337
  Lysis Time 85175
  Retraction 85170
  Thrombolytic Agents
    Tissue Plasminogen Activator (tPA) . . . 4077F
Carboxyhemoglobin 88740
Collection, for Autotransfusion
  Intraoperative 86891
  Preoperative 86890
Feces 82270, 82272-82274
Hemoglobin A1c (HbA1c) Level 3044F-3046F
Hemoglobin
  Carboxyhemoglobin 88740
  Concentration 85046
  Methemoglobin 88741
  Quantitative 88740
Injection
  Plasma 0232T
Methemoglobin 88741
Nuclear Medicine
  Flow Imaging 78445
  Red Cell 78140
  Red Cell Survival 78130-78135
Osmolality 83930
Plasma
  Exchange 36514-36516
  Frozen Preparation 86927
  Injection 0232T

Index

Reinfusion 0342T
Volume 78110, 78111
Platelet
Aggregation 85576
Automated Count 85049
Count 85008
Manual Count 85032
Neutralization 85597
Stem Cell
Count 86367
Donor Search 38204
Erythropoietin Therapy 3160F, 4090F-4095F
Harvesting 38205, 38206
Transplantation 38240-38242
Cell Concentration 38215
Cryopreservation 38207, 88240
Plasma Depletion 38214
Platelet Depletion 38213
Preparation 38207-38209
Red Blood Cell Depletion 38212
T-cell Depletion 38210
Thawing 38208, 38209, 88241
Tumor Cell Depletion 38211
Washing 38209
Transfusion 36430
Exchange 36455
Newborn 36450, 36456
Fetal 36460
Push
Infant to 2 years old 36440
Unlisted Services and Procedures 85999
Urine 83491
Viscosity 85810
Volume
Plasma 78110, 78111
Red Blood Cells 78120, 78121
Whole Blood 78122

Blood Banking
Frozen Blood Preparation 86930-86932, 88240
Frozen Plasma Preparation 86927
Physician Services 86077-86079

Blood Cell
CD4 and CD8
Including Ratio 86360
Apheresis 36511-36514, 36516
Enzyme Activity 82657
Photopheresis 36522
Sedimentation Rate
Automated 85652
Manual 85651

Blood Cell Count
Automated 85049
B Cells 86355
Blood Smear 85007, 85008
Complete (CBC) 85025-85027
Differential WBC Count 85004-85007, 85009
Hematocrit 85014
Hemoglobin 85018
Hemogram
Added Indices 85025-85027
Automated 85025-85027
Manual 85032
Microhematocrit 85013
Natural Killer (NK) Cells 86357
Red Blood Cells 85032-85041
Reticulocyte 85044-85046
Stem Cells 86367
T Cells 86359-86361
White Blood Cells 85032, 85048, 89055

Blood Cell Count, Red
See Red Blood Cell (RBC), Count

Blood Cell Count, White
See White Blood Cell, Count

Blood Cell, Red
See Red Blood Cell (RBC)

Blood Cell, White
See Leukocyte

Blood Coagulation
See Blood, Blood Clotting
Clot
See Clot
Defect
See Coagulopathy
Disorders
See Coagulopathy
Factor
See Clotting Factor
Test
See Blood, Blood Clotting

Blood Component Removal
See Apheresis

Blood Count, Complete
See Complete Blood Count (CBC)

Blood Flow
Graft Check 15860, 90940
Myocardial
Absolute Quantitation 0482T

Blood Gases
CO_2 82803
HCO_3 82803
O_2 Saturation 82805, 82810
pCO_2 82803
pH 82800, 82803, 82930
pO_2 .... 82803, 82820

Blood Letting
See Phlebotomy

Blood Lipoprotein
See Lipoprotein

Blood Pool Imaging
Cardiac
First Pass 78481-78483, 78496
Gated Equilibrium 78472, 78473, 78496
SPECT 78494

Blood Pressure
Baroreflex Activation Device
Implantation/Replacement 0266T-0273T
Determination
Central Arterial
Noninvasive WaveformAnalysis 93050
Monitoring, 24-Hour 93784, 93786, 93788, 93790
Ocular
Measurement 0198T
Monitoring 0329T
Performance Measures
Chronic Kidney Disease 0513F, 2000F, 3074F, 3075F, 3077F-3080F
Coronary Artery Disease 0001F, 3074F
Hypertension 3074F, 3075F, 3077F-3080F
Venous 93770

Blood Products
Irradiation 86945
Pooling 86965
Splitting 86985
Volume Reduction 86960

Blood Sample
Fetal 59030

Blood Serum
See Serum

Blood Smear
Microorganism Identification 87205-87207
Microscopic Examination 85007, 85008
Peripheral 85060
Sex Chromatin 88140
Surgical Pathology 88312, 88313, 88319

Blood Syndrome
Chromosome Analysis 88245, 88248, 88249

Blood Tests
Coagulation
See Blood, Blood Clotting
Cell Count
See Blood Cell Count
Culture, Bacteria
See Bacteria Culture
Gas Analysis
See Blood Gases
Iron Stores 3160F
Kt/V 3082F-3084F
Nuclear Medicine
Plasma Volume 78110, 78111
Platelet Survival 78191
Red Cell Survival 78130, 78135
Red Cell Volume 78120, 78121
Whole Blood Volume 78122
Panels
Acute Hepatitis 80074
Electrolyte 80051
General Health 80050
Hepatic Function 80076
Hepatitis, Acute 80074
Lipid 80061
Metabolic
Basic 80047, 80048
Comprehensive 80053
Obstetric 80055, 80081
Renal Function 80069
Typing
See Blood Typing, Serologic
Urea Nitrogen 84520-84525
Volume Determination 78122

Blood Transfusion, Autologous
See Autotransfusion

Blood Typing, Serologic
ABO Only 86900
Antigen Screen 86904
Antigen Testing, Donor Blood 86902
Compatibility 86920-86923
Other RBC Antigens 86905
Paternity Testing 86910, 86911
Rh (D) 86901
Rh Phenotype 86906

Blood Urea Nitrogen 84520-84525

Blood Vessels
Angioscopy 35400
Endoscopy 37500, 37501
Endothelial Function Assessment
Noninvasive 93998
Excision
See Arteriovenous Malformation; Bypass Graft
Exploration
Abdomen 35840
Carotid Artery 35701
Chest 35820
Extremity 35860
Femoral Artery 35721
Neck 35800

Popliteal Artery ... 35741
Vessel, Other ... 35761
Harvest
See Bypass Graft, Harvest
Repair
Aneurysm
See Aneurysm Repair
Aorta ... 33320-33322
Fistula
See Arteriovenous Fistula
Direct ... 35201-35226
Finger ... 35207
Hand ... 35207
Intra-abdominal ... 35221, 35281
Intrathoracic ... 35211, 35216, 35271, 35276
Lower Extremity ... 35226, 35286
Neck ... 35201, 35231, 35261
Great Vessel ... 33320-33322
Kidney ... 50100
Upper Extremity ... 35236, 35266
Malformation
See Arteriovenous Malformation
Shunt Creation
Direct ... 36818, 36821
Thomas Shunt ... 36835
with Bypass Graft ... 35686
with Graft ... 36825-36830
with Transposition ... 36818-36820
Shunt Revision
with Graft ... 36832

Blood, Occult
See Occult Blood

Bloom Syndrome
Chromosome Analysis ... 88245
Gene Analysis ... 81209

Blot Test, Ink
See Rorschach Test

Blotting, Western
See Western Blot

Blow-Out Fracture
Orbital Floor ... 21385-21395

Blue Dome Cyst
See Breast, Cyst

BMT
See Hematopoietic Progenitor Cell (HPC), Transplantation

Boarding Home Care
Established Patient ... 99334-99337
New Patient ... 99324-99328

Bodies
Acetone
See Drug Assay, Drug Procedure, Definitive Drug Class, Alcohols
Barr
See Barr Bodies
Carotid
See Carotid Body
Ciliary
See Ciliary Body
Heinz
See Heinz Bodies
Inclusion
See Inclusion Bodies
Ketone
See Ketone Body

Body Cast
See Cast

Body Fluid
Abdominal
See Paracentesis
Amniotic
See Amniotic Fluid
Blood
See Blood Tests
Cerebrospinal Fluid
See Cerebrospinal Fluid
Fetal
Procedures and Testing
See Fetal Procedure; Fetal Testing
Pleural
See Pleura
Semen
See Semen Analysis
Spinal
See Spinal Cord
Urine
See Urinalysis

Body of Vertebra
See Vertebral, Body

Boil
See Furuncle

Boil, Vulva
See Vulva, Incision and Drainage, Boil

Bone
Abscess
See Abscess, Bone
Biopsy
Needle ... 20220, 20225
Open ... 20240, 20245, 20250, 20251
Trocar ... 20220, 20225
with Vertebroplasty
Cervicothoracic ... 22510, 22512
Lumbosacral ... 22511, 22512
Cast
See Cast
Cyst
Drainage ... 20615
Injection ... 20615
Debridement ... 11044, 11047
Density Study
See Bone Density Study
Disease
Evaluation and Management
See Performance Measures, Osteoarthritis; Performance Measures, Osteoporosis
Excision
See Amputation; Arthrectomy
Fixation
See External Fixation; Fixation (Device)
Fracture
See Fracture
Implant Removal ... 20670, 20680
Insertion
Intraosseous Infusion ... 36680
Osseointegrated Implant ... 69714-69718
Marrow
See Bone Marrow
Nuclear Medicine
Density Study ... 78350, 78351
Imaging ... 78300-78320
SPECT ... 78320
Unlisted Services and Procedures ... 78399
Protein
Osteocalcin ... 83937
Radiography
Age Study ... 77072
Dual Energy X-ray Absorptiometry (DXA) ... 77080, 77081, 77085, 77086
Joint Stress ... 77071
Length Study ... 77073
Osseous Survey ... 77074-77077
Scan
See Bone, Nuclear Medicine
Skeletal Traction
See Skeletal Traction
Spur
See Exostosis
Tumor
Ablation
with Adjacent Soft Tissue ... 20982, 20983

Bone 4-Carboxyglutamic Protein
See Osteocalcin

Bone Conduction Hearing Device, Electromagnetic
Implantation/Replacement ... 69710
Removal/Repair ... 69711

Bone Density Study
Appendicular Skeleton ... 77081
Axial Skeleton ... 77078, 77080
Dual Energy X-ray Absorptiometry (DXA) ... 77080, 77081, 77085
Vertebral Fracture Assessment ... 77085, 77086
Ultrasound ... 0508T, 76977

Bone Graft
Allograft
See Allograft
Any Donor Area ... 20900, 20902
Autograft
See Autograft
Calcaneal Fracture ... 28420
Clavicle ... 23485
Cranium ... 61316, 61559, 62146-62148
Craniofacial Separation ... 21436
Femur ... 27170, 27177, 27470
Harvesting ... 20900-20902
Knee Drilling ... 29885
Malar Area ... 21210, 21366
Mandible ... 21127, 21194, 21215
Mandibular Ramus ... 21194
Maxilla ... 21210
Metacarpal Nonunion ... 26546
Metatarsal Nonunion ... 28322
Microvascular Anastomosis
Fibula ... 20955
Iliac Crest ... 20956
Metatarsal ... 20957
Other Site ... 20962
Nasal Area ... 21210
Nasomaxillary Complex Fracture ... 21348
Osteocutaneous Flap ... 20969-20973
Midface ... 21145-21147, 21150, 21151, 21154, 21155, 21159, 21160, 21182-21184, 21188
Orbit
Blowout Fracture ... 21395
Fracture ... 21408
Hypertelorism ... 21260
Repositioning ... 21267
Reconstruction ... 21182-21184, 21256
Palate, Cleft ... 42210
Phalanx Nonunion ... 26546
Spine Surgery ... 20930, 20931, 22586, 22899
Bone Marrow Aspiration ... 20939
Toe Transfer ... 26551
Ulna ... 25830
Vertebra ... 0222T
Cervical ... 0219T, 63051
Lumbar ... 0221T
Thoracic ... 0220T
Wrist ... 25810, 25825

Index

Bone Healing
Electrical Stimulation . . . 20974, 20975
Ultrasound Stimulation . . . 20979

Bone Infection
See Osteomyelitis

Bone Marrow
Aspiration . . . 38220, 38222
Biopsy . . . 38221, 38222, 88305
Blood-derived Peripheral Stem Cell
  See Hematopoietic Progenitor Cell (HPC)
Blood Supply Magnetic Resonance Imaging (MRI) . . . 77084
Cell Therapy . . . 0263T-0265T
Cryopreservation . . . 38207
Cytogenic Testing . . . 3155F
Donor Cell Acquisition . . . 38204
Harvesting . . . 0265T, 38230, 38232
Magnetic Resonance Imaging (MRI) . . . 77084
Nuclear Medicine
  Imaging . . . 78102-78104
Smear Interpretation . . . 85097
T-Cell Transplantation . . . 38240-38242
Transplant Preparation . . . 38207-38215

Bone Plate
Mandible . . . 21244

Bone Wedge Reversal
Osteotomy . . . 21122

Bordetella
Antibody . . . 86615
Antigen Detection
  Direct Fluorescence . . . 87265

Borrelia
Antibody Detection . . . 86617-86619

Borrelia burgdorferi ab
See Antibody, Detection, Lyme Disease

Borreliosis, Lyme
See Lyme Disease

Bost Fusion
See Arthrodesis, Wrist

Bosworth Operation
See Acromioclavicular Joint, Dislocation; Arthrodesis, Vertebra; Fasciotomy

Bottle Procedure
Repair of Tunica Vaginalis Hydrocele . . . 55060

Botulinum Toxin
See Chemodenervation

Boutonniere Deformity . . . 26426-26428

Bowel
See Intestines

Bowleg Repair . . . 27455-27457

Boyd Hip Disarticulation
See Amputation, Leg, Upper; Radical Resection; Replantation

Brace
See Cast
for Leg Cast . . . 29358
Vertebral Fracture . . . 22310, 22315

Brachial Arteries
See Artery, Brachial

Brachial Plexus
Anesthetic Injection . . . 64415, 64416
Decompression . . . 64713
Neuroplasty . . . 64708, 64713
Release . . . 64713
Repair/Suture . . . 64861

Brachiocephalic Artery
See Artery, Brachiocephalic

Brachycephaly
Reconstruction . . . 21175

Brachytherapy
High Dose Electronic . . . 0394T, 0395T
  Remote Afterloading . . . 77770-77772
Interstitial Application . . . 0395T, 77778
  Remote Afterloading . . . 77770-77772
  Device Placement
    Breast . . . 19296-19298
    Genitalia . . . 55920
    Head . . . 41019
    Intraocular . . . 67299
    Neck . . . 41019
    Pelvis . . . 55920
    Uterus . . . 57155
    Vagina . . . 57155, 57156
  Heyman Capsule Insertion . . . 58346
Intracavitary Application . . . 0395T, 77761-77763
Loading . . . 77790
Planning
  Isodose Plan . . . 77316-77318
  Prostate Volume Study . . . 76873
Radioelement Solution
  Infusion . . . 77750
  Instillation . . . 77750
Remote Afterloading
  Interstitial . . . 77770-77772
  Intracavitary . . . 77770-77772
  Surface . . . 77767, 77768
Surface Application . . . 0394T, 77789
  Remote Afterloading . . . 77767, 77768
Unlisted Clinical Procedures . . . 77799

Bradykinin
Blood or Urine . . . 82286

Brain
See Brainstem; Mesencephalon; Skull Base Surgery
Abscess
  Drainage . . . 61150, 61151
  Excision . . . 61514, 61522
  Incision and Drainage . . . 61320, 61321
Adhesions . . . 62161
Angiography . . . 36100, 70496
Biopsy . . . 61140
  Stereotactic . . . 61750, 61751
Catheter
  Insertion . . . 61210
  Irrigation . . . 62194, 62225
  Replacement . . . 62160, 62194, 62225
Catheter Placement
  for Radiation Source . . . 61770
Computer Assisted
  Procedure . . . 61781, 61782
Cortex
  Magnetic Stimulation . . . 64999, 90867-90869
  Mapping . . . 90867, 96020
    Motor Function . . . 64999
Cyst
  Drainage . . . 61150, 61151, 62161, 62162
  Excision . . . 61516, 61524, 62162
Debridement . . . 62010
Diagnostic Radiology
  CT Scan . . 0042T, 70450, 70460, 70470, 70496
  Imaging . . . 70010-70015, 78600, 78601, 78605-78610
    Cerebrospinal Fluid . . . 78630-78650
    Cisternography . . . 70015
    Vascular Flow . . . 78601, 78606, 78610
    Ventriculography . . . 78635
  Doppler Study . . . 93886, 93888, 93890, 93892, 93893
  Magnetic Resonance Imaging . . . 70551-70555, 70557-70559
  Perfusion Analysis . . . 0042T
  Positron Emission Tomography (PET) . . . 78608, 78609
Electrocorticography . . . 61536, 61538
Electroencephalography
  Cerebral Death Evaluation . . . 95824
  Monitored . . . 95812, 95813
  Recorded . . . 95816, 95819, 95822, 95827
Epileptogenic Focus
  Excision . . . 61534, 61536
  Monitoring . . . 61531, 61533, 61535, 61760
Excision
  Amygdala . . . 61566
  Choroid Plexus . . . 61544
  Craniopharyngioma . . . 61545
  Hemisphere . . . 61543
  Hippocampus . . . 61566
  Meningioma . . . 61512, 61519
  Other Lobe . . . 61323, 61539, 61540
  Temporal Lobe . . . 61537, 61538
  Tumor . . . 61510, 61518, 61520, 61521, 61526-61530, 61545, 62164
Exploration
  Infratentorial . . . 61305
  Supratentorial . . . 61304
Hematoma
  Drainage . . . 61154
  Incision and Drainage . . . 61312-61315
Implantation
  Chemotherapy Agent . . . 61517
  Electrode . . . 61210, 61533, 61850, 61860, 61863, 61864, 61867, 61868, 61870
  Pulse Generator . . . 61885, 61886
  Reservoir . . . 61210, 61215
Infusion . . . 95990, 95991
Lesion
  Aspiration, Stereotactic . . . 61750, 61751
  Excision . . . 61600, 61601, 61605-61608, 61615, 61616
Lobectomy . . . 61537-61540
Magnetoencephalography . . . 95965-95967
Mapping . . . 90867-90869, 95961, 95962, 96020
Meningioma
  Excision . . . 61512, 61519
Neurostimulation
  Analysis
    Brain . . . 95970, 95983, 95984
    Cranial Nerve . . . 95970, 95976, 95977
    Gastric . . . 95980-95982
    Peripheral Nerve . . . 95970-95972
    Spinal Cord . . . 95970-95972
    with Vagus Nerve Blocking Therapy . . 0317T
  Electrode
    Implantation . . . 61210, 61850, 61860, 61863, 61864, 61870
    Removal . . . 61880
    Revision . . . 61880
  Pulse Generator
    Insertion . . . 61885, 61886
    Removal . . . 61880
    Revision . . . 61880
Radiosurgery
  for Lesion . . . 61796-61800
  Radiation Treatment Delivery . . . 77371-77373
Removal
  Electrode . . . 61535, 61880
  Foreign Body . . . 61570, 62163

Index

Pulse Generator 61888
Shunt 62256-62258
Repair
Dura 61618
Wound 61571
Shunt
Creation 62190, 62192, 62200, 62223
Removal 62256-62258
Replacement 62160, 62194, 62225, 62230, 62256, 62258
Reprogramming 62252
Skull Surgery
See Skull Base Surgery
Stereotaxis-aided Procedures
Aspiration 61750, 61751
Biopsy 61750, 61751
Catheter Placement 61770
Create Lesion 61720, 61735, 61790, 61791
Navigation 61781, 61782
Procedure 61781, 61782
Radiation Treatment 77432
Radiosurgery 61796-61800, 77371-77373
Trigeminal Tract 61791
Transcranial Magnetic Stimulation (TMS) 90867-90869
Transection
Corpus Callosum 61541
Subpial 61567
Tumor
Excision
Cerebellopontine Angle 61520, 61526
Infratentorial 61518
Supratentorial 61510
Ventriculocisternostomy 62200, 62201
Torkildsen Type 62180

Brain Coverings
See Meninges

Brain Death
Determination 95824

Brain Stem
See Brainstem

Brain Stem Auditory Evoked Potential
See Evoked Potentials, Auditory Brainstem

Brain Surface Electrode
Stimulation 95961, 95962

Brain Tumor
Acoustic Neuroma
See Brain, Tumor, Excision
Craniopharyngioma
See Craniopharyngioma
Meningioma
See Meningioma

Brain Ventriculography
See Ventriculography

Brainstem
See Brain; Skull Base Surgery
Biopsy 61575, 61576
Decompression 61575, 61576
Diagnostic Tests
Auditory Implant 92640
Evoked Potentials 92585, 92586
Lesion
Excision 61575, 61576

Branchial Cleft
Cyst
Excision 42810-42815

Branchioma
See Branchial Cleft, Cyst

Breast
Ablation
Fibroadenoma 19105
Abscess
Incision and Drainage 19020
Aspiration
Cyst 19000, 19001
Augmentation 19324, 19325
Biopsy 19100, 19101
with Imaging of Specimen 19081-19086
with Localization Device Placement
Magnetic Resonance Guided .. 19085, 19086
Stereotactic Guidance 19081, 19082
Ultrasound Guided 19083, 19084
Cancer Gene Analysis
BRCA1 (BRCA1, DNA repair associate)
185delAG, 5385insC, 6174delT
Variants 81212
Duplication/Deletion 81162, 81164
Full Sequence 81162, 81165
Known Familial Variant 81215
BRCA2 (BRCA2, DNA repair associated)
185delAG, 5385insC, 6174delT
Variants 81212
Duplication/Deletion 81162, 81167
Full Sequence 81162, 81216
Known Familial Variant 81217
ERBB2 (HER2) 0009U
Cryosurgical Ablation 19105
Cyst
Excision 19120
Puncture Aspiration 19000, 19001
Diagnostic Imaging
Ductogram 19030, 77053, 77054
Galactogram 77053, 77054
Injection 19030
Magnetic Resonance Imaging (MRI)
with Computer-Aided Detection 77048, 77049
without Contrast 77046, 77047
Mammography, Diagnostic 77065, 77066
Mammogram, Screening 3014F, 77067
Ultrasound 76641, 76642
Excision
Biopsy 19100, 19101
Capsules 19371
Chest Wall Tumor 19260-19272
Cyst 19120
Lactiferous Duct 19110
Fistula 19112
Lesion 19120, 19125, 19126, 19301
by Needle Localization 19125, 19126
Mastectomy 19300-19307
Tissue 19120
Tumor 19120, 19260, 19271, 19272
Exploration
Abscess 19020
Nipple 19110
Imaging
Mammogram, Screening 3014F, 77067
Optical Coherence Tomography .. 0351T-0354T
Tactile 0422T
Implant
Biological
Insertion 19325, 19340, 19342
Preparation of Moulage 19396
Removal 19328, 19330
Soft Tissue Reinforcement 15777
Supply 19396
Lesion
Localization Device Placement
with Magnetic Resonance Guidance 19287, 19288
with Mammographic Guidance 19281, 19282
with Stereotactic Guidance ... 19283, 19284
with Ultrasound Guidance 19285, 19286
Mammaplasty
Augmentation 19324, 19325
Reduction 19318
Mastectomy
Complete 19303
Gynecomastia 19300
Modified Radical 19307
Partial 19301, 19302
Radical 19303-19306
Subcutaneous 19304
with Axillary Lymphadenectomy 19302
Mastopexy 19316
Axillary Lymph Node 0351T, 0352T
Periprosthetic Capsulectomy 19371
Periprosthetic Capsulotomy 19370
Radiation Therapy
Interstitial Radioelement Application
Catheter Placement 19296-19298
Preparation of Tumor Cavity 19294
Reconstruction
Augmentation 19324, 19325
Mammaplasty 19318-19325
Nipple 19350, 19355
Areola 19350
Revision 19380
with Free Flap 19364
with Latissimus Dorsi Flap 19361
with Other Techniques 19366
with Tissue Expander 19357
with Transverse Rectus Abdominis Myocutaneous Flap (TRAM) 19367-19369
Reduction 19318
Removal
Capsules 19371
Modified Radical 19307
Partial 19300-19302
Radical 19305, 19306
Simple, Complete 19303
Subcutaneous 19304
Suspension 19316
Tumor
Destruction/Reduction
Microwave Thermotherapy 19499
Excision
Benign 19120
Chest Wall 19260, 19271, 19272
Involving Ribs 19260, 19271, 19272
Malignant 19120
Unlisted Services and Procedures 19499

Breath Odor, Alcohol
See Alcohol, Breath

Breath Test
Alcohol, Ethyl 82075
Heart Transplant Rejection Detection 0085T
Helicobacter Pylori 78267, 78268, 83013
Hydrogen 91065
Methane 91065
Urea 78267, 78268

Breathing, Inspiratory Positive-Pressure
See Inhalation Treatment
Device
Intermittent Positive Pressure Breathing (IPPB)
Patient Utilization Demonstration/ Evaluation 94664

Bricker Procedure
Intestinal Anastomosis 50820

Bristow Procedure
See Capsulorrhaphy, Anterior

Brock Operation
See Valvotomy, Pulmonary Valve

Broken Nose
See Fracture, Nasal Bone

Bronchi
Allograft Preparation 32855, 32856
Aspiration
  Catheter 31720, 31725
  Endoscopic 31629, 31633, 31645, 31646
Biopsy 31625-31629, 31632, 31633
Bronchial Valve
  Insertion 31647, 31651
  Removal 31648, 31649
Bronchodilator
  Home Care 99503
  Spirometry 94012, 94060
Bronchoscopy
  Alveolar Lavage 31624
  Aspiration 31629, 31633, 31645, 31646
  Biopsy 31625-31629, 31632, 31633
  Catheter Placement for Radiotherapy . . . 31643
  Cell Brushing 31623
  Cell Washing 31622
  Computer-assisted/Image-guided Navigation 31627
  Dilation 31630, 31631, 31636, 31638
  Endobronchial Ultrasound (EBUS) 31652-31654
  Exploration 31622
    with Balloon Occlusion . . 31634, 31647, 31651
  Fiducial Marker Placement 31626
  Foreign Body Removal 31635
  Fracture Reduction 31630
  Stenosis Relief 31641
  Stent Placement 31631, 31636-31638
  Thermoplasty 31660, 31661
  Tumor Destruction 31641
  Tumor Excision 31640
  via Existing Tracheostomy 31615
Catheterization
  Aspiration 31725
  Bronchial Brush Biopsy 31717
  for Intracavitary Radioelement Application 31643
Endoscopy
  Ablation
    Photodynamic Therapy 96570, 96571
Exploration 31622, 31634, 31647, 31651
Fracture Reduction 31630
Insertion
  Bronchial Valve 31647, 31651
Needle Biopsy 31629, 31633
Reconstruction
  Anastomosis 31775, 32486
  Graft Repair 31770
  Stenosis 31775
Removal 32501
  Foreign Body 31635
Repair 32501
  Fistula 32815, 32906
  Stenosis 31641, 96570, 96571
Stent
  Placement 31636, 31637
  Revision 31638
Tests
  See Bronchial Challenge Test
  Air Leak Assessment 31647, 31651
  Airway Sizing 31647, 31651
  Bronchospasm Evaluation 94070, 94617
  Wheeze Rate 94799
  Thermoplasty 31660, 31661
Tumor
  Destruction 31641
  Excision 31640
Unlisted Services and Procedures 31899

Bronchial Allergen Challenge
See Bronchial Challenge Test

Bronchial Alveolar Lavage 31624

Bronchial Brush Biopsy
with Catheterization 31717

Bronchial Brushings/Protected Brushing 31623

Bronchial Challenge Test
See Allergy Tests
Bronchospasm Evaluation 94070, 94617
for Wheeze Rate 94799
with Antigens 95071
with Chemicals 95070
with Gases 95071
with Histamine 95070
with Methacholine 95070

Bronchial Provocation Tests
See Bronchial Challenge Test

Bronchial Thermoplasty 31660, 31661

Bronchioalveolar Lavage
See Lung, Lavage

Broncho-Bronchial Anastomosis . . 32486

Bronchoalveolar Lavage
See Lung, Lavage

Bronchoplasty 32501
See Reconstruction, Bronchi
Excision Stenosis and Anastomosis 31775
Graft Repair 31770

Bronchopneumonia, Hiberno-Vernal
See Q Fever

Bronchopulmonary Lavage
See Lung, Lavage

Bronchoscopy
Ablation
  Photodynamic Therapy 96570, 96571
Alveolar Lavage 31624
Aspiration 31629, 31633, 31645, 31646
Balloon Occlusion 31634, 31647, 31651
Biopsy 31625-31629, 31632, 31633
Brushing/Protected Brushing 31623
Catheter Placement
  Aspiration 31725
  Intracavitary Radioelement 31643
Computer-assisted Navigation 31627
Dilation 31630, 31631, 31636-31638
Exploration 31622, 31634, 31647, 31651
Fiducial Marker Placement 31626
Fracture Reduction 31630
Insertion of Bronchial Valve(s) 31647, 31651
Needle Biopsy 31629, 31633
Removal
  Bronchial Valve 31648, 31649
  Foreign Body 31635
  Tumor 31640, 31641
Stenosis 31641
Stent Placement 31631, 31636, 31637
Stent Revision 31638
with Airway Resizing 31647, 31648, 31649
with Assessment of Airway Leak 31647, 31648, 31649
with Balloon Occlusion 31647, 31648, 31649
with Bronchial Thermoplasty 31660, 31661
with Endobronchial Ultrasound (EBUS) 31652-31654
with Insertion of Bronchial Valves 31647, 31648, 31649

Bronchospasm Evaluation
See Pulmonology, Diagnostic, Spirometry

Bronkodyl
See Theophylline

Brow Ptosis
Repair 67900, 67909

Brucella
Antibody 86622
Antigen 86000

Bruise
See Hematoma

Brunschwig Operation
Pelvic Exenteration 58240

Brush Biopsy
See Biopsy; Needle Biopsy
Bronchi 31717

Brush Border Ab
See Antibody, Detection, Heterophile

Bucca
See Cheek

Buccal Mucosa
See Mouth, Mucosa

Bulbourethral Gland
Excision 53250

Bulla
Incision and Drainage
  Puncture Aspiration 10160
Lung
  Resection-plication 32141, 32655

BUN
See Blood Urea Nitrogen; Urea Nitrogen

Bunion Repair
Bunionectomy 28292
by Phalanx Osteotomy 28298, 28299
Chevron Procedure 28296
Concentric Procedure 28296
Keller Procedure 28292
Lapidus Procedure 28297
Mayo Procedure 28292
McBride Procedure 28292
Mitchell Procedure 28296
with Metatarsal Osteotomy 28295, 28296
with Sesamoidectomy 28292

Burgess Amputation
See Disarticulation, Ankle

Burkitt Herpesvirus
See Epstein-Barr Virus

Burns
Debridement . . 15002-15005, 16020, 16025, 16030
Dressings 16020, 16025, 16030
Escharotomy 15002-15005, 16035, 16036
Fenestration
  Body Surface 0479T, 0480T
First Degree, Initial Treatment 16000
Tissue Cultured Skin Grafts 15150-15152, 15155-15157
Total Body Surface Area (TBSA) Calculation . . 16000

Burr Hole
for Aspiration
Cyst 61156
Hematoma 61156
for Biopsy
Brain. 61140
Lesion. 61140, 61750, 61751
for Catheterization 61210
for Drainage
Abscess 61150, 61151
Cyst 61150, 61151
Hematoma 61154-61156
for Exploration
Infratentorial 61253
Supratentorial 61250
for Implantation
Catheter 61210
Cerebral Monitoring Device. 61210
EEG Electrode. 61210
Neurostimulator Array 61850, 61863, 61864, 61867, 61868
Pressure Recording Device 61210
Reservoir 61210
Strip Electrodes 61531
for Insertion
Pump 61210
Reservoir 61210
for Lesion Creation 61720
for Stereotactic Localization. 61770
for Ventricular Puncture 61020
with Injection, Contrast Media 61120
with Injection, Diagnostic or Therapeutic Substance 61026

Burrow's Operation
See Skin, Adjacent Tissue Transfer

Bursa
Ankle
Aspiration. 20605, 20606
Incision and Drainage 27604
Injection 20605, 20606
Arm, Lower
Aspiration. 20605, 20606
Incision and Drainage 25031
Injection 20605, 20606
Arm, Upper
Incision and Drainage 23931
Arthrocentesis
Intermediate. 20605, 20606
Major 20610, 20611
Small 20600, 20604
with Recording and Reporting. 20604, 20606, 20611
with Ultrasound Guidance. 20604, 20606, 20611
Elbow
Aspiration. 20605, 20606
Injection 20605, 20606
Excision 24105
Incision and Drainage 23931
Femur
Excision 27062
Finger
Aspiration. 20600, 20604
Injection 20600, 20604
Foot
Incision and Drainage 28001-28003
Hand
Incision and Drainage 26025, 26030
Hip
Aspiration. 20610, 20611
Injection 20610, 20611
Incision and Drainage 26991
Injection 20600, 20604-20606, 20610, 20611
Ischial
Excision 27060
Joint
Aspiration 20600, 20604-20606, 20610, 20611
Drainage. . 20600, 20604-20606, 20610, 20611
Injection . . 20600, 20604-20606, 20610, 20611
Knee
Aspiration. 20610, 20611
Excision 27340
Incision and Drainage 27301
Injection 20610, 20611
Leg, Lower. 27604
Leg, Upper
Incision and Drainage 27301
Palm
Incision and Drainage 26025, 26030
Pelvis
Incision and Drainage 26991
Shoulder
Aspiration. 20610, 20611
Drainage. 23031
Injection 20610, 20611
Toe
Aspiration. 20600, 20604
Injection 20600, 20604
Wrist
Aspiration. 20605, 20606
Incision and Drainage 25031
Injection 20605, 20606
Excision 25115, 25116

Bursectomy
See Excision, Bursa

Bursitis, Radiohumeral
See Tennis Elbow

Bursocentesis
See Aspiration, Bursa

Button
Bone Graft. 20900
Prosthesis
Nasal Septal 30220
Voice 31611

Butyrylcholine Esterase
See Cholinesterase

Bypass Graft
Arterial
Coronary. 33533-33536, 35600
Arterial-Venous
Coronary. . . 33517-33519, 33521-33523, 33530
Harvest
Artery 35600
Endoscopic. 33508
Vein 35500, 35572
In-Situ
See Bypass In-Situ
Placement
Vein Patch 35685
Reoperation. 35700
Repair
Abdomen 35907
Extremity 35903
Lower Extremity
with Composite Graft. 35681-35683
Neck. 35901
Thorax 35905
Revascularization
Extremity 35903
Neck. 35901
Thorax 35905
Revision
Lower Extremity
Femoral Artery 35883, 35884
with Angioplasty 35879
with Vein Interposition. 35881
Secondary Repair 35870
Thrombectomy
Coronary. 92973
Noncoronary. 37184-37186
Other than Hemodialysis Graft or Fistula. 35875, 35876
Venous
Aortobi-iliac 35538, 35638
Aortobifemoral. 35540, 35646
Aortocarotid. 35526, 35626
Aortoceliac. 35531, 35631
Aortofemoral 35539, 35647
Aortoiliac 35537, 35637
Aortoinnominate 35526, 35626
Aortomesenteric 35531, 35631
Aortorenal 35560, 35631
Aortosubclavian. 35526, 35626
Axillary-Axillary 35518, 35650
Axillary-Brachial. 35522
Axillary-Femoral. 35521, 35621
Axillary-Femoral-Femoral. 35533, 35654
Axillary-Popliteal 35623
Axillary-Tibial. 35623
Brachial-Brachial 35525
Brachial-Radial. 35523
Brachial-Ulnar 35523
Carotid-Brachial. 35510
Carotid-Contralateral Carotid 35509
Carotid-Subclavian. 35506, 35606
Carotid-Vertebral 35508, 35642
Common Carotid-Ipsilateral Internal Carotid 35501, 35601
Coronary. 33510-33514, 33516
Femoral-Femoral 35558, 35661
Femoral-Peroneal. 35566
Femoral-Popliteal. 35556, 35572, 35656
Femoral-Tibial 35566, 35666
Hepatorenal 35535
Ilioceliac. 35632
Iliofemoral 35565, 35665
Ilioiliac 35563, 35663
Iliomesenteric 35633
Iliorenal 35634
Mesenteric. 35531, 35631
Peroneal. 35566-35571, 35666-35671
Peroneal-Tibial. 35570
Popliteal-Peroneal 35571, 35671
Popliteal-Tibial. 35571, 35671
Splenorenal 35536, 35636
Subclavian-Axillary 35516, 35616
Subclavian-Brachial. 35512
Subclavian-Carotid. 35506
Subclavian-Subclavian. 35511, 35612
Subclavian-Vertebral 35515, 35645
Tibial/Peroneal Trunk-Tibial 35570
Tibial-Tibial 35570
with Composite Graft 35681

Bypass In-Situ
Femoral-Peroneal 35585
Femoral-Popliteal 35583
Femoral-Tibial. 35585
Popliteal-Peroneal. 35587
Popliteal-Tibial 35587
Tibial Artery 35585-35587
Ventricular Restoration. 33548

Bypass, Cardiopulmonary
See Cardiopulmonary Bypass

Index

C

C-13
Urea Breath Test . . . 83013, 83014
Urease Activity . . . 83013, 83014

C-14
Urea Breath Test . . . 78267, 78268
Urease Activity . . . 83013, 83014

C-Peptide . . . 80432, 84681

C-Reactive Protein . . . 86140, 86141

C-Section
See Cesarean Delivery

C Vitamin
See Ascorbic Acid

CABG
See Coronary Artery Bypass Graft (CABG)

Cadmium
Urine . . . 82300

Caffeine
Drug Assay . . . 80155
Halothane Contracture Test (CHCT) . . . 89049

Calcaneal Spur
See Heel Spur

Calcaneus
Bone Graft . . . 28420
Craterization . . . 28120
Cyst
  Excision . . . 28100-28103
Diaphysectomy . . . 28120
Excision . . . 28118-28120
Fracture
  Closed Treatment . . . 28400, 28405
  Open Treatment . . . 28415-28420
  Percutaneous Fixation . . . 28406
  with Bone Graft . . . 28420
  with Manipulation . . . 28405, 28406
Heel Spur . . . 28119
  Excision
Repair
  Osteotomy . . . 28300
Saucerization . . . 28120
Sequestrectomy . . . 28120
Tumor
  Excision . . . 28100-28103
  Radical Resection . . . 27647
X ray . . . 73650

Calcareous Deposits
Subdeltoid
  Removal . . . 23000

Calcifediol
See Vitamin, D

Calciferol
See Vitamin, D

Calcification
See Calcium, Deposits

Calciol
See Vitamin, D, Blood Serum Level, 25 hydroxy

Calcitonin
Blood or Urine . . . 82308
Stimulation Panel . . . 80410

Calcium
Blood
  Infusion Test . . . 82331
Deposits
  See Calculus, Removal
Ionized . . . 82330
Total . . . 82310
Urine . . . 82340

Calcium-Binding Protein, Vitamin K-Dependent
See Osteocalcin

Calcium-Pentagastrin Stimulation 80410

Calculus
Analysis . . . 82355, 82360, 82365, 82370
Destruction
  Bile Duct . . . 43265, 47544
  Extracorporeal Shock Wave Lithotripsy . . 50590
  Gallbladder . . . 47544
  Pancreatic Duct . . . 43265
Extraction
  Bladder . . . 51065
  Kidney . . . 50080, 50081
  Liver . . . 50080, 50081
  Transduodenal . . . 47460
Fragmentation
  Bile Duct . . . 43265
  Bladder . . . 52317, 52318
  Kidney . . . 50080, 50081
  Liver . . . 50080, 50081
  Ureter . . . 51065, 52325, 52353
Removal
  Bile Duct . . . 43264, 47544, 47554
  Biliary Tract . . . 47400, 47420, 47425, 47480
  Bladder . . . 51050, 52310, 52315, 52352
  Gallbladder . . . 47544
  Kidney . . . 50060, 50065, 50070, 50075, 50080, 50081, 50130, 50561, 50580, 52352
  Liver . . . 47400
  Pancreatic Duct . . . 43264, 48020
  Renal Pelvis . . . 50075, 50080, 50081, 50130
  Salivary Duct . . . 42330, 42335, 42340
  Ureter . . . 50610, 50620, 50630, 50945, 50961, 50980, 52310, 52315, 52320, 52352

Calculus of Kidney
See Calculus, Removal, Kidney

Caldwell-Luc Procedure
See Sinus/Sinuses, Maxillary; Sinusotomy
Orbital Floor Blowout Fracture . . . 21385

Caliper
Application/Removal . . . 20660

Callander Knee Disarticulation
See Disarticulation, Knee

Callosum, Corpus
See Corpus Callosum

Calmette-Guerin Bacillus Vaccine
See BCG Vaccine

Caloric Vestibular Test . . . 92533

Calprotectin
Fecal . . . 83993

Calycoplasty . . . 50405

Camey Enterocystoplasty . . . 50825

CAMP
See Cyclic AMP

Campbell Procedure . . . 27422

Campylobacter
Antibody . . . 86625

Campylobacter Pylori
See Helicobacter Pylori

Canal, Ear
See Auditory Canal

Canal, Semicircular
See Semicircular Canal

Canalith Repositioning . . . 95992

Canaloplasty . . . 69631, 69635

Candida
Antibody . . . 86628
Skin Test . . . 86485

Cannulation
Arterial . . . 36620, 36625
Arteriovenous . . . 36810, 36815
Common Bile Duct . . . 43273
Fallopian Tube . . . 58565
Pancreatic Duct . . . 43273
Sinus
  Maxillary . . . 31000
  Ostium . . . 31235
  Sphenoid . . . 31002
Thoracic Duct . . . 38794
Vas Deferens . . . 55200
Vein to Vein . . . 36800
Vertebral . . . 22513-22515
with Transcatheter Aortic Valve Replacement (TAVR/TAVI)
  Arterial and Venous . . . 33367-33369

Cannulation, Renoportal
See Anastomosis, Renoportal

Cannulization
See Cannulation; Catheterization
Arteriovenous . . . 36810-36815
Declotting . . . 36593, 36860, 36861
Dialysis Circuit . . . 36901-36903
ECMO
  See Extracorporeal Membrane Oxygenation (ECMO)
External
  Declotting . . . 36860, 36861
Vas Deferens . . . 55200
Vein to Vein . . . 36800

Canthocystostomy
See Conjunctivorhinostomy

Canthopexy
Lateral . . . 21282
Medial . . . 21280

Canthoplasty . . . 67950

Canthorrhaphy . . . 67880-67882

Canthotomy . . . 67715

Canthus
Reconstruction . . . 67950, 67961, 67966

Cap, Cervical
See Cervical Cap

Capsule
See Brachytherapy; Capsulectomy; Capsulodesis; Capsulorrhaphy; Capsulotomy; Cataract
Ankle . . . 27612, 27630
Biopsy . . . 44100
Drug Delivery Implants
  Contraceptive . . . 11976, 11981
  for Clinical Brachytherapy . . . 58346
Elbow . . . 24006, 24149
Eye . . . 66830
Finger . . . 26160, 26520

Foot . . . 28090, 28264, 28289, 28291
Hand . . . 26160, 26520
Heyman . . . 58346
Hip . . . 27036
Injection . . . 67515
Interphalangeal Joint . . . 26525, 28272
Knee . . . 27347, 27405, 27435
Leg . . . 27630
Shoulder . . . 23020
Tenon's . . . 67515
Toe . . . 28270, 28272
Wrist . . . 25320

Capsulectomy
Breast . . . 19371
Elbow . . . 24149
Foot . . . 28090
Hand . . . 26160, 26520
Hip . . . 27036
Knee . . . 27347
Metacarpophalangeal Joint . . . 26520

Capsulodesis
Metacarpophalangeal Joint . . . 26516-26518
Wrist . . . 25320

Capsulorrhaphy
Ankle . . . 27630
Anterior . . . 23450, 23455, 23460, 23462
Bankart Procedure . . . 23455
Bristow Procedure . . . 23460
Magnuson Type . . . 23450
Putti-Platt Procedure . . . 23450
Glenohumeral Joint . . . 23465, 23466
Multi-Directional Instability . . . 23466
Posterior . . . 23465
Shoulder . . . 29806
Thermal . . . 29999
Wrist . . . 25320

Capsulotomy
Breast . . . 19370
Eye . . . 66830
Foot . . . 28260-28262, 28264
Hip . . . 27036
Interphalangeal Joint . . . 28272
Knee . . . 27435
Leg . . . 27630
Metacarpophalangeal Joint . . . 26520
Metatarsophalangeal Joint . . . 28270
Shoulder . . . 23020
Toe . . . 28270-28272
Wrist . . . 25085, 25320

Captopril . . . 80416, 80417

Car Seat Testing . . . 94780, 94781

Carbamazepine
Assay . . . 80156, 80157

Carbazepin
See Carbamazepine

Carbinol
See Methanol

Carbohydrate Deficient Transferrin . . . 82373

Carbon Dioxide
Blood or Urine . . . 82374, 82803

Carboxycathepsin
See Angiotensin II

Carboxyhemoglobin . . . 82375, 82376, 88740

Carbuncle
Incision and Drainage . . . 10060, 10061

Carcinoembryonal Antigen
See Carcinoembryonic Antigen

Carcinoembryonic Antigen
Detection . . . 82378

Cardiac
Aorta
See Aorta
Arteries and Veins
See specific artery; Vein
Atrium
See Atria
Catheterization
See Cardiac Catheterization
Devices
See Cardiac Assist Devices
Diagnostic Imaging
See Cardiology, Diagnostic; Vascular Studies
Heart
See Heart
Myocardium
See Myocardium
Pacemaker
See Pacemaker, Heart
Pericardium
See Pericardium
Tumor
See Heart, Tumor
Valves
See Aortic Valve; Mitral Valve; Pulmonary Valve; Tricuspid Valve

Cardiac Arrhythmia, Tachycardia
See Tachycardia

Cardiac Assist Devices
Cardiac Contractility Modulation System
Device Evaluation . . . 0417T, 0418T
Insertion . . . 0408T-0411T
Relocation of Skin Pocket . . . 0416T
Removal . . . 0412T, 0413T
Replacement . . . 0414T
Repositioning . . . 0415T
Cardiovascular Physiologic Monitor System
Device Evaluation . . . 93290, 93297, 93299
Implantable Defibrillators
Subcutaneous Implantable Defibrillator (SICD)
Device Evaluation . . . 93260, 93261, 93287, 93295, 93296, 93644
Insertion
Electrode . . . 33202, 33203, 33271
Pulse Generator . . . 33230, 33231, 33240
System . . . 33270
Relocation of Skin Pocket . . . 33223
Removal . . . 33241, 33262, 33272
Repair, Electrode . . . 33218, 33220
Replacement, Pulse Generator . . . 33262
Repositioning, Electrode . . . 33215, 33273
Transvenous Implantable Pacing Defibrillator (ICD)
Device Evaluation . . . 93282-93284, 93287, 93289, 93295, 93296
Insertion
Electrode . . . 33202, 33203, 33216, 33217, 33224, 33225
Pulse Generator . . . 33230, 33231, 33249
System . . . 33249
Relocation of Skin Pocket . . . 33223
Removal
Electrodes . . . 33244
Pulse Generator . . . 33241, 33262-33264
Replacement, Pulse Generator 33262-33264
Repositioning, Electrode . . . 33215, 33273
Ischemia Monitoring System
Device Evaluation . . . 0528T, 0529T
Insertion or Replacement . . . 0525T-0527T
Removal . . . 0530T-0532T
Pacemaker System
Device Evaluation 93279-93281, 93286, 93288, 93293, 93294, 93296, 93724
Insertion
Electrode/Lead 33202, 33203, 33210, 33211, 33216, 33217, 33224, 33225, 33230, 33231, 33243, 33244, 33249, 93583
Pulse Generator . . . 33212, 33213, 33221
System . . . 33206-33208
Relocation of Skin Pocket . . . 33222
Removal . . . 33233-33237
Repair, Electrode . . . 33218-33220
Replacement
Catheter/Electrode . . . 33210, 33211
Pulse Generator . . . 33227-33229
Repositioning, Electrode . . . 33215, 33226
Single-to-Dual Chamber System
Upgrade . . . 33214
Pacemaker System, Leadless
Device Evaluation . . . 93279, 93286, 93288, 93294, 93296
Transcatheter Insertion . . . 33274
Transcatheter Removal . . . 33275
Transcatheter Replacement . . . 33274
Subcutaneous Cardiac Rhythm Monitor System
Device Evaluation . . . 93285, 93291, 93298, 93299
Insertion . . . 33285
Removal . . . 33286
Wireless Cardiac Stimulation System
Device Evaluation . . . 0521T, 0522T
Insertion . . . 0515T-0517T
Removal . . . 0518T
Replacement . . . 0519T, 0520T

Cardiac Atria
See Atria

Cardiac Catheterization
Combined Left and Right Heart . . . 93460, 93461
with Left Ventriculography . . . 93453, 93460, 93461
Combined Right and Retrograde Left
Congenital Cardiac Anomalies . . . 93531
Combined Right and Transseptal Left
Congenital Cardiac Anomalies . . 93532, 93533
Congenital Cardiac Anomalies . . . 93530-93533
for Angiography
Bypass Graft(s) . . . 93455, 93457, 93459, 93461
Congenital Heart . . . 93563, 93564
Coronary . . . 93454-93461, 93563, 93571
Left Atrial . . . 93565
Left Ventricular . . . 93565
Pulmonary . . . 93568
Right Atrial . . . 93566
Right Ventricular . . . 93566
for Biopsy . . . 93505
for Congenital Prosthetic Valve Implantation 33477
for Dilution Studies . . . 93561, 93562
for Flow Measurement . . . 93571, 93572
for Measurement of Oxygen/Cardiac Output 93451
for Opacification
Bypass Grafts . . . 93564
for Supravalvular Aortography . . . 93567
Imaging . . . 93452-93461, 93563-93568
Injection . . . 93454-93461, 93563-93568
Insertion
Flow Directed Catheter
Swan-Ganz . . . 93503

Index

Left Heart
by Transapical Puncture.............93462
by Transseptal Puncture through Intact Septum 93462
with Ventriculography.............93452, 93458, 93459, 93565
Pacemaker.............33210
Right Heart.............93451, 93456, 93503

Cardiac Electroversion
See Cardioversion

Cardiac Event Recorder
See Cardiac Assist Devices, Subcutaneous Cardiac Rhythm Monitor

Cardiac Magnetic Resonance Imaging (CMRI)
Morphology and Function.............75557, 75559, 75561, 75563
Stress.............75559, 75563
Velocity Flow Mapping.............75565

Cardiac Massage
Thoracotomy.............32160

Cardiac Output
Indicator Dilution.............93561, 93562

Cardiac Rehabilitation.............93797, 93798

Cardiac Transplantation
See Heart, Transplantation

Cardiectomy
Donor.............33930, 33940

Cardioassist.............92970, 92971

Cardiography
Acoustic.............93799
Arterial Pressure Waveform Analysis.............93050
Magnetocardiography.............0541T, 0542T

Cardiolipin Antibody.............86147

Cardiology
Diagnostic
Acoustic Cardiography.............93799
Arrhythmia Induction.............93618-93624, 93640, 93641, 93653-93656
Arterial Pressure Waveform Analysis.............93050
Atrial Electrogram.............93615, 93616
Esophageal Recording.............93615, 93616
Bioimpedance-derived Analysis.............93701
Echocardiography
See Echocardiography
Electrocardiography
See Electrocardiography
Ergonovine Provocation Test.............93024
External Heart Rate Data Recording for Nocturnal Epilepsy Seizure.............0381T-0386T
Intracardiac Pacing and Mapping
3-D Mapping.............93613, 93654
Follow-up Study.............93624
Localization.............93631
Slow Conduction Zone.............93631
Stimulation and Pacing.............93623
Tachycardia Sites.............93631
Intracardiac Pacing and Recording
Arrhythmia Induction.............93618-93624, 93653, 93654, 93656
Bundle of His.............93600, 93619, 93620, 93653, 93654, 93656
Comprehensive.............93619-93622
Intra-Atrial.............93602, 93610, 93616, 93656
Left Ventricular.............93654
Right Ventricular.............93603, 93653, 93656
Tachycardia Sites.............93609
Ventricular.............93612
Intravascular Ultrasound.............92978, 92979
Perfusion Imaging.............78451-78454
See Nuclear Medicine
Stress Tests
Cardiovascular.............93015-93018
Drug Induced.............93024
Multiple Gated Acquisition (MUGA).............78473
Temperature Gradient Studies.............93740
Tilt Table Evaluation.............93660
Venous Pressure Determination.............93784, 93786, 93788, 93790
Therapeutic
Ablation.............93650, 93653-93656
Cardioassist.............92970, 92971
Cardioversion.............92960, 92961
Intravascular Ultrasound.............92978, 92979
Pacing.............92953
Rehabilitation.............93668, 93797, 93798
Thrombolysis.............92975-92977
Thrombolysis, Coronary.............92977
Valvuloplasty.............92986-92990

Cardiomyotomy
See Esophagomyotomy

Cardioplasty.............43320

Cardiopulmonary Bypass
See Heart; Lung, Transplantation
Establishment.............34714, 34716, 34833
with Transcatheter Aortic Valve Replacement (TAVR/TAVI).............33367, 33368, 33369

Cardiopulmonary Resuscitation.............92950

Cardiotomy.............33310-33315

Cardiovascular Stress Test
See Exercise Stress Tests

Cardioversion.............92960, 92961

Care
Custodial
See Nursing Facility Services
Intensive
See Intensive Care
Neonatal Intensive
See Intensive Care, Neonatal
Self
See Self Care

Care Plan Oversight Services
See Physician Services

Carinal Reconstruction
See Trachea, Reconstruction

Carneous Mole
See Abortion

Carnitine.............82379

Carotene.............82380

Caroticum, Glomus
See Carotid Body

Carotid Artery
See Artery, Carotid

Carotid Body
Tumor
Excision.............60600-60605

Carpal Bone
See Wrist
Arthroplasty
with Implant.............25443
Cyst
Excision.............25130-25136
Dislocation
Closed Treatment.............25690
Open Treatment.............25695
Excision.............25210, 25215
Partial.............25145
Fracture
Closed Treatment.............25622, 25630, 25635, 25645
Open Treatment.............25628, 25645
with Manipulation.............25624, 25635
without Manipulation.............25630
Incision and Drainage.............26034
Insertion
Vascular Pedicle.............25430
Ligament Release.............29848
Osteoplasty
Shortening.............25394
Prosthetic Placement.............25443
Repair
Nonunion.............25431, 25440
with Fixation.............25628
with Styloidectomy.............25440
Scaphoid (Navicular)
Fracture.............25622, 25624, 25628
Nonunion Repair.............25440
Sequestrectomy.............25145
Tumor
Excision.............25130, 25135, 25136
Tunnel
See Carpal Tunnel

Carpal Tunnel
Injection
Therapeutic.............20526
Median Nerve Neuroplasty.............64721

Carpal Tunnel Syndrome
Decompression.............64721

Carpals
Incision and Drainage.............25035

Carpectomy.............25210, 25215

Carpometacarpal Joint
Arthrodesis.............25800
Finger.............26843, 26844
Thumb.............26841, 26842
Arthrotomy.............26070
Biopsy.............26100
Dislocation
Closed Treatment.............26670
with Manipulation.............26675, 26676
Open Treatment.............26685, 26686
Drainage.............26070
Exploration.............26070
Fusion
Hand.............26843, 26844
Thumb.............26841, 26842
Magnetic Resonance Imaging.............73221-73225
Removal
Foreign Body.............26070
Repair.............25447
Synovectomy.............26130

Cartilage Graft
Costochondral.............20910
Ear.............21235
for Mandibular Condyle Reconstruction.............21247
for Zygomatic Arch Reconstruction.............21255
Harvesting.............20910, 20912
Nasal Septum.............20912
Rib.............21230

Index

Cartilage, Arytenoid
See Arytenoid

Cartilage, Ear
See Ear Cartilage

Cartilaginous Exostoses
See Exostosis

Case Management Services
On-line . . . 98969, 99444
Team Conferences . . . 99366-99368
Telephone Calls . . . 98966-98968, 99441-99443

Cast
See Brace; Splint
Below Knee to Toes . . . 29405
Elbow to Finger . . . 29075
Finger . . . 29086
Hand and Lower Forearm . . . 29085
Hip Spica
- 1 and one-half . . . 29325
- 1 Leg . . . 29305
- Both Legs . . . 29325

Leg . . . 29445, 29450
Removal . . . 29700, 29705, 29710
Repair . . . 29720
Shoulder Spica . . . 29055
Shoulder to Hand . . . 29065
Shoulder to Hip . . . 29035
- with Head . . . 29040
- with 1 Thigh . . . 29044
- with Both Thighs . . . 29046

Thigh to Ankle . . . 29365
Thigh to Toes . . . 29345, 29355
Type
Ambulatory . . . 29355, 29425, 29440
- Club Foot . . . 29450, 29750
- Cylinder . . . 29365
- Figure-of-eight . . . 29049
- Gauntlet . . . 29085, 29750
- Halo
  - Body Cast . . . 29000
  - Cranial . . . 20661
  - for Thin Skull Osteology . . . 20664
  - Femur . . . 20663
  - Maxillofacial . . . 21100
  - Pelvic . . . 20662
  - Removal . . . 20665
- Long Arm . . . 29065
- Long Leg . . . 29358, 29450
- Minerva . . . 29040
- Patella Tendon Bearing (PTB) . . . 29435
- Rigid Total Contact . . . 29445
- Risser Jacket
  - Body . . . 29010
  - with Head . . . 29015
- Short Arm . . . 29075
- Short Leg . . . 29405, 29450
- Spica . . . 29055, 29305, 29720
- Velpeau . . . 29058
- Walker . . . 29355, 29425, 29440

Wedging . . . 29740, 29750
Windowing . . . 29730

Casting
Unlisted Services and Procedures . . . 29799

Castration
See Orchiectomy

Castration, Female
See Oophorectomy

CAT Scan
See CT Scan

Cataract
Discission . . . 66820, 66821
Excision . . . 66830
- Dilated Fundus Evaluation . . . 2020F

Extraction/Removal
- Extracapsular . . . 66982, 66984
- Intracapsular (ICCE) . . . 66983

Intraoperative Visual Axis Identification
- Patient Fixation . . . 0514T
- Presurgical Measurement and Calculations . . . 3073F

Incision . . . 66820, 66821
- Laser . . . 66821
- Stab Incision . . . 66820

Catecholamines . . . 80424, 82382-82384
Blood . . . 82383
Panel for Pheochromocytoma . . . 80424
Urine . . . 82382

Cathepsin-D . . . 82387

Catheter
See Cannulation; Catheterization; Venipuncture
Aspiration
- Nasotracheal . . . 31720
- Tracheobronchial . . . 31725

Balloon
- *See* Angioplasty, Transluminal, Balloon

Biopsy . . . 37200
Bladder . . . 51701-51703
- Irrigation . . . 51700

Blood Specimen Collection . . . 36592, 37799
Conversion
- Biliary Drainage
  - External to Internal-External . . . 47535
- Nephrostomy to Nephroureteral . . . 50434

Declotting . . . 36593, 36861
Drainage
- Biliary
  - Conversion . . . 47535
  - Exchange . . . 47536
  - Placement . . . 47533, 47534
  - Removal . . . 47537
- Peritoneal . . . 49406, 49407
- Pleural . . . 32556, 32557
- Retroperitoneal . . . 49406, 49407
- Spinal . . . 62272
- Ureteral . . . 50693
- Ventricular . . . 62162, 62164
- Visceral . . . 49405

Electrode Array . . . 63650
Embolization . . . 61624, 61626
- Peritoneal . . . 49423

Exchange
- Nephrostomy . . . 50435
- with Biliary Stent Placement . . . 47538-47540

for Cystourethroscopy . . . 52320-52356
for Embolectomy . . . 34001, 34051, 34101-34111, 34151, 34201, 34203
for Enteral Alimentation . . . 44015
for Placement
- Flow Directed . . . 93503
- Radiation Source . . . 61770
- Stent . . . 33621, 61635

for Thrombectomy . . . 34001, 34051, 34101-34111, 34151, 34201, 34203, 34401, 34421, 34451
for Infusion
- Brachial Plexus . . . 64416
- Femoral Nerve . . . 64448
- Lumbar Plexus . . . 64449
- Saline . . . 58340
- Sciatic Nerve . . . 64446
- Vertebral . . . 62324-62327

for Instillation
- Fibrinolysis . . . 32561, 32562
- Pleurodesis . . . 32560

Home Visit for Care . . . 99507
Intraperitoneal, Tunneled
- Insertion
  - Laparoscopic . . . 49324
  - Open . . . 49421
  - Percutaneous . . . 49418, 49419

Obstruction Clearance . . . 36595, 36596
Occlusion . . . 61624, 61626
Placement
- *See* Catheterization

Removal
- Central Venous . . . 36589
- Foreign Body . . . 37197
- Peritoneal . . . 49422
- Spinal Cord . . . 62355
- with Biliary Stent Placement . . . 47538-47540

Repair
- Central Venous . . . 36575
- Intraperitoneal . . . 49325

Replacement
- Central Venous . . . 36580, 36581, 36584
- Nephroureteral, Externally Accessible . . 50387
- Shunt System . . . 62230
- Subarachnoid . . . 62194
- Subdural . . . 62194
- Ventricular . . . 62225

Repositioning
- Central Venous . . . 36597

Transcatheter Therapy
- Arterial, for Chemotherapy . . . 36640
- Arterial, Intracranial . . . 61650, 61651
- Epidural or Subarachnoid . . . 62320-62327
- Newborn . . . 36660
- Thrombolysis . . . 37211-37214

Ureteral
- Manometric Studies . . . 50396, 50686
- Ureterography . . . 50684
- Ureteropyelography . . . 50684

Catheterization
See Catheter
Abdomen . . . 49421
Abdominal Artery . . . 36245-36248
Aorta . . . 36160, 36200
Arterial System . . . 36215, 36245-36248
- Cutdown . . . 36625
- Intracatheter/Needle . . . 36100-36140
- Percutaneous . . . 36620

Bile Duct
- Percutaneous
  - Conversion . . . 47535
  - Exchange . . . 47536
  - Placement . . . 47533, 47534
  - Removal . . . 47537

Bladder . . . 51045, 51102, 51702, 51703
Brachiocephalic Artery . . . 36215-36218
Brain . . . 61210
- Replacement . . . 62160, 62194, 62225

Breast
- for Interstitial Radioelement Application . . . 19296-19298, 20555, 41019

Bronchus
- for Intracavitary Radioelement Application . . . 31643

Cardiac
- *See* Cardiac Catheterization

Carotid Artery . . . 36100, 36221-36224, 36227, 36228
Central Venous
- *See* Central Venous Catheter Placement

Cerebral Artery . . . 36215

Cholecystostomy 47490
Coronary Artery 93455
Cystourethroscopy
Ejaculatory Duct 52010
Ureteral 52005
Dialysis 36901-36903, 49418, 49419, 49421
Electrode Array 63650
Extremity Artery 36140
Fallopian Tube 58345, 74742
Gastrointestinal 43241
Hepatic Vein 37182, 37183
Innominate Artery 36222, 36223, 36225
Intracardiac
Ablation 93650, 93653-93657
Intracranial Neuroendoscopic Ventricular ... 62160
Intraperitoneal Tunneled 49324, 49421
Jejunum
for Enteral 44015
Kidney
Percutaneous
for Nephrostomy 50432
Nephroureteral 50433
Legs 36245-36248
Nasotracheal 31720
Newborn
Umbilical Vein 36510
Pelvic Artery 36245-36248
Peripheral 36568-36573
Pleural Cavity 32550-32552
Portal Vein 36481, 37182, 37183
Pulmonary Artery 36013-36015
Radioelement Application 19296, 19297, 20555, 31643, 55875
Genitalia 55920
Head 41019
Neck 41019
Pelvic Organs 55920
Prostate 55875
Renal Artery 36251-36254
Salivary Duct 42660
Selective
See Selective Catheterization
Skull 61107
Spinal Cord 62350, 62351
Subclavian Artery 36225
Thoracic Artery 36215-36218
Tracheobronchial 31725
Umbilical Artery 36660
Umbilical Vein 36510
Ureter
Endoscopic 50553, 50572, 50953, 50972, 52005
Injection 50684
Manometric Studies 50396, 50686
via Kidney 50693
Uterus
Radiology 58340
Vena Cava 36010
Venous
Central Line
See Central Venous Catheter Placement
First Order 36011
for Organ Blood Sampling 36500
Intracatheter/Needle 36000
Second Order 36012
Umbilical Vein 36510
Vertebral Artery 36100, 36221, 36225, 36226, 36228
Ventricular 61020-61026, 61210-61215, 62160-62162, 62164, 62225

Cauda Equina
See Spinal Cord
Decompression
Cervical 63001, 63015, 63045, 63048
Lumbar .. 63005, 63012, 63017, 63087, 63088, 63091-63091, 63047, 63048, 63056, 63057
Sacral 63011, 63091-63091
Thoracic 63003, 63016, 63087, 63088, 63091-63091, 63046, 63048, 63055, 63057
Exploration
Cervical 63001, 63015
Thoracic 63003, 63016
Lumbar 63005, 63012, 63017
Sacral 63011

Cauterization
Anus
Control of Bleeding 46614
Fissure 46940, 46942
Hemorrhoid Destruction 46930
Tumor Removal 46610, 46612
Cervix 57522
Cryocautery 57511
Electro or Thermal 57510
Laser Ablation 57513
Chemical
Corneal Epithelium 65435, 65436
Granulation Tissue 17250
Colon
Control of Bleeding 45334, 45382
Lesion Removal 45384
Polyp Removal 45384
Tumor Removal 45333, 45384
Cornea 65450
Ectropion Repair 67915
Entropion Repair 67922
Esophagus
Tumor Removal 43216, 43250
Everted Punctum 68705
Intrarenal Stricture 52343, 52346
Iris 66155
Lacrimal Punctum Closure 68760
Nasopharyngeal Hemorrhage 42970
Nose
Hemorrhage 30901, 30903, 30905, 30906
Prostate Resection 52601
Rectum
Control of Bleeding 45317
Tumor Removal 45308, 45315
Skin Lesion 11055-11057, 17000-17004
Skin Tags 11200, 11201
Small Intestine
Control of Bleeding 44366, 44378, 44391
Tumor Removal 44365, 44392
Turbinate Mucosa
Electrocautery 30801, 30802
Ureteral Stricture 52341, 52344
Ureteropelvic Junction Stricture 52342, 52345
Urethral Caruncle 53265

Cavernitides, Fibrous
See Peyronie Disease

Cavernosography
Corpora 54230

Cavernosometry 54231

Cavities, Pleural
See Pleural Cavity

Cavus Foot Correction 28309

CBC
See Blood Cell Count; Complete Blood Count (CBC)

CCL4
See Carbon Tetrachloride

CCU Visit
See Critical Care Services

CD142 Antigens
See Thromboplastin

CD143 Antigens
See Angiotensin Converting Enzyme (ACE)

CD4 86360

CD8 86360

CEA
See Carcinoembryonic Antigen

Cecil Repair
See Urethroplasty

Cecostomy
Laparoscopic 44188
Obstructive Material Removal 49460
Skin Level 44320
Tube
Insertion
Open 44300
Percutaneous 49442
Radiological Evaluation 49465
Replacement 49450
with Colectomy 44141

Celiac Plexus
Destruction 64680
Injection
Anesthetic 64530
Neurolytic 64680

Celiac Trunk Artery
See Artery, Celiac

Celioscopy
See Endoscopy, Peritoneum

Celiotomy 49000
Abdomen
for Staging 49220

Cell Count
B Cells 86355
Bacterial Colony 87086
CD4 .... 86360, 86361
CD8 86360
CD34 86367
Chromosome Analysis
See Chromosome Analysis
Body Fluid 86152, 86153
Other than Blood 89050, 89051
Natural Killer (NK) 86357
Sperm 89310, 89320, 89322
Stem 86367
T Cells 86359-86361

Cell, Blood
See Blood Cell

Cell, Islet
See Islet Cell

Cell, Mother
See Stem Cell

Cell-Stimulating Hormone, Interstitial
See Luteinizing Hormone (LH)

Cellobiase
See Beta Glucosidase

Cellular Inclusion
See Inclusion Bodies

Central Shunt 33764

Central Venous Catheter Placement
Insertion
  Central
    Non-tunneled 36555, 36556
    Tunneled with Port 36560, 36561, 36566
    Tunneled with Pump 36563
    Tunneled without Port or Pump 36557, 36558, 36565
  Peripheral
    with Port 36570, 36571
    without Port or Pump 36568, 36569
Repair
  with Port or Pump 36576
  without Port or Pump 36575
Replacement
  Catheter Only 36578
  Complete
    Central 36580-36583
    Peripheral 36584, 36585
Repositioning 36597

Central Venous Catheter Removal 36589

Cephalic Version
of Fetus
  Anesthesia 01958
  External 59412

Cephalocele
See Encephalocele

Cephalogram, Orthodontic
See Orthodontic Cephalogram

Cerclage
Cervix 57700
  Abdominal 59325
  Removal under Anesthesia 59871
  Vaginal 59320
Femoral Fracture 27244, 27245, 27506, 27507
Humeral Shaft Fracture 24515, 24516
Tibial Shaft Fracture 27758, 27759

Cerebellopontine Angle Tumor
See Brain, Tumor, Excision; Brainstem; Mesencephalon; Skull Base Surgery

Cerebral Cortex Decortication
See Decortication

Cerebral Death
See Brain Death

Cerebral Hernia
See Encephalocele

Cerebral Perfusion Analysis
CT Scan 0042T

Cerebral Ventriculographies
See Ventriculography

Cerebral Vessels
Anastomosis 61711
Aneurysm Surgery
  Carotid Artery Occlusion 61705, 61708, 61710
  Cervical Approach 61703
  Intracranial Approach 61697, 61698, 61700, 61702
Angioplasty 61630
Arteriovenous Malformation Surgery
  Dural 61690, 61692
  Fistula 61705
  Infratentorial 61684, 61686
  Supratentorial 61680-61682
Dilation
  Intracranial Vasospasm 61640-61642
Occlusion 61623
Placement
  Stent
    Intravascular 61635
Thrombolysis 37195

Cerebrose
See Galactose

Cerebrospinal Fluid
Drainage
  Spinal Puncture 62272
Flow Imaging
  Cisternography 78630
  Leakage Detection and Localization 78650
  Shunt Evaluation 78645
  Tomographic (SPECT) 78647
  Ventriculography 78635
Leak
  See Cerebrospinal Fluid Leak
Shunt
  See Cerebrospinal Fluid Shunt
Test
  Cell Count 89050
  Immunoelectrophoresis 86325
  Myelin Basic Protein 83873
  Protein, Total 84157

Cerebrospinal Fluid Leak
Repair
  Craniotomy 62100
  Spinal Cord 63707-63709
  with Nasal/Sinus Endoscopy 31290, 31291
  with Skull Base Surgery 61618, 61619

Cerebrospinal Fluid Shunt
Creation 62190, 62192, 62220, 62223
  Lumbar 63740, 63741
Irrigation 62194, 62225
Removal 62256, 62258, 63746
Replacement 62160, 62258, 63744
  Catheter 62194, 62225, 62230
  Valve 62230
Reprogramming 62252
Torkildsen Operation 62180
Ventriculocisternostomy 62180, 62200, 62201

Ceruloplasmin 82390

Cerumen
Removal
  with Instrumentation 69210
  with Irrigation/Lavage 69209

Cervical Cap 57170

Cervical Lymphadenectomy 38720-38724

Cervical Mucus Penetration Test 89330

Cervical Plexus
Injection
  Anesthetic 64413

Cervical Pregnancy 59140

Cervical Puncture 61050-61055

Cervical Smears
Cytopathology
  Automated Screen 88174
  Hormone Evaluation 88155
  Manual Screen 88150, 88153, 88164, 88165
  Physician Interpretation 88141
  Partially Automated Screen 88147, 88148, 88152, 88166, 88167, 88175
Pap
  Any Reporting System 88174, 88175
  Bethesda System 88164-88167
  Non-Bethesda 88150, 88152, 88153

Cervical Spine
See Vertebra, Cervical
Chemodenervation, Muscles 64615

Cervical Sympathectomy
See Sympathectomy, Cervical

Cervicectomy
Amputation of Cervix 57530
Pelvic Exenteration 45126, 58240

Cervicocerebral Arch
Angiography
  See Angiography, Cervicocerebral Arch

Cervicoplasty 15819

Cervicothoracic Ganglia
See Stellate Ganglion

Cervix
See Cytopathology
Amputation
  Total 57530
Biopsy 57500, 57520
  Colposcopy 57454, 57455, 57460
Cauterization
  Cryocautery 57511
  Electro or Thermal 57510
  Laser Ablation 57513
Cerclage 57700
  Abdominal 59325
  Removal under Anesthesia 59871
  Vaginal 59320
Colposcopy 57452, 57454-57456, 57460, 57461
Conization 57461, 57520, 57522
Curettage
  Endocervical 57454, 57456, 57505
Dilation
  Canal 57800
  Stump 57558
Dilation and Curettage 57520, 57558
Ectopic Pregnancy 59140
Excision
  Radical 57531
  Stump
    Abdominal Approach 57540, 57545
    Vaginal Approach 57550, 57555, 57556
  Total 57530
Exploration
  Endoscopy 57452
Insertion
  Dilator 59200
  Laminaria 59200
  Prostaglandin 59200
Repair
  Cerclage 57700
    Abdominal 59325
    Suture 57720
    Vaginal 59320
Unlisted Nonobstetrical Services and Procedures 58999

Cesarean Delivery
Antepartum Care 59610, 59618
Delivery Only 59514
Delivery with Postpartum Care 59515
Routine Care 59510
Previous Cesarean Delivery
  Vaginal Delivery
    Delivery Only 59612
    Delivery with Postpartum Care 59614
    Routine Care 59610
  Unsuccessful Attempted Vaginal Delivery
    Cesarean Delivery Only 59620

Index

Delivery with Postpartum Care 59622
Routine Care 59618
with Tubal Ligation during Delivery 58611
with Hysterectomy 59525

Chalazion
Excision 67800
Multiple
Different Lids 67805
Same Lid 67801
Single 67800
under Anesthesia 67808

Challenge Tests
Bronchial Inhalation 95070, 95071
Cholinesterase Inhibitor 95857
Ingestion 95076, 95079

Chambers Procedure 28300

Change
Catheter
Percutaneous Drainage, with Contrast Monitoring 75984
Dressing, under Anesthesia 15852
Fetal Position
by Manipulation 59412
Stent
Bile or Pancreatic Duct 43276
Ureteral 50688
Tube
Percutaneous, with Contrast Monitoring 75984
Tracheotomy 31502
Ureterostomy 50688

Change of, Dressing
See Dressings, Change

CHCT
See Caffeine, Halothane Contracture Test (CHCT)

Cheek
Bone
Excision 21030, 21034
Fracture
Closed Treatment with Manipulation 21355
Open Treatment 21360-21366
Reconstruction 21270
Fascia Graft 15840
Muscle Graft 15841-15845
Muscle Transfer 15845
Rhytidectomy 15828
Skin Graft 15240, 15241
Tissue Transfer
Adjacent 14040, 14041
Flap 15574, 15620
Wound Repair 13131-13133

Cheilectomy
Metatarsophalangeal Joint Release 28289, 28291

Cheiloplasty
See Lip, Repair

Cheiloschisis
See Cleft Lip

Cheilotomy
See Incision, Lip

Chemical Cauterization
Corneal Epithelium 65435, 65436
Granulation Tissue 17250

Chemical Exfoliation 17360

Chemical Peel 15788-15793

Chemiluminescent Assay 82397

Chemistry Tests
See Pathology and Laboratory, Chemistry
Unlisted Chemistry Procedure 84999

Chemocauterization
Corneal Epithelium 65435
with Chelating Agent 65436

Chemodenervation
Anal Sphincter 46505
Bladder 52287
Eccrine Glands
Axillae 64650
Other Area 64653
Extraocular Muscle 67345
Extremity Muscle 64642-64645
Facial Muscle 64612, 64615
Guidance
Electrical Stimulation 95873
Needle Electromyography 64617, 95874
Larynx 64617
Neck Muscle 64615, 64616
Salivary Glands 64611
Trunk Muscle 64646, 64647

Chemonucleolysis 62292

Chemosurgery
Destruction of Benign Lesions 17110, 17111
Skin Lesion 17000-17004, 17110, 17111, 17270, 17280

Chemotaxis Assay 86155

Chemotherapy
Bladder Instillation 51720
Brain 61517
CNS 61517, 96450
Extracorporeal Circulation
Extremity 36823
Home Infusion Procedures 99601, 99602
Intra-Arterial
Cannulation 36823
Catheterization 36640
Infusion 96422, 96423, 96425
Insertion Infusion Pump 36260
Push 96420
Intralesional 96405, 96406
Intramuscular 96401, 96402
Intravenous
Infusion 96413, 96415, 96416, 96417
Infusion Pump 96416
Push 96409, 96411
Kidney Instillation 50391
Peritoneal Cavity 96446
Catheterization 49418
Pleural Cavity 96440
Pump Services
Implantable 96522
Maintenance 95990, 95991
Portable 96521
Reservoir Filling 96542
Subcutaneous 96401, 96402
Unlisted Procedure 96549
Ureteral Instillation 50391
Venous Cannulation 36823

Chest
See also Mediastinum; Thorax
Artery
Ligation 37616
Diagnostic Imaging
Angiography 71275
CT Angiography 71275
CT Scan 71250, 71260, 71270
Magnetic Resonance Angiography 71555
Magnetic Resonance Imaging (MRI) 71550-71552
PET Imaging 78811, 78814
Ultrasound 76604
X ray
See X ray, Chest
Exploration
Postoperative
Hemorrhage 35820
Infection 35820
Thrombosis 35820
Penetrating Wound 20101
Exit Site, Intraperitoneal Cannula/Catheter 49435
Repair
Blood Vessel 35211, 35216
with Other Graft 35271-35276
with Vein Graft 35241, 35246
Tube
See Thoracostomy
Tumor
See Chest Wall

Chest Cavity
Bypass Graft 35905
Thoracoscopy
See Thoracoscopy

Chest Wall
See Pulmonology, Therapeutic
Debridement 11044, 11047
Manipulation 94667, 94668
Mechanical Oscillation 94669
Reconstruction 49904
with Lung Tumor Resection 32504
Trauma 32820
Repair 32905
Closure 32810
Fistula 32906
Lung Hernia 32800
Resection 32503
Tumor
Ablation
Cryoablation 32994
Radiofrequency 32998
Excision 19260, 19271, 19272
Unlisted Services and Procedures 32999

Chest, Funnel
See Pectus Excavatum

Chevron Procedure 28296

Chiari Osteotomy of the Pelvis
See Osteotomy, Pelvis

Chicken Pox Vaccine
Varicella Virus (VAR) 90716

Child Procedure
Pancreatectomy 48146

Chimerism 81267, 81268

Chin
Cartilage Graft 21230
Repair
Augmentation 21120
Osteotomy 21121-21123
Rhytidectomy 15828
Skin Graft 15240, 15241
Tissue Transfer
Adjacent 14040, 14041
Flap 15574, 15620
Wound Repair 13131-13133

Chinidin
See Quinidine

Chiropractic Manipulation
See Manipulation, Chiropractic

Chiropractic Treatment
Spinal
Extraspinal 98940-98943

Chlamydia
Antibody 86631, 86632
Antigen Detection
Amplified Nucleic Acid Probe . . . 87486, 87491
Direct Nucleic Acid Probe 87485, 87490
Direct Optical 87810
Immunoassay 87320
Immunofluorescence 87270
Nucleic Acid Quantification 87487, 87492
Culture 87110

Chloramphenicol 82415

Chloride
Blood 82435
Other Source 82438
Panels
Basic Metabolic 80047, 80048
Comprehensive Metabolic 80053
Electrolyte 80051
Renal Function 80069
Spinal Fluid 82438
Urine 82436

Chloride, Methylene
See Dichloromethane

Chlorinated Hydrocarbons 82441

Chlorohydrocarbon
See Chlorinated Hydrocarbons

Choanal Atresia
Repair 30540-30545

Cholangiography
Injection 47531, 47532
Intraoperative 74300, 74301
Postoperative 47531
Repair
with Bile Duct Exploration 47700
with Cholecystectomy . . . 47563, 47605, 47620
Transhepatic
Laparoscopically Guided 47579
with Conversion of Drainage Catheter 47535
with Exchange of Drainage Catheter 47536
with Placement of Access to Small Bowel . . . 47541
with Placement of Drainage Catheter 47533, 47534
with Placement of Stent 47538-47540
with Removal of Drainage Catheter 47537

Cholangiopancreatography
See Bile Duct; Pancreatic Duct
Endoscopic Retrograde Cholangiopancreatography (ERCP)
with Ablation
Lesion 43278
Polyp 43278
Tumor 43278
with Biopsy 43261
with Collection of Specimen(s) 43260
with Exchange
Stent 43276
with Optical Endomicroscopy 0397T
with Papillotomy 43262
with Placement
Stent 43274
with Pressure Measurement Sphincter of Oddi 43263
with Removal
Foreign Body 43275
Stent 43275, 43276
with Removal/Destruction of Calculus 43264, 43265
with Sphincterotomy 43262, 43274, 43276, 43277
with Transendoscopic Balloon Dilation . . 43277
Intraoperative 74300, 74301
Postoperative 47531

Cholangiostomy
See Hepaticostomy

Cholangiotomy
See Hepaticostomy

Cholecalciferol
See Vitamin, D, Blood Serum Level, 25 hydroxy

Cholecystectomy
Any Method
with Cholangiography . . . 47563, 47605, 47620
with Choledochoenterostomy 47612
with Exploration Common Duct . . 47564, 47610
Donor Liver 47143
Excision 47600-47620
Laparoscopic 47562-47564

Cholecystenterostomy
Direct 47720
with Gastroenterostomy 47721, 47741
Laparoscopic 47570
Roux-en-Y 47740, 47741

Cholecystography 47490, 74290

Cholecystostomy
Open 47480
Percutaneous 47490
with Peripancreatic Drain Placement 48000

Cholecystotomy
Open 47480
with Choledochostomy 47420
with Choledochotomy 47420

Choledochoplasty
See Bile Duct, Repair

Choledochoscopy
Biliary Endoscopy 47550

Choledochostomy
Biliary Tract 47420, 47425

Choledochotomy
Biliary Tract 47420, 47425

Choledochus, Cyst
See Cyst, Choledochal

Cholera Vaccine
Live, for Oral Use 90625

Cholesterol
Measurement
HDL 83718
LDL 83721
Panel
Lipid 80061
Serum 82465
VLDL 83719

Choline Esterase I
See Acetylcholinesterase

Choline Esterase II
See Cholinesterase

Cholinesterase
Blood 82480, 82482

Cholylglycine
Blood 82240

Chondroitin Sulfate
Detection 82485

Chondromalacia Patella
Repair 27418

Chondropathia Patellae
See Chondromalacia Patella

Chopart Procedure 28800-28805
See Amputation, Foot; Radical Resection; Replantation

Chordotomies
See Cordotomy

Choriogonadotropin
See Chorionic Gonadotropin

Choriomeningitides, Lymphocytic
See Lymphocytic Choriomeningitis

Chorionic Gonadotropin 80414, 84702, 84703
Stimulation Panel 80414, 80415

Chorionic Growth Hormone
See Lactogen, Human Placental

Chorionic Tumor
See Hydatidiform Mole

Chorionic Villi
See Biopsy, Chorionic Villus

Chorionic Villus
Biopsy 59015

Choroid
Aspiration 67015
Lesion 67220, 67221, 67225
Neovascularization 67043

Choroid Plexus
Excision 61544

Christmas Factor 85250

Chromaffinoma, Medullary
See Pheochromocytoma

Chromatin, Sex
See Barr Bodies

Chromatography
Column
See specific analyte in Drug Assay; Pathology and Laboratory, Chemistry
Unspecified Non-Drug Analyte(s) 82542
Column/Mass Spectrometry
See specific analyte in Drug Assay; Pathology and Laboratory, Chemistry
Unspecified Non-Drug Analyte(s) 82542
Drug Screen 80305-80307, 80320-80377
Gas Liquid or HPLC
See specific analyte in Pathology and Laboratory, Chemistry
Typing 87143
Unspecified Non-Drug Analyte(s) 82542
Hemoglobin 83021, 83036
Paper
See specific analyte in Pathology and Laboratory, Chemistry
Sugars 84375
Unlisted Chemistry Procedure 84999

Thin-Layer
See specific analyte in Pathology and Laboratory, Chemistry
Unlisted Chemistry Procedure 84999

Chromium 82495

Chromogenic Substrate Assay 85130

Chromosome Analysis
See Amniocentesis
Added Study 88280, 88283, 88285, 88289
Amniotic Fluid 88267, 88269
Culture 88235
Biopsy Culture
Tissue 88233
Bone Marrow Culture 88237
Breakage Syndromes 88245, 88248, 88249
Ataxia Telangiectasia 88248
Clastogen Stress 88249
Fanconi Anemia 88248
Fragile-X 88248
Chorionic Villus 88267
5 Cells 88261
15-20 Cells 88262
20-25 Cells 88264
45 Cells 88263
Culture 88235
Cytogenomic Constitutional Microarray 81228, 81229
In Situ Hybridization 88272, 88273
Lymphocyte Culture 88230
Molecular Pathology, Level 5 81404
Pregnancy Associated Plasma Protein-A 84163
Tissue Culture
Amniotic Fluid Cells 88325
Blood Cells 88237
Bone Marrow Cells 88237
Chorionic Villus Cells 88235
Skin 88233
Tumor 88239
Unlisted Cytogenic Study 88299

Chromotubation
Oviduct 58350

Chronic Erection
See Priapism

Chronic Interstitial Cystitides
See Cystitis, Interstitial

Ciliary Body
Cyst
Destruction 66770
Excision 66500, 66505
Destruction
Cryotherapy 66720
Cyclodialysis 66740
Cyclophotocoagulation 66710, 66711
Diathermy 66700
Endoscopic 66711
Lesion
Destruction 66770
Excision 66500, 66505
Repair 66680
Suture 66682

Cimino Type Procedure 36821

Cinefluorographies
See Cineradiography

Cineplasty
Arm, Lower or Upper 24940

Cineradiography
Esophagus 74230
Pharynx 70371, 74230
Site Unspecified 76120, 76125
Speech Evaluation 70371
Swallowing Evaluation 74230

Circulation Assist
See Ventricular Assist Device (VAD)
Aortic 33967, 33970
Balloon 33967, 33970

Circulation, Extracorporeal
See Extracorporeal Circulation

Circulatory Assist
See Circulation Assist

Circumcision
Repair
Adhesions 54162
Incomplete 54163
Surgical Excision 54161
Neonate 54150, 54160

Cisternal Puncture 61050-61055

Cisternography
Cerebrospinal Fluid Flow Imaging 78630
Study 70015

Citrate
Blood or Urine 82507

Clagett Procedure
Chest Wall Closure 32810

Clavicle
Arthrocentesis
Acromioclavicular Joint 20605, 20606
Arthrotomy
Acromioclavicular Joint 23044, 23101
Sternoclavicular Joint . . . 23044, 23101, 23106
Bone Graft 23485
Craterization 23180
Cyst
Excision 23140
with Graft 23145, 23146
Diaphysectomy 23180
Dislocation
Acromioclavicular Joint
Closed Treatment 23540, 23545
Open Treatment 23550, 23552
Sternoclavicular Joint
Closed Treatment 23520, 23525
Open Treatment 23530, 23532
without Manipulation 23540
Excision 23170
Partial 23120, 23180
Total 23125
Fracture
Closed Treatment
with Manipulation 23505
without Manipulation 23500
Open Treatment 23515
Pinning, Wiring 23490
Prophylactic Treatment 23490
Repair
Osteotomy 23480
Malunion/Nonunion 23485
Saucerization 23180
Sequestrectomy 23170
Tumor
Excision 23140, 23145, 23146, 23200
with Graft 23145, 23146
Radical Resection 23200
X ray 73000

Clavicula
See Clavicle

Claviculectomy
Arthroscopic 29824
Open
Partial 23120
Total 23125

Claw Finger Repair 26499

Cleft Cyst, Branchial
See Branchial Cleft, Cyst

Cleft Foot
Reconstruction 28360

Cleft Hand
Repair 26580

Cleft Lip
Repair
Primary 40700-40702
Secondary 40720
with Pedicle Flap 40761
Rhinoplasty 30460-30462

Cleft Palate
Repair 42200-42225
Rhinoplasty 30460-30462

Cleft, Branchial
See Branchial Cleft

Clinical Act of Insertion
See Insertion

Clinical Chemistry Test
See Pathology and Laboratory, Chemistry

Clinical Pathology
Consultation 80500, 80502

Clitoroplasty
Intersex State 56805

Closed [Transurethral] Biopsy of Bladder
See Biopsy, Bladder, Cystourethroscopy

Clostridial Tetanus
See Tetanus

Clostridium Botulinum Toxin
See Chemodenervation

Clostridium Difficile
Antigen Detection
Immunoassay 87324
Immunoassay
with Direct Optical Observation 87803
Tissue Culture 87230
Toxin Genes Detection 87493

Clostridium Tetani ab
See Antibody, Detection, Tetanus

Closure 12001-13160
See Repair, Wound
Anal Fistula 46288
Atrioventricular Valve 33600
Cystostomy 51880
Enterostomy 44227, 44620, 44625, 44626
Laparoscopic 44227
Lacrimal Fistula 68770
Lacrimal Punctum
Plug 68761
Thermocauterization, Ligation or Laser Surgery 68760
Left Atrial Appendage
with Implant 33340

Paravalvular Leak
Percutaneous Transcatheter
Aortic Valve . . . 93591, 93592
Mitral Valve . . . 93590, 93592
Rectovaginal Fistula . . 57300, 57305, 57307, 57308
Semilunar Valve . . . 33602
Septal Defect
Ventricular . . . 33776, 33780, 93581
Ventricular Tunnel. . . 33722

Closure of Esophagostomy
See Esophagostomy, Closure

Closure of Gastrostomy
See Gastrostomy, Closure

Closure, Atrial Septal Defect
See Septal Defect, Atrial, Closure

Closure, Cranial Sutures, Premature
See Craniosynostosis

Closure, Fistula, Vesicouterine
See Fistula, Closure, Vesicouterine

Closure, Meningocele Spinal
See Meningocele Repair

Closure, Vagina
See Vagina, Closure

Clot . . . 34401-34490, 35875, 35876, 50230
See Thrombectomy; Thromboendarterectomy; Thrombolysis
Clotting
See Blood Coagulation, Test; Clotting Factor
Epidural Blood Patch . . . 62273
Declotting
Cystourethroscopic . . . 52001
External Cannula . . . 36860, 36861
Eye . . . 65930
Implanted Catheter . . . 36593
Pericardium . . . 32658, 33020
Vascular Access Device. . . 36593

Clot Lysis Time
Euglobin Lysis . . . 85360
Whole Blood Dilution . . . 85175

Clot Retraction
Coagulation Test. . . 85170

Clotting Disorder
See Coagulopathy

Clotting Factor
Factor I
See Fibrinogen
Factor II (Prothrombin). . . 85210
Factor III (Thromboplastin)
Factor IV
See Calcium
Factor VII (Proconvertin) . . . 85230
Factor VIII
AHG . . . 85240
Related Antigen. . . 85244
von Willebrand factor . . . 85247
VW factor. . . 85245, 85246
Factor IX (Christmas Factor. . . 85250
Factor X (Stuart-Prower). . . 85260
Factor X (Thrombokinase). . . 85260
Factor XI (Plasma Thromboplastin, Antecedent [PTA]). . . 85270
Factor XII (Hageman Factor) . . . 85280
Factor XIII (Fibrin Stabilizing) . . . 85290, 85291
Inhibition. . . 85705
Inhibition Test. . . 85347
Partial Time. . . 85730-85732

Clotting Inhibitors
Tests
Antithrombin III . . . 85300, 85301
Factor Inhibitor. . . 85335
Mixed Screen. . . 85611, 85732
Protein C. . . 85302, 85303, 85307
Protein S. . . 85305, 85306
Thrombomodulin . . . 85337
Thromboplastin Inhibition . . . 85705

Clotting Operation
See Excision, Nail Fold

Clotting Test
Protein C . . . 85303, 85307
Protein S . . . 85306
See Coagulation, Tests

Clotting Time
See Coagulation Time

Clozapine
Drug Assay . . . 80159

Clubfoot Cast . . . 29450
Wedging . . . 29750

CMG
See Cystometrogram

CMRI
See Cardiac Magnetic Resonance Imaging (CMRI)

CMV
See Cytomegalovirus

CNPB
See Continuous Negative Pressure Breathing (CNPB); Pulmonology, Therapeutic

Co-Factor I, Heparin
See Antithrombin III

CO2
See Carbon Dioxide

Coagulation
Tests
See Blood, Blood Clotting
Unlisted Services and Procedures . . . 85999

Coagulation Defect
See Coagulopathy

Coagulation Factor
See Clotting Factor

Coagulation Time . . . 85345-85348

Coagulation, Blood
See Coagulation

Coagulation, Light
See Photocoagulation

Coagulin
See Thromboplastin

Coagulopathy
Assay. . . 85130
Screen. . . 85390

Coccidioides
Antibody . . . 86635

Coccidioidin Test
See Streptokinase, Antibody

Coccidioidomycosis
Skin Test. . . 86490

Coccygeal Spine Fracture
See Coccyx, Fracture

Coccygectomy . . . 15920-15922, 27080

Coccyx
Excision. . . 27080
Coccygeal Approach, Rectal Tumor. . . 45160
Pressure Ulcer . . . 15920-15922
Fracture
Closed Treatment. . . 27200
Open Treatment. . . 27202
Tumor
Excision . . . 49215
X ray . . . 72220

Cochlear Device
Diagnostic Analysis . . . 92601, 92603
Implantation . . . 69930
Interface with Osseointegrated Implant. . . 69714, 69715, 69717
Programming. . . 92602, 92604

Cofactor Protein S
See Protein S

Coffey Operation
See Uterus, Repair, Suspension

Cognitive Function Tests
See Neurology, Diagnostic

Cognitive Skills Development
See Physical Medicine/Therapy/Occupational Therapy
One-on-one Patient Contact. . . 97127

Cold Agglutinin . . . 86156, 86157

Cold Pack Treatment. . . 97010

Cold Preservation
See Cryopreservation

Cold Therapies
See Cryotherapy

Colectomy
Partial . . . 44140
Laparoscopic . . . 44213
with Anastomosis . . . 44140
Laparoscopic. . . 44204, 44207, 44208
with Coloproctostomy . . . 44145, 44146
with Colostomy . . . 44141-44144
Laparoscopic. . . 44206, 44208
with Ileocolostomy
Laparoscopic. . . 44205
with Ileostomy . . . 44144
with Ileum Removal. . . 44160
with Splenic Flexure Mobilization. . . 44139
Laparoscopic. . . 44213
with Transanal Approach. . . 44147
Total
Laparoscopic . . . 44210-44212
with Creation of Ileal Reservoir . . . 44211
with Ileoanal Anastomosis. . . 44211
with Ileoproctostomy . . . 44210
with Ileostomy . . . 44210-44212
with Proctectomy . . . 44211, 44212
with Rectal Mucosectomy . . . 44211
without Proctectomy . . . 44210
Open
with Complete Proctectomy. . . 45121
with Ileoproctostomy . . . 44150
with Ileostomy . . . 44150, 44151
with Proctectomy . . . 44155-44158

Collagen Cross Links
Any Method . . . 82523
Cornea. . . 0402T

Collagen Injection . . . 11950-11954

Index

Collar Bone
See Clavicle

Collateral Ligament
Reconstruction
  Elbow 24346
  Interphalangeal Joint.......... 26545
  Metacarpophalangeal Joint 26541, 26542
Reduction
  Ulna 29902
Repair
  Ankle 27695, 27696, 27698
  Elbow 24345
  Interphalangeal Joint.......... 26540
  Knee.......... 27405, 27409
  Metacarpophalangeal Joint 26540

Collection and Processing
Aspirate
  See Aspiration
Brushings
  Abdomen 49320
  Anus.......... 46600, 46601
  Biliary Tract 47552
  Colon 44388, 45300, 45330, 45378
  Duodenum 43235, 44360, 44376
  Esophagus 43197, 43200, 43235
  Hepatobiliary System.......... 43260
  Ileum 44376, 44380
  Jejunum 43235
  Omentum 49320
  Peritoneum.......... 49320
  Rectum.......... 45300, 45330
  Small Intestine
    Pouch 44385
  Stomach.......... 43235
Radiological Guidance 75989
Specimen
  Capillary Blood.......... 36416
  Duodenum 43756, 43757
  for Dark Field Examination.......... 87164
  Ear 36416
  Hematoma 10140
  Sputum.......... 89220
  Stomach.......... 43754
  Sweat.......... 89230
  Tears 83861
  Venous Access Device.......... 36591
  Venous Blood.......... 36415, 36591, 36592
  Venous Catheter 36592
Stem Cells
  Harvesting
    Allogenic Blood 38205
    Autologous Blood..... 38206, 86890, 86891
  Processing 38210-38215
Washings
  Abdomen 49320
  Anus.......... 46600, 46601
  Biliary Tract 47552
  Colon 44388, 45300, 45330, 45378
  Duodenum 43235, 44360, 44376
  Esophagus 43197, 43200, 43235
  Hepatobiliary System.......... 43260
  Ileum 44376, 44380
  Jejunum.......... 43235
  Omentum 49320
  Peritoneum.......... 49320
  Rectum.......... 45300, 45330
  Small Intestine
    Pouch 44385
  Stomach.......... 43235

Colles Fracture 25600-25605

Colles Fracture Reversed
See Smith Fracture

Collins Syndrome, Treacher
See Treacher-Collins Syndrome

Collis Procedure
See Gastroplasty with Esophagogastric Fundoplasty

Colon
See Colon-Sigmoid
Ablation/Removal
  Lesion.... 44392, 44394, 44401, 45384, 45388
  Polyp..... 44392, 44394, 44401, 45384, 45388
  Tumor.... 44392, 44394, 44401, 45384, 45388
Biopsy 44025, 44100, 44322, 44389, 44407, 45380, 45392
  Endoscopic.......... 44389, 45380, 45392
Closure
  Fistula.......... 44650, 44660, 44661
  Stoma.......... 44620, 44625, 44626
Colonoscopy
  See Colonoscopy
Colostomy
  See Colostomy
Colotomy
  See Colotomy
CT Scan
  Colonography.......... 74261-74263
Endoscopy via Stoma
  Biopsy.......... 44389, 44407
  Decompression 44408
  Destruction
    Lesion.......... 44401
    Polyp.......... 44401
    Tumor 44401
  Dilation.......... 44405
  Exploration.......... 44388
  Hemorrhage Control.......... 44391
  Injection, Submucosal 44404
  Removal
    Foreign Body.......... 44390
    Lesion.......... 44392, 44394
    Polyp.......... 44392, 44394
    Tumor 44392, 44394
  Specimen Collection 44388
  Stent Placement.......... 44402
  Ultrasound 44406
Excision
  Partial.... 44140, 44141, 44143-44147, 44160
    Laparoscopic.......... 44204-44208
  Total.......... 44150, 44151, 44155-44158
    Laparoscopic.......... 44210-44212
Exploration 44025
Hemorrhage Control.......... 44391, 45382
Intraluminal Imaging.......... 0355T
Mucosal Resection 45390
Lavage
  Intraoperative.......... 44701
Lesion
  Ablation 45388
  Excision 44110, 44111
Lysis
  Adhesions 44005
Motility Study.......... 91117
Obstruction 44025-44050
Plication 44680
Reduction
  Hernia.......... 44050
  Volvulus 44050
Removal
  Foreign Body 44025, 44390, 45379
  Polyp.......... 44384
Repair
  Intussusception 44050
  Malrotation 44055
  Volvulus 44050
Splenic Flexure Mobilization
  Laparoscopic 44213
  Open.......... 44139
Suture
  Diverticula 44602-44605
  Injury 44602-44605
  Rupture.......... 44602-44605
  Ulcer.......... 44602-44605
  Wound 44602-44605
Tumor
  Ablation 45388
  Removal 45384, 45385
Ultrasound
  Endoscopic.......... 45391, 45392
Unlisted Procedure 45399
X ray with Contrast
  Barium Enema 74270, 74280

Colon-Sigmoid
See Colon
Biopsy
  Endoscopy 45331
Decompression.......... 45337
  Volvulus 45337
Endoscopy
  Ablation
    Lesion 45346
    Polyp.......... 45346
    Tumor 45346
  Band Ligation.......... 45350
  Biopsy.......... 45331
  Collection of Specimen 45330
  Dilation.......... 45340
  Exploration
    Transendoscopic Balloon 45330
  Hemorrhage Control.......... 45334
  Mucosal Resection 45349
  Needle Biopsy 45342
  Placement
    Decompresssion Tube 45337
    Stent.......... 45327, 45347
  Removal
    Foreign Body.......... 45332
    Polyp.......... 45333, 45338
    Tumor 45333, 45338
  Ultrasound 45341, 45342
Reconstruction
  Bladder from Sigmoid Colon 50810

Colonna Procedure
See Acetabulum, Reconstruction

Colonography
CT Scan
  Diagnostic 74261, 74262
  Screening.......... 74263

Colonoscopy
Flexible
  Ablation
    Lesion.......... 45388
    Polyp.......... 45388
    Tumor 45388
  Band Ligation.......... 45398
  Biopsy.......... 45380, 45392
  Collection of Specimen 45378
  Decompression 45393
  Diagnostic 45378
  Dilation.......... 45388
    Transendoscopic Balloon 45386
  Hemorrhage Control.......... 45382

Injection
Any Substance 45381
Mucosal Resection 45390
Placement
Stent 45389
Removal
Foreign Body 45379
Lesion 45384, 45385
Polyp 45384, 45385
Tumor 45384, 45385
Ultrasound 45391, 45392
Follow-up Intervals 0528F, 0529F
through Stoma
Ablation
Lesion 44401
Polyp 44401
Tumor 44401
Biopsy 44389, 44407
Decompression 44408
Diagnostic 44388
Dilation
Transendoscopic Balloon 44405
Exploration 44388
Hemorrhage Control 44391
Mucosal Resection 44403
Placement
Decompression Tube 44408
Stent 44402
Removal
Foreign Body 44390
Lesion 44392, 44394
Polyp 44392, 44394
Tumor 44392, 44394
Submucosal Injection 44404
Ultrasound
Biopsy 44407
Examination 44406

Color Vision Examination 92283

Colorrhaphy 44604

Colostomy
Abdominal 50810, 57307
Abdominoperineal 51597, 58240
External Fistulization 44320
Paracolostomy Hernia 44346
Revision 44340
Home Visit 99505
Ileocolostomy 44160, 44205
Laparoscopic 44188, 44206, 44208
Perineal 50810
Revision 44340, 44345, 44346
with Colorrhaphy 44605
with Partial Colectomy 44141, 44143, 44144, 44146
Hartmann Type 44143
Laparoscopic 44206, 44208
with Pelvic Exenteration 45126, 51597, 58240
with Proctectomy 45110
Laparoscopic 45395
with Rectal Repair 45563, 45805, 45825

Colotomy
Biopsy 44025
Exploration 44025
Foreign Body Removal 44025

Colpectomy
See Vaginectomy

Colpo-Urethrocystopexy
with Hysterectomy 58152, 58267, 58293
Marshall-Marchetti-Krantz Type 58152, 58267, 58293
Pereyra Type 58267, 58293

Colpoceliocentesis
See Colpocentesis

Colpocentesis 57020

Colpocleisis 57120

Colpocleisis Complete
See Vagina, Closure

Colpohysterectomies
See Hysterectomy, Vaginal

Colpoperineorrhaphy 57210

Colpopexy
Abdominal 57280
Laparoscopic 57425
Vaginal 57282, 57283

Colpoplasty
See Repair, Vagina

Colporrhaphy
Anterior 57240, 57289
with Insertion of Mesh 57267
with Insertion of Prosthesis 57267
Anteroposterior 57260-57265
with Enterocele Repair 57265
with Insertion of Mesh 57267
with Insertion of Prosthesis 57267
Nonobstetrical 57200
Posterior 57250
with Insertion of Mesh 57267
with Insertion of Prosthesis 57267

Colposcopy
Biopsy
Cervix 57420, 57421, 57454, 57455
Loop Electrode Biopsy 57460
Loop Electrode Conization 57461
Endometrium 58110
Vulva 56821
Cervix 57420, 57421, 57452, 57454-57456, 57460, 57461
Endometrium 58110
Exploration 57452
Vagina 57420, 57421, 57452
Vulva 56820
Biopsy 56821

Colpotomy
Exploration 57000
Pelvic Abscess Drainage 57010

Colprosterone
See Progesterone

Column Chromatography/Mass Spectrometry
See specific analyte in Pathology and Laboratory, Chemistry
Unspecified Non-Drug Analyte 82542

Columna Vertebralis
See Spine

Combined Heart-Lung Transplantation
See Transplantation, Heart-Lung

Combined Right and Left Heart Cardiac Catheterization
See Cardiac Catheterization, Combined Left and Right Heart

Comedones
Removal 10040

Commissurotomy
Right Ventricle 33476, 33478

Common Sensory Nerve
Repair/Suture 64834

Common Truncus
See Truncus Arteriosus

Communication Device
Non-Speech-Generating 92605, 92606, 92618
Speech-Generating 92607-92609

Community/Work Reintegration
Training 97537
See Physical Medicine/Therapy/Occupational Therapy

Comparative Analysis (Short Tandem Repeat)
Patient and Comparative Specimen .. 81265, 81266

Compatibility Test
Blood 86920, 86923
Specimen Pretreatment 86970-86972

Complement
Antigen 86160
Fixation Test 86171
Functional Activity 86161
Total Hemolytic 86162

Complete Blood Count (CBC)
See Blood Cell Count

Complete Colectomy
See Colectomy, Total

Complete Pneumonectomy
See Pneumonectomy, Completion

Complete Transposition of Great Vessels
See Transposition, Great Arteries

Complex, Factor IX
See Christmas Factor

Complex, Vitamin B
See B Complex Vitamins

Component Removal, Blood
See Apheresis

Composite Graft .. 15760-15770, 35681-35683

Compound B
See Corticosterone

Compound F
See Cortisol

Compression, Nerve, Median
See Carpal Tunnel Syndrome

Computed Tomographic Angiography
Abdomen 74174, 74175
Abdominal Aorta 75635
Arm 73206
Chest 71275
Head 70496
Heart 75574
Leg 73706
Neck 70498
Pelvis 72191, 74174

Computed Tomographic Scintigraphy
See Emission Computerized Tomography

Computed Tomography (CT)
See CT Scan

Computer Analysis
Acoustic Recording
Heart Sounds 93799

Index

Digital Image Data
Mammography . . . 77065-77067
Electrocardiographic Data . . . 93228
Motion Analysis . . . 96000-96004
Pediatric Home Apnea Monitor . . . 94776

Computer-Aided Detection (CAD)
Lesion
Chest Radiograph . . . 0174T, 0175T
Mammography . . . 77065-77067
Magnetic Resonance Imaging (MRI) . . . 77048, 77049

Computer-Assisted Navigation . . . 20985, 61781-61783
Bronchoscopy . . . 31627
Cranial Procedure . . . 67781-61782
Musculoskeletal Procedure . . 0054T, 0055T, 20985
Spinal Procedure . . . 61783

Computer-Assisted Testing . . . 96146
Cytopathology . . . 88121
Morphometric Analysis . . . 88121
Motion Analysis . . . 96000-96004
Neuropsychological . . . 96146
Psychological . . . 96146
Retinal Imaging . . . 0380T

Computer Data Analysis
Electrocardiographic . . . 0206T, 93228

Computerized Emission Tomography
See Emission Computerized Tomography

Concentration of Specimen
Cytopathology . . . 88108
Electrophoretic Fractionation and Quantitation . . . 84166
Immunoelectrophoresis . . . 86325
Immunofixation Electrophoresis . . . 86335
Infectious Agent . . . 87015
Ova and Parasites . . . 87177

Concentration, Hydrogen-Ion
See Blood Gases, pH

Concentration, Minimum Inhibitory
See Minimum Inhibitory Concentration

Concentric Procedure . . . 28296

Concha Bullosa Resection
with Nasal/Sinus Endoscopy . . . 31240

Conchae Nasale
See Nasal Turbinate

Conduction, Nerve
See Nerve Conduction

Conduit, Ileal
See Ileal Conduit

Condyle
Excision
See Condylectomy
Femur . . . 27508-27510, 27514
Knee . . . 27446
Femoral, Arthroplasty . . . 27442
Humerus
Fracture
Closed Treatment . . . 24576, 24577
Open Treatment . . . 24579
Percutaneous . . . 24582
Mandible
Reconstruction . . . 21247
Metatarsal
Excision . . . 28288
Toe
Resection . . . 28153

Condyle, Mandibular
See Mandibular Condyle

Condylectomy
Metatarsal Head . . . 28288
Posterior Cranial Fossa . . . 61597
Temporomandibular Joint . . . 21050

Condyloma
Anus . . . 46900
Penis . . . 54050, 54055-54057, 54060, 54065

Conference
Face-to-Face with Patient/Family . . . 99366
Interdisciplinary Medical Team . . . 99367, 99368

Congenital Arteriovenous Malformation
See Arteriovenous Malformation

Congenital Cardiac Anomaly
Catheterization . . . 93530-93533
Injection . . . 93563, 93564
Closure
Interatrial Communication . . . 93580
Ventricular Septal Defect . . . 93581
Echocardiography
Doppler, Fetal . . . 76827, 76828
Fetal . . . 76825, 76826
for Congenital Anomalies
Transesophageal . . . 93315-93317
Transthoracic . . . 93303, 93304
Ectopy
Ventricular
Treatment . . . 93654

Congenital Elevation of Scapula
See Sprengel's Deformity

Congenital Heart Septum Defect
See Congenital Cardiac Anomaly

Congenital Kidney Abnormality
Nephrolithotomy . . . 50070
Pyeloplasty . . . 50405
Pyelotomy . . . 50135

Congenital Laryngocele
See Laryngocele

Congenital Vascular Anomaly
See Vascular Malformation

Conisation
See Cervix, Conization

Conization
Cervix . . . 57461, 57520, 57522

Conjoint Psychotherapy
See Psychiatric Treatment, Family

Conjunctiva
Biopsy . . . 68100
Cyst
Incision and Drainage . . . 68020
Fistulization for Drainage . . . 68745, 68750
Follicle Expression . . . 68040
Graft . . . 65150, 65782
Harvesting, Living Donor . . . 68371
Injection . . . 68200
Insertion
Aqueous Drainage Device . . . 0449T, 0450T, 0474T
Stent . . . 68750
Lesion
Destruction . . . 68135
Excision . . . 68110, 68115
with Adjacent Sclera . . . 68130
Reconstruction . . . 68320, 68325, 68326, 68328
with Flap . . . 67971, 68360, 68362
Removal
Foreign Body . . . 65205, 65210
Repair
Eyelid Wound . . . 67961, 67966
Direct Closure . . . 65270, 67930, 67935
Mobilization and Rearrangement . . . 65272, 65273
Symblepharon
Division . . . 68340
with Graft . . . 68335
without Graft . . . 68330
Unlisted Services and Procedures . . . 68399

Conjunctivo-Tarso-Muller Resection . . . 67908

Conjunctivocystorhinostomy
See Conjunctivorhinostomy

Conjunctivodacryocystostomy
See Conjunctivorhinostomy

Conjunctivoplasty . . . 68320-68330
Reconstruction Cul-de-Sac
with Extensive Rearrangement . . . 68326
with Graft . . . 68326
Buccal Mucous Membrane . . . 68328
Repair of Symblepharon . . . 68330, 68335, 68340

Conjunctivorhinostomy
with Tube . . . 68750
without Tube . . . 68745

Conscious Sedation
See Sedation

Construction
Arterial
Conduit . . . 33920, 33608
Tunnel . . . 33505
Bladder from Sigmoid Colon . . . 50810
Eye Adhesions . . . 67880
Finger
Toe to Hand Transfer . . . 26551-26556
Gastric Tube . . . 43832
Neobladder . . . 51596
Tracheoesophageal Fistula . . . 31611
Vagina
with Graft . . . 57292
without Graft . . . 57291
Valve
Apical-Aortic Conduit . . . 33404

Consultation
Clinical Pathology . . . 80500, 80502
Inpatient . . . 99251-99255
New or Established Patient . . . 99251-99255
Interprofessional
Telephone/Internet Electronic Health Record . . . 99446-99449, 99451, 99452
Office and/or Other Outpatient . . . 99241-99245
New or Established Patient . . . 99241-99245
Psychiatric, with Family . . . 90887
Radiation Therapy
Radiation Physics . . . 77336, 77370
Surgical Pathology . . . 88321, 88323, 88325
Intraoperative . . . 88329, 88331-88334
X ray . . . 76140

Consumption Test, Antiglobulin
See Coombs Test

Contact Lens Services
Fittings and Prescription . . . 92071, 92072, 92310-92317
Modification . . . 92325
Prescription . . . 92314-92317
Replacement . . . 92326

Index

Continuous Negative Pressure Breathing (CNPB) 94662

Continuous Positive Airway Pressure (CPAP) 94660

Contouring
Cranial
  Bones 21181
  Sutures 61559
Forehead 21137, 21138
Frontal Sinus Wall 21139
Septoplasty 30520
Subcutaneous Injections 11950-11952, 11954
Tumor
  Facial Bone 21029

Contraception
Cervical Cap
  Fitting 57170
Diaphragm
  Fitting 57170
Intrauterine Device (IUD)
  Insertion 58300
  Removal 58301

Contraceptive Capsules, Implantable
Removal 11976

Contraceptive Device, Intrauterine
See Intrauterine Device (IUD)

Contracture
Bladder Neck
  Resection 52640
Elbow
  Release
    with Radical Resection of Capsule ... 24149
Finger Cast 29086
Palm
  Release 26121-26125
Scar
Shoulder
  Capsular Release 23020
Thumb
  Thenar Muscle Release 26508
Volkmann 25315
Wrist
  Capsulotomy 25085

Contracture of Palmar Fascia
See Dupuytren's Contracture

Contralateral Ligament
Repair
  Knee 27405

Contrast Aortogram
See Aortography

Contrast Bath Therapy
See Physical Medicine/Therapy/Occupational Therapy
Application of Modality 97034

Contrast Material
Injection
  Central Venous Access Device 36598
  Colonic Tube
    for Insertion 49440-49442
    for Radiological Evaluation 49465
    for Removal of Obstruction 49460
    for Replacement 49446, 49450-49452
  Cranial
    for Ventricular Puncture 61120
  Dacryocystography 68850
  Peritoneal
    for Assessment of Abscess or Cyst ... 49424
    for Evaluation of Venous Shunt 49427
    for Insertion of Tunneled Catheter 49418
  Peritoneal Cavity 49400
  Renal Angiography 36251-36254
  Saline Infusion Sonohysterography (SIS) 58340
  Spine
    for Localization 62263
  Urethrocystography 51605

Contrast Phlebogram
See Venography

Contusion
See Hematoma

Converting Enzyme, Angiotensin
See Angiotensin Converting Enzyme (ACE)

Coombs Test
Antihuman Globulin
Direct 86880
Indirect 86885, 86886
RBC Antibody Screen 86850, 86860

Copper 82525

Coprobilinogen
Feces Test 84577

Coproporphyrin 84119, 84120

Coracoacromial Ligament
Release 23415, 29826

Coracoid Process Transfer 23462

Cord, Spermatic
See Spermatic Cord

Cord, Spinal
See Spinal Cord

Cord, Vocal
See Vocal Cords

Cordectomy 31300

Cordocenteses
See Cordocentesis

Cordocentesis 59012

Cordotomy
Cervical 63194, 63196, 63198
Thoracic 63195, 63197, 63199

Corectomy
See Excision, Iris

Coreoplasty 66762

Cornea
Astigmatism
  Relaxing Incision 65772
  Wedge Resection 65775
Biopsy 65410
Collagen Cross Links 0402T
  with Pachymetry 0402T
  with Removal of Epithelium 0402T
Curettage 65435, 65436
  with Chelating Agent Application 65436
Epithelium
  Excision 65435, 65436
    with Chelating Agent 65436
Hysteresis Determination 92145
Implantation
  Corneal Ring Segments 65785
Incision
  for Astigmatism Correction 65772
  for Keratoplasty 0290T
Lesion
  Destruction 65450
  Excision 65400
    with Graft 65426
    without Graft 65420
Pachymetry 76514
Prosthesis 65770
Pterygium
  Excision 65420
Puncture 65600
Relaxing Incision 65772
Removal
  Foreign Body 65220, 65222
  Lesion 66600
Repair
  Incision 65772
  Wedge Resection 65775
  with Amniotic Membrane 65778-65780
  with Glue 65286
  Wound
    Nonperforating 65275
    Perforating 65280-65285
    Tissue Glue 65286
Reshape
  Epikeratoplasty 65767
  Keratomileusis 65760
  Keratophakia 65765
  Keratoprosthesis 65767
Scraping
  Smear 65430
Tattoo 65600
Tear Film Imaging 0330T
Tear Osmolarity 83861
Thickness Measurement 76514
Transplantation
  Amniotic Membrane 65780
  Autograft or Homograft
    Allograft Preparation 0290T, 65757
    Endothelial 65756
    Lamellar 65710
    Penetrating 65730, 65750, 65755
  for Aphakia 65750
Unlisted Procedures 66999

Coronary
Anomaly
  See Coronary Artery
Artery
  See Coronary Artery
Bypass Graft
  See Coronary Artery Bypass Graft (CABG)

Coronary Angioplasty, Transluminal Balloon
See Percutaneous Transluminal Angioplasty

Coronary Artery
Angiography 93454-93461
Angioplasty 92920, 92921
  with Atherectomy 92933, 92934, 92937, 92938, 92941, 92943, 92944
  with Stent Placement .. 92928, 92929, 92933, 92934, 92937, 92938, 92941, 92943, 92944
Atherectomy 92924-92295
  with Angioplasty 92933, 92934, 92937, 92938, 92941, 92943, 92944
  with Stent 92933, 92934, 92937, 92938, 92941, 92943, 92944
Endarterectomy 33572
Fractional Flow Reserve 0501T-0504T, 0523T
Graft
  Anomaly 33503, 33504
  Arterial Bypass 33533-33536
    Harvest 35600
  Arterial-Venous Bypass 33517-33519, 33521-33523

Index

Internal Mammary Artery Graft........4110F
Venous Bypass..............33510-33516
Harvest.........................35500
Insertion
Stent......................92928, 92929
Ligation..................................33502
Obstruction Severity Assessment..........0206T
Placement
Radiation Delivery Device............92974
Reconstruction..................33863, 33864
Repair
Anomaly....................33500-33507
Revascularization..............92937, 92938, 92941, 92943, 92944
Thrombectomy.......................92973
Thrombolysis....................92975, 92977
Translocation....................33506, 33507
Ventricular Restoration..................33548
Unroofing.................................33507

Coronary Artery Bypass Graft (CABG)
Anomalous Artery..................33503, 33504
Arterial Bypass..................33533-33536
Harvest..............................35600
Arterial-Venous Bypass...........33517-33519, 33521-33523
Harvest..............................35500
Beta Blocker Administered..............4115F
Harvest
Upper Extremity Artery..............35600
Upper Extremity Vein................35500
Internal Mammary Artery Graft...........4110F
Reoperation..............................33530
Revascularization..............92937, 92938, 92941, 92943, 92944
Spectroscopy
Catheter Based......................0205T
Venous Bypass..................33510-33516
Harvest.............................35500
Ventricular Restoration..................33548

Coronary Endarterectomy..........33572

Coroner's Exam....................88045

Coronoidectomy
Temporomandibular Joint.................21070

Corpectomy..................63101-63103

Corpora Cavernosa
Corpora Cavernosography................74445
Injection.............................54230
Corpus Spongiosum Shunt...............54430
Dynamic Cavernosometry................54231
Glans Penis Fistulization................54435
Injection
for Peyronie Disease...............54200
Pharmacologic Agent...............54235
Irrigation...............................54220
Peyronie Disease................54200-54205
Priapism.......................54220, 54430
Saphenous Vein Shunt..................54420

Corpora Cavernosa, Plastic Induration
See Peyronie Disease

Corpora Cavernosography
Imaging with Contrast.................74445
Injection.............................54230

Corpus Callosum
Transection..........................61541

Corpus Vertebrae (Vertebrale)
See Vertebral, Body

Correction of Cleft Palate
See Cleft Palate, Repair

Correction of Lid Retraction
See Repair, Eyelid, Retraction

Correction of Malrotation of Duodenum
See Ladd Procedure

Correction of Syndactyly
See Syndactyly, Repair

Correction of Ureteropelvic Junction
Stricture.........................52342, 52345

Cortex Decortication, Cerebral
See Decortication

Cortical Mapping
by Electric Stimulation............95961, 95962
Initial TMS Treatment.................90867
Noninvasive...........................96020

Corticoids
See Corticosteroids

Corticoliberin
See Corticotropic Releasing Hormone (CRH)

Corticosteroid Binding Globulin
See Transcortin

Corticosteroid Binding Protein
See Transcortin

Corticosteroids
Blood..................................83491
Urine..................................83491

Corticosterone
Blood or Urine.........................82528

Corticotropic Releasing Hormone (CRH)
Stimulation Panel......................80412

Cortisol...............80400, 80402, 80406, 80418, 80420, 80436, 82530
Stimulation............................80412
Total..................................82533

Cortisol Binding Globulin..........84449

Costectomy
See Rib, Excision

Costen Syndrome
See Temporomandibular Joint (TMJ)

Costotransversectomy............21610

Cothromboplastin
See Proconvertin

Cotte Operation
Uterine Suspension.............58400, 58410

Cotton Procedure
Bohler Procedure.......................28405

Counseling
See Preventive Medicine
Smoking and Tobacco Use
Cessation.......................99406, 99407

Counseling and/or Risk Factor Reduction Intervention, Preventive Medicine, Individual Counseling
See Preventive Medicine, Counseling, Individual, Risk Factor Reduction Intervention

Count
Blood Cell
See Blood Cell Count
Blood Platelet
See Blood, Platelet, Count
Cell
See Cell Count
Complete Blood
See Complete Blood Count (CBC)
Erythrocyte
See Red Blood Cell (RBC), Count
Leukocyte
See White Blood Cell, Count
Reticulocyte
See Reticulocyte, Count

Counters, Cell
See Cell Count

Countershock, Electric
See Cardioversion

Coventry Tibial Wedge Osteotomy
See Osteotomy, Tibia

Cowper's Gland
Excision...............................53250

Coxa
See Hip

Coxiella Burnetii
Antibody...............................86638

Coxsackie
Antibody...............................86658

CPAP
See Continuous Positive Airway Pressure (CPAP)

CPK
Blood.........................82550-82552

CPR (Cardiopulmonary Resuscitation)
Cardiac Arrest.........................92950

Cranial Bone
See Craniectomy; Craniotomy
Bone Graft
See Bone Graft
Burr Hole
See Burr Hole
Frontal Bone Flap...............61556, 61557
Halo Application
Thin Skull Osteology...............20664
Parietal Bone Flap.....................61556
Reconstruction
Extracranial...................21181-21184
Temporal Bone
Implantation
Cochlear Device.................69930
Hearing Device............69710, 69711
Osseointegrated Implant.....69714, 69715
Removal of Tumor...................69970
Resection..........................69535
Unlisted Procedure.................69979
Tumor
Excision.....................61563, 61564

Cranial Halo.........................20661

Cranial Nerve
Avulsion.................64732-64760, 64771
Cranial Nerve II
See Optic Nerve
Cranial Nerve V
See Trigeminal Nerve
Cranial Nerve VII
See Facial Nerve
Cranial Nerve X
See Vagus Nerve
Cranial Nerve XI
See Accessory Nerve, Spinal

Cranial Nerve XII
  See Hypoglossal Nerve
Decompression . . . 61458, 61460, 64716
Injection
  Anesthetic
    Trigeminal Nerve . . . 64400
    Vagus Nerve . . . 64408
  Neurolytic . . . 64600, 64605, 64610
Neuroplasty . . . 64716
Neurostimulator
  See Neurostimulators
Release . . . 64716
Repair
  Suture, with or without Graft . . . 64864, 64865
Transection . . . 64732-64760, 64771
Transposition . . . 64716

Cranial Tongs
Application/Removal . . . 20660
Removal . . . 20665

Craniectomy . . . 61501
See Craniotomy
Abscess Drainage . . . 61320, 61321
Anesthesia . . . 00211
Compression . . . 61450
Craniosynostosis
  Single Suture . . . 61550
  Multiple Sutures . . . 61552, 61558, 61559
Decompression . . . 61322, 61323, 61340, 61343
  Cranial Nerves . . . 61458
  Sensory Root of Gasserian Ganglion . . . 61450
Drainage . . . 61320, 61321
Evacuation of Hematoma . . . 61312-61315
Excision
  Abscess . . . 61514, 61522
  Bone Lesion . . . 61500
  Fenestration of Cyst . . . 61516, 61524
  Meningioma . . . 61512, 61519
  Tumor . . . 61500, 61510, 61518, 61520, 61521
Exploratory . . . 61304, 61305, 61458
for Electrode
  Cortical . . . 61860, 61870
  Subcortical . . . 61863, 61864, 61867, 61868
for Osteomyelitis . . . 61501
Release Stenosis . . . 61550-61552
Section . . . 61450, 61460
with Craniotomy . . . 61316, 61530
Wound Treatment . . . 61571

Craniofacial Procedures
Unlisted Services and Procedures . . . 21299

Craniofacial Separation
Bone Graft . . . 21436
Closed Treatment . . . 21431
External Fixation . . . 21435
Open Treatment . . . 21432, 21433, 21435, 21436
Wire Fixation . . . 21431, 21432

Craniomegalic Skull
Reduction . . . 62115, 62117

Craniopharyngioma
Excision . . . 61545

Cranioplasty
Autograft . . . 62146, 62147
Bone Graft . . . 61316, 62146, 62147
Bone Graft Retrieval . . . 62148
Encephalocele Repair . . . 62120
Skull Defect . . . 62140, 62141, 62145

Craniostenosis
See Craniosynostosis

Craniosynostosis
Bifrontal Craniotomy . . . 61557
Extensive Craniectomy . . . 61558, 61559
Front or Parietal . . . 61556
Multiple Sutures . . . 61552
Single Suture . . . 61550

Craniotomy
See Burr Hole; Craniectomy; Drill Hole
Anesthesia . . . 00211
Bifrontal . . . 61557
Decompression . . . 61322, 61323
Drainage . . . 61320, 61321
Evacuation of Hematoma . . . 61312-61315
Exploratory . . . 61304, 61305
for Craniosynostosis . . . 61556, 61557
for Encephalocele . . . 62121
for Excision
  Choroid Plexus . . . 61544
  Craniopharyngioma . . . 61545
  Epileptogenic Focus . . . 61534, 61536
  Foreign Body . . . 61570
  Tumor . . . 61546
for Hemispherectomy . . . 61543
for Implant of Neurostimulators . . . 61533, 61860, 61863, 61864, 61867, 61868, 61870
for Lobectomy . . . 61537-61540
for Transection of Corpus Callosum . . . 61541
for Wound Treatment . . . 61571
Frontal . . . 61556
Parietal . . . 61556
Removal
  Electrode Array . . . 61535
Skull Base Surgery . . . 61582, 61583, 61590, 61592
with Bone Flap . . . 61510-61516, 61526-61530, 61533-61545, 61566, 61567

Cranium
See Skull

Craterization
Calcaneus . . . 28120
Clavicle . . . 23180
Femur . . . 27070, 27071, 27360
Fibula . . . 27360, 27641
Hip . . . 27070
Humerus . . . 23184, 24140
Ileum . . . 27070
Metacarpal . . . 26230
Metatarsal . . . 28122
Olecranon Process . . . 24147
Phalanges
  Finger . . . 26235, 26236
  Toe . . . 28124
Pubis . . . 27070
Radius . . . 24145, 25151
Scapula . . . 23182
Symphysis Pubis . . . 27070, 27071
Talus . . . 28120
Tarsal . . . 28122
Tibia . . . 27360, 27640
Ulna . . . 25150

Creatine . . . 82553, 82554
Blood or Urine . . . 82540

Creatine Kinase
Total . . . 82550

Creatine Phosphokinase
Blood . . . 82552
Total . . . 82550

Creatinine
Blood . . . 82565
Clearance . . . 82575
Other Source . . . 82570
Urine . . . 82570-82575

Creation
Arteriovenous Fistula . . . 35686, 36825, 36830
Catheter Exit Site . . . 49436
Cavopulmonary Anastomosis . . . 33622
Colonic Reservoir . . . 45119, 45397
Complete Heart Block . . . 93650
Defect . . . 40720
Ileal Reservoir . . . 44158, 44211, 45113
Iliac Artery Conduit . . . 34833
Lesion . . . 61720, 61735, 61790, 63600
Mucofistula . . . 44144
Pericardial Window . . . 32659, 33025
Recipient Site . . . 15002-15005
Shunt
  Cerebrospinal Fluid
    See Cerebrospinal Fluid Shunt
Sigmoid Bladder . . . 50810
Speech Prosthesis . . . 31611
Stoma
  Bladder . . . 51980
  Tympanic Membrane . . . 69433, 69436
  Ureter . . . 50860
Subcutaneous Pocket
  with Glucose Sensor Insertion . . . 0446T, 0448T
Ventral Hernia . . . 39503
Vertebral Cavity . . . 22513-22515

CRF
See Corticotropic Releasing Hormone (CRH)

CRH
See Corticotropic Releasing Hormone (CRH)

Cricoid Cartilage Split
Laryngoplasty . . . 31587

Cricothyroid Membrane
Incision for Tracheostomy . . . 31605

Cristobalite
See Silica

Critical Care Services
See Emergency Department Services
Cardiopulmonary Resuscitation . . . 92950
Evaluation and Management . . . 99291, 99292
Interfacility Transport . . . 99466, 99467
Ipecac Administration for Poison . . . 99175
Neonatal
  Initial . . . 99468
  Intensive . . . 99477
  Low Birth Weight Infant . . . 99478, 99479
  Subsequent . . . 99469
Pediatric
  Initial . . . 99471, 99475
  Interfacility Transport . . . 99466, 99467
    Supervision . . . 99485, 99486
  Subsequent . . . 99472, 99476

Cross Finger Flap . . . 15574

Crossmatch . . . 86825, 86826, 86920-86923

Crossmatching, Tissue
See Tissue, Typing

Cruciate Ligament
Repair . . . 27407, 27409
  Arthroscopic Repair . . . 29888, 29889
  Knee
    with Collateral Ligament . . . 27409

Cryoablation
Nerve
  Percutaneous . . . 0440T-0442T

Cryofibrinogen . . . 82585

Cryofixation
See Cryopreservation

Cryoglobulin 82595

Cryopreservation
Bone Marrow 38207-38209
Cells 38207-38209, 88240, 88241
Embryo 89258, 89352
for Transplantation .. 32850, 33930, 33940, 44132, 47133, 47140, 48550, 50300-50320, 50547
Freezing and Storage
  Cells 88240
  Embryo 89258
  Reproductive Tissue
    Oocyte(s)................ 0357T, 89337
    Ovarian 0058T
    Sperm 89259
    Testicular 89335
  Stem Cells 38207
Thawing
  Cells 88241
  Embryo 89352
  Oocytes 89356
  Reproductive Tissue................ 89354
  Sperm.......................... 89353
  Stem Cells 38208, 38209

Cryosurgery 17000-17286, 47371, 47381
See Cryotherapy; Destruction
Ablation
  Fibroadenoma
    Breast 19105
  Lesion/Tumor
    Chest Wall 32994
    Liver 47371, 47381, 47383, 50250
    Pleura 32994
    Pulmonary...................... 32994
Bladder 52214
  Tumor............... 52234, 52235, 52240
Hemorrhoids 46999
Lesion
  Anus...................... 46916, 46924
  Bladder..................... 51030, 52224
  Ear 17280-17284, 17286
  Eyelid 17280-17284, 17286
  Face 17280-17284, 17286
  Lips................... 17280-17284, 17286
  Kidney 50250
  Mouth......... 40820, 17280-17284, 17286
  Nose.................. 17280-17284, 17286
  Penis...................... 54056, 54065
  Skin 17000, 17003, 17004, 17106-17108, 17110, 17111
  Urethra......................... 52224
  Vagina 57061, 57065
  Vulva 56501, 56515
Prostate...................... 52214, 55873
Trichiasis.......................... 67825
Tumor
  Bladder.............. 52234, 52235, 52240
  Rectum......................... 45190
Urethra 52214

Cryotherapy
Ablation
  Renal Tumor...................... 50593
Acne 17340
Bronchial Stenosis 31641
Destruction
  Bronchial Tumor................... 31641
  Ciliary Body 66720
  Retinopathy 67227
Lesion
  Cornea 65450
  Retina.......................... 67208
Retinal Detachment
  Prophylaxis....................... 67141
  Repair......... 67101, 67107, 67108, 67113
Retinopathy
  Destruction....................... 67227
  Treatment
    Preterm Infant.................. 67229
Trichiasis.......................... 67825

Cryptectomy
Unlisted Procedure, Anus 46999

Cryptococcus
Antibody 86641
Antigen Detection
  Immunoassay..................... 87327

Cryptococcus Neoformans
Antigen Detection
  Immunoassay..................... 87327

Cryptorchism
See Testis, Undescended

Cryptosporidium
Antigen Detection
  Immunofluorescence 87272
  Immunoassay..................... 87328

Crystal Identification
Any Body Fluid 89060
Tissue 89060

CSF
See Cerebrospinal Fluid

CT Scan
3-D Rendering................... 76376, 76377
  Not Requiring Independent Workstation...................... 76376
  Requiring Independent Workstation 76377
Bone
  Density Study..................... 77078
Brain 70450-70470
  Stroke Diagnosis 3110F-3112F
Computed Tomographic Angiography
  See Computed Tomographic Angiography
Drainage 75989
Follow-up Study 76380
Guidance
  Localization 77011
  Needle Placement.................. 77012
  Parenchymal Tissue Ablation 77013
  Radiation Therapy 77014
  Visceral Tissue Ablation 77013
Heart
  Evaluation
    Angiography 75574
    for Coronary Calcium 75571
    for Structure and Morphology 75572, 75573
Optical Coherence Tomography (OCT)
  Axillary Lymph Node 0351T, 0352T
  Breast.................... 0351T-0354T
  Intravascular 92978, 92979
Parathyroid Gland.................... 78072
Unlisted Services and Procedures 76497
with Contrast 70460
  Abdomen 74160, 74177
  Arm............................ 73201
  Brain..................... 0042T, 70460
  Cerebral Blood Flow/Volume.......... 0042T
  Ear 70481
  Face 70487
  Head........................... 70460
  Leg 73701
  Maxilla......................... 70487
  Neck........................... 70491
  Orbit........................... 70481
  Pelvis 72193, 74177
  Sella Turcica 70481
  Spine
    Cervical....................... 72126
    Lumbar 72132
    Thoracic 72129
  Thorax 71260
without and with Contrast
  Abdomen 74170, 74174, 74175, 74178, 75635
  Arm............................ 73202
  Brain...................... 70470, 70496
  Chest 71275
  Ear 70482
  Face 70488
  Head...................... 70470, 70496
  Leg 73702-73706, 75635
  Maxilla......................... 70488
  Neck...................... 70492, 70498
  Orbit........................... 70482
  Pelvis 72194, 74174, 74178
  Sella Turcica 70482
  Spine
    Cervical....................... 72127
    Lumbar 72133
    Thoracic 72130
  Thorax 71270
without Contrast..................... 70450
  Abdomen 74150, 74176, 74178
  Arm............................ 73200
  Brain........................... 70450
  Colon
    Colonography 74261-74263
  Ear 70480
  Face 70486
  Head........................... 70450
  Leg 73700
  Maxilla......................... 70486
  Neck........................... 70490
  Orbit........................... 70480
  Pelvis 72192, 74176, 74178
  Sella Turcica 70480
  Spine
    Cervical....................... 72125
    Lumbar 72131
    Thoracic 72128
  Thorax 71250

CT Scan, Radionuclide
See Emission Computerized Tomography

Cuff, Rotator
See Rotator Cuff

Culdocentesis
See Colpocentesis

Culture
Acid-Fast Bacilli 87116
Amniotic Fluid
  Chromosome Analysis............... 88235
Bacteria
  Aerobic.............. 87040-87071, 87077
  Anaerobic................... 87073-87076
  Blood 87040
  Other 87070-87075
  Screening 87081
  Stool...................... 87045, 87046
  Urine...................... 87086, 87088
Bone Marrow
  Chromosome Analysis............... 88237
  Neoplastic Disorders................ 88237
Chlamydia 87110

Chorionic Villus
  Chromosome Analysis 88235
Fertilized Oocytes
  for In Vitro Fertilization 89250
    Co-Culture of Embryo 89251
Fungus
  Blood 87103
  Hair 87101
  Nail 87101
  Skin 87101
  Source Other than Blood 87102
Lymphocyte
  Chromosome Analysis 88230
  HLA Typing 86821
Mold 87107
Mycobacteria 87118
Mycoplasma 87109
Oocyte/Embryo 89250
  Co-Culture of Oocyte/Embryo 89251
  Extended Culture 89272
Pathogen
  Presumptive 87081-87084
Skin
  Chromosome Analysis 88233
Tissue
  Homogenization 87176
  Infectious Agent Drug
  Resistance 87903, 87904
  Toxin/Antitoxin 87230
  Virus 87252, 87253
Tubercle Bacilli 87116
Tumor Tissue
  Chromosome Analysis 88239
Typing 87140-87158
Unlisted Services and Procedures 87999
Yeast 87106

Curettage
See Dilation and Curettage
Anal Fissure 46940
Cervix
  Endocervical 57454, 57456, 57505
Cornea 65435, 65436
Dentoalveolar 41830
Hydatidiform Mole 59870
Uterus
  Endometrial 58356
  Postpartum 59160

Curettage and Dilatation
See Dilation and Curettage

Curettage, Uterus
See Curettage, Uterus

Curettement
Skin Lesion
  Malignant . . 17270-17274, 17280-17284, 17286
  Premalignant 17000, 17003, 17004, 17110, 17111

Curietherapy
See Brachytherapy

Custodial Care
See Domiciliary Services; Nursing Facility Services

Cutaneolipectomy
See Lipectomy

Cutaneous Electrostimulation, Analgesic
See Application, Neurostimulation

Cutaneous Tag
See Skin, Tags

Cutaneous Tissue
See Integumentary System

Cutaneous-Vesicostomy
See Vesicostomy, Cutaneous

CVS
See Biopsy, Chorionic Villus

Cyanacobalamin
See Cyanocobalamin

Cyanide
Blood 82600
Tissue 82600

Cyanocobalamin 82607, 82608

Cyclic AMP 82030

Cyclic Somatostatin
See Somatostatin

Cyclocryotherapy
See Cryotherapy, Destruction, Ciliary Body

Cyclodialysis
Destruction
  Ciliary Body 66740

Cyclophotocoagulation
Destruction
  Ciliary Body 66710, 66711

Cyclosporine
Assay 80158

Cyst
See Pseudocyst
Abdomen
  Destruction/Excision 49203-49205
Abdominal Laparoscopy
  Aspiration 49322
Ankle
  Capsule 27630
  Tendon Sheath 27630
Bartholin's Gland
  Excision 56740
  Marsupialization 56440
Bile Duct 47715
Bladder
  Excision 51500
Bone
  Curettage
    Calcaneus 28100-28103
    Carpal 25130, 25135, 25136
    Clavicle 23140, 23145, 23146
    Femur 27355, 27356, 27357
    Finger 26210, 26215
    Humerus 24110, 24115, 24116
      Proximal 23150, 23155, 23156
    Mandible 21040
    Maxilla 21030
    Metacarpal 26200, 26205
    Olecranon Process 24120, 24125, 24126
    Radius 24120, 24125, 24126
    Talus 28100-28103
    Tibia 27635, 27637, 27638
    Toe 28108
    Zygoma 21030
  Drainage 20615, 63172
  Enucleation
    Mandible 21040
    Maxilla 21030
    Zygoma 21030
  Injection 20615
Brain
  Drainage . . 61150, 61151, 61156, 62161, 62162
  Excision 61516, 61524, 62162
Branchial Cleft
  Excision 42810, 42815
Breast
  Excision 19120
  Puncture Aspiration 19000, 19001
Calcaneus 28100-28103
Carpal 25130, 25135, 25136
Choledochal 47715
Ciliary Body
  Destruction 66770
Clavicle
  Excision 23140, 23145, 23146
Conjunctiva 68020
Dermoid
  Nose
    Excision 30124, 30125
Drainage
  Contrast Injection 49424
    with X ray 76080
Excision
  Cheekbone 21030
  Clavicle 23140
    with Allograft 23146
    with Autograft 23145
  Femur 27065-27067, 27355-27358
  Ganglion
    See Ganglion
  Humerus 23150, 24110
    with Allograft 23156
    with Autograft 23155
  Hydatid
    See Echinococcosis
  Lymphatic
    See Lymphocele
  Maxilla 21030
  Mediastinum 32662
  Olecranon Process 24120, 24125, 24126
    with Allograft 24126
    with Autograft 24125
  Ovarian 58925
  Pericardial 32661
  Pilonidal 11770-11772
  Radius 24120
    with Allograft 24126
    with Autograft 24125
  Salivary Gland 42408
  Scapula 23140
    with Allograft 23146
    with Autograft 23145
  Symphysis Pubis 27065-27067
Facial Bones
  Excision 21030
Femur 27065-27067, 27355-27358
Fibula 27635, 27637, 27638
Foot
  Excision 28090
Ganglion
  Aspiration/Injection 20612
Gums
  Incision and Drainage 41800
Hand
  Capsule 26160
  Tendon Sheath 26160
Hip 27065-27067
Humerus
  Excision 23150, 24110
    with Allograft 23156, 24116
    with Autograft 23155, 24115
Ilium 27065-27067
Incision and Drainage 10060, 10061
  Lung 32200
  Mouth
    Dentoalveolar 41800

Index

Lingual ... 41000
Masticator Space ... 41009, 41018
Sublingual ... 41005, 41006, 41015
Submandibular ... 41008, 41017
Submental ... 41007, 41016
Vestibular ... 40800, 40801
Ovarian ... 58800, 58805
Pilonidal ... 10080, 10081
Skin ... 10060, 10061
Spinal Cord ... 63172, 63173
Iris
Destruction ... 66770
Kidney
Ablation ... 50541
Aspiration ... 50390
Excision ... 50280, 50290
Injection ... 50390
X ray ... 74470
Knee
Baker's ... 27345
Excision ... 27347
Leg, Lower
Capsule ... 27630
Tendon Sheath ... 27630
Liver
Aspiration ... 47015
Drainage ... 47010
Marsupialization ... 47300
Lung
Incision and Drainage ... 32200
Removal ... 32140
Lymph Node
Axillary/Cervical
Excision ... 38550, 38555
Mandible
Excision ... 21040, 21046, 21047
Maxilla
Excision ... 21030, 21048, 21049
Mediastinal
Excision ... 32662
Resection ... 39200
Metacarpal ... 26200, 26205
Metatarsal ... 28104, 28106, 28107
Mouth ... 41000, 41005-41009, 41015-41018
Incision and Drainage ... 40800, 40801
Mullerian Duct
Excision ... 55680
Nose
Excision ... 30124, 30125
Olecranon ... 24120, 24125, 24126
Ovarian
Excision ... 58925
Incision and Drainage ... 58800, 58805
Pancreas ... 48500
Anastomosis ... 48520, 48540
Excision ... 48120
Marsupialization ... 48500
Pelvis
Aspiration ... 50390
Injection ... 50390
Pericardial
Excision ... 32661
Resection ... 33050
Phalanges
Finger ... 26210, 26215
Toe ... 28108
Pilonidal
Excision ... 11770-11772
Incision and Drainage ... 10080, 10081
Pubis ... 27065-27067
Radius ... 24120, 25120, 25125, 25126
Rathke's Pouch
See Craniopharyngioma
Removal
Skin ... 10040
Retroperitoneal
Destruction/Excision ... 49203-49205
Salivary Gland
Marsupialization ... 42409
Excision ... 42408
Scapula
Excision ... 23140, 23145, 23146
Seminal Vesicle
Excision ... 55680
Skene's Gland
Destruction ... 53270
Drainage ... 53060
Skin
Incision and Drainage ... 10060, 10061
Puncture Aspiration ... 10160
Removal ... 10040
Spinal Cord
Aspiration ... 62268
Incision and Drainage ... 63172, 63173
Sublingual Gland
Drainage ... 42409
Excision ... 42408
Symphysis Pubis ... 27065-27067
Talus ... 28100-28103
Tarsal ... 28104, 28106, 28107
Thyroglossal Duct
Excision ... 60280, 60281
Incision and Drainage ... 60000
Thyroid Gland
Aspiration ... 60300
Excision ... 60200
Injection ... 60300
Tibia ... 27635, 27637, 27638
Tongue ... 41000, 41005-41009
Ulna ... 24120, 25120, 25125, 25126
Urachal
Bladder
Excision ... 51500
Vaginal
Biopsy ... 57105
Excision ... 57135
Wrist
Excision ... 25111, 25112, 25130, 25135, 25136
Zygoma
Excision ... 21030

Cyst, Ovary
See Ovary, Cyst

Cystatin C
Blood ... 82610

Cystatins, Kininogen
See Kininogen

Cystectomy
Complete ... 51570
with Bilateral Pelvic Lymphadenectomy ... 51575, 51585, 51595
with Continent Diversion ... 51596
with Ureteroileal Conduit ... 51590
with Ureterosigmoidostomy ... 51580
Ovarian ... 58925
Laparoscopic ... 58662
Partial
Complicated ... 51555
Reimplantation of Ureters ... 51565
Simple ... 51550

Cystic Hygroma
See Hygroma

Cystine
Urine ... 82615

Cystitis
Interstitial ... 52260, 52265

Cystography
Bladder ... 74430
Injection ... 51600, 52281

Cystolithotomy ... 51050

Cystometrogram ... 51725-51729

Cystoplasty ... 51800

Cystorrhaphy ... 51860-51865

Cystoscopy
with Endopyelotomy ... 52000
with Ureteroneocystostomy ... 50947

Cystoscopy, with Biopsy
See Biopsy, Bladder, Cystourethroscopy

Cystostomy
Change Tube ... 51705, 51710
Closure ... 51880
Home Visit ... 99505
with Drainage ... 51040
with Fulguration ... 51020
with Insertion Radioactive Material ... 51020
with Tumor Destruction ... 51030
with Urethrectomy
Female ... 53210
Male ... 53215

Cystotomy
Excision
Bladder Diverticulum ... 51525
Bladder Tumor ... 51530
Vesical Neck ... 51520
Repair Ureterocele ... 51535
with Calculus Basket Extraction ... 51065
with Destruction Intravesical Lesion ... 51030
with Drainage ... 51040
with Fulguration ... 51020
with Insertion
Radioactive Material ... 51020
Ureteral Catheter ... 51045
with Removal Calculus ... 51050, 51065

Cystourethrogram, Retrograde
See Urethrocystography, Retrograde

Cystourethropexy
See Vesicourethropexy

Cystourethroplasty
Bladder/Vesical Neck ... 51800, 51820
Radiofrequency Micro-Remodeling ... 53860

Cystourethroscopy
Biopsy ... 52204, 52224, 52250, 52354
Brush ... 52007
Calibration and/or Dilation
Urethral Stricture or Stenosis ... 52281, 52630, 52647-52649
Catheterization
Ejaculatory Duct ... 52010
Ureteral ... 52005, 52320
Chemodenervation
Bladder ... 52287
Dilation
Bladder ... 52260, 52265
Intra-Renal Stricture ... 52343, 52346
Ureter ... 52341, 52342, 52344, 52345
Urethra ... 0499T, 52281, 52285
Drug Delivery
Urethral ... 0499T
Evacuation
Clot ... 52001

Examination 52000
Female Urethral Syndrome............... 52285
Incision
Bladder Neck 52285
Congenital Obstructive Hypertrophic Mucosal Folds.......................... 52400
Diverticulum...................... 52305
Urethral Valves 52400
Ejaculatory Duct................... 52402
Injection
for Cystography 52281
Implant Material 52327
Insertion
Indwelling Ureteral Stent 50947, 52332
Radioactive Substance 52250
Transprostatic Implant......... 52441, 52442
Ureteral Guide Wire................ 52334
Urethral Stent 52282
Instillation..................... 52005, 52010
Irrigation 52005, 52010
Lithotripsy.......................... 52353
Lysis
Urethra.......................... 53500
Urethrovaginal Septal Fibrosis 52285
Manipulation of Ureteral Calculus... 52330, 52352
Meatotomy
Ureteral 52290
Urethral .. 52281, 52285, 52630, 52647-52649
Removal
Calculus .. 52310, 52315, 52320, 52325, 52352
Foreign Body 52310, 52315
Urethral Stent 52310, 52315
Resection
Congenital Obstructive Hypertrophic Mucosal Folds.......................... 52400
Diverticulum...................... 52305
Ejaculatory Duct................... 52402
External Sphincter.................. 52277
Prostate 52601, 52630
Transurethral
Tumor......... 52234, 52235, 52240, 52355
Urethral Valves 52400
Ureterocele(s)............... 52300, 52301
Treatment
Lesion(s).......................... 52224
Ureteral Stricture.................. 52341
Urethral Syndrome 52285
Vasectomy
Transurethral 52402, 52630, 52647-52649
Vasotomy
Transurethral 52402
with Anterior Colporrhaphy .. 57240, 57260, 57265
with Direct Vision Internal Urethrotomy..... 52276
with Duct Radiography................. 52010
with Ejaculatory Duct Catheterization 52010
with Fulguration 52214
Lesion...................... 52224, 52354
Congenital Obstructive Hypertrophic Mucosal Folds.......................... 52400
Polyps.......................... 52285
Ureterocele(s)............... 52300, 52301
Urethral Valves 52400
Tumor.............. 52234, 52235, 52240
with Internal Urethrotomy ... 52630, 52647-52649
Female 52270, 52285
Male.......................... 52275
with Prostate
Laser Coagulation 52647
Laser Enucleation.................. 52649
Laser Vaporization 52648
with Pyeloscopy 52351
with Steroid Injection.................. 52283
with Ureteral Catheterization............ 52005
with Ureteral Meatotomy............... 52290
with Ureteropyelography 52005
with Ureteroscopy..................... 52351

Cytochrome Reductase, Lactic

See Lactic Dehydrogenase

Cytogenetic Study

Bone Marrow
Diagnostic 3155F
Neoplastic Disorder................ 88237
Breakage Syndromes
See Chromosome Analysis
Chromosome Analysis
See Chromosome Analysis
Interpretation and Report............... 88291
Molecular
DNA Probe 88271-88275, 88364-88366
Neoplastic Disorders
Bone Marrow...................... 88237
Tumor............................ 88239
Non-neoplastic Disorders
Amniotic Fluid 88235
Chorionic Villus Cells............... 88235
Lymphocyte 88230
Skin or Tissue Biopsy............... 88233
Unlisted Services and Procedures 88299

Cystoscopy

See Bladder, Endoscopy

Cytogenomic Constitutional (Genome-Wide) Microarray Analysis

Interrogation of Genomic Regions 81406, 81228, 81229

Cytomegalovirus

Antibody 86644, 86645
Antigen Detection
Direct Fluorescence................ 87271
Immunoassay...................... 87332
Nucleic Acid................ 87495-87497

Cytometries, Flow

See Flow Cytometry

Cytopathology

Cervical or Vaginal
Definitive Hormone Evaluation 88155
Pap 88164-88167
Requiring Interpretation by Physician ... 88141
Thin Layer Prep .. 88142, 88143, 88174, 88175
Evaluation..................... 88172, 88177
Needle Aspirate............. 88172, 88177
Flow Cytometry
See Flow Cytometry
Fluids, Washings, Brushings
Simple Filter...................... 88106
Smears........................... 88104
Forensic............................ 88125
Other Source................. 88160-88162
Sex Chromatin Identification
Barr Bodies....................... 88130
Polymorphonuclear Drumsticks........ 88140
Smears
Any Other Source............ 88160-88162
Brushings......................... 88104
Cervical or Vaginal
Automated Screen............... 88174
Hormone Evaluation.............. 88155
Manual Screen 88150, 88153, 88164, 88165
Partially Automated Screen........ 88147, 88148, 88152, 88166, 88167, 88175
Physician Interpretation........... 88141
Concentration Technique............ 88108
Fluids 88104
Washings......................... 88104
Techniques
See Saccomanno Technique
Concentration..................... 88108
In Situ Hybridization........... 88120, 88121
Morphometric Analysis
Computer-Assisted .. 88367, 88373, 88374
Manual 88368, 88369, 88377
Selective Cellular Enhancement 88112
Unlisted Cytopathology Procedure......... 88199
Urinary Tract Specimen 88120, 88121

Cytosol Aminopeptidase

See Leucine Aminopeptidase

Cytotoxic Screen

Lymphocyte..................... 86805, 86806
Percent Reactive Antibody (PRA) 86807, 86808
Serum Antibodies................ 86807, 86808

D

D & C Yellow No. 7

See Fluorescein

D-2, Vitamin

See Vitamin, D

D and C

See Dilation and Curettage

D and E

See Dilation and Evacuation

D Galactose

See Galactose

D Glucose

See Glucose

D, Vitamin

See Vitamin, D

D-Xylose Absorption Test.......... 84620

Dacryoadenectomy

Partial 68505
Total 68500
Dacryocystectomy................. 68520

Dacryocystogram

See Dacryocystography

Dacryocystography

Injection of Contrast................... 68850
Nuclear Imaging .. 78660 Radiological Examination 70170

Dacryocystorhinostomy

Lacrimal Sac/Nasal Cavity Fistulization..... 68720
with Nasal/Sinus Endoscopy 31239

Dacryocystostomies

See Dacryocystotomy
Dacryocystotomy 68420

Daily Living Activities

See Activities of Daily Living

Damus-Kaye-Stansel Procedure

See Anastomosis, Pulmonary

Dana Operation

See Rhizotomy

Dandy Operation

See Ventriculocisternostomy

Dark Adaptation Examination 92284

Dark Field Examination 87164-87166

Darkroom Test
See Glaucoma, Provocative Test

Darrach Procedure
See Excision, Ulna

David Procedure
See Aorta, Ascending, Graft

Day Test
See Blood, Feces

de Quervain's Disease Treatment .. 25000

Death, Brain
See Brain Death

Debridement
Ankle 29897, 29898
Bone 11044, 11047
with Open Fracture and/or Dislocation .. 11012
Brain 62010
Burns 01951-01953, 16020-16030
Cartilage 29862, 29877, 29880, 29881, 29885
Elbow 29837, 29838
with Prosthesis Removal 24160, 24164
Forearm 25023, 25025
Knee 27441, 27443, 27497, 27499
Leg 27892-27894
Lesion, Premalignant 96574
Liver 47361
Mastoid Cavity
Complex 69222
Simple 69220
Metatarsophalangeal Joint 28289, 28291, 29901, 29902
Muscle 11043, 11044, 11046, 11047
Infected 11004-11006, 11008
with Open Fracture and/or Dislocation 11011, 11012
Nails 11720, 11721
Nonviable Tissue 25023, 25025, 27497, 27892-27894
Nose
Endoscopic 31237
Pancreatic Tissue 48105
Penile Prosthesis Infected Field 54411, 54417
Shoulder 29822, 29823
with Prosthesis Removal 23334, 23335
Skin
Eczematous 11000, 11001
Excision 15920-15999
Infected 11000-11006
Subcutaneous Tissue 11042-11047
Infected 11004-11006, 11008
Necrotized 49568
with Open Fracture and/or Dislocation 11010-11012
Sternum 21627, 21750
Pathology Analysis 88304, 88305
Urethral/Bladder Infected Inflatable Sphincter Field 53448
Wound
Non-Selective 97602
Selective 97597, 97598
Thigh 27497, 27499
Wrist
Joint 29846
Nonviable Tissue 25023, 25025

Debulking Procedure
Ovary/Pelvis 58952-58958

Decompression
See Section
Arm, Lower 24495, 25020-25025
Auditory Canal, Internal 61591, 69960
Brainstem 61575, 61576
Carotid Artery 61590, 61591
Cauda Equina 63011, 63017, 63045-63048, 63056, 63057, 63087-63091
Colon 45337, 45393
Cranial Nerve 61458
Esophagogastric Varices 37181
Facial Nerve
Intratemporal 61590
Lateral to Geniculate Ganglion 69720, 69740
Medial to Geniculate Ganglion 69725, 69745
Total 69955
Transtemporal 61595
Fasciotomy
Leg 27892-27894
Pelvic/Buttock 27027
with Debridement 27057
Thigh/Knee 27496-27499
Finger 26035
Gasserian Ganglion
Sensory Root 61450
Hand 26035-26037
Intestines
Small 44021
Jejunostomy
Laparoscopic 44186, 44187
Leg
Fasciotomy 27600-27602
Nerve 64702-64727
Laminotomy/Laminectomy 0274T, 0275T
Root 22551, 22552, 63020-63048, 63055-63103
Nucleus Pulposus 62287
Optic Nerve 61564, 67570
Orbit 61330
Removal of Bone 67414, 67445
Pelvis/Buttock
Fasciotomy 27027
with Debridement 27057
Shoulder 29826-29828
Sigmoid Sinus 61595
Skull 61322, 61323, 61340-61345
Spinal Cord 0375T, 22856, 22858, 62287, 62380, 63001-63017, 63045-63103
with Arthrodesis 22551, 22552
Cauda Equina 63005
Osteophytectomy 0375T, 22551, 22552, 22856, 22858
Tarsal Tunnel Release 28035
Trachea 33800
Volvulus 45321, 45337
with Nasal/Sinus Endoscopy
Optic Nerve 31294
Orbit Wall 31292, 31293
Wrist 25020-25025

Decortication
Lung
Endoscopic 32651, 32652
Partial 32225
Total 32220
with Parietal Pleurectomy 32320

Decubiti
See Pressure, Ulcer (Decubitus)

Decubitus Ulcers
Excision
Coccygeal 15920, 15922
Ischial 15940, 15941, 15944-15946
Sacral 15931, 15933-15937
Trochanteric 15950-15953, 15956, 15958
Unlisted Procedure 15999

Deetjen's Body
See Blood, Platelet

Defect, Coagulation
See Coagulopathy

Defect, Heart Septal
See Septal Defect

Defect, Septal Closure, Atrial
See Septal Defect, Atrial, Closure

Deferens, Ductus
See Vas Deferens

Defibrillation
See Cardioversion

Defibrillator, Heart
Implantable Device
See Cardiac Assist Devices
Cardioverter-Defibrillator
See Cardiac Assist Devices
Wearable Device
Data Analysis 93292
Initial Set Up and Programming 93745

Deformity, Boutonniere
See Boutonniere Deformity

Deformity, Sprengel's
See Sprengel's Deformity

Degenerative, Articular Cartilage, Patella
See Chondromalacia Patella

Degradation Products, Fibrin
See Fibrin Degradation Products

Dehydroepiandrosterone 82626

Dehydroepiandrosterone Sulfate .. 82627

Dehydrogenase, 6-Phosphogluconate
See Phosphogluconate-6, Dehydrogenase

Dehydrogenase, Alcohol
See Antidiuretic Hormone

Dehydrogenase, Glucose-6-Phosphate
See Glucose-6-Phosphate, Dehydrogenase

Dehydrogenase, Glutamate
See Glutamate Dehydrogenase

Dehydrogenase, Isocitrate
See Isocitric Dehydrogenase

Dehydrogenase, Lactate
See Lactic Dehydrogenase

Dehydrogenase, Malate
See Malate Dehydrogenase

Dehydroisoandrosterone Sulfate
See Dehydroepiandrosterone Sulfate

Delay of Flap
Skin Graft 15600-15630

Deligation
Ureter 50940

Deliveries, Abdominal
See Cesarean Delivery

Delivery
See Cesarean Delivery; Vaginal Delivery

Delorme Operation
See Pericardiectomy

Denervation
Hip
Femoral 27035
Obturator 27035
Sciatic 27035

Denervation, Sympathetic
Chemodenervation 64650, 64653
Neurolytic Agent. 64680, 64681
Transcatheter Percutaneous. 0338T, 0339T

Dens Axis
See Odontoid Process

Denver Shunt
Patency Test 78291

Deoxycorticosterone
See Desoxycorticosterone

Deoxycortisol. 80436, 82634

Deoxyribonuclease
Antibody 86215

Deoxyribonuclease I
See DNAse

Deoxyribonucleic Acid (DNA)
Antibody 86225, 86226

Depilation
See Removal, Hair

Depletion
Bone Marrow/Stem Cells
Plasma 38214
Platelet. 38213
T-Cell 38210
Tumor Cell 38211

Deposit Calcium
See Calculus, Removal

Depth Electrode
Cerebral Implantation. 61760
Electrode Array Intracranial
See Neurostimulators

Derma-Fat-Fascia Graft. 15770

Dermabrasion 15780-15783

Dermatology
Actinotherapy 96900
Microscopic Examination of Hair 96902
Photochemotherapy
Ultraviolet A Treatment. 96912, 96913
Ultraviolet B Treatment 96910, 96913
Psoriasis Laser Treatment 96920-96922
Reflectance Confocal Microscopy (RCM)
Skin Imaging 96931-96936
Unlisted Services and Procedures 96999
Whole Body Photography 96904

Dermatoplasty
Intranasal 30620
Septal 30620

Dermoid
See Cyst, Dermoid

Derrick-Burnet Disease
See Q Fever

Descending Abdominal Aorta
See Aorta, Abdominal

Desmotomy
See Ligament, Release

Desoxycorticosterone 82633

Desoxycortone
See Desoxycorticosterone

Desoxyphenobarbital
See Primidone

Desquamation
See Exfoliation

Destruction
Ablation
See Ablation
Acne
See Acne Treatment
Calculus
See Calculus
Chemosurgery
See Chemosurgery
Cryosurgery
See Cryosurgery
Cyst
Abdomen 49203-49205
Ciliary Body 66770, 66740
Iris 66770
Electrosurgery
See Electrosurgery
Endometriomas
See Endometrioma
Hemorrhoids
Thermal 46930
Laser Surgery
See Laser Surgery
Lesion
Anal 46900-46917, 46924
Bladder. 51030
Choroid. 67220, 67221, 67225
Ciliary Body 66770
Conjunctiva 68135
Cornea 65450
Eyelid 67850
Facial 17000-17004, 17280-17286
Gums 41850
Iris 66770
Larynx. 31572
Mouth. 40820
Nerve
Plantar 64632
Nose
Intranasal 30117, 30118
Palate. 42160
Penis
Cryosurgery. 54056
Electrodesiccation 54055
Extensive 54065
Laser Surgery 54057
Simple. 54050-54060
Surgical Excision 54060
Pharynx. 42808
Prostate
Microwave Thermotherapy 53850
Radio Frequency Thermotherapy 53852, 53854
Retina
Cryotherapy, Diathermy 67208-67218, 67227
Photocoagulation 67210, 67228, 67229
Radiation by Implantation of Source . . 67218
Skin
Benign. 17110, 17111
Malignant. 17260-17286
Premalignant 17000-17004, 96567, 96573, 96574
Spinal Cord. 62280-62282
Uvula 42160
Vagina
Extensive 57065
Simple. 57061
Vascular, Cutaneous 17106-17108
Vulva
Extensive 56515
Simple. 56501
Nerve. . .64600-64610, 64620-64640, 64680, 64681
Neurofibroma
Extensive 0419T, 0420T
Polyp
See Ablation; Fulguration
Prostate. 55873
Prostate Tissue
Transurethral
Thermotherapy 53850, 53852, 53854
Sinus
Frontal 31080-31085
Tonsil
Lingual 42870
Tumor
Abdomen 49203-49205
Breast
Microwave Thermotherapy 19499
Colon 45388
Intestines
Large. 44401
Small. 44369
Mesentery 49203-49205
Peritoneum. 49203-49205
Rectum. 45190, 45320
Retroperitoneal 49203-49205
Urethra. 53220
Turbinate Mucosa. 30801, 30802
Ureter
See Fulguration
Urethra
See Fulguration
Warts
Flat. 17110, 17111
with Cystourethroscopy 52354

Determination, Blood Pressure
See Blood Pressure, Determination

Determination, Lung Volume. 94727, 94728

Developmental Cognitive Testing
Standardized Screening and Scoring 96110
by Physician. 96112, 96113

Device
Adjustable Gastric Band. 43770-43774
Cardiac
See Cardiac Assist Devices
Iliac Artery Occlusion Device
Insertion. 34808
Subcutaneous Port
for Gastric Restrictive Procedure. 43770, 43774, 43886-43888
Venous Access
Collection of Blood Specimen . . . 36591, 36592
Implanted Device 36591
Venous Catheter. 36592
Fluoroscopic Guidance. 36598, 77001
Insertion
Central 36560-36566
Peripheral 36570, 36571
Irrigation. 96523
Obstruction Clearance 36595, 36596
Imaging. 75901, 75902
Removal 36590
Repair. 36576

Index

Replacement 36582, 36583, 36585
Catheter 36578
Ventricular Assist
See Ventricular Assist Device (VAD)

Device Handling
Order Expediting 99002

Device, Intrauterine
See Intrauterine Device (IUD)

Device, Orthotic
See Orthotics

Dexamethasone
Suppression Panel 80420

DHA Sulfate
See Dehydroepiandrosterone Sulfate

DHEA
See Dehydroepiandrosterone

DHEA Sulfate
See Dehydroepiandrosterone Sulfate

Diagnosis, Psychiatric
See Psychiatric Diagnosis

Diagnostic Amniocentesis
See Amniocentesis

Diagnostic Aspiration, Eye
See Paracentesis, Eye, Anterior Chamber Fluid Removal

Diagnostic Radiological Examination
See X ray

Diagnostic Skin and Sensitization Tests
See Allergy Tests

Diagnostic Ultrasound
See Echography

Diagnostic Ultrasound of Heart
See Echocardiography

Dialyses, Peritoneal
See Dialysis, Peritoneal

Dialysis
Anesthesia 01844
Arteriovenous Fistula 36831-36833
End-Stage Renal Disease
See End-Stage Renal Disease Services, Dialysis
Hemodialysis
See Hemodialysis
Hemoperfusion 90997
Hepatitis B Vaccine (HepB) 90740, 90747
Introduction
Dialysis Circuit 36901-36903
with Transcatheter Placement of Stent 36906
Kt/V Level 3082F-3084F
Nephropathy Treatment Documented 3066F
Patient Training
Completed Course 90989
Per Session 90993
Peritoneal 90945, 90947, 4055F
Catheter Insertion 49418, 49419, 49421
Catheter Removal 49422
Home Infusion 99601, 99602
Plan of Care Documented 0507F
Thrombectomy
Dialysis Circuit 36904-36906
with Transcatheter Stent Placement
via Dialysis Circuit 36908
with Transluminal Balloon Angioplasy
via Dialysis Circuit 36907
with Vascular Embolization/Occlusion 36909
Unlisted Services and Procedures 90999

Dialysis, Extracorporeal
See Hemodialysis

Diaphragm
Assessment 58943, 58960
Contraception 57170
Imbrication
for Eventration 39545
Repair
Hernia 39540, 39541
Esophageal Hiatal 43280-43282, 43325
Neonatal 39503
Laceration 39501
Resection 39560, 39561
Unlisted Diaphragm Procedures 39599

Diaphragm Contraception
See Contraception, Diaphragm

Diaphysectomy
Calcaneus 28120
Clavicle 23180
Femur 27360
Fibula 27360, 27641
Humerus 23184, 24140
Metacarpal 26230
Metatarsal 28122
Olecranon Process 24147
Phalanges
Finger 26235, 26236
Toe 28124
Radius 24145, 25151
Scapula 23182
Talus 28120
Tarsal 28122
Tibia 27360, 27640
Ulna 24147, 25150

Diastase
See Amylase

Diastasis
See Separation
Pelvic Ring
Closed Treatment 27197, 27198

Diathermy
See Physical Medicine/Therapy/Occupational Therapy
Destruction
Ciliary Body 66700
Lesion
Retina 67208, 67227
Retinal Detachment
Prophylaxis 67141
Treatment 97024

Diathermy, Surgical
See Electrocautery

Dibucaine Number 82638

Dichloride, Methylene
See Dichloromethane

Dichlorides, Ethylene
See Dichloroethane

Diethylamide, Lysergic Acid
See Lysergic Acid Diethylamide

Diethylether 84600

Differential Count
See White Blood Cell, Count

Differentiation Reversal Factor
See Prothrombin

Diffusion Test, Gel
See Immunodiffusion

Digestive Tract
See Gastrointestinal Tract

Digit
See Finger; Toe
Destruction 64632
Injection 64455
Replantation 20816-20822

Digital Artery Sympathectomy 64820

Digital Slit-Beam Radiograph
See Scanogram

Digits
See Digit

Dihydroxyethanes
See Ethylene Glycol

Dihydroxyvitamin D 82652

Dilatation, Transluminal Arterial
See Angioplasty, Transluminal

Dilation
See Dilation and Curettage; Dilation and Evacuation
Anal
Endoscopy 46604
Sphincter 45905, 46940
Aortic Valve 33390, 33391
Bile Duct
Balloon 47542
Endoscopy 43277, 47555, 47556
Stricture 74363
with Stent Placement 47538-47540
Biliary Ampulla
Balloon 47542
Bladder
Cystourethroscopy 52260, 52265
Bronchi
Endoscopy 31630, 31636
Cerebral Vessels
Intracranial Vasospasm 61640-61642
Cervix
Canal 57800
Stump 57558
Colon
Endoscopy 45386
Colon-Sigmoid
Endoscopy 45340
Esophagus 43450, 43453
Balloon 43195, 43213, 43214, 43220, 43233, 43249
Endoscopy 43195, 43196, 43212, 43213, 43220, 43226, 43229, 43233, 43453
Gastric/Duodenal Stricture 43245
Surgical 43510
Intestines 44615
Endoscopy 44370
Stent Placement 44379, 44384, 44402
Kidney 50080, 50081
Intra-Renal Stricture 52343, 52346
Lacrimal Punctum 68801
Larynx
Endoscopy 31528, 31529
Nasolacrimal Duct
Balloon Catheter 68816
Nose
Balloon 31295-31297
Pancreatic Duct
Endoscopy 43277

Passage of Dilator
Esophagus 43248
Rectum
Endoscopy 45303, 45327, 45340, 45347, 45388, 45389
Transendoscopic Balloon 45386
Sphincter 45910
Renal Tract
Percutaneous 50436, 50437
Salivary Duct 42650, 42660
Sclera
Aqueous Outflow Canal 66174, 66175
Sinus Ostium 31295-31297
Sphincter of Oddi
Balloon 47542
Trachea
Endoscopy 31630, 31631, 31636, 31638
Ureter
Balloon 50706
Endoscopy 50553, 50572, 50575, 50953, 50972
with Cystourethroscopy 52341-52343
with Ureteroscopy 52344-52346
Urethra 52285, 52601, 52630, 52647-52649, 53660, 53661, 53665, 55801, 55821
Stenosis 52281
Stricture 52281, 53600, 53601, 53605, 53620, 53621, 53665
Vagina 57400

Dilation and Curettage
See Curettage; Dilation
Cervical Stump 57558
Cervix 57520, 57558
Corpus Uteri 58120
Induced Abortion 59840
with Amniotic Injections 59851
with Vaginal Suppository 59856
Postpartum 59160
with Amniotic Injections 59851
with Vaginal Suppositories 59856

Dilation and Evacuation 59841
Induced Abortion 59841
with Amniotic Injections 59851
with Vaginal Suppository 59856

Dioxide, Carbon
See Carbon Dioxide

Dioxide, Silicon
See Silica

Dipeptidyl Peptidase A
See Angiotensin Converting Enzyme (ACE)

Diphenylhydantoin
See Phenytoin

Diphosphate, Adenosine
See Adenosine Diphosphate

Diphtheria
See Vaccines and Toxoids
Antibody 86648

Dipropylacetic Acid
Assay 80164, 80165

Direct Pedicle Flap
Formation 15570, 15572, 15574, 15576
Transfer 15570, 15572, 15574, 15576, 15650

Disability Evaluation Services
Basic Life and/or Disability Examination 99450
Work-Related or Medical Disability Examination 99455, 99456

Disarticulation
Ankle 27889
Hip 27295
Knee 27598
Mandible 61590
Shoulder 23920
Wrist 25920

Disarticulation of Shoulder
See Shoulder, Disarticulation

Disc Chemolyses, Intervertebral
See Chemonucleolysis

Disc, Intervertebral
See Intervertebral Disc

Discectomies
See Arthroplasty; Discectomy

Discectomies, Percutaneous
See Discectomy, Percutaneous

Discectomy
Additional Segment 22226
Arthrodesis
Additional Interspace 22534, 22585, 22634
Cervical 22551, 22552, 22554, 22585
Lumbar 22533, 22534, 22558, 22585, 22630, 22899, 62380
Sacral 22586, 22899
Thoracic 22532, 22534, 22556, 22585, 63077, 63078
Cervical 0375T, 22220, 22551, 22552, 22554, 22856-22858, 63075, 63076
Lumbar 0163T, 0164T, 22224, 22630, 22633, 22634, 22857, 22899
Percutaneous 0274T, 0275T
Sacral 22586, 22899
Thoracic 22222
with End Plate Preparation 22856, 22858
with Osteophytectomy 0375T, 22856, 22858

Discharge Services
See Hospital Services
Hospital 99238, 99239
Newborn 99463
Nursing Facility 99315, 99316
Observation Care 99217, 99234, 99236

Discharge, Body Substance
See Drainage

Discission
Cataract
Laser Surgery 66821
Stab Incision 66820
Hyaloid Membrane 65810
Vitreous Strands 67030

Discography
Cervical Disc 72285
Injection 62290, 62291
Lumbar Disc 62287, 72295
Thoracic 72285

Discolysis
See Chemonucleolysis

Disease
Durand-Nicolas-Favre
See Lymphogranuloma Venereum
Erb-Goldflam
See Myasthenia Gravis
Heine-Medin
See Polio
Hydatid
See Echinococcosis
Lyme
See Lyme Disease
Ormond
See Retroperitoneal Fibrosis
Peyronie
See Peyronie Disease
Posada-Wernicke
See Coccidioidomycosis

Disease/Organ Panel
See Organ or Disease-Oriented Panel

Dislocated Elbow
See Dislocation, Elbow

Dislocated Hip
See Dislocation, Hip Joint

Dislocated Jaw
See Dislocation, Temporomandibular Joint

Dislocated Joint
See Dislocation

Dislocated Shoulder
See Dislocation, Shoulder

Dislocation
Acromioclavicular Joint
Closed Treatment 23540, 23545
Open Treatment 23550, 23552
Ankle
Closed Treatment 27840, 27842
Open Treatment 27846, 27848
Carpal
Closed Treatment 25690
Open Treatment 25695
Carpometacarpal Joint
Closed Treatment 26670, 26675
Open Treatment 26685, 26686
Percutaneous Fixation 26676
Thumb 26641
Bennett Fracture 26650, 26665
Elbow
Closed Treatment 24600, 24605
Monteggia 24620, 24635
Open Treatment 24586, 24587, 24615
Hip Joint
Closed Treatment 27250-27252, 27265, 27266
Congenital 27256-27259
Open Treatment 27253, 27254, 27258, 27259
without Trauma 27265, 27266
Interphalangeal Joint
Closed Treatment 26770, 26775, 28660, 28665
Open Treatment 26785, 28675
Percutaneous Fixation 26776, 28666
Knee 27560-27562
Closed Treatment 27550, 27552, 27560, 27562
Open Treatment 27556-27558, 27566, 27730
Recurrent 27420-27424
Leg
Knee 27560-27562
Closed Treatment 27550, 27552, 27560, 27562
Open Treatment 27556-27558, 27566, 27730
Recurrent 27420-27424
Patella
Closed Treatment 27560, 27562
Open Treatment 27566
Recurrent 27420, 27424
Tibiofibular Joint
Closed Treatment 27830, 27831
Open Treatment 27832

Index

Lunate
Closed Treatment . . . 25690
Open Treatment . . . 25695
with Manipulation . . . 25690
Metacarpophalangeal Joint
Closed Treatment . . . 26700-26706
Open Treatment . . . 26715
Percutaneous . . . 26705
Metatarsophalangeal Joint
Closed Treatment . . . 28630, 28635
Open Treatment . . . 28645
Percutaneous Fixation . . . 28636
Patella
Closed Treatment . . . 27560, 27562
Open Treatment . . . 27566
Recurrent . . . 27420, 27424
Pelvic Ring
Closed Treatment . . . 27197, 27198
Open Treatment . . . 27217, 27218
Percutaneous Fixation . . . 27216
with Manipulation . . . 27198
without Manipulation . . . 27197
Peroneal Tendons . . . 27675, 27676
Radiocarpal
Closed Treatment . . . 25660
Open Treatment . . . 25670
Radioulnar
Closed Treatment . . . 25675
Open Treatment . . . 25676
Radioulnar Joint
Closed Treatment . . . 25520
Galeazzi . . . 25520, 25525, 25526
Open Treatment . . . 25525, 25526
Radius
Closed Treatment . . . 24640
with Fracture
Closed Treatment . . . 24620
Open Treatment . . . 24635
Shoulder
Closed Treatment with Manipulation . . . 23650, 23655
Open Treatment . . . 23660
with Greater Tuberosity Fracture
Closed Treatment . . . 23665
Open Treatment . . . 23670
with Surgical or Anatomical Neck Fracture
Closed Treatment . . . 23675
Open Treatment . . . 23680
Skin
Debridement . . . 11010-11012
Sternoclavicular Joint
Closed Treatment
with Manipulation . . . 23525
without Manipulation . . . 23520
Open Treatment . . . 23530, 23532
Talotarsal Joint
Closed Treatment . . . 28570, 28575
Open Treatment . . . 28585
Percutaneous Fixation . . . 28576
Tarsal
Closed Treatment . . . 28540, 28545
Open Treatment . . . 28555
Percutaneous Fixation . . . 28546
Tarsometatarsal Joint
Closed Treatment . . . 28600, 28605
Open Treatment . . . 28615
Percutaneous Fixation . . . 28606
Temporomandibular Joint
Closed Treatment . . . 21480, 21485
Open Treatment . . . 21490
Thumb
Closed Treatment . . . 26641, 26645
Open Treatment . . . 26665
Percutaneous Fixation . . . 26650
with Fracture . . . 26645
Open Treatment . . . 26665
Percutaneous Fixation . . . 26650
with Manipulation . . . 26641, 26645, 26650
Tibiofibular Joint
Closed Treatment . . . 27830, 27831
Open Treatment . . . 27832
Toe
Closed Treatment . . . 26770, 26775, 28630-28635
Open Treatment . . . 28645
Percutaneous Fixation . . . 26776, 28636
Trans-Scaphoperilunar
Closed Treatment . . . 25680
Open Treatment . . . 25685
Vertebra
Additional Segment
Open Treatment . . . 22328
Cervical
Open Treatment . . . 22318, 22319, 22326
Closed Treatment
with Manipulation, Casting and/or Bracing . . . 22315
Lumbar
Open Treatment . . . 22325
Thoracic
Open Treatment . . . 22327
Wrist
Closed Treatment . . . 25660, 25675, 25680
Intercarpal . . . 25660
Open Treatment . . . 25670
Open Treatment . . . 25670, 25685
Percutaneous Fixation . . . 25671
Radiocarpal . . . 25660
Open Treatment . . . 25670
Radioulnar
Closed Treatment . . . 25675
Open Treatment . . . 25676
Percutaneous Fixation . . . 25671
with Fracture
Closed Treatment . . . 25680
Open Treatment . . . 25685
with Manipulation . . . 25660, 25675, 25680

Dislocation, Radiocarpal Joint
See Radiocarpal Joint, Dislocation

Disorder
Blood Coagulation
See Coagulopathy
Penis
See Penis
Retinal
See Retina

Displacement Therapy
Nose . . . 30210

Dissection
Axial Vessel
for Island Pedicle . . . 15740
Cavernous Sinus . . . 61613
Cranial Adhesions . . . 62161
Donor Organ
Heart . . . 33944
Heart/Lung . . . 33933
Kidney . . . 50323, 50325
Liver . . . 47143
Lung . . . 32855
Pancreas . . . 48551
Facial Nerve . . . 42420
for Debulking . . . 58952, 58953
Hygroma, Cystic
Axillary/Cervical . . . 38550, 38555
Infrarenal Aneurysm . . . 34701-34706, 34709-34711, 34830-34832
Lymph Nodes . . . 38542
Mediastinal . . . 60521, 60522
Neck
See Radical Neck Dissection
Neurovascular . . . 32503
Sclera . . . 67107
Urethra . . . 54328, 54332, 54336, 54348, 54352

Dissection, Neck, Radical
See Radical Neck Dissection

Distention
See Dilation

Diverticula, Meckel's
See Diverticulum, Meckel's

Diverticulectomy . . . 44800
Cervical Esophagus . . . 43180
Esophagus . . . 43130, 43135, 43180
Hypopharynx . . . 43180

Diverticulectomy, Meckel's
See Meckel's Diverticulum, Excision

Diverticulum
Bladder
See Bladder, Diverticulum
Large Intestine . . . 44604, 44605
Meckel's
Excision . . . 44800
Unlisted Procedure . . . 44899
Small Intestine . . . 44602, 44603
Urethra
Excision . . . 53230, 53235
Marsupialization . . . 53240
Urethroplasty . . . 53400, 53405

Division
Anal Sphincter . . . 46080
Flap . . . 15600, 15610, 15620, 15630
Intrauterine Septum . . . 58560
Muscle
Foot . . . 28250
Neck
Scalenus Anticus . . . 21700, 21705
Sternocleidomastoid . . . 21720, 21725
Plantar Fascia
Foot . . . 28250
Rectal Stricture . . . 45150
Saphenous Vein . . . 37700, 37722, 37735
Symblepharon . . . 68340

Division, Isthmus, Horseshoe Kidney
See Symphysiotomy, Horseshoe Kidney

Division, Scalenus Anticus Muscle . . . 21700, 21705

DNA
See Deoxyribonucleic Acid (DNA)

DNA Endonuclease
See DNAse

DNA Probe
See Cytogenetic Study, DNA Probe

DNAse
Antibody . . . 86215

Domiciliary Services
See Nursing Facility Services
Care Plan Oversight . . . 99339, 99340
Discharge Services . . . 99315, 99316
Established Patient . . . 99334-99337
New Patient . . . 99324-99328
Supervision . . . 99374, 99375

Donor Procedures
- *See* Harvesting
- Bone Harvesting . . . 20900-20902
- Bone Marrow Harvesting . . . 38230, 38232
- Conjunctival Graft . . . 68371
- Heart Excision . . . 33940
- Heart/Lung Excision . . . 33930
- Intestine Excision . . . 44132, 44133
- Kidney Excision . . . 50300, 50320
- Liver Excision . . . 47133
  - Segment . . . 47140-47142
- Lung Excision . . . 32850
- Mucosa of Vestibule of Mouth Excision . . . 40818
- Pancreas Excision . . . 48550
- Preparation of Fecal Microbiota . . . 44705
- Stem Cells . . . 38204
  - Donor Search . . . 38204
  - Harvesting . . . 38205, 38206

Dopamine
- *See* Catecholamines

Doppler Echocardiography . . . 76827, 76828, 93306-93308, 93320-93350
- Intracardiac . . . 93662
- Transesophageal . . . 93318
- Transthoracic . . . 93303-93317

Doppler Scan
- Arterial Studies
  - Coronary Flow Reserve . . . 93571, 93572
  - Extremities . . . 93922-93924
  - Fetal
    - Middle Cerebral Artery . . . 76821
    - Umbilical Artery . . . 76820
- Duplex
  - Transplanted Kidney . . . 76776
- Intracranial Arteries
  - Complete Study . . . 93886
  - Emboli Detection . . . 93892, 93893
  - Limited Study . . . 93888
  - Vasoreactivity Study . . . 93890
- Saline Infusion Sonohysterography (SIS) . . . 76831
- Transplanted Kidney . . . 76776

Dorsal Vertebra
- *See* Vertebra, Thoracic

Dose Plan
- *See* Dosimetry

Dosimetry
- Radiation Therapy
  - Basic Calculation . . . 77300
    - Oncology . . . 0520F
  - Brachytherapy . . . 77316-77318
  - Intensity Modulated Radiation Treatment (IMRT) . . . 77301, 77338, 77385, 77386
  - Special . . . 77331
  - Teletherapy . . . 77306, 77307, 77321
- Unlisted Radiation Dosimetry Procedure . . . 77399

Double-Stranded DNA
- *See* Deoxyribonucleic Acid (DNA)

DPH
- *See* Phenytoin

Drainage
- *See* Incision and Drainage; Paracentesis; Puncture Aspiration
- Abscess
  - Anal . . . 46045, 46050, 46060
  - Ankle . . . 27603
  - Appendix . . . 44900
  - Arm, Upper . . . 23930
  - Auditory Canal . . . 69020
  - Bartholin's Gland . . . 56420
  - Brain . . . 61150, 61151, 61320, 61321
  - Breast . . . 19020
  - Dentoalveolar Structures . . . 41800
  - Ear, External . . . 69000, 69005
  - Elbow . . . 23930
  - Eyelid . . . 67700
  - Finger . . . 26010, 26011
    - Tendon Sheath . . . 26020
  - Forearm . . . 25028
  - Knee . . . 27301
  - Leg . . . 27603
  - Liver . . . 47010
  - Lung . . . 31645, 31646, 32200
  - Lymph Node . . . 38300, 38305
  - Mouth
    - Lingual . . . 41000
    - Masticator Space . . . 41009, 41018
    - Sublingual . . . 41005, 41006, 41015, 42310
    - Submandibular Space . . . 41008, 41017
    - Submaxillary . . . 42310, 42320
    - Submental Space . . . 41007, 41016
  - Neck . . . 21501, 21502
  - Nasal . . . 30000
  - Nasal Septum . . . 30020
  - Ovary . . . 58820, 58822
  - Palate . . . 42000
  - Parotid . . . 42300, 42305
  - Pelvic . . . 45000
    - Supralevator . . . 45020
  - Perineal . . . 56405
  - Perirenal . . . 50020
  - Peritoneal . . . 49020
  - Peritonsillar . . . 42700
  - Pharyngeal . . . 42720, 42725
  - Prostate . . . 52700, 55720, 55725
  - Rectum . . . 45005, 46040
    - Supralevator . . . 45020
  - Renal . . . 50020
  - Retroperitoneal . . . 49060, 49323
  - Shoulder . . . 23030
  - Skene's Gland . . . 53060
  - Soft Tissue
    - Percutaneous . . . 10030
    - Subfascial . . . 22010, 22015
  - Subdiaphragmatic . . . 49040
  - Subphrenic . . . 49040
  - Spine
    - Subfascial . . . 22010, 22015
  - Thigh . . . 27301
  - Thorax . . . 21501, 21502
  - Urethra . . . 53040
  - Uvula . . . 42000
  - Vestibule of Mouth . . . 40800, 40801
  - Vulva . . . 56405
  - with X ray . . . 75989
  - Wrist . . . 25028
- Abscess, Superficial . . . 10060, 10061
- Bile Duct . . . 47533-47540
- Biliary Tract . . . 47400, 47420, 47425, 47480
  - Catheterization . . . 47533, 47534
- Bladder . . . 51040, 51080
- Brain . . . 62160, 62162, 62164
- Bursa
  - Arm, Upper . . . 23930
  - Elbow . . . 23930
  - Foot . . . 28001-28003
  - Forearm . . . 25028
  - Hip . . . 26990
  - Knee . . . 27301
  - Leg . . . 27604
  - Palm . . . 26025, 26030
  - Pelvis . . . 26990
  - Shoulder . . . 23031
  - Thigh . . . 27301
  - Wrist . . . 25028
- Catheter
  - *See* Catheter, Drainage
- Cyst
  - Brain . . . 61150, 61151, 62162
  - Breast . . . 19000, 19001
  - Conjunctiva . . . 68020
  - Dentoalveolar Structures . . . 41800
  - Intramedullary . . . 63172-63172
  - Liver . . . 47010
  - Lung . . . 32200
  - Mouth
    - Lingual . . . 41000
    - Masticator Space . . . 41009, 41018
    - Sublingual . . . 41005, 41006, 41015
    - Submandibular Space . . . 41008, 41017
    - Submental Space . . . 41007, 41016
  - Ovary . . . 58800, 58805
  - Pilonidal . . . 10080, 10081
  - Skene's Gland . . . 53060
  - Vestibule of Mouth . . . 40800, 40801
- Empyema
  - Chest . . . 32036, 32810
- Elbow . . . 23930
- Eye . . . 0191T, 0253T, 0376T, 66183
  - Lacrimal Gland . . . 68400
  - Lacrimal Sac . . . 68420
  - Paracentesis
    - *See* Paracentesis, Eye
- Fluid
  - Abdominal . . . 49082, 49083
  - Amniotic Fluid . . . 59001
  - Cerebrospinal . . . 62272
    - Spinal Cord . . . 62272
  - Fetal . . . 59074
  - Hand (Finger or Palm)
    - Tendon Sheath . . . 26020
  - Peritoneal
    - Percutaneous . . . 49406
    - Transrectal . . . 49407
    - Transvaginal . . . 49407
  - Retinal . . . 67108, 67113
  - Retroperitoneal
    - Percutaneous . . . 49406
    - Transrectal . . . 49407
    - Transvaginal . . . 49407
  - Visceral
    - Percutaneous . . . 49405
- Hematoma
  - Ankle . . . 27603
  - Brain . . . 61108, 61154, 61156
  - Dentoalveolar Structures . . . 41800
  - Ear, External . . . 69000, 69005
  - Forearm . . . 25028
  - Knee . . . 27301
  - Leg . . . 27603
  - Mouth
    - Lingual . . . 41000
    - Masticator Space . . . 41009, 41018
    - Sublingual . . . 41005, 41006, 41015
    - Submandibular Space . . . 41008, 41017
    - Submental Space . . . 41007, 41016
  - Nasal . . . 30000
  - Nasal Septum . . . 30020
  - Shoulder . . . 23030
  - Subungual . . . 11740
  - Vagina . . . 57022, 57023
  - Vestibule of Mouth . . . 40800, 40801
  - Wrist . . . 25028
- Hematoma, Superficial . . . 10140

Joint
Acromioclavicular . . . 23040
Ankle . . . 27610
Carpometacarpal . . . 26070
Glenohumeral . . . 23040
Hip . . . 26990, 27030
Interphalangeal . . . 26080, 28024
Intertarsal . . . 28022
Knee . . . 29871
Metacarpophalangeal . . . 26075
Metatarsophalangeal . . . 28022
Midcarpal . . . 25040
Pelvis . . . 26990
Radiocarpal . . . 25040
Sternoclavicular . . . 23044
Thigh . . . 27301
Wrist . . . 29843
Knee . . . 27310
Kidney . . . 50040
Lymph Node . . . 38300, 38305
Lymphocele
Peritoneal . . . 49062, 49323
Mediastinum . . . 39000
Onychia . . . 10060, 10061
Orbit . . . 67405, 67440
Pancreas
See Anastomosis, Pancreas to Intestines
Pseudocyst . . . 48510
Paronychia . . . 10060, 10061
Pelvis . . . 50125, 50433
Penis . . . 54015
Pericardial Sac . . . 32659
Pericardium . . . 33025
Peritonitis . . . 49020
Pleura . . . 32556, 32557
Postoperative Wound Infection . . . 10180
Pseudocyst
Gastrointestinal, Upper . . . 43240
Pancreas . . . 48510
Radiological Guidance . . . 75989
Rectum
Injury . . . 45562
Seroma
Skin . . . 10140
Syrinx
Intramedullary . . . 63172-63172
Ureter . . . 50600
Urethra
Extravasation . . . 53080-53085
Venous
Sinus Venosus . . . 33645
via Tube Thoracostomy . . . 32551

Drainage Implant, Glaucoma
See Aqueous Shunt

Dressings
Burns . . . 16020, 16025, 16030
Change
Anesthesia . . . 15852

DREZ Procedure
See Incision, Spinal Cord; Incision and Drainage

DRIL
See Revascularization, Distal Revascularization and Interval Ligation (DRIL)

Drill Hole
Skull . . . 61105
for Catheter . . . 61107
for Drainage of Hematoma . . . 61108
for Implantation of Electrode . . . 61850, 61863, 61864
for Implantation of Electrode Array . . . 61867, 61868
for Intracerebral Monitoring Device . . . 61107
for Pressure Recording Device . . . 61107

Drinking Test for Glaucoma
See Glaucoma, Provocative Test

Drug
Administration
Allergenic Extracts
See Allergen Immunotherapy
for Cancer
See Chemotherapy
for Cardiac Assessments . . . 93463
for Helicobacter Pylori Breath Test . . . 83014
Infusion
Epidural . . . 62360-62362
Home . . . 99601, 99602
Intravenous . . . 4100F, 96365-96368
Injection . . . 96372-96376
Instillation
See Instillation, Drugs
Unlisted Injection or Infusion . . . 96379
Analysis
See Pathology and Laboratory, Chemistry
Monitoring
Prescription Drug . . . 0011U, 0051U, 0054U
Procedure
See Drug Assay, Drug Procedure
Resistance Analysis
HIV 1 . . . 87903, 87904
Susceptibility Prediction
Infectious Agent . . . 87900
Quantitative
See Drug Assay

Drug Assay
Drug Procedure
Definitive Drug Class
6-Acetylmorphine . . . 80356
Acetylcodeine . . . 80356
Alcohols . . . 80320
Alcohol Biomarkers . . . 80321, 80322
Alkaloids, Not Otherwise Specified . . . 80323
Amphetamines . . . 80324-80326
Anabolic Steroids . . . 80327, 80328
Analgesics, Non Opioid . . . 80329-80331
Antidepressants
Not Otherwise Specified . . . 80338
Serotonergic Class . . . 80332-80334
Tricyclic and Other Cyclicals . 80335-80337
Antiepileptics, Not Otherwise Specified . . . 80339-80341
Antipsychotics, Not Otherwise Specified . . . 80342-80344
Barbiturates . . . 80345
Benzodiazepines . . . 80346, 80347
Buprenorphine; . . . 80348
Cannabinoids
Natural . . . 80349
Synthetic . . . 80350-80352
Cocaine . . . 80353
Codeine . . . 80361
Diacetylmorphine . . . 80356
Drug(s) or Substance(s), Definitive, Qualitative or Quantitative, Not Otherwise Specified . . . 80375-80377
Fentanyl . . . 80354
Gabapentin, Non-blood . . . 80355
Heroin Metabolite . . . 80356
Ketamine and Norketamine . . . 80357
Methadone . . . 80358
Methylenedioxyamphetamines (MDA, MDEA, MDMA) . . . 80359
Methylphenidate . . . 80360
Opiates, 1 or more . . . 80361
Opioids and Opiate Analogs . . . 80362-80364
Oxycodone . . . 80365
Pregabalin . . . 80366
Propoxyphene . . . 80367
Sedative Hypnotics (non benzodiazepines) . . . 80368
Skeletal Muscle Relaxants . . . 80369, 80370
Stimulants, Synthetic . . . 80371
Tapentadol . . . 80372
Tramadol . . . 80373
Stereoisomer (Enantiomer) Analysis, Single Drug Class . . . 80374
Presumptive Drug Class . . 80305-80307, 0007U
Interactions . . . 0006U
Therapeutic Drug Assay
See Therapeutic Drug Assay

Drug Delivery Implant
See Infusion Pump
Insertion . . . 11981
Irrigation . . . 96523
Maintenance and Refill
Brain . . . 95990, 95991
Epidural . . . 95990, 95991
Intra-arterial . . . 96522
Intrathecal . . . 95990, 95991
Intravenous . . . 96522
Intraventricular . . . 95990, 95991
Removal . . . 11982, 11983
with Reinsertion . . . 11983

Drug Instillation
See Instillation, Drugs

Drug Management
by Pharmacist . . . 99605-99607
Psychiatric . . . 90863

Drug Screen
See Drug Assay

Drugs, Anticoagulant
See Anticoagulant Management; Clotting Inhibitors

DST
See Dexamethasone, Suppression Panel

DT Shots
Diphtheria and Tetanus Toxoids (DT) . . . 90702
Diphtheria and Tetanus Toxoids, Acellular Pertussis, Haemophilus Influenza Type b, and Inactivated Poliovirus (DTaP-IPV/Hib) . . . 90698
Diphtheria and Tetanus Toxoids, Acellular Pertussis, Inactivated Poliovirus, Haemophilus Influenzae type b PRP-OMP Conjugate, and Hepatitis B (DTaP-IPV-Hib-HepB) . . . 90697

DTaP Immunization . . . 90700

DTaP-HepB-IPV Immunization . . . 90723

Dual Photon Absorptiometry
See Absorptiometry, X-ray, (DXA), Bone Density Study, Dual Energy

Dual X-ray Absorptiometry (DXA)
Appendicular . . . 77081
Axial Skeleton . . . 77080
Vertebral Fracture . . . 77085, 77086

Duct, Bile
See Bile Duct

Duct, Hepatic
See Hepatic Duct

Duct, Nasolacrimal
See Nasolacrimal Duct

Duct, Omphalomesenteric
See Omphalomesenteric Duct

Duct, Pancreatic
See Pancreatic Duct

Duct, Salivary
See Salivary Duct

Duct, Stensen
See Parotid Duct

Duct, Thoracic
See Thoracic, Duct

Ductogram, Mammary
See Galactogram

Ductus Arteriosus
Closure
  Transcatheter Percutaneous 93582
Repair 33820, 33824

Ductus Deferens
See Vas Deferens

Duhamel Procedure
See Proctectomy, Total

Dunn Operation
See Arthrodesis, Foot Joint

Duodenectomy
Partial 48153, 48154
Total 48150, 48152

Duodenostomy
Contrast Injection 49465
Insertion 49441
Obstructive Material Removal 49460
Radiological Evaluation 49465
Replacement 49451

Duodenotomy
Biopsy 43239, 44010
  Fine Needle Aspiration 43242
Exploration 44010
Foreign Body Removal 44010

Duodenum
Bariatric Surgery
  See Bariatric Surgery
Biopsy 43239, 44010
  Fine Needle Aspiration 43242
Donor Transplant 48550, 48551
Duodenostomy
  See Duodenostomy
Endoscopy 43233, 43235
  Catheter Placement 43241
  Cholangiopancreatography 43260
  Diagnostic 43235
  Dilation 43245
  Drainage, Pseudocyst 43240
  Examination 43259
    Ultrasound 43253
  Foreign Body Removal 43247, 43275
  with Control of Bleeding 43255
  with Injection
    Sclerotic Varix 43243
    Submucosal 43236, 43253
  with Ligation
    Sclerotic Varix 43244
  with Lithotripsy 43265
Excision 48150, 48152-48154
Exclusion 48547
Exploration 44010
Foreign Body Removal 44010
Incision 44010
Intubation and Aspiration 43756, 43757
Lysis 44055
Motility Study 91022
Naso- or Oro-gastric Feeding Tube
Repositioning 43761
Removal
  Lesion 43250, 43251
  Polyp 43250, 43251
  Tumor 43250, 43251
X ray 74260
Contrast Injection 49465

Duplex Scan
See Vascular Studies
Arterial Studies
  Aorta 93978, 93979
  Extracranial 93880-93882
  Lower Extremity 93925, 93926
  Penile 93980, 93981
  Upper Extremity 93930, 93931
  Visceral 93975-93979
Doppler
  See Doppler Scan, Duplex
Hemodialysis Access 93990
Venous Studies
  Extremity 93970, 93971
  Penile 93980, 93981

Dupuy-Dutemps Operation
See Reconstruction, Eyelid; Revision

Dupuytren's Contracture
Fasciotomy
  Open, Partial 26045
  Percutaneous 26040
Injection
  Enzyme 20527
Manipulation 26341
Palmar Fascial Cord
  Injection
    Enzyme 20527
  Manipulation 26341
Surgical Pathology 88304

Durand-Nicolas-Favre Disease
See Lymphogranuloma Venereum

Dust, Angel
See Phencyclidine

Duvries Operation
See Tenoplasty

Dwyer Procedure
See Osteotomy, Calcaneus

DXA
See Dual X-ray Absorptiometry (DXA)

Dynamometry
See Osteotomy, Calcaneus
Venous Studies
  See Osteotomy, Calcaneus
with Ophthalmoscopy 92260

E

E Antigens
See Hepatitis Antigen, Detection, Immunoassay, Be (HBeAg)

E B Virus
See Epstein-Barr Virus

E Vitamin
See Tocopherol

E1
See Estrone

E2
See Estradiol

E3
See Estriol

Ear
Collection of Blood 36416
Drum
  See Tympanic Membrane
External Ear
  Biopsy 69100, 69105
  Blood Specimen Collection 36416
  Debridement
    Mastoidectomy Cavity 69220-69222
  Drainage
    Abscess 69000, 69005
    Hematoma 69000, 69005
  Excision
    Partial 69110
    Total 69120
  Exostosis Excision 69140
  Graft
    See Graft, Ear
  Lesion
    Destruction, Malignant 17280
    Excision 11400-11444, 11446, 69145, 69150, 69155
    Excision, Malignant ... 11640-11644, 11646
    Shaving 11310
  Mastoid
    See Mastoid
  Piercing 69090
  Reconstruction
    External Auditory Canal 69310, 69320
    Protruding Ear 69300
    with Tissue Transfer 14060, 14061
  Prosthesis, Custom 21086
  Removal
    Foreign Body 69200, 69205
    Impacted Cerumen 69209, 69210
  Repair
    Complex 13151, 13152, 13153
    Intermediate 12051
    Simple 12011
    Superficial 12011
  Tympanic Membrane
    See Tympanic Membrane
  Unlisted Services and Procedures 69399
Inner Ear
  CT Scan 70480-70482
  Endolymphatic Sac 69805, 69806
  Insertion
    Cochlear Device 69930
  Labyrinth
    Excision 69905, 69910
    Incision for Perfusion 69801
  Unlisted Services and Procedures 69949
  Vertigo
    See Canalith Repositioning
  Vestibular Nerve Section 69915
Meatoplasty 69310
  for Congenital Atresia 69320
Middle Ear
  CT Scan 70480-70482
  Exploration 69440
  Excision
    Polyp 69540
    Glomus Tumor 69550, 69552, 69554
  Facial Nerve Decompression 69720, 69725
  Facial Nerve Suture 69740, 69745

Optical Coherence Tomography. . 0485T, 0486T
Repair
Fistula 69666, 69667
Stapes
Mobilization 69650
Stapedectomy.............. 69660-69662
Stapedotomy 69660-69662
Tumor
Excision............. 69550, 69552, 69554
Temporal Bone
Bone Conduction Hearing Device
Implantation 69710
Removal 69711
Repair.......................... 69711
Osseointegrated Implant
Implantation............... 69714, 69715
Removal 69717
Replacement..................... 69717
Resection 69535
Unlisted Services and Procedures...... 69799

Ear Canal
See Auditory Canal

Ear Cartilage
Graft
Autogenous
Ear Cartilage to Nose or Ear......... 21235
Rib Cartilage to Ear 21230

Ear Lobes
Pierce 69090

Ear Protector Attenuation
Measurements 92596
See Hearing Aid Services

Ear Wax
See Cerumen

Ear, Nose, and Throat
Audiologic Function Tests
See Audiologic Function Tests
Audiometry
See Audiometry
Binocular Microscopy 92504
Diagnostic Analysis
Auditory Brainstem Implant........... 92640
Cochlear Implant 92601-92604
Evaluation
Auditory Rehabilitation Status 92626, 92627, 92630, 92633
Language Comprehension and Expression 92523
Laryngeal Sensory Testing...... 92614-92617
Prescription of Communication Device
Non-speech-generating 92605, 92618
Speech-generating.......... 92607, 92608
Speech Fluency 92521
Speech Sound Production 92522
Swallowing 92610-92613, 92616
Voice and Resonance
Behavioral Analysis 92524
Examination under Anesthesia............ 92502
Facial Nerve Function Study............. 92516
Laryngeal Function Study 92520
Nasal Function Study 92512
Nasopharyngoscopy 92511
Treatment
Hearing, Language and Speech Disorder 92507, 92508
Oral Function for Feeding............. 92526
Swallowing Dysfunction 92526

Use and Programming of Communication Device
Non-speech-generating 92606
Speech-generating................ 92609
Vestibular Function Tests
See Vestibular Function Tests

Ebstein Anomaly Repair
Tricuspid Valve 33468

Eccrine Glands
Chemodenervation
Axillae 64650
Feet 64999
Hands............................ 64999
Other Area 64653

ECG
See Electrocardiography

Echinococcosis.............. 86171, 86280

Echocardiography
Doppler
See Doppler Echocardiography
Congenital Cardiac Anomaly
Fetal....................... 76825, 76826
Doppler, Fetal................ 76827, 76828
Transesophageal 93315-93317
Transthoracic 93303, 93304
Intracardiac........................... 93662
Myocardial
Contrast Perfusion.................. 0439T
Transesophageal........... 93312-93318, 93355
Transthoracic 93306-93308, 93350-93352
Congenital Cardiac Anomalies . . 93303, 93304
with Stress Test 93350-93352

Echoencephalography
Intracranial 76506

Echography
See Ultrasound

Echotomography
See Echography

Extracorporeal Life Support (ECLS)
See Extracorporeal Membrane Oxygenation (ECMO)

ECMO
See Extracorporeal Membrane Oxygenation (ECMO)

ECS
See Emission Computerized Tomography

ECSF (Erythrocyte Colony Stimulating Factor)
See Erythropoietin

ECT
See Emission Computerized Tomography

Ectasia
See Dilation

Ectopic Pregnancy
See Obstetrical Care
Abdominal............................ 59130
Cervix 59140
Laparoscopy 59150
with Salpingectomy and/or Oophorectomy 59151
Ovarian 59121
with Salpingectomy and/or Oophorectomy 59120
Tubal 59121
with Salpingectomy and/or Oophorectomy 59120

Uterine
with Hysterectomy.................. 59135
with Partial Uterine Resection......... 59136

Ectropion
Repair
Excision Tarsal Wedge 67916
Extensive 67917
Suture............................ 67914
Thermocauterization 67915

Education Services
Group.................... 98961, 98962, 99078
Individual
Pediatric Gastroenteritis Education..... 4058F

Education Supplies
Provided to Patient 99071

EEG
See Electroencephalography (EEG)

Egg
See Ova

Ehrlichia
Antibody 86666

EKG
See Electrocardiography

Elastase 82656

Elastography
Magnetic Resonance 76391
Ultrasound................ 76979, 76981-76983

Elbow
See Humerus; Radius; Ulna
Abscess
Incision and Drainage 23930, 23935
Anesthesia
See Anesthesia, Elbow
Arthrectomy 24155
Arthrocentesis.................. 20605, 20606
Arthrodesis 24800, 24802
Arthrography.......................... 73085
Contrast Injection.................. 24220
Arthroplasty 24360
Total Replacement............ 24361-24363, 24365, 24366
Prosthesis Removal 24160, 24164
Revision 24370, 24371
with Implant............... 24361, 24362
Arthroscopy
Diagnostic 29830
Surgical 29834-29838
Arthrotomy 24000
Capsular Release................... 24006
Drainage.......................... 24000
Exploration................. 24000, 24101
Removal of Foreign Body............. 24000
Synovectomy 24102
Synovial Biopsy 24100
Biopsy 24065, 24066, 24101
Synovial 24100, 29830
Bone Cortex Incision.................... 23935
Capsule
Excision 24006
Radical Resection 24149
Contracture Release.................... 24149
Dislocation
Closed Treatment....... 24600, 24605, 24640
Nursemaid Elbow.................. 24640
Open Treatment.................... 24615
Subluxate......................... 24640
Epicondylitis 24357-24359

Excision
Bursa . . . 24105
Synovium . . . 24102, 29835, 29836
Tumor
Soft Tissue . . . 24077, 24079
Subcutaneous . . . 24071, 24075
Subfascial . . . 24076
Exploration . . . 24000, 24101
Fracture
Monteggia . . . 24620, 24635
Open Treatment . . . 24586, 24587
Hematoma
Incision and Drainage . . . 23930
Incision and Drainage
Abscess, Deep . . . 23930
Bursa . . . 23931
Hematoma . . . 23930
Injection
Arthrography
Radiological . . . 24220
Magnetic Resonance Imaging (MRI) . . . 73221
Manipulation . . . 24300
Prosthesis
Removal
Humeral and Ulnar Components . . . 24160
Radial Head . . . 24164
Resection
Capsule . . . 24149
Heterotropic Bone . . . 24149
Joint . . . 24155
Soft Tissue . . . 24149
with Contracture Release . . . 24149
Removal
Foreign Body . . . 24000, 24101, 24200, 24201, 29834
Loose Body . . . 24101, 29834
Prosthesis . . . 24160
Repair
Advancement . . . 24330, 24331
Epicondylitis . . . 24357-24359
Flexorplasty . . . 24330
Graft . . . 24320
Hemiepiphyseal Arrest . . . 24470
Ligament . . . 24343-24346
Muscle . . . 24341
Muscle Transfer . . . 24301, 24320
Tendon . . . 24340-24342, 24357-24359
Lengthening . . . 24305
Repair . . . 24341, 24359
Tenodesis . . . 24340
Tenotomy . . . 24310, 24357-24359
Transfer . . . 24301
Tennis Elbow . . . 24357-24359
Seddon-Brookes Procedure . . . 24320
Steindler Advancement . . . 24330
Strapping . . . 29260
Tumor
Soft Tissue
Excision . . . 24071-24076
Radical Resection . . . 24077-24079
Ulnar Neuroplasty . . . 64718
Unlisted Elbow Procedure . . . 24999
X ray . . . 73070, 73080
with Contrast . . . 73085

Elbow, Golfer
See Elbow, Repair, Tendon; Tennis Elbow, Tenotomy

Elbows, Tennis
See Elbow, Repair, Tendon; Tennis Elbow, Tenotomy

Electric Countershock
See Cardioversion

Electric Stimulation
See Electrical Stimulation

Electric Stimulation, Transcutaneous
See Application, Neurostimulation

Electrical Modulation Pain Reprocessing, Transcutaneous . . . 0278T

Electrical Stimulation
Acupuncture . . . 97813, 97814
Arrhythmia Induction . . . 93618
Bone Healing
Invasive . . . 20975
Noninvasive . . . 20974
Brain Surface . . . 95961, 95962
Guidance
for Chemodenervation . . . 95873
Physical Therapy
Attended, Manual . . . 97032
Unattended . . . 97014
Spine . . 63650, 63655, 63661-63664, 63685, 63688

Electro-Hydraulic Procedure . . . 52325

Electro-Oculography . . . 92270

Electroanalgesia
See Application, Neurostimulation

Electrocardiography
12 Lead . . . 3120F, 93000
Evaluation . . . 93000, 93010, 93660
External Recording
Auto-Activated . . . 93268, 93270-93272
Holter Monitors
Up to 48 Hours of Continuous Monitoring . . . 93224-93227
Interpretation . . . 93272, 0295T, 0298T
Mobile
More than 24 Hours . . . 93228, 93229
More than 48 Hours up to 21 Days . . . 0295T-0298T
Patient-Activated . . . 0497T, 0498T, 93268, 93270-93272
Transmission and Evaluation . . . 93268, 93270, 93271
Up to 30 Days . . . 93268, 93270-93272
Up to 48 Hours Duration . . . 93224-93229
Rhythm
Evaluation . . . 93042
Microvolt T-wave Alternans . . . 93025
Recording . . . 0295T, 0296T
Scanning Analysis with Report . . 0295T, 0297T
Tracing . . . 93005, 93041
Tracing and Evaluation . . . 93040
Signal Averaged . . . 93278
Symptom-Related Memory Loop . . . 93268, 93270-93272

Electrocautery
Inferior Turbinates Soft Tissue . . . 30801, 30802
Prostate Resection . . . 52601
Ureteral Stricture . . . 52341-52346

Electrochemistry
See Electrolysis

Electroconvulsive Therapy . . . 90870

Electrocorticogram
from Implanted Brain Neurostimulator . . . 95836
Intraoperative . . . 61536, 61538, 95829

Electrode, Depth
See Depth Electrode

Electrodesiccation . . . 17000-17286
Lesion
Penis . . . 54055

Electroejaculation
Reproductive . . . 55870

Electroencephalography (EEG)
Brain Death . . . 95824
Coma . . . 95822
Digital Analysis . . . 95957
Electrode Placement . . . 95830
Intraoperative . . . 95955
Monitoring . . . 95812, 95813, 95950-95953, 95956
with Drug Activation . . . 95954
with Physical Activation . . . 95954
with WADA Activation . . . 95958
Standard . . . 95819

Electrogastrography . . . 91132, 91133

Electrogram, Atrial
Esophageal Recording . . . 93615, 93616

Electrolysis . . . 17380

Electromyographs
See Electromyography, Needle

Electromyography
Anorectal with Biofeedback . . . 90911
Fine Wire
Dynamic . . . 96004
Needle
Cranial Nerve Supplied Muscle . . 95867, 95868
Extremities . . . 95860-95864
Extremity . . . 95860, 95885, 95886
Face and Neck Muscles . . . 95867, 95868
Guidance
for Chemodenervation . . . 64617, 95874
Hemidiaphragm . . . 95866
Larynx . . . 95865
Non-extremity . . . 95887
Ocular . . . 92265
Other than Thoracic Paraspinal . . . 95870
Single Fiber Electrode . . . 95872
Thoracic Paraspinal Muscles . . . 95869
Sphincter Muscles
Anus . . . 51784, 51785
Needle . . . 51785
Urethra . . . 51784, 51785
Needle . . . 51785
Surface
Dynamic . . . 96002, 96004

Electron Microscopy
Diagnostic . . . 88348

Electronic Analysis
Cardiac Assist Devices
Cardiac Contractility Modulation System . . . 0417T, 0418T
Cardiovascular Physiologic Monitor System . . . 93290, 93297, 93299
Pacemaker System . . . 93279-93281, 93286, 93288, 93293, 93294, 93296, 93724
Pacemaker System, Leadless . . . 93279, 93286, 93288, 93294, 93296
Subcutaneous Cardiac Rhythm Monitor System . . . 93285, 93291, 93298, 93299
Subcutaneous Implantable Defibrillator (SICD) . . . 93260, 93261, 93287, 93295, 93296, 93644
Transvenous Implantable Pacing Defibrillator (ICD) . . . 93282-93284, 93287, 93289, 93295, 93296

Wireless Cardiac Stimulation System 0521T-0522T
Drug Infusion Pump 62367-62370
Gastric Neurostimulator 95980-95982
Neurostimulator
Brain 95970-95972, 95983, 95984
Cranial Nerve 95970, 95976, 95977
Gastric 95980-95982
Peripheral Nerve 95970-95972
Spinal Cord 95970-95972
with Vagus Nerve Blocking Therapy .. 0317T

Electrophoresis
Hemoglobin 83020
High Resolution 83701
Immuno- 86320, 86325, 86327
Immunofixation 86334, 86335
Protein 84165, 84166
Unlisted Electrophoretic Technique 82664

Electrophysiology Procedure 93600-93660

Electroretinogram
See Electroretinography

Electroretinography (ERG)
Full Field (ffERG, Flash ERG, Ganzfeld ERG) .. 92273
Multifocal (mfERG) 92274
Pattern (PERG) 0509T

Electrostimulation, Analgesic Cutaneous
See Application, Neurostimulation

Electrosurgery
Lesions
Anal 46924
Penile 54065
Proliferative 17106-17108
Skin, Benign 17110, 17111
Skin, Malignant 17266
Arms, Legs, or Trunk 17260-17264
Face, Ears, Eyelids, Nose, Lips, Mucous Membrane 17280-17284, 17286
Scalp, Neck, Hands, Feet, or Genitalia 17270-17274, 17276
Skin, Premalignant 17000, 17003, 17004
Vaginal 57061, 57065
Vulva 56501, 56515
Trichiasis
Epilation 67825
Tumor
Rectal 45190

Electroversion, Cardiac
See Cardioversion

Elevation, Scapula, Congenital
See Sprengel's Deformity

Elliot Operation
See Excision, Lesion, Sclera

Eloesser Procedure
See Thoracostomy, Empyema

Eloesser Thoracoplasty
See Thoracoplasty

Embolectomy
Aortoiliac Artery 34151, 34201
Axillary Artery 34101
Brachial Artery 34101
Carotid Artery 34001
Celiac Artery 34151
Femoral 34201
Iliac 34151-34201
Innominate Artery 34001-34101
Mesentery Artery 34151
Peroneal Artery 34203
Popliteal Artery 34201, 34203
Pulmonary Artery 33910, 33915, 33916
Radial Artery 34111
Renal Artery 34151
Subclavian Artery 34001, 34101
Tibial Artery 34203
Ulnar Artery 34111

Embolization
Central Nervous System 61624
Intra-arterial
for Aneurysm 61710
for Carotid-Cavernous Fistula 61710
for Vascular Malformation 61710
Non-Central Nervous System
Head or Neck 61626
Ureteral 50705
Vascular
Arterial 37242
Dialysis Circuit 36909
for Hemorrhage 37244
for Infarction 37243
for Lymphatic Extravasation 37244
for Organ Ischemia 37243
for Tumors 37243
Venous 37241

Embryo
Biopsy 89290, 89291
Carcinoembryonic Antigen 82378
Cryopreservation 89258
Thawing 89352
Culture 89250
with Co-Culture Oocyte 89251, 89272
Hatching, Assisted 89253
Implantation
See Implantation, Embryo
Preparation
for Transfer 89255
Storage 89342
Transfer
See Embryo Transfer

Embryo Implantation
See Implantation, Embryo

Embryo Transfer
In Vitro Fertilization 58970, 58974, 58976
Intrafallopian 58976
Intrauterine 58974
Preparation
for Transfer 89255

Embryo/Fetus Monitoring
See Monitoring, Fetal

Embryonated Eggs
Inoculation 87250

Emergency Department Services
Anesthesia 99140
Critical Care
See Critical Care Services
Physician Direction of Advanced Life Support 99288

Emesis Induction 99175

EMG
See Electromyography, Needle

EMI Scan
See CT Scan

Emission Computerized Tomography 78607

Emission-Computed Tomography, Single-Photon
See SPECT

Emmet Operation
Trachelorrhaphy 57720

Empyema
Drainage
Chest Wall Closure 32810
Thoracostomy 32035, 32036
Empyemectomy 32540
Enucleation 32540

Empyemectomy 32540

Encephalitis
Antibody
California 86651
Eastern Equine 86652
St. Louis 86653
Western Equine 86654

Encephalitis Virus Vaccine 90738

Encephalocele
Repair
Skull Base 62121
Skull Vault 62120

Encephalon
See Brain

End-Expiratory Pressure, Positive
See Pressure Breathing, Positive

End-Stage Renal Disease Services
Dialysis 90951-90970
Inpatient 90935, 90937, 90945, 90947
Home 90963-90966
Outpatient 90951-90962
Less Than a Full Month 90967-90970
Monthly 90951-90966

Endarterectomy
Aneurysm Repair
See Aneurysm Repair
Coronary Artery 33572
Anomaly 33500-33507
Pulmonary 33916
Thromboendarterectomy
See Thromboendarterectomy

Endemic Flea-Borne Typhus
See Murine Typhus

Endobronchial Challenge Tests
See Bronchial Challenge Test

Endobronchial Ultrasound (EBUS)
with Bronchoscopy 31652-31654

Endocavitary Fulguration
See Electrocautery

Endocrine System
Unlisted Services and Procedures ... 60699, 78099

Endocrine, Pancreas
See Islet Cell

Endolymphatic Sac
Exploration
with Shunt 69806
without Shunt 69805

Endometrial Ablation
Cryoablation . . . 58356
Curettage . . . 58356
Thermal . . . 58353
with Surgical Hysteroscopy . . . 58563

Endometrioma
Abdomen
Destruction/Excision . . . 49203-49205
Mesenteric
Destruction/Excision . . . 49203-49205
Peritoneal
Destruction/Excision . . . 49203-49205
Retroperitoneal
Destruction/Excision . . . 49203-49205

Endometriosis, Adhesive
See Adhesions, Intrauterine

Endometrium
Ablation . . . 58353, 58356, 58563
Biopsy . . . 58100, 58110, 58558
Curettage . . . 58356

Endomicroscopy
See Endoscopy, Endomicroscopy

Endomyocardial Biopsy . . . 93505

Endonuclease, DNA
See DNAse

Endoscopic Retrograde Cannulation of Pancreatic Duct
See Cholangiopancreatography

Endoscopies, Pleural
See Thoracoscopy

Endoscopy
See Arthroscopy; Thoracoscopy
Adrenal Gland
See Laparoscopy
Anus
Ablation
Polyp . . . 46615
Tumor . . . 46615
Biopsy . . . 46606
High-Resolution Magnification (HRA) . . . 46607
Collection of Specimen . . . 46600
High-Resolution Magnification (HRA) . . . 46601
Diagnostic . . . 46600, 46601
Dilation . . . 46604
Exploration . . . 46600
Hemorrhage . . . 46614
High Resolution Anoscopy (HRA) . . . 46601, 46607
Removal
Foreign Body . . . 46608
Polyp . . . 46610-46612
Tumor . . . 46610-46612
Atria
Surgical . . . 33265, 33266
Bile Duct . . . 43273
Biopsy . . . 47553
Cannulation . . . 43273
Catheterization . . . 47533-47537, 74328, 74330
Destruction
Calculi (Stone) . . . 43265
Dilation . . . 43277, 47555, 47556
Exploration . . . 47552
Intraoperative . . . 47550
Percutaneous . . . 47552-47556
Placement
Stent . . . 43274
Removal
Calculi (Stone) . . . 43264, 47554
Foreign Body . . . 43275
Specimen Collection . . . 43260
Sphincter Pressure . . . 43263
Sphincterotomy . . . 43262, 43274
Stent . . . 43275
Bladder . . . 52000
Biopsy . . . 52204, 52250, 52354
Catheterization . . . 52005, 52010
Destruction . . . 52214, 52354
Polyps . . . 52285
Dilation . . . 52260, 52265
Lesion . . 52224, 52234, 52235, 52240, 52400
Evacuation
Clot . . . 52001
Excision
Tumor . . . 52355
Exploration . . . 52351
Insertion
Radioactive Substance . . . 52250
Instillation . . . 52010
Irrigation . . . 52010
Litholapaxy . . . 52317, 52318
Lithotripsy . . . 52353
Removal
Calculus . . . 52310, 52315, 52352
Stent . . . 52310
Urethral Stent . . . 52282
Bladder Neck
Destruction . . . 52214
Polyps . . . 52285
Injection of Implant Material . . . 51715
Resection . . . 52500
Contracture . . . 52640
Brain
Catheterization . . . 62160
Dissection
Adhesions . . . 62161
Cyst . . . 62162
Drainage . . . 62162
Excision
Cyst . . . 62162
Brain Tumor . . . 62164
Pituitary Tumor . . . 62165
Removal
Foreign Body . . . 62163
Bronchi
Aspiration . . . 31645, 31646
Biopsy . . . 31625-31629, 31632, 31633
Computer-assisted Image-guided . . . 31627
Destruction
Lesion . . . 31641, 96570, 96571
Tumor . . . 31641, 96570, 96571
Dilation . . . 31630, 31631, 31636-31638
Excision
Tumor . . . 31640
Exploration . . . 31622
Lesion
Destruction . . . 31641, 96570, 96571
Needle Biopsy . . . 31629, 31633
Occlusion . . . 31634
Placement
Fiducial Markers . . . 31626
Radioelement Catheter . . . 31643
Stent . . . 31636, 31637
Removal
Foreign Body . . . 31635
Revision
Stent . . . 31638
Specimen Collection . . . 31623, 31624
Stenosis . . . 31641, 96570, 96571
through Tracheostomy . . . 31615
Tumor
Destruction . . . 31641, 96570, 96571
with Alveolar Lavage . . . 31624
with Brushing . . . 31623
with Cell Washing . . . 31622
with Endobronchial Ultrasound (EBUS)
Sampling . . . 31652, 31653
Cervix . . . 57452
Biopsy . . . 57421, 57454, 57455, 57460
Curettage . . . 57454, 57456
Exploration . . . 57452
Loop Electrode Biopsy . . . 57460
Loop Electrode Conization . . . 57461
Chest Cavity
Diagnostic . . . 32601, 32604, 32606
Surgical . . . 32650-32674
Colon
Ablation
Lesion . . . 45388
Polyp . . . 45388
Tumor . . . 45388
Biopsy . . . 44389, 45380, 45392
Band Ligation . . . 45350, 45398
Decompression . . . 45337
Destruction
Lesion . . . 44401
Tumor . . . 44401
Dilation . . . 45386, 45388
Transendoscopic Balloon . . . 45386
Exploration . . . 44388, 45378
Hemorrhage Control . . . 44391, 45382
Injection . . . 45381
Mucosal Resection . . . 45349
Placement
Decompression Tube . . . 45337
Stent . . . 45389
Removal
Foreign Body . . . 44390, 45379
Polyp . . . 44392, 45384, 45385
Tumor . . . 44392, 45384, 45385
Specimen Collection . . . 45380
Ultrasound . . . 45391, 45392
via Stoma . . . 44388-44394, 44402
Colon-Sigmoid
Ablation
Lesion . . . 45346
Polyp . . . 45346
Tumor . . . 45346
Band Ligation . . . 45350
Biopsy . . . 45331
Decompression . . . 45337
Dilation
Transendoscopic Balloon . . . 45340
Exploration . . . 45330
Hemorrhage . . . 45334
Injection . . . 45335
Mucosal Resection . . . 45349
Needle Biopsy . . . 45342
Placement
Decompression Tube . . . 45337
Stent . . . 45327, 45347
Removal
Foreign Body . . . 45332
Polyp . . . 45333, 45338
Tumor . . . 45333, 45338
Specimen Collection . . . 45330
Ultrasound . . . 45341, 45342
Volvulus . . . 45321, 45337
Duodenum
Ultrasound Examination . . . 43253
Endomicroscopy
Esophageal . . . 43206
Gastrointestinal . . . 43252

Index

Esophagus
- Biopsy . . . 43198, 43202
- Collection of Specimen . . . 43197, 43200
- Dilation . . . 43195, 43196, 43212-43214, 43220, 43226, 43229, 43233, 43248, 43249
- Exploration . . . 43200
- Hemorrhage . . . 43227
- Injection . . . 43192, 43201, 43204
- Injection Varices . . . 43243
- Insertion Stent . . . 43212
- Needle Biopsy . . . 43232
- Removal
  - Foreign Body . . . 43194, 43215
  - Polyp . . . 43216, 43217, 43229
  - Tumor . . . 43216, 43217, 43229
- Ultrasound . . . 43231, 43232, 43237, 43238, 43242, 43253
- Vein Ligation . . . 43205
- with Optical Endomicroscopy . . . 43206

Eye . . . 66990

Foot
- Plantar Fasciotomy . . . 29893

Gastrointestinal
- *See* Laparoscopy
- Ablation
  - Lesion . . . 43270
  - Polyp . . . 43270
  - Photodynamic Therapy . . . 96570, 96571
  - Tumor . . . 43270
- Capsule . . . 91110, 91111
- Upper . . . 3130F, 3132F, 3140F, 3141F
  - Biopsy . . . 43239
  - Catheterization . . . 43241
  - Dilation . . . 43245, 43248, 43249
  - Drainage of Pseudocyst . . . 43240
  - Exploration . . . 43235, 43252
  - Foreign Body . . . 43247
  - Hemorrhage . . . 43255
  - Inject Varices . . . 43243
  - Injection . . . 43236, 43253
  - Needle Biopsy . . . 43238, 43242
  - Referral . . . 3132F
  - Removal . . . 43247, 43250, 43251
  - Stent Placement . . . 43266
  - Thermal Radiation . . . 43257
  - Tube Placement . . . 43246
  - Ultrasound . . . 43237-43242, 43253, 43259, 76975
  - Vein Ligation . . . 43244
- with Optical Endomicroscopy . . . 43252

Heart
- Atria . . . 33265, 33266

Ileum
- Biopsy . . . 44382
- Stent Placement . . . 44384
- via Stoma . . . 44384

Intestines, Small
- Ablation
  - Polyp . . . 44369
  - Tumor . . . 44369
- Biopsy . . . 44361, 44377
- Destruction
  - Lesion . . . 44369
  - Tumor . . . 44369
- Diagnostic . . . 44376
- Exploration . . . 44360
- Hemorrhage . . . 44366, 44378
- Placement
  - Stent . . . 44370, 44379
  - Tube . . . 44372, 44373, 44379
- Removal
  - Foreign Body . . . 44363
  - Lesion . . . 44365
  - Polyp . . . 44364, 44365
  - Tumor . . . 44364, 44365
- Tube Placement . . . 44372
- Tube Revision . . . 44373
- via Stoma . . . 44380, 44382, 44384
  - Tumor . . . 44364, 44365

Intracranial . . . 62160-62165

Intraluminal Imaging
- Colon . . . 0355T
- Gastrointestinal Tract . . . 91110, 91111

Jejunum
- Ultrasound Examination . . . 43253

Kidney . . . 50551, 50570
- Biopsy . . . 50555, 50557, 50574-50576, 52354
- Catheterization . . . 50553, 50572
- Destruction . . . 50557, 50576, 52354
- Dilation
  - Stricture . . . 52343, 52346
- Excision
  - Tumor . . . 50562, 52355
- Exploration . . . 52351
- Lithotripsy . . . 52353
- Removal
  - Calculus . . . 50561, 50580, 52352
  - Foreign Body . . . 50561, 50580
- via Incision . . . 50570, 50572, 50574-50576, 50580
- via Stoma . . . 50551, 50553, 50555, 50557, 50561, 50562

Larynx
- Ablation, Lesion . . . 31572
- Arytenoidectomy . . . 31560, 31561
- Aspiration . . . 31515
- Biopsy . . . 31510, 31535, 31536
- Dilation . . . 31528, 31529
- Direct . . . 31515, 31520, 31525-31529
  - Diagnostic . . . 31520, 31525, 31526
  - Operative . . . 31530, 31531, 31535, 31536, 31540, 31541, 31545, 31546, 31560, 31561
- Epiglottis Stripping . . . 31540, 31541
- Excision
  - Tumor . . . 31540
- Flexible . . . 31575-31579
- Indirect . . . 31505, 31510-31513
- Insertion
  - Obturator . . . 31527
- Laser Destruction, Lesion . . . 31572
- Newborn, Diagnostic . . . 31525
- Reconstruction . . . 31545, 31546
- Removal
  - Foreign Body . . . 31511, 31530, 31531
  - Lesion . . . 31512, 31545, 31546
- Rigid Telescopic . . . 31579
- Vocal Cord
  - Injection . . . 31513, 31570, 31571
  - Lesion Removal . . . 31545
  - Stripping . . . 31540, 31541

Lung
- Biopsy . . . 31628, 31632

Mediastinoscopy
- Biopsy . . . 39401, 39402

Nose
- Diagnostic . . . 31231, 31233, 31235
- Surgical . . . 31237-31241, 31253-31257, 31259, 31267, 31276, 31287, 31288, 31290-31298
- Unlisted Services and Procedures . . . 31299

Otorhinolaryngologic Evaluation
- Cine or Video Recording
  - Laryngeal Sensory Testing . . . 92614-92617
  - Swallowing . . . 92612, 92613, 92616, 92617

Pancreatic Duct
- Cannulation . . . 43273
- Catheterization . . . 74329, 74330
- Destruction
  - Calculi (Stone) . . . 43265
- Dilation . . . 43277
- Placement
  - Stent . . . 43274
- Removal
  - Calculi (Stone) . . . 43264
  - Foreign Body . . . 43275
  - Stent . . . 43275
- Specimen Collection . . . 43260
- Sphincter Pressure . . . 43263
- Sphincterotomy . . . 43262, 43274

Pelvis . . . 52351
- Aspiration . . . 49322
- Destruction of Lesion . . . 52354, 58662
- Lysis of Adhesions . . . 58660
- Oviduct Surgery . . . 58670, 58671
- Removal of Adnexal Structures . . . 58661
- Resection
  - Tumor . . . 52355

Peritoneum
- Drainage
  - Lymphocele . . . 49323, 54690

Pleural Cavity
- Ablation
  - Photodynamic Therapy . . . 96570, 96571

Prostate
- Coagulation with Laser . . . 52647
- Incision . . . 52450
- Destruction . . . 52214
- Drainage
  - Abscess . . . 52700
- Enucleation with Laser . . . 52649
- Resection
  - Complete . . . 52601
  - Obstructive Tissue . . . 52630
- Vaporization with Laser . . . 52647

Rectum
- Ablation
  - Polyp . . . 45320
  - Tumor . . . 45320
- Biopsy . . . 45305
- Destruction
  - Tumor . . . 45320
- Dilation . . . 45303
- Exploration . . . 45300
- Hemorrhage . . . 45317
- Removal
  - Foreign Body . . . 45307
  - Polyp . . . 45308, 45309, 45315
  - Tumor . . . 45308, 45309, 45315
- Volvulus . . . 45321

Sinuses
- Diagnostic . . . 31233, 31235
- Surgical . . . 31237-31240, 31254-31256, 31267, 31276, 31287, 31288, 31290-31297
- Unlisted Services and Procedures . . . 31299

Spleen
- Removal . . . 38120

Spinal Cord Nerve Root
- Decompression . . . 62380

Stomach
- Ultrasound Examination . . . 43253

Testis
- Removal . . . 54690

Trachea
- *See* Bronchoscopy
- Biopsy . . . 31629
- Dilation . . . 31630, 31631, 31636-31638

Placement
Stent . . . 31631
via Tracheostomy . . . 31615
Ureter . . . 50575, 52351
Biopsy . . . 50955, 50957, 50974, 50976, 52007, 52354
Catheterization . . . 50572, 50953, 50972, 52005
Destruction . . . 50957, 50976, 52354
Lesion . . . 52354
Ureterocele . . . 52300, 52301
Dilation . . . 50572, 50575, 50953
Stricture . . . 52341, 52342, 52344, 52345
Excision
Tumor . . . 52355
Exploration . . . 52351
Incision . . . 52290
Injection of Implant Material . . . 52327
Insertion
Guide Wire . . . 52334
Transprostatic Implant . . . 52441, 52442
Lithotripsy . . . 52325, 52353
Manipulation of Ureteral Calculus . . . 52330
Placement
Stent . . . 50947, 52332
Removal
Calculus . . . 50961, 50980, 52320, 52352
Foreign Body . . . 50961, 50980
Resection . . . 52355, 52305
via Incision . . . 50970, 50972, 50974, 50976, 50980
via Stoma . . . 50951, 50953, 50955, 50957, 50961
Ureteral
Biopsy . . . 52007
Catheterization . . . 52005
Urethra . . . 52000
Biopsy . . . 52204, 52354
Catheterization . . . 52010
Destruction . . . 52214, 52354
Congenital Posterior Valves . . . 52400
Lesion . . 52214, 52224, 52234, 52235, 52240
Polyps . . . 52285
Dilation . . . 52281, 52285
Evacuation
Clot . . . 52001
Excision
Tumor . . . 52355
Exploration . . . 52351
Incision . . . 52285
Congenital Posterior Valves . . . 52400
Ejaculatory Duct . . . 52402
Internal . . . 52270, 52275, 52276
Meatotomy . . . 52281, 52285
Injection
for Cystography . . . 52281
Implant Material . . . 51715
Steroid . . . 52283
Insertion
Radioactive Substance . . . 52250
Stent . . . 52282
Lithotripsy . . . 52353
Removal
Calculus . . . 52310, 52315, 52352
Stent . . . 52310
Lysis
Fibrosis . . . 52285
Resection
Congenital Posterior Valves . . . 52400
Ejaculatory Duct . . . 52402
Sphincter . . . 52277
Vasectomy . . . 52402
Vasotomy . . . 52402
Uterus
See Laparoscopy
Vagina . . . 57420
Anesthesia . . . 00950
Biopsy . . . 57421, 57454
Exploration . . . 57452
Vascular
Surgical . . . 33508, 37500, 37501
Vulva . . . 56820
Biopsy . . . 56821

Endosteal Implant

Reconstruction
Mandible . . . 21248, 21249
Maxilla . . . 21248, 21249

Endothelioma, Dural

See Meningioma

Endotracheal Intubation

See Endotracheal Tube

Endotracheal Tube

Emergency Intubation . . . 31500

Endovascular Repair

Abdominal Aorta
See Aneurysm Repair, Abdominal Aorta
Angiography . . . 75956-75959
Delivery of Endograft . . . 34712, 34713
Delivery of Endovacular Prosthesis . . 34714-34716
Iliac Artery
with Endograft . . . 0254T, 34703-34708
with Prosthesis . . . 34709-34711
Infrarenal Abdominal Aorta
with Endograft . . . 34701-34706, 34845-34848
Revascularization
See Revascularization
Vena Cava
Filter Insertion . . . 37191
Repositioning . . . 37192
Retrieval . . . 37193
Thoracic Aorta
See Aorta, Thoracic, Repair
Visceral Aorta
with Fenestrated Endograft . . . 34839, 34841-34848

Endovascular Therapy

Ablation
Vein . . . 36473-36476, 36478, 36479, 36482, 36483
Balloon Angioplasty . . . 61630
Intracranial
Dilatation . . . 61640-61642
Infusion
for Other Than Thrombolysis . . 61650, 61651
for Thrombolysis . . . 61645
Injection . . . 61645
Thrombectomy . . . 61645
Occlusion
Arterial Balloon . . . 61623
Transcatheter . . . 61624, 61626
Vascular Catheterization . . . 61630, 61635

Enema

Contrast . . . 74270, 74280
Home Visit for Fecal Impaction . . . 99511
Therapeutic
for Intussusception . . . 74283

Energies, Electromagnetic

See Irradiation

ENT

See Ear, Nose, and Throat; Otorhinolaryngology

Entamoeba Histolytica

Antigen Detection
Immunoassay . . . 87336, 87337

Enterectomy

Donor . . . 44132, 44133
Partial . . . 44133
Laparoscopic . . . 44202, 44203
Small Intestine . . . 44120, 44121
for Congenital Atresia . . . 44126-44128
with Enterostomy . . . 44125
Transplanted Allograft . . . 44137

Enterocele

Repair
Abdominal Approach . . . 57270
Vaginal Approach . . . 57268, 57556
with Colporrhaphy . . . 57265
with Hysterectomy . . . 58263, 58270, 58280, 58292, 58294

Enterocystoplasty

Camey . . . 50825
with Intestinal Anastomosis . . . 51960

Enteroenterostomy

See Anastomosis, Intestines

Enterolysis . . . 44005

Laparoscopic . . . 44180

Enteropancreatostomy

See Anastomosis, Pancreas to Intestines

Enterorrhaphy . . . 44602, 44603, 44615

Enterostomy

Closure . . . 44227, 44620, 44625, 44626
Placement . . . 44300
with Enterectomy
Intestine, Small . . . 44125
with Enteroenterostomy . . . 44130
with Proctectomy . . . 45119, 45397

Enterotomy

Biopsy . . . 44020
Decompression . . . 44021
Excision
Lesion . . . 44110, 44111
Exploration . . . 44020
Foreign Body Removal . . . 44020
Intestinal Stricturoplasty . . . 44615

Enterovirus

Antibody . . . 86658, 87267, 87498

Entropion

Repair . . . 67921-67924
Excision Tarsal Wedge . . . 67923
Suture . . . 67921
Thermocauterization . . . 67922

Enucleation

Cyst
Mandible . . . 21040
Maxilla . . . 21030
Zygoma . . . 21030
Eye . . . 65101, 65103, 65105
Empyema
Pleural . . . 32540
Prostate . . . 52649
Tumor, Benign
Mandible . . . 21040
Maxilla . . . 21030
Zygoma . . . 21030

Enucleation, Cyst, Ovarian

See Cystectomy, Ovarian

Index

Enucleation, Prostate
See Prostate, Enucleation

Environmental Intervention
for Psychiatric Patients 90882

Enzyme Activity
Constituents 88319
Detection 87185
Incubation 86977
Immunoassay
See Infectious Agent, Antigen Detection, Immunoassay
Infectious Agent 87905
Ova and Parasites 87185
Specific Analytes
See Pathology and Laboratory, Enzymes

Enzyme, Angiotensin Converting
See Angiotensin Converting Enzyme (ACE)

Enzyme, Angiotensin-Forming
See Renin

EOG
See Electro-Oculography

Eosinocyte
See Eosinophils

Eosinophils
Nasal Smear 89190

Epicondylitises, Lateral Humeral
See Tennis Elbow

Epicondylitis, Radiohumeral
See Tennis Elbow

Epidemic Parotitis
See Mumps

Epididymectomy
Bilateral 54861
Unilateral 54860
with Excision of Spermatocele 54840

Epididymis
Anastomosis
to Vas Deferens
Bilateral 54901
Unilateral 54900
Biopsy 54800, 54865
Epididymography 74440
Excision
Bilateral 54861
Unilateral 54860
Exploration
Biopsy 54865
Incision and Drainage 54700
Lesion
Excision
Local 54830
Spermatocele 54840
Needle Biopsy 54800
Spermatocele
Excision 54840
Unlisted Services and Procedures 55899
X ray with Contrast 74440

Epididymograms 55300

Epididymography 74440

Epididymoplasty
See Repair, Epididymis

Epididymovasostomy
Bilateral 54901
Unilateral 54900

Epidural
Administration
Device 62360-62362, 62365
Analysis 62367
Drug 62320-62327
Hospital Management 01996
Anesthesia
See Epidural Anesthesia
Catheterization 62350, 62351
Removal 62355
Electrode
Insertion 61531, 63650, 63655
Removal 61535
Injection 62281, 62282, 62320-62327
Blood or Clot Patch 62273
Neurolytic Substance 62281, 62282
Transforaminal 64479, 64480, 64483, 64484
Ultrasound Guidance 0228T-0231T
with Disc Decompression 62287
Lysis 62263, 62264

Epidural Anesthesia
Infusion
with Imaging Guidance 62325, 62327
without Imaging Guidance 62324, 62326
Injection
with Imaging Guidance 62321, 62323
without Imaging Guidance 62320, 62322

Epidurography 72275

Epigastric
Hernia Repair 49570, 49572
Laparoscopic 49652

Epiglottidectomy 31420

Epiglottis
Excision 31420
Stripping 31540, 31541

Epikeratoplasty
Eye 65767

Epilation
See Removal, Hair

Epinephrine
See Catecholamines
Blood 82383, 82384
Urine 82384

Epiphyseal Arrest
Femur 20150, 27185, 27475, 27479-27485, 27742
Fibula 20150, 27477-27485, 27730-27742
Radius 20150, 25450-25455
Tibia 20150, 27477-27485, 27730, 27734-27742
Ulna 20150, 25450-25455

Epiphyseal Separation
Femur
Closed Treatment 27516, 27517
Open Treatment 27519
Percutaneous Treatment 27509
Radius
Closed Treatment 25600, 25605
Open Treatment 25607-25609
Percutaneous Treatment 25606

Epiphysiodesis
See Epiphyseal Arrest

Epiphysis
See Repair, Epiphysis

Epiploectomy 49255

Episiotomy 59610, 59612, 59300

Epispadias
Penis
Reconstruction 54385
Repair 54380, 54385, 54390
with Exstrophy of Bladder 54390
with Incontinence 54385, 54390

Epistaxis
See Hemorrhage, Control, Nasal (Epistaxis)

EPO
See Erythropoietin

Epstein-Barr Virus
Antibody 86663-86665

Equina, Cauda
See Cauda Equina

ERCP
See Bile Duct; Cholangiopancreatography; Pancreatic Duct

ERG
See Electroretinography

Ergocalciferol
See Vitamin, D

Ergocalciferols
See Vitamin, D

Ergonovine Provocation Test
Cardiovascular Assessment 93024

Erythrocyte
See Red Blood Cell (RBC)

Erythrocyte ab
See Antibody, Detection, Red Blood Cell

Erythrocyte Count
See Red Blood Cell (RBC), Count

Erythropoietin 82668

Escharotomy
Burns 16035, 16036
Graft Site 15002-15005

Escherichia coli 0157
Antigen Detection
Immunoassay 87335

ESD
See Endoscopy, Gastrointestinal, Upper

Esophageal Acid Infusion Test
See Acid Perfusion Study, Esophagus

Esophageal Polyp
See Polyp, Esophagus

Esophageal Tumor
See Tumor, Esophagus

Esophageal Varices
Decompression 37181
Ligation 43205, 43244, 43400
Sclerosis Injection 43204, 43243
Transection/Repair 43401

Esophagectomy
Ivor Lewis 43287
Laparoscopic Thoracoscopic 43287
Laparoscopic Transhiatal 43286
McKeown 43112, 43288
Partial 43116-43118, 43121-43124, 43287
Total 43107, 43108, 43112, 43113, 43124, 43286, 43288
Tri-incisional 43112, 43288

Esophagoenterostomy
with Total Gastrectomy 43620

Esophagogastroduodenoscopy
See Endoscopy, Gastrointestinal, Upper
Flexible Transoral
Ablation
Lesion . . . 43270
Polyp . . . 43270
Tumor . . . 43270
Band Ligation . . . 43244
Biopsy . . . 43239
Collection of Specimen . . . 43235
Control of Bleeding . . . 43255
Delivery of Thermal Energy . . . 43257
Dilation of Esophagus . . . 43233, 43249
Passage of Dilator over Guide Wire . . . 43248
Dilation of Gastric/Duodenal Stricture . . . 43245
Drainage of Pseudocyst . . . 43240
Esophagogastric Fundoplasty . . . 43210
Examination
Ultrasound Guided . . . 43237; 43238, 43253, 43259
Injection . . . 43236, 43243, 43253
Insertion
Catheter or Tube . . . 43241
Guide Wire . . . 43248
Needle Aspiration . . . 43238, 43242
Needle Biopsy . . . 43238, 43242
Placement
Gastrostomy Tube . . . 43246
Stent . . . 43266
Removal
Foreign Body . . . 43247
Lesion . . . 43250, 43251
Polyp . . . 43250, 43251
Tumor . . . 43250, 43251
Resection
Mucosal . . . 43254
with Optical Endomicroscopy . . . 43252

Esophagogastromyotomy
See Esophagomyotomy

Esophagogastrostomy . . . 43320

Esophagojejunostomy . . . 43340, 43341

Esophagomyotomy
Abdominal Approach . . . 43330
Heller Type . . . 32665, 43279, 43330
Laparoscopic . . . 43279
Thoracic Approach . . . 43331
Thoracoscopic . . . 32665
with Fundoplasty . . . 43279

Esophagorrhaphy
See Esophagus, Suture

Esophagoscopy
Transnasal
Biopsy . . . 43198
Collection of Specimen . . . 43197
Transoral
Ablation
Lesion . . . 43229
Biopsy . . . 43193, 43198, 43202
Collection of Specimen . . 43191, 43197, 43200
Dilation . . . 43195, 43196, 43212-43214, 43220, 43226, 43229, 43233
Exploration . . . 43200
Hemorrhage . . . 43227
Injection . . . 43192, 43201, 43204
Insertion Guide Wire . . . 43196, 43212, 43226, 43229
Ligation Varices . . . 43205
Mucosal Resection . . . 43211
Needle Biopsy . . . 43232
Removal
Foreign Body . . . 43194, 43215
Polyp . . . 43216, 43217, 43229
Tumor . . . 43216, 43217, 43229
Stent Placement . . . 43212
with Cricopharyngeal Myotomy . . . 43180
with Diverticulectomy . . . 43180
with Optical Endomicroscopy . . . 43206
with Ultrasound Examination . . . 43231, 43232
with Vein Ligation . . . 43205

Esophagostomy
Closure . . . 43420, 43425
External Fistulization . . . 43351, 43352
with Esophagectomy . . . 43124

Esophagotomy . . . 43020, 43045

Esophagotracheal Fistula
Repair . . . 43305, 43312, 43314

Esophagus
Ablation
Lesion . . . 43229
Polyp . . . 43229
Tumor . . . 43229
Acid Perfusion Test . . . 91030
Acid Reflux Tests . . . 91034, 91035, 91037, 91038
Balloon Distension Study . . . 91040
with Provocation . . . 91040
Biopsy
Endoscopy . . . 43198, 43202
Forceps . . . 3150F
Cricopharyngeal Myotomy . . . 43030, 43180
Dilation . . . 43450, 43453
Endoscopic . . . 43195, 43196, 43212-43214, 43220, 43226, 43229, 43233, 43248, 43249
Surgical . . . 43510
Endoscopy
See Endoscopy, Esophagus; Esophagoscopy; Esophagogastroduodenoscopy
Esophagoscopy
See Esophagoscopy
Excision
Diverticula . . . 43130, 43135
Ivor Lewis . . . 43287
Laparascopic Thoracoscopic . . . 43287
Laparascopic Transhiatal . . . 43286
McKeown . . . 43112, 43288
Partial . . . 43116-43118, 43121-43124, 43287
Total . . . 43107, 43108, 43112, 43113, 43124, 43286, 43288
Tri-incisional . . . 43112, 43288
Exploration
Endoscopy . . . 43200
Hemorrhage . . . 43227
Incision . . . 43020, 43045
Muscle . . . 43030
Imaging Studies . . . 91110, 91111
Motility . . . 78258
Obstructions . . . 74360
Reflux . . . 78262
Removal of Foreign Body . . . 74235
Strictures . . . 74360
Swallowing Function
Cineradiography . . . 74230
X ray . . . 74210, 74220
Injection
Sclerosis Agent . . . 43204
Submucosal . . . 43192, 43201
Insertion
Sengstaken Tamponade . . . 43460
Stent . . . 43212
Tamponade . . . 43460
Tube . . . 43510
Lengthening . . . 43283, 43338
Lesion
Excision . . . 43100, 43101
Ligation . . . 43405
Motility Study . . . 78258, 91010, 91013
with Perfusion . . . 91013
with Pressure Topography . . . 91299
with Stimulation . . . 91013
Mucosal Resection . . . 43211
Needle Biopsy
Endoscopy . . . 43232
Nuclear Medicine
Imaging (Motility) . . . 78258
Reflux Study . . . 78262
Reconstruction . . . 43300, 43310, 43313
Creation
Stoma . . . 43351, 43352
Esophagostomy . . . 43351, 43352
Fistula . . . 43305, 43312, 43314
Gastrointestinal . . . 43360, 43361
Removal
Foreign Bodies . . . 43020, 43045, 43194, 43215, 74235
Lesion . . . 43216
Polyp . . . 43216, 43217
Repair . . . 43300, 43310, 43313
Esophagogastric Fundoplasty . . . 43325, 43327, 43328
Esophagogastroduodenoscopic . . . 43210
Laparoscopic . . . 43280
Esophagogastroduodenoscopy . . 43235-43259
Esophagogastrostomy . . . 43320
Esophagojejunostomy . . . 43340, 43341
Esophagomyotomy . . . 43279
Esophagoplasty . . 43300, 43305, 43310, 43312
Fistula . . . 43305, 43312, 43314, 43420, 43425
Heller Esophagomyotomy . . . 32665
Muscle . . . 43330, 43331
Nissen Procedure . . . 43280
Paraesophageal Hernia
Laparoscopic . . . 43281, 43282
via Laparotomy . . . 43332, 43333
via Thoracoabdominal Incision . . . 43336, 43337
via Thoracotomy . . . 43334, 43335
Pre-existing Perforation . . . 43405
Thal-Nissen Procedure . . . 43325
Toupet Procedure . . . 43280
Varices . . . 43401
Wound . . . 43410, 43415
Sphincter Augmentation
Device Placement . . . 43284
Device Removal . . . 43285
Suture . . . 43405
Wound . . . 43410, 43415
Ultrasound
Endoscopy . . . 43231, 43232
Unlisted Services and Procedures . . . 43289, 43499
Vein
Ligation . . . 43205, 43400

Esophagus Neoplasm
See Tumor, Esophagus

Esophagus, Varix
See Esophageal Varices

Established Patient
Counseling
See Counseling
Critical Care . . . 99291, 99292
Domiciliary or Rest Home Visit . . . 99334-99337, 99339, 99340
Emergency Department Services . . . 99281-99285

Evaluation Services
  Basic Life and/or Disability 99450
  Work-related or Medical Disability 99455
Home Services 99347-99350, 99606
Hospital Inpatient Services......... 99221-99223, 99231-99236, 99238, 99239
Hospital Observation Services 99217-99220, 99224-99226, 99235, 99236
Inpatient Consultations............ 99251-99255
Nursing Facility.................. 99304-99310, 99315, 99316, 99318
Office and/or Other Outpatient
Consultations 99241-99245
Office Visit 99211-99215
Online Medical Evaluation 98969, 99444
Ophthalmological Services......... 92012, 92014
Outpatient Visit................. 99211-99215
Preventive Medicine.............. 99391-99397
Prolonged Services
  with Patient Contact 99354-99357
    with Physician Supervision ... 99415, 99416
  without Patient Contact......... 99358, 99359
Telephone Services.... 98966-98968, 99441-99443

Establishment
Colostomy
  Abdominal 50810
  Perineal 50810

Estes Operation
See Ovary, Transposition

Estlander Procedure 40525

Estradiol 82670
Response.......................... 80415

Estriol
Blood or Urine....................... 82677

Estrogen
Blood or Urine.................. 82671, 82672
Receptor Assay....................... 84233

Estrone
Blood or Urine....................... 82679

Ethanediols
See Ethylene Glycol

Ethanol
Breath.............................. 82075

Ethmoid
Artery Ligation 30915
Excision
  See Ethmoidectomy
Nasoethmoid
  See Nasoethmoid Complex
Repair
  Leak, Cerebrospinal Fluid............ 31290
Sinus
  See Sinus/Sinuses, Ethmoid

Ethmoid, Sinus
See Sinus/Sinuses, Ethmoid

Ethmoidectomy
Anterior............................ 31200
Endoscopic 31254, 31255
Partial 31254
Skull Base Surgery 61580, 61581
Total 31201, 31205, 31255

Ethosuccimid
See Ethosuximide

Ethosuximide
Assay............................... 80168

Ethyl Alcohol
See Ethanol

Ethylene Dichlorides
See Dichloroethane

Ethylene Glycol 82693

Ethylmethylsuccimide
See Ethosuximide

Etiocholanalone Measurement
See Etiocholanolone

Etiocholanolone 82696

ETOH
See Drug Assay, Drug Procedure, Definitive Drug Class, Alcohols

Euglobulin Lysis 85360

European Blastomycosis
See Cryptococcus

Eustachian Tube
Inflation
  Myringotomy 69420
    Anesthesia 69421

Eutelegenesis
See Artificial Insemination

Evacuation
Clots
  Endoscopic....................... 52001
Hematoma
  Brain........... 61108, 61154, 61312-61315
    Anesthesia 00211
  Subungual 11740
Hydatidiform Mole 59870
Intraspinal Lesion 63265
Meibomian Glands 0207T
Pregnancy
  See Dilation and Evacuation
  Cervical 59140
Stomach 43753

Evaluation
Cardiac Devices
  See Electronic Analysis, Cardiac Devices
Carotid Artery
  Atheroma 93895
  Intima Media Thickness............ 93895
Cine................................ 74230
Electrophysiologic.......... 93653, 93654, 93656
Physical Therapy................ 97161-97164
Treatment 92526
Video............................... 74230

Evaluation and Management
Advance Care Planning........... 99497, 99498
Assistive Technology
  Assessment 97755
Basic Life and/or Disability Evaluation
Services............................ 99450
Care Management
  Behavioral Health Conditions 99484
  Psychiatric Collaborative Care.. 99492-99494
Care Plan Oversight Services 0405T, 99339, 99340, 99374-99380
  Home Health Agency Care...... 99374, 99375
  Home or Rest Home Care 99339, 99340
  Hospice 99377, 99378
  Nursing Facility 99379, 99380
Care Planning
  Cognitive Impairment............... 99483
Case Management Services........ 99366-99368
Consultation 99241-99255
Chronic Care 99490, 99491
Complex Chronic Care............ 99487, 99489
Critical Care 99291, 99292
  Interfacility Pediatric Transport....... 99466, 99467, 99485, 99486
Domiciliary or Rest Home
  Established Patient 99334-99337
  New Patient.................. 99324-99328
Emergency Department 99281-99288
Health Behavior
  Assessment 96150
  Family Intervention 96154, 96155
  Group Intervention................ 96153
  Individual Intervention............. 96152
  Re-assessment.................... 96151
Home Services 99341-99350
Hospital....................... 99221-99233
  Discharge.................... 99238, 99239
Hospital Services
  Observation Care............ 99217-99220, 99224-99226, 99234-99236
Hyperbaric Oxygen Treatment Facility 99183
Insurance Exam.................. 99455, 99456
Internet Communication 98969, 99444
Low Birthweight Infant............ 99478, 99479
Medical Team Conferences 99366-99368
Neonatal Critical Care 99468, 99469
Newborn Care.................. 99460-99465
Nursing Facility
  See Nursing Facility Services
  Annual Assessment................ 99318
  Discharge.................... 99315, 99316
  Initial Care 99304-99306
  Other 99318
  Subsequent Care 99307-99310
Occupation Therapy Evaluation 97166, 97167
  Re-evaluation..................... 97168
Office and Other Outpatient........ 99201-99215
Online Services.................. 98969, 99444
Pediatric Critical Care............ 99471, 99472
Pediatric Interfacility Transport 99466-99476, 99485, 99486
Post-discharge Transitional Care 99495, 99496
Preventive Services.............. 99381-99429
Prolonged Services ... 99354-99360, 99415, 99416
Remote
  Physiologic Monitoring of Physiologic Parameters................. 99453, 99454
  Physiologic Monitoring Treatment Services......................... 99457
Standby Services 99360
Team Conferences 99366-99368
Telephone Services.... 98966-98968, 99441-99443
Transitional Care................ 99495, 99496
Unlisted Services and Procedures 99499
with Psychotherapy.......... 90833, 90836, 90838
Work-Related and/or Medical Disability
Evaluation........................... 99455

Evaluation Studies, Drug, Pre-Clinical
See Drug Screen

Everolimus
Drug Assay 80169

Evisceration
Ocular Contents
  with Implant...................... 65093
  without Implant 65091
Suture
  Abdominal Wall.................... 49900

Evisceration, Pelvic
See Exenteration, Pelvis

Evocative/Suppression Test 80400-80439
See Pathology and Laboratory, Evocative/ Suppression Test

Evoked Potentials
Auditory
See Audiometry
Auditory Brainstem 92585, 92586
Central Nervous System
Somatosensory Testing .. 95925-95927, 95938
Transcranial Motor Stimulation 95928, 95929, 95939
Visual 95930
Visual
Acuity 0333T
Central Nervous System 95930
Glaucoma Test 0464T

Evoked Potential, Auditory
See Audiometry

Ewart Procedure
See Palate, Reconstruction, Lengthening

Excavatum, Pectus
See Pectus Excavatum

Exchange
Drainage Catheter
under Radiological Guidance 49423
Fluid-Gas, Vitreous 67025
Intraocular Lens 66986
Strut
External Fixation System 20697

Exchange Transfusion
See Blood, Transfusion, Exchange

Excision
Abdomen
Tumor 49203-49205
Abdominal Wall
Tumor 22900-22903
Abscess
Brain 61514, 61522
Clavicle 23170
Facial Bones 21026
Femur 27070, 27071, 27360
Fibula 27360
Forearm 25145
Ilium 27070, 27071
Humerus 24134, 23174
Mandible 21025
Olecranon Process 24138
Pubic Symphysis 27070, 27071
Radial Head or Neck 24136
Scapula 23172
Tibia 27360
Wrist 25145
Acetabulum
Tumor 27076
Acromion 23130
Adenoids 42820, 42821, 42830, 42831, 42835, 42836
Adenoma
Thyroid Gland 60200
Adrenal Gland 60540, 60545, 60650
Ankle
Tumor 27618, 27619, 27632, 27634
Anus
Crypt 46999
Fissure 46200
Lesion 45108, 46922
Tag 46220, 46230
Aorta
Coarctation 33840-33851
Appendix 44950-44960
Arm, Lower
Tumor 25071, 25073, 25075, 25076
Arm, Upper
Tumor 24071, 24073, 24075, 24076
Arteriovenous Malformation
Spinal 63250-63252
Arytenoid Cartilage
See Arytenoidectomy
Atrial Septum 33735-33737
Back/Flank
Tumor 21930, 21933
Bartholin's Gland 56740
Auditory Canal, External
Lesion 69145, 69150, 69155
Bile Duct
Cyst 47715
Tumor 47711, 47712
Bladder
See Cystectomy
Cyst 51500
Diverticulum 51525
Neck Contracture 52640
Partial 51550-51565
Total 51570, 51580, 51590-51597
with Nodes 51575, 51585, 51595
Transurethral 52640
Tumor 51530
Bone
Abscess
Facial 21026
Mandible 21025
Epiphyseal Bar
Femur 20150
Fibula 20150
Radius 20150
Tibia 20150
Ulna 20150
Brain
Abscess 61514, 61522
Amygdala 61566
Cyst 61516, 61524, 62162
Epileptogenic Focus 61534, 61536
Hemisphere 61543
Hippocampus 61566
Lesion 61600-61608, 61615, 61616
Other Lobe 61323, 61539, 61540
Temporal Lobe 61537, 61538
Tumor 61510, 61518, 61520, 61521, 61526-61530, 61545, 62164
Brain Lobe
See Lobectomy, Brain
Brainstem
Lesion 61575, 61576
Breast
See Mastectomy
Chest Wall Tumor 19260-19272
Cyst 19120-19126
Fibroadenoma 19120-19126
Lactiferous Duct 19110
Fistula 19112
Lesion 19120-19126
Tumor 19120-19126
Bronchi
Tumor 31640
Bulbourethral Gland 53250
Burn Eschar 15002-15005
Bursa
Elbow 24105
Femur 27062
Forearm Tendon Sheath 25115, 25116
Hip 27060, 27062
Knee 27340
Synovium Wrist 25115, 25116
Bypass Graft 35901-35907
Calcaneus 28118-28120
Cyst 28100-28103
Tumor 28100-28103
Carotid Artery 60605
Carotid Body
Tumor 60600, 60605
Carpal 25210, 25215
Cyst 25130-25136
Tumor 25130-25136
Cartilage
Knee Joint 27332, 27333, 27335
Radioulnar Joint 25107
Shoulder Joint 23101
Caruncle
Urethra 53265
Cervix
Radical 57531
Stump
Abdominal Approach 57540, 57545
Vaginal Approach 57550, 57555, 57556
Total 57530
Tumor 58550, 58555
Chalazion
Multiple
Different Lids 67805
Same Lid 67801
Single 67800
with Anesthesia 67808
Cheekbone
Cyst 21030
Tumor 21030, 21034
Chest Wall
Tumor 19260-19272
Choroid Plexus 61544
Clavicle
Cyst 23140, 23145, 23146
Diaphysectomy 23180
Partial 23120, 23180
Sequestrectomy 23170
Total 23125
Tumor 23140, 23145, 23146
Coccyx 27080
Colon
See Colectomy
Colorectal
Tumor 45126
Condyle
See Condylectomy
Conjunctiva
Lesion 68110-68130
Constricting Ring
Finger 26596
Cornea
Lesion 65400
Pterygium 65420, 65426
Coronoid Process 21070
Cowper's Gland 53250
Cranial Bone
Tumor 61563, 61564
Cyst
See Ganglion, Cyst
Bile Duct 47715
Bladder 51500
Brain 61516, 61524, 62162
Breast 19120-19126
Calcaneus 28100-28103
Carpal 25130-25136
Cheekbone 21030
Clavicle 23140, 23145, 23146

Index

Epididymis 54840
Facial Bones 21030
Femur 27355-27358
Greater Trochanter 27065-27067
Fibula 27635-27638
Finger 26160, 26210, 26215
Foot
Tendon/Tendon Sheath 28090
Toe 28108
Hand 26160
Hip 27065-27067
Humerus 23150, 23155, 23156, 24110, 24115, 24116
Ileum
Wing 27065-27067
Kidney 50280, 50290
Knee 27345
Mandible 21040, 21046, 21047
Maxilla 21030, 21048, 21049
Mediastinum 32662, 39200
Metacarpal 26200, 26205
Metatarsal 28104, 28106, 28107
Mullerian Duct 55680
Nose 30124, 30125
Olecranon Process 24120, 24125, 24126
Ovary 58925
Pericardium 32661
Phalanges
Foot 28108
Hand 26210, 26215
Pharynx 42810-42815
Pilonidal 11770-11772
Pubic Symphysis 27065-27067
Radius 25120, 25125, 25126
Head or Neck 24120, 24125, 24126
Ranula 42408
Salivary Gland Duct 42408
Scapula 23140, 23145, 23146
Seminal Vesicle 55680
Sublingual 42408
Talus 28100-28103
Tarsal 28104, 28106, 28107
Thyroglossal Duct 60280, 60281
Thyroid Gland 60200
Tibia 27635, 27637, 27638
Toe
Tendon/Tendon Sheath 28092
Ulna 25120, 25125, 25126
Urachal 51500
Vaginal 57135
Zygoma 21030
Defect
Osteochondral 29891
Talus 29891
Tibia 29891
Dentoalveolar Structures
Alveolar Mucosa 41828
Alveolectomy 41830
Gingivectomy 41820
Operculectomy 41821
Tuberosities 41822, 41823
Tumor 41825-41827
Diverticulum
Bladder 51525
Esophagus 43130, 43135
Hypopharynx 43130, 43135
Mesentery (Meckel's) 44800
Urethra 53230, 53235, 53240
Ear
External 69110, 69120
Inner 69905, 69910
Vestibular Nerve 69915
Middle
Polyp 69540
Tumor 69550, 69552, 69554
Elbow
Tumor 24071, 24073, 24075, 24076
Elbow Joint 24155
Electrode 57522
Embolism
See Embolectomy
Epididymis 54860, 54861
Cyst 54840
Lesion 54830
Spermatocele 54840
Epiglottis 31420
Epiphyseal Bar 20150
Esophagus
See Esophagectomy
Lesion 43100, 43101
Eyelid
Lesion 67800, 67801, 67805, 67808, 67840
Face
Bone Tumor 21029, 21030, 21034-21040, 21044-21049
Cyst 21030
Soft Tissue Tumor 21011-21014
Fallopian Tube
Salpingectomy 58700
Salpingo-Oophorectomy 58720
Fascia
See Fasciectomy
Femur 27070, 27071, 27360
Cyst 27065-27067, 27355-27358
Tumor 27065-27067, 27327, 27328, 27337-27339, 27355-27358
Fibroadenoma
Breast 19120-19126
Fibula 27360, 27455, 27457, 27641
Cyst 27635-27638
Tumor 27635, 27637, 27638
Finger
Cyst 26160, 26210, 26215
Lesion 26160
Tumor 26111-26118, 26200, 26205
Vascular Malformation 26111, 26113, 26115, 26116
Fistula
Anal 46270, 46275, 46280, 46285, 46288
Lactiferous Duct 19112
Foot
Cyst 28090, 28100-28103, 28108
Fasciectomy 28060
Radical 28060-28062
Lesion 28090
Tumor 28039, 28041, 28043, 28045, 28100-28103
Forearm
Tumor 25071, 25073, 25075, 25076
Gallbladder
See Cholecystectomy
Ganglion
Finger or Hand 26160
Foot 28090
Toe 28092
Wrist 25111, 25112
Gingiva 41820
Gums 41820
Alveolus 41830
Lesion 41825-41827
Operculum 41821
Tumor 41825-41827
Hand
Cyst 26160
Lesion 26160
Tumor 26111, 26113, 26115, 26116
Vascular Malformation 26111, 26113, 26115, 26116
Heart
Donor 33940
Tumor 33210, 33130
Heart/Lung, Donor 33930
Hemorrhoids
See Hemorrhoidectomy
Hip 27070, 27071
Bone Cyst 27065-27067
Bursa 27060, 27062
Tumor 27043-27048, 27065-27067
Hippocampus 61566
Humerus
Cyst 23150, 23155, 23156, 24110, 24115, 24116
Diaphysectomy 23184, 24140
Head 23174, 23195
Sequestrectomy 24134
Tumor 23150, 23155, 23156, 24110, 24115, 24116
Hydrocele
Spermatic Cord 55500
Tunica Vaginalis 55040, 55041
Hygroma, Cystic 38550-38555
Hymenal Ring 56700
Ileum
Cyst 27065-27067
Ileoanal Reservoir 45136
Partial 27070, 27071
Ilium
Tumor 27065-27067, 27075, 27076
Innominate
Tumor 27077
Interphalangeal Joint
Toe, Proximal End 28160
Intervertebral Disc
See Discectomy
See Hemilaminectomy
Intestines
See Enterectomy
Lesion 44110, 44111
Iris
See Iridectomy
Ischium
Tumor 27075, 27076, 27078
Kidney
See Nephrectomy
Cyst 50280, 50290
Knee
Cyst 27345
Kneecap 27350
Lesion, Meniscus or Capsule 27347
Tumor 27327, 27328, 27337-27339
Labyrinth
Transcanal 69905
with Mastoidectomy 69910
Lacrimal Gland
See Dacryoadenectomy
Tumor 68540, 68550
Larynx
See Laryngectomy
Tumor 31300, 31540, 31541
with Pharynx
See Pharyngolaryngectomy
Leg, Lower
Tumor 27615, 27616, 27618, 27619, 27632, 27634, 27645, 27646
Leg, Upper
Tumor 27327-27329, 27337-27339, 27365

Lesion
Anal . . . 45108, 46922
Ankle Tendon Sheath . . . 27630
Auditory Canal, External . . . 69145, 69150, 69155
Exostosis . . . 69140
Brain . . . 61600-61608, 61615, 61616
Brainstem . . . 61575, 61576
Breast . . . 19120, 19125, 19126
Colon . . . 44110, 44111
Conjunctiva . . . 68110-68130
Cornea . . . 65400
Ear, Middle . . . 69540
Epididymis . . . 54830
Esophagus . . . 43100, 43101
Eyelid . . . 67840, 67800, 67801, 67805, 67808
Finger Tendon Sheath . . . 26160
Foot . . . 28080, 28090
Forearm Tendon Sheath . . . 25110
Gums . . . 41825-41827
Hand . . . 26160
Intestines . . . 44110, 44111
Intraspinal . . . 63300-63308
See Laminectomy
Knee Meniscus or Capsule . . . 27347
Leg Tendon/Sheath . . . 27630
Mesentery . . . 44820
Mouth . . . 40810-40816, 41116
Nerve . . . 64774-64792
Neuroma . . . 28080, 64774, 64776, 64778
Nose
Intranasal . . . 30117, 30118
Orbit . . . 61333, 67412, 67420
Palate . . . 42104, 42106, 42107
Pancreas . . . 48120
Penis . . . 54060
Pharynx . . . 42808
Rectum . . . 45108
Sclera . . . 66130
Skin
Benign . . . 11400-11404, 11406, 11420-11424, 11426, 11440-11444, 11446, 11450, 11451, 11462, 11463, 11470, 11471
Malignant . . . 11600-11604, 11606, 11620-11624, 11626, 11640-11644, 11646
Skull . . . 61500, 61615, 61616
Anterior . . . 61600, 61601
Base . . . 61575, 61576
Middle . . . 61605-61608
Posterior . . . 61615, 61616
Spermatic Cord . . . 55520
Spinal Cord
Intraspinal . . . 63265-63268, 63270-63273, 63300-63308
Upper . . . 61575, 61576
Tendon Sheath
Ankle and/or Leg . . . 27630
Forearm or Wrist . . . 25110
Testis . . . 54512
Toe . . . 28092
Tongue . . . 41110, 41112-41114
Urethra . . . 52224
Uterus
Uvula . . . 42104, 42106, 42107
Vertebral Column . . . 22100-22103
without Decompression . . . 22110, 22112, 22114, 22116
Wrist Tendon Sheath . . . 25110
Lip . . . 40500, 40510, 40520, 40525
Liver
See Hepatectomy
Lung
Bronchus Resection . . . 32486
Bullae
Completion . . . 32488
Lobe . . . 32480-32482
Pleurectomy . . . 32310, 32320
Pneumonectomy . . . 32440-32445
Segment . . . 32484
Tumor, Apical . . . 32503, 32504
Lung/Heart, Donor . . . 33930
Lymphatic System
See Lymphadenectomy
Hygroma, Cystic . . . 38550, 38555
Nodes . . . 38500, 38510, 38520, 38525, 38530, 38531
Mandible
Cyst . . . 21040, 21046, 21047
Mandibular Torus
Exostosis . . . 21031
Tumor . . . 21040, 21044-21047
Mass
Mediastinum . . . 32662
Pericardium . . . 32661
Mastoid Process
See Mastoidectomy
Maxilla
Cyst . . . 21030, 21048, 21049
Tumor . . . 21030, 21034, 21048, 21049
Maxillary Torus Palatinus . . . 21032
Mediastinum
Cyst . . . 32662, 39200
Tumor . . . 32662
Meningioma
Brain . . . 61512, 61519
Meniscus
Temporomandibular Joint . . . 21060
Mesentery
Lesion . . . 44820
Meckel's Diverticulum . . . 44800
Metacarpal . . . 26230
Cyst . . . 26200, 26205
Tumor . . . 26200-26205
Metatarsal
Cyst . . . 28104, 28106, 28107
Head . . . 28110-28114, 28122, 28140, 28288
Tumor . . . 28104, 28106, 28107
Mouth
Frenum . . . 40819, 41115
Lesion . . . 40810-40816, 41116
Mucosa . . . 40818
Ranula . . . 42408
Mucosa
Gums . . . 41828
Vestibule of Mouth . . . 40818
Nail Fold . . . 11765
Nails . . . 11750
Neck
Tumor . . . 21552, 21554-21556
Neoplasm
Spine . . . 63275-63290
Nerve
Foot . . . 28055
Hamstring Muscle . . . 27325
Neurofibroma . . . 64788-64792
Neurolemmoma . . . 64788-64792
Neuroma . . . 64774-64786
Popliteal . . . 27326
Sympathetic
See Sympathectomy
Neurofibroma . . . 64788-64790
Neurolemmoma . . . 64788-64792
Neuroma . . . 64774-64786
Nose
Cyst . . . 30124, 30125
Lesion . . . 30117, 30118
Polyp . . . 30110-30115
Rhinectomy . . . 30150, 30160
Skin . . . 30120
Turbinate, Inferior . . . 30130, 30140
Odontoid Process . . . 22548
Olecranon Process . . . 24147
Cyst . . . 24120, 24125, 24126
Tumor . . . 24120, 24125, 24126
Omentum . . . 49255
Operculum . . . 41821
Orbit
Lesion . . . 61333, 67412, 67420
Ovary
Cystectomy . . . 58925
Oophorectomy . . . 58940, 58943
Salpingo-oophorectomy . . . 58720
Wedge Resection/Bisection . . . 58920
Oviduct . . . 58700, 58720
Palate . . . 42120, 42145
Lesion . . . 42104, 42106, 42107
Pancreas
See Pancreatectomy
Ampulla of Vater . . . 48148
Lesion . . . 48120
Peripancreatic Tissue . . . 48105
Parathyroid Gland . . . 60500, 60502, 60505
Tumor . . . 42410, 42415, 42420, 42425, 42426
Parotid Gland
Partial . . . 42410-42415
Total . . . 42420-42426
Patella . . . 27350
Pelvis
Tumor . . . 27043, 27045, 27047, 27048, 27049, 27059
Penis
Amputation . . . 54120, 54125, 54130, 54135
Circumcision . . . 54150, 54160, 54161, 54163
Frenulotomy . . . 54164
Lesion . . . 54060
Plaque . . . 54110-54112
Post-Circumcision Adhesion . . . 54162
Pericardium . . . 33030, 33031
Cyst . . . 32661
Mass . . . 32661
Tumor . . . 32661
Peritoneum
Tumor . . . 49203-49205
Petrous Temporal Apex . . . 69530
Phalanges
Cyst
Finger . . . 26210, 26215
Toe . . . 28108
Finger . . . 26235, 26236
Toe . . . 28124, 28126, 28150, 28153
Hemiphalangectomy . . . 28160
Tumor . . . 26210, 26215, 26260, 26262, 28108, 28175
Pharynx . . . 42145, 42890, 42892, 42894
Cyst . . . 42810, 42815
Lesion . . . 42808
with Larynx . . . 31390, 31395
Pituitary Gland . . . 61546, 61548
Tumor . . . 61546, 61548, 62165
Plaque
Penis . . . 54110-54112
Pleura . . . 32310-32320
Thoracoscopic . . . 32656
Polyp
Nose . . . 30110, 30115
Endoscopic . . . 31237
Urethra . . . 53260
Caruncle . . . 53265

Index

Presacral
  Tumor . . . 49215
Prostate
  See Proctectomy
Pterygium . . . 65420, 65426
Pulmonary Artery . . . 33910, 33915, 33916
Pubic Symphysis . . . 27070, 27071
  Cyst . . . 27065-27067
  Tumor . . . 27065-27067
Radius . . . 24130, 24145, 25151
  Cyst . . . 24120, 24125, 24126, 25120, 25125, 25126
  Styloid Process . . . 25230
  Tumor . . . 24120, 24125, 25120, 25125, 25126
Rectum
  See Proctectomy
  Lesion . . . 45108
  Prolapse . . . 45130, 45135
  Stricture . . . 45150
  Tumor . . . 45160, 45171, 45172
Redundant Skin of Eyelid
  See Blepharoplasty
Retroperineal
  Tumor . . . 49203-49205
Ribs . . . 21600, 21610, 21615, 21616
Sacrococcygeal
  Tumor . . . 49215
Salivary Gland Duct
  Cyst . . . 42408
Scalp
  Tumor . . . 21011-21014
Scapula . . . 23172, 23182, 23190
  Cyst . . . 23140, 23145, 23146
  Tumor . . . 23140, 23145, 23146
Sclera . . . 66150, 66155, 66160, 66170
  Lesion . . . 66130
Scrotum . . . 55150
Semilunar Cartilage of Knee
  See Knee, Meniscectomy
Seminal Vesicle . . . 55650
  Mullerian Duct Cyst . . . 55680
Sesamoid Bone
  Toe . . . 28315
  Shoulder
  Tumor . . . 23071, 23073, 23075, 23076
Sinus
  Ethmoid . . . 31200, 31201, 31205
  Maxilla . . . 31225, 31230
Skene's Glands . . . 53270
Skin
  Excess . . . 15830, 15832-15839, 15847
  Lesion, Benign . . . 11400-11404, 11406, 11420-11424, 11426, 11440-11444, 11446, 11450, 11451, 11462, 11463, 11470, 11471
  Lesion, Malignant . . . 11600-11604, 11606, 11620-11624, 11626, 11640-11644, 11646
  Nose . . . 30120
Skin Graft
  Infected
    Abdomen . . . 35907
    Extremity . . . 35903
    Neck . . . 35901
    Thorax . . . 35905
  Site Preparation . . . 15002-15005
Skull . . . 61501
  Lesion . . . 61500
    Anterior . . . 61600, 61601
    Base . . . 61575, 61576
    Middle . . . 61605-61608
    Posterior . . . 61615, 61616
  Tumor . . . 61500
Spermatic Cord
  Lesion . . . 55520
  Variocele . . . 55530, 55535, 55540
Spermatocele . . . 54840
Spine
  Lesion . . . 63300-63308
  Neoplasm . . . 63275-63278, 63280-63283, 63285-63287, 63290
Spinal Cord
  Lesion . . . 61575, 61576, 63265-63268, 63270-63273, 63300-63308
Spleen . . . 38100-38102
Stapes . . . 69660, 69661
Sternum . . . 21620, 21627, 21630, 21632
Stomach
  See Gastrectomy
  Tumor . . . 43610, 43611
Sublingual Gland . . . 42450
  Cyst . . . 42408
Submandibular (Submaxillary) Gland 42440, 42509
Sweat Glands
  Axillary . . . 11450, 11451
  Inguinal . . . 11462, 11463
  Perianal . . . 11470, 11471
  Perineal . . . 11470, 11471
  Umbilical . . . 11470, 11471
Synovium
  See Synovectomy
Talus . . . 28120, 28130
  Cyst . . . 28100, 28102, 28103
  Osteochondral Defect . . . 29891
  Tumor . . . 28100, 28102, 28103
Tarsal . . . 28116, 28122
  Cyst . . . 28104, 28106, 28107
  Tumor . . . 28104, 28106, 28107
Temporal Bone . . . 69530, 69535
Tendon
  Finger . . . 26180, 26390, 26415
  Forearm . . . 25109
  Hand . . . 26390, 26415
  Palm . . . 26170
  Wrist . . . 25109
Tendon Sheath
  Cyst . . . 28092
  Finger . . . 26145
  Foot . . . 28086-28088
  Forearm . . . 25115, 25116
    Bursa . . . 25115, 25116
    Cyst . . . 25120, 25125, 25126
    Lesion . . . 25110
    Synovia . . . 25115, 25116
    Tumor . . . 25120, 25125, 25126
  Leg
    Lesion . . . 27630
  Palm . . . 26145
  Wrist
    Ganglion . . . 25111, 25112
    Lesion . . . 25110
    Bursa . . . 25115, 25116
    Synovectomy . . . 25118, 25119
    Synovia . . . 25115, 25116
Testis
  See Orchiectomy
  Lesion . . . 54512
  Tumor . . . 54530, 54535
Thigh
  Tumor . . . 27327, 27328, 27337, 27339
Thorax
  Tumor . . . 21552, 21554-21556
Thrombus
  See Thrombectomy
Thromboendarterectomy
  See Thromboendarterectomy
Thymus Gland . . . 60520-60522
Thyroglossal Duct
  Cyst . . . 60280, 60281
Thyroid Gland
  See Thyroidectomy
  Lobectomy
    Partial . . . 60210, 60212
    Total . . . 60220, 60225
  Tumor . . . 60200
Tibia . . . 27360, 27640
  Cyst . . . 27635, 27637, 27638
  Osteochondral Defect . . . 29891
  Tumor . . . 27635, 27637, 27638
Toe
  Lesion . . . 28092
  Tumor . . . 28039, 28041, 28043, 28045, 28175
Tongue
  See Glossectomy
  Lesion . . . 41110, 41112-41114
  Lingual Frenum . . . 41115
Tonsils . . . 42820, 42821, 42825, 42826
  Lingual . . . 42870
  Radical Resection . . . 42842, 42844, 42845
  Tag . . . 42860
Torus Mandibularis . . . 21031
Trachea
  Stenosis and Anastomosis . . . 31780, 31781
  Tumor . . . 31785, 31786
Tricuspid Valve . . . 33460
Tumor
  Abdomen . . . 49203-49205
  Abdominal Wall . . . 22900-22903
  Acetabulum . . . 27076
  Ankle . . . 27618, 27619, 27632, 27634
  Arm, Lower . . . 25071, 25073, 25075, 25076
  Arm, Upper . . . 24071, 24073, 24075, 24076
  Back/Flank . . . 21930, 21933
  Bile Duct . . . 47711, 47712
  Bladder . . . 51530
  Brain . . . 61510, 61518, 61520, 61521, 61526-61530, 61545, 62164
  Breast . . . 19120, 19125, 19126
    Chest Wall . . . 19260, 19271, 19272
  Bronchi . . . 31640
  Calcaneus . . . 28100-28103
  Carpal . . . 25130-25136
  Carotid Body . . . 60600, 60605
  Cervix . . . 58550, 58555
  Cheekbone . . . 21030, 21034
  Clavicle . . . 23140, 23145, 23146
  Colorectal . . . 45126
  Cranial Bone . . . 61563, 61564
  Dentoalveolar Structures . . . 41825-41827
  Ear, Middle . . . 69550, 69552, 69554
  Elbow . . . 24071, 24073, 24075, 24076
  Face
    Bone . . . 21029, 21030, 21034, 21040, 21046-21049
    Soft Tissue . . . 21011-21014
  Femur . . . 27065-27067, 27327, 27328, 27337-27339, 27355-27358
  Fibula . . . 27635, 27637, 27638
  Finger . . . 26111-26118
  Flank
    See Excision, Tumor, Back/Flank
  Foot
    Soft Tissue . . . 28039, 28041, 28043, 28045
  Forearm . . . 25071, 25073, 25075, 25076
  Greater Trochanter, Femur . . . 27065-27067
  Gums . . . 41825-41827
  Hand . . . 26111-26118
  Heart . . . 33120-33130
  Hip . . . 27043-27048, 27065-27067

Index

Humerus . . . 23150, 23155, 23156, 24110, 24115, 24116
Ilium . . . 27065-27067, 27075, 27076
Innominate . . . 27077
Ischium
Radical Resection Including
Acetabulum . . . 27076
Ramus
Radical Resection . . . 27075
Tuberosity
Radical Resection . . . 27078
Knee . . . 27327, 27328, 27337-27339
Lacrimal Gland . . . 68540, 68550
Larynx . . . 31300, 31540, 31541
Leg, Lower . . . 27615-27619, 27632, 27634, 27645, 27646
Leg, Upper . . . 27327-27329, 27337-27339, 27365
Lung . . . 32503, 32504
Mandible . . . 21040, 21044-21047
Maxilla . . . 21030, 21034, 21048, 21049
Mediastinum . . . 32662
Mesentery . . . 49203-49205
Metacarpal . . . 26200-26205
Metatarsal . . . 28104, 28106, 28107
Neck . . . 21552, 21554-21556
Olecranon Process . . . 24120, 24125, 24126
Parotid Gland . . . 42410-42426
Pelvis . . . 27043, 27045, 27047, 27048, 27049, 27059
Pericardium . . . 32661
Peritoneum . . . 49203-49205
Phalanges . . . 26210-26215, 26260, 26262
Toe . . . 26215, 28108, 28175
Pituitary Gland . . . 61546, 61548, 62165
Presacral . . . 49215
Pubis . . . 27065-27067, 27075, 27076
Radius . . . 24120-24125, 25120, 25125, 25126
Rectum . . . 45160-45172
Retroperineal . . . 49203-49205
Sacrococcygeal . . . 49215
Scalp . . . 21011-21016
Scapula . . . 23140, 23145, 23146
Shoulder . . . 23071-23078
Skull . . . 61500
Stomach . . . 43610, 43611
Talus . . . 28100, 28102, 28103
Tarsal Bones . . . 28104, 28106, 28107
Testis . . . 54530, 54535
Thigh . . . 27327, 27328, 27337, 27339
Thorax . . . 21552, 21554-21556
Thyroid . . . 60200
Tibia . . . 27635, 27637, 27638
Toe . . . 28039-28045, 28175
Trachea . . . 31785, 31786
Ulna . . . 25120, 25125, 25126
Ureter
Radical Resection . . . 52355
Urethra . . . 53220
Uterus
Fibroid . . . 58140, 58145, 58146
Hydatidiform Mole . . . 59100
Intramural Myoma . . . 58545, 58546
Leiomyomata . . . 58561
Ulna
Darrach Procedure . . . 25240
Tumor . . . 25120, 25125, 25126
Ureter
Urethra
Tumor . . . 53220
Uterus
Fibroid . . . 58140, 58145, 58146
Hydatidiform Mole . . . 59100
Intramural Myoma . . . 58545, 58546
Leiomyomata . . . 58561
Uvula
Lesion . . . 42104, 42106, 42107
Vagina . . . 57135
Vertebra, Cervical . . . 22100
Vertebra, Lumbar . . . 22102
Vertebra, Thoracic . . . 22101
Wrist . . . 25071-25076
Zygoma . . . 21030, 21034
Turbinate, Inferior . . . 30130, 30140
Tympanic Nerve . . . 69676
Ulcer
Pressure
Coccyx . . . 15920, 15922
Ischium . . . 15940, 15941, 15944-15946
Sacrum . . . 15931, 15933-15937
Trochanter . . . 15950-15953, 15956, 15958
Stomach . . . 43610
Ulna . . . 24147, 25150, 25240
Darrach Procedure . . . 25240
Cyst . . . 25120, 25125, 25126
Umbilicus . . . 49250
Urachus
Cyst . . . 51500
Ureter
See Ureterectomy
Ureterocele . . . 51535
Urethra
Bulbourethral Gland . . . 53250
Diverticulum . . . 53230, 53235, 53240
Lesion . . . 52224
Prolapse . . . 53275
Skene's Glands . . . 53270
Urethrectomy . . . 53210, 53215
Uterus
See Hysterectomy
Myoma . . . 58545, 58546
Tumor . . . 58140, 58145, 58146
Uvula . . . 42140, 42145
Vagina
Cyst . . . 57135
Lumen . . . 57120
Septum . . . 57130
Vaginectomy
Complete . . . 57110-57112, 58275, 58280
Partial . . . 57106, 57107, 57109
Varicocele
Spermatic Cord . . . 55530, 55535, 55540
Vas Deferens . . . 55250
Vascular Malformation
Finger . . . 26111, 26113, 26115, 26116
Hand . . . 26111, 26113, 26115, 26116
Vein
Varicose . . . 37765, 37766
Vertebra
Additional Segment . . . 22103, 22116
Cervical . . . 22110
for Tumor . . . 22100, 22110
Lumbar . . . 22102
for Tumor . . . 22114
Thoracic . . . 22112
for Tumor . . . 22101
Vertebral Body . . . 63081-63103
Corpectomy . . . 63081, 63082, 63085-63088, 63090, 63091
Vitreous
See Vitrectomy
Vulva
See Vulvectomy
Wrist
Radial Styloidectomy . . . 25230
Tendon Sheath . . . 25109
Zygoma
Cyst . . . 21030

Exclusion

Duodenum . . . 48547
Small Intestine . . . 44700

Exenteration

Orbit
Anterior Cranial Fossa
Craniofacial . . . 61581
Orbitocranial . . . 61585
Removal Orbital Contents . . . 65110
with Muscle or Myocutaneous Flap . . . 65114
with Therapeutic Removal of Bone . . . 65112
with Maxillectomy . . . 31230
Pelvis . . . 45126, 51597, 58240

Exercise Stress Tests

Cardiovascular . . . 93015-93018, 93464
Pulmonary . . . 94617, 94618

Exercise Test

See Electromyography, Needle
Cardiopulmonary . . . 94621
Ischemic Limb . . . 95875

Exercise Therapy

See Physical Medicine/Therapy/Occupational Therapy

Exfoliation

Chemical . . . 17360

Exocrine, Pancreas

See Pancreas

Exomphalos

See Omphalocele

Exostectomy

Foot . . . 28288

Exostosis

Excision
External Auditory Canal . . . 69140
Fibula . . . 27635
Foot . . . 28288
Palate . . . 21031, 21032
Tibia . . . 27635

Expander, Skin, Inflatable

See Tissue, Expander

Expired Gas Analysis

See Pulmonology, Diagnostic, Expired Gas Analysis

Exploration

Abdomen . . . 49000, 49002, 54535, 54560
Penetrating Wound . . . 20102
Staging . . . 58960
Adrenal Gland . . . 60540, 60545, 60650
Anal
Endoscopy . . . 46600
Ankle . . . 27610, 27620
Anus
Surgical . . . 45990
Arm, Lower . . . 25248
Artery
Brachial . . . 24495
Carotid . . . 35701
Femoral . . . 35721
Other . . . 35761
Popliteal . . . 35741
Back
Penetrating Wound . . . 20102

Bile Duct . . . 47420, 47425, 47480
  Atresia . . . 47700
  Endoscopy . . . 47552
Blood Vessel
  Abdomen . . . 35840
  Chest . . . 35820
  Extremity . . . 35860
  Neck . . . 35800
Brain
  Infratentorial . . . 61305
  Supratentorial . . . 61304
  via Burr Hole
    Infratentorial . . . 61253
    Supratentorial . . . 61250
Breast . . . 19020
  Nipple . . . 19110
Bronchi
  Endoscopy . . . 31622
Bronchoscopy . . . 31622
Cardiotomy . . . 33310, 33315
Cauda Equina . . . 63005, 63011, 63017
Chest . . . 32100, 32601
  Penetrating Wound . . . 20101
Colon
  Colotomy . . . 44025
  Endoscopic . . . 44388, 45378
Colon-Sigmoid
  Endoscopic . . . 45330, 45335
Common Bile Duct
  with Cholecystectomy . . . 47564, 47610
Duodenum . . . 44010
Ear, Middle . . . 69440
Elbow . . . 24000, 24101
Epididymis . . . 54865
Esophagus
  Endoscopy . . . 43200
Extremity
  Penetrating Wound . . . 20103
Finger Joint . . . 26075-26080
Flank
  Penetrating Wound . . . 20102
Forearm . . . 25248
Gallbladder . . . 47480
Gastrointestinal Tract, Upper
  Endoscopy . . . 43235, 43252
Hand Joint . . . 26070
Heart . . . 33310, 33315
Hepatic Duct . . . 47400
Hip . . . 27033
Intestines, Small
  Endoscopy . . . 44360
  Enterotomy . . . 44020
Joint
  See Joint, Exploration
Kidney . . . 50010, 50045, 50120
Lacrimal Duct . . . 68810, 68811, 68815, 68816
  Canaliculi . . . 68840
  Endoscopy . . . 31505, 31510-31513, 31520, 31525, 31526, 31575
Laparoscopic
  Surgical
    Pelvis . . . 49321-49327
Liver . . . 47400
  Wound . . . 47361, 47362
Mediastinum . . . 39000, 39010, 60505
Nasolacrimal Duct . . . 68810, 68811, 68815, 68816
Neck
  Penetrating Wound . . . 20100
Nerves
  Cranial . . . 61458, 61460
Nose
  Endoscopy . . . 31231, 31233, 31235
Ocular
  for Strabismus . . . 67340
Orbit . . . 61333
  with/without Biopsy . . . 67450
  without Bone Flap . . . 67400
Parathyroid Gland . . . 60500, 60502, 60505
Pelvis . . . 49320
Rectum
  Injury . . . 45562, 45563
  Surgical . . . 45990
Retroperitoneal Area . . . 49010
Scrotum . . . 55110
Shoulder Joint . . . 23040-23044, 23107
Sinus
  Frontal . . . 31070-31075, 31255
  Maxillary . . . 31020-31030
Spinal Cord . . . 63001, 63003, 63005, 63011, 63015-63017, 63040, 63042-63044
Spine Fusion . . . 22830
Stomach . . . 43500
Testis
  Undescended . . . 54550, 54560
Toe Joint . . . 28024
Ureter . . . 50600
Vagina . . . 57000
  Endocervical . . . 57452
Wound
  See Wound, Exploration
Wrist . . . 25101, 25248
  Joint . . . 25040

Exploration, Larynx by Incision
See Laryngotomy, Diagnostic

Exploratory Laparotomy
See Abdomen, Exploration

Expression
Conjunctiva . . . 68040

Exteriorization, Small Intestine
See Enterostomy

External Auditory Canal
See Auditory Canal

External Cephalic Version . . . 59412

External Ear
See Ear, External Ear

External Extoses
See Exostosis

External Fixation
Adjustment/Revision . . . 20693
Application
  Multiplane . . . 20692
  Stereotactic Computer Assisted 20696, 20697
  Uniplane . . . 20690
  with Stereotaxis . . . 20696, 20697
Craniofacial Separation Treatment . . . 21435
Mandibular Fracture
  Open Treatment . . . 21454
  Percutaneous Treatment . . . 21452
Nasoethmoid Fracture . . . 21339
Removal . . . 20670, 20680, 20694
Spine
  See Spinal Instrumentation

Extirpation, Lacrimal Sac
See Dacryocystectomy

Extracorporeal Circulation
Cannulation
  Chemotherapy Perfusion . . . 36823
  Extremity . . . 36823

Extracorporeal Dialyses
See Hemodialysis

Extracorporeal Membrane Oxygenation (ECMO)
Arterial Exposure with Graft Conduit Creation . . . 33987
Insertion of Cannula(e)
  Open . . . 33953, 33954
  Percutaneous . . . 33951, 33952
  Sternotomy/Thoracotomy . . . 33955, 33956
Daily Management
  Veno-Arterial . . . 33949
  Veno-Venous . . . 33948
Initiation
  Veno-Arterial . . . 33947
  Veno-Venous . . . 33946
Left Heart Vent
  Insertion . . . 33988
  Removal . . . 33989
Removal of Cannula(e)
  Open . . . 33969, 33984
  Percutaneous . . . 33965, 33966
  Sternotomy/Thoracotomy . . . 33985, 33986
Repositioning of Cannula(e)
  Open . . . 33959, 33962
  Percutaneous . . . 33957, 33958
  Sternotomy/Thoracotomy . . . 33963, 33964
    Birth through 5 years
    Six Years and Older . . . 33964

Extracorporeal Photochemotherapies
See Photopheresis

Extracorporeal Shock Wave Therapy
Calculus
  See Lithotripsy
Humeral Epicondyle . . . 0102T
Integumentary . . . 0512T, 0513T
Musculoskeletal . . . 0101T, 0102T
Plantar Fascia . . . 28890

Extracranial
Catheterization
  See Angiography
Intracranial . . . 61623

Extraction
Calculus
  See Calculus, Extraction
Cataract . . . 66983, 66984
Foreign Body
  Eye . . . 65260, 65265
Thrombus
  Mechanical . . . 36904

Extraction, Cataract
See Cataract, Extraction/Removal

Extradural Anesthesia
Infusion
  with Imaging Guidance . . . 62325, 62327
  without Imaging Guidance . . . 62324, 62326
Injection
  with Imaging Guidance . . . 62321, 62323
  without Imaging Guidance . . . 62320, 62322

Extradural Injection
See Epidural, Injection

Extraocular Muscle
See Eye Muscles

Extrauterine Pregnancy
See Ectopic Pregnancy

Extravasation Blood
See Hemorrhage

Extremity
Lower
Harvest of Vein for Bypass Graft....... 35500
Harvest of Vein for Vascular Reconstruction.................... 35572
Revision................... 35879-35881
Upper
Harvest of Artery for Coronary Artery Bypass Graft.............................. 35600
Harvest of Vein for Bypass Graft....... 35500
Repair
Blood Vessel.................... 35206
Wound Exploration
Penetrating Wound................ 20103

Eye
See Ciliary Body; Conjunctiva; Cornea; Iris; Lens; Orbit; Retina; Sclera; Vitreous
Age-Related Eye Disease Study (AREDS)
Counseling.......................... 4177F
Aspiration
Orbital Contents.................... 67415
Biopsy
Cornea..................... 65410, 65430
Extraocular Muscle................ 67346
Orbit............................ 67400
Chemodenervation
Extraocular Muscle................ 67345
Contact Lens
See Contact Lens Services
Decompression
Orbit
See Orbit, Decompression
Destruction
Ciliary Body
See Ciliary Body
Cyst
Ciliary Body..................... 66770
Iris............................. 66770
Lesion
Choroid............ 67220, 67221, 67225
Ciliary Body..................... 66770
Cornea........................... 65450
Iris............................. 66770
Retina............. 67208, 67210, 67218
Retinopathy................. 67227-67229
Diagnostic and Monitoring Studies
Biometry............. 76516, 76519, 92136
Blood Flow Measurement........... 0198T
Corneal Hysteresis Determination...... 92145
Corneal Pachymetry................ 76514
Computerized Corneal Topography..... 92025
Dilated Fundus Evaluation...... 2020F, 2021F
Dilated Macular Exam......... 2019F, 2021F
Dilated Retinal Exam.............. 2022F
Field Stereoscopic Photos........... 2024F
Eye Imaging Validation............. 2026F
Foreign Body Localization........... 76529
Heterochromatic Flicker Photometry.... 0506T
Interferometry
Biometry......................... 92136
Intraocular Pressure
Measurement............. 0198T, 92100
Monitoring....................... 0329T
Optic Nerve Head Evaluation.......... 2027F
Pupillometry...................... 0341T
Retinal Imaging................... 0380T
Tear Film Imaging................. 0330T
Tear Osmolarity................... 83861
Ultrasound................. 76510-76514
Biometry................ 76516-76519
Foreign Body.................... 76529
Visual Field
Assessment.............. 0378T, 0379T
Exam.................... 92081-92083
X ray............................ 70030
Diagnostic Ophthalmology
See Ophthalmology, Diagnostic
Dilation
Outflow Canal............. 66174, 66175
Discission
Anterior Hyaloid Membrane.......... 65810
Cataract
Laser Surgery.................... 66821
Stab Incision.................... 66820
Vitreous Strands.................. 67030
Drainage
Anterior Segment 0191T, 0253T, 0376T, 66183
Orbit.................... 67405, 67440
with Aqueous Removal............. 65800
with Aspiration
Choroidal Fluid.................. 67015
Subretinal Fluid................. 67015
Vitreous......................... 67015
with Discission of Anterior Hyaloid Membrane........................ 65810
with Removal
Blood............................ 65815
Vitreous......................... 65810
Endoscopy........................ 66990
Enucleation................. 65101-65105
with Implant..... 65103, 65105, 65135, 65140
Evaluation
Dilated Fundus.................... 2021F
Evisceration
Ocular.................. 65091, 65093
with Implant............. 65093, 65130
Excision
Iris
See Iridectomy
Lesion............... 65400, 65900, 66130
Pterygium................. 65420, 65426
Vitreous
See Vitrectomy
Exenteration
Orbital............... 65110, 65112, 65114
Exploration
Orbit
See Orbit, Exploration
Fistulization
Sclera.......... 66150, 66155, 66160, 66170
Goniotomy........................ 65820
Implant
Lacrimal Canaliculus.............. 0356T
Ocular
Insertion........... 65093, 65103, 65105, 65130, 65135, 65140
Modification..................... 65125
Reinsertion............... 65150, 65155
Removal............ 65175, 65920, 67120
Orbital
See Orbit
Incision
Adhesions
Anterior Synechiae......... 65860, 65870
Corneovitreal Adhesions.......... 65880
Goniosynechiae................... 65865
Posterior Synechiae.............. 65875
Cornea, Relaxing.................. 65772
to Reposition Lens Prosthesis......... 66825
Iris................. 66500, 66505, 66761
Laser..... 65860, 66821, 66761, 66821, 67031
Orbit
See Orbitotomy
Trabeculae................ 65820, 65850
Injection
Air or Liquid..................... 66020
Alcohol.......................... 67505
into Tenon's Capsule.............. 67515
Medication................. 66030, 67500
Pharmacologic Agent.......... 0465T, 67028
Vitreous Substitute................ 67025
Insertion
Aqueous Drainage Device
to Extraocular Reservoir...... 66179, 66180
without Extraocular Reservoir...... 0376T, 0449T, 0450T, 66183
Drug-Eluting Ocular Insert
Eyelid................... 0444T, 0445T
Implantation
Corneal Ring Segments............ 65785
Drainage Device........... 0191T, 0253T
Drug Delivery System............. 67027
Electrode Array.................. 0100T
Foreign Material for Reinforcement... 65155
Ganciclovir Implant.............. 67027
Muscles, Attached................ 65140
Muscles, Not Attached............ 65135
Reinsertion...................... 65150
Scleral Shell.................... 65130
Prosthetic Lens
See Lens, Prosthesis
Keratomileusis.................... 65760
Lesion
Choroid
Destruction.......... 67220, 67221, 67225
Ciliary Body
Destruction...................... 66770
Cornea
Destruction...................... 65450
Excision.................. 65400, 65900
Iris
Destruction...................... 66770
Orbit
Removal................... 67412, 67420
Retina
Destruction.......... 67208, 67210, 67218
Sclera
Excision......................... 66130
Meibomian Glands
Evacuation....................... 0207T
Near Infrared Dual Imaging........... 0507T
Nerve
Destruction...................... 67345
Paracentesis
with Aqueous Removal............. 65800
with Discission of Anterior Hyaloid Membrane........................ 65810
with Removal
Blood............................ 65815
Vitreous......................... 65810
Placement
Amniotic Membrane Graft...... 65778-65780
Limbal Conjunctival Graft........... 65782
Limbal Stem Cell Graft.............. 65781
Radiation Source Applicator.......... 67299
Prophylaxis
Retinal Detachment.......... 67141, 67145
Prosthesis
Custom Preparation................ 21077
Intraocular Lens
Exchange......................... 66986
Insertion........................ 66985
Removal.......................... 0308T
Repositioning.................... 66825
Ocular Telescope.................. 0308T

Retinal Receiver and Pulse Generator
Placement 0100T
Implantation Electrode Array 0100T
Pterygium
Excision 65420, 65426
Transposition 65420, 65426
Puncture
Cornea 65600
Radial Keratotomy 65771
Reconstruction
Graft
Conjunctiva 65782
Stem Cell 65781
Transplantation
Amniotic Membrane 65778-65780
Removal
Blood 65815
Blood Clot 65930
Bone 65112, 67445
Cataract
See Cataract, Extraction/Removal
Epithelial Downgrowth 65900
Foreign Body
Conjunctival Embedded 65210
Conjunctival Superficial 65205
Corneal 65220, 65222, 65275
Corneal Epithelium 65435, 65436
Intraocular 65235, 65260, 65265
Orbit 67413, 67430
Implant
Anterior Segment 65920
Ocular 65175
Posterior Segment 67120, 67121
Lens Material
See Lens, Removal
Lesion
Orbit 67412, 67420
Membrane 65810
Vitreous
See Vitreous, Removal
Repair
Astigmatism, Surgical 65772, 65775
Conjunctiva 65270, 65272, 65273
Cornea
See Cornea, Repair
Iris 66680, 66682
See Iridoplasty
Muscles 65290
Retina
See Retina, Repair
Sclera
See Sclera, Repair
Trabeculae 65855
Wound
Direct Closure 65270
Operative 66250
Rearrangement 65272, 65273
Scraping
Cornea, Diagnostic 65430
Severing
Vitreous 67031
Adhesions 67031
Membranes 67031
Opacities 67031
Strands 67031
Shunt, Aqueous
to Extraocular Reservoir 66179, 66180
Revision 66184, 66185
without Extraocular Reservoir . . . 0376T, 66183
Strabismus Surgery
See Strabismus
Transluminal Dilation
Aqueous Outflow Canal 66174, 66175
Trabeculectomy Ab Externo
See Trabeculectomy ab Externo
Transplant
See Keratoplasty
Epikeratoplasty 65767
Keratophakia 65765
Unlisted Services and Procedures
Anterior Segment 66999
Extraocular Muscle 67399
Posterior Segment 67299

Eye Allergy Test
See Allergy Tests

Eye Evisceration
See Evisceration, Ocular Contents

Eye Exam
Established Patient 92012-92014
New Patient 92002-92004
Radiological 70030
with Anesthesia 92018, 92019

Eye Exercises
Training 92065

Eye Muscles
Attached to Implant 65105, 65140, 65155
Biopsy 67346
Chemodenervation 67345
Flap Graft 65114
Repair
Strabismus
See Strabismus
Wound 65290
Transposition 67320
Unlisted Services and Procedures 67399

Eye Prosthesis
See Prosthesis, Ocular; Prosthesis, Orbital

Eye Socket
See Orbit; Orbital Contents; Orbital Floor; Periorbital Region

Eyebrow
Repair
Ptosis 67900
Osteoplastic Flap Incision . . . 31080, 31084, 31086

Eyeglasses
See Spectacle Services

Eyelashes
Trichiasis Correction
Epilation
by Forceps Only 67820
by Other than Forceps 67825
Incision of Lid Margin 67830, 67835
for Biopsy 67810

Eyelid
Abscess
Incision and Drainage 67700
Biopsy
Incisional 67810
Blepharoplasty 15820-15823, 67914
Chalazion
Excision
Multiple 67801, 67805
Single 67800
with Anesthesia 67808
Closure by Suture 67875
Evacuation
Meibomian Glands 0207T
Incision
Canthus 67715
Severing of Tarsorrhaphy 67710
Injection
Subconjunctival 68200
Lesion
Destruction 67850
Excision 67840
Skin, Benign 11440-11444, 11446
Skin, Malignant 11640-11644, 11646, 17280-17284, 17286
Shaving
Dermal/Epidermal 11310-11313
Meibomian Glands
Evacuation 0207T
Near Infrared Dual Imaging 0507T
Placement
Drug-Eluting Ocular Insert 0444T, 0445T
Reconstruction
Canthus 67950
Superficial
Adjacent Tissue Transfer 14060, 14061
Total 67973-67975
Total Eyelid
Lower 67973-67975
Second Stage 67975
Upper 67974
Transfer of Tarsoconjunctival Flap from Opposing Eyelid 67971
Removal
Foreign Body 67938
Repair 21280-21282
Blepharoptosis
See Blepharoptosis
Ectropion
Blepharoplasty 15820-15823, 67914
Suture 67914
Entropion
Excision Tarsal Wedge 67923
Extensive 67924
Suture 67921
Thermocauterization 67922
Excisional 67961
over One-Fourth of Lid Margin 67966
Lagophthalmos 67912
Lashes
Epilation, by Forceps Only 67820
Epilation, by Other than Forceps 67825
Lid Margin 67830, 67835
Lid Retraction 67911
Overcorrection of Ptosis 67909
Skin
Complex 13151-13153
Intermediate 12051-12057
Wound
Full Thickness 67935
Partial Thickness 67930
Superficial 12011, 12013-12018
Repair with Graft
Retraction 67911
Skin Graft
Delayed/Sectioned Flap 15630
Dermal Autograft 15135, 15136
Epidermal Autograft 15115, 15116
Full-Thickness 15260, 15261, 67961
Pedicle 15576
Skin Substitute 15275-15278
Split-Thickness 15120, 15121, 67961
Superficial
Recipient Site Preparation 15004, 15005
Tissue-cultured Autograft 15155-15157
Suture
for Intermarginal Adhesions 67880
for Temporary Closure of Eyelids 67875
with Transposition of Tarsal Plate 67882

Tissue Transfer, Adjacent 67961
Unlisted Services and Procedures 67999

Eyelid Ptoses
See Blepharoptosis

F

Face
CT Scan 70486-70488
Lesion
Destruction 17000-17004, 17280-17286
Magnetic Resonance Imaging (MRI) 70540-70543
Reconstruction
Facial Bones
Secondary 21275
Forehead 21172-21180, 21182-21184
Lip 40525-40527, 40761
Malar Augmentation 21210, 21270
Mandible 21244-21246, 21248, 21249
Mandibular Condyle 21247
Mandibular Rami 21193-21196
Maxilla 21245, 21246, 21248, 21249
Midface
Forehead Advancement 21159, 21160
with Bone Graft 21145-21160, 21188
without Bone Graft 21141-21143
LeFort I 21141-21147, 21155, 21160
LeFort II 21150, 21151
LeFort III 21154, 21155, 21159, 21160
Mouth 40840-40845
Nose 30400-30420, 30430-30450, 30620
Cleft Lip/Cleft Palate 30460-30462
Septum 30520
Orbit 21172-21180, 21182-21184, 21256, 21275
Orbitocraniofacial 21275
Periorbital Region 21267, 21268
Tumor Resection 21011-21016

Face Lift 15824-15826, 15828

Facial Asymmetries
See Hemifacial Microsomia

Facial Bone
See Mandible; Maxilla
Tumor
Excision 21034

Facial Bones
Abscess
Excision 21026
Excision 21026
Reconstruction
Augmentation 21208
Reduction 21209
Secondary 21275
Repair 21208, 21209
Tumor
Contouring 21029
Excision 21029, 21030
X ray 70140-70150

Facial Nerve
Anastomosis
to Hypoglossal 64868
to Spinal Accessory 64866
Avulsion 64742
Chemodenervation, Muscles 64615
Decompression 61590, 61596
Intratemporal
Lateral to Geniculate Ganglion 69720, 69740
Medial to Geniculate Ganglion 69725, 69745
Total 69955
Function Study 92516
Incision 64742
Injection
Anesthetic 64402
Mobilization 61590, 61595, 61596
Repair
Lateral to Geniculate Ganglion 69740
Medial to Geniculate Ganglion 69745
Repair/Suture
with or without Graft 64864, 64865
Suture
Lateral to Geniculate Ganglion 69740
Medial to Geniculate Ganglion 69745
Transection 64742

Facial Nerve Paralysis
Graft 15840-15842, 15845
Repair 15840-15842, 15845

Facial Prosthesis
Impression 21088

Facial Rhytidectomy
See Face Lift

Factor, ACTH-Releasing
See Corticotropic Releasing Hormone (CRH)

Factor, Antinuclear
See Antinuclear Antibodies (ANA)

Factor, Blood Coagulation
See Clotting Factor

Factor, Fitzgerald
See Fitzgerald Factor

Factor, Fletcher
See Fletcher Factor

Factor, Hyperglycemic-Glycogenolytic
See Glucagon

Factor Inhibitor Tests
See Pathology and Laboratory, Factor Inhibitor Tests

Factor, Intrinsic
See Intrinsic Factor

Factor, Rheumatoid
See Rheumatoid Factor

Factor, Sulfation
See Somatomedin

Fallopian Tube
Anastomosis 58750
Biopsy 49321
Cannulation 58565
Catheterization 58345, 74742
Destruction
Endoscopic 58670
Ectopic Pregnancy 59121
with Salpingectomy and/or Oophorectomy 59120, 59151
Excision 58661, 58700, 58720, 58943, 58950, 58953, 58956
Ligation 58600, 58611
Lysis
Adhesions 58740
Occlusion 58615
Endoscopic 58671
Placement
Implant for Occlusion 58565
Repair 58752
Anastomosis 58750
Create Stoma 58673, 58770
Tumor
Resection . . 58950, 58952-58954, 58956-58958
Unlisted Services and Procedures 58999
X ray
Hysterosalpingography 74740

Fallopian Tube Pregnancy
See Ectopic Pregnancy, Tubal

Fallot, Tetralogy of
See Tetralogy of Fallot

Family Adaptive Behavior Treatment Guidance
See Adaptive Behavior Services, Treatment Guidance

Family Psychotherapy
See Psychotherapy, Family of Patient

Fanconi Anemia
Chromosome Analysis 81242, 88248

Farnsworth-Munsell Color Test
See Color Vision Examination

Farr Test
See Gammaglobulin, Blood

Fasanella-Servat Procedure 67908

Fascia Graft 15840

Fascia Lata Graft
Harvesting 20920-20922

Fascial Defect
Leg 27656
Urostomy 50728

Fascial Graft
Cheek 15840
Fascia and Skin
Flap 15733, 15734, 15736, 15738
Free
Microvascular Anastomosis 15758
Harvest 20920, 20922
Reconstruction
Collateral Ligament 26541
Hamstring Muscle 27386
Infrapatellar Tendon 27381
Quadriceps Muscle 27386
Tendon Pulley 26502
Sternoclavicular Dislocation 23532

Fasciectomy
Foot 28060-28062
Palm 26121-26125

Fasciocutaneous Flaps
Muscle 15733-15738
Pharyngeal Wall 42894

Fasciotomy
Arm, Lower 24495, 25020-25025
Buttock
Decompression 27027
with Debridement 27057
Foot 28008
Hand Decompression 26037
Hip 27025
Knee 27305, 27496-27499
Leg, Lower 27600-27602, 27892-27894
Leg, Upper 27305, 27496-27499, 27892-27894
Palm 26040-26045
Pelvis
Decompression 27027
with Debridement 27057
Plantar
Endoscopic 29893
Thigh 27025

Index

Toe 28008
Wrist 25020-25025

FAST
See Allergen Immunotherapy

Fat
Feces 82705-82715
Removal
  Lipectomy 15876-15879

Fat Stain
Feces 89125
Respiratory Secretions 89125
Sputum 89125
Urine 89125

Fatty Acid
Blood 82725
Long-Chain Omega-3
  Red Blood Cell (RBC) Membranes 0111T
Very Long Chain 82726

Favre-Durand Disease
See Lymphogranuloma Venereum

FDP
See Fibrin Degradation Products

Fecal Microbiota Transplant 44705

Feedback, Psychophysiologic
See Biofeedback; Training, Biofeedback

Female Castration
See Oophorectomy

Female Gonad
See Ovary

Femoral Arteries
See Artery, Femoral

Femoral Nerve
Injection
  Anesthetic 64447, 64448

Femoral Stem Prosthesis
See Arthroplasty, Hip

Femoral Vein
See Vein, Femoral

Femur
See Hip; Knee; Leg, Upper
Abscess
  Incision 27303
Amputation 27590
Bone Graft 27170, 27177, 27470
Bursa
  Excision 27062
Craterization 27070, 27071, 27360
Cyst
  Excision 27065-27067, 27355-27358
Diaphysectomy 27360
Drainage 27303
Excision 27070, 27071, 27360
Femoroplasty 29914
Fracture 27244
  Closed Treatment 27501-27503, 27267, 27268
  Distal 27508, 27510, 27514
  Distal, Medial or Lateral Condyle 27509
    Open Treatment 27514
  Epiphysis 27516-27519
    Open Treatment 27519
  Intertrochanteric 27244
    Closed Treatment 27238
    Treatment with Implant 27244
    with Implant 27245
    with Manipulation 27240
  Neck
    Closed Treatment 27230-27232
    Open Treatment 27236, 27177-27179, 27181
    Percutaneous Fixation 27235
  Open Treatment 27245, 27269, 27506,
    27507, 27511-27513
  Percutaneous Fixation 27509
  Peritrochanteric 27244
    Closed Treatment 27238
    Open Treatment 27236, 27269
    Treatment with Implant 27244
    with Implant 27245
    with Manipulation 27240
  Proximal End, Head
    Closed Treatment 27267, 27268
  Shaft 27500, 27502, 27506, 27507
  Subtrochanteric 27244
    Closed Treatment 27238
    Treatment with Implant 27244
    with Implant 27245
    with Manipulation 27240
  Supracondylar 27501-27503,
    27509, 27511-27513
    Open Treatment 27511, 27513
    with Manipulation 27503
    without Manipulation 27501
  Transcondylar 27501-27503,
    27509, 27511-27513
    Open Treatment 27511, 27513
    with Manipulation 27503
    without Manipulation 27501
  Trochanteric
    Closed Treatment 27246
    Open Treatment 27248
Halo 20663
Hemiepiphyseal Arrest 27485
Osteoplasty
  Lengthening 27466-27468
  Shortening 27465, 27468
Osteotomy
  without Fixation 27448
Prophylactic Treatment 27187, 27495
Radiostereometric Analysis (RSA) 0350T
Realignment 27454
Reconstruction 27468
  at Knee 27442, 27443, 27446
  Lengthening 27466-27468
  Shortening 27465, 27468
Repair 27470-27472
  Epiphysis 27181, 27475-27479, 27742
    Arrest 27185
  Muscle Transfer 27110, 27400
  Osteotomy 27140, 27151-27156,
    27161-27165, 27450-27454
  with Graft 27170
Saucerization 27070, 27071, 27360
Tumor
  Excision 27065-27067, 27078,
    27355-27358, 27365
Unlisted Procedure 27599
X ray 73551, 73552

Fenestration Procedure
Skin
  Laser 0479T, 0480T
Tracheostomy 31610

Fenestration, Pericardium
See Pericardiostomy

Ferric Chloride
Urine 81005

Ferrihemoglobin
See Methemoglobin

Ferritin
Blood or Urine 82728

Ferroxidase
See Ceruloplasmin

Fertility Control
See Contraception

Fertility Test
Huhner Test 89310
Male Infertility
  Gene Analysis
    CFTR intron 8 poly-T Analysis 81224
    DAZ/SRY Deletion 81403
Semen Analysis 89300, 89310, 89320-89322
Sperm Analysis 89331
  Antibodies 89325
  Cervical Mucus Penetration Test 89330
  Hamster Penetration 89329
Sperm Evaluation 89331

Fertilization
Assisted
  Oocyte
    Microtechnique 89280, 89281
In Vitro
  See In Vitro Fertilization
Oocyte Culture 89250
  with Co-Culture 89251

Fertilization in Vitro
See In Vitro Fertilization

Fetal Biophysical Profile 76818, 76819

Fetal Contraction Stress Test 59020

Fetal Hemoglobin
for Fetal-Maternal Hemorrhage 85460, 85461
Hemoglobin F 83030, 83033
Kleihauer-Betke 85460

Fetal Lung Maturity Assessment; Lecithin Sphingomyelin Ratio 83661

Fetal Monitoring
See Monitoring, Fetal

Fetal Non-Stress Test
Antepartum 59025
Ultrasound 76815-76818

Fetal Procedure
Amniocentesis 59000
Amnioinfusion 59070
Amniotic Fluid Reduction 59001
Cord Occlusion 59072
Cordocentesis 59012
  Ultrasound Guidance 76941
Fluid Drainage 59074
Intrauterine Transfusion 36460
  Ultrasound Guidance 76941
Magnetic Cardiac Signal Recording 0475T-0478T
Magnetic Resonance Imaging (MRI) 74712, 74713
Non-stress Test 59025
Shunt Placement 59076
Stress Test 59020
Unlisted Fetal Invasive Procedure 59897
Unlisted Laparoscopy Procedure 59898
Unlisted Procedure, Maternity Care and Delivery 59899

Fetal Testing
Amniocentesis 59000
Amniotic Fluid
  Lung Maturity 83661, 83663, 83664
Blood 59030

Index

Heart . . . 76825, 76826
Doppler
Complete . . . 76827
Follow-up or Repeat Study . . . 76828
Hemoglobin . . . 83030-83033, 85460
Home Visit . . . 99500
Magnetic Resonance Imaging (MRI) . . . 74712, 74713
Non-Stress Test . . . 59025
Ultrasound . . . 76815-76818
Ultrasound
Biophysical Profile . . . 76818, 76819
Fetal . . . 76813-73816
Fetal and Maternal . . . 76801, 76802, 76805, 76810-76812, 76817
Heart . . . 76825-76828
Middle Cerebral Artery . . . 76821
Umbilical Artery . . . 76820

Fetuin
See Alpha-Fetoprotein (AFP)

Fever, Australian Q
See Q Fever

Fever, Japanese River
See Scrub Typhus

Fibrillation
Atrial
Performance Measures . . . 1060F, 1061F
Documentation . . . 1060F, 1061F
Treatment . . . 93656, 93657

Fibrillation, Heart
See Fibrillation, Atrial

Fibrin Degradation Products
See Pathology and Laboratory, Fibrin Degradation Products

Fibrin Deposit
Removal . . . 32150, 32653

Fibrin Stabilizing Factor
Clotting Test . . . 85290, 85291

Fibrinase
See Plasmin

Fibrinogen
Activity . . . 85384
Antigen . . . 85385

Fibrinolysin
See Plasmin

Fibrinolysins
Screen . . . 85390

Fibrinolysis
Alpha-2 Antiplasmin . . . 85410
Assay . . . 85396
Activity . . . 85397
ADAMTS-13 . . . 85397
Plasmin . . . 85400
Plasminogen . . . 85420, 85421
Plasminogen Activator . . . 85415
Pleural Cavity
Instillation of Agent . . . 32561, 32562

Fibroadenoma
Ablation
Cryosurgical . . . 19105
Excision . . . 19120

Fibroblastoma, Arachnoidal
See Meningioma

Fibrocutaneous Tags
Removal . . . 11200, 11201

Fibromatosis, Dupuytren's
See Dupuytren's Contracture

Fibromatosis, Penile
See Peyronie Disease

Fibromyoma
See Leiomyomata

Fibronectin, Fetal . . . 82731

Fibrosis, Penile
See Peyronie Disease

Fibrosis, Retroperitoneal
See Retroperitoneal Fibrosis

Fibrous Cavernitides
See Peyronie Disease

Fibrous Dysplasia
Cranial Bone . . . 21181-21184
Facial Bone . . . 21029

Fibula
See Ankle; Knee; Tibia
Amputation . . . 27880-27882, 27884, 27886, 27888
Bone Graft with Microvascular Anastomosis . . . 20955
Craterization . . . 27360, 27641
Cyst
Excision . . . 27635, 27637, 27638
Diaphysectomy . . . 27360, 27641
Excision . . . 27360, 27455, 27457, 27641
Proximal . . . 27832
Epiphyseal Bar . . . 20150
Fracture
Malleolus . . . 27786, 27788, 27792, 27814
Shaft . . . 27780, 27781, 27784
with Distal Tibia Fracture . . . 27826, 27828
with Tibial Shaft Fracture . . . 27750, 27752, 27756, 27758, 27759
Proximal
Open Treatment . . . 27784
Incision . . . 27607
Tibiofibular Joint
Arthrodesis . . . 27871
Dislocation . . . 27830-27832
Disruption . . . 27829
Osteoplasty
Lengthening . . . 27715
Shortening . . . 27715
Repair
Epiphysis . . . 27477, 27479, 27485, 27732, 27734, 27740, 27742
Nonunion or Malunion . . . 27726
Osteotomy . . . 27707, 27709, 27712, 27676
Saucerization . . . 27360, 27641
Tumor
Excision
Bone . . . 27635, 27637, 27638
Radical Resection . . . 27646
Soft Tissue . . . 27615, 27616
Subcutaneous . . . 27618, 27632
Subfascial . . . 27619, 27634
X ray . . . 73590

Figure of Eight Cast
Application . . . 29049

Filariasis . . . 86280, 86682

Filtering Operation
See Incision, Sclera, Fistulization; Incision and Drainage

Filtration Implant, Glaucoma
See Aqueous Shunt

Fimbrioplasty
Uterus . . . 58760
Laparoscopic . . . 58672

Fine Needle Aspiration
Diagnostic . . . 10021
Evaluation . . . 88172, 88173, 88177
Orbital Contents . . . 67415
Transendoscopic . . . 43232, 43242
Colon . . . 45392
Esophagus . . . 43238

Fine Needle Aspiration (FNA) Biopsy
Lesion
with CT Guidance . . . 10009, 10010
with Fluoroscopic Guidance . . . 10007, 10008
with MR Guidance . . . 10011, 10012
with Ultrasound Guidance . . . 10005, 10006
without Guidance . . . 10004, 10021

Finger
Abscess
Incision and Drainage . . . 26010, 26011
Amputation . . . 26910, 26951, 26952
Blood Specimen, Finger Stick . . . 36416
Blood Vessel Repair . . . 35207
Bone
Bone Graft . . . 26546
Craterization . . . 26235, 26236
Cyst
Excision . . . 26210-26215
Diaphysectomy . . . 26235, 26236
Excision . . . 26235, 26236
Partial . . . 28114, 28285
Fracture
Articular
Closed Treatment . . . 26740
Open Treatment . . . 26746
with Manipulation . . . 26742
Distal . . . 26755, 26756
Closed Treatment . . . 26750
Open Treatment . . . 26765
Percutaneous Fixation . . . 26756
Open Treatment . . . 26735
Distal . . . 26765
Shaft . . . 26720-26727
Open Treatment . . . 26735
Incision and Drainage . . . 26034
Nonunion . . . 26546
Ostectomy
Radical
for Tumor . . . 26260-26262
Repair
Lengthening . . . 26568
Nonunion . . . 26546
Osteotomy . . . 26567
Saucerization . . . 26235, 26236
Sesamoidectomy . . . 26185
Thumb
Fracture
Shaft . . . 26720-26727
Tumor
Excision . . . 26210-26215
Radical Resection . . . 26260, 26262
Cast . . . 29086
Claw Finger Correction . . . 26499
Collateral Ligament
Reconstruction . . . 26541, 26542, 26545
with Graft . . . 26541, 26545
Repair . . . 26540
Decompression . . . 26035
Diagnostic Imaging
Joint, Magnetic Resonance Imaging (MRI) . . . 73221
X ray . . . 73140

Index

Excision
  Constricting Ring ... 26596
  Fascia ... 26123, 26125
  Vascular Malformation ... 26111, 26113, 26115-26118
Fracture, Phalanges
  See Fracture, Phalanges
Implant
  Removal ... 26320
Joint
  Arthrocentesis ... 20600, 20604
  Arthrodesis
    Interphalangeal Joint ... 26860-26863
    Metacarpophalangeal Joint ... 26850-26852
  Arthroplasty
    Interphalangeal Joint ... 26535
      with Prosthetic Implant ... 26536
    Metacarpophalangeal Joint ... 26530
      with Prosthetic Implant ... 26531
  Aspiration ... 20600, 20604
  Biopsy ... 26105, 26110
  Capsulectomy ... 26520-26525
  Capsulodesis ... 26516-26518
  Capsulotomy ... 26520-26525
  Dislocation ... 26770, 26775, 26785
  Drainage ... 26075, 26080
  Exploration ... 26075, 26080
  Fracture ... 26740, 26742, 26746
  Injection ... 20600, 20604
  Lesion Excision ... 26160
  Manipulation ... 26340
  Release ... 26123, 26125
  Removal of Foreign Body ... 26075, 26080
  Synovectomy ... 26140, 26145
  Tenodesis ... 26471, 26474
Macrodactylia Repair ... 26590
Pollicization ... 26550
Polydactylous Digit Reconstruction ... 26587
Replantation ... 20816, 20822
Reposition ... 26555
Skin Replacement
  Dermal Autograft ... 15135, 15136
  Epidermal Autograft ... 15115, 15116
  Filleted Flap ... 14350
  Recipient Site Preparation ... 15004, 15005
  Skin Substitute ... 15275-15278
  Split-Thickness ... 15120, 15121
  Tissue-cultured Autograft ... 15155-15157
Splint ... 29130, 29131
Strapping ... 29280, 29584
Syndactyly Repair ... 26560-26562
Tendon
  Extensor
    Delayed Tendon Graft ... 26416
    Excision ... 26180, 26415
    Lengthening ... 26476
    Reconstruction ... 26140
    Repair ... 26418, 26420, 26426, 26428, 26432-26434
    Shortening ... 26477
    Synthetic Rod Implantation ... 26415
    Tenolysis ... 26445, 26449
    Tenotomy ... 26460
  Flexor
    Delayed Tendon Graft ... 26392
    Excision ... 26180, 26390
    Lengthening ... 26478
    Repair ... 26350, 26352, 26356-26358
    Shortening ... 26479
    Synthetic Rod Implantation ... 26390
    Tenolysis ... 26440, 26442
    Tenosynovectomy ... 26145
    Tenotomy ... 26455
  Grafts ... 26502
    Extensor ... 26412, 26420, 26428, 26434
    Flexor ... 26352, 26358
    Profundus ... 26372
    Replace Rod Implant ... 26392, 26416
  Profundus
    Repair ... 26370, 26372, 26373
  Pulley Reconstruction ... 26500, 26502
  Sheath
    Incision ... 26055, 26060
    Incision and Drainage ... 26020
    Lesion Excision ... 26160
  Tenotomy ... 26060
  Transfer ... 26497, 26498, 26510
Transfer
  Finger to Another Position ... 26555
  Toe Joint ... 26556
  Toe to Hand ... 26551, 26553, 26554
Tumor, Soft Tissue
  Excision ... 26111, 26113, 26115-26118
  Radical Resection ... 26117, 26118, 26260, 26262
Unlisted Services and Procedures ... 26989
Volar Plate Reconstruction ... 26548
Web Finger Repair ... 26560-26562

Finger Flap
Filleted ... 14350

Finger Joint
See Finger, Joint

Finney Operation
See Gastroduodenostomy

FISH
See Fluorescent In Situ Hybridization (FISH)

Fissure in Ano
See Anus, Fissure

Fissurectomy
Anus ... 46200
  with Hemorrhoidectomy ... 46257, 46261
    with Fistulectomy ... 46258, 46262

Fissurectomy, Anal
See Fissurectomy, Anus

Fistula
Closure
  Anal ... 46288
  Bronchi ... 32815
  Bronchopleural ... 32906
  Enterocolic ... 44650
  Enteroenteric ... 44650
  Enterovesical ... 44660, 44661
  Esophageal ... 43420, 43425
  Gastrocolic ... 43880
  Intestinal Cutaneous ... 44640
  Kidney ... 50520-50526
  Lacrimal ... 68770
  Nephrocutaneous ... 50520
  Nephrovisceral ... 50525, 50526
  Postauricular Mastoid ... 69700
  Pyelocutaneous ... 50520
  Rectourethral ... 45820, 45825
  Rectovesical ... 45800, 45805
  Rectovaginal ... 57300, 57305, 57307, 57308
  Renocolic ... 50525, 50526
  Salivary ... 42600
  Trachea ... 31820
  Ureter ... 50920-50930
  Ureterocutaneous ... 50920, 53520
  Ureterovisceral ... 50930
  Urethrorectal ... 45820, 45825
  Urethrovaginal ... 57310, 57311
  Vesicoenteric ... 44660, 44661
  Vesicouterine ... 51920, 51925
  Vesicovaginal ... 51900, 57320, 57330
Creation
  See Fistulization
Excision
  Anal ... 46270, 46275, 46280, 46285
  Branchial Cleft ... 42815
  Lactiferous Duct ... 19112
Repair
  Anal ... 46288, 46706
  Anorectal ... 46707
  Anovestibular ... 46716
  Arteriovenous
    See Arteriovenous Fistula
  Carotid-Cavernous ... 61613, 61705, 61708, 61710
  Esophageal ... 43360
  Esophagotracheal ... 43305, 43312, 43314
  Graft-enteric ... 35870
  Ileoanal Pouch ... 46710, 46712
  Mouth ... 30580, 30600
  Nasolabial ... 42260
  Nose ... 30580, 30600
  Oval Window, Ear ... 69666
  Penis ... 54340, 54344, 54348
  Round Window, Ear ... 69667
  Tracheoesophageal ... 43305, 43312, 43314
  Urethra ... 53400, 53405
Suture
  Kidney ... 50520-50526
  Ureter ... 50920-50930
Ultrasound ... 76936
X ray ... 76080

Fistula Arteriovenous
See Arteriovenous Fistula

Fistulectomy
Anal ... 46060, 46270-46285
  with Hemorrhoidectomy ... 46258, 46262

Fistulization
Anoperineal ... 46715, 46716
Arteriovenous
  See Arteriovenous Fistula
Colon
  See Colostomy
Conjunctiva to Nasal Cavity ... 68745, 68750
Dacryocystorhinostomy ... 68720
Esophagus ... 43351, 43352
Intestinal ... 44144
  See Enterostomy
Penis ... 54435
Pharynx ... 42955
Rectourethral ... 46740, 46742
Rectovaginal ... 46740, 46742
Sclera
  See Sclera, Fistulization
Tracheopharyngeal ... 31755
Tracheoesophageal ... 43305, 43312, 43314

Fistulization, Interatrial
See Septostomy, Atrial

Fistulotomy
Anal ... 46270, 46280

Fitting
Amputation
  Leg ... 27881
  Thigh ... 27591
Cervical Cap ... 57170
Contact Lens ... 92071, 92072, 92310-92317
  See Contact Lens Services
Diaphragm ... 57170

Intravaginal Support Device 57160
Low Vision Aid 92354, 92355
See Spectacle Services
Orthotics 97760
Spectacle Prosthesis 92352, 92353
Spectacles 92340-92342
Voice Prosthetic 92597
Wheelchair 97542

Fitzgerald Factor
Kininogen Assay 85293

Fixation
Arthrodesis
Finger 26843, 26850, 26860
Thumb 26841, 26850, 26860
Dislocation
Ankle 27842, 27846, 27848
Finger 26706, 26715
Finger Joint 26776, 26785
Foot
Interphalangeal 28675
Metatarsophalangeal 28636, 28645
Talotarsal 28576, 28585
Tarsal 28546, 28555
Tarsometatarsal 28606, 28615
Hip 27216-27218
Knee 27556
Pelvis 27216-27218
Temporomandibular 21485
Thumb 26650, 26665
Thumb Joint 26776, 26785
Fracture
Ankle
Bimalleolar 27814
Malleolar 27766, 27769
Manipulation 27860
Trimalleolar 27822, 27823
Bennett Fracture 26650, 26665
Carpal Scaphoid
Clavicle 23515
Craniofacial 21432, 21435, 21436
Elbow 24635
Femur
Head Fracture 27254, 27269
Neck Fracture 27235, 27236
Shaft Fracture 27506
Trochanteric Fracture 27248
Fibula 27826, 27828, 27780, 27792
Finger 26607, 26608, 26615, 26756, 26765
Finger Joint 26746
Foot
Calcaneus 28406, 28415
Great Toe 28496, 28505
Metatarsal 28476, 28485
Sesamoid 28531
Talus 28436, 28445
Tarsus 28456, 28465
Hand
Carpometacarpal 26676, 26685, 26706, 26715
Hip 27226-27228
Interdental 21421, 21431
Knee 27524, 27540, 29850
Larynx 31584
Malar 21365
Mandibular 21196, 21452-21454, 21462, 21470
Maxillofacial 21100, 21110, 21345, 21346, 21421, 21435
Nasal 21330, 21339, 21340, 21345, 21346
Odontoid Process 22318
Pelvis 27216-27218
Radius 24665, 25606-25609, 25671
Shaft . . . 25515, 25525, 25526, 25574, 25575
Rib 21811-21813
Scapula 23585
Shoulder 23670, 23680, 23700
Spine
See Spinal Instrumentation
Sternum 21825
Thumb 26756, 26765, 26727, 26735
Thumb Joint 26746
Tibia 27535, 27536, 27827, 27828, 29855, 29856
Tibial Shaft 27756, 27758
Ulna 24685, 25671
Ulnar Shaft 25545, 25574, 25575
Wrist 29847
Osteotomy
Femur 27165, 27181, 27450
Foot
Calcaneus 28300
Talar 28302
Tarsal 28304
Repair of Nonunion 25628
Carpal Bone 25431, 25440
Clavicle 23485
Fibula 27726
without Fracture
Interdental 21497

Fixation (Device)
See Spinal Instrumentation
Ankle
Dislocation 27842, 27846, 27848
Fracture
Bimalleolar 27814
Malleolar 27766, 27769
Trimalleolar 27822, 27823
Manipulation 27860
Bennett Fracture 26650, 26665
Carpal Bone 25431, 25440, 25628
Clavicle 23485, 23515
Craniofacial 21432, 21435, 21436
Elbow 24635
External
See External Fixation
Femur
Condylar Fracture 27509, 27511, 27513, 27514
Curettage 27358
Cyst Excision 27358
Epiphyseal Separation 27519, 27509
Head Fracture 27254, 27269
Neck Fracture 27235, 27236
Osteotomy 27165, 27181, 27450
Shaft Fracture 27506
Trochanteric Fracture 27248
Tumor Excision 27358
Fibula
Fracture 27826, 27828, 27780, 27792
Nonunion or Malunion 27726
Tibiofibular Syndesmosis 27829, 27832
Finger
Arthrodesis 26843, 26850, 26860
Dislocation 26706, 26715
Fracture . . 26607, 26608, 26615, 26756, 26765
Joint Dislocation 26776, 26785
Joint Fracture 26746
Nonunion 26546
Shaft 26727, 26735
Foot
Dislocation
Interphalangeal 28675
Metatarsophalangeal 28636, 28645
Talotarsal 28576, 28585
Tarsal 28546, 28555
Tarsometatarsal 28606, 28615
Fracture
Calcaneus 28406, 28415
Great Toe 28496, 28505
Metatarsal 28476, 28485
Sesamoid 28531
Talus 28436, 28445
Tarsus 28456, 28465
Osteotomy
Calcaneus 28300
Talar 28302
Tarsal 28304
Hand
Carpometacarpal 26676, 26685, 26706, 26715
Harrington Rod 22840, 22850
Hip
Acetabular Fracture 27226-27228
Dislocation 27216-27218
Humerus 23615, 23630, 24400, 24538
Condylar . . 24545, 24546, 24566, 24579, 24582
Interdental 21110, 21421, 21431, 21462
without Fracture 21497
Knee
Dislocation 27556
Fracture 27524, 27540, 29850
Joint Manipulation 29887, 29892
Osteochondritis Dissecans 29885, 29887
Malar 21365
Mandibular . . . 21196, 21452-21454, 21462, 21470
Maxillofacial 21100, 21110, 21345, 21346, 21421, 21435
Nasal 21330, 21339, 21340, 21345, 21346
Odontoid Process 22318
Pelvis
Dislocation 27216-27218
Fracture 27216-27218
Spinal Instrumentation 22848
Radius 24665, 25606-25609, 25671
Shaft 25515, 25525, 25526, 25574, 25575
Removal 20670, 20680
Rib 21811-21813
Scapula 23585
Shoulder 23670, 23680, 23700
Sternum 21825
Temporomandibular Dislocation 21485
Thumb
Arthrodesis 26841, 26850, 26860
Dislocation 26650, 26665
Fracture 26756, 26765
Joint Dislocation 26776, 26785
Joint Fracture 26746
Shaft Fracture 26727, 26735
Tibia
Fracture 27535, 27536, 27827, 27828, 29855, 29856
Shaft Fracture 27756, 27758
Tibiofibular Syndesmosis 27829, 27832
Ulnar Fracture 24685, 25671
Shaft 25545, 25574, 25575
Styloid 25651
Wrist
Fracture 29847
Arthroplasty 25332
Caliper 20660
Cranial Tong 20660
Interdental 21110
Multiplane 20692
Stereotactic Computer Assisted 20696, 20697
Pin/Wire 20650
Skeletal
Humeral Epicondyle
Percutaneous 24566

Index

Stereotactic Frame 20660
Uniplane 20690
Vertebral with Arthroplasty 0202T
Spinal
See Spinal Instrumentation

Fixation Test, Complement
See Complement, Fixation Test

Fixation, External
See External Fixation

Fixation, Kidney
See Nephropexy

Fixation, Rectum
See Proctopexy

Fixation, Tongue
See Tongue, Fixation

Flank
See Back/Flank

Flap
See Skin Graft and Flap

Flatfoot Correction 28735

Flea Typhus
See Murine Typhus

Fletcher Factor 85292

Flow Cytometry 88182-88189
Diagnostic/Pretreatment 3170F

Flow-Volume Loop
See Pulmonology, Diagnostic

Flu Vaccines
See Vaccines and Toxoids, Influenza

Fluid Collection
Amniocentesis
See Amniocentesis
Arterial Catheter 37799
Catheter
Percutaneous 10030
Image Guided 10030
Percutaneous 49405, 49406
Transrectal 49407
Transvaginal 49407
Incision and Drainage
Cerebrospinal Fluid 62272
Hematoma 10140
Skin 10140
Soft Tissue
Percutaneous 10030
Sputum 89220
Sweat 89230
Tears 83861
Venipuncture 36415
Venous Access Device 36591
Venous Catheter 36592

Fluid, Amniotic
See Amniotic Fluid

Fluid, Body
See Body Fluid

Fluid, Cerebrospinal
See Cerebrospinal Fluid

Fluorescein
Angiography, Ocular .. 92230, 92235, 92242, 92287
Intravenous Injection
Vascular Flow Check, Graft 15860

Fluorescein Angiography
See Angiography, Fluorescein

Fluorescent In Situ Hybridization (FISH)
Probe 88364-88366
Morphometric Analysis
Computer-Assisted 88367, 88373, 88374
Manual 88368, 88369, 88377
Cytogenetics 88271-88275
Cytopathology 88120, 88121

Fluoride
Chemistry 82735
Varnish
Application 99188

Fluoroscopy
Examination
Angiography 36901, 36902, 36903
Central Venous Access Device 36598
GI Tract 74340
Larynx 70370
Pharynx 70370
Guidance
Abscess Drainage 75989
Bile Duct
Calculus Removal 47544
Guide Catheter 74328, 74330
Catheterization
Central Venous 36597
Dialysis Circuit 36901, 36902, 36903
Renal Artery 36251-36254
Spine/Paraspinous 77003
Chest
Bronchoscopy 31622-31638, 31640, 31641, 31643, 31645, 31646, 31647-31649, 31651, 31660, 31661
Disc Decompression 62287
Electrothermal Annuloplasty 22526, 22527
Esophagoscopy 43213, 43214
Intubation
Colonic 49442, 49450
Duodenostomy 49441, 49451
Gastro-jejunostomy 49446, 49452
Gastrostomy 49440, 49446, 49450
GI Tract 74340
Jejunostomy 49441, 49446, 49451
Nasogastric 43752
Nephrostomy 50389
Orogastric 43752
Nephroureteral Catheter
Replacement 50387
Spinal Neurostimulator Electrode
Removal 63661, 63662
Revision/Replacement 63663, 63664
Stoma
Creation 49465
Removal of Foreign Body 49460
Thrombectomy
Arterial
Coronary 92973
Intracranial 61645
Noncoronary 37184-37186
Venous 37187, 37188
Vena Cava Filter
Insertion 37191
Removal 37193
Repositioning 37192
Venous Access Device 36598, 77001
Hourly 76000
Needle Biopsy 77002
Unlisted Services and Procedures 76496

FNA
See Fine Needle Aspiration (FNA) Biopsy

Foam Stability Test 83662

Fold, Vocal
See Vocal Cords

Foley Operation Pyeloplasty
See Pyeloplasty

Foley Y-Pyeloplasty 50400-50405

Folic Acid
Blood 82746
Serum 82747

Follicle Stimulating Hormone (FSH) 80418, 80426, 83001

Folliculin
See Estrone

Follitropin
See Follicle Stimulating Hormone (FSH)

Follow-up Inpatient Consultations
See Consultation, Inpatient

Follow-up Services
See Hospital Services; Office and/or Other Outpatient Services
Post-Op 99024

Fontan Procedure
See Repair, Heart, Anomaly; Revision

Food Allergy Test
Allergen-specific IgE 86003, 86005, 86008
Challenge Test 95076, 95079

Foot
See Metatarsal; Tarsal
Abscess
Bone Cortex 28005
Amputation 28800-28805
Bone
See Metatarsal; Tarsal
Bursa
Incision and Drainage 28001
Capsulotomy 28260-28262
Casts and Strapping
Clubfoot Cast 29450
Compression System 29581
Strapping 29540
Unna Boot 29580
Cleft Foot Reconstruction 28360
Clubfoot Repair 28262
Cast 29450
Wedging 29750
Fasciectomy 28060
Radical 28060-28062
Fasciotomy 28008
Endoscopic 29893
Incision 28002, 28003, 28005
Joint
See Talotarsal Joint; Tarsal Joint; Tarsometatarsal Joint
Capsulotomy 28260-28262, 28264
Drainage 28020, 28022, 28024
Exploration 28020, 28022, 28024
Magnetic Resonance Imaging (MRI) 73721-73723
Removal of Foreign Body 28020, 28022, 28024
Synovectomy 28070, 28072
Lesion
Excision 28080, 28090
Magnetic Resonance Imaging (MRI) 73718-73720
Nerve
Destruction
Neurolytic 64632
Excision 28055

Graft 64890, 64891, 64895, 64896
Incision 28035
Neuroma
Excision 28080, 64782
Injection of Anesthetic or Steroid 64455
Morton's 64632, 64455
Neuroplasty 64702
Suture
Common Sensory 64834
Digital 64831, 64832
Each Additional 64837
Median Motor Thenar 64835
Ulnar Motor 64836
Removal
Foreign Body 28190, 28192, 28193
Muscle 28250
Tendon 28200-28230, 28234-28238
Replantation 20838
Sesamoid
Excision 28315
Skin Graft
Dermal Autograft 15135, 15136
Epidermal Autograft 15115, 15116
Recipient Site Preparation 15004, 15005
Skin Substitute 15275-15278
Split-Thickness 15120, 15121
Tissue-cultured Autograft 15155-15157
Suture
Tendon 28200-28210
Tendon
Extensor
Repair 28208, 28210
Tenolysis 28225, 28226
Tenotomy 28234
Flexor
Repair 28200, 28202
Tenolysis 28220, 28222
Tenotomy 28230, 28232
Lengthening 28621-28262
Lesion Excision 28090
Tendon Sheath
Synovectomy 28086, 28088, 28090
Tenotomy 28010, 28011, 28230, 28234
Transfer 27690-27692
Tissue Transfer
Adjacent 14040, 14041
Flap 15574, 15620
Tumor
Soft Tissue
Excision 28039, 28041, 28043, 28045
Radical Resection 28046, 28047
Unlisted Services and Procedures 28899
Wound Repair 13131-13133
X ray 73620, 73630

Foot Abscess
See Abscess, Bone, Foot

Foot Navicular Bone
See Navicular Bone, Tarsal

Forearm 20805
See Arm, Lower

Forehead
Flap 15731
Reconstruction 21179, 21180, 21182-21184
Midface 15730, 21159, 21160
Reduction 21137-21139

Forehead and Orbital Rim
Reconstruction 21172-21180

Forensic Exam
Autopsy 88040
Cytopathology 88125

Foreskin of Penis
See Penis, Prepuce

Formycin Diphosphate
See Fibrin Degradation Products

Fournier's Gangrene
See Debridement, Skin, Subcutaneous Tissue, Infected

Fowler-Stephens Orchiopexy
See Orchiopexy

Fowler-Stephens Procedure 54650

Fraction, Factor IX
See Christmas Factor

Fracture
Acetabulum
Closed Treatment 27220-27222
Open Treatment 27226-27228
with Manipulation 27222
without Manipulation 27220
Alveolar Ridge
Closed Treatment 21440
Open Treatment 21445
Ankle
Bimalleolar 27808, 27810, 27814
Lateral 27786, 27788, 27792, 27808, 27810, 27814
Medial 27760, 27762, 27766, 27808, 27810, 27814
Posterior 27767-27769, 27808, 27810, 27814
Trimalleolar 27816, 27818, 27822, 27823
Ankle Bone
Medial 27760-27762
Bennett's
See Thumb, Fracture
Blow-Out Fracture
Orbital Floor 21385-21387, 21390, 21395
Bronchi
Reduction 31630
Calcaneus
Closed Treatment 28400-28405
Open Treatment 28415-28420
Percutaneous Fixation 28406
with Manipulation 28405, 28406
without Manipulation 28400
Carpal
Closed Treatment
with Manipulation 25624, 25635
without Manipulation 25622, 25630
Open Treatment 25628, 25645
Carpal Scaphoid
Closed Treatment 25622
Open Treatment 25628
Cheekbone
Open Treatment 21360-21366
with Manipulation 21355
Clavicle
Closed Treatment
with Manipulation 23505
without Manipulation 23500
Open Treatment 23515
Closed Treatment 27520
Coccyx
Closed Treatment 27200
Open Treatment 27202
Colles
See Colles Fracture
Colles-Reversed
See Smith Fracture
Elbow
Monteggia
Closed Treatment 24620
Open Treatment 24635
Open Treatment 24586, 24587
Femur
Closed Treatment 27230, 27238-27240, 27246, 27267, 27268, 27500-27503, 27508, 27510, 27516, 27517
with Manipulation 27232
without Manipulation 27267
Open Treatment 27269
Distal 27508, 27510, 27514
Epiphysis 27516-27519
Intertrochanteric
Closed Treatment 27238
Intramedullary Implant 27245
Plate/Screw Implant 27244
Treatment with Implant 27244, 27245
with Manipulation 27240
Neck
Closed Treatment 27230
Open Treatment 27236
Percutaneous Fixation 27235
with Manipulation 27232
Open Treatment 27245, 27248, 27506, 27507, 27511-27514, 27519
Percutaneous Fixation 27235, 27509
Peritrochanteric
Closed Treatment 27238
Intramedullary Implant Shaft 27245, 27500, 27502, 27506, 27507
Open Treatment 27244, 27245
with Manipulation 27240
Proximal
Closed Treatment 27267, 27268
Open Treatment 27269
Subtrochanteric
Closed Treatment 27238
Intramedullary Implant 27245
Open Treatment 27244, 27245
with Manipulation 27240
Supracondylar 27501-27503, 27509, 27511-27513
Transcondylar 27501-27503, 27509, 27511-27513
Trochanteric
Closed Treatment 27246
Open Treatment 27248
with Manipulation 27232, 27502, 27503, 27510
without Manipulation 27230, 27238, 27246, 27500, 27501, 27508, 27516, 27517, 27520
Fibula
Bimalleolar
Closed Treatment 27808-27810
Open Treatment 27814
Closed Treatment 27780, 27781, 27786-27788, 27808-27810
Malleolus 27786-27814
Open Treatment 27784, 27792, 27814
Shaft 27780-27786, 27808
Open Treatment 27784
with Manipulation 27788, 27810
without Manipulation 27780, 27781
Fixation
See Fixation, Fracture
Frontal Sinus
Open Treatment 21343, 21344
Great Toe
Closed Treatment 28490
without Manipulation 28490

Heel
Open Treatment 28415-28420
with Manipulation 28405, 28406
without Manipulation 28400
Humerus
Closed Treatment 24500-24505
with Manipulation 23605
without Manipulation 23600
Condyle
Closed Treatment 24576, 24577
Open Treatment 24579
Percutaneous 24582
Epicondyle
Closed Treatment 24560-24565
Open Treatment 24575
Skeletal Fixation
Percutaneous 24566
Greater Tuberosity Fracture
Closed Treatment with
Manipulation 23625
Closed Treatment without
Manipulation 23620
Open Treatment 23630
Open Treatment 23615, 23616
Shaft 24500-24505, 24516
Open Treatment 24515
Supracondylar
Closed Treatment 24530-24535
Open Treatment 24545, 24546
Percutaneous Fixation 24538
Transcondylar
Closed Treatment 24530-24535
Open Treatment 24545, 24546
Percutaneous Fixation 24538
with Dislocation
Closed Treatment 23665
Open Treatment 23670
with Shoulder Dislocation
Closed Treatment 23675
Open Treatment 23680
Hyoid Bone
Open Treatment 31584
Ilium
Open Treatment 27215, 27218
Percutaneous Fixation 27216
Knee 27520
Arthroscopic Treatment 29850, 29851
Open Treatment 27524
Larynx
Fixation 31584
Open Treatment 31584
Malar Area
Open Treatment 21360-21366
with Bone Graft 21366
with Manipulation 21355
Mandible
Closed Treatment
Interdental Fixation 21453
with Manipulation 21451
without Manipulation 21450
Open Treatment 21454-21470
External Fixation 21454
with Interdental Fixation 21462
without Interdental Fixation 21461
Percutaneous Treatment 21452
Maxilla
Closed Treatment 21421
Open Treatment 21422, 21423
Metacarpal
Closed Treatment 26600-26605
with Fixation 26607
Open Treatment 26615
Percutaneous Fixation 26608
with Manipulation 26605-26607
without Manipulation 26600
Metatarsal
Closed Treatment 28470-28475
Open Treatment 28485
Percutaneous Fixation 28476
with Manipulation 28475, 28476
without Manipulation 28450, 28470
Monteggia
See Fracture, Ulna; Monteggia Fracture
Nasal Bone
Closed Treatment 21310-21320
Open Treatment 21325-21335
with Manipulation 21315-21320
without Manipulation 21310
Nasal Septum
Closed Treatment 21337
Open Treatment 21336
Nasal Turbinate
Therapeutic 30930
Nasoethmoid
Open Treatment 21338, 21339
Percutaneous Treatment 21340
with Fixation 21340
Nasomaxillary
Closed Treatment 21345
Open Treatment 21346-21348
with Bone Grafting 21348
with Fixation 21345-21347
Navicular
Closed Treatment 25622
Open Treatment 25628
with Manipulation 25624
Odontoid
Open Treatment
with Graft 22319
without Graft 22318
Orbit
Closed Treatment
with Manipulation 21401
without Manipulation 21400
Open Treatment 21406-21408
Blowout Fracture 21385-21395
Orbital Floor
Blow Out 21385-21395
Palate
Closed Treatment 21421
Open Treatment 21422, 21423
Patella
Closed Treatment
without Manipulation 27520
Open Treatment 27524
Pelvic Ring
Closed Treatment 27197, 27198
Open Treatment
Anterior 27217
Posterior 27218
Percutaneous Fixation 27216
with Manipulation 27198
without Manipulation 27197
Phalanges
Articular
Closed Treatment 26740
Open Treatment 26746
with Manipulation 26742
Closed Treatment 26742, 28510
Articular 26740
Distal 26750
with Manipulation 26755
Distal 26755, 26756
Closed Treatment 26750
Finger or Thumb 26765
Percutaneous Fixation 26756
Finger/Thumb
Closed Treatment 26720-26725
Shaft 26720, 26727
with Manipulation 26725-26727
Great Toe 28490
Closed Treatment 28495
Distal 26765
Open Treatment 28505
Percutaneous Fixation 28496
with Manipulation 28495, 28496
Shaft
Closed Treatment 26725
Open Treatment 26735
Percutaneous Fixation 26727
Toe
Closed Treatment 28515
Open Treatment 28525
with Manipulation 28515
without Manipulation 28510
with Manipulation 26742, 26755
without Manipulation 26740, 26750
Radius
Closed Treatment 25560-25565
Colles 25600-25605
Distal 25600-25609
Open Treatment 25607-25609
Smith 25600-25605
Head/Neck
Closed Treatment 24650-24655
Open Treatment 24665, 24666
Open Treatment 25515, 25607-25609
Internal Fixation 25607-25609
Percutaneous Fixation 25606
Shaft 25500, 25525, 25526
Closed Treatment 25500-25505, 25520
Open Treatment 25515, 25525,
25526, 25574
with Manipulation 25565, 25605
with Radioulnar Joint
Dislocation 25525, 25526
with Ulna 25560-25565
Open Treatment 25574, 25575
without Manipulation 25560, 25600
Rib
with Internal Fixation 21811-21813
Scaphoid
Closed Treatment 25622
Open Treatment 25628
with Dislocation
Closed Treatment 25680
Open Treatment 25685
with Manipulation 25624
Scapula
Closed Treatment
with Manipulation 23575
without Manipulation 23570
Open Treatment 23585
Sesamoid
Closed Treatment 28530
Foot 28530, 28531
Open Treatment 28531
Skeletal Traction 20650
Acetabulum Fracture 27220
Femoral Fracture 27232, 27240,
27502, 27503, 27517
Hip Socket 27220
Humerus Fracture 23605, 24505, 24535
Phalangeal Fracture 26725
Scapula Fracture 23575
Tibia Fracture 27532, 27752, 27762, 27825
Skin
Debridement 11010-11012
Skull 62000-62010

Sternum
  Closed Treatment . . . 21820
  Open Treatment . . . 21825
Talus
  Closed Treatment . . . 28430-28435
  Open Treatment . . . 28445
  with Manipulation . . . 28435, 28436
  without Manipulation . . . 28430
Tarsal
  Open Treatment . . . 28465
  Percutaneous Fixation . . . 28456
  with Manipulation . . . 28455, 28456
Thumb
  with Dislocation . . . 26645-26650
    Open Treatment . . . 26665
      with Manipulation . . . 26650
Tibia . . . 27759
  Arthroscopic Treatment . . . 29855, 29856
    Plateau
      Bicondylar . . . 29856
      Unicondylar . . . 29855
  Bimalleolar
    Closed Treatment . . . 27808-27810
    Open Treatment . . . 27814
  Closed Treatment . . . 27530-27532, 27538, 27750-27752, 27760-27762, 27808-27810, 27824, 27825
  Distal . . . 27824-27828
    Articular . . . 27826-27828
  Intercondylar . . . 27538-27540
  Malleolus . . . 27760-27769, 27808-27814
  Open Treatment . . . 27535, 27536, 27540, 27758, 27766, 27814, 27826-27828
  Percutaneous Fixation . . . 27756
  Plateau . . . 27530-27536
    Arthroscopic Treatment . . . 29855, 29856
    Unicondylar
      Open Treatment . . . 27535
  Shaft . . . 27750-27759
  with Manipulation 27752, 27760-27762, 27810
  without Manipulation . . . 27530, 27750, 27760-27762, 27808, 27825
Trachea
  Endoscopy . . . 31630
Ulna
  See Elbow; Humerus; Radius
  Closed Treatment . . . 25560-25565
  Olecranon
    Closed Treatment . . . 24670-24675
    Open Treatment . . . 24685
  Open Treatment . . . 25574, 25575
  Shaft
    Closed Treatment . . . 25530-25535
    Open Treatment . . . 25545, 25574
  Styloid Process
    Closed Treatment . . . 25650
    Open Treatment . . . 25652
    Percutaneous Fixation . . . 25651
  with Dislocation
    Closed Treatment . . . 24620
    Monteggia . . . 24620-24635
    Open Treatment . . . 24635
  with Manipulation . . . 25535, 25565
  with Radius . . . 25560-25565
    Open Treatment . . . 25575
  without Manipulation . . . 25530, 25560
Ulna and Radius
  Open Treatment . . . 25574, 25575
Vertebra
  Additional Segment
    Open Treatment . . . 22328
  Cervical
    Open Treatment . . . 22326
  Closed Treatment
    with Manipulation, Casting and/or Bracing . . . 22315
    without Manipulation . . . 22310
  Lumbar
    Open Treatment . . . 22325
  Posterior
    Open Treatment . . . 22325-22327
  Thoracic
    Open Treatment . . . 22327
  with Shoulder Dislocation
    Closed Treatment . . . 23675
    Open Treatment . . . 23680
Vertebral Fracture Assessment . . . 77085, 77086
Vertebral Process
Wrist
  with Dislocation
    Closed Treatment . . . 25680
    Open Treatment . . . 25685
Zygomatic Arch
  Open Treatment . . . 21356-21366
  with Manipulation . . . 21355

Fractured Catheter Retrieval . . . 37197

Fragile-X
Chromosome Analysis . . . 88248
FMR1 Gene Analysis . . . 81243

Fragility
Red Blood Cell
  Mechanical . . . 85547
  Osmotic . . . 85555, 85557

Frames, Stereotactic
See Stereotactic Frame

Francisella . . . 86000
Antibody . . . 86668

Fredet-Ramstedt Procedure . . . 43520

Free E3
See Estriol

Free Skin Graft
See Skin, Grafts, Free

Free T4
See Thyroxine, Free

Frei Disease
See Lymphogranuloma Venereum

Frenectomy
Lip . . . 40819
Tongue . . . 41115

Frenectomy, Lingual
Tongue . . . 41115

Frenotomy
Lip . . . 40806
Tongue . . . 41010

Frenulectomy
See Frenectomy

Frenuloplasty . . . 41520

Frenum
Lip
  Excision . . . 40819
  Incision . . . 40806
Tongue
  Excision . . . 41115
  Incision . . . 41010
Revision . . . 41520

Frenumectomy . . . 40819

Frickman Operation
See Proctopexy

Frontal Craniotomy . . . 61556

Frontal Sinus
See Sinus/Sinuses, Frontal

Frontal Sinusotomy
See Exploration, Sinus, Frontal

Frost Suture
Temporary Closure of Eyelids . . . 67875

Frozen Blood Preparation
Freezing . . . 86930, 86932
Thawing . . . 86931

Fructose
Semen . . . 82757
TLC Screen . . . 84375

Fructose Intolerance Breath Test . . . 91065

Fruit Sugar
See Fructose

FSF . . . 85290, 85291

FSH
See Follicle Stimulating Hormone (FSH)

FSP
See Fibrin Degradation Products

FT-4 . . . 84439

Fulguration
Bladder . . . 51020, 52285
Cervix . . . 57500, 57520
Cystourethroscopy with . . . 52214, 52400
  Lesion . . . 52224
  Tumor . . . 52234, 52235, 52240, 52250
Kidney
  Endoscopic . . . 50557, 50576
Lesion
  Ovary . . . 58662
  Pelvis . . . 58662
  Peritoneal . . . 58662
Oviducts . . . 58670
Ureter . . . 50957, 50976, 52354
Ureterocele
  Ectopic . . . 52301
  Orthotopic . . . 52300
Urethra . . . 52285, 53220, 53260

Fulguration, Endocavitary
See Electrocautery

Full Thickness Graft . . . 15200-15261

Function Test, Lung
See Pulmonology, Diagnostic

Function Test, Vestibular
See Vestibular Function Tests

Function, Study, Nasal
See Nasal Function Study

Functional Ability
See Activities of Daily Living

Fundoplasty
Esophagogastric . . . 43325
Esophagogastroduodenoscopic . . . 43210
  Laparoscopic . . . 43279, 43280, 43283
  Laparotomy . . . 43327
  Thoracotomy . . . 43328
Esophagomyotomy
  Laparoscopic . . . 43279

Index

Paraesophageal Hiatal Hernia Repair
  Laparoscopic ... 43281, 43282
  with Fundoplication
    Laparotomy ... 43332, 43333
    Thoracoabdominal Incisional ... 43336, 43337
    Thoracotomy ... 43334, 43335

Fundoplication
Paraesophageal Hiatal Hernia Repair
  via Laparotomy ... 43332, 43333
  via Thoracoabdominal Incision ... 43336, 43337
  via Thoracotomy ... 43334, 43335

Fungus
Antibody ... 86671
Culture
  Blood ... 87103
  Hair ... 87101
  Identification ... 87106
  Nail ... 87101
  Other ... 87102
  Skin ... 87101
Tissue Exam ... 87220

Funnel Chest
See Pectus Excavatum

Furuncle
Incision and Drainage ... 10060, 10061

Furuncle, Vulva
See Vulva, Incision and Drainage, Furuncle

Fusion
Great Toe ... 28760
Interphalangeal ... 28285
Metatarsocuneiform ... 28297
Pleural Cavity
  Instillation of Agent for Pleurodesis ... 32560
Thumb
  in Opposition ... 26820
Vertebrae
See Arthrodesis

Fusion, Epiphyseal-Diaphyseal
See Epiphyseal Arrest

Fusion, Joint
See Arthrodesis

Fusion, Joint, Ankle
See Ankle, Arthrodesis

Fusion, Joint, Interphalangeal, Finger
See Arthrodesis, Finger Joint, Interphalangeal

G

Gabapentin
Assay ... 80171

Gait Training ... 97116

Galactogram ... 77053, 77054
Injection ... 19030

Galactokinase
Blood ... 82759

Galactose
Blood ... 82760
Urine ... 82760

Galactose-1-Phosphate
Uridyl Transferase ... 82775, 82776

Galeazzi Fracture/Dislocation
Radial Shaft ... 25520, 25525, 25526

Gall Bladder
See Gallbladder

Gallbladder
See Bile Duct
Anastomosis
  with Intestines ... 47720, 47721, 47740, 47741
Biopsy ... 43261
Diagnostic Imaging
  Nuclear Medicine ... 78226, 78227
  X ray with Contrast ... 74290
Destruction
  Calculi (Stone) ... 47544
Excision
  See Cholecystectomy
Exploration ... 47480
  Endoscopic Retrograde
  Cholangiopancreatography (ERCP) ... 43260
Fistulization ... 47480, 47490
Incision ... 47480
Incision and Drainage ... 47480
Pharmacologic Intervention ... 78227
Removal
  Calculi (Stone) ... 47480, 47544
Repair
  with Gastroenterostomy ... 47741
  with Intestines ... 47720, 47721, 47740, 47741
Stimulation ... 43757
Unlisted Services and Procedures ... 47999

Galvanocautery
See Electrocautery

Galvanoionization
See Iontophoresis

Gamete Intrafallopian Transfer (GIFT) ... 58976

Gamete Transfer
In Vitro Fertilization ... 58976

Gamma Camera Imaging
See Nuclear Medicine, Diagnostic

Gamma Glutamyl Transferase ... 82977

Gamma Seminoprotein
See Antigen, Prostate Specific

Gammacorten
See Dexamethasone

Gammaglobulin
Blood ... 82784, 82785, 82787

Gamulin Rh
See Immune Globulins, Rho(D)

Ganglia, Trigeminal
See Gasserian Ganglion

Ganglion
Cyst
  Aspiration/Injection ... 20612
  Drainage ... 20612
  Wrist
    Excision ... 25111, 25112
Gasserian
  See Gasserian Ganglion
Geniculate
  Facial Nerve
    Decompression ... 69720, 69725
    Suture ... 69740, 69745
Injection
  Anesthetic
    Sphenopalatine ... 64505
    Stellate ... 64510
Stellate
  See Stellate Ganglion

Ganglion Cervicothoracicum
See Stellate Ganglion

Ganglion Pterygopalatinum
See Sphenopalatine Ganglion

Ganglion, Gasser's
See Gasserian Ganglion

Gardner Operation
See Meningocele Repair

Gardnerella Vaginalis Detection ... 87510-87512

Gasser Ganglion
See Gasserian Ganglion

Gasserian Ganglion
Sensory Root
  Compression ... 61450
  Decompression ... 61450
  Section ... 61450
Creation of Lesion
  Stereotactic ... 61790

Gastrectomy
Longitudinal ... 43775
Partial ... 43631-43635, 43845, 48150, 48152
  with Gastrojejunostomy ... 43632
Proximal ... 43117, 43118, 43121-43123
Sleeve ... 43775
Total ... 43620-43622
  with Esophagoenterostomy ... 43620
with Gastroduodenostomy ... 43631

Gastric Acid
Analysis ... 82930

Gastric Analysis Test
Secretory Study ... 43754, 43755

Gastric Electrodes
Neurostimulator
  Implantation
    Laparoscopic ... 43647
    Open ... 43881
  Removal
    Laparoscopic ... 43648
    Open ... 43882
  Replacement
    Laparoscopic ... 43647
    Open ... 43881
  Revision
    Laparoscopic ... 43648
    Open ... 43882

Gastric Intubation
Diagnostic ... 43754-43757
Therapeutic ... 43753

Gastric Lavage, Therapeutic
Intubation ... 43753

Gastric Tests
Acid Reflux ... 91034, 91035, 91037, 91038
Motility ... 91020

Gastric Ulcer Disease
See Stomach, Ulcer

Gastrin ... 82938-82941

Gastrocnemius Recession
Leg, Lower ... 27687

Gastroduodenostomy
Establishment 43810
Revision 43850, 43855
with Gastrectomy 43631

Gastroenterology, Diagnostic
Breath Test
Hydrogen 91065
Methane 91065
Urea 78267, 78268
Motility Study
Colon 91117
Esophagus 91010, 91013
Gastric 91020
Esophagus Tests
Acid Perfusion 91030
Acid Reflux 91034-91038
Balloon Distension Study 91040
with Provocation 91040
Intubation with Specimen
Collection 43754, 43755
Motility Study 91010, 91013
Gastric Tests
Emptying Imaging Study 78264
with Small Bowel Transit 78265
with Small Bowel and Colon Transit .. 78266
Motility 91020
Gastroesophageal Reflux Test
See Acid Reflux Test, Gastroesophageal
Imaging
Gastrointestinal Tract
See Gastrointestinal Tract
Manometry 91010, 91013, 91020, 91022
Rectum
Sensation, Tone, and Compliance Test .. 91120
Rectum/Anus
Manometry 91122
Stomach
Stimulation of Secretion 43755
Unlisted Services and Procedures 91299

Gastroenterostomy
for Obesity
Laparoscopic 43644, 43645
for Repair 47721, 47741

Gastroesophageal Reflux Test
with Electrode Placement 91034, 91035, 91037, 91038

Gastrointestinal Endoscopies
See Endoscopy, Gastrointestinal

Gastrointestinal Exam
Capsule Endoscopy
Colon 0355T
Esophagus 91110, 91111
CT Scan
Colon 74261-74263
Endoscopic Imaging
Intraluminal
Colon 0355T
Esophagus 91110, 91111
Radiological Imaging
Bile Ducts 47531, 47532, 74300, 74301
Colon 74270, 74280
Duodenum 74260
Esophagus 74210, 74220
Swallowing Function 74230
Gallbladder 74290, 78226
Gastrointestinal Tract
See Gastrointestinal Tract, Imaging, Radiological
Pharynx 74210
Protein Loss 78282
Small Intestine 74249-74251
Nuclear Medicine
Blood Loss Study 78278
Esophageal Motility 78258
Gastric Emptying Imaging Study 78264
with Small Bowel Transit 78265
with Small Bowel and Colon Transit .. 78266
Gastric Mucosa Imaging 78261
Gastroesophageal Reflux Study 78262
Hepatobiliary 78226, 78227
Intestine 78290
Liver 78201, 78215, 78216
SPECT 78205
with Vascular Flow 78202, 78206
Peritoneal-Venous Shunt Patency 78291
Protein Loss Study 78282
Salivary Gland 78230-78232
Spleen 78215
Unlisted Diagnostic Nuclear Medicine Procedure 78299
Ultrasound
Endoscopic 76975

Gastrointestinal Pathogen ... 87505-87507

Gastrointestinal Tract
Imaging
CT Scan
Colon 74261-74263
Endoscopic
Esophagus 91110, 91111
Radiological 74340
Colon 74270, 74280
Duodenum 74260
Small Intestine 74245, 74249-74251
Upper .. 74240, 74241, 74245-74247, 74249
Measurements
Transit 91112
Pressure 91112
Reconstruction 43360, 43361
Upper
Dilation 43249, 74360
X ray 74240, 74241, 74245
Guide Dilator 74360
Guide Intubation 74340
with Contrast 74246-74249

Gastrointestinal, Upper
Biopsy 43239
Dilation
Endoscopy 43245
Esophagus 43249
Passage of Dilator 43248
Endoscopy
Ablation
Lesion 43270
Polyp 43270
Tumor 43270
Biopsy 43239
Catheterization 43241
Collection of Specimen 43235
Dilation 43245, 43248, 43249
Drainage
Pseudocyst 43240
Esophageal Ultrasound .. 43237, 43238, 43253
Examination 43235, 43252
Ultrasound 43253
Hemorrhage 43255
Injection 43236, 43253
Injection, Varices 43243
Ligation, Varices 43244
Mucosal Resection 43254
Needle Biopsy 43238, 43242
Removal
Foreign Body 43247
Lesion 43251
Polyp 43251
Tumor 43251
Stent Placement 43266
Thermal Radiation 43257
Tube Placement 43246
Ultrasound 43237, 43238, 43242, 43253, 43259, 76975
Exploration
Endoscopy 43235, 43252
Hemorrhage
Endoscopic Control 43255
Imaging
Radiological 74240, 74241, 74245-74247, 74249
Ultrasound Endoscopy 43237, 43238, 43242, 43259, 76975
Injection
Submucosal 43236
Transmural 43253
Varices 43243
Lesion
Ablation 43270
Ligation of Vein 43244
Needle Biopsy
Endoscopy 43238, 43242
Reconstruction
Esophageal 43360
Removal
Foreign Body 43247
Lesion 43250
Polyp 43250, 43251
Tumor 43250
Tube Placement
Endoscopy 43246
Ultrasound
Endoscopy 43237, 43238, 43242, 43259, 76975

Gastrojejunostomy
Conversion from Gastrostomy Tube 49446
Contrast Injection 49465
Removal of Obstructive Material 49460
Replacement of Tube 49452
Revision of Gastrojejunal Anastomosis 43860, 43865
Whipple Procedure 48150
with Duodenal Exclusion 48547
with Pancreatectomy 48150
with Partial Gastrectomy 43632
with Vagotomy 43825
without Vagotomy 43820

Gastroplasty
Collis 43338
Esophageal Lengthening 43283, 43338
Laparoscopic 43279, 43280, 43283
Revision
for Obesity 43644, 43645, 43842, 43843, 43845-43848
Wedge 43338

Gastroplasty with Esophagogastric Fundoplasty
Laparoscopic 43820

Gastrorrhaphy
Injury 43840
Perforated Ulcer 43840
Wound 43840

Gastroschises
See Gastroschisis

Gastroschisis
Repair 49605
with Prosthesis 49605
Removal of Prosthesis 49606

Index

Gastrostomy
Closure 43870
Laparoscopic
Temporary 43653
Laparoscopic 43653
Neonatal 43831
Radiological Assessment 49465
Revision of Tract
with Replacement of Gastrostomy Tube. . 43763
Temporary............................ 43830
Tube
See Gastrostomy Tube
with Pancreatic Drain.................. 48001
with Pyloroplasty 43640
with Vagotomy 43640, 43641

Gastrostomy Tube
Contrast Injection 49465
Conversion
to Gastro-jejunostomy Tube 49446
to Jejunostomy Tube 44373
Obstructive Material Removal 49460
Placement
Endoscopic 43246
Percutaneous 49440
with Conversion to Gastro-jejunostomy
Tube 49446
Replacement.......................... 49450
Percutaneous
Requiring Revision of Gastrostomy
Tract 43763
with Fluoroscopic Guidance......... 49450
without Imaging/Endoscopic
Guidance.................. 43762, 43763
Repositioning
Feeding Tube 43761

Gastrotomy
Exploration 43500
Foreign Body Removal 43500
Suture Repair
Bleeding Ulcer 43501
Esophagogastric Laceration.......... 43502
with Esophageal Tube Insertion........... 43510

GDH
See Glutamate Dehydrogenase

Gel Diffusion
Detection............................. 86331

Gel Diffusion Test
See Immunodiffusion

Gene Analysis
Analytes
ABCA4 (ATP-binding cassette, sub-family A [ABC1], member 4).................. 81408
ABCC8 (ATP-binding cassette, sub-family C [CFTR/MRP], member 8). . 81400, 81401, 81407
ABCD1 (ATP-binding cassette, sub-family D [ALD], member 1).................. 81405
ABL1 (ABL proto-oncogene 1, non-receptor tyrosine kinase) 81170, 81401
ACADM (acyl-CoA dehydrogenase, C-4 to C-12 straight chain) 81400, 81401
ACADS (acyl-CoA dehydrogenase, C-2 to C-3 short chain) 81404, 81405
ACADVL (acyl-CoA dehydrogenase, very long chain)......................... 81406
ACE (angiotensin I converting enzyme [peptidyl-dipeptidase A] 1)........... 81400
ACTA2 (actin, alpha 2, smooth muscle, aorta) 81405
ACTC1 (actin, alpha, cardiac muscle 1). . 81405
ACTN4 (actinin, alpha 4) 81406
ADRB2 (adrenergic, beta-2-, receptor, surface) 81401
AFF2 (AF4/FMR2 family, member 2 [FMR2])..................... 81171, 81172
AFG3L2 (AFG3 ATPase family gene 3 like 2 [S. cerevisiae]) 81406
AGL (amylo-alpha-1, 6-glucosidase, 4-alpha-glucanotransferase) 81407
AHI1 (Abelson helper integration site 1) 81407
AIRE (autoimmune regulator).......... 81406
ALDH7A1 (aldehyde dehydrogenase 7 family, member A1) 81406
ANG (angiogenin, ribonuclease, RNase A family, 5) 81403
ANKRD1 (ankyrin repeat domain 1)..... 81405
ANO5 (anoctamin 5)................ 81406
ANOS1 (anosmin-1) 81406
APOB (apolipoprotein B) 81401
APOE (apolipoprotein E)............. 81401
APP (amyloid beta [A4] precursor protein)......................... 81406
AGTR1 (angiotensin II receptor, type 1). . 81400
APC (adenomatous polyposis coli)...................... 81201, 81202
APTX (aprataxin) 81405
AQP2 (aquaporin 2 [collecting duct]).... 81404
AR (androgen receptor) . . 81173, 81174, 81204
ARSA (arylsulfatase A) 81405
ARX (aristaless related homeobox)................. 81403, 81404
ASPA (aspartoacylase)............... 81200
ASPM (asp [abnormal spindle] homolog, microcephaly associated [Drosophila]) . . 81407
ASS1 (argininosuccinate synthase 1) . . . 81406
ASXL1 (additional sex combs like 1, transcriptional regulator)....... 81175, 81176
ATL1 (atlastin GTPase 1)............ 81406
ATM (ataxia telangiectasia mutated) . . . 81408
ATN1 (atrophin 1)................. 81177
ATP1A2 (ATPase, Na+/K+ transporting, alpha 2 polypeptide) 81406
ATP7B (ATPase, Cu++ transporting, beta polypeptide)...................... 81406
ATXN1 (ataxin 1) 81178
ATXN2 (ataxin 2) 81179
ATXN3 (ataxin 3) 81180
ATXN7 (ataxin 7) 81181
ATXN8OS (ATXN8 opposite strand [non-protein coding]) 81182
ATXN10 (ataxin 10) 81183
AVPR2 (arginine vasopressin receptor 2) 81404
BBS1 (Bardet-Biedl syndrome 1)....... 81406
BBS2 (Bardet-Biedl syndrome 2)....... 81406
BBS10 (Bardet-Biedl syndrome 10) 81404
BCKDHA (branched chain keto acid dehydrogenase E1, alpha polypeptide)................ 81400, 81405
BCKDHB (branched chain keto acid dehydrogenase E1, beta polypeptide)................ 81205, 81406
BCL1/IgH, t(11;14) 81401
BCR/ABL1 (chronic myelogenous leukemia) Translocation 81206-81208
BCS1L (BCS1-like [S. cerevisiae]) 81405
BEST1 (bestrophin 1) 81406
BLM (Bloom syndrome, RecQ helicase-like) 81209
BMPR2 (bone morphogenetic protein receptor, type II [serine/threonine kinase])................... 81405, 81406
BRAF (B-Raf proto-oncogene, serine/threonine kinase) 81210, 81406
BRCA1 (BRCA1, DNA repair associated)...... 81162-81166, 81212, 81215
BRCA2 (BRCA2, DNA repair associated)........... 81162-81164, 81167, 81212, 81216, 81217
BSCL2 (Berardinelli-Seip congenital lipodystrophy 2 [seipin]).............. 81406
BTD (biotinidase) 81404
BTK (Bruton agammaglobulinemia tyrosine kinase) 81406
BTK (Bruton's tyrosine kinase)......... 81233
C10orf2 (chromosome 10 open reading frame 2) 81404
CACNA1A (calcium voltage-gated channel subunit alpha 1A)............ 81184-81186
CACNB2 (calcium channel, voltage-dependent, beta 2 subunit)..................... 81406
CALR (calreticulin) (eg, myeloproliferative disorders) 81219
CAPN3 (calpain 3) 81406
CASQ2 (calsequestrin 2 [cardiac muscle]) 81405
CASR (calcium-sensing receptor) 81405
CAV3 (caveolin 3).................. 81404
CBFB/MYH11 (inv (16)) 81401
CBS (cystathionine-beta-synthase) 81401, 81406
CD40LG (CD40 ligand) 81404
CCND1/IGH (BCL1/IgH, t(11;14))....... 81401
CCR5 (chemokine C-C motif receptor 5) 81400
CDH1 (cadherin 1, type 1, E-cadherin [epithelial])....................... 81406
CDH23 (cadherin-related 23).......... 81408
CDKL5 (cyclin-dependent kinase-like 5) 81405, 81406
CDKN2A (cyclin-dependent kinase inhibitor 2A)...................... 81404
CEBPA (CCAAT/enhancer binding protein [C/EBP], alpha).................... 81218
CEL (carboxyl ester lipase [bile salt stimulated lipase]) 81403
CEP290 (centrosomal protein 290kDa) . . 81408
CFH/ARMS2 (complement factor H/age-related maculopathy susceptibility 2) 81401
CFTR (cystic fibrosis transmembrane conductance regulator) 81220-81224
CHD7 (chromodomain helicase DNA binding protein 7) 81407
CHRNA4 (cholinergic receptor, nicotinic, alpha 4) 81405
CHRNB2 (cholinergic receptor, nicotinic, beta 2 [neuronal]).................. 81405
Chromosome 1p-/19q-............... 81402
Chromosome 18q- 81402
CLCN1 (chloride channel 1, skeletal muscle)........................... 81406
CLCNKB (chloride channel, voltage-sensitive Kb)...................... 81406
CLRN1 (clarin 1) 81400, 81404
CNBP (CCHC-type zinc finger nucleic acid binding protein) 81187
CNTNAP2 (contactin associated protein-like 2)..................... 81406
COL1A1 (collagen, type I, alpha 1)...... 81408
COL1A1/PDGFB (t(17;22)).............. 81402
COL1A2 (collagen, type I, alpha 2)...... 81408
COL4A1 (collagen, type IV, alpha 1) 81408
COL4A3 (collagen, type IV, alpha 3 [Goodpasture antigen]) 81408
COL4A4 (collagen, type IV, alpha 4) 81407
COL4A5 (collagen, type IV, alpha 5) 81407, 81408
COL6A1 (collagen, type VI, alpha 1) 81407

COL6A2 (collagen, type VI, alpha 2) 81406, 81407
COL6A3 (collagen, type VI, alpha 3) 81407
COX6B1 (cytochrome c oxidase subunit VIb polypeptide 1) 81404
COX10 (COX10 homolog, cytochrome c oxidase assembly protein). 81405
COX15 (COX15 homolog, cytochrome c oxidase assembly protein). 81405
CPOX (coproporphyrinogen oxidase) 81405
CPT1A (carnitine palmitoyltransferase 1A [liver]) 81406
CPT2 (carnitine palmitoyltransferase 2) 81404
CRB1 (crumbs homolog 1 [Drosophila]).. 81406
CREBBP (CREB binding protein). . 81406, 81407
CRX (cone-rod homeobox) 81404
CSTB (cystatin B) 81188-81190
CTNNB1 (catenin [cadherin-associated protein], beta 1, 88kDa) 81403
CTRC (chymotrypsin C) (eg, hereditary pancreatitis). 81405
CYP1B1 (cytochrome P450, family 1, subfamily B, polypeptide 1) 81404
CYP21A2 (cytochrome P450, family 21, subfamily A, polypeptide 2)..... 81402, 81405
CYP2C19 (cytochrome P450, family 2, subfamily C, polypeptide 19) 81225
CYP2C9 (cytochrome P450, family 2, subfamily C, polypeptide 9) 81227
CYP2D6 (cytochrome P450, family 2, subfamily D, polypeptide 6) 81226
CYP3A4 (cytochrome P450, family 3, subfamily A member 4). 81230
CYP3A5 (cytochrome P450, family 3, subfamily A member 5). 81231
CYP11B1 (cytochrome P450, family 11, subfamily B, polypeptide 1) 81405
CYP17A1 (cytochrome P450, family 17, subfamily A, polypeptide 1). 81405
CYP21A2 (cytochrome P450, family 21, subfamily A, polypeptide2) 81402, 81405
Constitution 81228, 81229
Neoplasia 81406
DAZ/SRY (deleted in azoospermia and sex determining region Y) 81403
DBT (dihydrolipoamide branched chain transacylase E2) 81405, 81406
DCX (doublecortin). 81405
DEK/NUP214 (t(6;9)). 81401
DES (desmin) 81405
DFNB59 (deafness, autosomal recessive 59) 81405
DGUOK (deoxyguanosine kinase) 81405
DHCR7 (7-dehydrocholesterol reductase) 81405
DLAT (dihydrolipoamide S-acetyltransferase). 81406
DLD (dihydrolipoamide dehydrogenase) . 81406
DMD (dystrophin). 81161, 81408
DMPK (DM1 protein kinase) 81234, 81239
DNMT3A (DNA [cytosine-5-]-methyltransferase 3 alpha) 81403
DPYD (dihydropyrimidine dehydrogenase) 81232
DSC2 (desmocollin) 81406
DSG2 (desmoglein 2). 81406
DSP (desmoplakin). 81406
DYSF (dysferlin, limb girdle muscular dystrophy 2B [autosomal recessive]) 81408
E2A/PBX1 (t(1;19)). 81401
EFHC1 (EF-hand domain [C terminal] containing 1) 81406
EGFR (epidermal growth factor receptor) 81235
EGR2 (early growth response 2) 81404
EIF2B2 (eukaryotic translation initiation factor 2B, subunit 2 beta, 39kDa). 81405
EIF2B3 (eukaryotic translation initiation factor 2B, subunit 3 gamma, 58kDa) 81406
EIF2B4 (eukaryotic translation initiation factor 2B, subunit 4 delta, 67kDa) 81406
EIF2B5 (eukaryotic translation initiation factor 2B, subunit 5 epsilon, 82kDa) 81406
EMD (emerin) 81404, 81405
EML4/ALK (inv(2)) 81401
ENG (endoglin) 81405, 81406
EPCAM (epithelial cell adhesion molecule) 81403
EPM2A (epilepsy, progressive myoclonus type 2A, Lafora disease [laforin]). 81404
ESR1/PGR (receptor 1/progesterone receptor) 81402
ETV6/NTRK3 (t(12;15)). 81401
ETV6/RUNX1 (t(12;21)). 81401
EWSR1/ATF1 (t(2;22)) 81401
EWSR1/ERG (t(21;22)) 81401
EWSR1/FLI1 (t(11;22)) 81401
EWSR1/WT1 (t(11;22)). 81401
EYA1 (eyes absent homolog 1 [Drosophila]). 81405, 81406
EZH2 (enhancer of zeste 2 polycomb repressive complex 2 subunit). 81236, 81237
F2 (prothrombin, coagulation factor II) 81240, 81400
F5 (coagulation factor V) 81241, 81400
F7 (coagulation factor VII [serum prothrombin conversion accelerator]). 81400
F8 (coagulation factor VIII). 81403, 81406, 81407
F9 (coagulation factor IX). 81238
F11 (coagulation factor XI). 81401
F12 (coagulation factor XII [Hageman factor]) 81403
F13B (coagulation factor XIII, B polypeptide) 81400
FAH (fumarylacetoacetate hydrolase [fumarylacetoacetase]) 81406
FANCC (Fanconi anemia, complementation group C) 81242
FASTKD2 (FAST kinase domains 2) 81406
FBN1 (fibrillin 1). 81408
FGB (fibrinogen beta chain) 81400
FGF23 (fibroblast growth factor 23). 81404
FGFR1 (fibroblast growth factor receptor 1) 81400, 81405
FGFR2 (fibroblast growth factor receptor 2) 81404
FGFR3 (fibroblast growth factor receptor 3) 81400, 81401, 81403, 81404
FH (fumarate hydratase) 81405
FHL1 (four and a half LIM domains 1) ... 81404
FIG4 (FIG4 homolog, SAC1 lipid phosphatase domain containing [S. cerevisiae]). 81406
FIP1L1/PDGFRA (del(4q12)) 81401
FKRP (fukutin related protein) 81404
FKTN (fukutin) 81400, 81405
FLG (filaggrin). 81401
FLT3 (fms-related tyrosine kinase 3). 81245, 81246
FMR1 (fragile X mental retardation 1) 81243, 81244
FOXG1 (forkhead box G1). 81404
FOXO1/PAX3 (t(2;13)). 81401
FOXO1/PAX7 (t(1;13)). 81401
FSHMD1A (facioscapulohumeral muscular dystrophy 1A). 81404
FTSJ1 (FtsJ RNA methyltransferase homolog 1 [E. coli]). 81405, 81406
FUS (fused in sarcoma) 81406
FUS/DDIT3 (t(12;16)) 81401
FXN (frataxin). 81284-81286, 81289
G6PC (glucose-6-phosphatase, catalytic subunit) 81250
G6PD (glucose-6-phosphate dehydrogenase) 81247-81249
GAA (glucosidase, alpha; acid) 81406
GABRG2 (gamma-aminobutyric acid [GABA] A receptor, gamma 2) 81405
GALC (galactosylceramidase) ... 81401, 81406
GALT (galactose-1-phosphate uridylyltransferase) 81401, 81406
GARS (glycyl-tRNA synthetase). 81406
GBA (glucosidase, beta, acid) 81251
GCDH (glutaryl-CoA dehydrogenase). ... 81406
GCH1 (GTP cyclohydrolase 1). 81405
GCK (glucokinase [hexokinase 4]) 81406
GDAP1 (ganglioside-induced differentiation-associated protein 1). 81405
GFAP (glial fibrillary acidic protein). 81405
GH1 (growth hormone 1) 81404
GHR (growth hormone receptor) 81405
GHRHR (growth hormone releasing hormone receptor). 81405
GJB1 (gap junction protein, beta 1). 81403
GJB2 (gap junction protein, beta 2, 26kDa, connexin 26). 81252, 81253
GJB6 (gap junction protein, beta 6, 30kDa, connexin 30). 81254
GLA (galactosidase, alpha) 81405
GLUD1 (glutamate dehydrogenase 1) 81406
GNAQ (guanine nucleotide-binding protein G[q] subunit alpha) 81403
GNE (glucosamine [UDP-N-acetyl]-2-epimerase/N-acetylmannosamine kinase) 81400, 81406
GP1BB (glycoprotein Ib [platelet], beta polypeptide) 81404
GRN (granulin) 81406
H19 (imprinted maternally expressed transcript [non-protein coding]) 81401
HADHA (hydroxyacyl-CoA dehydrogenase/3-ketoacyl-CoA thiolase/enoyl-CoA hydratase [trifunctional protein] alpha subunit). ... 81406
HADHB (hydroxyacyl-CoA dehydrogenase/3 ketoacyl-CoA thiolase/enoyl-CoA hydratase [trifunctional protein], beta subunit) 81406
HBA1/HBA2 (alpha globin 1 and alpha globin 2). 81257-81259, 81269
HBB (hemoglobin, beta, beta-Globin) 81361-81364
HEXA (hexosaminidase A [alpha polypeptide]) 81255, 81406
HFE (hemochromatosis) 81256
HLA Class I and II Typing, Low Resolution 81370, 81371
HLA Class I Typing, Low Resolution 81372-81374
HLA Class II Typing, Low Resolution 81375-81377
HLA Class I and II Typing, High Resolution 81378
HLA Class I Typing, High Resolution 81379-81381
HLA Class II Typing, High Resolution 81382, 81383
HLCS (HLCS holocarboxylase synthetase). 81406
HMBS (hydroxymethylbilane synthase). . 81406
HNF1A (HNF1 homeobox A). 81405
HPA (Human Platelet Antigen). .. 81105-81112
HNF1B (HNF1 homeobox B). 81404, 81405

Index

HNF4A (hepatocyte nuclear factor 4, alpha) . . . 81406
HRAS (v-Ha-ras Harvey rat sarcoma viral oncogene homolog) . . . 81403, 81404
HSD3B2 (hydroxyl-delta-5-steroid dehydrogenase, 3 beta- and steroid-delta isomerase 2) . . . 81404
HSD11B2 (hydroxysteroid [11-beta] dehydrogenase 2) . . . 81404
HSPB1 (heat shock 27kDa protein 1) . . . 81404
HTRA1 (HtrA serine peptidase 1) . . . 81405
HTT (huntingtin) . . . 81271, 81274
Human Erythrocyte Antigen . . . 81403
Human Platelet Antigen 1 (HPA-1) . . . 81105
Human Platelet Antigen 2 (HPA-2) . . . 81106
Human Platelet Antigen 3 (HPA-3) . . . 81107
Human Platelet Antigen 4 (HPA-4) . . . 81108
Human Platelet Antigen 5 (HPA-5) . . . 81109
Human Platelet Antigen 6 (HPA-6w) . . . 81110
Human Platelet Antigen 9 (HPA-9w) . . . 81111
Human Platelet Antigen 15 (HPA-15) . . . 81112
IDH1 (isocitrate dehydrogenase 1 [NADP+], soluble) . . . 81120
IDH2 (isocitrate dehydrogenase 2 [NADP+], mitochondrial) . . . 81121
IDS (iduronate 2-sulfatase) . . . 81405
IDUA (iduronidase, alpha L-) . . . 81406
IFNL3 (interferon, lambda 3) . . . 81283
IGH@ (immunoglobulin heavy chain locus) . . . 81261-81263
IGH@/BCL2 (t(14;18)) . . . 81401, 81402
IGK@ (immunoglobulin kappa light chain locus) . . . 81264
IKBKAP (inhibitor of kappa light polypeptide gene enhancer in B-cells, kinase complex-associated protein) . . . 81260
IL2RG (interleukin 2 receptor, gamma) . . . 81405
INF2 (inverted formin, FH2 and WH2 domain containing) . . . 81406
INS (insulin) . . . 81404
ISPD (isoprenoid synthase domain containing) . . . 81405
ITPR1 (inositol 1,4,5-trisphosphate receptor, type 1) . . . 81408
IVD (isovaleryl-CoA dehydrogenase) . . . 81400, 81406
JAG1 (jagged 1) . . . 81406, 81407
JAK2 (Janus kinase 2) . . . 81270, 81403
JUP (junction plakoglobin) . . . 81406
KCNC3 (potassium voltage-gated channel, Shaw-related subfamily, member 3) . . . 81403
KCNH2 (potassium voltage-gated channel, subfamily H [eag-related], member 2) . . . 81406
KCNJ2 (potassium inwardly-rectifying channel, subfamily J, member 2) . . . 81403
KCNJ1 (potassium inwardly-rectifying channel, subfamily J, member 1) . . . 81404
KCNJ10 (potassium inwardly-rectifying channel, subfamily J, member 10) . . . 81404
KCNJ11 (potassium inwardly-rectifying channel, subfamily J, member 11) . . . 81403
KCNQ1 (potassium voltage-gated channel, KQT-like subfamily, member 1) . . . 81406
KCNQ1OT1 (KCNQ1 overlapping transcript 1 [non-protein coding]) . . . 81401
KCNQ2 (potassium voltage-gated channel, KQT-like subfamily, member 2) . . . 81406
KDM5C (lysine [K]-specific demethylase 5C) . . . 81407
KIAA0196 (KIAA0196) . . . 81407
Killer cell immunoglobulin-like receptor (KIR) gene family . . . 81403
KIT (v-kit Hardy-Zuckerman 4 feline sarcoma viral oncogene homolog) . . . 81272, 81273
Known familial variant not otherwise specified . . . 81403
KRAS (Kirsten rat sarcoma viral oncogene homolog) . . . 81275, 81276, 81405
L1CAM (L1 cell adhesion molecule) . . . 81407
LAMA2 (laminin, alpha 2) . . . 81408
LAMB2 (laminin, beta 2 [laminin S]) . . . 81407
LAMP2 (lysosomal-associated membrane protein 2) . . . 81405
LCT (lactase-phlorizin hydrolase) . . . 81400
LDB3 (LIM domain binding 3) . . . 81406
LDLR (low density lipoprotein receptor) . . . 81405, 81406
LEPR (leptin receptor) . . . 81406
LHCGR (luteinizing hormone/choriogonadotropin receptor) . . . 81406
LINC00518 (long intergenic non-protein coding RNA 518) . . . 81401
LITAF (lipopolysaccharide-induced TNF factor) . . . 81404
LMNA (lamin A/C) . . . 81406
LRP5 (low density lipoprotein receptor-related protein 5) . . . 81406
LRRK2 (leucine-rich repeat kinase 2) . . . 81401, 81408
MAP2K1 (mitogen-activated protein kinase 1) . . . 81406
MAP2K2 (mitogen-activated protein kinase 2) . . . 81406
MAPT (microtubule-associated protein tau) . . . 81406
MC4R (melanocortin 4 receptor) . . . 81403
MCCC1 (methylcrotonoyl-CoA carboxylase 1 [alpha]) . . . 81406
MCCC2 (methylcrotonoyl-CoA carboxylase 2 [beta]) . . . 81406
MCOLN1 (mucolipin 1) . . . 81290
MECP2 (methyl CpG binding protein 2 [Rett syndrome]) . . . 81302-81304
MED12 (mediator complex subunit 12) . . . 81401
MEFV (Mediterranean fever) . . . 81402, 81404
MEG3/DLK1 (maternally expressed 3 [non-protein coding]/delta-like 1 homolog [Drosophila]) . . . 81401
MEN1 (multiple endocrine neoplasia I) . . . 81404, 81405
MFN2 (mitofusin 2) . . . 81406
MGMT (O-6-methylguanine-DNA methyltransferase) . . . 81287
MICA (MHC class I polypeptide-related sequence A) . . . 81403
MLH1 (mutL homolog 1, colon cancer, nonpolyposis type 2) . . . 81288, 81292-81294
MLL/AFF1 (t(4;11)) . . . 81401
MLL/MLLT3 (t(9;11)) . . . 81401
MMAA (methylmalonic aciduria [cobalamine deficiency] type A) . . . 81405
MMAB (methylmalonic aciduria [cobalamine deficiency] type B) . . . 81405
MMACHC (methylmalonic aciduria [cobalamin deficiency] cblC type, with homocystinuria) . . . 81404
MPI (mannose phosphate isomerase) . . . 81405
MPL (myeloproliferative leukemia virus oncogene, thrombopoietin receptor, TPOR) . . . 81402, 81403
MPV17 (MpV17 mitochondrial inner membrane protein) . . . 81404, 81405
MPZ (myelin protein zero) . . . 81405
MSH2 (mutS homolog 2, colon cancer, nonpolyposis type 1) . . . 81295-81297
MSH6 (mutS homolog 6 [E. coli]) 81298-81300
MT-ATP6 (mitochondrially encoded ATP synthase 6) . . . 81401
MT-ND4, MT-ND6 (mitochondrially encoded NADH dehydrogenase 4, mitochondrially encoded NADH dehydrogenase 6) . . . 81401
MT-RNR1 (mitochondrially encoded 12S RNA) . . . 81401, 81403
MT-TK (mitochondrially encoded tRNA lysine) . . . 81401
MT-TL1 (mitochondrially encoded tRNA leucine 1 [UUA/G]) . . . 81401
MT-TL1, MT-ND5 (mitochondrially encoded tRNA leucine 1 [UUA/G], mitochondrially encoded NADH dehydrogenase 5) . . . 81401
MT-TS1 (mitochondrially encoded tRNA serine 1) . . . 81403
MT-TS1, MT-RNR1 (mitochondrially encoded tRNA serine 1 [UCN], mitochondrially encoded 12S RNA) . . . 81401
MTM1 (myotubularin 1) . . . 81405, 81406
MTHFR (5, 10-methylenetetrahydrofolate reductase) . . . 81291
MUT (methylmalonyl CoA mutase) . . . 81406
MUTYH (mutY homolog [E. coli]) 81401, 81406
MYD88 (myeloid differentiation primary response 88) . . . 81305
MYBPC3 (myosin binding protein C, cardiac) . . . 81407
MYH6 (myosin, heavy chain 6, cardiac muscle, alpha) . . . 81407
MYH7 (myosin, heavy chain 7, cardiac muscle, beta) . . . 81407
MYH11 (myosin, heavy chain 11, smooth muscle) . . . 81408
MYL2 (myosin, light chain 2, regulatory, cardiac, slow) . . . 81405
MYL3 (myosin, light chain 3, alkali, ventricular, skeletal, slow) . . . 81405
MYO7A (myosin VIIA) . . . 81407
MYOT (myotilin) . . . 81405
NDP (Norrie disease [pseudoglioma]) . . . 81403, 81404
NDUFA1 (NADH dehydrogenase [ubiquinone] 1 alpha subcomplex, 1, 7.5kDa) . . . 81404
NDUFAF2 (NADH dehydrogenase [ubiquinone] 1 alpha subcomplex, assembly factor 2) . . . 81404
NDUFS1 (NADH dehydrogenase [ubiquinone] Fe-S protein 1, 75kDa [NADH-coenzyme Q reductase]) . . . 81406
NDUFS4 (NADH dehydrogenase [ubiquinone] Fe-S protein 4, 18kDa [NADH-coenzyme Q reductase]) . . . 81404
NDUFS7 (NADH dehydrogenase [ubiquinone] Fe-S protein 7, 20kDa [NADH-coenzyme Q reductase]) . . . 81405
NDUFS8 (NADH dehydrogenase [ubiquinone] Fe-S protein 8, 23kDa [NADH-coenzyme Q reductase]) . . . 81405
NDUFV1 (NADH dehydrogenase [ubiquinone] flavoprotein 1, 51kDa) . . . 81405
NEB (nebulin) . . . 81400, 81408
NEFL (neurofilament, light polypeptide) . . 81405
NF1 (neurofibromin 1) . . . 81408
NF2 (neurofibromin 2 [merlin]) . . . 81405, 81406
NHLRC1 (NHL repeat containing 1) . . . 81403
NIPA1 (non-imprinted in Prader-Willi/Angelman syndrome 1) . . . 81404
NLGN3 (neuroligin 3) . . . 81405
NLGN4X (neuroligin 4, X-linked) . . 81404, 81405
NOD2 (nucleotide-binding oligomerization domain containing 2) . . . 81401
NOTCH1 (notch 1) . . . 81407

Gene Analysis, Analytes

NOTCH3 (notch 3) 81406
NPC1 (Niemann-Pick disease, type C1) . . 81406
NPC2 (Niemann-Pick disease, type C2 [epididymal secretory protein E1]) 81404
NPHP1 (nephronophthisis 1 [juvenile]) 81405, 81406
NPHS1 (nephrosis 1, congenital, Finnish type [nephrin]) 81407
NPHS2 (nephrosis 2, idiopathic, steroid resistant [podocin]) 81405
NPM1 (nucleophosmin [nucleolar phosphoprotein B23, numatrin]) 81310
NPM1/ALK (t(2;5)) 81401
NRAS (neuroblastoma RAS viral [v-ras] oncogene homolog) 81311
NR0B1 (nuclear receptor subfamily 0, group B, member 1) 81404
NSD1 (nuclear receptor binding SET domain protein 1) 81405, 81406
NUDT15 (nudix hydrolase 15) 81306
OPA1 (optic atrophy 1) 81406, 81407
OPTN (optineurin) 81406
OTC (ornithine carbamoyltransferase) . . . 81405
PABPN1 (poly[A] binding protein nuclear 1) 81312
PAFAH1B1 (platelet-activating factor acetylhydrolase 1b, regulatory subunit 1 [45kDa]) 81405, 81406
PAH (phenylalanine hydroxylase) 81406
PALB2 (partner and localizer of BRCA2) 81406
PARK2 (Parkinson protein 2, E3 ubiquitin protein ligase [parkin]) 81405, 81406
PAX2 (paired box 2) 81406
PAX8/PPARG (t(2;3) (q13;p25)) 81401
PC (pyruvate carboxylase) 81406
PCA3/KLK3 (prostate cancer antigen 3 [non protein coding]/kallikrein related peptidase 3 [prostate specific antigen]) 81313
PCCA (propionyl CoA carboxylase, alpha polypeptide) 81405, 81406
PCCB (propionyl CoA carboxylase, beta polypeptide) 81406
PCDH15 (protocadherin-related 15) 81400, 81406, 81407
PCDH19 (protocadherin 19) 81405
PCSK9 (proprotein convertase subtilisin/kevin type 9) 81406
PDGFRA (platelet-derived growth factor receptor, alpha polypeptide) 81314
PDHA1 (pyruvate dehydrogenase [lipoamide] alpha 1) 81405, 81406
PDHB (pyruvate dehydrogenase [lipoamide] beta) 81405
PDHX (pyruvate dehydrogenase complex, component X) 81406
PDX1 (pancreatic and duodenal homeobox 1) 81404
PHEX (phosphate regulating endopeptidase homolog, X-linked) 81406
PHOX2B (paired-like homeobox 2b) 81403, 81404
PIK3CA (phosphatidylinositol-4,5-bisphosphate 3-kinase, catalytic subunit alpha) 81404
PINK1 (PTEN induced putative kinase 1) 81405
PKD1 (polycystic kidney disease 1 [autosomal dominant]) 81407
PKD2 (polycystic kidney disease 2 [autosomal dominant]) 81406
PKHD1 (polycystic kidney and hepatic disease 1) 81408
PKLR (pyruvate kinase, liver and RBC) (eg, pyruvate kinase deficiency) 81405
PKP2 (plakophilin 2) 81406
PLCE1 (phospholipase C, epsilon 1) 81407
PLCG2 (phospholipase C gamma 2) 81320
PLN (phospholamban) 81403
PLP1 (proteolipid protein 1) 81404, 81405
PML/RARalpha, (t(15;17)) (promyelocytic leukemia/retinoic acid receptor alpha) 81315, 81316
PMP22 (peripheral myelin protein 22) 81324-81326
PMS2 (PMS2 postmeiotic segregation increased 2 [S. cerevisiae]) 81317-81319
PNKD (paroxysmal nonkinesigenic dyskinesia) 81406
POLG (polymerase [DNA directed], gamma) 81406
POMGNT1 (protein O-linked mannose beta1, 2-N-acetylglucosaminyltransferase) 81406
POMT1 (protein-O-mannosyltransferase 1) 81406
POMT2 (protein-O-mannosyltransferase 2) 81406
POU1F1 (POU class 1 homeobox 1) 81405
PPOX (protoporphyrinogen oxidase) 81406
PPP2R2B (protein phosphatase 2 regulatory subunit Bbeta) 81343
PQBP1 (polyglutamine binding protein 1) 81404, 81405
PRAME (preferentially expressed antigen in melanoma) 81401
PRKAG2 (protein kinase, AMP-activated, gamma 2 non-catalytic subunit) 81406
PRKCG (protein kinase C, gamma) 81406
PRNP (prion protein) 81404
PROP1 (PROP paired-like homeobox 1) . . 81404
PRPH2 (peripherin 2 [retinal degeneration, slow]) 81404
PRSS1 (protease, serine, 1 [trypsin 1]) 81401, 81404
PRX (periaxin) 81405
PSEN1 (presenilin 1) 81405
PSEN2 (presenilin 2 [Alzheimer disease 4]) 81406
PTEN (phosphatase and tensin homolog) 81321-81323
PTPN11 (protein tyrosine phosphatase, non-receptor type 11) 81406
PYGM (phosphorylase, glycogen, muscle) 81401, 81406
RAB7A (RAB7A, member RAS oncogene family) 81405
RAF1 (v-raf-1 murine leukemia viral oncogene homolog 1) 81404, 81406
RAI1 (retinoic acid induced 1) 81405
REEP1 (receptor accessory protein 1) . . . 81405
RET (ret proto-oncogene) 81404-81406
RHD (Rh blood group, D antigen) 81403
RHO (rhodopsin) 81404
RP1 (retinitis pigmentosa 1) 81404
RPE65 (retinal pigment epithelium specific protein 65kDa) 81406
RPS19 (ribosomal protein S19) 81405
RRM2B (ribonucleotide reductase M2 B [TP53 inducible]) 81405
RUNX1 (runt related transcription factor 1) 81334
RUNX1/RUNX1T1(t(8;21)) 81401
RYR1 (ryanodine receptor 1, skeletal) 81406, 81408
RYR2 (ryanodine receptor 2 [cardiac]) . . . 81408
SCN1A (sodium channel, voltage-gated, type I, alpha subunit) 81407
SCN1B (sodium channel, voltage-gated, type I, beta) 81404
SCN4A (sodium channel, voltage-gated, type IV, alpha subunit) 81406
SCN5A (sodium channel, voltage-gated, type V, alpha subunit) 81407
SCNN1A (sodium channel, nonvoltage-gated 1 alpha) 81406
SCNN1B (sodium channel, nonvoltage-gated 1, beta) 81406
SCNN1G (sodium channel, nonvoltage-gated 1, gamma) 81406
SCO1 (SCO cytochrome oxidase deficient homolog 1) 81405
SCO2 (SCO cytochrome oxidase deficient homolog 2 [SCO1L]) 81404
SDHA (succinate dehydrogenase complex, subunit A, flavoprotein [Fp]) 81406
SDHB (succinate dehydrogenase complex, subunit B, iron sulfur) 81405
SDHC (succinate dehydrogenase complex, subunit C, integral membrane protein, 15kDa) 81404, 81405
SDHD (succinate dehydrogenase complex, subunit D, integral membrane protein) . . 81404
SEPT9 (Septin9) 81327
SERPINA1 (serpin peptidase inhibitor, clade A [alpha-1 antiproteinase, antitrypsin], member 1) 81332
SERPINE1 (serpine peptidase inhibitor clade E, member 1, plasminogen activator inhibitor 1, PAI 1) 81400
SETX (senataxin) 81406
SGCA (sarcoglycan, alpha [50kDa dystrophin-associated glycoprotein]) 81405
SGCB (sarcoglycan, beta [43kDa dystrophin-associated glycoprotein]) 81405
SGCD (sarcoglycan, delta [35kDa dystrophin-associated glycoprotein]) 81405
SGCE (sarcoglycan, epsilon) 81405, 81406
SGCG (sarcoglycan, gamma [35kDa dystrophin-associated glycoprotein]) 81404, 81405
SH2D1A (SH2 domain containing 1A) 81403, 81404
SH3TC2 (SH3 domain and tetratricopeptide repeats 2) 81406
SHOC2 (soc-2 suppressor of clear homolog) 81400, 81405
SHOX (short stature homeobox) 81405
SIL1 (SIL1 homolog, endoplasmic reticulum chaperone [S. cerevisiae]) 81405
SLC9A6 (solute carrier family 9 [sodium/hydrogen exchanger], member 6) 81406
SLC2A1 (solute carrier family 2 [facilitated glucose transporter], member 1) 81405
SLC12A1 (solute carrier family 12 [sodium/potassium/chloride transporters], member 1) 81407
SLC12A3 (solute carrier family 12 [sodium/chloride transporters], member 3) 81407
SLC16A2 (solute carrier family 16, member 2 [thyroid hormone transporter]) . . . 81404, 81405
SLC22A5 (solute carrier family 22 [organic cation/carnitine transporter], member 5) 81405
SLC25A4 (solute carrier family 25 [mitochondrial carrier; adenine nucleotide translocator], member 4) 81404
SLC25A20 (solute carrier family 25 [carnitine/acylcarnitine translocase], member 20) 81404, 81405
SLC26A4 (solute carrier family 26, member 4) 81406

Index

SLC37A4 (solute carrier family 37 [glucose-6-phosphate transporter], member 4) ... 81406
SLCO1B1 (solute carrier organic anion transporter family, member 1B1) ... 81328
SMAD4 (SMAD family member 4) ... 81405, 81406
SMN1 (survival of motor neuron 1, telomeric) ... 81329, 81336, 81337
SMN2 (survival of motor neuron 2, centromeric) ... 81329, 81336, 81337
SMPD1 (sphingomyelin phosphodiesterase 1, acid lysosomal) ... 81330
SNRPN/UBE3A (small nuclear ribonucleoprotein polypeptide N/ubiquitin protein ligase E3A) ... 81331
SOD1 (superoxide dismutase 1, soluble) ... 81404
SOS1 (son of sevenless homolog 1) ... 81406
SPAST (spastin) ... 81405, 81406
SPG7 (spastic paraplegia 7 [pure and complicated autosomal recessive]) ... 81405, 81406
SPG11 (spastic paraplegia 11 [autosomal recessive]) ... 81407
SPINK1 (serine peptidase inhibitor, Kazal type 1) ... 81404
SPRED1 (sprouty-related, EVH1 domain containing 1) ... 81405
SPTBN2 (spectrin, beta, non-erythrocytic 2) ... 81407
SRY (sex determining region Y) ... 81400
SS18/SSX1 (t(X;18)) ... 81401
SS18/SSX2 (t(X;18)) ... 81401
STAT3 (signal transducer and activator of transcription 3 [acute-phase response factor]) ... 81405
STK11 (serine/threonine kinase 11) ... 81404, 81405
STXBP1 (syntaxin binding protein 1) ... 81406
SURF1 (surfeit 1) ... 81405
TACO1 (translational activator of mitochondrial encoded cytochrome c oxidase I) ... 81404
TARDBP (TAR DNA binding protein) ... 81405
TAZ (tafazzin) ... 81406
TBP (TATA box binding protein) ... 81344
TBX5 (T-box 5) ... 81405
TCF4 (transcription factor 4) ... 81405, 81406
TERT (telomerase reverse transcriptase) ... 81345
TGFBR1 (transforming growth factor, beta receptor 1) ... 81405
TGFBR2 (transforming growth factor, beta receptor 2) ... 81405
TGFBI (transforming growth factor beta-induced) ... 81333
TH (tyrosine hydroxylase) ... 81406
THAP1 (THAP domain containing, apoptosis associated protein 1) ... 81404
THRB (thyroid hormone receptor, beta) ... 81405
TK2 (thymidine kinase 2, mitochondrial) 81405
TMEM43 (transmembrane protein 43) ... 81406
TMEM67 (transmembrane protein 67) ... 81407
TNNC1 (troponin C type 1 [slow]) ... 81405
TNNI3 (troponin I, type 3 [cardiac]) ... 81405
TNNT2 (troponin T, type 2 [cardiac]) ... 81406
TOR1A (torsin family 1, member A [torsin A]) ... 81400, 81404
TP53 (tumor protein 53) ... 81404, 81405
TPM1 (tropomyosin 1 [alpha]) ... 81405
TPMT (thiopurine S-methyltransferase) ... 81335
TRB@ (T cell receptor beta locus) ... 81340, 81341
TRD@ (T cell antigen receptor, delta) Rearrangement ... 81402
TRG@ (T cell receptor gamma locus) ... 81342
TRPC6 (transient receptor potential cation channel, subfamily C, member 6) ... 81406
TSC1 (tuberous sclerosis 1) ... 81405, 81406
TSC2 (tuberous sclerosis 2) ... 81406, 81407
TTPA (tocopherol [alpha] transfer protein) ... 81404
TTR (transthyretin) ... 81404
TWIST1 (twist homolog 1 [Drosophila]) ... 81403, 81404
TYMP (thymidine phosphorylase) ... 81405
TYMS (thymidylate synthetase) ... 81346
TYR (tyrosinase [oculocutaneous albinism IA]) ... 81404
UBA1 (ubiquitin-like modifier activating enzyme 1) ... 81403
UBE3A (ubiquitin protein ligase E3A) ... 81406
UGT1A1 (UDP glucuronosyltransferase 1 family, polypeptide A1) ... 81350
UMOD (uromodulin) ... 81406
Uniparental disomy (UPD) ... 81402
USH1C (Usher syndrome 1C [autosomal recessive, severe]) ... 81407
USH1G (Usher syndrome 1G [autosomal recessive]) ... 81404
USH2A (Usher syndrome 2A [autosomal recessive, mild]) ... 81408
VHL (von Hippel-Lindau tumor suppressor) ... 81403, 81404
VKORC1 (vitamin K epoxide reductase complex, subunit 1) ... 81355
VPS13B (vacuolar protein sorting 13 homolog B [yeast]) ... 81407, 81408
VWF (von Willebrand factor) ... 81401, 81403-81406, 81408
WAS (Wiskott-Aldrich syndrome [eczema-thrombocytopenia]) ... 81406
WDR62 (WD repeat domain 62) ... 81407
WT1 (Wilms tumor 1) ... 81405
ZEB2 (zinc finger E-box binding homeobox 2) ... 81404, 81405
ZNF41 (zinc finger protein 41) ... 81404

Chimerism Analysis ... 81267, 81268
Comparative Analysis Using Short Tandem Repeat (STR) Markers ... 81265, 81266
Cytogenomic Constitutional Targeted Microarray Analysis
  Chromosome 22q13 ... 81405
Cytogenomic Microarray Analysis, Neoplasia ... 81406
HLA Class I and II Typing, Low Resolution ... 81370, 81371
HLA Class I Typing, Low Resolution ... 81372-81374
HLA Class II Typing, Low Resolution ... 81375-81377
HLA Class I and II Typing, High Resolution ... 81378
HLA Class I Typing, High Resolution 81379-81381
HLA Class II Typing, High Resolution ... 81382, 81383
Human Platelet Antigen Genotyping 81105-81112
Microsatellite Instability Analysis ... 81301
Short Tandem Repeat (STR) Analysis ... 81265, 81266, 81402
Translocation Analysis
  BCR/ABL1 (t(9;22)) ... 81206-81208
  CCND1/IGH (BCL1/IgH, t(11;14)) ... 81401
  COL1A1/PDGFB (t(17;22)) ... 81402
  E2A/PBX1 (t(1;19)) ... 81401
  EML4/ALK (inv(2)) ... 81401
  ETV6/NTRK3 (t(12;15)) ... 81401
  ETV6/RUNX1 (t(12;21)) ... 81401
  EWSR1/ATF1 (t(12;22)) ... 81401
  EWSR1/ERG (t(21;22)) ... 81401
  EWSR1/FLI1 (t(11;22)) ... 81401
  EWSR1/WT1 (t(11;22)) ... 81401
  FOXO1/PAX3 (t(2;13)) ... 81401
  FOXO1/PAX7 (t(1;13)) ... 81401
  FUS/DDIT3 (t(12;16)) ... 81401
  IGH@/BCL2 (t(14;18) ... 81402
  MLL/AFF1 (t(4;11)) ... 81401
  MLL/MLLT3 (t(9;11)) ... 81401
  NPM1/ALK (t(2;5)) ... 81401
  PAX8/PPARG (t(2;3)) (q13;p25)) ... 81401
  PML/RARalpha (t(15;17)) ... 81315, 81316
  RUNX1/RUNX1T1 (t(8;21)) ... 81401
  SS18/SSX1 (t(X;18)) ... 81401
  SS18/SSX2 (t(X;18)) ... 81401

Gene Product
See Protein

Genioplasty
Augmentation ... 21120, 21123
Osteotomy ... 21121-21123

Genitourinary Sphincter, Artificial
See Prosthesis, Urethral Sphincter

Genomic Sequencing Procedures (GSPs) and Other Molecular Multianalyte Assays
Acute Myelogenous Leukemia ... 0023U
Aortic Dysfunction or Dilation ... 81410, 81411
Ashkenazi Jewish Associated Disorders ... 81412
Cardiac Ion Channelopathies ... 81413, 81414
COMT (catechol-O-methyltransferase) ... 0032U
CYP1A2 (cytochrome P450 family 1, subfamily A, member 2) ... 0031U
CYP2D6 (cytochrome P450, family 2, subfamily D, polypeptide 6) ... 0028U
Drug Metabolism ... 0029U, 0030U
Exome ... 0036U, 81415-81417
Fetal Chromosomal Aneuploidy ... 81420
Fetal Chromosomal Microdeletion(s) ... 81422
Gene Rearrangement Detection ... 0012U
Genome ... 81425-81427
Germline Disorders ... 0012U
Hearing Loss ... 81430, 81431
Helicobacter Pylori Detection and Antibiotic Resistance ... 0008U
Hematolymphoid Neoplasia . 0014U, 0016U, 0017U
Hereditary Breast Cancer-Related Disorders ... 81432, 81433
Hereditary Cardiomyopathy ... 81439
Hereditary Colon Cancer Disorders ... 81435, 81436
Hereditary Neuroendocrine Tumor Disorders ... 81437, 81438
Hereditary Peripheral Neuropathies ... 81448
Hereditary Retinal Disorders ... 81434
HTR2A (5-hydroxytryptamine receptor 2A) ... 0033U
HTR2C (5-hydroxytryptamine receptor 2C) ... 0033U
JAK2 (Janus kinase 2) ... 0027U
Non-small Cell Lung Neoplasia ... 0022U
NUDT15 (nudix hydroxlase 15) ... 0034U
Noonan Spectrum Disorders ... 81442
Nuclear Encoded Mitochondrial Genes ... 81440
Severe Inherited Conditions ... 81443
Solid Organ Neoplasia ... 0013U, 0037U
Targeted Genomic Sequence Analysis Panel ... 81445, 81450, 81455
Thyroid DNA and RNA ... 0026U
TPMT (thiopurine S-methyltransferase) ... 0034U
Whole Mitochondrial Genome ... 81460, 81465
X-linked Intellectual Disability (XLID) ... 81470, 81471

Genotype Analysis
by Nucleic Acid
  Hepatitis C Virus ... 87902
  HIV-1 ... 87901, 87906
    Protease/Reverse Transcriptase Regions ... 87901
    Vancomycin Resistance ... 87500
Human Platelet Antigen ... 81105-81112

Gentamicin
Assay ... 80170

Gentamycin Level
See Gentamicin

Gentiobiase
See Beta Glucosidase

Genus: Human Cytomegalovirus Group
See Cytomegalovirus

GERD
See Gastroesophageal Reflux Test

German Measles
See Rubella

Gestational Trophoblastic Tumor
See Hydatidiform Mole

GGT
See Gamma Glutamyl Transferase

GI Tract
See Gastrointestinal Tract

Giardia
Antigen Detection
  Immunoassay ... 87329
  Immunofluorescence ... 87269

Giardia Lamblia
Antibody ... 86674

Gibbons Stent
Ureteral ... 52332

GIF
See Somatostatin

GIFT
See Gamete Intrafallopian Transfer (GIFT)

Gill Operation
Laminectomy ... 63012

Gillies Approach
Fracture
  Zygomatic Arch ... 21356

Gingiva
See Gums

Gingiva, Abscess
Incision and Drainage ... 41800

Gingivectomy
Each Quadrant ... 41820

Gingivoplasty
Each Quadrant ... 41872

Girdlestone Laminectomy
See Laminectomy

Girdlestone Procedure
See Acetabulum, Reconstruction

Gla Protein (Bone)
See Osteocalcin

Gland
See Specific Gland

Gland, Adrenal
See Adrenal Gland

Gland, Bartholin's
See Bartholin's Gland

Gland, Bulbourethral
See Bulbourethral Gland

Gland, Lacrimal
See Lacrimal Gland

Gland, Mammary
See Breast

Gland, Parathyroid
See Parathyroid Gland

Gland, Parotid
See Parotid Gland

Gland, Pituitary
See Pituitary Gland

Gland, Salivary
See Salivary Glands

Gland, Sublingual
See Sublingual Gland

Gland, Sweat
See Sweat Glands, Excision

Gland, Thymus
See Thymus Gland

Gland, Thyroid
See Thyroid Gland

Glasses
See Spectacle Services

Glaucoma
Counseling ... 4174F
Cryotherapy ... 66720
Cyclophotocoagulation ... 66710, 66711
Diathermy ... 66700
Filtration Implant
  See Aqueous Shunt
Fistulization of Sclera ... 66150
  Through Ciliary Body ... 66999
Iridectomy ... 66625, 66630
Plan of Care ... 0517F

Glaucoma Drainage Implant
See Aqueous Shunt

Glenn Procedure ... 33766, 33767

Glenohumeral Joint
Arthrodesis ... 23800, 23802
Arthroplasty ... 23470, 23472-23474
Arthrotomy ... 23040
  with Biopsy ... 23100
  with Drainage ... 23040
  Foreign Body Removal ... 23040
  with Exploration ... 23040, 23107
  with Synovectomy ... 23105
Capsulorrhaphy ... 23465, 23466
Exploration ... 23040, 23107
Removal
  Foreign or Loose Body ... 23040, 23107

Glenoid Fossa
Allograft ... 23473, 23474
Arthroplasty ... 23473, 23474
Reconstruction ... 21255

Globulin
Antihuman
  Coombs Test
    Direct ... 86880, 86885, 86886
    Indirect ... 86850, 86870
Immune
  Administration ... 96365-96368
  Product
    Botulinum Antitoxin ... 90288
    Botulism ... 90288
    Cytomegalovirus (CMV-IgIV) ... 90291
    Diphtheria Antitoxin ... 90296
    Gammaglobulin ... 82784, 82785
    Hepatitis B (HBIg) ... 90371
    Ig ... 90281
    IgIV ... 90283
    Rabies (RIg/RIg-HT)) ... 90375, 90376
    Respiratory Syncytial Virus ... 90378
    Rho(D) (RhIg/RhIgIV) ... 90384-90386
    SCIg ... 90284
    Tetanus (TIg) ... 90389
    Unlisted ... 90399
    Vaccinia ... 90393
    Varicella-zoster ... 90396
Sex Hormone Binding ... 84270

Globulin, Corticosteroid-Binding
See Transcortin

Globulin, Rh Immune
See Immune Globulins, Rho(D)

Globulin, Thyroxine-Binding
See Thyroxine Binding Globulin

Glomerular Procoagulant Activity
See Thromboplastin

Glomus Caroticum
See Carotid Body

Glossectomy
Complete ... 41140, 41145
Composite ... 41150, 41153, 41155
Partial ... 41135
  Half ... 41130
  Less than Half ... 41120

Glossopexy
See Tongue, Fixation

Glossorrhaphy
See Suture, Tongue

Glucagon
Measurement ... 82943
Tolerance Panel ... 80422, 80424
Tolerance Test ... 82946

Glucose
Blood Test ... 82947, 82948, 82950
  Home Test ... 82962
Body Fluid ... 82945
Interstitial Fluid
  Continuous Monitoring ... 95249-95251
    Data Interpretation ... 99091
Panel
  Basic Metabolic ... 80047, 80048
  Comprehensive Metabolic ... 80053
  Glucagon Tolerance ... 80422, 80424
  Growth Hormone Suppression ... 80430
  Insulin Tolerance ... 80434, 80435
  Insulin-induced C-peptide Suppression .. 80432
  Renal Function ... 80069
Sensor
  Insertion
    Subcutaneous Pocket ... 0446T, 0448T
  Removal ... 0447T, 0448T
Tolerance Test ... 82951, 82952
  Intravenous Push ... 96374
Urinalysis ... 81000-81003, 81005

Glucose Phosphate Isomerase
See Phosphohexose Isomerase

Glucose Phosphate Isomerase Measurement
See Phosphohexose Isomerase

Glucose-6-Phosphate
Dehydrogenase ... 82955-82960

Glucosidase ... 82963

Index

Glucuronide Androstanediol 82154

Glue
Anal Fistula Repair 46706
Bronchoscopy
  Balloon Occlusion 31634
Cornea Wound 65286
Sclera Wound 65286

Glukagon
See Glucagon

Glutamate Dehydrogenase
Blood 82965

Glutamate Pyruvate Transaminase
See Transaminase, Glutamic-Pyruvic

Glutamic Alanine Transaminase
See Transaminase, Glutamic-Pyruvic

Glutamic Aspartic Transaminase
See Transaminase, Glutamic-Oxaloacetic

Glutamic Dehydrogenase
See Glutamate Dehydrogenase

Glutamyltransferase, Gamma 82977

Glutathione 82978

Glutathione Reductase 82979

Glycanhydrolase, N-Acetylmuramide
See Lysozyme

Glycated Hemoglobins
See Glycohemoglobin

Glycated Protein 82985

Glycerol Phosphoglycerides
See Phosphatidylglycerol

Glycerol, Phosphatidyl
See Phosphatidylglycerol

Glycerophosphatase
See Alkaline Phosphatase

Glycinate, Theophylline Sodium
See Theophylline

Glycocholic Acid
See Cholylglycine

Glycohemoglobin
Glycosylated Hemoglobin 83036

Glycosaminoglycan
See Mucopolysaccharides

Goeckerman Treatment
Photochemotherapy 96910, 96912, 96913

Gol-Vernet Operation
See Pyelotomy, Exploration

Goldwaite Procedure
Knee 27422

Golfer's Elbow
See Tennis Elbow

Gonadectomy, Female
See Oophorectomy

Gonadectomy, Male
See Excision, Testis

Gonadotropin
Chorionic 84702-84704
  Stimulation Panel 80414
FSH 83001
ICSH 83002
LH 83002
Stimulation Panel 80426

Gonadotropin Panel
Stimulation 80426

Gonioscopy
Ophthalmic 92020

Goniotomy
Congenital Glaucoma 65820

Gonococcus
See Neisseria Gonorrhoeae

GOTT
See Transaminase, Glutamic-Oxaloacetic

GPUT
See Galactose-1-Phosphate, Uridyl Transferase

Graft
Allograft
  See Allograft
Anal 46753
Aorta
  See Aorta, Graft
Artery
  Bypass Graft
    See Bypass Graft, Arterial; Bypass Graft, Arterial-Venous
  Coronary 33503
Bone
See Bone Graft
Bone Marrow
  Aspiration 20939
  Transplantation
    See Hematopoietic Progenitor Cell (HPC), Transplantation
Bone and Skin 20969, 20970, 20972, 20973
Cartilage
  See Cartilage Graft
Conjunctiva 65782
  Harvesting 68371
Cornea
  with Lesion Excision 65426
Cornea Transplant
  See Cornea, Transplantation
Dura
  Cranial
    Craniectomy 61343
    Anterior Cranial Fossa 61601
    Middle Cranial Fossa 61606, 61608
    Posterior Cranial Fossa 61616
  Spinal Cord 63710
    Laminectomy 63180, 63182
Ear
  Dermal Autograft 15135, 15136
  Epidermal Autograft 15115, 15116
  Full-thickness Graft, Free 15260, 15261
  Preparation of Recipient Site 15004, 15005
  Skin Substitute Graft 15275-15278
  Split-thickness Autograft 15120, 15121
  Tissue Cultured Skin Autograft . . 15155-15157
Eye
  Amniotic Membrane 65778-65780
  Conjunctiva 65782
  Stem Cell 65781
for Facial Nerve Paralysis
  Fascia 15840
  Muscle 15841, 15842, 15845
Fascia
  See Fascial Graft
Fascia Lata
  Harvesting 20920, 20922
Gum Mucosa 41870
Intestine 43116, 46748
Muscle
  See Muscle Flaps; Muscle Grafts
Nail Bed
  Reconstruction 11762
Nerve
  See Nerve Graft
Oral Mucosa 40818
Organ
  See Transplantation
Pancreas
  See Pancreas, Transplantation
Patency
  Blood Flow Check 15860
  Vascular Flow Check 15860
Skin
  See Skin Graft and Flap
Skin Substitute
  See Skin Substitute Graft
Tendon
  Finger 26392, 26416, 26420, 26428, 26434
  Hand 26392, 26412, 26416
  Harvesting 20924
Tissue
  Harvesting 20926
Vein
  Bypass Graft
    See Bypass Graft, Venous
  Cross-Over 34520

Grain Alcohol
See Drug Assay, Drug Procedure, Definitive Drug Class, Alcohols

Granulation Tissue
Cauterization, Chemical 17250

Gravis, Myasthenia
See Myasthenia Gravis

Gravities, Specific
See Specific Gravity

Great Toe
Arthrodesis
  Interphalangeal Joint 28755
    with Tendon Transfer 28760
  Metatarsophalangeal Joint 28750
Fracture
  Closed Treatment 28490
  Open Treatment 28505
  Skeletal Fixation 28496
Osteocutaneous Flap 20973
Toe-to-Hand Transfer 20973
  Wrap-around with Bone Graft 26551

Great Vessels
Graft Insertion 33330, 33335
Shunt
  Aorta to Pulmonary Artery
    Ascending 33755
    Descending 33762
  Central 33764
  Subclavian to Pulmonary Artery 33750
  Vena Cava to Pulmonary Artery . . 33766, 33767
Suture Repair 33320-33322
Translocation
  Aortic Root 33782, 33783
Transposition Repair
  Aortic Pulmonary Artery
  Reconstruction 33778-33781
  Atrial Baffle Procedure 33774-33777
  with Subpulmonary Stenosis 33770, 33771
  with Ventricular Septal Defect . . 33770, 33771
Unlisted Services and Procedures 33999

Great Vessels Transposition
See Transposition, Great Arteries

Greater Tuberosity Fracture
Humeral
Closed Treatment 23620, 23625, 23665
Open Treatment 23630, 23670
with Shoulder Dislocation
Closed Treatment 23665
Open Treatment 23670

Greater Vestibular Gland
See Bartholin's Gland

Green Operation
See Scapulopexy

Grippe, Balkan
See Q Fever

Gritti Operation
See Amputation, Leg, Upper; Radical Resection; Replantation

Groin Area
Incision
Femoral Artery Exposure 34812
Repair
Hernia 49550-49557
Revision
Femoral Arterial Bypass Graft 35883

Group Adaptive Behavior Treatment
See Adaptive Behavior Services, Treatment, Group

Group Health Education
Genetic 98961, 98962, 99078
Physical 99078
Preventive Medicine 99411
Self-Management, Condition or Treatment 98961, 98962

Grouping, Blood
See Blood Typing, Serologic

Growth Factors, Insulin-Like
See Somatomedin

Growth Hormone 83003
Human
Antibody 86277
Measurement 83003
Growth Hormone Stimulation Panel 80428
Growth Hormone Suppression Panel 80430
Insulin Tolerance Panel 80435
Pituitary Evaluation Panel 80418

Growth Hormone Release Inhibiting Factor
See Somatostatin

Growth Stimulation Expressed Gene 2 83006

GTT
See Glucose, Tolerance Test
See Hydatidiform Mole

Guaiac Test
See Blood, Feces

Guard Stain
Special Stain, Group II 88313

Gullet
See Esophagus

Gums
Abscess
Incision and Drainage 41800
Alveolus
Excision 41830
Cyst
Incision and Drainage 41800
Excision
Gingiva 41820
Operculum 41821
Graft
Mucosa 41870
Hematoma
Incision and Drainage 41800
Lesion
Destruction 41850
Excision 41825-41827
Mucosa
Excision 41828
Graft 41870
Reconstruction
Alveolus 41874
Gingiva 41872
Removal
Bone 41806
Foreign Body 41805
Tuberosities
Excision 41822, 41823
Tumor
Excision 41825-41827
Unlisted Services and Procedures 41899

Gunning-Lieben Test
See Drug Assay, Drug Procedure, Definitive Drug Class, Alcohols

Guthrie Test
Phenylalanine (PKU) 84030

H

H Flu
See Haemophilus Influenza (H Flu)

H1N1
Immunization
See Vaccines and Toxoids

HAA (Hepatitis Associated Antigen)
See Hepatitis Antigen, Detection, Immunoassay, B Surface (HBsAg)

HAAb
See Antibody, Detection, Hepatitis A (HAAb)

Haemoglobin F
See Fetal Hemoglobin

Haemophilus Influenza (H Flu)
Antibody 86684
Antigen Detection 87275
Immunoassay 87804
Nucleic Acid Detection
Reverse Transcription, Amplified Probe 87501-87503
Vaccines
Hib-HepB 90748
Hib-MenCY 90644
Hib, PRP-OMP Conjugate 90647
Hib, PRP-T Conjugate 90648, 90748

Haemorrhage
See Hemorrhage

Haemorrhage Rectum
See Hemorrhage, Endoscopic Control, Rectum

Hageman Factor
Clotting Factor XII 85280

HAI Test
See Hemagglutination Inhibition Test

Hair
Cell
Ear, Function Analysis 92588
Electrolysis 17380
Fungi Isolation 87101
KOH Examination 87220
Microscopic Evaluation 96902
Transplant
Punch Graft 15775, 15776
Strip Graft 15220, 15221

Hair Removal
See Removal, Hair

Hallux
See Great Toe

Halo
Body Cast 29000
Cranial 20661
for Thin Skull Osteology 20664
Femur 20663
Maxillofacial 21100
Pelvic 20662
Removal 20665

Haloperidol
Assay 80173

Halstead-Reitan Neuropsychological Battery
Administration and Scoring 96139
Evaluation Services 96132, 96133

Halsted Mastectomy
See Mastectomy, Radical

Halsted Repair
See Hernia Repair, Inguinal

Ham Test
See Hemolysins

Hammertoe Repair
Correction 28285, 28286

Hamster Penetration Test
Sperm Evaluation 89329

Hand
Amputation
at Metacarpal 25927, 26910
at Wrist 25920
Revision 25922
Ray Amputation 26910
Revision 25924, 25929, 25931
Bone
Cyst
Curettage 26210, 26215
Excision 26210, 26215
Osteotomy, Metacarpal 26565
Incision and Drainage 26034
Casts, Splints, and Strapping 29065, 29085
Compression System 29584
Gauntlet Cast 29085
Long Arm Cast 29065
Long Arm Splint 29105
Short Arm Cast 29075
Short Arm Splint 29125, 29126
Strapping 29280
Decompression 26035
Diagnostic Imaging
Magnetic Resonance Imaging (MRI) 73218-73220
Angiography 73225
X ray 73120, 73130

Drainage
Bursa . . . 26025, 26030
Fasciectomy . . . 26121, 26123, 26125
Fasciotomy
Decompressive . . . 26037
Injection, Enzyme . . . 20527, 26341
Open . . . 26045
Percutaneous . . . 26040
Fracture
Carpometacarpal . . . 26645, 26650
Interphalangeal
See Interphalangeal Joint, Fracture
Metacarpal
Closed Treatment . . . 26600, 26605, 26607
Open Treatment . . . 26615
Skeletal Fixation . . . 26608
Metacarpophalangeal . . . 26740-26746
Phalangeal . . . 26720-26735, 26750-26765
Injection
Cell Therapy for Scleroderma . . . 0490T
Insertion
Tendon Graft . . . 26392
Joint
See Carpometacarpal Joint; Intercarpal Joint
Manipulation
Carpometacarpal Fracture . . . 26645, 26650
Dupuytren's Cord . . . 26341
Joint Dislocation
See Carpometacarpal Joint; Intercarpal Joint
Metacarpal Fracture . . . 26605, 26607
Palmar Fascial Cord . . . 26341
Nerve
Graft . . . 64890, 64891, 64895, 64896
Neuroma, Excision . . . 64782, 64783
Neuroplasty . . . 64704
Suture
Additional Nerve . . . 64837
Common Sensory . . . 64834
Digital . . . 64831
Reconstruction
Tendon Pulley . . . 26500-26502
Removal
Implantation . . . 26320
Tube/Rod . . . 26390-26392, 26416
Repair
Blood Vessel . . . 35207
Cleft Hand . . . 26580
Muscle . . . 26591-26593
Release, Thenar . . . 26508
Transfer, Hypothenar . . . 26494
Non-Union, Metacarpal . . . 26546
Tendon
Extensor
Delayed Tendon Graft . . . 26416
Excision . . . 26170, 26415
Lengthening . . . 26476
Realignment . . . 26437
Reconstruction
Repair . . . 26410
Shortening . . . 26477
Synthetic Rod Implantation . . . 26415
Tenolysis . . . 26445
Tenotomy . . . 26460
Flexor
Delayed Tendon Graft . . . 26392
Excision . . . 26390
Lengthening . . . 26478
Repair
Shortening . . . 26479
Synthetic Rod Implantation . . . 26390
Tenolysis . . . 26440, 26442
Tenosynovectomy . . . 26145
Tenotomy . . . 26450
Grafts . . . 26502
Extensor . . . 26412, 26420, 26428, 26434
Flexor . . . 26352, 26358
Profundus . . . 26372
Replace Rod Implant . . . 26392, 26416
Opponensplasty . . 26490, 26492, 26494, 26496
Profundus
Repair . . . 26370, 26372, 26373
Pulley Reconstruction . . . 26500, 26502
Sheath
Incision and Drainage . . . 26020
Lesion Excision . . . 26160
Synovectomy . . . 26145
Tenotomy . . . 26060
Transfer
Carpometacarpal Area . . . 26480, 26483
Cross Intrinsic . . . 26510
Dorsum . . . 26480, 26483
Palmar . . . 26485, 26489
Superficialis . . . 26490
with Graft . . . 26492
Replantation . . . 20808
Skin Graft . . . 15240, 15241
Strapping . . . 29280
Tendon
Excision . . . 26390
Extensor . . . 26415
Tenotomy . . . 26450, 26460
Tissue Transfer
Adjacent . . . 14040, 14041
Flap . . . 15574, 15620
Toe-to-Hand Transfer . . . 20973
Wound Repair . . . 13131-13133
Tumor
Excision . . 26111, 26113, 26115, 26116, 26200
Radical Resection . . . 26117, 26118, 26250
Unlisted Services and Procedures . . . 26989
Vascular Malformation
Excision . . . 26111, 26113, 26115, 26116

Hand Abscess
See Abscess, Tissue, Hand

Hand Phalanges
See Phalanx, Finger

Hand(s) Dupuytren's Contracture(s)
See Dupuytren's Contracture

Handling
Device Order Implementation . . . 99002
Radioelement . . . 77790
Specimen Transport . . . 99000, 99001

Hanganutziu-Deicher Antibodies
See Antibody, Detection, Heterophile

Haptoglobin
Measurement . . . 83010-83012

Hard Palate
See Palate

Harelip Operation
See Cleft Lip, Repair

Harii Procedure
Carpal Bone . . . 25430

Harrington Rod
Insertion . . . 22840
Removal . . . 22850

Hartmann Procedure
Colectomy with Colostomy
Closure . . . 44626
Laparoscopic . . . 44206
Open . . . 44143

Harvest of Upper Extremity Artery for Coronary Artery Bypass . . . 35600
See Coronary Artery Bypass Graft (CABG)

Harvesting
Adipose Tissue Cells
Cell Therapy for Scleroderma . . . 0489T
Bone Graft . . . 20900-20902
Spine Surgery
Allograft . . . 20930-20934
Autograft . . . 20936-20938
Bone Marrow
Allogeneic . . . 38230
Autologous . . . 0265T, 20939, 38232
Cartilage Graft
Ear . . . 21235
Glenoid Fossa . . . 21255
Mandibular Condyle . . . 21247
Rib . . . 21230
Zygomatic Arch . . . 21255
Conjunctival Graft . . . 68371
Eggs
In Vitro Fertilization . . . 58970
Fascia Lata Graft . . . 20920-20922
Lower Extremity Vein
for Vascular Reconstruction . . . 35572
Mucosa . . . 40818
Organs
Duodenum . . . 48550
Heart . . . 33940
Heart/Lung . . . 33930
Intestines . . . 44132, 44133
Kidney . . . 50300, 50320, 50547
Liver . . . 47133, 47140-47142
Lung . . . 32850
Pancreas . . . 48550
Skin
for Tissue-Cultured Autograft . . . 15040
Stem Cell
Blood-derived . . . 38205, 38206
Limbal . . . 65781
Tendon Graft . . . 20924
Tissue Grafts, Other . . . 20926
Upper Extremity Artery
for Coronary Artery Bypass Graft . . . 35600
Upper Extremity Vein
for Bypass Graft . . . 35500
Endoscopic . . . 33508
Multiple . . . 35681-35683

Hauser Procedure
Patella . . . 27420

Hayem's Elementary Corpuscle
See Blood, Platelet

Haygroves Procedure . . . 27120

HBcAb
See Antibody, Detection, Hepatitis B, Core (HBcAb)

HBeAb
See Antibody, Detection, Hepatitis Be (HBeAb)

HBeAg
See Hepatitis Antigen, Detection, Immunoassay, Be (HBeAg)

HBsAb
See Antibody, Detection, Hepatitis B, Surface (HBsAb)

HBsAg (Hepatitis B Surface Antigen)
See Hepatitis Antigen, Detection, Immunoassay, B Surface (HBsAg)

HCG
See Chorionic Gonadotropin

HCO_3
See Bicarbonate

HCV Antibodies
See Antibody, Detection, Hepatitis C Virus (HCV)

HDL
See Lipoprotein

Head
Excision
Bone, Facial 21025, 21026
Tumor, Soft Tissue. 21011-21016
Fracture and/or Dislocation
See Fracture; Dislocation
Halo Appliance 21100
Imaging
Angiography. 70496, 70544-70546
CT Scan 70450, 70460, 70470, 70496
Magnetic Resonance Angiography (MRA). 70544-70546
Positron Emission Tomography (PET) 78811, 78814
Ultrasound Exam 76506, 76536
X ray. 70350
Prosthesis
Custom Preparation
See Impression, Maxillofacial
Introduction or Removal
Cheekbone
Malar Augmentation. 21270
Chin. 21120
Cornea 65770
Ear
Ossicle Reconstruction 69633, 69637
Facial
Osteoplasty. 21208
Lens 66825, 66982-66985
Mandible 21125
Ocular. 65770, 66982-66985
Telescope Prosthesis 0308T
Temporary. 92358
Nasal Septum. 30220
Orbital. 21179
Ossicle Reconstruction
Chain. 69633
Palate 42280, 42281
Retina 0100T
Skull Plate. 62142, 62143
Spectacle
Fitting 92352, 92353
Repair 92371
Speech Aid 31611
Temporomandibular Joint 21243
Voice. 31611
Unlisted Maxillofacial Prosthetic Procedure. 21089
Lipectomy, Suction Assisted. 15876
Nerve
Graft. 64885, 64886
Other Procedures 21299, 21499
Repair/Revision and/or Reconstruction
See Cranioplasty; Face; Mandible
Rhytidectomy
See Rhytidectomy
Unlisted Services and Procedures 21499

Head Rings, Stereotactic
See Stereotactic Frame

Headbrace
See Halo

Heaf Test
See TB Test

Health Behavior
See Evaluation and Management, Health Behavior

Health Risk Assessment Instrument
Administration
Caregiver-Focused 96161
Patient-Focused 96160

Hearing Aid
Device
Attenuation Measurements. 92596
Check 92592, 92593
Evaluation, Electroacoustic 92594, 92595
Examination and Selection 92590, 92591
Implants
Bone Conduction
Implantation 69710
Removal 69711
Repair 69711
Replacement. 69710
Brainstem
Implantation 61863, 61867
Programming 92640
Cochlear
Implantation 69930
Programming 92601-92604
Rehabilitation 92626, 92627
Osseointegrated
Implantation 69714, 69715
Replacement. 69717, 69718

Hearing Aid Check 92592, 92593

Hearing Aid Services
Attenuation Measurements
Ear Protector 92596
Electroacoustic Test 92594, 92595
Examination 92590, 92591

Hearing Tests
See Audiologic Function Tests

Hearing Therapy
Evaluation 92626, 92627
for Hearing Loss
Postlingual 92633
Prelingual 92630
Individual. 92507
Group. 92508
Cochlear Implant
Analysis and Programming 92601-92604
Rehabilitation. 92626, 92627

Heart
Ablation
Arrhythmogenic Focus . . . 33250, 33251, 33261
Atrial Tissue. 33254-33259
Endoscopic 33265, 33266
Anomaly
Repair. 33615, 33617
Aorta
See Aorta
Arrhythmia
See Tachycardia
Artificial Heart
Implantation. 33927
Removal. 33929
Replacement 33928
Atria
See Atria
Balloon Device
Insertion. 33973
Removal. 33974
Biopsy 93505
UltrasonicGuidance 76932
Blood Vessel
Repair. 33320-33322
Cardiac Contractility Modulation
Electrode
Reposition. 0415T
Cardiac Output Measurements. 93451, 93561, 93562
Cardiac Rehabilitation 93797, 93798
Cardioassist
Circulation 92970, 92971
Cardiopulmonary Bypass
with Aortic Aneurysm Repair. 33877
with Ascending Aorta Graft. 33860, 33863, 33864
with Atrial Septectomy/Septostomy 33736
with Chamber Fistula Repair 33500
with Descending Thoracic Aorta Graft . . 33875
with Lung Transplant. 32852, 32854
with Operative Ablation. 33251, 33256, 33259, 33261
with Pericardiectomy. 33031
with Pulmonary Artery Repair . . 33910, 33916, 33922, 33926
with Replacement of Ventricular Assist Device 33983
with Septal Defect Repair
See Septal Defect
with Sinus of Valsalva Repair . . . 33720, 33702
with Transcatheter Aortic Valve Replacement (TAVR/TAVI). 33367-33369
with Transverse Arch Graft 33870
with Tumor Excision/Resection 33120
with Valve Repair
See Aortic Valve; Mitral Valve; Tricuspid Valve; Pulmonary Valve
with Wound Repair 33305
Cardioversion 92960, 92961
Catheterization
See Cardiac Catheterization
Cardiac Event Recorder
See Cardiac Assist Devices, Subcutaneous Cardiac Rhythm Monitor
Coronary Artery Bypass Graft
See Coronary Artery Bypass Graft (CABG)
Cor Triatriatum
Repair. 33732
Cyst
Pericardial
Resection 33050
Diagnostic Imaging
Acoustic Cardiography. 93799
Angiography
See Angiography, Heart
Blood Pool 78472, 78473, 78481, 78483, 78496
SPECT 78494
CT Scan 75571-75573
Angiography 75574
Magnetic Resonance
See Cardiac Magnetic Resonance Imaging (CMRI)
Myocardial Imaging
Magnetocardiography 0541T, 0542T
Quantitative Assessment of Mechanics 0399T
Infarct Avid 78466, 78468, 78469
Perfusion. 78451-78454
Perfusion Study 78491, 78492
PET Metabolic Evaluation 78459
SPECT. 0332T, 78451, 78452, 78469
Sympathetic Innervation 0331T, 0332T

Shunt Detection....................78428
Unlisted Cardiovascular Diagnostic Nuclear Medicine Procedure.................78499
Ventriculography
See Ventriculography
Electrical Recording
See Electrophysiology Procedure
Electrode
Insertion....... 33202, 33203, 33210, 33211, 33216, 33217, 33224, 33225
Removal.............................33238
Single/Dual Chamber........33243, 33244
Electrophysiologic Study
See Electrophysiology Procedure
Exploration......................33310-33315
External Heart Rate Data Recording
for Nocturnal Epilepsy Seizure .. 0381T-0386T
Foreign Body Removal 33310
Great Vessels
See Great Vessels
Heart-Lung Bypass
See Cardiopulmonary Bypass
Heart-Lung Transplantation
See Transplantation, Heart-Lung
Hemodynamic Monitoring
Noninvasive................ 93880, 93882, 93922-93931, 93970-93990, 93998
with Pharmacologic Agent............93463
with Physiologic Exercise Study 93464
Infundibular Stenosis 33476-33478
Injection
Radiological
See Cardiac Catheterization, Injection
Intraoperative Pacing and Mapping........93631
Ischemia Monitoring System 0525T-0532T
Ligation
Fistula.............................37607
Myocardium
Imaging 78466-78469
Quantitative Assessment of Mechanics .. 0399T
SPECT........0332T, 78451, 78452, 78469
Sympathetic Innervation 0331T, 0332T
Infarction
Revascularization.....92941, 92943, 92944
Tissue Plasminogen Activator (tPA)
Therapy.........................4077F
Perfusion Study 78451-78454
Revascularization.............33140, 33141
Open Chest Massage 32160
Output
See Cardiac Output
Pacemaker
See Cardiac Assist Devices
Pacing
Arrhythmia Induction................93618
Atria..............................93610
Left Ventricular Wireless Stimulator System
See Cardiac Assist Devices
Rate Increase
See Tachycardia
Transcutaneous
Temporary.......................92953
Ventricular 33224-33226, 93612
Implantable Defibrillator System
See Cardiac Assist Devices
Pericardium
Drainage..........................33025
Pericardiectomy 33030, 33031
Pericardiocentesis 33010, 33011
Tube Pericardiostomy 33015
for Removal of Clot.................33020
for Removal of Foreign Body 33020
Wound 33300-33305
Resuscitation 92950
Septal Defect
See Septal Defect
Sinus of Valsalva
Repair..................... 33702-33722
Sinus Venosus
Repair.............................33645
Sounds
See Heart Sounds
Tetralogy of Fallot
Repair................ 33692-33697, 33924
Thrombectomy
See Thrombectomy
Total Replacement Heart System
Implantation.......................33927
Removal...........................33929
Replacement 33928
Transplantation..................33935, 33945
Allograft Preparation..........33933, 33944
Harvest............................33940
Tumor
Cardiac
Excision...................33120-33130
Pericardial
Resection 33050
Unlisted Services and Procedures 33999
Valve
Aortic
See Aortic Valve
Bicuspid
See Mitral Valve
Mitral
See Mitral Valve
Pulmonary
See Pulmonary Valve
Tricuspid
See Tricuspid Valve
Valve Closure
Atrioventricular 33600
Semilunar..........................33602
Vena Cava
Reconstruction.....................34502
Ventricle
Commissurotomy
Right Ventricle 33476-33478
Leadless Pacemaker System
Device Evaluation
Interrogation.......93288, 93294, 93296
Peri-procedural 93286
Programming...................93279
Transcatheter Insertion 33274
Transcatheter Removal 33275
Transcatheter Replacement.........33274
Obstruction Removal 33619
Pacing................33224-33226, 93612
Repair................33548, 33611, 33612
Ventricular Tunnel Repair 33722
Ventriculomyectomy 33416
Ventricular Assist Device (VAD)
See Ventricular Assist Device (VAD)
Wound
Repair......................33300-33305

Heart Sounds

Acoustic Cardiography 93799
Acoustic Recording
with Computer Analysis..............93799

Heart Vessels

See Great Vessels
Angioplasty
See Angioplasty; Percutaneous Transluminal Angioplasty

Heat Unstable Haemoglobin

See Hemoglobin, Thermolabile

Heavy Lipoproteins

See Lipoprotein

Heavy Metal

Qualitative.............................83015
Quantitative 83018

Heel

Bone
See Calcaneus
Dual-energy X-ray Absorptiometry.........77080
Fracture
See Calcaneus, Fracture
Spur
Excision 28119
Stick, for Collection of Blood 36416
X ray 73650

Heel Bone

See Calcaneus

Heel Fracture

See Calcaneus, Fracture

Heel Spur

Excision...............................28119

Heine-Medin Disease

See Polio

Heinz Bodies

Assessment.....................85441, 85445

Helicobacter Pylori

Antibody 86677
Antigen Detection
Immunoassay................87338, 87339
Blood Test.............................83009
Breath Test
Urea, Liquid Scintillation Counter
Acquisition 78267
Analysis 78268
Urease Activity....................83013
Injection for Breath Test............83014
Stool 87338
Urease Activity 83009, 83013, 83014

Heller Operation

See Heller Procedure

Heller Procedure

Esophagomyotomy
Open.......................43330, 43331
Laparoscopic 43279
Thoracoscopic 32665

Helminth

Antibody 86682

Hemagglutination Inhibition Test

by Antibody............................86280

Hemangioma

See Lesion, Skin; Tumor

Hemapheresis

See Apheresis

Hematochezia

See Blood, Feces

Hematologic Test

See Blood Tests

Hematology

Unlisted Services and Procedures 85999

Hematoma
Ankle
Incision and Drainage . . . 27603
Arm, Lower
Incision and Drainage . . . 25028
Arm, Upper
Incision and Drainage . . . 23930
Brain
Aspiration via Burr Hole. . . . 61156
Drainage via Burr Hole. . . . 61154-61156
Evacuation via Burr Hole . . . 61108, 61154
Evacuation via Craniotomy . . . 61312-61315
Chest
Incision and Drainage . . . 21501, 61154
Ear, External
Incision and Drainage . . . 69000, 69005
Elbow
Incision and Drainage . . . 23930
Endovascular
See Endovascular Repair
Epididymis
Incision and Drainage . . . 54700
Gums
Incision and Drainage . . . 41800
Hip. . . . 26990
Integumentary System/Superficial
Incision and Drainage . . . 10140
Puncture Aspiration. . . . 10160
Knee . . . 27301
Leg, Lower
Incision and Drainage . . . 27603
Leg, Upper. . . . 27301
Mouth . . . 41015-41018
Incision and Drainage
Dentoalveolar. . . . 41800
Lingual . . . 41000
Masticator Space. . . . 41009, 41018
Sublingual. . . . 41005, 41006, 41015
Submandibular. . . . 41008, 41017
Submental . . . 41007, 41016
Vestibular. . . . 40800, 40801
Nail
Evacuation. . . . 11740
Nasal Septum
Incision and Drainage . . . 30020
Neck
Incision and Drainage . . . 21501, 21502
Nose
Incision and Drainage . . . 30000, 30020
Pelvis
Incision and Drainage . . . 26990
Scrotum
Incision and Drainage . . . 54700
Shoulder
Incision and Drainage . . . 23030
Skin
Incision and Drainage . . . 10140
Puncture Aspiration. . . . 10160
Subdural . . . 61108
Subungual
Evacuation . . . 11740
Testis
Incision and Drainage . . . 54700
Thigh
Incision and Drainage . . . 27301
Thorax
Incision and Drainage . . . 21501
Tongue . . . 41000, 41005, 41006, 41015
Vagina
Incision and Drainage . . . 57022, 57023
Wrist. . . . 25028

Hematopoietic Progenitor Cell (HPC)
Donor Search and Cell Acquisition. . . . 38204
Harvesting. . . . 38205, 38206
HPC Boost. . . . 38243
Transplant Preparation
Cell Concentration. . . . 38215
Cell Depletion . . . 38210-38214
Cryopreservation and Storage. . . . 38207
Thawing. . . . 38208, 38209
Transplantation. . . . 38240-38242

Hematopoietic Stem Cell Transplantation
See Stem Cell, Transplantation

Hematopoietin
See Erythropoietin

Hematuria
See Blood, Urine

Hemic System
Unlisted Procedure, Hemic System . . . 38999
Unlisted Procedure, Spleen
Laparoscopic . . . 38129

Hemiepiphyseal Arrest
Elbow . . . 24470

Hemifacial Microsomia
Reconstruction
Mandibular Condyle. . . . 21247

Hemilaminectomy . . . 63020-63044

Hemilaryngectomy. . . . 31370-31382

Hemipelvectomies
See Amputation, Interpelviabdominal

Hemiphalangectomy
Toe . . . 28160

Hemispherectomy
Brain
Partial. . . . 61543

Hemocytoblast
See Stem Cell

Hemodialyses
See Hemodialysis

Hemodialysis. . . . 90935-90937
Access
Anastomosis
Arteriovenous. . . . 36818-36821
Cannulation
Arteriovenous. . . . 36810
Closure. . . . 36815
Revision . . . 36815
Vein to Vein . . . 36800
Blood Flow Study . . . 90940
Duplex Scan of Access . . . 93990
Home Visit. . . . 99512
Kt/V Level . . . 3082F-3084F
Plan of Care Documented. . . . 0505F
Procedure
via Catheter . . . 4054F
via Functioning Arteriovenous Fistula . . . 4052F
Thrombectomy . . . 36831
via Functioning Arteriovenous Graft . . . 4053F
with Evaluation . . . 90935, 90937

Hemofiltration
Dialysis Procedure . . . 90945, 90947

Hemoglobin
Analysis
O_2 Affinity. . . . 82820
A1c (HbA1c) Level. . . . 3044F, 3045F
Carboxyhemoglobin . . . 82375, 82376, 88740
Chromatography . . . 83021
Concentration . . . 85046
Electrophoresis . . . 83020
Fetal . . . 83030-83033, 85460, 85461
Fractionation and Quantitation. . . . 83020
Glycosylated (A1C) . . . 83036, 83037
Hgb
Transcutaneous Testing. . . . 88738
Methemoglobin. . . . 83045-83050
Transcutaneous . . . 88741
Non-Automated . . . 83026
Plasma. . . . 83051
Sulfhemoglobin. . . . 83060
Thermolabile . . . 83065-83068
Transcutaneous. . . . 88740
Urine . . . 83069

Hemoglobin F
Fetal Hemoglobin
Copper Sulfate. . . . 83030-83033
Differential Lysis . . . 85460, 85461

Hemoglobin, Glycosylated
See Glycohemoglobin

Hemogram
Complete Blood Count
Added Indices . . . 85025-85027
Automated . . . 85025-85027
Manual. . . . 85014-85018, 85032

Hemolysins
Acid. . . . 85475
with Agglutinins . . . 86940, 86941

Hemolytic Complement
See Complement, Total Hemolytic

Hemolytic Complement, Total
See Complement, Total Hemolytic

Hemoperfusion
Dialysis . . . 90997

Hemophil
See Clotting Factor

Hemorrhage
Control
Gastrointestinal . . . 43753
Liver . . . 47350
Lung . . . 32110
Nasal (Epistaxis)
Complex . . . 30903
Initial. . . . 30905
Simple. . . . 30901
Subsequent. . . . 30906
Nasopharynx . . . 42970-42972
Neck. . . . 35800
Oropharynx. . . . 42960-42962
Prostate, Transurethral Fulguration. . . . 52214
Throat. . . . 42960-42962
Uterus
Postpartum . . . 59160
Vagina . . . 57180
Endoscopic Control
Anus. . . . 46614
Chest Cavity. . . . 32654
Colon . . . 44391, 45382
Colon-Sigmoid . . . 45334
Esophagus . . . 43227, 43460
Gastrointestinal, Upper . . . 43255
Intestines, Small . . . 44366, 44378
Nose. . . . 31238
Rectum. . . . 45317
Vascular . . . 37244

Hemorrhoidectomy
Complex 46260
with Fissurectomy 46261, 46262
External Complete 46250
Ligation 46221, 46945, 46946
Simple 46255
with Fissurectomy 46257, 46258

Hemorrhoidopexy
Stapling 46947

Hemorrhoids
Band Ligation
with Colonoscopy 45398
with Sigmoidoscopy 45350
Destruction 46930
Excision
See Hemorrhoidectomy
Incision
External 46083
Injection
Sclerosing Solution 46500
Ligation 0249T, 46945, 46946
Stapling 46947
Suture 46945, 46946

Hemosiderin
Qualitative 83070

Heparin
Assay 85520
Neutralization 85525
Protamine Tolerance Test 85530

Heparin Cofactor I
See Antithrombin III

Hepatectomy
Extensive 47122
Left Lobe 47125
Partial
Donor 47140-47142
Lobe 47120
Right Lobe 47130
Total
Donor 47133

Hepatic Abscess
See Abscess, Tissue, Liver

Hepatic Arteries
See Artery, Hepatic

Hepatic Artery Aneurysm
See Artery, Hepatic, Aneurysm

Hepatic Duct
Anastomosis
with Gastrointestinal Tract 47765
U-Tube Hepaticoenterostomy 47802
Exploration 43260, 47400
Incision and Drainage 47400
Nuclear Medicine
Imaging 78226, 78227
Pharmacologic Intervention 78227
Removal
Calculi (Stone) 47400
Repair
with Intestines 47765, 47802
Unlisted Services and Procedures 47999

Hepatic Haemorrhage
See Hemorrhage, Control, Liver

Hepatic Portal Vein
See Vein, Hepatic Portal

Hepatic Portoenterostomies
See Hepaticoenterostomy

Hepatic Transplantation
See Liver, Transplantation

Hepaticodochotomy
See Hepaticostomy

Hepaticoenterostomy
U-Tube 47802

Hepaticostomy
Drainage 47400
Exploration 47400
Removal of Calculus 47400

Hepaticotomy
Drainage 47400
Exploration 47400
Removal of Calculus 47400

Hepatitis A and Hepatitis B
Antibody
See Hepatitis Antibody
Vaccine
HepA-HepB 90636

Hepatitis A Vaccine (HepA)
Adolescent/Pediatric
2 Dose Schedule 90633
3 Dose Schedule 90634
and Hepatitis B Vaccine 90636
Adult Dosage 90632

Hepatitis Antibody
A (HAAb) 86708, 86709
B
B Core (HBcAb) 86704, 86705
B Surface (HBsAb) 86706
Be (HBeAb) 86707
C 86803, 86804
Delta Agent 86692
IgG 86704
IgM 86704, 86705, 86709
Panel
Acute Hepatitis 80074
Obstetric 80055, 80081

Hepatitis Antigen
Detection
Immunoassay
B Surface (HBsAg) 87340, 87341
Be (HBeAg) 87350
Delta Agent 87380
Nucleic Acid
B 87516, 87517
C 87520-87522
Drug Susceptibility 87902
G 87525-87527

Hepatitis B and Hib Vaccine (Hib-HepB)
Intramuscular 90748

Hepatitis B Vaccine (HepB)
Dosage
Adolescent 90743
Adult 90739, 90746
Immunosuppressed 90740, 90747
Pediatric/Adolescent 90744
and Haemophilus Influenza b Vaccine (Hib-HepB) 90748
and Hepatitis A Vaccine 90636

Hepatitis B Virus E Antigen
Hepatitis Be Antigen (HBeAg) 87350

Hepatitis B Virus Surface ab
See Antibody, Detection, Hepatitis B, Surface (HBsAb)

Hepatorrhaphy
See Liver, Repair

Hepatotomy
Drainage
Abscess
Open 47010
Cyst 47010

Hernia Repair
Abdominal
Reduction by Laparotomy 44050
Diaphragmatic 39540, 39541
Neonatal 39503
Transthoracic 43334, 43335
Epigastric 49570
Incarcerated 49572
Laparoscopic 49652
Incarcerated 49653
Strangulated 49653
Strangulated 49572
Femoral
Initial 49550
Incarcerated 49553
Strangulated 49553
Recurrent 49555
Incarcerated 49557
Strangulated 49557
Incisional
Implantation, Mesh or Prosthesis 49568
Initial 49560
Incarcerated 49561
Strangulated 49561
Laparoscopic 49654-49657
Incarcerated 49655, 49657
Strangulated 49655, 49657
Recurrent 49565
Incarcerated 49566
Strangulated 49566
Thoracoabdominal 43336, 43337
Inguinal
Incarcerated 49492, 49496, 49501, 49507, 49521
Infant Gestation, Surgery Age
Full Term, Birth to 6 Months 49495, 49496
Preterm, 37 Weeks Gestational Age to 50 Weeks 49491, 49492
Preterm, 50 Weeks Gestational Age to 6 Months 49495, 49496
Initial, Child 5 Years or Older 49505, 49507
Initial, Child under 5 Years 49500, 49501
Laparoscopic
Initial 49650
Recurrent 49651
Recurrent, Any Age 49520, 49521
Sliding, Any Age 49525
Strangulated 49492, 49496, 49507, 49521
with Orchiopexy 54640
Intestinal 44050
Lumbar 49540
Lung 32800
Neonatal 39503
Paracolostomy 44346
Paraesophageal
Hiatal
Laparotomy 43332, 43333
Thoracoabdominal Incision 43336, 43337
Thoracotomy 43334, 43335
Laparoscopic 43281, 43282
Spigelian 49590
Laparoscopic 49652
Incarcerated 49653
Strangulated 49653

Umbilicus
  Child, 5 Years and Up 49585
    Incarcerated 49587
    Strangulated..................... 49587
  Child, under 5 Years................. 49580
    Incarcerated 49582
    Strangulated..................... 49582
  Laparoscopic 49652
    Incarcerated 49653
    Strangulated..................... 49653
  Reducible.................. 49580, 49585
    Laparoscopic.............. 49652, 49653
  with Urachal Cyst or Sinus Excision 51500
Ventral
  Implantation, Mesh or Prosthesis 49568
  Initial 49560
    Incarcerated 49561
    Strangulated..................... 49561
  Laparoscopic 49654-49657
    Incarcerated 49655, 49657
    Strangulated.............. 49655, 49657
  Recurrent 49565
    Incarcerated 49566
    Strangulated..................... 49566
  Laparoscopic 49652
    Incarcerated 49653
    Strangulated..................... 49653
with Spermatic Cord Repair 55540

Hernia, Cerebral
See Encephalocele

Hernia, Rectovaginal
See Rectocele

Hernia, Umbilical
See Omphalocele

Heroin Screen
See Drug Assay

Herpes Simplex
Antibody 86694-86696
Antigen Detection
  Immunofluorescence 87273, 87274
  Nucleic Acid................ 87528-87530
Identification
  Smear and Stain 87207

Herpes Smear and Stain
Inclusion Bodies 87207

Herpes Virus-4 (Gamma), Human
See Epstein-Barr Virus

Herpes Virus-6
Detection.................... 87531, 87532
Quantification......................... 87533

Herpetic Vesicle
Destruction
  Anus............... 46900, 46910, 46916, 46917, 46922, 46924
  Penis..... 54050, 54055-54057, 54060, 54065

Heteroantibodies
See Antibody, Detection, Heterophile

Heterophile Antibody
Screening 86308-86310

Heterotropia
See Strabismus

Hex B
See b-Hexosaminidase

Hexadecadrol
See Dexamethasone

Hexosephosphate Isomerase
See Phosphohexose Isomerase

Heyman Procedure
Femoral Neck 27179
Midtarsal............................. 28264

Hg Factor
See Glucagon

HGB
See Hemoglobin, Concentration

HGH
See Growth Hormone, Human

HHV-4
See Epstein-Barr Virus

HIAA
See Hydroxyindoleacetic Acid, Urine

Hib Vaccine
4 Dose Schedule
  PRP-T 90648
PRP-OMP
  3 Dose Schedule 90647

Hibb Operation 22610, 22612, 22614

Hidradenitis
Excision....................... 11450-11471
Suppurative
  Incision and Drainage 10060, 10061

High Altitude Simulation Test
HAST........................ 94452, 94453

High Density Lipoprotein
See Lipoprotein

High Molecular Weight Kininogen
See Fitzgerald Factor

High Resolution Anoscopy (HRA)
Diagnostic............................ 46601
Biopsy................................ 46607

Highly Selective Vagotomy
See Vagotomy, Highly Selective

Highmore Antrum
See Sinus/Sinuses, Maxillary

Hill Procedure
See Gastroplasty with Esophagogastric Fundoplasty

Hinton Positive
See RPR

Hip
See Femur; Pelvis
Abscess
  Incision and Drainage 26990, 26991
Arthrocentesis................ 20610, 20611
Arthrodesis 27284-27286
Arthrography.......................... 73525
Arthroplasty 27130-27132
Arthroscopy.......... 29860-29863, 29914-29916
Arthrotomy 27030-27033
Biopsy........................ 27040-27045
Bone
  Drainage.......................... 26992
Bursa
  Incision and Drainage 26990, 26991
Capsulectomy
  with Release, Flexor Muscles 27036
Cast........................ 29305-29325
Craterization 27070
Cyst
  Excision 27065-27067
Denervation........................... 27035
Echography
  Infant 76885, 76886
Endoprosthesis
  See Prosthesis, Hip
Excision............................... 27070
Exploration 27033
Fasciotomy 27025
Fusion 27284-27286
Hematoma
  Incision and Drainage 26990
Injection
  Radiological 27093-27096
Radiostereometric Analysis (RSA) 0350T
Reconstruction
  Total Replacement.................. 27130
Removal
  Cast 29710
  Foreign Body 27033, 27086, 27087
    Arthroscopic............... 29861-29863
  Loose Body
    Arthroscopic............... 29861-29863
  Prosthesis.................. 27090, 27091
Repair
  Muscle Transfer.. 27100-27105, 27110, 27111
  Osteotomy 27146-27156
  Tendon............................ 27097
Replacement
  Partial........................... 27125
  Total...................... 27130, 27132
Saucerization 27070
Stem Prostheses
  See Arthroplasty, Hip
Strapping............................. 29520
Tenotomy
  Abductor Tendon 27006
  Adductor Tendon 27000-27003
  Iliopsoas......................... 27005
Total Replacement 27130-27132
Tumor
  Excision 27047, 27048, 27065-27067
  Radical Resection 27049, 27059
Ultrasound
  Infant 76885, 76886
X ray
  Bilateral 73521-73523
  Unilateral 73501-73503
  with Contrast 73525

Hip Joint
Arthroplasty 27132
  Revision 27134-27138
Arthrotomy 27052, 27054
Biopsy................................ 27052
Capsulotomy
  with Release, Flexor Muscles 27036
Dislocation 27250-27252
  Congenital 27256-27259
  Open Treatment.............. 27253, 27254
  without Trauma 27265, 27266
Manipulation........................... 27275
Reconstruction
  Revision 27134-27138
Synovium
  Excision 27054
    Arthroscopic............... 29860-29863
Total Replacement 27132

Hip Stem Prostheses
See Arthroplasty, Hip

Hippocampus
Excision............................... 61566

Histamine
Measurement 83088

Histamine Release Test
Leukocyte 86343

Histochemistry
Stain on Frozen Tissue Block 88314
Enzyme Constituents 88319

Histocompatibility Testing
See Tissue, Typing

Histoplasma
Detection
Immunoassay
Antibody 86698
Antigen 87385

Histoplasma capsulatum
Antigen Detection
Immunoassay 87385

Histoplasmin Test
See Histoplasmosis, Skin Test

Histoplasmoses
See Histoplasmosis

Histoplasmosis
Skin Test 86510

History and Physical
See Evaluation and Management, Office and Other Outpatient

HIV
Antibody 86701-86703
Confirmation Test 86689

HIV-1
Antibody Detection
Immunoassay 86701, 86703, 87389
Immunoassay with Direct Optical Observation 87806
Antigen Detection
Immunoassay 87389, 87390
Immunoassay with Direct Optical Observation 87806
Genotype Analysis 87901, 87906
Infectious Agent Detection
Amplified Probe 87535
Direct Probe 87534
Quantification 87536

HIV-2
Antibody Detection
Immunoassay 86702, 86703, 87389
Immunoassay with Direct Optical Observation 87806
Antigen Detection
Immunoassay 87389, 87391
Infectious Agent Detection
Amplified Probe 87538
Direct Probe 87537
Quantification 87539

HK3 Kallikrein
See Antigen, Prostate Specific

HLA
See Human Leukocyte Antigen (HLA)

HMRK
See Fitzgerald Factor

HMW Kininogen
See Fitzgerald Factor

Hoffman Apparatus 20690

Hofmeister Operation
See Gastrectomy, Total

Holotranscobalamin
Quantitative 84999

Holten Test
See Creatinine, Urine

Holter Monitor 93224-93227

Home Services
Activities of Daily Living 99509
Anticoagulant Management 93793
Apnea Monitoring 94774-94777
Catheter Care 99507
Enema Administration 99511
Established Patient 99347-99350
Hemodialysis 99512
Home Infusion Procedures 99601, 99602
Individual or Family Counseling 99510
Intramuscular Injections 99506
Mechanical Ventilation 99504
New Patient 99341-99345
Newborn Care 99502
Postnatal Assessment 99501
Prenatal Monitoring 99500
Respiratory Therapy 99503
Sleep Studies 95805-95811
Actigraphy Testing 95803
Stoma Care 99505
Unlisted Services and Procedures 99600
Ventilation Assist 94005

Home Visit
See House Calls

Homocyst(e)ine 83090
Urine 82615

Homogenization, Tissue
for Culture 87176

Homograft
Cornea
Amniotic Membrane 65780
Autograft or Homograft
Allograft Preparation 0290T, 65757
Endothelial 65756
Lamellar 65710
Penetrating 65730, 65750, 65755
for Aphakia 65750
Skin Substitute
Arms 15271-15274
Digits 15275-15278
Eyelids 15275-15278
Face 15275-15278
Feet 15275-15278
Genitalia 15275-15278
Hands 15275-15278
Legs 15271-15274
Mouth 15275-15278
Orbits 15275-15278
Scalp 15275-15278
Trunk 15271-15274

Homologous Grafts
See Graft

Homologous Transplantation
See Allograft

Homovanillic Acid
Urine 83150

Hormone Assay
ACTH 82024
Aldosterone
Blood or Urine 82088
Androstenedione
Blood or Urine 82157
Androsterone
Blood or Urine 82160
Angiotensin II 82163
Corticosterone 82528
Cortisol
Total 82533
Dehydroepiandrosterone 82626
Estradiol 82670
Estriol 82677
Estrogen 82671, 82672
Estrone 82679
Follicle Stimulating Hormone
Gonadotropin 83001
Gonadotropin Releasing Hormone Panel 80426
Pituitary Evaluation Panel 80418
Growth Hormone 83003
Hydroxyprogesterone 83498
Luteinizing Hormone 83002
Somatotropin 83003
Testosterone
Bioavailable 84410
Free 84402
Total 84403
Response 80414
Total 84403
Vasopressin 84588

Hormone Pellet Implantation
Estradiol 11980
Testosterone 11980

Hormone, Adrenocorticotrophic
See Adrenocorticotropic Hormone (ACTH)

Hormone, Corticotropin-Releasing
See Corticotropic Releasing Hormone (CRH)

Hormone, Growth
See Growth Hormone

Hormone, Human Growth
See Growth Hormone, Human

Hormone, Interstitial Cell-Stimulating
See Luteinizing Hormone (LH)

Hormone, Parathyroid
See Parathormone

Hormone, Pituitary Lactogenic
See Prolactin

Hormone, Placental Lactogen
See Lactogen, Human Placental

Hormone, Somatotropin Release-Inhibiting
See Somatostatin

Hormone, Thyroid-Stimulating
See Thyroid Stimulating Hormone (TSH)

Hormone-Binding Globulin, Sex
See Globulin, Sex Hormone Binding

Hormones, Adrenal Cortex
See Corticosteroids

Hormones, Antidiuretic
See Antidiuretic Hormone

Hospital Discharge Services
See Discharge Services, Hospital

Hospital Services
Advance Care Planning 99497, 99498
Inpatient Services 99238, 99239
Chronic Care Management 99490, 99491
Complex 99487, 99489

Discharge Services 99238, 99239, 1110F, 1111F
Initial Care
New or Established Patient ... 99221-99233
Initial Hospital Care 99221-99223
Newborn 99460-99462, 99477
Prolonged Services 99356, 99357
Subsequent Hospital Care 99231-99233
Observation
Discharge Services 99234-99236
Initial Care 99218-99223
Same Day Admission
Discharge Services 99234-99236
Subsequent Newborn Care 99462
Post-discharge Transitional Care Management Services 99495, 99496

Hot Pack Treatment
Application 97010

House Calls
Established Patient 99347-99350
New Patient 99341-99345

HPC
See Hematopoietic Progenitor Cell (HPC)

HPL
See Lactogen, Human Placental

HTLV-I
Antibody
Confirmatory Test 86689
Detection 86687

HTLV-II
Antibody 86688

HTLV-III
See HIV

HTLV-III Antibodies
See Antibody, Detection, Human Immunodeficiency Virus (HIV)

HTLV-IV
See HIV-2

Hubbard Tank Therapy
Each 15 minutes 97036

Hue Test
Color Vision Exam 92283

Huggin Operation
See Orchiectomy, Simple

Huhner Test
Semen Analysis 89300, 89320

Human Chorionic Gonadotropin
See Chorionic Gonadotropin

Human Chorionic Somatomammotropin
See Lactogen, Human Placental

Human Cytomegalovirus Group
See Cytomegalovirus

Human Epididymis Protein 86305

Human Growth Hormone (HGH)
Anterior Pituitary Evaluation Panel 80418
Antibody 86277
Insulin Tolerance Panel 80435
Measurement 83003
Stimulation Panel 80428
Suppression Panel 80430

Human Herpes Virus 4
See Epstein-Barr Virus

Human Immunodeficiency Virus
See HIV

Human Immunodeficiency Virus 1
See HIV-1

Human Immunodeficiency Virus 2
See HIV-2

Human Leukocyte Antigen (HLA)
Antibody Analysis 86828-86835
Crossmatch 86825, 86826
Molecular Pathology 81370-81383
Tissue Typing 86812, 86813, 86816, 86817, 86821

Human Papillomavirus
Vaccine
See Vaccines and Toxoids, Human Papillomavirus (HPV)

Human Papillomavirus Detection
Nucleic Acid Probe 0500T, 87623-87625

Human Placental Lactogen
See Lactogen, Human Placental

Human T Cell Leukemia Virus I
See HTLV-I

Human T Cell Leukemia Virus I Antibodies
See Antibody, Detection, HTLV-I

Human T Cell Leukemia Virus II
See HTLV-II

Human T Cell Leukemia Virus II Antibodies
See Antibody, Detection, HTLV-II

Humeral Epicondylitises, Lateral
See Tennis Elbow

Humeral Fracture
See Fracture, Humerus

Humerus
See Arm, Upper; Shoulder
Abscess
Incision and Drainage 23935
Craterization 23184, 24140
Cyst
Excision 23150, 24110
with Allograft 23156, 24116
with Autograft 23155, 24115
Diaphysectomy 23184, 24140
Excision 23174, 23184, 23195, 24134, 24140, 24150
Fracture
Closed Treatment 24500-24505
with Manipulation 23605
without Manipulation 23600
Condyle
Closed Treatment 24576, 24577
Open Treatment 24579
Percutaneous Fixation 24582
Epicondyle
Closed Treatment 24560-24565
Open Treatment 24575
Skeletal Fixation
Percutaneous 24566
Greater Tuberosity Fracture
Closed Treatment with Manipulation 23625
Closed Treatment without Manipulation 23620
Open Treatment 23630
Open Treatment 23615, 23616
Shaft 24500-24505, 24516
Open Treatment 24515
Supracondylar
Closed Treatment 24530-24535
Open Treatment 24545, 24546
Percutaneous Fixation 24538
Transcondylar
Closed Treatment 24530-24535
Open Treatment 24545, 24546
Percutaneous Fixation 24538
with Dislocation 23665-23670
Osteomyelitis 24134
Pinning, Wiring 23491, 24498
Prophylactic Treatment 23491, 24498
Radical Resection 23220, 24150
Radial Head or Neck 24152
Repair 24430
Nonunion, Malunion 24430-24435
Osteoplasty 24420
Osteotomy 24400-24410
with Graft 24435
Resection Head 23195
Saucerization 23184, 24140
Sequestrectomy 23174, 24134
Tumor
Excision .. 23150, 23220, 24071-24076, 24110
with Allograft 23156, 24116
with Autograft 23155, 24115
X ray 73060

Hummelshein Operation
See Strabismus, Repair

Humor Shunt, Aqueous
See Aqueous Shunt

HVA
See Homovanillic Acid

Hybridization Probes, DNA
See Nucleic Acid Probe

Hydatid Disease
See Echinococcosis

Hydatid Mole
See Hydatidiform Mole

Hydatidiform Mole
Evacuation and Curettage 59870
Excision 59100

Hydration
Intravenous 96360, 96361
Rehydration Oral Solution 4056F
Status 2030F, 2031F

Hydrocarbons, Chlorinated
See Chlorinated Hydrocarbons

Hydrocele
Aspiration 55000
Excision
Bilateral
Tunica Vaginalis 55041
Unilateral
Spermatic Cord 55500
Tunica Vaginalis 55040
Repair 55060

Hydrochloric Acid, Gastric
See Acid, Gastric

Hydrochloride, Vancomycin
See Vancomycin

Hydrocodon
See Dihydrocodeinone

Hydrogen Ion Concentration
See Blood Gases, pH

Index

Hydrolase, Acetylcholine
See Acetylcholinesterase

Hydrolase, Triacylglycerol
See Lipase

Hydrolases, Phosphoric Monoester
See Phosphatase

Hydrotherapy (Hubbard Tank)
Application 97036
See Physical Medicine/Therapy/Occupational Therapy

Hydrotubation
See Chromotubation

Hydroxycorticosteroid 83491

Hydroxyindoleacetic Acid
Urine 83497
  Qualitative 81005

Hydroxypregnenolone
3 Beta-hydroxydehydrogenase Deficiency Panel 80406
Quantitative 84143

Hydroxyprogesterone
ACTH Stimulation Panel 80402, 80406
Quantitative 83498

Hydroxyproline
Free 83500
Total 83505

Hydroxytyramine
See Dopamine

Hygroma
Cystic
  Axillary/Cervical
    Excision 38550-38555

Hymen
Excision 56700
Incision 56442

Hymenal Ring
Revision 56700

Hymenectomy 56700

Hymenotomy 56442

Hyoid
Muscle
  Incision and Suspension 21685

Hyperbaric Oxygen Pressurization 99183

Hypercycloidal X ray 76101, 76102

Hyperdactylies
See Supernumerary Digit

Hyperglycemic Glycogenolytic Factor
See Glucagon

Hyperhidrosis 64650-64653

Hypertelorism of Orbit
See Orbital Hypertelorism

Hyperthermia Therapy
See Thermotherapy

Hyperthermia Treatment 77600-77620

Hypnotherapy 90880

Hypodermis
See Subcutaneous Tissue

Hypogastric Plexus
Destruction 64681
Injection
  Anesthetic 64517
  Neurolytic 64680, 64681

Hypoglossal Nerve
Anastomosis
  Facial-Hypoglossal 64868
  Facial-Spinal 64866

Hypoglossal-Facial Anastomosis
See Hypoglossal Nerve, Anastomosis, Facial-Hypoglossal

Hypopharynges
See Hypopharynx

Hypopharynx
Diverticulectomy 43130, 43180

Hypophysectomy 61546-61548, 62165

Hypophysis
See Pituitary Gland

Hypopyrexia
See Hypothermia

Hypospadias
Repair 54300, 54352
  Complications 54340-54348
  First Stage 54304
    Proximal Penile or Penoscrotal 54332
  One Stage
    Meatal Advancement 54322
    Perineal 54336
  Urethroplasty
    Local Skin Flaps 54324
    Local Skin Flaps and Mobilization of Urethra 54326
    Local Skin Flaps, Skin Graft Patch and/or Island Flap 54328
  Urethroplasty for Second Stage 54308, 54312, 54316
    Free Skin Graft 54316
  Urethroplasty for Third Stage 54318

Hypothermia
Treatment
  Neonatal
    Selective 99184
    Total 99184

Hypoxia
Breathing Response 94450
High Altitude Simulation Test 94452, 94453

Hysterectomy
Abdominal
  Radical 58210
  Resection of Ovarian Malignancy 58951, 58953, 58954, 58956
  Supracervical 58180
  Total 58150, 58200, 58956
    with Colpo-Urethrocystopexy 58152
    with Omentectomy 58956
    with Partial Vaginectomy 58200
Cesarean
  after Cesarean Delivery 59525
  with Closure of Vesicouterine Fistula 51925
Laparoscopic 58541-58544
  Radical 58548
  Total 58570-58573, 58575
Removal
  Lesion 59100
Supracervical
  Laparoscopic 58541-58544
Vaginal 58260-58270, 58290-58294, 58550-58554
  Laparoscopic 58550, 58570-58573, 58575
  Radical 58285
  Removal Tubes/Ovaries 58262, 58263, 58291, 58292, 58552, 58554
    Repair of Enterocele 58263, 58292, 58294
  with Colpectomy 58275-58280
  with Colpo-Urethrocystopexy 58267, 58293

Hysterolysis
See Lysis, Adhesions, Uterus

Hysteroplasty 58540

Hysterorrhaphy 58520, 59350

Hysterosalpingography 74740
Catheterization 58345
Injection Procedure 58340

Hysterosalpingostomy
See Implantation, Tubouterine

Hysteroscopy
Ablation
  Endometrial 58563
Diagnostic 58555
Lysis
  Adhesions 58559
Placement
  Fallopian Tube Implants 58565
Removal
  Impacted Foreign Body 58562
  Leiomyomata 58561
Resection
  of Intrauterine Septum 58560
Surgical with Biopsy 58558
Unlisted Services and Procedures 58578, 58579

Hysterosonography
See Ultrasound; Sonohysterography

Hysterotomy
See Cesarean Delivery
Abdominal 59100
with Failed Abortion 59852, 59857
with Tubal Ligation 58611

Hysterotrachelectomy
See Amputation, Cervix

I

I Antibodies, HTLV
See Antibody, Detection, HTLV-I

I, Angiotensin
See Angiotensin I

I, Coagulation Factor
See Fibrinogen

I, Heparin Co-Factor
See Antithrombin III

ICCE
See Cataract, Extraction/Removal, Intracapsular (ICCE)

Ichthyosis, Sex Linked
See Syphilis Test

ICSH
See Luteinizing Hormone (LH)

Identification
Antibody
  See Antibody Identification
Antigen
  See Antigen Detection

Axial Vessel
for Island Pedicle . . . 15740
Crystal, Light Microscopy . . . 89060
Microbe
See Infectious Agent; Bacteria Culture; Ova; Parasites
Oocyte
from Follicular Fluid . . . 89254
Sex Chromatin . . . 88130, 88140
Sperm
from Aspiration . . . 89257
from Tissue . . . 89264
Medicolegal . . . 88125
Urate Crystal . . . 89060

IDH
See Isocitric Dehydrogenase, Blood

IG
See Immune Globulins

IgA . . . 82784

IgD . . . 82784

IgE . . . 82785, 86003, 86005, 86008

IgG . . . 82784, 82787, 86001

IgM . . . 82784

II, Coagulation Factor
See Prothrombin
See Gene Analysis

II, Cranial Nerve
See Optic Nerve

Ileal Conduit
Visualization . . . 50690

Ileoscopy
via Stoma . . . 44380-44382, 44384

Ileostomy . . . 45136
Continent (Kock Procedure) . . . 44316
Ileoanal Reservoir . . . 45136
Laparoscopic . . . 44186, 44187
Non-Tube . . . 44310, 44187
Revision . . . 44312-44314

Iliac Arteries
See Artery, Iliac

Iliac Crest
Microvascular Anastomosis
Bone Graft . . . 20956
Free Osteocutaneous Flap . . . 20970

Iliohypogastric Nerve
Injection
Anesthetic . . . 64425

Ilioinguinal Nerve
Injection
Anesthetic . . . 64425

Ilium
Craterization . . . 27070
Cyst
Excision . . . 27065-27067
Excision . . . 27070
Fracture
Open Treatment . . . 27215, 27218
Saucerization . . . 27070
Tumor
Excision . . . 27065-27067, 27075, 27076

Ilizarov Procedure
Monticelli Type . . . 20692
See Application, Bone Fixation Device

IM Injection
See Injection, Intramuscular

Imaging
See Vascular Studies

Imaging, Gamma Camera
See Nuclear Medicine, Diagnostic

Imaging, Magnetic Resonance
See Magnetic Resonance Imaging (MRI)

Imaging, Ultrasonic
See Echography

Imbrication
Diaphragm . . . 39545

Immune Complex Assay . . . 86332

Immune Globulin Administration
Intravenous Infusion . . 96365-96368, 96374, 96375
Injection . . . 96372

Immune Globulin E
See IgE

Immune Globulins
Antitoxin
Botulinum . . . 90287
Diphtheria . . . 90296
Botulism . . . 90288
Cytomegalovirus . . . 90291
Hepatitis B . . . 90371
Human . . . 90281, 90283, 90284
Rabies . . . 90375, 90376
Respiratory Syncytial Virus . . . 90378
Rho(D) . . . 90384-90386
Tetanus . . . 90389
Unlisted Immune Globulin . . . 90399
Vaccinia . . . 90393
Varicella-Zoster . . . 90396

Immunization Administration
Each Additional Vaccine/Toxoid . . . 90472, 90474
with Counseling . . . 90461
One Vaccine/Toxoid . . . 90471, 90473
with Counseling . . . 90460

Immunization, Mumps
See Mumps, Immunization

Immunoassay
Amniotic Fluid Protein . . . 84112
Analyte . . . 83516, 83518-83520
Calprotectin, Fecal . . . 83993
Hemoglobin, Fecal . . . 82274
Cellular Function
Detection of Biomarker . . . 86352
Infectious Agent
See Infectious Agent
Other than Infectious Agent
Antibody/Antigen . . . 83516, 83518, 83519
Tumor Antigen
Qualitative/Semiquantitative . . . 86294
Quantitative
CA-125 . . . 86304
CA 15-3 . . . 86300
CA 19-9 . . . 86301
Other Antigen . . . 86316
Human Epididymis Protein 4 (HE4) . . . 86305

Immunoblotting, Western
See Western Blot

Immunochemical, Lysozyme (Muramidase)
See Lysozyme

Immunocytochemistry
Antibody . . . 88341, 88342, 88344

Immunodeficiency Virus Type 1, Human
See HIV-1

Immunodeficiency Virus Type 2, Human
See HIV-2

Immunodeficiency Virus, Human
See HIV

Immunodiffusion
Gel Diffusion
Antibody or Antigen . . . 86331
Ouchterlony . . . 86331
Unspecified . . . 86329

Immunoelectrophoresis
Crossed/2-dimensional Assay . . . 86320
Fluids Other Than Serum . . . 86325
Serum . . . 86320

Immunofixation Electrophoresis
Fluids Other Than Serum . . . 86335
Serum . . . 86334

Immunofluorescence Microscopy
Antibody Stain Procedure . . . 88346, 88350
Antiserum Culture Typing . . . 87140
Infectious Agent Antigen Detection
See Infectious Agent, Antigen Detection, Immunofluorescence

Immunogen
See Antigen

Immunoglobulin . . . 82784-82787
Platelet Associated Antibody . . . 86023
Thyroid Stimulating . . . 84445

Immunoglobulin E
See IgE

Immunologic Skin Test
See Skin, Tests

Immunohistochemistry
Antibody . . . 88341, 88342, 88344

Immunology . . . 86000-86849
Tissue Typing
See Tissue, Typing
Unlisted Immunology Procedure . . . 86849

Immunotherapies, Allergen
See Allergen Immunotherapy

Impedance Testing
Tympanometry . . . 92567, 92570
See Audiologic Function Tests

Imperfectly Descended Testis
See Testis, Undescended

Implant Removal
See Removal, Implant

Implant, Breast
See Breast, Implant

Implant, Glaucoma Drainage
See Aqueous Shunt

Implant, Orbital
See Orbital Implant

Implant, Penile
See Penile Prosthesis

Implant, Penile Prosthesis, Inflatable
See Penile Prosthesis, Insertion, Inflatable

Index

Implant, Subperiosteal
See Subperiosteal Implant

Implant, Ureters into, Bladder
See Anastomosis, Ureter, to Bladder

Implantable Defibrillator
See Cardiac Assist Devices, Implantable Defibrillators

Implantable Loop Recorder System
See Cardiac Assist Devices, Subcutaneous Cardiac Rhythm Monitor

Implantation
Abdominal Wall
  Non-biologic or Synthetic Implant . . . 0437T
Aortic Valve
  Transcatheter . . . 33361-33369
Artificial Heart . . . 33927
Baroreflex Activation Device . . . 0266T-0268T
  Lead . . . 0267T
  Pulse Generator . . . 0268T
  Total System . . . 0266T
Biological Implant
  Soft Tissue Reinforcement . . . 15777
Bone
  for External Speech Processor/Cochlear Stimulator . . . 69714-69718
Brain
  Chemotherapy . . . 61517
Cochlear Device . . . 69930
Drug Delivery Device . . . 11981, 11983, 61517
Drug-Eluting Device
  Lacrimal Canaliculus . . . 0356T
Embryo . . . 58974
Ethmoid Sinus
  Drug-Eluting Implant . . . 31237, 31299
Eye
  Anterior Segment . . . 65920
  Aqueous Shunt to Extraocular Placement or Replacement of Pegs . . . 65125
  Corneal Ring Segments . . . 65785
  Posterior Segment
    Extraocular . . . 67120
    Intraocular . . . 67121
  Replacement of Pegs . . . 65125
  Reservoir . . . 66179, 66180
  Vitreous
    Drug Delivery System . . . 67027
Fallopian Tube . . . 58565
Hearing Aid Hormone Pellet(s)
  Bone Conduction . . . 69710
Hip Prosthesis
  See Arthroplasty, Hip
Hormone Pellet . . . 11980
Intraocular Lens
  See Insertion, Intraocular Lens
Joint
  See Arthroplasty
Left Atrial Appendage . . . 33340
Load
  Upper Eyelid . . . 67912
Mesh . . . 49568
  Hernia Repair . . . 43333, 43335, 43337, 49568, 49652-49657
  Vaginal Repair . . . 57267
Nerve
  into Bone . . . 64787
  into Muscle . . . 64787
Neurostimulator Systems
  See Neurostimulators
Ovum . . . 58976
Pressure Sensor
  Pulmonary Artery . . . 33289
Pulmonary Valve
  Transcatheter Percutaneous . . . 33477
Removal . . . 20670-20680
  Ankle . . . 27704
  Breast . . . 19328-19330
  Contraceptive Capsules . . . 11976
  Disc . . . 22865
  Eye . . . 67120, 67121
  Finger . . . 26320
  Hand . . . 26320
  Wrist . . . 25449
Reservoir Vascular Access Device
  Declotting . . . 36593
Radiotereometric Analysis (RSA)
  Interstitial . . . 0347T
Retinal Electrode Array . . . 0100T
Total Replacement Heart System . . . 33927
Trunk
  Biological Implant . . . 15777
  Soft Tissue Reinforcement . . . 15777
Tubouterine . . . 58752
Ventricular Assist Device
  See Ventricular Assist Device (VAD)

Impression, Maxillofacial
Auricular Prosthesis . . . 21086
Definitive Obturator Prosthesis . . . 21080
Facial Prosthesis . . . 21088
Interim Obturator . . . 21079
Mandibular Resection Prosthesis . . . 21081
Nasal Prosthesis . . . 21087
Oral Surgical Splint . . . 21085
Orbital Prosthesis . . . 21077
Palatal Augmentation Prosthesis . . . 21082
Palatal Lift Prosthesis . . . 21083
Speech Aid Prosthesis . . . 21084
Surgical Obturator . . . 21076

IMRT
See Intensity Modulated Radiation Treatment (IMRT)

IMT
See Intima-Media Thickness (IMT) Study

In Situ Hybridization
Chromosome Analysis . . . 88272, 88273
Cytopathology . . . 88120, 88121
Fluorescent
  See Fluorescent In Situ Hybridization (FISH)
Nucleic Acid Probe . . . 88120, 88121, 88364-88366

In Vitro Fertilization . . . 58321, 58322

In Vivo Laboratory Procedures
Unlisted Service . . . 88749

In Vivo NMR Spectroscopy
See Magnetic Resonance Spectroscopy

Incision
See Incision and Drainage
Abdomen . . . 49000
  Exploration . . . 58960
Accessory Nerve . . . 63191
Anal
  Fistula . . . 46270, 46280
  Septum . . . 46070
  Sphincter . . . 46080
Ankle . . . 27607
  Tendon . . . 27605, 27606
Anus
  See Anus, Incision
Aortic Valve
  for Stenosis . . . 33415
Artery
  Nose . . . 30915-30920
Atrial Septum . . . 33735-33737
Bile Duct
  Sphincter . . . 43262, 47460
Bladder
  Catheterization . . . 51045
  with Destruction . . . 51020-51030
  with Radiotracer . . . 51020
Bladder Diverticulum . . . 52305
Brachial Artery
  Exposure . . . 34834
Brain
  Amygdalohippocampectomy . . . 61566
  Subpial . . . 61567
Breast
  Capsules . . . 19370
Burn Scab . . . 16035, 16036
Buttock . . . 27027, 27057
Cataract
  Secondary
    Laser Surgery . . . 66821
    Stab Incision Technique . . . 66820
Chest
  Biopsy . . . 32096-32098
  with Therapeutic Wedge
  Resection . . . 32505, 32506
Colon
  Exploration . . . 44025
  Stoma
    Creation . . . 44320-44322
    Revision . . . 44340-44346
Cornea
  for Astigmatism . . . 65772
  Laser
    for Keratoplasty . . . 0290T
Corpus Callosum . . . 61541
Cricothyroid Membrane . . . 31605
Dentate Ligament . . . 63180-63182
Duodenum . . . 44010
Ear, Inner
  Labyrinth
    Transcanal . . . 69801
Elbow . . . 24000
Esophagus . . . 43020, 43045
  Muscle . . . 43030
Exploration
  Heart . . . 33310-33315
  Kidney . . . 50010
Eye
  Adhesions . . . 65880
    Anterior Segment . . . 65860-65865
    Anterior Synechiae . . . 65870
    Corneovitreal . . . 65880
    Posterior . . . 65875
  Anterior Chamber . . . 65820
  Trabeculae . . . 65850
Eyelid
  Canthus . . . 67715
  Margin
    for Biopsy . . . 67810
  Sutures . . . 67710
Femoral Artery
  Exposure . . . 34812, 34813
Fibula . . . 27607
Finger
  Decompression . . . 26035
  Tendon . . . 26060, 26455-26460
  Tendon Sheath . . . 26055
Foot . . . 28005
  Capsule . . . 28260-28264
  Fasciotomy . . . 28008
  for Infection . . . 28002, 28003
  Tendon . . . 28230, 28234
Gallbladder . . . 47490

Hand Decompression 26035-26037
Tendon 26450, 26460
Heart
Exploration 33310-33315
Hemorrhoids
External 46083
Hepatic Ducts
See Hepaticostomy
Hip
Denervation 27035
Exploration 27033
Fasciotomy 27025
Joint Capsule
for Flexor Release 27036
Tendon
Abductor 27006
Adductor 27000-27003
Iliopsoas 27005
Hymen
See Hymen, Incision
Hymenotomy 56442
Hyoid
Muscle 21685
Iliac Artery
Exposure 34820, 34833
Intercarpal Joint
Dislocation 25670
Interphalangeal Joint
Capsule 26525
Intestines (Except Rectum)
See Enterotomy
Intestines, Small 44010
Biopsy 44020
Creation
Pouch 44316
Stoma 44300-44310, 44314
Decompression 44021
Exploration 44020
Incision 44020
Removal
Foreign Body 44020
Revision
Stoma 44312
Iris 66500-66505
Kidney 50010, 50045
Knee
Capsule 27435
Exploration 27310
Fasciotomy 27305
Removal of Foreign Body 27310
Lacrimal Punctum 68440
Lacrimal Sac
See Dacryocystotomy
Larynx 31300
Leg, Lower
Fasciotomy 27600-27602
Leg, Upper
Fasciotomy 27305
Tenotomy 27306, 27307, 27390-27392
Lip
Frenum 40806
Liver
See Hepatotomy
Lung
Biopsy 32096, 32097
Decortication
Partial 32225
Total 32220
Lymphatic Channels 38308
Mastoid
See Mastoidotomy
Metacarpophalangeal Joint
Capsule 26520
Mitral Valve 33420-33422
Muscle
See Myotomy
Nerve. . . 64568, 64575-64580, 64595, 64702-64772
Foot 28035
Root 63185-63190
Sacral 64581
Vagus 43640, 43641
Nose
See Rhinotomy
Orbit
See Orbitotomy
Palm
Fasciotomy 26040-26045
Pancreas
Sphincter 43262
Pelvis
Fasciotomy 27027, 27057
Penis
Prepuce 54000, 54001
Newborn 54000
Pericardium
with Clot Removal 33020
with Foreign Body Removal 33020
with Tube 33015
Pharynx
Stoma 42955
Pleura
Biopsy 32098
Pleural Cavity
Empyema 32035, 32036
Prostate
Exposure
Bilateral Pelvic Lymphadenectomy . . . 55865
Insertion Radioactive Substance 55860
Lymph Node Biopsy 55862
Transurethral 52450
Pterygomaxillary Fossa 31040
Pulmonary Valve 33470, 33471, 33474
Pyloric Sphincter 43520
Retina
Encircling Material 67115
Sclera
Fistulization
Sclerectomy with Punch or Scissors with
Iridectomy 66160
Thermocauterization with Iridectomy . 66155
Trabeculectomy ab Externo in Absence
Previous Surgery 66170
Trephination with Iridectomy 66150
Seminal Vesicle 55600-55605
Complicated 55605
Shoulder
Bone 23035
Capsular Contracture Release 23020
Removal
Calcareous Deposits 23000
Tenomyotomy 23405, 23406
Shoulder Joint 23040-23044
Sinus
Frontal 31070-31087
Maxillary 31020-31032
Endoscopic 31256-31267
Multiple 31090
Sphenoid
Sinusotomy 31050, 31051
Skin 10040, 10060, 10061,
10080, 10081, 10120-10180
Skull 61316, 62148
Suture 61550-61552
Spinal Cord 63200
Tract 63170, 63194-63199
Stomach
Creation
Stoma 43830-43832
Exploration 43500
Pyloric Sphincter 43520
Synovectomy 26140
Temporomandibular Joint 21010
Tendon
Arm, Upper 24310
Thigh
Fasciotomy 27025
Thoracoabdominal
Paraesophageal Hiatal Hernia
Repair 43336, 43337
Thorax
Empyema 32035, 32036
Thyroid Gland
See Thyrotomy
Tibia 27607
Toe
Capsule 28270-28272
Fasciotomy 28008
Tendon 28232-28234
Tenotomy 28010, 28011
Tongue
Frenum 41010
Trachea
Emergency 31603-31605
Planned 31600, 31601
Fenestration with Flaps 31610
Tympanic Membrane 69420
with Anesthesia 69421
Ureter 50600
Ureterocele 51535
Urethra 53000-53010
Meatus 53020-53025
Uterus
Remove Lesion 59100
Vagina
Exploration 57000
Vas Deferens 55200
for X ray 55300
Vestibule of the Mouth
See Mouth, Vestibule, Incision and Drainage
Vitreous Strands
Laser Surgery 67031
Pars Plana Approach 67030
Wrist 25100-25105
Capsule 25085
Decompression 25020-25025
Tendon Sheath 25000, 25001

Incision and Drainage

See Drainage; Incision
Abdomen
Fluid 49082, 49083
Pancreatitis 48000
Abscess
Abdomen 49020, 49040
Open 49040
Soft Tissue
Anal 46045-46050
Ankle 27603
Appendix 44900
Arm, Lower 25028
Arm, Upper 23930, 23931
Auditory Canal, External 69020
Bartholin's Gland 56420
Bladder 51080
Brain 61320, 61321
Breast 19020
Ear, External
Complicated 69005
Simple 69000

Elbow . . . 23930
Epididymis . . . 54700
Eyelid . . . 67700
Finger . . . 26010, 26011
Gums . . . 41800
Hip . . . 26990
Kidney . . . 50020
Knee . . . 27301
Leg, Lower . . . 27603
Leg, Upper . . . 27301
Liver . . . 47010
Lung . . . 32200
Lymph Node . . . 38300-38305
Mouth . . . 40800, 40801, 41005-41009, 41015-41018
Nasal Septum . . . 30020
Neck . . . 21501, 21502
Nose . . . 30000-30020
Ovary . . . 58820-58822
Abdominal Approach . . . 58822
Palate . . . 42000
Paraurethral Gland . . . 53060
Parotid Gland . . . 42300-42305
Pelvis . . . 26990, 45000
Perineum . . . 56405
Peritoneum . . . 49020
Prostate . . . 55720-55725
Rectum . . . 45005-45020, 46040, 46050-46060
Retroperitoneal . . . 49060
Open . . . 49060
Salivary Gland . . . 42300-42320
Scrotum . . . 54700, 55100
Skene's Gland . . . 53060
Skin . . . 10060, 10061
Subdiaphragmatic . . . 49040
Sublingual Gland . . . 42310-42320
Submaxillary Gland . . . 42310-42320
Subphrenic . . . 49040
Testis . . . 54700
Thorax . . . 21501, 21502
Throat . . . 42700-42725
Tongue . . . 41000-41006, 41015
Tonsil . . . 42700
Urethra . . . 53040
Uvula . . . 42000
Vagina . . . 57010
Vulva . . . 56405
Wrist . . . 25028
Ankle . . . 27610
Bile Duct . . . 47420-47425
Bladder . . . 51040
Bulla
Skin
Puncture Aspiration . . . 10160
Bursa
Ankle . . . 27604
Arm, Lower . . . 25031
Elbow . . . 23931
Foot . . . 28001
Hip . . . 26991
Knee . . . 27301
Leg, Lower . . . 27604
Leg, Upper . . . 27301
Palm . . . 26025-26030
Pelvis . . . 26991
Wrist . . . 25031
Carbuncle
Skin . . . 10060, 10061
Carpals . . . 25035, 26034
Comedones
Skin . . . 10040
Cyst
Conjunctiva . . . 68020
Gums . . . 41800
Liver . . . 47010
Lung . . . 32200
Mouth . . . 40800, 40801, 41005-41009, 41015-41018
Ovarian . . . 58800-58805
Skin . . . 10040, 10060, 10061
Pilonidal . . . 10080, 10081
Puncture Aspiration . . . 10160
Spinal Cord . . . 63172, 63173
Thyroid Gland . . . 60000
Tongue . . . 41000-41006, 41015, 60000
Elbow
Abscess . . . 23935
Arthrotomy . . . 24000
Femur . . . 27303
Fluid Collection
Skin . . . 10140
Foreign Body
Skin . . . 10120, 10121
Furuncle . . . 10060, 10061
Gallbladder . . . 47480
Hematoma
Ankle . . . 27603
Arm, Lower . . . 25028
Arm, Upper . . . 23930
Brain . . . 61312-61315
Ear, External
Complicated . . . 69005
Simple . . . 69000
Elbow . . . 23930
Epididymis . . . 54700
Gums . . . 41800
Hip . . . 26990
Knee . . . 27301
Leg, Lower . . . 27603
Leg, Upper . . . 27301
Mouth . . . 40800, 40801, 41005-41009, 41015-41018
Nasal Septum . . . 30020
Neck . . . 21501, 21502
Nose . . . 30000-30020
Pelvis . . . 26990
Scrotum . . . 54700
Skin . . . 10140
Puncture Aspiration . . . 10160
Skull . . . 61312-61315
Testis . . . 54700
Thorax . . . 21501, 21502
Tongue . . . 41000-41006, 41015
Vagina . . . 57022, 57023
Wrist . . . 25028
Hepatic Duct . . . 47400
Hip
Bone . . . 26992, 27030
Humerus
Abscess . . . 23935
Interphalangeal Joint
Toe . . . 28024
Intertarsal Joint . . . 28020
Kidney . . . 50040, 50125
Knee . . . 27303, 27310
Lacrimal Gland . . . 68400
Lacrimal Sac . . . 68420
Liver
Abscess or Cyst . . . 47010
Mediastinum . . . 39000-39010
Metatarsophalangeal Joint . . . 28022
Milia, Multiple . . . 10040
Onychia . . . 10060, 10061
Orbit . . . 67405, 67440
Paronychia . . . 10060, 10061
Pelvic
Bone . . . 26992
Penis . . . 54015
Pericardium . . . 33025
Phalanges
Finger . . . 26034
Pilonidal Cyst . . . 10080, 10081
Pustules
Skin . . . 10040
Radius . . . 25035
Seroma
Skin . . . 10140
Shoulder
Abscess . . . 23030
Arthrotomy
Acromioclavicular Joint . . . 23044
Sternoclavicular Joint . . . 23044
Bursa . . . 23031
Hematoma . . . 23030
Shoulder Joint
Arthrotomy
Glenohumeral Joint . . . 23040
Spine
Abscess . . . 22010-22015
Tarsometatarsal Joint . . . 28020
Tendon Sheath
Finger . . . 26020
Palm . . . 26020
Thorax
Deep . . . 21510
Toe . . . 28024
Ulna . . . 25035
Ureter . . . 50600
Vagina . . . 57020
Wound Infection
Skin . . . 10180
Wrist . . . 25028, 25040

Incisional Hernia Repair
See Hernia Repair, Incisional

Inclusion Bodies
Fluid . . . 88106
Smear . . . 87207, 87210

Incomplete Abortion
See Abortion, Incomplete

Indicator Dilution Studies
Cardiac Output . . . 93562
Thermodilution . . . 93561

Induced Abortion
See Abortion

Induced Hyperthermia
See Thermotherapy

Induced Hypothermia
See Hypothermia

Induratio Penis Plastica
See Peyronie Disease

Indwelling Catheter
Percutaneous, Lung
See Pleural Cavity, Catheterization

Infant, Newborn, Intensive Care
See Intensive Care, Neonatal

Infantile Paralysis
See Polio

Infection
Diagnosis
Group A Strep Test . . . 3210F
Immunoassay . . . 86317, 86318

Rapid Test 86403, 86406
Treatment
Antibiotic Prescribed 4045F

Infection, Actinomyces
See Actinomycosis

Infection, Bone
See Osteomyelitis

Infection, Filarioidea
See Filariasis

Infection, Postoperative Wound
See Postoperative Wound Infection

Infection, Wound
See Wound, Infection

Infectious Agent
Antibody Detection
Immunoassay, Multistep
Actinomyces 86602
Adenovirus 86603
Aspergillus 86606
Bacterium 86609
Bartonella 86611
Blastomyces 86612
Bordetella 86615
Borrelia 86617-86619
Brucella 86622
Campylobacter 86625
Candida 86628
Chlamydia 86631, 86632
Coccidioides 86635
Coxiella Burnetii 86638
Cryptococcus 86641
Cytomegalovirus (CMV) 86644, 86645
Diphtheria 86648
Ehrlichia 86666
Encephalitis 86651-86654
Enterovirus 86658, 87498
Epstein-Barr Virus 86663-86665
Francisella Tularensis 86668
Fungus, Other 86671
Giardia Lamblia 86674
Helicobacter Pylori 86677
Helminth 86682
Haemophilus Influenzae 86684
Hepatitis
Delta Agent 86692
Hepatitis A (HAAb) 86708, 86709
Hepatitis B
Core 86704
IgM 86705
Surface 86706
Hepatitis Be 86707
Hepatitis C 86803, 86804
Herpes Simplex 86694-86696
Histoplasma 86698
HIV 86689, 86701-86703
HIV-1 . . . . . 86701, 86703, 87389, 87806
HIV-2 . . . . . 86702, 86703, 87389, 87806
HTLV-I 86687, 86689
HTLV-II 86688
Influenza Virus 86710
Legionella 86713
Leishmania 86717
Leptospira 86720
Listeria Monocytogenes 86723
Lyme Disease 86617
Lymphocytic Choriomeningitis 86727
Malaria 86750
Mucormycosis 86732
Mumps 86735
Mycoplasma 86738
Neisseria Meningitidis 86741
Nocardia 86744
Parvovirus 86747
Plasmodium 86750
Protozoa 86753
Respiratory Syncytial Virus 86756
Rickettsia 86757
Rotavirus 86759
Rubella 86762
Rubeola 86765
Salmonella 86768
Shigella 86771
Tetanus 86774
Thyroglobulin 86800
Toxoplasma 86777, 86778
Treponema Pallidum 86780
Trichinella 86784
Tuberculosis 86580
Varicella-Zoster 86787
Virus, Other 86790
West Nile Virus 86788, 86789
Yersinia 86793
Immunoassay, Other Antibody
Quantitative 86317
Immunoassay, Single Step
Qualitative/Semiquantitative 86318
Antigen Detection
Direct Fluorescence
Bordetella 87265
Chlamydia Trachomatis 87270
Cryptosporidium 87272
Cytomegalovirus 87271
Enterovirus 87267
Giardia 87269
Influenza A 87276
Legionella Pneumophila 87278
Respiratory Syncytial Virus 87280
Treponema Pallidum 87285
Varicella-Zoster 87290
Immunoassay
Adenovirus 87301, 87809
Aspergillus 87305
Chlamydia Trachomatis 87320
Clostridium Difficile 87324
Cryptococcus Neoformans 87327
Cryptosporidium 87328
Cytomegalovirus 87332
Entamoeba Histolytica Dispar Group . . 87336
Entamoeba Histolytica Group 87337
Escherichia coli 0157 87335
Giardia 87329
Helicobacter Pylori 87338, 87339
Hepatitis B Surface Antigen (HBsAg) . . 87340
Hepatitis B Surface Antigen (HBsAg)
Neutralization 87341
Hepatitis Be Antigen (HBeAg) 87350
Hepatitis, Delta Agent 87380
Histoplasma capsulatum 87385
HIV-1 . . . . . 87389, 87390
HIV-2 87391
Influenza A 87400
Influenza B 87400
Multiple Step Method 87301-87449, 87451
Not Otherwise Specified 87449, 87450
Polyvalent 87451
Respiratory Syncytial Virus 87420
Rotavirus 87425
Shiga-like Toxin 87427
Single Step Method 87450
Streptococcus, Group A 87430
Immunofluorescence
Adenovirus 87260
Herpes Simplex 87273, 87274
Influenza B 87275
Not Otherwise Specified 87299
Parainfluenza Virus 87279
Pneumocystis Carinii 87281
Polyvalent 87300
Rubeola 87283
Immunoassay, with Direct Optical Observation
Chlamydia Trachomatis 87810
Clostridium Difficile 87803
Gonorrhea 87850
HIV-1 87806
Influenza 87804
Neisseria Gonorrhoeae 87850
Not Otherwise Specified 87899
Respiratory Syncytial Virus 87807
Streptococcus, Group A 87880
Streptococcus, Group B 87802
Trichomonas Vaginalis 87808
Nucleic Acid Probe
Bartonella Henselae 87471-87472
Bartonella Quintana 87471-87472
Borrelia Burgdorferi 87475, 87476
Candida Species 87480-87482
Chlamydia Pneumoniae 87485-87487
Chlamydia Trachomatis 87490-87492
Clostridium Difficile 87493
Cytomegalovirus 87495-87497
Enterovirus 87498, 87500
Gardnerella Vaginalis 87510-87512
Gastrointestinal Pathogen 87505-87507
Gonorrhea 87850
Hepatitis B Virus 87516, 87517
Hepatitis C 87520-87522
Hepatitis G 87525-87527
Herpes Simplex Virus 87528-87530
Herpes Virus-6 87531-87533
HIV-1 87534-87536
HIV-2 87537-87539
Influenza 87501-87503
Legionella Pneumophila 87540-87542
Multiple Organisms 87800, 87801
Mycobacteria Avium-
Intracellulare 87560-87562
Mycobacteria Species 87550-87552
Mycobacteria Tuberculosis . . . 87555-87557
Mycoplasma Pneumoniae 87580-87582
Neisseria Gonorrhoeae 87590-87592
Not Otherwise Specified 87797-87799
Papillomavirus, Human 0500T, 87623-87625
Respiratory Virus 87631-87634
Staphylococcus Aureus 87640, 87641
Streptococcus, Group A 87650-87652
Streptococcus, Group B 87653
Trichomonas Vaginalis 87660, 87661
Vancomycin Resistance 87500
Zika Virus 87662
Concentration 87015
Detection by Nucleic Acid Probe
Central Nervous System Pathogen 87483
Enzymatic Activity 87905
Genotype Analysis
by Nucleic Acid
Cytomegalovirus 87910
Hepatitis B Virus 87912
Hepatitis C Virus 87902
HIV-1 Regions 87901, 87906
Phenotype Analysis
by Nucleic Acid
HIV-1 Drug Resistance 87903, 87904
Phenotype Prediction
by Genetic Database 87900

Infectious Mononucleosis Virus
See Epstein-Barr Virus

Index

Inflammatory Process
Localization
  Nuclear Medicine 78805-78808

Inflation
Eustachian Tube
  Myringotomy 69420
    Anesthesia 69424

Influenza A
Antigen Detection
  Direct Fluorescence 87276
  Immunoassay 87400

Influenza B
Antigen Detection
  Immunoassay 87400
  Immunofluorescence 87275

Influenza Vaccine
See Vaccines and Toxoids

Influenza Virus
Antibody 86710
Detection
  by Immunoassay
    with Direct Optical Observation 87804
  by Nucleic Acid 87501-87503

Infraorbital Nerve
Avulsion 64734
Incision 64734
Transection 64734

Infrared Light Treatment
Application 97026

Infratentorial Craniectomy
Drainage of Abscess 61321
Evacuation of Hematoma 61314, 61315
Excision of Tumor 61518, 61519, 61521
Excision of Abscess 61522
Excision of Cyst 61524
Exploratory 61305

Infusion
Amnion
  Transabdominal 59070
Anesthetic
  Paravertebral Block (PVB) 64463
Cerebral
  for Other Than Thrombolysis 61650, 61651
  for Thrombolysis
    Intravenous 37195
    Percutaneous Transluminal 61645
for Thrombolysis
  Percutaneous Transluminal 61645
  Transcatheter Therapy 37211-37214
Hydration 96360, 96361
  Status Documented 2030F, 2031F
Intra-Arterial 96373
  Unlisted 96379
Intraosseous 36680
Intravenous Unlisted 96379
  Diagnostic/Prophylactic/
  Therapeutic 96365-96368, 96379
  Hydration 96360, 96361
Radioelement 77750
Subcutaneous 96369-96371
Spinal
  Diagnostic/Therapeutic 62324-62327
    Device Implantation/
    Replacement 62360-62362
Transcatheter Therapy 37211-37214

Infusion Pump
Electronic Analysis
  Spinal Cord 62367-62370
Insertion
  Intra-Arterial 36260
Intra-Arterial
  Removal 36262
  Revision 36261
Intravenous
  Insertion 36563
  Repair 36576
  Replacement 36583
Maintenance 95990, 95991, 96521, 96522
  See Chemotherapy, Pump Services
Refill 62369, 62370
Reprogramming 62368-62370
Spinal Cord 62361, 62362
Ventricular Catheter 61215

Infusion Therapy
Arterial Catheterization 36640
by Pump
  See Infusion Pump
Hydration 96360, 96361
  Status Documented 2030F, 2031F
Home Infusion Procedures 99601, 99602
Intravenous 96365-96368, 96379
  Chemotherapy 96413, 96415-96417, 96422, 96423, 96425
Spinal 62324-62327, 62350, 62351
  Device Implantation/
  Replacement 62360-62362
Subcutaneous 96369-96371, 96379
Unlisted Therapeutic Infusion 96379

Ingestion Challenge Test
Incremental/Sequential 95076, 95079
See Allergy Tests

Inguinal Hernia Repair
See Hernia Repair, Inguinal

INH
See Drug Assay

Inhalation
Pentamidine 94642

Inhalation Provocation Tests
See Bronchial Challenge Test

Inhalation Treatment
Continuous 94644, 94645
for Airway Obstruction
  Pressurized or Nonpressurized 94640
Nebulizer 94664
Home Visit 99503

Inhibin A 86336

Inhibition Test, Hemagglutination
See Hemagglutination Inhibition Test

Inhibition, Fertilization
See Contraception

Inhibitor, Alpha 1-Protease
See Alpha-1 Antitrypsin

Inhibitor, Alpha 2-Plasmin
See Alpha-2 Antiplasmin

Inhibitory Concentration, Minimum
See Minimum Inhibitory Concentration

Initial Inpatient Consultations
New or Established Patient 99251-99255

Injection
See Allergen Immunotherapy; Infusion
Abdomen
  Air 49400
  Contrast Material 49400
Anesthetic Agent
  Paravertebral Block (PVB) 64461, 64462
  Sacroiliac Joint 27096
  Spine
    Cervical 0228T, 0229T, 62320, 62321, 62324, 62325
    Lumbar 0230T, 0231T, 62322, 62323, 62326, 62327
    Sacral 0230T, 0231T, 62322, 62323, 62326, 62327
    Thoracic 0228T, 0229T, 62320, 62321, 62324, 62325
Angiography
  Pulmonary 75746
Ankle
  Radial 27648
Antibiotic
  See Antibiotic Administration
Antigen (Allergen) 95115-95125
Anus
  Bulking Agent 0377T
  Sclerosing Solution 46500
Aorta (Aortography)
  Radiological 93567
Aponeurosis 20550
Arthrography
  Sacroiliac Joint 27096
Bile Duct
  Cholangiography 47531, 47532
Bladder
  for Chemodenervation 52287
  Radiological 51600-51610
Brain Canal 61070
Bursa 20600, 20604, 20605, 20610, 20611
Cardiac Catheterization 93454-93464, 93563-93568
Carpal Tunnel
  Therapeutic 20526
Chemotherapy 96401-96542, 96549
Cistern
  Medication or Other 61055
Contrast 49465
  via Catheter 36598, 49424
Corpora Cavernosa 54235
Cyst
  Bone 20615
  Kidney 50390
  Pelvis 50390
  Thyroid 60300
Diagnostic
  Additional Sequential, Each Push 96376
Elbow
  Arthrography
    Radiological 24220
Epidural
  See Epidural, Injection
Esophageal Varices
  Endoscopy 43204, 43243
Esophagus
  Sclerosing Agent 43204
  Submucosal 43192, 43201, 43236
Extremity
  Pseudoaneurysm 36002
Eye
  Anterior Segment
    Air 66020
    Medication 66030
  Pharmacologic Agent 0465T, 67028
  Posterior Segment
    Intravitreal 67028
    Suprachoroidal 0465T
Eyelid
  Subconjunctival 68200

Foot
Nerve . . . 64455
Fluid Collection
Sclerosant . . . 49185
Ganglion
Anesthetic . . . 64505, 64510
Ganglion Cyst . . . 20612
Gastric Secretion Stimulant . . . 43755
Gastric Varices
Endoscopy . . . 43243
Hand
Cell Therapy for Scleroderma . . . 0490T
Heart Vessels
Cardiac Catheterization . . . 93454-93464, 93563-93568
See Catheterization, Cardiac
Radiological . . . 93454-93461
Hemorrhoids
Sclerosing Solution . . . 46500
Hip
Radiological . . . 27093-27095
Insect Venom . . . 95130-95134
Intervertebral Disc
Chemonucleolysis Agent . . . 62292
Radiological . . . 62290, 62291
Intra-amniotic . . . 59852
Intra-arterial . . . 96373, 96379
Thrombolytic . . . 37184-37186, 61645
Intradermal
for Tattooing . . . 11920-11922
Intralesional
Skin . . . 11900, 11901
Intramuscular . . . 96372
Therapeutic . . . 96372, 99506
Intravenous . . . 96379
Nuclear Diagnostic Localization . . . 78808
Thrombolytic . . . 37187, 37188
Unlisted . . . 96379
Vascular Flow Check, Graft . . . 15860
Intravenous Push . . . 96374-96376
Joint . . . 20600, 20604-20606, 20610, 20611
Kidney
Drugs . . . 50391
for Nephrostogram . . . 50430, 50431
Knee
Radiological . . . 27369
Lacrimal Gland
Radiological . . . 68850
Larynx
Endoscopic . . . 31570, 31573, 31574
Left Heart
Radiological . . . 93565
Lesion
Skin . . . 11900, 11901
Ligament . . . 20550
Liver . . . 47015
Mammary Ductogram/Galactogram . . . 19030
Muscle Endplate
Facial . . . 64612
Nerve
Anesthetic . . . 01991, 01992, 64400-64530
Neurolytic Agent 64600-64640, 64680, 64681
Orbit
Retrobulbar
Alcohol . . . 67505
Medication . . . 67500
Tenon's Capsule . . . 67515
Pancreatography . . . 48400
Paravertebral Facet Joint/Nerve
with Image Guidance . . . 64490-64495
with Ultrasound Guidance . . . 0213T-0218T
Penis
for Erection . . . 54235
Peyronie Disease . . . 54200
with Surgical Exposure of Plague . . . 54205
Radiology . . . 54230
Vasoactive Drugs . . . 54231
Peritoneal Cavity Air
See Pneumoperitoneum
Platelet Rich Plasma . . . 0232T
Prophylactic
Additional Sequential, Each Push . . . 96376
Radiological
Breast . . . 19030
Cholangiography . . . 47531, 47532
Rectum
Sclerosing Solution . . . 45520
Right Heart
See Cardiac Catheterization, Injection
Radiological . . . 93566
Sacroiliac Joint
for Arthrography . . . 27096
Salivary Duct . . . 42660
Salivary Gland
Radiological . . . 42550
Sclerosant
Esophagus . . . 43204
Intravenous . . . 36465, 36466, 36468, 36470, 36471
Sentinel Node
Identification . . . 38792, 38900
Shoulder
Arthrography
Radiological . . . 23350
Shunt
Peritoneal
Venous . . . 49427
Sinus Tract . . . 20500
Diagnostic . . . 20501
Spider Veins
Sclerosant . . . 36468
Spinal Artery . . . 62294
Spinal Cord
Anesthetic . . . 62320-62327
Blood . . . 62273
Neurolytic Agent . . . 62280-62282
Other . . . 62320-62327
Radiological . . . 62284
Steroids
Spine
Cervical . . . 0228T, 0229T, 62320, 62321, 62324, 62325
Lumbar . . . 0230T, 0231T, 62322, 62323, 62326, 62327
Sacral . . . 0230T, 0231T, 62322, 62323, 62326, 62327
Thoracic . . . 0228T, 0229T, 62320, 62321, 62324, 62325
Urethral Stricture . . . 52283
Subcutaneous . . . 96372
Silicone . . . 11950-11954
Therapeutic . . . 96372
Timed
Application of On-Body Injection Device . . . 96377
Temporomandibular Joint
Arthrography . . . 21116
Tendon Origin, Insertion . . . 20551
Tendon Sheath . . . 20550
Therapeutic
Additional Sequential, Each Push . . . 96376
Extremity Pseudoaneurysm . . . 36002
Lung . . . 32960
Thyroid . . . 60300
Turbinate . . . 30200
Thoracic Cavity
See Pleurodesis
Trachea . . . 31612
Puncture . . . 31612
Trigger Point(s)
One or Two Muscles . . . 20552
Three or More Muscles . . . 20553
Turbinate . . . 30200
Ureter
Drugs . . . 50391
for Ureterogram . . . 50430, 50431
Radiological . . . 50684
Vein
Sclerosant . . . 36465, 36466, 36468, 36470, 36471
Venography . . . 36005
Ventricle
Dye . . . 61120
Medication or Other . . . 61026
Vitreous . . . 67028
Fluid Substitute . . . 67025
Vocal Cords
Therapeutic . . . 31513, 31570, 31571
White Blood Cells
Autologous Concentrate . . . 0481T
Wrist
Carpal Tunnel
Therapeutic . . . 20526
Radiological . . . 25246

Inner Ear
See Ear, Inner Ear

Innominate
Artery
See Artery, Brachiocephalic
Bone
Osteotomy . . . 27146
Tumor Excision . . . 27077

Innominate Arteries
See Artery, Brachiocephalic

Inorganic Sulfates
See Sulfate

Inpatient Consultations
See Consultation, Inpatient

INR Test Review
with Anticoagulant Management . . . 93793

Insemination
Artificial
Intra-cervical . . . 58321
Intra-uterine . . . 58322
of Oocytes . . . 89268
Sperm Washing . . . 58323

Insertion
See also Implantation; Intubation; Transplantation
Aqueous Drainage Device
to Extraocular Reservoir . . . 66179, 66180
without Extraocular Reservoir . . . 0376T, 0449T, 0450T, 66183
Balloon
Intra-Aortic . . . 33967, 33973
Breast
Implants . . . 19340-19342
Bronchial Valve . . . 31647, 31651
Cannula
Arteriovenous . . . 36810-36815
ECMO
See Extracorporeal Membrane Oxygenation (ECMO)

Extra Corporeal Circulation
for Regional Chemotherapy of
Extremity........................36823
for On-Body Injector.................96377
Thoracic Duct.......................38794
Vein to Vein........................36800
Cardiac Contractility Modulation System
See Cardiac Assist Devices
Catheter
Abdomen.................. 49324, 49418, 49419, 49421, 49435
Abdominal Artery............ 36245-36248
Aorta..............................36200
Bladder............... 51045, 51701-51703
Brachiocephalic Artery......... 36215-36218
Brain......................61210, 61770
for Interstitial Radioelement
Application.... 19296-19298, 20555, 41019
Bronchi............................31717
Bronchus
for Intracavitary Radioelement
Application........................31643
Cardiac
See Catheterization, Cardiac
Flow Directed.....................93503
Gastrointestinal, Upper..............43241
Jejunum...........................44015
Lower Extremity Artery........ 36245-36248
Nasotracheal.......................31720
Pelvic Artery................ 36245-36248
Pleural Cavity................32550, 32556
with Imaging Guidance............32557
Portal Vein........................36481
Prostate...........................55875
Pulmonary Artery............ 36013-36015
Right Heart........................36013
Skull..............................61107
Spinal Cord.................62350, 62351
Suprapubic.................51045, 51102
Thoracic Artery.............. 36215-36218
Tracheobronchial...................31725
Transthoracic......................33621
Urethra..................... 51701-51703
Vena Cava.........................36010
Venous.........36011, 36012, 36400-36410, 36420-36425, 36500-36510, 36555-36558, 36568-36573
Cecostomy Tube.....................49442
Cervical Dilation....................59200
Cochlear Device.....................69930
Colonic Tube........................49442
Defibrillator System
See Cardiac Assist Devices, Implantable
Defibrillators
Distraction Device
Interlaminar/Interspinous Process,
Lumbar...................... 22867-22870
Drug Delivery Implant............11981, 11983
Drug-Eluting Implant
Lacrimal Canaliculus................0356T
Duodenostomy Tube..................49441
Electrode
Brain..........61531-61533, 61760, 61863, 61864, 61867, 61868
Chest Wall
Respiratory Sensor................0466T
Heart......... 33202, 33203, 33210, 33211, 33216, 33217, 33224, 33225, 33271, 93620-93622
Nerve..................... 64553-64581
Retina............................0100T
Sphenoidal........................95830
Spinal Cord.................. 63650-63655
Stomach
Laparoscopic
Neurostimulator................43647
Stimulation
Open
Neurostimulator................43881
Endotracheal Tube
Emergency Intubation...............31500
Filter
Vena Cava........................37191
Gastrostomy Tube
Laparoscopic.......................43653
Percutaneous......................43246
Glucose Sensor
with Subcutaneous Pocket
Creation...................0446T, 0448T
Graft
Aorta...................... 33330-33335
Heart Vessel................ 33330-33335
Guide Wire
Endoscopy.........................43248
Esophagoscopy.....................43248
with Dilation... 43196, 43212, 43226, 43229
Heyman Capsule
Uterus
for Brachytherapy.................58346
Iliac Artery
Occlusion Device...................34808
Implant
Bone
for External Speech Processor/Cochlear
Stimulator................ 69714-69718
Implantable Cardioverter-Defibrillator (ICD)
See Cardiac Assist Devices, Implantable
Defibrillators
Infusion Pump
Intra-Arterial......................36260
Intravenous........................36563
Spinal Cord.................62361, 62362
Intracatheter/Needle
Aorta.............................36160
Dialysis Circuit.............. 36901-36903
Intra-Arterial................ 36100-36140
Intravenous........................36000
Intraocular Lens.....................66983
Manual or Mechanical
Technique..................66982, 66984
Not Associated with Concurrent Cataract
Removal..........................66985
Intrauterine Device (IUD)..............58300
Ischemia Monitoring System....... 0525T-0527T
Jejunostomy Tube
Endoscopy.........................44372
Percutaneous......................49441
Keel
Laryngoplasty......................31580
Laminaria...........................59200
Left Ventricular Wireless Stimulator
System..................... 0515T-0517T
Mesh
Pelvic Floor.......................57267
Needle
Bone..............................36680
Intraosseous.......................36680
Prostate...........................55875
Needle Wire
Trachea..........................31730
Neurostimulator
See Neurostimulators
Nose
Septal Prosthesis...................30220
Obturator
Larynx............................31527
Ocular Implant
in Scleral Shell....................65130
Muscles, Attached.................65140
Muscles, Not Attached.............65135
with Foreign Material...............65155
with/without Conjunctival Graft.......65150
Orbital Transplant...................67550
Oviduct
Chromotubation....................58350
Hydrotubation.....................58350
Ovoid
Vagina
for Brachytherapy.................57155
Pacemaker, Heart
See Cardiac Assist Devices
Packing
Vagina...........................57180
Penile Prosthesis, Inflatable
See Penile Prosthesis, Insertion, Inflatable
Pessary
Vagina...........................57160
Pin
Skeletal Traction..................20650
Probe
Brain............................61770
Prostaglandin.......................59200
Prostate
Radioactive Substance.............55860
Prosthesis
Knee.....................27438, 27445
Nasal Septal......................30220
Palate............................42281
Pelvic Floor.......................57267
Penis
Inflatable................. 54401-54405
Noninflatable.....................54400
Speech...........................31611
Testis............................54660
Urethral Sphincter............ 53444, 53445
Pulse Generator
See Cardiac Assist Devices; Neurostimulators
Radioactive Material
Bladder...........................51020
Cystourethroscopy.................52250
Radiation Afterloading Apparatus.........57156
Vagina
for Brachytherapy.................57156
Receiver
Brain.....................61885, 61886
Spinal Cord.......................63685
Reservoir
Brain.................... 61210-61215
Spinal Cord.......................62360
Subcutaneous......................49419
Shunt..............................36835
Abdomen
Vein............................49425
Venous..........................49426
Eye
to Suprachoroidal Space..........0253T
Intrahepatic Portosystemic...........37182
Spinal Instrument....................22849
Spinous Process....................22841
Spinal Instrumentation
Anterior................... 22845-22847
Biomechanical Device... 22853, 22854, 22859
Internal Spinal Fixation..............22841
Pelvic Fixation.....................22848
Posterior Nonsegmental
Harrington Rod Technique..........22840
Posterior Segmental.......... 22842-22844
Stabilization/Distraction Device 22869, 22870

Stent
- Bile Duct 43274, 47801
- Bladder 51045
- Conjunctiva 68750
- Coronary 92928, 92929
- Esophagus 43212
- Gastrointestinal, Upper 43266
- Ileum 44384
- Indwelling 50605
- Lacrimal Duct 68815
- Larynx 31580
- Pancreatic Duct 43274
- Small Intestines 44370, 44379
- Ureter 50688
- Ureter via Kidney 50693
- Ureteral 50947, 52332
- Urethral 52282

Subcutaneous Cardiac Rhythm Monitor
- *See* Cardiac Assist Devices

Tamponade
- Esophagus 43460

Tandem
- Uterus
  - for Brachytherapy 57155

Tendon Graft
- Finger 26392
- Hand 26392

Testicular Prosthesis
- *See* Prosthesis, Testis

Tissue Expanders
- Skin 11960-11971

Transprostatic Implant 52441, 52442

Tube
- Esophagus 43510
- Gastrointestinal, Upper 43241
- Ileum 44384
- Small Intestines 44379
- Trachea 31730
- Ureter 50688

Ureteral Guide Wire 52334

Valve
- Bronchial 31647, 31651

Vascular Pedicle
- Carpal Bone 25430

Venous Access Device
- Central 36560-36566
- Peripheral 36570, 36571

Ventilating Tube 69433

Ventricular Assist Device
- *See* Ventricular Assist Device (VAD)

Wire
- Skeletal Traction 20650

Inspiratory Positive Pressure Breathing

See Intermittent Positive Pressure Breathing (IPPB)

Instillation

Agent for Fibrinolysis 32561, 32562

Agent for Pleurodesis 32560

Contrast Material

Drugs
- Bladder 51700
  - Anticarcinogenic Agent 51720
- Endoscopic
  - Bladder 52005, 52010
  - Kidney 50551, 50570
  - Renal Pelvis 50551, 50570
  - Ureter 50951, 50970
  - Urethra 52005, 52010, 53660
- Kidney 50391
- Ureter 50391

Instillation, Bladder

See Bladder, Instillation

Instrumentation

See Application; Bone, Fixation; Spinal Instrumentation

Spinal
- Insertion 22840-22848, 22853, 22854, 22859, 22869, 22870
- Reinsertion 22849
- Removal 22850, 22852, 22855
- with Arthrodesis 22586

Insufflation, Eustachian Tube

See Eustachian Tube, Inflation

Insulin

Antibody 86337

Blood 83525

Free 83527

Panels
- for ACTH Insufficiency 80434
- for Insulinoma 80422
- Glucagon Tolerance 80422
- Insulin-induced C-peptide Suppression 80432
- Insulin Tolerance 80434, 80435

Insulin C-Peptide Measurement

See C-Peptide

Insulin-Like Growth Factors

See Somatomedin

Insurance

Basic Life and/or Disability Evaluation Services 99450

Disability Examination
- Basic Life and/or Disability 99450
- Work Related or Medical Disability 99455, 99456

Integumentary System

Ablation
- Breast 19105
- Photodynamic Therapy 96570, 96571

Biopsy
- Lesion
  - Fine Needle Aspiration (FNA) 10004-10012, 10021
  - Incisional 11106, 11107
  - Punch 11104, 11105
  - Tangential 11102, 11103
  - with Imaging of Specimen 19081-19086

Breast
- *See* Breast

Burns
- *See* Burns

Debridement 11000-11006, 11010-11047

Destruction
- *See* Dermatology
- Actinotherapy 96900
- Benign Lesion 17000, 17003, 17004, 17110, 17111
- Chemical Exfoliation 17360
- Cutaneous Vascular Proliferative Lesion 17106-17108
- Cryotherapy 17340
- Electrolysis Epilation 17380
- Malignant Lesion 17260-17286
- Mohs Micrographic Surgery 17311-17315
- Premalignant Lesion 17000, 17003, 17004
  - by Photodynamic Therapy 96567, 96573, 96574
- Unlisted Services and Procedures 17999

Drainage
- Image Guided 10030

Dressing Change
- with Anesthesia 15851

Excision
- Benign Lesion 11400-11404, 11406, 11420-11424, 11426, 11440-11444, 11446
- Excessive Skin/Tissue 15830, 15832-15839
- for Hidradenitis
  - Axillary 11450, 11451
  - Inguinal 11462, 11463
  - Perianal 11470, 11471
  - Perineal 11470, 11471
  - Umbilical 11470, 11471
- Lipectomy 15830, 15832-15839
  - Suction Assisted 15876-15879
- Malignant Lesion 11600-11604, 11606, 11620-11624, 11626, 11640-11644, 11646
- Nail 11750
- Pressure Ulcer
  - Coccygeal 15920, 15922
  - Ischial 15940, 15941, 15944-15946
  - Sacral 15931, 15933-15937
  - Trochanteric 15950-15953, 15956, 15958
  - Unlisted Procedure 15999

Fluid Collection
- Image Guided 10030

Implantation
- Hormone Pellet, Subcutaneous 11980

Incision and Drainage
- Abscess 10060, 10061
- Acne 10040
- by Puncture Aspiration
  - Abscess 10160
  - Bulla 10160
  - Cyst 10160
  - Hematoma 10160
- Fluid 10140
- Hematoma 10140
- Pilonidal Cyst 10080, 10081
- Postoperative Wound Infection 10180
- Seroma 10140

Insertion
- Tissue Expander 11960
- Prosthesis 11970

Introduction
- Drug Delivery Implant 11981, 11983
- Filling Material 11950-11954
- Pigment for Tattooing 11920-11922

Nail 11720-11765
- *See* Nails

Paring
- Benign Hyperkeratotic Lesion 11055-11057

Photography 96904

Pilonidal Cyst
- Excision 11770-11772
- Incision 10080, 10081

Pressure Ulcers 15920-15999

Removal
- Contraceptive Capsules Implant 11976
- Drug Delivery Implant 11982, 11983
- Foreign Body 10120, 10121
- Sutures
  - with Anesthesia 15850-15852
- Tissue Expander 11970, 11971

Repair
- Adjacent Tissue Transfer/Rearrangement
  - *See* Tissue, Transfer, Adjacent
- Other Procedures 15780-15879
- with Grafts and Flaps
  - *See* Skin Graft and Flap
- Wounds
  - *See* Wound, Repair
- Skin and/or Deep Tissue 15570-15738

Rhytidectomy
- *See* Face Lift

Index

Shaving
  Epidermal or Dermal Lesion. 11300-11313
Skin Replacement Surgery and Skin Substitutes
  Autograft/Tissue Cultured
  Autograft 15040-15157
  Skin Substitute Graft
    See Skin Substitute Graft
  Surgical Preparation 15002-15005
Skin Tags
  Removal 11200, 11201
Tattooing. 11920-11922
Treatment
  Superficial Wound Dehiscence . . 12020, 12021
Trunk
  Biological Implant
  Soft Tissue Reinforcement 15777
Unlisted Skin, Mucous Membrane, Subcutaneous
Tissue Procedure. 17999

Integumentum Commune
See Integumentary System

Intensity Modulated Radiation Treatment (IMRT)
Complex 77386
Simple. 77385

Intensive Care
Low Birthweight Infant
  Subsequent Care 99478-99480
Neonate
  Initial 99477

Interbody
Arthrodesis
  Presacral 22586

Intercarpal Joint
Arthrodesis . . . 25800, 25805, 25810, 25820, 25825
Dislocation
  Closed Treatment. 25660
  Open Treatment. 25670
Magnetic Resonance Imaging 73221-73225
Repair 25447

Intercostal Nerve
Destruction 64620
Injection
  Anesthetic 64420, 64421
  Neurolytic. 64620

Interdental Fixation
Craniofacial Separation
  Closed Treatment. 21431
  Open Treatment. 21432
Device
  Application. 21110
  Removal 20670, 20680
Mandibular Fracture
  Closed Treatment. 21453, 21470
  Open Treatment. 21462
Maxillary Fracture
  Closed Treatment. 21421
Nasomaxillary Complex Fracture
  Closed Treatment. 21345
Palatal Fracture
  Closed Treatment. 21421
without Fracture 21497

Interdental Papilla
See Gums

Interdental Wire Fixation
Craniofacial Separation
  Closed Treatment. 21431
Mandibular Fracture
  Open Treatment. 21470
Maxillary Fracture
  Closed Treatment. 21421
Nasomaxillary Complex Fracture
  Closed Treatment. 21345
Palatal Fracture
  Closed Treatment. 21421
without Fracture 21110, 21497

Interferometry
Ophthalmic Biometry 92136

Intermediate Care Facilities (ICFs)
See Nursing Facility Services

Intermittent Positive Pressure Breathing (IPPB)
Device
  Inhalation Treatment for Airway
  Obstruction. 94640
  Patient Utilization
    Demonstration 94664
    Evaluation. 94664

Internal Breast Prostheses
See Prosthesis, Breast

Internal Ear
See Ear, Inner Ear

Internal Rigid Fixation
Femoral Neck Fracture 27236
Reconstruction
  Mandibular Rami 21196

International Normalized Ratio
Patient/Caregiver Training 93792
Test Review 93793

Internet E/M Service
Interprofessional Consultation. 99446-99449,
  99451, 99452
Online Evaluation and Management 98969, 99444

Interphalangeal Joint
Amputation 28825
Arthrodesis 26860-26863, 28755, 28760
Arthroplasty 26535, 26536
Arthrotomy 26080
  with Biopsy 28054
  with Drainage 28024
  with Exploration. 28024
  with Removal of Foreign Body. 28024
Biopsy 28054
  Synovium 26110
Capsule
  Excision 26525
  Incision. 28272
Dislocation
  Closed Treatment. 26770, 26775
    with Anesthesia 28665
    without Anesthesia 28660
  Open Treatment. 26785
    with Internal Fixation. 28675
  Percutaneous Fixation 26776, 28666
  with Manipulation 26340, 28666
Excision
  Toe, Proximal End 28160
Exploration 26080, 28024
Fasciectomy with Release 26123, 26125
Fracture
  Closed Treatment. 26740
  Open Treatment. 26746
  with Manipulation 26742
Fusion 26860-26863
Great Toe
  Arthrodesis. 28755
    with Tendon Transfer. 28760
  Fusion. 28755
    with Tendon Transfer. 28760
Removal of Foreign Body 26080
Repair
  Collateral Ligament 26540, 26545
  Volar Plate 26548
Synovectomy. 26140
Toe 28272
  Arthrotomy. 28024
  Dislocation. 28660-28665, 28675
    Percutaneous Fixation 28666
  Excision 28160
  Exploration. 28024
  Removal
    Foreign Body. 28024
    Loose Body 28024
  Synovial
    Biopsy 28054

Interprofessional Telephone/ Internet/Electronic Health Record Consultation 99446-99449, 99451, 99452

Interruption
Vein
  Femoral 37650
  Iliac. 37660
  Lower Leg. 37735
  Saphenous Vein 37700

Intersex State
Clitoroplasty 56805
Vaginoplasty 57335

Intersex Surgery
Female to Male. 55980
Male to Female. 55970

Interspace
Arthrodesis
  Presacral
    See Arthrodesis, Vertebra, Lumbar

Interstitial Cell Stimulating Hormone
See Luteinizing Hormone (LH)

Interstitial Cystitides, Chronic
See Cystitis, Interstitial

Interstitial Cystitis
See Cystitis, Interstitial

Interstitial Fluid Pressure
Monitoring 20950

Interstitial Cell Stimulating Hormone
See Luteinizing Hormone (LH)

Interstitial Radiation Therapy
See Brachytherapy, Interstitial Application
Radioelement Application 77778
  Device Placement
    Breast 19296-19298
    Genitalia 55920
    Head 41019
    Neck 41019
    Pelvis 55920
    Uterus. 57155
    Vagina. 57155, 57156
  Heyman Capsules Insertion. 58346
  Ultrasonic Guidance. 76965

Intertarsal Joint
Arthrotomy 28020, 28050
Biopsy 28050
Drainage 28020
Exploration 28020

Removal
Foreign Body 28020
Loose Body 28020
Synovectomy 28070

Interthoracoscapular Amputation
See Amputation, Interthoracoscapular

Intertrochanteric Femur Fracture
See Femur, Fracture, Intertrochanteric

Intervertebral Chemonucleolysis
See Chemonucleolysis

Intervertebral Disc
Annuloplasty 22526, 22527
Arthroplasty
Artificial Disc 0163T, 0375T, 22856-22858
Removal 0095T, 0164T, 22864, 22865
Revision 0098T, 0165T, 22861, 22862
Aspiration 62267
Biopsy 62267
Decompression 63075-63078
by Needle 62287
Discectomy
See Discectomy
Discography
Cervical 72285
Injection 62291
Lumbar 62292, 72295
Injection 62290
Thoracic 72285
Injection 62291
Herniated
Excision
Cervical 63020, 63035, 63040, 63043
Lumbar 62380, 63030, 63035, 63042-63044, 63056, 63057
Thoracic 63055, 63057, 63064, 63066
Injection
Chemonucleolysis Agent 62292
X ray 62290, 62291
Insertion
Biomechanical Device . . . 22853, 22854, 22859
Removal
Artificial Disc 0095T, 0164T, 22864, 22865
by Needle 62287
Revision
Artificial Disc Arthroplasty 0098T, 0165T, 22861, 22862

Intestinal Anastomosis
See Anastomosis, Intestines

Intestinal Invagination
See Intussusception

Intestinal Peptide, Vasoactive
See Vasoactive Intestinal Peptide

Intestines
Alimentation 44015
Allotransplantation 44135, 44136
Removal 44137
Anastomosis 44130, 44625, 44626
Camey Enterocystoplasty 50825
Closure 44227
Koch Pouch 50825
Laparoscopic 44227
with Cystectomy 51590
with Intestinal Replacement of Ureter . . 50840
Biopsy 44100
Closure
Enterostomy 44620, 44625, 44626
Large or Small 44227, 44625, 44626
Fistula 44640, 44650, 44660
with Resection 44661
Stoma 44620-44625
Construction
Neobladder 51596
Ureter 50840
Enteroenterostomy 44130
Enterolysis 44005
Laparoscopic 44180
Enterostomy
Closure 44620, 44625, 44626
Laparoscopic 44227, 44625, 44626
Excision
Donor 44132, 44133
Fecal Microbiota Transplantation
Preparation of Specimen 44705
Graft 43116, 46748
Ladd Procedure 44055
Laparoscopic Resection
with Anastomosis 44202, 44203
Exteriorization 44602-44605
Lesion
Excision 44110, 44111
Lysis
Laparoscopic 44180
of Adhesions 44005
of Duodenal Bands 44050
Malrotation
Correction 44055
Mobilization 43108, 43113, 43118, 43123, 43361
Nuclear Medicine
Imaging 78290
Obstruction
Stricturoplasty 44615
Plication 44680
Reconstruction
Bladder 50820
Colonic Reservoir 45119
for Obstruction 44615
Pouch 43622, 43634
Resection 44661
Laparoscopic 44227
Transplantation
Allograft Preparation 44715-44721
Donor Enterectomy 44132, 44133
Removal of Allograft 44137
Unlisted Services and Procedures 44799
Laparoscopic 44238
Ureteroenterostomy 50800
Volvulus
Reduction 44050

Intestines, Large
See Anus; Colon; Rectum

Intestines, Small
Anastomosis 43845, 44130
Closure 44227
Laparoscopic Resection 44202, 44203
Biopsy 44020
Endoscopy 44361
Catheterization
Jejunum 44015
Decompression 44021
Destruction
Lesion 44369
Tumor 44369
Endoscopy 44364
Ablation
Lesion 44369
Polyp 44369
Tumor 44369
Biopsy 44361, 44377, 44382, 44386
Collection of Specimen 44360, 44376, 44380, 44385
Control of Bleeding 44366, 44378
via Stoma 44382
Destruction
Lesion 44369
Tumor 44369
Diagnostic 44360, 44376, 44380
Evaluation
Pouch
Ileal Reservoir 44385
Kock 44385, 44386
Exploration 44360
Hemorrhage 44366, 44378
Ileal Reservoir 44385, 44386
Insertion
Stent 44370, 44379
Tube 44372
Kock Pouch 44385, 44386
Removal
Foreign Body 44363
Lesion 44364, 44365
Polyp 44364, 44365
Tumor 44364, 44365
Repair
Fistula 46707
Tube Placement 44372
Tube Revision 44373
via Stoma
Balloon Dilation 44381
Biopsy 44382
Diagnostic 44380
Stent Placement 44384
Enterostomy
Placement 44300
Excision 44120, 44121, 44125-44128
Partial with Anastomosis 44140
Exclusion 44700
Exploration 44020
Gastrostomy Tube 44373
Hemorrhage 44378
Hemorrhage Control 44366
Ileostomy 44310-44314, 45136
Continent 44316
Incision 44020
Creation
Pouch 44316
Stoma 44300-44310, 44314
Decompression 44021
Exploration 44020
Revision
Stoma 44312
Stoma Closure 44620-44626
Insertion
Catheter 44015
Duodenostomy Tube 49441
Jejunostomy Tube 44372, 49441
Jejunostomy 44310
Lysis
Adhesions 44005
Removal
Foreign Body 44020, 44363
Repair
Diverticula 44602, 44603
Enterocele
Abdominal Approach 57270
Vaginal Approach 57268
Fistula 44640-44661
Hernia 44050
Malrotation 44055
Obstruction 44050
Ulcer 44602, 44603

Index

Volvulus 44050
Wound 44602, 44603
Revision
Jejunostomy Tube 44373, 49451, 49452
Specimen Collection 43756, 43757
Suture
Diverticula 44602, 44603
Fistula 44640-44661
Plication 44680
Ulcer 44602, 44603
Wound 44602, 44603
X ray 74245, 74249-74251
Guide Intubation 74355

Intestinovesical Fistula
Enterovesical
Closure 44660, 44661

Intima-Media Thickness (IMT) Study
Artery
Carotid, Common 0126T

Intimectomy
See Endarterectomy

Intra-Arterial Injections
See Injection, Intra-arterial

Intra-Abdominal Voiding Pressure Studies
Gastric 51797
Intraperitoneal 51797
Rectal 51797

Intra-Osseous Infusion
See Infusion, Intraosseous

Intracapsular Extraction of Lens
See Lens, Removal, Lens Material, Intracapsular

Intracardiac Echocardiography
See Echocardiography, Intracardiac

Intracranial
Biopsy 61140
Extracranial 61623
Microdissection 69990

Intracranial Arterial Perfusion
Thrombolysis 61624

Intracranial Neoplasm, Acoustic Neuroma
See Brain, Tumor, Excision

Intracranial Neoplasm, Craniopharyngioma
See Craniopharyngioma

Intracranial Neoplasm, Meningioma
See Meningioma

Intrafallopian Transfer, Gamete
See GIFT

Intraluminal Angioplasty
See Angioplasty

Intramuscular Injection
See Injection, Intramuscular

Intraocular Lens
Cataract Removal
See Cataract
Exchange 66986
Insertion 66983
Manual or Mechanical
Technique 66982, 66984
Not Associated with Concurrent Cataract
Removal 66985

Intraoperative Visual Axis Identification
Patient Fixation 0514T

Intratracheal Intubation
See Insertion, Endotracheal Tube

Intrauterine Contraceptive Device
See Intrauterine Device (IUD)

Intrauterine Device (IUD)
Insertion 58300
Removal 58301

Intrauterine Synechiae
See Adhesions, Intrauterine

Intravascular Foreign Body Removal (Fractured Catheter) 37197

Intravascular Stent
Placement
See Transcatheter, Placement, Intravascular Stent

Intravascular Ultrasound
Coronary Vessel or Graft
Endoluminal Imaging 92978, 92979
Noncoronary Vessel 37252, 37253

Intravenous Infusion
Diagnostic 96365-96368, 96379
Hydration 96360, 96361
Status Documented 2030F, 2031F
Intravenous Unlisted 96379
Prophylactic 96365-96368, 96379
Therapeutic 96365-96368, 96379
Cerebral
for Thrombolysis 37195
Chemotherapy 96413, 96415-96417, 96422, 96423, 96425
Device Implantation/Replacement 62360-62362
Unlisted Therapeutic Infusion 96379

Intravenous Injection
See Injection, Intravenous

Intravenous Pyelogram
See Urography, Intravenous

Intravenous Therapy
See Injection, Chemotherapy
Cerebral
for Thrombolysis 37195
Chemotherapy 96413, 96415-96417, 96422, 96423, 96425
Infusion 96365-96368, 96379
Pain Management 96365-96368, 96374, 96379
Spinal
Device Implantation/Replacement 62360-62362
Unlisted Intravenous 96379

Intravesical Instillation
See Bladder, Instillation

Intravitreal Injection
Pharmacologic Agent 67028

Intrinsic Factor
Quantitative 83528
Antibody 86340

Introduction
Breast
Localization Device Placement .. 19081-19086
Drug Delivery Implant 11981, 11983
Gastrointestinal Tube 44500
with Fluoroscopic Guidance 74340
Tissue Expanders
Skin 11960-11971

Intubation
See Insertion
Endotracheal Tube 31500
Esophageal
with Laparotomy 43510
Eustachian Tube
See Eustachian Tube, Inflation
Gastric
Diagnostic 43754-43757
Therapeutic 43753
Specimen Collection
Duodenal 43756, 43757
Gastric 43754-43757

Intubation Tube
See Endotracheal Tube

Intussusception
Reduction
Enema 74283
Laparotomy 44050

Invagination, Intestinal
See Intussusception

Inversion, Nipple
See Nipples, Inverted

Iodide Test
Thyroid Uptake 78012, 78014

Ionization, Medical
See Iontophoresis

Iontophoreses
See Iontophoresis

Iontophoresis
Application 97033
Sweat Collection 89230

Ipecac Administration
for Poisoning 99175

IPPB
See Intermittent Positive Pressure Breathing (IPPB)

Iridectomy
by Laser Surgery 66761
for Glaucoma 66625, 66630
Optical 66635
with Cataract Removal 66830
with Corneoscleral or Corneal Section 66600
with Cyclectomy 66605
with Sclerectomy 66160
with Thermocauterization 66155
with Trephination 66150

Iridodialysis
Ciliary Body Repair 66680

Iridoplasty
Photocoagulation 66762

Iridotomy
by Laser Surgery 66761
by Stab Incision 66500
with Transfixion as for Iris Bombe 66505

Iris
Cyst
Destruction 66770
Excision
Optical 66635
Peripheral 66625
Sector 66630
with Cataract Removal 66830
with Corneoscleral or Corneal Section .. 66600
with Cyclectomy 66605
with Sclerectomy 66160

with Thermocauterization 66155
with Trephination.................. 66150
Incision
by Laser Surgery 66761
Stab 66500
with Transfixion as for Iris Bombe...... 66505
Lesion
Destruction....................... 66770
Repair
Suture........................... 66682
with Ciliary Body 66680
Revision
Laser Surgery..................... 66761
Photocoagulation.................. 66762
Suture
with Ciliary Body 66682

Iron
Blood............................. 83540

Iron Binding Capacity
Blood............................. 83550

Iron Hematoxylin Stain
for Microorganisms.............. 87209, 88312

Iron Stain
Blood......................... 85536, 88313

Irradiation
Blood Products 86945

Irrigation
Bladder 51700, 52005, 52010, 53448
Bronchus 31624
Caloric Vestibular Test 92537, 92538
Catheter
Brain...................... 62194, 62225
Corpora Cavernosa
for Priapism 54220
Eye
Anterior Chamber.................. 65815
Lacrimal Punctum.................. 68801
Nasolacrimal Duct 68810
Lung 32997
Penis 54411, 54417
for Priapism 54220
Peritoneal
See Peritoneal Lavage
Shunt
Cerebrospinal Fluid 61070
Spinal Cord....................... 63744
Sinus
Maxillary 31000
Sphenoid 31002
Ureter
Endoscopic................. 50951, 50970
Vagina............................ 57150
Venous Access Device 96523
Ventricular Catheter 62225
Wrist
Arthroscopy 29843

Irving Sterilization
See Ligation, Fallopian Tube, Oviduct

Ischemic Stroke
History of Onset 1065F, 1066F
Tissue Plasminogen Activator (tPA)
Administration 4077F

Ischium
Biopsy 20245
Bursa
Excision 27060
Pressure Ulcer
Excision 15940, 15941, 15944-15946

Tumor
Radical Resection 27075, 27076, 27078

Ischiectomy
with Pressure Ulcer Excision 15941

Island Pedicle Flaps
Graft 15740

Islands of Langerhans
See Islet Cell

Islet Cell
Antibody 86341

Isocitrate Dehydrogenase
See Isocitric Dehydrogenase

Isocitric Dehydrogenase
Blood.............................. 83570

Isolation
Sperm 89260, 89261
Virus
Centrifuge Enhanced 87254
Inoculation 87250, 87252
Non-immunologic Method............ 87255
Tissue Culture 87253

Isomerase, Glucose 6 Phosphate
See Phosphohexose Isomerase

Isthmusectomy
Thyroid Gland 60210, 60212, 60220, 60225

IUD
See Intrauterine Device (IUD)

IV
See Injection, Chemotherapy; Intravenous Therapy

IV Infusion Therapy
See Intravenous Infusion, Therapeutic

IV Injection
See Injection, Intravenous

IV, Coagulation Factor
See Calcium

IVF
See Artificial Insemination; In Vitro Fertilization

Ivy Bleeding Time
Bleeding Time....................... 85002

IX Complex, Factor
See Christmas Factor

J

Jaboulay Operation
See Gastroduodenostomy

Jaboulay Operation Gastroduodenostomy
See Gastroduodenostomy

Jannetta Procedure
See Decompression, Cranial Nerve; Section

Japanese Encephalitis Virus
See Vaccines and Toxoids

Japanese, River Fever
See Scrub Typhus

Jatene Type Procedure 33770-33781

Jaw Joint
See Facial Bones; Mandible; Maxilla

Jaws
Muscle Reduction............... 21295, 21296
Orthopantogram X ray
for Orthodontics.................. 70355

Jejunostomy
Catheterization 44015
Contrast........................... 49465
Conversion
from Gastrostomy Tube 44373
Endoscopic 44373
Percutaneous 49446
Insertion
Catheter......................... 44015
Endoscopic....................... 44372
Percutaneous..................... 49441
Laparoscopic................. 44186, 44187
Non-Tube 44187, 44310
Obstructive Material Removal 49460
Replacement........................ 49451
with Pancreatic Drain 48001

Jejunum
Creation
Stoma
See Jejunostomy
Endoscopy
Examination...................... 43242
Needle Aspiration 43242
Needle Biopsy 43242
Ultrasound 43259
Transfer
with Microvascular Anastomosis
Free............................ 43496

Johannsen Procedure
Urethroplasty 53400

Joint
Acromioclavicular
See Acromioclavicular Joint
Arthrocentesis
Bursa.................... 20600, 20604
Intermediate Joint........... 20605, 20606
Large Joint................. 20610, 20611
Small Joint................. 20600, 20604
Aspiration 20600, 20604, 20605, 20606, 20610, 20611
Dislocation
See Dislocation
Drainage 20600, 20604, 20605, 20606, 20610, 20611
Exploration
Acromioclavicular 23044
Ankle 27610, 27620
Carpometacarpal 26070
Elbow........................... 24101
Finger 26075-26080
Glenohumeral.............. 23040, 23107
Hand............................ 26070
Hip 27033
Interphalangeal
Finger 26080
Toe 28024
Intertarsal........................ 28020
Knee...................... 27310, 27331
Metacarpophalangeal 26070
Metatarsophalangeal 28022
Midcarpal........................ 25040
Radiocarpal 25040
Sternoclavicular................... 23044
Tarsometatarsal................... 28020
Wrist 25101
Finger
See Finger, Joint

Index

Fixation (Surgical)
  See Arthrodesis
Foot
  See Talotarsal Joint; Tarsal Joint; Tarsometatarsal Joint
Hip
  See Hip Joint
Injection 0213T-0218T, 20600, 20604, 20605, 20610, 20611
Intertarsal
  See Intertarsal Joint
Knee
  See Knee Joint
Ligament
  See Ligament
Magnetic Resonance Imaging
  Extremity, Lower 73721
  Extremity, Upper 73221
Metacarpophalangeal
  See Metacarpophalangeal Joint
Metatarsophalangeal
  See Metatarsophalangeal Joint
Nuclear Medicine
  Imaging 78300, 78305, 78306, 78315
  SPECT 78320
Radiology
  Stress Views 77071
  Survey Views 77077
Replacement
  Temporomandibular 21243
  Vertebral 0202T, 20931, 20938, 22554, 22556, 22854, 63081, 63085, 63087, 63090
Sacroiliac
  See Sacroiliac Joint
Shoulder
  See Glenohumeral Joint
Sternoclavicular
  See Sternoclavicular Joint
Survey 77077
Temporomandibular
  See Temporomandibular Joint (TMJ)
  Arthrography 70332
  Dislocation Temporomandibular
    See Dislocation, Temporomandibular Joint
  Implant
    See Prosthesis, Temporomandibular Joint
  Magnetic Resonance Imaging 70336
  Radiology 70328
Wrist
  See Radiocarpal Joint

Joint Syndrome, Temporomandibular
See Temporomandibular Joint (TMJ)

Jones and Cantarow Test
See Blood Urea Nitrogen; Urea Nitrogen, Clearance

Jones Procedure
Arthrodesis 28760

Jugal Bone
See Zygomatic Arch

Jugular Vein
See Vein, Jugular

K

Kader Operation
See Incision, Stomach, Creation, Stoma; Incision and Drainage

Kala Azar Smear 87207

Kallidin I /Kallidin 9
See Bradykinin

Kallikrein HK3
See Antigen, Prostate Specific

Kallikreinogen
See Fletcher Factor

Kasai Procedure 47701

Kedani Fever
See Scrub Typhus

Keel
Insertion/Removal
  Laryngoplasty 31580

Kelikian Procedure 28280

Keller Procedure 28292

Kelly Urethral Plication 57220

Keratectomy
Partial
  for Lesion 65400

Keratomileusis 65760

Keratophakia 65765

Keratoplasty
Endothelial 65756
  Allograft Preparation 65757
Lamellar
  Anterior 65710
  Laser Preparation 0290T
Penetrating 65730
  in Aphakia 65750
  Laser Preparation 0290T
  in Pseudophakia 65755

Keratoprosthesis 65770

Keratotomy
Radial 65771

Ketogenic Steroids 83582

Ketone Body 82009, 82010

Ketosteroids 83586, 83593

Kidner Procedure 28238

Kidney
Abscess
  Incision and Drainage 50020
    Open 50020
Anesthesia 00862
Biopsy 50200, 50205
  Endoscopic 50555, 50557, 52354
Catheterization
  Endoscopic 50572
  Nephroureteral 50387
Cyst
  Ablation 50541
  Aspiration 50390
  Excision 50280, 50290
  Injection 50390
  X ray 74470
Destruction
  Calculus 50590
  Endoscopic 50557, 50576, 52354
Endoscopy
  Biopsy 50555, 50574-50576, 52354
  Catheterization 50553, 50572
  Destruction 50557, 50576, 52354
  Dilation
    Intra-Renal Stricture 52343, 52346
    Ureter 50553
  Excision
    Tumor 52355
  Exploration 52351
  Lithotripsy 52353
  Removal
    Calculus 50060-50075
    Foreign Body 50561, 50580
  via Incision 50562, 50570, 50572, 50574-50576, 50580
  via Stoma 50551, 50553, 50555, 50557, 50561
Excision
  Donor 50300, 50320, 50547
  Partial 50240
    Laparoscopic 50543
  Laparoscopic 50545-50548
  Recipient 50340
  Transplantation 50370
  with Ureters 50220, 50225, 50230, 50234, 50236
Exploration 50010, 50045, 50120
Incision 50010, 50045
Incision and Drainage 50040, 50125
Injection
  Drugs 50391
  for Nephrostogram 50430, 50431
Insertion
  Stoma 50400
Instillation
  Drugs 50391
Lithotripsy 50590
Manometry
  Pressure 50396
Mass
  Ablation 50542
    Cryosurgical 50250
    Radiofrequency 50592
Needle Biopsy 50200
Nuclear Medicine
  Function Study 78725
  Imaging 78700, 78701, 78707-78710
  Unlisted Services and Procedures 78799
Placement
  Catheter
    Nephrostomy 50432
    Nephroureteral 50433
Removal
  Calculus 50060, 50065, 50070, 50075, 50080, 50130, 50561
  Foreign Body 50561, 50580
  Tube
    Nephrostomy 50389
Repair
  Blood Vessels 50100
  Fistula 50520, 50525, 50526
  Fixation 50400, 50405
  Horseshoe Kidney 50540
  Wound 50500
Solitary 50405
Suture
  Fistula 50520, 50525, 50526
  Horseshoe Kidney 50540
Transplantation
  Allograft Preparation 50323-50329
  Anesthesia
    Donor 00862
    Recipient 00868
  Donor 00862
  Donor Nephrectomy 50300, 50320, 50547
  Implantation of Graft 50360
  Recipient Nephrectomy 50340, 50365
  Reimplantation Kidney 50380
  Removal Transplant Renal Autograft ... 50370

Index

Tumor
  Ablation
    Cryotherapy 50593
Ultrasound 76770, 76775, 76776
X ray with Contrast
  Guide Catheter 50433

Kidney Stone
See Calculus, Removal, Kidney

Killian Operation
See Sinusotomy, Frontal Sinus

Kinase, Creatine
See CPK

Kineplasty
See Cineplasty

Kinetic Therapy 97530
See Physical Medicine/Therapy/Occupational Therapy

Kininase A
See Angiotensin Converting Enzyme (ACE)

Kininogen 85293

Kininogen, High Molecular Weight
See Fitzgerald Factor

Kleihauer-Betke Test 85460

Kloramfenikol
See Chloramphenicol

Knee
See Femur; Fibula; Patella; Tibia
Abscess 27301
Arthrocentesis 20610, 20611
Arthrodesis 27580
Arthroplasty 27440-27445, 27447
  Revision 27486, 27487
Arthroscopy
  Diagnostic 29870
  Surgical 29866-29868, 29871, 29873-29877, 29879-29889
Arthrotomy 27310, 27330-27335, 27403
Autograft, Osteochondral, Open 27416
Biopsy 27323, 27324, 27330, 27331
  Synovium 27330
Bone
  Drainage 27303
  Graft 29885
Bone Graft 29885
Bursa 27301
  Excision 27340
Cyst
  Excision 27345-27347
Disarticulation 27598
Dislocation 27550-27552, 27556-27558, 27560-27562, 27566
  Open Treatment 27556-27558, 27566
Drainage 27310
Excision
  Cartilage 27332, 27333
  Ganglion 27347
  Lesion 27347
  Patella 27350, 27424
  Synovium 27334, 27335
Exploration 27310, 27331
Fasciotomy 27305, 27496-27499
Fracture 27520-27524, 27538, 27540
  Arthroscopic Treatment 29850, 29851
Fusion 27580
Hematoma 27301
Incision
  Capsule 27435
Injection
  X ray, CT-MRI 27369
Magnetic Resonance Imaging (MRI) 73721-73723
Manipulation 27570
Meniscectomy 27332, 27333
Patella
  See Patella
Radiostereometric Analysis (RSA) 0350T
Reconstruction 27437, 27438
  Ligament 27427-27429
  with Prosthesis 27445
Removal
  Foreign Body 27310, 27331, 27372
  Loose Body 27331
  Prosthesis 27488
Repair
  Ligament 27405-27409
    Collateral 27405
    Collateral and Cruciate 27409
    Cruciate 27407-27409
  Meniscus 27403
  Tendon 27380, 27381
Replacement 27447
  Intraoperative Use, Kinetic Balance Sensor 0396T
Retinacular
  Release 27425
Strapping 29530
Suture
  Tendon 27380, 27381
Transplantation
  Chondrocytes 27412
  Meniscus 29868
  Osteochondral
    Allograft 27415, 29867
    Autograft 27412, 29866
Tumor
  Excision 27327, 27328, 27337-27339
  Radical Resection 27329, 27364, 27365
Unlisted Services and Procedures 27599
X ray 73560-73564
  Arthrography 73580
  Bilateral 73565
X ray with Contrast
  Arthrography 73580
  Injection, Contrast 27369

Knee Joint
Arthroplasty 27437, 27438, 27440-27443, 27445-27447
  Revision 27486
Biopsy 27331
Debridement 27441
Disarticulation 27598
Drainage 27310
Exploration 27310, 27331
Excision
  Semilunar Cartilage 27332, 27333
  Synovium 27334, 27335
Fusion 27580
Manipulation 27570
Removal
  Foreign Body 27310, 27331
Repair
  Condyle 27446, 27447
  Debridement 27441
  Dislocation
    Patella 27420, 27424, 27425
    Plateau 27446, 27447
  Resurfacing 27447
  Synovectomy
    Partial 27443
  with Prosthesis
    See Prosthesis, Knee

Knee Prosthesis
See Prosthesis, Knee

Kneecap
Excision 27350, 27424
Repair
  Instability 27420-27424
  Arthroplasty 27437, 27438
    with Prosthesis 27438

Knock-Knee Repair 27455-27457

Kocher Operation
See Dislocation, Shoulder

Kocher Pylorectomy
See Gastrectomy, Partial

Kock Pouch 44316
Endoscopic Evaluation 44385, 44386
Formation 50825

Kock Procedure 44316

KOH
Slide Tissue Examination
  Ectoparasite Ova 87220
  Fungus 87220
  Mite 87220

Kraske Procedure 45116

Kroenlein Procedure 67420

Krukenberg Procedure 25915

Kyphectomy
More than Two Segments 22819
Up to Two Segments 22818

Kyphoplasty 22513-22515

L

L Ascorbic Acid
See Ascorbic Acid

L Aspartate 2 Oxoglutarate Aminotransferase
See Transaminase, Glutamic-Oxaloacetic

L-Alanine
See Aminolevulinic Acid (ALA)

L-Leucylnaphthylamidase
See Leucine Aminopeptidase

L/S Ratio
Amniotic Fluid 83661

Labial Adhesions
Lysis 56441

Labyrinth
See Ear, Inner Ear

Labyrinthectomy 69905
with Mastoidectomy 69910
with Skull Base Surgery 61596

Labyrinthotomy
Transcanal 69801

Laceration Repair
See Repair, Laceration

Lacrimal Duct
Balloon 68816
Canaliculi
  Insertion
    Drug-Eluting Implant 0356T
  Repair 68700

Dilation ... 68816
Exploration ... 68810
Canaliculi ... 68840
Stent ... 68815
with Anesthesia ... 68811
Insertion
Stent ... 68815
Nasolacrimal Duct Probing ... 68816
Removal
Dacryolith ... 68530
Foreign Body ... 68530
X ray with Contrast ... 70170

Lacrimal Gland
Biopsy ... 68510
Close Fistula ... 68770
Excision
Partial ... 68505
Total ... 68500
Fistulization ... 68720
Incision and Drainage ... 68400
Injection
X ray ... 68850
Tear Flow Diagnostic Procedure
Microfluidic Analysis ... 83861
Nuclear Medicine ... 78660
Removal
Dacryolith ... 68530
Foreign Body ... 68530
Repair
Fistula ... 68770
Tumor
Excision
Frontal Approach ... 68540
with Osteotomy ... 68550
X ray ... 70170

Lacrimal Punctum
Closure
by Plug ... 68761
by Thermocauterization, Ligation or Laser Surgery ... 68760
Dilation ... 68801
Incision ... 68440
Repair ... 68705

Lacrimal Sac
Biopsy ... 68525
Excision ... 68520
Incision and Drainage ... 68420

Lacrimal System
Unlisted Services and Procedures ... 68899

Lactase Deficiency Breath Test ... 91065

Lactate ... 83605

Lactate Dehydrogenase ... 83615-83625

Lactic Acid ... 83605

Lactic Cytochrome Reductase
See Lactate Dehydrogenase

Lactic Dehydrogenase
See Lactate Dehydrogenase

Lactiferous Duct
See Mammary Duct; Mammary Ductogram
Excision ... 19112
Exploration ... 19110

Lactoferrin
Fecal ... 83630, 83631

Lactogen, Human Placental ... 83632

Lactogenic Hormone
See Prolactin

Lactose
Urine ... 83633

Ladd Procedure ... 44055

Lagophthalmos
Correction ... 67912

Laki-Lorand Factor
See Fibrin Stabilizing Factor

Lamblia Intestinalis
See Giardia Lamblia

Lambrinudi Operation
See Arthrodesis, Foot Joint

Lamellar Keratoplasties
See Keratoplasty, Lamellar

Laminaria
Insertion
for Cervical Dilation ... 59200
for Abortion ... 59855

Laminectomy
Arthrodesis ... 22630, 22632-22634
for Decompression
Cervical ... 0274T, 61343, 63001, 63015, 63045, 63048
Lumbar ... 0275T, 63005, 63012, 63017, 63047, 63048
Sacral ... 63011
Thoracic ... 0274T, 63003, 63016, 63046, 63048
for Excision
Arteriovenous Malformation ... 63250-63252
Intraspinal Lesion ... 63300-63308
Neoplasm ... 63275-63278, 63280-63283, 63285-63287, 63290
Other than Neoplasm ... 63265-63268, 63270-63273
for Implantation of Electrodes ... 63655
Lumbar ... 0202T, 22630, 63012
with Cordotomy ... 63194-63199
with Creation of Shunt ... 63740
with Diagnostic/Therapeutic Injection ... 62351
with Discectomy ... 0274T, 0275T, 63020
with Drainage ... 63172, 63173
with Dural/Cerebrospinal Fluid Leak Repair ... 63709
with Exploration
Cervical ... 63001, 63015, 63045, 63048
Lumbar ... 63005, 63017, 63047, 63048
Thoracic ... 63003, 63016, 63046, 63048
Sacral ... 63011
with Facetectomy ... 0202T, 0274T, 0275T, 63045-63048
with Foraminotomy ... 0202T, 0274T, 0275T, 63045-63048
with Ligamentous Resection ... 0274T, 0275T, 63180, 63182
with Myelotomy ... 63170
with Nerve Resection ... 63191
with Rhizotomy ... 63185, 63190
with Spinal Cord Release ... 63200

Laminoplasty
Cervical ... 63050, 63051

Lamotrigine
Drug Assay ... 80175

Langerhans Islands
See Islet Cell

Language Evaluation
Language Comprehension and Expression ... 92523
Speech Fluency ... 92521
Speech Sound Production ... 92522
Voice and Resonance
Behavioral Analysis ... 92524

Language Therapy
Individual ... 92507
Group ... 92508

LAP
See Leucine Aminopeptidase

Laparoscopic Appendectomy
See Appendectomy, Laparoscopic

Laparoscopic Biopsy of Ovary
See Biopsy, Ovary

Laparoscopy
Abdomen
Aspiration
Cavity ... 49322
Cyst ... 49322
Biopsy ... 49321
Collection of Specimen ... 49320
Diagnostic ... 49320
Drainage
Lymphocele ... 49323
Placement
Interstitial Radiation Device ... 49327
Unlisted Procedures ... 49329
Adrenal Gland
Biopsy ... 60650
Excision ... 60650
Appendix
Appendectomy ... 44970
Aspiration ... 49322
Biopsy ... 49321
Lymph Nodes ... 38570
Biliary Tract
Cholangiography ... 47563
with Biopsy ... 47579
Cholecystectomy ... 47562-47564
Cholecystenterostomy ... 47570
Bladder
Repair
Sling Operation ... 51992
Urethral Suspension ... 51990
Unlisted ... 51999
Laparoscopic ... 44188
Colon
Cecostomy ... 44188
Colectomy
Partial ... 44204-44208, 44213
Total ... 44210-44212
Colostomy ... 44188
Destruction
Lesion ... 58662
Ectopic Pregnancy ... 59150
with Salpingectomy and/or Oophorectomy ... 59151
Esophagus
Esophagogastric Fundoplasty ... 43280
Esophagomyotomy Fundoplasty ... 43279
Heller Type Esophagomyotomy ... 43279
Hernia Repair ... 43281, 43282
Lengthening ... 43283
Sphincter Augmentation
Device Placement ... 43284
Device Removal ... 43285
Gastric Restrictive Procedures ... 43644, 43645, 43770-43775
Hernia Repair
Epigastric
Incarcerated or Strangulated ... 49653
Reducible ... 49652

Incisional
Incarcerated or Strangulated 49655
Reducible 49654
Incisional Recurrent
Incarcerated or Strangulated 49657
Reducible 49656
Inguinal
Initial. 49650
Recurrent 49651
Paraesophageal 43281, 43282
Spigelian
Incarcerated or Strangulated 49653
Reducible 49652
Umbilical
Incarcerated or Strangulated 49653
Reducible 49652
Ventral
Incarcerated or Strangulated 49653
Reducible 49652
Unlisted Procedures. 49659
Intestines
Enterectomy. 44202, 44203
Enterolysis 44180
Enterostomy
Closure 44227
Ileostomy 44187
Jejunostomy. 44186, 44187
Reconstruction with Gastric Bypass 43645
Resection
with Anastomosis. 44202, 44203
Kidney
Ablation
Cysts 50541
Lesions 50542
Allograft Preparation 50325
Nephrectomy 50544-50548
Donor 50547
Liver
Ablation
Tumor 47370, 47371
Lymph System
Biopsy. 38570
Lymphadenectomy 38571-38573
Lysis of Adhesions 58660
Lysis of Intestinal Adhesions 44180
Nephrectomy. 50545-50548
Partial. 50543
Omentum
Collection of Specimen 49320
Diagnostic 49320
Omentopexy 49326
Unlisted Procedures. 49329
Ovary/Oviduct
Ectopic Pregnancy 59150
with Salpingectomy and/or
Oophorectomy 59151
Excision of Lesions. 58662
Fimbrioplasty 58672
Fulguration
Lesions 58662
Oviducts 58670
Lysis of Adhesions. 58660
Occlusion of Oviducts 58671
Oophorectomy 58661
Oviduct Surgery 58670, 58671, 58679
Removal
Ovary(s). 58544, 58552, 58554
Tube(s) 58544, 58552, 58554
Salpingectomy 58661
Salpingostomy 58673
Unlisted Procedure. 58679
Pelvis. 49320
Placement
Interstitial Radiation Device. 49327
Pyeloplasty. 50544
Peritoneum
Collection of Specimen 49320
Diagnostic 49320
Catheter Insertion 49324
Placement
Interstitial Radiation Device. 49327
Removal of Obstructive Material. 49325
Unlisted Procedures. 49329
Prostate
Prostatectomy 55866
Rectum
Proctectomy
Complete 45395
with Creation of Colonic Reservoir . . . 45397
Proctopexy
for Prolapse 45400, 45402
Unlisted 45499
Removal
Fallopian Tube 58661
Leiomyomata 58545, 58546
Ovaries 58661
Spleen 38120
Testis 54690
Spermatic Cord
Ligation
Veins. 55550
Unlisted Procedure. 55559
Spleen
Splenectomy 38120, 38129
Splenic Flexure
Mobilization 44213
Stomach
Gastrectomy
Longitudinal/Sleeve 43775
Gastric Bypass 43644, 43645
Gastric Restrictive Procedures. . . 43770-43775, 43848, 43886-43888
Gastroenterostomy 43644, 43645
Gastrostomy, Temporary 43653
Neurostimulator Electrode
Implantation 0312T, 43647
Removal 0314T, 43648
Replacement. 0313T, 43647
Revision 0313T, 43648
Vagus Nerves Transection. 43651, 43652
Roux-En-Y. 43644
Testis
Orchiectomy 54690
Orchiopexy 54692
Unlisted Procedures. 54699
Transplantation
Donor Allograft Preparation
Kidney. 50325
Uterus
Ablation
Fibroids. 58674
Unlisted Services and Procedures
Abdomen, Peritoneum, and Omentum. . . 49329
Appendix 44979
Biliary Tract 47579
Bladder. 51999
Endocrine System 60659
Esophagus 43289
Hernioplasty, Herniorrhaphy,
Herniotomy. 49659
Intestine 44238
Liver 47379
Lymphatic System 38589
Maternity Care and Delivery 59898, 59899
Oviduct, Ovary 58679
Rectum. 45499
Renal 50549
Spermatic Cord. 55559
Spleen 38129
Stomach. 43659
Testis 54699
Ureter. 50949
Uterus. 58578, 58579
Ureter
Ureterectomy 50546, 50548
Ureterolithotomy 50945
Ureteroneocystostomy. 50947, 50948
Unlisted Procedure. 50949
Urethra
Incontinence Repair. 51990, 51992
Urethral Suspension 51990
Uterus
Biopsy. 57421
Endometrium 58558
Hysteroscopy
Diagnostic. 58555
with Endometrial Ablation 58563
with Endometrial Biopsy 58558
with Division/Resection Intrauterine
Septum 58560
with Lysis of Intrauterine Adhesions . . 58559
with Polypectomy 58558
with Removal
Impacted Foreign Body 58562
Leiomyomata. 58561
Unlisted Hysteroscopy Procedure 58578
Hysterectomy. 58541-58544
Radical 58548
Total 58570-58573, 58575
Vaginal 58550, 58552-58554
In Vitro Fertilization 58976
Retrieve Oocyte 58970
Transfer Embryo 58974
Transfer Gamete. 58976
Myomectomy 58545, 58546
Placement
Fallopian Tube Cannulation 58565
Unlisted Procedure. 58579
Vagina
Biopsy. 57421
Colpopexy. 57425
Colposcopy. 57420
Paravaginal Defect Repair. 57423
Prosthetic Graft Revision. 57426
Vaginal Hysterectomy 58550-58554
Vaginal Suspension 57425

Laparotomy

Abdominal
Exploration. 49000, 49002
Esophagogastric
Fundoplasty 43327, 43328
Hiatal Hernia Repair 43332, 43333
Gastric
Electrode
Implantation 43881
Removal 43882
Replacement. 43881
Revision 43882
Intestinal
Reduction
Internal Hernia 44050
Intussusception 44050
Volvulus 44050
Liver
Aspiration/Injection
Parasitic Abscess 47015
Parasitic Cyst 47015

Staging
  Hodgkin's Disease ... 49220
  Lymphoma ... 49220
  Ovarian Malignancy ... 58960
  Peritoneal Malignancy ... 58960
  Tubal Malignancy ... 58960
Stomach
  Biopsy ... 43605

Laparotomy, Exploratory
See Abdomen, Exploration

Lapidus Procedure ... 28297

Large Bowel
See Anus; Rectum

Laroyenne Operation
See Vagina, Abscess, Incision and Drainage

Larval Therapy ... 97602

Laryngeal Function Study ... 92520

Laryngeal Sensory Testing ... 92614-92617

Laryngectomy ... 31360-31382
Partial ... 31367-31382
Subtotal ... 31367, 31368
Total ... 31360, 31365

Laryngocele
Removal ... 31300

Laryngofissure ... 31300

Laryngography
Contrast ... 76499

Laryngopharyngectomy
See Excision, Larynx, with Pharynx

Laryngopharynx
See Hypopharynx

Laryngoplasty
Cricoid Split ... 31587
for Fracture
  Fixation ... 31584
  Open Reduction ... 31584
for Laryngeal Stenosis ... 31551-31554
Laryngeal Web ... 31580
Medialization ... 31591

Laryngoscopy
Direct ... 31515-31571
  Aspiration ... 31515
  Biopsy ... 31535, 31536
  Diagnostic ... 31525, 31526
  Dilation ... 31528, 31529
  Exploration ... 31520-31526, 31575
  Newborn ... 31520
Flexible ... 31575-31579
  Ablation, Lesion ... 31572
  Biopsy ... 31576
  Diagnostic ... 31575
  Injection
    Vocal Cord ... 31570, 31571, 31573, 31574
  Laser Destruction, Lesion ... 31572
  Removal
    Foreign Body ... 31577
    Lesion ... 31578
  Removal
    Foreign Body ... 31530, 31531
    Lesion ... 31545, 31546
  Operative ... 31530-31561
    Arytenoidectomy ... 31560, 31561
    Excision of Tumor ... 31540, 31541
    Stripping of Vocal Cords ... 31540, 31541
Indirect ... 31505-31513
  Biopsy ... 31510
  Diagnostic ... 31505
  Exploration ... 31505
  Injection
    Vocal Cord ... 31513
Insertion
  Obturator ... 31527
  Removal
    Foreign Body ... 31511
    Lesion ... 31512
Newborn ... 31520
Rigid Telescopic ... 31579
with Operating Microscope or Telescope ... 31526, 31531, 31536, 31541, 31545, 31546, 31561, 31571
with Stroboscopy ... 31579

Laryngotomy ... 31300

Larynx
Aspiration
  Endoscopy ... 31515
Biopsy
  Endoscopy ... 31510, 31535, 31536, 31576
Dilation
  Endoscopic ... 31528, 31529
Electromyography
  Needle ... 95865
Endoscopy
  Ablation, Lesion ... 31572
  Direct ... 31515-31571
  Excision ... 31545, 31546
  Exploration ... 31505, 31520-31526, 31575
  Flexible ... 31575-31579
    with Stroboscopy ... 31579
  Indirect ... 31505-31513
  Laser Destruction, Lesion ... 31572
  Operative ... 31530-31561
  Removal, Lesion ... 31512, 31578
Excision
  Lesion ... 31512, 31578
    Endoscopic ... 31545, 31546
  Partial ... 31367-31382
  Total ... 31360-31365
  with Pharynx ... 31390-31395
Exploration
  Endoscopic ... 31505, 31520-31526, 31575
Fracture
  Fixation ... 31584
  Open Reduction ... 31584
Insertion
  Keel ... 31580
  Obturator ... 31527
  Stent ... 31580
Lesion
  Ablation ... 31572
  Laser Destruction ... 31572
  Removal ... 31512, 31578
Medialization ... 31591
Muscle
  Chemodenervation ... 64617
Reconstruction
  Cricoid Split ... 31587
  Stenosis ... 31551-31554
  Web ... 31580
Removal
  Foreign Body
    Endoscopic ... 31511, 31530, 31531, 31577
  Lesion
    Endoscopic ... 31512, 31545, 31546, 31578
Repair
  Reinnervation Neuromuscular Pedicle ... 31590
Stroboscopy ... 31579
Tumor
  Excision ... 31300
    Endoscopic ... 31540, 31541
Unlisted Services and Procedures ... 31599
Vocal Cord(s)
  Injection ... 31513, 31570, 31571, 31573, 31574
    Stripping ... 31540, 31541
X ray ... 70370

Laser Surgery
Anus ... 46614, 46917
Bladder ... 52214, 52224
Bronchi
  Stenosis ... 31641
  Tumor ... 31641
Cataract ... 66821
Cautery
  Anus ... 46614
  Cervix ... 57513, 57520
  Colon ... 44391, 45317, 45382
  Esophagus ... 43227
  Hemorrhoids ... 46930
  Rectum ... 45317, 45334
  Small Intestine ... 44366, 44378
Fenestration
  Body Surface ... 0479T, 0480T
Incompetent Vein ... 0524T, 36478, 36479
Iridectomy ... 66761
Iridotomy ... 66761
Lacrimal Punctum ... 68760
Lens, Posterior ... 66821
Lesion
  Anus ... 46917, 46924
  Bladder ... 52224
  Choroid ... 67220
  Colon ... 45320
  Larynx ... 31572
  Mouth ... 40820
  Nose ... 30117, 30118
  Penis ... 54057, 54065
  Rectum ... 45320
  Skin ... 17000-17111, 17260-17286
  Vagina ... 57061, 57065
  Vulva ... 56501, 56515
Myocardium ... 33140, 33141
Ocular Adhesion ... 65860
Polyp
  Colon ... 45320
Prostate ... 52647, 52648, 52649
Retina ... 67108, 67113, 67145
Revascularization ... 33140, 33141
Trabeculoplasty ... 65855
Trichiasis ... 67825
Tumors
  Bladder ... 52234, 52235, 52240
  Bronchi ... 31641
  Colon ... 45320
  Rectum ... 45190
Ureter ... 52341-52346
Urethra and Bladder ... 52214
Vitreous ... 67031, 67039, 67040, 67043

Laser Treatment
See Laser Surgery
Inflammatory Skin Disease ... 96920-96922

Lateral Epicondylitis
See Tennis Elbow

Latex Fixation ... 86403-86406

LATS
See Thyrotropin Releasing Hormone (TRH)

Latzko Operation
See Repair, Vagina, Fistula; Revision

LAV
See HIV

LAV Antibodies
See Antibody, Detection, Human Immunodeficiency Virus (HIV)

LAV-2
See HIV-2

Lavage
Bladder . . . 51700
Colon . . . 44701
Knee Joint . . . 29871
Lung
  Bronchial . . . 31624
  Total . . . 32997
Gastrointestinal . . . 43753
Maxillary Sinus . . . 31000
Peritoneal . . . 49084
Sphenoid Sinus . . . 31002
Stomach . . . 43753
Wrist Joint . . . 29843

LCM
See Lymphocytic Choriomeningitis

LD
See Lactate Dehydrogenase

LDH . . . 83615-83625

LDL
See Lipoprotein, LDL

Lead . . . 83655

Leadbetter Procedure . . . 53431

Lecithin-Sphingomyelin Ratio . . . 83661

Lecithinase C
See Tissue, Typing

Lee and White Test . . . 85345

LEEP Procedure . . . 57460
Loop Electrode Conization . . . 57461
Loop Electrode Excision . . . 57522

LeFort Procedure
Vagina . . . 57120

LeFort I Procedure
Midface Reconstruction . . . 21141-21147, 21155, 21160
Palatal or Maxillary Fracture . . . 21421-21423

LeFort II Procedure
Midface Reconstruction . . . 21150, 21151
Nasomaxillary Complex Fracture . . . 21345-21348

LeFort III Procedure
Craniofacial Separation . . . 21431-21436
Midface Reconstruction . . . 21154-21160

Left Atrioventricular Valve
See Mitral Valve

Left Heart Cardiac Catheterization
See Cardiac Catheterization, Left Heart

Leg
Bone Procedures
  See Specific Bone
Cast
  Full Leg . . . 29705
  Rigid Total Contact . . . 29445
Dislocation
  See Dislocation, Leg
Fracture
  See Fracture, specific bone
Incision
  Embolectomy . . . 34201, 34203
  Thrombectomy . . . 34201, 34203, 34421, 34451
Injection
  Sclerosant . . . 36465, 36466, 36468, 36470, 36471
Joint
  See Joint, Knee
Lipectomy . . . 15833
Lower
  See Ankle; Fibula; Knee; Tibia
  Abscess
    Incision and Drainage . . . 27603
  Amputation . . . 27598, 27880-27882
    Revision . . . 27884-27886
  Angiography . . . 73706
  Artery
    Ligation . . . 37618
  Biopsy . . . 27613, 27614
  Bursa
    Incision and Drainage . . . 27604
  Bypass Graft . . . 35903
  Cast . . . 29405-29435, 29450
  CT Scan . . . 73700-73706
  Decompression . . . 27600-27602, 27892-27894
  Exploration
    Blood Vessel . . . 35860
  Fasciotomy . . . 27600-27602, 27892-27894
  Hematoma
    Incision and Drainage . . . 27603
  Incision . . . 27607
  Lesion
    Excision . . . 27630
  Neurectomy . . . 27325, 27326
  Repair
    Blood Vessel . . . 35226
    Blood Vessel with Other Graft . . . 35286
    Blood Vessel with Vein Graft . . . 35256
    Fascia . . . 27656
    Tendon . . . 27612, 27650, 27652, 27654, 27656, 27658-27692
  Revascularization . . . 37228-37235
  Splint . . . 29515
  Strapping
    Compression . . . 29581
    Unna Boot . . . 29580
  Suture
    Tendon . . . 27658-27665
    Nerve . . . 64856, 64857, 64859
  Tenotomy . . . 27605, 27606
  Tumor
    Excision . . . 27618, 27619, 27632, 27634
    Radical Resection . . . 27615, 27616
  Ultrasound
    Complete . . . 76881
    Limited . . . 76882
  Unlisted Services and Procedures . . . 27899
  Unna Boot . . . 29580
  Vein
    Ligation . . . 37718, 37760, 37761
    Division . . . 37718
    Stripping . . . 37718
  X ray . . . 73592
Magnetic Resonance Imaging (MRI) . . . 73718-73720
Neuroplasty . . . 64708, 64712
Nerve Graft . . . 64892, 64897, 64898
Splint . . . 29505
Strapping
  Multi-layer Compression System . . . 29581
Upper
  See Femur
  Abscess
    Incision and Drainage . . . 27301
  Amputation . . . 27590-27592
    at Hip . . . 27290-27295
    Revision . . . 27594-27596
  Angiography . . . 73706, 75635
  Artery
    Ligation . . . 37618, 37650
  Biopsy . . . 27323, 27324
  Body Cast . . . 29044, 29046
  Bursa . . . 27301
    Incision and Drainage . . . 27301
  Bypass Graft . . . 35903
  Cast . . . 29345-29355, 29365, 29450
  Cast Brace . . . 29358
  CT Scan . . . 73700-73706, 75635
  Exploration
    Blood Vessel . . . 35860
  Fasciotomy . . . 27025, 27305, 27496-27499, 27892-27894
  Halo Application . . . 20663
  Hematoma . . . 27301
    Incision and Drainage . . . 27301
  Lipectomy . . . 15832
  Neurectomy . . . 27325, 27326
  Removal
    Cast . . . 29705
    Foreign Body . . . 27372
  Repair
    Blood Vessel with Other Graft . . . 35286
    Blood Vessel with Vein Graft . . . 35256
    Muscle . . . 27385, 27386, 27400, 27430
    Tendon . . . 27393-27400
  Revascularization . . . 37224-37227
  Splint . . . 29505
  Strapping
    Unna Boot . . . 29580
  Suture
    Muscle . . . 27385, 27386
    Nerve . . . 64856-64859
  Tendon Transfer/Transplant . . . 27396, 27397, 27400
  Tenotomy . . . 27306, 27307, 27390-27392
  Transplantation
    Testis to Thigh . . . 54680
  Tumor
    Excision . . . 27327, 27328, 27337-27339
    Resection . . . 27329, 27364, 27365
  Ultrasound
    Complete . . . 76881
    Limited . . . 76882
  Unlisted Services and Procedures . . . 27599
  Unna Boot . . . 29580
  X ray . . . 73592
Varicose Vein
  Division . . . 37785
  Excision . . . 37785
  Ligation . . . 37785
  Phlebectomy . . . 37765, 37766
Vein
  Ligation
    Great Saphenous . . . 37700, 37722, 37735
    Perforator . . . 37760, 37761
  Division . . . 37700, 37722, 37735
  Stripping . . . 37722, 37735
Wound Exploration
  Penetrating . . . 20103

Leg Length Measurement X ray
See Scanogram

Legionella
Antibody . . . 86713
Antigen . . . 87278, 87540-87542

Legionella Pneumophila
Antigen Detection
Amplified Probe 87541
Direct Fluorescence 87278
Direct Probe 87540
Quantification 87542

Leiomyomata
Removal 58140, 58145, 58545, 58546, 58561

Leishmania
Antibody 86717

Lengthening, Tendon
See Tendon, Lengthening

Lens
Contact
See Contact Lens Services
Extracapsular 66940
Incision 66821, 66825
Intracapsular 66920
Dislocated 66930
Intraocular
Exchange 66986
Reposition 66825
Laser 66821
Prosthesis
Insertion 66983
Manual or Mechanical Technique 66982, 66984
Not Associated with Concurrent Cataract Removal 66985
Ocular Telescope 0308T
Removal
Crystalline 0308T
Intraocular Lens 0308T
Repositioning 66825
Removal 67108, 67113
Cataract
See Cataract
Foreign Body 65235
Lens Material
Aspiration Technique 66840
Extracapsular 66940
Intracapsular 66920-66930
Pars Plana Approach 66852
Phacofragmentation Technique 66850

Lens Material
Removal
Aspiration Technique 66840
Extracapsular 66940
Intracapsular 66920-66930
Pars Plana Approach 66852
Phacofragmentation Technique 66850

Leptomeningioma
See Meningioma

Leptospira
Antibody 86720

Leriche Operation 64809
See Sympathectomy, Thoracolumbar

Lesion
See also Tumor
Ablation
Endoscopic Retrograde Cholangiopancreatography (ERCP) 43278
Stereotactic
Magnetic Resonance Image Guided High Intensity Focused Ultrasound (MRgFUS) 0398T
Anal
Destruction 46900-46917, 46924
Excision 45108, 46922
Ankle
Tendon Sheath
Excision 27630
Arm, Lower
Tendon Sheath
Excision 25110
Auditory Canal, External
Excision
Exostosis 69140
Radical with Neck Dissection 69155
Radical without Neck Dissection 69150
Soft Tissue 69145
Biopsy
Fine Needle Aspiration
See Fine Needle Aspiration (FNA) Biopsy
Incisional 11106, 11107
Punch 11104, 11105
Tangential 11102, 11103
Bladder
Destruction 51030
Fulguration 52224, 52234, 52235, 52240
Resection 52234, 52235, 52240
Treatment 52224
Brain
Excision 61534, 61536, 61600-61608, 61615, 61616
Brainstem
Excision 61575, 61576
Breast
Detection
Mammography 77065-77067
Excision 19120-19126
Localization Device Placement
with Magnetic Resonance Guidance 19085, 19086, 19287, 19288
with Mammographic Guidance 19281, 19282
with Stereotactic Guidance 19081, 19082, 19283, 19284
with Ultrasound Guidance 19083, 19084, 19285, 19286
Chemotherapy 96405, 96406
Choroid 67220, 67221, 67225
Ciliary Body
Destruction 66770
Colon
Ablation 44401, 45388
Excision 44110, 44111
Conjunctiva
Destruction 68135
Excision 68110-68130
Over 1 cm 68115
with Adjacent Sclera 68130
Cornea
Destruction 65450
Excision 65400
of Pterygium 65420-65426
Cranium
Radiosurgery 61796-61800
Stereotactic Radiation Therapy 77432
Ear, Middle
Excision 69540
Epididymis
Excision 54830
Esophagus
Ablation 43229
Excision 43100, 43101
Removal 43216, 43217
Eyelid
Destruction 67850
Excision
Multiple, Different Lids 67805
Multiple, Same Lid 67801
Single 67800
under Anesthesia 67808
without Closure 67840
Facial
Destruction 17000-17004, 17280-17286
Finger
Tendon Sheath
Excision 26160
Foot
Excision 28080, 28090
Gums
Destruction 41850
Excision 41825-41828
Hand Tendon Sheath 26160
Intestines
Excision 44110
Intestines, Small
Ablation 44369
Excision 44111
Iris
Destruction 66770
Larynx
Ablation 31572
Laser Destruction 31572
Removal 31512, 31545, 31546, 31578
Leg, Lower
Tendon Sheath
Excision 27630
Mesentery
Excision 44820
Mouth
Destruction 40820
Excision 40810-40816, 41116
Vestibule
Destruction 40820
Repair 40830
Nose
Intranasal
Excision 30117, 30118
Orbit
Excision 61333, 67412, 67420
Ovary
Excision 58662
Palate
Destruction 42160
Excision 42104, 42106, 42107
Pancreas
Excision 48120
Pelvis
Excision 58662
Penis
Destruction
Cryosurgery 54056
Electrodesiccation 54055
Extensive 54065
Laser Surgery 54057
Simple 54050-54060
Surgical Excision 54060
Excision 54060
Penile Plaque 54110-54112
Peritoneum
Excision 58662
Pharynx
Destruction 42808
Excision 42808
Radiosurgery
Cranial 61796-61800

Rectum
Excision 45108
Renal Pelvis
Biopsy.......................... 52354
Fulguration....................... 52354
Retina
Destruction
Extensive 67227, 67228
Localized................. 67208-67210
Radiation by Implantation of Source.... 67218
Sclera
Excision 66130
Skin
Abrasion................... 15786, 15787
Biopsy
Fine Needle Aspiration
(FNA)............. 10004-10012, 10021
Incisional 11106, 11107
Punch 11104, 11105
Tangential................ 11102, 11103
with Imaging of Specimen 19081-19086
Destruction
Benign............ 17110, 17111, 17250
Malignant................ 17260-17286
Premalignant 17000-17004
Excision
Benign.................... 11400-11471
Malignant................ 11600-11646
Injection.................. 11900, 11901
Multi-spectral Analysis 0400T, 0401T
Paring or Curettement 11055-11057
Reflectance Confocal Microscopic
Imaging 96931
Shaving 11300-11313
Skin Tags
Removal................... 11200, 11201
Skull
Excision .. 61500, 61600-61608, 61615, 61616
Spermatic Cord
Excision 55520
Spinal Cord
Destruction................. 62280-62282
Excision 61575, 61576,
63265-63273, 63300-63308
Stereotactic Radiation Therapy 77432, 77435
Testis
Excision 54512
Toe
Excision 28092
Tongue
Excision 41110-41114
Ureter
Biopsy.......................... 52354
Destruction................. 52341, 52342,
52344, 52345, 52354
Fulguration....................... 52354
Urethra
Fulguration................ 52224, 53265
Treatment....................... 52224
Uvula
Destruction....................... 42160
Excision 42104-42107
Vagina
Destruction................ 57061-57065
Vulva
Destruction
Extensive 56515
Simple.......................... 56501
Wrist Tendon
Excision 25110

Leu 2 Antigens
See CD8

Leucine Aminopeptidase 83670

Leukemia Lymphoma Virus I Antibodies, Human T Cell
See Antibody, Detection, HTLV-I

Leukemia Lymphoma Virus I, Adult T Cell
See HTLV-I

Leukemia Lymphoma Virus II Antibodies, Human T Cell
See Antibody, Detection, HTLV-II

Leukemia Virus II, Hairy Cell Associated, Human T Cell
See HTLV-II

Leukoagglutinins 86021

Leukocyte
See White Blood Cell
Alkaline Phosphatase.................. 85540
Antibody 86021
Count.................... 85032, 85048, 89055
Fecal Assessment...................... 89055
Histamine Release Test 86343
Human Leukocyte Antigen (HLA)
See HLA
Phagocytosis......................... 86344
Transfusion.......................... 86950
Urinalysis 81000

Levarterenol
See Noradrenalin

Levator Muscle Repair
See Blepharoptosis, Repair

LeVeen Shunt
Insertion 49425
Patency Test......................... 78291
Revision............................. 49426

Levetiracetam
Drug Assay 80177

Levulose
See Fructose

LGV
See Lymphogranuloma Venereum

LH
See Luteinizing Hormone (LH)

LHR
See Leukocyte, Histamine Release Test

Lid Suture
See Blepharoptosis, Repair

Lidocaine
Assay................................ 80176

Lift, Face
See Face Lift

Ligament
Ankle
Collateral Ligament Repair 27695, 27696
Augmentation
Knee..................... 29888, 29889
Collateral
Reconstruction
Elbow 24344, 24346, 24362
Interphalangeal Joint............ 26545
Metacarpophalangeal Joint... 26541, 26542
Reduction
Ulna 29902
Repair
Ankle.............. 27695, 27696, 27698
Elbow 24343, 24345
Interphalangeal Joint............. 26540
Knee 27405, 27409
Metacarpophalangeal Joint......... 26540
Coracoacromial
Release 23130, 23415, 29826
Cruciate
Repair
Knee 27407, 27409, 29888, 29889
Dentate
Section.................... 63180, 63182
Elbow
Collateral Ligament
Reconstruction 24344, 24346, 24362
Repair.................... 24343, 24345
Injection 20550
Knee 27557, 27558
Collateral Ligament Repair 27405, 27409
Cruciate Ligament Repair 27407, 27409
Reconstruction.............. 27427-27429
Reconstruction
Elbow 24344, 24346, 24362
Knee........... 27427-27429, 29888, 29889
Reduction
Ulna
Collateral Ligament 29902
Release
Coracoacromial 23130, 23415, 29826
Transverse Carpal 29848
Repair
Ankle 27695, 27696, 27698
Elbow 24343-24346
Knee Joint 27405-27409
Wrist 25320
Transverse Carpal
Release 29848
Ulna
Collateral Ligament Reduction 29902
Wrist
Release 29848
Repair........................... 25320

Ligation
Artery
Abdomen 37617
Carotid 37600-37606, 61611
Chest 37616
Coronary.......................... 33502
Ethmoidal......................... 30915
Extremity 37618
Fistula........................... 37607
Hepatic........................... 47360
Maxillary 30920
Neck............................. 37615
Temporal 37609
Cranial Sinus......................... 61598
Esophageal Varices......... 43205, 43244, 43400
Fallopian Tube
Oviduct.............. 58600-58611, 58670
Gastric Varices 43244
Gastroesophageal...................... 43405
Hemorrhoids 46945, 46946
with Ultrasound 0249T
Lacrimal Punctum 68760
Oviducts 59100
Salivary Duct......................... 42665
Shunt
Aorta
Pulmonary........................ 33924
Peritoneal
Venous 49428
Submandibular Duct.................... 42510

Thoracic Duct . . . 38380
Abdominal Approach . . . 38382
Thoracic Approach . . . 38381
Tubal . . . 58600
Vein
Clusters . . . 37785
Esophagus . . . 43205, 43244, 43400
Femoral . . . 37650
Gastric . . . 43244
Iliac . . . 37660
Jugular, Internal . . . 37565
Perforate . . . 37500, 37760, 37761
Saphenous . . . 37700-37735, 37780
Spermatic . . . 55530, 55535, 55540, 55550
Vena Cava . . . 37619
Wharton's Ducts . . . 42510

Ligature Strangulation
Skin Tags . . . 11200, 11201

Light Coagulation
See Photocoagulation

Light Scattering Measurement
See Nephelometry

Light Therapy, UV
See Actinotherapy

Limb
See Extremity

Limited Lymphadenectomy for Staging
See Lymphadenectomy, Limited, for Staging

Limited Neck Dissection
with Thyroidectomy . . . 60252

Limited Resection Mastectomies
See Breast, Excision, Lesion

Lindholm Operation
See Tenoplasty

Lingual Bone
See Hyoid, Bone

Lingual Frenectomy
See Excision, Mouth, Frenum

Lingual Nerve
Avulsion . . . 64740
Transection . . . 64740

Lingual Tonsil
See Tonsils, Lingual

Linton Procedure . . . 37760

Lip
Abbe-Estlander Procedure . . . 40527
Biopsy . . . 40490
Excision
Abbe-Estlander Procedure . . . 40527
Estlander Procedure . . . 40525
Frenum . . . 40819
Full Thickness . . . 40525, 40527
Transverse Wedge . . . 40510
V . . . 40520
Incision
Frenum . . . 40806
Malleolus
Fixation . . . 27823
Reconstruction . . . 40525-40527
Repair . . . 40650-40654
Cleft Lip . . . 40700-40761
Complex . . . 13151-13153
Fistula . . . 42260
Resection . . . 40530
Shave . . . 40500
Suture
Tongue to Lip . . . 41510
Unlisted Services and Procedures . . . 40799
Vermilionectomy . . . 40500

Lip, Cleft
See Cleft Lip

Lipase . . . 83690

Lipectomy
Excision . . . 15830-15839, 15847
Suction Assisted . . . 15876-15879

Lipectomy, Aspiration
See Liposuction

Lipids
Feces . . . 82705-82710
Panel . . . 80061
Phospholipid
Antibody . . . 86147, 86148
Neutralization . . . 85597, 85598

Lipo-Lutin
See Progesterone

Lipolysis, Aspiration
See Liposuction

Lipophosphodiesterase I
See Tissue, Typing

Lipoprotein
(a) . . . 83695
Apolipoprotein . . . 82172
Blood . . . 83695, 83700-83721
Delipidation
HDL . . . 0342T
HDL . . . 83718
LDL . . . 83700-83704, 83721, 83722
Phospholipase A2 . . . 83698
VLDL . . . 83719

Lipoprotein, Alpha
See Lipoprotein

Lipoprotein, Pre-Beta
See Lipoprotein, Blood

Liposuction . . . 15876-15879

Lisfranc Operation
See Amputation, Foot; Radical Resection; Replantation

Listeria Monocytogenes
Antibody . . . 86723

Lithium
Assay . . . 80178

Litholapaxy . . . 52317, 52318

Lithotripsy
See Extracorporeal Shock Wave Therapy
Bile Duct Calculi (Stone)
Endoscopy . . . 43265
Bladder . . . 52353
Kidney . . . 50080, 50081, 50590, 52353
Pancreatic Duct Calculi (Stone)
Endoscopy . . . 43265
Ureter . . . 52353
Urethra . . . 52353
with Cystourethroscopy . . . 52353
with Indwelling Ureteral Stent Insertion . . . 52356

Lithotrity
See Litholapaxy

Liver
See Hepatic Duct
Ablation
Tumor . . . 47380-47383
Laparoscopic . . . 47370, 47371
Abscess
Aspiration . . . 47015
Incision and Drainage
Open . . . 47010
Injection . . . 47015
Aspiration . . . 47015
Biopsy . . . 47700
Needle . . . 47000, 47001
Wedge . . . 47100
with Staging Laparotomy . . . 49220
Assist System
Care Plan Oversight . . . 0405T
Cyst
Aspiration . . . 47015
Incision and Drainage
Open . . . 47010
Injection . . . 47015
Drainage . . . 47400
Image Guided Fluid Collection . . . 49405
Excision
Extensive . . . 47122
Partial . . . 47120, 47125-47130
Donor . . . 47140-47142
Total
Donor . . . 47133
Exploration . . . 47400
Hemorrhage . . . 47350-47362
Injection . . . 47015
Lobectomy . . . 47125-47130
Partial . . . 47120
Needle Biopsy . . . 47000, 47001
Nuclear Medicine
Imaging . . . 78201-78216
Vascular Flow . . . 78206
Removal
Calculus . . . 47400
Repair
Abscess . . . 47300
Cyst . . . 47300
Wound . . . 47350-47362
Suture
Wound . . . 47350-47362
Transplantation
Partial . . . 47135, 47144, 47145
Whole . . . 47135
Allograft Preparation . . . 47143-47147
Lobe Split . . . 47145
Trisegment Split . . . 47144
Trisegmentectomy . . . 47122
Ultrasound
Elastography, Shear Wave . . . 91200
Unlisted Services and Procedures . . . 47379, 47399

Living Activities, Daily
See Activities of Daily Living

Lobectomy
Brain . . . 61323, 61537-61540
Partial . . . 61539, 61540
Temporal Lobe . . . 61537, 61538
Contralateral Subtotal
Thyroid Gland . . . 60212, 60225
Liver . . . 47120-47130
Donor . . . 47141, 47142
Lung . . . 32480-32482
Sleeve . . . 32486
Thoracoscopic . . . 32663, 32670
Parotid Gland . . . 42410-42415
Sleeve . . . 32486

Temporal Lobe 61537, 61538
Thoracoscopic
  Lung 32663, 32670
Thyroid Gland
  Partial 60210-60212
  Total 60220-60225

Local Excision Mastectomies
See Breast, Excision, Lesion

Local Excision of Lesion or Tissue of Femur
See Tumor, Femur

Localization of Nodule
Breast
  Device Placement
    with Magnetic Resonance Guidance 19085, 19086, 19287, 19288
    with Mammographic Guidance 19281, 19282
    with Stereotactic Guidance 19081, 19082, 19283, 19284
    with Ultrasound Guidance 19083, 19084, 19285, 19286
Soft Tissue
  Device Placement 10035, 10036

Log Hydrogen Ion Concentration
See Blood Gases, pH

Long Acting Thyroid Stimulator
See Thyrotropin Releasing Hormone (TRH)

Long-Term Care Facility Visits
See Nursing Facility Services

Longmire Operation
See Anastomosis, Hepatic Duct to Intestines

Loop Recorder System, Implantable
See Cardiac Assist Devices, Subcutaneous Cardiac Rhythm Monitor

Loopogram
See Urography, Antegrade

Loose Body
Removal
  Ankle Joint 27620, 29894
  Carpometacarpal Joint 26070
  Elbow Joint 24101, 29834
  Glenohumeral Joint 23107
  Hip Joint 27033
  Interphalangeal Joint 28024
  Intertarsal Joint 28020
  Knee Joint 27331
  Metatarsophalangeal Joint 28022
  Shoulder Joint 29819
  Subtalar Joint 29904
  Tarsometatarsal Joint 28020
  Toe 28022
  Wrist Joint 25101

Lord Procedure
See Anal Sphincter, Dilation

Louis Bar Syndrome
See Ataxia Telangiectasia

Low Birth Weight Intensive Care Services 99478-99480

Low Density Lipoprotein
See Lipoprotein, LDL

Low Frequency Ultrasound 97610

Low Vision Aids
See Spectacle Services
Fitting 92354, 92355

Lower Extremities
See Extremity, Lower

Lower GI Series
See Barium Enema

LRH
See Luteinizing Releasing Factor

LSD
See Lysergic Acid Diethylamide

LTH
See Prolactin

Lumbar
See Spine

Lumbar Plexus
Decompression 64714
Infusion
  Anesthetic 64449
Neuroplasty 64714
Repair/Suture 64862

Lumbar Puncture
See Spinal Tap

Lumbar Spine Fracture
See Fracture, Vertebra, Lumbar

Lumbar Sympathectomy
See Sympathectomy, Lumbar

Lumbar Vertebra
See Vertebra, Lumbar

Lumen Dilation 74360

Lumpectomy 19301, 19302

Lunate
Arthroplasty
  with Implant 25444
Dislocation
  Closed Treatment 25690
  Open Treatment 25695

Lung
Ablation
  Tumor 32994, 32998
Abscess
  Incision and Drainage
    Open 32200
Air Leak Assessment 31647, 31651
Airway Sizing 31647, 31651
Biopsy 32096, 32097
  Bronchoscopic 31628, 31629, 31632, 31633
  Thoracoscopic 32607, 32608
    Infiltrate 32607
    Mass 32608
    Nodule 32608
Bullae
  Resection-Plication
    Thoracoscopic 32655
    Thoracotomy 32141
Collapse
  See Lung Collapse Therapy
Cyst
  Incision and Drainage
    Open 32200
  Removal 32140
Decortication
  Endoscopic 32651, 32652
  Partial 32225, 32651
  Total 32220, 32652
  with Parietal Pleurectomy 32320
Drainage
  Image Guided Fluid Collection 49405
  Empyema 32035, 32036
    Closure, Chest Wall 32810
Empyema
  Drainage 32035, 32036
  Excision 32540
  Thoracostomy 32035-32026
Excision
  Bronchus Resection 32486
  Completion 32488
  Donor
    Heart-Lung 33930
    Lung 32850
  Empyema 32540
  Lobe 32480-32482
  Pneumonectomy 32440-32445
  Segment 32484
  Tumor 32503, 32504
Exploration 32100
Foreign Body
  Removal 32151
Hemorrhage Control 32110
  Thoracoscopic 32654
Insertion
  Bronchial Valve 31647, 31651
Lavage
  Bronchial 31624
  Total 32997
Lysis
  Adhesions 32124, 32940
Needle Biopsy 32405
Nuclear Medicine
  Imaging, Perfusion 78580, 78597, 78598
  Imaging, Ventilation 78579, 78582, 78598
  Unlisted Services and Procedures 78599
Placement
  Interstitial Device 32553
Pleura
  See Pleura
Pneumolysis 32652, 32940
Pneumonostomy 32200
Pneumothorax
  Repeat 32215
  Therapeutic 32960
Removal 32440-32445
  Bilobectomy 32482
    Thoracoscopic 32670
  Bronchial Valve 31648, 31649
  Bronchoplasty 32501
  Completion Pneumonectomy 32488
  Extrapleural 32445
  Pneumonectomy 32440-32445
    Thoracoscopic 32671
  Segmentectomy
    Thoracoscopic 32669
  Single Lobe 32480
  Single Segment 32484
  Sleeve Lobectomy 32486
  Sleeve Pneumonectomy 32442
  Two Lobes 32482, 32670
  Volume Reduction 32491
Repair
  Hernia 32800
Resection
  Anatomic Lung 32507
  Diagnostic Wedge 32507
  Pancoast Tumor 32503, 32504
  Therapeutic Wedge 32505, 32506
  Tumor 32503, 32504

Index

Resection-Plication
  Bullae 32141, 32655
    Thoracoscopic 32672
  Emphysematous 32491
    Thoracoscopic 32672
Segmentectomy 32484, 32669
Tear
  Repair 32110
Thoracoscopy
  See Thoracoscopy
Thoracostomy
  Empyema 32035-32026
Thoracotomy
  Biopsy 32096, 32097
  Cardiac Massage 32160
  Exploration 32100
  for Post-Op Complications 32120
  Hemorrhage Control 32110
  Removal
    Bullae 32141
    Cyst 32140
    Fibrin Deposit 32150
    Intrapleural Foreign Body 32150
    Intrapulmonary Foreign Body 32151
  Repair 32110
  with Open Intrapleural Pneumonolysis .. 32124
  with Resection-Plication of Bullae 32141
Transplantation
  Allograft Preparation
    Heart/Lung 33933
    Lung 32855, 32856
    Marginal (Extended) Lung 0494T-0496T
  Donor Pneumonectomy
    Heart/Lung 33930
    Lung 32850
  Heart/Lung 33935
  Lung 32851-32854
Tumor
  Resection 32503, 32504
Unlisted Services and Procedures 32999
Volume Reduction 32491
  Thoracoscopic 32672

Lung Collapse Therapy
Air Injection 32960
Pneumonolysis 32940
Rib Resection 32900
Schede Thoracoplasty 32905
Thoracoplasty 32905
  Closure, Bronchopleural Fistula 32906

Lung Function Tests
See Pulmonology, Diagnostic

Lung Volume Reduction (LVRS)
Emphysematous 32491, 32672

Lupus Anticoagulant Assay 85705

Lupus Band Test
See Immunofluorescence Microscopy, Antibody Stain Procedure

Luteinizing Hormone (LH)
Gonadotropin 83002
Ovulation Tests 84830
Panels
  Gonadotropin Releasing Hormone Stimulation 80426
  Pituitary Evaluation 80418

Luteinizing Releasing Factor 83727

Luteotropic Hormone
See Prolactin

Luteotropin
See Prolactin

Luteotropin, Placental
See Lactogen, Human Placental

Lyme Disease 86617, 86618

Lyme Disease ab
See Antibody, Detection, Lyme Disease

Lyme Disease Vaccine
See Vaccines and Toxoids

Lymph Duct
Injection
  for Lymphangiography 38790
Thoracic
  Cannulation 38794
  Ligation 38380-38382
  Suture 38380-38382

Lymph Nodes
Abdominal
  Excision 38747
Abscess
  Incision and Drainage 38300-38305
Aortic
  Excision 38780
Axillary
  Hygroma, Cystic
    Excision 38550-38555
  Lymphadenectomy
    Complete 19305-19307, 38745
    Superficial 38740
  Optical Coherence Tomography .. 0351T, 0352T
  Ultrasound 76641, 76642
Biopsy
  Needle 38505
  Open 38500, 38510, 38520, 38525, 38530, 38531
Celiac
  Excision 38747
Cervical
  Hygroma, Cystic
    Excision 38550-38555
  Lymphadenectomy
    Complete 38720
    Modified 38724
Dissection
  Jugular 38542
Drainage
  Manual 97140
Excision 38500, 38510, 38520, 38525, 38530, 38531
  Abdominal 38747
  Aortic 38780
  Celiac 38747
  Gastric 38747
  Hypogastric 38770, 55845, 55865
  Iliac 38770, 55845, 55865
  Inguinofemoral 38760-38765, 38531
  Laparoscopic 38571-38573
  Limited, for Staging
    Para-Aortic 38562, 38747
  Mediastinal 21632, 32674, 38746
  Obturator 38770, 55845, 55865
    Pelvic 38562
    Retroperitoneal 38564
  Pelvic 38562, 38770, 38780, 57531
  Peripancreatic 38747
  Portal 38747
  Radical
    Axillary 19305-19307, 38740-38745
    Cervical 38720-38724
    Suprahyoid 38700
  Renal 38780
  Retroperitoneal Transabdominal 38780
  Thoracic 38746
  Vena Caval 38747
Exploration
  Jugular 38542
Gastric
  Excision 38747
Hilar
  Sampling
    Endobronchial Ultrasound (EBUS) Guided 31652, 31653
Hygroma
  Axillary/Cervical
    Excision 38550-38555
Hypogastric
  Excision 38770, 55845, 55865
Identification
  Sentinel
    Injection, Radioactive Tracer 38792
    Intraoperative 38900
Iliac
  Excision 38770, 55845, 55865
Inguinofemoral
  Excision 38760-38765
Jugular
  Dissection 38542
Mediastinal
  Excision 21632
    Thoracoscopic 32674
    by Thoracotomy 38746
  Mediastinoscopy 39402
  Sampling
    Endobronchial Ultrasound (EBUS) Guided 31652, 31653
Nuclear Medicine
  Imaging 78195
Obturator
  Excision 38770, 55845, 55865
Para-Aortic
  Biopsy 57112, 57531, 58200, 58210, 58548, 58943
  Excision .. 38562, 38747, 58951, 58954, 58960
Pelvic
  Biopsy 55812, 55842, 55862, 58200, 58943, 58954
  Excision 38562, 38770, 38780, 55845, 55865, 58210, 58548, 58951, 58954, 58960
Peripancreatic
  Excision 38747
Portal
  Excision 38747
Renal
  Excision 38780
Removal
  Regional
    with Nephrectomy 50545
Suprahyoid
  Excision 38700
Therapy 97140
Thoracic
  Excision 38746
Vena Caval
  Excision 38747

Lymph Vessels
Imaging
  Lymphangiography
    Abdomen 75805-75807
    Arm 75801-75803
    Leg 75801-75803
    Pelvis 75805-75807
  Nuclear Medicine 78195
Incision 38308

Lymphadenectomy
Abdominal 38747
Aortic 38780
Axillary 38740-38745
Bilateral Inguinofemoral 54130, 56632, 56637
Bilateral Pelvic 51575, 51585, 51595, 54135, 55845, 55865
Total 38571-38573, 57531, 58210
Celiac 38747
Cervical 38720-38724
Diaphragmatic Assessment 58960
Gastric 38747
Hypogastric 38770, 55845, 55865
Iliac 38770, 55845, 55865
Inguinofemoral 38760-38765
Inguinofemoral, Iliac and Pelvic 56640
Injection
Sentinel Node 38792, 38900
Limited
Para-Aortic, Resection of Ovarian Malignancy 58951, 58954
Pelvic 55842, 55862, 58954
for Staging
Para-Aortic 38562
Pelvic 38562
Retroperitoneal 38564
Mediastinal 21632
Thoracoscopic 32674
by Thoracotomy 38746
Obturator 38770, 55845, 55865
Para-Aortic 58958
Pelvic 38770, 38780, 55845, 55865, 57531, 58210, 58548, 58958
Peripancreatic 38747
Portal 38747
Radical
Axillary 38740-38745
Cervical 38720-38724
Pelvic 54135, 55845, 58548
Suprahyoid 38700
Regional 50230
Thoracoscopic 32674
by Thoracotomy 38746
Renal 38780
Retroperitoneal Transabdominal 38780
Suprahyoid 38700
Thoracic
by Thoracotomy 38746
Unilateral Inguinofemoral 56631, 56634
Vena Caval 38747

Lymphadenitis
Incision and Drainage 38300-38305

Lymphadenopathy Associated Antibodies/Virus
See Antibody, Detection, Human Immunodeficiency Virus (HIV)

Lymphangiogram
See Lymphangiography

Lymphangiography
Abdomen 75805-75807
Arm 75801-75803
Injection 38790
Leg 75801-75803
Pelvis 75805-75807

Lymphangioma, Cystic
See Hygroma; Lymph Nodes, Hygroma

Lymphangiotomy 38308

Lymphatic Channels
Incision 38308

Lymphatic Cyst
See Lymphocele

Lymphatic System
Unlisted Procedure 38999

Lymphatics
See Lymph Nodes; Lymph Vessels
Imaging
Nuclear Medicine 78195

Lymphoblast Transformation
See Blastogenesis

Lymphocele
Drainage
Laparoscopic 49323
Open 49062

Lymphocoele
See Lymphocele

Lymphocyte
Culture 86821
Tissue 88230
Toxicity Assay 86805, 86806
Transformation 86353

Lymphocyte, Thymus-Dependent
See T Cells

Lymphocytes, CD4
See CD4

Lymphocytes, CD8
See CD8

Lymphocytic Choriomeningitis
Antibody 86727

Lymphocytotoxicity 86805, 86806

Lymphoma Virus, Burkitt
See Epstein-Barr Virus

Lynch Procedure 31075

Lysergic Acid Diethylamide
Drug Assay
Alkaloids, Not Otherwise Specified 80323

Lysis
Adhesions
Epidural 62263, 62264
Fallopian Tube 58660, 58740
Foreskin 54450
Intestinal 44005, 44180
Labial 56441
Lung 32124, 32940
Nose 30560
Ovary 58660, 58740
Oviduct 58660, 58740
Penile
Post-Circumcision 54162
Ureter 50715-50725
Urethra 53500
Uterus 58559
Clot
Time 85175
Euglobulin 85360
Fibrosis
Urethral 52285
Hemoglobin 85460, 85461
Intranasal Synechia 30560

Lysozyme 85549

M

Macrodactylia
Repair 26590

Macroscopic Examination
Arthropod 87168
Parasite 87169
Tissue 88387, 88388

Magnesium 83735

Magnet Operation
See Ciliary Body; Cornea; Eye, Removal, Foreign Body; Iris; Lens; Retina; Sclera; Vitreous

Magnetic Resonance Angiography (MRA)
Abdomen 74185
Arm 73225
Chest 71555
Head 70544-70546
Leg 73725
Neck 70547-70549
Pelvis 72198
Spine 72159

Magnetic Resonance Imaging (MRI)
Diagnostic
3-D Rendering 76376, 76377
Not Requiring Independent Workstation 76376
Requiring Independent Workstation 76377
Abdomen 74181-74183
Ankle 73721-73723
Arm 73218-73220
Joint 73221-73223
Bone Marrow Study 77084
Brain 70551-70555
Intraoperative 70557-70559
Chest 71550-71552
Elbow 73221
Face 70540-70543
Fetal 74712, 74713
Finger Joint 73221-73223
Foot 73718, 73719
Foot Joints 73721-73723
Hand 73218-73220, 73223
Heart 75557-75565
Joint
Lower Extremity 73721-73723
Upper Extremity 73221-73223
Knee 73721-73723
Leg 73718-73720
Joint 73721-73723
Obstetrical
Maternal Pelvis 74712, 74713
Neck 70540-70543
Orbit 70540-70543
Pelvis 72195-72197
Spectroscopy 76390
Spine
Cervical 72141, 72142, 72156
Lumbar 72148, 72149, 72158
Thoracic 72146, 72147, 72157
Temporomandibular Joint (TMJ) 70336
Toe 73721-73723
Wrist 73221
Guidance
Arthrography, Enhanced
Shoulder
Injection 23350

Index

Brain
Stereotactic Lesion Ablation
Magnetic Resonance Image Guided High Intensity Focused Ultrasound (MRgFUS) 0398T
Stereotactic Lesion Biopsy 61751
Breast
with Computer-Aided Detection 77048, 77049
without Contrast 77046, 77047
Biopsy 19085, 19086
Lesion Localization Device Placement 19085, 19086, 19287, 19288
Needle Placement 77021
Orthopedic Procedure
Computer-assisted Navigation 0055T
Parenchymal Tissue Ablation 77022
Unlisted Procedure 76498

Magnetic Resonance Spectroscopy 76390

Magnetic Stimulation
Transcranial 90867-90869

Magnetoencephalography (MEG) 95965-95967

Magnuson Procedure 23450

MAGPI Operation 54322

MAGPI Procedure
See Hypospadias, Repair

Major Vestibular Gland
See Bartholin's Gland

Malar Area
Augmentation 21270
Bone Graft 21210
Fracture
Open Treatment 21360-21366
with Bone Graft 21366
with Manipulation 21355
Reconstruction 21270

Malar Bone
See Cheek, Bone

Malaria Antibody 86750

Malaria Smear 87207

Malate Dehydrogenase 83775

Maldescent, Testis
See Testis, Undescended

Male Circumcision
See Circumcision

Malformation, Arteriovenous
See Arteriovenous Malformation

Malic Dehydrogenase
See Malate Dehydrogenase

Malignant Hyperthermia Susceptibility
Caffeine Halothane Contracture Test (CHCT) 89049

Malleolus
See Ankle; Fibula; Leg, Lower; Tibia; Tibiofibular Joint

Mallet Finger Repair 26432, 26433

Maltose
Tolerance Test 82951, 82952

Malunion Repair
Clavicle 23485
Femur
with Graft 27472
without Graft 27470
Fibula 27726
Humerus
with Graft 24435
without Graft 24430
Metatarsal Bone 28322
Radius
with Graft 25405, 25420
without Graft 25400, 25415
Tarsal Bone 28320
Tibia
by Synostosis with Fibula 27725
with Graft 27722, 27724
without Graft 27720
Ulna
with Graft 25405, 25420
without Graft 25400, 25415

Mammalian Oviduct
See Fallopian Tube

Mammaplasty
Augmentation 19324, 19325
Reduction 19318

Mammary Abscess
See Abscess, Tissue, Breast

Mammary Arteries
See Artery, Mammary

Mammary Duct
X ray 77053, 77054
Contrast Injection 19030

Mammary Ductogram
X ray 77053, 77054
Contrast Injection 19030

Mammary Stimulating Hormone
See Prolactin

Mammillaplasty
See Nipples, Reconstruction

Mammogram 77065-77067

Mammography 77065-77067
Localization, Lesion
Device Placement 19281, 19282
Magnetic Resonance Imaging (MRI)
with Computer-Aided Detection 77048, 77049
without Contrast 77046, 77047
Screening Mammography 77067
Tomosynthesis 77061-77063
with Computer-Aided Detection (CAD) 77065-77067

Mammoplasty
See Mammaplasty

Mammotomy
Mastotomy
Drainage of Abscess 19020
Exploration 19020

Mammotropic Hormone, Pituitary
See Prolactin

Mammotropic Hormone, Placental
See Lactogen, Human Placental

Mammotropin
See Prolactin

Mandated Services
On Call Services 99026, 99027

Mandible
See Facial Bones; Maxilla; Temporomandibular Joint (TMJ)
Abscess
Excision 21025
Bone Graft 21215
Condyle
See Mandibular Condyle
Cyst
Excision 21040, 21046, 21047
Disarticulation 61590
Excision
Abscess 21025
Bone 21025
Cyst 21040, 21046, 21047
Torus Mandibularis 21031
Tumor 21040, 21044, 21045, 21046, 21047
Fracture
Closed Treatment
Alveolar Ridge 21440
with Interdental Fixation 21453
with Manipulation 21451
without Manipulation 21450
Open Treatment 21454-21470
Alveolar Ridge 21445
Condylar Fracture 21465
External Fixation 21454
with Interdental Fixation 21462
without Interdental Fixation 21461
Percutaneous Treatment 21452
Osteotomy 21198, 21199
with Cyst Excision 21046, 21047
with Tumor Excision 21046, 21047
Prosthesis
Impression 21081
Rami
See Mandibular Rami
Reconstruction
with Implant 21244-21246, 21248, 21249
Removal
Foreign Body 41806
Resection
with Glossectomy 41150, 41155
Splitting 61576
Torus Mandibularis
Excision 21031
Tumor
Excision 21040-21047
X ray 70100-70110

Mandibular Body
Augmentation
with Bone Graft 21127
with Prosthesis 21125

Mandibular Condyle
Fracture
Open Treatment 21465
Reconstruction 21247

Mandibular Condylectomy
See Condylectomy

Mandibular Fracture
See Fracture, Mandible

Mandibular Rami
Reconstruction
with Bone Graft 21194
with Internal Rigid Fixation 21196
without Bone Graft 21193
without Internal Rigid Fixation 21195

Mandibular Resection Prosthesis 21081

Mandibular Staple Bone Plate
Reconstruction
Mandible 21244

Manganese 83785

Manipulation
Chest Wall 94667, 94668
Chiropractic.................... 98940-98943
Clubfoot Cast Application................ 29450
Dislocation and/or Fracture
Acetabulum 27222
Acromioclavicular 23545
Ankle 27810, 27818, 27860
Bennett Fracture 26645, 26650
Calcaneal 28405, 28406
Carpal 25635
Carpal Scaphoid.................. 25624
Carpometacarpal 26670-26676
Thumb Dislocation 26641, 26645, 26650
Clavicular 23505
Elbow 24300, 24620, 24640
Femoral .. 27232, 27268, 27503, 27510, 27517
Peritrochanteric 27240
Femoral Shaft..................... 27502
Fibula 27781, 27788
Finger 26725-26727, 26742, 26755
Joint 26340
Greater Tuberosity
Humeral 23625
Hand...................... 26670-26676
Heel 28405, 28406
Hip 27257
Hip Socket 27222
Humeral 23605, 24505, 24535
Condyle.................. 24577, 24582
Epicondyle 24565, 24566
Tuberosity...................... 23625
Intercarpal 25660
Interphalangeal Joint........ 26340, 26742, 26770-26776, 28666
Knee...................... 27538, 29850
Lunate 25690
Malar Area........................ 21355
Mandibular........................ 21451
Metacarpal.................. 26605-26607
Metacarpophalangeal ... 26700-26706, 26742
Metacarpophalangeal Joint 26700-26706, 26340, 26742
Metatarsal................. 28475, 28476
Metatarsophalangeal Joint........... 28636
Monteggia 24620
Navicular 25624
Orbit 21401
Pelvis 27275
Pelvic Ring 27198
Phalangeal Shaft.................. 26727
Distal, Finger or Thumb 26755
Finger/Thumb............. 26725, 26727
Phalanges............ 28495, 28496, 28510
Finger 26742, 26755, 26770-26776
Finger/Thumb.................... 26727
Great Toe 28495, 28496
Toes 28515
Radial............... 24655, 25565, 25605
Radial Shaft............... 25505, 25565
Radiocarpal 25660
Radioulnar 25675
Scapular 23575
Shoulder.................... 23650-23655
Joint 23700
with Greater Tuberosity........... 23665
Sternoclavicular................... 23525
with Neck Fracture............... 23675
Talotarsal........................ 28576
Talus...................... 28435, 28436
Tarsal................ 28455, 28456, 28546
Tarsometatarsal Joint 28606
Thumb 26641-26650
Tibial 27532, 27752, 27762, 27768, 27825
Trans-Scaphoperilunar.............. 25680
Ulnar...................... 24675, 25605
Ulnar Shaft................ 25535, 25565
Vertebral 22315
Wrist 25259, 25624, 25635, 25660, 25675, 25680, 25690
Dupuytren's Cord 26341
Slipped Epiphysis
Femur 27178
Foreskin........................... 54450
Globe....................... 92018, 92019
Hip................................ 27275
Interphalangeal Joint
Finger 26340
Proximal 26742
Knee Joint......................... 27570
Adhesions 29884
Lymphatic Drainage 97140
Manual Therapy 97140
Osteopathic..................... 98925-98929
Palmar Fascial Cord 26341
Rectal
Dilation.................... 45905, 45910
Reduction, Procidentia.............. 45900
Removal, Fecal Impaction 45915
Shoulder
Adhesions 29825
Application of Fixation Apparatus...... 23700
Spine
with Anesthesia................... 22505
without Anesthesia................ 97140
Temporomandibular Joint(s) (TMJ) 21073
Ureter 52330, 52352

Manometric Studies
Abdominal Voiding Pressure............. 51797
Bladder Voiding Pressure 51728, 51729
Blood Pressure
See Blood Pressure
Colon.............................. 91117
Cranial Pressure 61107, 61210
Duodenal Motility.................... 91022
Esophagus.......................... 91010
with Perfusion 91013
with Stimulation 91013
Gastric Motility...................... 91020
Gastrointestinal Tract.................. 91112
Intraocular Pressure 0198T, 92100
Interstitial Fluid Pressure 20950
Kidney Pressure 50396
Plantar Pressure 96001-96004
Pulmonary Pressure 94750
Rectum/Anus 91122
Sphincter of Oddi 43263
Ureter Pressure...................... 50686
Ureterostomy 50686
Urethra Voiding Pressure 51727, 51729

Manometry
Anorectal.......................... 91122
Rectum 90911
with Biofeedback Training 90911

Mantoux Test
See TB Test, Skin Test

Manual Therapy 97140

Maquet Procedure................... 27418

Marcellation Operation
See Hysterectomy, Vaginal

Marrow, Bone
See Bone Marrow

Marshall-Marchetti-Krantz Procedure 51840, 51841, 58152, 58267, 58293

Marsupialization
Abscess
Liver 47300
Acne 10040
Cyst
Bartholin's Gland.................. 56440
Liver 47300
Pancreatic 48500
Sublingual Salivary 42409
Urethral Diverticulum.................. 53240

Mass
Abdomen
Biopsy........................... 49180
Kidney
Ablation 50542
Cryosurgical 50250
Lung
Biopsy.................... 32097, 32608
Resection 32505, 32506, 32666, 32667
Mediastinum
Excision 32662
Surgical Pathology................. 88307
Pericardium
Excision 32661
Renal
Ablation 50250, 50542
Retroperitoneal
Biopsy........................... 49180
Soft Tissue
Surgical Pathology................. 88307

Mass Spectrometry and Tandem Mass Spectrometry
Analyte
See specific analyte in Drug Assay; Pathology and Laboratory, Chemistry
Unspecified Non-Drug Analyte 83789

Massage
Cardiac 32160
Therapy 97124
See Physical Medicine/Therapy/Occupational Therapy

Masseter Muscle/Bone
Bone and Muscle
Reduction.................. 21295, 21296
Muscle Flap......................... 15733

Massively Parallel Sequencing (MPS)
See Next Generation Sequencing (NGS) and Other Molecular Multianalyte Assays

Mastectomy
Gynecomastia........................ 19300
Modified Radical...................... 19307
Partial 19301, 19302
Radical 19303-19306
Simple, Complete 19303
Subcutaneous 19304
with Axillary Lymphadenectomy.......... 19302

Mastectomy, Halsted
See Mastectomy, Radical

Index

Mastoid
Excision
Complete . . . 69502
Debridement . . . 69220
Radical . . . 69511
Modified . . . 69505
Petrous Apicectomy . . . 69530
Simple . . . 69501
Obliteration . . . 69670
Repair
by Excision . . . 69601-69603
Fistula . . . 69700
with Apicectomy . . . 69605
with Tympanoplasty . . . 69604

Mastoid Cavity
Debridement . . . 69220-69222

Mastoidectomy
Osseointegrated Implant
for External Speech Processor/Cochlear Stimulator . . . 69715, 69718
with Apicectomy . . . 69605
with Labyrinthectomy . . . 69910
with Skull Base Surgery . . . 61591, 61597
Decompression . . . 61595
Facial Nerve . . . 61595
with Tympanoplasty . . . 69604, 69641-69646
Cochlear Device Implantation . . . 69930
Complete . . . 69502
Revision . . . 69601
Ossicular Chain Reconstruction . . . 69605
Radical . . . 69511
Modified . . . 69505
Revision . . . 69602, 69603
Simple . . . 69501
with Labyrinthectomy . . . 69910
with Petrous Apicectomy . . . 69530

Mastoidotomy . . . 69635-69637
with Tympanoplasty . . . 69635
Ossicular Chain Reconstruction . . . 69636
and Synthetic Prosthesis . . . 69636

Mastoids
Polytomography . . . 76101, 76102
X ray . . . 70120-70130

Mastopexy . . . 19316

Mastotomy
Drainage of Abscess . . . 19020
Exploration . . . 19020

Maternity Care
See Abortion; Cesarean Delivery; Ectopic Pregnancy; Obstetrical Care

Maternity Care and Delivery . . . 59612-59622, 59898

Maxilla
See Facial Bones; Mandible
Bone Graft . . . 21210, 21348
CT Scan . . . 70486-70488
Cyst
Excision . . . 21030, 21048, 21049
Excision . . . 21030, 21032-21034
Cyst . . . 21030, 21048, 21049
Torus Palatinus . . . 21032
Tumor . . . 21030, 21034, 21048, 21049
Fracture
Closed Treatment . . . 21345, 21421
Open Treatment . . 21346-21348, 21422, 21423
with Fixation . . . 21345-21347, 21435, 21485
Osteotomy . . . 21206
Reconstruction
with Implant . . . 21245, 21246, 21248, 21249
Tumor
Excision . . . 21030, 21048, 21049

Maxillary Arteries
See Artery, Maxillary

Maxillary Sinus
See Sinus/Sinuses, Maxillary

Maxillary Torus Palatinus
Excision . . . 21032

Maxillectomy . . . 31225-31230
Partial . . . 21049
with Craniofacial Procedures . . . 61581

Maxillofacial Fixation
See Fixation (Device), Maxillofacial

Maxillofacial Impressions
Auricular Prosthesis . . . 21086
Facial Prosthesis . . . 21088
Mandibular Resection Prosthesis . . . 21081
Nasal Prosthesis . . . 21087
Obturator Prosthesis
Definitive . . . 21080
Interim . . . 21079
Surgical . . . 21076
Oral Surgical Splint . . . 21085
Orbital Prosthesis . . . 21077
Palatal Prosthesis
Augmentation . . . 21082
Lift . . . 21083
Speech Aid Prosthesis . . . 21084

Maxillofacial Procedures
Fixation
See Fixation (Device), Maxillofacial
Reconstruction
See Face, Reconstruction
Unlisted Services and Procedures . . . 21299

Maxillofacial Prosthetics . . . 21076-21088
Impressions
See Maxillofacial Impressions
Unlisted Services and Procedures . . . 21089

Maydl Operation . . . 45563, 50810
See Colostomy

Mayo Hernia Repair . . . 49582

Mayo Procedure . . . 28292

Maze Procedure
Endoscopic . . . 33265, 33266
Open . . . 33254-33256

McBride Procedure . . . 28292

McBurney Operation . . . 49582

McCannel Procedure . . . 66682

McKissock Surgery . . . 19318

McVay Operation . . . 49582

Measles Uncomplicated
See Rubeola

Measles Vaccine
See Vaccines and Toxoids

Measles, German
See Rubella

Meat Fibers
Feces . . . 89160

Meatoplasty
External Auditory Canal . . . 69310
Urethra . . . 53450, 53460

Meatotomy
Cystourethroscopy . . . 52281
Infant . . . 53025
Prostate
Laser Coagulation . . . 52647
Laser Enucleation . . . 52649
Laser Vaporization . . . 52648
Transurethral Resection . . . 52630
Electrosurgical . . . 52601
with Prostatectomy . . . 55801, 55821
Ureter . . . 52290
Urethral . . . 52285, 53020
Infant . . . 53025

Meckel's Diverticulum
Excision . . . 44800
Unlisted Services and Procedures . . . 44899

Median Nerve
Decompression . . . 64721
Neuroplasty . . . 64721
Release . . . 64721
Repair/Suture
Motor Thenar . . . 64835
Transposition . . . 64721

Median Nerve Compression
See Carpal Tunnel Syndrome

Mediastinal Cyst
See Cyst, Mediastinal; Mediastinum, Cyst

Mediastinoscopy
Biopsy
Mediastinal Lymph Node . . . 39402
Mediastinal Mass . . . 39401

Mediastinotomy
Cervical Approach . . . 39000
Transthoracic Approach . . . 39010

Mediastinum
Cyst
Excision . . . 32662
Resection . . . 39200
Drainage
Image Guided Fluid Collection . . . 49405
Endoscopy
Biopsy . . . 39401, 39402
Excision
Cyst . . . 32662
Mass . . . 32662
Lymph Node . . . 19272, 21632, 32674, 38746
Tumor . . . 32662
Exploration . . . 39000-39010, 60505
Incision and Drainage . . . 39000-39010
Lymph Node
Biopsy
Medianoscopy . . . 39402
Lymphadenectomy . . . 19272, 21632, 32674, 38746
Sampling
Endobronchial Ultrasound (EBUS) Guided . . . 31652, 31653
Mass
Biopsy
Medianoscopy . . . 39401
Needle Biopsy . . . 32405
Excision . . . 32662
Radical Dissection . . . 60522
Removal
Foreign Body . . . 39000-39010

Resection
- Cyst ... 39200
- Tumor ... 39220

Thoracoscopy
- Biopsy ... 32606
- Diagnostic ... 32601
- Excision
  - Cyst ... 32662
  - Mass ... 32662
  - Tumor ... 32662

Tumor
- Excision ... 32662
- Resection ... 39220

Unlisted Procedure ... 39499

Medical Disability Evaluation Services ... 99455, 99456

Medical Genetics ... 96040
Genetic Counseling ... 96040

Medical Team Conference ... 99366-99368

Medical Testimony ... 99075

Medication Therapy Management
Pharmacist Provided ... 99605-99607
Psychiatric ... 90863

Medicine, Preventive
See Preventive Medicine

Medicine, Pulmonary
See Pulmonology

Medulla
Creation of Lesion
- Stereotactic ... 61791

Decompression
- Craniectomy ... 61343

Megacolon
Decompression
- with Colonoscopy ... 45393
- with Sigmoidoscopy ... 45337

Meibomian Cyst
See Chalazion

Membrane Oxygenation, Extracorporeal
See Extracorporeal Membrane Oxygenation (ECMO)

Membrane, Mucous
See Mucosa

Membrane, Tympanic
See Tympanic Membrane

Meninges
Excision
- Tumor ... 61512, 61519

Meningitis, Meningococcal
- Antibody ... 86741
- Vaccine ... 90620, 90621, 90644, 90733, 90734

Repair
- Meningocele ... 63700, 63702
- Myelomeningocele ... 63704, 63706
- Pseudomeningocele ... 63709

Meningioma
Excision ... 61512, 61519

Meningitis, Lymphocytic Benign
See Lymphocytic Choriomeningitis

Meningocele Repair
Meningocele ... 63700, 63702
Myelomeningocele ... 63704, 63706
Pseudomeningocele ... 63709

Meningococcal
See Meninges, Meningitis, Meningococcal

Meningococcal Vaccine
See Meninges, Meningitis, Meningococcal, Vaccine

Meningococcus
See Neisseria Meningitidis

Meningomyelocele
See Myelomeningocele

Meniscectomy
Knee Joint ... 27332, 27333
- Arthroscopic ... 29880, 29881

Temporomandibular Joint ... 21060

Meniscus
Knee
- Excision ... 27332, 27333
  - Arthroscopic ... 29880, 29881
- Lesion
  - Excision ... 27347
- Repair ... 27403
  - Arthroscopic ... 29882, 29883
- Transplantation ... 29868

Mental Nerve
Avulsion ... 64736
Incision ... 64736
Transection ... 64736

Mercury
Qualitative ... 83015
Quantitative ... 83825

Mesenteric Arteries
See Artery, Mesenteric

Mesentery
Lesion
- Excision ... 44820

Repair ... 44850
Suture ... 44850
Unlisted Services and Procedures ... 44899

Mesh
for Exclusion
- Small Intestine from Pelvis ... 44700

Implantation
- Hernia Repair ... 43282, 43333, 43335, 43337, 49652-49654, 49568, 49652-49657

Insertion
- Pelvic Floor ... 57267

Removal
- Abdominal, Infected ... 11008

Metabisulfite Test
See Red Blood Cell (RBC), Sickling

Metabolite
Thromboxane ... 84431

Metacarpal
Amputation ... 26910
Graft ... 26546
Craterization ... 26230
Cyst
- Excision ... 26200, 26205

Diaphysectomy ... 26230
Excision
- Bone ... 26230
- Cyst ... 26200-26205
- Tumor ... 26200-26205

Fracture
- Closed Treatment ... 26600, 26605
  - with Fixation ... 26607
- Open Treatment ... 26615
- Percutaneous Fixation ... 26608
- with Manipulation ... 26605-26607
- without Manipulation ... 26600

Ray Amputation ... 26910
Repair
- Lengthening ... 26568
- Non-union ... 26546
- Osteotomy ... 26565

Resection
- Tumor ... 26250

Saucerization ... 26230
Tumor
- Excision ... 26200-26205
- Radical Resection ... 26250

Metacarpophalangeal Joint
Arthrodesis ... 26850-26852
Arthroplasty ... 26530, 26531
Arthroscopy
- Diagnostic ... 29900
- Surgical ... 29901, 29902
- with Debridement ... 29901

Arthrotomy ... 26075
Biopsy
- Synovium ... 26105, 29900

Capsule
- Excision ... 26520
- Fixation ... 26516-26518
- Incision ... 26520

Capsulodesis ... 26516-26518
Dislocation
- Closed Treatment ... 26700, 26705
- Open Treatment ... 26715
- Percutaneous Fixation ... 26706
- with Manipulation ... 26340

Drainage ... 26075
Exploration ... 26075
Fracture, Articular
- Closed Treatment ... 26740
- Open Treatment ... 26746
- with Manipulation ... 26742

Fusion ... 26516-26518, 26850-26852
Implantation
- Prosthetic
  - Joint ... 26531

Reconstruction
- Collateral Ligament ... 26541, 26542

Removal of Foreign Body ... 26075
Repair
- Collateral Ligament ... 26540

Synovectomy ... 26135

Metadrenaline
See Metanephrines

Metals, Heavy
See Heavy Metal

Metanephrines ... 83835

Metatarsal
See Foot
Amputation ... 28810
Bone Graft ... 20957
- Osteocutaneous ... 20972

Condyle
- Excision ... 28288

Craterization ... 28122
Cyst
- Excision ... 28104-28107

Diaphysectomy ... 28122
Excision ... 28110-28114, 28122, 28140

Index

Fracture
  Closed Treatment
    with Manipulation 28475, 28476
    without Manipulation 28470
  Open Treatment 28485
  Percutaneous Fixation 28476
Microvascular Anastomosis
  Bone Graft 20957
  Free Osteocutaneous Flap 20972
  Repair
    Lengthening 28306-28309
    Nonunion or Malunion 28322
    Osteotomy 28306-28309
    Shortening 28306-28309
  Saucerization 28122
  Sequestrectomy 28122
  Tumor
    Excision 28104-28107
    Radical Resection 28173

Metatarsectomy 28140

Metatarsophalangeal Joint
Amputation 28820
Arthrotomy 28022, 28052
Biopsy 28052
Capsulotomy 28270
Cheilectomy 28289, 28291
Dislocation
  Closed Treatment 28630-28635
  Open Treatment 28645
  Percutaneous Fixation 28636
Drainage 28022
Exploration 28022
Great Toe
  Arthrodesis 28750
  Fusion 28750
Removal
  of Foreign Body 28022
  of Loose Body 28022
Repair
  Hallux Rigidus 28289, 28291
Synovial
  Biopsy 28052
  Excision 28072

Methaemoglobin
See Methemoglobin

Methane Test 91065

Methbipyranone
See Metyrapone

Methemalbumin 83857

Methemoglobin 83045-83050

Methenamine Silver Stain 88312

Methopyrapone
See Metyrapone

Methoxyhydroxymandelic Acid
See Vanillylmandelic Acid

Methyl Alcohol
See Methanol

Methylene Bichloride
See Dichloromethane

Methylfluorprednisolone
See Dexamethasone

Metroplasty
See Hysteroplasty

Metyrapone
Panel 80436

MIC
See Minimum Inhibitory Concentration

Micro-ophthalmia
Orbit Reconstruction 21256

Microalbumin
Urine 82043, 82044

Microbiology 87003-87999

Microbiota, Transplantation Fecal Matter 44705

Microdissection 88380, 88381

Microfluidic Analysis 83861

Microfluorometries, Flow
See Flow Cytometry

Microglobulin, Beta 2
Blood 82232
Urine 82232

Micrographic Surgery
Mohs Technique 17311-17315

Micrographic Surgery, Mohs
See Mohs Micrographic Surgery

Micropigmentation
Correction 11920-11922

Microsatellite Instability Analysis 81301

Microscope, Surgical
See Operating Microscope

Microscopic Evaluation
Blood Smear 85007, 85008
Hair 96902
Necropsy 88020, 88025, 88027-88029, 88036, 88037
Surgical Pathology 88302, 88304, 88305, 88307, 88309, 88399
Urinalysis 81015

Microscopies, Electron
See Electron Microscopy

Microscopy
Binocular
  Ear Exam 92504
Reflectance Confocal Microscopy (RCM)
  Lesion 96932
  Skin Imaging 96931-96936
Specular
  Endothelial Cell Analysis 92286

Microsomal Antibody 86376

Microsomia, Hemifacial
See Hemifacial Microsomia

Microsurgery
Operating Microscope 69990

Microvascular Anastomosis
Bone Graft
  Fibula 20955
  Iliac Crest 20956
  Metatarsal 20957
  Other Site 20962
Fascial Flap, Free 15758
Finger Transfer 26555
Intestinal Graft, Free 43116
Jejunum Transfer, Free 43496
Muscle Flap, Free 15756
Myocutaneous Flap
  Breast Reconstruction 19368
  Pharyngeal Wall Resection with Closure 42894
Omental Flap, Free 49906
Osteocutaneous Flap 20969
  Iliac Crest 20970
  Metatarsal 20972
  Great Toe with Web 20973
Skin Flap, Free 15757
Toe Joint, Free 26556
Toe-to-Hand Transfer 26551, 26553, 26554

Microvite A
See Vitamin, A

Microwave Therapy 97024
See Physical Medicine/Therapy/Occupational Therapy

Midbrain
See Brain; Brainstem; Mesencephalon; Skull Base Surgery

Midcarpal Medioccipital Joint
Arthrotomy 25040

Middle Cerebral Artery Velocimetry 76821

Middle Ear
See Ear, Middle Ear

Midface
Reconstruction
  Forehead
    Advancement 21159, 21160, 21172, 21175, 21263
    Alteration 21175
    Entire/Majority 21179, 21180
    with Bone Graft 21145-21160, 21188
    without Bone Graft 21141-21143
  LeFort I 21141-21143, 21145-21147, 21155, 21160
  LeFort II 21150, 21151
  LeFort III 21154, 21155, 21159, 21160

Mile Operation
See Colectomy, Total, Laparoscopic, with Proctectomy

Milia, Multiple
Removal 10040

Miller Procedure 28737

Miller-Abbott Intubation
Introduction 44500
  with Radiological Guidance 74340

Minerva Cast
Application 29040
Removal 29710

Minimum Inhibitory Concentration 87186

Minimum Lethal Concentration 87187

Minnesota Multiphasic Personality Inventory
See MMPI

Miscarriage
Incomplete Abortion 59812
Missed Abortion
  First Trimester 59820
  Second Trimester 59821
Septic Abortion 59830

Missed Abortion
See Abortion

Mitchell Procedure 28296

Mitogen Blastogenesis 86353

Mitral Valve
Closure
Paravalvular Leak . . . 93590, 93592
Incision . . . 33420, 33422
Occlusion
Paravalvular Leak . . . 93590, 93592
Repair . . . 33425-33427
Transcatheter . . . 0345T, 33418, 33419
Replacement . . . 33430
Transcatheter Mitral Valve Implantation/Replacement (TMVI) . . . 0483T, 0484T

Mitrofanoff Operation . . . 50845

Miyagawanella
See Chlamydia

MLC
See Lymphocyte, Culture

MMR Shots . . . 90707
See Vaccines and Toxoids

Mobilization
Conjunctiva . . . 65272, 65273
Cranium . . . 61595-61597, 61590, 61591
Intestine . . . 43108, 43113, 43118, 43123, 43361
Nerve . . . 64874
Splenic Flexure . . . 44139
Laparoscopic . . . 44213
Stapes . . . 69650
Urethra . . . 54300, 54326, 54344

Moderate Sedation
See Sedation

Modified Radical Mastectomy
See Mastectomy, Modified Radical

Mohs Micrographic Surgery 17311-17315

Molar Pregnancy
See Hydatidiform Mole

Mold
Cast . . . 29450
Culture . . . 87107

Mole, Carneous
See Abortion

Mole, Hydatid
See Hydatidiform Mole

Molecular Cytogenetics . . . 88271-88275
Interpretation and Report . . . 88291

Molecular Diagnostics
Reverse Transcription and Amplified Probe
Central Nervous System Pathogen . . . 87483
Enterovirus . . . 87498
Hepatitis C . . . 87521
HIV-1 . . . 87535
HIV-2 . . . 87538
Reverse Transcription and Quantification
Hepatitis C . . . 87522
HIV-1 . . . 87536
HIV-2 . . . 87539

Molecular Oxygen Saturation
See Oxygen Saturation

Molecular Pathology . . . 81161, 81200-81383, 81400-81408
See Gene Analysis
Unlisted Procedure . . . 81479

Molecular Probes . . . 88120

Molluscum Contagiosum
Destruction . . . 17110, 17111, 46900, 46910, 46916, 46917, 54050-54065
Excision
Anus . . . 46922
Penis . . . 54060

Monilia
See Candida

Monitoring
Ablation Therapy
Incompetent Vein . . . 0524T, 36473-36476, 36478, 36479, 36482, 36483
Parenchymal Tissue
Computed Tomography . . . 77013
Magnetic Resonance . . . 77022
Ultrasound . . . 76940
Renal Mass . . . 50250, 50542
ACE/ARB Therapy . . . 4188F
Anticonvulsant Therapy . . . 4191F
Blood Pressure, 24 Hour . . . 93784-93790
by Arterial Catheterization . . . 36620
Cardiac
Cardiovascular Physiologic Monitor System . . . 93290, 93297
Ischemia Monitoring System . . . 0525T-0532T
Subcutaneous Cardiac Rhythm Monitor System . . . 93285, 93291, 93298, 93299
Digoxin Therapy . . . 4189F
Diuretic Therapy . . . 4190F
ESRD . . . 90951-90959, 90963-90965
Electrocardiogram
See Electrocardiography
Electroencephalogram . . . 95812, 95813, 95950-95953, 95956
with Drug Activation . . . 95954
with Physical Activation . . . 95954
with WADA Activation . . . 95958
Fetal
During Labor . . . 59050, 59051, 99500
Interpretation Only . . . 59051
Magnetic Cardiac Signal . . . 0475T-0478T
Glucose
Home Device . . . 82962
Interstitial Fluid . . . 95249-95251
Tolerance Test . . . 82951, 82952
Hemodynamic
Pulmonary Artery Pressure . . . 33289, 93264
Interstitial Fluid Pressure . . . 20950
Intraocular Pressure . . . 0329T
Neurological
Arterial Occlusion . . . 61623
Neurophysiologic
Intraoperative . . . 95940, 95941
Pediatric Apnea . . . 94774-94777
Physiologic Parameters
Remote . . . 99453, 99454
Treatment Management Services . . . 99457
Retinal Disease . . . 92228
Seizure . . . 0381T-0386T, 61531-61533, 61760
with Contrast
Biliary Drainage . . . 47533-47540
Catheter . . . 75984, 93503

Monitoring, Sleep . . . 95800, 95801
See Polysomnography

Monoethylene Glycol
See Ethylene Glycol

Mononuclear Cell Antigen . . . 86356

Mononucleosis Virus, Infectious
See Epstein-Barr Virus

Monophosphate, Adenosine
See Adenosine Monophosphate (AMP)

Monophosphate, Adenosine Cyclic
See Cyclic AMP

Monospot Test
See Rapid Test for Infection

Monoxide, Carbon
Diffusing Capacity . . . 94729

Monteggia Fracture . . . 24620-24635

Monticelli Procedure
See Application, Bone Fixation Device

Morbilli
See Rubeola

Morphometric Analysis
Computer-Assisted . . . 88367, 88373, 88374
Manual . . . 88368, 88369, 88377
Nerve . . . 88356
Skeletal Muscle . . . 88355
Tumor . . . 88358-88361
Urinary Tract Specimen . . . 88120, 88121

Morton's Neuroma
Excision . . . 28080

Mosaicplasty . . . 27416

Mosenthal Test
See Urinalysis, Routine

Mother Cell
See Stem Cell

Motility Study
Colon . . . 91117
Duodenal . . . 91022
Esophagus . . . 91010
with Perfusion . . . 91013
with Stimulation . . . 91013
Imaging . . . 78258
Sperm . . . 89300

Motion Analysis
by Video and 3-D Kinematics . . . 96000, 96004
Computer-based . . . 96000, 96004
Movement Disorder Monitoring . . . 0533T-0536T

Motion Management Simulation
Respiratory . . . 77293

Mouth
Abscess
Incision and Drainage . . . 40800, 40801, 41005-41009, 41015-41018
Biopsy . . . 40808, 41108
Cyst
Incision and Drainage . . . 40800, 40801, 41005-41009, 41015-41018
Excision
Frenum . . . 40819
Gums
See Gums
Hematoma
Incision and Drainage . . . 40800, 40801, 41005-41009, 41015-41018
Lesion
Destruction . . . 40820
Excision . . . 40810-40816, 41116
Vestibule
Destruction . . . 40820
Lips
See Lip
Mucosa
Donor Excision . . . 40818
Lesion
Excision . . . 40810, 40812, 40814, 40816
Reconstruction . . . 40840-40845

Removal
Foreign Body 40804, 40805
Repair
Laceration 40830, 40831, 41250, 41252
Resection
with Glossectomy 41150, 41153, 41155
Skin Graft
Dermal Autograft 15135, 15136
Epidermal Autograft 15115, 15116
Recipient Site Preparation 15004, 15005
Skin Substitute 15275-15278
Split-Thickness 15120, 15121
Tissue-cultured Autograft 15155-15157
Tongue
See Tongue
Unlisted Services and Procedures . . . 40899, 41599
Vestibule
Biopsy 40808
Destruction
Lesion 40820
Scar 40820
Excision
Frenum 40819
Incision and Drainage
Abscess 40800, 40801
Cyst 40800, 40801
Hematoma 40800, 40801
Removal
Foreign Body 40804, 40805
Repair 40830-40845
Unlisted Procedures 40899
Wound Repair 13131-13133

Move
See Transfer
Finger 26555
Toe Joint 26556
Toe to Hand 26551-26554

MPD Syndrome
See Temporomandibular Joint (TMJ)

MPR
See Multifetal Pregnancy Reduction

MR Spectroscopy
See Magnetic Resonance Spectroscopy

MRA
See Magnetic Resonance Angiography (MRA)

MRI
See Magnetic Resonance Imaging (MRI)
See Multiple Sleep Latency Testing (MSLT)

Mucin
Synovial Fluid 83872

Mucocele
Sinusotomy
Frontal 31075

Mucopolysaccharides 83864

Mucormycoses
See Mucormycosis

Mucormycosis
Antibody 86732

Mucosa
Ablation
Turbinates 30801, 30802
Advancement
Lip 40500
Urethra 53450
Biopsy
Vaginal 57100-57105
Gross and Microscopic Examination
Oral 88305
Nasal 88305
Vaginal 88302
Ectopic Gastric Imaging 78290
Excision
Alveolar, Hyperplastic 41828
Vestibule of Mouth, Donor 40818
Fulguration
Hypertrophic Folds
Urethra 52400
Lesion
Ablation
Vestibule of Mouth 40810-40818
Photodynamic Therapy . . . 96567, 96573, 96574
Periodontal Grafting 41870
Polyp
Sinus
Removal 31051
Stripping
Sinus 31051
Resection
Endoscopy 43211
Hypertrophic Folds
Urethra 52400
Turbinates
Ablation 30801, 30802
Vaginal
Biopsy 57100, 57105

Mucosa, Buccal
See Mouth, Mucosa

Mucous Cyst
Tendon Sheath/Joint Capsule
Excision
Hand or Finger 26160

Mucous Membrane
See Mouth, Mucosa
Excision
Benign Lesion 11440-11446
Malignant Lesion 11640-11646
Layer Closure, Wounds 12051-12057
Simple Repair, Wounds 12011-12018
Excision
Sphenoid Sinus 31288
Graft
Buccal 67835, 68325, 68328, 68335
Lesion
Destruction 17000-17004, 17280-17286
Excision
Benign 11440-11446
Malignant 11640-11646
Shaving 11310-11313
Rectum
Proctoplasty for Prolapse 45505
Repair
Trichiasis 67835
Wound
Superficial 12011, 12013-12018
Intermediate 12051-12057
Tests
Nasal 95065
Ophthalmic 95060
Unlisted Procedure 17999

Mucus Cyst
See Mucous Cyst

MUGA (Multiple Gated Acquisition) 78472, 78473, 78483

Muller Procedure
See Sleep Study

Multianalyte Assays with Algorithmic Analyses
Autoimmune
DNA Antibody, High Avidity 0039U
Rheumatoid Arthritis 81490
Cardiology
Heart Transplant 0055U, 81595
Chemistry
Glycosylated Acute Phase Proteins 0024U
Tenofovir 0025U
Vitamin D, 25 Hydroxy D2 and D3 . . . . . 0038U
Coronary Artery Disease 81493
Drug Testing
Interactions 0006U
Prescription Drug Monitoring 0011U, 0051U, 0054U
Drug Metabolism 0029U, 0030U
Drug Test, Presumptive 0007U, 0020U
Endocrinology 81506
Fetal
Congenital Abnormalities 81508-81512
Fetal Aneuploidy 0009M, 81507
Twin Zygosity 0060U
Germline Disorders
COMT (catechol-O-methyltransferase) . . 0032U
CYP1A2 (cytochrome P450 family 1, subfamily A, member 2) 0031U
CYP2D6 (cytochrome P450, family 2, subfamily D, polypeptide 6) 0028U
Exome (Somatic Mutations) 0036U
FLT3 (fms-related tyrosine kinase 3) 0046U
Gene Rearrangement Detection 0012U
HTR2A (5-hydroxytryptamine receptor 2A) 0033U
JAK2 (Janus kinase 2) 0027U
NPM1 (nucleophosmin) 0049U
TPMT (thiopurine S-methyltransferase) 0034U
Hematology
Hematolymphoid Neoplasia 0014U
Red Blood Cell Antigen Typing 0001U
ctHb1, ctHb2, ctHbO2, ctHbR, StO2 . . . . . 0061U
Infectious Disease
Bacterial, Strain Typing 0010U
Borrelia burgdorferi, Antibody Detection 0041U-0044U
Hepatitis C Virus 81596
Lipoprotein 0052U
Liver Disease 0002M, 0003M
Microbiology
Helicobacter Pilori Detection 0008U
Oncology
Acute Myelogenous Leukemia 0023U, 0050U, 0056U
Breast . . . 0009U, 0040U, 0045U, 81518-81521
Colon 81525
Colorectal 0002U, 81528
Gastrointestinal Neuroendocrine 0007M
Gynecologic 81535, 81536
Hematolymphoid Neoplasia 0016U
Hematolymphoidneoplasia 0017U
Liver 0006M
Lung 0022U, 81538
Merkel Cell Carcinoma 0058U, 0059U
Ovarian 0003U, 81500, 81503
Prostate 0005U, 0011M, 0021U, 0047U, 0053U, 81539, 81541, 81551
RNA 0019U
Solid Organ Neoplasm . . 0037U, 0048U, 0057U
Thyroid 0018U, 0026U, 81545
Tissue of Origin 81504

Tumor of Unknown Origin 81540
Urothelial 0012M, 0013M
Neurology
Prion Disease 0035U
Scoliosis 0004M
Unlisted Multianalyte Assay with Algorithmic Analysis 81599

Multifetal Pregnancy Reduction ... 59866

Multiple Sleep Latency Testing (MSLT) 95805

Multiple Valve Procedures
See Valvuloplasty

Mumford Operation
See Claviculectomy, Open, Partial

Mumford Procedure 29824

Mumps
Antibody 86735
Immunization 90707, 90710
Vaccine
MMR 90707
MMRV 90710

Muramidase 85549

Murine Typhus 86000

Muscle
See specific muscle
Abdomen
See Abdomen, Abdominal Wall
Biofeedback Training
Perineal 90911
Biopsy 20200-20206
Extraocular 67346
Needle 20206
Chemodenervation 64612, 64615-64617, 64642-64647, 67345
Guidance 95873, 95874
Compartment Syndrome
Detection 20950
Cutting
Pyloric 43520
Debridement 11011, 11012, 11043, 11044, 11046, 11047
Infected 11004-11006
Nonviable 25023, 25025, 27057, 27497, 27499
Leg 27892-27894
Delivery
Thermal Energy
for Gastroesophageal Reflux Disease 43257
Division
See Muscle Division
Excision
Lip 40816
Pectoral 19305-19307
Fasciotomy
See Fasciotomy
Flaps
Fasciocutaneous 15733, 15734, 15736, 15738
Muscle, Free 15842
with Microvascular
Anastomosis 15756, 42894
Myocutaneous 15733, 15734, 15736, 15738, 61619
Grafts
Muscle, Free 15841, 25265, 25274
Heart
See Myocardium
Imbrication
Anus 46761
Implantation
Eye 65105, 65140, 65155
Nerve to Muscle 64787
Incision
Esophagus 32665, 43130, 43279, 43330, 43331
Hyoid 21685
Pharynx 43030, 43130
Pylorus 43520
Injection 20552, 20553
Masseter, Reduction
See Masseter Muscle/Bone
Interstitial Fluid Pressure
Monitoring 20950
Neck
See Neck Muscle
Neurectomy
Hamstring 27325
Placement
Catheter
Interstitial Radioelement Application .. 20555
Range of Motion
See Range of Motion Test
Redirection/Rerouting/Repositioning
Extraocular 67320
Leg, Lower 27690, 27691
Leg, Upper 27396, 27397
Mouth 40845
Release
Foot 28240
Hand 26508, 26593
Hip 27036
Knee 27422
Removal
Foreign Body 20520-20525
Repair
Arm, Upper 24341
Blepharoptosis 67901-67908
Elbow 24341
Extraocular 65290, 67311-67316, 67334, 67340, 67346
Forearm 25260-25274
Frontalis Technique 67901, 67902
Hand 26591, 26593
Wrist 25260-25274
Revision
Arm, Upper 24330, 24331
Suspension
Hyoid 21685
Suture
Hamstring 27385
Quadriceps 27385
Testing
See Muscle Testing
Transfer
Arm, Upper 24301, 24320
Elbow 24301
Femur 27110
Hand 26494
Hip 27100-27105, 27111
Regional 15845
Rotator Cuff 23410, 23412
Shoulder 23395-23397, 24301, 24320, 23410, 23412
Thigh 27400
Transplant
Anus 46760
Unlisted Extraocular Muscle Procedure 67399

Muscle Compartment Syndrome
Detection 20950

Muscle Denervation
See Denervation

Muscle Division
Plantar 28250
Scalenus Anticus 21700-21705
Sternocleidomastoid 21720-21725

Muscle Flaps 15731-15738
Fasciocutaneous 15733, 15734, 15736, 15738
Muscle, Free 15842
with Microvascular
Anastomosis 15756, 42894
Myocutaneous 15733, 15734, 15736, 15738, 61619

Muscle Grafts
Free 15841, 25265, 25274

Muscle Testing
Dynamometry, Eye 92260
Electromyography
See Electromyography
Extraocular Multiple Muscles 92265
Ischemic Limb 95875
Manual 95831-95834
Range of Motion
See Range of Motion Test
Reflex
See Reflex Test

Muscle, Oculomotor
See Eye Muscles

Muscles
See Muscle

Musculo-Skeletal System
See Musculoskeletal System

Musculoplasty
See Muscle, Repair

Musculoskeletal System
Computer-Assisted Surgical Navigation 0054T, 0055T, 20985
Unlisted Services and Procedures 20999, 24999, 25999, 26989, 27299, 27599, 27899
Unlisted Services and Procedures, Head 21499

Musculotendinous (Rotator) Cuff
Repair 23410-23412

Mustard Procedure
See Repair, Great Arteries; Revision

Myasthenia Gravis
Cholinesterase Inhibitor Challenge Test 95857

Myasthenic, Gravis
See Myasthenia Gravis

Mycobacteria
Culture 87116
Identification 87118
Detection 87550-87562
Sensitivity Studies 87190

Mycophenolate (mycophenolic acid)
Drug Assay 80180

Mycoplasma
Antibody 86738
Culture 87109
Detection 87580-87582

Mycota
See Fungus

Myectomy, Anorectal
See Myomectomy, Anorectal

Myelencephalon
See Medulla

Myelin Basic Protein
Cerebrospinal Fluid 83873

Index

Myelography
Brain 70010
Injection Procedure 62284
Spine
Cervical 62302, 62305, 72240
Lumbosacral 62304, 62305, 72265
Thoracic 62303, 62305, 72255
Total 72270

Myelomeningocele
Repair 63704-63706

Myeloperoxidase (MPO) 83876

Myelotomy 63170

Myocardium
Blood Flow
Absolute Quantitation 0482T
Ischemia Assessment
Echocardiography 0439T
Perfusion Imaging 78451-78454
Echocardiography 0439T
Positron Emission Tomography (PET) 78459
Resection 33542
Revascularization 33140, 33141

Myocardial Imaging
Blood Flow
Absolute Quantitation 0482T
Echocardiography
Contrast Perfusion 0439T
for Strain
Quantitative Assessment of Myocardial Mechanics 0399T
Infarct Avid 78466-78469
Magnetocardiography 0541T, 0542T
Metabolic Evaluation
PET 78459
Perfusion Study
Nuclear Medicine
Planar 78453, 78454
PET 78491, 78492
SPECT 78451, 78452
Repair
Postinfarction 33542
Sympathetic Innervation 0331T, 0332T

Myocutaneous Flaps 15731-15738, 15756

Myofascial Pain Dysfunction Syndrome
See Temporomandibular Joint (TMJ)

Myofibroma
See Leiomyomata

Myoglobin 83874

Myomectomy
Anorectal 45108
Uterus 58140-58146
Laparoscopic 58545, 58546

Myoplasty
See Muscle, Repair

Myotomy
Cricopharangeal 43180
Esophagus 32665, 43130, 43180, 43279, 43330, 43331
Hyoid 21685
Pharynx 43030, 43130
Pylorus 43520

Myringoplasty 69620

Myringostomy
See Myringotomy

Myringotomy 69420, 69421

Myxoid Cyst
See Ganglion

N

N. Meningitidis
See Neisseria Meningitidis

Naffziger Operation
See Decompression, Orbit; Section

Nagel Test
See Color Vision Examination

Nail Bed
Reconstruction 11762
Repair 11760

Nail Fold
Excision
Wedge 11765

Nail Plate Separation
See Nails, Avulsion

Nails
Avulsion 11730-11732
Biopsy 11755
Debridement 11720, 11721
Drainage 10060, 10061
Evacuation
Hematoma, Subungual 11740
Excision 11750
KOH Examination 87220
Reconstruction 11762
Removal 11730-11732, 11750
Trimming 11719

Narcosynthesis
Diagnostic and Therapeutic 90865

Nasal Abscess
See Nose, Abscess

Nasal Area
Bone Graft 21210

Nasal Bleeding
See Epistaxis

Nasal Bone
Bone Graft 21210
Fracture
Closed Treatment 21310-21320
Open Treatment 21325-21335
with Manipulation 21315-21320
without Manipulation 21310
Reconstruction
See Rhinoplasty
X ray 70160

Nasal Deformity
Repair 40700-40761

Nasal Function Study 92512

Nasal Polyp
See Nose, Polyp

Nasal Prosthesis
Impression 21087

Nasal Septum
Abscess
Incision and Drainage 30020
Fracture
Closed Treatment 21337
Open Treatment 21336
Hematoma
Incision and Drainage 30020
Insertion
Button Prosthesis 30220
Repair 30630
Septoplasty 30520
Submucous Resection 30520

Nasal Sinuses
See Sinus/Sinuses

Nasal Smear
Eosinophils 89190

Nasal Turbinate
Fracture
Therapeutic 30930

Nasoethmoid Complex
Fracture
Open Treatment 21338, 21339
Percutaneous Treatment 21340
Reconstruction 21182-21184

Nasogastric Tube
Placement 43752

Nasolacrimal Duct
Dilation 68816
Exploration 68810
with Anesthesia 68811
Insertion
Catheter 68816
Stent 68815
Tube 68815
Repair 21340
X ray
with Contrast 70170

Nasomaxillary
Fracture
Closed Treatment 21345
Open Treatment 21346-21348
with Bone Grafting 21348

Nasopharynges
See Nasopharynx

Nasopharyngoscopy 92511

Nasopharynx
See Pharynx
Biopsy
Lesion 42804-42806
Hemorrhage 42970-42972
Unlisted Services and Procedures 42999

Natriuretic Peptide 83880

Natural Killer (NK) Cells
Count 86357

Natural Ostium
Sinus
Maxillary 31000
Sphenoid 31002

Navicular Bone
Carpal
Arthroplasty
with Implant 25443
Fracture
Closed Treatment 25622
Open Treatment 25628
with Manipulation 25624
Repair
Nonunion 25431, 25440
Tarsal
Arthrodesis 28737
Excision 28238

Navigation
Computer Assisted Procedures
Bronchoscopy 31627
Cranial 61781, 61782
Musculoskeletal. . . . 20985
Orthopedic 0054T, 0055T
Spinal. . . . 61783

Neck
Angiography 70498, 70547-70549
Artery
Ligation 37615
Biopsy 21550
Bypass Graft 35901
CT Scan. . . . 70490-70492, 70498
with PET Scan 78814
Dissection, Radical
See Radical Neck Dissection
Exploration
Blood Vessel 35800
Lymph Nodes 38542
Incision and Drainage
Abscess 21501, 21502
Hematoma 21501, 21502
Lipectomy, Suction Assisted. . . . 15876
Magnetic Resonance Angiography (MRA) 70547-70549
Magnetic Resonance Imaging (MRI) 70540-70543
Muscle
Chemodenervation. . . . 64616
Nerve
Graft. . . . 64885, 64886
Nuclear Medicine
Thyroid Carcinoma Imaging. . . . 78015
PET Scan 78811
with CT Scan 78814
Repair
Blood Vessel 35201
with Other Graft. . . . 35261
with Vein Graft. . . . 35231
Rhytidectomy 15828
Skin
Graft 15240, 15241
Revision 15819
Tissue Transfer
Adjacent. . . . 14040, 14041
Flap. . . . 15574, 15620
Tumor
Excision 21552-21558
Radical Resection 21557, 21558
Ultrasound Exam. . . . 76536
Unlisted Services and Procedures, Surgery . . 21899
Urinary Bladder
See Bladder, Neck
Wound
Exploration. . . . 20100
Repair. . . . 13131-13133
X ray 70360

Neck Muscle
Division
Scalenus Anticus 21700-21705
Sternocleidomastoid 21720-21725

Necropsy
Coroner's Exam. . . . 88045
Forensic Exam. . . . 88040
Gross and Micro Exam 88020-88029
Gross Exam. . . . 88000-88016
Organ. . . . 88037
Regional 88036
Unlisted Services and Procedures 88099

Needle Biopsy
See Biopsy
Abdomen Mass. . . . 49180
Bone 20220-20225
Bone Marrow 38221, 38222
Breast 19100
Bronchi 31629, 31633
Colon
Endoscopy 45392
Colon-Sigmoid
Endoscopy 45342
CT Scan Guidance. . . . 77012
Epididymis. . . . 54800
Esophagus
Endoscopy 43232
Fluoroscopic Guidance 77002
Gastrointestinal, Upper
Endoscopy 43238, 43242
Intervertebral Disc 62267
Kidney 50200
Liver. . . . 47000, 47001
Lung. . . . 32405
Lymph Nodes 38505
Mediastinum. . . . 32405
Muscle 20206
Nucleus Pulposus 62267
Pancreas 48102
Paravertebral Tissue. . . . 62267
Pleura 32400
Prostate. . . . 55700
Transperineal. . . . 55706
Retroperitoneal Mass. . . . 49180
Salivary Gland. . . . 42400
Spinal Cord 62269
Testis. . . . 54500
Thyroid Gland 60100
Transbronchial 31629, 31633

Needle Localization
Breast
with Lesion Excision 19125, 19126
CT Guidance 77012
Fluoroscopic Guidance 77002
Spine 77003
Magnetic Resonance Imaging Guidance 77021
Ultrasonic Guidance 76942

Needle Manometer Technique 20950

Needle Wire
Introduction
Trachea 31730

Neer Procedure. . . . 23470

Negative Pressure Wound Therapy. . . . 97605-97608

Neisseria Gonorrhoeae . . 87590-87592, 87850

Neisseria Meningitidis
Antibody 86741

Neobladder
Construction 51596

Neonatal Critical Care
See Newborn Care
Initial. . . . 99468
Subsequent. . . . 99469

Neoplasm
Cancer Photoradiation Therapy
See Photochemotherapy
Cardiac
See Heart, Tumor
Colon
See Colon, Tumor
Esophageal
See Tumor, Esophagus
Spinal Cord
See Spinal Cord, Neoplasm
Unspecified Nature of Brain
See Brain, Tumor

Neoplastic Growth
See Tumor

Nephelometry 83883

Nephrectomy
Donor. . . . 50300-50320, 50547
Laparoscopic. . . . 50545-50548
Partial 50240
Laparoscopic 50543
Recipient. . . . 50340
with Ureters 50220-50236, 50546, 50548

Nephrolith
See Calculus, Removal, Kidney

Nephrolithotomy. . . . 50060-50075

Nephropexy 50400-50405

Nephroplasty
See Kidney, Repair

Nephropyeloplasty
See Pyeloplasty

Nephrorrhaphy 50500

Nephroscopy
See Endoscopy, Kidney

Nephrostogram
Injection Procedure. . . . 50430, 50431
with Catheter Conversion
Nephrostomy to Nephroureteral 50434
with Nephrostomy Catheter Exchange. . . . 50435
with Placement of Ureteral Stent. . . . 50693-50695

Nephrostolithotomy
Percutaneous 50080, 50081

Nephrostomy
Change Catheter. . . . 50434, 50435
Insertion
Guide Wire. . . . 52334
Placement of Catheter 50432
with Drainage. . . . 50040
with Pyeloplasty 50400

Nephrostomy Tract
Establishment. . . . 52334

Nephrotomogram
See Nephrotomography

Nephrotomography. . . . 74415

Nephrotomy 50040-50045
with Drainage. . . . 50040
with Exploration 50045

Nerve
Axillary
See Axillary Nerve
Biopsy. . . . 64795
Block
See Injection, Anesthetic Agent
Cryoablation
Percutaneous 0440T-0442T
Cranial
See Cranial Nerve
Facial
See Facial Nerve
Intercostal
See Intercostal Nerve

Lingual
  See Lingual Nerve
Median
  See Median Nerve
Neuroma
  Excision
    Cutaneous....64774
    Digital....64776, 64778
    Foot, Other than Digital....64782, 64783
    Hand, Other than Digital....64782, 64783
    Peripheral....64784
    Sciatic....64786
Obturator
  See Obturator Nerve
Peripheral
  See Peripheral Nerve
Phrenic
  See Phrenic Nerve
Sciatic
  See Sciatic Nerve
Spinal
  See Spinal Nerve
Tibial
  See Tibial, Nerve
Ulnar
  See Ulnar Nerve
Vestibular
  See Vestibular Nerve

Nerve Block
See Injection, Anesthetic Agent

Nerve Conduction
Motor/Sensory Nerve....95905, 95907-95913

Nerve Graft
Additional Nerve....64901, 64902
Arm or Leg....64892, 64893, 64897, 64898
Foot or Hand....64890, 64891, 64895, 64896
Head or Neck....64885, 64886
Neurovascular Pedicle....15750
Pedicle....64905, 64907

Nerve Root
See Cauda Equina; Spinal Cord
Decompression....0375T, 22856, 22858, 63020-63048, 63055-63103
Incision....63185-63190
Section....63185-63190

Nerve Stimulation, Transcutaneous
See Application, Neurostimulation

Nerve Teasing....88362

Nerve II, Cranial
See Optic Nerve

Nerve V, Cranial
See Trigeminal Nerve

Nerve VII, Cranial
See Facial Nerve

Nerve X, Cranial
See Vagus Nerve

Nerve XI, Cranial
See Accessory Nerve, Spinal

Nerve XII, Cranial
See Hypoglossal Nerve

Nerves
Anastomosis
  Facial to Hypoglossal....64868
  Facial to Spinal Accessory....64866
Avulsion....64732-64772
Biopsy....64795
Closure
  Amputation, Ankle....27888
Decompression....64702-64727
  Cranial....61458, 61460
  Laminotomy/Laminectomy....0274T, 0275T
Denervation....27035
Destruction....64600-64681
Excision
  See Neurectomy
Graft....64885-64902
Implantation
  Electrode Array....64553-64581
  to Bone....64787
  to Muscle....64787
Incision....28035, 43640, 43641, 64732-64772
Injection
  Anesthetic....01991, 01992, 64400-64530
Diagnostic Agent....0213T, 64493-64495
  Neurolytic Agent....64600-64681
  Therapeutic Agent....0213T, 64490-64495
Insertion
  Electrode Array....64553-64581
Lesion
  Excision....64774-64792
Neurofibroma
  Excision....64788-64792
Neurolemmoma
  Excision....64788-64792
Neurolytic
  Internal....64727
Neuroma
  Destruction....64632
  Excision....64774-64786
  Injection....64455
Neuroplasty....64702-64721
Pedicle Transfer....64905, 64907
Removal
  Electrode Array....64585
Repair
  Allograft....64910, 64912, 64913
  Autogenous Graft....64911
  Microdissection....69990
  Suture....64831-64876
  Synthetic Conduit....64910
Revision
  Electrode Array....64585
Spinal Accessory
  Incision....63191
  Section....63191
Suture....64831-64876
Sympathectomy
  Excision....64802-64818
Transection....64732-64772
Vagus Nerve....43640, 43641
  Laparoscopic....43651, 43652
Transposition....64718-64721
Unlisted Services and Procedures....64999

Nervous System
Central Nervous System Pathogen
  Nucleic Acid Detection....87483
Extracranial, Peripheral Nerves and Autonomic Nervous System
  Avulsion....64732-64772
  Destruction....64600-64681
  Excision....64774-64823
  Injection....64400-64530
  Neurorrhaphy....64831-64911
  Neuroplasty....64702-64727
  Neurostimulation
    See Neurostimulators
  Transection....64732-64772
Nuclear Medicine
  Unlisted Services and Procedures....78699
Skull, Meninges, and Brain....61000-62258
Spine and Spinal Cord....62263-63746
Unlisted Procedure....64999

Nesidioblast
See Islet Cell

Neural Conduction
See Nerve Conduction

Neural Ganglion
See Ganglion

Neurectomy
Foot....28055
Gastrocnemius....27326
Hamstring Muscle....27325
Hip
  Obturator....27003
Leg, Lower....27326
Leg, Upper....27325
Morton....28080
Popliteal....27326
Tympanic....69676

Neuroendoscopy
Intracranial....62160-62165

Neurofibroma
Destruction
  Extensive....0419T, 0420T
Excision
  Cutaneous Nerve....64788
  Extensive....64792
  Peripheral Nerve....64790

Neurolemmoma
Excision
  Cutaneous Nerve....64788
  Extensive....64792
  Peripheral Nerve....64790

Neurologic System
See Nervous System

Neurology
Brain Cortex Magnetic Stimulation....90867-90869
Brain Mapping....90867, 96020
Brain Surface Electrode Stimulation....95961, 95962
Central Motor
  Motor Function Mapping....64999
  Transcranial Motor Stimulation....95928, 95929
Cognitive Performance....96125
Diagnostic
  Anal Sphincter....51785
  Autonomic Function Tests
    Heart Rate Response....95921, 95943
    Parasympathetic....95943
    Pseudomotor Response....95921-95924
    Sympathetic Function....95921-95924, 95943
    Valsalva Maneuvers....95922, 95943
Electrocorticogram
  from Implanted Brain Neurostimulator....95836
  Intraoperative....61536, 61538, 95829
Electroencephalogram (EEG)
  Brain Death....95824
  Electrode Placement....95830
  Intraoperative....95955
  Monitoring....95812, 95813, 95950-95953, 95956
  Physical or Drug Activation....95954
  Sleep....95800, 95801, 95822, 95827
  Standard....95819
  WADA Activation....95958
Electroencephalography (EEG)
  Digital Analysis....95957

Electromyography
Fine Wire
Dynamic....96004
Ischemic Limb Exercise Test....95875
Needle....51785, 95860-95872
Surface
Dynamic....96002-96004
Evoked Potentials
Auditory....92585, 92586
Central Motor....95928, 95929, 95939
Somatosensory Testing..95925-95927, 95938
Visual....0333T, 0464T, 95930
Higher Cerebral Function
Aphasia Test....96105
Cognitive Performance....96125
Developmental Tests....96110, 96112, 96113
Neurobehavioral Status....96116, 96121
Neuropsychological Testing
Administration and Scoring....96139
Automated Testing and Result....96146
Evaluation Services....96132, 96133
Neurobehavioral Status....96116, 96121
Magnetoencephalography (MEG)....95965-95967
Motion Analysis
by Video and 3-D Kinematics....96000, 96004
Computer-based....96000, 96004
Movement Disorder Monitoring 0533T-0536T
Muscle Testing
Manual....95831-95834
Nerve Conduction
Motor and Sensory Nerve....95905-95913
Neurofunctional Testing....96020
Neuromuscular Junction Tests....95937
Neurophysiological Monitoring
Intraoperative....95940, 95941
Plantar Pressure Measurements
Dynamic....96001, 96004
Polysomnography....95782, 95783, 95808-95811
Range of Motion....95851, 95852
Reflex
Blink Reflex....95933
Sleep Study....95800, 95801, 95805-95811
Actigraphy Testing....95803
Somatosensory Testing....95925-95927, 95938, 95939
Cholinesterase Inhibitor Challenge Test....95857
Therapeutic
Magnetic Stimulation
Transcranial....90867-90869
Unlisted Services and Procedures....95999
Urethral Sphincter....51785

Neurolysis
Internal....64727
with Neuroplasty....64702-64721

Neuroma
Acoustic
See Brain, Tumor, Excision
Excision
Cutaneous Nerve....64774
Digital Nerve....64776-64778
Foot....28080
Foot Nerve....64782, 64783
Hand Nerve....64782, 64783
Peripheral Nerve....64784
Sciatic Nerve....64786
Injection
Anesthetic Agent....64455
Steroid....64455
Interdigital
Morton
Excision....28080

Neuromuscular Junction Tests....95937

Neuromuscular Pedicle
Reinnervation
Larynx....31590

Neuromuscular Reeducation....97112
See Physical Medicine/Therapy/Occupational Therapy

Neurophysiologic Testing
Autonomic Nervous Function
Heart Rate Response....95921-95924
Pseudomotor Response....95921-95924
Sympathetic Function....95921-95924
Intraoperative....95940, 95941

Neuroplasty
Cranial Nerve....64716
Digital Nerve....64702, 64704
Peripheral Nerve....64708, 64712-64714, 64716, 64718, 64719, 64721
Arm....64708
Brachial Plexus....64713
Cranial....64716
Leg....64708
Lumbar Plexus....64714
Median at Carpal Tunnel....64721
Sciatic....64712
Ulnar at Elbow....64718
Ulnar at Wrist....64719

Neuropsychological Testing
Administration and Scoring....96139
Automated Testing and Result....96146
Evaluation Services....96130-96133
Computer-Assisted....96146

Neurorrhaphy....64831-64876
Peripheral Nerve
Conduit....64910
with Graft....64885-64907

Neurostimulators
Brain
Electronic Analysis....95970, 95983, 95984
Implantation....61863, 61864, 61867, 61868, 61885, 61886
Removal....61880
Replacement....61885, 61886, 61888
Revision....61880, 61888
Cranial Nerve
Electronic Analysis....95970, 95977
Implantation....64553, 64568
Removal....64570
Replacement....64569
Revision....64569
Gastric Nerve
Electronic Analysis....95980-95982
Implantation/Replacement....43647, 43881, 64590
Revision/Removal....43648, 43882, 64595
Peripheral Nerve
Electronic Analysis....95970-95972
Implantation....64555, 64575, 64580
Removal....64585, 64595
Replacement....64590
Revision....64585, 64595
Sacral Nerve
Electronic Analysis....95970-95972
Implantation....64561, 64581
Spinal Cord
Electronic Analysis....95970-95972
Implantation....63650, 63655
Removal....63661, 63662, 63688
Replacement....63663, 63664, 63685
Revision....63663, 63664, 63688

Phrenic Nerve System for Sleep Apnea
Device Evaluation....0434T-0436T
Insertion....0424T-0427T
Removal....0428T-0430T
Replacement....0424T-0427T, 0431T
Repositioning....0432T, 0433T
Tibia
Percutaneous....64566
Vagus Nerve System for Morbid Obesity
Electronic Analysis/Programming....0317T
Implantation....0312T
Replacement....0313T, 0316T
Removal....0314T, 0315T
Revision....0313T

Neurotomy, Sympathetic
See Gasserian Ganglion, Sensory Root, Decompression

Neurovascular Pedicle Flaps....15750

Neutralization Test
Virus....86382

New Patient
Domiciliary or Rest Home Visit....99324-99328
Emergency Department Services....99281-99288
Home Services....99341-99345
Hospital Inpatient Services....99221-99239
Hospital Observation Services....99217-99220
Initial Office Visit....99201-99205
Inpatient Consultations....99251-99255
Office and/or Other Outpatient Consultations....99241-99245

Newborn Care....99460-99465, 99502
Attendance at Delivery....99464
Blood Transfusion
Exchange....36450, 36456
Push....36440
Circumcision
Clamp or Other Device....54150
Surgical Excision....54160
History and Examination....99460, 99463
Home Visit....99502
Initial Care
Birthing Room....99460, 99463
Hospital....99460, 99463
Other Site....99461
Laryngoscopy....31520
Normal....99460-99463
Prepuce Slitting....54000
Preventive
Office....99461
Resuscitation....99465
Standby for Cesarean Delivery....99360
Subsequent Hospital Care....99462
Umbilical Artery Catheterization....36660

Next Generation Sequencing (NGS) and Other Molecular Multianalyte Assays
Aortic Dysfunction or Dilation....81410, 81411
Exome....81415-81417
Fetal Chromosomal Aneuploidy....81420
Genome....81425-81427
Hearing Loss....81430, 81431
Hereditary Breast Cancer-Related Disorders....81432, 81433
Hereditary Colon Cancer Disorders..81435, 81436
Hereditary Neuroendocrine Tumor Disorders....81437, 81438
Hereditary Retinal Disorders....81434
Noonan Spectrum Disorders....81442
Nuclear Encoded Mitochondrial Genes....81440
Severe Inherited Conditions....81443

Index

Targeted Genomic Sequence Analysis
Panel . . . 81445, 81450, 81455
Whole Mitochondrial Genome . . . 81460, 81465
X-linked Intellectual Disability (XLID) . . . 81470, 81471

Nickel . . . 83885

Nicolas-Durand-Favre Disease
See Lymphogranuloma Venereum

Nidation
See Implantation

Nikaidoh Procedure
Aortic Root Translocation . . . 33782, 33783

Nipples
See Breast
Exploration . . . 19110
Inverted . . . 19355
Lesion
  Excision . . . 19120
Reconstruction . . . 19350

Nissen Operation
See Fundoplasty, Esophagogastric

Nissen Procedure
See Gastroplasty with Esophagogastric Fundoplasty

Nitrate Reduction Test
See Urinalysis

Nitric Oxide
Administration . . . 93463
Expired Gas Determination . . . 95012

Nitroblue Tetrazolium Dye Test . . . 86384

Nitrogen, Blood Urea
See Blood Urea Nitrogen

NMR Imaging
See Magnetic Resonance Imaging (MRI)

NMR Spectroscopies
See Magnetic Resonance Spectroscopy

No Man's Land
Tendon Repair . . . 26356-26358

Noble Procedure
See Repair; Suture

Nocardia
Antibody . . . 86744

Nocturnal Penile Rigidity Test . . . 54250

Nocturnal Penile Tumescence Test . . . 54250

Node Dissection, Lymph
See Dissection, Lymph Nodes

Node, Lymph
See Lymph Nodes

Nodes
See Lymph Nodes

Non-Invasive Vascular Imaging
See Vascular Studies

Non-Office Medical Services . . . 99056
Emergency Care . . . 99060

Non-Stress Test, Fetal . . . 59025
with Biophysical Profile . . . 76818

Nonunion Repair
Carpal . . . 25431, 25440
Clavicle . . . 23485
Femur
  with Graft . . . 27472
  without Graft . . . 27470
Fibula . . . 27726
Humerus . . . 24430-24435
Metacarpal . . . 26546
Metatarsal . . . 28322
Phalanx . . . 26546
Radius . . . 25400-25405, 25415-25420
Tarsal . . . 28320
Tibia . . . 27720, 27722, 27724, 27725
Ulna . . . 25400, 25415, 25415, 25415, 25420
with Bone Graft . . . 23485, 25405, 25415, 26546, 27470, 27722, 27724, 28322

Noradrenalin
Blood . . . 82383, 82384
Urine . . . 82384

Norepinephrine
See Catecholamines
Blood . . . 82383, 82384
Urine . . . 82384

Norwood Procedure . . . 33611, 33612, 33619
See Repair, Heart, Ventricle; Revision

Nose
Abscess
  Incision and Drainage . . . 30000-30020
Artery
  Ligation . . . 30915-30920
Biopsy
  Intranasal . . . 30100
  Endoscopic . . . 31237
Debridement
  Endoscopic . . . 31237
Dermoid Cyst
  Excision
    Complex . . . 30125
    Simple . . . 30124
Displacement Therapy . . . 30210
Endoscopy
  Diagnostic . . . 31231-31235
  Surgical . . 31237-31241, 31253-31257, 31259, 31267, 31276, 31287, 31288, 31290-31298
Excision
  Rhinectomy . . . 30150-30160
  Turbinate . . . 30140
Fracture
  Closed Treatment . . . 21345
  Open Treatment . . . 21325-21336, 21338, 21339, 21346, 21347
  Percutaneous Treatment . . . 21340
  with Fixation . . . 21330, 21340, 21345-21347
Hematoma
  Incision and Drainage . . . 30000-30020
Hemorrhage Control
  Cauterization . . . 30901-30906
  Packs . . . 30901-30906
    Endoscopic . . . 31237
Insertion
  Septal Prosthesis . . . 30220
Lesion
  Destruction or Excision
    External Approach . . . 30118
    Internal Approach . . . 30117
Lysis of Adhesions . . . 30560
Polyp
  Excision
    Endoscopic . . . 31237
    Extensive . . . 30115
    Simple . . . 30110
Reconstruction
  Cleft Lip/Cleft Palate . . . 30460-30462
  Complete . . . 30410
  Dermatoplasty . . . 30620
  Primary . . . 30400, 30420
  Secondary . . . 30430-30450
  Septum . . . 30520
Removal
  Foreign Body . . . 30300
    by Lateral Rhinotomy . . . 30320
    with Anesthesia . . . 30310
Repair
  Adhesions . . . 30560
  Cleft Lip . . . 40700-40761
  Choanal Atresia . . . 30540, 30545
  Complex . . . 13151-13153
  Fistula . . . 30580-30600, 42260
  Rhinophyma . . . 30120
  Septum . . . 30540-30545, 30630
  Synechia . . . 30560
  Vestibular Stenosis . . . 30465
Skin
  Excision . . . 30120
  Surgical Planing . . . 30120
Submucous Resection Turbinate
  Excision . . . 30140
Turbinate
  Excision . . . 30130-30140
  Fracture . . . 30930
  Injection . . . 30200
Turbinate Mucosa
  Cauterization . . . 30801, 30802
Unlisted Services and Procedures . . . 30999

Nose Bleed
Cauterization . . . 30901-30906
Packs . . . 30901-30906
  Endoscopic . . . 31237

NTD . . . 86384
See Nitroblue Tetrazolium Dye Test

Nuclear Antigen
Antibody . . . 86235

Nuclear Imaging
See Nuclear Medicine
Planar
  Parathyroid Gland . . . 78070
Subtraction
  Parathyroid Gland . . . 78070

Nuclear Magnetic Resonance Imaging
See Magnetic Resonance Imaging (MRI)

Nuclear Magnetic Resonance Spectroscopy
See Magnetic Resonance Spectroscopy

Nuclear Matrix Protein 22 . . . 86386

Nuclear Medicine
Diagnostic
  Adrenal Gland Imaging . . . 78075
  Bile Duct
    Imaging . . . 78226, 78227
  Bladder
    Residual Study . . . 78730
  Blood
    Blood pool imaging . . . 78472, 78473, 78481, 78483
  Bone and Joint
    Bone Density Study . . . 78350, 78351
    Imaging . . . 78300-78320
    SPECT . . . 78320
    Ultrasound . . . 76977
  Bone Marrow
    Imaging . . . 78102-78104

Brain
Blood Flow 78610
Cerebrospinal Fluid Imaging . . . 78630-78650
Imaging 78600-78609
PET Imaging 78608, 78609
Vascular Flow 78601, 78606, 78610
Endocrine System
Parathyroid Gland Imaging 78070-78072
Unlisted Services and Procedures 78099
Esophagus
Imaging (Motility) 78258
Reflux Study 78262
Flow Imaging 78445
Plasma Volume 78110-78121
Platelet Survival 78191
Red Cell Sequestration 78140
Red Cell Survival 78130-78135
Red Cells Volume 78120, 78121
Unlisted Services and Procedures 78199
Whole Blood Volume 78122
Gallbladder
Imaging 78226, 78227
Gastric
Emptying Imaging Study 78264-78266
Mucosa Imaging 78261
Urea Breath Test 78267, 78268
Gastroesophageal Reflux Study 78262
Gastrointestinal
Blood Loss Imaging 78278
Intestine Imaging 78290
Peritoneal-Venous Shunt Patency 78291
Protein Loss Study 78282
Unlisted Services and Procedures 78299
Genitourinary System
Unlisted Services and Procedures 78799
Heart
Angiography 78445
Blood Flow 78414
Blood Pool Imaging 78472, 78473, 78481-78483
Blood Pool SPECT Imaging 78494-78496
Myocardial Imaging . . . 78459, 78466-78469
Myocardial PET Imaging 78459, 78491, 78492
Myocardial Perfusion Imaging 78451-78454
Shunt Detection 78428
Vascular Flow Imaging 78445
Venography 78445
Venous Thrombosis Imaging . . 78456-78458
Unlisted Services and Procedures 78499
Hepatic Duct
Imaging 78226, 78227
Inflammatory Process 78805-78807
Injection Procedure 78808
Intestines
Imaging 78290
Kidney
Function Study 78725
Imaging 78700-78710
Imaging, SPECT 78710
Vascular Flow 78701-78709
Lacrimal Gland Tear Flow 78660
Liver
Imaging 78201-78216
Vascular Flow 78202, 78206, 78216
Lung
Imaging, Perfusion 78580, 78597, 78598
Imaging, Ventilation . . . 78579, 78582, 78598
Unlisted Respiratory Procedure 78599
Lymphatics and Lymph Nodes
Imaging 78195
Positron Emission Tomography (PET) 78811-78816
with Computed Tomography . . 78814-78816
Pulmonary Perfusion 78580, 78597, 78598
Pulmonary Ventilation 78579, 78582
Salivary Gland
Function Study 78232
Imaging 78230, 78231
Spleen
Imaging 78185, 78215, 78216
Unlisted Services and Procedures 78199
Testes
Imaging 78761
Thyroid
Imaging for Metastases 78015-78018
Imaging with Flow 78013
Metastases Uptake 78020
Uptake 78012, 78014
Tumor Localization
Radiopharmaceutical . . 78800-78804, 78808
SPECT 78803, 78807
Urea Breath Test 78267, 78268
Ureter
Reflux Study 78740
Vein
Thrombosis Imaging 78456-78458
Unlisted Procedures
Cardiovascular 78499
Endocrine 78099
Gastrointestinal 78299
Genitourinary 78799
Hemopoietic 78199
Lymphatic 78199
Miscellaneous 78999
Musculoskeletal 78399
Nervous System 78699
Respiratory 78599
Reticuloendothelial 78199
Unlisted Diagnostic Procedures
Cardiovascular 78499
Endocrine 78099
Gastrointestinal 78299
Genitourinary 78799
Hematopoietic, Reticuloendothelial, and Lymphatic 78199
Miscellaneous 78999
Musculoskeletal 78399
Nervous System 78699
Respiratory 78599
Therapeutic
Radiopharmaceutical, Administration
Interstitial Radioactive Colloid 79300
Intra-Arterial 79445
Intra-Articular 79440
Intracavitary 79200
Intravenous 79101
Intravenous Infusion 79403
Oral 79005
Thyroid 79200-79300
Unlisted Radiopharmaceutical Procedure 79999

Nucleases, DNA
See DNAse

Nucleic Acid Probe
Amplified Probe Detection
Infectious Agent
Bartonella Henselae 87471
Bartonella Quintana 87471
Borrelia Burgdorferi 87476
Candida Species 87481
Central Nervous System Pathogen . . . 87483
Chlamydia Pneumoniae 87486
Chlamydia Trachomatis 87491
Cytomegalovirus 87496
Enterovirus 87498, 87500
Gardnerella Vaginalis 87511
Hepatitis B Virus 87516
Hepatitis C 87521, 87522
Hepatitis G 87526
Herpes Simplex Virus 87529
Herpes Virus-6 87532
HIV-1 . . . . . 87535, 87536
HIV-2 . . . . . 87538, 87539
Legionella Pneumophila 87541
Multiple Organisms 87801
Mycobacteria Avium-Intracellulare . . . 87561
Mycobacteria Species 87551
Mycobacteria Tuberculosis 87556
Mycoplasma Pneumoniae 87581
Neisseria Gonorrhoeae 87591
Not Otherwise Specified 87798, 87801
Staphylococcus Aureus 87640, 87641
Streptococcus, Group A 87651
Streptococcus, Group B 87653
Zika Virus 87662
Direct Probe Detection
Infectious Agent
Borrelia Burgdorferi 87475
Candida Species 87480
Chlamydia Pneumoniae 87485
Chlamydia Trachomatis 87490
Clostridium Difficile 87493
Cytomegalovirus 87495
Gardnerella Vaginalis 87510
Gastrointestinal Pathogen 87505-87507
Hepatitis C 87520
Hepatitis G 87525
Herpes Simplex Virus 87528
Herpes Virus-6 87531
HIV-1 87534
HIV-2 87537
Legionella Pneumophila 87540
Multiple Organisms 87800
Mycobacteria Avium-Intracellulare . . . 87560
Mycobacteria Species 87550
Mycobacteria Tuberculosis 87555
Mycoplasma Pneumoniae 87580
Neisseria Gonorrhoeae 87590
Not Otherwise Specified 87797
Papillomavirus, Human 0500T, 87623-87625
Streptococcus, Group A 87650
Trichomonas Vaginalis 87660, 87661
Genotype Analysis
Infectious Agent
Hepatitis C Virus 87902
HIV-1 Regions 87901, 87906
In Situ Hybridization . . 88120, 88121, 88364-88366
Morphometric Analysis
Computer-Assisted 88367, 88373, 88374
Manual 88368, 88369, 88377
Phenotype Analysis
Infectious Agent
HIV-1 Drug Resistance 87903, 87904
Quantification
Infectious Agent
Bartonella Henselae 87472
Bartonella Quintana 87472
Candida Species 87482
Chlamydia Pneumoniae 87487
Chlamydia Trachomatis 87492
Cytomegalovirus 87497
Gardnerella Vaginalis 87512
Hepatitis B Virus 87517

Hepatitis C 87522
Hepatitis G 87527
Herpes Simplex Virus 87530
Herpes Virus-6 87533
HIV-1 87536
HIV-2 87539
Legionella Pneumophila 87542
Mycobacteria Avium-Intracellulare . . . 87562
Mycobacteria Species 87552
Mycobacteria Tuberculosis 87557
Mycoplasma Pneumoniae 87582
Neisseria Gonorrhoeae 87592
Not Otherwise Specified 87799
Streptococcus, Group A 87652

Nucleolysis, Intervertebral Disc
See Chemonucleolysis

Nucleotidase 83915

Nursemaid Elbow 24640

Nursing Facility Discharge Services
See Discharge Services, Nursing Facility

Nursing Facility Services
Annual Assessment 99318
Care Plan Oversight Services 99379, 99380
Comprehensive Assessments
Discharge Services . . . 99315, 99316, 1110F, 1111F
Initial Care 99304-99306
Subsequent Care 99307-99310

Nuss Procedure
with Thoracoscopy 21743
without Thoracoscopy 21742

Nutrition Therapy
Group 97804
Home Infusion 99601, 99602
Initial Assessment 97802
Reassessment 97803

Nystagmus Tests
See Vestibular Function Tests
Optokinetic 92534, 92544
Positional 92532, 92542
Spontaneous 92531, 92541

O

O_2 Saturation
See Oxygen Saturation

Ober-Yount Procedure 27025
See Fasciotomy, Hip

Obliteration
Mastoid 69670
Vagina
Total 57110-57112
Vault 57120

Oblongata, Medulla
See Medulla

Observation 99217-99220, 99224-99226, 99234-99236
See Evaluation and Management; Hospital Services

Observational Behavioral Follow-Up Assessment
Behavior Identification
Assessment 97151, 97152

Obstetrical Care
Abortion
Induced
by Amniocentesis Injection . . . 59850-59852
See Abortion; Cesarean Delivery; Ectopic Pregnancy
by Dilation and Curettage 59840
by Dilation and Evaluation 59841
Missed
First Trimester 59820
Second Trimester 59821
Spontaneous 59812
Therapeutic 59840-59852
Antepartum Care 59425, 59426
Cesarean Delivery 59618-59622
Only 59514
Routine 59510
with Hysterectomy 59525
Curettage
Hydatidiform Mole 59870
Diagnostic Imaging
Fetal
Biophysical Profile 76818, 76819
Doppler Velocimetry 76820, 76821
Echocardiography 76825-76828
Fetal and Maternal
Magnetic Resonance Imaging (MRI) 74712, 74713
Pregnant Uterus
Ultrasound 76801, 76802, 76805, 76810-76817
Evacuation
Hydatidiform Mole 59870
External Cephalic Version 59412
Miscarriage
Surgical Completion 59812-59821
Placenta Delivery 59414
Postpartum Care 59430, 59514
Septic Abortion 59830
Total (Global) 59400, 59610, 59618
Unlisted Services and Procedures . . . 59898, 59899
Vaginal
after Cesarean (VBAC) 59610-59614
Vaginal Delivery 59409, 59410
Delivery after Cesarean 59610-59614

Obstruction
See Occlusion

Obstruction Clearance
Venous Access Device 36595, 36596

Obstruction Colon
See Colon, Obstruction

Obturator Nerve
Avulsion 64763-64766
Incision 64763-64766
Transection 64763-64766

Obturator Prosthesis 21076
Definitive 21080
Insertion
Larynx 31527
Interim 21079

Occipital Nerve, Greater
Avulsion 64744
Incision 64744
Injection
Anesthetic 64405
Transection 64744

Occlusion
Bronchi
Balloon 31634, 31647, 31651
Fallopian Tube
Oviduct 58565, 58615, 58671
Paravalvular Leak
Aortic Valve 93591, 93592
Mitral Valve 93590, 93592
Penis
Vein 37790
Umbilical Cord 59072
Ureteral 50705
Vascular
Arterial, other than Hemorrhage or Tumor 37242
Carotid Artery 37606, 61705
Dialysis Circuit 36909
during Endovascular Therapy 34820
for Hemorrhage 37244
for Infarction 37243
for Lymphatic Extravasation 37244
for Organ Ischemia 37243
for Tumors 37243
Nervous System
Cranial 61623, 61624, 61626
Spinal . . 61624, 61626, 62294, 63250-63252
Placement of Occlusion Device 34808
Veinous, other than Hemorrhage 37241
with Ligation 37606

Occlusive Disease of Artery
See Repair, Artery; Revision

Occult Blood 82270-82272
by Hemoglobin Immunoassay 82274

Occupational Therapy
Evaluation 97165, 97166, 97167
Procedures
See Physical Medicine/Therapy/Occupational Therapy, Procedures
Re-evaluation 97168

Ocular Implant
See Orbital Implant
Insertion
Drainage Device 0191T, 0253T, 0376T, 66183
Drug-Eluting Insert
Eyelid 0444T, 0445T
Scleral Shell 65130
Muscles, Attached 65140
Muscles, Not Attached 65135
Modification 65125
Reinsertion 65150
with Foreign Material 65155
Removal 65175

Ocular Muscle
See Eye Muscles

Ocular Orbit
See Orbit

Ocular Screening
Instrument Based 99174, 99177
Retinal Polarization Scan 0469T

Ocular Prostheses
See Prosthesis, Ocular

Oculomotor Muscle
See Eye Muscles

Oddi Sphincter
See Sphincter of Oddi

Odontoid Dislocation
Open Treatment/Reduction 22318
with Grafting 22319

Odontoid Fracture
Open Treatment/Reduction 22318
with Grafting 22319

Odontoid Process
Excision 22548

Oesophageal Neoplasm
See Tumor, Esophagus

Oesophageal Varices
See Esophageal Varices

Oesophagus
See Esophagus

Oestradiol
See Estradiol

Office and/or Other Outpatient Services
Consultation
See Consultation
Established Patient 99211-99215
New Patient 99201-99205
Normal Newborn 99461
Office Visit
Established Patient 99211-99215
New Patient 99201-99205
Outpatient Visit
Established Patient 99211-99215
New Patient 99201-99205
Prolonged Services 99354, 99355, 99415, 99416

Office Medical Services
After Hours 99050
Emergency Care 99058
Extended Hours 99051

Office or Other Outpatient Consultations
See Consultation, Office and/or Other Outpatient

Olecranon
See Elbow; Humerus; Radius; Ulna
Bursa
Arthrocentesis 20605, 20606
Cyst
Excision 24125, 24126
Tumor
Cyst 24120
Excision 24125, 24126

Olecranon Process
Craterization 24147
Diaphysectomy 24147
Excision 24147
Abscess 24138
Fracture
See Elbow; Humerus; Radius
Closed Treatment 24670-24675
Open Treatment 24685
Osteomyelitis 24138, 24147
Saucerization 24147
Sequestrectomy 24138

Oligoclonal Immunoglobulins 83916

Omentectomy
Separate Procedure 49255
with Laparotomy 58960
with Lymph Node Laparoscopy 38573
with Oophorectomy 58943
with Tumor Debulking 58575, 58950-58954, 58956-58958, 58960

Omentum
Excision 49255, 58950-58958
Flap 49904, 49905
Free
with Microvascular Anastomosis 49906
Omentopexy 49326
Unlisted Services and Procedures 49999

Omphalectomy 49250

Omphalocele
Repair 49600-49611

Omphalomesenteric Duct
Excision 44800

Omphalomesenteric Duct, Persistent
See Diverticulum, Meckel's

Oncoprotein
Des-gamma-carboxyprothrombin (DCP) 83951
HER-2/neu 83950

Online Internet Assessment and Management
Nonphysician 98969
Physician 99444

One Stage Prothrombin Time . . 85610, 85611
See Prothrombin Time

Onychectomy
See Excision, Nails

Onychia
Drainage 10060, 10061

Oocyte
Assisted Fertilization
Microtechnique 89280, 89281
Biopsy 89290, 89291
Cryopreservation
Immature Oocyte(s) 0357T
Culture
Extended 89272
Less than 4 Days 89250
with Co-Culture 89251
Identification
Follicular Fluid 89254
Insemination 89268
Retrieval
for In Vitro Fertilization 58970
Storage 89346
Thawing 89356

Oophorectomy 58262, 58263, 58291, 58292, 58552, 58554, 58661, 58940-58943
Ectopic Pregnancy
Laparoscopic Treatment 59120
Surgical Treatment 59120

Oophorectomy, Partial
See Excision, Ovary

Oophorocystectomy
See Cystectomy, Ovarian

Open Biopsy, Adrenal Gland
See Adrenal Gland, Biopsy

Operating Microscope 69990

Operation/Procedure
Abbe-Estlander 00102, 40527, 40761
Akin 28298
Bankart 23455
Barker 28120, 28130
Batch-Spittler-McFadden 01404, 27598
Bischof 63170
Blalock-Hanlon 33735-33737
Blalock-Taussig 33750
Bohler 28405
Bristow 23460
Brunschwig operation 58240
Burrow's 14000-14350
Camey Enterocystoplasty 50825
Campbell 27422
Chambers 28300
Chevron 28296
Clagett 32810
Colles Fracture 25600
Conjunctivo-Tarso-Muller Resection 67908
Coombs Test 86880
Cotte Operation 58400-58410
Damus-Kaye-Stansel Procedure 33606
Dandy Operation 62180, 62200, 62201
Darrach Procedure 25240
de Quervain's Disease Treatment 25000
Dunn
See Arthrodesis, Foot Joint
Dupuytren's Contracture 26040-26045
Duvries
See Tenoplasty
Dwyer-type Procedure 28300
Ebstein Anomaly Repair 33468
Estes
See Ovary, Transposition
Estlander Procedure 40525
Fasanella-Servat Procedure 67908
Foley Y-pyeloplasty 50400-50405
Fontan
See Repair, Heart, Anomaly
Fowler-Stephens Orchiopexy 54650
Fowler-Stephens Procedure 54650
Fredet-Ramstedt Procedure 43520
Frost Suture 67875
Gibbons Stent 52332
Gill Operation 63012
Glenn Procedure 33766, 33767
Goeckerman Treatment 96910-96913
Goldwaite Procedure 27422
Green
See Scapulopexy
Halsted Operation 49491
Harii Procedure 25430
Harrington Rod Technique 00670
Hauser Procedure 27420
Haygroves Procedure 27120
Heller Operation 32665
Heller Procedure 32665, 43330, 43331
Heyman Procedure 27179, 28264
Hibb Operation 22610, 22612, 22614
Ilizarov Procedure, Monticelli type 20692
Jaboulay Operation Gastroduodenostomy . . . 43810
Jaboulay Operation 43810
Jannetta Procedure 61458
Jatene type 33770-33781
Johannsen Procedure 53400
Jones Procedure 28760
Kasai Procedure 47701
Kelikian Procedure 28280
Keller Procedure 28292
Kelly Urethral Plication 57220
Kocher Operation 23650-23680
Kocher pylorectomy 43631
Kock Pouch 44316
Kock Procedure 44316
Kraske Procedure 45116
Kroenlein Procedure 67420
Krukenberg Procedure 25915
Ladd Procedure 44055
Lapidus Procedure 28297, 28297
Leadbetter Procedure 53431
Leriche Operation 64809

Index

Linton Procedure . . . 37760
Lisfranc Operation . . . 28600-28615
Lynch Procedure . . . 31075
Magnuson Procedure . . . 23450
Maquet Procedure . . . 27418
Marcellation Operation . . . 00944
Marshall-Marchetti-Krantz Procedure . . . 51840, 51841, 58152, 58267, 58293
Maydl Operation . . . 45563, 50810
Mayo Hernia Repair . . . 49582
Mayo Procedure . . . 28292
Maze Procedure . . . 33254-33256, 33265, 33266
McBride Procedure . . . 28292
McBurney Operation . . . 49582
McCannel Procedure . . . 66682
McKissock Surgery . . . 19318
McVay Operation . . . 49582
Meckel's Diverticulum . . . 44899
Meckel's Excision . . . 44800
Miller Procedure . . . 28737
Miller-Abbott Intubation . . . 44500, 74340
Mitchell Procedure . . . 28296, 28296
Mitrofanoff Operation . . . 50845
Mohs Micrographic Surgery . . . 17311-17315
Monteggia Fracture . . . 24620-24635
Monticelli Procedure . . . 20690
Mumford Procedure . . . 29824
Nissen Procedure . . . 43327, 43328
Norwood Procedure . . . 33611, 33612, 33619
Nuss Procedure . . . 21742, 21743
Ober-Yount Procedure . . . 27025
Péans' Operation . . . 27290, 27295
Pemberton Osteotomy of Pelvis . . . 27158
Pereyra Procedure . . . 51845, 57289, 58267, 58293
Pirogoff Procedure . . . 27888
Polya Gastrectomy . . . 43631-43635, 43845
Potts-Smith Procedure . . . 33762
Puestow Procedure . . . 48548
Putti-Platt Procedure . . . 23450
Ramstedt
  See Pyloromyotomy
Rashkind Procedure . . . 33735-33737
Raz Procedure . . . 51845
Richardson Procedure . . . 53460
Ripstein Operation . . . 45540, 45541
Ross-Konno Procedure . . . 33440
Ross Procedure . . . 33413
Roux-En-Y Procedure . . . 43621, 43633, 43634, 43644, 43846, 47740, 47741, 47780-47785, 48540
Sang-Park Procedure . . . 33735-33737
Schanz
  See Femur, Osteotomy
Schede Procedure . . . 32905, 32906
Scheie Procedure . . . 00147, 66155
Schlatter Operation Total Gastrectomy . . . 43620-43622
Scribner Cannulization . . . 36810
Seddon-Brookes Procedure . . . 24320
Sengstaaken Tamponade, Esophagus . . . 43460
Senning Procedure . . . 33774-33777
Senning Type . . . 33774-33777
Smith-Robinson Operation . . . 22614
Soave Procedure . . . 45120
Sofield Procedure . . . 24410
Ssbanejew-Frank Operation . . . 43830-43832
Stamey Procedure . . . 51845
Steindler Stripping . . . 28250
Stenger Test . . . 92565, 92577
Stookey-Scarff Procedures . . . 62200
Strassman Procedure . . . 58540
Strayer Procedure . . . 01474
Sturmdorf Procedure . . . 57520
Swanson Procedure . . . 28309
Swenson Procedure . . . 45120
Syme Procedure . . . 27888
Takeuchi Procedure . . . 33505
Tenago Procedure . . . 53431
Thal-Nissen Procedure . . . 43325
Thiersch Operation . . . 15050
Thiersch Procedure . . . 46753
Thompson Procedure . . . 27430
Tompkins Metroplasty . . . 58540
Torek Procedure . . . 00930
Torkildsen Procedure . . . 62180
Touroff Operation . . . 37615
Tuffier Vaginal Hysterectomy . . . 00944, 58260
Von Kraske Proctectomy . . . 45111
Waldius Procedure . . . 27445
Walsh Modified Radical . . . 00865
Waterston Procedure . . . 33755
Watson-Jones Procedure . . . 27695-27698
Wertheim Operation . . . 00846
Whipple Procedure . . . 48150
Whitman Astragalectomy . . . 28120, 28130
Whitman Procedure . . . 27120
Winiwater Operation . . . 47720-47740
Winter Procedure . . . 54435
Witzel Operation . . . 43500, 43520, 43830-43832

Operation Microscopes
See Operating Microscope

Operculectomy . . . 41821

Operculum
See Gums

Ophthalmic Mucous Membrane Test . . . 95060
See Allergy Tests

Ophthalmology
Unlisted Services and Procedures . . . 92499
  See Ophthalmology, Diagnostic

Ophthalmology, Diagnostic
Color Vision Exam . . . 92283
Computerized Scanning
  Anterior . . . 92132
  Posterior . . . 92133, 92134
Dark Adaptation . . . 92284
Electro-oculography . . . 92270
Electromyography, Needle . . . 92265
Electroretinography . . . 0509T, 92273, 92274
Endoscopy . . . 66990
Evoked Potentials
  Acuity . . . 0333T
  Central Nervous System . . . 95930
  Glaucoma Test . . . 0464T
Eye Exam
  Established Patient . . . 92012-92014
  New Patient . . . 92002-92004
  with Anesthesia . . . 92018, 92019
Gonioscopy . . . 92020
Heterochromatic Flicker Photometry . . . 0506T
Instrument-based Screening . . . 99172, 99174
Ocular Photography
  External . . . 92285
Ophthalmoscopy . . . 92225, 92226
  with Dynamometry . . . 92260
  with Fluorescein Angiography . . . 92235, 92242
  with Fluorescein Angioscopy . . . 92230
  with Fundus Photography . . . 92250
  with Indocyanine-Green Angiography . . . 92240, 92242
  Remote Imaging . . . 92227, 92228
Refractive Determination . . . 92015
Retinal Imaging . . . 0380T
Sensorimotor Exam . . . 92060
Tear Film Imaging . . . 0330T
Tonometry
  Serial . . . 92100
Ultrasound . . . 76511-76529
Visual Acuity Screen . . . 99172, 99173
Visual Field Exam . . . 0378T, 0379T, 92081-92083
Visual Function Screen . . . 99172, 99174, 99177

Ophthalmoscopy . . . 92225, 92226
See Ophthalmology, Diagnostic

Optic Nerve
Decompression . . . 67570
  with Nasal/Sinus Endoscopy . . . 31294
Diagnostic Imaging
  Computerized Scanning . . . 92133
Head Evaluation . . . 2027F

Optical Coherence Tomography (OCT)
Axillary Lymph Node . . . 0351T, 0352T
Breast . . . 0351T-0354T
Intravascular . . . 92978, 92979
Middle Ear . . . 0485T, 0486T
Skin Lesion . . . 0470T, 0471T

Optical Endomicroscopy
Esophageal . . . 43206
Gastrointestinal . . . 43252
with Endoscopic Retrograde Cholangiopancreatography (ERCP) . . . 0397T

Optokinetic Nystagmus Test
See Nystagmus Tests, Optokinetic

Oral Lactose Tolerance Test 82951, 82952
See Glucose, Tolerance Test

Oral Mucosa
See Mouth, Mucosa

Oral Surgical Splint . . . 21085

Orbit
See Orbital Contents; Orbital Floor; Periorbital Region
Biopsy
  Exploration . . . 67450
  Fine Needle Aspiration or Orbital Contents . . . 67415
  Orbitotomy without Bone Flap . . . 67400
Bone Graft . . . 21182-21184, 21256, 21260, 21267, 21395, 21408
CT Scan . . . 70480-70482
Decompression . . . 61330
  Bone Removal . . . 67414, 67445
Exploration . . . 67400, 67450
  Lesion
    Excision . . . 61333
Fracture
  Closed Treatment
    with Manipulation . . . 21401
    without Manipulation . . . 21400
  Open Treatment . . . 21406-21408
    Blowout Fracture . . . 21385-21395
Incision and Drainage . . . 67405, 67440
Injection
  Retrobulbar . . . 67500-67505
  Tenon's Capsule . . . 67515
Insertion
  Implant . . . 67550
Lesion
  Excision . . . 67412, 67420
Magnetic Resonance Imaging (MRI) 70540-70543
Removal
  Bone . . . 67445
  Foreign Body . . . 67413, 67430
  Implant . . . 67560
  Lesion . . . 61333

Sella Turcica 70482
Unlisted Services and Procedures 67599
X ray 70190-70200

Orbit Area
Reconstruction
Secondary 21275

Orbit Wall
Decompression
with Nasal/Sinus Endoscopy.... 31292, 31293

Orbital Contents
Aspiration 67415

Orbital Floor
See Orbit; Periorbital Region
Fracture
Blow Out 21385-21395

Orbital Hypertelorism
Osteotomy
Periorbital.................. 21260-21263

Orbital Implant
See Ocular Implant
Insertion 67550
Removal 67560

Orbital Prosthesis 21077

Orbital Rim and Forehead
Reconstruction 21172-21180

Orbital Rims
Reconstruction 21182-21184

Orbital Transplant 67560

Orbital Walls
Reconstruction 21182-21184

Orbitocraniofacial Reconstruction
Secondary........................ 21275

Orbitotomy
with Bone Flap
for Exploration 67450
Lateral Approach 67420
with Drainage 67440
with Removal Foreign Body.......... 67430
with Removal of Bone for
Decompression 67445
with Removal Foreign Body 67413
with Removal of Bone for Decompression... 67414
without Bone Flap
for Exploration 67400
with Drainage Only 67405
with Removal Lesion 67412

Orchidectomies
See Excision, Testis

Orchidopexy
See Orchiopexy

Orchidoplasty
See Repair, Testis

Orchiectomy
Laparoscopic........................ 54690
Partial 54522
Radical
Abdominal Exploration.............. 54535
Inguinal Approach 54530
Simple........................ 54520

Orchiopexy
Abdominal Approach 54650
Inguinal Approach.................. 54640
Intra-Abdominal Testis................ 54692

Orchioplasty
See Repair, Testis

Organ Grafting
See Transplantation

Organ or Disease-Oriented Panel
Acute Hepatitis...................... 80074
Electrolyte........................ 80051
General Health Panel 80050
Hepatic Function Panel.............. 80076
Hepatitis Panel 80074
Lipid Panel........................ 80061
Metabolic
Basic.................... 80047, 80048
Comprehensive 80053
Obstetric Panel 80055, 80081
Renal Function 80069

Organ System, Neurologic
See Nervous System

Organic Acids 83918-83921

Ormond Disease
See Retroperitoneal Fibrosis

Orogastric Tube
Placement........................ 43752

Oropharynx
Biopsy 42800

Orthodontic Cephalogram 70350

Orthomyxoviridae
See Influenza Virus

Orthomyxovirus
See Influenza Virus

Orthopantogram 70355

Orthopedic Cast
See Cast

Orthopedic Surgery
Computer Assisted Navigation........... 20985
Stereotaxis
Computer Assisted................. 20985

Orthoptic Training 92065

Orthoroentgenogram 77073

Orthosis
See Orthotics

Orthotics
Fitting 97760
Management and Training......... 97760, 97763

Os Calcis Fracture
See Calcaneus, Fracture

Oscillation
Chest Wall 94669

Osmolality
Blood........................ 83930
Urine 83935

Osseous Survey............. 77074-77076

Osseous Tissue
See Bone

Ossicles
Excision
Stapes
with Footplate Drill Out 69661
without Foreign Material 69660, 69661
Mobilization
Stapes 69650

Reconstruction
Ossicular Chain
Tympanoplasty with Antrotomy or
Mastoidotomy 69636, 69637
Tympanoplasty with
Mastoidectomy....... 69642, 69644, 69646
Tympanoplasty without
Mastoidectomy............ 69632, 69633
Replacement
with Prosthesis 69633, 69637
Revision
Stapedectomy 69662
Stapedotomy 69662

Ostectomy
Calcaneus 28118-28120
Metacarpal........................ 26250
Metatarsal ... 28110-28114, 28122, 28140, 28288
Phalanges
Finger..................... 26260-26262
Toe....................... 28124, 28150
Pressure Ulcer
Coccygeal........................ 15920
Ischial................ 15941, 15945, 15946
Sacral................ 15933, 15935, 15937
Trochanteric........... 15951, 15953, 15958
Rib........................ 21502
Scapula 23190
Sternum........................ 21620
Talus 28120, 28130
Tarsal 28116, 28122

Osteocalcin........................ 83937

Osteocartilaginous Exostoses
See Exostosis

Osteochondroma
See Exostosis

Osteocutaneous Flap
with Microvascular Anastomosis.... 20969-20973

Osteoma
Sinusotomy
Frontal 31075

Osteomyelitis
Calcaneus
Partial Excision.................... 28120
Clavicle
Partial Excision.................... 23180
Craterization
See Craterization
Diaphysectomy
See Diaphysectomy
Elbow
Incision and Drainage 23935
Excision
Facial 21026
Mandible 21025
Skull 61501
Femur/Knee
Incision and Drainage 27303
Partial Excision.................... 27360
Finger
Incision........................ 26034
Partial Excision.............. 26235, 26236
Hand Incision 26034
Hip
Incision, Deep 26992
Partial Excision.............. 27070, 27071
Humerus 24134
Incision and Drainage 23935
Partial Excision.............. 23184, 24140

Index

Index

Incision
Ankle ... 27607
Elbow ... 23935
Femur ... 27303
Finger ... 26034
Foot ... 28005
Forearm ... 25035
Hand ... 26034
Hip ... 26992, 27070, 27071
Humerus ... 23935
Knee ... 27303
Leg ... 27607
Shoulder ... 23035
Thorax ... 21510
Wrist ... 25035
Metacarpal
Partial Excision ... 26230
Metatarsal
Partial Excision ... 28122
Olecranon Process
Partial Excision ... 24138, 24147
Pelvis
Incision, Deep ... 26992
Radius ... 24136, 24145
Partial Excision ... 24145, 25150
Saucerization
See Saucerization
Scapula
Partial Excision ... 23182
Sequestrectomy
Calcaneus ... 28120
Clavicle ... 23170
Forearm ... 24145
Humerus ... 23174, 24134
Metatarsal ... 28122
Olecranon Process ... 24138
Radius ... 24136
Scapula ... 23172
Skull ... 61501
Talus ... 28120
Tarsal ... 28122
Wrist ... 24145
Talus
Partial Excision ... 28120
Tarsal
Partial Excision ... 28122
Tibia
Partial Excision ... 27360, 27640
Ulna
Partial Excision ... 25150

Osteopathic Manipulation ... 98925-98929

Osteoplasty
Carpal Bone ... 25394
Facial Bones
Augmentation ... 21208
Reduction ... 21209
Femoral Neck ... 27179
Femur ... 27179
Lengthening ... 27466-27468
Shortening ... 27465, 27468
Fibula
Lengthening ... 27715
Humerus ... 24420
Metacarpal ... 26568
Phalanges, Finger ... 26568
Radius ... 25390-25393
Tibia
Lengthening ... 27715
Ulna ... 25390-25393
Vertebra
Cervicothoracic ... 22510, 22512
Lumbosacral ... 22511, 22512

Osteotomy
Calcaneus ... 28300
Chin ... 21121-21123
Clavicle ... 23480-23485
Femur ... 27140, 27151
Femoral Neck ... 27161
for Slipped Epiphysis ... 27181
with Fixation ... 27165
with Open Reduction of Hip ... 27156
with Realignment ... 27454
without Fixation ... 27448-27450
Fibula ... 27707-27712
Hip ... 27146-27151
Femoral
with Open Reduction ... 27156
Femur ... 27151
Humerus ... 24400-24410
Mandible ... 21198, 21199
Extra-Oral ... 21047
Intra-Oral ... 21046
Mandibular Rami ... 21193, 21194
Maxilla ... 21206
Extra-Oral ... 21049
Intra-Oral ... 21048
Metacarpal ... 26565
Metatarsal ... 28306-28309
with Bunionectomy ... 28295, 28296
Orbit Reconstruction ... 21256
Pelvis ... 27158
Periorbital
Orbital Hypertelorism ... 21260-21263
Osteotomy with Graft ... 21267, 21268
Phalanges
Finger ... 26567
Toe ... 28299, 28310-28312
with Bunionectomy ... 28298
Radius
and Ulna ... 25365, 25375
Distal Third ... 25350
Middle or Proximal Third ... 25355
Multiple ... 25370
Skull Base ... 61582-61585, 61592
Spine
Anterior ... 22220-22226
Posterior
Posterolateral ... 22210-22214
Posterior or Posterolateral
Three-Column ... 22206-22208
Talus ... 28302
Tarsal ... 28304, 28305
Tibia ... 27455-27457, 27705, 27709-27712
Ulna ... 25360
and Radius ... 25365, 25375
Multiple ... 25370
Vertebra
Additional Segment
Anterior Approach ... 22226
Posterior/Posterolateral Approach ... 22216
Cervical
Anterior Approach ... 22220
Posterior/Posterolateral Approach ... 22210
Lumbar
Anterior Approach ... 22224
Posterior/Posterolateral Approach ... 22214
Thoracic
Anterior Approach ... 22222
Posterior/Posterolateral Approach ... 22212
with Bunionectomy ... 28295, 28296, 28298, 28299 with Graft
Reconstruction
Periorbital Region ... 21267, 21268

Otolaryngology
Diagnostic
Exam under Anesthesia ... 92502

Otomy
See Incision

Otoplasty ... 69300

Otorhinolaryngology
Unlisted Services and Procedures ... 92700

Ouchterlony Immunodiffusion ... 86331

Outer Ear
See Ear, External Ear

Outpatient Visit
See History and Physical; Office and/or Other Outpatient Services

Output, Cardiac
See Cardiac Output

Ova
Smear ... 87177

Oval Window
Repair Fistula ... 69666

Oval Window Fistula
Repair ... 69666

Ovarian Cyst
See Cyst, Ovarian; Ovary, Cyst

Ovarian Vein Syndrome
Ureterolysis ... 50722

Ovariectomies
See Oophorectomy

Ovariolysis ... 58740

Ovary
Abscess
Incision and Drainage ... 58820-58822
Abdominal Approach ... 58822
Biopsy ... 49321, 58900
Cryopreservation ... 0058T
Cyst
Excision ... 58925
Incision and Drainage ... 58800-58805
Excision ... 58662, 58720
Cyst ... 58925
Partial
Oophorectomy 58661, 58940, 58953, 58954
Ovarian Malignancy ... 58943
Peritoneal Malignancy ... 58943
Tubal Malignancy ... 58943
Wedge Resection ... 58920
Total ... 58940-58943
Laparoscopy ... 58660-58662, 58679
Lesion
Excision ... 58662
Fulguration ... 58662
Lysis
Adhesions ... 58660, 58740
Malignancy
Resection ... 58950-58952, 58957, 58958
Staging Laparotomy ... 58960
Oncology
Biochemical Assay
Apolipoprotein A1 ... 81503
Beta-2 Microglobulin ... 81503
CA-125 ... 81500, 81503
HE4 ... 81500
Menopausal Status ... 81500
Pre-albumin ... 81503
Transferrin ... 81503

Pregnancy
  Surgical Treatment 59120, 59121
Radical Resection 58950-58952
Removal
  with Pelvic Exenteration 45126, 58240
  with Radical Trachelectomy 57531
  with Hysterectomy
  Abdominal 58150, 58152, 58180, 58200, 58210
  Laparoscopic ... 58542, 58544, 58548, 58554, 58552, 58571, 58573, 58575
  Vaginal......... 58262, 58263, 58291, 58292
Transposition 58825
Tumor
  Resection.................. 58950-58958
Unlisted Services and Procedures ... 58679, 58999
Wedge Resection 58920

Oviduct
Anastomosis 58750
Chromotubation 58350
Ectopic Pregnancy................ 59120, 59121
Excision........................ 58700-58720
Fulguration
  Laparoscopic 58670
Hysterosalpingography.................. 74740
Laparoscopy 58679
Ligation........................ 58600-58611
Lysis
  Adhesions 58740
Occlusion............................ 58615
  Laparoscopic 58671
Repair 58752
  Anastomosis 58750
  Create Stoma........................ 58770
Unlisted Services and Procedures ... 58679, 58999
X ray with Contrast.................... 74740

Ovocyte
See Oocyte

Ovulation Tests 84830

Ovum Implantation
See Implantation

Ovum Transfer Surgery
See Gamete Intrafallopian Transfer (GIFT)

Oxalate 83945

Oxcarbazepine
Drug Assay 80183

Oxidase, Ceruloplasmin
See Ceruloplasmin

Oxidoreductase, Alcohol-Nad+
See Antidiuretic Hormone

Oximetry (Noninvasive)
See Pulmonology, Diagnostic
Blood O2 Saturation Determination
  Ear or Pulse 94760-94762
  Pulse, Recording
    Car Seat/Bed Testing........ 94780, 94781
  with Pulmonary Stress Testing 94618

Oxoisomerase
See Phosphohexose Isomerase

Oxosteroids
See Ketosteroids

Oxygen Saturation........... 82805-82810

Oxygenation, Extracorporeal Membrane
See Extracorporeal Membrane Oxygenation (ECMO)

Oxyproline
See Hydroxyproline

Oxytocin Stress Test, Fetal 59020

P

P&P
See Proconvertin

P B Antibodies
See Antibody, Detection, Heterophile

Pacemaker
See Cardiac Assist Devices

Pachymetry
Cornea.............................. 76514
  with Collagen Cross-Linking 0402T

Packing
Nasal Hemorrhage 30901-30906

Pain Management
Electrical Reprocessing.................. 0278T
Epidural/Intrathecal 62350, 62351, 62360-62362, 99601, 99602
Intravenous Therapy ... 96365-96368, 96374-96379

Palate
Abscess
  Incision and Drainage 42000
Biopsy 42100
Bone Graft........................... 42210
Excision
  Lesion.............................. 42120
Fracture
  Closed Treatment..................... 21421
  Open Treatment............... 21422, 21423
Lesion
  Destruction......................... 42160
  Excision 42104-42120
Prosthesis
  Augmentation 21082
  Impression 42280
  Insertion........................... 42281
  Lift 21083
Reconstruction
  Lengthening 42226, 42227
Repair
  Cleft Palate 42200-42225
  Laceration 42180-42182
  Vomer Flap.......................... 42235
Unlisted Services and Procedures 42299

Palate, Cleft
See Cleft Palate

Palatoplasty 42145, 42200-42225

Palatoschisis
See Cleft Palate

Palm
Arch
  Sympathectomy....................... 64823
Bursa
  Incision and Drainage 26025-26030
Dupuytren's Contracture
  Injection 20527
  Manipulation 26341
Fascial Cord
  Enzyme Injection 20527
  Manipulation 26341
Fasciectomy 26121-26123
Fasciotomy 26040-26045
Injection, Enzyme
  Fascial Cord 20527
  Dupuytren's Contracture 20527
Tendon
  Excision 26170
  Incision............................ 26450
  Lysis 26440, 26442
  Transfer 26485, 26489
Tendon Sheath
  Excision 26145
  Incision and Drainage 26020

Palsy, Seventh Nerve
See Facial Nerve Paralysis

Pancreas
Anastomosis
  with Intestines......... 48520-48540, 48548
Biopsy 48100
  Needle Biopsy 48102
Cyst
  Anastomosis 48520-48540
  Repair.............................. 48500
Debridement
  Peripancreatic Tissue................ 48105
Dilation
  Ampulla of Vater 47542, 43277
Endoscopy
  See Endoscopy, Pancreatic Duct
Excision
  Ampulla of Vater 48148
  Duct 48148
  Partial.... 48140-48146, 48150, 48154, 48160
  Peripancreatic Tissue................ 48105
  Total 48155-48160
Lesion
  Ablation 43278
  Excision 48120
Needle Biopsy......................... 48102
Placement
  Drainage.................... 48000, 48001
Polyp
  Ablation............................ 43278
Pseudocyst
  Drainage
    Open 48510
    Percutaneous 49405
Removal
  Calculi (Stone) 43264, 48020
Removal Transplanted Allograft........... 48556
Repair
  Cyst 48500
Resection 48105
Suture 48545
Transplantation...... 48160, 48550, 48554-48556
  Allograft Preparation 48550-48552
Tumor
  Ablation 43278
Unlisted Services and Procedures 48999
X ray 74300, 74301
  Injection Procedure 48400

Pancreas, Endocrine Only
See Islet Cell

Pancreatectomy
Donor................................ 48550
Partial 48140-48146, 48150-48154, 48160
Total 48155-48160
with Transplantation................... 48160

Pancreatic DNAse
See DNAse

Pancreatic Duct
Destruction
  Calculi (Stone) 43265
Dilation
  Endoscopy 43277
Endoscopic Retrograde Cholangiopancreatography (ERCP)
  with Optical Endomicroscopy 0397T
Endoscopy 43273
  Ablation 43278
  Collection
    Specimen 43260
  Destruction
    Calculi (Stone) 43265
  Dilation 43277
  Placement
    Stent 43274
  Removal (Endoscopic)
    Calculi (Stone) 43264
    Foreign Body 43275
    Stent 43275
  Sphincter Pressure 43263
  Sphincterotomy 43262
  Tube Placement 43274
Incision
  Sphincter 43262
Removal
  Calculi (Stone) 43264
  Foreign Body 43275
  Stent 43275
Tube Placement
  Nasopancreatic 43274
  Stent 43274
Tumor
  Ablation 43278
X ray
  Guide Catheter 74329, 74330
  Injection Procedure 47531, 47532, 48400
  Intra-operative 74300, 74301

Pancreatic Elastase 1 (PE1) 82656

Pancreatic Islet Cell AB
See Antibody, Detection, Islet Cell

Pancreaticojejunostomy 48145, 48150, 48153, 48548

Pancreatography
Injection Procedure 48400
Intraoperative 74300, 74301
Postoperative 47531, 47532

Pancreatorrhaphy 48545

Pancreatotomy
See Incision, Pancreas

Pancreozymin-Secretin Test 82938

Panel
See Blood Tests; Organ or Disease-Oriented Panel

Panniculectomy
See Lipectomy

Pap Smears
Any Reporting System 88174, 88175
Bethesda System 88164-88167
Non-Bethesda 88150, 88152, 88153

Paper, Chromatography
See Chromatography, Paper

Papilla, Interdental
See Gums

Papilloma
Destruction
  Anus 46900-46924
  Penis 54050-54065
Excision
  Breast 19110

PAPP D
See Lactogen, Human Placental

Para-Tyrosine
See Tyrosine

Paracentesis
Abdomen 49082, 49083
Eye
  Anterior Chamber Fluid Removal 65800
  with Aqueous Removal 65800
  with Discission of Anterior Hyaloid Membrane 65810
  with Removal
    Blood 65815
    Vitreous 65810
Fetal 59074
Thorax 32554, 32555
  with Imaging Guidance 32555

Paracervical Nerve
Injection
  Anesthetic 64435

Paraffin Bath Therapy 97018
See Physical Medicine/Therapy/Occupational Therapy

Paraganglioma, Medullary
See Glucagon, Tolerance Panel; Pheochromocytoma

Parainfluenza Virus
Antigen Detection
  Immunofluorescence 87279

Paralysis, Facial Nerve
See Facial Nerve Paralysis

Paralysis, Infantile
See Polio

Paranasal Sinuses
See Sinus/Sinuses

Parasites
Blood 87206-87209
Macroscopic Examination 87169
Smear 87177
  from Primary Source 87206, 87207
  Stain 87207, 87209
Tissue 87220

Parasitic Worms
See Helminth

Parathormone 83970

Parathyrin
See Parathormone

Parathyroid Autotransplantation .. 60512

Parathyroid Gland
Autotransplant 60512
Excision 60500-60502
Exploration 60500-60505
Nuclear Medicine
  Imaging, Planar 78070-78072
    with SPECT 78071
    with SPECT and CT Scan 78072

Parathyroid Hormone 83970

Parathyroid Transplantation
See Parathyroid Gland, Autotransplant; Transplantation, Parathyroid

Parathyroidectomy 60500-60505

Paraurethral Gland
See Skene's Gland

Paravertebral Nerve
Destruction 64633-64636
Injection
  Anesthetic 64461, 64462, 64490-64495
  Diagnostic Agent 64490-64495
    with Ultrasound Guidance 0213T-0218T
  Neurolytic 64633-64636
  Therapeutic Agent 64490-64495
    with Ultrasound Guidance 0213T-0218T
Infusion
  Anesthetic 64463

Parietal Cell Vagotomies
See Vagotomy, Highly Selective

Parietal Craniotomy
for Craniosynostosis 61556, 61557

Paring
Skin Lesion
  Benign Hyperkeratotic 11055-11057

Paronychia
Incision and Drainage 10060, 10061

Parotid Duct
Diversion 42507-42510
Reconstruction 42507-42510

Parotid Gland
Abscess
  Incision and Drainage 42300-42305
Calculi (Stone)
  Excision 42330, 42340
Chemodenervation 64611
Excision
  Partial 42410-42415
  Total 42420-42426
Tumor
  Excision 42410-42426

Parotitises, Epidemic
See Mumps

Pars Abdominalis Aortae
See Aorta, Abdominal

Partial
Colectomy
  See Colectomy, Partial
Cystectomy
  See Cystectomy, Partial
Esophagectomy
  See Esophagectomy, Partial
Gastrectomy
  See Gastrectomy, Partial
Glossectomy
  See Glossectomy, Partial
Hepatectomy
  See Hepatectomy, Partial
Mastectomy
  See Mastectomy, Partial
Nephrectomy
  See Nephrectomy, Partial
Pancreatectomy
  See Pancreatectomy, Partial
Splenectomy
  See Splenectomy, Partial

Thromboplastin Time
See Thromboplastin, Partial Thromboplastin Time (PTT)
Ureterectomy
See Ureterectomy, Partial

Particle Agglutination 86403-86406

Particle Beam 61796, 63620
Stereotactic Radiosurgery (Cranial) (Spinal) 61796-61799, 63620, 63621

Parvovirus
Antibody 86747

Patch
Allergy Tests 95044
See Allergy Tests

Patella
See Knee
Application
Patellar Tendon Bearing Cast 29435
Dislocation 27560-27566
Repair................ 27420, 27422, 27424
Excision 27350
Prepatellar Bursa 27340
with Reconstruction................. 27424
Fracture
Closed Treatment....... 27520, 27560, 27562
with Anesthesia 27562
Open Treatment............. 27524, 27566
with Internal Fixation 27524
with Patellectomy.......... 27524, 27566
Reconstruction 27437, 27438
Repair
Arthroplasty................ 27437, 27438
Chondromalacia 27418
Instability 27420-27424
with Prosthesis 27438
Resurfacing 27447
Suture
Infrapatellar Tendon 27380, 27381

Patella, Chondromalacia
See Chondromalacia Patella

Patellar Tendon Bearing (PTB) Cast
Application 29435

Patellectomy
Complete........................ 27524, 27566
Partial 27524, 27566
with Reconstruction 27424, 27524, 27566

Patent Ductus Arteriosus (PDA)
Repair 33820, 33822, 33824, 93582

Paternity Testing............. 86910, 86911

Patey's Operation
See Mastectomy, Radical

Pathologic Dilatation
See Dilation

Pathology and Laboratory
Anatomic Pathology
See Autopsy
Antibody Identification
See Antibody; Antibody Identification
Antigen Detection
See Antigen Detection
Atomic Absorption Spectroscopy 82190
Blood Tests
Cell Count
See Blood Cell Count
Coagulation
See Coagulation, Tests
Gas Analysis
See Blood Gases
Smear
See Blood Smear
Typing
See Blood Typing, Serologic
Urea Nitrogen 84520-84525
Breath Test
Alcohol, Ethyl...................... 82075
Heart Transplant Rejection Detection... 0085T
Helicobacter Pylori............ 78267, 78268, 83013, 83014
Hydrogen 91065
Methane............................ 91065
Urea 78267, 78268
Caffeine Halothane Contracture Test (CHCT) 89049
Cell Count
Blood
See Blood Cell Count, Complete (CBC)
Body Fluid....... 86152, 86153, 89050, 89051
Crystal Identification 89060
with Immunologic Selection and Identification 86152, 86153
Cerebrospinal Fluid
Cell Count......................... 89050
Immunoelectrophoresis 86325
Myelin Basic Protein 83873
Protein, Total 84157
Cervical Smears
See Cervical Smears
Chemiluminescent Assay 82397
Chemistry 82009-84999
Acetaminophen 80329-80331
Acetic Anhydride 84600
Acetylcholinesterase
Blood or Urine.................... 82013
Acetylsalicylic Acid 80329-80331
Acid
Bile 82239
Gastric 82930
Acid Phosphatase 84060, 84066
Acid Probes, Nucleic
See Nucleic Acid Probe
Acylcarnitines 82016, 82017
Adenosine Diphosphate
Blood........................... 82030
Adenosine Monophosphate (AMP)
Blood........................... 82030
Adrenalin
See Catecholamines
Blood........................... 82383
Urine.................... 82382, 82384
Adrenaline-Noradrenaline...... 82382-82384
Adrenocorticotropic Hormone (ACTH) ... 80400-80406, 80412, 80418, 82024
Blood or Urine.................... 82024
Alanine Amino Transferase........... 84460
Albumin
Ischemia modified 82045
Other Source..................... 82042
Serum, Plasma or Whole Blood 82040
Urine.................... 82043, 82044
Alcohol
Ethanol
Any Specimen, Except Breath 80320-80322
Breath 82075
Urine 80320-80322
Ethylene Glycol 82693
Alcohol Dehydrogenase
See Antidiuretic Hormone
Alcohol, Isopropyl
See Isopropyl Alcohol
Alcohol, Methyl
See Methanol
Aldolase
Blood............................ 82085
Aldosterone
Blood............................ 82088
Suppression Evaluation 80408
Urine............................ 82088
Alkaline Phosphatase ... 84075, 84078, 84080
Alkaloids
See Specific Drug
Not Otherwise Specified 80323
Alpha-1 Antitrypsin 82103, 82104
Alpha-Fetoprotein (AFP)
Amniotic Fluid.................... 82106
Serum 82105, 82107
Alpha-tocopherol 84446
Aluminum
Blood............................ 82108
Amine
Vaginal Fluid..................... 82120
Amino Acids................. 82127-82139
Aminolevulinic Acid (ALA)
Blood or Urine.................... 82135
Aminotransferase
See Transaminase
Aminotransferase, Alanine
See Transaminase, Glutamic-Pyruvic
Aminotransferase, Aspartate
See Transaminase, Glutamic-Oxaloacetic
Ammonia
Blood............................ 82140
Amniotic Fluid 82143
Amobarbital 80345
Amphetamine................ 80324-80326
Amylase
Blood............................ 82150
Urine............................ 82150
Androstanediol Glucuronide 82154
Androstenedione
Blood or Urine.................... 82157
Androstenolone
See Dehydroepiandrosterone
Androsterone
Blood or Urine.................... 82160
Angiotensin I-converting Enzyme 82164
Angiotensin Forming Enzyme.......... 82164
Angiotensin II........................ 82163
Antimony 83018
Qualitative 83015
Apolipoprotein
Blood or Urine.................... 82172
Arsenic.................... 82175, 83018
Qualitative 83015
Aspartate Aminotransferase (AST) 84450
Ascorbic Acid
Blood............................ 82180
Aspirin 80329-80331
Atomic Absorption Spectroscopy 82190
b-Hexosaminidase 83080
B-1 Vitamin
See Vitamin
B-6 Vitamin
See Vitamin
B-12 Vitamin
See Vitamin
Barbiturates 80345
Barium 83018
Qualitative 83015
Beryllium 83018
Qualitative 83015
Beta Glucosidase 82963

Index

Beta-2-Microglobulin
Blood. 82232
Urine. 82232
b-Hexosaminidase 83080
Bicarbonate 82374
Bile Acids. 82239
Bilirubin
Blood. 82247, 82248
Feces. 82252
Total
Direct. 82247, 82248
Biotinidase. 82261
Bismuth 83018
Qualitative 83015
Blood Gases
CO_2 82803
HCO_3 82803
O_2 Saturation 82805, 82810
pCO_2 82803
pH 82800, 82803, 82930
pO_2 . . . . . 82803, 82820
Blood Urea Nitrogen 84520-84525
Blood, Occult 82270-82274
See Occult Blood
Bone g1a Protein 83937
Bradykinin
Blood or Urine Test. 82286
C-13
Urea Breath Test 83013, 83014
Urease Activity. 83013, 83014
C-14
Urea Breath Test 78267, 78268
Urease Activity. 83013, 83014
C-Peptide 84681
Cadmium 82300
Calcitonin. 82308
Calcium
Blood
Infusion Test. 82331
Ionized 82330
Total 82310
Urine. 82340
Calculus
Analysis 82355, 82360, 82365, 82370
Calprotectin
Fecal 83993
Carbohydrate Deficient Transferrin. 82373
Carbon Dioxide. 82374, 82803
Carbon Tetrachloride 82441
Carboxyhemoglobin 82375, 82376
Carcinoembryonic Antigen. 82378
Carnitine. 82379
Carotene. 82380
Catecholamines 80424, 82382-82384
Blood. 82383
Panel for Pheochromocytoma. 80424
Urine. 82382
Cathepsin-D 82387
Ceruloplasmin 82390
Cervicovaginal Fluid Evaluation
Amniotic Fluid Proteins 84112
Chemiluminescent Assay. 82397
Chloride
Blood. 82435
Other Source. 82438
Spinal Fluid. 82438
Urine. 82436
Chloride, Methylene
See Dichloromethane
Chlorinated Hydrocarbons 82441
Chlorohydrocarbon
See Chlorinated Hydrocarbons
Cholesterol
HDL. 83718
LDL 83721, 83722
Serum or Whole Blood 82465
Choline Esterase I
See Acetylcholinesterase
Choline Esterase II
See Cholinesterase
Cholinesterase
Blood. 82480, 82482
Cholylglycine 82240
Chondroitin B Sulfate. 82485
VLDL 83719
Chorionic Gonadotropin (hCG) 84702-84704
Chorionic Growth Hormone
See Lactogen, Human Placental
Chromatography
See specific analyte in Pathology and Laboratory, Chemistry
Unspecified Non-Drug Analyte(s). 82542
Hemoglobin 83021, 83036
Sugars. 84375
Chromium. 82495
Citrate 82507
Cocaine 80353
Screen. 80305-80307
Collagen Cross Links 82523
Copper 82525
Coproporphyrin
Blood. 84119, 84120
Feces. 84126
Corticosteroids
Blood or Urine. 83491
Corticosterone 82528
Cortisol
Free. 82530
Total 82533
Cortisol Binding Globulin 84449
Creatine 82540
Creatine Kinase (CK), (CPK) 82550-82554
Creatinine
Blood. 82565
Other Source. 82570
Screen. 82575
Cristobalite
See Silica
CRF
See Corticotropic Releasing Hormone (CRH)
CRH
See Corticotropic Releasing Hormone (CRH)
Cryofibrinogen 82585
Cryoglobulin. 82784, 82785
Qualitative 82595
Cyanacobalamin
See Cyanocobalamin
Cyanide 82600
Cyanocobalamin. 82607, 82608
Cyclic AMP. 82030
Cyclic Somatostatin
See Somatostatin
Cyclosporine. 80158
Cystatin C
Blood. 82610
Cystatins, Kininogen
See Kininogen
Cystine
Urine. 82615
Dehydroepiandrosterone 82626
Dehydroepiandrosterone Sulfate. 82627
Delta-aminolevulinic Acid (ALA) 82135
Deoxycortisol 82634
Des-Gamma-Carboxy-Prothrombin (DCP)
Oncoprotein 83951
Desoxycorticosterone 82633
Diastase
Blood or Urine. 82150
Dibucaine Number 82638
Dichloroethane. 82441
Dichloromethane 82441
Diethylether 84600
Dihydrocodeinone 80361
Dihydrotestosterone (DHT) 80327, 80328, 82642
Dihydroxyvitamin D 82652
Dimethadione. 80339-80341
Dopamine. 82383, 82384
D-Xylose Absorption Test 84620
Elastase 82656
Electrophoresis
Electrophoretic Technique, Unspecified. 82664
Hemoglobin 83020
High Resolution 83701
Protein 84165, 84166
Enzyme Activity
Infectious Agent 87905
Unspecified
Nonradioactive Substrate. 82657
Radioactive Substrate. 82658
Epiandrosterone. 80327, 80328
Epinephrine
Blood or Urine. 82382-82384
Erythropoietin. 82668
Estradiol 82670
Estriol 82677
Estrogen Receptor Assay. 84233
Estrogens
Blood or Urine. 82671, 82672
Estrone 82679
Ethanol
Any Source, Except Breath. 80320-80322
Breath 82075
Ethyl Alcohol 80320
Breath 82075
Ethchlorvynol
Blood or Urine. 80320
Ethylene Glycol 82693
Etiocholanolone 82696
Fat Differential, Fecal 82715
Fat or Lipids, Fecal 82710
Qualitative 82705
Fatty Acids, Nonesterified 82725
Fatty Acids, Very Long Chain 82726
C20-22 Omega-3. . . . . 0111T
Ferritin 82728
Fetal Fibronectin 82731
Fetal Hemoglobin
See Hemoglobin
Fetal Lung Maturity Assessment
Fluorescence Polarization. 83663
Foam Stability Test. 83662
Lamellar Body Density 83664
Lecithin Sphingomyelin (L/S) Ratio 83661
Fetoprotein, Alpha-1
Serum 82105
Amniotic Fluid. 82106
Fibronectin, Fetal 82731
Fluoride 82735
Flurazepam. 80346, 80347
Folic Acid
RBC 82747
Serum 82746
Follicle Stimulating Hormone (FSH). 83001
Fructosamine 82985

Pathology and Laboratory, Chemistry

Fructose
Semen. 82757
TLC Screen 84375
FT-4 84439
Galactokinase
RBC. 82759
Galactose. 82760
Galactose-1-Phosphate Uridyl
Transferase 82775
Screen. 82776
Galectin-3. 82777
Gamma-Glutamyltransferase (GGT). 82977
Gammaglobulin, IgA 82784, 82787
Gammaglobulin, IgD 82784, 82787
Gammaglobulin, IgE. 82785, 82787
Allergen Specific 86003, 86005, 86008
Gammaglobulin, IgG 82784, 82787
Gammaglobulin, IgM. 82784, 82787
Gases, Blood
CO_2 82803
HCO_3 82803
O_2 . . . . . 82803, 82805, 82810
pCO_2 82803
pH 82800, 82803, 82930
pO_2 . . . . . 82803, 82820
Gastric Acid Analysis. 82930
Gastrin 82941
Post Secretin Stimulation. 82938
Gentamicin. 80170
GGT 82977
Glucagon 82943
Tolerance 82946
Glucose
Blood. 82947, 82948
Home Monitoring Device 82962
Other than Blood 82945
Post Glucose Dose 82950
Tolerance 82951, 82952
Glucose-6-Phosphate Dehydrogenase
(G6PD) 82955
Screen. 82960
Glucosidase 82963
Glucuronide Androstanediol 82154
Glutamine. 82127, 82128, 82131
Glutamate Dehydrogenase 82965
Glutamyltransferase, Gamma 82977
Glutathione 82978
Glutathione Reductase
RBC. 82979
Glycated Protein. 82985
Glycohemoglobin 83036
Glycosylated (A1c) Hemoglobin. 83021, 83036, 83037
Gonadotropin, Chorionic 84702
Qualitative 84703
Free Beta Chain 84704
Follicle Stimulating Hormone (FSH) . . . 83001
Luteinizing Hormone (LH) 83002
Growth Stimulation Expressed Gene 2 . . 83006
Haptoglobin 83010
Phenotypes 83012
H. (Helicobacter) Pylori
Blood, Urease Activity 83009
Breath, Urease Activity 83013, 83014
Infectious Agent Antigen 87339
Stool 87338
HDL Cholesterol 83718
Heavy Metal. 83015, 83018
HGH (Human Growth Hormone). 83003
Hemoglobin
Chromatography. 83021
Copper Sulfate Method 83026, 83030, 83033, 83036
Electrophoresis. 83020
Fecal, Immunoassay. 82274
Plasma 83051
Thermolabile. 83065
Unstable 83068
Urine. 83069
Hemoglobin F. 83030, 83033
Hemoglobin A1c (Glycosylated). 83021, 83036, 83037
Hemoglobin-Oxygen Affinity 82820
Hemosiderin
Qualitative 83070
HER-2/neu Oncoprotein. 83950
Heroin. 80305-80307, 80356
HIAA (5-Hydroxyindolacetic Acid) 83497
Urine, Qualitative 81005
Histamine. 83088
Holotranscobalamin. 84999
Homocysteine 83090
Homocystine
Urine. 82615
Homovanillic Acid (HVA) 83150
Human Growth Hormone (HGH). 83003
HVA (Homovanillic Acid) 83150
Hydroxycorticosteroid, 17- (17-OHCS) . . . 83491
Hydroxyindoleacetic Acid, 5- (HIAA) 83497
Urine, Qualitative 81005
Hydroxypregnenolone, 17-. 84143
Hydroxyprogesterone
17-d. 83498
Hydroxyproline
Free. 83500
Total 83505
Hydroxytryptamine, 5-. 84260
IgA 82784
IgD 82784
IgE 82785, 82787, 86003, 86005, 86008
IgG 82784, 82787
IgM. 82784, 82787
Immunoassay, Unspecified Analyte . . . 83516, 83518-83520
Immunoglobulins 82784, 82785
Insulin. 83525, 83527
Insulin Tolerance Test 80434, 80435
Intrinsic Factor 83528
Iron 83540
Binding Capacity. 83550
Isocitric Dehydrogenase (IDH) 83570
Isopropyl Alcohol 80320
Ketogenic Steroids. 83582
Ketone Body. 82009, 82010
Ketosteroids, 17- (17-KS). 83586, 83593
Lactate 83605
Lactate Dehydrogenase. 83615, 83625
Lactic Acid 83605
Lactoferrin, Fecal 83631
Qualitative 83630
Lactogen, Human Placental 83632
Lactose, Urine
Qualitative 83633
LAP 83670
LD 83615-83625
LDH. 83615-83625
LDL Cholesterol 83721, 83722
Lead 83655
Lecithin-Sphingomyelin Ratio 83661
Leucine Aminopeptidase (LAP) 83670
LH 83002
Lipase. 83690
Lipoprotein (a), Blood
Electrophoretic Fractionation 83700
High-resolution Fractionation. 83701
Quantitation 83704
HDL Cholesterol 83718
LDL Cholesterol 83721, 83722
VLDL Cholesterol 83719
Lipoprotein-associated Phospholipase
A2 (Lp-PLA2). 83698
LRH. 83727
Luteinizing Hormone (LH). 83002
Luteinizing Releasing Factor (LRH) 83727
Macroglobulins, Alpha-2 86329
Magnesium 83735
Malate Dehydrogenase 83775
Maltose Tolerance. 82951, 82952
Mammotropin 84146
Manganese 83785
Marijuana. 80305-80307
Mass Spectrometry, Unspecified
Analyte. 83789
Qualitative 80305-80307
Mercury 83018, 83825
Qualitative 83015
Metanephrines. 83835
Methadone. 80358
Methamphetamine 80324-80326
Methanol 80320
Methemalbumin. 83857
Methemoglobin 83050
Qualitative 83045
Methsuximide 80339-80341
Methyl Alcohol. 80320
Microalbumin. 82043, 82044
Microfluidic Analysis. 83861
Microglobulin, Beta-2 82232
MPO 83876
Mucin
Synovial Fluid 83872
Mucopolysaccharides, Acid. 83864
Myelin Basic Protein
Cerebrospinal Fluid. 83873
Myeloperoxidase (MPO) 83876
Myoglobin 83874
Natriuretic Peptide. 83880
Nephelometry, Unspecified Analyte 83883
Nickel. 83885
Nicotine 80323
Nucleotidase 83915
Occult Blood. 82270-82272
Oligoclonal Bands 83916
Oligoclonal Immunoglobulins 83916
Oncoprotein 83950, 83951
Des-Gamma-Carboxy-Prothrombin
(DCP). 83951
HER-2/neu 83950
Opiates. 80361-80364
Oral Lactose Tolerance Test 82951, 82952
Organic Acids. 83918-83921
Osmolality
Blood. 83930
Urine. 83935
Osteocalcin 83937
Ovulation Tests 84830
Oxalate. 83945
Oxygen Saturation 82805, 82810
Pancreatic Elastase 1 (PE1) 82656
Pancreozymin-Secretin Test 82938
PAMG-1 84112
Parathormone. 83970
Parathyroid Hormone 83970
pH
Blood. 82800, 82803
Body Fluid 83986
Exhaled Breath Condensate. 83987
Phencyclidine (PCP) 83992
Phenobarbital. 80345

Phenothiazine ... 80342-80344
Phenylalanine (PKU)
  Blood ... 84030
Phenylalanine-Tyrosine Ratio ... 84030, 84510
Phenylketones
  Qualitative ... 84035
Phosphatase, Acid ... 84060, 84066
Phosphatase, Alkaline ... 84075, 84078, 84080
Phosphates, Inorganic ... 84100
Phosphates, Organic
  See specific method
Phosphatidylglycerol ... 84081
Phosphogluconate, 6-, Dehydrogenase
  RBC ... 84085
Phospholipase A2
  Lipoprotein-associated (Lp-PLA2) ... 83698
  Secretory Type II (sPLA2-IIA) ... 0423T
Phosphohexose Isomerase ... 84087
Phosphorus, Inorganic ... 84100
  Urine ... 84105
Pituitary Gonadotropins ... 83001, 83002
PKU ... 84030
Placenta Alpha Microglobulin-1 (PAMG-1) ... 84112
Plasma Protein-A, Pregnancy-Associated (PAPP-A) ... 84163
Porphobilinogen, Urine ... 84110
  Qualitative ... 84106
Porphyrin Precursors ... 82135, 84106, 84110
Porphyrins
  Feces, Quantitative ... 84126
  Urine, Qualitative ... 84119
  Urine, Quantitation and Fractionation ... 84120
Potassium
  Blood ... 84132
  Urine ... 84133
Prealbumin ... 84134
Pregnancy Test
  Blood ... 84702-84704
  Urine ... 81025
Pregnancy Associated Plasma Protein-A ... 84163
Pregnanediol ... 84135
Pregnanetriol ... 84138
Pregnenolone ... 84140
Procalcitonin (PCT) ... 84145
Progesterone ... 84144
Progesterone Receptors ... 84234
Proinsulin ... 84206
Prolactin ... 84146
Prostaglandin ... 84150
Prostate Specific Antigen ... 84152-84154
Protein
  See Protein
Protoporphyrin
  RBC ... 84202
  RBC, Screen ... 84203
Pyridoxal Phosphate ... 84207
Pyruvate ... 84210
Pyruvate Kinase ... 84220
Quinine ... 84228
Receptor Assay
  Estrogen ... 84233
  Non-endocrine ... 84238
  Progesterone ... 84234
  Unspecified Hormone ... 84235
Reinsch Test ... 83015
Renin ... 84244
Renin-Converting Enzyme ... 82164
Riboflavin ... 84252
Ropes Test ... 83872
Salicylates ... 80329-80331
Selenium ... 84255
Serotonin ... 84260
Sex Hormone Binding Globulin ... 84270
Serum Glutamic Oxalacetic Transaminase (SGOT) ... 84450
Serum Glutamic Pyruvate Transaminase (SGPT) ... 84460
Sialic Acid ... 84275
Sickle Hemoglobin ... 85660
Silica ... 84285
Sodium
  Blood ... 84295
  Unspecified Source ... 84302
  Urine ... 84300
Somatomammotropin, Chorionic ... 83632
Somatomedin ... 84305
Somatostatin ... 84307
Somatotropin ... 83003
Specific Gravity
  Other than Urine ... 84315
  Urine ... 81000-81003
Spectrophotometry
  Unspecified Analyte ... 84311
Stone Analysis ... 82355, 82360, 82365, 82370
Sugars ... 84375-84379
Sulfate
  Urine ... 84392
Sulfhemoglobin ... 83060
Sweat Test ... 82435
T-3 ... 84479-84482
T-4 ... 84436, 84437, 84439, 84479
Tear Osmolarity ... 83861
Testosterone ... 84402, 84403, 84410
Thiamine ... 84425
Thiocyanate ... 84430
Thromboxane
  Urine ... 84431
Thyroglobulin ... 84432
Thyroid Hormone Binding Ratio ... 84479
Thyroid Hormone Uptake ... 84479
Thyroid Stimulating Hormone (TSH) ... 84443
Thyroid Stimulating Immune Globulins (TSI) ... 84445
Thyroxine ... 84436, 84437, 84439
Thyroxine Binding Globulin (TBG) ... 84442
Tobramycin ... 80200
Tocopherol, Alpha ... 84446
Transcortin ... 84449
Transferase
  Alanine Amino ... 84460
  Aspartate Amino ... 84450
Transferrin ... 84466
Triglycerides ... 84478
Triiodothyronine ... 84480-84482
Troponin ... 84484
  Qualitative ... 84512
Trypsin
  Duodenal Fluid ... 84485
  Feces ... 84488, 84490
Tyrosine ... 84510
Unlisted Chemistry Procedure ... 84999
Urea Nitrogen ... 84520, 84525
  Screen ... 84545
  Urine ... 84540
Uric Acid
  Blood ... 84550
  Other Source ... 84560
Urobilinogen
  Feces ... 84577
  Urine ... 84578, 84580, 84583
Uroporphyrin ... 84120
Valproic Acid (Dipropylacetic Acid) ... 80164, 80165
Vanillylmandelic Acid (VMA)
  Urine ... 84585
Vasoactive Intestinal Peptide (VIP) ... 84586
Vasopressin ... 84588
Vitamins
  See Vitamin
Volatiles ... 84600
Xylose Absorption ... 84620
Zinc ... 84630
Cholesterol
  HDL ... 83718
  LDL ... 83721
  Lipid Panel ... 80061
  Serum ... 82465
  VLDL ... 83719
Chorionic Gonadotropin
  Detection ... 84703
  Free Beta Chain ... 84704
  Measurement ... 84702
  Stimulation Panel ... 80414, 80415
Chromatography
  See Chromatography
Chromium ... 82495
Chromogenic Substrate Assay
  Coagulation Test ... 85130
Chromosome Analysis
  See Chromosome Analysis
Clinical Consultation ... 80500-80502
Coagulation
  See Coagulation, Tests
Cryopreservation
  Cells ... 88240, 88241
  Oocyte(s)
    Immature ... 0357T
    Mature ... 89337
  Ovarian Tissue ... 0058T
  Testicular ... 89335
Cytogenetic Studies ... 88230-88299
Cytopathology ... 88104-88140
  Cervical or Vaginal
    Requiring Interpretation by Physician ... 88141
    Thin Layer Prep ... 88142, 88143, 88174, 88175
  Concentration Technique ... 88108
    See Saccomanno Technique
  Evaluation ... 88172, 88177
    Immediate Cytohistologic Study ... 88172, 88177
  Fluids, Washings, Brushings ... 46600, 46601, 88104-88108
  Forensic ... 88125
  Other Source ... 88160-88162
  Selective Cellular Enhancement Technique ... 88112
  Smears
    Cervical or Vaginal ... 88141-88167, 88174, 88175
    Nasal ... 89190
  Unlisted Services and Procedures ... 88199
  Urinary Tract Specimen
    In Situ Hybridization Technique ... 88120, 88121
Drug Assay (Testing)
  See Drug Assay
Enzymes
  Specific Analytes
    3 Beta-Hydroxydehydrogenase ... 80406
    6-Phosphoglutonate Dehydrogenase ... 84085
    21 Hydroxylase ... 80402, 81402, 81405
    Acetylcholinesterase ... 82013
    Acetylglucosaminyltransferase ... 81406
    Aldolase ... 82085

Index

Alpha-1 Antiproteinase 81332
Amylase 82150
Angiotensin Converting Enzyme (ACE). 81400, 82164
Antistreptokinase. 86590
Aspartoacylase. 81200
Biotinidase 81404, 82261
b-Hexosaminidase 83080
Cholinesterase 82480, 82482
Creatine Kinase 82550, 82552-82554
Dehydrogenase. 81205, 81400, 81401, 81404, 81405
Deoxyribonuclease Antibody 86215
Diastase 82150
Elastase 82656
Galactokinase. 82759
Galactose-1-phosphate Uridyl Transferase. 82775, 82776
Gamma-glutamyltransferase 82977
Glucose-6-phosphate Dehydrogenase. 82955, 82960
Glucosidase 81251, 82963
Glucuronosyltransferase 1 81350
Glutamate Dehydrogenase. 82965
Glutamyltransferase. 82977
Glutathione Reductase 82979
Hexosaminidase. 81255, 81406
Hydroxylase 81406
Isocitric Dehydrogenase. 83570
Kinase. . 81270, 81245, 81246, 81401, 81404
Lactate Dehydrogenase 83615
Leucine Aminopeptidase 83670
Leukocyte Alkaline Phosphatase 85540
Ligase 81331
Lipase 83690
Lipoprotein-associated Phospholipase A2 83698
Malate Dehydrogenase 83775
Mannosyltransferase 81406
Methyltransferase 81401
Muramidase 85549
Myeloperoxidase 83876
Peptidase 81400
Peroxidase 82270-82272
Phosphatase . . 80053, 80076, 81250, 84060, 84066, 84075, 84078, 84080
Phosphodiesterase 81330
Phosphohexose Isomerase. 84087
Polymerase 81406
Pseudocholinesterase 82480
Pyruvate Kinase 84220
Reductase. 81355, 81291
Reptilase. 85635
Streptokinase Antibody 86590
Transferase. . . . 80053, 80076, 84450, 84460
Urease 83009, 83013, 83014
Uridylyltransferase. 81401, 81406
Evocative/Suppression Test
Agent Administration. 96360, 96361, 96372-96375
Analytes
Evaluation Panel
Anterior Pituitary. 80418
Metyrapone Panel 80436
Stimulation Panel
ACTH 80400, 80402, 80406
Calcitonin 80410
Corticotropic Releasing Hormone (CRH). 80412
Chorionic Gonadotropin 80414, 80415
Gonadotropin Releasing Hormone . . 80426
Growth Hormone. 80428
Renin, Peripheral Vein 80417
Renin, Renal Vein 80416
Thyrotropin Releasing Hormone (TRH). 80438, 80439
Suppression Panel
Dexamethasone 80420
Growth Hormone. 80430
Insulin-induced C-peptide. 80432
Tolerance Panel
Glucagon 80422, 80424
Insulin 80434, 80435
Physician Monitoring
See Evaluation and Management
Factor Inhibitor Tests
Activated Protein C Resistance Assay. . . 85307
Antithrombin III Activity. 85300
Antithrombin III Antigen Assay 85301
Factor Inhibitor Test. 85335
Protein C
Activity 85303
Antigen. 85302
Protein S
Free. 85306
Total 85305
Fibrin Degradation Products
Agglutination. 85362
Paracoagulation. 85366
Quantitative 85379
D-dimer 85378, 85379
Fibrinolysis
See Fibrinolysis
Flow Cytometry. 88182-88189
See Flow Cytometry
Gene Analysis
Analytes
See Gene Analysis, Analytes
Chimerism Analysis. 81267, 81268
Comparative Analysis Using Short Tandem Repeat (STR) Markers 81265, 81266
Cytogenomic Microarray Analysis. 81406
HLA Class I and II Typing, Low Resolution 81370, 81371
HLA Class I Typing, Low Resolution 81372-81374
HLA Class II Typing, Low Resolution 81375-81377
HLA Class I and II Typing, High Resolution 81378
HLA Class I Typing, High Resolution 81379-81381
HLA Class II Typing, High Resolution 81382, 81383
Human Platelet Antigen Genotyping. 81105-81112
Microsatellite Instability Analysis. 81301
Translocation
See Gene Analysis, Translocation
Genetic Testing
See Gene Analysis
Genomic Sequencing Procedure
See Genomic Sequencing Procedure
Globulin
See Globulin
Hematology and Coagulation 85002-85999
Blood Cell Count
See Blood Cell Count
Blood Tests
See Blood Tests
Blood Typing
See Blood Typing, Serologic Compatibility. 86920-86923
Coagulation
See Coagulation
Disorders
Anemia 0516F
Coagulopathy
See Coagulopathy
Hemodynamic Evaluation
Central Cardiovascular. 78414
Exercise Study 93464
Pharmacologic Agent Study. 93463
Portography 37182, 37183, 75885
Venography. 75889
Unlisted Services and Procedures. 85999
Hemoglobin
See Hemoglobin
Hormone Assay
See Hormone Assay
Human Growth Hormone (HGH)
See Human Growth Hormone (HGH)
Immunology
See Immunology
Infectious Agent
Amplified Probe Detection
See Nucleic Acid Probe, Amplified Probe Detection, Infectious Agent
Analytes
See Infectious Agent
Antibody Detection
See Antibody; Antibody Identification
Antigen Detection
See Antigen Detection
Concentration. 87015
Enzyme Activity 87905
Genotype Analysis
See Infectious Agent, Genotype Analysis
Immunoassay Detection
See Infectious Agent, Antibody Detection
Nucleic Acid Detection
See Infectious Agent, Antigen Detection, Nucleic Acid Probe
Phenotype Analysis
See Infectious Agent, Phenotype Analysis
Quantification
See Nucleic Acid Probe, Quantification, Infectious Agent
Iontophoresis
Sweat Collection 89230
In Vivo Procedures 88720-88749
Meat Fibers
Feces 89160
Microbiology. 87003-87999
Microorganism Identification
by Animal Inoculation
See Animal Inoculation
by Culture
See Bacteria Culture; Culture, Bacteria
by Dark Field Examination 87164-87166
by Examination. 87168-87172
by Nucleic Acid Probe
See Nucleic Acid Probe
by Nucleic Acid Sequencing 87153
by Smear or Stain 87177, 87205-87210
by Tissue Culture 87230, 87252, 87253
Sensitivity Studies. 87181-87190
Serum Bactericidal Titer 87197
Virus Isolation 87250-87255
Molecular Pathology. 81200-81099
Multianalyte Assays with Algorithmic Analyses
Adoponectin. 81506
Apoliproprotein A1. 81503
AFP. 81510-81512
Beta-2 Microglobulin. 81503
CA-125. 81500, 81503
DIA 81509, 81511, 81512

Ferritin ... 81506
Glucose ... 81506
HbA1c ... 81506
hCG ... 81508-81512
HE4 ... 81500
hs-CRP ... 81506
Insulin ... 81506
Interleukin 2-receptor Alpha ... 81506
mRNA ... 81518-81521
Oncological Gene Profiling ... 81504
PAPP-A ... 81508, 81509
Prealbumin ... 81503
Trisomy 21, 18, and 13 ... 81507
Transferrin ... 81503
uE3 ... 81510-81512
Unlisted ... 81599
Nucleic Acids
See Nucleic Acid Probe
Optical Endomicroscopy ... 88375
Organ or Disease-Oriented Panel
See Organ or Disease-Oriented Panel
Ovulation Tests ... 84830
Panels
See Blood Tests, Panels; Organ or Disease-Oriented Panel
Particle Agglutination ... 86403-86406
Paternity Testing ... 86910, 86911
pH
See pH
Protein
See Protein
Postmortem ... 88000-88099
Radioimmunoassay ... 82009-84999
Receptor Assay
See Receptor Assay
Red Blood Cell (RBC)
See Red Blood Cell (RBC)
Respiratory Syncytial Virus
See Respiratory Syncytial Virus
Reticulocyte
Count ... 85044-85046
Reproductive Medicine ... 89250-89398
Cryopreservation
See Cryopreservation
Embryo
See Embryo
Oocyte
See Oocyte
Reproductive Tissue
See Reproductive Tissue
Sperm Analysis/Evaluation
See Pathology and Laboratory, Sperm
Smear and Stain
See Smear and Stain
Spectrometry, Mass
Non-drug Analytes ... 83789
See specific analyte in Drug Assay; Pathology and Laboratory, Chemistry
Column Chromatography
Unspecified Non-drug Analyte(s) ... 82542
Spectrophotometry ... 84311
Spectroscopy
Atomic Absorption ... 82190
Bioimpedance Spectroscopy (BIS) ... 93702
Fluorescent
Advanced Glycation Endproducts (AGE) ... 88749
Infrared ... 82365
Intravascular ... 0205T
Magnetic Resonance ... 76390
Lipoprotein ... 83704
Sperm
Analysis
Antibodies ... 89325
Cervical Mucus Penetration Test ... 89330
Evaluation from Semen
Count ... 89310, 89320, 89322
Motility ... 89300, 89310, 89320-89322
Differential ... 89320, 89322
Presence ... 89300, 89321
for Retrograde Ejaculation ... 89331
Forensic ... 88125
Hamster Penetration Test ... 89329
Huhner Test ... 89300
Cryopreservation ... 89259
Storage ... 89343
Thawing ... 89353
Identification
Aspiration ... 89257
from Testis Tissue ... 89264
Isolation ... 89260, 89261
Sputum ... 89220
Stem Cell
See Stem Cell
Storage
See Storage
Streptococcus, Group A
Antigen Detection
Immunoassay ... 87430
Nucleic Acid ... 87650-87652
Direct Optical Observation ... 87880
Streptococcus, Group B
by Immunoassay
with Direct Optical Observation ... 87802
Sugars ... 84375-84379
Surgical Pathology ... 88300-88399
Antibody Stain Procedure
Immunofluorescence ... 88346, 88350
Archived Tissue Examination ... 88363
Consultation ... 88321-88325
Intraoperative ... 88329-88334
Decalcification Procedure ... 88311
Electron Microscopy ... 88348
Gross and Micro Exam
Level II ... 88302
Level III ... 88304
Level IV ... 88305
Level V ... 88307
Level VI ... 88309
Gross Exam
Level I ... 88300
Histochemistry ... 88313-88319
Immunocytochemistry ... 88313, 88341, 88342, 88344
Immunofluorescent Study ... 88346, 88350
Immunohistochemistry ... 88341, 88342, 88344
Macroscopic Tissue Examination 88387, 88388
Microdissection ... 88380, 88381
Morphometry
See Morphometric Analysis
Nerve Teasing ... 88362
Optical Endomicroscopy ... 88375
Protein Analysis ... 88371, 88372
Special Stain ... 88312-88314, 88319
Staining ... 88312-88314
Tissue Hybridization ... 88364-88366
Unlisted Services and Procedures 88399, 89240
Sweat Collection
Iontophoresis ... 89230
Syphilis Test ... 86592, 86593
T Cells
See T Cells
Therapeutic Drug Assay
See Therapeutic Drug Assay
Thrombin Time ... 85670-85675
Thrombomodulin ... 85337
Thromboplastin
See Thromboplastin
Tolerance Test
See Tolerance Test
Toxicology Screen ... 80305-80307
Transfusion Medicine
Antibody
Elution ... 86860
Identification ... 86870
Screen ... 86850
Antihuman Globulin Test
See Coombs Test
Blood Processing
Autologous ... 86890, 86891
Frozen ... 86927, 86930-86932
Irradiation ... 86945
Pooling ... 86965
Pretreatment ... 86970-86972, 86975-86978
Splitting ... 86985
Volume Reduction ... 86960
Blood Typing
See Blood Typing, Serologic
Leukocyte Transfusion ... 86950
Unlisted Procedure ... 86999
Urea Nitrogen
Blood ... 84520-84525
Clearance ... 84545
Quantitative ... 84520
Semiquantitative ... 84525
Urine ... 84540
Urinalysis
See Urinalysis
Vitamin
See Vitamin
Western Blot
HIV ... 86689
Protein ... 84181, 84182
Tissue Analysis ... 88371, 88372
White Blood Cell
Alkaline Phosphatase ... 85540
Antibody ... 86021
Count ... 85032, 85048, 89055
Differential ... 85004-85007, 85009
Histamine Release Test ... 86343
Phagocytosis ... 86344
Transfusion ... 86950

PBG
See Porphobilinogen

PCP
See Phencyclidine

PCR
See Genomic Sequencing Procedures (GSPs) and Other Molecular Multianalyte Assays

Péans' Operation
See Amputation, Leg, Upper, at Hip; Radical Resection; Replantation

Pectoral Cavity
See Chest Cavity

Pectus Carinatum
Reconstructive Repair ... 21740-21743
with Thoracoscopy ... 21743

Pectus Excavatum
Reconstructive Repair ... 21740-21742
with Thoracoscopy ... 21743

Pediatric Critical Care ... 99471, 99472

Pediatric Intensive Care ... 99478

Pedicle Fixation
- Insertion 22840, 22842-22844

Pedicle Flap
- Abbe-Estlander Type 40761
- for Breast Reconstruction
  - Double 19369
  - Single 19367
- for Cerebrospinal Fluid Leak 61619
- for Eyelid Repair 67961
- for Lip Repair 40761
- for Vaginal Lengthening 46748
- Formation 15570-15576
- Island 15740
- Neurovascular 15750
- Transfer 15650
- Vascular 15730, 15731, 15733
- Zygomaticofacial Flap 15730

PEEP
See Pressure Breathing, Positive

Pelvi-Ureteroplasty
See Pyeloplasty

Pelvic Adhesions
See Adhesions, Pelvic

Pelvic Exam
- Preventive 99397
- under Anesthesia 57410

Pelvic Exenteration 45126, 51597, 58240

Pelvic Fixation
See Spinal Instrumentation

Pelvic Lymphadenectomy 38770, 38780, 55845, 55865, 57531, 58210, 58210, 58548, 58958

Pelvimetry 74710

Pelviolithotomy 50130

Pelvis
See Hip
- Abscess
  - Incision and Drainage 26990, 45000
- Angiography 72191, 74174
- Biopsy 27040, 27041
- Bone
  - Drainage 26992
- Brace Application 20662
- Bursa
  - Incision and Drainage 26991
- CT Scan 72191-72194, 74174, 74176-74178
- Destruction
  - Lesion 58662
- Endoscopy
  - Destruction of Lesion 58662
  - Lysis of Adhesions 58660
- Exclusion
  - Small Intestine 44700
- Exenteration 45126, 51597, 58240
- Fasciotomy
  - Decompression 27027
    - with Debridement 27057
- Halo 20662
- Hematoma
  - Incision and Drainage 26990
- Lysis
  - Adhesions 58660
- Magnetic Resonance Angiography 72198
- Magnetic Resonance Imaging (MRI) 72195-72197
  - Obstetric 74712, 74713
- Removal
  - Foreign Body 27086, 27087
- Repair
  - Osteotomy 27158
  - Tendon 27098
- Ring Dislocation/Fracture
  - Closed Treatment 27197, 27198
    - with Manipulation 27198
    - without Manipulation 27197
  - Open Treatment 27217, 27218
    - with Internal Fixation 27217, 27218
  - Percutaneous Skeletal Fixation 27216
- Tumor
  - Excision 27043-27048
  - Radical Resection 27049, 27059
- Ultrasound 76856, 76857
- Unlisted Services and Procedures for Hips and Hip Joint 27299
- X ray 72170-72190
  - Manometry 74710
  - with Hip(s) 73501-73503, 73521-73523

Pemberton Osteotomy of Pelvis 27158

Penectomy
See Amputation, Penis

Penetrating Keratoplasties
See Keratoplasty, Penetrating

Penile Induration
See Peyronie Disease

Penile Prosthesis
- Insertion
  - Inflatable 54401-54405
  - Noninflatable 54400
- Removal
  - Inflatable 54406, 54410-54417
  - Semi-rigid 54415-54417
- Repair
  - Inflatable 54408
- Replacement
  - Inflatable 54410, 54411, 54416, 54417
  - Semi-rigid 54416, 54417

Penile Rigidity Test 54250

Penile Tumescence Test 54250

Penis
- Amputation
  - Complete 54125
  - Partial 54120
  - Radical 54130-54135
  - Replanted 54438
- Biopsy 54100-54105
- Circumcision
  - Lysis of Adhesions 54162
  - Repair 54163
  - Surgical Excision
    - Newborn 54150, 54160, 54161
- Destruction
  - Lesion 54050, 54055-54057, 54060, 54065
- Drainage 54015
- Excision
  - Partial 54120
  - Prepuce 54150-54161, 54163
  - Total 54125-54135
- Frenulotomy 54164
- Incision
  - Frenulum 54164
  - Prepuce 54000, 54001
- Incision and Drainage 54015
- Injection
  - for Erection 54235
  - Peyronie Disease 54200
    - Surgical Exposure Plaque 54205
  - Vasoactive Drugs 54231
  - X ray 54230
- Insertion
  - Prosthesis
    - Inflatable 54401-54405
    - Noninflatable 54400
- Irrigation
  - Priapism 54220
- Lesion
  - Destruction
    - Cryosurgery 54056
    - Electrodesiccation 54055
    - Extensive 54065
    - Laser Surgery 54057, 54065
    - Simple 54050-54060
    - Surgical Excision 54060
  - Excision 54060
    - Penile Plaque 54110-54112
- Nocturnal Penile Tumescence Test 54250
- Occlusion
  - Vein 37790
- Plaque
  - Excision 54110-54112
- Plethysmography 54240
- Prepuce
  - Adhesions
    - Lysis 54450
  - Slitting 54000, 54001
  - Stretching 54450
- Removal
  - Foreign Body 54115
  - Prosthesis
    - Inflatable 54406, 54410-54417
    - Semi-rigid 54415-54417
- Repair
  - Angulation 54360
  - Chordee 54300-54304, 54328
  - Complications 54340-54348
  - Epispadias 54380-54390
  - Fistulization 54435
  - Hypospadias 54328-54352
  - Injury 54440
  - Priapism with Shunt 54420-54430
  - Prosthesis
    - Inflatable 54408
  - Corporeal Tear(s) 54437
- Replacement
  - Prosthesis
    - Inflatable 54410, 54411, 54416, 54417
    - Semi-rigid 54416, 54417
- Replantation 54438
- Revascularization 37788
- Rigidity Test 54250
- Suture
  - Urethral Injury 53505
- Test Erection 54250
- Unlisted Services and Procedures 55899
- Venous Studies 93980, 93981

Penis Adhesions
- Lysis
  - Post-circumcision 54162

Penis Prostheses
See Penile Prosthesis

Pentagastrin Test
See Gastric Analysis Test

Pentamidine
See Inhalation Treatment

Peptidase P
See Angiotensin Converting Enzyme (ACE)

Peptidase S
See Leucine Aminopeptidase

Peptide, Connecting
See C-Peptide

Peptide, Vasoactive Intestinal
See Vasoactive Intestinal Peptide

Peptidyl Dipeptidase A
See Angiotensin Converting Enzyme (ACE)

Percutaneous Abdominal Paracentesis
See Abdomen, Drainage

Percutaneous Atherectomies
See Artery, Atherectomy

Percutaneous Biopsy, Gallbladder/Bile Ducts
See Bile Duct, Biopsy

Percutaneous Catheter Retrieved . . 37197

Percutaneous Discectomies
See Discectomy, Percutaneous

Percutaneous Electric Nerve Stimulation
See Application, Neurostimulation

Percutaneous Insertion—Ventricular Assist Device 33990, 33991

Percutaneous Lumbar Discectomy
See Decompression

Percutaneous Lysis
Epidural Adhesions 62263, 62264

Percutaneous Nephrostomies
See Nephrostomy, Percutaneous

Percutaneous Pleural Fluid Drainage
with Imaging 32557
without Imaging 32556

Percutaneous Transluminal Angioplasty
Artery
  Aortic 37246, 37247
  Brachiocephalic 37246, 37247
  Coronary 92920, 92921
  Pulmonary 92997, 92998
  Renal 37246, 37247
  Visceral 37246, 37247
Vein 36902, 36905, 36907, 37248, 37249

Percutaneous Transluminal Coronary Angioplasty
See Percutaneous Transluminal Angioplasty

Pereyra Procedure 51845, 57289, 58267, 58293

Performance Measures
Aortic Aneurysm 9001F-9004F
Acute Bronchitis
  Interventions
    Antibiotic Prescribed 4120F-4124F
Acute Otitis Externa/Otitis Media with Effusion
  Diagnostic/Screening Processes or Results
    Hearing Testing 3230F
  History
    Auricular Pain 1116F
    Periauricular Pain 1116F
  Interventions
    Antimicrobial Therapy 4131F, 4132F
    Effusion Antihistamines/
    Decongestants 4133F, 4134F
    Systemic Antimicrobials 4131F, 4132F
    Systemic Steroids 4135F, 4136F
    Topical Therapy 4130F
  Physical Examination
    Membrane Mobility 2035F
Amyotrophic Lateral Sclerosis (ALS)
  Diagnostic/Screening Processes or Results
    Cognitive Behavioral Impairment
    Screening 3755F
    Dysarthria Evaluation 3762F, 3763F
    Impaired Nutrition Screening . . . 3759F-3761F
    Pulmonary Function Testing 3758F
    Symptom Evaluation 3756F, 3757F
  Interventions
    End-of-Life Planning Assistance 4553F
    Nutritional Support Offered 4551F
    Pharmacotherapy 4540F, 4541F
    Respiratory Support Options 4550F
    Speech Pathologist Referral 4552F
  Patient History
    Respiratory Insufficiency 1503F-1505F
  Patient Management
    Care Planning 0580F
Anesthesiology/Critical Care
  Interventions
    Active Warming 4250F
    Anesthesia 4255F, 4256F
    Head of Bed Elevation 4167F
    Mechanical Ventilation 4168F, 4169F
  Patient Safety
    Maximal Sterile Barrier Technique . . . 6030F
Annual Monitoring
  Interventions
    Angiotensin Converting Enzyme
    (ACE)/Angiotensin Receptor Blockers
    (ARB) 4188F, 4210F
    Anticonvulsant 4191F, 4230F
    Digoxin 4189F, 4220F
    Diuretic 4190F, 4221F
Asthma
  Follow-up or Other Outcomes
    Discharge Plan 5250F
  History 1005F
    Assessment of Tobacco Use or Exposure
    to Second-hand Smoke 1031F-1033F
    Intermittent 1039F
    Persistent 1038F
  Interventions
    Alternative Long-term Control Medication
    Prescribed 4144F
    Inhaled Corticosteroids 4140F
    Pharmacologic Therapy 4015F
  Physical Examination
    Impairment Assessment 2015F
    Risk Assessment 2016F
  Therapeutic, Preventive or Other Interventions
    Tobacco Use Cessation
      Counseling 4000F, 4004F
      Pharmacologic Therapy 4001F, 4004F
Atrial Fibrillation/Flutter
  Diagnostic/Screening Processes or Results
    International Normalized Ratio (INR)
    Measured 3555F
    Thromboembolism Risk 3550F-3552F
  History
    Thromboembolism Risk Assessed 1180F
  Interventions
    Warfarin Therapy 4300F, 4301F
Back Pain
  Diagnostic/Screening Processes or Results
    Imaging Study 3330F, 3331F
  History
    Back Pain and Function 1130F
    Employment Status 1130F
    Exercise 1136F, 1137F
    Mental Health Assessment 1134F, 1135F
    Prior Treatment Response 1130F
    Warning Signs 1130F
  Interventions
    Bed Rest Counseling 4248F
    Exercise Regimen 4240F, 4242F
    Range of Activity Counseling 4245F
  Patient Management
    Episode Initial Visit 0525F
    Episode Subsequent Visit 0526F
  Physical Examination
    Initial Visit 2040F
    Mental Health Documented 2044F
Care for Older Adults
  History
    Advance Care Plan 1157F, 1158F
    Functional Status Assessment 1170F
    Medication Review . . . 1111F, 1159F, 1160F
    Pain Severity Assessed 1125F, 1126F
  Patient Management
    Pain Plan of Care 0521F
Carotid Stenosis 9005F-9007F
Chronic Kidney Disease
  Diagnostic/Screening Processes or Results
    Blood Pressure, Diastolic 3078F-3080F
    Blood Pressure, Systolic 3074F-3079F
    Hemoglobin 3279F-3281F
    Serum Levels 3278F
  Interventions
    Erythropoieses-Stimulating Agents (ESA)
    Therapy 4171F, 4172F
  Patient Management
    Blood Pressure Management 0513F
    Elevated Hemoglobin 0514F
Chronic Obstructive Pulmonary Disease
  Diagnostic/Screening Processes or Results
    Functional Expiratory Volume . . . 3040F-3042F
    Oxygen Saturation 3035F
    Spirometry 3023F, 3025F
  History
    Dyspnea 1018F, 1019F
    Pneumococcus Immunization 1022F
    Symptom Assessment 1015F
    Tobacco Use 1034F-1036F
  Interventions
    Angiotensin Converting Enzyme
    (ACE)/Angiotensin Receptor Blockers
    (ARB) 4188F, 4210F
    Bronchodilator Prescription 4025F
    Influenza Immunization 4035F, 4037F
    Oxygen Therapy 4030F
    Pharmacologic Therapy 4001F
    Pneumococcus Immunization 4040F
    Pulmonary Rehabilitation 4033F
    Tobacco Use Cessation Intervention
      Counseling 4000F, 4004F
      Pharmacologic Therapy 4001F, 4004F
Chronic Wound Care
  Interventions
    Compression Therapy 4267F, 4268F
    Diabetic Foot Care 4305F
    Dressings 4265F, 4266F
    Pressure Offloading 4269F
    Wound Surface Culture 4260F, 4261F
  Physical Examination
    Blood Pressure 2000F
    Wound Characteristics 2050F
Community Acquired Bacterial Pneumonia
  Diagnostic/Screening Processes or Results
    Chest X ray 3006F
    Oxygen Saturation 3028F

History
Co-Morbid Conditions 1026F
Influenza Immunization 1030F
Pneumococcus Immunization........ 1022F
Pneumonia Assessment........... 0012F
Tobacco Use.........1000F, 1034F-1036F
Interventions
Antibiotic Prescription 4045F
Counseling 4000F
Pharmacologic Therapy 4001F
Tobacco Use Cessation Intervention
Counseling 4000F, 4004F
Pharmacologic Therapy..... 4001F, 4004F
Patient Safety
Level of Care Rationale 6005F
Physical Examination
Hydration Status................. 2018F
Mental Status................... 2014F
Vital Signs 2010F
Composite Codes
Community-acquired Bacterial Pneumonia
Assessment 0012F
Heart Failure Assessment 0001F
Intraocular Lens (IOL) Placement
Assessment 0014F
Melanoma Follow-up............... 0015F
Osteoarthritis Assessment 0005F
Coronary Artery Bypass Graft
Interventions
Mammary Artery Graft....... 4110F, 4115F
Coronary Artery Disease
Diagnostic/Screening Processes or Results
Blood Pressure, Diastolic......3078F-3080F
Blood Pressure, Systolic.......3074F-3079F
Left Ventricular Ejection
Fraction................... 3021F, 3022F
Lipid Panel 3011F, 3048F-3050F
History
Angina Occurrence.......... 1011F, 1012F
Angina Assessed by Activity .. 1002F, 1010F
Qualifying Cardiac Event 1460F, 1461F
Smokeless Tobacco Use........... 1035F
Tobacco Use.................... 1000F
Tobacco Smoker.................. 1034F
Tobacco Non-Use................. 1036F
Interventions
Angiotensin Converting Enzyme (ACE)/
Angiotensin Receptor Blockers
(ARB).......................... 4010F
Anti-Hypertensive Agents 4145F
Aspirin or Clopidogrel............. 4086F
Antiplatelet Therapy.............. 4011F
Beta-Blocker Therapy............. 4008F
Cardiac Rehabilitation
Program 4500F, 4510F
Counseling 4000F
Pharmacologic Therapy 4001F
Statin Therapy 4013F
Tobacco Use Cessation
Counseling 4000F, 4004F
Pharmacologic Therapy..... 4001F, 4004F
Patient Management
Anginal Symptoms Plan of Care...... 0557F
Lipid Control Plan of Care.......... 0556F
Physical Examination
Blood Pressure 2000F
Dementia
History
Advance Care Plan................ 1123F
Cognition Assessment 1494F
Functional Status Assessment....... 1175F
Neuropsychiatric Symptoms
Assessment 1181F-1183F
Severity Classification 1490F-1493F
Diagnostic/Screening Processes or Results
Depression Screening 3725F
Interventions
Caregiver Education and Support..... 4322F
Counseling on Symptoms, End of Life
Decisions 4350F
Neuropsychiatric
Intervention 4525F, 4526F
Patient Safety
Safety Counseling 6101F, 6102F, 6110F
Diabetes
Diagnostic/Screening Processes or Results
Blood Pressure, Diastolic......3078F-3080F
Blood Pressure, Systolic.......3074F-3079F
Hemoglobin
A1c 3046F
Lipids 3048F-3050F
Macroalbuminuria 3060F-3062F
Nephropathy Treatment............ 3066F
Retinopathy Risk................. 3072F
Urine Protein..............3060F-3062F
Distal Symmetric Polyneuropathy
(DSP)......................3751F-3754F
Electrodiagnostic Studies..... 3751F, 3752F
Screening Test 3754F
Symptom and Signs Present 3753F
History
Tobacco Use...............1034F-1036F
Interventions
Pharmacologic 4001F
Tobacco Use Cessation Intervention
Counseling 4000F, 4004F
Pharmacologic Therapy..... 4001F, 4004F
Physical Examination
Eye 2022F, 2024F, 2026F
Foot............................ 2028F
Distal Symmetric Polyneuropathy
(DSP) 3751F-3754F
Emergency Medicine
Diagnostic/Screening Processes or Results
Electrocardiogram 3120F
Oxygen Saturation 3028F
Interventions
Antibiotic 4045F
Aspirin at Arrival 4084F
Physical Examination
Mental Status.................... 2014F
Vital Signs 2010F
Endoscopy and Polyp Surveillance
Colonoscopy Intervals 0528F, 0529F
End Stage Renal Disease
Diagnostic/Screening Processes or Results
Hemoglobin Level...........3279F-3281F
Kt/V Level.................3082F-3084F
Interventions
Arteriovenous (AV) Fistula Referral ... 4051F
Hemodialysis 4052F-4054F
Influenza Immunization 4037F
Peritoneal Dialysis 4055F
Patient Management
Anemia Plan of Care.............. 0516F
Hemodialysis Plan of Care.......... 0505F
Peritoneal Dialysis Plan of Care...... 0507F
Epilepsy
Diagnostic/Screening Processes or Results
Electroencephalogram (EEG) 3650F
MRI/CT Scan 3324F
Follow-Up or Other Outcomes
Surgical Therapy Considered........ 5200F
History
Etiology Reviewed and Documented .. 1205F
Seizure Type and Frequency
Documented 1200F
Interventions
Childbearing Counseling 4340F
Safety Counseling 4330F
Patient Safety
Anti-Epileptic Drug (AED) Side Effects
Counseling 6070F
Eye Care
Diagnostic/Screening Processes or Results
Intraocular Pressure (IOP)..... 3284F, 3285F
Presurgical Calculations...... 3073F, 3325F
Interventions
Age Related Eye Disease Study (AREDS)
Formulation...................... 4177F
Glaucoma Counseling.............. 4174F
Visual Acuity..................... 4175F
Patient Management
Glaucoma Plan of Care............. 0517F
Physical Examination
Dilated Fundus 2020F
Gastroesophageal Reflux Disease (GERD)
Diagnostic/Screening Processes or Results
Barium Swallow............ 3140F-3142F,
3150F, 3200F
Barrett's Esophagus
Biopsy......... 3140F-3142F, 3150F, 3200F
Upper Endoscopy 3130F, 3132F
History
Alarm Symptoms 1070F, 1071F
Assessment of Therapy at 12
months 1118F
Interventions
Histamine H2 Receptor Antagonist
(H2RA).................... 4185F, 4186F
Proton Pump Inhibitor (PPI).... 4185F, 4186F
Geriatrics
Diagnostic/Screening Processes or Results
Falls Risk........................ 3288F
History
Advance Care Plan.......... 1123F, 1124F
Medication Reconciliation 1111F
Patient Discharge................ 1110F
Urinary Incontinence 1090F, 1091F
Patient Management
Falls Plan 0518F
Urinary Incontinence Plan 0509F
Physical Examination
Fall Screening.............. 1100F, 1101F
Heart Failure
Composite Measures
Heart Failure Assessment 0001F
Diagnostic/Screening Processes or Results
Activity Level Evaluation 3115F, 3119F
Clinical Symptoms
Evaluation................. 3115F, 3119F
Disease-specific Structured Assessment
Tool Completed 3117F
Left Ventricular Ejection Fraction.....3019F,
3021F, 3022F, 3055F, 3056F
New York Heart Association (NYHA) Class
Documented 3118F
History
Activity Level 1003F
Status of Symptoms......... 1450F, 1451F
Symptoms of Volume Overload 1004F
Interventions
Angiotensin Converting Enzyme
(ACE)/Angiotensin Receptor Blockers
(ARB)............... 4010F, 4480F, 4481F

Beta-Blocker Therapy 4008F
Implantable Defibrillator Counseling . . 4470F
Patient Education 4003F, 4450F
Warfarin Therapy 4012F
Patient Management
Symptom Management Plan of Care . . 0555F
Physical Examination
Blood Pressure 2000F
Clinical Signs of Volume Overload 2002F
Weight 2001F
Hematology
Diagnostic/Screening Processes or Results
Bone Marrow 3155F
Flow Cytometry Studies 3170F
Iron Stores 3160F
Interventions
Erythropoietin Therapy 4090F, 4095F
Multiple Myeloma: Treatment with Bisphosphonates 4100F
Hepatitis C
Diagnostic/Screening Processes or Results
Genotype Testing 3266F
Hepatitis A Immunity 3215F
Hepatitis B Immunity 3216F
RNA Testing 3218F, 3220F, 3265F
History
Initial Evaluation 1119F
Subsequent Evaluation 1121F
Interventions
Antiviral Therapy 4150F, 4151F
Counseling 4158F, 4159F
Education, Alcohol 4158F
Education, Contraception 4159F
Hepatitis A Vaccination 4148F, 4155F
Hepatitis B Vaccination 4149F, 4157F
Peginterferon and Ribavirin Therapy . . 4153F
RNA Testing 4150F, 4151F
Hydration 2030F, 2031F
HIV/AIDS
Diagnostic/Screening Processes or Results
CD4+ Cell Count 3492F-3500F
Chlamydia Screening 3511F
Gonorrhea Screening 3511F
Hepatitis B Screening 3216F, 3513F
Hepatitis C Screening 3514F, 3515F
History of AIDS-defining Condition . . . 3490F
Infants of Undetermined HIV Status . . 3491F
Nadir CD4+ Cell Count 3492F, 3493F
RNA Viral Load 3502F, 3503F
Syphilis Screening 3512F
Tuberculosis Screening 3510F
Interventions
Antiretroviral Therapy 4276F
Antiviral Therapy 4270F, 4271F
High Risk Sexual Behavior Screening 4293F
Influenza Immunization 4274F
Injection Drug Use Screening 4290F
Pneumococcal Immunization 4040F
Pneumocystis Jiroveci Pneumonia Prophylaxis 4279F, 4280F
Patient Management
RNA Control Plan of Care 0575F
Hypertension
Diagnostic/Screening Processes or Results
Blood Pressure, Diastolic 3078F-3080F
Blood Pressure, Systolic 3074F-3079F
Plan of Care 3074F, 3075F, 3077F-3080F
Interventions
Anti-Hypertensive Agents 4145F
Hypertension Plan of Care 4050F
Physical Examination
Blood Pressure 2000F
Inflammatory Bowel Disease
Diagnostic/Screening Processes or Results
Clostridium Difficile Testing 3520F
Corticosteroid Dose Monitoring 3750F
Hepatitis B Virus Status Assessed 3517F
X-ray Absorptiometry (DXA) . . . 3095F, 3096F
History
Assessment of Type, Location, Activity 1052F
Patient Safety
First Course of Anti-TNF (Tumor Necrosis Factor) Therapy Not Received 6150F
Interventions
Corticosteroid Sparing Therapy 4142F
Venous Thromboembolism (VTE) Prophylaxis 4069F
Lung Cancer/Esophageal Cancer
Diagnostic/Screening Processes or Results
Pre-Surgery Performance Status Review 3328F
Pulmonary Function Test 3038F
Tumor, Node and Metastases (TNM) Staging Documented 3323F
Major Depressive Disorder
Diagnostic/Screening Processes or Results
Depression 3351F-3354F
Severity Classification 3088F-3093F
Suicide Risk 3085F, 3092F
History
Diagnostic Status 1040F
Interventions
Electroconvulsive Therapy 4066F, 4067F
Psychotherapy 4060F-4062F
Psychotropic Medication 4063F-4065F
Patient Management
Plan of Follow-up Care Documented . . 0545F
Physical Examination
Clinical Interview 2060F
Melanoma
Diagnostic/Screening Processes or Results
Cancer Stage 3321F, 3322F
Imaging Studies 3319F, 3320F
History
Moles 1050F
Outcomes
Counseling 5005F
Scheduled Patient Follow Up 7010F
Treatment Plan 5050F
Physical Examination
Skin Exam 2029F
Nuclear Medicine
Diagnostic/Screening Processes or Results
Bone Scintigraphy Study Report 3570F
Fracture Risk Assessment 3572F, 3573F
Follow-up or Other Outcomes
Fracture Risk Conveyed to Referring Physician 5100F
Oncology
Diagnostic/Screening Processes or Results
Cancer Stage 3370F-3390F
Estrogen Receptor 3315F, 3316F
Malignancy Report 3317F, 3318F
Progesterone Receptor 3315F, 3316F
Interventions
Adjuvant Chemotherapy for Colon Cancer 4180F
Aromatase Inhibitor (AI) 4179F
Tamoxifen Inhibitor 4179F
Outcomes
Oncological Treatment Summary Report 5020F
Patient Management
Chemotherapy Regimen 0519F
Pain Plan of Care 0521F
Radiation Dose Limits 0520F
Physical Examination
Pain Level 1125F, 1126F
Osteoarthritis
History
Anti-inflammatory Risk 1008F
Assessment 0005F
Symptom and Functional 1006F
OTC Medication Use 1007F
Interventions
Anti-inflammatory/Analgesic 4016F
Gastrointestinal Prophylaxis 4017F
Therapeutic Exercise 4018F
Therapy 4016F
Physical Examination
Involved Joint 2004F
Osteoporosis
Diagnostic/Screening Processes or Results
Screening 3095F, 3096F
Interventions
Counseling 4019F
Pharmacologic 4005F
Outcomes
Care Coordination 5015F
Palliative/End of Life Care
Diagnostic/Screening Processes or Results
Dyspnea Screening 3450F-3452F
History
Advance Care Plan 1123F, 1124F
Disease Prognosis 1152F, 1153F
Risk of Death Assessment 1150F, 1151F
Patient Management
Dyspnea Plan of Care 0535F
Parkinson Disease
Diagnostic/Screening Processes or Results
Cognitive Impairment/Dysfunction Assessed 3720F
Psychiatric Disorders/Disturbances Assessed 3700F
Interventions
Autonomic Dysfunction Symptoms Queried with Patient 4326F
Medication-related Motor Complications 4324F
Rehabilitation Options Discussed with Patient 4400F
Sleep Disturbances Queried with Patient 4328F
Treatment Options Reviewed with Patient 4325F
Patient History
Diagnosis Reviewed 1400F
Patient Safety
Falls Incidence Queried with Patient . . 6080F
Stage-Specific Safety Counseling 6090F
Pathology
Diagnostic/Screening Processes or Results
Cancer Resection (Colon/Breast) 3260F
Esophageal Biopsy Report for Dysplasia 3126F
Gleason Score Pathology Report 3267F
Histologic Grade 3260F
Immunohistochemistry (IHC) Evaluation of HER2 . . . . 3394F, 3395F
Margin Status Pathology Report 3267F
pN Category Report 3260F, 3267F
pT Category Report 3260F, 3267F
Specimen Site Other than Primary Tumor Site 3250F

Patient Management
Cytopathology Report........ 0550F, 0551F
Patient Safety
Timeout Verification 6100F
Pediatric Acute Gastroenteritis
Interventions
Education 4058F
Oral Rehydration.................. 4056F
Physical Examination
Hydration Status........... 2030F, 2031F
Oral Rehydration........... 2030F, 2031F
Weight Measurement 2001F
Pediatric End Stage Renal Disease
Diagnostic/Screening Processes or Results
Kt/V Level..................3082F-3084F
Interventions
Influenza Immunization 4274F
Patient Management
Hemodialysis Plan of Care.......... 0505F
Pediatric Pharyngitis
Diagnostic/Screening Processes or Results
Strep Test as Appropriate 3210F
Interventions
Antibiotic 4120F, 4124F
Perioperative Care 2
Interventions
Antibiotic Prophylaxis
Discontinuation...........4042F, 4043F, 4046F, 4049F
Selection...................... 4041F
Timing.................. 4047F, 4048F
Aspirin Prophylaxis................ 4563F
Coronary Artery Stent Status
Confirmed 4561F, 4562F
Body Temperature Recorded .. 4559F, 4560F
Inhalational Anesthetic 4554F, 4555F
Postoperative Nausea and Emesis
Assessment............... 4556F, 4557F
Administration of Anti-Emetic 4558F
Venous Thromboembolism.......... 4044F
Patient Management
Transfer of Care............0581F-0584F
Prenatal Care
Diagnostic/Screening Processes or Results
ABO and Rh Typing................ 3293F
D RH Status 3290F, 3291F
Interventions
Anti-D Immune Globulin Received.... 4178F
Prenatal-Postpartum Care
Diagnostic/Screening Processes or Results
Anti-D Immune Globulin
Status.................... 3290F, 3291F
HIV 3292F
Interventions
Anti-D Immune Globulin............ 4178F
Influenza Immunization 4037F
Patient Management...........0500F-0503F
Preventive Care and Screening
Diagnostic/Screening Processes or Results
Alcohol Misuse.................... 3016F
Body Mass Index (BMI) Documented.. 3008F
Cervical Cancer Screening 3015F
Colorectal Screening 3017F
Screening Mammography 3014F
History
Tobacco Use.........1000F, 1034F-1036F
Interventions
Influenza Immunization 4037F
Pharmacologic Therapy 4001F
Pneumococcal Vaccination.......... 4040F
Tobacco Use Cessation Intervention
Counseling 4000F, 4004F
Pharmacologic Therapy..... 4001F, 4004F
Prostate Cancer
Diagnostic/Screening Processes or Results
Bone Scan................ 3269F, 3270F
Gleason Score 3268F
Primary Tumor Stage 3268F
Prostate-Specific Antigen (PSA)...... 3268F
Risk of Recurrence 3271F-3274F
Interventions
Counseling on Treatment Options 4163F
External Beam Radiotherapy .. 4200F, 4201F
Hormonal Therapy Adjuvant......... 4164F
Intensity Modulated Radiation
Therapy.......................... 4165F
3D Conformal Radiotherapy.......... 4165F
Radiology
Diagnostic/Screening Processes or Results
Mammogram Assessment
Documented..........3340F-3345F, 3350F
Outcomes
Diagnostic Mammogram 5062F
Patient Safety
Controlled Dosage 6040F
Fluoroscopic Radiation Exposure 6045F
Structural Measures
Mammogram Assessment Categories 7020F
Mammogram Reminder 7025F
Rheumatoid Arthritis
Diagnostic/Screening Processes or Results
Post-therapy TB Screening.......... 3455F
Rheumatoid Arthritis Disease Activity
Assessment 3470F-3472F
Rheumatoid Arthritis Prognosis
Assessment 3475F, 3476F
Interventions
Anti-Rheumatic Drug Therapy 4187F, 4195F, 4196F
Glucocorticoid Therapy.........4192F-4194F
Screening Colonoscopy Adenoma Detection Rate
Diagnostic/Screening Processes or Results
Adenoma/Neoplasm
Detection 3775F, 3776F
Stroke and Stroke Rehabilitation
Diagnostic/Screening Processes or Results
Carotid Imaging 3100F
CT/MRI Assessment.......... 3111F, 3112F
Lesion Screening 3110F-3112F
History
Anticoagulant Therapy....... 1060F, 1061F
Tissue Plasminogen 1065F, 1066F
Interventions
Anticoagulant Therapy............ 4075F
Antiplatelet Therapy.............. 4073F
Rehabilitation Services 4079F
Thrombosis Prophylaxis 4070F
Tissue Plasminogen 4077F
Patient Safety
Dysphagia Screening 6010F
NPO Order....................... 6020F
Swallowing Eligibility.............. 6015F
Substance Abuse Disorders
Interventions
Alcohol Dependency Treatment
Options 4320F
Opioid Addiction Treatment Options .. 4306F
Upper Respiratory Infection in Children
Interventions
Antibiotic Prescribed 4120F-4124F

Performance Test
See Physical Medicine/Therapy/Occupational Therapy
Cognitive........................... 96125
Performance Test, Physical Therapy........ 97750

Perfusion
Imaging
Brain
CT Scan......................... 0042T
PET Scan........................ 78609
Myocardial.................. 78451-78454
PET Scan.................. 78491, 78492
Pulmonary 78580, 78582, 78597, 78598
for Esophageal Motility Study 91013
Test
Esophageal Acid 91030
Therapeutic
Hemoperfusion, Dialysis 90997
Vestibuloactive Drugs 69801

Perfusion Pump
See Infusion Pump

Perfusion, Intracranial Arterial
Thrombolysis.......................... 61624

Pericardectomies
See Excision, Pericardium

Pericardial Cyst
See Cyst, Pericardial

Pericardial Sac
Drainage 32659
Thoracoscopy
Biopsy............................ 32604
Diagnostic 32601
Removal
Clot 32658
Foreign Body..................... 32658

Pericardial Window
Creation
for Drainage................. 32659, 33025

Pericardial Window Technic
See Pericardiostomy

Pericardiectomy
Complete...................... 33030, 33031
Subtotal....................... 33030, 33031

Pericardiocentesis 33010, 33011
Ultrasound Guidance 76930

Pericardiostomy
Tube 33015

Pericardiotomy
Removal
Clot.............................. 33020
Foreign Body 33020

Pericardium
Biopsy
Endoscopic........................ 32604
Cyst
Excision 32661
Resection......................... 33050
Diagnostic Thoracoscopy 32601
Excision...................... 33030, 33031
Window, for Drainage......... 32659, 33025
Incision
Removal
Clot............................ 33020
Foreign Body.................... 33020
Pericardiostomy.................... 33015
Incision and Drainage.................. 33025
Mass
Excision 32661
Puncture Aspiration 33010, 33011

Index

Removal
Endoscopic
Clot 32658
Foreign Body 32658
Tumor
Excision 32661
Resection 33050

Peridural Anesthesia
Infusion 62324-62327
Injection 62320-62323

Peridural Injection
See Epidural, Injection

Perineal Prostatectomy
See Prostatectomy, Perineal

Perineoplasty 56810

Perineorrhaphy
Repair
Rectocele 57250

Perineum
Abscess
Incision and Drainage 56405
Biopsy
Lesion 56605, 56606
Colostomy 50810
Anogenital Examination
with Magnification and Image Recording 99170
Debridement
Infected 11004, 11006
Removal
Prosthesis 53442
Repair 56810
X ray with Contrast 74775

Perionychia
See Paronychia

Periorbital Region
Reconstruction
Osteotomy with Graft 21267, 21268
Repair, Osteotomy 21260-21263
Treatment
Orbital Floor Blowout Fracture 21386, 21390, 21395

Peripheral Artery Disease (PAD) Rehabilitation 93668

Peripheral Nerve
Repair/Suture
Major 64856, 64857, 64859

Peripherally Inserted Central Catheter (PICC)
See Central Venous Catheter Placement, Insertion, Peripheral

Periprosthetic Capsulectomy
Breast 19371

Peristaltic Pumps
See Infusion Pump

Peritoneal Dialysis 90945-90947, 4055F
Catheter Insertion 49418, 49419, 49421
Catheter Removal 49422
Home Infusion 99601, 99602
Kt/V Level 3082F-3084F
Plan of Care Documented 0507F

Peritoneal Free Air
See Pneumoperitoneum

Peritoneal Lavage 49084

Peritoneoscopy
See Peritoneum, Endoscopy

Peritoneum
Abscess
Incision and Drainage 49020
Percutaneous 49406
Chemotherapy Administration 96446
See Chemotherapy
Drainage
Image Guided Fluid Collection 49406, 49407
Intramedullary Cyst/Syrinx 63173
Lymphocele 49062, 49323
Endoscopy
Biopsy 49321
Diagnostic 49320
Drainage
Lymphocele 49323
Insertion
Catheter 49324
Revision
Cannula/Catheter 49326
Exchange
Drainage Catheter 49423
Injection
Air 49400
Contrast 49400
via Catheter 49424
Insertion
Catheter 49418, 49419
for Dialysis 49421
Shunt
Peritoneal-Venous 49425
Subarachnoid/Subdural-Peritoneal 62192, 63740, 63741
Ventriculo-Peritoneal 62223
Lavage 49084
Lesion
Excision
Laparoscopic 58662
Fulguration
Laparoscopic 58662
Ligation
Shunt 49428
Removal
Catheter 49422
Foreign Body 49402
Shunt 49429
Shunt, Peritoneal-Venous
Insertion 49425
Ligation 49428
Radiological Evaluation 78291
Injection, Contrast 49427
Removal 49429
Revision 49426
Tumor
Destruction 49203-49205
Excision 49203-49205
Resection 58950-58958
Unlisted Services and Procedures 49999
Laparoscopic 49329
Venous Shunt
Injection 49427
X ray 74190
Injection
Air/Contrast 49400

Persistent Truncus Arteriosus
See Truncus Arteriosus

Persistent, Omphalomesenteric Duct
See Diverticulum, Meckel's

Personal Care
See Self Care

Pessary
Insertion 57160

Pesticides
Chlorinated Hydrocarbons 82441

PET
See Positron Emission Tomography (PET)

Petrous Temporal
Excision
Apex 69530

Peyronie Disease
Excision
Penile Plaque 54110-54112
Excision with Graft 54110-54112
Injection 54200
Surgical Exposure 54205

pH
Blood Gases 82800, 82803
Exhaled Breath Condensate 83987
Gastric Acid 82930
Other Fluid 83986
Urine 81000-81003, 83986

Phacoemulsification
Removal
Extracapsular Cataract 66982, 66984
Secondary Membranous Cataract 66850

Phagocytosis
White Blood Cells 86344

Phalangectomy
Toe 28150
Partial 28160

Phalanges (Hand)
See Phalanx, Finger

Phalanx, Finger
Abscess
See Finger, Abscess
Amputation 26910, 26951, 26952
Bone
See Finger, Bone
Collateral Ligament
See Finger, Collateral Ligament
Excision
See Finger, Excision
Fracture
See Fracture, Phalanges
Joint
See Interphalangeal Joint

Phalanx, Great Toe
Arthrodesis 28750, 28755, 28760
Fracture 28490
Open Treatment 28505
with Manipulation 28495, 28496
Osteocutaneous Flap with Web 20973
Percutaneous Fixation 28496
without Manipulation 28490
Toe-to-Hand Transfer 20973
Wrap-around with Bone Graft 26551

Pharmaceutic Preparations
See Drug

Pharmacotherapies
See Chemotherapy

Pharyngeal Tonsil
See Adenoids

Pharyngectomy
Limited 42890

Pharyngolaryngectomy 31390-31395

Pharyngoplasty 42950

Pharyngorrhaphy
See Pharynx, Suture

Pharyngostomy 42955

Pharyngotomy
See Incision, Pharynx

Pharyngotympanic Tube
See Eustachian Tube

Pharynx
See Nasopharynx; Throat
Abscess
  Incision and Drainage 42720, 42725
Biopsy 42800-42806
Cineradiography 70371, 74230
Creation
  Stoma 42955
Cyst, Brachial Cleft
  Excision 42815
Excision
  Partial 42890
  Resection 42892-42894
  with Larynx 31390-31395
Fistulization
  External for Feeding 42955
Hemorrhage Control 42960-42962
Lesion
  Destruction 42808
  Excision 42808
Reconstruction 42950
  with Palate 42145
Removal
  Foreign Body 42809
Repair
  with Esophagus 42953
Suture
  Wound 42900
Unlisted Services and Procedures 42999
Video Study 70371, 74230
X ray 70370, 74210

Phencyclidine 80305-80307, 83992

Phenobarbital 80345

Phenothiazine 80342-80344

Phenotype Analysis
Alpha-1-antitrypsin 82104
by Genotypic Bioinformatics 87900
by Nucleic Acid 87901-87904, 87906
  Infectious Agent
    HIV-1 Drug Resistance 87903, 87904, 87906

Phenotype Prediction
by Genetic Database
  HIV-1 Drug Susceptibility 87900

Phenylalanine 84030

Phenylalanine-Tyrosine Ratio 84030

Phenylketones 84035

Phenylketonuria
See Phenylalanine

Phenytoin
Assay 80185, 80186

Pheochromocytoma 80424

Pheresis
See Apheresis

Phlebectasia
See Varicose Vein

Phlebectomy
Varicose Veins 37765, 37766

Phlebographies
See Venography

Phleborrhaphy
See Suture, Vein

Phlebotomy
Therapeutic 99195

Phoria
See Strabismus

Phosphatase
Alkaline 84075, 84080
  Blood 84078

Phosphatase Acid 84060
Blood 84066

Phosphate, Pyridoxal
See Pyridoxal Phosphate

Phosphatidyl Glycerol
See Phosphatidylglycerol

Phosphatidylcholine Cholinephosphohydrolase
See Tissue, Typing

Phosphatidylglycerol 84081

Phosphocreatine Phosphotransferase, ADP
See CPK

Phosphogluconate-6
Dehydrogenase 84085

Phosphoglycerides, Glycerol
See Phosphatidylglycerol

Phosphohexose Isomerase 84087

Phosphohydrolases
See Phosphatase

Phosphokinase, Creatine
See CPK

Phospholipase C
See Tissue, Typing

Phospholipid Antibody 86147

Phospholipid, Neutralization 85597, 85598

Phosphomonoesterase
See Phosphatase

Phosphoric Monoester Hydrolases
See Phosphatase

Phosphorus 84100
Urine 84105

Phosphotransferase, ADP Phosphocreatine
See CPK

Photo Patch
Allergy Test 95052
  See Allergy Tests

Photochemotherapies, Extracorporeal
See Photopheresis

Photochemotherapy 96910-96913
See Dermatology
Endoscopic Light 96570, 96571

Photocoagulation
Endolaser Panretinal
  Vitrectomy 67040
Focal Endolaser
  Retinal Detachment 67108, 67113
  Vitrectomy 67040
Iridoplasty 66762
Lesion
  Choroid 67220
  Cornea 65450
  Retina 67210, 67227, 67228
Retinal Detachment
  Prophylaxis 67145
  Repair 67105, 67107
Treatment
  Retinopathy 67228, 67229
    Preterm Infant, at Birth 67229

Photodynamic Therapy
for Lesion 67221, 67225, 96567, 96573, 96574
for Tissue Ablation 96570, 96571

Photography
Fundus 92250
Ocular 92285
Skin
  Monitoring 96904

Photography, Ocular 92285

Photon Beam Therapy
See Radiation Therapy, Treatment Delivery

Photopheresis
Blood 36522

Photoradiation Therapies
See Actinotherapy

Photosensitivity Testing 95056
See Allergy Tests

Phototherapies
See Actinotherapy

Phototherapy, Ultraviolet
See Actinotherapy

Phrenic Nerve
Anastomosis
Avulsion 64746
Incision 64746
Injection
  Anesthetic 64410
Neurostimulator System for Sleep Apnea
  Device Evaluation 0434T-0436T
  Insertion 0424T-0427T
  Removal 0428T-0430T
  Replacement 0424T-0427T, 0431T
  Repositioning 0432T, 0433T
Transection 64746

Physical Medicine/Therapy/ Occupational Therapy
See Neurology, Diagnostic
Activities of Daily Living 97535, 99509
Aquatic Therapy
  with Exercises 97113
Athletic Training
  Evaluation 97169-97171
  Re-Evaluation 97172
  Orthotic/Prosthetic 97763
Cognitive Skills Development 97127
Community/Work Reintegration 97537

Evaluation
Athletic Training 97169-97171
Re-evaluation 97172
Occupational Therapy 97165-97167
Re-evaluation 97168
Physical Therapy 97161-97163
Re-evaluation 97164
Kinetic Therapy 97530
Manual Therapy 97140
Modalities
Contrast Baths 97034
Diathermy Treatment 97024
Electric Stimulation
Attended, Manual 97032
Unattended 97014
Hot or Cold Pack 97010
Hydrotherapy (Hubbard Tank) 97036
Infrared Light Treatment 97026
Iontophoresis 97033
Microwave Therapy 97024
Paraffin Bath 97018
Traction 97012
Ultrasound 97035
Ultraviolet Light 97028
Unlisted Modality 97039
Vasopneumatic Device 97016
Whirlpool Therapy 97022
Orthotics Training 97760, 97763
Osteopathic Manipulation 98925-98929
Procedures
Aquatic Therapy 97113
Direct 97032-97039
Gait Training 97116
Group Therapeutic 97150
Massage Therapy 97124
Neuromuscular Reeducation 97112
Physical Performance Test 97750
Supervised 97010-97028
Therapeutic Exercises 97110
Traction Therapy 97140
Work Hardening 97545, 97546
Prosthetic Training 97761
Self-care Training 97535
Sensory Integration 97533
Therapeutic Activities
One-on-one Patient Contact 97530
Unlisted Services and Procedures 97139, 97799
Wheelchair Management 97542
Work Reintegration 97537

Physical Therapy
See Physical Medicine/Therapy/Occupational Therapy
Evaluation 97161-97163
Re-evaluation 97164

Physician Services
Care Management
Behavioral Health Conditions 99484
Psychiatric Collaborative Care 99492-99494
Care Planning
Cognitive Impairment 99483
Care Plan Oversight Services
Domiciliary Facility 99339, 99340
Home Health Agency 99374, 99375
Home or Rest Home 99339, 99340
Hospice 99377, 99378
Liver Assist System Patient 0405T
Nursing Facility 99379, 99380
Case Management Services 99366-99368
Consultation, Interprofessional
Electronic Health Record Assessment and Report 99446-99449, 99451, 99452
Telephone/Internet Assessment and Report 99446-99449, 99451, 99452
Direction, Advanced Life Support 99288
Online 99444
Prolonged
with Direct Patient Contact 99354-99357
Inpatient 99356, 99357
Outpatient/Office 99354, 99355, 99415, 99416
without Direct Patient Contact 99358, 99359
Standby 99360
Supervision, Care Plan Oversight 99339, 99340, 99374-99380
Team Conference 99367
Telephone 99441-99443

PICC Line
See Central Venous Catheter Placement, Insertion, Peripheral

Piercing of Ear Lobe 69090

Piles
See Hemorrhoids

Pilonidal Cyst
Excision 11770-11772
Incision and Drainage 10080, 10081

Pin
See Wire
Application, Uniplane External Fixation System
See External Fixation
Insertion/Removal
Skeletal Traction 20650
Retention, Palatal Prosthesis 42281
Prophylactic Treatment
Femur 27187
Humerus 24498
Shoulder 23490, 23491
Removal 20670, 20680

Pinch Graft 15050

Pinna
See Ear, External Ear

Pinworms
Examination 87172

Pirogoff Procedure 27888

Pituitary Epidermoid Tumor
See Craniopharyngioma

Pituitary Gland
Excision 61546-61548
Tumor
Excision 61546-61548, 62165

Pituitary Growth Hormone
See Growth Hormone

Pituitary Lactogenic Hormone
See Prolactin

Pituitectomy
See Pituitary Gland, Excision

PKU
See Phenylalanine

Placement
Adjustable Gastric Restrictive Device 43770
Biodegradable Material
Peri-prostatic 55874
Breast Localization Device
Imaging Guided
with Biopsy 19081-19086
without Biopsy 19281-19288
Catheter
Aneurysm Sac
Breast
for Interstitial Radioelement Application 19296-19298, 20555, 41019
Bronchus
for Intracavitary Radioelement Application 31643
See Catheterization
Head
Interstitial Radioelement Application 41019
Kidney
Nephrostomy 50432
Nephroureteral 50433
Neck
Interstitial Radioelement Application 41019
Pelvic Organs
Interstitial Radioelement Application 55920
Prostate 55875
Renal Artery
Selective 36251, 36252
Superselective 36253, 36254
Ureter via Kidney 50695
Catheter, Cardiac 93503
See Catheterization, Cardiac
Cecostomy Tube 44300, 49442
Dosimeter
Prostate 55876
Drainage
Pancreas 48001
Drug-Eluting Ocular Insert
Eyelid 0444T, 0445T
Duodenostomy Tube 49441
Endoscopic Access
Biliary Tract 47541
Endovascular Prosthesis
Aorta 33883-33886, 34709-34711
Iliac Artery 34709-34711
Enterostomy Tube 44300
Esophageal Sphincter Augmentation Device 43284
Fiducial Markers
Bronchus 31626
Prostate 55876
Gastrostomy Tube 43246, 49440
Guidance
Catheter
Abscess 75989
Specimen 75989
Prosthesis
Thoracic Aorta 75958, 75959
Implant
Vertebra
Intrafacet 0219T-0222T
Interstitial Device
Abdomen 49411, 49412
Lungs 32553
Omentum 49411, 49412
Pelvis 49411, 49412
Pleura 32553
Peritoneum 49411, 49412
Prostate 55876
Retroperitoneum 49411, 49412
Jejunostomy Tube
Endoscopic 44372
Percutaneous 49441
Lesion Localization Device
Breast
Imaging Guided 19081-19086, 19281-19288
Soft Tissue 10035, 10036
Nasogastric Tube 43752

Needle
Bone 36680
Interstitial Radioelement Application
Genitalia 55920
Head 41019
Muscle 20555
Neck 41019
Pelvic Organs 55920
Soft Tissue 20555
Prostate 55875
Orogastric Tube 43752
Osteopromotive Material 20930
Radiation Delivery Device
Intracoronary Artery 92974
Pleural Cavity 32553
Radiation Therapy Applicator
Breast 19294
Seton
Anal 46020
Stent
Biliary 47538-47540
Bronchial 31636, 31637
Cardiac 33621
Colonic 44402, 45327, 45347, 45389
Intravascular
Coronary 92928, 92929
Intracranial 61635
Tracheal 31631
Ureteral 50947
Subconjunctival Retinal Prosthesis 0100T
Synthetic Device
Vertebra 0220T-0222T

Placenta
Delivery 59414

Placenta Alpha Microglobulin-1 . . 84112

Placental Lactogen
See Lactogen, Human Placental

Placental Villi
See Chorionic Villus

Plagiocephaly 21175

Planing
Nose
Skin 30120

Plantar Common Digital Nerve
Destruction
Neurolytic 64632
Injection
Anesthetic Agent 64455

Plantar Digital Nerve
Decompression 64726

Plantar Pressure Measurements
Dynamic 96001, 96004

Plasma
Exchange 36514-36516
Frozen Preparation 86927
Injection 0232T
Volume 78110, 78111

Plasma Prokallikrein
See Fletcher Factor

Plasma Protein-A, Pregnancy-Associated (PAPP-A) 84163

Plasma Test
Volume Determination 78110, 78111

Plasma Thromboplastin
Antecedent 85270
Component 85250

Plasmin 85400

Plasmin Antiactivator
See Alpha-2 Antiplasmin

Plasminogen 85420, 85421

Plasmodium
Antibody 86750

Plastic Repair of Mouth
See Mouth, Repair

Plate, Bone
See Bone Plate

Platelet
See Blood Cell Count, Complete (CBC)
Aggregation 85576
Antibody 86022, 86023
Assay 85055
Blood 85025, 85027
Count 85032, 85049
Human Platelet Antigen
Genotyping 81105-81112
Neutralization 85597

Platelet Cofactor I
See Clotting Factor

Platelet Test
Survival Test 78191

Platysmal Flap 15825

PLC
See Lymphocyte, Culture; Tissue, Typing

Pleoptic Training 92065

Plethysmography
See Vascular Studies
Extremities 93922, 93923
Penis 54240
Pulmonary 94726, 94750

Pleura
Biopsy 32098, 32400, 32609
Decortication 32320
Empyema
Excision 32540
Excision 32310-32320
Thoracoscopic 32656
Fibrinolysis
Agent 32561, 32562
Foreign Body
Removal 32150, 32151
Insertion
Catheter 32550
Tube 32551
Needle Biopsy 32400
Placement
Interstitial Device 32553
Pleurodesis
by Agent 32560
Thoracoscopic 32650
Removal
Catheter 32552
Fibrin Deposit 32653
Foreign Body 32653
Repair 32215
Scarification 32215
Thoracoscopy
Biopsy 32609
Exploration 32601
Pleurodesis 32650
Removal
Fibrin Deposit 32653
Foreign Body 32653
Thoracotomy 32098, 32100
Biopsy 32098
Excision 32656
Exploration 32100
Lysis 32124
Removal
Cyst 32140
Foreign Body 32150, 32151
Tumor
Cryoablation 32994
Unlisted Services and Procedures 32999

Pleural Cavity
Ablation
Photodynamic Therapy 96570, 96571
Aspiration 32554
with Imaging Guidance 32555
Catheterization 32550-32552
Chemotherapy Administration 96440
See Chemotherapy
Incision
Empyema 32035, 32036
Instillation of Agent for Fibrinolysis . . 32561, 32562
Instillation of Agent for Pleurodesis 32560
Puncture and Drainage 32554-32557
with Imaging Guidance 32555, 32557
Thoracostomy 32035, 32036

Pleural Endoscopies
See Thoracoscopy

Pleural Scarification
for Repeat Pneumothorax 32215

Pleural Tap
See Thoracentesis

Pleurectomy
Parietal 32310-32320
Endoscopic 32656

Pleuritis, Purulent
See Pleural Cavity, Incision, Empyema

Pleurocentesis
See Thoracentesis

Pleurodesis
Thoracoscopic 32650
Instillation of Agent 32560

Pleurosclerosis
See Pleurodesis

Pleurosclerosis, Chemical
See Pleurodesis, Instillation of Agent

Plexectomy, Choroid
See Choroid Plexus, Excision

Plexus
Brachialis
See Brachial Plexus
Cervicalis
See Cervical Plexus
Choroid
See Choroid Plexus
Coeliacus
See Celiac Plexus
Lumbalis
See Lumbar Plexus

PLGN
See Plasminogen

Plication, Sphincter, Urinary Bladder
See Bladder, Repair, Neck

Pneumocisternogram
See Cisternography

Pneumococcal Vaccine
See Vaccines and Toxoids

Pneumocystis Carinii
Antigen Detection
　Immunofluorescence ... 87281

Pneumogastric Nerve
See Vagus Nerve

Pneumogram
Infant ... 94772

Pneumolysis
See Pneumonolysis

Pneumonectomy ... 32440-32445
Thoracoscopic ... 32671
Completion ... 32488
Donor ... 32850, 33930
Sleeve ... 32442

Pneumonology
See Pulmonology

Pneumonolysis ... 32940
Intrapleural ... 32652
Open Intrapleural ... 32124

Pneumonostomy ... 32200

Pneumonotomy
See Incision, Lung

Pneumoperitoneum
Injection of Air ... 49400

Pneumothorax
Pleurodesis ... 32560
Pleural Scarification for Repeat ... 32215
Therapeutic
　Injection Intrapleural Air ... 32960

Polio
Antibody Detection ... 86658
Vaccine ... 90713

Poliovirus Vaccine
See Vaccines and Toxoids

Pollicization
Digit ... 26550

Polya Gastrectomy
See Gastrectomy, Partial

Polydactylism
See Polydactyly; Supernumerary Digit

Polydactyly
Finger
　Reconstruction ... 26587
　Repair ... 26587
Toe ... 28344

Polyp
Ablation
　Endoscopic
　　Anus ... 46615
　　Colon ... 44401, 45388
　　Esophagus ... 43229
　　Rectum ... 45320, 45346
　　Small Intestine ... 44369
　　Upper Gastrointestinal Tract .. 43270, 43278
Antrochoanal
　Removal ... 31032
Anus
　Ablation
　　Endoscopic ... 46615
　Removal
　　Endoscopic ... 46610-46612
Colon
　Ablation ... 44401, 45388
　Removal ... 44392, 44394, 45384, 45385
Esophagus
　Ablation ... 43229
　Removal ... 43216, 43217
Excision
　Ear ... 69540
　Nose
　　Endoscopic ... 31237-31240
　　Extensive ... 30115
　　Simple ... 30110
　Urethra ... 53260
　Uterus ... 58558
Fulguration
　Urethra ... 53260
　Endoscopic
　　Bladder ... 52285
　　Urethra ... 52285
Nose
　Excision
　　Endoscopic ... 31237-31240
　　Extensive ... 30115
　　Simple ... 30110
Rectum
　Ablation
　　Endoscopic ... 45320, 45346
　Removal
　　Endoscopic ... 45308, 45309, 45315, 45333
Removal
　Endoscopic
　　Anus ... 46610-46612
　　Colon ... 44392, 44394, 45384, 45385
　　Esophagus ... 43216, 43217
　　Rectum ... 45308, 45309, 45315, 45333
　　Small Intestine ... 44364, 44365
　　Upper Gastrointestinal Tract .. 43250, 43251
Small Intestine
　Ablation
　　Endoscopic ... 44369
　Removal
　　Endoscopic ... 44364, 44365
Sphenoid Sinus
　Removal ... 31051
Urethra
　Excision ... 53260
　Fulguration ... 53260
Uterus
　Excision ... 58558

Polypectomy
Nose
　Endoscopic ... 31237-31240
　Extensive ... 30115
　Simple ... 30110
Urethra ... 53260
Uterus ... 58558

Polypeptide, Vasoactive Intestinal
See Vasoactive Intestinal Peptide

Polysomnography ... 95782, 95783, 95808-95811

Pomeroy's Operation
See Tubal Ligation

Pooling
Blood Products ... 86965
Cardiac Blood Pool Imaging
　See Blood Pool Imaging

Popliteal Arteries
See Artery, Popliteal

Popliteal Synovial Cyst
See Baker's Cyst

Poradenitistras
See Lymphogranuloma Venereum

PORP (Partial Ossicular Replacement Prosthesis) ... 69633, 69637

Porphobilinogen
Urine ... 84106-84110

Porphyrin Precursors ... 82135

Porphyrins
Feces ... 84126
Urine ... 84119, 84120

Port Image(s) ... 77417

Portal Vein
See Vein, Hepatic Portal

Portoenterostomies, Hepatic
See Hepaticoenterostomy

Portoenterostomy ... 47701

Positional Nystagmus Test
See Nystagmus Tests, Positional

Positive End Expiratory Pressure
See Pressure Breathing, Positive

Positive-Pressure Breathing, Inspiratory
See Intermittent Positive Pressure Breathing (IPPB)

Positron Emission Tomography (PET)
Brain ... 78608, 78609
Chest ... 78811
Head/Neck ... 78811
Heart ... 78459
Myocardial Imaging
　Blood Flow Absolute Quantitation ... 0482T
　Perfusion Study ... 78491, 78492
Skull Base to Mid-thigh ... 78812
Whole Body ... 78813
with Computed Tomography (CT) ... 78814, 78815

Post-Op Visit ... 99024

Postauricular Fistula
Closure ... 69700

Postcaval Ureter
See Retrocaval Ureter

Postmortem
See Autopsy

Postop Vas Reconstruction
See Vasovasorrhaphy

Postoperative Wound Infection
Incision and Drainage ... 10180

Postpartum Care
Cesarean Delivery ... 59515
　after Attempted Vaginal Delivery ... 59622
　Previous ... 59610, 59614-59618, 59622
Vaginal Delivery ... 59430
　after Previous Cesarean Delivery ... 59614

Potassium ... 84132
Urine ... 84133

Potential, Auditory Evoked
See Auditory Evoked Potentials

Potential, Evoked
See Evoked Potentials

Potts-Smith Procedure ... 33762

Pouch, Kock
See Kock Pouch

Index

PPP
See Fibrin Degradation Products

PRA
See Cytotoxic Screen

Prealbumin 84134

Prebeta Lipoproteins
See Lipoprotein, Blood

Pregnancy
Abortion
  Induced 59855-59857
    by Amniocentesis Injection 59850-59852
    by Dilation and Curettage 59840
    by Dilation and Evaluation 59841
  Septic 59830
  Therapeutic
    by Dilation and Curettage 59851
    by Hysterectomy 59852
    by Saline 59850
Cesarean Delivery 59618-59622
  Only 59514
  Postpartum Care 59514, 59515
  Routine Care 59510
  Vaginal Birth After 59610-59614
  with Hysterectomy 59525
Ectopic
  Abdominal 59130
  Cervix 59140
  Interstitial
    Partial Resection Uterus 59136
    Total Hysterectomy 59135
  Laparoscopy
    with Salpingectomy and/or Oophorectomy 59151
    without Salpingectomy and/or Oophorectomy 59150
  Tubal 59121
    with Salpingectomy and/or Oophorectomy 59120
Imaging
  See Obstetrical Care, Diagnostic Imaging
Miscarriage
  Surgical Completion
    Any Trimester 59812
    First Trimester 59820
    Second Trimester 59821
Molar
  See Hydatidiform Mole
Multifetal Reduction 59866
Placenta Delivery 59414
Vaginal Delivery 59409, 59410
  after Cesarean Delivery 59610-59614
  Antepartum Care 59425, 59426
  Postpartum Care 59430
  Total Obstetrical Care 59400, 59610, 59618

Pregnancy Test 84702-84704
Urinalysis 81025

Pregnanediol 84135

Pregnanetriol 84138

Pregnenolone 84140

Prekallikrein
See Fletcher Factor

Prekallikrein Factor 85292

Premature, Closure, Cranial Suture
See Craniosynostosis

Prenatal Procedure 59897
Amnioinfusion
  Transabdominal 59070
Drainage
  Fluid 59074
Occlusion
  Umbilical Cord 59072
Shunt 59076

Prenatal Testing
Amniocentesis 59000
  with Amniotic Fluid Reduction 59001
Amniotic Fluid Proteins
  Cervicovaginal Fluid Evaluation 84112
Chorionic Villus Sampling 59015
Congenital Abnormalities
  Biochemical Assays 81508-81512
Cordocentesis 59012
Fetal Blood Sample 59030
Fetal Monitoring 59050
  Interpretation Only 59051
Magnetic Resonance Imaging (MRI) 74712, 74713
Non-Stress Test, Fetal 59025, 99500
Oxytocin Stress Test 59020
Stress Test
  Oxytocin 59020
Placental Alpha Microglobulin-1 (PAMG-1) 84112
Ultrasound 76801-76817
  Fetal Biophysical Profile 76818, 76819
  Fetal Heart 76825

Preparation
Custom Breast Implant 19396
Custom Prostheses
  See Impression, Maxillofacial
for Transfer
  Embryo 89255
for Transplantation
  Fecal Microbiota 44705
  Heart 33933, 33944
  Heart/Lung 33933
  Intestines 44715-44721
  Kidney 50323-50329
  Liver 47143-47147
  Lung 32855, 32856, 33933
  Pancreas 48551, 48552
  Renal 50323-50329
  Stem Cells 38207-38215
Recipient Site
  Skin Graft 15002-15005
Thawing
  Embryo
    Cryopreserved 89352
  Oocytes
    Cryopreserved 89356
  Reproductive Tissue
    Cryopreserved 89354
  Sperm
    Cryopreserved 89353

Presacral
Arthrodesis
  See Arthrodesis, Vertebra, Lumbar

Presacral Sympathectomy
See Sympathectomy, Presacral

Prescription
Contact Lens 92310-92317
  See Contact Lens Services

Pressure Breathing
See Pulmonology, Therapeutic
Negative
  Continuous (CNP) 94662
Positive
  Continuous (CPAP) 94660

Pressure
Anorectal 91122
Blood
  See Blood Pressure
Esophageal Pressure Topography
Study 91013, 91299
Gastrointestinal Tract
  Measurement 91112
Interstitial Fluid 20950
Intraocular
  Measurement 0198T, 0329T, 92100
  Monitoring 0329T
Sphincter of Oddi
  See Sphincter of Oddi, Pressure Measurement
Pulmonary 94750
Ulcer (Decubitus)
  Excision
    Coccygeal 15920, 15922
    Ischial 15940, 15941, 15944-15946
    Sacral 15931, 15933-15937
    Trochanteric 15950-15953, 15956, 15958
    Unlisted Procedure 15999
Venous
  See Blood Pressure, Venous
Voiding
  See Voiding Pressure Studies

Pretreatment
Red Blood Cell
  Antibody Identification 86970-86972
Serum
  Antibody Identification 86975-86978

Prevention & Control
See Prophylaxis

Preventive Medicine
Behavior Change Intervention
  Group
    Diabetes Prevention 0403T
    Risk Factor Reduction 99411, 99412
  Individual
    Diabetes Prevention 0488T
    Substance Abuse Other Than Tobacco 99408, 99409
    Tobacco Use Cessation 99406, 99407
Comprehensive
Established Patient 99382-99397
New Patient 99381-99387
Counseling
  Group Counseling 99411, 99412
  Individual
    Behavior Change 99406-99408
    Exercise 4019F
    Risk Factor Reduction Intervention 99401-99404
    Self-Examination for Moles 5005F
Fluoride Varnish Application 99188
Health Risk Assessment 96160, 96161
Immunization
  See Immunization Administration; Vaccines and Toxoids
Interventions
  See Performance Measures, Preventive Care and Screening
Newborn Care
  See Newborn Care, Normal
Unlisted Services and Procedures 99429

Index

Priapism
Repair
  Fistulization 54435
  with Shunt 54420-54430

Primidone
Assay 80188

PRL
See Prolactin

Procalcitonin (PCT) 84145

Pro-Insulin C Peptide
See C-Peptide

Proalbumin
See Prealbumin

Probes, DNA
See Nucleic Acid Probe

Probes, Nucleic Acid
See Nucleic Acid Probe

Procainamide
Assay 80190-80192

Procalcitonin (PCT) 84145

Process
Coracoid
  Transfer 23462
Coronoid
  Coronoidectomy 21070
Odontoid
  Excision 22548
  Fracture 22318
Olecranon
  Craterization 24147
  Diaphysectomy 24147
  Excision, Cyst or Tumor . . 24120, 24125, 24126
  Saucerization 24147
  Sequestrectomy 24138
Spinous
  Wiring 22841
Styloid
  Fracture 25650, 25652
  Styloidectomy 25230, 25440
Vertebral
  Excision 22100-22103, 22110, 22116

Procidentia
Rectum
  Excision 45130-45135
  Reduction 45900

Procoagulant Activity, Glomerular
See Thromboplastin

Proconvertin 85230

Proctectasia
See Dilation, Rectum

Proctectomy
Partial
  Open 45113-45116, 45123
Total 45110-45112, 45119-45121
  Laparoscopic 45395-45397
  Open 45110, 45112, 45119, 45120
with Colectomy 44155-44158, 45121
  Laparoscopic 44211, 44212
with Colectomy/Ileostomy
  Laparoscopic 44212
  Open 44155
with Pelvic Exenteration 45126

Proctocele
See Rectocele

Proctopexy
Laparoscopic 45400-45402
  with Sigmoid Resection 45402
Open 45540, 45541
  with Sigmoid Excision 45550

Proctoplasty 45500-45505

Proctorrhaphy
See Rectum, Suture

Proctoscopies
See Anoscopy

Proctosigmoidoscopy
Ablation
  Polyp or Lesion 45320
Biopsy 45305
Collection of Specimen 45300
Destruction
  Tumor 45320
Diagnostic 45300
Dilation 45303
Exploration 45300
Hemorrhage Control 45317
Placement
  Stent 45327
Removal
  Foreign Body 45307
  Polyp 45308-45315
  Tumor 45315
Volvulus Repair 45321

Products, Gene
See Protein

Proetz Therapy
Nose 30210

Profibrinolysin
See Plasminogen

Progenitor Cell
See Stem Cell

Progesterone 84144

Progesterone Receptors 84234

Progestin Receptors
See Progesterone Receptors

Proinsulin 84206

Projective Test
Psychiatric Evaluation 90885

Prokallikrein
See Fletcher Factor

Prokallikrein, Plasma
See Fletcher Factor

Prokinogenase
See Fletcher Factor

Prolactin 80418, 84146

Prolapse
See Procidentia

Prolapse, Rectal
See Procidentia, Rectum

Prolastin
See Alpha-1 Antitrypsin

Prolonged Services 99354-99360
with Direct Patient Contact 99354-99357
  Inpatient 99356, 99357
  Outpatient/Office 99354, 99355
    Clinical Staff with Physician Supervision 99415, 99416

Prophylactic Treatment
See Preventive Medicine
Antibiotic 4042F, 4045F, 4046F-4049F
Antimicrobial
  Cefazolin or Cefuroxime 4041F, 4043F
Clavicle
  Methylmethacrylate 23490
  Nailing 23490
  Pinning 23490
  Plating 23490
  Wiring 23490
Deep Vein Thrombosis 4070F
Femoral Neck and Proximal Femur
  Methylmethacrylate 27187
  Nailing 27187
  Pinning 27187
  Wiring 27187
Femur 27495
  Methylmethacrylate 27495
  Nailing 27495
  Pinning 27495
  Wiring 27495
Humerus
  Methylmethacrylate 23490, 24498
  Pinning, Wiring 23491, 24498
NSAID 4017F
Pneumocystis Jiroveci Pneumonia . . . 4279F, 4280F
Radius 25490, 25492
  Methylmethacrylate 25490, 25492
  Nailing 25490, 25492
  Pinning 25490, 25492
  Plating 25490, 25492
  Wiring 25490, 25492
Retinal Detachment 67141, 67145
Shoulder
  Clavicle 23490
  Humerus 23491
Tibia 27745
  Methylmethacrylate 27745
  Nailing 27745
  Pinning 27745
  Plating 27745
  Wiring 27745
Ulna 25491, 25492
  Methylmethacrylate 25491, 25492
  Nailing 25491, 25492
  Pinning 25491, 25492
  Plating 25491, 25492
  Wiring 25491, 25492
Venous Thromboembolism (VTE) 4044F

Prophylaxis
Anticoagulant Therapy 4075F
Deep Vein Thrombosis (DVT) 4070F
Retina
  Detachment
    Cryotherapy, Diathermy 67141
    Photocoagulation 67145

Prostaglandin 84150
Insertion 59200, 59855

Prostanoids
See Prostaglandin

Prostate
Ablation
  Cryosurgery 55873
  Waterjet 0421T
Abscess
  Drainage 52700
  Incision and Drainage 55720-55725
Biopsy
  Incisional 55705
  Needle or Punch 55700, 55706

Stereotactic 55706
Transperineal 55706
Brachytherapy
Needle Insertion 55875
Cancer Performance Measures
See Performance Measures, Prostate Cancer
Coagulation
Laser 52647
Destruction
Cryosurgery 55873
Thermotherapy
Microwave 53850
Radio Frequency 53852, 53854
Enucleation
Laser 52649
Excision
Partial 55801, 55821-55831
Perineal 55801-55815
Radical 55810-55815, 55840-55845
Retropubic 55831-55845
Laparoscopic 55866
Suprapubic 55821
Transurethral 52402, 52601, 52630
Exploration
Exposure 55860
with Nodes 55862-55865
Incision
Exposure 55860-55865
Transurethral 52450
Insertion
Catheter 55875
Needle 55875
Radioactive Substance 55860
Transprostatic Implant 52441, 52442
Needle Biopsy 55700
Transperineal 55706
Placement
Biodegradable Material
Transperineal 55874
Catheter 55875
Dosimeter 55876
Fiducial Marker 55876
Interstitial Device 55876
Needle 55875
Resection
Transurethral 52601, 52630
Spectral Analysis, Real-Time 0443T
Thermotherapy
Transurethral 53850, 53852, 53854
Ultrasound 76872, 76873
Unlisted Services and Procedures 55899
Urinary System 53899
Vaporization
Laser 52648

Prostate Specific Antigen ... 84152-84154

Prostatectomy
Electrosurgical 52601
Laparoscopic 55866
Perineal
Partial 55801
Radical 55810-55815
Retropubic
Partial 55831
Radical 55840-55845, 55866
Suprapubic
Partial 55821
Transurethral 52601, 52630

Prostatic Abscess
See Abscess, Tissue, Prostate

Prostatotomy 55720-55725

Prosthesis
Arm
Removal 24160, 24164
Breast
Insertion 19325, 19340-19342
with Tissue Expander 19357
Removal 19328-19330
Supply 19396
Button
Bone Graft 20900
Nasal Septum 30220
Voice 31611
Cheekbone
Malar Augmentation 21270
Chin 21120
Cornea 65770
Diaphragm
Complex Repair 39561
Ear
Ossicle Reconstruction 69633, 69637
PORP 69633, 69637
TORP 69633, 69637
Elbow
Removal
Humeral and Ulnar Components 24160
Radial Head 24164
Endovascular
Bypass
Composite, with Vein 35681
Endoprosthesis
Abdominal Aortic 34845-34848
Aorto-bi-iliac 34831
Aorto-bifemoral 34832
Brachial 34834
Celiac Artery 34841-34848
Femoral 34812, 34813
Iliac 0254T, 34709, 34710, 34711, 34820, 34833
Ilio-iliac 34707, 34708
Infrarenal Abdominal Aortic 34709, 34710, 34711, 34845-34848
Infrarenal Aortic 34830, 35697
Mesenteric 34841-34848
Renal Artery 34841-34848
Visceral Aortic 34841-34848
Visceral Artery 34841-34848
Thoracic Aorta 33883-33886
Facial
Osteoplasty 21208
Femur 27236
Finger Joint 26531, 26536
Forehead 21138
Head
Impression and Custom Preparation
See Impression, Maxillofacial
Heart
Aortic Arch Repair 33852
Aortic Enlargement 33851
Aortic Valve 33361-33365, 33367-33369, 33405
Atrioventricular Valve 33670
Mitral Valve 33426
Repair 0345T, 33418, 33419
Pulmonary Valve 33475, 33477
Shunt 33764
Valve Prosthesis Repair 33496
Ventricular Patch 33548
Hernia
Gastroschisis 49605, 49606
Hiatal 43333, 43335, 43337
Omphalocele 49605, 49606
Ventral 49568, 49652-49657
Hip
Insertion 27125, 27130, 27236
Removal 27090, 27091
Infected
Removal
Abdominal Wall 11008
Intestines 44700
Joint
Humeral 23616, 24361, 24363
Revision 24370, 24371
Lunate 25444
Radial Head 24666
Radius, Distal 25441, 25446
Scaphoid Carpal 25443
Trapezium 25445
Ulnar 25442, 24363
Revision 24370, 24371
Wrist 25446
Knee
Arthroplasty
Insertion 27438, 27445
Intraoperative Use, Kinetic Balance Sensor 0396T
Removal 27488
Lens
Insertion 66982-66985
Repositioning 66825
without Cataract Removal 66985
Mandible 21125
Nasal Septum
Insertion 30220
Ocular 65770, 66982-66985
Removal
Intraocular Lens 0308T
Telescope Prosthesis 0308T
Temporary 92358
Orbital 21179
Orthotic
Training 97761
Ossicle Reconstruction
Chain 69633
Palate 42280, 42281
Penis
Insertion 54400-54405
Removal 54406, 54415
Repair 54408
Replacement 54410, 54411, 54416, 54417
Perineum
Removal 53442
Retina
Placement
Pulse Generator 0100T
Receiver 0100T
Shoulder
Removal 23334, 23335
Skull Plate
Removal 62142
Replacement 62143
Spectacle
Fitting 92352, 92353
Repair 92371
Speech Aid
Insertion 31611
Spine
Insertion 22853, 22854, 22859
Synthetic 69633, 69637
Temporomandibular Joint
Arthroplasty 21243
Testis
Insertion 54520, 54660

Index

Tissue Expander, Other than Breast
Insertion ... 11960
Removal without Prosthesis Insertion ... 11971
Replacement with Prosthesis ... 11970
Training ... 97761
Unlisted Maxillofacial Prosthetic Procedure 21089
Urethral Sphincter
Insertion ... 53444, 53445
Removal ... 53446, 53447
Repair ... 53449
Replacement ... 53448
Vagina
Insertion ... 57267
Removal ... 57295, 57296, 57426
Revision ... 57295, 57296, 57426
Wrist
Insertion ... 25443-25446
Removal ... 25250, 25251

Prosthetic Valve, Aortic Valve Replacement
See Aortic Valve Replacement, with Prosthesis

Protease F
See Plasmin

Protein
A, Plasma (PAPP-A) ... 84163
Apoliproprotein A1 ... 81503
Analysis, Tissue
Western Blot ... 88371
Beta-2 Microglobulin ... 81503
C
Activated (APC) ... 85307
Activator ... 85337
Activity ... 85303
Antigen ... 85302
Reactive ... 86140, 86141
Resistance Assay ... 85307
CA-125 ... 81500, 81503
Cerebrospinal Fluid ... 83873
DIA ... 81509
Electrophoresis ... 84165, 84166
Other Fluids ... 84166
Western Blot ... 84181, 84182
Glycated ... 82985
hCG ... 81508, 81509
HE4 ... 81500
Human Epididymis Protein 4 ... 86305
Myelin Basic ... 83873
Nuclear Matrix Protein 22 (NMP22) ... 86386
Osteocalcin ... 83937
PAPP-A ... 81508, 81509
Prealbumin ... 81503, 84134
S
Free ... 85306
Total ... 85305
Serum, Plasma or Whole Blood ... 84155, 84165
Total ... 84155-84157
by Refractometry ... 84160
Transferrin ... 81503
Urine ... 84156
Urine ... 84156
Dipstick ... 81000
Western Blot ... 84181, 84182, 88371, 88372

Protein Analysis, Tissue
Western Blot ... 88371

Protein Blotting
See Western Blot

Protein C Activator ... 85337

Protein C Antigen ... 85302

Protein C Assay ... 85303

Protein C Resistance Assay ... 85307

Protein S
Assay ... 85306
Total ... 85305

Prothrombase
See Thrombokinase

Prothrombin ... 85210

Prothrombin Time ... 85610, 85611

Prothrombinase
See Thromboplastin

Prothrombokinase ... 85230

Protime
See Prothrombin Time

Proton Treatment Delivery
Complex ... 77525
Intermediate ... 77523
Simple ... 77520-77522

Protoporphyrin ... 84202, 84203

Protozoa
Antibody ... 86753

Provitamin A
See Vitamin, A

Provocation Test
Allergy
See Allergy Tests
Bronchospasm, Evaluation ... 94070
Ergonovine ... 93024
Esophageal Balloon Distension Study ... 91040
with Electrogastrography ... 91133

Prower Factor
See Stuart-Prower Factor

PSA
See Prostate Specific Antigen

Pseudocyst
Esophagus
Drainage ... 43240
Pancreas
Drainage ... 48510

Pseudophakia
See Keratoplasty

PSG
See Polysomnography

Psoriasis Treatment ... 96910-96922
See Dermatology; Photochemotherapy

Psychiatric Diagnosis
Assessment
Brief Emotional/Behavioral ... 96127
Behavior Identification ... 0362T, 97151, 97152
Evaluation of Records or Reports ... 90885
Evaluation ... 90791
with Medical Services ... 90792
Interactive Complexity ... 90785
Performance Measures
Dementia
See Performance Measures, Dementia
Major Depressive Disorder (MDD)
See Performance Measures, Major Depressive Disorder
Suicide Risk Assessment ... 3085F
Unlisted Services and Procedures ... 90899

Psychiatric Treatment
Adaptive Behavior
See Adaptive Behavior Services
Biofeedback Training ... 90875, 90876
Consultation with Family ... 90887
Drug Management ... 90863
Electroconvulsive Therapy ... 4066F, 90870
Referral, Documented ... 4067F
Environmental Intervention ... 90882
Family ... 90846-90849, 99510
Group ... 90853
Hypnotherapy ... 90880
Narcosynthesis Analysis ... 90865
Pharmacotherapy
Antidepressant ... 4063F, 4064F
Antipsychotic ... 4065F
Drug Management ... 90863
Psychoanalysis ... 90845
Psychotherapy
See Psychotherapy
Report Preparation ... 90889
Suicide Risk Assessment ... 3085F
Transcranial Magnetic Stimulation (TMS) ... 90867-90869
Unlisted Services and Procedures ... 90899

Psychoanalysis ... 90845

Psychophysiologic Feedback
See Biofeedback

Psychotherapy
Family of Patient ... 90846, 90847
for Crisis ... 90839, 90840
Group Other Than Multifamily ... 90853
Individual Patient ... 90832-90834, 90836-90838
Interactive Complexity ... 90785
Major Depressive Disorder ... 4060F-4062F
Multifamily ... 90849
Prolonged Services, Outpatient
with Patient Contact ... 99354, 99355
Referral, Documented ... 4062F
with Pharmacologic Management ... 90863

PTA ... 85270

PTA (Factor XI)
See Clotting Factor

PTC Factor ... 85250

PTCA
See Percutaneous Transluminal Angioplasty

Pteroylglutamic Acid
See Folic Acid

Pterygium
Excision ... 65420
with Graft ... 65426

Pterygomaxillary Fossa
Incision ... 31040

Pterygopalatine Ganglion
See Sphenopalatine Ganglion

PTH
See Parathormone

Ptosis
See Blepharoptosis; Procidentia

PTT
See Thromboplastin, Partial Thromboplastin Time (PTT)

Ptyalectasis
See Dilation, Salivary Duct

Pubic Symphysis
Arthrodesis . . . 27282
Craterization . . . 27070, 27071
Cyst
Excision . . . 27065-27067
Dislocation/Fracture
Open Treatment . . . 27217
Excision
Partial . . . 27070, 27071
Saucerization . . . 27070, 27071
Tumor
Radical Resection . . . 27075

Pubis
See Pubic Symphysis

Pudendal Nerve
Destruction . . . 64630
Injection
Anesthetic . . . 64430
Neurolytic . . . 64630

Puestow Procedure . . . 48548

Pulled Elbow
See Nursemaid Elbow

Pulmonary Artery
Angiography . . . 75741, 75743, 75746
Banding . . . 33690
Application . . . 33620
Removal . . . 33622
Catheterization . . . 36013-36015
Embolism . . . 33910-33916
Excision . . . 33910-33916
Monitoring
with Pressure Sensor . . . 33289, 93264
Percutaneous Transluminal
Angioplasty . . . 92997, 92998
Reimplantation . . . 33788
Repair . . . 33620, 33690, 33917-33920
Shunt
from Aorta . . . 33755-33762, 33924
from Vena Cava . . . 33766, 33767
Subclavian . . . 33750
Transection . . . 33922

Pulmonary Function Test
See Pulmonology, Diagnostic

Pulmonary Hemorrhage
See Hemorrhage, Control, Lung

Pulmonary Perfusion Imaging . . . 78580, 78582, 78597, 78598

Pulmonary Valve
Implantation
Prosthesis
Transcatheter . . . 33477
Incision . . . 33470, 33471, 33474
Repair . . . 33470, 33471, 33474
Replacement . . . 33475
with Aortic Valve . . . 33440

Pulmonary Vein
Isolation . . . 93656
Repair
Complete . . . 33730
Partial . . . 33724
Stenosis . . . 33726
Stenosis
Repair . . . 33726

Pulmonology
Diagnostic
Air Leak Assessment . . . 31647, 31651
Airway Closing Volume . . . 94727
Airway Obstruction
Inhalation Treatment . . . 94640
Airway Sizing . . . 31647, 31651
Apnea Monitoring
Pediatric . . . 94774-94777
Bronchodilation . . . 94060, 94664
Bronchospasm Provocation . . . 94070
Bed Testing
Infant through 12 months . . . 94780, 94781
Car Seat Testing
Infant through 12 months . . . 94780, 94781
Carbon Dioxide Response Curve . . . 94400
Carbon Monoxide Diffusion Capacity . . . 94729
Circadian Respiratory Pattern . . . 94772
Exercise Test . . . 94621
Expired Gas Analysis
CO_2 . . . 94770
NO . . . 95012
O_2 and CO_2 . . . 94681
O_2 Update, Direct . . . 94680
O_2 Uptake, Indirect . . . 94690
Quantitative . . . 94250
Flow-Volume Loop . . . 94375
Hemoglobin O_2 Affinity . . . 82820
High Altitude Simulation Test
(HAST) . . . 94452, 94453
Hypoxia Response Curve . . . 94450
Maximum Breathing Capacity . . . 94200
Maximum Voluntary Ventilation . . . 94200
Membrane Compliance . . . 94750
Membrane Diffusion Capacity . . . 94729
Oximetry
Ear or Pulse . . . 94760-94762
Pediatric Pneumogram . . . 94772
Plethysmography . . . 94726
Resistance to Airflow . . . 94726, 94728
Spirometry
Evaluation . . . 94010-94015, 94060, 94070
Evaluation Only . . . 94016
Patient Initiated . . . 94014
Sputum Mobilization with Inhalants . . . 94664
Stress Test, Pulmonary . . . 94618
Vital Capacity . . . 94150
Wheeze Rate . . . 94799
Therapeutic
Airway Obstruction
Inhalation Treatment . . . 94640
Expired Gas Analysis . . . 94250
Inhalation
Pentamidine . . . 94642
Inhalation Treatment
See Inhalation Treatment
Intrapulmonary Surfactant
Administration . . . 94610
Manipulation of Chest Wall . . . 94667, 94668
Mechanical Oscillation of Chest Wall . . . 94669
Pressure Ventilation
Negative (CNP) . . . 94662
Positive (CPAP) . . . 94660
Unlisted Services and Procedures . . . 94799
Ventilation Assist . . . 94002-94005, 99504
Unlisted Services and Procedures . . . 94799

Pulse Generator
Baroreflex Activation Device
Implantation/Replacement . . . 0268T
Revision/Removal . . . 0271T
Respiratory Sensor Electrode/Electrode Array
Insertion . . . 0466T
Removal . . . 0468T
Replacement . . . 0467T
Revision . . . 0467T
Implantable Defibrillator
Insertion . . . 33230, 33231, 33240
Removal . . . 33241
Removal with Replacement . . . 33262-33264
Pacemaker
Insertion . . . 33212, 33213, 33221
Removal . . . 33233
Replacement . . . 33227-33229
Neurostimulator
Insertion . . . 61885, 61886, 64568, 64590
Removal/Revision . . . 61888, 64570, 64595
Systems
See Baroreflex Activation Device; Implantable Defibrillator; Neurostimulators; Pacemaker, Heart

Pulse Rate Increased
See Tachycardia

Pump
See Chemotherapy, Pump Services; Infusion Pump

Pump Services
Oxygenator/Heat Exchanger . . . 99190-99192
Maintenance
Drug Delivery Pump . . 95990, 95991, 96521-96523

Pump, Infusion
See Infusion Pump

Punch Graft . . . 15775, 15776

Puncture
Artery
Diagnosis . . . 36600
Chest
Drainage . . . 32554-32557
with Imaging Guidance . . . 32555, 32557
Cisternal
See Cisternal Puncture
Cornea . . . 65600
Follicle
Oocyte Retrieval . . . 58970
Lumbar
See Spinal Tap
Pericardium . . . 33010, 33011
Pleural Cavity
Drainage . . . 32556, 32557
Sinus
for Endoscopy . . . 31233, 31235
Skull
Drain Fluid . . . 61000-61020
Cistern . . . 61050
Inject Cistern . . . 61055
Inject Ventricle . . . 61026
Shunt
Drain Fluid . . . 61070
Injection . . . 61070
Spinal Cord
Diagnostic . . . 62270
Drain Fluid . . . 62272
Lumbar . . . 62270
Tracheal
Aspiration and/or Injection . . . 31612
Vein
See Venipuncture
Ventricle
See Ventricular Puncture

Puncture Aspiration
Abscess
Skin . . . 10160
Bulla . . . 10160
Cyst
Breast . . . 19000, 19001
Skin . . . 10160
Hematoma . . . 10160
Hydrocele . . . 55000

Index

Pleural Cavity . . . 32554
    with Imaging Guidance . . . 32555
Tunica Vaginalis . . . 55000

Puncturing
See Puncture

Pupillometry . . . 0341T

Pure-Tone Audiometry
See Audiometry, Pure Tone

Pustules
Removal . . . 10040

Putti-Platt Procedure . . . 23450

PUVA
See Dermatology; Photochemotherapy; Ultraviolet Light Therapy

Pyelogram
See Urography, Intravenous; Urography, Retrograde

Pyelography . . . 74400, 74425

Pyelolithotomy . . . 50130
Anatrophic . . . 50075
Coagulum . . . 50130

Pyeloplasty . . . 50400-50405, 50544
Foley-Y . . . 50400
Repair
    Horseshoe Kidney . . . 50540
Secondary . . . 50405

Pyeloscopy
with Cystourethroscopy . . . 52351
    Biopsy . . . 52354
    Destruction . . . 52354
    Lithotripsy . . . 52353
    Removal
        Calculus . . . 52352
    Tumor Excision . . . 52355

Pyelostolithotomy
Percutaneous . . . 50080, 50081

Pyelostomy
Change Tube . . . 50435
with Drainage . . . 50125
with Pyeloplasty . . . 50400, 50405

Pyelotomy
Complicated . . . 50135
Exploration . . . 50120
with Drainage . . . 50125
with Removal of Calculus . . . 50130
with Renal Endoscopy . . . 50570

Pyeloureteroplasty
See Pyeloplasty

Pyloric Sphincter
Incision . . . 43520
Reconstruction . . . 43800

Pyloromyotomy . . . 43520

Pyloroplasty . . . 43800
with Vagotomy . . . 43640

Pyothorax
See Abscess, Bone, Thorax

Pyridoxal Phosphate . . . 84207

Pyrophosphate, Adenosine
See Adenosine Diphosphate

Pyrophosphorylase, Udp Galactose
See Galactose-1-Phosphate, Uridyl Transferase

Pyruvate . . . 84210-84220

Q

Q Fever . . . 86000, 86638

Q Fever ab
See Antibody, Detection, Coxiella Burnetii

QST
See Quantitative Sensory Testing (QST)

Quadrantectomy . . . 19301, 19302

Quadriceps Repair . . . 27430
Suture . . . 27385, 27386

Quantitative Sensory Testing (QST)
Cooling Stimuli . . . 0108T
Heat-Pain Stimuli . . . 0109T
Other Stimuli . . . 0110T
Touch Pressure Stimuli . . . 0106T
Vibration Stimuli . . . 0107T

Quick Test
See Prothrombin Time

Quinidine
Assay . . . 80194

Quinine . . . 84228

R

Rabies Vaccine
See Vaccines and Toxoids

Rachicentesis
See Spinal Tap

Radial Artery
See Artery, Radial

Radial Head, Subluxation
See Nursemaid Elbow

Radial Keratotomy . . . 65771
Intraoperative Visual Axis Identification
    Patient Fixation . . . 0514T

Radiation
See Irradiation

Radiation Physics
Consultation . . . 77336-77370
Unlisted Services and Procedures . . . 77399

Radiation Therapy
Consultation
    Radiation Physics . . . 77336-77370
Dose Plan . . . 77300, 77301, 77306, 77307, 77331
    Brachytherapy . . . 0394T, 0395T, 77316-77318
    Intensity Modulated Radiation Treatment (IMRT) . . . 77338
        Multi-leaf Collimator (MLC) Device . . . 77338
    Radiotherapy
        3-Dimensional . . . 77295
    Teletherapy . . . 77306, 77307, 77321
Field Set-up . . . 77280, 77285, 77290
Guidance
    CT . . . 77014
    for Localization of Target Volume . . . 77387
    Interstitial Devices, Placement . . 49411, 49412
Intraoperative Radiation Therapy
    Breast
        Preparation of Tumor Cavity . . . 19294
Planning . . . 77261-77263, 77299
Port Image(s) . . . 77417
Radiosurgery . . . 77371-77373
Respiratory Motion Management
    Simulation . . . 77293
Special Treatment Procedure . . . 77470
Stereotactic Body . . . 77373
    Target Delineation
        Thoracic . . . 32701
    Cerebral Lesions . . . 77371, 77372
    Guidance . . . 77387
Treatment Delivery . . . 77401, 77402, 77407, 77412
    Brachytherapy
        See Brachytherapy
    High Energy Neutron Radiation . . . 77423
    Intensity Modulation . . . 77385, 77386
    Interstitial Radiation Therapy
        See Interstitial Radiation Therapy
    Intraoperative . . . 77424, 77425
    Localization . . . 77387
    Proton Beam . . . 77520-77525
    Stereotactic . . . 77371-77373
        Body . . . 77373
    Superficial . . . 77401
    Tracking . . . 77387
Treatment Device . . . 77332-77334
Treatment Management
    1 or 2 Fractions Only . . . 77431
    Intraoperative . . . 77469
    Stereotactic
        Body . . . 77435
        Cerebral . . . 77432
    Unlisted Services and Procedures . . . 77499
    Weekly . . . 77427

Radiation, X
See X ray

Radical Excision of Lymph Nodes
See Lymph Nodes, Excision, Radical

Radical Mastectomies, Modified
See Mastectomy, Modified Radical

Radical Neck Dissection
Laryngectomy . . . 31365-31368
Pharyngolaryngectomy . . . 31390-31395
with Auditory Canal Surgery . . . 69155
with Thyroidectomy . . . 60254
with Tongue Excision . . . 41135, 41145, 41153-41155

Radical Resection
See Resection, Radical
Abdomen . . . 51597
Elbow
    Capsule, Soft Tissue, Bone
        with Contracture Release . . . 24149
Mediastinum . . . 60522
Sternum . . . 21630-21632
Tonsil . . . 42842-42845
Tumor
    Abdominal Wall . . . 22904, 22905
    Acetabulum . . . 27076
    Ankle . . . 27615, 27616
    Arm, Lower . . . 25077, 25078
    Arm, Upper . . . 24077, 24079
    Back/Flank . . . 21935, 21936
    Calcaneus . . . 27647
    Clavicle . . . 23200
    Elbow . . . 24077, 24079
    Face . . . 21015, 21016
    Femur . . . 27078, 27365
    Fibula . . . 27646
    Finger . . . 26117, 26118
    Foot . . . 28046, 28047
    Forearm . . . 25077, 25078
    Hand . . . 26117, 26118

Hip . . . 27075, 27076
Humerus . . . 23220, 24150
Ilium . . . 27076
Ischial Ramus . . . 27075, 27076
Knee . . . 27329, 27364, 27365
Leg, Lower . . . 27615, 27616
Leg, Upper . . . 27329, 27364, 27365
Lymph Nodes
See Lymphadenectomy
Mandible . . . 21045
Metacarpal . . . 26250
Metatarsal . . . 28173
Neck . . . 21557, 21558
Ovarian . . . 58950-58954, 58957
Pelvis . . . 27049, 27059
Peritoneal . . . 58950-58954, 58957
Phalanges
Finger . . . 26260, 26262
Toe . . . 28175
Pubic Ramus . . . 27075, 27076
Radius . . . 24152, 25170
Scalp . . . 21015, 21016
Scapula . . . 23210
Shoulder . . . 23077, 23078
Symphysis Pubis . . . 27075
Talus . . . 27647
Tarsal . . . 28171
Thigh . . . 27329, 27364
Thorax . . . 21557, 21558
Tibia . . . 27645
Toe . . . 28046, 28047
Ulna . . . 25170
Wing of Ilium . . . 27075, 27076
Wrist . . . 25077, 25078

Radical Vaginal Hysterectomy
See Hysterectomy, Vaginal, Radical

Radical Vulvectomy
See Vulvectomy, Radical

Radio-Cobalt B-12 Schilling Test
See Vitamin, B-12, Absorption Study

Radioactive Colloid Therapy . . . 79300

Radioactive Substance
Injection
Sentinel Node . . . 38792
Insertion
Bladder . . . 51020, 52250
Prostate . . . 55860
Urethra . . . 52250

Radiocarpal Joint
Arthrotomy . . . 25040
Dislocation
Closed Treatment . . . 25660
Open Treatment . . . 25670

Radiocinematographies
See Cineradiography

Radioelement
Application . . . 77761-77763, 77767, 77768, 77770-77772, 77778, 77789
Device Placement
Breast . . . 19296-19298
Genitalia . . . 55920
Head . . . 41019
Intracavitary . . . 31643
Muscle . . . 20555
Neck . . . 41019
Pelvis . . . 55920
Prostate . . . 55875
Soft Tissue . . . 20555
Uterus . . . 57155
Vagina . . . 57155, 57156
Heyman Capsules Insertion . . . 58346
Ultrasound Guidance . . . 76965
Handling . . . 77790
Infusion . . . 77750

Radioelement Substance
Catheter Placement
Breast . . . 19296-19298
Bronchus . . . 31643
Muscle . . . 20555
Prostate . . . 55875
Soft Tissue . . . 20555
Needle Placement
Muscle . . . 20555
Prostate . . . 55875
Soft Tissue . . . 20555

Radiography
See Radiology; X ray

Radioimmunosorbent Test
See Gammaglobulin, Blood

Radioisotope Brachytherapy
See Brachytherapy

Radioisotope Scan
See Nuclear Medicine

Radiological Marker
Preoperative Placement
Excision of Breast Lesion . . . 19125, 19126

Radiology
Bone/Joint Studies
Computed Tomography . . . 77078
Dual-Energy X-ray Absorptiometry (DXA) . . . 77080, 77081, 77085, 77086
Radiography . . . 77071-77077
Diagnostic Imaging
Abdomen . . . 74018, 74019, 74021
Abscess, Fistula or Sinus Tract, Study . . 76080
Chest . . . 71045-71048
Cineoradiography . . . 76120, 76125
Complex Body Motion Section . . 76101, 76102
Computed Tomography Follow-up Study . . . 76380
X-ray Examination Consultation . . . 76140
Fluoroscopy . . . 76000, 76496
Gastrointestinal Tract . . . 74210-74363
Gynecological and Obstetrical Imaging . . . 74710-74775
Head and Neck . . . 70010-70559
Heart . . . 75557-75524
Lower Extremities . . . 73501-73725
Magnetic Resonance Spectroscopy . . . 76390
Nose to Abdomen, for Foreign Body . . . 76010
Single Plane Body Section . . . 76100
Spine and Pelvis . . . 72020-72295
Surgical Specimen . . . 76098
3D Rendering, Tomographic . . . 76376, 76377
Upper Extremities . . . 73000-73225
Urinary Tract . . . 74018-74485
Vascular Procedures
Aorta and Arteries . . . 36901-36906, 75600-75774
Transcatheter Procedures . . . 75894-75989
Veins and Lymphatics . . . 75801-75893
Videoradiography . . . 76120, 76125
Diagnostic Ultrasound
See Ultrasound
Mammography
See Mammography
Nuclear Medicine
See Nuclear Medicine
Radiation Oncology
Device Design/Construction . . . 77332-77334, 77338
Dosimetry
See Dosimetry
Medical Physics Consultation . . . 77336, 77370
Treatment Delivery
See Radiation Therapy, Treatment Delivery
Treatment Planning . . . 77261-77263, 77299
Field Setting . . . 77280, 77285, 77290, 77293
Radiation Therapy
See Radiation Therapy
Radiological Guidance
Computed Tomography . . . 77011-77014
Fluoroscopy . . . 77001-77003
Magnetic Resonance Imaging . . . 77021, 77022
Unlisted Services and Procedures
Brachytherapy . . . 77799
Computed Tomography . . . 76497
Fluoroscopy . . . 76496
Magnetic Resonance . . . 76498
Nuclear Medicine . . . 78099, 78199, 78299, 78399, 78499, 78599, 78699, 78799, 78999
Radiation Physics . . . 77399
Radiographic . . . 76499
Radiopharmaceutical . . . 79999
Treatment Management . . . 77499
Treatment Planning . . . 77299
Ultrasound . . . 76999
X ray
See X ray

Radionuclide CT Scan
See Emission Computerized Tomography

Radionuclide Imaging
See Nuclear Medicine, Diagnostic

Radionuclide Therapy
See Radiopharmaceutical Therapy

Radionuclide Tomography, Single-Photon Emission-Computed
See SPECT

Radiopharmaceutical Localization
Inflammatory Process . . . 78805-78807
Injection . . . 78808

Radiopharmaceutical Therapy
Interstitial . . . 79300
Intra-Arterial . . . 79445
Intra-Articular . . . 79440
Intracavitary . . . 79200
Intravenous . . . 79101, 79403
Oral . . . 79005
Unlisted Services and Procedures . . . 79999

Radiostereometric Analysis (RSA) . . . 0347T-0350T

Radiosurgery
Brain
Lesion . . . 61796-61800
Treatment Delivery . . . 77371, 77372

Radiotherapeutic
See Radiation Therapy

Radiotherapies
See Irradiation

Radiotherapy, Surface
See Application, Radioelement, Surface

Radioulnar Joint
Arthrodesis
with Resection of Ulna . . . 25830
Arthrotomy . . . 25107

Index

Dislocation
Closed Treatment. 25520, 25525
with Manipulation 25675
Open Treatment. 25526, 25676
Percutaneous Fixation 25671
Reconstruction 25337

Radius
See Arm, Lower; Elbow; Ulna
Amputation
See Amputation, Arm, Lower
Arthroplasty 24365
with Implant. 24366, 25441
Craterization 24145, 25151
Cyst
Excision 24125, 24126, 25120-25126
Diaphysectomy 24145, 25151
Dislocation
Partial. 24640
Subluxate. 24640
with Fracture
Closed Treatment. 24620
Open Treatment 24635
Excision
Epiphyseal Bar 20150
Head. 24130
Partial. 24136, 25145, 25151
Styloid Process. 25230, 25440
Fracture
Colles
Treatment. 25600
Distal 25600-25609
Closed Treatment. 25600-25605
Open Treatment 25607-25609
Percutaneous Fixation 25606
Head/Neck
Closed Treatment. 24650-24655
Open Treatment 24665, 24666
Shaft
Closed Treatment. 25500-25505, 25520, 25560, 25565
Open Treatment 25515, 25525, 25526, 25574, 25575
Manipulation 25505, 25565
with Ulna 25560-25565, 25574, 25575
Smith Type
Closed Treatment. 25600, 25605
with Ulna
Open Treatment 25575
Implant
Removal 24164
Incision and Drainage. 25035
Osteomyelitis 24136, 24145
Osteoplasty
Lengthening 25391, 25393
Shortening 25390, 25392
Osteotomy. . . . 25350, 25355, 25365, 25370, 25375
Sofield Type 25370
Prophylactic Treatment. 25490, 25492
Repair
Defect, with Graft 25425, 25426
Epiphyseal Arrest. 25450-25455
Epiphyseal Separation
Closed. 25600
Closed with Manipulation 25605
Open Treatment 25607-25609
Percutaneous Fixation 25606
Malunion or Nonunion. 25400, 25405, 25415, 25420
Osteotomy 25350-25355, 25370-25375
and Ulna 25365
with Graft. 25405, 25420-25426
Replacement with Prosthesis
Distal 25441, 25446
Radial Head 24666
Replantation 20805
Saucerization 24145, 25151
Sequestrectomy 24136, 25145
Styloidectomy. 25230, 25440
Tumor
Cyst 24120
Excision . . 24125, 24126, 25120-25126, 25170
Radical Resection 24152, 25170

Ramstedt Operation
See Pyloromyotomy

Ramus Anterior, Nervus Thoracicus
See Intercostal Nerve

Range of Motion Test
Body, Total
with Hands. 95834
without Hands 95833
Cholinesterase Inhibitor Challenge 95857
Extremities or Trunk
with Hand. 95852
without Hand 95851
Eye. 92018, 92019
for Myasthenia Gravis 95857
Hand 95832, 95834, 95852
Muscle 95831

Rapid Heart Rate
See Tachycardia

Rapid Plasma Reagin Test . . . 86592, 86593

Rapid Test for Infection 86308, 86403-86406
Monospot Test 86308

Rapoport Test 52005

Rashkind Procedure 33735-33737

Rat Typhus
See Murine Typhus

Rathke Pouch Tumor
See Craniopharyngioma

Rays, Roentgen
See X ray

Raz Procedure 51845
See Repair, Bladder, Neck

RBC
See Red Blood Cell (RBC)

RBC ab
See Antibody, Detection, Red Blood Cell

Reaction, Polymerase Chain
See Genomic Sequencing Procedures (GSPs) and Other Molecular Multianalyte Assays

Realignment
Femur
Shaft. 27454
Hand
Extensor Tendon 26437
Humeral Shaft
Intramedullary Rod. 24410
Knee
Extensor Tendon 27422
Radius
Intramedullary Rod. 25370, 25375
Tibia
Intramedullary Rod. 27712
Ulna
Intramedullary Rod. 25370, 25375

Receptor
See CD4; Estrogen, Receptor Assay; Fc Receptor; Progesterone Receptors

Receptor Assay
Hormone
Estrogen. 84233
Progesterone 84234
Unspecified 84235
Nonendocrine 84238

Recession
Gastrocnemius
Leg, Lower 27687
Hamstring 27097
Strabismus Surgery. . . 67311-67314, 67316, 67334

Reconstruction
See Revision
Abdominal Wall
Omental Flap 49905
Acetabulum. 27120-27122
Anal
Congenital Absence. 46730-46740
Fistula. 46742
Graft. 46753
Sphincter 46750, 46751, 46760-46761
Ankle. 27700-27703
Apical-Aortic Conduit 33404
Atrial 33257-33259
Endoscopic. 33265, 33266
Open. 33254-33259
Auditory Canal, External. 69310-69320
Bile Duct
Anastomosis 47800
Bladder
and Urethra 51800-51820
Radiofrequency Micro-Remodeling . . . 53860
from Colon 50810
from Intestines. 50820, 51960
Breast 19357-19369
Augmentation 19324, 19325
Mammaplasty 19318-19325
Nipple. 19350-19355
Revision 19380
Transverse Rectus Abdominis Myocutaneous Flap. 19367-19369
with Free Flap 19364
with Latissimus Dorsi Flap. 19361
with Other Techniques. 19366
with Tissue Expander. 19357
Bronchi 32501
Anastomosis 31775, 32486
Graft Repair 31770
Stenosis 31775
Canthus. 67950
Carpal 25443
Carpal Bone. 25394, 25430
Cheekbone 21270
Chest Wall 19271, 19272, 32504
Omental Flap 49904
Trauma 32820
Cleft Palate 42200-42225
Conduit
Apical-Aortic 33404
Conjunctiva 68320-68335
with Flap
Bridge or Partial 68360
Total 68362
Cranial Bone
Extracranial 21181-21184

Ear, Middle
Tympanoplasty with Antrotomy or Mastoidotomy
with Ossicular Chain Reconstruction 69636, 69637
Tympanoplasty with Mastoidectomy . . . 69641
Radical or Complete 69644, 69645
with Intact or Reconstructed Wall 69643, 69644
with Ossicular Chain Reconstruction . . 69642
Tympanoplasty without Mastoidectomy 69631
with Ossicular Chain Reconstruction 69632, 69633
Elbow 24360
Collateral Ligament 24344, 24346
Fascia Lata Ligament 24362
Total Replacement 24363
Revision 24370, 24371
with Implant 24361, 24362
Esophagus 43300, 43310, 43313
Creation
Stoma 43351, 43352
Esophagostomy 43351, 43352
Fistula 43305, 43312, 43314
Gastrointestinal 43360, 43361
Eye
Graft
Conjunctiva 65782
Stem Cell 65781
Transplantation
Amniotic Membrane 65778-65780
Eyelid
Canthus 67950
Second Stage 67975
Total 67973-67975
Total Eyelid
Lower, One Stage 67973
Upper, One Stage 67974
Tarsoconjunctival Flap Transfer 67971
Facial Bones
Secondary 21275
Fallopian Tube
See Repair
Femur
Lengthening 27466-27468
Shortening 27465, 27468
Fibula
Lengthening 27715
Finger 26548
Polydactylous 26587
Foot
Cleft 28360
Forehead 21172-21180, 21182-21184
Glenoid Fossa 21255
Gums
Alveolus 41874
Gingiva 41872
Hand
Tendon Pulley 26390, 26500-26502
Toe to Finger Transfer 26551-26556
Heart
Atrial 33257-33259
Endoscopic 33265, 33266
Open 33254-33256
Atrial Septum 33735-33737
for Hypoplasia 33622
for Obstruction 33622
Pulmonary Artery Shunt 33924
Vena Cava 34502
Hip
Replacement 27130-27132
Secondary 27134-27138
Hip Joint
with Prosthesis 27125
Interphalangeal Joint 26535, 26536
Collateral Ligament 26545
Intestines, Small
Anastomosis 43845, 44130
Knee 27437, 27438
Femur 27442, 27443, 27446
Ligament 27427-27429
Replacement 27447
Revision 27486, 27487
Tibia 27440-27443, 27446
with Prosthesis 27438, 27445
Kneecap
Instability 27420-27424
Larynx
Cricoid Split 31587
Medialization 31591
Stenosis 31551-31554
Web 31580
with Fracture Repair 31584
LeFort I 21141-21147, 21155, 21160
LeFort II 21150, 21151
LeFort III 21154, 21155, 21159, 21160
Lip 40525-40527, 40761
Lunate 25444
Malar Augmentation
Prosthetic Material 21270
with Bone Graft 21210
Mandible
with Implant 21244-21246, 21248, 21249
Mandibular Condyle 21247
Mandibular Rami
with Bone Graft 21194
with Internal Rigid Fixation 21196
without Bone Graft 21193
without Internal Rigid Fixation 21195
Maxilla
with Implant 21245, 21246, 21248, 21249
Metacarpophalangeal Joint 26135, 26140, 26530, 26531, 26541
Midface
Forehead Advancement 21159, 21160
with Bone Graft 21145-21160, 21188
without Bone Graft 21141-21143
Mouth 40840-40845
Nail Bed 11762
Nasoethmoid Complex 21182-21184
Navicular 25443
Nose
Cleft Lip/Cleft Palate 30460-30462
Dermatoplasty 30620
Primary 30400-30420
Secondary 30430-30450
Septum 30520
Orbit 21256
Orbit Area
Secondary 21275
Orbit with Bone Grafting 21182-21184
Orbital Rim 21172-21180
Orbital Rims 21182-21184
Orbital Walls 21182-21184
Orbitocraniofacial
Secondary Revision 21275
Oviduct
Fimbrioplasty 58760
Palate
Cleft Palate 42200-42225
Lengthening 42226, 42227
Parotid Duct
Diversion 42507-42510
Patella 27437, 27438
Instability 27420-27424
Penis
Angulation 54360
Chordee 54300-54304
Complications 54340-54348
Epispadias 54380-54390
Hypospadias 54332, 54352
One Stage Distal with Urethroplasty 54324-54328
One Stage Perineal 54336
Periorbital Region
Osteotomy with Graft 21267, 21268
Pharynx 42950
Pyloric Sphincter 43800
Radioulnar Joint 25337
Radius 24365, 25390-25393, 25441
Arthroplasty
with Implant 24366
Shoulder
Rotator Cuff 23420
Joint
with Implant 23470, 23472-23474
Skull 21172-21180
Defect 62140, 62141, 62145
Spinal Elements 63051, 63295
Sternum 21740-21742
with Thoracoscopy 21743
Stomach
for Obesity 43644, 43645, 43845-43848
Gastric Bypass 43644, 43645, 43846
Roux-En-Y 43644, 43846
with Duodenum . . 43810, 43850-43855, 43865
with Jejunum 43820-43825, 43860
Superior-Lateral Orbital Rim and Forehead 21172-21175
Supraorbital Rim and Forehead 21179, 21180
Symblepharon 68335
Temporomandibular Joint
Arthroplasty 21240-21243
Throat 42950
Thumb
from Finger 26550
Opponensplasty 26490-26496
Tibia
Lengthening 27715
Tubercle 27418
Toe
Angle Deformity 28313
Extra Toes 28344
Hammertoe 28285, 28286
Macrodactyly 28340, 28341
Polydactylous 26587
Syndactyly 28345
Webbed Toe 28345
Tongue
Frenum 41520
Trachea
Carina 31766
Cervical 31750
Fistula 31755
Intrathoracic 31760
Trapezium 25445
Tympanic Membrane 69620
Ulna 25390-25393, 25442
Radioulnar 25337
Ureter 50700
with Intestines 50840
Urethra 53410-53440, 53445
Complications 54340-54348
Hypospadias
One Stage Distal with Meatal Advancement 54322
One Stage Distal with Urethroplasty 54324-54328

Index

Suture to Bladder . . . 51840, 51841
Urethroplasty for Second Stage 54308-54316
Urethroplasty for Third Stage . . . 54318
Uterus . . . 58540
Vas Deferens
See Vasovasorrhaphy
Vena Cava . . . 34502
with Resection . . . 37799
Wound Repair . . . 13100-13160
Wrist . . . 25320
Zygomatic Arch . . . 21255

Rectal Bleeding
See Hemorrhage, Endoscopic Control, Rectum

Rectal Prolapse
See Procidentia, Rectum

Rectal Sphincter
Dilation . . . 45910

Rectocele
Repair . . . 45560, 57250

Rectopexy
See Proctopexy

Rectoplasty
See Proctoplasty

Rectorrhaphy
See Rectum, Suture

Rectovaginal Fistula
Closure . . . 57300, 57305, 57307, 57308

Rectovaginal Hernia
See Rectocele

Rectum
See Anus
Abscess
Incision and Drainage . . . 45005-45020, 46040, 46060
Advancement Flap . . . 46288
Biopsy . . . 45100
Dilation
Endoscopy . . . 45303
Endoscopy
Biopsy . . . 45305
Destruction
Tumor . . . 45320
Dilation . . . 45910
Endoscopic . . . 45303
Exploration . . . 45300
Hemorrhage . . . 45317
Removal
Foreign Body . . . 45307
Polyp . . . 45308-45315
Tumor . . . 45308-45315
Volvulus Decompression . . . 45321
Excision
Muscularis Propria . . . 45172
Partial . . . 45111, 45113-45116, 45123
Total . . . 45110, 45112, 45119, 45120
with Colon . . . 45121
Exploration
Endoscopic . . . 45300
Surgical . . . 45990
Hemorrhage
Endoscopic . . . 45317
Hemorrhoid
See Hemorrhoids
Incontinence
Graft . . . 46753
Thiersch Procedure . . . 46753
Injection
Sclerosing Solution . . . 45520
Laparoscopy . . . 45499
Lesion
Excision . . . 45108
Manometry . . . 91122
Mucosectomy . . . 44157, 44158, 44211, 45113
Procidentia
Excision . . . 45130-45135
Prolapse
Excision . . . 45130-45135
Injection, Sclerosing Solution . . . 45520
Removal
Fecal Impaction . . . 45915
Foreign Body . . . 45307, 45915
Repair
Fistula . . . 45800-45825, 46707
Incontinence . . . 46753
Injury . . . 45562, 45563
Prolapse . . . 45505-45541, 45900
Rectocele . . . 45560
Stenosis . . . 45500
with Sigmoid Excision . . . 45550
Sensation, Tone, and Compliance Test . . . 91120
Stricture
Dilation . . . 45910
Division . . . 45150
Excision . . . 45150
Suture
Fistula . . . 45800-45825
Prolapse . . . 45540, 45541
Tumor
Destruction . . . 45190, 45320
Excision . . . 45160-45172
Transanal Endoscopic . . . 0184T
Unlisted Services and Procedures . . . 45999
Laparoscopic . . . 45499
Voiding Pressure
See Voiding Pressure Studies, Rectum

Red Blood Cell (RBC)
Antibody . . . 86850-86870
Pretreatment . . . 86970-86972
Count . . . 85032-85041
Fetal . . . 85460, 85461
Fetomaternal Hemorrhage . . . 85460, 85461
Fragility
Mechanical . . . 85547
Osmotic . . . 85555-85557
Hematocrit . . . 85014
Omega-3 Fatty Acids . . . 0111T
Sedimentation Rate
Automated . . . 85652
Manual . . . 85651
Sequestration . . . 78140
Sickling . . . 85660
Survival Test . . . 78130-78135
Volume Determination . . . 78120, 78121

Red Blood Cell ab
See Antibody, Detection, Red Blood Cell

Reductase, Glutathione
See Glutathione Reductase

Reductase, Lactic Cytochrome
See Lactic Dehydrogenase

Reduction
Amniotic Fluid . . . 59001
Collateral Ligament
Ulnar . . . 29902
Craniomegalic Skull . . . 62115, 62117
Ear, Protruding . . . 69300
for Dislocation
Carpometacarpal . . . 26686
for Fracture
Laryngeal . . . 31584
Odontoid . . . 22318, 22319
Tracheal . . . 31630
Vertebral . . . 22325-22328
Forehead . . . 21137-21139
Internal Hernia
Mesentery . . . 44050
Intussusception . . . 44050
Mammaplasty . . . 19318
Masseter Muscle/Bone . . . 21295, 21296
Osteoplasty
Facial Bones . . . 21209
Overcorrection of Ptosis . . . 67909
Pregnancy
Multifetal . . . 59866
Procidentia . . . 45900
Skull
Craniomegalic . . . 62115, 62117
Tissue . . . 30801
Torsion
Testis . . . 54600
Tumor
Bone
Ablation Therapy . . . 20982, 20983
Breast
Pulmonary . . . 32994, 32998
Volume
Blood Products . . . 86960
Lung . . . 32491
Volvulus . . . 44050, 44055
with Reconstruction
Hip . . . 27147, 27156
Radioulnar Joint . . . 25337
Wrist . . . 25230

Reflex Test
Blink Reflex . . . 95933

Reflux Study . . . 78262
Gastroesophageal . . . 91034-91038

Refraction
Ophthalmological . . . 92015

Rehabilitation
Artery
Occlusive Disease . . . 93668
Auditory
Post-Lingual Hearing Loss . . . 92633
Pre-Lingual Hearing Loss . . . 92630
Status Evaluation . . . 92626, 92627
Cardiac . . . 93797, 93798

Rehabilitation Facility
Discharge Services . . . 1110F, 1111F

Rehabilitative
See Rehabilitation

Reimplantation
Arteries
Aorta
Prosthesis . . . 35697
Carotid . . . 35691, 35694, 35695
Coronary Ostium . . . 33783
Subclavian . . . 35693-35695
Vertebral . . . 35691-35693
Visceral . . . 35697
Kidney . . . 50380
Pulmonary Artery . . . 33788
Ureters . . . 51565

Reinnervation
Larynx
Neuromuscular Pedicle . . . 31590

Reinsch Test . . . 83015

Reinsertion
Drug Delivery Implant . . . 11983
Ocular Implant . . . 65150, 65155
Spinal Fixation Device . . . 22849
Tendon
Biceps . . . 24342
Triceps . . . 24342

Relative Density
See Specific Gravity

Release
Capsule
Ankle . . . 27612
Elbow . . . 24149
Foot . . . 28260
Knee . . . 27435
Metatarsophalangeal Joint . . . 28289, 28291
Shoulder . . . 23020
Carpal Tunnel . . . 64721
Choroidal Fluid . . . 67015
Fascia
Finger/Thumb . . . 26123
Heel . . . 28119
Flexor Muscles
Hip . . . 27036
Knee Joint . . . 29873
Ligament
Coracoacromial . . . 23130, 23415, 29826
Knee
Retinacular . . . 27425
Transverse Carpal . . . 29848
Metacarpophalangeal Joint . . . 26135
Muscle
Abductor Hallucis . . . 28240
Hamstring . . . 27097
Hand . . . 26508, 26593
Hip . . . 27036
Knee . . . 27422
Nerve . . . 64702-64726
Neurolytic . . . 64727
Penis
Chordee . . . 54352
from Scrotum . . . 54318
Retina
Encircling Material . . . 67115
Fluid . . . 67015
Scar . . . 11042, 14040, 14041
Colostomy . . . 44340
Eye . . . 67343
Ileostomy . . . 44312
Spinal Cord . . . 63200
Stapes . . . 69650
Tarsal Tunnel . . . 28035
Tendon . . . 24332, 25295
Vitreous . . . 67015

Release-Inhibiting Hormone, Somatotropin
See Somatostatin

Relocation
Skin Pocket
Implantable Defibrillator . . . 33223
Pacemaker . . . 33222

Removal
Adjustable Gastric Restrictive Device 43772-43774
Allograft
Intestinal . . . 44137
Artificial Heart . . . 33929
Artificial Intervertebral Disc
Cervical Interspace . . . 0095T, 22864
Lumbar Interspace . . . 0164T, 22865
Balloon
Intra-Aortic . . . 33974
Balloon Assist Device
Intra-Aortic . . . 33968, 33971
Baroreflex Activation Device . . . 0269T-0271T
Blood Clot
Eye . . . 65930
Blood Component
Apheresis . . . 36511-36516
Breast
See Mastectomy
Bronchial Valve . . . 31648, 31649
Calcareous Deposits
Subdeltoid . . . 23000
Calculi (Stone)
See Calculus, Removal
Capsules
Breast . . . 19371
Cardiac Event Recorder
See Cardiac Assist Devices, Subcutaneous Cardiac Rhythm Monitor
Cast . . . 29700, 29705, 29710
Cataract
See Cataract, Extraction/Removal
Catheter
Central Venous . . . 36589
Peritoneum . . . 49422
Pleural Cavity . . . 32552
Spinal Cord . . . 62355
Cerclage
Cervix . . . 59871
Cerumen
Auditory Canal, External . . . 69209, 69210
Clot
Pericardium . . . 33020
Endoscopic . . . 32658
Comedones . . . 10040
Contraceptive Capsules . . . 11976
Cranial Tongs . . . 20665
Cyst . . . 10040
Dacryolith
Lacrimal Duct . . . 68530
Lacrimal Gland . . . 68530
Drug Delivery Implant . . . 11982, 11983
Ear Wax
Auditory Canal, External . . . 69209, 69210
Electrode
Array
Nerve . . . 64585
Brain . . . 61535, 61880
Chest Wall
Respiratory Sensor . . . 0468T
Heart . . . 33238
Spinal Cord . . . 63661-63664
Stomach . . . 43648, 43882
Embolus
See Embolectomy
Esophageal Sphincter Augmentation Device . . . 43285
External Fixation System . . . 20694
Eye
Bone . . . 67414, 67445
Epithelium . . . 65435, 65436
Ocular Contents
with Implant . . . 65093
without Implant . . . 65091
Orbital Contents Only . . . 65110
with Bone . . . 65112
with Implant
Muscles Attached . . . 65105
Muscles, Not Attached . . . 65103
with Muscle or Myocutaneous Flap . . . 65114
without Implant . . . 65101
Fallopian Tube
Laparoscopy . . . 58661
with Hysterectomy . . . 58542, 58544, 58548
Fat
Lipectomy . . . 15876-15879
Fecal Impaction
Rectum . . . 45915
Fibrin Deposit . . . 32150
Filter
Vena Cava . . . 37193
Fixation Device . . . 20670-20680
Foreign Body
Anal . . . 46608
Ankle Joint . . . 27610, 27620
Arm
Lower . . . 25248
Upper . . . 24200, 24201
Auditory Canal, External . . . 69200
with Anesthesia . . . 69205
Bile Duct . . . 43275
Bladder . . . 52310-52315
Brain . . . 61570, 62163
Bronchi . . . 31635
Colon . . . 44025, 44390, 45379
Colon-Sigmoid . . . 45332
Conjunctival Embedded . . . 65210
Cornea
with Slit Lamp . . . 65222
without Slit Lamp . . . 65220
Duodenum . . . 44010
Elbow . . . 24000, 24101, 24200, 24201
Esophagus . . . 43020, 43045, 43215, 74235
Eye
Anterior Chamber . . . 65235
Corneal . . . 65220, 65222
Eyelid . . . 67938
External Eye . . . 65205-65222
Posterior Segment . . . 65260, 65265
Finger . . . 26075-26080
Foot . . . 28190-28193
Gastrointestinal, Upper . . . 43247
Gum . . . 41805
Hand . . . 26070
Hip . . . 27033, 27086, 27087
Hysteroscopy . . . 58562
Interphalangeal Joint
Toe . . . 28024
Intertarsal Joint . . . 28020
Intestines, Small . . . 44020, 44363
Intraocular . . . 65235-65265
Kidney . . . 50561, 50580
Knee Joint . . . 27310, 27331, 27372
Lacrimal Duct . . . 68530
Lacrimal Gland . . . 68530
Larynx . . . 31511, 31530, 31531, 31577
Leg, Upper . . . 27372
Lung . . . 32151
Mandible . . . 41806
Mediastinum . . . 39000-39010
Metatarsophalangeal Joint . . . 28022
Mouth . . . 40804, 40805
Muscle . . . 20520, 20525
Nose . . . 30300
Anesthesia . . . 30310
Lateral Rhinotomy . . . 30320
Orbit . . . 67413, 67430
with Bone Flap . . . 67430
without Bone Flap . . . 67413
Pancreatic Duct . . . 43275
Patella
See Patellectomy
Pelvis . . . 27086, 27087
Penile Tissue . . . 54115

Penis . . . 54115
Pericardium . . . 33020
Endoscopic . . . 32658
Peritoneum . . . 49402
Pharynx . . . 42809
Pleura . . . 32150, 32151
Endoscopic . . . 32653
Rectum . . . 45307, 45915
Scrotum . . . 55120
Shoulder . . . 23040-23044
Deep . . . 23333
Subcutaneous . . . 23330
Skin
with Debridement . . . 11010-11012
Stomach . . . 43500
Subcutaneous Tissue . . . 10120, 10121
with Debridement . . . 11010-11012
Tarsometatarsal Joint . . . 28020
Tendon Sheath . . . 20520-20525
Toe . . . 28022
Ureter . . . 50961, 50980
Urethra . . . 52310-52315
Uterus . . . 58562
Vagina . . . 57415
Wrist . . . 25040, 25101, 25248
Hair
Electrolysis . . . 17380
Halo . . . 20665
Hearing Aid
Bone Conduction . . . 69711
Hematoma
Brain . . . 61312-61315
Implant . . . 20670-20680
Ankle . . . 27704
Breast . . . 19328-19330
Contraceptive Capsules . . . 11976
Disc . . . 22865
Eye . . . 67120, 67121
Finger . . . 26320
Hand . . . 26320
Radius . . . 24164
Shoulder . . . 23334, 23335
Wrist . . . 25449
Infusion Pump
Intra-Arterial . . . 36262
Intravenous . . . 36590
Spinal Cord . . . 62365
Interstitial Glucose Sensor . . . 0447T, 0448T
Intra-Aortic Balloon . . . 33974
Assist Device . . . 33968, 33971
Intrauterine Device (IUD) . . . 58301
Ischemia Monitoring System . . . 0530T-0532T
Keel
Laryngoplasty . . . 31580
Lacrimal Gland
Partial . . . 68505
Total . . . 68500
Lacrimal Sac
Excision . . . 68520
Laryngocele . . . 31300
Leiomyomata . . . 58545, 58546, 58561
Lens . . . 66920-66940
Lens Material . . . 66840-66852
Lesion
Conjunctiva . . . 68040
Larynx . . . 31512, 31578
Endoscopic . . . 31545, 31546
Small Intestine . . . 43250
Loose Body
See Loose Body, Removal
Lung
Apical Tumor . . . 32503, 32504
Bronchial Valve . . . 31648, 31649
Bronchoplasty . . . 32501
Completion Pneumonectomy . . . 32488
Cyst . . . 32140
Extrapleural . . . 32445
Pneumonectomy . . . 32440-32445
Single Lobe . . . 32480
Single Segment . . . 32484
Sleeve Lobectomy . . . 32486
Sleeve Pneumonectomy . . . 32442
Two Lobes . . . 32482
Volume Reduction . . . 32491
Lymph Nodes
Abdominal . . . 38747
Inguinofemoral . . . 38760-38765
Pelvic . . . 38770
Retroperitoneal
Transabdominal . . . 38780
Thoracic . . . 38746
Mammary Implant . . . 19328-19330
Mastoid
Air Cells . . . 69670
Mesh
Abdominal Wall . . . 11008
Milia, Multiple . . . 10040
Nails . . . 11730-11732, 11750
Neurostimulators
Pulse Generator . . . 64595
Receiver . . . 64595
Ocular Implant . . . 65175, 65920
Orbital Implant . . . 67560
Ovary
Laparoscopy . . . 58661
with Hysterectomy . . . 58542, 58544, 58548
Pacemaker System
Electrodes
by Thoracotomy . . . 33236
Pulse Generator Only . . . 33233
Implantable Defibrillator System
See Cardiac Assist Devices
Patella, Complete . . . 27424
Percutaneous Ventricular Assist Device . . . 33992
Plate
Skull . . . 62142
Polyp
Anal . . . 46610, 46612
Antrochoanal . . . 31032
Colon . . . 44392, 45385
Colon-Sigmoid . . . 45333
Endoscopy . . . 44364, 44365, 44394
Esophagus . . . 43217, 43250
Gastrointestinal, Upper . . . 43250, 43251
Rectum . . . 45315
Sinus . . . 31032, 31051
Prosthesis
Abdomen . . . 49606
Abdominal Wall . . . 11008
Elbow
Humeral and Ulnar Components . . . 24160
Radial Head . . . 24164
Glenoid Component . . . 23334, 23335
Hip . . . 27090, 27091
Humeral Component . . . 23334, 23335, 24160
Knee . . . 27488
Penis . . . 54406, 54410-54417
Perineum . . . 53442
Radial Head . . . 24164
Shoulder . . . 23334, 23335
Skull . . . 62142
Ulnar Component . . . 24160
Urethral Sphincter . . . 53446, 53447
Wrist . . . 25250, 25251
Pulse Generator
Brain . . . 61888
Spinal Cord . . . 63688
Pustules . . . 10040
Receiver
Brain . . . 61888
Spinal Cord . . . 63688
Reservoir
Spinal Cord . . . 62365
Seton
Anal . . . 46030
Shoulder Joint
Foreign or Loose Body . . . 23107
Shunt
Brain . . . 62256-62258
Heart . . . 33924
Peritoneum . . . 49429
Spinal Cord . . . 63746
Skin Tags . . . 11200, 11201
Sling
Urethra . . . 53442
Vagina . . . 57287
Spinal Instrumentation
Anterior . . . 22855
Posterior Nonsegmental
Harrington Rod . . . 22850
Posterior Segmental . . . 22852
Stent
Bile Duct . . . 43275
Pancreatic Duct . . . 43275
Ureteral . . . 50382-50386
Subcutaneous Port
for Gastric Restrictive
Procedure . . . 43887, 43888
Suture
Anal . . . 46754
Anesthesia . . . 15850, 15851
Thrombus
See Thrombectomy
Tissue Expanders
Skin . . . 11971
Total Replacement Heart System . . . 33929
Transplant
Intestines . . . 44137
Kidney . . . 50370
Tube
Ear, Middle . . . 69424
Nephrostomy . . . 50389
Tumor
Larynx . . . 31578
Small Intestine . . . 43250
Temporal Bone . . . 69970
Ureter
Ligature . . . 50940
Urethral Stent
Bladder . . . 52310-52315
Urethra . . . 52310-52315
Uterus
Laparoscopy . . . 58541, 58543, 58548
Vein
Clusters . . . 37785
Perforation . . . 37760, 37761
Saphenous . . . 37718-37735, 37780
Varicose . . . 37765, 37766
Venous Access Device . . . 36590
Obstruction . . . 75901, 75902
Ventilating Tube
Ear, Middle . . . 69424
Ventricular Assist Device . . . 33977, 33978
Intracorporeal . . . 33980
Vitreous
Anterior Approach . . . 67005-67010

Wire
Anal ... 46754

Renal Abscess
See Abscess, Tissue, Kidney

Renal Arteries
See Artery, Renal

Renal Autotransplantation
See Autotransplantation, Renal

Renal Calculus
See Calculus, Removal, Kidney

Renal Cyst
See Cyst, Kidney

Renal Dialyses
See Hemodialysis

Renal Disease Services
See Dialysis

Renal Transplantation
See Kidney, Transplantation

Renin ... 80408, 80416, 80417, 84244

Renin-Converting Enzyme ... 82164

Reoperation
Carotid
Thromboendarterectomy ... 35390
Coronary Artery Bypass
Valve Procedure ... 33530
Distal Vessel Bypass ... 35700

Repair
See Revision
Abdomen ... 49900
Hernia ... 49491-49525, 49565, 49570, 49582-49590
Omphalocele ... 49600-49611
Suture ... 49900
Abdominal Wall ... 15830, 15847
Anal
Anomaly ... 46744-46748
Fistula ... 46288, 46706, 46715, 46716
Stricture ... 46700-46705
Aneurysm
Aorta
Abdominal ... 34845-34848
Infrarenal ... 34830-34832
Thoracic ... 33877-33886
Intracranial Artery ... 61697-61708
Ankle
Ligament ... 27695-27698
Tendon ... 27612, 27650-27654, 27680-27687
Aorta ... 33320-33322, 33802, 33803
Coarctation ... 33840-33851
Graft ... 33860-33877
Infrarenal Abdominal
Endovascular ... 34701-34706, 34845-34848
Sinus of Valsalva ... 33702-33720
Thoracic ... 75956-75959
Endovascular ... 33880-33891
Visceral
Endovascular ... 34841-34848
Physician Planning ... 34839
Anorectum
Fistula ... 46707
Aortic Arch
with Cardiopulmonary Bypass ... 33853
without Cardiopulmonary Bypass ... 33852
Aortic Valve ... 33390, 33391
Obstruction
Outflow Tract ... 33414
Septic Hypertrophy ... 33416
Stenosis ... 33415
Arm
Lower ... 25260-25263, 25270
Fasciotomy ... 24495
Secondary ... 25265, 25272-25274
Tendon ... 25290
Tendon Sheath ... 25275
Muscle ... 24341
Tendon ... 24332, 24341, 25280, 25295, 25310-25316
Upper
Muscle Revision ... 24330, 24331
Muscle Transfer ... 24301, 24320
Tendon Lengthening ... 24305
Tendon Revision ... 24320
Tendon Transfer ... 24301
Tenotomy ... 24310
Arteriovenous Fistula
Abdomen
Acquired or Traumatic ... 35189
Congenital ... 35182
Extremity
Acquired or Traumatic ... 35190
Congenital ... 35184
Head
Acquired or Traumatic ... 35188
Congenital ... 35180
Neck
Acquired or Traumatic ... 35188
Congenital ... 35180
Thorax
Acquired or Traumatic ... 35189
Congenital ... 35182
Arteriovenous Malformation
Iliac
Endograft ... 0254T
Intracranial ... 61680-61692
Intracranial Artery ... 61705-61708
Spinal Artery ... 62294
Spinal Cord ... 63250-63252
Artery
Angioplasty
Aorta ... 37246-37247
Axillary ... 37246-37247
Brachiocephalic ... 37246-37247
Bypass Graft ... 35501-35571, 35601-35683, 35691-35695, 35700
Bypass In-Situ ... 35583-35587
Bypass Venous Graft ... 33510-33516, 35510-35525
Coronary ... 33507
Femoral ... 37224
Iliac ... 37220-37222, 37227
Endograft ... 0254T
Occlusive Disease ... 35001, 35005-35021, 35045-35081, 35091, 35102, 35111, 35121, 35131, 35141, 35151, 37220-37235, 92941, 92943, 92944
Popliteal ... 37224
Pulmonary ... 33690
Renal ... 37246, 37247
Renal or Visceral ... 37246, 37247
Subclavian ... 37246-37247
Thromboendarterectomy ... 35301-35321, 35341-35390
Tibioperoneal ... 37228-37235
Viscera ... 37246, 37247
Arytenoid Cartilage ... 31400
Atria
Laparoscopic ... 33265, 33266
Open ... 33254-33256
Bile Duct ... 47701
with Intestines ... 47760, 47780-47785
Wound ... 47900
Bladder
Exstrophy ... 51940
Fistula ... 44660, 44661, 45800-45805, 51880-51925
Neck ... 51845
Resection ... 52500
Wound ... 51860-51865
Blepharoptosis
Frontalis Muscle Technique with Fascial Sling ... 67902
Blood Vessel
Abdomen ... 35221
with Other Graft ... 35281
with Vein Graft ... 35251
Chest ... 35211-35216
with Other Graft ... 35271-35276
with Vein Graft ... 35241-35246
Finger ... 35207
Graft Defect ... 35870
Hand ... 35207
Kidney ... 50100
Lower Extremity ... 35226
with Other Graft ... 35286
with Vein Graft ... 35256
Neck ... 35201
with Other Graft ... 35261
with Vein Graft ... 35231
Upper Extremity ... 35206
with Other Graft ... 35266
with Vein Graft ... 35236
Body Cast ... 29720
Brain
Wound ... 61571
Breast
Suspension ... 19316
Bronchi
Fistula ... 32815
Brow Pyrosis ... 67900
Bunion ... 28292, 28295-28299
Bypass Graft ... 35901-35907
Fistula ... 35870
Calcaneus
Osteotomy ... 28300
Cannula ... 36860, 36861
Carpal ... 25440
Carpal Bone ... 25431
Cervix
Cerclage ... 57700
Abdominal ... 59320-59325
Suture ... 57720
Chest Wall ... 32905
Closure ... 32810
Fistula ... 32906
Chin
Augmentation ... 21120, 21123
Osteotomy ... 21121-21123
Clavicle
Osteotomy ... 23480-23485
Cleft Hand ... 26580
Cleft Lip ... 40525-40527, 40700-40761
Nasal Deformity ... 40700, 40701, 40720-40761
Cleft Palate
See Cleft Palate, Repair
Colon
Fistula ... 44650-44661
Hernia ... 44050
Malrotation ... 44055
Obstruction ... 44050

Cornea
  See Cornea, Repair
Coronary Chamber Fistula . . . 33500, 33501
Cyst
  Bartholin's Gland . . . 56440
  Liver . . . 47300
Diaphragm
  for Eventration . . . 39545
  Hernia . . . 39503, 39540, 39541
  Laceration . . . 39501
Ductus Arteriosus . . . 33820-33824, 93582
Ear, Middle
  Oval Window Fistula . . . 69666
  Round Window Fistula . . . 69667
Elbow
  Hemiepiphyseal Arrest . . . 24470
  Ligament . . . 24343-24346
  Muscle . . . 24341
  Muscle Transfer . . . 24301
  Tendon . . . 24340-24342
    Each . . . 24341
  Tendon Lengthening . . . 24305
  Tendon Transfer . . . 24301
  Tennis Elbow . . . 24357-24359
Encephalocele . . . 62121
Endovascular
  See Endovascular Repair
Enterocele
  Hysterectomy . . . 58270, 58294
Epididymis . . . 54900, 54901
Epiphysis
  Femur . . . 27177-27181, 27475, 27479, 27485, 27742, 27516-27519
  Fibula . . . 27477, 27479, 27485, 27732, 27734, 27740, 27742
  Tibia . . . 27477-27485, 27730-27742
Epispadias . . . 54380-54390
Esophagus . . . 43300, 43310, 43313
  Esophagogastrostomy . . . 43320
  Esophagojejunostomy . . . 43340, 43341
  Fistula . . . 43305, 43312, 43314, 43420-43425
  Fundoplasty . . . 43210, 43325
    Laparotomy . . . 43327
    Thoracotomy . . . 43328
  Lengthening . . . 43283, 43338
  Muscle . . . 43330, 43331
  Pre-Existing Perforation . . . 43405
  Varices . . . 43401
  Wound . . . 43410-43415
Eye
  Ciliary Body . . . 66680
    Suture . . . 66682
  Conjunctiva . . . 65270-65273
    Wound . . . 65270-65273
  Cornea . . . 65275
    with Amniotic Membrane . . . 65778-65780
    Astigmatism . . . 65772-65775
    with Glue . . . 65286
    Wound . . . 65275-65285
  Fistula
    Lacrimal Gland . . . 68770
  Iris
    Suture . . . 66682
    with Ciliary Body . . . 66680
  Lacrimal Duct
    Canaliculi . . . 68700
  Lacrimal Punctum . . . 68705
  Retina
    Detachment . . . 67101, 67105, 67107, 67108, 67110, 67113
  Sclera
    Reinforcement . . . 67250-67255
    Staphyloma . . . 66225
    with Glue . . . 65286
    with Graft . . . 66225
    Wound . . . 65286, 66250
  Strabismus
    Chemodenervation . . . 67345
  Symblepharon
    Division . . . 68340
    with Graft . . . 68335
    without Graft . . . 68330
  Trabeculae . . . 65855
Eye Muscles
  Strabismus
    Adjustable Sutures . . . 67335
    One Horizontal Muscle . . . 67311
    One Vertical Muscle . . . 67314
    Posterior Fixation Suture Technique . . . 67334, 67335
    Previous Surgery, Not Involving Extraocular Muscles . . . 67331
    Release Extensive Scar Tissue . . . 67343
    Superior Oblique Muscle . . . 67318
    Two Horizontal Muscles . . . 67312
    Two or More Vertical Muscles . . . 67316
  Wound
    Extraocular Muscle . . . 65290
Eyebrow
  Ptosis . . . 67900
Eyelashes
  Epilation
    by Forceps . . . 67820
    by Other than Forceps . . . 67825
  Incision of Lid Margin . . . 67830
    with Free Mucous Membrane Graft . . . 67835
Eyelid . . . 21280-21282
  Ectropion . . . 67916, 67917
    Suture . . . 67914
    Thermocauterization . . . 67915
  Entropion . . . 67924
    Excision Tarsal Wedge . . . 67923
    Suture . . . 67921-67924
    Thermocauterization . . . 67922
  Excisional . . . 67961-67966
  Lagophthalmos . . . 67912
  Ptosis
    Conjunctivo-Tarso-Muller's Muscle-Levator Resection . . . 67908
    Frontalis Muscle Technique . . . 67901, 67902
    Levator Resection . . . 67903, 67904
  Reduction of Overcorrection . . . 67909
    Superior Rectus Technique . . . 67906
  Retraction . . . 67911
  Wound
    Suture . . . 67930-67935
Facial Bones . . . 21208, 21209
Facial Nerve
  Paralysis . . . 15840-15845
  Suture
    Intratemporal, Lateral to Geniculate Ganglion . . . 69740
    Intratemporal, Medial to Geniculate Ganglion . . . 69745
Fallopian Tube . . . 58752
  Anastomosis . . . 58750
  Create Stoma . . . 58770
Fascial Defect . . . 50728
Femur . . . 27470-27472
  Epiphysis . . . 27475-27485, 27742
    Arrest . . . 27185
    by Pinning . . . 27176
    by Traction . . . 27175
    Open Treatment . . . 27177, 27178
    Osteoplasty . . . 27179
    Osteotomy . . . 27181
  Muscle Transfer . . . 27110
  Osteotomy . . . 27140, 27151, 27450-27454
    Femoral Neck . . . 27161
    with Fixation . . . 27165
    with Open Reduction . . . 27156
  with Graft . . . 27170
Fibula
  Epiphysis . . . 27477-27485, 27730-27742
  Nonunion or Malunion . . . 27726
  Osteotomy . . . 27707-27712
Finger
  Claw Finger . . . 26499
  Macrodactylia . . . 26590
  Polydactylous . . . 26587
  Syndactyly . . . 26560-26562
  Tendon
    Extensor . . . 26415-26434, 26445-26449
    Flexor . . . 26356-26358, 26440-26442
    Joint Stabilization . . . 26474
    PIP Joint . . . 26471
  Toe Transfer . . . 26551-26556
  Trigger . . . 26055
  Volar Plate . . . 26548
  Web Finger . . . 26560-26562
Fistula
  Anorectal . . . 46707
  Carotid-Cavernous . . . 61710
  Ileoanal Pouch . . . 46710-46712
  Mastoid . . . 69700
  Rectovaginal . . . 57308
Foot
  Fascia . . . 28250
  Muscle . . . 28250
  Tendon . . . 28200-28226, 28238
Gallbladder
  with Gastroenterostomy . . . 47741
  with Intestines . . . 47720-47740
Great Arteries . . . 33770-33781
Great Vessel . . . 33320-33322
Hallux Valgus . . . 28292, 28295-28299
Hamstring . . . 27097
Hand
  Cleft Hand . . . 26580
  Muscle . . . 26591-26593
  Tendon
    Extensor . . . 26410-26416, 26426-26428, 26433-26437
    Flexor . . . 26350-26358, 26440
    Profundus . . . 26370-26373
Hearing Aid
  Bone Conduction . . . 69711
Heart
  Anomaly . . . 33600-33617
  Aortic Sinus . . . 33702-33722
  Atria
    Laparoscopic . . . 33265, 33266
    Open . . . 33254-33256
  Atrioventricular Canal . . . 33660-33665
    Complete . . . 33670
  Atrioventricular Valve . . . 33660-33665
  Blood Vessel . . . 33320-33322
  Cor Triatriatum . . . 33732
  Infundibular . . . 33476-33478
  Mitral Valve . . . 0345T, 33418-33420, 33422, 33425-33427
  Myocardium . . . 33542
  Outflow Tract . . . 33476-33478
  Patent Ductus Arteriosus . . . 33820, 33822, 33824, 93582
  Postinfarction . . . 33542-33545
  Prosthetic Valve . . . 33670, 33852, 33853
  Prosthetic Valve Dysfunction . . . 33496
  Pulmonary Artery Shunt . . . 33924

Pulmonary Valve 33470-33474
Septal Defect 33545, 33608-33610, 33681-33688, 33692-33697, 33782, 33783
Atrial and Ventricular 33647
Atrium 33641
Septal Reduction Therapy 93583
Sinus of Valsalva 33702-33722
Sinus Venosus 33645
Tetralogy of Fallot 33692-33697
Tricuspid Valve 33465
Ventricle 33548, 33611, 33612
Obstruction 33619
Ventricular Tunnel 33722
Wound 33300-33305
Hepatic Duct
with Intestines 47765, 47802
Hernia
Epigastric
Incarcerated 49572
Reducible 49570
Femoral
Initial
Incarcerated 49553
Reducible 49550
Recurrent
Incarcerated 49557
Reducible 49555
Incisional
Initial
Reducible 49560
Incarcerated or Strangulated 49561
Recurrent
Reducible 49565
Incarcerated or Strangulated 49566
Inguinal 49491-49525
Intestinal 44025-44050
Lumbar 49540
Lung 32800
Orchiopexy 54640
Paraesophageal Hiatal 43332-43337
Sliding 49525
Spigelian 49590
Incarcerated or Strangulated 49653
Reducible 49652
Umbilical 49580, 49585
Incarcerated 49582, 49587, 49653
Reducible 49580, 49652
Ventral
Incarcerated or Strangulated 49653
Reducible 49652
with Spermatic Cord 54640
Hip
Muscle Transfer 27100-27105, 27111
Osteotomy 27146-27156
Tendon 27097
Humerus 24420-24430
Osteotomy 24400-24410
with Graft 24435
Ileostomy
See Ileostomy
Integumentary System
See Integumentary System, Repair
Interphalangeal Joint
Volar Plate 26548
Intestine
Large
Ulcer 44605
Wound 44605
Intestines
Enterocele
Abdominal Approach 57270
Vaginal Approach 57268
Large
Closure Enterostomy 44620-44626
Diverticula 44605
Obstruction 44615
Intestines, Small
Closure Enterostomy 44620-44626
Diverticula 44602, 44603
Fistula 44640-44661
Hernia 44050
Malrotation 44055
Obstruction 44025-44050
Ulcer 44602, 44603
Wound 44602, 44603
Introitus
Vagina 56800
Iris, Ciliary Body 66680
Jejunum
Free Transfer
with Microvascular Anastomosis 43496
Kidney
Fistula 50520-50526
Horseshoe 50540
Renal Pelvis 50400-50405
Wound 50500
Knee
Cartilage 27403
Instability 27420
Ligament 27405-27409
Collateral 27405
Collateral and Cruciate 27409
Cruciate 27407-27409
Meniscus 27403
Tendon 27380, 27381
Laceration
Diaphragm 39501
Esophagogastric 43502
Mouth 40830, 40831
Palate 42180, 42182
Stomach 43501, 43502
Tongue 41250, 41252
Larynx
Fracture 31584
Reinnervation
Neuromuscular Pedicle 31590
Leg
Lower
Fascia 27656
Tendon 27658-27692
Upper
Muscle 27385, 27386, 27400, 27430
Tendon 27393-27400
Ligament
See Ligament, Repair
Lip 40650-40654
Cleft Lip 40700-40761
Fistula 42260
Liver
Abscess 47300
Cyst 47300
Wound 47350-47361
Lung
Hernia 32800
Pneumolysis 32940
Tear 32110
Mastoidectomy
Complete 69601
Modified Radical 69602
Radical 69603
with Apicectomy 69605
with Tympanoplasty 69604
Maxilla
Osteotomy 21206
Mesentery 44850
Metacarpal
Lengthening 26568
Nonunion 26546
Osteotomy 26565
Metacarpophalangeal Joint
Capsulodesis 26516-26518
Collateral Ligament 26540-26542
Fusion 26516-26518
Metatarsal 28322
Osteotomy 28306-28309
Microsurgery 69990
Mitral Valve 0345T, 33418-33420, 33422, 33425-33427
Mouth
Laceration 40830, 40831
Vestibule of 40830-40845
Musculotendinous Cuff 23410-23412
Nail Bed 11760
Nasal Deformity
Cleft Lip 40700-40761
Nasal Septum 30630
Navicular 25440
Neck Muscles
Scalenus Anticus 21700-21705
Sternocleidomastoid 21720-21725
Nerve 64876
Graft 64885-64902, 64910-64913
Microrepair 69990
Pedicle Transfer 64905, 64907
Suture 64831-64876
Synthetic Conduit 64910
Nose
Adhesions 30560
Fistula 30580-30600, 42260
Rhinophyma 30120
Septum 30540-30545, 30630
Synechia 30560
Vestibular Stenosis 30465
Omphalocele 49600-49611
Osteotomy
Femoral Neck 27161
Radius
and Ulna 25365
Ulna
and Radius 25365
Vertebra
Additional Segment 22216, 22226
Cervical 22210, 22220
Lumbar 22214, 22224
Thoracic 22212, 22222
Oviduct 58752
Create Stoma 58770
Pacemaker
Heart
Electrode 33218-33220
Palate
Laceration 42180-42182
Vomer Flap 42235
Pancreas
Cyst 48500
Pseudocyst 48510
Percutaneous 49405
Paravaginal Defect 57284, 57285, 57423
Pectus Carinatum 21740-21742
with Thoracoscopy 21743
Pectus Excavatum 21740-21742
with Thoracoscopy 21743
Pelvic Floor
Prosthetic Insertion 57267
Pelvis
Osteotomy 27158
Tendon 27098

Index

Penis
- Corporeal Tear(s) 54437
- Fistulization 54435
- Injury 54440
- Priapism 54420-54435
- Shunt 54420-54430

Perineum 56810
Periorbital Region
- Osteotomy 21260-21263

Phalanx
- Finger
  - Lengthening 26568
  - Osteotomy 26567
- Nonunion 26546
- Toe
  - Osteotomy 28310-28312

Pharynx
- with Esophagus 42953

Pleura 32215
Prosthesis
- Penis 54408

Pulmonary Artery 33917-33920, 33925, 33926
- Reimplantation 33788

Pulmonary Valve 33470, 33471, 33474
Pulmonary Venous Return 33724
Pulmonary Venous Stenosis 33726
Quadriceps
- *See* Quadriceps Repair

Radius
- Epiphyseal 25450-25455
- Malunion or Nonunion 25400, 25415, 25415, 25420
- Osteotomy 25350-25355, 25370-25375
- with Graft 25405, 25420-25426

Rectocele
- *See* Rectocele, Repair

Rectovaginal Fistula 57308
Rectum
- Fistula 45800-45825
- Injury 45562, 45563
- Prolapse 45505-45541, 45900
- Rectocele 45560
- Stenosis 45500
- with Sigmoid Excision 45550

Retinal Detachment with Diathermy
- *See* Diathermy, Retinal Detachment, Repair

Rotator Cuff
- *See* Rotator Cuff, Repair

Salivary Duct 42500-42505
- Fistula 42600

Scapula
- Fixation 23400
- Scapulopexy 23400

Sclera
- *See* Sclera, Repair

Scrotum 55175-55180
Septal Defect 33782, 33783, 33813, 33814
Shoulder
- Capsule 23450-23466
- Cuff 23410-23412
- Ligament Release 23415
- Muscle Transfer 23395-23397
- Musculotendinous Rotator Cuff . . 23415-23420
- Tendon 23410-23412, 23430-23440
- Tenomyotomy 23405, 23406

Sinus
- Ethmoid
  - Cerebrospinal Fluid Leak 31290
- Sphenoid
  - Cerebrospinal Fluid Leak 31291

Sinus of Valsalva 33702-33722
Skin
- Wound
  - Complex 13100-13160
  - Intermediate 12031-12057
  - Simple 12020, 12021

Skull
- Cerebrospinal Fluid Leak 62100
- Encephalocele 62120

Spica Cast 29720
Spinal Cord 63700
- Cerebrospinal Fluid Leak 63707-63709
- Meningocele 63700-63702
- Myelomeningocele 63704-63706

Spinal Meningocele
- *See* Meningocele Repair

Spine
- Lumbar Vertebra 22514, 22515
- Osteotomy 22210-22226
- Thoracic Vertebra 22513, 22515

Spleen 38115
Stomach
- Esophagogastrostomy 43320
- Fistula 43880
- Fundoplasty 43325, 43327, 43328
- Laceration 43501, 43502
- Stoma 43870
- Ulcer 43501

Talus
- Osteotomy 28302

Tarsal 28320
- Osteotomy 28304, 28305

Testis
- Injury 54670
- Suspension 54620-54640
- Torsion 54600

Throat
- Pharyngoesophageal 42953
- Wound 42900

Thumb
- Muscle 26508
- Tendon 26510

Tibia 27720-27725
- Epiphysis 27477-27485, 27730-27742
- Osteotomy 27455-27457, 27705, 27709-27712
- Pseudoarthrosis 27727

Toe
- Bunion 28292, 28295-28299
- Muscle 28240
- Tendon 28240
- Webbing 28280, 28345

Toes
- Macrodactylia 26590
- Polydactylous 26587

Tongue 41250-41252
- Laceration 41250-41252
- Suture 41510

Trachea
- Fistula 31755
  - with Plastic Repair 31825
  - without Plastic Repair 31820
- Stenosis 31780, 31781
- Stoma 31613, 31614
  - Scar 31830
  - with Plastic Repair 31825
  - without Plastic Repair 31820
- Wound
  - Cervical 31800
  - Intrathoracic 31805

Tricuspid Valve 33463-33465
Truncus Arteriosus
- Rastelli Type 33786

Tunica Vaginalis
- Hydrocele 55060

Tympanic Membrane 69450, 69610
Ulna
- Epiphyseal 25450-25455
- Malunion or Nonunion 25400, 25415, 25415, 25420
- Osteotomy 25360, 25370-25375, 25425, 25426
- with Graft 25405, 25420

Umbilicus
- Omphalocele 49600-49611

Ureter
- Anastomosis 50740-50825
- Continent Diversion 50825
- Deligation 50940
- Fistula 50920-50930
- Lysis Adhesions 50715-50725
- Suture 50900
- Urinary Undiversion 50830

Ureterocele 51535
Urethra
- Artificial Sphincter 53449
- Diverticulum 53240, 53400-53405
- Fistula 45820-45825, 53400-53405, 53520
- Stoma 53520
- Stricture 53400-53405
- Urethrocele 57230
- with Replantation of Penis 54438
- Wound 53502-53515

Urethral Sphincter 57220
Urinary Incontinence 53431-53440, 57284, 57285, 57423
Uterus
- Fistula 51920-51925
- Rupture 58520, 59350
- Suspension 58400-58410

Vagina
- Anterior
  - *See* Colporrhaphy, Anterior
- Cystocele 57240, 57260, 57284, 57285, 57423
- Enterocele 57265
- Fistula 46715, 46716, 51900
  - Rectovaginal 57300-57307
  - Transvesical and Vaginal Approach . . . 57330
  - Urethrovaginal 57310, 57311
  - Vesicovaginal 57320-57330
- Hysterectomy 58267, 58293
- Incontinence 57284, 57285, 57288, 57423
- Pereyra Procedure 57289
- Postpartum 59300
- Prolapse 57282, 57284
- Rectocele 57250-57260
- Suspension 57280-57284
  - Laparoscopic 57423, 57425
- Wound 57200-57210

Vaginal Wall Prolapse
- *See* Colporrhaphy

Vas Deferens
- Suture 55400

Vein
- Angioplasty 37248, 37249
- Femoral 34501
- Graft 34520
- Pulmonary 33730
- Transposition 34510

Vulva
- Postpartum 59300

Wound
- Complex 13100-13160
- Intermediate 12031-12057
- Simple 12001-12021

Wound Dehiscence
- Complex 13160
- Simple 12020, 12021

Wrist 25260-25263, 25270, 25447
Bone 25440
Carpal Bone 25431
Cartilage 25107
Removal
Implant 25449
Secondary 25265, 25272-25274
Tendon 25280-25316
Tendon Sheath 25275
Total Replacement 25446

Repeat Surgeries
See Reoperation

Replacement
Adjustable Gastric Band 43773
Aortic Valve 33361-33365, 33367-33369, 33405, 33406, 33410-33413
Arthroplasties, Hip
See Arthroplasty, Hip
Artificial Heart
Intracorporeal 33928
Baroreflex Activation Device 0266T-0268T
Cardiac Devices, Implanted
See Cardiac Assist Devices
Catheter
See Catheter, Replacement
Cecostomy Tube 49450
Cerebrospinal Fluid Shunt 62160, 62194, 62225-62230
Colonic Tube 49450
Contact Lens
See Contact Lens Services
Duodenostomy Tube 49451
Elbow
Total 24363
Revision 24370, 24371
Electrode
Chest Wall
Respiratory Sensor 0467T
Heart 33210, 33211, 33216, 33217
Stomach 43647, 43881
Eye
Drug Delivery System 67121
Gastro-Jejunostomy Tube 49452
Gastrostomy Tube 43762, 43763, 49450
Hearing Aid
Bone Conduction 69710
Hip 27130-27132
Revision 27134-27138
Implant
Bone
for External Speech Processor/Cochlear Stimulator 69717, 69718
Intervertebral Disc
Cervical Interspace 0098T, 22861
Lumbar Interspace 0165T, 22862
Ischemia Monitoring System 0525T-0527T
Jejunostomy Tube 49451
Joint
See Prosthesis, Joint
Knee
Arthroplasty
Intraoperative Use, Kinetic Balance Sensor 0396T
Partial 27446
Total 27447
Mitral Valve 33430
Nephrostomy Tube
See Nephrostomy, Change Catheter
Nerve 64726
Neurostimulator
Pulse Generator/Receiver
Intracranial 61885
Peripheral Nerve 64590
Spinal 63685
Ossicles
with Prosthesis 69633, 69637
Ossicular Replacement
See TORP (Total Ossicular Replacement Prosthesis)
Pacemaker
See Cardiac Assist Devices
Implantable Defibrillator
See Cardiac Assist Devices
Penile
Prosthesis 54410, 54411, 54416, 54417
Prosthesis
Skull 62143
Urethral Sphincter 53448
Pulmonary Valve 33475
Pulse Generator
See Pulse Generator
Receiver
Brain 61885
Peripheral Nerve 64590
Spinal Cord 63685
Shoulder 23472
Revision 23473, 23474
Skin
Skin Substitute Graft 15271-15278
Skull Plate 62143
Spinal Cord
Reservoir 62360
Stent
Nephroureteral 50387
Ureteral 50382-50386
Strut
External Fixation System 20697
Subcutaneous Port
for Gastric Restrictive Procedure 43888
Tissue Expanders
Skin 11970
Total Replacement
See Hip, Total Replacement
Total Replacement Heart System
Intracorporeal 33928
Tricuspid Valve 33465
Ureter
with Intestines 50840
Valve
Aortic 33405, 33406, 33410-33413
Mitral 33430
Pulmonary 33413, 33475
Tricuspid Valve 33465
Venous Access Device 36582, 36583, 36585
Catheter 36578
Venous Catheter
Central 36580, 36581, 36584
Ventricular Assist Device
Pump 33981-33983

Replantation
Arm
Lower 20805
Upper 20802
Digit 20816-20822
Foot 20838
Forearm 20805
Hand 20808
Penis 54438
Thumb 20824-20827

Report Preparation
Arthrocentesis
Intermediate Joint 20605, 20606
Major Joint 20610, 20611
Small Joint 20600, 20604
Extended, Medical 99080
Performance Measures
Bone Scintigraphy Study 3570F
Esophageal Biopsy 3126F
Carotid Image Study 3100F
Oncology Treatment Summary 5020F
Pathology 0550F, 0551F
Prenatal 0500F, 0501F
Psychiatric 90889

Repositioning
Baroreflex Activation Device 0266T-0271T
Central Venous Catheter 36597
Electrode
Cardiac Contractility Modulation 0415T
Heart 33215, 33226
Epidural Catheter 62350
Filter
Vena Cava 37192
Gastrostomy Tube 43761
Heart
Defibrillator
Leads 33215, 33226
Intraocular Lens Prosthesis 66825
Intrathecal Catheter 62350
Muscle
Vestibule of Mouth 40845
Orbital 21267, 21268
Renal Vessels 50100
Tricuspid Valve 33468
Ureter 50715
Uveal Tissue 65285
Ventricular Assist Device 33993

Reproductive Tissue
Ovarian
Cryopreservation 89240
Storage 89344
Thawing 89354
Testicular
Cryopreservation 89335
Sperm Identification 89264
Storage 89344
Thawing 89354

Reprogramming
Cardiac Pacing Device
Implantable Defibrillator 33270, 93642
Cochlear Implant 92602, 92604
Implanted Drug Infusion Pump 62368-62370
Implanted Neurostimulator Pulse Generator System 95971, 95982
Shunt
Cerebrospinal 62252

Reptilase Test 85635

Reptilase Time
See Thrombin Time

Resection
Anatomic
Lung 32668
Aortic Valve
Stenosis 33415
Bladder Diverticulum 52305
Bladder Neck
Transurethral 52500
Brain Lobe
See Lobectomy, Brain

Index

Chest
Diagnostic Wedge 32507, 32668
Therapeutic Wedge 32505, 32506, 32666, 32667
Chest Wall 19260-19272
Clavicle
Tumor 23200
Cricotracheal 31592
Cyst
Mediastinal 39200
Pericardial 33050
Diaphragm 39560, 39561
Endaural
See Ear, Inner Ear
Esophagus
Mucosal 43211
Gastrointestinal
Mucosal 43254
Humeral Head 23195
Intestines, Small
Laparoscopic 44202, 44203
Lip 40530
Lung 32503, 32504
Anatomic 32507, 32668
Bullae 32141, 32655
Emphysematous 32491, 32672
Mouth
with Tongue Excision 41153
Myocardium
Aneurysm 33542
Septal Defect 33545
Nasal Septum Submucous
See Nasal Septum, Submucous Resection
Nose
Septum 30520
Ovary, Wedge
See Ovary, Wedge Resection
Palate 42120
Pericardium
Cyst 33050
Sac 32659
Tumor 33050
Phalangeal Head
Toe 28153
Prostate Transurethral
See Prostatectomy, Transurethral
Radical
Tumor
Soft Tissue
Abdominal Wall 22904, 22905
Ankle 27615, 27616
Arm, Lower 25077, 25078
Arm, Upper 24077, 24079
Back 21935, 21936
Elbow 24077
Face 21015, 21016
Femur 27329, 27364
Fibula 27646
Finger 26117, 26118
Foot 28046, 28047
Hand 26117, 26118
Hip 27049, 27059
Knee 27329, 27364
Leg, Lower 27615, 27616
Leg, Upper 27329, 27364
Neck 21557, 21558
Pelvis 27049, 27059
Scalp 21015, 21016
Shoulder 23077, 23078
Thigh 27329, 27364
Toe 28046, 28047
Wrist 25077, 25078
Synovial Membrane
See Synovectomy
Temporal Bone 69535
Thymus
Thoracoscopic 32673
Trachea
Cricotracheal 31592
Tumor
Bladder 52234, 52235, 52240
Calcaneus 27647
Cardiac 33130
Clavicle 23200
Fallopian Tube 58957, 58958
Femur 27365
Fibula 27646
Finger 26260, 26262
Humerus 23220
Kidney 52355
Knee 27365
Mediastinum 39220
Metatarsal 28173
Ovary 58957, 58958
Pericardium 33050
Peritoneum 58957, 58958
Radius 25170
Scapula 23210
Sternum 21630
Talus 27647
Tarsal 28171
Tibia 27645
Toe 28175
Ulna 25170
Ureter 52355
Urethra 52334-52235, 52240, 52355
Ulna
Arthrodesis
Radioulnar Joint 25830
Ureterocele
Ectopic 52301
Orthotopic 52300
Vena Cava
with Reconstruction 37799

Resonance Spectroscopy, Magnetic
See Magnetic Resonance Spectroscopy

Respiration, Positive-Pressure
See Pressure Breathing, Positive

Respiratory Motion Management Simulation
for Radiation Treatment 77293

Respiratory Pattern Recording
Preventive
Home Apnea Monitoring 94774, 94775
Infant 94772
Sleep Study . . . 94799, 95800, 95801, 95806, 95807
Wheeze Rate 94799

Respiratory Syncytial Virus
Antibody 86756
Antigen Detection
Direct Fluorescence 87280
Direct Optical Observation 87807
Immunoassay 87420
Nucleic Acid 87631-87634

Respiratory Syncytial Virus Immune Globulin
See Immune Globulins
Antigen Detection
See Immune Globulins, Respiratory Syncytial Virus

Response, Auditory Evoked
See Auditory Evoked Potentials

Rest Home Visit
See Domiciliary Services

Resuscitation
Cardiac
See Cardiac Massage
Cardiopulmonary 92950
Newborn 99465

Reticulocyte
Count 85044-85046

Retina
Diagnostic Imaging
Computerized Scanning 92134
Electroretinography 0509T, 92273, 92274
Fluorescein Angiography 92235, 92242
Ophthalmoscopy 92225, 92226
Remote 92227, 92228
Incision
Encircling Material 67115
Intra-Ocular Retinal Electrode Array
Device Evaluation 0472T, 0473T
Initial Programming 0472T
Interrogation 0472T, 0473T
Lesion
Destruction
Extensive 67227, 67228
Localized 67208-67218
Macular/Fundus Exam, Dilated 2019F-2021F
Findings Communicated for Diabetes Management 5010F
Monitoring
Time Series Images
Computer Aided Animation, Analysis 0380T
Prophylaxis
Retinal Detachment 67141, 67145
Prosthesis 0100T
Release
Encircling Material 67115
Removal
Implanted Material 67120
Repair
Detachment 67113
by Scleral Buckling 67107, 67108, 67113
Cryotherapy . . . 67101, 67107, 67108, 67113
Encircling 67107
Imbrication 67107
Injection of Air 67110
Photocoagulation 67105, 67107, 67108
Scleral Dissection 67107
Tamponade 67108, 67113
with Drainage of Subretinal Fluid . . . 67101, 67105, 67107, 67108, 67113
with Removal of Lens 67113
with Vitrectomy 67108, 67113
Prophylaxis
Detachment 67141-67145
Retinopathy
Destruction
Cryotherapy, Diathermy 67227
Detection 92225-92228
Macular Degeneration
Dilated Macular Exam 2019F
Treatment
Cryotherapy 67229
Photocoagulation 67228, 67229
Preterm Infant 67229
Time Series Images
Computer Aided Animation, Analysis . . . 0380T

Retinacular
Knee
Release 27425

Retinopathy
Detection....................... 92225-92228
Destruction
  Cryotherapy, Diathermy.............. 67227
Treatment
  Cryotherapy....................... 67229
  Photocoagulation............. 67228, 67229
  Preterm Infant..................... 67229
Macular Degeneration
  Dilated Macular Exam............... 2019F

Retraction, Clot
See Clot Retraction

Retrieval
Cranial Bone Graft..................... 62148
Filter
  Vena Cava......................... 37193
Foreign Body
  Intracranial........................ 62163
  Intravascular...................... 37197
Oocyte................................ 58970
Suture
  from Iris.......................... 66682

Retrocaval Ureter
Ureterolysis........................... 50725

Retrograde Cholangiopancreatographies, Endoscopic
See Cholangiopancreatography

Retrograde Cystourethrogram
See Urethrocystography, Retrograde

Retrograde Pyelogram
See Urography, Retrograde

Retroperitoneal Area
Abscess
  Incision and Drainage
    Open........................... 49060
    Percutaneous.................... 49406
Biopsy................................ 49010
Cyst
  Destruction/Excision.......... 49203-49205
Endometriomas
  Destruction/Excision.......... 49203-49205
Exploration............................ 49010
Needle Biopsy
  Mass.............................. 49180
Tumor
  Destruction/Excision.......... 49203-49205

Retroperitoneal Fibrosis
Ureterolysis........................... 50715

Retropubic Prostatectomies
See Prostatectomy, Retropubic

Revascularization
Artery
  Coronary.. 92937, 92938, 92941, 92943, 92944
  Femoral/Popliteal....... 0505T, 37224-37227
  Iliac......................... 37220-37223
  Tibial/Peroneal............... 37228-37235
Coronary Artery Bypass Graft...... 92937, 92938, 92941, 92943, 92944
Distal Revascularization and Interval Ligation (DRIL).............................. 36838
Distal Upper Extremity
  with Interval Ligation................ 36838
Interval Ligation
  Distal Revascularization and Interval Ligation (DRIL)........................... 36838
Penis................................. 37788
Transmyocardial................. 33140, 33141

Reversal, Vasectomy
See Vasovasorrhaphy

Reverse T3
See Triiodothyronine, Reverse

Reverse Triiodothyronine
See Triiodothyronine, Reverse

Revision
See Reconstruction
Abdomen
  Intraperitoneal Catheter............. 49325
Adjustable Gastric Restrictive Device...... 43771
Aorta................................. 33404
Baroreflex Activation Device....... 0269T-0271T
Blepharoplasty................. 15820-15823
Bronchial Stent........................ 31638
Bronchus.............................. 32501
Bypass Graft
  Vein Patch......................... 35685
Cervicoplasty.......................... 15819
Colostomy
  See Colostomy, Revision
Cornea
  Prosthesis......................... 65770
  Reshaping
    Epikeratoplasty.................. 65767
    Keratomileusis.................. 65760
    Keratophakia.................... 65765
Ear, Middle............................ 69662
Electrode
  Chest Wall
    Respiratory Sensor............... 0467T
External Fixation System................ 20693
Eye
  Aqueous Shunt.............. 66184, 66185
Gastric Restrictive Procedure
  Other than Adjustable Gastric Restrictive Device.............................. 43848
Gastrostomy Tube...................... 44373
Hip Replacement
  See Replacement, Hip, Revision
Hymenal Ring.......................... 56700
Ileostomy
  See Ileostomy, Revision
Infusion Pump
  Intra-arterial...................... 36261
  Intravenous..... 36576-36578, 36582, 36583
Iris
  Iridoplasty........................ 66762
  Iridotomy......................... 66761
Jejunostomy Tube...................... 44373
Lower Extremity Arterial Bypass.... 35879-35881
Rhytidectomy................... 15824-15829
Shoulder
  See Arthroplasty, Shoulder Joint
Shunt
  Intrahepatic Portosystemic........... 37183
Sling................................. 53442
Stapedectomy
  See Stapedectomy, Revision
Stomach
  for Obesity........................ 43848
Subcutaneous Port
  for Gastric Restrictive Procedure....... 43886
Tracheostomy
  Scar.............................. 31830
Urinary-Cutaneous Anastomosis.... 50727, 50728
Vagina
  Prosthetic Graft........ 57295, 57296, 57426
  Sling
    Stress Incontinence............... 57287
Venous Access Device............ 36576-36578, 36582, 36583, 36585
Ventricle
  Ventriculomyectomy................ 33416
  Ventriculomyotomy................. 33416

Rh (D)
See Blood Typing, Serologic

Rh Immune Globulin
See Immune Globulins, Rho(D)

Rheumatoid Factor........... 86430, 86431

Rhinectomy
Partial................................ 30150
Total................................. 30160

Rhinomanometry.................. 92512

Rhinopharynx
See Nasopharynx

Rhinophyma
Repair................................ 30120

Rhinoplasty
Cleft Lip/Cleft Palate............. 30460-30462
Primary....................... 30400-30420
Secondary..................... 30430-30450

Rhinoscopy
See Endoscopy, Nose

Rhinotomy
Lateral........................ 30118, 30320

Rhizotomy................... 63185-63190

Rho Variant Du.................... 86905

Rhomboid Flap.............. 14000-14302

Rhytidectomy................ 15824-15829

Rhytidoplasties
See Face Lift

Rib
Excision................. 21600-21616, 32900
Fracture
  External Fixation................... 21899
  Open Treatment
    with Internal Fixation........ 21811-21813
Graft
  to Face............................ 21230
Resection............... 19260-19272, 32900
X ray......................... 71100-71111

Riboflavin......................... 84252

Richardson Operation Hysterectomy
See Hysterectomy, Abdominal, Total

Richardson Procedure............. 53460

Rickettsia
Antibody.............................. 86757

Ridell Operation
See Sinusotomy, Frontal Sinus

Ridge, Alveolar
See Alveolar Ridge

Right Atrioventricular Valve
See Tricuspid Valve

Right Heart Cardiac Catheterization
See Cardiac Catheterization, Right Heart

Ripstein Operation.......... 45540, 45541
See Proctopexy

Index

Risk Factor Reduction Intervention
Group . . . 99411, 99412
  Diabetes Prevention . . . 0403T
Individual . . . 99401-99404
  Diabetes Prevention . . . 0488T

Risisser Jacket
Application . . . 29010-29015
Removal . . . 29710

Rocky Mountain Spotted Fever . . . 86000

Roentgen Rays
See X ray

Roentgenographic
See X ray

Roentgenography
See X ray

Ropes Test . . . 83872

Ross Information Processing Assessment . . . 96125

Ross Procedure . . . 33413

Rotation Flap
See Skin, Adjacent Tissue Transfer

Rotator Cuff
Repair . . . 23410-23420

Rotavirus
Antibody . . . 86759
Antigen Detection
  Immunoassay . . . 87425

Rotavirus Vaccine
3 Dose . . . 90680
2 Dose . . . 90681

Round Window
Repair Fistula . . . 69667

Round Window Fistula
Repair . . . 69667

Roux-En-Y Procedure . . . 43621, 43633, 43634, 43644, 43846, 47740, 47741, 47780-47785, 48540

RPR
See Syphilis Test

RSV
See Immune Globulins; Respiratory Syncytial Virus

RT3
See Triiodothyronine, Reverse

Rubbing Alcohol
See Isopropyl Alcohol

Rubella
Antibody . . . 86762
Vaccine . . . 90707, 90710

Rubella HI Test
See Hemagglutination Inhibition Test

Rubella/Mumps
See Vaccines and Toxoids

Rubeola
Antibody . . . 86765
Antigen Detection
  Immunofluorescence . . . 87283

Rubeolla
See Rubeola

Russell Viper Venom Time . . . 85612, 85613

S

Sac, Endolymphatic
See Endolymphatic Sac

Saccomanno Technique . . . 88108

Sacral Nerve
Implantation
  Electrode Array . . . 64561, 64581

Sacral, Pre-
Arthrodesis
  See Arthrodesis, Vertebra, Lumbar

Sacroiliac Joint
Arthrodesis
  Open . . . 27280
  Percutaneous . . . 27279
Arthrotomy . . . 27050
Biopsy . . . 27050
Dislocation
  Open Treatment . . . 27218
Fusion . . . 27280
Injection for Arthrography . . . 27096
X ray . . . 72200-72202

Sacrum
Augmentation
  Percutaneous . . . 0200T, 0201T
Bone Biopsy . . . 0200T, 0201T
Sacroplasty
  Percutaneous . . . 0200T, 0201T
Tumor
  Excision . . . 49215
X ray . . . 72220

Sahli Test
See Gastroenterology, Diagnostic, Stomach

Salicylate
Assay . . . 80329-80331

Saline-Solution Abortion
See Abortion, Induced, by Saline

Salivary Duct
Catheterization . . . 42660
Dilation . . . 42650-42660
Diversion . . . 42507-42510
Ligation . . . 42665, 42510
Repair . . . 42500-42505
  Fistula . . . 42600

Salivary Gland Virus
See Cytomegalovirus

Salivary Gland
Abscess
  Incision and Drainage
    Parotid . . . 42300-42305
    Sublingual . . . 42310
    Submaxillary . . . 42310-42320
Biopsy . . . 42405
Calculi (Stone)
  Excision . . . 42330-42340
Chemodenervation . . . 64611
Cyst
  Marsupialization . . . 42409
  Excision . . . 42408
Duct
  See Salivary Duct
Excision
  Parotid Gland . . . 42410, 42415, 42420, 42425, 42426
  Sublingual Gland . . . 42450
  Submandibular Gland . . . 42440, 42509
Injection
  X ray . . . 42550
Needle Biopsy . . . 42400
Nuclear Medicine
  Function Study . . . 78232
  Imaging . . . 78230, 78231
Tumor
  Parotid
    Excision . . . 42410, 42415, 42420, 42425, 42426
Unlisted Services and Procedures . . . 42699
X ray . . . 70380-70390
  with Contrast . . . 70390

Salmonella
Antibody . . . 86768

Salpingectomy
Complete or Partial . . . 58700
  Laparoscopic . . . 58661
for Ectopic Pregnancy . . . 59120
  Laparoscopic . . . 59151
with Vaginal Hysterectomy . . . 58262, 58263, 58291, 58292
  Laparoscopic . . . 58552, 58554
with Oophorectomy . . . 58943

Salpingo-Oophorectomy . . . 58720
Laparoscopic . . . 58571, 58573, 58575
Resection Ovarian Malignancy . . . 58950-58958
Resection Peritoneal Malignancy . . . 58950-58958
Resection Tubal Malignancy . . . 58950-58958

Salpingohysterostomy
See Implantation, Tubouterine

Salpingolysis . . . 58740
Laparoscopic . . . 58660

Salpingoneostomy . . . 58673, 58770

Salpingoplasty
See Fallopian Tube, Repair

Salpingostomy . . . 58673, 58770
Laparoscopic . . . 58673

Salter Osteotomy of the Pelvis
See Osteotomy, Pelvis

Sampling
See also Biopsy; Brush Biopsy; Needle Biopsy
Blood
  Arterial . . . 36620
  Fetal Scalp . . . 59030
  Ocular . . . 0198T
  Organ . . . 36500
  Plasma . . . 78110, 78111
  Red Cell . . . 78120, 78121
  Venous . . . 75893
Chorionic Villus . . . 59015, 76945
Endometrium . . . 58100, 58558
Lymph Node
  Endobronchial Ultrasound (EBUS) Guided
    Hilar . . . 31652, 31653
    Mediastinal . . . 31652, 31653
  Para-Aortic . . . 57109, 57112, 57531, 58200, 58210, 58548
  Pelvic . . . 58200
  Periaortic . . . 38572, 38573
  Retroperitoneal . . . 38570
Stereotactic Template Guided . . . 55706

Sang-Park Procedure . . . 33735-33737

Sao Paulo Typhus
See Rocky Mountain Spotted Fever

Saucerization
Calcaneus 28120
Clavicle 23180
Femur 27070, 27360
Fibula 27360, 27641
Hip 27070
Humerus 23184, 24140
Ileum 27070
Metacarpal 26230
Metatarsal 28122
Olecranon Process 24147
Phalanges
  Finger 26235, 26236
  Toe 28124
Pubis 27070
Radius 24145, 25151
Scapula 23182
Symphysis Pubis 27070, 27071
Talus 28120
Tarsal 28122
Tibia 27360, 27640
Ulna 25150

Saundby Test
See Blood, Feces

Scabies
See Tissue, Examination for Ectoparasites

Scalenotomy
See Muscle Division, Scalenus Anticus

Scalenus Anticus
Division 21700-21705

Scaling
See Exfoliation

Scalp
Lesion
  Destruction 17270-17274, 17276
  Excision
    Benign 11420-11424, 11426
    Malignant 11620-11624, 11626
  Shaving 11305-11308
Skin Graft
  Dermal Autograft 15135, 15136
  Epidermal Autograft 15115, 15116
  Flap 15610
  Pedicle Formation 15572
  Recipient Site Preparation .. 15004, 15005
  Skin Substitute 15275-15278
  Split-Thickness 15120, 15121
  Tissue-cultured Autograft .. 15155-15157
Tissue Transfer
  Adjacent 14020, 14021
Tumor
  Excision 21011-21014
  Radical Resection 21015, 21016
Venipuncture
  Child 36405
Wound
  Repair 12001, 12002, 12004-12007, 12031, 12032, 12034-12037, 13120-13122

Scalp Blood Sampling
Fetal 59030

Scan
See Nuclear Medicine, Diagnostic
Abdomen
  See Abdomen, CT Scan
CT
  See CT Scan
MRI
  See Magnetic Resonance Imaging (MRI)
PET
  See Positron Emission Tomography (PET)
Radionuclide
  See Emission Computerized Tomography
SPECT
  See SPECT

Scanning, Radioisotope
See Nuclear Medicine, Diagnostic

Scanogram 77073

Scaphoid
Fracture
  Closed Treatment 25622
  Open Treatment 25628
  with Manipulation 25624
Nonunion
  Repair 25440
Replacement 25443

Scapula Bone
Craterization 23182
Cyst
  Excision 23140
    with Allograft 23146
    with Autograft 23145
Diaphysectomy 23182
Excision
  Partial 23172, 23182, 23190
Fracture
  Closed Treatment
    with Manipulation 23575
    without Manipulation 23570
  Open Treatment 23585
Ostectomy 23190
Repair
  Fixation 23400
  Scapulopexy 23400
Saucerization 23182
Sequestrectomy 23172
Tumor
  Excision 23140, 23210
    with Allograft 23146
    with Autograft 23145
  Radical Resection 23210
X ray 73010

Scapulopexy 23400

Scarification
Pleural 32215

Scarification of Pleura
See Pleurodesis

Schanz Operation
See Femur, Osteotomy

Schauta Operation
See Hysterectomy, Vaginal, Radical

Schede Procedure 32905, 32906

Scheie Procedure 66155

Schlatter Operation Total Gastrectomy 43620-43622

Schlicter Test 87197
See Bactericidal Titer, Serum

Schuchard Procedure
Osteotomy
  Maxilla 21206

Schwannoma, Acoustic
See Brain, Tumor, Excision

Sciatic Nerve
Administration, Anesthetic
  Infusion 64446
  Injection 64445, 64446
Decompression 64712
Neuroma
  Excision 64786
Neuroplasty 64712
Release 64712
Repair/Suture 64858

Scintigraphy
See Nuclear Medicine, Diagnostic
Computed Tomographic
  See Emission Computerized Tomography

Scissoring
Skin Tags 11200, 11201

Sclera
Aqueous Drainage Device
  to Extraocular Reservoir 66179, 66180
  without Extraocular Reservoir ... 0376T, 66183
Excision
  Sclerectomy with Punch or Scissors 66160
Fistulization
  for Glaucoma
    Through Ciliary Body 66999
  Sclerectomy with Punch or Scissors with Iridectomy 66160
  Thermocauterization with Iridectomy ... 66155
  Trabeculectomy ab Externo 66170, 66172
  Trephination with Iridectomy 66150
Lesion
  Excision 66130
Repair
  Reinforcement
    with Graft 67255
    without Graft 67250
  Staphyloma
    with Graft 66225
  with Glue 65286
  Wound
    Operative 66250
    Tissue Glue 65286

Scleral Buckling Operation
See Retina, Repair, Detachment

Scleral Ectasia
See Staphyloma, Sclera

Sclerectomy 66160

Sclerotherapy
Esophageal Varices 43204, 43243
Fluid Collection 49185
Gastric Varices 43243
Hemorrhoids 46500
Perirectal 45520
Venous 36465, 36466, 36468, 36470, 36471

Sclerotomy
See Incision, Sclera

Screening, Drug
See Drug Screen
Alcohol and/or Substance Abuse 99408, 99409

Scribner Cannulization 36810

Scrotal Varices
See Varicocele

Scrotoplasty 55175-55180

Index

Scrotum
Abscess
Incision and Drainage 54700, 55100
Exploration 55110
Hematoma
Incision and Drainage 54700
Removal
Foreign Body 55120
Repair 55175-55180
Resection 55150
Ultrasound 76870
Unlisted Services and Procedures 55899

Scrub Typhus 86000

Second Look Surgery
See Reoperation

Section
See Decompression
Cesarean
See Cesarean Delivery
Cranial Nerve 61460
Spinal Access 63191
Dentate Ligament 63180-63182
Gasserian Ganglion
Sensory Root 61450
Nerve Root 63185-63190
Spinal Accessory Nerve 63191
Spinal Cord Tract 63194-63199
Vestibular Nerve
Transcranial Approach 69950
Translabyrinthine Approach 69915

Sedation
Moderate 99151-99153, 99155-99157
with Independent Observation .. 99151-99153

Seddon-Brookes Procedure 24320

Sedimentation Rate
Blood Cell
Automated 85652
Manual 85651

Segmentectomy
Breast 19301, 19302
Lung 32484
Thoracoscopic 32669

Seidlitz Powder Test
See X ray, with Contrast

Selective Catheterization
Arterial
First Order
Abdominal 36245
Brachiocephalic Branch 36215
Lower Extremity 36245
Pelvic 36245
Renal 36251, 36252
Thoracic Branch 36215
Second Order
Abdominal 36246
Brachiocephalic Branch 36216
Lower Extremity 36246
Pelvic 36246
Thoracic Branch 36216
Superselective
Abdominal 36247, 36248
Brachiocephalic Branch 36217, 36218
Lower Extremity 36247, 36248
Pelvic 36247, 36248
Renal 36253, 36254
Thoracic Branch 36217, 36218
Pulmonary 36014, 36015
Venous
First Order Branch 36011
Second Order Branch 36012
with Angiography
Carotid Arch 36223, 36224
Carotid Artery 36222-36224, 36227, 36228
Cervicocerebral Arch 36222-36226
Innominate Artery 36222, 36223, 36225
Subclavian Artery 36225
Vertebral Vessels 36225, 36226, 36228

Selective Cellular Enhancement Technique 88112

Selenium 84255

Self Care
See Physical Medicine/Therapy/Occupational Therapy
Training 97535, 98960-98962, 99509

Sella Turcica
CT Scan 70480-70482
X ray 70240

Semen
See Sperm

Semen Analysis 89300-89322
Sperm Analysis 89331
Antibodies 89325
with Sperm Isolation 89260, 89261

Semenogelase
See Antigen, Prostate Specific

Semilunar
Bone
See Lunate
Ganglion
See Gasserian Ganglion

Seminal Vesicle
Cyst
Excision 55680
Excision 55650
Incision 55600-55605
Mullerian Duct
Excision 55680
Unlisted Services and Procedures 55899
Vesiculography 74440
X ray with Contrast 74440

Seminin
See Antigen, Prostate Specific

Semiquantitative 81005

Sengstaken Tamponade
Esophagus 43460

Senning Procedure 33774-33777
See Repair, Great Arteries; Revision

Senning Type 33774-33777

Sensitivity Study
Antibiotic
Agar 87181
Disc 87184
Enzyme Detection 87185
Macrobroth 87188
MIC 87186
Microtiter 87186
MLC 87187
Mycobacteria 87190
Antiviral Drugs
HIV-1
Tissue Culture 87904

Sensorimotor Exam 92060

Sensory Nerve
Common
Repair/Suture 64834

Sentinel Node
Excision
See Lymph Nodes, Excision
Identification
Injection of Radioactive Tracer 38792
Intraoperative Identification 38900

Separation
Craniofacial
Closed Treatment 21431
Open Treatment 21432-21436

Septal Defect
Ablation 93583
Atrial
Closure 33615, 33647
Repair 33641, 33660
Closure
Atrial 33615, 33647
Percutaneous Transcatheter 93583
Ventricular 33647, 33675-33688, 93581
Obliteration
Aortopulmonary 33813, 33814
Repair
Atrial 33641, 33660
Nikaidoh Procedure 33782, 33783
Ventricular 33782, 33783
Ventricular
Closure 33647, 33675-33688, 93581
Repair 33782, 33783

Septectomy
Atrial 33735-33737
Balloon (Rashkind Type) 92992
Blade Method (Sang-Park) 92993
Closed
See Septostomy, Atrial
Submucous Nasal
See Nasal Septum, Submucous Resection

Septic Abortion
See Abortion, Septic

Septoplasty 30520

Septostomy
Atrial 33735-33737
Balloon (Rashkind Type) 92992
Blade Method (Park) 92993

Septum, Nasal
See Nasal Septum

Sequestrectomy
Carpal 25145
Clavicle 23170
Humeral Head 23174
Humerus 24134
Olecranon Process 24138
Radius 24136, 25145
Scapula 23172
Skull 61501
Ulna 24138, 25145

Serialography
Aorta 75605, 75625, 75630

Serodiagnosis, Syphilis
See Serologic Test for Syphilis

Serologic Test for Syphilis ... 86592, 86593

Seroma
Incision and Drainage
Skin 10140

Serotonin . . . 84260

Serum
Albumin
See Albumin, Serum, Plasma or Whole Blood
Antibody Identification
Pretreatment . . . 86975-86978
CPK
See Creatine Kinase, Total
Serum Immune Globulin . . . 90281-90284

Sesamoid Bone
Finger
Excision . . . 26185
Foot
Excision . . . 28292, 28295-28299
Fracture . . . 28530, 28531
Thumb
Excision . . . 26185
Toe
Excision . . . 28315

Sesamoidectomy
Finger . . . 26185
Foot . . . 28292, 28295-28299
Thumb . . . 26185
Toe . . . 28315

Severing of Blepharorrhaphy
See Tarsorrhaphy, Severing

Sex Change Operation
Female to Male . . . 55980
Male to Female . . . 55970

Sex Chromatin
See Barr Bodies

Sex Chromatin Identification . . . 88130-88140

Sex Hormone Binding Globulin . . . 84270

Sex-Linked Ichthyoses
See Syphilis Test

SGOT . . . 84450

SGPT . . . 84460

Shaving
Skin Lesion . . . 11300-11313

SHBG
See Sex Hormone Binding Globulin

Shelf Procedure
See Osteotomy, Hip

Shiga-like Toxin
Antigen Detection
Immunoassay . . . 87427

Shigella
Detection
Antibody . . . 86771
by Nucleic Acid . . . 87505-87507

Shirodkar Operation
See Repair, Cervix, Cerclage, Abdominal

Shock Wave (Extracorporeal) Therapy
See Extracorporeal Shock Wave Therapy

Shock Wave Lithotripsy . . . 50590

Shop Typhus of Malaya
See Murine Typhus

Short Tandem Repeat (STR) Analysis . . . 81265, 81266, 81402

Shoulder
Abscess
Drainage . . . 23030
Amputation . . . 23900-23921
Anesthesia
See Anesthesia, Shoulder
Arthrocentesis . . . 20610, 20611
Arthrodesis . . . 23800
with Autogenous Graft . . . 23802
Arthrography
Injection
Radiological . . . 23350
Arthroscopy
Diagnostic . . . 29805
Surgical . . . 29806-29828
Biceps Tenodesis . . . 29828
Arthrotomy . . . 23035, 23040, 23044
with Removal Loose or Foreign Body . . . 23107
Biopsy
Deep . . . 23066
Soft Tissue . . . 23065
Blade
See Scapula Bone
Bone
Excision
Acromion . . . 23130
Clavicle . . . 23120-23125
Incision . . . 23035
Tumor
Excision . . . 23140-23146
Bursa
Aspiration . . . 20610, 20611
Drainage . . . 23031
Injection . . . 20610, 20611
Capsular Contracture Release . . . 23020
Cast/Splint
Figure Eight . . . 29049
Long Arm Cast . . . 29065
Long Arm Splint . . . 29105
Removal . . . 29710
Shoulder to Hips . . . 29035
Spica . . . 29055
Velpeau . . . 29058
Clavicle
See Clavicle
Disarticulation . . . 23920, 23921
Dislocation
Closed Treatment
with Manipulation . . . 23650-23655, 23665, 23675
Open Treatment . . . 23660, 23670, 23680
Exploration . . . 23107
Hematoma
Drainage . . . 23030
Joint
See Acromioclavicular Joint; Glenohumeral Joint; Sternoclavicular Joint
Manipulation
Application of Fixation Apparatus . . . 23700
Prophylactic Treatment . . . 23490, 23491
Removal
Calcareous Deposits . . . 23000
Cast . . . 29710
Foreign Body
Intramuscular . . . 23333
Subcutaneous . . . 23330
Subfascial . . . 23333
Foreign or Loose Body . . . 23107
Repair
Capsule . . . 23450-23466
Ligament Release . . . 23415
Muscle Transfer . . . 23395-23397
Rotator Cuff . . . 23410-23420
Seddon-Brookes Procedure . . . 24320
Tendon . . . 23410-23412, 23430-23440
Tenomyotomy . . . 23405, 23406
Replacement . . . 23472
Revision . . . 23473, 23474
Scapula
See Scapula Bone
Strapping . . . 29240
Surgery
Unlisted Services and Procedures . . . 23929
Tumor
Soft Tissue
Excision . . . 23071-23076
Radical Resection . . . 23077, 23078
Unlisted Services and Procedures . . . 23929
X ray . . . 73020-73030
X ray with Contrast . . . 73040
Injection . . . 23350

Shoulder Joint
See Glenohumeral Joint
Arthroplasty
with Implant . . . 23470, 23472-23474
Arthrotomy
with Biopsy . . . 23100, 23101
with Synovectomy . . . 23105, 23106
Dislocation
Open Treatment . . . 23660
with Greater Tuberosity Fracture
Closed Treatment . . . 23665
Open Treatment . . . 23670
with Surgical or Anatomical Neck Fracture
Closed Treatment with Manipulation . . . 23675
Open Treatment . . . 23680
Excision
Torn Cartilage . . . 23101
Exploration . . . 23040-23044
Incision and Drainage . . . 23040-23044
Removal
Foreign Body . . . 23040-23044
X ray . . . 73050

Shunt(s)
Aqueous
to Extraocular Reservoir . . . 66179, 66180
Revision . . . 66184, 66185
without Extraocular Reservoir . . . 0376T, 66183
Arteriovenous
See Arteriovenous Shunt
Brain
Creation . . . 62180-62223
Removal . . . 62256-62258
Replacement . . . 62160, 62194, 62225-62230, 62258
Reprogramming . . . 62252
Cerebrospinal Fluid
See Cerebrospinal Fluid Shunt
Creation
Arteriovenous
Direct . . . 36821
ECMO
See Extracorporeal Membrane Oxygenation (ECMO)
Thomas Shunt . . . 36835
Transposition . . . 36818-36820
with Bypass Graft . . . 35686
with Graft . . . 36825-36830
Cerebrospinal Fluid . . . 62200
Fetal . . . 59076
Great Vessel
Aorta . . . 33321
Pulmonary . . . 33924

Index

Aorta to Pulmonary Artery
Ascending 33755
Descending 33762
Central 33764
Subclavian to Pulmonary Artery 33750
Vena Cava to Pulmonary Artery . . 33766-33768
Intra-Atrial 33735-33737
LeVeen
See LeVeen Shunt
Nonvascular
X ray 75809
Peritoneal
Venous
Injection 49427
Ligation 49428
Removal 49429
X ray 75809
Pulmonary Artery
See Pulmonary Artery, Shunt
Revision
Arteriovenous 36832
Spinal Cord
Creation 63740, 63741
Irrigation 63744
Removal 63746
Replacement 63744
Superior Mesenteric-Caval
See Anastomosis, Caval to Mesenteric
Thomas Shunt 36835
Ureter to Colon 50815
Ventriculocisternal with Valve
See Ventriculocisternostomy

Shuntogram 75809

Sialic Acid 84275

Sialodochoplasty 42500-42505

Sialogram
See Sialography

Sialography 70390

Sickling
Electrophoresis 83020

Siderocytes 85536

Siderophilin
See Transferrin

Sigmoid
See Colon-Sigmoid

Sigmoid Bladder
Creation 50810
Cystectomy 51590

Sigmoidoscopy
Ablation
Lesion 45346
Polyp 45346
Tumor 45346
Band Ligation 45350
Biopsy 45331
Collection
Specimen 45330
Decompression 45337
Diagnostic 45330
Dilation, balloon 45340
Exploration 45330, 45335
Hemorrhage Control 45334
Hemorrhoid Ligation 45350
Injection
Submucosal 45335
Mucosal Resection 45349
Needle Biopsy 45342
Placement
Decompression Tube 45337
Stent 45347
Removal
Foreign Body 45332
Polyp 45333, 45338
Tumor 45333, 45338
Repair
Volvulus 45337
Resection 45349
Ultrasound 45341, 45342

Signal-Averaged Electrocardiography
See Electrocardiography, Signal Averaged

Silica 84285

Silicon Dioxide
See Silica

Silicone
Contouring Injections 11950-11954

Silver Operation
See Keller Procedure

Simple Mastectomies
See Mastectomy

Single Photon Absorptiometry
See Absorptiometry, X-ray (DXA), Bone Density Study, Single Photon

Single Photon Emission Computed Tomography
See SPECT

Sinus, Sphenoid
See Sinus/Sinuses, Sphenoid

Sinus/Sinuses
Carotid
Baroreflex Activation Device
See Baroreflex Activation Device
Cranial
Decompression 61595
Excision of Lesion 61607
Ligation 61598
Resection 61591
Dilation 31295-31297
Endoscopy
Nasal
Diagnostic 31231, 31233, 31235
Biopsy 31237
Debridement 31237
Decompression 31292-31294
Dilation 31295-31297
Exploration 31276
Hemorrhage Control 31238
Polypectomy 31237
Surgical 31237-31241, 31253-31257, 31259, 31267, 31276, 31287, 31288, 31290-31298
Ethmoid
Drug-Eluting Implant
Placement 31237, 31299
Excision 31200-31205
with Nasal/Sinus Endoscopy . . 31254, 31255
Repair of Cerebrospinal Leak 31290
Ethmoidectomy 31254, 31255
Excision
See Excision, Sinus
Frontal
Destruction 31080-31085
Dilation 31296
Exploration 31070-31075
with Nasal/Sinus Endoscopy 31276
Fracture
Open Treatment 21343, 21344
Incision 31070-31087
Injection 20500
Diagnostic 20501
Maxillary
Antrostomy 31256-31267
Caldwell-Luc Operation 21385
Dilation 31295
Excision 31225-31230
Exploration 31020-31032
with Nasal/Sinus Endoscopy 31233
Incision 31020-31032, 31256-31267
Irrigation 31000
Skull Base 61581
Surgery 61581
Multiple
Incision 31090
Paranasal
Incision 31090
Nasal
Endoscopy
Diagnostic 31231, 31233, 31235
Surgical 31237-31241, 31253-31257, 31259, 31267, 31276, 31287, 31288, 31290-31298
Pilonidal
See Cyst, Pilonidal
Pyriform
Resection 42892
Sinus of Valsalva
Repair 33702-33722
Sinus Venosus
Repair 33645
Sphenoid
Biopsy 31050, 31051
Dilation 31295-31298
Exploration 31050, 31051
with Nasal/Sinus Endoscopy . . 31235, 31253
Incision 31050, 31051
with Nasal/Sinus Endoscopy 31257, 31259, 31287, 31288
Irrigation 31002
Repair of Cerebrospinal Leak 31291
Sinusotomy 31050, 31051
Skull Base Surgery 61580, 61581
Unlisted Services and Procedures 31299
X ray 70210-70220

Sinusectomy, Ethmoid
See Sinus/Sinuses, Ethmoidectomy

Sinusoidal Rotational Testing
See Ear, Nose, and Throat

Sinusoscopy
Sinus
Maxillary 31233
Sphenoid 31235

Sinusotomy
Combined 31090
Frontal Sinus
Exploratory 31070-31075
Nonobliterative 31086, 31087
Obliterative 31080-31085
Maxillary 31020-31032
Caldwell-Luc Operation 21385
Multiple
Paranasal 31090
Sphenoid Sinus 31050, 31051

Sirolimus
Drug Assay 80195

SISI Test 92564

Sistrunk Operation
See Cyst, Thyroid Gland, Excision

Six Minute Walk Test 94618

Size Reduction, Breast
See Breast, Reduction

Skeletal Fixation
Ankle Dislocation 27842, 27846
Bennett Fracture 26650
Calcaneal Fracture 28406
Carpometacarpal Fracture
Dislocation 26650, 26676
Femoral Fracture 27235, 27509
Humeral Fracture 24538, 24566, 24582
Interphalangeal Joint Dislocation ... 26776, 28666
Metacarpal Fracture 26608
Metacarpophalangeal Dislocation 26706
Metatarsal Fracture 28476
Metatarsophalangeal Dislocation 28636
Pelvic Bone Fracture/Dislocation 27216
Phalangeal Fracture 26727, 26756, 28496
Radial Fracture 25525, 25606
Radioulnar Dislocation 25671
Sternal Fracture 21825
Talar Fracture 28436
Talotarsal Joint Dislocation 28576
Tarsal Dislocation 28546
Tarsal Fracture 28456
Tarsometatarsal Joint Dislocation 28606
Tibial Fracture 27756
Ulnar Fracture 25651

Skeletal Traction
Insertion/Removal
Pin/Wire 20650
Acetabulum Fracture 27220
Femoral Fracture 27232, 27240, 27502, 27503, 27517
Hip Socket 27220
Humerus Fracture 23605, 24505, 24535
Phalangeal Fracture 26725
Scapula Fracture 23575
Tibia Fracture 27532, 27752, 27762, 27825

Skene's Gland
Abscess
Incision and Drainage 53060
Destruction 53270
Excision 53270

Skilled Nursing Facilities (SNFs)
See Nursing Facility Services

Skin
Abrasion 15786, 15787
Chemical Peel 15788-15793
Dermabrasion 15780-15783
Abscess
See Abscess, Tissue, Skin/Superficial
Adjacent Tissue Transfer 14000-14350
Allografts
See Allograft, Skin Substitute
Biopsy
Breast 19100, 19101
Chemical Exfoliation 17360
Complete Physical Examination 2029F
Cyst
See Cyst, Skin
Debridement 11000-11006, 11010-11012, 11042-11047
Eczematous 11000, 11001
Infected 11000-11006
Subcutaneous Tissue 11042-11047
Infected 11004-11006
with Open Fracture and/or
Dislocation 11010-11012
Decubitus Ulcer(s)
See Pressure, Ulcer (Decubitus)
Desquamation
See Exfoliation
Destruction
Benign Lesions
One to Fourteen 17110
Fifteen or More 17111
Flat Warts 17111
Lesions 17106-17108
Malignant Lesions 17260-17286
Premalignant Lesions
by Photodynamic Therapy ... 96567, 96573, 96574
Fifteen or More Lesions 17004
First Lesion 17000
Two to Fourteen Lesions 17003
Diagnostic
Advanced Glycation Endproducts (AGE) . 88749
Excision
Debridement 11000-11006, 11010-11012, 11042-11045
Excess Skin 15830-15839, 15847
Hemangioma 11400-11446
Lesion
Benign 11400-11446
Malignant 11600-11646
Expanders
See Tissue, Expander
Fasciocutaneous Flaps 15730, 15731, 15733, 15734, 15736, 15738
Grafts
Free 15050-15157, 15200-15261, 15757
Harvesting
for Tissue Culture 15040
Homografts
See Skin Substitute Graft
Incision and Drainage 10040, 10060, 10061, 10080, 10081, 10120-10140, 10160-10180
See Incision, Skin
Lesion
See Lesion; Tumor
Multi-spectral Analysis 0400T, 0401T
Verrucous
See Warts
Mole
Melanoma Performance Measures
Follow-up Assessment 0015F
History 1050F
Patient Self-Examination Counseling ... 5005F
Muscle Flaps 15731-15738
Myocutaneous Flaps 15731-15738
Nose
Surgical Planing 30120
Paring 11055-11057
Photography
Diagnostic 96904
Removal
Skin Tags 11200, 11201
Revision
Blepharoplasty 15820-15823
Cervicoplasty 15819
Rhytidectomy 15824-15829
Shaving 11300-11313
Tags
Removal 11200, 11201
Tests
See Allergy Tests
Candida 86485
Coccidioidomycosis 86490
Histoplasmosis 86510
Other Antigen 86486
Tuberculosis 86580
Treatments
See Dermatology
Unlisted Services and Procedures 17999
Wound Repair
Complex 13100-13160
Intermediate 12031-12057
Simple 12001-12021

Skin Graft and Flap
Composite Graft 15760-15770
Cross Finger Flap 15574
Delay 15600-15630
Delay of Flap 15600-15630
Derma-Fat-Fascia 15770
Dermal Autograft 15130-15136
Epidermal Autograft 15110-15116
Fascial
Free 15758
Fasciocutaneous 15733, 15734, 15736, 15738
Fillet Flap, Finger or Toe 14350
Formation 15570-15576
Free
Microvascular Anastomosis 15756-15758
Free Skin Graft
Full Thickness 15200-15261
Island Pedicle Flap 15740
Muscle 15733, 15734, 15736, 15738, 15842
Free 15756
Myocutaneous 15731, 15733, 15734, 15736, 15756
Pedicle Flap
Abbe-Estlander Type 40761
for Breast Reconstruction
Double 19369
Single 19367
for Cerebrospinal Fluid Leak 61619
for Eyelid Repair 67961
for Lip Repair 40761
for Vaginal Lengthening 46748
Formation 15570-15576
Island 15740
Neurovascular 15750
Transfer 15650
Vascular 15731
Pinch Graft 15050
Platysmal 15825
Punch Graft 15775, 15776
Punch Graft for Hair Transplant 15775, 15776
Recipient Site Preparation 15002-15005
Skin
Free 15757
Skin Autograft 15150-15157
Skin Substitute Graft 15271-15278
SMAS Flap 15829
Split Graft 15100, 15101, 15120, 15121
Superficial Musculoaponeurotic System 15829
Tissue Transfer 14000-14350
Tissue-Cultured 15040, 15150-15157
Transfer 15650
Vascular Flow Check 15860
Zygomaticofacial Flap 15730

Skin Substitute Graft
Arms 15271-15274
Digits 15275-15278
Eyelids 15275-15278
Face 15275-15278
Feet 15275-15278
Genitalia 15275-15278
Hands 15275-15278
Legs 15271-15274
Mouth 15275-15278
Orbits 15275-15278

Scalp 15275-15278
Trunk 15271-15274

Skull
Bone Graft 61316, 61559, 62146-62148
Burr Hole
  Biopsy Brain 61140
  Drainage
    Abscess 61150, 61151
    Cyst 61150, 61151
    Hematoma 61154-61156
  Exploration
    Infratentorial 61253
    Supratentorial 61250
  Insertion
    Catheter 61210
    EEG Electrode 61210
    Reservoir 61210
  Intracranial
    Biopsy 61140
  with Injection 61120
Decompression 61322, 61323, 61340-61345
  Orbit 61330
Drill Hole
  Catheter 61107
  Drainage Hematoma 61108
  Exploration 61105
Excision 61501
Exploration
  Drill Hole 61105
Fracture 62000-62010
Halo Application/Removal
  Thin Skull Osteology 20664
Hematoma
  Drainage 61108
Incision
  Suture 61550-61552
Insertion
  Catheter 61107
Lesion
  Excision .. 61500, 61600-61608, 61615, 61616
Orbit
  Excision
    Lesion 61333
Puncture
  Cervical 61050
  Cisternal 61050
  Drain Fluid 61070
  Injection 61070
  Subdural 61000, 61001
  Ventricular Fluid 61020
Reconstruction 21172-21180
  Defect 62140, 62141, 62145
Reduction
  Craniomegalic 62115, 62117
Removal
  Plate 62142
  Prosthesis 62142
Repair
  Cerebrospinal Fluid Leak 62100
  Encephalocele 62120
Replacement
  Plate 62143
  Prosthesis 62143
Thin Skull Osteology
  Halo Application/Removal 20664
Tumor
  Excision 61500
X ray 70250-70260

Skull Base Surgery
Anterior Cranial Fossa
  Bicoronal Approach 61586
  Craniofacial Approach 61580-61583
  Extradural 61600, 61601
  Intradural 61583
  LeFort I Osteotomy Approach 61586
  Orbitocranial Approach 61584, 61585
  Transzygomatic Approach 61586
Biopsy 61575, 61576
Carotid Aneurysm 61613
Carotid Artery
  Transection/Ligation 61611
Craniotomy 62121
Decompression 61575, 61576
Dura
  Repair of Cerebrospinal Fluid
  Leak 61618, 61619
Lesion Excision 61575, 61576
Middle Cranial Fossa
  Extradural 61605, 61607
  Infratemporal Approach 61590, 61591
  Intradural 61606, 61608
Midline Tumor
  Excision 61521
  Orbitocranial Zygomatic Approach 61592
Posterior Cranial Fossa
  Extradural 61615
  Intradural 61616
  Transcochlear Approach 61596
  Transcondylar Approach 61597
  Transpetrosal Approach 61598
  Transtemporal Approach 61595
Repair
  Encephalocele 62121

Sleep Study 95800, 95801, 95806, 95807
Actigraphy 95803

Sliding Inlay Graft, Tibia
See Ankle; Tibia, Repair

Sling Operation
Incontinence 53440
  Removal 53442
Stress Incontinence 51992, 57287
Vagina 57287, 57288

Small Bowel
See Intestines, Small
Neoplasm
  See Tumor, Intestines, Small

SMAS Flap 15829

Smear
Cervical
  See Cervical Smears
Papanicolaou
  See Pap Smears

Smear and Stain
Blood Smears
  Microorganism Identification ... 87205-87207
  Microscopic Examination 85007, 85008
  Peripheral 85060
  Sex Chromatin 88140
  Surgical Pathology 88312, 88313, 88319
Bone Marrow Smear 85097
Cervical or Vaginal Smears
  Automated Screen 88174
  Hormone Evaluation 88155
  Physician Interpretation 88141
  Partially Automated Screen 88147, 88148, 88152, 88166, 88167, 88175
  Manual Screen... 88150, 88153, 88164, 88165
  Pap
    Any Reporting System 88174, 88175
    Bethesda System 88164-88167
    Non-Bethesda 88150, 88152, 88153
Concentration Smear Technique 88108
Nasal Smear 89190
Other Cytopathology Smear Source .. 88160, 88161
Ova and Parasites Smear 87177, 87209
Selective Cellular Enhancement Smear
Technique 88112
Stains
  Acid-Fast 87206
  Complex Special 87209
  Fluorescent 87206
  Gram or Giemsa 87205
  for Bacteria 87205, 87206
  for Cell Types 87205, 87206
  for Fungi 87205, 87206
  for Inclusion Bodies 87207
  for Ova/Parasites 87177, 87209
  for Parasites 87206-87209
  for Viruses 87206
Wet Mount Smear 87210

Smith Fracture 25600-25605

Smith-Robinson Operation 22614

Smoking and Tobacco Use Cessation
Counseling 99406, 99407
Performance Measures 4001F, 4004F

SO4
See Sulfate

Soave Procedure 45120

Sodium 84295, 84302
Urine 84300

Sodium Glycinate, Theophylline
See Theophylline

Sofield Procedure 24410, 25370, 27712

Soft Tissue
See Tissue, Soft

Solar Plexus
See Celiac Plexus

Solitary Cyst
See Bone, Cyst

Somatomammotropin, Chorionic .. 83632

Somatomedin 84305

Somatosensory Testing
Lower Limbs 95926, 95938, 95939
Trunk or Head 95927
Upper Limbs 95925, 95938, 95939

Somatostatin 84307

Somatotropin 83003

Somatotropin Release Inhibiting Hormone
See Somatostatin

Somatropin
See Growth Hormone, Human

Somnographies
See Polysomnography

Somophyllin T
See Theophylline

Sonography
See Echography

Sonohysterography 76831
Saline Infusion
  Injection Procedure 58340

Sore, Bed
See Pressure, Ulcer (Decubitus)

Spasm Eyelid
See Blepharospasm

Special Services
After Hours Medical Services. 99050
Analysis
Computer Data Analysis, Remote
Electrocardiographic 0206T
Physiologic Data 99091
Device Handling 99002
Emergency Care In Office 99058
Emergency Care Out of Office 99060
Extended Hours Medical Services . . . 99051-99053
Group Education 99078
Self-Management 98961, 98962
Hyperbaric Oxygen 99183
Individual Education
Self-management 98960
Medical Testimony 99075
Non-Office Medical Services 99056
On Call Services 99026, 99027
Phlebotomy 99199
Post-Op Visit 99024
Pump Services. 99190-99192
Reports and Forms
Medical, Extended 99080
Psychiatric 90889
Specimen Handling. 99000, 99001
Supply of Materials 99070
Educational 99071
Unlisted Services and Procedures 99199
Unusual Travel 99082

Specific Gravity
Body Fluid 84315

Specimen Collection
Aspirate
See Aspiration
Brushings
Abdomen 49320
Anus. 46600, 46601
Biliary Tract 47552
Colon 44388, 45300, 45330, 45378
Duodenum 43235, 44360, 44376
Esophagus 43191, 43197, 43200, 43235
Hepatobiliary System. 43260
Ileum 44376, 44380
Omentum 49320
Peritoneum. 49320
Rectum. 45300, 45330
Small Intestine. 44385
Stomach. 43235
Radiological Guidance 75989
Specimen
Capillary Blood. 36416
Duodenum 43756, 43757
for Dark Field Examination. 87164
Ear 36416
Hematoma 10140
Imaging 19081-19086
Sputum. 89220
Stomach. 43754
Sweat. 89230
Tears 83861
Venous Access Device. 36591
Venous Blood. 36415, 36591, 36592
Venous Catheter 36592
Washings
Abdomen 49320
Anus. 46600, 46601
Biliary Tract 47552
Colon 44388, 45300, 45330, 45378
Duodenum 43235, 44360, 44376
Esophagus 43191, 43197, 43200, 43235
Hepatobiliary System. 43260
Ileum 44376, 44380
Omentum 49320
Peritoneum. 49320
Rectum. 45300, 45330
Small Intestine. 44385
Stomach. 43235

Specimen Concentration 87015

Specimen Handling. 99000, 99001

SPECT
Bone/Joint Imaging 78320
Brain Imaging 78607
Cerebrospinal Fluid Flow Imaging 78647
Heart
Blood Pool Imaging 78494
Myocardial Imaging. 78469
Sympathetic Innervation 0332T
Perfusion Imaging 78451; 78452
Multiple 78452, 78454
Single 78451, 78453
Kidney Imaging 78710
Liver Imaging. 78205
Localization
Inflammatory Process 78807
Parathyroid Gland 78072
Tumor. 78803
Parathyroid Gland 78071, 78072

Spectacle Services
Fitting
Low Vision Aid 92354, 92355
Spectacle Prosthesis 92352, 92353
Spectacles 92340-92342
Repair 92370, 92371

Spectrometry
Mass
Analyte
See specific analyte in Drug Assay; Pathology and Laboratory, Chemistry
Unspecified Non-Drug Analyte 83789
Column Chromatography
See specific analyte in Pathology and Laboratory, Chemistry
Unspecified Non-Drug Analyte(s). 82542

Spectrophotometry
Atomic Absorption
See Atomic Absorption Spectroscopy
Unspecified Analyte 84311

Spectroscopy
Atomic Absorption 82190
Bioimpedance Spectroscopy (BIS) 93702
Fluorescent
Advanced Glycation Endproducts (AGE) 88749
Real-Time Spectral Analysis
Prostate Tissue. 0443T
Infrared 82365
Intravascular 0205T
Magnetic Resonance 76390
Lipoprotein. 83704
Near-Infrared
Wound Study 0493T

Spectrum Analyses
See Spectrophotometry
Digital Multi-spectral
Skin Lesion 0400T, 0401T

Speech Evaluation
Behavioral and Qualitative Analysis. 92524
Cine. 70371
Comprehension. 92523
Expression. 92523
Fluency 92521
for Prosthesis 92597, 92607, 92608
Sound Production 92522, 92523
Video. 70371

Speech Prosthesis. 21084, 92609
Creation. 31611
Evaluation 92597, 92607, 92608
Insertion 31611

Speech Therapy
Evaluation 92521-92524
Group. 92508
Individual. 92507

Sperm
Cryopreservation. 89259
Preparation. 58323
Storage. 89343
Thawing 89353
Evaluation 89329-89331

Sperm Analysis
Antibodies. 89325
Cervical Mucus Penetration Test 89330
Evaluation from Semen
Count 89310, 89320, 89322
Motility. 89300, 89310, 89320-89322
Differential. 89320, 89322
Presence. 89300, 89321
for Retrograde Ejaculation 89331
Forensic. 88125
Hamster Penetration Test. 89329
Huhner Test. 89300
Identification
Aspiration. 89257
from Testis Tissue 89264
Isolation 89260, 89261

Sperm Washing. 58323

Spermatic Cord
Hydrocele
Excision 55500
Laparoscopy
Ligation, Vein. 55550
Lesion
Excision 55520
Repair
Veins 55530-55540
Abdominal Approach 55535
with Hernia Repair 55540
Unlisted Procedure 55559
Varicocele
Excision 55530-55540

Spermatic Veins
Excision. 55530-55540
Ligation. 55550

Spermatocele
Excision. 54840

Spermatocystectomy
See Spermatocele, Excision

Sphenoid Sinus
See Sinus/Sinuses, Sphenoid

Sphenoidotomy
Excision
with Nasal/Sinus Endoscopy. . . . 31287, 31288

Sphenopalatine Ganglion
Injection
Anesthetic 64505

Index

Sphincter
Anal
See Anal Sphincter
Artificial Genitourinary
See Prosthesis, Urethral Sphincter
Common Bile Duct
Incision 47420, 47425, 47460, 47620
Electromyography 51784, 51785
Esophageal
Delivery, Thermal Energy 43257
Excision 43262
Pyloric
See Pyloric Sphincter
Rectal
See Rectal Sphincter
Sphincter of Oddi
See Sphincter of Oddi
Urethral
See Urethral, Sphincter

Sphincter of Oddi
Dilation 47542
Excision 43262
Pressure Measurement
Endoscopy 43263

Sphincteroplasty
Ampulla of Vater 47542
Anal 46750, 46751, 46760, 46761
Bile Duct 47420, 47425, 47460, 47620
Bladder Neck
See Bladder, Repair, Neck

Sphincterotomy
Anal 46080, 46200
Bile Duct 43274, 47420, 47425, 47460, 47620

Spica Cast
Hip 29305-29325
Repair 29720
Shoulder 29055

Spinal Accessory Nerve
Anastomosis
to Facial Nerve 64866
Laminectomy 63191
Injection
Anesthetic 64999
Section 63191

Spinal Column
See Spine

Spinal Cord
See Cauda Equina; Nerve Root
Biopsy 63275-63290
Cyst
Aspiration 62268
Incision and Drainage 63172, 63173
Decompression 63001-63003, 63055-63057, 63064, 63066, 63101-63103, 62380, 0274T, 0275T
with Cervical Laminoplasty 63050, 63051
with Craniectomy 61343
with Discectomy 62380
with Facetectomy 62380
with Foraminotomy 0202T, 62380
with Laminotomy 62380
Drain Fluid 62272
Exploration
Cervical 63001, 63015
Thoracic 63003, 63016
Lumbar 63005, 63012, 63017
Sacral 63011
Graft
Dura 63710
Implantation
Electrode 63650-63655
Pulse Generator 63685
Receiver 63685
Incision 63200
Dentate Ligament 63180-63182
Tract 63170, 63194-63199
Injection
Anesthetic 62320-62327
Blood 62273
CT Scan 62284
Neurolytic Agent 62280-62282
Other 62320-62327
X ray 62284
Insertion
Electrode 63650-63655
Pulse Generator 63685
Receiver 63685
Lesion
Creation 63600
Destruction 62280-62282
Excision 63265-63273, 63300-63308
Needle Biopsy 62269
Neoplasm
Excision 63275-63290
Neurostimulator Pulse Generator System
Electronic Analysis 95972
Puncture (Tap)
Diagnostic 62270
Drain Fluid 62272
Lumbar 62270
Radiosurgery
Stereotactic 63620, 63621
Reconstruction
Dorsal Spine Elements 63295
Release 63200
Removal
Catheter 62355
Electrode 63661-63664
Pulse Generator 63688
Pump 62365
Receiver 63688
Reservoir 62365
Repair
Cerebrospinal Fluid Leak 63707-63709
Meningocele 63700-63702
Myelomeningocele 63704-63706
Section
Dentate Ligament 63180-63182
Tract 63194-63199
Shunt
Create 63740, 63741
Irrigation 63744
Removal 63746
Replacement 63744
Stereotaxis
Computer-Assisted Procedure 61783
Creation Lesion 63600
Stimulation 63610
Syrinx
Aspiration 62268
Tumor
Excision 63275-63290

Spinal Cord Neoplasms
See Spinal Cord
Tumor
See Spinal Cord, Tumor; Tumor

Spinal Fluid
See Cerebrospinal Fluid

Spinal Fracture
See Fracture, Vertebra

Spinal Instrumentation
Anterior 22845-22847
Removal 22855
Biomechanical Device 22853, 22854, 22859
Harrington Rod Technique
Insertion 22840
Removal 22850
Internal Fixation 22841
Pelvic Fixation 22848
Posterior Nonsegmental 22840
Removal 22850
Posterior Segmental 22842-22844
Removal 22852
Reinsertion of Spinal Fixation Device 22849

Spinal Manipulation
See Manipulation, Chiropractic

Spinal Nerve
Avulsion 64772
Decompression
Root 62380
Transection 64772

Spinal Tap
See Cervical Puncture; Cisternal Puncture; Subdural Tap; Ventricular Puncture
Drainage Fluid 62272
Lumbar 62270

Spine
See Intervertebral Disc; Spinal Cord; Vertebra; Vertebral, Body; Vertebral, Process
Allograft
Morselized 20930
Structural 20931
Arthroplasty
Cervical . . 0375T, 22856, 22858, 22861, 22864
Lumbar . . . 0163T, 0164T, 22857, 22862, 22865
Aspiration 62267
Augmentation
Lumbar Vertebra 22514, 22515
Thoracic Vertebra 22513, 22515
Autograft
Bone Marrow Aspiration 20939
Local 20936
Morselized 20937
Structural 20938
Biopsy
Open 20250, 20251
Percutaneous 22510-22512
CT Scan
Bone Density Study 77078
Cervical 72125-72127
Lumbar 72131-72133
Thoracic 72128-72130
Decompression 62287, 62380, 0274T, 0275T
Deformity
Arthrodesis 22800-22812
Exposure 22818, 22819
Scoliosis X-ray Study 72081-72084
Fixation 22842
Foraminotomy 0202T
Fusion
Anterior 22808-22812
Anterior Approach 22548-22585, 22812
Exploration 22830
Lateral Extracavitary 22532-22534
Posterior Approach 22590-22802
Posterior/Posterolateral and/or Lateral Transverse Technique . . . 22612, 22633, 22634
Presacral Interbody Technique 22586
Transverse Technique . . . 22612, 22633, 22634
Incision and Drainage
Abscess 22010-22015

Injection
Cervical 0228T, 0229T, 62320, 62321, 62324, 62325
Lumbar 0230T, 0231T, 62322, 62323, 62326, 62327
Sacral 0230T, 0231T, 62322, 62323, 62326, 62327
Thoracic 0228T, 0229T, 62320, 62321, 62324, 62325
with Fluoroscopic Guidance........... 77003
Insertion
Instrumentation 22840-22848, 22853, 22854, 22859
Kyphectomy................ 22818, 22819
Magnetic Resonance Angiography......... 72159
Magnetic Resonance Imaging
Cervical 72141, 72142, 72156, 72159
Lumbar 72148, 72149, 72158, 72159
Thoracic 72146, 72147, 72157, 72159
Manipulation
with Anesthesia.................... 22505
Myelography
Cervical 72240
Lumbosacral....................... 72265
Thoracic 72255
Total............................. 72270
Placement of Osteopromotive Material..... 20930
Radiosurgery
Stereotactic 63620, 63621
Computer Assisted (Navigational).... 61783
Reconstruction
Dorsal Spine Elements............... 63295
Reinsertion
Instrumentation 22849
Removal
Instrumentation 22850, 22852-22855
Repair, Osteotomy
Anterior 22220-22226
Posterior......... 22206-22208, 22210-22214
Cervical Laminoplasty 63050, 63051
Posterolateral..................... 22216
Ultrasound.......................... 76800
Unlisted Services and Procedures 22899
X ray 72020
Absorptiometry .. 77080, 77081, 77085, 77086
Cervical 72040, 72050, 72052
Lumbosacral..... 72100, 72110, 72114, 72120
Scoliosis Study............... 72081-72084
Radiostereometric Analysis (RSA)...... 0348T
Thoracic 72070, 72072, 72074
Thoracolumbar...................... 72080
Total........................ 72081-72084
with Contrast
Cervical......................... 72240
Lumbosacral..................... 72265
Thoracic 72255
Total 72270

Spine Chemotherapy
Administration 96450
See Chemotherapy

Spirometry.................. 94010-94070
See Pulmonology, Diagnostic
Patient Initiated 94014-94016

Splanchnicectomy
See Nerves, Sympathectomy, Excision

Spleen
Drainage
Image Guided Fluid Collection......... 49405
Excision....................... 38100-38102
Laparoscopic 38120
Injection
Radiological 38200
Nuclear Medicine
Imaging 78185, 78215, 78216
Repair 38115
Unlisted Procedure
Laparoscopic 38129

Splenectomy
Laparoscopic......................... 38120
Partial 38101
Partial with Repair, Ruptured Spleen....... 38115
Total 38100
En bloc 38102

Splenoplasty
See Repair, Spleen

Splenoportography 75810
Injection Procedures.................. 38200

Splenorrhaphy..................... 38115

Splint
See Casting; Strapping
Arm
Long 29105
Short..................... 29125, 29126
Finger 29130, 29131
Leg
Long 29505
Short............................. 29515
Oral Surgical 21085
Ureteral
See Ureteral, Splinting

Split Grafts 15100, 15101, 15120, 15121

Split Renal Function Test
See Cystourethroscopy, Catheterization, Ureteral

Splitting
Blood Products 86985

Spontaneous Abortion
See Abortion

Sprengel's Deformity 23400

Spring Water Cyst
See Cyst, Pericardial

Spur, Bone
See Exostosis
Calcaneal
See Heel Spur

Sputum Analysis.................. 89220

SRIH
See Somatostatin

SRS/SBRT (Stereotactic Body Radiation Therapy)
Thoracic
See Radiation Therapy, Stereotactic Body, Target Delineation, Thoracic

Ssabanejew-Frank Operation.................. 43830-43832

ST2
Growth Stimulation Expressed Gene 2...... 83006

Stabilizing Factor, Fibrin
See Fibrin Stabilizing Factor

Stable Factor 85230

Stallard Procedure
See Conjunctivorhinostomy

Stamey Procedure................ 51845

Standby Services................. 99360

Stanford-Binet Test
See Psychiatric Diagnosis, Psychological Testing

Stapedectomy
Revision............................ 69662
with Footplate Drill Out 69661
without Foreign Material 69660

Stapedotomy
Revision............................ 69662
with Footplate Drill Out 69661
without Foreign Material 69660

Stapes
Excision
with Footplate Drill Out............. 69661
without Foreign Material............ 69660
Mobilization 69650
Release 69650
Revision............................ 69662

Staphyloma
Sclera
Repair
with Graft....................... 66225

Statin Therapy
Performance Measures
Coronary Heart Disease.............. 4013F

Statistics/Biometry
See Biometry

Steindler Stripping 28250

Stellate Ganglion
Injection
Anesthetic 64510

Stem Cell
Cell Concentration 38215
Count............................... 86367
Cryopreservation................ 38207, 88240
Donor Search 38204
Harvesting..................... 38205, 38206
Hematopoietic Progenitor Cells
See Hematopoietic Progenitor Cell (HPC)
Limbal
Allograft......................... 65781
Plasma Depletion 38214
Platelet Depletion..................... 38213
Red Blood Cell Depletion 38212
T-Cell Depletion 38210
Thawing 38208, 38209, 88241
Transplantation................. 38240-38242
Tumor Cell Depletion 38211
Washing 38209

Stem, Brain
See Brainstem

Stenger Test 92565, 92577
See Audiologic Function Tests

Stenosis
Aortic
See Aortic Stenosis
Auditory Canal, External
Reconstruction.................... 69310
Bronchi 96570, 96571
Reconstruction.................... 31775
Relief 31641
Laryngeal
Repair.................... 31551-31554
Nasal
Repair........................... 30465

Index

Pulmonary Artery
  Repair . . . 33782, 33917
Pulmonary Vein
  Repair . . . 33726
Tracheal
  Excision . . . 31780, 31781
Urethral
  See Urethral, Stenosis
Ventricular
  Resection . . . 33476

Stensen Duct
See Parotid Duct

Stent
Exchange
  Biliary Duct . . . 43276
  Pancreatic Duct . . . 43276
for Revascularization
  Intracoronary . . . 92937, 92938, 92941, 92943, 92944
Placement
  Arterial
    See Artery, Stent Placement
  Bronchial . . . 31631, 31636, 31637
  Cardiac . . . 33621
  Colonoscopy . . . 45397
    via Stoma . . . 44402
  Endoscopy
    Bile Duct . . . 43274
    Gastrointestinal, Upper . . . 43266
    Intestinal . . . 44379
    Pancreatic Duct . . . 43274
  Enteroscopy . . . 44370
  Esophagoscopy . . . 43212
  Ileoscopy . . . 44384
  Larynx . . . 31553, 31554, 31580
  Proctosigmoidoscopy . . . 45327
  Sigmoidoscopy . . . 45347
  Tracheal . . . 31631
  Ureter . . . 50605, 52282, 52356, 53855
  Ureteroneocystostomy . . . 50947, 50948
Removal
  Biliary . . . 43276
  Ureteral . . . 50382-50386
Replacement
  Nephroureteral . . . 50387
  Ureteral . . . 50382
Revision
  Bronchoscopy . . . 31638
Urethra . . . 52282

Stent, Intravascular
See Transcatheter, Placement, Intravascular Stent

Stents, Tracheal
See Tracheal, Stent

Stereotactic Body Radiation Therapy (SRS/SBRT)
Thoracic
  See Radiation Therapy, Stereotactic Body, Target Delineation

Stereotactic Frame
Application/Removal . . . 20660

Stereotactic Radiosurgery
Cranial . . . 61796-61800
  Headframe Application . . . 61800
Spinal . . . 63620, 63621

Stereotaxis
Aspiration
  Brain Lesion . . . 61750
    with CT Scan and/or MRI . . . 61751
Biopsy
  Aspiration
    Brain Lesion . . . 61750
  Brain . . . 61750
    with CT Scan and/or MRI . . . 61751
  Breast . . . 19081, 19283, 19284
  Prostate . . . 55706
Catheter Placement
  Brain
    Radiation Source . . . 61770
Computer Assisted
  Cranial Procedure . . . 61781, 61782
  Orthopedic Surgery . . . 20985
  Spinal Procedure . . . 61783
Creation Lesion
  Brain
    Deep . . . 61720, 61735
    Percutaneous . . . 61790
  Gasserian Ganglion . . . 61790
  Spinal Cord . . . 63600
  Trigeminal Tract . . . 61791
CT Scan
  Aspiration . . . 61751
  Biopsy . . . 61751
Excision Lesion
  Brain . . . 61750
Focus Beam
  Radiosurgery . . . 77371-77373
    Cranial . . . 61796-61799
    Spinal . . . 63620, 63621
    Stereotactic Frame Application 20660, 61800
Lesion Ablation, Intracranial
  Magnetic Resonance Image Guided High Intensity Focused Ultrasound (MRgFUS) . . . 0398T
Placement
  Localization Device
    Breast . . . 19081, 19082, 19283, 19284
Radiation Therapy . . . 77432-77435
Stimulation
  Spinal Cord . . . 63610

Sterile Coverings
See Dressings

Sternal Fracture
See Fracture, Sternum

Sternoclavicular Joint
Arthrotomy . . . 23044
  with Biopsy . . . 23101
  with Synovectomy . . . 23106
Dislocation
  Closed Treatment
    with Manipulation . . . 23525
    without Manipulation . . . 23520
  Open Treatment . . . 23530-23532
    with Fascial Graft . . . 23532

Sternocleidomastoid
Division . . . 21720-21725

Sternotomy
Closure . . . 21750

Sternum
Debridement . . . 21627
Excision . . . 21620, 21630-21632
Fracture
  Closed Treatment . . . 21820
  Open Treatment . . . 21825
Ostectomy . . . 21620
Radical Resection . . . 21630-21632
Reconstruction . . . 21740-21742, 21750
  with Thoracoscopy . . . 21743
X ray . . . 71120-71130

Steroid-Binding Protein, Sex
See Globulin, Sex Hormone Binding

Steroids
Anabolic
  See Androstenedione
Injection
  Foot Neuroma . . . 64455, 64632
  Urethral Stricture . . . 52283
Ketogenic
  Urine . . . 83582

STH (Somatotropic Hormone)
See Growth Hormone

Stimulating Antibody, Thyroid
See Immunoglobulin, Thyroid Stimulating

Stimulation
Electric
  See Electrical Stimulation
Lymphocyte
  See Blastogenesis
Spinal Cord
  Stereotaxis . . . 63610
Transcutaneous Electric
  See Application, Neurostimulation

Stimulator, Long-Acting Thyroid
See Thyrotropin Releasing Hormone (TRH)

Stimulators, Cardiac
See Heart, Pacemaker

Stimulus Evoked Response . . . 51792

Stoffel Operation
See Rhizotomy

Stoma
Creation
  Bladder . . . 51980
  Kidney . . . 50551-50561
  Stomach
    Neonatal . . . 43831
    Temporary . . . 43830, 43831
  Ureter . . . 50860
Ureter
  Endoscopy via . . . 50951-50961

Stomach
Anastomosis
  with Duodenum . . . 43810, 43850-43855
  with Jejunum . . . 43820-43825, 43860-43865
Biopsy . . . 43605
Creation
  Stoma
    Temporary . . . 43830, 43831
  Temporary Stoma
    Laparoscopic . . . 43653
Electrode
  Removal . . . 43882
Electrogastrography . . . 91132, 91133
Excision
  Partial . . . 43631-43635, 43845
  Total . . . 43620-43622
Exploration . . . 43500
Gastric Bypass . . . 43644, 43645, 43846
  Revision . . . 43848
Gastric Restrictive Procedures . . . 43770-43775, 43848, 43886-43888
Implantation
  Electrodes . . . 43647, 43881
Incision . . . 43830-43832
  Exploration . . . 43500
  Pyloric Sphincter . . . 43520
  Removal
    Foreign Body . . . 43500

Laparoscopy 43647, 43648
Nuclear Medicine
Blood Loss Study 78278
Gastric Emptying Imaging Study 78264
with Small Bowel Transit........... 78265
with Small Bowel and Colon Transit . . 78266
Gastric Mucosa Imaging 78261
Protein Loss Study................. 78282
Reflux Study...................... 78262
Reconstruction
for Obesity 43644, 43645, 43842-43847
Roux-En-Y................... 43644, 43846
Removal
Foreign Body 43500
Repair 48547
Fistula........................... 43880
Fundoplasty 43325, 43327, 43328
Laparoscopic............... 43280-43282
Laceration 43501, 43502
Stoma............................ 43870
Ulcer............................. 43501
Replacement
Electrodes 43647, 43881
Specimen Collection............. 43754, 43755
Stimulation of Secretion................ 43755
Suture
Fistula........................... 43880
for Obesity 43842, 43843
Stoma............................ 43870
Ulcer............................. 43840
Wound 43840
Tumor
Excision 43610, 43611
Ulcer
Excision 43610
Unlisted Services and Procedures . . . 43659, 43999

Stomatoplasty
See Mouth, Repair

Stone, Kidney
See Calculus, Removal, Kidney

Stookey-Scarff Procedure
See Ventriculocisternostomy

Stool Blood
See Blood, Feces

Storage
Embryo 89342
Oocyte............................. 89346
Reproductive Tissue 89344
Sperm.............................. 89343

Strabismus
Chemodenervation 67345
Repair
Adjustable Sutures 67335
Extraocular Muscles 67340
One Horizontal Muscle 67311
One Vertical Muscle 67314
Posterior Fixation Suture
Technique.................. 67334, 67335
Previous Surgery, Not Involving Extraocular
Muscles.......................... 67331
Release Extensive Scar Tissue 67343
Superior Oblique Muscle............ 67318
Transposition..................... 67320
Two Horizontal Muscles 67312
Two or More Vertical Muscles 67316

Strapping
See Cast; Splint
Ankle.............................. 29540
Compression 29581
Arm
Compression 29584
Chest.............................. 29200
Elbow 29260
Finger 29280
Compression 29584
Foot............................... 29540
Compression 29581
Hand 29280
Compression 29584
Hip................................ 29520
Knee 29530
Leg
Compression 29581
Shoulder 29240
Thorax............................. 29200
Toes............................... 29550
Unlisted Services and Procedures 29799
Unna Boot.......................... 29580
Wrist.............................. 29260

Strassman Procedure............. 58540

Strayer Procedure
Leg, Lower.......................... 27687

Streptococcus pneumoniae Vaccine
See Vaccines and Toxoids

Streptococcus, Group A
Antigen Detection
Immunoassay...................... 87430
Nucleic Acid................. 87650-87652
Direct Optical Observation 87880

Streptococcus, Group B
by Immunoassay
with Direct Optical Observation 87802

Streptokinase, Antibody 86590

Stress Tests
Cardiovascular 93015-93024
Multiple Gated Acquisition (MUGA). . 78472, 78473
Myocardial Perfusion Imaging 78451-78454
Pulmonary.......................... 94618
See Pulmonology, Diagnostic

Stricture
Dilation
Gastric/Duodenal.................. 43245
Ureteral
Balloon 50706
Endoscopy............... 50553, 50572,
50575, 50953, 50972
with Cystourethroscopy 52341-52343
with Ureteroscopy 52344-52346
Repair
Urethra.................... 53400-53405
Urethra
See Urethral, Stenosis

Stricturoplasty
Intestines 44615

Stroboscopy
Larynx 31579

STS 86592, 86593
See Syphilis Test

Stuart-Prower Factor 85260

Study, Color Vision
See Color Vision Examination

Sturmdorf Procedure 57520

Styloid Process
Radial
Excision 25230

Styloidectomy
Radial 25230

Stypven Time
See Russell Viper Venom Time

Subacromial Bursa
Arthrocentesis.................. 20610, 20611

Subclavian Arteries
See Artery, Subclavian

Subcutaneous Cardiac Rhythm Monitor
Insertion 33285
Removal 33286

Subcutaneous Infusion
See Infusion, Subcutaneous

Subcutaneous Injection
See Injection, Subcutaneous

Subcutaneous Mastectomies
See Mastectomy, Subcutaneous

Subcutaneous Tissue
Excision................. 15830-15839, 15847

Subdiaphragmatic Abscess
See Abscess, Tissue, Subdiaphragmatic

Subdural Electrode
Insertion 61531-61533
Removal 61535

Subdural Hematonia
See Hematoma, Subdural

Subdural Puncture........... 61105-61108

Subdural Tap................. 61000, 61001

Sublingual Gland
Abscess
Incision and Drainage 42310-42320
Calculi (Stone)
Excision 42330
Cyst
Drainage......................... 42409
Excision 42408
Excision............................ 42450

Subluxation
Elbow
Closed Treatment.................. 24640
Pelvic Ring
Closed Treatment............. 27197, 27198

Submandibular Gland
Calculi (Stone)
Excision 42330-42335
Excision............................ 42440

Submaxillary Gland
Abscess
Incision and Drainage 42310-42320

Submucous Resection of Nasal Septum
See Nasal Septum, Submucous Resection

Subperiosteal Implant
Reconstruction
Mandible 21245, 21246
Maxilla.................... 21245, 21246

Subphrenic Abscess
See Abscess, Tissue, Subphrenic

Subtrochanteric Fracture
See Femur, Fracture, Subtrochanteric

Sucrose Hemolysis Test
See Red Blood Cell (RBC), Fragility, Osmotic

Suction Lipectomies
See Liposuction

Sudoriferous Gland
See Sweat Glands, Excision

Sugar Water Test
See Red Blood Cell (RBC), Fragility, Osmotic

Sugars 84375-84379

Sugiura Procedure
See Esophagus, Repair, Varices

Sulfate
Chondroitin
See Chondroitin Sulfate
DHA
See Dehydroepiandrosterone Sulfate
Urine 84392

Sulfation Factor
See Somatomedin

Sulphates
See Sulfate

Sumatran Mite Fever
See Scrub Typhus

Superficial Musculoaponeurotic System (SMAS) Flap
Rhytidectomy 15829

Supernumerary Digit
Reconstruction 26587
Repair 26587

Supply
See Chemotherapy
Educational Materials 99071
Low Vision Aids
See Spectacle Services
Materials 99070
Prosthesis
Breast 19396

Suppositories, Vaginal
See Pessary

Suppression 80400-80408

Suppression/Testing
See Evocative/Suppression Test

Suppressor T Lymphocyte Marker
See CD8

Suppurative Hidradenitis
See Hidradenitis, Suppurative

Suprahyoid
Lymphadenectomy 38700

Supraorbital
Nerve
Avulsion 64732
Incision 64732
Transection 64732
Reconstruction
Forehead 21179, 21180
Rim 21179, 21180

Suprapubic Prostatectomies
See Prostatectomy, Suprapubic

Suprarenal
Gland
See Adrenal Gland
Vein
See Vein, Adrenal

Suprascapular Nerve
Injection
Anesthetic 64418

Suprasellar Cyst
See Craniopharyngioma

Surface CD4 Receptor
See CD4

Surface Radiotherapy
See Application, Radioelement, Surface

Surgeries
Breast-Conserving
See Breast, Excision, Lesion
Conventional
See Celiotomy
Laser
See Laser Surgery
Mohs
See Mohs Micrographic Surgery
Repeat
See Reoperation

Surveillance
See Monitoring

Suspension
Aorta 33800
Kidney
See Nephropexy
Muscle
Hyoid 21685
Tongue Base 41512
Vagina
See Colpopexy

Suture
See Repair
Abdomen 49900
Aorta 33320-33322
Bile Duct
Wound 47900
Bladder
Fistulization 44660, 44661, 45800-45805, 51880-51925
Vesicouterine 51920-51925
Vesicovaginal 51900
Wound 51860-51865
Cervix 57720
Colon
Diverticula 44604, 44605
Fistula 44650-44661
Plication 44680
Stoma 44620-44625
Ulcer 44604, 44605
Wound 44604, 44605
Esophagus
Wound 43410-43415
Eyelid 67880
Closure of 67875
with Transposition of Tarsal Plate 67882
Wound
Full Thickness 67935
Partial Thickness 67930
Facial Nerve
Intratemporal
Lateral to Geniculate Ganglion 69740
Medial to Geniculate Ganglion 69745
Foot
Tendon 28200-28210
Gastroesophageal 43405
Great Vessel 33320-33322
Hemorrhoids 46945, 46946
Hepatic Duct
See Hepatic Duct, Repair
Intestine
Large
Diverticula 44605
Ulcer 44605
Wound 44605
Intestines
Large
Diverticula 44604
Ulcer 44604
Wound 44604
Small
Diverticula 44602, 44603
Fistula 44640-44661
Plication 44680
Ulcer 44602, 44603
Wound 44602, 44603
Stoma 44620-44625
Iris
with Ciliary Body 66682
Kidney
Fistula 50520-50526
Horseshoe 50540
Wound 50500
Leg, Lower
Tendon 27658-27665
Leg, Upper
Muscle 27385, 27386
Liver
Wound 47350-47361
Mesentery 44850
Nerve 64831-64876
Pancreas 48545
Pharynx
Wound 42900
Rectum
Fistula 45800-45825
Prolapse 45540, 45541
Removal
Anesthesia 15850, 15851
Spleen
See Splenorrhaphy
Stomach
Fistula 43880
Laceration 43501, 43502
Stoma 43870
Ulcer 43501, 43840
Wound 43840
Tendon
Foot 28200-28210
Knee 27380, 27381
Testis
Injury 54670
Suspension 54620-54640
Thoracic Duct
Abdominal Approach 38382
Cervical Approach 38380
Thoracic Approach 38381
Throat
Wound 42900
Tongue
Base Suspension 41512
to Lip 41510
Trachea
Fistula
with Plastic Repair 31825
without Plastic Repair 31820
Stoma
with Plastic Repair 31825
without Plastic Repair 31820

Wound
Cervical 31800
Intrathoracic 31805
Ulcer 44604, 44605
Ureter 50900
Deligation 50940
Fistula 50920-50930
Urethra
Fistula 45820-45825, 53520
Stoma 53520
to Bladder 51840, 51841
Wound 53502-53515
Uterus
Fistula 51920-51925
Rupture 58520, 59350
Suspension 58400-58410
Vagina
Cystocele 57240, 57260
Enterocele 57265
Fistula
Rectovaginal 57300-57307
Transvesical and Vaginal Approach . . . 57330
Urethrovaginal 57310, 57311
Vesicovaginal 51900, 57320-57330
Rectocele 57250-57260
Suspension 57280, 57283
Wound 57200-57210
Vas Deferens 55400
Vein
Femoral 37650
Iliac 37660
Wound 44604, 44605

Swallowing
Evaluation 92610-92613, 92616, 92617
Imaging 74230
Treatment 92526

Swan-Ganz Catheter
Insertion 93503

Swanson Procedure 28309

Sweat Collection
Iontophoresis 89230

Sweat Glands
Excision
Axillary 11450, 11451
Inguinal 11462, 11463
Perianal 11470, 11471
Perineal 11470, 11471
Umbilical 11470, 11471

Sweat Test 82435
See Chloride, Blood

Swenson Procedure 45120

Syme Procedure 27888

Sympathectomy
Artery
Digital 64820
Radial 64821
Superficial Palmar Arch 64823
Ulnar 64822
Cervical 64802
Cervicothoracic 64804
Digital Artery
with Magnification 64820
Lumbar 64818
Presacral 58410
Thoracic 32664
Thoracolumbar 64809
with Rib Excision 21616

Sympathetic Nerve
Excision 64802-64818
Injection
Anesthetic 64520-64530

Sympathins
See Catecholamines

Symphysiotomy
Horseshoe Kidney 50540

Symphysis, Pubic
See Pubic Symphysis

Syncytial Virus, Respiratory
See Respiratory Syncytial Virus

Syndactylism, Toes
See Webbed, Toe

Syndactyly
Repair 26560-26562

Syndesmotomy
See Ligament, Release

Syndrome
Adrenogenital
See Adrenogenital Syndrome
Ataxia-Telangiectasia
See Ataxia Telangiectasia
Bloom
See Bloom Syndrome
Carpal Tunnel
See Carpal Tunnel Syndrome
Costen's
See Temporomandibular Joint (TMJ)
Erb-Goldflam
See Myasthenia Gravis
Ovarian Vein
See Ovarian Vein Syndrome
Synechiae, Intrauterine
See Adhesions, Intrauterine
Treacher Collins
See Treacher-Collins Syndrome
Urethral
See Urethral, Syndrome

Syngesterone
See Progesterone

Synostosis (Cranial)
See Craniosynostosis

Synovectomy
Ankle 27625, 27626
Partial 29895
Carpometacarpal Joint 26130
Elbow 24102, 29836
Partial 29835
with Prosthesis Removal
Humeral and Ulnar Components 24160
Radial Head 24164
Finger
Joint 26135-26140
Tendon Sheath 26145
Foot
Tendon Sheath 28086, 28088, 28090
Glenohumeral Joint 23105
Hip Joint 27054, 29863
Interphalangeal Joint 26140
Intertarsal Joint 28070
Knee Joint 27334, 27335
Partial 27441, 27443, 29875, 29876
Metacarpophalangeal Joint 26135
Metatarsophalangeal Joint 28072
Palm
Tendon Sheath 26145
Shoulder
with Prosthesis Removal 23334, 23335
Shoulder Joint 29821
Partial 29820
Sternoclavicular Joint 23106
Subtalar Joint 29905
Tarsometatarsal Joint 28070
Wrist
Joint 25105, 29845
Partial 29844
Radical 25115, 25116
Tendon Sheath 25118, 25119

Synovial
Bursa
See Bursa
Cyst
See Ganglion
Membrane
See Synovium
Popliteal Space
See Baker's Cyst

Synovium
Biopsy
Carpometacarpal Joint 26100
Interphalangeal Joint 26110
Knee Joint 27330
Metacarpophalangeal Joint
with Synovial Biopsy 26105
Excision
Carpometacarpal Joint 26130
Finger Joint 26135-26140
Hip Joint 27054
Interphalangeal Joint 26140
Knee Joint 27334, 27335

Syphilis ab
See Antibody, Detection, Treponema Pallidum

Syphilis Test 86592, 86593

Syrinx
Spinal Cord
Aspiration 62268

System
Endocrine
See Endocrine System
Hemic
See Hemic System
Lymphatic
See Lymphatic System
Musculoskeletal
See Musculoskeletal System
Nervous
See Nervous System

T

T Cell Leukemia Virus I Antibodies, Adult
See Antibody, Detection, HTLV-I

T Cell Leukemia Virus I, Human
See HTLV-I

T Cell Leukemia Virus II Antibodies, Human
See Antibody, Detection, HTLV-II

T Cell Leukemia Virus II, Human
See HTLV-II

Index

T Cells
CD4
Absolute . . . 86361
Chimeric Antigen Receptor (CAR-T)
Therapy . . . 0537T-0540T
Count . . . 86359
Gene Rearrangement . . . 81340-81342
Ratio . . . 86360

T Lymphotropic Virus Type III Antibodies, Human
See Antibody, Detection, Human Immunodeficiency Virus (HIV)

T-3
See Triiodothyronine

T3 Free
See Triiodothyronine, Free

T-4 . . . 84436-84439, 86360

T4 Molecule
See CD4

T4 Total
See Thyroxine, Total

T-7 Index
See Thyroxine, Total

T-8
See CD8; T Cells, Ratio

T-Cell T8 Antigens
See CD8

T-Phyl
See Theophylline

Taarnhoj Procedure
See Decompression, Gasserian Ganglion, Sensory Root; Section

Tachycardia
Mapping of Sites . . . 93609, 93654
Treatment
Ventricular . . . 93653, 93654

Tacrolimus
Drug Assay . . . 80197

Tag, Skin
See Skin, Tags

Tail Bone
Excision . . . 27080
Fracture . . . 27200-27202

Takeuchi Procedure . . . 33505

Talectomy
See Astragalectomy

Talotarsal Joint
Dislocation . . . 28570-28575, 28585
Percutaneous Fixation . . . 28576

Talus
Arthrodesis
Pantalar . . . 28705
Subtalar . . . 28725
Triple . . . 28715
Arthroscopy
Surgical . . . 29891, 29892
Subtalar . . . 29904-29907, 29915, 29916
Autograft, Osteochondral . . . 28446
Craterization . . . 28120
Cyst
Excision . . . 28100-28103
Diaphysectomy . . . 28120
Excision . . . 28120, 28130
Fracture
Open Treatment . . . 28445
Percutaneous Fixation . . . 28436
with Manipulation . . . 28435, 28436
without Manipulation . . . 28430
Repair
Osteochondritis Dissecans . . . 29892
Osteotomy . . . 28302
Saucerization . . . 28120
Subtalar Joint
Sinus Tarsi Implant
Insertion . . . 0335T
Removal . . . 0510T
Removal and Reinsertion . . . 0511T
Tumor
Excision . . . 28100-28103
Radical Resection . . . 27647

TAP (Transversus Abdominis Plane) Block
Cisternal
See Cisternal Puncture
Lumbar Diagnostic
See Spinal Tap
Somatic Nerves . . . 64486-64489

Tarsal
Fracture
Percutaneous Fixation . . . 28456

Tarsal Bone
See Repair, Tarsal

Tarsal Joint
See Foot
Arthrodesis . . . 28730-28735, 28740
with Advancement . . . 28737
with Lengthening . . . 28737
Craterization . . . 28122
Cyst
Excision . . . 28104-28107
Diaphysectomy . . . 28122
Dislocation . . . 28540-28545, 28555
Percutaneous Fixation . . . 28545, 28546
Excision . . . 28116, 28122
Fracture
Open Treatment . . . 28465
with Manipulation . . . 28455, 28456
without Manipulation . . . 28450
Fusion . . . 28730-28735, 28740
with Advancement . . . 28737
with Lengthening . . . 28737
Repair
Nonunion or Malunion . . . 28320
Osteotomy . . . 28304, 28305
Saucerization . . . 28122
Tumor
Excision . . . 28104-28107
Radical Resection . . . 28171

Tarsal Strip Procedure . . . 67917-67924

Tarsal Tunnel Release . . . 28035

Tarsal Wedge Procedure . . . 67916, 67923

Tarsometatarsal Joint
Arthrodesis . . . 28730-28735, 28740
Arthrotomy . . . 28020, 28050
Dislocation . . . 28600-28605, 28615
Percutaneous Fixation . . . 28606
Exploration . . . 28020
Fusion . . . 28730-28735, 28740
Removal
Foreign Body . . . 28020
Loose Body . . . 28020
Synovial
Biopsy . . . 28050
Excision . . . 28070

Tarsorrhaphy . . . 67875
Median . . . 67880
Severing . . . 67710
with Transposition of Tarsal Plate . . . 67882

Tattoo
Cornea . . . 65600
Skin . . . 11920-11922

TAVR/TAVI
See Transcatheter Aortic Valve Replacement (TAVR/TAVI)

TB Test
Antigen Response . . . 86480, 86481
Skin Test . . . 86580

TBG
See Thyroxine Binding Globulin

TBS
See Bethesda System

TCT
See Thrombin Time

Td Shots
See Tetanus

Team Conference
Case Management Services . . . 99366-99368

Tear Duct
See Lacrimal Duct

Tear Film Imaging . . . 0330T

Tear Gland
See Lacrimal Gland

Technique
Pericardial Window
See Pericardiostomy
Projective
See Projective Test

Teeth
X ray . . . 70300-70320

Telangiectasia
Chromosome Analysis . . . 88248
Sclerotherapy . . . 36465, 36466, 36468, 36470, 36471

Telangiectasia, Cerebello-Oculocutaneous
See Ataxia Telangiectasia

Telephone
Consultation
Interprofessional . . . 99446-99449, 99451, 99452
Evaluation and Management
Nonphysician . . . 98966-98968
Physician . . . 99441-99443
Pacemaker Analysis . . . 93293

Teletherapy
Dose Plan . . . 77306, 77307

Temperature Gradient Studies . . . 93740

Temporal Arteries
See Artery, Temporal

Temporal Bone
Electromagnetic Bone Conduction Hearing Device
Implantation/Replacement . . . 69710
Removal/Repair . . . 69711

Excision ... 69535
Resection ... 69535
Tumor
  Removal ... 69970
Unlisted Services and Procedures ... 69979

Temporal, Petrous
Excision
  Apex ... 69530

Temporomandibular Joint (TMJ)
Arthrocentesis ... 20605, 20606
Arthrography ... 70328-70332
  Injection ... 21116
Arthroplasty ... 21240-21243
Arthroscopy
  Diagnostic ... 29800
  Surgical ... 29804
Arthrotomy ... 21010
Cartilage
  Excision ... 21060
Condylectomy ... 21050
Coronoidectomy ... 21070
Dislocation
  Closed Treatment ... 21480-21485
  Open Treatment ... 21490
Injection
  Radiological ... 21116
Magnetic Resonance Imaging (MRI) ... 70336
Manipulation ... 21073
Meniscectomy ... 21060
Prostheses
  See Prosthesis, Temporomandibular Joint
Reconstruction
  See Reconstruction, Temporomandibular Joint
X ray with Contrast ... 70328-70332

Tenago Procedure ... 53431

Tendinosuture
See Suture, Tendon

Tendon
Achilles
  See Achilles Tendon
Arm, Upper
  Revision ... 24320
Biceps
  Reinsertion ... 24342
  Resection ... 23440
  Tenodesis ... 23430, 29828
  Transplantation ... 23440
Excision
  Finger ... 26180
  Forearm ... 25109
  Palm ... 26170
  Wrist ... 25109
Finger
  Excision ... 26180
Forearm
  Excision ... 25109
  Repair ... 25260-25274
Fixation
  Biceps ... 23430, 29828
Graft
  Harvesting ... 20924
Insertion
  Biceps Tendon ... 24342
Lengthening
  Ankle ... 27685, 27686
  Arm, Upper ... 24305
  Elbow ... 24305
  Finger ... 26476, 26478
  Forearm ... 25280
  Hand ... 26476, 26478
  Leg, Lower ... 27685, 27686
  Leg, Upper ... 27393-27395
  Toe ... 28240
  Wrist ... 25280
Palm
  Excision ... 26170
Release
  Arm, Lower ... 25295
  Arm, Upper ... 24332
  Wrist ... 25295
Resection
  Biceps ... 23440
Shortening
  Ankle ... 27685, 27686
  Finger ... 26477, 26479
  Hand ... 26477, 26479
  Leg, Lower ... 27685, 27686
Transfer
  Arm, Lower ... 25310-25312, 25316
  Arm, Upper ... 24301
  Elbow ... 24301
  Finger ... 26497, 26498
  Hand ... 26480-26489
  Leg, Lower ... 27690-27692
  Leg, Upper ... 27400
  Pelvis ... 27098
  Thumb ... 26490-26492, 26510
  Wrist ... 25310-25312, 25316
Transplant
  Biceps ... 23440
  Leg, Upper ... 27396, 27397
Wrist
  Excision ... 25109
  Repair ... 25260-25274

Tendon Origin
Insertion
  Injection ... 20551

Tendon Pulley Reconstruction of Hand
See Hand, Reconstruction, Tendon Pulley

Tendon Sheath
Arm
  Lower
    Repair ... 25275
Finger
  Incision ... 26055
  Incision and Drainage ... 26020
  Lesion ... 26160
Foot
  Excision ... 28086-28088
Hand Lesion ... 26160
Injection ... 20550
Palm
  Incision and Drainage ... 26020
Removal
  Foreign Body ... 20520-20525
Wrist
  Excision, Radical ... 25115, 25116
  Incision ... 25000, 25001
  Repair ... 25275

Tenectomy, Tendon Sheath
See Excision, Lesion, Tendon Sheath

Tennis Elbow
Tenotomy ... 24357-24359

Tenodesis
Biceps Tendon
  Arthroscopic ... 29828
  at Elbow ... 24340
  Shoulder ... 23430
Finger ... 26471-26474
Wrist ... 25300, 25301

Tenolysis
Ankle ... 27680, 27681
Arm, Lower ... 25295
Arm, Upper ... 24332
Finger
  Extensor ... 26445-26449
  Flexor ... 26440-26442
Foot ... 28220-28226
Hand Extensor ... 26445-26449
  Flexor ... 26440-26442
Leg, Lower ... 27680, 27681
Wrist ... 25295

Tenomyotomy
Shoulder ... 23405, 23406

Tenon's Capsule
Injection ... 67515

Tenoplasty
Anesthesia ... 01714

Tenorrhaphy
See Suture, Tendon

Tenosuspension
See Tenodesis

Tenosuture
See Suture, Tendon

Tenotomy
Achilles Tendon ... 27605, 27606
Ankle ... 27605, 27606
Arm, Lower ... 25290
Arm, Upper ... 24310
Elbow ... 24357-24359
Finger ... 26060, 26455-26460
Foot ... 28230, 28234
Hand ... 26450, 26460
Hip
  Abductor ... 27006
  Adductor ... 27000-27003
  Iliopsoas Tendon ... 27005
Leg, Upper ... 27306, 27307, 27390-27392
Toe ... 28010, 28011, 28232-28234, 28240
Wrist ... 25290

TENS
See Application, Neurostimulation; Physical Medicine/Therapy/Occupational Therapy

Tension, Ocular
See Glaucoma

Termination, Pregnancy
See Abortion

Test
Antiglobulin
  See Coombs Test
Aphasia
  See Aphasia Testing
Bender Visual-Motor Gestalt
  See Bender-Gestalt Test
Binet
  See Binet Test
Blood
  See Blood Tests
Blood Coagulation
  See Coagulation
Breath
  See Breath Test
Cervical Mucus Penetration
  See Cervical Mucus Penetration Test
Clinical Chemistry
  See Pathology and Laboratory, Chemistry

Index

Complement Fixation
See Complement, Fixation Test
Exercise
See Exercise Stress Tests
Fern
Cervical Smear....88155
Fetal
Amniotic Fluid....84112
Nonstress
See Fetal Non-Stress Test
Function, Vestibular
See Vestibular Function Tests
Gel Diffusion
See Immunodiffusion
Glucose Tolerance
See Glucose, Tolerance Test
Hearing
See Audiologic Function Tests
Hemagglutination Inhibition
See Hemagglutination Inhibition Test
Ink Blot
See Rorschach Test
Intelligence
See Intelligence Test
Lung Function
See Pulmonology, Diagnostic
Neutralization
See Neutralization Test
Papanicolaou
See Pap Smears
Pregnancy
See Pregnancy Test
Quick
See Prothrombin Time
Radioimmunosorbent
See Gammaglobulin, Blood
Rorschach
See Rorschach Test
Schilling
See Schilling Test
Skin
See Skin, Tests
Stanford-Binet
See Psychiatric Diagnosis
Tuberculin
See Skin, Tests, Tuberculosis

Test Tube Fertilization
See In Vitro Fertilization

Tester, Color Vision
See Color Vision Examination

Testes
Cryopreservation....89335
Nuclear Medicine
Imaging....78761
Undescended
See Testis, Undescended

Testicular Vein
See Spermatic Veins

Testimony, Medical....99075

Testing, Histocompatibility
See Tissue, Typing

Testing, Neuropsychological
See Neuropsychological Testing

Testing, Range of Motion
See Range of Motion Test

Testis
Abscess
Incision and Drainage....54700
Biopsy....54500-54505
Excision
Laparoscopic....54690
Partial....54522
Radical....54530-54535
Simple....54520
Hematoma
Incision and Drainage....54700
Insertion
Prosthesis....54660
Lesion
Excision....54512
Needle Biopsy....54500
Repair
Injury....54670
Suspension....54620-54640
Torsion....54600
Suture
Injury....54670
Suspension....54620-54640
Transplantation
to Thigh....54680
Tumor
Excision....54530-54535
Undescended
Exploration....54550-54560
Unlisted Services and Procedures....54699, 55899

Testosterone....84402
Response....80414
Stimulation....80414, 80415
Total....84403

Testosterone Estradiol Binding Globulin
See Globulin, Sex Hormone Binding

Tetanus....86280
Antibody....86774
Immunoglobulin....90389
Vaccine
See Vaccines and Toxoids

Tetrachloride, Carbon
See Carbon Tetrachloride

Tetralogy of Fallot....33692-33697, 33924

Thal-Nissen Procedure....43325

Thawing
See Frozen Blood Preparation
Cryopreserved
Embryo....89352
Oocytes....89356
Reproductive Tissue....89354
Sperm....89353
Previously Frozen Cells....38208, 38209

Thawing and Expansion
of Frozen Cell....88241

THBR
See Thyroid Hormone Binding Ratio

Theleplasty
See Nipples, Reconstruction

Theophylline
Assay....80198

Therapeutic
Abortion
See Abortion, Therapeutic
Apheresis
See Apheresis, Therapeutic
Drug Assay
See Therapeutic Drug Assay
Mobilization
See Mobilization
Photopheresis
See Photopheresis
Radiology
See Radiation Therapy

Therapeutic Drug Assay
Amikacin....80150
Amitriptyline....80335-80337
Benzodiazepine....80346, 80347
Caffeine....80155
Carbamazepine....80156, 80157
Clozapine....80159
Cyclosporine....80158
Desipramine....80335-80337
Digoxin....80162, 80163
Dipropylacetic Acid....80164, 80165
Doxepin....80335-80337
Ethosuximide....80168
Everolimus....80169
Gabapentin....80171
Gentamicin....80170
Gold....80375
Haloperidol....80173
Imipramine....80335-80337
Lamotrigine....80175
Levetiracetam....80177
Lidocaine....80176
Lithium....80178
Mycophenolate (mycophenolic acid)....80180
Nortriptyline....80335-80337
Oxcarbazepine....80183
Phenobarbital....80184
Phenytoin....80185, 80186
Primidone....80188
Procainamide....80190-80192
Quantitative
Other....80299
Quinidine....80194
Salicylate....80329-80331
Sirolimus....80195
Tacrolimus....80197
Theophylline....80198
Tiagabine....80199
Tobramycin....80200
Topiramate....80201
Vancomycin....80202
Zonisamide....80203

Therapies
Cold
See Cryotherapy
Exercise
See Exercise Therapy
Family
See Psychotherapy, Family of Patient
Language
See Language Therapy
Milieu
See Environmental Intervention
Occupational
See Occupational Therapy
Photodynamic
See Photochemotherapy
Photoradiation
See Actinotherapy
Physical
See Physical Medicine/Therapy/Occupational Therapy
Speech
See Speech Therapy

Tocolytic
See Tocolysis
Ultraviolet
See Actinotherapy

Therapy
ACE Inhibitor Therapy
See Performance Measures
Beta Blocker Therapy
See Performance Measures
CAR-T Cell. 0537T-0540T
Desensitization
See Allergen Immunotherapy
Hemodialysis
See Hemodialysis
Hot Pack
See Hot Pack Treatment
Pharmacologic; for Cessation of Tobacco Use
See Performance Measures
Radiation
Brachytherapy 77767, 77768, 77770-77772, 0394T, 0395T
Speech
See Speech Therapy
Statin Therapy, Prescribed
See Performance Measures

Thermocauterization
Ectropion
Repair. 67922
Lesion
Cornea 65450

Thermocoagulation
See Electrocautery

Thermotherapy
Microwave
Prostate Tissue 53850
Radiofrequency. 53852, 53854
Prostate Tissue 53852

Thiamine. 84425

Thiersch Operation 15050
See Pinch Graft

Thiersch Procedure 46753

Thigh
Fasciotomy 27025
See Femur; Leg, Upper

Thin Layer Chromatographies
See Chromatography, Thin-Layer

Thiocyanate 84430

Third Disease
See Rubella

Thompson Procedure. 27430

Thoracectomy
See Thoracoplasty

Thoracentesis 32554, 32555
with Imaging Guidance. 32555

Thoracic
Anterior Ramus
See Intercostal Nerve
Aorta
See Aorta, Thoracic
Arteries
See Artery, Thoracic
Cavity
See Chest Cavity
Duct
See Lymphatics
Cannulation 38794
Ligation 38380
Abdominal Approach 38382
Thoracic Approach 38381
Suture
Abdominal Approach 38382
Cervical Approach 38380
Thoracic Approach 38381
Empyema
See Pleural Cavity, Incision, Empyema
Surgery
Video-Assisted
See Thoracoscopy
Vertebra
See Vertebra, Thoracic
Wall
See Chest Wall

Thoracocentesis
See Thoracentesis

Thoracoplasty 32905
with Closure Bronchopleural Fistula. 32906

Thoracoscopy
Diagnostic
with Biopsy 32604, 32606, 32607-32609
without Biopsy. 32601
Surgical. 32650-32674
with Control Traumatic Hemorrhage. . . . 32654
with Creation Pericardial Window 32659
with Diagnostic Wedge Resection 32668
with Esophagomyotomy. 32665
with Excision Mediastinal Cyst, Tumor and/or Mass. 32662
with Excision Pericardial Cyst, Tumor and/or Mass. 32661
with Lobectomy 32663
with Mediastinal Lymphadenectomy . . . 32674
with Open Treatment of Rib Fracture
Internal Fixation Placement . . . 21811-21813
with Parietal Pleurectomy 32656
with Partial Pulmonary Decortication . . . 32651
with Pleurodesis 32650
with Regional Lymphadenectomy 32674
with Removal Intrapleural Foreign Body. 32653
with Removal of Clot/Foreign Body. 32658
with Resection of Thymus 32673
with Resection-Plication of Bullae 32655
with Sternum Reconstruction 21743
with Therapeutic Wedge Resection. 32666, 32667
with Thoracic Sympathectomy 32664
with Total Pulmonary Decortication 32652

Thoracostomy
Drainage 32551
Empyema. 32035, 32036
Hemothorax. 32551
Tube 32551

Thoracotomy
Cardiac Massage 32160
Lymphadenectomy
Thoracic 38746
for Post-Op Complications 32120
Hemorrhage 32110
Removal
Bullae. 32141
Cyst 32140
Defibrillator 33243
Electrodes 33238
Foreign Body
Intrapleural. 32150
Intrapulmonary. 32151
Pacemaker. 33236, 33237
Repair
Paraesophageal Hiatal Hernia. . . 43334, 43335
Resection
Diagnostic Wedge. 32507
Therapeutic Wedge 32505, 32506
Transmyocardial Laser
Revascularization 33140, 33141
with Biopsy. 32096, 32097
with Lung Repair. 32110
with Open Intrapleural Pneumolysis. 32124
with Resection-Plication of Bullae 32141

Thorax
See Chest; Chest Cavity; Mediastinum
Angiography 71275
Biopsy 21550
CT Scan. 71250-71275
Incision
Empyema 32035, 32036
Incision and Drainage
Abscess 21501, 21502
Deep. 21510
Hematoma 21501, 21502
Stereotactic Body Radiation Therapy
Target Delineation. 32701
Strapping. 29200
Tube Thoracostomy. 32551
Tumor
Excision 21552-21558
Excision/Resection. 21557, 21558
Unlisted Services and Procedures, Surgery . . 21899

Three Glass Test
See Urinalysis, Glass Test

Three-Day Measles
See Rubella

Throat
See Pharynx
Abscess
Incision and Drainage 42700-42725
Biopsy 42800-42806
Hemorrhage 42960-42962
Reconstruction 42950
Removal
Foreign Body 42809
Repair
Pharyngoesophageal 42953
Wound 42900
Suture
Wound 42900
Unlisted Services and Procedures 42999

Thrombectomy
See Thromboendarterectomy
Aortoiliac Artery 34151-34201
Arteriovenous Fistula
Graft. 36830-36833
Axillary Artery. 34101
Axillary Vein 34490
Brachial Artery 34101
Bypass Graft
Other than Hemodialysis Graft or Fistula. 35875, 35876
Carotid Artery 34001
Celiac Artery 34151
Dialysis Graft 36831, 36833
Femoral 34201
Femoropopliteal Vein 34421-34451
Iliac 34151-34201
Iliac Vein 34401-34451

Innominate Artery 34001-34101
Mesentery Artery 34151
Percutaneous
  Coronary Artery 92973
  Dialysis Circuit 36904-36906
  Fluoroscopic Guidance 37184-37188
  Intracranial Artery 61645
  Mechanical Arterial 37184-37186
  Mechanical Venous 37187, 37188
  Noncoronary Artery 37184-37186
Peroneal Artery 34203
Popliteal Artery 34201-34203
Radial Artery 34111
Renal Artery 34151
Subclavian Artery 34001-34101
Subclavian Vein 34471-34490
Tibial Artery 34203
Ulnar Artery 34111
Vena Cava 34401-34451
Vena Caval 50230

Thrombin Inhibitor I
See Antithrombin III

Thrombin Time 85670-85675

Thrombocyte (Platelet)
See Blood, Platelet

Thrombocyte ab
See Antibody, Detection, Platelet

Thromboendarterectomy
See Thrombectomy
Aorta, Abdominal 35331
Aortoiliofemoral Artery 35363
Axillary Artery 35321
Brachial Artery 35321
Carotid Artery 35301, 35390
Celiac Artery 35341
Femoral Artery 35302, 35371, 35372
Iliac Artery 35351, 35361-35363
Iliofemoral Artery 35355, 35363
Innominate Artery 35311
Mesenteric Artery 35341
Peroneal Artery 35305, 35306
Popliteal Artery 35303
Renal Artery 35341
Subclavian Artery 35301, 35311
Superficial Femoral Artery 35302
Tibial Artery 35305, 35306
Tibioperoneal Trunk Artery 35304
Vertebral Artery 35301

Thrombokinase 85260

Thrombolysin
See Plasmin

Thrombolysis
See also Clot, Declotting
Arterial
  Intracranial
    Transcatheter Infusion 37211, 37195
    Percutaneous Transluminal 61645
  Other Than Coronary
    Transcatheter Infusion 37211, 37213
Cerebral
  Infusion
    Intravenous 37195
Cessation 37214
Coronary Vessels
  Infusion 92975, 92977
Cranial Vessels
  Infusion 37195
Dialysis Circuit 36904-36906
Infusion
  Arterial 37211-37214, 37195
  Dialysis Circuit 36904-36906
Transcatheter Therapy 37211-37214

Thrombolysis Biopsy Intracranial
Arterial Perfusion 61624

Thrombolysis Intracranial 65205
See Ciliary Body; Cornea; Eye, Removal, Foreign Body; Iris; Lens; Retina; Sclera; Vitreous

Thrombomodulin 85337

Thromboplastin
Inhibition 85705
Inhibition Test 85347
Partial Thromboplastin Time (PTT) ... 85730-85732

Thromboplastin Antecedent, Plasma
See Plasma Thromboplastin, Antecedent

Thromboplastinogen
See Clotting Factor

Thromboplastinogen B
See Christmas Factor

Thromboxane
Urine 84431

Thumb
Amputation 26910-26952
Arthrodesis
  Carpometacarpal Joint 26841, 26842
Dislocation
  with Fracture 26645-26650
    Open Treatment 26665
Fracture
  with Dislocation 26645-26650
    Open Treatment 26665
Fusion
  in Opposition 26820
Reconstruction
  from Finger 26550
  Opponensplasty 26490-26496
Repair
  Muscle 26508
  Muscle Transfer 26494
  Tendon Transfer 26510
Replantation 20824-20827
Sesamoidectomy 26185
Unlisted Services and Procedures 26989

Thymectomy
Partial 60520-60522
Sternal Split/Transthoracic Approach 60521, 60522
Total 60520-60522
Transcervical Approach 60520

Thymotaxin
See Beta-2-Microglobulin

Thymus Gland
Excision 60520, 60521
Resection
  Thoracoscopic 32673

Thyrocalcitonin
See Calcitonin

Thyroglobulin 84432
Antibody 86800

Thyroglossal Duct
Cyst
  Excision 60280, 60281

Thyroid Gland
Cyst
  Aspiration 60300
  Excision 60200
  Incision and Drainage 60000
  Injection 60300
Excision
  for Malignancy
    Limited Neck Dissection 60252
    Radical Neck Dissection 60254
  Partial 60210-60225
  Secondary 60260
  Total 60240, 60271
    Cervical Approach 60271
    Removal All Thyroid Tissue 60260
    Sternal Split/Transthoracic Approach 60270
    Transcervical Approach 60520
Metastatic Cancer
  Nuclear Imaging 78015-78018
Needle Biopsy 60100
Nuclear Medicine
  Imaging for Metastases 78015-78018
  Imaging with Flow 78013
  Metastases Uptake 78020
  Uptake 78012, 78014
Procalcitonin 84145
Tumor
  Excision 60200

Thyroid Hormone Binding Ratio 84479

Thyroid Hormone Uptake 84479

Thyroid Stimulating Hormone (TSH) 80418, 80438, 80439, 84443

Thyroid Stimulating Hormone Receptor ab
See Thyrotropin Releasing Hormone (TRH)

Thyroid Stimulating Immune Globulins 84445

Thyroid Stimulator, Long Acting
See Thyrotropin Releasing Hormone (TRH)

Thyroid Suppression Test
Nuclear Medicine
  Thyroid, Uptake 78012, 78014

Thyroidectomy
Partial 60210-60225
Secondary 60260
Total 60240, 60271
  Cervical Approach 60271
  for Malignancy
    Limited Neck Dissection 60252
    Radical Neck Dissection 60254
  Removal All Thyroid Tissue 60260
  Sternal Split/Transthoracic Approach ... 60270

Thyrolingual Cyst
See Cyst, Thyroglossal Duct

Thyrotomy 31300

Thyrotropin Receptor Ab
See Thyrotropin Releasing Hormone (TRH)

Thyrotropin Releasing Hormone (TRH) 80438, 80439

Thyroxine
Free 84439
Neonatal 84437
Total 84436
True 84436

Thyroxine Binding Globulin 84442

Tiagabine
Drug Assay ... 80199

Tibia
See Ankle
Arthroscopy Surgical ... 29891, 29892
Artery
  Thrombectomy ... 34203
  Thromboendarterectomy ... 35305, 35306
Axial Bone Density
  Pulse-Echo Ultrasound ... 0508T
Craterization ... 27360, 27640
Cyst
  Excision ... 27635-27638
Diaphysectomy ... 27360, 27640
Excision ... 27360, 27640
  Epiphyseal Bar ... 20150
Fracture
  Arthroscopic Treatment ... 29855, 29856
    Plafond ... 29892
  Closed Treatment ... 27824, 27825
  Distal ... 27824-27828
  Intercondylar ... 27538-27540
  Malleolus ... 27760-27766, 27808-27814
  Open Treatment ... 27535, 27536, 27758, 27759, 27826-27828
  Plateau ... 29855, 29856
    Closed Treatment ... 27530-27536
  Shaft ... 27752-27759
  with Manipulation ... 27825
  without Manipulation ... 27824
Incision 27607, 27455-27457, 27705, 27709-27712
Manipulation .. 27532, 27752, 27762, 27768, 27825
Neurostimulation
  Posterior ... 64566
Osteoplasty
  Lengthening ... 27715
Prophylactic Treatment ... 27745
Reconstruction ... 27418
  at Knee ... 27440-27443, 27446
Repair ... 27720-27725
  Epiphysis ... 27477-27485, 27730-27742
  Malunion/Nonunion ... 27720, 27722, 27724, 27725
  Osteochondritis Dissecans
  Arthroscopy ... 29892
  Osteotomy 27455-27457, 27705, 27709-27712
  Pseudoarthrosis ... 27727
  Realignment ... 27712
  Skeletal Traction
    See Skeletal Traction, Tibia Fracture
  Tubercleplasty ... 27418
Revascularization ... 37228-37235
Saucerization ... 27360, 27640
Tibiofibular Joint
  Arthrodesis ... 27871
  Dislocation ... 27830-27832
  Disruption ... 27829
Tumor
  Excision ... 27635-27638
  Radical Resection ... 27645
X ray ... 73590

Tibial
Arteries
  See Artery, Tibial
Nerve
  Repair/Suture
    Posterior ... 64840

Tibiofibular Joint
Arthrodesis ... 27871
Dislocation ... 27830-27832
Disruption
  Open Treatment ... 27829
Fusion ... 27871

TIG
See Immune Globulins, Tetanus

Time
Bleeding
  See Bleeding, Time
Prothrombin
  See Prothrombin Time
Reptilase
  See Thrombin Time

Tinnitus
Assessment ... 92625

Tissue
Crystal Identification ... 89060
Culture
  Chromosome Analysis ... 88230-88239
  Homogenization ... 87176
  Non-neoplastic Disorder ... 88230, 88237
  Skin Grafts ... 15100, 15101, 15120, 15121
    Harvesting ... 15040
  Solid Tumor ... 88239
  Toxin/Antitoxin ... 87230
  Virus ... 87252, 87253
Dissection, Macroscopic ... 88387, 88388
Examination, Macroscopic ... 88387, 88388
Enzyme Activity ... 82657
Examination for Ectoparasites ... 87220
Examination for Fungi ... 87220
Expander
  Breast Reconstruction with ... 19357
  Insertion
    Skin ... 11960
  Removal
    Skin ... 11971
  Replacement
    Skin ... 11970
Grafts
  Harvesting ... 20926
Granulation
  See Granulation Tissue
Homogenization ... 87176
Hybridization In Situ ... 88364-88366
  Morphometric Analysis
    Computer-Assisted ... 88367, 88373, 88374
    Manual ... 88368, 88369, 88377
Implant
  Biological ... 15777
Mucosal
  See Mucosa
Preparation
  Macroscopic ... 88387, 88388
Previously Diagnosed/Archived
  Retrieved/Selected for Examination ... 88363
Skin Harvest for Culture ... 15040
Soft
  Drainage ... 10030
  Fluid Collection ... 10030
  Tumor
    See Tumor
Substitute ... 15271-15278
Transfer
  Adjacent
    Eyelids ... 67961
    Skin ... 14000-14350
  Facial Muscles ... 15845
  Finger Flap ... 14350
  Toe Flap ... 14350
Typing
  Culture ... 87140-87158
  Human Leukocyte Antigen (HLA)
    Antibodies ... 86812-86817
    Crossmatch ... 86825, 86826
  Lymphocyte Culture ... 86821

Tissue Culture
from Skin Harvest ... 15040
Skin Grafts ... 15150-15157

Tissue Factor
See Thromboplastin

TLC
See Chromatography, Thin-Layer
Screen ... 84375

TMJ
See Temporomandibular Joint (TMJ)
Manipulation, Therapeutic
  See Manipulation, Temporomandibular Joint(s) (TMJ)
Prostheses
  See Prosthesis, Temporomandibular Joint

TMS
See Psychiatric Treatment, Transcranial Magnetic Stimulation (TMS)

Tobacco
See Performance Measures

TMVR
See Transcatheter, Mitral Valve Repair

Tobramycin
Assay ... 80200

Tocolysis ... 59412

Tocopherol ... 84446

Toe
Amputation ... 28810-28825
Arthrocentesis ... 20600, 20604
Bone
  Condyle
    Excision ... 28126
  Craterization ... 28124
  Cyst
    Excision ... 28108
  Diaphysectomy ... 28124
  Excision ... 28150, 28810, 28820
    Joint ... 28160, 28825
    Partial ... 28124
    Proximal End ... 28160
  Fracture
    Closed Treatment ... 28510, 28515
    Open Treatment ... 28525
    with Manipulation ... 28515
    without Manipulation ... 28510
  Repair
    Osteotomy ... 28310-28312
  Resection
    Base ... 28126
    Condyle ... 28153
    with Macrodactyly Reconstruction ... 28341
  Saucerization ... 28124
  Transfer
    Joint ... 26556
    Toe-to-Hand ... 26553, 26554
  Tumor
    Excision ... 28108
    Radical Resection ... 28175
Capsulotomy ... 28270-28272
Dislocation
  See Dislocation, Toe
Fasciotomy ... 28008
Graft
  Bone ... 26551
  Flap ... 14350, 20973

Tendon 20974
Lesion
Excision 28092
Reconstruction
Angle Deformity 28313
Extra Toes 28344
Hammertoe 28285, 28286
Macrodactyly 28340, 28341
Polydactyly 28344
Syndactylization 28280
Syndactyly 28345
Webbed Toe 28345
Repair
Bunion 28292, 28295-28299
Cock-up Fifth 28286
Muscle 28240
Tendon 28232-28234, 28240
Webbed 28280
Webbed Toe 28345
Strapping 29550
Tendon
Graft 20924
Incision 28010, 28011, 28232-28234
Transfer
Toe-to-hand 26551, 26553, 26554
Tumor
Excision 28039, 28041, 28043, 28045
Radical Resection 28046, 28047
Unlisted Services and Procedures 28899

Toe Flap
Osteocutaneous with Web Space 20973
Tissue Transfer 14350

Tolerance Test
Glucagon 82946
Glucose 82951, 82952
Heparin-Protamine 85530
Insulin 80434, 80435
Maltose 82951, 82952

Tomodensitometries
See CT Scan

Tomographic Scintigraphy, Computed
See Emission Computerized Tomography

Tomographic SPECT
Myocardial Imaging 78469

Tomographies, Computed X ray
See CT Scan

Tomography, Computerized Axial
See CT Scan

Tomography, Emission Computed
See Positron Emission Tomography (PET)
Single Photon
See SPECT

Tomosynthesis, Breast, Digital 77061-77063

Tompkins Metroplasty 58540

Tongue
Abscess
Incision and Drainage 41000-41006, 41015
Base Suspension 41512
Biopsy 41100-41105
Cyst
Incision and Drainage 41000-41006, 41015, 60000
Excision
Complete 41140-41155
Frenum 41115
Partial 41120-41135
with Mouth Resection 41150-41153
with Radical Neck 41135, 41145, 41153-41155
Hematoma
Incision and Drainage 41000-41006, 41015
Incision
Frenum 41010
Lesion
Excision 41110-41114
Reconstruction
Frenum 41520
Repair
See Repair, Tongue
Laceration 41250-41252
Suture 41510
Suture 41510
Unlisted Services and Procedures 41599

Tonometry, Serial 92100

Tonsil, Pharyngeal
See Adenoids

Tonsillectomy 42820-42826

Tonsils
Abscess
Incision and Drainage 42700
Excision 42825, 42826
Lingual 42870
Radical 42842-42845
Tag 42860
with Adenoids 42820, 42821
Lingual
Destruction 42870
Unlisted Services and Procedures 42999

Topiramate
Assay 80201

Torek Procedure
See Orchiopexy

Torkildsen Procedure 62180

TORP (Total Ossicular Replacement Prosthesis) 69633, 69637

Torsion Swing Test 92546

Torula
See Cryptococcus

Torus Mandibularis
Tumor Excision 21031

Total
Abdominal Hysterectomy
See Hysterectomy, Abdominal, Total
Bilirubin Level
See Bilirubin, Total
Catecholamines
See Catecholamines, Urine
Cystectomy
See Bladder, Excision, Total
Dacryoadenectomy
See Dacryoadenectomy, Total
Elbow Replacement
See Replacement, Elbow, Total
Esophagectomy
See Esophagectomy, Total
Gastrectomy
See Gastrectomy
Hemolytic Complement
See Complement, Total Hemolytic
Hip Arthroplasty
See Hip, Total Replacement
Knee Arthroplasty
See Prosthesis, Knee
Mastectomies
See Mastectomy
Ostectomy of Patella
See Patellectomy
Splenectomy
See Splenectomy, Total

Total Body Surface Area (TBSA) Calculation
Initial Burn Treatment 16000

Touroff Operation 37615

Toxicology Screen 80305-80307

Toxin Assay 87230

Toxin, Botulinum
See Chemodenervation

Toxoplasma
Antibody 86777, 86778

Trabeculectomies
See Trabeculoplasty

Trabeculectomy ab Externo
in Absence of Previous Surgery 66170
with Scarring Previous Surgery 66172

Trabeculoplasty
by Laser Surgery 65855

Trabeculotomy
ab Externo 65850
Goniotomy 65820

Trachea
Aspiration 31612, 31629, 31720
Catheter 31720-31725
Decompression 33800
Dilation 31630, 31631, 31636-31638
Endoscopy
via Tracheostomy 31615
Excision
Stenosis 31780, 31781
Fistula 31755
with Plastic Repair 31825
without Plastic Repair 31820
Fracture
Endoscopy 31630
Incision
Emergency 31603-31605
Planned 31600, 31601
Fenestration with Flaps 31610
Introduction
Emergency Intubation 31500
Needle Wire 31730
Puncture
Aspiration and/or Injection 31612
Reconstruction
Carina 31766
Cervical 31750
Fistula 31755
Intrathoracic 31760
Repair
Cervical 31750
Fistula 31755
Intrathoracic 31760
Stoma 31613, 31614
Resection
Cricotracheal 31592
Revision
Stoma
Scars 31830
Scar
Revision 31830

Stenosis
  Excision . . . 31780, 31781
  Repair . . . 31780, 31781
Stent
  Placement . . . 31631
Stoma
  Repair
    with Plastic Repair . . . 31825
    without Plastic Repair . . . 31820
  Revision
    Scars . . . 31830
Tumor
  Excision
    Cervical . . . 31785
    Thoracic . . . 31786
Unlisted Services and Procedures
  Bronchi . . . 31899
Wound
  Suture
    Cervical . . . 31800
    Intrathoracic . . . 31805

Tracheal
Stent
  Placement . . . 31631
Tubes
  See Endotracheal Tube

Trachelectomy . . . 57530
Radical . . . 57531

Tracheloplasty
See Cervicoplasty

Trachelorrhaphy . . . 57720

Tracheo-Esophageal Fistula
Repair . . . 43305, 43312, 43314

Tracheobronchoscopy
through Tracheostomy . . . 31615

Tracheoplasty
Cervical . . . 31750
Intrathoracic . . . 31760
Tracheopharyngeal Fistulization . . . 31755

Tracheostoma
Revision . . . 31613, 31614

Tracheostomy
Emergency . . . 31603-31605
Fenestration with Flaps . . . 31610
Planned . . . 31600, 31601
Revision
  Scar . . . 31830
Surgical Closure
  with Plastic Repair . . . 31825
  without Plastic Repair . . . 31820
Tracheobronchoscopy through . . . 31615
with Laryngoplasty . . . 31584

Tracheotomy
Tube Change . . . 31502

Tracking Tests (Ocular) . . . 92545
See Ear, Nose, and Throat

Tract, Urinary
See Urinary Tract

Traction Therapy
See Physical Medicine/Therapy/Occupational Therapy
Manual . . . 97140
Mechanical . . . 97012

Training
Activities of Daily Living . . . 97535, 99509
Biofeedback . . . 90875, 90901-90911
Cognitive Skills . . . 97127
Community/Work Reintegration . . . 97537
Compensatory . . . 97127, 97535
Home Management . . . 97535, 99509
Orthoptic/Pleoptic . . . 92065
Orthotics . . . 97760, 97763
Prosthetics . . . 97761
Self Care . . . 97535, 98960-98962, 99509
Sensory Integration . . . 97533
Walking (Physical Therapy) . . . 97116
Wheelchair Management . . . 97542

TRAM Flap
Breast Reconstruction . . . 19367-19369

Trans-Scaphoperilunar
Fracture/Dislocation
  Closed Treatment . . . 25680
  Open Treatment . . . 25685

Transaminase
Glutamic-Oxaloacetic . . . 84450
Glutamic-Pyruvic . . . 84460

Transanal Endoscopic Microsurgery (TEMS)
See Rectum, Tumor, Excision, Transanal Endoscopic

Transcatheter Procedures
Aortic Valve Replacement
  See Transcatheter Aortic Valve Replacement (TAVR/TAVI)
Biopsy . . . 37200
Closure
  Cranial . . . 61624-61626
  Ductus Arteriosus . . . 93582
  Left Atrial Appendage . . . 33340
  Heart . . . 93580-93582
  Paravalvular Leak . . . 93590-93592
Delivery
  Chemical Adhesive . . . 36482, 36483
  Endograft Fixation Device . . . 34712
Denervation
  Renal Sympathetic . . . 0338T, 0339T
Embolization
  Cranial . . . 61624-61626
  Vascular . . . 37241-37244
Implantation
  Pulmonary Artery Pressure Sensor . . . 33289
Insertion
  Leadless Pacemaker System . . . 33274
Mitral Valve Implantation/Replacement (TMVI) . . . 0483T, 0484T
Mitral Valve Repair . . . 0345T, 33418, 33419
Occlusion
  Cranial . . . 61624-61626
  Paravalvular Leak
    Aortic Valve . . . 93591, 93592
    Mitral Valve . . . 93590, 93592
  Vascular . . . 37241-37244
Pulmonary Valve Implantation . . . 33477
Removal
  Leadless Pacemaker System . . . 33275
Replacement
  Leadless Pacemaker System . . . 33274
Retrieval
  Foreign Body (Fractured Catheter) . . . 37197
Stent Placement
  See Stent, Placement, Transcatheter
Therapy
  Embolization . . . 75894, 75898
  Infusion (Arterial or Venous) . . . 37211-37214, 61650, 61651
    Radiological Supervision . . . 75898
Perfusion
  Cranial . . . 61624-61626
Septal Reduction . . . 93583

Transcatheter Aortic Valve Replacement (TAVR/TAVI)
Axillary Artery Approach . . . 33363
Femoral Artery Approach . . . 33361, 33362
Iliac Artery Approach . . . 33364
Transaortic Approach . . . 33365
Transapical Exposure . . . 33366
with Cardiopulmonary Bypass Support . . . 33367-33369
with Arterial/Venous Cannulation . . . 33367-33369

Transcatheter Foreign Body
Retrieval . . . 37197

Transcortin . . . 84449

Transcranial
Doppler Study (TCP) . . . 93886-93893
Stimulation, Magnetic . . . 90867-90869
Stimulation, Motor . . . 95928, 95929

Transcutaneous Testing
Bilirubin . . . 88720
Carboxyhemoglobin . . . 88740
Hemoglobin (Hgb) . . . 88738
Unlisted In Vivo Procedure . . . 88749
Methemoglobin . . . 88741

Transcutaneous Electric Nerve Stimulation
See Application, Neurostimulation

Transdermal Electrostimulation
See Application, Neurostimulation

Transcutaneous Electrical Modulation Pain Reprocessing . . . 0278T

Transection
Artery
  Carotid . . . 61611
Blood Vessel
  Kidney . . . 50100
Brain
  Subpial . . . 61567
Nerve . . . 64732-64772
  Vagus . . . 43640, 43641
Pulmonary Artery . . . 33922

Transesophageal
Doppler Echocardiography . . . 93312-93318, 93355
  during Heart Procedure . . . 93355

Transfer
Blastocyst
  See Embryo Transfer
Gamete Intrafallopian
  See GIFT
Jejunum
  with Microvascular Anastomosis
    Free . . . 43496
Preparation
  Embryo . . . 89255
    Cryopreserved . . . 89352
Surgical
  See Transposition
Tendon
  See Tendon, Transfer
Finger . . . 26555
Toe Joint . . . 26556
Toe to Hand . . . 26551-26556

Transferase
Alanine Amino . . . 84460
Aspartate Amino . . . 84450

Index

Glutamic Oxaloacetic 84450

Transferrin 84466

Transformation
Lymphocyte 86353

Transfusion
Blood 36430
  Exchange 36455
    Newborn 36450, 36456
  Fetal 36460
  Push
    Infant 36440
Blood Parts
  Apheresis 36511-36516
Unlisted Services and Procedures 86999
White Blood Cells 86950

Transfusion of, Blood, Autologous
See Autotransfusion

Transluminal
Angioplasty
  Arterial
    Radiological Supervision 37246, 37247
Atherectomies
  See Artery, Atherectomy
Coronary Balloon Dilatation
  See Percutaneous Transluminal Angioplasty
Stent Placement
  See Stent, Transluminal Placement

Transmyocardial Laser Revascularization 33140, 33141

Transosteal Bone Plate
Reconstruction
  Mandible 21244

Transpeptidase, Gamma-Glutamyl
See Gamma Glutamyl Transferase

Transplant
See Graft
Bone
  See Bone Graft
Hair
  See Hair, Transplant

Transplantation
See Graft
Allogeneic
  Cornea
    See Homograft, Cornea
  Skin
    See Homograft, Skin Substitute
Autologous
  See Autograft
Bone Marrow 38240-38242
Cartilage
  Knee
    Allograft 27415, 29867
    Autograft 27412, 29866
Chondrocytes
  Knee 27412
Conjunctiva 65782
Cornea
  Autograft/Homograft
    Allograft Preparation 0290T, 65757
    Endothelial 65756
    Epikeratoplasty 65767
    Keratophakia 65765
    Lamellar 65710
    Penetrating 65730-65755
Eye
  Amniotic Membrane 65778-65780
  Conjunctiva 65782
  Stem Cell 65781
Fecal Microbiota
  Preparation of Specimen 44705
Hair
  Punch Graft 15775, 15776
  Strip 15220, 15221
Heart 33945
  Allograft Preparation 33933, 33944
Heart-Lung 33935
Heterologous
  See Allograft, Skin Substitute
Intestines
  Allograft Preparation 44715-44721
  Donor Enterectomy 44132, 44133
  Removal of Allograft 44137
Liver 47135
  Allograft Preparation 47143-47147
  Allotransplantation 47135
    Heterotopic 47399
Lung
  Allograft Preparation 0494T, 32855, 32856, 33933
  Anesthesia 00580
  Donor Pneumonectomy 32850
  Double, with Cardiopulmonary Bypass 32854
  Double, without Cardiopulmonary Bypass 32853
  Initiation and Monitoring, Cadaver 0495T-0496T
  Single, with Cardiopulmonary Bypass 32852
  Single, without Cardiopulmonary Bypass 32851
Meniscus
  Knee 29868
Muscle
  See Muscle Flaps
Pancreas 48160, 48550, 48554-48556
  Allograft Preparation 48551, 48552
Parathyroid 60512
Renal
  Allograft Preparation 50323-50329
  Allotransplantation 50360
    with Recipient Nephrectomy 50365
  Autotransplantation 50380
  Donor Nephrectomy 50300-50320, 50547
  Recipient Nephrectomy 50340
  Removal Transplanted Renal Allograft 50370
Skin
  See Homograft, Skin Substitute
Stem Cells 38240-38242
  Cell Concentration 38215
  Cryopreservation 38207
  Harvesting 38205, 38206
  Plasma Depletion 38214
  Platelet Depletion 38213
  Red Blood Cell Depletion 38212
  T-Cell Depletion 38210
  Thawing 38208, 38209
  Tumor Cell Depletion 38211
  Washing 38209
Testis
  to Thigh 54680
Tendon 23440, 24301, 25310-25312
Tissue, Harvesting
  See Graft, Tissue, Harvesting

Transpleural Thoracoscopy
See Thoracoscopy

Transposition
Arteries
  Carotid 33889, 35691, 35694, 35695
  Subclavian 33889, 35693-35695
  Vertebral 35691-35693
Cranial Nerve 64716
Eye Muscles 67320
Great Arteries
  Aortic Root (Nikaidoh Procedure) 33782, 33783
  Repair 33770-33781
Nerve 64718-64721
Ovary 58825
Peripheral Nerve
  Major 64856
Vein Valve 34510

Transthoracic Echocardiography
See Echocardiography

Transthyretin
See Prealbumin

Transureteroureterostomy 50770

Transurethral Procedure
Bladder Neck
  Resection 52500
Cystourethroscopy
  See Cystourethroscopy
Female Bladder Neck
  Radiofrequency Remodeling 53860
Litholapaxy 52317, 52318
Prostate
  Abscess Drainage 52700
  Destruction
    Microwave Thermotherapy 53850
    Radiofrequency 53852, 53854
  Incision 52450
  Resection 52601, 52630
Renal Pelvis
  Ureteral Stent Removal/Replacement 50385, 50386

Trapezium
Arthroplasty
  with Implant 25445

Travel, Unusual 99082

Treacher-Collins Syndrome
Midface Reconstruction 21150, 21151

Treatment, Tocolytic
See Tocolysis

Tremor Measurement
Monitor 0533T-0536T
with Accelerometer(s), Gyroscopes 95999

Trendelenburg Operation
See Leg, Vein, Ligation

Trephine Procedure
Sinusotomy
  Frontal 31070

Treponema Pallidum 86780
Antigen Detection
  Direct Fluorescence 87285

TRH
See Thyrotropin Releasing Hormone (TRH)

Triacylglycerol
See Triglycerides

Triacylglycerol Hydrolase
See Lipase

Tributyrinase
See Lipase

Trichiasis
Repair 67825
  Epilation, by Forceps 67820
  Epilation, by Other than Forceps 67825

Incision of Lid Margin 67830
with Free Mucous Membrane Graft. . . 67835

Trichina
See Trichinella

Trichinella
Antibody 86784
Trichogram 96902

Trichomonas Vaginalis
Antigen Detection
by Immunoassay with Direct Optical
Observation 87808
Nucleic Acid. 87660, 87661

Trichrome Stain. 88313

Tricuspid Valve
Excision 33460
Repair 33463-33465
Replacement 33465
Repositioning 33468

Tridymite
See Silica

Trigeminal Ganglia
See Gasserian Ganglion

Trigeminal Nerve
Chemodenervation 64615
Destruction 64600-64610
Injection
Anesthetic 64400
Neurolytic. 64600-64610

Trigeminal Tract
Stereotactic
Create Lesion 61791

Trigger Finger Repair 26055

Trigger Point
Injection
One or Two Muscles 20552
Two or More Muscles 20553

Triglyceridase
See Lipase

Triglyceride Lipase
See Lipase

Triglycerides. 84478

Trigonocephaly 21175

Triiodothyronine
Free 84481
Reverse 84482
Total 84480
True 84480

Triolean Hydrolase
See Lipase

Trioxopurine
See Uric Acid

Tripcellim
See Trypsin

Trisegmentectomy 47122

Trocar Biopsy
Bone 20220, 20225
Renal 50200

Trochanteric Femur Fracture
See Femur, Fracture, Trochanteric

Trophoblastic Tumor GTT
See Hydatidiform Mole

Troponin 84484
Qualitative. 84512
Quantitative 84484

Truncal Vagotomies
See Vagotomy, Truncal

Truncus Arteriosus
Repair 33786

Truncus Brachiocephalicus
See Artery, Brachiocephalic

Trunk, Brachiocephalic
See Artery, Brachiocephalic

Trypanosomiases
See Trypanosomiasis

Trypanosomiasis. 86171, 86280

Trypsin
Duodenum. 84485
Feces. 84488-84490

Trypsin Inhibitor, Alpha 1-Antitrypsin
See Alpha-1 Antitrypsin

Trypure
See Trypsin

Tsalicylate Intoxication
See Salicylate

TSH
See Thyroid Stimulating Hormone (TSH)

TSI
See Thyroid Stimulating Immune Globulins

Tsutsugamushi Disease
See Scrub Typhus

TT
See Thrombin Time

TT-3
See Triiodothyronine, True

TT-4
See Thyroxine, True

Tuba Auditoria (Auditiva)
See Eustachian Tube

Tubal Embryo Stage Transfer
See Embryo Transfer

Tubal Ligation 58600
Laparoscopic. 58670
with Cesarean Delivery. 58611

Tubal Occlusion
See Fallopian Tube, Occlusion
Create Lesion

Tubal Pregnancy. 59121
with Salpingectomy and/or Oophorectomy . . 59120

Tube Change
Colonic 49450
Duodenostomy 49451
Gastro-Jejunostomy 49452
Gastrostomy 43762, 43763, 49446
Jejunostomy 49451
Tracheostomy 31502

Tube Placement
Cecostomy Tube 44300, 49442
Duodenostomy Tube. 49441
Endoscopic
Bile Duct, Pancreatic Duct. 43274
Jejunostomy Tube
Percutaneous 49441

Nasobiliary, Nasopancreatic
for Drainage 43274
Enterostomy Tube 44300
Gastrostomy Tube. 43246, 49440
Nasogastric Tube 43752
Orogastric Tube. 43752
Renal Pelvis
with Tract Dilation 50436, 50437

Tube, Fallopian
See Fallopian Tube

Tubectomy
See Excision, Fallopian Tube

Tubed Pedicle Flap
Formation 15570-15576

Tubercle Bacilli
Culture. 87116

Tubercleplasty
Tibia
Anterior 27418

Tuberculin Test
See Skin, Tests, Tuberculosis

Tuberculosis
Antigen Response Test. 86480, 86481
Culture. 87116
Skin Test 86580

Tuberculosis Vaccine (BCG) . . 90585, 90586

Tubes
Colonic
See Colon
Duodenostomy
See Duodenostomy
Endotracheal
See Endotracheal Tube
Gastrostomy
See Gastrostomy Tube
Jejunostomy
See Jejunostomy

Tudor' Rabbit Ear'
See Urethra, Repair

Tummy Tuck
See Abdominoplasty

Tumor
See Craniopharyngioma
Abdomen
Destruction/Excision 49203-49205
Abdominal Wall
Excision 22900-22903
Radical Resection 22904, 22905
Acetabulum
Excision 27076
Ankle
Excision 27618, 27619, 27632, 27634
Radical Resection. 27615, 27616
Arm, Lower
Soft Tissue
Excision. 25071-25076
Radical Resection. 25077, 25078
Arm, Upper
Soft Tissue
Excision. 24071-24076
Radical Resection. 24077, 24079
Back/Flank
Excision 21930-21933
Radical Resection 21935, 21936
Bile Duct
Ablation 43278
Excision 47711, 47712

Index

Bladder 52234-52240
  Excision .. 51530, 52234, 52235, 52240, 52355
  Fulguration 52234, 52235, 52240
Bone
  Ablation
    with Adjacent Soft Tissue 20982, 20983
Brain 61510
  Excision 61518, 61520, 61521, 61526-61530, 61545, 62164
    Cerebellopontine Angle 61520, 61526, 61530
    Infratentorial 61518
    Midline 61521
    Supratentorial 61510
Breast
  Excision 19120-19126
  Intraoperative Radiation Therapy (IORT)
    Preparation of Tumor Cavity 19294
Bronchi
  Excision 31640
Calcaneus
  Excision 28100-28103
  Radical Resection 27647
Carpal
  Excision 25130-25136
Carotid Body
  Excision 60600, 60605
Cervix
  Excision 58550, 58555
Cheekbone 21030, 21034
Chest Wall
  Cryoablation 32994
  Excision 19260-19272
Clavicle
  Excision 23140, 23200
    with Allograft 23146
    with Autograft 23145
Coccyx 49215
Colon
  Destruction 44401, 45388
Colorectal
  Excision 45126
Cranial Bone
  Excision 61563, 61564
  Reconstruction 21181-21184
Dentoalveolar Structures
  Excision 41825-41827
Ear, Middle
  Excision 69550, 69552, 69554
Elbow
Excision 24071-24076
  Radical Resection 24077, 24079
Esophagus
  Ablation 43229
Face or Scalp
  Excision 21011-21014
  Radical Resection 21015, 21016
Facial Bone 21029, 21030, 21034-21040, 21046-21049
Fallopian Tube
  Resection 58950, 58952-58958
Femur 27065-27067
  Excision 27065-27067, 27327, 27328, 27337-27339, 27355-27358
  Resection 27365
Fibroid
  See Leiomyomata
Fibula
  Excision 27635-27638
  Radical Resection 27646
Finger
  Excision 26111-26116
  Radical Resection 26117, 26118
Foot
  Excision 28039-28045
  Radical Resection 28046, 28047
Forearm
  Excision 25071-25076
  Radical Resection 25077, 25078
Gastrostomy
  See Lesion
Gums
  Excision 41825-41827
Hand
  Excision 26111-26116
  Radical Resection 26117, 26118
Head
  Excision 21011-21016
Heart
  Excision 33120-33130
Hip
  Excision 27043-27048
  Radical Resection 27049, 27059, 27075, 27076
Humerus
  Excision 23150, 24110
  Radical Resection 23220, 24150, 27075-27078
    with Allograft 23156, 24116
    with Autograft 23155, 24115
Ileum 27065-27067
Immunoassay for Antigen 86294, 86316
  CA-125 86304
  CA 15-3 86300
  CA 19-9 86301
Innominate
  Excision 27077
Intestines, Small
  Destruction 44369
Ischial
  Radical Resection 27075, 27076, 27078
Kidney
  Ablation
    Radiofrequency 50592
  Excision 50562, 52355
Knee
  Excision 27327, 27328, 27337, 27339
  Radical Resection 27329, 27364
Lacrimal Gland
  Excision
    Frontal Approach 68540
    with Osteotomy 68550
Larynx
  Excision 31300
    Endoscopic 31540, 31541, 31578
  Incision 31300
Leg, Lower
  Excision 27618, 27619, 27632-27634
  Radical Resection 27615, 27616
Leg, Upper
  Excision 27327, 27328, 27337-27339
Localization
  Nuclear Medicine 78800-78804
Lung
  Excision 32503, 32504
Mandible
  Excision 21044-21047
Maxilla
  Excision 21030, 21034, 21048, 21049
Mediastinal
  Resection 39220
Mediastinum 32662
Meningioma 61512
  Excision 61519
Metacarpal
  Excision 26200-26205
  Radical Resection 26250
Metatarsal
  Excision 28104-28107
  Radical Resection 28173
Neck
  Excision 21552-21556
  Radical Resection 21557, 21558
Olecranon
  Excision 24120
Olecranon Process
  with Allograft
    Excision 24126
  with Autograft
    Excision 24125
Ovary
  Resection 58950-58958
Pancreatic Duct
  Ablation 43278
Parotid Gland
  Excision 42410-42426
Pelvis
  Excision 27043-27048
  Radical Resection 27049, 27059
Pericardial
  Endoscopic 32661
  Resection 33050
Peritoneum
  Excision 49203-49205
  Debulking 58575, 58950-58958
Phalanges
  Finger 26210-26215, 26260-26262
  Toe
    Excision 28108
    Radical Resection 28175
Pituitary Gland
  Excision 61546-61548, 62165
Pleura
  Cryoablation 32994
Positron Emission Tomography (PET) 78811-78816
Pubis 27065-27067
Pulmonary
  Ablation
  Cryoablation 32994
  Radiofrequency 32998
Radiation Therapy
  See Brachytherapy; Interstitial Radiation Therapy
Radius 25120-25126, 25170
  Excision 24120
  with Allograft
    Excision 24126
  with Autograft
    Excision 24125
Rectum
  Destruction 45190, 45320
  Excision 45160-45172
Renal
  Ablation 50593
Retroperitoneal
  Destruction/Excision 49203-49205
Sacrum 49215
Scapula
  Excision 23140, 23210
    with Allograft 23146
    with Autograft 23145
Shoulder
  Soft Tissue
    Excision 23071-23076
    Radical Resection 23077, 23078
Skin
  Mohs Micrographic Surgery 17311-17315
Skull
  Excision 61500

Spinal Cord
Excision 63275-63290
Stomach
Excision 43610, 43611
Talus
Excision 28100-28103
Radical Resection 27647
Tarsal
Excision 28104-28107
Radical Resection 28171
Temporal Bone
Removal 69970
Testis
Excision 54530-54535
Thigh
Excision 27327, 27328, 27337, 27339
Radical Resection 27329, 27364, 27365
Thorax
Excision 21552-21558
Radical Resection 21557, 21558
Thyroid
Excision 60200
Tibia 27365, 27635-27638
Radical Resection 27645
Toe
Excision 28039-28045
Radical Resection 28046, 28047
Torus Mandibularis 21031
Trachea
Excision
Cervical 31785
Thoracic 31786
Ulna 25120-25126, 25170
Excision 24120
with Allograft
Excision 24126
with Autograft
Excision 24125
Ureter
Excision 52355
Urethra
Excision 53220, 52355
Fulguration 52234-52240
Uterus
Excision 58140-58146
Resection 58950-58958
Vagina
Excision 57135
Vertebra
Additional Segment
Excision 22116
Cervical
Excision 22100
Lumbar 22102
Thoracic
Excision 22101
Wrist
Bone
Curettage 25130, 25135, 25136
Excision 25130, 25135, 25136
Radical Resection 25077, 25078
Subcutaneous
Excision 25071, 25075
Subfascial
Excision 25073, 25076

Tunica Vaginalis
Hydrocele
Aspiration 55000
Excision 55040, 55041
Repair 55060

Turbinate
Excision 30130-30140
Fracture
Therapeutic 30930
Injection 30200
Submucous Resection
Nose Excision 30140

Turbinate Mucosa
Cauterization 30801, 30802

Turcica, Sella
See Sella Turcica

TURP
See Prostatectomy, Transurethral

Tylectomy
See Breast, Excision, Lesion

Tympanic Membrane
Create Stoma 69433, 69436
Myringoplasty 69620
Myringotomy 69421
Neurectomy 69676
Repair 69610
Tympanolysis 69450
Tympanoplasty
See Tympanoplasty
Tympanostomy 69433, 69436
Removal of Tube 69424

Tympanic Nerve
Excision 69676

Tympanolysis 69450

Tympanomastoidectomy
See Tympanoplasty

Tympanometry 92550, 92567, 92570
See Audiologic Function Tests

Tympanoplasty
See Myringoplasty
with Ossicular Chain Reconstruction 69646
with Antrotomy or Mastoidotomy 69635
with Ossicular Chain Reconstruction 69636
and Synthetic Prosthesis 69637
with Mastoidectomy 69641
Radical or Complete 69645
with Intact or Reconstructed Wall 69643
and Ossicular Chain Reconstruction . . 69644
with Ossicular Chain Reconstruction 69642
without Mastoidectomy 69631
with Ossicular Chain Reconstruction 69632
and Synthetic Prosthesis 69633

Tympanostomy
Local Anesthetic 69433
General Anesthesia 69436
Removal of Tube 69424

Tympanotomy
See Myringotomy

Typhoid Vaccine
Oral 90690
Intramuscular 90691

Typhus
Endemic
See Murine Typhus
Mite-Borne
See Scrub Typhus
Sao Paulo
See Rocky Mountain Spotted Fever
Tropical
See Scrub Typhus

Typing, Blood
See Blood Typing, Serologic

Typing, HLA
See Human Leukocyte Antigen (HLA), Tissue Typing

Typing, Tissue
See Tissue, Typing

Tyrosine 84510

Tzank Smear 88160, 88161

U

UDP Galactose Pyrophosphorylase
See Galactose-1-Phosphate, Uridyl Transferase

UFR
See Uroflowmetry

Ulcer
Anal
See Anus, Fissure
Decubitus
Excision
Coccygeal 15920, 15922
Ischial 15940, 15941, 15944-15946
Sacral 15931, 15933-15937
Trochanteric . . . 15950-15953, 15956, 15958
Unlisted Procedure 15999
Pinch Graft 15050
Pressure 15920-15999
Stomach
Excision 43610

Ulcerative, Cystitis
See Cystitis, Interstitial

Ulna
See Arm, Lower; Elbow; Humerus; Radius
Arthrodesis
Radioulnar Joint
with Bone Graft 25830
with Resection 25830
Arthroplasty
with Implant 25442
Bone Graft 25830
Centralization or Wrist 25335
Craterization 24147, 25150, 25151
Cyst
Excision 24125, 24126, 25120-25126
Diaphysectomy 24147, 25150, 25151
Excision 24147
Abscess 24138
Complete 25240
Epiphyseal Bar 20150
Partial 25145-25151, 25240
Fracture
Closed Treatment 25530-25535
Olecranon 24670-24675
Open Treatment 24685, 25545
Shaft 25530-25545
Open Treatment 25574
Styloid
Closed Treatment 25650
Open Treatment 25652
Percutaneous Fixation 25651
with Dislocation
Closed Treatment 24620
Open Treatment 24635
with Manipulation 25535
with Radius 25560-25565
Open Treatment 25575
without Manipulation 25530
Incision and Drainage 25035

Index

Osteoplasty 25390-25393
Prophylactic Treatment 25491, 25492
Realignment 25370, 25375
Reconstruction
Radioulnar Joint 25337
Repair
Collateral Ligament 29902
Epiphyseal Arrest 25450-25455
Malunion or Nonunion 25400, 25415, 25415, 25420
Osteotomy 25360, 25370-25375
and Radius 25365
with Graft 25405, 25420-25426
Saucerization 24147, 25150, 25151
Sequestrectomy 24138, 25145
Tumor
Cyst 24120
Excision .. 24125, 24126, 25120-25126, 25170

Ulnar Arteries
See Artery, Ulnar

Ulnar Nerve
Decompression 64718
Neuroplasty 64718, 64719
Reconstruction 64718, 64719
Release 64718, 64719
Repair/Suture
Motor 64836
Transposition 64718, 64719

Ultrasonic
See Ultrasound

Ultrasonic Cardiography
See Echocardiography

Ultrasonic Procedure 52325

Ultrasonography
See Echography

Ultrasound
See Echocardiography; Ultrasound
3-D Rendering 76376, 76377
Not Requiring Independent Workstation .. 76376
Requiring Independent Workstation 76377
Abdomen 76700-76706
Aortic Aneurysm Screening 76706
Arm
Complete 76881
Limited 76882
Artery
Intracranial 93886-93893
Middle Cerebral 76821
Umbilical 76820
Bladder 51798
Bone Density Study 0508T, 76977
Breast 76641, 76642
Bronchi
Endobronchial Ultrasound (EBUS) 31652-31654
Chest 76604
Colon
Endoscopic 45391, 45392
Colon-Sigmoid
Endoscopic 45341, 45342
Computer-assisted Surgical Navigation
CT/MRI 0055T
Fluoroscopic 0054T
Drainage
Abscess 75989
Echoencephalography
See Echoencephalography
Elastography 76981-76983
Esophagus
Endoscopy 43231, 43232
Ultrasound Guided 43237, 43238, 43253
Eye 76510-76513
Biometry 76516-76519
Foreign Body 76529
Pachymetry 76514
Fetus 76818-76828
Follow-Up 76970
for Physical Therapy 97035
Gastrointestinal 76975
Gastrointestinal, Upper
Endoscopic 43237, 43238, 43242, 43259
Guidance
Amniocentesis 59001, 76946
Amnioinfusion 59070
Arteriovenous Fistulae 76936
Arthrocentesis
Intermediate Joint 20606
Major Joint 20611
Small Joint 20604
Biopsy
Breast 19083, 19084
Bone Marrow Cell Therapy 0263T-0265T
Chorionic Villus Sampling 76945
Cryosurgery 55873
Drainage
Fetal Fluid 59074
Endometrial Ablation 58356
Endoscopic Examination
Esophagus 43253
Stomach 43253
Fetal Cordocentesis 76941
Fetal Transfusion 76941
Heart Biopsy 76932
Needle Biopsy 43232, 43238, 43242, 45342, 45392, 76942
Occlusion
Umbilical Cord 59072
Ova Retrieval 76948
Pericardiocentesis 76930
Placement of Lesion Localization Device
Breast 19083, 19084, 19285, 19286
Pseudoaneurysm 76936
Radioelement 76965
Shunt Placement
Fetal 59076
Thoracentesis 76942
Tissue Ablation 76940
Uterine Fibroid Ablation 58674
Vascular Access 76937
Head 76506, 76536
Heart
Fetal 76825
Hips
Infant 76885, 76886
Hysterosonography 76831
Intraoperative 76998
Intravascular
Coronary Vessel or Graft
Endoluminal Imaging 92978, 92979
Noncoronary 37252, 37253
Kidney 76770-76776
Liver
Elastography, Shear Wave 91200
Magnetic Resonance Image Guided High Intensity Focused Ultrasound (MRgFUS) 0398T
Stereotactic Lesion Ablation
Intracranial 0398T
Neck 76536
Needle or Catheter Placement 20555
Noncoronary
Intravascular 37252, 37253
Obstetrical
Pregnant Uterus 76801, 76802, 76805, 76810-76817
Pelvis 76856, 76857
Prostate 76856, 76873
Rectal 76872, 76873
Retroperitoneal 76770-76775
Scrotum 76870
Sonohysterography 76831
Spine 76800
Therapy
to Aid Bone Healing 20979
to Aid Wound Healing 97605-97608
Umbilical Artery 76820
Unlisted Services and Procedures 76999
Uterus
Nonobstetrical ... 76830, 76831, 76856, 76857
Obstetrical 76801, 76802, 76805, 76810-76817
Tumor Ablation 0071T, 0072T
Vagina 76830
Wound Therapy 97610

Ultraviolet Light Therapy
Dermatology
Ultraviolet A 96912
Ultraviolet B 96910
for Dermatology 96900
for Physical Medicine 97028

Umbilectomy 49250

Umbilical
Artery Ultrasound 76820
Hernia
See Omphalocele
Vein Catheterization
See Catheterization, Umbilical Vein

Umbilical Cord
Occlusion 59072

Umbilicus
Excision 49250
Repair
Hernia 49580-49587
Omphalocele 49600-49611

Undescended Testicle
See Testis, Undescended

Unfertilized Egg
See Ova

Unguis
See Nails

Unilateral Simple Mastectomy
See Mastectomy

Unlisted Services and Procedures 99499, 99600
Abdomen 22999, 49329, 49999
Allergy/Immunology 95199
Anal 46999
Anesthesia 01999
Arm 25999
Arthroscopy 29999
Autopsy 88099
Bile Duct 47999
Bladder 51999
Brachytherapy 77799
Breast 19499
Bronchi 31899
Cardiac 33999
Cardiovascular Studies 93799
Casting 29799
Cervix 58999

Chemistry Procedure 84999
Chemotherapy 96549
Chest 32999
Coagulation 85999
Colon 45399
Conjunctiva Surgery 68399
Craniofacial 21299
CT Scan 76497
Cytogenetic Study 88299
Cytopathology 88199
Dermatology 96999
Dialysis 90999
Diaphragm 39599
Ear
　External 69399
　Inner 69949
　Middle 69799
Endocrine System 60699
Epididymis 55899
Esophagus 43289, 43499
Evaluation and Management Services 99499
Eye
　Extraocular Muscle 67399
Eye Surgery
　Anterior Segment 66999
　Posterior Segment 67299
Eyelid 67999
Fluoroscopy 76496
Forearm 25999
Gallbladder 47999
Gastroenterology Test 91299
Gum 41899
Hand 26989
Hemic System 38999
Hepatic Duct 47999
Hip Joint 27299
Home Services 99600
Hysteroscopy 58579
Immunization 90749
Immunology 86849
Infusion 96379
Injection 96379
Injection of Medication 96379
Intestine
　Laparoscopic 44238
　Small 44799
Kidney 53899
Lacrimal System 68899
Laparoscopy 38129, 38589, 43289, 43659, 44238, 44979, 47379, 47579, 49329, 49659, 50549, 50949, 54699, 55559, 58578, 58679, 59898, 60659
Larynx 31599
Lip 40799
Liver 47379, 47399
Lungs 32999
Lymphatic System 38999
Magnetic Resonance 76498
Maxillofacial 21299
Maxillofacial Prosthetics 21089
Meckel's Diverticulum 44899
Mediastinum 39499
Mesentery Surgery 44899
Microbiology 87999
Mouth 40899, 41599
Musculoskeletal 25999, 26989
Musculoskeletal Surgery
　Abdominal Wall 22999
　Neck 21899
　Spine 22899
　Thorax 21899
Musculoskeletal System 20999
　Ankle 27899
　Arm, Upper 24999
　Elbow 24999
　Head 21499
　Knee 27599
　Leg, Lower 27899
　Leg, Upper 27599
Necropsy 88099
Nervous System Surgery 64999
Neurology/Neuromuscular Testing 95999
Noninvasive Vascular Study 93998
Nose 30999
Nuclear Medicine 78999
　Blood 78199
　Bone 78399
　Endocrine System 78099
　Genitourinary System 78799
　Heart 78499
　Hematopoietic System 78199
　Lymphatic System 78199
　Musculoskeletal System 78399
　Nervous System 78699
　Therapeutic 79999
Obstetrical Care 59898, 59899
Omentum 49329, 49999
Ophthalmology 92499
Orbit 67599
Otorhinolaryngology 92700
Ovary 58679, 58999
Oviduct 58679, 58999
Palate 42299
Pancreas Surgery 48999
Pathology 89240
Pelvis 27299
Penis 55899
Peritoneum 49329, 49999
Pharynx 42999
Physical Therapy 97039, 97139, 97799
Pleura 32999
Pressure Ulcer 15999
Preventive Medicine 99429
Prostate 55899
Psychiatric 90899
Pulmonology 94799
Radiation Physics 77399
Radiation Therapy 77499
　Planning 77299
Radiology, Diagnostic 76499
Radionuclide Therapy 79999
Radiopharmaceutical Therapy 79999
Rectum 45499, 45999
Reproductive Medicine
　Laboratory Procedure 89398
Salivary Gland 42699
Scrotum 55899
Seminal Vesicle 55899
Shoulder Surgery 23929
Sinuses 31299
Skin 17999
Special Services and Reports 99199
Spine 22899
Stomach 43659, 43999
Strapping 29799
Surgical Pathology 88399
Temporal Bone 69979
Testis 54699, 55899
Throat 42999
Tongue 41599
Tonsil/Adenoid 42999
Toxoid 90749
Trachea 31899
Transfusion 86999
Ultrasound 76999
Ureter 50949
Urinary System 53899
Uterus 58578, 58579, 58999
Uvula 42299
Vaccine 90749
Vagina 58999
Vas Deferens 55899
Vascular 37799
Vascular Endoscopy 37501
Vascular Injection 36299
Vascular Studies 93799, 93998
Wrist 25999

Unna Paste Boot 29580
Removal 29700

UPP
See Urethra, Pressure Profile

Upper
Digestive System Endoscopy
　See Endoscopy, Gastrointestinal, Upper
Extremity
　See Arm, Upper; Elbow; Humerus
Gastrointestinal Bleeding
　See Gastrointestinal, Upper, Hemorrhage
Gastrointestinal Endoscopy, Biopsy
　See Biopsy
GI Tract
　See Gastrointestinal Tract, Upper

Urachal Cyst
See Cyst, Urachal

Urea Breath Test 78267, 78268, 83014

Urea Nitrogen
Blood 84520-84525
Clearance 84545
Quantitative 84520
Semiquantitative 84525
Urine 84540

Urea Nitrogen, Blood
See Blood Urea Nitrogen

Urecholine Supersensitivity Test
See Cystometrogram

Ureter
Anastomosis
　to Bladder 50780-50785
　to Colon 50810-50815
　to Intestine 50800, 50820-50825
　to Kidney 50740-50750
　to Ureter 50760-50770
Biopsy
　Endoluminal, Non-endoscopic 50606
　Endoscopic 50955, 50957, 50974, 50976, 52007
Catheterization 52005
　Construction 50840
　via Kidney 50693
Continent Diversion 50825
Creation
　Stoma 50860
Cystectomy 51580, 51590
Deligation 50940
Destruction
　Endoscopic 50957, 50976, 52354
Dilation 52341, 52342, 52344, 52345
　Balloon 50706
　Endoscopic 50553, 50572, 50953, 50972
Drainage 50600
Embolization 50705
Endoscopy
　Biopsy 50955-50957, 50974-50976, 52007, 52354
　Catheterization 50953, 50972, 52005

Index

Destruction 50957, 50976, 52354
Dilation 50572, 50575, 50953
Stricture 52341, 52342, 52344, 52345
Excision
Tumor 52355
Exploration 52351
Injection of Implant Material 52327
Insertion
Guide Wire 52334
Stent . . . 50947, 52282, 52332-52334, 53855
Irrigation 50951, 50970
Lithotripsy 52353
Manipulation of Ureteral Calculus 52330
Removal
Calculus 50961, 50980, 52320-52325, 52352
Foreign Body 50961, 50980
Resection 52355
Ureterocele(s) 52300, 52301
via Incision 50970-50980
via Stoma 50951-50961
with Indwelling Stent Insertion 52356
Exploration 50600
Incision and Drainage 50600
Injection
Drugs 50391
Radiological
for Ureterography 50430, 50431, 50684
for Ureteropyelography 50684, 50690
Insertion
Stent 50688, 50693, 50695, 50947, 52332
Tube 50688
Instillation
Drugs 50391
Lesion
Destruction 52354
Lithotripsy 52353
Lysis
Adhesions 50715-50725
Manometric Studies
Pressure 50686
Meatotomy 52290
Nuclear Medicine
Reflux Study 78740
Occlusion 50705
Postcaval
See Retrocaval Ureter
Reconstruction 50700
with Intestines 50840
Reflux Study 78740
Reimplantation 51565
Removal
Anastomosis 50830
Calculus 50610-50630, 50961, 51060-51065, 52320-52325
Foreign Body 50961
Stent 50382-50386
Repair 50900
Anastomosis 50740-50825
Continent Diversion 50825
Deligation 50940
Fistula 50920-50930
Lysis Adhesions 50715-50725
Ureterocele 51535
Ectopic 52301
Orthotopic 52300
Urinary Undiversion 50830
Replacement
Nephroureteral Catheter, Externally Accessible 50387
Stent 50382, 50385
with Intestines 50840
Resection 52355
Revision
Anastomosis 50727, 50728
Stent
Change 50688
Insertion 50688
Placement
with Nephrostogram 50693-50695
with Ureterogram 50693-50695
Suture 50900
Deligation 50940
Fistula 50920-50930
Tube
Change 50688
Insertion 50688
Tumor Resection 52355
Unlisted Services and Procedures . . . 50949, 53899
X ray with Contrast
Guide Dilation 74485

Ureteral
Catheterization
See Catheterization, Ureter
Guide Wire Insertion 52334
Meatotomy
See Meatotomy, Ureter
Splinting 50400-50405
Stent Insertion 52332

Ureterectomy 50650-50660
Partial 50220, 50546
Total 50548

Ureterocalycostomy 50750

Ureterocele
Excision 51535
Fulguration
Ectopic 52301
Orthotopic 52300
Incision 51535
Repair 51535
Resection
Ectopic 52301
Orthotopic 52300

Ureterocolon Conduit 50815

Ureteroenterostomy 50800
Revision 50830

Ureterography
Injection Procedure 50430, 50431, 50684
with Catheter Conversion
Nephrostomy to Nephroureteral 50434
with Nephrostomy Catheter Exchange 50435
with Placement of Ureteral Stent 50693-50695

Ureteroileal Conduit 50820
Cystectomy 51590
Removal 50830

Ureterolithotomy 50610-50630
Laparoscopy 50945
Transvesical 51060

Ureterolysis
for Ovarian Vein Syndrome 50722
for Retrocaval Ureter 50725
for Retroperitoneal Fibrosis 50715

Ureteroneocystostomy 50780-50785, 50830, 51565
Laparoscopic 50947, 50948

Ureteroplasty 50700

Ureteropyelography . . . 50951, 50970, 52005
Injection Procedure 50684, 50690

Ureteropyelostomy 50740

Ureteroscopy
Dilation
Intra-Renal Stricture 52346
Ureter 52344, 52345
Third Stage with Cystourethroscopy 52351
Biopsy 52354
Destruction 52354
Lithotripsy 52353
Removal
Calculus 52352
Tumor Excision 52355

Ureterosigmoidostomy 50810
Revision 50830

Ureterostomy 50860, 50951
Injection Procedure 50684
Manometric Studies 50686

Ureterostomy Stent
Change 50688

Ureterostomy Tube
Change 50688

Ureterotomy 50600
Insertion Indwelling Stent 50605

Ureteroureterostomy . . 50760-50770, 50830

Urethra
Abscess
Incision and Drainage 53040
Adhesions
Lysis 53500
Artificial Sphincter
Repair 53449
Biopsy 52204, 53200
Destruction 52214-52224
Dilation 52260-52265, 53600-53621
General 53665
Suppository and/or Instillation . . 53660, 53661
Diverticulum
See Urethral, Diverticulum
Drainage
Extravasation 53080-53085
Endoscopy 52000
Biopsy 52204, 52354
Catheterization 52010
Destruction 52354, 52400
Evacuation
Clot 52001
Excision
Tumor 52355
Exploration 52351
Incision
Ejaculatory Duct 52402
Injection of Implant Material 51715
Lithotripsy 52353
Removal
Calculus 52352
Resection
Ejaculatory Duct 52402
Vasectomy 52402
Vasotomy 52402
Excision
Diverticulum 53230-53235
Total
Female 53210
Male 53215
Incision 53000-53010
Meatus 53020-53025

Incision and Drainage . . . 53060
Insertion
Stent . . . 52282
Lesion
Destruction . . . 53265
Excision . . . 53260
Paraurethral Gland
Incision and Drainage . . . 53060
Polyp
Destruction . . . 53260
Excision . . . 53260
Pressure Profile . . . 51727, 51729
Prolapse
Destruction . . . 53275
Excision . . . 53275
Repair . . . 53275
Radiotracer . . . 52250
Reconstruction . . . 53410-53440, 53445
and Bladder . . . 51800-51820
Radiofrequency Micro-Remodeling . . . 53860
Complications . . . 54340-54348
Hypospadias
One Stage . . . 54322-54328
Second Stage . . . 54308-54316
Third Stage . . . 54318
Meatus . . . 53450-53460
Removal
Calculus . . . 52310-52315
Foreign Body . . . 52310-52315
Sling . . . 53442
Urethral Stent . . . 52310-52315
Repair
Diverticulum . . . 53240, 53400-53405
Fistula . . . 45820-45825, 53400-53405, 53520
Sphincter . . . 57220
Stricture . . . 53400-53405
Urethrocele . . . 57230
with Replantation of Penis . . . 54438
Wound . . . 53502-53515
Skene's Gland
Incision and Drainage . . . 53060
Sphincter . . . 52277
Electromyography . . . 51784, 51785
Needle . . . 51785
Insertion
Prosthesis . . . 53444
Reconstruction . . . 53445
Removal
Prosthesis . . . 53446, 53447
Repair
Prosthesis . . . 53449
Replacement
Prosthesis . . . 53448
Suture
Fistula . . . 45820-45825, 53520
to Bladder . . . 51840, 51841
Wound . . . 53502-53515
Tumor
Destruction . . . 53220
Excision . . . 53220
Unlisted Services and Procedures . . . 53899
Urethrocystography . . . 74450-74455
Urethrotomy . . . 52270-52276
X ray with Contrast . . . 74450-74455

Urethral
Diverticulum
Marsupialization . . . 53240
Meatus, Dorsal
See Epispadias
Sphincter
Biofeedback Training . . . 90911
Electromyography . . . 51784, 51785
Prosthesis
Insertion . . . 53444
Removal . . . 53446, 53447
Replacement . . . 53448
Resection . . . 52277
Stenosis
Dilation . . . 52281
Stent
Insertion . . . 52282
Removal
Bladder . . . 52310-52315
Urethra . . . 52310-52315
Stricture
Dilation . . . 52281, 53600-53621
Injection
Steroids . . . 52283
Syndrome
Cystourethroscopy . . . 52285

Urethrectomy
Total
Female . . . 53210
Male . . . 53215

Urethrocele
See Urethra, Prolapse

Urethrocystography . . . 74450-74455
Contrast and/or Chain . . . 51605
Retrograde . . . 51610
Voiding . . . 51600

Urethrocystopexy
See Vesicourethropexy

Urethromeatoplasty . . . 53450-53460

Urethropexy . . . 51840, 51841

Urethroplasty . . . 46744-46746
First Stage . . . 53400
One Stage
Hypospadias . . . 54322-54328
Reconstruction
Female Urethra . . . 53430
Male Anterior Urethra . . . 53410
Prostatic/Membranous Urethra
First Stage . . . 53420
One Stage . . . 53415
Second Stage . . . 53425
Second Stage . . . 53405
Hypospadias . . . 54308-54316
Third Stage
Hypospadias . . . 54318

Urethrorrhaphy . . . 53502-53515

Urethroscopy
See Endoscopy, Urethra

Urethrostomy . . . 53000-53010

Urethrotomy . . . 53000-53010
Direct Vision
with Cystourethroscopy . . . 52276
Internal . . . 52601, 52647, 52648
with Cystourethroscopy
Female . . . 52270
Male . . . 52275

Uric Acid
Blood . . . 84550
Other Source . . . 84560
Urine . . . 84560

Uridyltransferase, Galactose-1-Phosphate
See Galactose-1-Phosphate, Uridyl Transferase

Uridylyltransferase, Galactosephosphate
See Galactose-1-Phosphate, Uridyl Transferase

Urinalysis
Automated . . . 81001, 81003
Glass Test . . . 81020
Microalbumin . . . 82043, 82044
Microscopic . . . 81015
Pregnancy Test . . . 81025
Qualitative . . . 81005
Routine . . . 81002
Screen . . . 81007
Semiquantitative . . . 81005
Unlisted Services and Procedures . . . 81099
Volume Measurement . . . 81050
without Microscopy . . . 81002

Urinary Bladder
See Bladder

Urinary Catheter Irrigation
See Irrigation, Catheter

Urinary Sphincter, Artificial
See Prosthesis, Urethral Sphincter

Urinary Tract
X ray with Contrast . . . 74400-74425

Urine
Albumin . . . 82042-82044
Blood . . . 83491
Colony Count . . . 87086
Pregnancy Test . . . 81025
Tests . . . 81001

Urobilinogen
Feces . . . 84577
Urine . . . 84578-84583

Urodynamic Tests
Bladder Capacity
Ultrasound . . . 51798
Cystometrogram . . . 51725-51729
Electromyography Studies
Needle . . . 51785
Residual Urine
Ultrasound . . . 51798
Stimulus Evoked Response . . . 51792
Urethra Pressure Profile . . . 51727
Uroflowmetry . . . 51736-51741
Voiding Pressure Studies
Bladder . . . 51728, 51729
Intra-Abdominal . . . 51797
Rectal . . . 51797

Uroflowmetry . . . 51736-51741

Urography
Antegrade . . . 74425
Infusion . . . 74410-74415
Intravenous . . . 74400-74415
Retrograde . . . 74420

Uroporphyrin . . . 84120

Urothromboplastin
See Thromboplastin

Uterine
Adhesion
See Adhesions, Intrauterine
Cervix
See Cervix
Endoscopies
See Endoscopy, Uterus

Index

Hemorrhage
Postpartum
Control 59160

Uterus
Ablation
Endometrium 58353-58356
Fibroid
Laparoscopic..................... 58674
Radiofrequency.................. 0404T
Tumor
Ultrasound, Focused......... 0071T, 0072T
Biopsy
Endometrium 58100-58110
Endoscopic....................... 58558
Catheterization
X ray........................... 58340
Chromotubation 58350
Curettage 58356
Postpartum........................ 59160
Dilation and Curettage 58120
Postpartum........................ 59160
Ectopic Pregnancy
Interstitial
Partial Resection Uterus............ 59136
Total Hysterectomy 59135
Endoscopy
Ablation
Endometrial 58563
Fibroid........................... 58674
Exploration......................... 58555
Surgery..................... 58558-58565
Treatment.................. 58558-58565
Excision
Laparoscopic 58541-58544, 58550
with Removal of Ovaries 58262, 58263, 58291-58293, 58552, 58554, 58575
Total 58570-58573, 58575
Partial............................ 58180
Radical
Laparoscopic..................... 58548
Open..................... 58210, 58285
Removal of Tubes and/or
Total................58150-58152, 58200, 58570-58573, 58575, 58953-58956
Vaginal.....................58260-58270, 58290-58294, 58550-58554
with Colpectomy............ 58275-58280
with Colpo-Urethrocystopexy........ 58267
with Repair of Enterocele..... 58270, 58294
Hemorrhage
Postpartum........................ 59160
Hydatidiform Mole
Excision 59100
Hydrotubation 58350
Hysterosalpingography................... 74740
Incision
Remove Lesion..................... 59100
Insertion
Heyman Capsule
for Brachytherapy................. 58346
Intrauterine Device (IUD)............. 58300
Tandem
for Brachytherapy................. 57155
Laparoscopy 58578
Lesion
Excision 58545, 58546, 59100
Reconstruction 58540
Removal
Intrauterine Device (IUD)............. 58301
Repair
Fistula..................... 51920-51925
Rupture.................... 58520, 59350
Suspension........................ 58400
with Presacral Sympathectomy 58410
Sonohysterography..................... 76831
Suture
Rupture........................... 59350
Tumor
Ablation
Ultrasound, Focused......... 0071T, 0072T
Excision
Abdominal Approach 58140, 58146
Vaginal Approach................ 58145
Unlisted Services and Procedures ... 58578, 58999
X ray with Contrast..................... 74740

UTP Hexose 1 Phosphate Uridylyltransferase
See Galactose-1-Phosphate, Uridyl Transferase

UV Light Therapy
See Actinotherapy

Uvula
Abscess
Incision and Drainage 42000
Biopsy 42100
Excision....................... 42140-42145
Lesion
Destruction........................ 42145
Excision 42104-42107
Unlisted Services and Procedures 42299

Uvulectomy........................ 42140

V

V Flap Procedure
One Stage Distal Hypospadias Repair 54322

V, Cranial Nerve
See Trigeminal Nerve

V-Y Operation, Bladder, Neck
See Bladder, Repair, Neck

V-Y Plasty
See Skin, Adjacent Tissue Transfer

Vaccination
Vaccine Administration
See Immunization Administration
Vaccines and Toxoids
See Vaccines and Toxoids

Vaccines and Toxoids
Adenovirus 90476, 90477
Anthrax 90581
Chicken Pox
Varicella Virus (VAR) 90716
Cholera
Live, for Oral Use.................. 90625
Dengue Vaccine 90587
Diphtheria and Tetanus Toxoids (DT)......... 90702
Diphtheria, Tetanus, Acellular Pertussis (DtaP) (Tdap) 90700, 90715
Diphtheria, Tetanus Toxoids, Acellular Pertussis, Haemophilus Influenza type b, and Inactivated Poliovirus (DTaP-IPV/Hib) 90698
Diphtheria, Tetanus, Acellular Pertussis, and Inactivated Poliovirus (DtaP-IPV) 90696
Diphtheria, Tetanus, Acellular Pertussis, Hepatitis B, and Inactivated Poliovirus (DtaP-HepB-IPV) 90723
Diphtheria, Tetanus Toxoids, Acellular Pertussis, Inactivated Poliovirus, Haemophilus Influenzae type b PRP-OMP Conjugate, and Hepatitis B (DTaP-IPV-Hib-HepB).................... 90697
Encephalitis, Japanese.................... 90738
Haemophilus Influenza B (Hib) 90647, 90648
and Meningococcal Conjugate, Serogroups C and Y (Hib-MenCY)................ 90644
Hepatitis A (HepA) 90632-90634
Hepatitis A and Hepatitis B (HepA-HepB) ... 90636
Hepatitis B (HepB)
Adolescent Dose 90743
Adult Dose 90739, 90746
Dialysis or Immunosuppressed Dose.................... 90740, 90747
Pediatric/Adolescent Dose 90744
Hepatitis B and Haemophilus Influenza B (Hib-HepB)........................... 90748
Human Papillomavirus (HPV)
Bivalent (2vHPV).................. 90650
Nonavalent (9vHPV)................ 90651
Quadrivalent (4vHPV)............... 90649
Influenza
Antibiotic Free 90756
Cell Cultured 90661, 90674, 90756
DNA Derived (RIV3) 90673
Enhanced Immunogenicity (IIV) 90662
for Intradermal Use 90630, 90654
for Intramuscular Use ... 90653, 90655-90658, 90661, 90662, 90666-90668, 90673, 90674, 90685-90689, 90756
for Intranasal Use 90660, 90664, 90672
Inactivated (IIV) 90653
Pandemic
Live (LAIV) for Intranasal Use........ 90664
Split (IIV) for Intramuscular Use 90666-90668
Preservative Free 90630, 90654, 90655, 90656, 90661, 90662, 90666, 90673, 90674, 90685, 90686
Quadrivalent
ccIIV3 90661
ccIIV4 .... 90674, 90756
IIV4 .... 90630, 90685-90689
LAIV4 90672
RIV4 90682
Trivalent, DNA Derived (RIV3).......... 90673
Trivalent, Live Virus (LAIV3)........... 90660
Trivalent, Split Virus (IIV3)........... 90654-90658, 90660, 90673
for Intradermal Use 90654
for Intramuscular Use ..... 90655-90658 with Increased Antigen Content 90662
Measles, Mumps, and Rubella (MMR)...... 90707
Measles, Mumps, Rubella, and Varicella (MMRV)............................. 90710
Meningococcus
Meningococcal Conjugate, Serogroups A, C, Y, W-135 (MCV4, MenACWY)........... 90734
Meningococcal Conjugate, Serogroups C and Y, Haemophilus Influenza type b (Hib-MenCY)....................... 90644
Meningococcal Polysaccharide Quadrivalent (MPSV4) 90733
Meningococcal Recombinant Lipoprotein Vaccine, Serogroup B (MenB-FHbp) 90621
Meningococcal Recombinant Protein Vaccine, Serogroup B (MenB-4C)............. 90620
Pneumococcal
13-valent (PCV13).................. 90670
23-valent (PPSV23).................. 90732
Poliovirus, Inactivated
Intramuscular...................... 90713

Subcutaneous 90713
Rabies 90675, 90676
Rotavirus
Attenuated (RV1) 90681
Pentavalent (RV5) 90680
Tetanus and Diphtheria Toxoids (Td) 90714
Tetanus, Diphtheria, and Acellular Pertussis (Tdap) 90715
Tuberculosis (BCG) 90585, 90586
Typhoid 90690
Unlisted Vaccine/Toxoid 90749
Varicella (Chicken Pox) (VAR) 90716
Yellow Fever 90717
Zoster (Shingles) (HZV) 90736, 90750

Vagina
Abscess
Incision and Drainage 57010
Amines Test 82120
Biopsy
Colposcopy 57421
Endocervical 57454
Extensive 57105
Simple 57100
Brachytherapy
Insertion of Afterloading Apparatus 57156
Closure 57120
Colposcopy ... 57420, 57421, 57455, 57456, 57461
Construction
with Graft 57292
without Graft 57291
Cyst
Excision 57135
Dilation 57400
Endocervical
Biopsy 57454
Exploration 57452
Excision
Closure 57120
Complete
with Removal of Paravaginal Tissue 57111, 57112
with Removal of Vaginal Wall 57110
Partial
with Removal of Paravaginal Tissue 57107
with Lymphadenectomy 57109
with Removal of Vaginal Wall 57106
Total 57110
with Hysterectomy 58275-58280
with Repair of Enterocele 58280
Exploration
Endocervical 57452
Incision 57000
Fluid
Sialidase Activity 87905
Hematoma
Incision and Drainage 57022, 57023
Hemorrhage 57180
Hysterectomy 58290, 58550-58554
Incision and Drainage 57020
Insertion
Afterloading Apparatus
for Brachytherapy 57156
Ovoid
for Brachytherapy 57155
Packing for Bleeding 57180
Pessary 57160
Irrigation 57150
Lesion
Destruction 57061-57065
Extensive 57065
Simple 57061
Prolapse
Sacrospinous Ligament Fixation 57282
Removal
Foreign Body 57415
Prosthetic Graft 57295, 57296, 57426
Sling
Stress Incontinence 57287
Repair 56800
Cystocele 57240, 57260
Combined Anteroposterior 57260-57265
Posterior 57240
Enterocele 57265
Fistula 51900
Rectovaginal 57300-57308
Transvesical and Vaginal Approach 57330
Urethrovaginal 57310, 57311
Vesicovaginal 51900, 57320-57330
Hysterectomy 58267, 58293
Incontinence 57284, 57285, 57288
Obstetric 59300
Paravaginal Defect 57284, 57285, 57423
Pereyra Procedure 57289
Prolapse 57282-57285, 57423
Prosthesis Insertion 57267
Rectocele
Combined Anteroposterior 57260-57265
Posterior 57250
Suspension 57280-57283
Laparoscopic 57425
Urethral Sphincter 57220
Wound 57200-57210
Colpoperineorrhaphy 57210
Colporrhaphy 57200
Revision
Prosthetic Graft 57295, 57296, 57426
Sling
Stress Incontinence 57287
Septum
Excision 57130
Suspension 57280-57283
Laparoscopic 57425
Suture
Cystocele 57240, 57260
Enterocele 57265
Fistula 51900, 57300-57330
Rectocele 57250-57260
Wound 57200-57210
Tumor
Excision 57135
Ultrasound 76830
Unlisted Services and Procedures 58999
X ray with Contrast 74775

Vaginal Delivery 59400, 59610-59614
after Previous Cesarean Delivery 59610-59612
Attempted 59618-59622
Antepartum Care 59400
Cesarean Delivery after Attempted 59618
Delivery Only 59620
Postpartum Care 59622
Delivery after Previous
Vaginal Delivery Only
Postpartum Care 59614
Delivery Only 59409
External Cephalic Version 59412
Placenta 59414
Postpartum Care 59410
Routine Care 59400

Vaginal Hysterectomy 58552-58554

Vaginal Smear
See Pap Smears

Vaginal Suppositories
Induced Abortion 59855
with Dilation and Curettage 59856
with Hysterectomy 59857

Vaginectomy
Partial 57106
with Abdominal Hysterectomy 58200
with Vaginal Hysterectomy 58275
Radical 57107, 57109, 57111, 57112
Total 57110

Vaginoplasty
Intersex State 57335

Vaginorrhaphy
See Colporrhaphy

Vaginoscopy
Biopsy 57454
Exploration 57452

Vaginotomy
See Colpotomy

Vagotomy
Abdominal 64760
Highly Selective 43641
Parietal Cell 43641, 64755
Selective 43640
Truncal 43640
with Gastroduodenostomy Revision, Reconstruction 43855
with Gastrojejunostomy Revision, Reconstruction 43865
with Partial Distal Gastrectomy 43635

Vagus Nerve
Avulsion
Abdominal 64760
Selective 64755
Blocking Therapy 0312T-0317T
Incision 43640, 43641
Abdominal 64760
Selective 64755
Injection
Anesthetic 64408
Transection 43640, 43641
Abdominal 64760
Selective 43652, 64755
Truncal 43651

Valproic Acid
See Dipropylacetic Acid

Valproic Acid Measurement
See Dipropylacetic Acid

Valsalva Sinus
See Sinus/Sinuses, Sinus of Valsalva

Valva Atrioventricularis Sinistra (Valva Mitralis)
See Mitral Valve

Valve
Aortic
See Aortic Valve
Bicuspid
See Mitral Valve
Bronchial
See Bronchi, Bronchial Valve
Mitral
See Mitral Valve
Pulmonary
See Pulmonary Valve
Tricuspid
See Tricuspid Valve

Index

Valve Stenoses, Aortic
See Aortic Stenosis

Valvectomy
Tricuspid Valve 33460

Valvotomy
Mitral Valve 33420, 33422
Pulmonary Valve 33470, 33471, 33474
Reoperation 33530

Valvuloplasty
Aortic Valve 33390, 33391
Femoral Vein 34501
Mitral Valve 33425-33427
Percutaneous Balloon
  Aortic Valve 92986
  Mitral Valve 92987
  Pulmonary Valve 92990
Prosthetic Valve 33496
Reoperation 33530
Tricuspid Valve 33463-33465

Van Den Bergh Test
See Bilirubin, Blood

Vancomycin
Assay 80202
Resistance 87500

Vanillylmandelic Acid
Urine 84585

Vanilmandelic Acid
See Vanillylmandelic Acid

Varicella (Chicken Pox)
See Vaccines and Toxoids

Varicella-Zoster
Antibody 86787
Antigen Detection
  Direct Fluorescence 87290

Varices Esophageal
See Esophageal Varices

Varicocele
Spermatic Cord
  Excision 55530-55540

Varicose Vein
Ablation
  Chemical Adhesive 36482, 36483
  Laser 36478, 36479
  Mechanochemical 36473, 36474
  Radiofrequency 36475, 36476
Cluster
  Division 37785
  Excision 37788
  Ligation 37785
Stab Phlebectomy 37765, 37766

Vas Deferens
Anastomosis
  to Epididymis 54900, 54901
Excision 55250
Incision 55200
  for X ray 55300
Repair
  Suture 55400
Unlisted Services and Procedures 55899
Vasography 74440
X ray with Contrast 74440

Vascular Flow Check, Graft 15860

Vascular Injection
Unlisted Services and Procedures 36299

Vascular Lesion
Cranial
  Excision 61600-61608, 61615, 61616
Cutaneous
  Destruction 17106-17108

Vascular Malformation
Cerebral
  Obliteration 61613
  Repair 61680, 61682, 61684, 61686, 61690, 61692, 61705, 61708, 61710
Finger
  Excision 26111-26116
Hand
  Excision 26111-26116
Spine
  Occlusion 62294, 63250-63252

Vascular Procedures
Angioscopy
  Noncoronary Vessels 35400
Brachytherapy
  Intracoronary Artery 92974
Embolization 37241-37244
Endoscopy
  Surgical 37500
Harvest
  Lower Extremity Vein 35572
Intravascular Ultrasound
  Coronary Vessels 92978, 92979
  Noncoronary Vessels 37252, 37253
Ligation
  Vena Cava 37619
Occlusion 37241-37244
Optical Coherence Tomography 92978, 92979
Spectroscopy
  Catheter Based 0205T
Stent Placement
  Intracoronary 92928, 92929
Thrombolysis
  Cerebral 37195
  Coronary 92975-92977
  Intracranial 61645
  Noncoronary 37211-37214

Vascular Rehabilitation
See Peripheral Artery Disease (PAD) Rehabilitation

Vascular Studies
Angioscopy
  Noncoronary Vessels 35400
Aorta 93978, 93979
Arterial Studies (Non-Invasive)
  Extracranial 93880-93882
  Extremities 93922-93924
  Intracranial 93886-93890
  Lower Extremity 93925, 93926
  Middle Cerebral Artery, Fetal 76821
  Umbilical Artery, Fetal 76820
Artery Studies
  Upper Extremity 93930, 93931
Bioimpedance Cardiovascular Analysis 93701
Blood Pressure Monitoring, 24 Hour 93784-93790
Cardiac Catheterization
  Imaging 93452-93461
Endothelial Function Assessment
  Noninvasive 93998
Hemodialysis Access 93990
Kidney
  Multiple Study
    with Pharmacological Intervention 78709
  Single Study
    with Pharmacological Intervention 78708
Penile Vessels 93980, 93981
Spectroscopy
  Catheter Based 0205T
Temperature Gradient 93740
Unlisted Services and Procedures 93799, 93998
Venous Studies
  Extremity 93970, 93971
  Venous Pressure 93770
Visceral Studies 93975-93979

Vascular Surgery
Arm, Upper
  Anesthesia 01770-01782
Elbow
  Anesthesia 01770-01782
Endoscopy 37500
Unlisted Services and Procedures 37799

Vasectomy 55250
Laser Coagulation of Prostate 52647
Laser Vaporization 52648
Reversal
  See Vasovasorrhaphy
Transurethral
  Cystourethroscopic 52402
Transurethral Electrosurgical Resection of Prostate 52601
Transurethral Resection of Prostate 52648

Vasoactive Drugs
Injection
  Penis 54231

Vasoactive Intestinal Peptide 84586

Vasogram
See Vasography

Vasography 74440

Vasointestinal Peptide
See Vasoactive Intestinal Peptide

Vasopneumatic Device Therapy 97016
See Physical Medicine/Therapy/Occupational Therapy

Vasopressin 84588

Vasotomy 55200, 55300
Transurethral
  Cystourethroscopic 52402

Vasovasorrhaphy 55400

Vasovasostomy 55400

VATS
See Thoracoscopy

VDRL
See Syphilis Test

Vein
Ablation Therapy
  Endovenous
    Chemical Adhesive 36482, 36483
    Laser 36478, 36479
    Mechanochemical 36473, 36474
    Radiofrequency 36475, 36476
Adrenal
  Venography 75840-75842
Anastomosis
  Caval to Mesenteric 37160
  Intrahepatic Portosystemic 37182, 37183
  Portocaval 37140
  Reniportal 37145
  Saphenopopliteal 34530
  Splenorenal 37180, 37181
  to Vein 37140-37160, 37182, 37183

Index

Angioplasty
Transluminal 37248, 37249
Arm
Harvest of Vein for Bypass Graft 35500
Venography 75820-75822
Axillary
Thrombectomy 34490
Biopsy 37200
Transcatheter 75970
Cannulization
to Artery 36810-36815
to Vein 36800
Catheterization
Central Insertion 36555-36558
Organ Blood 36500
Peripheral Insertion 36568-36573
Removal 36589
Repair 36575
Replacement 36578-36581, 36584
Umbilical 36510
Division
Saphenous 37718-37722
Endoscopic Harvest
for Bypass Graft 33508
External Cannula
Declotting 36860, 36861
Extremity
Non-Invasive Studies 93970, 93971
Femoral
Repair 34501
Femoropopliteal
Thrombectomy 34421-34451
Guidance
Fluoroscopic 77001
Ultrasound 76937
Hepatic Portal
Splenoportography 75810
Venography 75885-75887
Iliac
Thrombectomy 34401-34451
Injection
Sclerosant 36465, 36466, 36468, 36470, 36471
Interrupt
Femoral 37650
Iliac 37660
Jugular
Venography 75860
Leg
Harvest for Vascular Reconstruction 35572
Venography 75820-75822
Ligation
Clusters 37785
Esophagus 43205
Jugular 37565
Perforation 37760, 37761
Saphenous 37700-37735, 37780
Secondary 37785
Liver
Venography 75889-75891
Neck
Venography 75860
Nuclear Medicine
Thrombosis Imaging 78456-78458
Orbit
Venography 75880
Portal
Catheterization 36481
Pulmonary
Isolation 93656
Repair 33730
Removal
Clusters 37785
Varicose 37765, 37766
Renal
Venography 75831-75833
Repair
Angioplasty 37248, 37249
Graft 34520
Sampling
Venography 75893
Sinus
Venography 75870
Skull
Venography 75870-75872
Spermatic
Excision 55530-55540
Ligation 55550
Splenic
Splenoportography 75810
Stripping
Saphenous 37718-37735
Subclavian
Thrombectomy 34471-34490
Thrombectomy 37187, 37188
Other than Hemodialysis Graft or Fistula 35875, 35876
Thrombolysis
Transcatheter Infusion 37212-37214
Unlisted Services and Procedures 37799
Valve Transposition 34510
Varicose
See Varicose Vein
Vena Cava
Thrombectomy 34401-34451
Venography 75825-75827

Velpeau Cast 29058

Vena Cava
Catheterization 36010
Filter
Insertion 37191
Repositioning 37192
Retrieval 37193
Ligation 37619
Reconstruction 34502
Resection with Reconstruction 37799

Vena Caval
Thrombectomy 50230

Venereal Disease Research Laboratory
See VDRL

Venesection
See Phlebotomy

Venipuncture
See Cannulation; Catheterization
Child/Adult
Cutdown 36425
Percutaneous 36410
Infant
Cutdown 36420
Percutaneous 36400-36406
Routine 36415

Venography
Adrenal 75840-75842
Arm 75820-75822
Epidural 75872
Hepatic Portal 75885-75887
Injection 36005
Jugular 75860
Leg 75820-75822
Liver 75889-75891
Neck 75860
Nuclear Medicine 78445, 78457, 78458
Orbit 75880
Renal 75831-75833
Sagittal Sinus 75870
Vena Cava 75825-75827
Venous Sampling 75893

Venorrhaphy
See Suture, Vein

Venotomy
See Phlebotomy

Venous Access Device
Blood Collection 36591, 36592
Declotting 36593
Fluoroscopic Guidance 77001
Insertion
Central 36560-36566
Peripheral 36570, 36571
Irrigation 96523
Obstruction Clearance 36595, 36596
Guidance 75901, 75902
Removal 36590
Repair 36576
Replacement 36582, 36583, 36585
Catheter Only 36578

Venous Blood Pressure
See Blood Pressure, Venous

Venovenostomy
See Anastomosis, Vein

Ventilating Tube
Insertion 69433
Removal 69424

Ventilation Assist
Home, Domiciliary or Rest Home 94005, 99504
Hospital Inpatient/Observation 94002, 94003
Nursing Facility 94004

Ventricular Assist Device (VAD)
Implantable Counterpulsation Aortic System
Insertion 0451T-0454T
Interrogation Device Evaluation 0463T
Programming Device Evaluation 0462T
Relocation 0459T
Removal 0455T-0458T
Repositioning 0460T, 0461T
Replacement 0451T-0454T
Insertion
Extracorporeal 33975, 33976, 33978
Implantable 33979
Percutaneous 33990, 33991
Removal 33977, 33980, 33992
Replacement 33981, 33982
Repositioning 33993
Interrogation and Programming 93750

Ventricular Puncture 61020-61026, 61105-61120

Ventriculocisternostomy 62180, 62200, 62201

Ventriculography
Anesthesia
Brain 00214
Cardiac 01920
Nuclear Imaging 78635
Injection 61026, 61055, 93452, 93453, 93458-93461

Ventriculomyectomy 33416

Ventriculomyotomy 33416

Vermiform Appendix
See Appendix

Vermilionectomy 40500

Verruca Plana
See Warts, Flat

Verruca(e)
See Warts

Version, Cephalic
See Cephalic Version

Vertebra
See Intervertebral Disc; Spinal Cord; Spine; Vertebral, Body; Vertebral, Process
Arthrodesis
  Anterior 22548-22585
  Exploration 22830
  Lateral Extracavitary 22532-22534
  Posterior 22590-22802
  Sacral 22586, 22899
  Spinal Deformity
    Anterior Approach 22808-22812
    Posterior Approach 22800-22804
Aspiration 62267
Bone Graft 0222T
  Cervical 0219T
  Lumbar 0221T
  Thoracic 0220T
Cervical
  Excision
    for Tumor 22100, 22110
  Fracture 23675-23680
Decompression 62287
  Laminotomy/Laminectomy 0274T, 0275T
Excision
  Partial 22100-22103, 22110, 22112, 22114, 22116
Facetectomy
  Partial 62380, 63020
Fracture/Dislocation
  Open Treatment
    Additional Segment 22328
    Cervical 22326
    Lumbar 22325
    Thoracic 22327
Kyphectomy 22818, 22819
Lumbar
  Distraction Device 22867-22870
  Excision
    for Tumor 22102, 22114
Foraminotomy 0202T
Osteoplasty
  with Image Guidance
    Cervicothoracic 22510, 22512
  Lumbosacral 22511, 22512
Osteotomy
  Additional Segment
    Anterior Approach 22226
    Posterior/Posterolateral Approach 22216
  Cervical
    Anterior Approach 22220
    Posterior/Posterolateral Approach 22210
  Lumbar
    Anterior Approach 22224
    Posterior/Posterolateral Approach 22214
  Thoracic
    Anterior Approach 22222
    Posterior/Posterolateral Approach 22212
Placement
  Intrafacet Implant 0222T
    Cervical 0219T
    Lumbar 0221T
    Thoracic 0220T
Thoracic
  Excision
    for Tumor 22101, 22112

Vertebrae
See Vertebra
Arthrodesis
  Anterior 22548-22585
  Lateral Extracavitary 22532-22534
  Spinal Deformity 22818, 22819

Vertebral
Arteries
  See Artery, Vertebral
Body
  Biopsy
    Open 20250, 20251
    Percutaneous 22510-22512
  Excision
    Decompression 63081-63103
    Lesion 63300-63308
    with Skull Base Surgery 61597
  Fracture/Dislocation
    Closed Treatment
      without Manipulation 22310
  Insertion
    Stabilization/Distraction Device 22869, 22870
  Kyphectomy 22818, 22819
  Repair
    Injection
      Cervicothoracic 22510, 22512
      Lumbosacral 22511, 22512
Column
  See Spine
Corpectomy 63081-63103, 63300-63308
  with Insertion of Biomechanical Device 22854
Disc
  See Intervertebral Disc
Fracture
  See Fracture, Vertebra
Joint Replacement
  Lumbar Spine 0202T
Process
  Fracture/Dislocation
    Closed Treatment
      with Manipulation, Casting and/or Bracing 22315

Very Low Density Lipoprotein
See Lipoprotein, Blood

Vesication
See Bulla

Vesicle, Seminal
See Seminal Vesicle

Vesico-Psoas Hitch 50785

Vesicostomy
Cutaneous 51980

Vesicourethropexy 51840, 51841

Vesicovaginal Fistula
Closure 51900, 57320, 57300

Vesiculectomy 55650

Vesiculogram, Seminal
See Vesiculography

Vesiculography 55300, 74440

Vesiculotomy 55600-55605
Complicated 55605

Vessel, Blood
See Blood Vessels

Vessels Transposition, Great
See Transposition, Great Arteries

Vestibular Function Tests
See Ear, Nose, and Throat
Additional Electrodes 92547
Caloric Vestibular Test
  with Recording 92537, 92538
  without Recording 92533
Foveal Stimulation 92540
Nystagmus
  Optokinetic 92534, 92540, 92544
  Positional 92532, 92540, 92542
  Spontaneous 92531, 92540, 92541
Peripheral Stimulation 92540
Posturography 92548
Sinusoidal Rotational Testing 92546
Torsion Swing Test 92546
Tracking Test 92540, 92545

Vestibular Nerve
Section
  Transcranial Approach 69950
  Translabyrinthine Approach 69915

Vestibule of Mouth
See Mouth, Vestibule

Vestibuloplasty 40840-40845

Vidal Procedure
See Varicocele, Spermatic Cord, Excision

Video
Esophagus 74230
Pharynx 70371, 74230
Speech Evaluation 70371
Swallowing Evaluation 74230

Video-Assisted Thoracoscopic Surgery
See Thoracoscopy

Videoradiography
Esophagus 74230
Pharynx 70371, 74230
Site Unspecified 76120-76125
Speech Evaluation 70371
Swallowing Evaluation 74230

VII, Coagulation Factor
See Proconvertin

VII, Cranial Nerve
See Facial Nerve

VIII, Coagulation Factor
See Clotting Factor

Villus, Chorionic
See Chorionic Villus

Villusectomy
See Synovectomy

VIP
See Vasoactive Intestinal Peptide

Viral Antibodies 86280

Viral Warts
See Warts

Virus
AIDS
  See HIV-1
Burkitt Lymphoma
  See Epstein-Barr Virus
Human Immunodeficiency
  See HIV
Influenza
  See Influenza Virus

Respiratory Syncytial
See Respiratory Syncytial Virus
Salivary Gland
See Cytomegalovirus

Virus Identification
Immunofluorescence . . . 87254

Virus Isolation . . . 87250-87255

Visceral Larval Migrans . . . 86280

Viscosities, Blood
See Blood, Viscosity

Visit, Home
See House Calls

Visual Acuity Screen
Automated . . . 99172, 99173
Evoked Potentials . . . 0333T

Visual Field
Assessment . . . 0378T, 0379T
Exam . . . 92081-92083

Visual Function Screen . . . 1055F, 99172

Visual Reinforcement Audiometry . . 92579
See Audiologic Function Tests

Visualization
Ileal Conduit . . . 50690

Vital Capacity Measurement . . . 94150

Vitamin
A . . . 84590
B Complex
See B Complex Vitamins
B-1 . . . 84425
B-12 . . . 82607, 82608
Holotranscobalamin . . . 84999
B-2 . . . 84252
B-6 . . . 84207
B-6 Measurement
See Pyridoxal Phosphate
BC
See Folic Acid
C . . . 82180
D
Blood Serum Level
25 hydroxy . . . 82306
1, 25 dihydroxy . . . 82652
Counseling . . . 4019F
E . . . 84446
K . . . 84597
K Dependent Bone Protein
See Osteocalcin
K-Dependent Protein S
See Protein S
Other, Unspecified . . . 84591

Vitelline Duct
See Omphalomesenteric Duct

Vitrectomy
Anterior Approach
Partial . . . 67005
Subtotal . . . 67010
for Retinal Detachment . . . 67108, 67113
by Sampling . . . 0198T
Pars Plana Approach . . . 67036-67043
with Endolaser Panretinal Photocoagulation 67040
with Focal Endolaser Photocoagulation . . . 67039
with Implantation or Replacement
Drug Delivery System . . . 67027
Retinal Electrodes . . . 0100T
with Lens Material Removal . . . 66852
with Retinal Prosthesis Placement . . . 0100T

Vitreous
Aspiration . . . 67015
Excision
Pars Plana Approach . . . 67036, 67041-67043
Implantation
Drug Delivery System . . . 67027
Incision
Strands . . . 67030, 67031
Injection
Fluid Substitute . . . 67025
Pharmacologic Agent . . . 67028
Photocoagulation
with Endolaser . . . 67039, 67040
Placement
Radiation Source . . . 67299
Release . . . 67015
Removal . . . 67005, 67010, 67027
Anterior Approach . . . 67005
Subtotal . . . 67010
Strands
Discission . . . 67030
Severing . . . 67031
Subtotal . . . 67010

VLDL
See Lipoprotein, Blood

VMA
See Vanillylmandelic Acid

Vocal Cords
Injection
Endoscopy . . . 31513
Augmentive . . . 31574
Therapeutic . . . 31570, 31571, 31573
Laryngeal Medialization . . . 31591

Voice
See Speech Evaluation

Voice Box
See Larynx

Voice Button . . . 31611

Voiding Pressure Studies
Abdominal . . . 51797
Bladder . . . 51728, 51729
Rectum . . . 51797
Urethra . . . 51729

Volatiles . . . 84600

Volkman Contracture . . . 25315, 25316

Volume Reduction
Blood Products . . . 86960
Lung . . . 32491

Volume Reduction, Lung
See Lung Volume Reduction (LVRS)

Von Kraske Proctectomy . . . 45111

VP
See Voiding Pressure Studies

Vulva
Biopsy
Endoscopic . . . 56821
Lesion . . . 56605, 56606
Colposcopy . . . 56820
Excision
See Vulvectomy
Incision and Drainage
Abscess . . . 56405
Boil . . . 10060, 10061
Furuncle . . . 10060, 10061
Lesion
Biopsy . . . 56605, 56606
Destruction . . . 56501-56515
Repair
Obstetric . . . 59300

Vulvectomy
Complete . . . 56625, 56633-56640
Partial . . . 56620, 56630-56632
Radical . . . 56630, 56631, 56633-56640
Complete
with Bilateral Inguinofemoral
Lymphadenectomy . . . 56637
with Inguinofemoral, Iliac, and Pelvic
Lymphadenectomy . . . 56640
with Unilateral Inguinofemoral
Lymphadenectomy . . . 56634
Partial
with Bilateral Inguinofemoral
Lymphadenectomy . . . 56632
with Unilateral Inguinofemoral
Lymphadenectomy . . . 56631
Simple
Complete . . . 56625
Partial . . . 56620

VZIG
See Immune Globulins, Varicella-Zoster

W

W-Plasty
See Skin, Adjacent Tissue Transfer

WADA Activation Test . . . 95958
See also Electroencephalography (EEG)

Waldius Procedure . . . 27445

Wall, Abdominal
See Abdomen, Abdominal Wall

Walsh Modified Radical Prostatectomy
See Prostatectomy

Warts
Flat
Destruction . . . 17110, 17111

Washing
Sperm . . . 58323

Wassmund Procedure
Osteotomy
Maxilla . . . 21206

Water Wart
See Molluscum Contagiosum

Waterston Procedure . . . 33755

Watson-Jones Procedure . . . 27695-27698

Wave, Ultrasonic Shock
See Ultrasound

WBC
See White Blood Cell

Webbed
Toe
Repair . . . 28280

Wechsler Memory Scales
See Neuropsychological Testing

Wedge Excision
Lip . . . 40510
Liver Biopsy . . . 47100

Index

Nail Fold 11765
Osteotomy 21122
Tarsal 67916, 67923

Wedge Resection
Cornea 65775
Lung 32505-32507, 32666-32668
Ovary 58920
Vesical Neck 51800

Well-Baby Care 99381, 99391, 99461

Wellness Behavior
See Evaluation and Management, Health Behavior

West Nile Virus
Antibody 86788, 86789

Westergren Test
See Sedimentation Rate, Blood Cell

Western Blot
HIV 86689
Protein 84181, 84182
Tissue Analysis 88371, 88372

Wheelchair Management
Training 97542

Wheelchair Management/Propulsion
See Physical Medicine/Therapy/Occupational Therapy

Wheeler Procedure
Discission Secondary Membranous Cataract 66820

Wheeze Rate
See Acoustic Respiratory Measurements

Whipple Procedure 48150

Whirlpool Therapy 97022

White Blood Cell
Alkaline Phosphatase 85540
Antibody 86021
Count 85032, 85048, 89055
Differential 85004-85007, 85009
Histamine Release Test 86343
Injection
Autologous Concentrate 0481T
Phagocytosis 86344
Transfusion
See Leukocyte, Transfusion

Whitman Astragalectomy
See Talus, Excision

Whitman Procedure 27120

Wick Catheter Technique 20950

Window
Oval
See Oval Window
Round
See Round Window

Window Technic, Pericardial
See Pericardiostomy

Windpipe
See Trachea

Winiwarter Operation
See Anastomosis, Gallbladder to Intestines

Winter Procedure 54435

Wintrobe Test
See Sedimentation Rate, Blood Cell

Wire
See Pin
Fixation
Insertion/Removal
Skeletal Traction 20650
Interdental
without Fracture 21497
Guide
Dilation over 43196, 43212, 43226, 43229, 43248, 43453, 45303, 46604
Insertion
Endoscopic 43196, 43212, 43226, 43229, 43248, 52334
Needle
See Needle Wire
Thiersch
Removal 46754

Wiring
Prophylactic Treatment
Humerus 24498

Wirsung Duct
See Pancreatic Duct

Wisconsin Card Sorting Test
See Neuropsychological Testing

Witzel Operation 43500, 43520, 43830-43832
See Incision, Stomach, Creation, Stoma; Incision and Drainage

Womb
See Uterus

Wood Alcohol
See Methanol

Work Hardening 97545, 97546
See Physical Medicine/Therapy/Occupational Therapy

Work Related Evaluation Services 99455, 99456

Worm
See Helminth

Wound
Ablation
Laser 0491T, 0492T
Care
Debridement
Non-Selective 97602
Selective 97597, 97598
Negative Pressure Therapy 97605-97608
Ultrasound Application 97610
Dehiscence
Repair 12020, 12021, 13160
Exploration
Penetrating
Abdomen/Flank/Back 20102
Chest 20101
Extremity 20103
Neck 20100
Penetrating Trauma 20100-20103
Healing
Extracorporeal Shock Wave
Therapy 0512T, 0513T
Infection
Incision and Drainage
Postoperative 10180
Near-Infrared Spectroscopy Studies 0493T
Negative Pressure Therapy 97605-97608
Repair
Axillae
Complex 13131-13133
Intermediate 12031, 12032, 12034-12037
Simple 12001, 12002, 12004-12007
Arms
Complex 13120-13122
Intermediate 12031, 12032, 12034-12037
Simple 12001, 12002, 12004-12007
Cheeks
Complex 13131-13133
Chin
Complex 13131-13133
Ears
Complex 13151-13153
Intermediate 12051, 12052, 12054-12057
Simple 12011, 12013-12018
Eyelids
Complex 13151-13153
Intermediate 12051, 12052, 12054-12057
Simple 12011, 12013-12018
Face
Intermediate 12051, 12052, 12054-12057
Simple 12011, 12013-12018
Feet
Complex 13131-13133
Intermediate 12041, 12042, 12044-12047
Simple 12001, 12002, 12004-12007
Forehead
Complex 13131-13133
Genitalia
Complex 13131-13133
Intermediate 12041, 12042, 12044-12047
Simple 12001, 12002, 12004-12007
Hands
Complex 13131-13133
Intermediate 12041, 12042, 12044-12047
Simple 12001, 12002, 12004-12007
Legs
Complex 13120-13122
Intermediate 12031, 12032, 12034-12037
Simple 12001, 12002, 12004-12007
Lips
Complex 13153
Intermediate 12051, 12052, 12054-12057
Simple 12011, 12013-12018
Mouth
Complex 13131-13133
Mucous Membranes
Intermediate 12051, 12052, 12054-12057
Simple 12011, 12013-12018
Neck
Intermediate 12041, 12042, 12044-12047
Simple 12001, 12002, 12004-12007
Nose
Complex 13151-13153
Intermediate 12051, 12052, 12054-12057
Simple 12011, 12013-12018
Scalp
Complex 13120-13122
Intermediate 12031, 12032, 12034-12037
Simple 12001, 12002, 12004-12007
Trunk
Complex 13100-13102
Intermediate 12031, 12032, 12034-12037
Simple 12001, 12002, 12004-12007
Urethra 53502-53515
with Secondary Closure 13160
Strapping
Suture
Bladder 51860-51865
Kidney 50500
Trachea
Cervical 31800
Intrathoracic 31805
Urethra 53502-53515
Ultrasound Therapy 97610

Vagina
Repair 57200-57210

Wrist
See Arm, Lower; Carpal Bone
Abscess 25028
Arthrocentesis 20605, 20606
Arthrodesis 25800
with Graft 25805, 25810, 25825
Arthrography 73115
Arthroplasty 25332, 25443, 25447
Revision 25449
Total Replacement 25446
with Implant 25441, 25442, 25444, 25445
Arthroscopy
Diagnostic 29840
Surgical 29843-29848
Arthrotomy 25040, 25100-25105
for Repair 25107
Biopsy 25065, 25066, 25100, 25101
Bone Graft 25810, 25825
Bursa
Aspiration 20605, 20606
Excision 25115, 25116
Incision and Drainage 25031
Injection 20605, 20606
Capsule
Incision 25085
Cast 29085
Cyst 25130-25136
Decompression 25020-25025
Disarticulation 25920
Reamputation 25924
Revision 25922
Dislocation
Closed Treatment 25660
Intercarpal 25660
Open Treatment 25670
Open Treatment 25670, 25676
Percutaneous Fixation 25671
Radiocarpal 25660
Open Treatment 25670
Radioulnar
Closed Treatment 25675
Percutaneous Fixation 25671
with Fracture
Closed Treatment 25680
Open Treatment 25685
with Manipulation 25259, 25660, 25675
Excision
Carpal 25210-25215
Cartilage 25107
Exploration 25040, 25101
Fasciotomy 25020-25025
Fracture 25645
Closed Treatment 25622, 25630
Open Treatment 25628
with Dislocation 25680-25685
with Manipulation 25259, 25624, 25635
Ganglion Cyst
Excision 25111, 25112
Hematoma 25028
Incision 25040, 25100-25105
Tendon Sheath 25000, 25001
Injection
Carpal Tunnel
Therapeutic 20526
X ray 25246
Joint
See Radiocarpal Joint
Lesion, Tendon Sheath
Excision 25110
Magnetic Resonance Imaging (MRI) 73221
Reconstruction
Capsulectomy 25320
Capsulorrhaphy 25320
Carpal Bone 25394, 25430
Realign 25335
Removal
Foreign Body 25040, 25101, 25248
Implant 25449
Loose Body 25101
Prosthesis 25250, 25251
Repair 25447
Bone 25440
Carpal Bone 25431
Muscle 25260, 25270
Secondary 25263-25265, 25272-25274
Tendon 25260, 25270, 25280-25316
Secondary 25263-25265, 25272-25274
Tendon Sheath 25275
Strapping 29260
Synovium
Excision 25105, 25115-25119
Tendon
Excision 25109
Tendon Sheath
Excision 25115, 25116
Tenodesis 25300, 25301
Tenotomy 25290
Tumor 25130-25136
Bone
Curettage 25130, 25135, 25136
Excision 25130, 25135, 25136
Soft Tissue
Radical Resection 25077, 25078
Subcutaneous
Excision 25071, 25075
Subfascial
Excision 25073, 25076
Unlisted Services and Procedures 25999
X ray 73100-73110
with Contrast 73115

X

X, Coagulation Factor
See Stuart-Prower Factor

X, Cranial Nerve
See Vagus Nerve

X-Linked Ichthyoses
See Syphilis Test

X ray
Abdomen 74018, 74019, 74021, 74022
Abscess 76080
Acromioclavicular Joint 73050
Ankle 73600-73610
Radiostereometric Analysis (RSA) 0350T
Arm, Lower 73090
Arm, Upper 73092
Auditory Meatus 70134
Barium Swallow Test 3142F, 3200F
Bile Duct
Guide Dilation 74360
Body Section 76100
Motion 76101, 76102
Bone
Age Study 77072
Dual Energy Absorptiometry 77080, 77081
Length Study 77073
Osseous Survey 77074-77077
Ultrasound 76977
Breast 77065-77067
Tomosynthesis 77061-77063
with Computer-aided
Detection 77065-77067
Calcaneus 73650
Chest 71045-71048
with Computer-Aided Detection 0174T, 0175T
Clavicle 73000
Coccyx 72220
Consultation 76140
Duodenum 74260
Elbow 73070-73080
Radiostereometric Analysis (RSA) 0349T
Esophagus 74220
Eye 70030
Facial Bones 70140-70150
Fallopian Tube 74742
Femur 73551, 73552
Radiostereometric Analysis (RSA) 0350T
Fibula 73590
Finger 73140
Fistula 76080
Foot 73620-73630
Gastrointestinal Tract
See Gastrointestinal Tract, Imaging, Radiological
Guide Dilation 74360
Guide Intubation 74340
Hand 73120-73130
Head 70350
Heel 73650
Hip
Bilateral 73521-73523
Unilateral 73501-73503
Radiostereometric Analysis (RSA) 0350T
Humerus 73060
Intestines, Small 74245, 74249-74251
Guide Intubation 74355
Jaws 70355
Joint
Stress Views 77071
Knee 73560-73564, 73580
Bilateral 73565
Radiostereometric Analysis (RSA) 0350T
Larynx 70370
Leg 73592
Lumen Dilator 74360
Mandible 70100-70110
Mastoids 70120-70130
Nasal Bone 70160
Neck 70360
Nose to Rectum
Foreign Body 76010
Orbit 70190-70200
Orthopantogram 70355
Panoramic 70355
Pelvis 72170-72190
Manometry 74710
with Hip(s) 73501-73503, 73521-73523
Peritoneum 74190
Pharynx 70370, 74210
Radiostereometric Analysis (RSA) 0348T-0350T
Ribs 71100-71111
Sacroiliac Joint 72200-72202
Sacrum 72220
Salivary Gland 70380
Scapula 73010
Sella Turcica 70240
Shoulder 73020-73030, 73050
Radiostereometric Analysis (RSA) 0349T
Sinus Tract 76080

Sinuses 70210-70220
Skull 70250, 70260
with Spine 72081-72084
Specimen/Surgical 76098
Spine 72020
Cervical .. 72040, 72050, 72052, 72081-72084
Lumbosacral 72100-72120, 72081-72084
Thoracic 72070-72074, 72081-72084
Thoracolumbar 72080, 72081-72084
Total 72081-72084
Standing
Radiostereometric Analysis (RSA) 0348T
Sternum 71120-71130
Teeth 70300-70320
Tibia 73590
Toe 73660
Total Body
Foreign Body 76010
Unlisted Services and Procedures ... 76120-76125
Upper Gastrointestinal Series
(Upper GI Series) 3142F, 3200F
with Contrast
Ankle 73615
Aorta 75600-75630
Artery
Abdominal 75726
Additional Vessels 75774
Adrenal 75731-75733
Arm 75710-75716
Leg 75710-75716
Mammary 75756
Pelvic 75736
Pulmonary 75741-75746
Spine 75705
Transcatheter Therapy 75894-75898
Bile Duct 47531, 47532, 74300, 74301
Catheterization 75984
Drainage 47533-47540
Guide Catheter 74328, 74330
Bladder 74430, 74450-74455
Brain 70010-70015
Central Venous Access Device 36598
Colon
Barium Enema 74270-74280
Corpora Cavernosa 74445
Elbow 73085
Epididymis 74440
Gallbladder 74290
Gastrointestinal Tract 74246-74249
Hip 73525
Iliofemoral Artery 75630
Intervertebral Disc
Cervical 72285
Lumbar 72295
Thoracic 72285
Joint
Stress Views 77071
Kidney
Cyst 74470
Guide Catheter 50433
Knee 73560-73564, 73580
Lacrimal Duct 70170
Lymph Vessel
Abdomen 75805-75807
Arm 75801-75803
Leg 75801-75803
Mammary Duct 77053, 77054
Nasolacrimal Duct 70170
Oviduct 74740
Pancreas 47531, 74300, 74301
Pancreatic Duct
Guide Catheter 74329, 74330
Perineum 74775
Peritoneum 74190
Salivary Gland 70390
Seminal Vesicles 74440
Shoulder 73040
Spine
Cervical 72240
Lumbosacral 72265
Thoracic 72255
Total 72270
Temporomandibular Joint
(TMJ) 70328-70332
Ureter
Guide Dilation 74485
Urethra 74450-74455
Guide Dilation 74485
Urinary Tract 74400-74425
Uterus 74740
Vas Deferens 74440
Vein
Adrenal 75840-75842
Arm 75820-75822
Hepatic Portal 75810, 75885-75887
Jugular 75860
Leg 75820-75822
Liver 75889-75891
Neck 75860
Orbit 75880
Renal 75831-75833
Sampling 75893
Sinus 75870
Skull 75870-75872
Splenic 75810
Vena Cava 75825-75827
Wrist 73115
Wrist 73100-73110
Radiostereometric Analysis (RSA) 0349T

X ray Tomography, Computed
See CT Scan

Xa, Coagulation Factor
See Thrombokinase

Xenoantibodies
See Antibody, Detection, Heterophile

Xenografts, Skin
See Allograft, Skin Substitute

Xenotransplantation
See Allograft

XI, Coagulation Factor
See Plasma Thromboplastin, Antecedent

XI, Cranial Nerve
See Accessory Nerve, Spinal

XII, Coagulation Factor
See Hageman Factor

XII, Cranial Nerve
See Hypoglossal Nerve

XIII, Coagulation Factor
See Fibrin Stabilizing Factor

Xylose Absorption Test
Blood 84620
Urine 84620

Y

Yacoub Procedure
See Heart, Cardiopulmonary Bypass, with Ascending Aorta Graft

Yeast
Culture 87106

Yellow Fever Vaccine 90717

Yersinia
Antibody 86793

YHrium-Aluminum-Garnet (YAG) Laser
See Eye, Incision

Z

Ziegler Procedure
Discission Secondary Membranous
Cataract 66820

Zinc 84630

Zinc Manganese Leucine Aminopeptidase
See Leucine Aminopeptidase

Zonisamide
Drug Assay 80203

Zygoma
See Zygomatic Arch

Zygomatic Arch
Fracture
Open Treatment 21356-21366
with Manipulation 21355
Reconstruction 21255

Notes

Notes